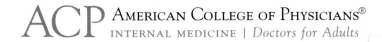

MKSAP® 16

Medical Knowledge Self-Assessment Program®

Endocrinology and Metabolism

Welcome to the Endocrinology and Metabolism Section of MKSAP 16!

Here, you will find updated information on diabetes mellitus, disorders of the pituitary gland, disorders of the thyroid gland, disorders of the adrenal glands, reproductive disorders, and calcium and bone disorders. All of these topics are uniquely focused on the needs of generalists and subspecialists *outside* of endocrinology and metabolism.

The publication of the 16th edition of Medical Knowledge Self-Assessment Program heralds a significant event, culminating 2 years of effort by dozens of leading subspecialists across the United States. Our authoring committees have strived to help internists succeed in Maintenance of Certification, right up to preparing for the MOC examination, and to get residents ready for the certifying examination. MKSAP 16 also helps you update your medical knowledge and elevates standards of self-learning by allowing you to assess your knowledge with 1,200 all-new multiple-choice questions, including 84 in Endocrinology and Metabolism.

MKSAP began more than 40 years ago. The American Board of Internal Medicine's examination blueprint and gaps between actual and preferred practices inform creation of the content. The questions, refined through rigorous face-to-face meetings, are among the best in medicine. A psychometric analysis of the items sharpens our educational focus on weaknesses in practice. To meet diverse learning styles, we offer MKSAP 16 online and in downloadable apps for PCs, tablets, laptops, and smartphones. We are also introducing the following:

High-Value Care Recommendations: The Endocrinology and Metabolism section starts with several recommendations based on the important concept of health care value (balancing clinical benefit with costs and harms) to address the needs of trainees, practicing physicians, and patients. These recommendations are part of a major initiative that has been undertaken by the American College of Physicians, in collaboration with other organizations.

Content for Hospitalists: This material, highlighted in blue and labeled with the familiar hospital icon (🏥), directly addresses the learning needs of the increasing number of physicians who work in the hospital setting. MKSAP 16 Digital will allow you to customize quizzes based on hospitalist-only questions to help you prepare for the Hospital Medicine Maintenance of Certification Examination.

We hope you enjoy and benefit from MKSAP 16. Please feel free to send us any comments to mksap_editors@acponline.org or visit us at the MKSAP Resource Site (mksap.acponline.org) to find out how we can help you study, earn CME, accumulate MOC points, and stay up to date. I know I speak on behalf of ACP staff members and our authoring committees when I say we are honored to have attracted your interest and participation.

Sincerely,

Patrick Alguire, MD, FACP
Editor-in-Chief
Senior Vice President
Medical Education Division
American College of Physicians

Endocrinology and Metabolism

Committee

Silvio E. Inzucchi, MD, FACP, Editor[2]
Professor of Medicine
Clinical Chief, Section of Endocrinology
Yale University School of Medicine
Director, Yale Diabetes Center
Yale-New Haven Hospital
New Haven, Connecticut

Howard H. Weitz, MD, FACP, Associate Editor[1]
Professor of Medicine
Director, Jefferson Heart Institute
Director, Division of Cardiology
Jefferson Medical College of Thomas Jefferson University
Philadelphia, Pennsylvania

Baha M. Arafah, MD, FACP[1]
Professor of Medicine
Chief, Division of Endocrinology
Case Western Reserve University
Case Medical Center
Cleveland, Ohio

Kenneth D. Burman, MD, MACP[2]
Chief, Endocrine Section
Washington Hospital Center
Professor, Department of Medicine
Georgetown University
Washington, DC

Elizabeth Holt, MD, PhD[2]
Assistant Professor of Medicine
Department of Internal Medicine, Section of Endocrinology
Yale University School of Medicine
New Haven, Connecticut

Laurence Katznelson, MD[2]
Professor of Medicine and Neurosurgery
Stanford University School of Medicine
Medical Director, Pituitary Center
Stanford Hospital and Clinics
Stanford, California

David K. McCulloch, MD[2]
Clinical Professor of Medicine
Department of Endocrinology and Metabolism
University of Washington
And Diabetologist and Medical Director of Clinical Improvement
Group Health Cooperative
Seattle, Washington

Maria A. Yialamas, MD, FACP[1]
Associate Program Director, Internal Medicine Residency
Department of Medicine
Brigham and Women's Hospital
Boston, Massachusetts

Editor-in-Chief

Patrick C. Alguire, MD, FACP[1]
Senior Vice President, Medical Education
American College of Physicians
Philadelphia, Pennsylvania

Deputy Editor-in-Chief

Philip A. Masters, MD, FACP[1]
Senior Medical Associate for Content Development
American College of Physicians
Philadelphia, Pennsylvania

Senior Medical Associate for Content Development

Cynthia D. Smith, MD, FACP[2]
American College of Physicians
Philadelphia, Pennsylvania

Endocrinology and Metabolism Clinical Editor

Cynthia A. Burns, MD, FACP[1]

Endocrinology and Metabolism Reviewers

Amindra S. Arora, MD[1]
Arnold A. Asp, MD, FACP[1]
Lee R. Berkowitz, MD, FACP[1]
Lara Hume, MD[1]
Lia Logio, MD, FACP[1]

Endocrinology and Metabolism Reviewers Representing the American Society for Clinical Pharmacology & Therapeutics

Linda A. Hershey, MD, PhD[2]
L. Amy Sun, MD, PhD[1]

Endocrinology and Metabolism ACP Editorial Staff

Ellen McDonald, PhD[1], Senior Staff Editor
Sean McKinney[1], Director, Self-Assessment Programs
Margaret Wells[1], Managing Editor
Linnea Donnarumma[1], Assistant Editor

ACP Principal Staff

Patrick C. Alguire, MD, FACP[1]
Senior Vice President, Medical Education

D. Theresa Kanya, MBA[1]
Vice President, Medical Education

Sean McKinney[1]
Director, Self-Assessment Programs

Margaret Wells[1]
Managing Editor

Valerie Dangovetsky[1]
Program Administrator

Becky Krumm[1]
Senior Staff Editor

Ellen McDonald, PhD[1]
Senior Staff Editor

Katie Idell[1]
Senior Staff Editor

Randy Hendrickson[1]
Production Administrator/Editor

Megan Zborowski[1]
Staff Editor

Linnea Donnarumma[1]
Assistant Editor

John Haefele[1]
Assistant Editor

Developed by the American College of Physicians

---

1. Has no relationships with any entity producing, marketing, re-selling, or distributing health care goods or services consumed by, or used on, patients.

2. Has disclosed relationships with entities producing, marketing, re-selling, or distributing health care goods or services consumed by, or used on, patients. See below.

Conflicts of Interest

The following committee members, reviewers, and ACP staff members have disclosed relationships with commercial companies:

Kenneth D. Burman, MD, MACP
Research Grants/Contracts
Pfizer, Amgen, Exelixis, Innovative Technologies
Board Member
American Thyroid Association; FDA, Endocrine Advisory Committee
Other
UpToDate, Medscape, Endocrine Society

Linda A. Hershey, MD, PhD
Research Grants/Contracts
Reviewer for AAAS Research Competitiveness Program
Honoraria
Medlink Neurology
Speakers Bureau
Medical Education Speakers Network

Elizabeth Holt, MD, PhD
Consultantship
Merck

Silvio E. Inzucchi, MD, FACP
Consultantship
Takeda, Merck, Amylin, Medtronic, Boehringer Ingelheim
Honoraria
NovoNordisk
Research Grants/Contracts
Boehringer Ingelheim, Eli Lilly
Other
Endocrine Society, UpToDate

Laurence Katznelson, MD
Research Grants/Contracts
Novartis, Ipsen, Pfizer, Genentech
Consultantship
Pfizer
Speakers Bureau
Ipsen

David K. McCulloch, MD
Royalties
UpToDate

Cynthia D. Smith, MD, FACP
Stock Options/Holdings
Merck and Company

Acknowledgments

The American College of Physicians (ACP) gratefully acknowledges the special contributions to the development and production of the 16th edition of the Medical

Knowledge Self-Assessment Program® (MKSAP® 16) made by the following people:

Graphic Services: Michael Ripca (Technical Administrator/Graphic Designer) and Willie-Fetchko Graphic Design (Graphic Designer).

Production/Systems: Dan Hoffmann (Director, Web Services & Systems Development), Neil Kohl (Senior Architect), and Scott Hurd (Senior Systems Analyst/Developer).

MKSAP 16 Digital: Under the direction of Steven Spadt, Vice President, ACP Digital Products & Services, the digital version of MKSAP 16 was developed within the ACP's Digital Product Development Department, led by Brian Sweigard (Director). Other members of the team included Sean O'Donnell (Senior Architect), Dan Barron (Senior Systems Analyst/Developer), Chris Forrest (Senior Software Developer/Design Lead), Jon Laing (Senior Web Application Developer), Brad Lord (Senior Web Developer), John McKnight (Senior Web Developer), and Nate Pershall (Senior Web Developer).

The College also wishes to acknowledge that many other persons, too numerous to mention, have contributed to the production of this program. Without their dedicated efforts, this program would not have been possible.

Introducing the MKSAP Resource Site (mksap.acponline.org)

The MKSAP Resource Site (mksap.acponline.org) is a continually updated site that provides links to MKSAP 16 online answer sheets for print subscribers; access to MKSAP 16 Digital, Board Basics® 3, and MKSAP 16 Updates; the latest details on Continuing Medical Education (CME) and Maintenance of Certification (MOC) in the United States, Canada, and Australia; errata; and other new information.

ABIM Maintenance of Certification

Check the MKSAP Resource Site (mksap.acponline.org) for the latest information on how MKSAP tests can be used to apply to the American Board of Internal Medicine for Maintenance of Certification (MOC) points.

RCPSC Maintenance of Certification

In Canada, MKSAP 16 is an Accredited Self-Assessment Program (Section 3) as defined by the Maintenance of Certification Program of The Royal College of Physicians and Surgeons of Canada (RCPSC) and approved by the Canadian Society of Internal Medicine on December 9, 2011. Approval of Part A sections of MKSAP 16 extends from July 31, 2012, until July 31, 2015. Approval of Part B sections of MKSAP 16 extends from December 31, 2012, to December 31, 2015. Fellows of the Royal College may earn three credits per hour for participating in MKSAP 16 under Section 3. MKSAP 16 will enable Fellows to earn up to 75% of their required 400 credits during the 5-year MOC cycle. A Fellow can achieve this 75% level by earning 100 of the maximum of 174 *AMA PRA Category 1 Credits*™ available in MKSAP 16. MKSAP 16 also meets multiple CanMEDS Roles for RCPSC MOC, including that of Medical Expert, Communicator, Collaborator, Manager, Health Advocate, Scholar, and Professional. For information on how to apply MKSAP 16 CME credits to RCPSC MOC, visit the MKSAP Resource Site at mksap.acponline.org.

The Royal Australasian College of Physicians CPD Program

In Australia, MKSAP 16 is a Category 3 program that may be used by Fellows of The Royal Australasian College of Physicians (RACP) to meet mandatory CPD points. Two CPD credits are awarded for each of the 174 *AMA PRA Category 1 Credits*™ available in MKSAP 16. More information about using MKSAP 16 for this purpose is available at the MKSAP Resource Site at mksap.acponline.org and at www.racp.edu.au. CPD credits earned through MKSAP 16 should be reported at the MyCPD site at www.racp.edu.au/mycpd.

Continuing Medical Education

The American College of Physicians is accredited by the Accreditation Council for Continuing Medical Education (ACCME) to provide continuing medical education for physicians.

The American College of Physicians designates this enduring material, MKSAP 16, for a maximum of 174 *AMA PRA Category 1 Credits*™. Physicians should claim only the credit commensurate with the extent of their participation in the activity.

Up to 12 *AMA PRA Category 1 Credits*™ are available from December 31, 2012, to December 31, 2015, for the MKSAP 16 Endocrinology and Metabolism section.

Learning Objectives

The learning objectives of MKSAP 16 are to:
- Close gaps between actual care in your practice and preferred standards of care, based on best evidence
- Diagnose disease states that are less common and sometimes overlooked and confusing
- Improve management of comorbid conditions that can complicate patient care
- Determine when to refer patients for surgery or care by subspecialists

- Pass the ABIM Certification Examination
- Pass the ABIM Maintenance of Certification Examination

Target Audience

- General internists and primary care physicians
- Subspecialists who need to remain up-to-date in internal medicine
- Residents preparing for the certifying examination in internal medicine
- Physicians preparing for maintenance of certification in internal medicine (recertification)

Earn "Same-Day" CME Credits Online

For the first time, print subscribers can enter their answers online to earn CME credits in 24 hours or less. You can submit your answers using online answer sheets that are provided at mksap.acponline.org, where a record of your MKSAP 16 credits will be available. To earn CME credits, you need to answer all of the questions in a test and earn a score of at least 50% correct (number of correct answers divided by the total number of questions). Take any of the following approaches:

1. Use the printed answer sheet at the back of this book to record your answers. Go to mksap.acponline.org, access the appropriate online answer sheet, transcribe your answers, and submit your test for same-day CME credits. There is no additional fee for this service.

2. Go to mksap.acponline.org, access the appropriate online answer sheet, directly enter your answers, and submit your test for same-day CME credits. There is no additional fee for this service.

3. Pay a $10 processing fee per answer sheet and submit the printed answer sheet at the back of this book by mail or fax, as instructed on the answer sheet. Make sure you calculate your score and fax the answer sheet to 215-351-2799 or mail the answer sheet to Member and Customer Service, American College of Physicians, 190 N. Independence Mall West, Philadelphia, PA 19106-1572, using the courtesy envelope provided in your MKSAP 16 slipcase. You will need your 10-digit order number and 8-digit ACP ID number, which are printed on your packing slip. Please allow 4 to 6 weeks for your score report to be emailed back to you. Be sure to include your email address for a response.

If you do not have a 10-digit order number and 8-digit ACP ID number or if you need help creating a username and password to access the MKSAP 16 online answer sheets, go to mksap.acponline.org or email custserv@acponline.org.

Disclosure Policy

It is the policy of the American College of Physicians (ACP) to ensure balance, independence, objectivity, and scientific rigor in all of its educational activities. To this end, and consistent with the policies of the ACP and the Accreditation Council for Continuing Medical Education (ACCME), contributors to all ACP continuing medical education activities are required to disclose all relevant financial relationships with any entity producing, marketing, re-selling, or distributing health care goods or services consumed by, or used on, patients. Contributors are required to use generic names in the discussion of therapeutic options and are required to identify any unapproved, off-label, or investigative use of commercial products or devices. Where a trade name is used, all available trade names for the same product type are also included. If trade-name products manufactured by companies with whom contributors have relationships are discussed, contributors are asked to provide evidence-based citations in support of the discussion. The information is reviewed by the committee responsible for producing this text. If necessary, adjustments to topics or contributors' roles in content development are made to balance the discussion. Further, all readers of this text are asked to evaluate the content for evidence of commercial bias and send any relevant comments to mksap_editors@acponline.org so that future decisions about content and contributors can be made in light of this information.

Resolution of Conflicts

To resolve all conflicts of interest and influences of vested interests, the ACP precluded members of the content-creation committee from deciding on any content issues that involved generic or trade-name products associated with proprietary entities with which these committee members had relationships. In addition, content was based on best evidence and updated clinical care guidelines, when such evidence and guidelines were available. Contributors' disclosure information can be found with the list of contributors' names and those of ACP principal staff listed in the beginning of this book.

Hospital-Based Medicine

For the convenience of subscribers who provide care in hospital settings, content that is specific to the hospital setting has been highlighted in blue. Hospital icons (🏥) highlight where the hospital-only content begins, continues over more than one page, and ends.

Educational Disclaimer

The editors and publisher of MKSAP 16 recognize that the development of new material offers many opportunities for error. Despite our best efforts, some errors may persist in print. Drug dosage schedules are, we believe, accurate and in accordance with current standards. Readers are advised, however, to ensure that the recommended dosages in MKSAP 16 concur with the information provided in the product information material. This is especially important in cases of new, infrequently used, or highly toxic drugs. Application of the information in MKSAP 16 remains the professional responsibility of the practitioner.

The primary purpose of MKSAP 16 is educational. Information presented, as well as publications, technologies, products, and/or services discussed, is intended to inform subscribers about the knowledge, techniques, and experiences of the contributors. A diversity of professional opinion exists, and the views of the contributors are their own and not those of the ACP. Inclusion of any material in the program does not constitute endorsement or recommendation by the ACP. The ACP does not warrant the safety, reliability, accuracy, completeness, or usefulness of and disclaims any and all liability for damages and claims that may result from the use of information, publications, technologies, products, and/or services discussed in this program.

Publisher's Information

Unauthorized Use of This Book Is Against the Law

MKSAP 16 ISBN: 978-1-938245-00-8
(Endocrinology and Metabolism) ISBN: 978-1-938245-07-7

Printed in the United States of America.

For order information in the U.S. or Canada call 800-523-1546, extension 2600. All other countries call 215-351-2600. Fax inquiries to 215-351-2799 or email to custserv@acponline.org.

Errata and Norm Tables

Errata for MKSAP 16 will be available through the MKSAP Resource Site at mksap.acponline.org as new information becomes known to the editors.

MKSAP 16 Performance Interpretation Guidelines with Norm Tables, available July 31, 2013, will reflect the knowledge of physicians who have completed the self-assessment tests before the program was published. These physicians took the tests without being able to refer to the syllabus, answers, and critiques. For your convenience, the tables are available in a printable PDF file through the MKSAP Resource Site at mksap.acponline.org.

Table of Contents

Endocrinology and Metabolism High-Value Care Recommendations

The American College of Physicians, in collaboration with multiple other organizations, is embarking on a national initiative to promote awareness about the importance of stewardship of health care resources. The goals are to improve health care outcomes by providing care of proven benefit and reducing costs by avoiding unnecessary and even harmful interventions. The initiative comprises several programs that integrate the important concept of health care value (balancing clinical benefit with costs and harms) for a given intervention into various educational materials to address the needs of trainees, practicing physicians, and patients.

To integrate discussion of high-value, cost-conscious care into MKSAP 16, we have created recommendations based on the medical knowledge content that we feel meet the below definition of high-value care and bring us closer to our goal of improving patient outcomes while conserving finite resources.

High-Value Care Recommendation: A recommendation to choose diagnostic and management strategies for patients in specific clinical situations that balances clinical benefit with cost and harms with the goal of improving patient outcomes.

Below are the High-Value Care Recommendations for the Endocrinology and Metabolism section of MKSAP 16.

- The older diabetic agents, such as insulin, the sulfonylureas, and metformin, have proven long-term glycemic control and cost effectiveness (see Item 35).
- For most patients with type 2 diabetes mellitus, lifestyle modifications and metformin therapy are the best initial treatments (see Item 11).
- Cost concerns are a factor in determining which pharmacologic agents for diabetes mellitus are used because the newer insulin preparations (insulin glargine, detemir, aspart, lispro, and glulisine) are far more expensive than regular insulin or neutral protamine Hagedorn (NPH) insulin (see Item 35).
- Repeated or serial measurements of antithyroid antibody titers are not recommended in the management of thyroid disorders in most persons because the degree of a titer's elevation does not indicate a need for treatment; only an abnormal TSH level does.
- A thyroid scan and radioactive iodine uptake test are not useful in the evaluation of patients with hypothyroidism.
- Ultrasonography is recommended for imaging thyroid nodules, with fine-needle aspiration biopsy reserved for nodules larger than 1 cm in diameter.
- Patients with asymptomatic stable simple goiters can be serially monitored clinically; serial ultrasonography is not recommended for these goiters.
- The best initial test for male hypogonadism is a morning (8 AM) measurement of the total testosterone level; if this level is normal, then hypogonadism is excluded (see Item 21 and Item 51).
- Screening woman for osteoporosis with bone mineral density measurements (using dual-energy x-ray absorptiometry [DEXA]) should not begin before age 65 years unless the patient has a particularly high risk for osteoporosis (risk factors such as a previous fracture, glucocorticoid use, a family history of hip fracture, current tobacco use, alcoholism, or secondary osteoporosis).
- Do not screen women who are premenopausal for osteoporosis.
- Do not repeat bone mineral density testing before 10 years in patients with normal or low normal values on previous testing.
- No clear benefit of newer bisphosphonate drugs has been demonstrated compared with older agents, which are available in generic form and may be more cost-effective for long-term therapy.

Endocrinology and Metabolism

Diabetes Mellitus

Classification and Diagnosis of Diabetes

Overview

Diabetes mellitus occurs when inadequate glycemic control results in elevated blood glucose levels. An inadequate production of the hormone insulin, resistance to the actions of insulin, or some combination of both mechanisms can cause this state. Patients with diabetes have a significantly increased risk of developing macrovascular disease (coronary artery, cerebrovascular, and peripheral vascular disorders) and microvascular disease (retinopathy, nephropathy, and neuropathy).

The two major forms of diabetes are type 1 and type 2 (**Table 1**). Diabetes not only can develop from autoimmunity or genetic predisposition, but also can result from use of drugs that damage the pancreas or cause resistance to the actions of insulin. Drug-induced diabetes is becoming more common because of the increasing use of immunosuppressive drugs (such as cyclosporine and tacrolimus) that can inhibit insulin secretion and of HIV protease inhibitors and atypical antipsychotic drugs (such as clozapine and olanzapine) that can induce weight gain, central obesity, elevated triglyceride levels, and insulin resistance.

> **KEY POINT**
>
> - Patients with diabetes mellitus have a significantly increased risk of developing macrovascular disease (coronary artery, cerebrovascular, and peripheral vascular disorders) and microvascular disease (retinopathy, nephropathy, and neuropathy).

Insulin Resistance

When the body becomes resistant to the effects of insulin, the pancreas compensates by secreting more insulin. Because the pancreas secretes one C-peptide molecule with each insulin

TABLE 1. Classification of Diabetes Mellitus
Type 1 Diabetes[a]
Immune mediated
Idiopathic (seronegative)
Type 2 Diabetes[b]
Ketosis Prone[c]
Gestational Diabetes
Other Types
Genetic defects in beta-cell function (including six distinct MODY syndromes)
Genetic defects in insulin action
Diseases of the exocrine pancreas (pancreatitis, trauma/pancreatectomy, neoplasia, cystic fibrosis, hemochromatosis, fibrocalculous pancreatopathy)
Endocrinopathies (acromegaly, Cushing syndrome, glucagonoma, pheochromocytoma, hyperthyroidism)
Drug related (glucocorticoids, thiazides, β-blockers, diazoxide, tacrolimus, cyclosporine, niacin, HIV protease inhibitors, atypical antipsychotics [clozapine, olanzapine])
Infections (congenital rubella, cytomegalovirus)
Rare forms of immune-mediated diabetes ("stiff man" syndrome, anti–insulin receptor autoantibodies)
Genetic syndromes (Down, Klinefelter, Turner, Wolfram [DIDMOAD], and Prader-Willi syndromes; myotonic dystrophy)

DIDMOAD = diabetes insipidus, diabetes mellitus, optic atrophy, and deafness; MODY = maturity-onset diabetes of the young.

[a]Beta-cell destruction usually leading to absolute insulin deficiency.

[b]Insulin resistance with progressive relative insulin deficiency.

[c]More common in nonwhite patients who present with diabetic ketoacidosis but become non–insulin dependent over time.

molecule, endogenous insulin production can be determined by measuring the amount of insulin or C-peptide in the blood. Although this method may be useful in diagnosing causes of hypoglycemia in persons without diabetes, it may not help determine the degree of insulin resistance or reliably distinguish between type 1 and type 2 diabetes. In the early stages of both types of diabetes, obese persons secrete high levels of insulin and C-peptide. Therefore, the most useful test in determining whether obese patients have type 1 or type 2 diabetes is to determine whether they have pancreatic autoantibodies (such as islet cell antibodies or glutamic acid decarboxylase antibodies) in their blood. This determination is essential because in patients with type 1 diabetes, treatment with insulin should begin as soon as possible.

Screening for Diabetes

After reviewing the available literature, the U.S. Preventive Services Task Force has found no direct evidence of future health benefits from mass screening and treatment of diabetes mellitus in asymptomatic individuals. Screening is recommended in asymptomatic adults who have treated or untreated sustained blood pressure greater than 135/80 mm Hg. In contrast, the American Diabetes Association (ADA) suggests a more comprehensive recommendation for screening that focuses on asymptomatic adults who either are at increased risk for developing diabetes or are age 45 years or older (**Table 2**).

Diagnostic Criteria for Diabetes

The diagnosis of diabetes is usually based on elevated (in the diabetes range) hemoglobin A_{1c} values, fasting or random plasma glucose levels, or oral glucose tolerance test results on

two separate occasions or on a single random plasma glucose level of 200 mg/dL (11.1 mmol/L) or greater while a patient is experiencing classic symptoms of hyperglycemia, such as polyuria, polydipsia, or blurred vision (**Table 3**). Patients whose results on these tests are above normal but less than the diabetes range are considered to be at increased risk for diabetes.

Type 1 Diabetes

Type 1 diabetes usually presents dramatically with severe hyperglycemic symptoms, such as fatigue, polyuria, polydipsia, polyphagia, visual blurring, weight loss, nausea, vomiting, and dehydration. This type, which comprises approximately 5% of all diabetes, most commonly results from slow autoimmune destruction of insulin-producing pancreatic beta cells by autoantibodies in persons with particular *HLA* susceptibility genes in the DQA and DQB regions of chromosome 6. Age of onset and rate of beta-cell destruction depend on the particular combination of susceptibility and protective genes a person has and on exposure to one or more environmental triggers (possibly viral). Left untreated, patients with type 1 diabetes may rapidly develop diabetic ketoacidosis (DKA), which has a high morbidity and mortality (see later discussion).

Although most common in children and lean young adults, type 1 diabetes can present less dramatically in obese persons and in older adults. At the time of disease presentation, 60% to 80% of the affected person's pancreatic beta cells are already destroyed, and the remaining beta cells are not functioning well because of the hyperglycemia and metabolic dysfunction associated with the untreated disease. After insulin therapy (and fluid and electrolyte replacement, if needed) has begun, the residual beta-cell function may

---

TABLE 2.   American Diabetes Association Screening Guidelines for Diabetes Mellitus

Overweight persons (BMI ≥25) with one (or more) additional risk factor(s):

   Physical inactivity

   First-degree relative with diabetes

   High-risk ethnicity (black, Latin American, American Indian, Asian American, Pacific Islander)

   Delivered an infant weighing >4500 g (158.7 oz) (women)

   Gestational diabetes (women)

   Hypertension

   HDL cholesterol level <35 mg/dL (0.90 mmol/L) and/or triglyceride level >250 mg/dL (2.82 mmol/L)

   Polycystic ovary syndrome (women)

   Hemoglobin A_{1c} value ≥5.7% and IGT or IFG on previous testing

   Acanthosis nigricans

   History of cardiovascular disease

In the absence of the above criteria, anyone age 45 years or older

If results are normal, repeat testing every 3 years

IFG = impaired fasting glucose; IGT = impaired glucose tolerance.

Adapted with permission of American Diabetes Association, from Standards of Medical Care in Diabetes—2011. Diabetes Care. 2011;34(Suppl 1):S14. [PMID: 21193625]; permission conveyed through Copyright Clearance Center, Inc.

TABLE 3. Diagnostic Criteria for Diabetes Mellitus[a]

Criteria No.	Test	Normal Range	Increased Risk for Diabetes	Diabetes
1	—	—	—	Classic hyperglycemic symptoms plus a random plasma glucose ≥200 mg/dL (11.1 mmol/L)
2	Fasting plasma glucose	<100 mg/dL (5.6 mmol/L)	100-125 mg/dL (5.6-6.9 mmol/L)	≥126 mmol/L (7.0 mmol/L)
3	Random plasma glucose or during a 2-hour 75-g OGTT	<140 mg/dL (7.8 mmol/L)	140-199 mg/dL (7.8-11.0 mmol/L)	≥200 mg/dL (11.1 mmol/L)
4	Hemoglobin A$_{1c}$	<5.7%	5.7%-6.4%	≥6.5%

OGTT = oral glucose tolerance test.

[a]In the absence of hyperglycemic symptoms, criteria 2 through 4 should be confirmed by repeat testing. If two tests are performed and only one has abnormal results, the American Diabetes Association recommends repeating the test with abnormal results.

Data from American Diabetes Association. Standards of Medical Care in Diabetes—2011. Diabetes Care. 2011;34(Suppl 1):S13. [PMID: 21193625]

improve sufficiently for the insulin dosage to be reduced. This "honeymoon" period may persist for several weeks to months. Although insulin was routinely discontinued during this period in the past, the standard practice now is continuous insulin therapy after diagnosis to preserve endogenous insulin secretion for many months (or years) longer. This makes the goal of maintaining good glycemic control much more attainable.

Although DKA is usually considered a hallmark of type 1 diabetes, certain patients (most often nonwhite patients) with DKA at presentation who are initially treated with insulin and fluid replacement can stop taking insulin and be treated with lifestyle changes and oral hypoglycemic agents for many years. They do not have autoantibodies or the characteristic *HLA* gene associations of typical type 1 diabetes.

KEY POINT

- Left untreated, patients with type 1 diabetes may rapidly develop diabetic ketoacidosis.

Type 2 Diabetes

Type 2 diabetes (approximately 90% of all diabetes) occurs because of a slow decline in pancreatic beta-cell function. This process results in decreasing insulin secretion over decades, although most patients continue to produce some insulin throughout their lives. Besides progressive insulin deficiency, patients with type 2 diabetes develop varying degrees of insulin resistance. The severity of the insulin resistance and insulin deficiency determines when in life frank hyperglycemia develops to a degree that the patient meets diagnostic criteria for diabetes. Although type 2 diabetes most often affects middle-aged and older patients, the disorder can occur much earlier in life, especially in an era of increasing obesity and inactivity among children and adolescents.

Although the genetic association of type 2 diabetes is much stronger than that of type 1 and the penetrance of type 2 diabetes in families is high, the specific genes involved have not yet been identified. Because some insulin secretion continues in type 2 diabetes, lipolysis is suppressed, DKA is rare, and the presenting symptoms usually are much less dramatic. Because the onset can be so insidious, some patients already have evidence of microvascular complications at the time of diagnosis, which suggests the presence of hyperglycemia for many years before diagnosis.

In addition to abnormal glucose metabolism and insulin resistance, many patients with type 2 diabetes have central obesity, hypertension, and hyperlipidemia, features often collectively called "the metabolic syndrome." Although these features individually confer additional cardiovascular risk, it is unknown if their combination does so. Consensus is lacking about the exact way to diagnose the metabolic syndrome and whether doing so is clinically valuable.

Prediction and Prevention of Type 2 Diabetes

Many features listed in Table 2 identify persons with a high risk of developing type 2 diabetes. Several studies have randomized persons at high risk (for example, those with impaired glucose tolerance or women who have had gestational diabetes) to interventions aimed at preventing them from later developing diabetes (**Table 4**). Whether diabetes has been prevented or simply delayed for a few years is still unclear. No long-term studies have shown whether early treatment prolongs life or delays long-term complications. However, counseling persons to eat a healthier diet, exercise more, maintain normal weight, and stop smoking—all of which help prevent type 2 diabetes—should be a public health imperative in the twenty-first century.

TABLE 4. Strategies to Prevent or Delay Onset of Type 2 Diabetes Mellitus

Intervention	Effectiveness
Diet and exercise	Sustained weight loss of 7%, with at least 150 minutes of moderate exercise per week, shown to delay onset of diabetes by up to 3 years
Smoking cessation	Modestly effective as long as it does not cause weight gain
Bariatric surgery	Effective if used in obese persons (BMI >40)
Metformin	Shown to delay onset of diabetes by up to 3 years
Lipase inhibitors (orlistat)	Shown to delay onset of diabetes by up to 3 years
α-Glucosidase inhibitors (acarbose, voglibose)	Shown to delay onset of diabetes by up to 3 years
Thiazolidinediones (troglitazone, rosiglitazone, pioglitazone)	Shown to delay onset of diabetes by up to 3 years
Insulin and insulin secretagogues (sulfonylureas, meglitinides)	Ineffective
ACE-inhibitors (such as ramipril) and angiotensin receptor blockers (such as valsartan)	Ineffective
Estrogen-progestin	Modest effect only

KEY POINTS

- In addition to abnormal glucose metabolism and insulin resistance, patients with type 2 diabetes also often have central obesity, hypertension, and hyperlipidemia, features that often are collectively called "the metabolic syndrome."
- Counseling persons to eat a healthier diet, exercise more, maintain a normal weight, and stop smoking can help delay or prevent onset of type 2 diabetes.

Gestational Diabetes

Gestational diabetes occurs when a woman's pancreas cannot increase insulin secretion enough to overcome the acute insulin resistance of pregnancy. This condition affects at least 7% of pregnancies in the United States; this number may be higher when women with overt diabetes at their first prenatal visit are included. Untreated gestational diabetes is associated with large babies (macrosomia); premature delivery; an increased risk of preeclampsia, stillbirth, and more complex delivery (including cesarean section); and neonatal respiratory compromise, jaundice, hypoglycemia, and hypocalcemia. The International Association of Diabetes and Pregnancy Study Group (IADPSG) recommends screening women for previously undiagnosed diabetes at the first obstetric visit using the criteria in Table 3. If a woman does not have diabetes by these criteria, then screening for gestational diabetes is recommended at 24 to 28 weeks of gestation by performing a 75-g oral glucose tolerance test (**Table 5**). Women at low risk for gestational diabetes (age <25 years, thin body habitus, no family history of diabetes, white race) can be excluded from this screening. Screening should be considered earlier than 24 weeks in women at increased risk for gestational diabetes (BMI >30, history of previous gestational diabetes or polycystic ovary syndrome, previous newborn with excessive birth weight [>4500 g {158.7 oz}], family history of diabetes, or high-risk race/ethnicity [black, Hispanic, American Indian, South Asian, Pacific Islander]).

The mainstays of gestational diabetes treatment are diet and exercise to maintain fasting and premeal plasma glucose levels less than 95 mg/dL (5.3 mmol/L) and 1-hour postprandial values less than 130 to 140 mg/dL (7.2-7.8 mmol/L). Most women can meet these goals with lifestyle changes alone. If they cannot, then insulin should be started. Although glyburide and metformin have been used successfully in pregnancy and are options for women who refuse to take insulin, their safety in pregnancy relative to insulin has not been definitively established.

Although gestational diabetes usually resolves after delivery, it is likely to recur in future pregnancies. Women with a history of gestational diabetes are at high risk for type 2 diabetes in the decade after pregnancy. Therefore, they should be

TABLE 5. Screening for Gestational Diabetes

When to Screen[a]	Test	Result[b]
At 24-28 weeks' gestation (after a minimum 8-hour fast)	Oral glucose tolerance test using a 75-g glucose load followed by plasma glucose measurement 1 and 2 hours after the glucose load	Fasting, ≥92 mg/dL (5.1 mmol/L) At 1 h, ≥180 mg/dL (10 mmol/L) At 2 h, ≥153 mg/dL (8.5 mmol/L)

[a]It is reasonable to exclude women at low risk from screening and to screen earlier in women at high risk.

[b]Gestational diabetes is diagnosed if one or more of these values is equaled or exceeded.

advised to lose weight (if BMI is >25), continue healthy diet and exercise patterns, and undergo annual screening for diabetes (see Table 3). It has been recently recognized that the offspring of mothers with prepregnancy obesity who develop gestational diabetes during pregnancy are at increased risk for childhood obesity. The reason for this is not clear but may involve a combination of genetic factors and maternal imprinting of genes during intrauterine life.

KEY POINT

- Gestational diabetes, which occurs when a woman's pancreas cannot increase insulin secretion enough to overcome the acute insulin resistance of pregnancy, develops in approximately 7% of pregnancies in the United States.

Other Types of Diabetes

Rare genetic forms of type 2 diabetes caused by defects in beta-cell function are grouped together as maturity-onset diabetes of the young (*MODY* genes 1-6) or as genetic defects in insulin action (such as type A insulin resistance). Diseases of the exocrine pancreas, such as pancreatitis and cystic fibrosis, can lead to diabetes if enough of the pancreas is destroyed or removed. Similarly, endocrine conditions in which excessive amounts of hormones antagonistic to insulin action are secreted (acromegaly, Cushing syndrome, and glucagonoma) can lead to diabetes (see Table 1).

Management of Diabetes

Glycemic Monitoring

Chronic hyperglycemia causes significant microvascular and macrovascular damage, and strategies to lower blood glucose levels remain the mainstay of diabetes management, with the exact target level individualized for each patient. The effectiveness of self-monitoring in patients with type 2 diabetes who take only oral medications that do not predispose to hypoglycemia is not clear. Self-monitoring of eating and exercise habits and blood glucose levels is crucial for patients taking multiple injections of insulin or using continuous infusion insulin pumps and for those taking medications that increase the risk of hypoglycemia, such as sulfonylureas. This step not only gives all patients with diabetes a tool with which to understand how their lifestyle choices and responses to different life situations can affect their blood glucose level, but also provides physicians with a tool with which to discuss a patient's status and recommend changes to his or her diabetes regimen.

Testing blood glucose levels 1 or 2 hours after meals can show the different effects of portion size and type of food being consumed and is necessary for a complete picture of a patient's glycemic status. Testing before, during, and after exercise can show the impact of exercise on glycemic control. Testing blood glucose levels at times when a patient experiences symptoms possibly due to a high or low level (such as sweating, nausea, or anxiety) provides useful insights into a patient's daily glycemic control, whether the finding is hypoglycemia, hyperglycemia, or euglycemia. The most common cause of day-to-day variability of blood glucose levels is variability in a patient's eating and exercise habits. Finally, testing in the middle of the night can identify nocturnal hypoglycemia.

Erythrocytes circulate for approximately 120 days before being destroyed, and glucose attaches to hemoglobin during periods of sustained hyperglycemia. The percentage of hemoglobin that has been glycosylated (the hemoglobin A_{1c} value) is thus a surrogate indicator of the average blood glucose level during the previous 3 months. The hemoglobin A_{1c} value should thus be obtained at regular intervals, with patients whose diabetes treatment is being adjusted tested at 3-month intervals and patients at goal receiving a stable treatment regimen tested every 6 months. In patients receiving hemodialysis, those with hemolytic anemia or certain hemoglobinopathies, or those with recent blood transfusions, hemoglobin A_{1c} values may be falsely lowered because of the presence of erythrocytes less than 120 days old in the sample.

The findings from the Diabetes Control and Complications Trial (DCCT) led to the creation of a table showing the estimated average plasma glucose level for any given hemoglobin A_{1c} level (**Table 6**). A hemoglobin A_{1c} goal of less than 7.0% is appropriate for many nonpregnant adults with a long life expectancy, no cardiovascular disease, and a short duration of diabetes because studies have shown reductions in microvascular and neuropathic complications and long-term macrovascular disease in such patients who reached this goal. For patients with a long duration of diabetes, known cardiovascular disease, multiple comorbid conditions, or a history of severe hypoglycemia, hemoglobin A_{1c} goals

TABLE 6. Comparison of Hemoglobin A_{1c} Value and Estimated Average Plasma Glucose Level		
Hemoglobin A_{1c} Value	**Estimated Average Plasma Glucose Level**	
	mg/dL	**mmol/L**
5.0	97	5.0
6.0	126	6.0
7.0	154	7.0
8.0	183	8.0
9.0	212	9.0
10.0	240	10.0
11.0	269	14.9
12.0	298	16.5

Adapted with permission of American Diabetes Association, from Translating the A1C assay into estimated average glucose values. Nathan DM, Kuenen J, Borg R, Zheng H, Schoenfeld D, Heine RJ; A1C-derived average glucose study group. [erratum in Diabetes Care. 2009;32(1):207]. Diabetes Care. 2008;31(8):1476. [PMID: 18540046]; permission conveyed through Copyright Clearance Center, Inc.

should be less stringent because of the risk of hypoglycemia and because studies of intensive hemoglobin A_{1c}–lowering regimens have shown no correlation with reduction in macrovascular outcomes in these patients.

Many blood glucose monitors have a memory function that provides the average reading for the past 7, 14, or 30 days, and this meter average can be compared with the estimated average plasma glucose level. If the meter average is lower or higher than the estimated average plasma glucose level, hyperglycemia or hypoglycemia is likely occurring when the patient is not testing (such as postprandially or during sleep). Real-time continuous glucose monitoring is available and has the potential to improve glycemic control while decreasing the incidence of hypoglycemia. Thus far, however, clinical trials testing the efficacy of real-time continuous glucose monitoring systems have had mixed results.

KEY POINTS

- Because erythrocytes circulate for approximately 120 days before being destroyed and because glucose becomes attached to hemoglobin during periods of hyperglycemia, the hemoglobin A_{1c} value provides an estimate of the average blood glucose level during the previous 3 months.

- The hemoglobin A_{1c} value should be obtained at regular intervals, every 6 months for patients with diabetes receiving a stable treatment regimen whose previous values were at goal and every 3 months for those whose diabetes regimens are being adjusted because their previous values were not at goal.

Cardiovascular Risk

Because diabetes is associated with a significantly increased risk of macrovascular complications, especially atherosclerotic vascular disease, reducing future cardiovascular risk is a priority in diabetes management. Ten measures that should be considered for patients with diabetes appear below:

1. Stopping smoking
2. Maintaining a normal weight
3. Eating a healthy diet
4. Exercising moderately for at least 150 minutes per week
5. Using a statin
6. Using an ACE inhibitor or angiotensin receptor blocker (ARB)
7. Using aspirin
8. Maintaining an LDL cholesterol level of less than 100 mg/dL (2.59 mmol/L)
9. Maintaining a blood pressure of less than 130/80 mm Hg
10. Maintaining a hemoglobin A_{1c} level of less than 7.0%

The health benefits of smoking cessation and maintaining a normal weight are not controversial. However, what

constitutes a healthy diet, how often to exercise, at what age to start medication, and what to recommend as blood pressure, hemoglobin A_{1c} level, and lipid level targets have been debated. Regarding statins, the Heart Protection Study showed significant benefit with simvastatin, 40 mg/d, in all patients with diabetes who were older than 40 years and had at least one other risk factor for heart disease, even for patients whose cholesterol level was not elevated at baseline. Regarding blood pressure medication, the Heart Outcomes Prevention Evaluation (HOPE) study found that ramipril was beneficial in patients with diabetes who were older than 55 years, even those who did not have hypertension. The ADA and American Heart Association recommend that LDL cholesterol levels be less than 100 mg/dL (2.59 mmol/L) for all persons with diabetes and that a target of less than 70 mg/dL (1.81 mmol/L) be considered for those who already have heart disease or macrovascular disease of any type, including stroke and peripheral vascular disease.

Whether all patients with diabetes should have a blood pressure less than 130/80 mm Hg is unclear. The ACCORD study group compared a conservative systolic blood pressure target (<140 mm Hg) with a more aggressive one (<120 mm Hg) in more than 4700 patients with type 2 diabetes (mean age, 62 years) who had evidence of preexisting cardiovascular disease. No difference in the annual rate of fatal and nonfatal cardiovascular disease events was found over 8 years of follow-up, although more adverse events related to drug side effects occurred in those trying to achieve the more aggressive target. Although treatment efforts have traditionally focused on achieving hemoglobin A_{1c} levels close to the normal range, recent evidence suggests that values approaching normal in older patients with preexisting cardiovascular disease may be associated with increased all-cause mortality. This information underscores the need to establish individualized treatment goals in this population.

KEY POINTS

- Because diabetes is associated with a significantly increased risk of macrovascular complications, especially atherosclerotic vascular disease, reducing future cardiovascular risk is a priority in diabetes management.

- Statins have significant benefit in patients with diabetes who are older than 40 years and have at least one other risk factor for heart disease.

Lowering Blood Glucose Levels in Type 2 Diabetes

Nonpharmacologic Approaches

Lifestyle changes (such as weight loss, increased exercise, and decreased carbohydrate intake) are the cornerstone of type 2 diabetes treatment and should be considered in every person with the disease. For patients with type 2 diabetes and obesity, a slow, steady weight loss—achieved by eating a diet with moderate amounts of complex high-fiber carbohydrates, protein, and fat and engaging in moderate exercise on a daily basis—should be a goal. Only approximately 5% to 10% of patients with type 2 diabetes will be able to control their blood glucose levels with lifestyle measures alone. Even if pharmacologic agents must be added later, these drugs will be much more effective and will require lower doses if patients also focus on lifestyle measures. Although exercise usually lowers the blood glucose level in patients with diabetes, this level may increase if exercise is attempted when the patient's insulin level is low, such as first thing in the morning before any insulin is taken, as a result of exercise-induced hepatic gluconeogenesis; in the absence of sufficient plasma insulin (hypoinsulinemia), the glucose cannot be absorbed by the muscles and other tissues, and the blood glucose level continues to increase.

For patients with diabetes and morbid obesity, various forms of weight-loss surgery (bariatric surgery) are available. Bariatric surgery causes weight loss by restriction, malabsorption, or a combination of the two and has resulted in a significant rate of remission of diabetes in some studies. For more information on bariatric surgery and its complications, see MKSAP 16 Gastroenterology and Hepatology and MKSAP 16 General Internal Medicine.

Pharmacologic Agents

At the time of diabetes diagnosis, lifestyle changes should be encouraged and a noninsulin agent started. In the past decade, agents to help lower blood glucose levels in patients with diabetes have proliferated, with no fewer than 12 different drug classes now available (**Table 7**). The available drugs vary markedly in cost, route and frequency of administration, effect on body weight, mechanism of action, adverse effect profile, and known effects on serious outcomes (microvascular and macrovascular events, morbidity, and mortality). Much is now known about older diabetes agents, such as insulin, the sulfonylureas, and metformin, that provide proven long-term glycemic control and cost effectiveness. Newer agents offer the potential advantage of targeting different metabolic pathways, and adding or combining these agents can lower blood glucose levels by different mechanisms. However, the long-term efficacy and safety of these drugs relative to older drugs are not as well established, and the newer drugs tend to be considerably more expensive.

The natural history of type 2 diabetes is of progressive loss of pancreatic beta-cell function in addition to underlying insulin resistance; as pancreatic beta-cell function continues to decline, postprandial blood glucose levels increase. Therefore, most patients will require more than one pharmacologic agent over time to maintain their plasma glucose level at goal. No consensus exists among experts about which combination of agents works best. Options are to add oral agents that help lower postprandial blood glucose levels (sulfonylureas, α-glucosidase inhibitors, meglitinides, or dipeptidyl peptidase-4

inhibitors), injectable agents that slow gastric emptying and suppress glucagon (pramlintide, exenatide, or liraglutide), or insulin. For most patients, metformin is the best agent to add to lifestyle modifications as an initial therapy.

The sulfonylureas vary mostly in dose and half-life. Those with long half-lives, such as chlorpropamide and glyburide, can cause profound, prolonged hypoglycemia, especially in older patients and patients with impaired kidney function. Therefore, these drugs should be avoided in these two populations. For the past 40 years, concern has existed that treatment with certain sulfonylureas increases myocardial damage after coronary artery occlusion because first- and second-generation sulfonylureas (such as glyburide) bind to myocardial and pancreatic adenosine triphosphate–sensitive potassium channels, thus blocking myocardial preconditioning mechanisms. Third-generation sulfonylureas (such as gliclazide and glimepiride) bind exclusively to pancreatic beta-cell potassium channels. One study showed that in-patient mortality of patients with diabetes who sustained acute ST-elevation and non–ST-elevation myocardial infarctions was significantly lower for those taking gliclazide or glimepiride (2.7%) than those taking glyburide (7.5%; $P<0.02$).

KEY POINT

- For most patients with type 2 diabetes, lifestyle modifications and metformin therapy are the best initial treatments; as their disease progresses, many will need to use additional pharmacologic agents.

Insulin Therapy for Diabetes

Basal insulin generally is used in type 2 diabetes if a patient is unable to achieve a target fasting plasma glucose level with lifestyle modification and oral hypoglycemic agents alone. Adding a longer-acting form of insulin (such as neutral protamine Hagedorn [NPH] insulin, insulin detemir, or insulin glargine) either at bedtime or first thing in the morning also can be effective. (Of note, insulin detemir and insulin glargine are two- to four-times more expensive than NPH insulin and, in randomized controlled trials, generally achieve the same hemoglobin A_{1c} values and only modestly less hypoglycemia than does NPH insulin.) A basal insulin usually is combined with an oral hypoglycemic agent (such as a long-acting insulin at bedtime combined with daytime metformin) to achieve adequate control.

Premixed insulins (**Table 8**), which combine different insulin types with differing pharmacokinetic profiles, can minimize the number of daily injections a patient takes. The size and timing of the peak insulin effect can be altered by using different proportions of a rapid-acting insulin analogue, short-acting regular insulin, and long-acting insulin (**Figure 1**). Although twice-daily premixed insulins can be used quite effectively in patients with type 2 diabetes who have stable daily routines of what and when they eat and how much they exercise, the day-to-day variability of insulin absorption means that

TABLE 7.	Pharmacologic Agents Used to Lower Blood Glucose Levels in Type 2 Diabetes Mellitus				
Class	**Route of Administration**	**Mechanism of Action**	**Effect on Weight**	**Risks and Concerns**	**Long-Term Studies on Definitive Outcomes**
Insulin	Injection	Decreases hepatic glucose production, increases peripheral glucose uptake, and supports anabolism	Increase	Hypoglycemia; insulin allergy (rare)	Decrease in both microvascular and macrovascular events
Sulfonylureas (tolbutamide, chlorpropamide, glipizide, glyburide, gliclazide, glimepiride)	Oral	Stimulate insulin secretion from pancreatic beta cells	Increase	Hypoglycemia (especially in drugs with long half-lives); weight gain; skin rashes (including photosensitivity)	Decrease in microvascular events but possible increase in macrovascular events with tolbutamide, chlorpropamide, glyburide, and glipizide; not seen with gliclazide or glimepiride
Biguanides (metformin)	Oral	Decrease hepatic glucose production, decrease free fatty acids, increase insulin-mediated uptake of glucose in muscles	Neutral	Diarrhea and abdominal discomfort; lactic acidosis (exceedingly rare); contraindicated in presence of progressive liver, kidney, or cardiac failure	Decrease in both microvascular and macrovascular events and decreased risk of cancer
α-Glucosidase inhibitors (acarbose, miglitol, voglibose)	Oral	Inhibit polysaccharide absorption	Neutral	Flatulence; abdominal discomfort	May reduce CVD events (acute MI and hypertension)
Thiazolidine-diones (rosiglitazone, pioglitazone)	Oral	Activate nuclear PPARγ receptors to regulate gene expression in numerous tissues, increase peripheral uptake of glucose, decrease hepatic glucose production	Increase	Fluid retention; heart failure; macular edema; osteoporosis (possible increased risk of bladder cancer with pioglitazone)	Increase in CVD events (heart failure, acute MI) and mortality with rosiglitazone; unclear whether pioglitazone causes net harm or good
Meglitinides (repaglinide, nateglinide)	Oral	Stimulate insulin release from pancreatic beta cells	Increase	Hypoglycemia	None
Lipase inhibitors (orlistat)	Oral	Inhibit dietary fat absorption	Decrease	Flatulence; abdominal discomfort; oily feces; occasional fecal incontinence; reduced absorption of fat-soluble vitamins	None
Amylino-mimetics (pramlintide)	Injection	Slow gastric emptying, suppress glucagon secretion, increase satiety	Decrease	Nausea; vomiting; increased hypoglycemic risk of insulin	None
GLP-1 mimetics (exenatide and liraglutide)	Injection	Slow gastric emptying, suppress glucagon secretion, increase satiety	Decrease	Hypoglycemia when used in combination with sulfonylureas; nausea and vomiting; possible increased risk of pancreatitis and chronic kidney disease	None

(continued on next page)

TABLE 7. Pharmacologic Agents Used to Lower Blood Glucose Levels in Type 2 Diabetes Mellitus (*continued*)

Class	Route of Administration	Mechanism of Action	Effect on Weight	Risks and Concerns	Long-Term Studies on Definitive Outcomes
DPP-4 inhibitors (sitagliptin, saxagliptin, vildagliptin)	Oral	Slow gastric emptying, suppress glucagon secretion	Neutral	Hypoglycemia when used in combination with sulfonylureas; nausea; skin rashes; increased risk of infections; possible increased risk of pancreatitis	None
Bile acid sequestrants (colesevelam)	Oral	Unclear	Neutral	Constipation; dyspepsia; increased triglyceride level; possible increase in LDL cholesterol level; reduced absorption of fat-soluble vitamins	None
Dopamine agonists (bromocriptine)	Oral	Unclear central nervous system effects	Neutral	Nausea; headache; orthostatic hypotension; inhibition of lactation; potential exacerbation of psychosis	None

CVD = cardiovascular disease; DPP-4 = dipeptidyl peptidase–4; GLP-1 = glucagon-like peptide-1; MI = myocardial infarction; PPARγ = peroxisome proliferator-activated receptor-γ.

TABLE 8. Pharmacokinetic Properties of Insulin Products[a]

Insulin Type	Onset	Peak	Duration
Rapid-acting (lispro, aspart, glulisine)	5-15 min	45-90 min	2-4 h
Short-acting (regular)	0.5-1 h	2-4 h	4-8 h
NPH insulin	1-3 h	4-10 h	10-18 h
Detemir	1-2 h	None[b]	12-24 h[c]
Glargine	2-3 h	None[b]	20-24+ h
Premixed insulins			
70% NPH/30% regular	0.5-1 h	2-10 h	10-18 h
50% NPH/50% regular	0.5-1 h	2-10 h[d]	10-18 h
75% NPL/25% lispro	10-20 min	1-6 h	10-18 h
50% NPL/50% lispro	10-20 min	1-6 h[d]	10-18 h
70% NPA/30% aspart	10-20 min	1-6 h	10-18 h

NPA = neutral protamine aspart; NPH = neutral protamine Hagedorn; NPL = neutral protamine lispro.

[a]The time course of each insulin varies significantly between persons and within the same person on different days. Therefore, the time periods listed should be considered general guidelines only.

[b]Both insulin detemir and insulin glargine can produce a peak effect in some persons, especially at higher doses.

[c]The duration of action for insulin detemir varies depending on the dose given.

[d]Premixed insulins containing a larger proportion of rapid- or short-acting insulin tend to have larger peaks occurring at an earlier time than mixtures containing smaller proportions of rapid- or short-acting insulin.

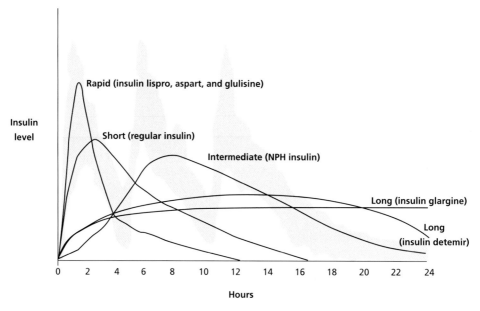

FIGURE 1. Plasma insulin profiles of different types of insulin preparations. The shaded areas represent the range of normal insulin responses to three meals in persons without diabetes. NPH = neutral protamine Hagedorn.

patients may experience unpredictable episodes of hypoglycemia during the middle of the day or night with these preparations. An alternative strategy is to use an intensified insulin regimen of basal and preprandial insulins, similar to approaches used by patients with type 1 diabetes. Cost concerns are a factor in determining which pharmacologic choices are made (see Table 8) because the newer insulin preparations (insulin glargine, detemir, aspart, lispro, and glulisine) are far more expensive than regular insulin and NPH insulin.

Insulin treatment is essential for all patients with type 1 diabetes and for many patients with type 2 diabetes who have significant insulin deficiency in addition to their underlying insulin resistance. The degree of complexity in the regimen should be decided collaboratively with each patient. Although once or twice daily regimens with long- or intermediate-acting or premixed insulins offer the convenience and lower cost of fewer injections and fewer blood glucose tests, concern has been raised that these agents may lead to higher plasma insulin levels throughout the day, which may cause unpredictable hypoglycemia and weight gain. Intensified insulin regimens with three to five insulin injections per day or a continuous subcutaneous insulin infusion, although more complicated, allow for more precise control of blood glucose levels between meals, overnight, after food intake or exercise, and with stress. This approach separates insulin delivery into basal and prandial components.

Most patients require 0.5 to 1.5 units/kg/d of insulin, although this may vary greatly depending on the patient's degree of insulin resistance or sensitivity. Most persons with type 1 diabetes are quite sensitive to insulin, and thus 0.5 units/kg/d is a good initial dose. In contrast, most persons with type 2 diabetes have significant insulin resistance and

thus may require upward titration from this starting dose to 1 to 1.5 units/kg/d, depending on their individual response. Approximately half the daily dose is given as a basal insulin (one or two injections of NPH insulin, insulin glargine, or insulin detemir, or a continuous basal subcutaneous infusion from an insulin pump). Before each meal, a bolus of rapid-acting insulin is given, and these three injections account for the other half of the day's total insulin use. Ideally, the total bolus amount is determined by the amount of carbohydrates about to be consumed (typically, 1 unit for every 10 [or 15] grams of carbohydrate) plus a correction factor predicated on the preprandial blood glucose level. A typical correction factor for a patient with type 1 diabetes is 1 additional unit for every 40 (or 50) mg/dL (2.2 [or 2.8] mmol/L) above 100 mg/dL (5.6 mmol/L) the preprandial glucose level is; for patients with type 2 diabetes, the correction factor is 1 additional unit for every 25 mg/dL (1.4 mmol/L) above 100 mg/dL (5.6 mmol/L) the preprandial glucose level is. These preprandial bolus injections must be given as separate injections and not mixed with the basal insulin. When short-acting or rapid-acting insulin is mixed with longer-acting insulin, the pharmacokinetics change to cause a significantly delayed single peak (as seen with premixed insulins) (see Figure 1).

For patients trying to achieve hemoglobin A_{1c} levels less than 7.0%, fasting and premeal glucose targets usually are set at approximately 80 to 130 mg/dL (4.4-7.2 mmol/L). If these levels are not being attained or postprandial levels are consistently greater than 200 mg/dL (11.1 mmol/L) despite using these calculations, the formulae can be changed (for example, to take 1 unit for every 10 grams of carbohydrates consumed and 1 additional unit for every 30 mg/dL [1.7 mmol/L] above target the preprandial blood glucose level is).

- Although more convenient and less costly, once or twice daily regimens with intermediate-acting or pre-mixed insulins can cause more frequent and unpredictable hypoglycemia and weight gain in patients with diabetes.
- Most patients with diabetes who take daily insulin receive an intensified regimen of basal and preprandial insulins, with the dosage of the latter varying depending on the amount of carbohydrates about to be consumed and on what the preprandial blood glucose level is.

Inpatient Management of Hyperglycemia and Diabetes

When patients with type 1 or type 2 diabetes are admitted to a hospital for treatment of diabetes or other conditions, glycemic control is likely to deteriorate. Additionally, when patients with previously undiagnosed diabetes are admitted to a hospital, their outcomes and length of stay are likely to be much worse if the diabetes remains undiagnosed or untreated. For these reasons, measurement of plasma glucose and hemoglobin A_{1c} levels should be routine when most adults are admitted.

The main goals for patients with diabetes during hospitalization are to (1) avoid hypoglycemia; (2) avoid severe hyperglycemia, volume depletion, and electrolyte abnormalities; (3) ensure adequate nutrition; (4) address diabetes education needs; and (5) facilitate smooth transition back to the ambulatory setting. Success and ease in achieving these goals depend on the type of diabetes and the severity of the underlying illness precipitating the admission. The key is to perform frequent blood glucose testing during hospitalization (either before meals and bedtime or every 6 hours if the patient is receiving nothing by mouth).

For patients with type 2 diabetes who follow dietary therapy and take oral agents, continuing their oral agents may be reasonable if they are still eating. If patients are not able or allowed to eat, then oral agents should be stopped. Oral agents should also be stopped in the presence of specific contraindications:

- Metformin should be stopped if intravenous contrast dye will be used or if the reason for admission could cause lactic acidosis.
- Thiazolidinediones (pioglitazone, rosiglitazone) should be stopped in patients admitted with prevalent or suspected cardiovascular disease, peripheral edema, heart failure, ventricular dysfunction, or osteoporosis.
- Both metformin and thiazolidinediones should be discontinued in patients with either acute or chronic liver dysfunction.

- Sulfonylureas and meglitinides, which increase the risk of hypoglycemia, should be stopped if food intake may be unpredictable.

A plasma glucose range of 140 to 180 mg/dL (7.8-10.0 mmol/L) is recommended for critically ill hospitalized patients with hyperglycemia. The glycemic targets for noncritically ill hospitalized patients have not been adequately determined by research trials, but current recommendations from a consensus statement by the ADA and the American Association of Clinical Endocrinologists are to maintain fasting and premeal glucose levels of less than 140 mg/dL (7.8 mmol/L) but no lower than 90 mg/dL (5.0 mmol/L) and random or postprandial levels of less than 180 mg/dL (10.0 mmol/L).

All patients with type 1 diabetes and many with type 2 will require insulin treatment while in the hospital. The use of sliding-scale insulin without basal insulin generally is discouraged. When sliding-scale regular or rapid-acting insulin is used without basal insulin, the likelihood of wide swings from hyperglycemia to hypoglycemia is much stronger. If the blood glucose level is at target and no insulin is given, then the glucose level is almost certain to be much higher when next checked; at that time, a large dose of rapid-acting insulin most likely will be given, which will result in hypoglycemia. A better approach is to give basal insulin subcutaneously and then add a preprandial rapid-acting insulin in a variable dose based on the amount of carbohydrate the patient is planning to eat, with an additional amount to correct for the degree of preprandial hyperglycemia. For patients who are more critically ill or whose blood glucose level cannot be maintained in the target range with subcutaneous insulin, an intravenous glucose infusion, which allows much more rapid adjustments, should be considered, provided adequate skilled staff is available for safe administration.

- A plasma glucose range of 140 to 180 mg/dL (7.8-10.0 mmol/L) is recommended for critically ill hospitalized patients with hyperglycemia.
- In noncritically ill hospitalized patients with hyperglycemia, a consensus statement recommends fasting and premeal glucose levels of less than 140 mg/dL (7.8 mmol/L) but no lower than 90 mg/dL (5.0 mmol/L) and random or postprandial levels of less than 180 mg/dL (10.0 mmol/L).

Acute Complications of Diabetes
Diabetic Ketoacidosis and Hyperglycemic Hyperosmolar Syndrome

Insulin-deficient states, whether absolute or relative, can result in DKA or hyperglycemic hyperosmolar syndrome (HHS), which are both serious and life-threatening conditions. The most common causes of DKA are new-onset type 1 diabetes, inappropriate underdosing of insulin or missed insulin dosing (alone or in combination with infection or other serious illnesses), and myocardial ischemia. A spectrum of metabolic decompensation occurs in DKA (**Figure 2**). The degree of hyperglycemia and acidosis depends on several factors, including the severity of insulin deficiency, diet, kidney function, and any additional inciting factor. A patient with type 1 diabetes who has complete insulin deficiency can develop acidosis in a matter of hours, frequently with plasma glucose levels in excess of 400 to 500 mg/dL (22.2-27.8 mmol/L). In certain patients, however, only relatively mild hyperglycemia (200-250 mg/dL [11.1-13.9 mmol/L]) is seen. For example, if the patient is not eating or drinking, severe ketoacidosis may occur before the plasma glucose level has increased by very much. Alternatively, patients with impaired hepatic function or ongoing use of alcohol may have a relatively dampened degree of hepatic glucose production, which is the primary driver of hyperglycemia in DKA. In contrast, an older patient with only partial insulin deficiency might develop hyperglycemia and dehydration subacutely over days or even weeks. If the patient still produces enough endogenous insulin to prevent lipolysis,

but not enough to control the plasma glucose level, he or she will remain nonketotic. However, if sugary liquids are consumed to quench thirst, if the patient has impaired renal clearance of glucose, or if a coexisting infection or other inciting factor is present, HHS—a severe hyperosmolar nonketotic hyperglycemia—can develop.

The earliest symptoms of severe hyperglycemia are polyuria, polydipsia, and weight loss. As hyperglycemia worsens, neurologic symptoms appear, including lethargy, drowsiness, focal deficits, and coma. As the acidosis and electrolyte disturbance worsen, patients experience nausea, vomiting, abdominal pain, and hyperventilation. Total-body loss of electrolytes, especially potassium, can be severe but may not be apparent initially because potassium leaks out of cells, which causes the serum potassium level to appear falsely "normal." After insulin is administered, the available potassium moves rapidly back inside the cells, which results in a precipitous decrease in the serum potassium level.

The initial evaluation of a patient with suspected DKA or HHS should include laboratory studies, such as measurement of plasma glucose, serum electrolyte, serum creatinine, and

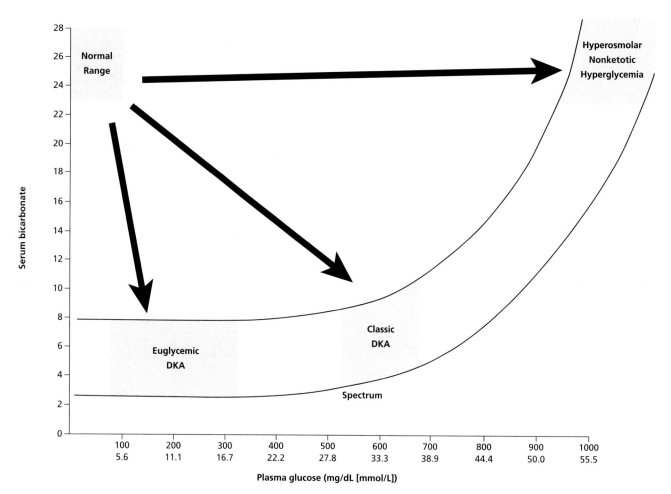

FIGURE 2. Spectrum of metabolic decompensation that occurs in DKA. DKA = diabetic ketoacidosis.

blood urea nitrogen levels; a complete blood count with leukocyte differential; urinalysis, including urine ketones; determination of plasma osmolality and the presence of serum ketones (if urine ketones are present); and an arterial blood gas analysis (if the serum bicarbonate level is substantially reduced). Electrocardiography is also recommended. The plasma glucose level should be measured every hour, whereas the other serum and plasma levels should be measured every 2 to 4 hours, depending on the severity of the acidosis and the clinical response. Unless profound acidemia is detected, repeat arterial blood gas measurement is usually unnecessary if the venous pH or serum bicarbonate level can be obtained every 2 to 4 hours.

DKA and HHS are best managed in an intensive care unit, especially if the patient has signs of clinical instability (such as hypotension, bradycardia, increased work of breathing, altered mental status, or a pH less than 7.0). Treatment includes careful replacement of fluids, electrolytes, and insulin (with intravenous infusion of regular insulin) and correction of acidosis, if present (**Table 9**). Although the appropriate additional testing to identify the underlying causes of the DKA or HHS will depend on clinical circumstances, a few points are worth noting. In the absence of infection, the leukocyte count may be greater than 20,000/microliter (20×10^9/L) in DKA because of ketoacidosis alone. Because metabolic decompensation also can suppress temperature, the lack of a fever does not rule out infection. Additionally, abdominal pain in the setting of diabetic ketoacidosis is typically generalized and usually seen when the serum bicarbonate level is substantially less than 15 meq/L (15 mmol/L); focal abdominal pain, especially if the acidosis is not severe (>15 meq/L [15 mmol/L]), more likely represents an intra-abdominal problem. Because metabolic decompensation also can cause an increased serum amylase level (to >1000 units/L), a high amylase level is not a reliable indicator of acute pancreatitis.

KEY POINTS

- The initial evaluation of a patient with suspected diabetic ketoacidosis or hyperglycemic hyperosmolar syndrome should include frequent measurement of plasma glucose, serum electrolyte, serum creatinine, and blood urea nitrogen levels and plasma osmolality; a complete blood count; urinalysis; an arterial blood gas analysis (if the serum bicarbonate level is substantially reduced); and electrocardiography.

- Management of diabetic ketoacidosis and hyperglycemic hyperosmolar syndrome should include careful replacement of fluids, electrolytes, and insulin (with intravenous infusion of regular insulin) and correction of acidosis, preferably in an intensive care unit if the patient is unstable clinically.

Hypoglycemia

The brain uses glucose as its preferred fuel. When a person's plasma glucose level is less than 70 mg/dL (3.9 mmol/L), signals are sent from the brain to the pancreas, liver, and

TABLE 9.	Management of Hyperglycemic Crisis (DKA and HHS)		
Fluids	**Insulin (Regular)**	**Potassium**	**Correction of Acidosis**
Assess for volume status, then give 0.9% saline at 1 L/h initially in all patients, and continue if patient is severely hypovolemic. Switch to 0.45% normal saline at 250-500 mL/h if corrected serum sodium level becomes normal or high. When the plasma glucose level reaches 200 mg/dL (11.1 mmol/L) in patients with DKA or 300 mg/dL (16.7 mmol/L) in HHS, switch to 5% dextrose with 0.45% normal saline at 150-250 mL/h.	Give regular insulin, 0.1 unit/kg, as an intravenous bolus followed by 0.1 unit/kg/h as an intravenous infusion; if the plasma glucose level does not decrease by 10% in the first hour, give an additional bolus of 0.14 unit/kg and resume previous infusion rate; when the plasma glucose level reaches 200 mg/dL (11.1 mmol/L) in DKA and 300 mg/dL (16.7 mmol/L) in HHS, reduce to 0.02-0.05 unit/kg/h, and maintain the plasma glucose level between 150-200 mg/dL (8.3 mmol/L) until anion gap acidosis is resolved in DKA.	Assess for adequate kidney function, with adequate urine output (approximately 50 mL/h). If serum potassium is <3.3 meq/L (3.3 mmol/L), do not start insulin but instead give intravenous potassium chloride, 20-30 meq/h, through a central line catheter until the serum potassium level is >3.3 meq/L (3.3 mmol/L); then add 20-30 meq of potassium chloride to each liter of intravenous fluids to keep the serum potassium level in the 4.0-5.0 meq/L (4.0-5.0 mmol/L) range. If the serum potassium level is >5.2 meq/L (5.2 mmol/L), do not give potassium chloride but instead start insulin and intravenous fluids and check the serum potassium level every 2 hours.	If pH is <6.9, give sodium bicarbonate, 100 mmol in 400 mL of water, and potassium chloride, 20 meq, infused over 2 hours. If pH is 6.9 or greater, do not give sodium bicarbonate.

DKA = diabetic ketoacidosis; HHS = hyperglycemic hyperosmolar syndrome.

adrenal glands that collectively raise the plasma glucose level. The hormones involved are glucagon, epinephrine, norepinephrine, cortisol, and growth hormone; hepatic gluconeogenesis also occurs. Hyperadrenergic symptoms (sweating, rapid heartbeat, anxiety, hunger, and tremor) are usually experienced first. If the plasma glucose level continues to decline, brain function becomes impaired, and neuroglycopenic signs and symptoms (cognitive impairment, somnolence, dizziness, slurred speech, and change in personality) develop. If these signs and symptoms are not recognized and treated and the plasma glucose level continues to decrease, the patient may lose consciousness, develop focal neurologic signs (such as hemiparesis), or have seizures.

Although most common in type 1 diabetes, severe hypoglycemia also can occur in type 2 diabetes in patients who are taking insulin or drugs (such as sulfonylureas and meglitinides) that stimulate the release of insulin. The situations in which hypoglycemia most commonly develops involve patients taking too large a dose of insulin, delaying or skipping a meal, eating fewer carbohydrates than normally, or exercising more than usual. Older patients who take sulfonylureas with long half-lives or who develop heart failure or kidney impairment can have high drug levels in their blood due to decreased clearance, which results in profound and prolonged hypoglycemia. Prolonged exercise that is not followed by consumption of complex carbohydrates can lead to hypoglycemia several hours later as the muscles and the liver continue to remove glucose from the blood to replenish their glycogen stores. This is especially problematic if exercise occurs in the evening before bedtime. Excess alcohol consumption also can cause hypoglycemia by suppressing hepatic glucose production. Alcohol additionally may blunt a person's ability to recognize hypoglycemic symptoms (slurred speech, altered personality), and these symptoms may be wrongly attributed by others to his or her alcohol use.

Distinguishing between the following four hypoglycemic situations can be useful:

1. Severe hypoglycemia, which requires the assistance of another person to administer a carbohydrate (preferably glucose sublingually or intravenously) or subcutaneous glucagon

2. Documented symptomatic hypoglycemia, which occurs when a patient feels typical hyperadrenergic hypoglycemic symptoms and verifies that the blood glucose level is less than 70 mg/dL (3.9 mmol/L) before self-treating with 15 grams of a carbohydrate

3. Asymptomatic hypoglycemia (or hypoglycemic unawareness), in which a patient does not develop typical hyperadrenergic symptoms but has a measured plasma glucose level of less than 70 mg/dL (3.9 mmol/L); this situation occurs most often in type 1 diabetes in patients striving for excellent glycemic control

(hemoglobin A_{1c} value <7.0%) who have chronic, frequent episodes of hypoglycemia. The body's ability to recognize hypoglycemia and secrete counterregulatory hormones in response to hypoglycemia deteriorates and leaves these patients vulnerable to further episodes of severe hypoglycemia. Treatment for this hypoglycemic unawareness is to reduce the insulin dosage and eat more carbohydrates both at meals and between meals to ensure a blood glucose level of 150 to 200 mg/dL (8.3-11.1 mmol/L) at all times for several weeks. This step allows the body to "reset" so that hypoglycemia is recognized and the counterregulatory response to hypoglycemia is improved.

4. Relative hypoglycemia, in which a patient experiences hyperadrenergic hypoglycemic symptoms but has a measured plasma glucose level greater than 70 mg/dL (3.9 mmol/L); this situation occurs most often in patients who have had months (or longer) of hyperglycemia (plasma glucose levels >200 mg/dL [11.1 mmol/L] at all times) whose plasma glucose levels are then lowered by medication or lifestyle changes closer to the normal range. Hyperadrenergic hypoglycemic symptoms can occur when the plasma glucose level in these patients is 120 mg/dL (6.7 mmol/L) or even higher. If these patients continue to keep their plasma glucose level substantially less than 200 mg/dL (11.1 mmol/L), the threshold at which they manifest hypoglycemic symptoms will fall to more typical levels (<70 mg/dL [3.9 mmol/L]).

Patients vary in how well they tolerate the hyperadrenergic symptoms of hypoglycemia psychologically. Fear of the symptoms and of the hypoglycemia itself is a common barrier to achieving hemoglobin A_{1c} goals. Although the human brain can tolerate recurrent episodes of hypoglycemia relatively well, cognitive deficits can be found among children and adults who have had years of repeated episodes of severe hypoglycemia. In older patients and those whose livelihood would be jeopardized by hypoglycemia (commercial vehicle drivers, persons who work with dangerous equipment), it is reasonable (and indeed preferable) to set hemoglobin A_{1c} targets at higher levels and to adjust treatment regimens to reduce the chance of hypoglycemia.

KEY POINTS

- Although most common in type 1 diabetes mellitus, hypoglycemia also occurs in patients with type 2 diabetes who are taking insulin or drugs that stimulate the release of insulin.

- In relative hypoglycemia, a patient experiences typical hypoglycemic symptoms but has a measured plasma glucose level greater than 70 mg/dL (3.9 mmol/L).

Chronic Complications of Diabetes

Diabetic Retinopathy

Because the retina is highly vascular and can be viewed directly through an ophthalmoscope, it gives the earliest indication of microvascular damage from hyperglycemia. Diabetic retinopathy generally develops and progresses slowly and predictably. Chronic hyperglycemia causes edema, hard exudates, and tiny hemorrhages in the retinal layers. Microaneurysms in the vessel wall may result in retinal infarcts (soft exudates or "cotton wool" spots). These features are collectively called background or nonproliferative diabetic retinopathy. As the retina becomes more ischemic, proliferative retinopathy can occur, in which blood vessels rupture and often cause extensive intraocular bleeding. Fibrosis and contraction follow, leading to retinal detachment. This severe proliferative retinopathy may thus result in a substantial loss of vision.

Management of diabetic retinopathy consists of regular retinal evaluation by direct visual examination through an ophthalmoscope or by high-quality retinal photographs. Screening guidelines are shown in **Table 10**. This screening does not need to be started until 5 years after diagnosis of type 1 diabetes because of the general lack of retinopathy seen in the early years of the disease. Because type 2 diabetes usually develops slowly, undetected hyperglycemia may be present for many years before diagnosis. Therefore, retinal screening should start immediately in patients with this type of diabetes; approximately 10% of these patients have evidence of diabetic retinopathy at diagnosis. In patients with background retinopathy and poor glycemic control, a rapid improvement in glycemic control can result in a temporary worsening of retinopathy (particularly retinal infarcts). This pattern also is seen in pregnant women with diabetes in whom diabetic retinopathy can appear suddenly and progress rapidly. Therefore, pregnant women with diabetes should be screened for retinopathy during the first trimester and in each trimester thereafter.

The risk of retinopathy can be reduced (or the progression slowed) by excellent glycemic control (hemoglobin A_{1c} value <7.0%), lowering blood pressure, smoking cessation, or use of ACE inhibitors. The mainstay of treatment for advanced diabetic retinopathy is laser photocoagulation. In patients with macular edema, focal laser therapy in the surrounding retina can reduce the edema and restore vision. When proliferative retinopathy develops, more widespread laser therapy (often several thousand tiny laser burns delivered to the periphery of the retina) is used. As these burns scar and become avascular, the total retinal area is reduced by approximately one third; the remaining retina thus receives more blood, and new vessels involute. As a result, the risk of major intraocular bleeding or retinal detachment is reduced and central vision is preserved, but at the expense of a loss of peripheral vision. After widespread (panretinal) laser photocoagulation, many patients notice a significant worsening of their peripheral vision while driving, which can be especially noticeable and troubling at night.

In addition to laser photocoagulation therapy, an alternative or complementary management of proliferative diabetic retinopathy is intraocular injections of inhibitors of vascular endothelial growth factors, such as bevacizumab or ranibizumab, every 4 to 8 weeks.

KEY POINT

- The mainstay of treatment of advanced diabetic retinopathy is laser photocoagulation.

Diabetic Nephropathy

Chronic hyperglycemia causes progressive damage to the glomerular basement membranes of the kidneys in patients with diabetes. The kidneys then begin to release excessive amounts of protein into the urine. This proteinuria is associated with an increased serum creatinine level, worsening hypertension, and progression to end-stage kidney disease requiring dialysis or kidney transplantation. Although diabetes remains the leading cause of chronic kidney failure in the United States and is the most common reason for dialysis and kidney transplantation, the overall incidence of diabetic nephropathy has declined significantly in the past two decades. Improved glycemic and blood pressure control, the use of ACE inhibitors or ARBs, and smoking cessation programs are largely responsible for this decrease. Some research

TABLE 10. Screening Recommendations for Diabetic Retinopathy

Clinical Situation	When to Start Screening	Screening Frequency
Type 1 diabetes	At 5 years after diagnosis	Annually[a]
Type 2 diabetes	At diagnosis	Annually[a]
In pregnant women with either type of diabetes	First trimester	Every trimester and then closely for 1 year postpartum
In women with either type of diabetes planning to conceive	During preconception planning	Same as recommendations for pregnant women once conception occurs

[a]It is reasonable to screen every 2 years if no diabetic retinopathy is present and to screen more often than annually if diabetic retinopathy is advanced or progressing rapidly.

evidence suggests that intensive glucose management may prevent or delay the onset and progression of diabetic nephropathy. Patients with type 1 diabetes who have no detectable proteinuria 20 years after diagnosis are unlikely to develop end-stage kidney disease. Although the incidence of diabetic nephropathy is somewhat lower in type 2 diabetes, significant genetic and ethnic variation exists.

Protein in the urine can be measured by determining the albumin-creatinine ratio. Values between 30 and 300 mg/g indicate microalbuminuria, and values greater than 300 mg/g indicate macroalbuminuria (or overt proteinuria). Patients with type 2 diabetes should be tested annually for microalbuminuria from the time of diagnosis, and patients with type 1 diabetes should begin annual testing 5 years after diagnosis. Persistent microalbuminuria suggests not only that a patient is at significantly increased risk of developing overt diabetic nephropathy in the future, but also that the risk of future cardiovascular disease is at least four times higher than that of age- and gender-matched patients with no microalbuminuria. Vigorous exercise, menstruation, illness, and acute hyperglycemia can cause false elevations in the urine albumin-creatinine ratio.

For more information on diabetic nephropathy, see MKSAP 16 Nephrology.

Diabetic Neuropathy

Nerve cells (sensory, motor, and autonomic) are vulnerable to damage from chronic hyperglycemia, and clinical manifestations of neuropathy tend to appear as a later complication of diabetes, particularly diabetes that is not optimally controlled. Also, an acute distal symmetric diabetic neuropathy may occur after an episode of severe hyperglycemia and cause segmental demyelination in a stocking-glove distribution. Peripheral diabetic neuropathy results in sharp, stabbing, or burning pain in the toes, feet, lower legs, and hands. Patients also may feel discomfort when the skin is touched (dysesthesia) and a heaviness and clumsiness in their feet and legs. Symptoms often are worse at night. Immediate relief often is obtained by topical application of capsaicin cream and relatively low oral doses of tricyclic antidepressants or partial serotonin and norepinephrine reuptake inhibitors. If this approach does not relieve symptoms, adding an antiseizure medication (gabapentin, pregabalin, carbamazepine, or phenytoin) may help, but opiates should be avoided. Patients also should be encouraged to try to reduce their hemoglobin A_{1c} levels to less than 7.0%, which may help remyelinate the nerves and reverse the neuropathy.

Acute ocular or truncal mononeuropathies can occur. No specific treatment for these mononeuropathies is effective, but they usually resolve spontaneously over a few months. Diabetic amyotrophy should be considered in patients with recently diagnosed or well-controlled diabetes who develop acute proximal leg pain or weakness and weight loss. The nerves of patients with diabetes are more vulnerable to entrapment neuropathies, including carpal tunnel syndrome or meralgia paresthetica.

The combination of nerve damage and impaired peripheral vascular circulation places patients with chronic diabetic neuropathy at high risk for foot ulcers and amputations. All patients with diabetes should have their feet examined at least annually to assess for decreased sensation and detect ulcers, calluses, foot deformities, pain, abnormal pressure sensation, and peripheral pulses. These patients should be strongly encouraged to inspect their feet daily and seek help at the earliest signs of ulceration or infection. Charcot foot deformity may develop over time in patients with seemingly minor foot trauma, axonal loss, and small muscle atrophy.

Damage to autonomic nerves elsewhere in the body can present as erectile dysfunction (present in 50% of men with diabetes who are older than 50 years), gastroparesis (see MKSAP 16 Gastroenterology and Hepatology), chronic diarrhea or constipation, orthostatic hypotension, resting sinus tachycardia, postprandial hypotension, abnormal hidrosis, and neurogenic bladder. Patients with manifestations of cardiovascular neuropathy are at increased risk of sudden cardiac death, and thus cardiac risk reduction should be strongly encouraged.

For more information on diabetic neuropathy, see MKSAP 16 Neurology.

KEY POINT

- All patients with diabetes should have their feet examined at least annually to assess for decreased sensation and detect ulcers, calluses, foot deformities, pain, abnormal pressure sensation, and peripheral pulses.

Hypoglycemia in Patients Without Diabetes

Hypoglycemia is rare in persons without diabetes because the healthy body has robust mechanisms for maintaining glucose homeostasis. As the plasma glucose falls to less than the normal range, the pancreatic islet cells turn off insulin secretion and hepatic glycogenolysis supplies glucose to maintain the plasma glucose level above 70 mg/dL (3.9 mmol/L). When this level is less than 70 mg/dL (3.9 mmol/L), glucagon and epinephrine secretion increases, and when it is less than 60 mg/dL (3.3 mmol/L), cortisol and growth hormone secretion increases. When hepatic glycogen stores are exhausted (in approximately 8 hours), hepatic gluconeogenesis becomes the sole source of glucose production. Hypoglycemia can occur when hepatic glycogen stores are depleted as a result of extreme starvation, sepsis, or hepatic dysfunction; when alcohol ingestion suppresses hepatic glucose production; and when cortisol is deficient (as in untreated Addison disease and adrenocorticotropic hormone deficiency [secondary glucocorticoid deficiency]).

In apparently healthy persons without diabetes, hypoglycemic symptoms usually occur either in the fasting or postprandial state.

Fasting Hypoglycemia

When hypoglycemic symptoms occur in the fasting state or at least not in the immediate postprandial period, the differential diagnosis includes the presence of an insulin-secreting tumor (insulinoma), which is exceedingly rare; the surreptitious injection of insulin; or the ingestion of a sulfonylurea or meglitinide (see Table 7). Because symptoms of hypoglycemia are nonspecific and can be caused by anxiety or stress, one must document that the plasma glucose level is actually low at the times when symptoms are experienced. Therefore, hypoglycemia is best diagnosed when three conditions coexist (Whipple triad): (1) hypoglycemic symptoms are present, (2) a low plasma glucose level is documented by a laboratory (because self–blood glucose monitors may be unreliable at low glucose levels), and (3) prompt resolution of symptoms occurs after glucose ingestion. When Whipple triad is observed, further evaluation for the cause of pathologic hypoglycemia should include an inpatient 72-hour fast with regular measurement of simultaneous plasma glucose, proinsulin, insulin, C-peptide (a measure of endogenous insulin secretion), β-hydroxybutyrate (a ketone body produced in the absence of insulin), and sulfonylurea levels (to rule out surreptitious ingestion) (**Table 11**). If the results are consistent with insulinoma, only then should CT imaging of the pancreas be performed to localize the tumor and direct its surgical resection by an endocrine surgeon. Because insulinomas are often small, further testing (with, for example, endoscopic ultrasonography) may be necessary for localization. If the results indicate exogenous injection of insulin or surreptitious ingestion of sulfonylureas, a psychiatric evaluation may be appropriate, especially in patients with a history of a mood or psychiatric disorder.

Postprandial Hypoglycemia

The occurrence of true postprandial hypoglycemia among persons without diabetes who have no history of gastric bypass surgery is extremely uncommon although frequently misdiagnosed. A patient may report feeling sleepy, shaky, or weak 1 to 3 hours after a large meal rich in simple carbohydrates, and a tentative diagnosis of hypoglycemia may be made. Using an oral glucose tolerance test to confirm the diagnosis should be avoided because of the high incidence of hypoglycemia in healthy persons given a 75-g glucose load.

A better way to establish the diagnosis is to observe the patient and measure the plasma glucose level when symptoms occur. Most of the time, euglycemia will be detected. Whether or not symptoms are due to hypoglycemia, the best treatment is to recommend smaller and more frequent meals.

Disorders of the Pituitary Gland

Hypothalamic Disease

The hypothalamus produces multiple hormones that control pituitary function, especially anterior pituitary gland function. These include corticotropin-releasing hormone, which stimulates the release of adrenocorticotropic hormone (ACTH); gonadotropin-releasing hormone (GnRH), which stimulates the release of luteinizing hormone (LH) and follicle-stimulating hormone (FSH); thyrotropin-releasing hormone, which stimulates the release of thyroid-stimulating hormone (TSH); and growth hormone (GH)–releasing hormone, which stimulates the release of GH. These hormones travel from the hypothalamus through the pituitary stalk and are then released into the pituitary gland. Pathologic disruption of the pituitary stalk may disrupt the flow of these hypothalamic hormones and thus cause a decrease in hormone secretion, which leads to a reduction in pituitary gland function. An exception to this process occurs with the hormone prolactin, an anterior pituitary gland hormone under the tonic inhibitory control of dopamine released from the pituitary stalk; disruption of dopamine delivery from the pituitary stalk causes the prolactin level to increase.

The posterior pituitary gland consists mainly of neuronal axons that extend from the supraoptic and paraventricular

TABLE 11.	Differential Diagnosis of Spontaneous Fasting Hypoglycemia in a Person Without Diabetes			
Diagnosis	**Plasma Glucose Level**	**Serum Insulin Level**	**Plasma C-Peptide Level**	**Urine or Blood Metabolites of Sulfonylureas or Meglitinides**
Insulinoma	↓	↑	↑	Negative
Surreptitious use of sulfonylureas or meglitinides	↓	↑	↑	Positive
Surreptitious use of insulin	↓	↑	↓	Negative

nuclei of the hypothalamus through the stalk. The two major hormones associated with the posterior pituitary gland are antidiuretic hormone and oxytocin.

Most causes of hypothalamic disorders are acquired, although rare genetic causes of hypothalamic dysfunction exist. Causes of acquired hypothalamic disease include trauma due to brain injury, neurosurgery, or cranial irradiation; infiltrative diseases, including sarcoidosis, Langerhans cell histiocytosis, lymphoma, and metastatic cancer (most commonly from breast and lung cancer); and compression by pituitary tumors with suprasellar extension, particularly tumors with a cystic composition or (rarely) associated with cancer. Acquired hypothalamic structural diseases (such as craniopharyngioma) present with signs and symptoms related to the anatomic location of the lesion and the rapidity of the increase in lesion size. Besides its role in pituitary function, the hypothalamus is involved in the regulation of various behaviors and functions, such as satiety and body temperature. Hypothalamic dysfunction may lead to excessive eating, profound hypothermia, hypersexuality, or somnolence. Hypothalamic lesions also often cause central diabetes insipidus by disrupting antidiuretic hormone production.

KEY POINT

- Hypothalamic lesions often cause diabetes insipidus by disrupting antidiuretic hormone production.

Hypopituitarism

Causes and General Management

Hypopituitarism results from disorders of the pituitary gland or hypothalamus that lead to decreased secretion of pituitary gland hormones (**Table 12**). Pituitary tumors and their treatment (surgery and radiation therapy) are the most common causes of hypopituitarism in adults (>75%), followed by extrapituitary lesions (<15%), such as a craniopharyngioma or

TABLE 12. Acquired Causes of Hypopituitarism

Tumors (pituitary adenomas, craniopharyngiomas, dysgerminomas, meningiomas, gliomas, metastatic tumors, Rathke cleft cysts)

Irradiation

Trauma (neurosurgery, external blunt trauma)

Infiltrative disease (sarcoidosis, Langerhans cell histiocytosis, tuberculosis)

Empty sella syndrome

Vascular (apoplexy, Sheehan syndrome, subarachnoid hemorrhage)

Lymphocytic hypophysitis

Metabolic causes (hemochromatosis, critical illness, malnutrition, anorexia nervosa, psychosocial deprivation)

Idiopathic causes

Rathke cleft cyst. Other mass lesions that can lead to hypopituitarism include nonpituitary neoplasms (such as germinoma and meningioma), metastatic cancers, Langerhans cell histiocytosis, and lymphocytic hypophysitis (an autoimmune disorder characterized by symmetric enlargement of the sellar contents that occurs mostly during or after pregnancy and is commonly associated with ACTH deficiency). The presence of a sellar mass in the setting of diabetes insipidus suggests the presence of a lesion of nonpituitary origin. Neurosurgical removal or debulking of the tumor may reduce the pressure on the pituitary gland and thus result in improved pituitary function. However, neurosurgery performed on the pituitary gland also may result in resection of normal gland, which can lead to hypopituitarism.

Pituitary tumor apoplexy, which denotes hemorrhagic infarction of the tumor, causes sudden onset of headache, possible diplopia (from compression of cranial nerves within the cavernous sinus[es]), and acute hypopituitarism. Pituitary tumor apoplexy is a neurosurgical emergency. In addition to neurosurgical decompression of the pituitary gland, urgent replacement of glucocorticoids may be necessary because of acute ACTH deficiency. Replacement of thyroid hormone, sex hormones, and GH is typically not urgent but may be necessary. Sheehan syndrome in pregnancy involves pituitary gland infarction in the setting of severe blood loss and hypotension at delivery and presents with subacute, progressive hypopituitarism, an inability to lactate because of prolactin deficiency, and amenorrhea. Central adrenal insufficiency is the primary cause of mortality in Sheehan syndrome.

Cranial irradiation causes progressive hypopituitarism in approximately 40% of patients. Some degree of hypopituitarism also has been reported in approximately 25% of patients after severe traumatic brain injury, ischemic stroke, and subarachnoid hemorrhage. Hormonal deficiencies are typically noted acutely, although rarely they may be detected more than 1 year after injury. The more severe the injury, the more likely are hormone deficiencies. GH deficiency is the most commonly noted, is usually seen together with at least one other pituitary deficiency, and has been associated with reduced quality of life after injury.

Infiltrative lesions that can lead to hypopituitarism include hemochromatosis, lymphocytic hypophysitis, and granulomatous diseases (such as sarcoidosis). Hypopituitarism is managed with replacement of the hormones secreted directly from the pituitary gland (GH or vasopressin) or those normally secreted under pituitary control (hydrocortisone, levothyroxine, testosterone, or estrogen-progesterone), with adjustment of daily replacement doses determined clinically by whether the hormone has been over- or underreplaced (**Table 13**). Because ACTH deficiency can be life threatening in light of the associated cortisol deficiency, the hypothalamic-pituitary-adrenal axis should be assessed acutely in patients in whom hypopituitarism is suspected.

TABLE 13.	Hormonal Replacement Therapy in Hypopituitarism
Hormone Deficiency	**Therapeutic Replacement Regimen**
TSH	Levothyroxine, 50-200 mg/d; adjust by measuring free T_4 levels; obtaining TSH levels is not indicated because these levels are uninterpretable in patients known to be TSH deficient.
ACTH	Hydrocortisone, 10-20 mg in AM and 5-10 mg in PM *or* prednisone, 2.5-5 mg in AM and 2.5 mg in PM; adjust clinically.
	Stress dosing for hydrocortisone, 50-100 mg IV every 8 hours.
LH/FSH	
Men	Testosterone: 1% gel, 1-2 packets (5-10 g) or 1.62% gel, 2-4 pumps (40.5-81 mg) daily; transdermal patch, 5 g daily; or testosterone enanthate or cypionate, 50-300 mg IM every 1-4 weeks. Adjust by measuring testosterone levels. Will need injectable gonadotropins (LH, FSH) or GnRH for spermatogenesis (if fertility is desired).
Women	Cyclic conjugated estrogens (0.3–0.625 mg) and medroxyprogesterone acetate (5-10 mg) *or* low-dose oral contraceptive pills. Estrogen patches also available. Will need injectable gonadotropins (LH, FSH) if fertility is desired.
GH	Adults start at 200-300 µg subcutaneously daily and increment by 100-200 µg at bimonthly intervals. Adjust to maintain IGF-1 levels in the midnormal range. Women receiving oral estrogens require higher doses.
Vasopressin	Desmopressin: metered nasal spray, 10-20 µg once or twice daily; or tablets, 0.1-0.4 mg every 8-12 h; or injected, 1-2 µg subcutaneously or IV, every 6-12 h

ACTH = adrenocorticotropic hormone; FSH = follicle-stimulating hormone; GH = growth hormone; GnRH = gonadotropin-releasing hormone; IGF-1 = insulin-like growth factor 1; IM = intramuscularly; IV = intravenously; LH = luteinizing hormone; µg = microgram(s); T_4 = thyroxine; TSH = thyroid-stimulating hormone.

KEY POINTS

- Pituitary tumors and their treatment are the most common causes of hypopituitarism in adults; neurosurgical removal or debulking of these tumors may reduce the pressure on the pituitary gland and result in improved pituitary function.

- Urgent glucocorticoid replacement is necessary in patients with pituitary tumor apoplexy.

Growth Hormone Deficiency

GH deficiency in adults may reflect either persistence of childhood-onset disease or newly acquired disease and typically occurs with other pituitary deficiencies. In children, GH deficiency causes short stature. In adults, however, acquired GH deficiency causes reduced lean muscle mass and increased fat mass, reduced strength and stamina, decreased bone mineral density, an increased cardiovascular risk profile, and a decreased quality of life. Adult-onset GH deficiency is the most common pituitary deficiency associated with a structural sellar or suprasellar lesion that has been treated with neurosurgical intervention and/or cranial irradiation.

Biochemical testing includes demonstration of a low serum insulin-like growth factor 1 (IGF-1) level and a test for GH reserve based on a stimulation test that uses insulin (to induce hypoglycemia), glucagon, arginine, or GH-releasing hormone. GH replacement therapy should be considered in patients with other pituitary deficiencies and in those with unequivocal evidence of deficiency, with resultant benefits in lean body and fat mass, improvement in lipid profiles, and improvement in the sense of well being.

Isolated idiopathic adult-onset GH deficiency is rare, and the utility of replacing GH in adults with idiopathic GH deficiency is debatable given the lack of robust data showing that treatment results in resolution of ill effects. Because of this uncertainty, consultation with an endocrinologist is appropriate if treatment is being considered.

KEY POINT

- Adult-onset growth hormone (GH) deficiency is the most common pituitary deficiency associated with a structural sellar or suprasellar lesion that has been treated with neurosurgical intervention and/or cranial irradiation; isolated idiopathic adult-onset GH deficiency is rare.

Gonadotropin Deficiency

In hypogonadotropic hypogonadism, the pituitary gland produces less LH and FSH, which leads to hypogonadism (reduced estrogen production and ovulatory capacity by the ovary or diminished testosterone secretion and spermatogenesis by the testis). Clinical features of hypogonadotropic hypogonadism include amenorrhea, breast atrophy, vaginal dryness, and diminished libido in women and decreased libido, erectile dysfunction, loss of skeletal muscle mass, and anemia in men. Acquired hypogonadotropic hypogonadism in women commonly results from weight loss, severe dietary restriction, anorexia nervosa, stress, heavy exercise, or severe illness, although it also may be idiopathic. MRI or CT is recommended in patients with hypogonadotropic hypogonadism to rule out structural disease. In both sexes, loss of gonadal hormones can lead to loss of bone density. Of note, hyperprolactinemia can suppress GnRH secretion and also lead to hypogonadotropic hypogonadism.

Features, diagnosis, and treatment of hypogonadism is addressed in Reproductive Disorders.

Adrenocorticotropic Hormone Deficiency

ACTH deficiency causes hypocortisolism, and low or normal ACTH levels are seen in the presence of a low measured cortisol level, in contrast to the elevated ACTH values seen in primary adrenal insufficiency. Whereas patients with primary adrenal insufficiency have increased skin pigmentation due to elevated ACTH levels, patients with ACTH deficiency do not. Symptoms of nausea, vomiting, malaise, weakness, dizziness, fatigue, fever, and hypotension can occur with ACTH deficiency, although often subacutely, with malaise and weakness being most prominent. In ACTH deficiency, adrenal production of mineralocorticoids and potassium homeostasis remain intact because the hypothalamic-pituitary-adrenal axis is controlled separately by the renin-angiotensin system. This contrasts with the frequent finding of hyperkalemia in primary adrenal insufficiency. The presentation of ACTH deficiency may be variable, and some patients may be asymptomatic, but affected patients typically exhibit symptoms of hypocortisolemia during physiologically stressful events, such as surgery or sepsis. Details regarding symptoms, diagnosis, and therapy of primary and secondary adrenal insufficiency are provided in Disorders of the Adrenal Gland.

The most common cause of ACTH deficiency is suppression of corticotropin-releasing hormone and ACTH secretion by exogenous corticosteroids for longer than 2 to 3 weeks. Similarly, megestrol acetate, which is used for appetite stimulation in cachetic patients with cancer or AIDS, has some glucocorticoid activity and can suppress ACTH secretion. Although patients who take megestrol acetate do not usually show clinical evidence of hypercortisolism (Cushing syndrome), patients should be monitored for hypocortisolism after the drug is discontinued.

When not due to medication, ACTH deficiency frequently is detected in combination with the loss of other pituitary hormones.

Thyroid-Stimulating Hormone Deficiency

In central hypothyroidism, TSH deficiency leads to reduced secretion of thyroxine (T_4), and thus a measurement of the patient's serum T_4 level is necessary to establish the diagnosis. The signs and symptoms of central hypothyroidism are similar to those of primary hypothyroidism, namely, fatigue, weight gain, cold intolerance, and constipation. In contrast to the elevated TSH level seen in primary hypothyroidism, TSH deficiency is associated with a low free T_4 level and an inappropriately normal or low TSH level. This distinction is important because a normal TSH level may be associated with significant hypothyroidism in a patient with central hypothyroidism and TSH deficiency. Acquired central

hypothyroidism usually is associated with deficiencies of other pituitary hormones. Because both serum free T_4 and TSH levels can be low in central hypothyroidism, distinguishing between central hypothyroidism and the euthyroid sick syndrome may be difficult in patients with severe illness or starvation. Generally, those with euthyroid sick syndrome have elevated levels of reverse triiodothyronine (T_3), unlike those with central hypothyroidism.

Thyroid hormone dosing in patients with central hypothyroidism should be adjusted on the basis of clinical symptoms to maintain free T_4 levels within the midnormal reference range, unless doing so causes iatrogenic hyperthyroidism or hypothyroidism. TSH levels cannot be used as a measure of adequacy of replacement in these patients as they can in patients with an intact hypothalamic-pituitary axis.

Diabetes Insipidus

Diabetes insipidus is characterized by excessive urination due to a deficiency of antidiuretic hormone (also known as arginine vasopressin [AVP]) secretion, as in central diabetes insipidus, or a defect in AVP's ability to act on the kidney, as in nephrogenic diabetes insipidus. In either situation, the kidney does not concentrate urine, which results in excretion of dilute urine relative to plasma. The resultant increase in plasma osmolality leads to both polydipsia through stimulation of central osmoreceptors and polyuria because of the inability to retain free water and concentrate the urine. If patients have an adequate thirst mechanism and access to water, the serum sodium level should remain normal to high normal, although accompanied by significant polyuria and polydipsia. In partial central diabetes insipidus, the patient is largely asymptomatic because of adequate compensation through an intact thirst mechanism and ready access to water. However, with a stressor—such as water deprivation, a central nervous system event that alters the set point for stimulation of thirst, or pregnancy with degradation of AVP caused by placental vasopressinase—diabetes insipidus may become clinically apparent.

Causes of central diabetes insipidus include rare familial syndromes. In acquired cases, causes are usually mass lesions (neoplasms, such as craniopharyngioma, germinoma, and metastatic cancer), trauma (neurosurgery or traumatic brain injury), and infiltrative disorders (sarcoidosis or Langerhans cell histiocytosis) that compromise hypothalamic function. Transient central diabetes insipidus commonly occurs immediately after pituitary surgery but may resolve rapidly after the procedure.

As with polyuria, the differential diagnosis of central diabetes insipidus includes primary polydipsia due to a psychiatric disorder, medications (such as phenothiazines that cause dry mouth), or hypothalamic lesions that affect the thirst center (such as sarcoidosis); osmotic diuresis, as in uncontrolled diabetes mellitus and postobstructive diuresis; and hypercalcemia. A serum chemistry panel should be obtained to rule out osmotic causes. If the baseline serum sodium level is high normal or elevated, particularly if the urine osmolality is lower than the plasma osmolality, then diabetes insipidus is likely. If the baseline serum sodium level is less than 136 meq/L [136 mmol/L]) and urine osmolality is high, then diabetes insipidus is unlikely. (In fact, the syndrome of inappropriate antidiuretic hormone secretion is likely present.) If the baseline serum sodium level is within the normal range, a water deprivation test should be performed to differentiate diabetes insipidus from primary polydipsia.

In a water deprivation test, the serum sodium level and plasma osmolality are measured every 2 hours, and the urine volume, urine osmolality, and body weight are measured every hour. The test is finished when (1) the urine osmolality is greater than 600 mosm/kg H_2O (appropriately concentrated), (2) urine osmolality fails to concentrate for 2 consecutive hours, (3) plasma osmolality is greater than 295 mosm/kg H_2O, (4) serum sodium level is greater than 145 meq/L (145 mmol/L), or (5) the patient has lost greater than 5% body weight. The patient is then given desmopressin acetate. If any of the five parameters are met before the test begins, the water deprivation test is not recommended, and desmopressin can be administered first, followed by measurement of urine volume and osmolality every 30 minutes for 2 hours. During water deprivation and before desmopressin administration, healthy persons will increase their urine osmolality to greater than 800 mosm/kg H_2O, but those with diabetes insipidus will not increase theirs above 300 mosm/kg H_2O. In response to desmopressin, patients with central diabetes insipidus will increase their urine osmolality by at least 50%, but those with nephrogenic diabetes insipidus will not respond appreciably.

Treatment of central diabetes insipidus includes desmopressin—administered orally, by a metered nasal spray, or (if needed) by subcutaneous or intravenous injection—and the instruction to drink until no longer thirsty. Water intoxication can be avoided as long as the patient drinks only when thirsty. In the unconscious patient or someone whose thirst mechanisms are not operative, extreme care must be exerted to avoid undertreatment and overtreatment. Accurate determination of daily body weight, fixed dosages of fluid intake, and frequent monitoring of the serum sodium level are necessary.

KEY POINTS

- In the presence of polyuria, diabetes insipidus is likely if the baseline serum sodium level is high normal or clearly elevated, particularly when the urine osmolality is lower than the plasma osmolality.

- If the baseline serum sodium level is within the normal range in the setting of polyuria, a water deprivation test should be performed to differentiate diabetes insipidus from primary polydipsia.

Pituitary Tumors

Pituitary tumors (adenomas) arise from monoclonal neoplasms of the cells comprising the pituitary gland, including somatotrophs (GH), corticotrophs (ACTH), gonadotrophs (LH and FSH), lactotrophs (prolactin), and thyrotrophs (TSH). These tumors also are defined by size, with microadenomas being less than 10 mm in diameter and macroadenomas being 10 mm in diameter or greater. The most common pituitary tumor is a nonfunctioning adenoma; the most common functional pituitary tumor is a prolactinoma. Most pituitary adenomas are sporadic, although some (<5%) occur as part of the familial multiple endocrine neoplasia type 1 syndrome, which is associated with endocrine tumors of the pituitary gland, parathyroid glands, and pancreas (the three "Ps"). Although most pituitary adenomas are benign, they can be locally invasive and lead to significant compressive symptoms because of their proximity to adjacent critical structures, such as the optic chiasm. Pituitary tumors, therefore, can lead to local problems (such as visual field deficits and headaches) and also have systemic effects due to hormone hypersecretion or compression of the normal gland with resultant hypopituitarism.

Approach to a Sellar Mass

A sellar mass may be detected incidentally, for example during the evaluation of trauma, headache, sinusitis, or another disorder. If the lesion is detected on a CT scan, then MRI should be performed because an MRI provides better anatomic definition. After it is detected, the sellar mass should be characterized further by determining if hormone hypersecretion is present. Additionally, the serum prolactin level should be determined in all patients with a sellar mass to exclude a prolactinoma. If the history or physical examination is suggestive of either acromegaly or Cushing syndrome, the appropriate biochemical test should be performed. If the evaluation shows no evidence of pituitary hypersecretion, the lesion is either a clinically nonfunctioning adenoma or a nonpituitary lesion. Further evaluation for local mass effects, such as the presence of visual field compromise or hypopituitarism due to compression of the optic chiasm or normal pituitary gland, respectively, should then be performed, particularly in the setting of a macroadenoma. Therapy is warranted if the lesion is functional (such as a hormone-secreting adenoma) or if hypopituitarism or other local mass effects are found. If the lesion is nonfunctional and no accompanying mass effects are detected, serial follow-up evaluation is advised.

Mass Effects of Pituitary Tumors

Because the clinical manifestation of pituitary tumors is often insidious and slow in onset, these tumors are often large when detected. As a result, these enlarging tumors can cause mass effects on local structures. Macroadenomas with suprasellar extension compressing the optic chiasm can cause visual field defects, including bitemporal hemianopia, and invasion of the cavernous sinus area can result in cranial nerve palsies, with manifestations such as diplopia. Headaches are frequently described, and the sudden explosive onset of headache suggests possible hemorrhagic infarction of the tumor (apoplexy). Compression of the adjacent normal pituitary gland can cause hypopituitarism. Notably, diabetes insipidus is rarely caused by pituitary tumors and should instead raise the suspicion of a nonpituitary lesion, such as a cystic tumor (craniopharyngioma or Rathke cleft cyst) or a metastatic neoplasm.

Treatment of Pituitary Tumors

The goals of treating pituitary tumors are to remove or reduce the tumor mass (to decompress the local mass effects), correct pituitary hormone hypersecretion, maintain normal pituitary gland function, and prevent recurrence. Surgery is first-line therapy for macroadenomas and hypersecretory pituitary tumors, except prolactinomas. The neurosurgical approach is primarily transsphenoidal by way of an endonasal route. In experienced hands, transsphenoidal surgery is extremely safe. Permanent hypopituitarism, significant hemorrhage, and optic nerve injury occur in less than 5% of patients.

Radiation therapy is used primarily as adjuvant treatment for patients with residual disease or continued hormone hypersecretion after surgery. Irradiation is used as primary therapy only for patients who cannot undergo surgery. Because of the prolonged time needed to normalize hypersecretory states and shrink tumors, which often do not change in size after irradiation, surgery is preferred. Conventional, fractionated radiation therapy may take as long as 6 weeks. In contrast, stereotactic radiosurgery, intensity-modulated radiation therapy, and proton beam therapy may take only one or a few sessions and may be preferable from the standpoint of convenience. Complications of radiation therapy include long-term hypopituitarism in approximately 40% of treated patients and secondary neoplasms in approximately 1.5%.

Medical therapy is generally used adjuvantly after unsuccessful surgery, except with prolactinomas for which dopamine agonist therapy is first-line treatment.

KEY POINTS

- Surgery is first-line therapy for macroadenomas and hypersecretory pituitary tumors, except prolactinomas for which medical therapy with a dopamine agonist is preferred.

- Radiation therapy is used primarily as adjuvant treatment for patients with residual disease after pituitary tumor removal or continued hormone hypersecretion after surgery and as primary therapy for patients who cannot undergo surgery.

Hyperprolactinemia and Prolactinomas

Causes

Prolactin is secreted by the pituitary lactotroph cells under tonic inhibition by dopamine. This hormone is secreted in a pulsatile fashion, with the highest mean levels produced during sleep. Physiologic causes of hyperprolactinemia include pregnancy, nipple stimulation, exercise, and food intake. Therefore, in a woman with modest hyperprolactinemia, pregnancy should first be excluded, and the prolactin test should be repeated in a fasting state, with no strenuous exercise before testing. A routine breast examination usually does not raise serum prolactin levels enough to cause concern.

The most common cause of hyperprolactinemia is a prolactinoma, which is a benign adenoma. Microprolactinomas are less than 10 mm in diameter, and macroprolactinomas are 10 mm or greater in diameter. Although prolactinomas are the most common type of secretory pituitary adenoma (25%-40%), not all patients with hyperprolactinemia have prolactinomas (**Table 14**). Hyperprolactinemia is present in hypothyroidism, liver disease, and kidney failure, with a serum creatinine level typically less than 2 mg/dL (177 micromoles/L).

Many medications increase prolactin secretion by blocking dopamine release or action. This occurs most commonly with antipsychotic medications (including haloperidol, risperidone, and other antidopaminergic drugs), opiates, gastric motility drugs (metoclopramide and domperidone), and the calcium channel blocker verapamil. Estrogens increase prolactin secretion in a dose-response fashion, but the usual estrogen dose in oral contraceptives rarely causes symptomatic hyperprolactinemia.

Any hypothalamic or sellar mass that impinges on the pituitary stalk and disrupts dopamine flow can increase serum prolactin levels. Because serum prolactin levels correspond to prolactinoma size, the presence of a large sellar or suprasellar mass with only a modest increase in serum prolactin level (<150 ng/mL [150 micrograms/L]) usually indicates a cause other than a prolactinoma. Smaller prolactinomas also can result in a modest elevation of prolactin levels.

A patient with hyperprolactinemia without a clear secondary or drug-induced cause should be assessed by an imaging study (preferably, MRI of the pituitary gland) to exclude a mass lesion.

KEY POINT

- The most common cause of hyperprolactinemia is a prolactinoma.

Clinical Features and Therapy of Hyperprolactinemia and Prolactinomas

Common signs and symptoms of hyperprolactinemia include galactorrhea, oligomenorrhea, amenorrhea, and hirsutism in premenopausal women; erectile dysfunction in men; and decreased libido, infertility, headache, and osteopenia in both sexes. The presence of an underlying sellar, suprasellar, or hypothalamic mass may cause headache

TABLE 14.	Causes of Hyperprolactinemia
Cause	**Result**
Pituitary disease	Prolactinomas
	Growth hormone–secreting tumors (cosecretion of prolactin or pituitary stalk effects)
	Nonfunctioning pituitary tumors (pituitary stalk effects)
	Lymphocytic hypophysitis (pituitary stalk effects)
	Empty sella syndrome (pituitary stalk effects)
	Cushing disease (cosecretion of prolactin or pituitary stalk effects)
Nonpituitary sellar and parasellar lesions	Craniopharyngioma
	Hypothalamic disease (sarcoidosis, Langerhans cell histiocytosis, lymphoma)
	Metastatic tumors to pituitary/hypothalamus
	Meningiomas
	Dysgerminomas
	Irradiation
Neurogenic	Chest wall or spinal cord disease
	Breast stimulation/lesions
Drugs	Psychotropic agents (butyrophenones and phenothiazines, monoamine oxidase inhibitors, tricyclic antidepressants, fluoxetine, molindone, risperidone, cocaine)
	Antihypertensive agents (verapamil, methyldopa, reserpine)
	Metoclopramide
	(Estrogen in conventionally used doses does not cause hyperprolactinemia.)
Other	Pregnancy
	Physiologic cause (coitus, nipple stimulation, strenuous exercise, stress)
	Hypothyroidism
	Chronic kidney failure
	Cirrhosis
	Macroprolactinoma
	Idiopathic
	Adrenal insufficiency
	Ectopic secretion

and mass effects, including peripheral visual field loss and ophthalmoplegia.

The indications to treat hyperprolactinemia in women include estrogen deficiency (in a premenopausal patient with amenorrhea and oligomenorrhea), infertility, bothersome galactorrhea, and hirsutism. In men, indications to treat include symptomatic testosterone deficiency, with symptoms such as erectile dysfunction, reduced libido, or gynecomastia. Headache, mass effects in patients with underlying sellar and suprasellar lesions, and osteopenia and osteoporosis due to gonadal insufficiency are indications to treat in both men and women.

When treatment is necessary, medical therapy with a dopamine agonist is the treatment of choice for most symptomatic patients (**Table 15**). A dopamine agonist can cause a rapid decrease in the serum prolactin level and shrinkage of the prolactinoma. More specifically, in as many as 90% of

patients, it can normalize prolactin levels, reverse hypogonadism, and shrink tumors by at least 50%. Because of these rapid decreases in tumor size, dopamine agonists can be used as first-line therapy, even in patients with mild visual field defects, as long as visual acuity is not threatened by rapid progression of the tumor or recent tumor hemorrhage. Secondary causes of hyperprolactinemia must first be excluded because treatment of underlying conditions, such as hypothyroidism, should normalize the serum prolactin level. In patients with drug-induced hyperprolactinemia (prolactin levels rarely >200 ng/mL [200 micrograms/L]), especially those with psychiatric disorders, a change to a different medication is preferable but not always advisable, and dopamine agonists may be contraindicated because of reported worsening of psychiatric disease. When dopamine agonists are used in this setting, close consultation with the patient's psychiatrist is warranted. In women with

TABLE 15. Medical Therapies for Pituitary Adenomas

Type of Pituitary Adenoma	Medication
Prolactinoma	Cabergoline
	Bromocriptine
Adenomas causing acromegaly	Somatostatin analogues (octreotide, lanreotide)
	Cabergoline
	Pegvisomant
Adenomas causing Cushing disease	Ketoconazole
	Mifepristone
	Cabergoline
	Mitotane
	Etomidate (parenteral)
TSH-secreting adenomas	Somatostatin analogues (octreotide, lanreotide)
Nonfunctioning adenomas	Cabergoline
	Somatostatin analogues (octreotide, lanreotide)

TSH = thyroid-stimulating hormone.

prolactinomas who do not desire pregnancy, estrogen deficiency may be treated by estrogen replacement (in the form of an oral contraceptive, for example) alone to maintain normal vaginal health and bone mass. Although estrogen replacement may result in a modest increase in the serum prolactin level, the dose of estrogens used in most oral contraceptives poses little risk of prolactinoma enlargement. Nevertheless, the serum prolactin level should be monitored in these women.

Bromocriptine and cabergoline are the two oral dopamine agonists available in the United States to treat prolactin disorders: Bromocriptine is administered daily, and cabergoline is administered once or twice weekly. Although the more expensive drug, cabergoline is associated with more tumor shrinkage and normalization of prolactin levels and generally is better tolerated than bromocriptine. Adverse effects of dopamine agonists include gastrointestinal upset, nasal congestion, headache, and dizziness. Some studies have associated cabergoline with cardiac valve abnormalities, primarily in patients with Parkinson disease for which the cabergoline dosage is much higher than that used for prolactin disorders. Most subsequent studies have not shown a definitive connection between cabergoline use and cardiac valvular disease in prolactinoma management.

Permanent withdrawal of the dopamine agonist can be considered in some patients. The current recommendation is to consider withdrawal of the agonist if the prolactin level has been normal for at least 2 years and no visible tumor is seen on a pituitary MRI. Patients with these findings still require close follow-up evaluation with serial measurement of prolactin levels to assess for recurrence. Recurrence rates of up to 50% have been reported.

Neurosurgery is considered in patients with prolactinomas who are unresponsive to or poorly tolerant of dopamine agonist therapy and always should be considered in patients with a cystic prolactinoma because the cystic component will be unresponsive to medical therapy. Remission rates after transsphenoidal surgery have been reported to be as high as 80% for microprolactinomas but no more than 40% for macroprolactinomas. In patients with surgical remission, the long-term recurrence rate is approximately 20%. Radiation therapy, including stereotactic radiosurgery, is used less commonly for prolactinomas but is indicated for macroprolactinomas that do not respond to either medical or surgical treatment.

KEY POINTS

- Common signs and symptoms of hyperprolactinemia include galactorrhea, oligomenorrhea, amenorrhea, and hirsutism in premenopausal women; erectile dysfunction in men; and decreased libido, infertility, headache, and osteopenia in both sexes.
- For most symptomatic patients with hyperprolactinemia and prolactinomas, medical therapy with a dopamine agonist is usually the treatment of choice; permanent withdrawal of the drug can be considered in some patients, particularly those whose serum prolactin level has normalized (for at least 2 years) or whose tumor is no longer visible.

Pregnancy in a Patient with a Prolactinoma

Dopamine agonists have no documented risks of fetal malformations or other adverse outcomes in pregnancy; the collection of available data on the safety of bromocriptine is significantly larger than that for cabergoline. Nevertheless, in women taking a dopamine agonist, the standard management is to stop the drug after conception, except for women with a history of optic chiasmal compression with visual field compromise.

In normal women, the pituitary gland triples in size during pregnancy. Prolactinomas also may increase in size during pregnancy. Therefore, concern exists that the growing prolactinoma may cause worsening symptoms, including visual field defects and headache; pregnant women with prolactinomas are typically seen every 2 to 3 months for clinical assessment. If clinical evidence suggests symptomatic prolactinoma growth, then reinstitution of a dopamine agonist (with bromocriptine being the preferred agent in this setting), transsphenoidal surgical decompression, or delivery if the pregnancy is sufficiently advanced should be considered. Otherwise, dopamine agonist therapy is reinstituted after nursing is completed. Serial visual field testing may be useful to ensure maintenance of chiasmal function, although routine pituitary MRI is not necessary. Prolactin level measurement has no value during pregnancy.

KEY POINT

- Because prolactinomas may increase in size in pregnant women and lead to visual field loss, close clinical monitoring should be performed during pregnancy.

Other Disorders Involving Adenomas

Acromegaly

Causes and Diagnosis

Acromegaly is a disorder characterized by GH hypersecretion, most commonly by a GH-secreting pituitary adenoma. Like other pituitary tumor syndromes, acromegaly is usually sporadic, although it may occur in the setting of multiple endocrine neoplasia type 1 or familial acromegaly. When GH hypersecretion occurs before epiphyseal closure (in a child or adolescent), exaggerated linear growth of the long bones occurs, with resultant pituitary gigantism. When it occurs in adults after epiphyseal closure, acromegaly results. Clinical features include frontal bossing; prognathism, with dental malocclusion and increased spacing between the teeth; enlargement of the nose, lips, and tongue; skin tags; arthritis; carpal tunnel syndrome; sleep apnea; and excess sweating.

Patients with acromegaly have an increased incidence of type 2 diabetes mellitus, cardiovascular disease, hypertension, hypertrophic cardiomyopathy, and atherosclerotic arterial disease; they also have a two- to threefold increase in premature mortality. Because of an increased risk of premalignant polyps and colon cancer, screening with colonoscopy is recommended for all persons with GH excess.

The diagnosis of acromegaly is based on biochemical evidence of GH hypersecretion, typically with an elevated IGF-1 level. A random GH value is not useful because of the pulsatile nature of GH secretion. GH stimulates the liver to produce IGF-1, which serves as an integrated marker of GH levels. Measuring the IGF-1 level is a simple test and may be done randomly. Results correlate well with clinical symptoms. An oral glucose tolerance test also can be useful in a patient in whom the diagnosis of acromegaly is not clear. A nadir GH level of less than 1 ng/mL (1 microgram/L) excludes the disease.

A pituitary MRI can reveal the size and location of the pituitary adenoma and confirm the presence of mass effects. Approximately 80% of patients with acromegaly have macroadenomas. Patients with acromegaly should be referred to an endocrinologist for definitive diagnostic testing and therapy.

Treatment

The goals of therapy for acromegaly are to normalize the IGF-1 level, control the GH levels, reduce tumor bulk, prevent or decrease the number of comorbidities, and reduce the risk of premature death. Reduction of GH hypersecretion will lead to lessening of soft tissue abnormalities, but bony changes will persist. In addition, normalization of biochemical parameters will result in improvements in cardiac function, glucose control, hypertension, and sleep apnea and will help decrease the risk of premature mortality. The primary therapy is transsphenoidal surgery by an experienced neurosurgeon, which will normalize biochemical parameters in as many as 90% of patients with microadenomas and 40% of patients with macroadenomas.

Medical therapy is used mostly in the adjuvant setting in patients with residual disease after surgery (such as a residual tumor outside of the sella in the cavernous sinus, which is not surgically accessible). Somatostatin analogues are commonly used and normalize GH and IGF-1 levels in approximately 40% to 65% of patients. Long-acting preparations of octreotide and lanreotide are administered as monthly injections. Somatostatin analogues can shrink tumors modestly but usually not to the extent that dopamine agonists can shrink prolactinomas. Adverse effects of somatostatin analogues include diarrhea, abdominal bloating, and an increased risk of cholelithiasis. Cabergoline, a dopamine agonist, also may be considered because it is administered orally and is relatively inexpensive (compared with a somatostatin analogue). This drug normalizes biochemical parameters in 30% to 40% of patients with acromegaly, particularly those with modest disease activity.

A third type of drug used for medical therapy is a GH receptor antagonist, specifically pegvisomant, which blocks GH and thus causes a decline in IGF-1 values. Pegvisomant administered as a daily or twice weekly injection normalizes the IGF-1 level in more than 90% of patients and has associated clinical benefits. Safety monitoring of pegvisomant includes serial liver chemistry testing (elevations in serum values are uncommonly detected) and brain MRI (to monitor for tumor growth, which has been described with use of this drug). Pegvisomant is generally recommended as second-line medical therapy, either as a substitution for or in combination with a somatostatin analogue.

Radiation therapy also is used adjuvantly for management of residual disease after surgery, for disease unresponsive to medical therapy, or for patients in whom medical therapy is poorly tolerated.

KEY POINTS

- An elevated insulin-like growth factor 1 level in the setting of signs or symptoms of growth hormone excess is consistent with acromegaly.
- The primary therapy for acromegaly is transsphenoidal surgery to remove the causative growth hormone–secreting pituitary adenoma.
- Somatostatin analogues and dopamine agonists can be used adjuvantly in patients with acromegaly who have residual disease after surgery.

Cushing Disease

Cushing disease is Cushing syndrome caused by excess production of ACTH by a pituitary adenoma. Cushing syndrome is discussed in Disorders of the Adrenal Glands.

Clinically Nonfunctioning and Gonadotropin-Producing Adenomas

Clinically nonfunctioning adenomas are pituitary tumors that have no clinical manifestation of pituitary hormone hypersecretion. Because these tumors are not associated with a pituitary hormone hypersecretory syndrome, such as Cushing disease or acromegaly, they often are detected later and are macroadenomas at diagnosis. Therefore, these tumors often manifest with signs and symptoms of mass effects, such as headache, visual field loss, or hypopituitarism, but also may be detected incidentally. Occasionally, serum LH or FSH is produced at high levels, which results in high serum levels, and these tumors are referred to as LH- or FSH-producing gonadotroph adenomas.

Therapy of clinically nonfunctioning and gonadotropin-producing adenomas is largely surgical, with the goal of decompressing local structures, maintaining or improving pituitary function, and removing tumor mass. Indications for surgery include visual field loss, compression of adjacent structures, headache, hemorrhage into the tumor (apoplexy), and hypopituitarism. Visual field defects and pituitary dysfunction may improve after successful surgery, depending on the extent and duration of compromise. Radiation therapy is often used adjuvantly to control residual tumor after surgery. Medical therapy has been largely unsuccessful in tumor shrinkage in affected patients.

Incidentalomas

A pituitary incidentaloma refers to a sellar lesion that is detected during imaging for other reasons. Most incidentalomas are pituitary in origin, followed by cystic lesions, such as small craniopharyngiomas or Rathke cleft cysts (see Disorders of the Adrenal Gland, Incidentaloma). As with a sellar mass, a thorough history, physical examination, and laboratory evaluation should be performed for assessment of pituitary hormone hypersecretion (see Pituitary Tumors, Approach to a Sellar Mass). Notably, serum prolactin levels are often modestly elevated with any mass that causes pituitary stalk compression and disruption of dopamine flow. Macroincidentalomas should be evaluated with imaging studies for the presence of local mass effects and hypopituitarism. If the imaging study reveals that the lesion abuts the optic chiasm, then visual field testing should be performed.

Treatment (usually surgery) is indicated for patients with visual field compromise, oculomotor palsies, optic chiasm compression, or evidence of hormone hypersecretion. Surgery should be considered in the setting of tumor growth or loss of pituitary function. Therefore, monitoring with pituitary MRI at 6- to 12-month intervals for at least 3 years is warranted for a microadenoma to detect an enlarging tumor that may require surgery, with more frequent and protracted monitoring of any macroadenoma.

KEY POINT

- Treatment (usually surgery) is indicated for patients with pituitary incidentalomas causing visual field compromise, oculomotor palsies, optic chiasm compression, or hormone hypersecretion; surgery also should be considered in the setting of tumor growth or loss of pituitary function

Thyroid-Stimulating Hormone–Secreting Tumors

TSH- or thyrotropin-secreting pituitary adenomas are the least common type of pituitary tumor and reflect overproduction of TSH by the pituitary thyrotroph cells. The diagnosis usually is made during the evaluation of hyperthyroidism. In contrast to patients with primary hyperthyroidism, whose TSH level is suppressed, biochemical testing of patients with a TSH-secreting adenoma reveals an elevated T_4 level and an elevated or nonsuppressed TSH level. The diagnosis should be confirmed with a pituitary MRI. TSH-secreting pituitary adenomas are often macroadenomas, and the primary therapy is neurosurgical resection. For residual disease after surgery, medical therapy with a somatostatin analogue is highly effective in lowering the TSH level and controlling the hyperthyroidism in as many as 80% of patients. Adjuvant radiation therapy also may be needed for control of any residual tumor.

Disorders of the Thyroid Gland

Thyroid Physiology

The hypothalamic-pituitary axis controls thyroid hormone synthesis, production, and secretion by releasing thyrotropin-releasing hormone and thyroid-stimulating hormone (TSH) through a negative feedback loop involving thyroxine (T_4) and triiodothyronine (T_3). The thyroid gland primarily produces T_4 and a small amount of T_3. Approximately 85% of the body's circulating T_3 is produced by extrathyroidal peripheral conversion of T_4 by 5′-deiodinase enzymes, mainly in the liver and kidney. Most ambulatory patients with thyroid dysfunction have a normal hypothalamic-pituitary axis with either low serum TSH levels (indicating thyrotoxicosis) or elevated TSH levels (indicating primary hypothyroidism). Occasionally, a patient will have disease mediated by pituitary or hypothalamic dysfunction.

Only relatively small, unbound concentrations of T_4 and T_3 are biologically active (free T_4 and T_3). When bound to circulating proteins (primarily thyroxine-binding globulin [TBG] and, to a lesser extent, transthyretin and albumin), these hormones are inactive and act as large storage reservoirs.

Conditions affecting protein binding of thyroid hormone can significantly affect measured levels of total thyroid hormone, which makes measurement of total T_4 and T_3 levels inaccurate and relatively uninterpretable (see later discussion).

Iodide is required for thyroid hormone synthesis, and adequate dietary iodine intake (from, for example, seafood, dairy products, iodized salt, or other iodine-rich food sources) is essential for thyroid hormone production. Although iodine deficiency is a worldwide health problem, iodine intake in the United States is generally adequate, according to the National Health and Nutrition Examination Survey (NHANES) study. The recommended iodine intake for persons older than 13 years is 150 micrograms/d but is higher for pregnant and lactating women (220 and 290 micrograms/d, respectively).

KEY POINT

- Adequate iodine intake is critical for thyroid hormone production.

Evaluation of Thyroid Function

Although various tests exist for evaluating thyroid function (**Table 16**), the serum TSH level is the most sensitive

TABLE 16. Common Tests of Thyroid Function

Measurement	Normal Range	Indication	Comment
Serum TSH	0.5-5.0 µU/mL (0.5-5.0 mU/L)	Suspected thyroid dysfunction	Misleading results in central hypothyroidism in which TSH level is inappropriately low or normal
Serum free T_4	0.9-2.4 ng/dL (12-31 pmol/L)	Suspected thyroid dysfunction with concern for pituitary dysfunction; or evidence of TSH abnormality	Variable normal ranges depending on assay
Serum free T_3	3.6-5.6 ng/L (5.6-8.6 pmol/L)	T_3 thyrotoxicosis	May substitute with total T_3 (In contrast to free thyroid hormone assays, total T_4 or T_3 measurement is affected by the serum-binding protein level.)
Serum thyroglobulin	3-40 ng/mL (3-40 µg/L)	Suspected subacute thyroiditis or suspected surreptitious ingestion of thyroid hormone or analogues; followed as a tumor marker in patients with well-differentiated thyroid cancer	Goal of an undetectable level in patients with prior thyroidectomy and radioactive iodine remnant therapy for differentiated thyroid cancer; difficult to interpret serum thyroglobulin levels in the presence of thyroglobulin antibodies
Serum TSI	0-125%	Graves disease; (euthyroid) ophthalmopathy	Not generally needed to diagnose Graves disease
Serum TBII	<10%	Similar to TSI	Not generally needed to diagnose Graves disease; detection of both blocking and stimulating antibodies against the TSH receptor
Anti–thyroid peroxidase antibodies	<2 units/mL	Suspected Hashimoto thyroiditis	Not generally needed; has predictive value for determining risk of development of overt hypothyroidism
RAIU	10%-30% of dose at 24 hours	Determination of the cause of thyrotoxicosis	Contraindicated in pregnancy and breast feeding

µg = microgram(s); µU = microunit(s); mU = milliunit(s); RAIU = radioactive iodine uptake; T_3 = triiodothyronine; T_4 = thyroxine; TBII = thyrotropin-binding inhibitory immunoglobulin; TSH = thyroid-stimulating hormone; TSI = thyroid-stimulating immunoglobulin.

indicator of thyroid function in ambulatory patients with a normal pituitary gland. Therefore, determination of the TSH level should be the first test used for patients with symptoms or signs that may be due to thyroid dysfunction. A free T_4 level may be measured concurrently with the TSH level if the clinical suspicion of thyroid or pituitary disease is high. In patients with a risk of pituitary gland dysfunction, such as those with a history of cranial irradiation, pituitary surgery, or massive head trauma, TSH and free T_4 levels should be measured to determine if central hypothyroidism is present.

Because levels of total T_4, which comprises both bound and free T_4, are affected by variations in binding protein levels, they may not accurately reflect free T_4 levels. Free T_4 is available for conversion to active T_3 but represents only a small fraction of the total T_4. Present techniques are able to estimate the free T_4 level with relatively high accuracy by determining the direct free T_4 level, by using equilibrium dialysis, or by using analogue assays.

If the TSH level is abnormal, measurement of other thyroid hormone levels is then recommended. For example, measurement of the free T_4 level is recommended to ascertain the severity of the patient's hypothyroidism if the TSH level is elevated. If the TSH level is suppressed, then measurement of free T_4 and T_3 levels is recommended to ascertain the severity of the patient's thyrotoxicosis. Most patients with thyrotoxicosis will have elevations of both levels; only rarely is the T_3 level alone elevated (T_3 thyrotoxicosis). Measurement of the T_3 level is not indicated in patients with hypothyroidism because the T_3 level is conserved and may remain within the normal range, even in patients with significant hypothyroidism.

The major thyroid antibodies are anti–thyroid peroxidase (anti-TPO) antibodies, antithyroglobulin antibodies, and anti-TSH receptor antibodies (thyroid-stimulating immunoglobulins [TSIs] and thyrotropin-binding inhibitory immunoglobulins [TBIIs]). Elevated titers of anti-TPO and antithyroglobulin antibodies are associated with autoimmune hypothyroidism (Hashimoto thyroiditis), and elevated levels of TSI or TSII antibodies are associated with autoimmune hyperthyroidism (Graves disease). In the presence of a normal TSH level, a positive thyroid antibody titer does not indicate the need for treatment but instead confers an increased risk for future thyroid dysfunction. In a person with a strong family history of autoimmune thyroid disease, measurement of anti-TPO antibody titers assesses future risk of developing hypothyroidism. Measurement of antithyroglobulin antibody titers is not as sensitive and thus is not the preferred test. Repeated or serial measurements of antithyroid antibody titers are not recommended because the degree of a titer's elevation does not indicate a need for treatment; only an abnormal TSH level does. An exception to this recommendation is in women who are or wish to become pregnant whose anti-TPO titer is positive and whose TSH level is in the normal range. This special population has a higher risk of infertility, preterm delivery, and miscarriage, and thus serial measurements are appropriate.

TSIs and TBIIs are highly associated with Graves disease. When the diagnosis of Graves disease cannot be made clinically in a patient with hyperthyroidism, measurement of the serum level of these antibodies is recommended, especially if radioactive iodine uptake studies are not available or if radioactive iodine exposure is contraindicated, as in pregnancy and breastfeeding.

Thyroglobulin is a glycoprotein that stores thyroid hormone within the thyroid gland. This glycoprotein is released into the blood stream, and serum levels can be elevated in both hyperthyroidism and destructive thyroiditis and decreased in factitious thyrotoxicosis after ingestion of exogenous thyroid hormone. Obtaining a serum thyroglobulin level is thus helpful diagnostically in patients who are euthyroid when assessing for factitious ingestion of thyroid hormone. Measurement of the serum thyroglobulin level also is recommended in patients with a history of well-differentiated thyroid cancer (papillary or follicular thyroid cancer) because the glycoprotein is an effective tumor marker used to detect thyroid cancer recurrence or persistence at the earliest possible stage. In patients who have undergone thyroidectomy and radioactive iodine ablation as initial treatment for thyroid cancer, detectable serum thyroglobulin levels likely indicate the presence of thyroid cancer cells. In most immunometric assays, thyroglobulin antibodies interfere with accurate measurement and lead to falsely low serum thyroglobulin levels. Therefore, whenever the serum thyroglobulin level is measured, thyroglobulin antibodies also are measured; if antibodies are present, the serum thyroglobulin level may not be reliable.

In clinical settings, calcitonin, which is secreted by C cells of the thyroid gland, is used primarily as a tumor marker in patients with a history of medullary thyroid cancer. Although routine measurement of the serum calcitonin level is not recommended in all patients with thyroid nodules or thyroid dysfunction, its measurement is recommended in patients with thyroid nodules who are at higher risk for medullary thyroid cancer, such as those with a positive family history of medullary thyroid cancer, with features of multiple endocrine neoplasia type 2 (MEN2), or with thyroid biopsy results suggestive of medullary thyroid cancer.

The radioactive iodine uptake (RAIU) test measures iodine uptake by the thyroid gland over a specified time period (for example, at 4 and 24 hours after iodine injection). Patients with thyrotoxicosis (hyperthyroidism) typically have an elevated (higher than 30% at 24 hours) or high-normal RAIU, which indicates endogenous production of thyroid hormones. In patients with subacute, silent, or postpartum thyroiditis or exposure to exogenous thyroid hormones, the RAIU will be very low (<5% at 24 hours), which indicates very little endogenous production. A thyroid scan will show diffuse uptake of the radioactive iodine in Graves disease or more focal uptake in toxic multinodular goiter or toxic adenoma. These radionuclide studies are contraindicated during pregnancy and in women who are breast feeding. Postpartum thyroiditis occurs in approximately 30% of women with an elevated serum thyroid peroxidase antibody level.

Functional Thyroid Disorders

Thyrotoxicosis

The term thyrotoxicosis denotes thyroid hormone excess from any cause (**Figure 3**). Hyperthyroidism specifically refers to endogenous thyroid gland overactivity, most commonly caused by Graves disease, toxic multinodular goiter, or toxic adenoma. Fatigue, anxiety, insomnia, weight loss (despite increased appetite), tremulousness, tremor, heat intolerance, oligo- or amenorrhea, hyperdefecation, palpitations, shortness of breath or dyspnea on exertion, and muscle weakness are among the diverse signs and symptoms of thyrotoxicosis. The severity of symptoms may not correlate with the extent of thyroid hormone elevation. Older patients with apathetic hyperthyroidism, for example, may have minimal hyperadrenergic symptoms and instead may have atrial fibrillation or heart failure at presentation. Thyrotoxicosis may be associated with stare (due to lid retraction), dry itchy eyes, and tearing.

A thorough history and physical examination should be performed, as should appropriate laboratory and anatomic studies (**Table 17**). Typical laboratory findings of thyrotoxicosis include a suppressed TSH level and an elevated free T_4 and/or T_3 level; the TSH level is undetectable when the patient has overt hyperthyroidism. Anti-TPO and antithyroglobulin antibody levels also may be elevated with thyrotoxicosis. Thyroid ultrasonography is recommended for patients with thyrotoxicosis if a palpable nodule, a hypofunctioning area on an isotope scan, or a personal or family history of thyroid cancer is present.

Rarely, a patient may have a TSH-secreting pituitary tumor that stimulates the thyroid gland to secrete excessive T_4 and/or T_3. In contrast to more common causes of hyperthyroidism, TSH-secreting pituitary tumors may be associated with a detectable or even normal TSH level in the context of an elevated free T_4 or T_3 level. A pituitary MRI will show a pituitary tumor, and the α-subunit to serum TSH ratio will be greater than 1. Treatment is directed at the pituitary adenoma because thyroid gland–directed treatment typically is ineffective.

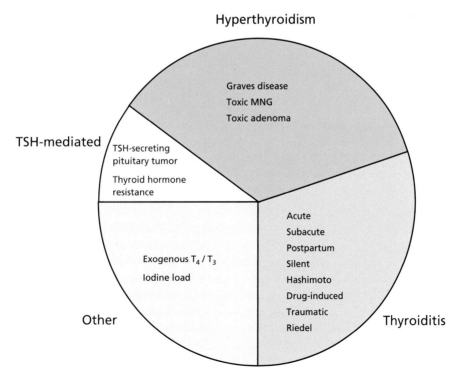

FIGURE 3. Types of thyrotoxicosis. MNG = multinodular goiter; T_3 = triiodothyronine; T_4 = thyroxine; TSH = thyroid-stimulating hormone.

TABLE 17. Classic Test Result Patterns in Thyrotoxicosis

Test	Graves Disease	Toxic Adenoma/ MNG	SAT Thyrotoxic Phase	Postpartum Thyroiditis	Exogenous T_4	Exogenous T_3	TSH-Secreting Pituitary Tumor	Reference Range
TSH	↓	↓	↓	↓	↓	↓	Normal or elevated	0.5-5.0 µU/mL (0.5-5.0 mU/L)
FT_4	↑	↑	↑	↑	↑	Normal/↓	↑	0.9-2.4 ng/dL (12-31 pmol/L)
FT_3	↑	↑	↑	↑	Normal/↑	↑	Normal/↑	3.6-5.6 ng/dL (5.6-8.6 pmol/L)
TPO Ab	+/–	+/–	+/–	+/–				<35 units/mL
TSI	+							<125%
TBII	+							<16%
RAIU	↑	↑	<5%	<5%	<5%	<5%	Normal/↑	10%-30% at 24 h

Ab = antibody; FT_3 = free triiodothyronine; FT_4 = free thyroxine; µU = microunit(s); mU = milliunits; MNG = multinodular goiter; RAIU = radioactive iodine uptake; SAT = subacute thyroiditis; TBII = thyrotropin-binding inhibitory immunoglobulin; TG = thyroglobulin; TPO = anti–thyroid peroxidase; TSH = thyroid-stimulating hormone; TSI = thyroid-stimulating immunoglobulin; ↓ = decreased; ↑ = increased; + = present; – = absent.

KEY POINTS

- Typical laboratory findings of thyrotoxicosis include a suppressed thyroid-stimulating hormone level (usually undetectable) and an elevated free thyroxine and/or triiodothyronine level.

- Radioactive iodine uptake by the thyroid gland is elevated in hyperthyroidism and decreased in destructive thyroiditis and exogenous thyroid hormone exposure.

Graves Disease

Graves disease is an autoimmune disease that can affect the thyroid gland, ocular muscles, orbital fat, and skin. Hyperthyroidism is by far its most common manifestation. In Graves disease, antibodies against the TSH receptor are produced. These antibodies stimulate autonomous thyroid gland function and secretion of excess T_4 and T_3.

Graves disease of the eye (ophthalmopathy) involves infiltration of the fibroblastic tissues of the ocular musculature, which leads to hypertrophy. Although the basic pathophysiology of Graves ophthalmopathy is not well understood, it is thought to involve stimulation of TSH receptors in orbital tissues (such as fibroblasts and adipose tissue), which results in increased cellular proliferation and local production of glycosaminoglycans. These processes result in inflammation and edema of extraocular muscles and an increase in retro-orbital tissues that causes proptosis, diplopia, chemosis, and, rarely, decreased visual acuity. Severity varies from mild to severe. Exophthalmos, orbital muscle dysfunction (as in diplopia), and conjunctival irritation may be important manifestations. Diagnosed clinically or with orbital CT or MRI,

ophthalmopathy occurs in as many as 25% of patients with Graves hyperthyroidism but also may occur in patients with normal findings on thyroid function tests who have elevated TSH receptor antibodies.

Graves disease of the skin (pretibial myxedema) involves infiltration of the dermis (usually of the anterior shin). Graves disease of the skin occurs in less than 5% of patients but almost always in patients who already have Graves hyperthyroidism and eye disease.

The main risk factor for Graves disease is a family history of autoimmune thyroid disease. Physical examination of the thyroid gland may reveal the classic smooth, rubbery, firm goiter, often characterized by a bruit.

Adrenergic symptoms from thyrotoxicosis should be treated promptly with β-blocker therapy; cardioselective β-blockers, such as atenolol, are preferred. Propranolol decreases (minimally) T_4 to T_3 conversion, but the decreased amount of T_3 is thought to be relatively clinically insignificant. The benefits of the cardioselective action of β-blockers are considered more clinically relevant, and once-daily administration of atenolol leads to increased adherence to the medical regimen.

Graves hyperthyroidism can be treated with antithyroid drugs, radioactive iodine (^{131}I) ablation, or thyroid surgery. Two antithyroid drugs are available in the United States, namely, methimazole and propylthiouracil. Methimazole is the first choice because of its increased potency, once-daily dosing regimen, and lower incidence of serious adverse effects (mainly hepatic). Propylthiouracil is used in women in the first trimester of pregnancy (because of the teratogenicity of methimazole) or patients unable to tolerate methimazole.

Antithyroid drugs can be used either for short-term control of hyperthyroidism before thyroidectomy or radioactive iodine treatment or for longer periods (12-24 months) to achieve spontaneous disease remission. Whether this remission is due to the natural history of Graves hyperthyroidism or to treatment with antithyroid drugs is unknown, but 30% to 50% of treated patients will experience a remission. Patients with small goiters, mild elevations in their T_4 and T_3 levels, and lower initial drug doses are more likely to have a remission. Although most patients will have a recurrence of hyperthyroidism, prolonged remission occurs in 20% to 30% of patients with remission induced by antithyroid agents. Methimazole and propylthiouracil may start to lower free T_4 and T_3 levels within several days, but the full beneficial effect may not be seen for several weeks, depending on the severity of the hyperthyroidism and on the medication dosage. TSH suppression may persist even after a decrease in or normalization of free T_4 and/or T_3 levels. Therefore, serial TSH measurements should not be used to routinely monitor patients with hyperthyroidism.

Although generally well tolerated, antithyroid drugs have some notable adverse effects. Approximately 5% to 10% of patients taking antithyroid drugs develop drug rashes. Of more serious concern, these drugs are associated (albeit rarely) with agranulocytosis and hepatotoxicity. Propylthiouracil has been associated with elevated aminotransferase levels and a higher rate of serious hepatic injury than methimazole, and for that reason methimazole is preferred. A mild and usually reversible cholestatic pattern on liver chemistry tests can be seen with methimazole. Baseline liver chemistry studies and a complete blood count (with leukocyte differential) are thus recommended before initiation of antithyroid drugs. Patients taking antithyroid drugs who develop high fever, sore throat, prominent flulike symptoms, rash, jaundice, icterus, or other symptoms of serious illness should be immediately assessed for an adverse reaction to the medication.

A single appropriate dose of radioactive iodine can ablate an overactive thyroid in Graves disease in greater than 90% of patients. Adverse effects are uncommon, but patients may develop transient anterior neck pain or tenderness from radiation thyroiditis. An exacerbation of the thyrotoxic state for several weeks can occur because of the release of preformed hormone. The expected and desired outcome is permanent hypothyroidism, which typically occurs within 2 to 3 months of therapy, at which time thyroid hormone replacement therapy is begun.

Graves ophthalmopathy occurs more commonly in smokers and persons with a family history of the disorder. Its severity varies from mild to severe and may involve exophthalmos, inflammatory eye changes (chemosis, conjunctival injection, periorbital edema, or iritis), extraocular muscle palsies causing double vision, and optic nerve compression causing reduced visual acuity and (rarely) blindness. A primary focus in managing Graves ophthalmopathy should be to establish a euthyroid state. Because radioactive iodine treatment has been associated with (at least transient) worsening of Graves ophthalmopathy, its use is not recommended in patients with severe Graves ophthalmopathy. A thyroidectomy is preferred when definitive therapy for hyperthyroidism is required in a patient with severe Graves ophthalmopathy. Patients with advanced ophthalmopathy should be cared for by an experienced ophthalmologist, who may treat with local measures (such as artificial tears), corticosteroids, orbital irradiation, or orbital decompression, as necessary.

KEY POINT

- Radioactive iodine can effectively ablate an overactive thyroid in Graves disease in greater than 90% of patients, usually after a single dose; this treatment should be avoided in patients with significant Graves ophthalmopathy.

Toxic Multinodular Goiter and Toxic Adenoma

Toxic multinodular goiter and toxic adenoma result from an activating somatic mutation in the TSH receptor gene, which leads to autonomy of function and secretion of excess T_4 and T_3 from the nodule(s) affected. Recent iodine exposure from acute iodine loads, usually from iodinated contrast dye used in CT scans and angiographic procedures (such as cardiac catheterization), can induce thyrotoxicosis in patients with preexisting autonomy of thyroid function (Jod-Basedow phenomenon). MRI and ultrasonography should be used preferentially in patients with autonomy of thyroid function to avoid iodine exposure from iodinated contrast.

Physical examination usually reveals one or more palpable nodule(s) or overall gland enlargement. Therefore, obtaining a thyroid ultrasound is recommended to assess any detected nodule for cancer risk and the need for biopsy. Thyroid cancer is not often diagnosed in a patient with hyperthyroidism, but any nodule found should be considered for biopsy on the basis of its size and imaging characteristics (see later discussion of thyroid nodules). A multinodular goiter associated with hyperthyroidism can be treated with either radioactive iodine or surgery depending on multiple factors, including the size of the thyroid gland, evidence of obstruction (such as hoarseness with recurrent laryngeal nerve impairment), dyspnea, or local symptoms suggestive of cervical venous obstruction (such as engorgement of neck veins, especially when raising the hands above the head). Radioactive iodine therapy may effectively treat the hyperthyroidism, but surgery usually is indicated for large goiters with local compressive symptoms, except in patients who are not good surgical candidates. Radioactive iodine generally results in a modest decrease in goiter size (approximately 30% to 50%) over many months.

With toxic adenoma, a thyroid scan with radioactive iodine (^{131}I) will reveal a solitary overactive ("hot") nodule with suppression of the rest of the gland. With toxic multi-nodular goiter, the scan will reveal patchy uptake of radioactive iodine that is increased in autonomous regions and reduced outside those areas. In areas of decreased uptake, if a distinct "cold" nodule is present (confirmed as a nodule on a thyroid ultrasound), a biopsy is recommended before any treatment with radioactive iodine. Close monitoring with thyroid function tests is indicated approximately every 6 to 8 weeks.

Radioactive iodine ablation is the treatment of choice. Ideally, the hyperactive nodule(s) is(are) ablated over several months, and the normal thyroid tissue returns to normal function, which negates the need for lifelong thyroid hormone replacement therapy. The limitation of this treatment is the avidity of the nodule(s) for iodine. If the radioactive iodine uptake is not sufficiently high, the nodule(s) will not be ablated and the hyperthyroidism will persist. Surgical removal of the involved lobe (in patients with toxic adenoma) and total thyroidectomy (in patients with toxic multinodular goiter) is usually offered to those whose gland is not sufficiently avid for the radioactive iodine to result in ablation or who have proven thyroid cancer by biopsy. Antithyroid drugs modulate thyroid hormone production in toxic multinodular goiter and toxic adenoma and thus must be administered continuously to control hyperthyroidism.

KEY POINT

• Radioactive iodine ablation is the preferred treatment of toxic multinodular goiter and toxic adenoma.

Destructive Thyroiditis

Thyroiditis involves transient destruction of thyroid tissue, which disrupts follicles and causes the release of preformed thyroid hormone into the circulation. Forms of destructive thyroiditis include subacute (de Quervain), silent, and postpartum thyroiditis. Subacute thyroiditis most commonly occurs after a viral infection and usually involves severe thyroid and neck pain; fever, fatigue, malaise, anorexia, and myalgia are common. Silent thyroiditis is painless. Postpartum thyroiditis is a subset of painless autoimmune thyroiditis and can occur up to 12 months after parturition. It affects 5% to 8% of pregnant women in the United States and can recur with each pregnancy.

Subacute thyroiditis is associated with systemic signs of inflammation (such as an elevated erythrocyte sedimentation rate or C-reactive protein level), elevated serum free T_4 and T_3 levels, and a low serum TSH level. The disorder usually follows a classic course of approximately 6 weeks of thyrotoxicosis, a shorter period of euthyroidism, 4 to 6 weeks of hypothyroidism, and then restoration of euthyroidism. The severity and duration of an episode of destructive thyroiditis vary among patients. The clinical courses of silent and postpartum thyroiditis are more variable than that of subacute thyroiditis. Those who have had any type of thyroiditis are at increased risk for subsequent bouts. The hypothyroid phase

is usually mild but can be prolonged or permanent and require thyroid hormone replacement. This more severe presentation is more likely to occur in patients with postpartum thyroiditis. When necessary, levothyroxine generally is given for approximately 6 months to allow time for thyroid gland recovery and then is tapered and stopped, with ongoing monitoring for recurrent hypothyroidism.

Figure 4 shows typical results of thyroid function and RAIU tests in patients with destructive thyroiditis. Antithyroid agents, such as methimazole or propylthiouracil, have no role in the treatment of destructive thyroiditis because endogenous production of thyroid hormone is very low. β-Adrenergic blocker therapy is recommended in specific patients during the thyrotoxic phase. NSAIDs are the first line of therapy for the neck pain of subacute thyroiditis; corticosteroid therapy is indicated in patients with severe pain unresponsive to NSAIDs and in patients with markedly elevated free T_4 or T_3 levels.

KEY POINT

• The hypothyroid phase of destructive thyroiditis can be so severe that replacement therapy with levothyroxine should be considered; this therapy is most commonly necessary in postpartum thyroiditis.

Drug-Induced Thyrotoxicosis

Multiple agents can cause thyrotoxicosis, including amiodarone (most common), interferon alfa, interleukin-2, and lithium carbonate. Iodine loads from drugs, iodinated contrast, or, in rare cases, significant povidone-iodine exposure can trigger hyperthyroidism in persons with preexisting or

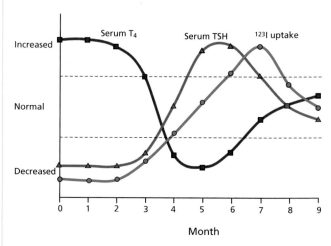

FIGURE 4. Triphasic changes in thyroid hormone levels associated with destructive thyroiditis. Measurement of serum T_4, serum TSH, and radioactive iodine (^{123}I) uptake shows thyrotoxicosis during the first 3 months, followed by hypothyroidism for 3 months, and then by euthyroidism. ^{123}I = radioactive iodine; T_4 = thyroxine; TSH = thyroid-stimulating hormone.

underlying thyroid autonomy. Lithium is more commonly associated with hypothyroidism than hyperthyroidism. Although the average diet in the United States contains approximately 150 to 200 micrograms/d of iodine, amiodarone contains 75 mg (75,000 micrograms) of iodine per tablet and has a half-life of months while stored in tissues. Persistent effects on thyroid function can be seen for up to 1 year after drug discontinuation.

Iodine-induced hyperthyroidism (type 1) and destructive thyroiditis (type 2) are the two forms of amiodarone-induced thyrotoxicosis. Type 1 thyrotoxicosis is more common in iodine-deficient geographic areas in patients with multinodular goiter and is treated with antithyroid agents. Type 2 thyrotoxicosis generally occurs in iodine-sufficient regions, such as the United States, and is treated with corticosteroid therapy. In practice, however, the distinction between the two types of disease is not clear, and many patients have overlapping disease, which is treated with both antithyroid agents and corticosteroids. In patients who are unresponsive to antithyroid drugs and corticosteroid therapy, a thyroidectomy may be recommended. These patients typically have multiple clinical issues and also are hyperthyroid. Therefore, the decision regarding thyroidectomy must be based on individual circumstances.

Because the management of amiodarone-induced thyrotoxicosis can be complex, involvement of an endocrinologist is appropriate. If possible, discontinuation of amiodarone should be attempted, although stopping the drug may (rarely) not be possible from a cardiac perspective. Consultation with the patient's cardiologist is thus important.

KEY POINT

- The most common cause of drug-induced thyrotoxicosis is amiodarone, which has high iodine content and can cause an iodine-induced thyrotoxicosis or destructive thyroiditis.

Subclinical Hyperthyroidism

Subclinical hyperthyroidism is characterized by a suppressed serum TSH level with concomitant T_4 and T_3 levels within the reference range. Repeat thyroid hormone levels should be obtained in 3 or 6 months to confirm that this is a continuing problem. Symptoms are mild, and most patients are asymptomatic.

Persistent mild hyperthyroidism has potential negative effects on cardiac function, the central nervous system, and bone mass. Which patients should receive treatment remains a matter of debate, but consensus supports intervention when the TSH level is less than 0.1 microunit/mL (0.1 milliunit/L), especially in patients who are 65 years and older, have tachyarrhythmias or heart disease, are postmenopausal with low bone mass, or are markedly symptomatic. The management of TSH levels less than the normal range but 0.1 microunit/mL (0.1 milliunit/L) or greater is less certain.

Data suggest an increased risk of atrial fibrillation when the TSH level is less than 0.3 microunit/mL (0.3 milliunit/L). Postmenopausal patients with a TSH level less than 0.1 microunit/mL (0.1 milliunit/L) also have a higher risk of bone loss. When treatment is warranted, radioactive iodine ablation may be preferred. Often, however, the gland is not avid enough to trap sufficient iodine, and methimazole must be used to normalize the TSH level.

Hypothyroidism

A common disorder, hypothyroidism has a higher prevalence in women than men (2% versus 0.2%) and in persons with other underlying autoimmune diseases. The most frequent cause is Hashimoto thyroiditis, followed distantly by iatrogenic hypothyroidism (which can occur after radioactive iodine ablation for Graves disease, external beam radiation to the thyroid bed, or surgical removal of the thyroid gland). Amiodarone, lithium carbonate, interferon alfa, interleukin-2, and other medications can cause hypothyroidism; amiodarone causes hypothyroidism in approximately 10% of North Americans who take it chronically. Pituitary disease, pituitary tumors, and pituitary surgery can cause central hypothyroidism. Congenital forms of hypothyroidism, such as thyroid agenesis or dyshormonogenesis (a genetic defect in the synthesis of thyroid hormone), are rarer causes of hypothyroidism. Celiac disease, which occurs more frequently in patients with autoimmune thyroid disease than in the general population, is sometimes associated with inadequate levothyroxine absorption and resultant increased levothyroxine dosing requirements in patients with established hypothyroidism.

The numerous and largely nonspecific clinical manifestations of hypothyroidism include fatigue, reduced endurance, weight gain, cold intolerance, constipation, impaired concentration and short-term memory, dry skin, edema, mood changes, depression, psychomotor retardation, muscle cramps, myalgia, menorrhagia, and reduced fertility. Physical examination findings can include a reduced basal temperature, diastolic hypertension, an enlarged thyroid gland, bradycardia, pallor, dry and cold skin, brittle hair, hoarseness, and a delayed recovery phase of deep tendon reflexes. Some patients with mild hypothyroidism will exhibit few or none of these signs and symptoms. Results of laboratory studies can confirm hypothyroidism (**Table 18**). Measurement of serum TSH and total or free T_4 levels is required, but measurement of the serum T_3 level is generally not needed. Anti-TPO or thyroglobulin antibodies in the serum suggest Hashimoto thyroiditis as the cause of hypothyroidism. A thyroid scan and RAIU test are not useful. In patients with hypothyroidism in whom a goiter or nodule is palpated, imaging the gland with ultrasonography to evaluate for nodular disease requiring biopsy is appropriate.

Levothyroxine therapy is the mainstay of thyroid hormone replacement. The drug should be taken on an empty

TABLE 18. Classic Test Result Patterns in Hypothyroidism

	Hashimoto Thyroiditis	Subclinical Hypothyroidism	SAT Recovery Phase	Postpartum Thyroiditis Hypothyroid Phase	Central Hypothyroidism	Reference Range
TSH	↑	↑	↑	↑	↓/Normal	0.5-5.0 µU/mL (0.5-5.0 mU/L)
FT$_4$	Normal/↓	Normal	Normal/↓	Normal/↓	↓/Normal	0.9-2.4 ng/dL (12-31 pmol/L)
FT$_3$	Normal/↓	Normal	Normal/↓	Normal/↓	Normal/↓	3.6-5.6 ng/dL (5.6-8.6 pmol/L)
TPO Ab	+	+/−	+/−	+/−		<35 units/mL
TG Ab	+/−	+/−	+/−	+/−		<20 units/mL

Ab = antibody; FT$_3$ = free triiodothyronine; FT$_4$ = free thyroxine; µU = microunit(s); mU = milliunit(s); SAT = subacute thyroiditis; TG = thyroglobulin; TPO = anti–thyroid peroxidase; TSH = thyroid-stimulating hormone; ↓ = decreased; ↑ = increased; + = present; − = absent.

stomach 1 hour before or 2 to 3 hours after intake of food or calcium- or iron-containing supplements. Although attention recently has focused on liothyronine therapy and combination T$_3$-T$_4$ therapy that uses either thyroid hormone extract or synthetic T$_3$-T$_4$ combinations, most evidence to date shows that neither has a clinical advantage over traditional levothyroxine treatment. T$_3$ preparations have a short half-life and have been associated with acute spikes in serum T$_3$ levels, which are of particular concern in older adult patients or patients with cardiac abnormalities.

For patients receiving thyroid hormone replacement therapy, an appropriate target for the TSH level is 0.5 to 4.3 microunits/mL (0.5-4.3 milliunits/L). Discussion of the utility of aiming for a TSH level of 1.0 to 3.0 microunits/mL (1.0-3.0 milliunits/L) in most patients has occurred because of concerns that older patients and patients with positive antithyroid antibodies or a family history of thyroid disease tend to have higher TSH levels. However, no robust evidence supports this lower TSH goal. Patients age 80 years and older with subclinical or overt hypothyroidism are more likely to survive to age 89 years than their peers with normal or low serum TSH values. Increasing evidence suggests that the normal reference range for persons age 80 years and older is approximately 1 to 7 microunits/mL (1-7 milliunits/L), although further studies in this area are required. It is now recognized that patients in this age range generally should not be placed on exogenous levothyroxine solely for an elevated TSH level but that a complete consideration of the patient and the clinical context is necessary.

KEY POINT

- A target range of 0.5 to 4.3 microunits/mL (0.5-4.3 milliunits/L) for the thyroid-stimulating hormone level is appropriate for most patients with defined thyroid disease taking levothyroxine; a higher range may be appropriate for persons age 80 years and older.

Subclinical Hypothyroidism

In subclinical hypothyroidism, the serum TSH level is greater than the reference range, with concomitant serum T$_4$ and T$_3$ levels in the reference range. Patients typically have mild or no symptoms of hypothyroidism. The causes of subclinical hypothyroidism are the same as for overt hypothyroidism. Patients with subclinical hypothyroidism may have mild elevations in total cholesterol, LDL cholesterol, and even C-reactive protein levels, and some meta-analyses have shown an increased risk for atherosclerosis and cardiac events. However, evidence is insufficient to conclude that treatment with levothyroxine minimizes risks or improves outcomes when the TSH level is 10 microunits/mL (10 milliunits/L) or less. Treatment is recommended when serum TSH levels are greater than 10 microunits/mL (10 milliunits/L). Levothyroxine therapy also can be considered for patients who are markedly symptomatic, have a goiter, are pregnant or are planning to become pregnant, or have positive anti–TPO antibodies. The evidence currently is most compelling for treating pregnant patients with subclinical hypothyroidism; the normal ranges of the TSH level in patients who are pregnant are 0.1 to 2.5 microunits/mL (0.1-2.5 milliunits/L) in the first trimester, 0.2 to 3.0 microunits/mL (0.2-3.0 milliunits/L) in the second trimester, and 0.3 to 3.0 microunits/mL (0.3-3.0 milliunits/L) in the third trimester. Patients desirous of becoming pregnant should have a TSH level between 0.5 and 2.5 microunits/mL (0.5-2.5 milliunits/L).

KEY POINT

- Pregnant women or women desirous of becoming pregnant who have subclinical hypothyroidism should receive thyroid hormone replacement therapy if their thyroid-stimulating hormone level is greater than the normal range for their condition.

Structural Disorders of the Thyroid Gland

The primary structural disorders of the thyroid gland are nodules, goiters, and cancers. Rarer causes include aberrant or ectopic structural disorders, such as agenesis, hemiagenesis, substernal and lingual abnormalities, and struma ovarii.

Thyroid Nodules

Palpable thyroid nodules have a prevalence of approximately 5% in women and 1% in men in iodine-sufficient areas, such as the United States, and the prevalence increases with age. The differential diagnosis of thyroid nodules is varied (**Table 19**). Because most thyroid nodules are benign, the clinician's task is to identify malignant lesions (5%-15%) in the most accurate, efficient, and cost-effective manner (**Figure 5**). Factors associated with an increased cancer risk include age less than 20 or greater than 60 years, male gender, previous head or neck irradiation, a family history of thyroid (especially medullary) cancer, rapid nodule growth, and hoarseness. Pain is uncommon and is more often associated with benign than malignant nodules. The presence of a hard palpable nodule (or nodules), local cervical lymphadenopathy, fixation to adjacent tissue, and vocal cord paralysis increases the likelihood of cancer.

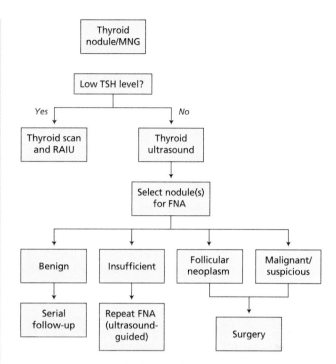

FIGURE 5. Evaluation of a thyroid nodule. Algorithm showing the suggested evaluation of a thyroid nodule. FNA = fine-needle aspiration; MNG = multinodular goiter; RAIU = radioactive iodine uptake; TSH = thyroid-stimulating hormone.

TABLE 19.	Differential Diagnosis of Thyroid Nodules
Diagnosis	**Notes**
Benign	
Thyroid nodule	Adenomatoid hyperplasia, colloid nodule, adenomatoid nodule, follicular or Hürthle cell adenoma, and hyalinizing trabecular adenoma
Thyroglossal duct cyst	Midline cystic mass at level of hyoid bone; moves upward with protrusion of the tongue; may become infected; rarely malignant
Pyramidal lobe of thyroid	Cephalad projection of thyroid tissue from isthmus; may be palpable in autoimmune thyroid disease
Lipoma	Benign focal subcutaneous accumulation of fat
Dermoid cyst	Soft mass in the suprasternal notch
Teratoma	Type of germ cell tumor that may contain several different types of tissue (such as hair, muscle, and bone); mediastinal location at times
Branchial cyst	Soft lateral neck mass anterior to upper third of sternocleidomastoid muscle; usually seen in adults; cholesterol crystals in cyst fluid
Cervical lymphadenopathy	Possibly benign or may be associated with malignancy, including thyroid cancer
Malignant	
Thyroid cancer (primary)	Papillary (variants: follicular, diffuse sclerosing, columnar, tall cell)
	Follicular (variants: Hürthle cell [oncocytic])
	Medullary
	Anaplastic
Thyroid lymphoma	Rapidly enlarging, firm neck mass; often bilateral; classically seen in older women with a history of Hashimoto thyroiditis
Metastatic cancer	Metastases of other primary cancer to thyroid (breast, melanoma, kidney)
Sarcoma	Tumors usually arising from connective tissue, with most being malignant

Measurement of the serum TSH level should be the first test performed in a patient with a thyroid nodule. If the level is suppressed, free T_4 and T_3 levels should be measured and a radionuclide scan considered. Treatment for incidentally discovered hyperthyroidism should then be undertaken. Less than 1% of hyperfunctioning nodules contain malignancy. If the TSH level is normal or elevated, thyroid ultrasonography should be performed as soon as possible to allow for timely fine-needle aspiration (FNA) biopsy, if indicated. Measurement of thyroid antibody levels is also appropriate, especially in patients with multinodular goiters or patients in whom autoimmune thyroid disease is suspected. Routine calcitonin measurement is not recommended for patients with thyroid nodules but is used to follow disease activity in patients with medullary thyroid cancer and should be considered in persons with a family history of medullary thyroid cancer. This test also should be considered in patients with MEN2 (or related disorders) or symptoms suggestive of this disease. The serum thyroglobulin level is the primary tumor marker in patients with well-differentiated thyroid cancer who have had thyroidectomy and radioactive iodine ablation.

Thyroid ultrasonography is the imaging test of choice in patients with palpable thyroid nodules and enables accurate detection and sizing of all nodules in the thyroid gland. Ultrasound characteristics are used to further delineate cancer risk in any detected nodule (**Table 20**). Additional characteristics suggestive of malignancy include size greater than 3 cm, hypoechogenicity, shape taller than wide, irregular infiltrative margins, microcalcifications within the nodule, and high intranodular vascular flow. Nodules that are purely cystic with a surrounding hypolucency (halo) or peripheral vascular flow are less likely to harbor cancer. Although ultrasound findings have reasonable specificity, they have poor sensitivity for predicting thyroid cancer and cannot by themselves be used to determine the presence or absence of cancer. CT and MRI without contrast are not routinely used but may sometimes be indicated, as in the presence of a substernal goiter, cervical lymphadenopathy, or tracheal compression. Use of intravenous dye with CT scans should be avoided, if possible, because this dye may induce hyperthyroidism in a patient with a multinodular goiter or interfere with other tests (such as an isotope radionuclide scan) or treatments.

A thyroid scan and RAIU test are appropriate in the presence of a suppressed serum TSH level because a toxic nodule (or toxic multinodular goiter) may be present.

FNA biopsy, performed either by nodule palpation or under ultrasonographic guidance, is essential in the evaluation of thyroid nodules. This procedure, when performed correctly, is a safe, simple, and relatively inexpensive method of determining the presence of cancer in a nodule. Its sensitivity is approximately 95%, with a false-negative rate of approximately 4%, depending to some extent on the nodule size. FNA biopsy is recommended for any nodule greater than 1 cm in diameter that is solid and hypoechoic on ultrasonography and for any nodule 2 cm or greater that is mixed cystic-solid without worrisome sonographic characteristics Consideration of biopsy may be appropriate for smaller nodules (at least 5 mm in diameter) in patients with risk factors, such as a history of radiation exposure, a family or personal history of thyroid cancer, cervical lymphadenopathy, or suspicious ultrasound characteristics. FNA biopsy is not routinely recommended for thyroid nodules less than 1 cm in diameter. Because large nodules (>4 cm) may be associated with sampling error, resampling of such nodules in the future is prudent, even when the nodule remains stable in size.

Patients with nodules greater than 4 cm who have associated worrisome clinical findings (such as abnormal cervical lymphadenopathy or hoarseness), radiologic features (such as a history of external radiation to the neck; see also Table 20), or laboratory findings but benign results of FNA biopsy can be considered for thyroidectomy. The Bethesda classification system has six possible cytopathologic diagnoses: (1) benign nodule, (2) malignant nodule, (3) nondiagnostic sample, (4) nodule suspicious for malignancy, (5) follicular neoplasm, and (6) follicular lesion of undetermined significance. The last three diagnoses imply an increased risk of malignancy, even though clearly malignant cells were not detected, and surgery is typically recommended to allow for histologic evaluation. Histopathologic analysis yields a diagnosis of frank malignancy in approximately 15% to 30% of these surgical samples.

Benign nodules should be monitored by periodic neck examination and ultrasonography (every 6-18 months), with repeat FNA biopsy recommended if the nodule has significant growth in the interval (50% by volume or 20% in two dimensions) or when subsequent ultrasound or clinical findings are suspicious. If the nodules are stable in both size and ultrasound characteristics after at least 18 months, the timing of clinical evaluation and ultrasonography could be extended to longer intervals (every 3-5 years).

Malignant nodules require prompt surgical removal. Surgical complications of thyroidectomy include hypoparathyroidism and recurrent laryngeal nerve paresis. The lowest complication rates are associated with thyroid surgery

TABLE 20. Ultrasound Characteristics of Thyroid Nodules

Cancerous Nodules	Benign Nodules
Microcalcifications	Comet tail
Increased intranodular vascularity	Increased peripheral nodule vascularity
Hypoechogenicity	Hyperechogenicity
Irregular border	Halo present
Taller than wide (sagittal view)	Pure cyst

performed by experienced thyroid surgeons at large-volume medical centers.

The previous practice of giving patients levothyroxine to shrink thyroid nodules has been abandoned because of its inefficacy, the usefulness of FNA biopsy, and the morbidities associated with iatrogenic thyrotoxicosis.

KEY POINT

- In the evaluation of thyroid nodules that may be malignant, ultrasonography is recommended for imaging, followed by fine-needle aspiration biopsy for nodules larger than 1 cm in diameter.

Goiters

Multinodular Goiter

Multinodular goiters are more frequent with advancing age, iodine deficiency, and Hashimoto disease. Cancer risk is the same for a thyroid gland with a solitary nodule or with multiple nodules (approximately 5%-10%), and thus evaluation and management of multiple nodules also is basically the same as for a solitary nodule. In a multinodular gland, nodules with suspicious ultrasound characteristics are preferentially chosen for biopsy; in the absence of suspicious characteristics (see Table 20), the largest nodules are chosen for biopsy. Large multinodular goiters, especially those with a substernal extension, may present with local compressive symptoms, such as dysphagia, hoarseness, or even dyspnea. To confirm the presence and quantify the severity of mass effect caused by a multinodular goiter, barium swallow, direct vocal cord visualization, spirometry with flow volume loops, or neck and chest CT without contrast may be necessary. In select circumstances, radioactive iodine can be used to shrink (to a limited degree) a multinodular goiter but is not the first-line option in the United States, except in patients with thyrotoxicosis due to autonomous function. Thyroid surgery may be indicated if (1) local compressive symptoms are prominent and clinically significant, (2) malignancy is suspected, or (3) cosmetic intervention is desired by the patient.

Simple Goiter

A simple goiter is the presence of an enlarged thyroid gland without nodules. Dyshormonogenesis occasionally causes a simple goiter. On ultrasound, simple goiters can be homogeneous or heterogeneous. Patients with asymptomatic, stable simple goiters can be serially monitored clinically, but serial ultrasound in not recommended because of the lack of nodular disease. Primary thyroid lymphoma, which is rare and more likely to occur in older patients with Hashimoto thyroiditis, can present as a symptomatic rapidly enlarging goiter, usually with a very firm texture and often with systemic symptoms associated with temperature elevation. FNA biopsy of rapidly expanding firm goiters is recommended.

KEY POINT

- Barium swallow, direct vocal cord visualization, spirometry with flow volume loops, or neck and chest CT without contrast may be necessary to confirm the presence of and quantify the severity of mass effect caused by a multinodular goiter.

Thyroid Cancer

More than 95% of thyroid cancer is well differentiated and typically associated with long-term survival and low morbidity. The major forms of thyroid cancer are papillary (85%), follicular (10%), and medullary (4%); approximately 1% consists of poorly differentiated aggressive types, like anaplastic. Even less frequent are primary thyroid lymphoma and metastases to the thyroid of other cancers, such as breast cancer, kidney cancer, and melanoma. Medullary thyroid cancer can be a component of MEN2A and can be associated with hyperparathyroidism with hypercalcemia and hypertension due to a pheochromocytoma. Medullary thyroid cancer typically is characterized by plasmacytoid, spindle, round, or polygonal cells on biopsy. All patients with medullary thyroid cancer should have *RET* proto-oncogene sequencing after other appropriate evaluation, including measurement of plasma free metanephrine and normetanephrine levels to detect or exclude the presence of a pheochromocytoma.

Staging and prognosis of well-differentiated thyroid cancer (papillary and follicular) are based on American Joint Committee on Cancer criteria, which include age (<45 or ≥45 years), primary tumor size, local and distant metastases, and capsular and lymphovascular invasion. In brief, in patients younger than 45 years, stage I disease includes thyroid cancer of any size, with or without cervical lymph node involvement and without distant spread; stage II refers to patients who have distant spread of disease. In patients 45 years and older, stage I thyroid cancer denotes tumors 2 cm or less in size without local invasion or positive cervical lymph nodes, stage II denotes tumors greater than 2 cm but no more than 4 cm in size without local invasion or positive cervical lymph nodes, stage III denotes tumors larger than 4 cm in size with slight local invasion with or without cervical lymph node involvement, and stage IV denotes thyroid cancer that either has invaded nearby neck structures or superior mediastinal lymph nodes or may or may not have invaded local tissues or lymph nodes but has spread to distant sites.

Patients with stage I and II disease tend to do very well, with patients younger than 40 years having a less than 2% mortality rate at 30 years. Patients with stage III and IV disease have 10-year survival rates of approximately 82% and 38%, respectively. Treatment of well-differentiated thyroid cancer involves a combination of thyroidectomy, radioactive iodine therapy, and suppression of TSH secretion with levothyroxine therapy. Radioactive iodine therapy frequently is administered for stage III and IV disease, especially with lymph node involvement, to decrease the risk of recurrence and death.

The extent of thyroid gland removal required varies and generally depends on tumor size, with solitary tumors less than 1 cm in diameter generally effectively managed by lobectomy. Patients with larger tumors, multifocal disease, known cervical lymph node metastasis, and a history of irradiation are best treated with total or near-total thyroidectomy. Suppression of TSH secretion has been associated with long-term improvement in morbidity and mortality in patients with stage III and IV disease. The degree of TSH suppression targeted varies with risk of recurrence and is based on several factors, including stage of disease, presence of residual tumor, time since original diagnosis, and patient tolerance of TSH suppression.

The 2009, American Thyroid Association Guidelines regarding thyroid cancer recommended that patients with persistent disease should have a goal TSH level of less than 0.1 microunit/mL (0.1 milliunit/L). Patients who are currently disease free but at high risk of recurrence should have a goal TSH level of 0.1 to 0.5 microunit/mL (0.1-0.5 milliunit/L) for 5 to 10 years, and those who are disease free and at low risk of recurrence should have a goal TSH level of 0.3 to 2.0 microunits/mL (0.3-2.0 milliunits/L).

KEY POINT

- Treatment of well-differentiated thyroid cancer involves a combination of thyroidectomy, radioactive iodine therapy, and suppression of TSH secretion with levothyroxine therapy.

Effects of Nonthyroidal Illness on Thyroid Function Tests

Nonthyroidal illness can alter the results of thyroid function tests, an effect referred to as the euthyroid sick syndrome, which is more common in critically ill patients but can occur in more stable hospitalized patients. Most commonly, T_3 levels decline sharply, and reverse T_3 (an inactive thyroid hormone metabolite) levels increase. Free T_4 levels typically decrease but remain in the reference range. A frankly low free T_4 level is usually seen in critical illness and is a poor prognostic indicator. The TSH response is less consistent, with low, normal, and elevated levels reported. However, in a patient with a nonthyroidal illness only, it is unusual for TSH levels to become undetectable or increase to greater than approximately 10 microunits/mL (10 milliunits/L) because these elevated TSH levels suggest the presence of primary hypothyroidism.

Cytokines and various other inflammatory mediators released during systemic illness also play a role in euthyroid sick syndrome. The thyroid hormone patterns seen in nonthyroidal illness appear to be an adaptive response to mitigate catabolism associated with severe physiologic stress and provide a protective effect by way of transient central hypothyroidism. Intervention with thyroid hormone therapy has not proved beneficial and is not indicated in patients with altered thyroid function test results most likely caused by nonthyroidal illness. Almost all patients have a normal TSH level after their recovery, and all thyroid hormone levels typically normalize by 8 weeks after recovery. H

KEY POINT

- Nonthyroidal illness (usually severe) can alter thyroid function test results, an effect known as euthyroid sick syndrome; results usually normalize by 8 weeks after recovery from the illness.

Thyroid Function and Disease in Pregnancy

Abnormal thyroid function during pregnancy can greatly affect the health of both mother and fetus. Elevated estrogen levels increase the TBG level, which increases the total T_4 and T_3 levels. To compensate for the increase in the TBG level and altered T_4 and T_3 kinetics and to keep the free T_4 level stable, women who take levothyroxine for hypothyroidism usually require an increased dosage (approximately 30%-50%) during pregnancy. Increasing the levothyroxine dosage at the start of pregnancy or early in pregnancy is recommended to anticipate this increased requirement, maintain normal maternal thyroid function, and provide adequate thyroid hormone to the fetus.

During the first trimester of pregnancy, increased levels of human chorionic gonadotropin (HCG) can stimulate thyroid hormone production by way of cross-reactivity with the TSH receptor because of the common α-subunit shared by HCG and TSH. Serum TSH levels may decrease to low-normal or even below-normal ranges in the first trimester, but this is rarely associated with thyrotoxicosis. The TSH level slowly increases to normal by 16 weeks' gestation.

Maternal or fetal thyroid hormone deficiency can negatively affect fetal neurocognitive development. The goal TSH level during the first trimester is approximately 0.1 to 2.5 microunits/mL (0.1-2.5 milliunits/L); in the second and third trimesters, it is approximately 0.1 to 3.0 microunits/mL (0.1-3.0 milliunits/L). The value of general prenatal maternal evaluation of thyroid function is still debated. At a minimum, thyroid function tests should be obtained in patients with strong risk factors for thyroid disease, and close monitoring is required in those with a known history of a thyroid disorder. In women planning pregnancy who have known hypothyroidism, the TSH level should be maintained at 0.5 to 2.5 microunits/mL (0.5-2.5 milliunits/L) during the preconception period.

Pregnant women receiving thyroid replacement therapy should have their thyroid hormone status monitored frequently to assess the effect of levothyroxine dose adjustments. Levothyroxine requirements increase in most patients with hypothyroidism during pregnancy. The levothyroxine dosage can be increased by giving two extra doses a week. Another reasonable approach is to attempt to maintain the TSH level at less than 2.5 microunits/mL (2.5 milliunits/L) by making frequent adjustments to the dosage, as dictated by the results of laboratory studies every 2 weeks during the first half of pregnancy and every 4 to 6 weeks during the second half. The increased levothyroxine requirements occur mainly in the first trimester of pregnancy.

Because some symptoms of thyrotoxicosis (tachycardia, heat intolerance, fatigue) overlap with symptoms of normal pregnancy, changes in thyroid function test results associated with normal pregnancy may be difficult to discern from true thyrotoxicosis. Compounding this difficulty is the contraindication during pregnancy (and in women who are breastfeeding) to some diagnostic techniques, such as thyroid scans and radioiodine uptake tests, to avoid radiation exposure of the fetus. The presence of a moderate goiter or ophthalmopathy can indicate the presence of Graves disease. Although HCG–mediated TSH receptor stimulation tends to resolve by 16 weeks' gestation, changes of primary thyroid disease persist longer, albeit with some improvement. When true hyperthyroidism is diagnosed during pregnancy, prompt referral to an endocrinologist and a high-risk obstetrician is recommended.

KEY POINT

- Thyroid scans and radioactive iodine uptake testing are contraindicated in pregnant patients and in patients who are breastfeeding or have done so recently.

Thyroid Emergencies

Whereas most thyroid conditions are not urgent, thyroid storm and myxedema coma are life-threatening conditions that require prompt diagnosis and intervention, typically in consultation with an endocrinologist.

Thyroid Storm

Thyroid storm is a life threatening condition that presents as severe thyrotoxicosis, coupled with secondary systemic decompensation. This disorder can be differentiated from other forms of thyrotoxicosis by the presence of temperature elevation, significant tachycardia, heart failure, gastrointestinal disorders, diarrhea, nausea, vomiting, and sometimes jaundice. Neurologically, agitation and disorientation can occur. Thyroid storm most commonly occurs in Graves disease and has a higher frequency in younger women, but it also can be due to a toxic adenoma or multinodular goiter. This disorder can occur in long-standing, untreated hyperthyroidism but usually is precipitated by an underlying condition,

such as surgery, infection, trauma, parturition, acute iodine exposure, radioactive iodine (^{131}I) therapy, or ingestion of medications, including salicylates and pseudoephedrine. Signs include marked hyperthermia, marked sinus and supraventricular tachycardia, severe mental status changes (from psychosis to coma), features of heart failure (such as pulmonary edema), and gastrointestinal and hepatic abnormalities (such as nausea and vomiting, jaundice, hepatic failure).

Successful treatment of thyroid storm reduces thyroid hormone production and secretion by the thyroid gland, decreases peripheral conversion of T_4 to bioactive T_3, addresses associated adrenergic and thermoregulatory changes, treats all precipitating factors, and aggressively reverses any systemic decompensation. Definitive therapy for the causative thyroid disorder should be considered when the patient is stable. A combination of antithyroid drugs (propylthiouracil or methimazole), iodine solution, high-dose corticosteroids, β-blockers, and (rarely) lithium are used for treatment. Compared with atenolol and methimazole, propranolol and propylthiouracil have a slight added benefit of reducing T_4 to T_3 conversion, although the clinical benefits of this advantage are not clear because high-dose corticosteroid therapy is a potent inhibitor of this conversion. Intravenous corticosteroids also are routinely administered until it is clear that endogenous adrenal function is adequate to ensure that adrenal insufficiency is not present or has not been precipitated by levothyroxine therapy. Even with aggressive therapy and supportive measures, mortality rates are as high as 15% to 20%.

KEY POINT

- Therapeutic interventions for thyroid storm are a combination of antithyroid drugs, iodine solution, corticosteroids, β-blockers, and (rarely) lithium.

Myxedema Coma

A severe manifestation of hypothyroidism, often to the point of systemic decompensation, myxedema coma is potentially life threatening, especially without prompt diagnosis and treatment. Myxedema coma occurs more frequently in women than men and in older adult patients. Onset is usually insidious. This disorder usually is seen in patients with a history of hypothyroidism, thyroidectomy, or radioactive iodine therapy. Primary hypothyroidism accounts for greater than 95% of all occurrences, but episodes also have been reported in patients with central hypothyroidism. Precipitating factors are numerous and varied, including chronic poor (or no) adherence to daily thyroid hormone replacement therapy, stroke, heart failure, myocardial infarction, infection, metabolic disturbances, cold exposure (more common in the winter), trauma, gastrointestinal bleeding, acidosis, and hypoglycemia.

The two most common findings of myxedema coma are mental status changes and hypothermia. Mental status changes occur in greater than 90% of patients and can manifest as lethargy, stupor, coma, or sometimes psychosis ("myxedema madness"). Hypothermia (temperature less than 34.4 °C [94.0 °F]) occurs in 88% of patients; the lower the temperature, the worse the prognosis. Virtually all organ systems and biochemical pathways are slowed by myxedema coma. Hypoventilation leading to hypoxemia and hypercapnia are also common findings, as are (to a lesser degree) bradycardia, hypotension, hyponatremia, and hypoglycemia. The mortality rate of myxedema coma is high (20% or greater). Older patients generally do worse, as do patients with evidence of severe illness (high Acute Physiology and Chronic Health Evaluation [APACHE] Scale score, low Glasgow Coma Scale score).

If myxedema coma is suspected, the TSH and free T_4 levels should be checked promptly. The diagnosis is made clinically, but the TSH level is typically markedly elevated and the free T_4 level is usually low. A random cortisol level also should be obtained to assess for concomitant adrenal insufficiency.

No consensus exists about the most effective thyroid hormone replacement regimen for myxedema coma. Intravenous levothyroxine has traditionally been administered, with an initial bolus of 200 to 500 micrograms followed by daily doses between 50 and 100 micrograms until transition to oral administration is feasible. These relatively high doses of levothyroxine are recommended to replenish the depleted tissue stores of thyroid hormone. However, they may be associated with cardiac irregularities and should be used cautiously, with a more common starting dose of 100 to 200 micrograms used, especially in patients with known or suspected cardiac disorders. Supplementation with liothyronine (oral or intravenous) at doses between 5 and 10 micrograms twice daily has been proposed but is controversial, especially because a definitive benefit of this therapy has not been shown. If liothyronine is used, it should be administered cautiously in lower doses and in combination with levothyroxine. If high doses of levothyroxine are administered for myxedema coma (or any severe hypopituitarism), concurrent treatment with high-dose glucocorticoids (such as hydrocortisone) is recommended until adrenal insufficiency is excluded and appropriate adrenal function is confirmed. As with thyroid storm, all underlying precipitating conditions must be addressed. ▪

Disorders of the Adrenal Glands

Adrenal Insufficiency

Physiologic Regulation of Adrenal Function

The three layers of the adrenal cortex secrete three distinct classes of corticosteroids under separate regulatory mechanisms (**Figure 6**). Cortisol is the primary glucocorticoid and is produced by the zona fasciculata; dehydroepiandrosterone

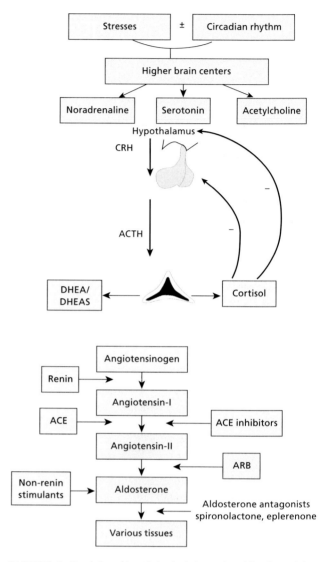

FIGURE 6. Regulation of hypothalamic-pituitary-adrenal function and the renin-angiotensin system. *Top,* hypothalamic secretion of CRH is mediated by several neurotransmitters in response to changes in stress levels and circadian rhythm. ACTH stimulates the zona fasciculata of the adrenal cortex to synthesize cortisol, which in turn feeds back centrally by negatively inhibiting CRH and ACTH secretion. ACTH also stimulates zona reticularis to synthesize the adrenal androgens DHEA and DHEAS, but these hormones do not participate in the feedback mechanism. *Bottom,* regulation of the renin-angiotensin system involves aldosterone being secreted by the outermost layer of the adrenal cortex (zona glomerulosa) as a result of angiotensin II stimulation. The site of action of commonly used drugs that interfere with the system is shown. ACTH = adrenocorticotropic hormone; ARB = angiotensin receptor blocker; CRH = corticotropin-releasing hormone; DHEA = dehydroepiandrosterone; DHEAS = DHEA sulfate.

(DHEA) and its sulfated form, DHEA sulfate (DHEAS), are the primary adrenal androgens and are produced by the zona reticularis. The production of these corticosteroids is tightly controlled by pituitary secretion of adrenocorticotropic hormone (ACTH), which, in turn, is regulated by hypothalamic secretion of corticotropin-releasing hormone (CRH).

Secreted cortisol provides negative feedback on pituitary synthesis of ACTH and hypothalamic synthesis of CRH. This integrated system keeps cortisol secretion tightly controlled. The adrenal androgens DHEA and DHEAS do not participate in negative feedback on pituitary and hypothalamic secretion. Aldosterone, the primary adrenal mineralocorticoid, is produced by the zona glomerulosa and is regulated by the renin-angiotensin system. Renin, an enzyme secreted by the kidney, regulates the conversion of angiotensinogen to angiotensin I. Angiotensin I is converted into angiotensin II, which stimulates aldosterone secretion.

Description, Causes, and Diagnosis of Adrenal Insufficiency

Adrenal insufficiency is a clinical and biochemical entity characterized by partial or complete loss of secretion of adrenocortical steroids (corticosteroids). Diseases involving the adrenal glands themselves, such as autoimmune adrenalitis, lead to primary adrenal insufficiency, in which secretion of all corticosteroids (aldosterone, cortisol, DHEA, and DHEAS) is impaired. In contrast, central adrenal insufficiency is caused either by ACTH secretion by a disease process that destroys the pituitary corticotrophs (secondary adrenal insufficiency) or by a hypothalamic disease that destroys the cells secreting CRH (tertiary adrenal insufficiency). Distinguishing between the secondary and tertiary forms of the disease can be difficult.

The most common cause of adrenal insufficiency in adults is the use of exogenous glucocorticoids administered chronically for their anti-inflammatory effect in the treatment of other medical conditions. Chronic glucocorticoid use leads to suppression of CRH and ACTH secretion centrally and, ultimately, to atrophy of the zona fasciculata and zona reticularis in the adrenal glands, with impairment of their ability to secrete physiologically regulated cortisol, particularly under stress conditions. Secretion of aldosterone from the zona glomerulosa is not affected because it is under control of the renin-angiotensin system. Common causes of primary and central adrenal insufficiency are shown in **Table 21**.

The clinical manifestations of adrenal insufficiency are often insidious, with fatigue and malaise being the dominant symptoms (**Table 22**); a high degree of clinical suspicion may be needed to pursue the diagnosis in the presence of subtle

TABLE 21. Causes of Adrenal Insufficiency	
Primary Adrenal Insufficiency	**Central Adrenal Insufficiency**
Autoimmune adrenalitis	Exogenous glucocorticoid therapy
Infection (tuberculosis, mycosis, bacterial, HIV-associated)	Hypothalamic/pituitary diseases or surgery
Metastatic cancer	Cranial irradiation
Adrenal hemorrhage (acute disease)	Chronic administration of drugs with glucocorticoid activity (such as megestrol)
Medications (such as etomidate, ketoconazole, mitotane, and metyrapone)	

TABLE 22. Characteristics of Adrenal Insufficiency					
Deficiency	**Type of Adrenal Insufficiency**	**Symptoms**	**Signs**	**Crucial Laboratory Findings**	**Additional Laboratory Findings**
Cortisol	Primary and central	Fatigue, nausea, anorexia, weight loss, abdominal pain, arthralgias, low-grade fever	Hyperpigmentation (in primary disease only),[a] slight decrease in blood pressure (unless cortisol deficiency is complete)	Low basal serum cortisol level (<5 µg/dL [138 nmol/L]) with suboptimal response (<18.0 µg/dL [497 nmol/L]) to cosyntropin; high plasma ACTH level (in primary disease only)	Hyponatremia; normal potassium level; azotemia; anemia; leukopenia, with high percentage of eosinophils and lymphocytes; hypoglycemia
Aldosterone	Primary	Salt craving, postural dizziness	Hypotension, dehydration	Low serum aldosterone level and high plasma renin activity	Hyponatremia; hyperkalemia
Adrenal androgen	Primary and central	Decreased libido	Decreased pubic/axillary hair (only in women)	Low serum DHEA and DHEAS levels	—

ACTH = adrenocorticotropic hormone; DHEA = dehydroepiandrosterone; DHEAS = dehydroepiandrosterone sulfate; µg = microgram(s).

[a]Results from increased secretion of ACTH and its precursor, pro-opiomelanocortin. An increase in the latter leads to increased secretion of one of its products, melanocortin-stimulating hormone, which causes the hyperpigmentation.

systemic symptoms. However, adrenal insufficiency also may present dramatically, as in addisonian crisis, in which hypotension and vascular collapse predominate. This presentation can be precipitated by severe stresses, such as concurrent illnesses or surgical procedures. Adrenal crisis is most common with primary adrenal insufficiency in which loss of both glucocorticoids and mineralocorticoids occurs and leads to vascular instability; it is less common in patients with secondary adrenal insufficiency (except under extreme circumstances) because the renin-aldosterone system is usually intact and profound hypotension and hypovolemia do not occur.

Adrenal insufficiency should be suspected in patients with suggestive signs or symptoms, especially those at increased risk for the disease (see Table 22). Adrenal insufficiency is diagnosed by demonstrating a low basal serum cortisol level that does not increase appropriately after stimulation with the ACTH analogue cosyntropin. Random serum cortisol levels vary, depending on the time of day, because of the pulsatile nature of ACTH secretion and the normal diurnal variation of cortisol levels (with the highest levels occurring in the morning and lowest in the evening). Random levels also fluctuate with the degree of physical stress present at the time of measurement. Assays for serum cortisol measurement determine the total (protein-bound and free) cortisol level. Because greater than 90% of the cortisol in the circulation is protein bound (to corticosteroid-binding globulin and albumin), an increase in binding proteins (as occurs during pregnancy or with estrogen therapy) results in increased serum cortisol levels without altering the physiologically important free hormone levels. Similarly, patients with hypoproteinemia have lower total serum cortisol levels despite having normal serum free cortisol levels. This becomes clinically relevant in critically ill patients who are hypoproteinemic (see later discussion).

When primary adrenal insufficiency is present, serum cortisol and aldosterone levels are low, but plasma renin activity and ACTH levels are increased. A minimal or no increase in the serum cortisol level from baseline in response to cosyntropin stimulation, preferably performed in the morning, confirms the diagnosis. Healthy persons increase their serum cortisol levels to greater than 18.0 micrograms/dL (497 nmol/L) after cosyntropin, 250 micrograms intravenously, is administered. Patients with central adrenal insufficiency have low plasma ACTH levels and normal aldosterone levels. Using a lower dose of cosyntropin (1 microgram instead of 250 micrograms) results in a modest increase in the plasma ACTH level that is similar to that achieved during insulin-induced hypoglycemia and, therefore, improves the diagnostic accuracy of the test in patients with central adrenal insufficiency. Serum levels of DHEA and DHEAS are characteristically low in both primary and central adrenal insufficiency.

If a diagnosis of central adrenal insufficiency is suspected on the basis of biochemical findings, imaging of the pituitary gland (preferably with MRI) should be performed to exclude other possible causes, such as a pituitary adenoma and any other sellar or perisellar mass.

Treatment of Adrenal Insufficiency

The goal of adrenal insufficiency treatment is to offer appropriate hormone replacement that closely mimics physiologic conditions, whenever possible, and to educate patients about their disease and the need to adjust their dosages with concurrent illnesses in order to avoid repeated hospital admissions and potential development of adrenal crises. Patients with primary adrenal insufficiency require glucocorticoid and mineralocorticoid replacement, but those with central disease need glucocorticoid replacement only. **H**

Although several agents are available for glucocorticoid replacement (**Table 23**), many endocrinologists prefer using hydrocortisone. The advantages of hydrocortisone are that it is identical to the natural product, has a shorter half-life, and

TABLE 23. Glucocorticoid Replacement Therapy in Adrenal Insufficiency			
Condition	**Hydrocortisone**	**Prednisone**	**Dexamethasone**
Physiologic daily dosing	15-25 mg/d orally in three divided doses at 8 AM (7.5-12.5 mg), 12 PM (5-7.5 mg) and 6 PM (2.5-5 mg)	3-5 mg/d orally in two divided doses at 8 AM (2-3 mg) and 3 PM (1-2 mg)	0.375 to 0.75 mg/d orally in one dose or preferably as two divided doses
Minor stress (such as cold symptoms)	30-50 mg/d orally in three doses for 2-3 days	8-15 mg/d orally in two divided doses for 2-3 days	1-2 mg/d orally in two divided doses for 2-3 days
Moderate stress (such as a minor/moderate surgical procedure)	45-75 mg/d orally or IV in three to four divided doses for 2-3 days	15-20 mg/d orally or IV (as prednisolone) in two or three divided doses for 2-3 days; hydrocortisone can be used instead	2-3 mg/d orally in two divided doses for 2-3 days; hydrocortisone can be used instead
Severe stress (such as a major surgical procedure, sepsis)	100-150 mg/d IV in four divided doses for 1 day; taper to physiologic dose over 3-5 days	Follow hydrocortisone regimen	Follow hydrocortisone regimen
Septic shock, severe inflammatory process	150-200 mg/d IV in four divided doses; taper as clinically tolerated	Follow hydrocortisone regimen	Follow hydrocortisone regimen

IV = intravenously.

can be tightly titrated more easily to mimic normal cortisol secretion (with higher morning doses and lower afternoon and evening doses). Longer-acting medications, such as prednisone and dexamethasone, are often given once daily and are more convenient for patients, although they are susceptible to metabolism that may vary from one patient to the next, which makes optimal dosing more difficult. Whichever preparation is used, daily replacement doses should be titrated to minimize symptoms of underreplacement and adjusted to avoid overreplacement, which leads to iatrogenic Cushing syndrome. Educating patients about their illness and the need for dose adjustments (increases) with intercurrent illnesses ("sick day rules"; see Table 23) is crucial, and they should be advised to wear medical alert identification indicating their diagnosis and dependence on glucocorticoid replacement therapy.

The standard drug for mineralocorticoid replacement therapy in patients with primary adrenal insufficiency is fludrocortisone, 0.05 to 0.1 mg/d. Patients with either primary or central adrenal insufficiency are deficient in adrenal androgen, but androgen replacement therapy is not essential for survival, and the data are not clear that replacement offers a clear benefit.

Adrenal Function During Critical Illness

In healthy persons, glucocorticoid secretion is increased during critical illness, generally in proportion to the degree of stress associated with the illness. In patients with adrenal insufficiency, therefore, glucocorticoid replacement doses should be increased during stressful events (see Table 23).

Testing for adrenal insufficiency during critical illness occasionally can be difficult. In patients with critical illness and hypoproteinemia, measured serum cortisol levels often appear lower than they would be otherwise. Despite this limitation, adrenal function testing in these patients continues to rely on serum total cortisol measurements because determination of the free fraction is not available for clinical use in a timely manner. True adrenal insufficiency is not common in critically ill patients but should always be considered in those at increased risk. Because no agreed upon diagnostic criteria or indications for treatment of adrenal insufficiency in critical illness exist, establishing the diagnosis is difficult, as is knowing when to treat. A random serum cortisol level greater than 15 micrograms/dL (414 nmol/L) in a critically ill patient and a level greater than 12 micrograms/dL (331 nmol/L) in a critically ill patient who has hypoproteinemia (serum albumin level <2.5 g/dL [25 g/L]) make the diagnosis of adrenal insufficiency unlikely.

A stimulation test, with cosyntropin for example, is not necessary in patients during critical illness because they are already stimulated by their stressful illnesses. Some critically ill patients, such as those with septic shock, might develop severe protracted hypotension that is unresponsive to standard therapy. Most, if not all, of these patients have elevated serum total and free cortisol levels and lack other biochemical features of adrenal insufficiency. The term "relative" adrenal insufficiency continues to be mistakenly used by some to refer to a presentation such as this. High-dose hydrocortisone therapy given to patients with septic shock has not been shown to influence mortality but may result in a faster reversal of shock. This therapy, which may be associated with adverse effects, is thus directed not at treating adrenal dysfunction, but rather at controlling the associated overwhelming inflammatory response.

KEY POINTS

- The most common cause of central adrenal insufficiency is adrenocorticotropic hormone suppression resulting from exogenous glucocorticoid replacement therapy.

- Primary adrenal insufficiency should be suspected when serum cortisol and aldosterone levels are low and plasma renin activity and adrenocorticotropic hormone levels are increased; a minimal or no increase in serum cortisol level after cosyntropin stimulation confirms the diagnosis.

- Glucocorticoid replacement therapy in primary or central adrenal insufficiency involves the use of a glucocorticoid (hydrocortisone, prednisone, or dexamethasone), whereas fludrocortisone is used for mineralocorticoid replacement therapy in primary adrenal insufficiency only.

Cushing Syndrome

Cushing syndrome comprises the constellation of signs and symptoms occurring after prolonged exposure to supraphysiologic doses of glucocorticoids. Although patients with various illnesses may have cushingoid features, some that should raise concern for true Cushing syndrome include proximal muscle weakness, multiple ecchymoses, prominent supraclavicular fat pads, violaceous striae, hypokalemia, unexplained osteoporosis, new-onset hypertension, and diabetes mellitus (**Figure 7**). Causes of Cushing syndrome are outlined in **Table 24**, with the most common being oral, intra-articular, intramuscular, inhalational, or topical administration of exogenous glucocorticoids for the treatment of various illnesses.

When the diagnosis of Cushing syndrome is suspected, it should be confirmed or satisfactorily ruled out because of its association with increased morbidity and mortality. The diagnosis is made by demonstrating unequivocal evidence of hypercortisolism, usually through the combination of initial tests and confirmatory studies, if needed (**Figure 8**). The three approaches most often used to evaluate for hypercortisolism are (1) assessment of urine free cortisol excretion in a 24-hour period, (2) documentation of loss of feedback inhibition of cortisol on the hypothalamic-pituitary axis with dexamethasone suppression testing, and (3) documentation of the loss of normal diurnal variation in cortisol secretion with late-night salivary cortisol measurement.

In evaluating patients with clinical features suggestive of Cushing syndrome, starting with any of the previously

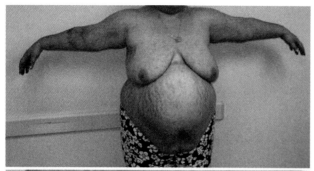

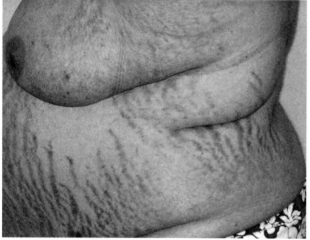

FIGURE 7. Classic features of Cushing syndrome in a patient with an adrenocorticotropic hormone–secreting pituitary adenoma. Central obesity and striae are evident (*top*). A close-up view of the striae (*bottom*) reveals their wide, violaceous nature.

mentioned approaches is appropriate. In general, however, two of the three tests are needed to confirm the diagnosis. Measurement of 24-hour urine free cortisol excretion is the gold standard test for diagnosing Cushing syndrome. A threefold to fourfold increase over normal values is diagnostic

of Cushing syndrome; if this increase is present, no additional testing is required. For less dramatic increases, another diagnostic approach for hypercortisolism is required, such as the overnight dexamethasone suppression test or measurement of a late-night salivary cortisol level. The overnight dexamethasone suppression test is performed by obtaining a morning (8 or 9 AM) serum cortisol level after 1 mg of dexamethasone has been administered at 11 PM the night before; a normal response is generally considered to be a level less than 2 micrograms/dL (55 nmol/L) in healthy persons. Serum cortisol levels greater than 5 micrograms/dL (138 nmol/L) after dexamethasone administration the previous night are highly suggestive of Cushing syndrome. However, values of 2 to 5 micrograms/dL (55-138 nmol/L) require additional testing. In interpreting test results, one should consider factors that may increase corticosteroid-binding globulin levels and thus falsely increase the serum cortisol level (such as estrogen therapy or pregnancy). Caution also should be exercised in interpreting data from this test in patients taking medications that induce the cytochrome P-450 enzyme system, such as phenytoin or phenobarbital, and thereby increase the metabolism of dexamethasone.

In healthy persons, cortisol secretion exhibits a diurnal rhythm whereby serum cortisol levels reach a nadir late at night and peak in the early morning. Because loss of this diurnal rhythm is a central feature of Cushing syndrome, measurement of the nighttime cortisol level can be used as a diagnostic test. Salivary cortisol is in equilibrium with the free cortisol in the circulation. Thus, the finding of an elevated midnight salivary cortisol level on at least two separate occasions should raise concern about the possibility of Cushing syndrome, if the saliva sample was taken on a quiet, restful night.

Confirmatory testing also is needed when initial studies are suggestive of but equivocal for hypercortisolism. If not performed as an initial study, the 24-hour urine free cortisol

TABLE 24. Causes of Cushing Syndrome (Hypercortisolism)	
Type of Cushing Syndrome[a]	**Cause**
Endogenous	
ACTH dependent (75%-80% of patients)	ACTH-secreting pituitary adenoma (60%-65% of patients)
	Ectopic ACTH secretion by tumors, such as carcinoid tumors (10%-15% of patients)
	CRH-secreting tumors (rare)
ACTH independent (20%-25% of patients)	Adrenal adenoma (10%-15% of patients)
	Adrenal carcinoma (5%-10% of patients)
Exogenous	Prolonged administration of supraphysiologic doses of glucocorticoid therapy (such as prednisone, dexamethasone, or hydrocortisone)
	Administration of drugs with glucocorticoid activity (progestational agents, such as megestrol)

ACTH = adrenocorticotropic hormone; CRH = corticotropin-releasing hormone.

[a]Patients with ACTH-dependent Cushing syndrome have hypercortisolism associated with normal or elevated plasma ACTH levels; those with ACTH-independent Cushing syndrome have hypercortisolism associated with low or undetectable plasma ACTH levels. Patients with exogenous Cushing syndrome have low or undetectable plasma ACTH levels, and their serum cortisol levels often are low unless the glucocorticoid used cross reacts in the cortisol assay.

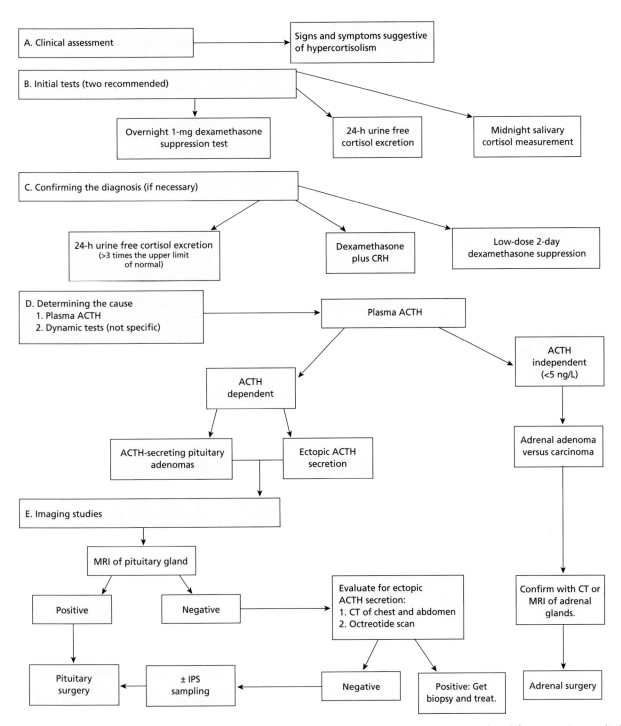

FIGURE 8. Evaluation of patients with suspected Cushing syndrome. After the diagnosis is suspected, the evaluation goes through five consecutive steps (A-E). In patients with ACTH-dependent Cushing syndrome who have normal MRIs of the pituitary gland, ectopic ACTH secretion is possible. Inferior petrosal sinus catheterization can confirm the central source of ACTH secretion in those with negative pituitary MRIs. ACTH = adrenocorticotropic hormone; CRH = corticotropin-releasing hormone; IPS = inferior petrosal sinus catheterization.

test remains the gold standard confirmatory study. The standard (as opposed to the overnight) low-dose dexamethasone suppression test also may also be used as a confirmatory study. Dexamethasone (0.5 mg) administered every 6 hours for 48 hours typically causes suppression of serum cortisol levels to

less than 2 micrograms/dL (55 nmol/L) and of 24-hour urine free cortisol excretion to less than 20 micrograms/24 h (55 nmol/24 h), with higher levels consistent with Cushing syndrome. Using a CRH plus desmopressin stimulation test may be helpful in selected patients with multiple equivocal studies for hypercortisolism; however, doing so is expensive and not a routine test for diagnosing Cushing syndrome.

After hypercortisolism is firmly established, further evaluation should explore the cause, whether adrenal, pituitary, or ectopic. For example, measurement of the plasma ACTH level can differentiate ACTH-dependent hypercortisolism (ACTH level is inappropriately normal or elevated, as with a pituitary adenoma) from ACTH-independent hypercortisolism (ACTH level is low [<5 pg/mL {1.1 pmol/L}] or undetectable, as with adrenal neoplasms). The ACTH level should be measured simultaneously with the cortisol level. Other approaches used to determine the cause of hypercortisolism include dynamic testing with higher doses of dexamethasone (for example, 8 mg/d). The value of the high-dose dexamethasone suppression test is limited, however, because of significant overlap in responses observed among patients with different forms of Cushing syndrome.

Imaging studies should be obtained only after biochemical documentation of hypercortisolism is established. These studies offer no diagnostic information relevant to Cushing syndrome but instead aid in localizing any associated tumor. An MRI of the sella turcica should be obtained in patients with ACTH-dependent hypercortisolism. However, MRIs are normal in 40% to 50% of patients with documented ACTH-secreting pituitary adenomas because of the small size of these adenomas. This makes it difficult to differentiate patients with ACTH-secreting adenomas (75%) from others with ectopic ACTH secretion on the basis of an MRI. Dynamic contrast-enhanced pituitary MRI imaging can improve detection in some cases. Additionally, a significant overlap exists between these two entities in terms of their biochemical features and responsiveness to dexamethasone suppression or other dynamic testing (such as with CRH). An approach used to evaluate for a central source of ACTH secretion in patients with true-negative pituitary MRIs is bilateral inferior petrosal sinus catheterization with central and peripheral measurements of plasma ACTH levels simultaneously from both sides before and after CRH stimulation. This test is technically difficult and should only be performed at experienced centers. Instead of performing the inferior petrosal sinus catheterization, some centers with extensive experience in managing Cushing syndrome opt to proceed to surgical exploration of the pituitary gland in patients with normal MRIs who also have normal CT scans of the abdomen and chest.

In patients with hypercortisolism associated with suppressed plasma ACTH levels, a dedicated CT scan of the adrenal glands often shows a tumor (a smaller, homogeneous, more lipid-rich adenoma versus a larger, more irregular, vascular carcinoma). Although differentiating between a cortisol-secreting adrenal adenoma and a carcinoma is sometimes possible using clinical, biochemical, and imaging features, histologic confirmation of capsular invasion is necessary for larger lesions. The evaluation and management of suspected Cushing syndrome should be performed by an experienced endocrinologist.

The treatment of exogenous Cushing syndrome is to discontinue exogenous glucocorticoid replacement therapy whenever possible by using alternative therapy to treat the condition in question. Alternatively, if glucocorticoid replacement is necessary, then the smallest dose possible should be administered either once daily or every other day in the morning (9-10 AM). The treatment of endogenous Cushing syndrome depends on its cause, with ACTH-secreting pituitary adenomas (Cushing disease) best treated with pituitary adenomectomy. Immediately after this surgery, patients develop ACTH deficiency requiring daily glucocorticoid replacement therapy until endogenous ACTH production resumes, which can take as long as a year. Patients with residual disease after pituitary surgery might benefit from stereotactic radiosurgery and adjuvant medical therapy with drugs that inhibit glucocorticoid synthesis (such as ketoconazole or metyrapone) or are cytotoxic to adrenocortical cells (such as mitotane).

The preferred treatment of Cushing syndrome caused by cortisol-producing adrenal adenomas and carcinomas is surgical resection of the tumor, preferably through a laparoscopic approach. Postoperatively, most patients have resultant adrenal insufficiency lasting as long as 12 months that requires daily glucocorticoid replacement for several months. Although cortisol-secreting adenomas are generally curable with surgical resection, adrenal carcinomas might not be totally resectable and can recur. Further treatment of patients with adrenal carcinomas is discussed later. The treatment of Cushing syndrome caused by ectopic ACTH secretion should be directed at the cause, which often is difficult because many of the tumors secreting ACTH ectopically are malignant. Patients with these tumors typically have signs and symptoms of malignancy (weight loss, cachexia, and temporal wasting) and biochemical features of mineralocorticoid activity. When cortisol is secreted in large quantities, the mineralocorticoid activity becomes much more apparent and is associated with classic features, such as hypertension, hypokalemia, and excessive urine potassium loss. Most patients will require medical therapy to control their hypercortisolism and may require bilateral adrenalectomy if medical therapy is ineffective.

KEY POINTS

- The diagnosis of Cushing syndrome involves demonstration of persistent hypercortisolism associated with poor suppressibility with dexamethasone or loss of the normal diurnal variation in cortisol secretion.

- For Cushing disease caused by an adrenocorticotropic hormone–secreting pituitary adenoma, adenomectomy is the treatment of choice.

- Patients with Cushing syndrome develop transient adrenal insufficiency (lasting up to 12 months) immediately after surgical removal of any causative tumor (adrenocorticotropic hormone–secreting tumor or cortisol-producing adrenal tumor).

Adrenal Incidentaloma

The increasing use of imaging studies for various medical indications has revealed otherwise unrecognized adrenal masses in less than 1% of the population younger than 30 years and up to 7% of the population older than 70 years (**Figure 9**). Adrenal masses in younger patients are more likely to be functional and/or malignant than those found in older patients. Evaluating adrenal masses should address their potential for malignancy (whether primary or metastatic) and their functional status. Functional tumors originate from any of the three layers of the adrenal cortex or from the adrenal medulla and secrete products of the respective portion of the glands.

Initial assessment should include a thorough history and physical examination to detect any indications of malignant disease and any clinical evidence of hormone hypersecretion (**Figure 10**). Most patients with metastatic cancer of the adrenal glands have clinical evidence of disease elsewhere. Imaging characteristics and the phenotype of the mass (size, CT attenuation, and contrast washout) also provide important information relative to the risk of malignancy. The risk of malignancy (primary or metastatic) is only 2% for masses less than 4 cm in size but increases to 25% for those 6 cm or larger. Benign adrenal adenomas generally have a low CT attenuation (<10 Hounsfield units) and exhibit rapid contrast medium washout (>50% at 10 minutes). In contrast, a high CT attenuation (>20 Hounsfield units) and a delay in contrast medium washout (<50%) are typical of pheochromocytomas

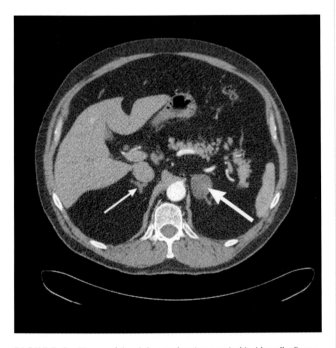

FIGURE 9. CT scan of the abdomen showing a typical incidentally discovered left adrenal mass (*thick white arrow*) in an asymptomatic man. The normal right adrenal gland is shown as an inverted Y shape (*thin white arrow*). The mass is lipid-rich and has a low attenuation factor (<10 Hounsfield units).

or malignant lesions. Primary adrenocortical carcinomas are typically large, have irregular borders, and may include areas of necrosis. Although imaging characteristics and phenotype do not predict function, they reliably predict biologic behavior. Similarly, T2-weighted MRIs are usually isointense to the liver in benign adenomas and hyperintense in adrenocortical carcinoma, pheochromocytoma, and metastatic disease. For the up to 15% of adrenal incidentalomas that are bilateral, the differential diagnosis includes bilateral adrenal hyperplasia and metastatic cancer.

Nearly 10% of adrenal incidentalomas are functional, although most have no overt clinical manifestations. Therefore, testing is usually necessary to identify functional tumors secreting catecholamines, cortisol, or aldosterone. Measurements of urine excretion or plasma levels of catecholamine metabolites (fractionated metanephrines) are good initial tests for pheochromocytoma, and further testing is reasonable when results are abnormal (see later discussion of pheochromocytoma). Notably, some patients with incidental adrenal tumors could have early-stage pheochromocytoma and thus may have negative results on biochemical testing. These patients will have imaging characteristics (high CT attenuation, delay in contrast medium washout) that raise concern for pheochromocytoma. Measurements of plasma ACTH and serum cortisol levels before and after the overnight administration of dexamethasone (1 mg) are appropriate initial tests to evaluate for possible cortisol production. Plasma ACTH levels are low in patients with cortisol-secreting adrenal tumors. Urine free cortisol measurement may also be used, either as an initial study or to confirm abnormal or equivocal results of a dexamethasone suppression test. Although the optimal upper range for the serum cortisol level after dexamethasone administration is debatable in this clinical setting, most authorities consider a value of 5 micrograms/dL (138 nmol/L) or greater to be clearly abnormal. Evaluation for aldosterone-secreting adenomas should be carried out in patients with hypertension or those with spontaneous hypokalemia by determining the plasma aldosterone level and plasma renin activity. Excess adrenal androgen production can be seen in patients with adrenal cancer and should be evaluated with determination of plasma DHEA and DHEAS levels, if suggested by the clinical presentation.

Management of an adrenal incidentaloma depends on its size, imaging characteristics (phenotype), and functional abilities (see Figure 10). Almost all adrenal tumors that are overtly functional, are larger than 6 cm in size, or have unfavorable imaging characteristics should be considered for surgical removal. The one exception is aldosterone-secreting adenomas, which may not need to be surgically removed because hyperaldosteronism often can be treated medically. Pre- and postoperative management of an adrenal incidentaloma in patients treated surgically is directed at the functionality of the tumor (see sections on Cushing Syndrome, Pheochromocytoma, and Primary Hyperaldosteronism).

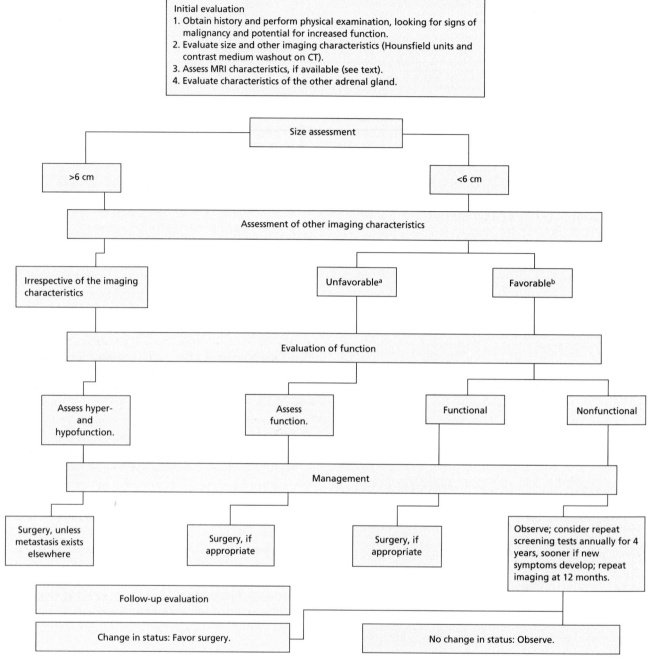

FIGURE 10. Flow sheet showing the evaluation and management of an incidentally discovered adrenal mass. Masses larger than 6 cm are more likely to be malignant.

[a]Unfavorable imaging characteristics: high CT attenuation (>20 Hounsfield units), irregular border, delayed contrast (<50%) washout.

[b]Favorable imaging characteristics: low CT attenuation (<10 Hounsfield units), smooth contour, rapid (≥50%) contrast washout.

Consensus exists that patients who have nonfunctional tumors smaller than 4 cm with favorable imaging characteristics should be followed, although agreement is lacking about how often tests (hormonal and imaging) should be repeated, if at all. CT scans of the adrenal glands (with and without contrast) provide anatomic details that are considered by many to be superior to those obtained by MRI. However, MRI's lack of radiation exposure offers some advantage. Most authorities suggest CT for follow-up studies unless concerns about exposure to radiation or contrast material exist. Although some experts recommend that hormonal evaluation be performed annually for 3 to 4 years, others advocate repeat biochemical testing only when signs or symptoms of hormonal excess are discovered. A reasonable compromise is to reevaluate patients for Cushing syndrome and pheochromocytoma at 1 year or at any time a change in clinical manifestations or imaging characteristics occurs. Regarding imaging, a repeat CT scan should be obtained at least once 6 to 12 months after the initial finding, with some advocating repeat imaging at 6, 12, and 24 months after the tumor is detected.

Testing should be repeated if significant changes in size or imaging characteristics are noted. Controversy surrounds the management of nonfunctional adrenal incidentalomas that are 4 to 6 cm in size with favorable imaging characteristics. Whereas some advocate surgical removal, others favor a management scheme similar to that for incidentalomas less than 4 cm in size.

KEY POINTS

- Assessment of incidentally discovered adrenal masses should address whether the mass is benign or malignant, primary or metastatic, and functional or nonfunctional.

- All adrenal tumors that are functional, are larger than 6 cm in size, or have unfavorable imaging characteristics should be considered for surgical removal.

Pheochromocytoma

Pheochromocytomas are rare tumors (0.1%-0.6% of persons with hypertension) composed of chromaffin cells that can secrete biogenic amines (norepinephrine, epinephrine, and dopamine) and their metabolites. Most pheochromocytomas secrete predominantly norepinephrine, which results in sustained or episodic hypertension. Less commonly, these tumors might secrete predominantly epinephrine, which can cause hypotension. Nearly 90% of pheochromocytomas arise in the adrenal medulla, and 10% are extra-adrenal, located primarily along the sympathetic chain (paragangliomas). Approximately 25% of pheochromocytomas are familial and associated with genetic disorders (such as multiple endocrine neoplasia type 2, neurofibromatosis 1, and von Hippel-Lindau disease), 10% are asymptomatic, and 10% are malignant. The familial forms of pheochromocytoma tend to occur in multiple sites, are more likely to recur after surgical resection, and are associated with other benign or malignant tumors. Genetic testing should thus be considered in patients with a family history of this tumor, in those with bilateral or extra-adrenal disease, and in younger persons with other tumors.

The clinical manifestations of pheochromocytoma vary, with hypertension (episodic or sustained) observed in greater than 90% of patients. Other signs and symptoms include episodes of diaphoresis, pallor, palpitations, headache, hyperglycemia, weight loss, arrhythmias (atrial and ventricular fibrillation), and (rarely) catecholamine-induced cardiomyopathy. The classic triad of severe headache, diaphoresis, and palpitations is highly suggestive of pheochromocytoma. Because some (10%) pheochromocytomas are diagnosed in asymptomatic patients evaluated for adrenal incidentalomas, the diagnosis should be suspected in any patient at risk (**Table 25**). Patients suspected of having a pheochromocytoma should not receive β-blockers until treated with adequate α-adrenergic blockade to avoid the potential sequela of worsened hypertension due to unopposed α stimulation.

The diagnosis of pheochromocytoma relies on the documentation of excessive secretion of catecholamines or their metabolites as measured in the plasma or in a 24-hour urine collection. Because significant catecholamine metabolism is intratumoral, measurement of catecholamine metabolites (metanephrines) is the most appropriate approach in defining catecholamine secretion. A positive test often is defined as an elevation in the plasma value or 24-hour urine excretion that is greater than twice the upper limit of normal. The upper limits of normal may vary between laboratories, with some laboratories using a hypertensive population to establish their normal value; in such assays, the distinction between patients with and without pheochromocytomas becomes easier.

In approaching the diagnosis of pheochromocytoma, one can start with measurement of either the plasma level or urine metanephrine excretion as long as the sensitivity, specificity, and limitations of the approach used are considered. There are many instances of discordance between urine and plasma measurements of catecholamine metabolites, in which case the urine levels are more specific and thus more reliable. Because the management of pheochromocytoma may involve imaging studies, it is essential first to evaluate for and then confirm the diagnosis biochemically. When clinical suspicion of pheochromocytoma is high, measurement of the plasma free metanephrine level is preferred because of the higher sensitivity of this test. When that test is positive, the 24-hour urine catecholamine metabolite excretion should be determined to confirm the diagnosis. When clinical suspicion is low, measurement of the 24-hour urine excretion of catecholamines and metanephrines is preferred because of the lower false-positive rate (higher specificity); further testing would not be necessary unless convincing clinical, familial, or genetic predisposing factors for the disease exist.

TABLE 25. Patient History Prompting Screening for Pheochromocytoma

Suggestive (hyperadrenergic) cyclic spells of hypertension, diaphoresis, palpitations, or headache
Familial predisposing syndrome (neurofibromatosis 1, MEN2, succinate dehydrogenase B mutation)
Previous vasopressor response to anesthesia or angiography
Adrenal incidentaloma
Hypertension at a young age (<20 years)
Drug-resistant hypertension
Unexplained cardiomyopathy and atrial fibrillation

MEN2 = multiple endocrine neoplasia type 2.

The preference is that patients not receive any medications during testing, but this often is not practical. Tricyclic antidepressants and other drugs with similar pharmacologic features (such as cyclobenzaprine) are among the drugs that interfere with measurement of catecholamines and metanephrines. Other interfering drugs include antihypertensive agents (such as reserpine), medications with adrenergic receptor agonist activity (such as decongestants), psychoactive drugs with dopamine or norepinephrine reuptake inhibition properties (such as buspirone), but not other selective serotonin reuptake inhibitors. In addition, acetaminophen intake can interfere with the measurement of plasma metanephrine levels in some assays. The use of medications that interfere with catecholamine and metanephrine assays should be discontinued at least 2 weeks before testing. Catecholamine and metanephrine levels that are elevated but are less than twice the upper limit of normal can occur in patients in a hyperadrenergic state, in those with anxiety disorders or high levels of psychological stress, and sometimes in those with essential hypertension. Additionally, catecholamine secretion is appropriately increased in stressful conditions, such as critical illness, and thus testing patients for pheochromocytoma in these circumstances may lead to misleading conclusions. In situations in which equivocal results are obtained, repeat testing and other biochemical studies for pheochromocytoma, such as the clonidine suppression test, may be indicated.

After the diagnosis of pheochromocytoma is biochemically confirmed, imaging studies should be performed to determine the tumor's location. Either adrenal CT with and without contrast or MRI without contrast is a reasonable option. The anatomic details are better appreciated on a CT scan, although exposure to radiation is avoided with MRI. Metaiodobenzylguanidine (MIBG), a compound with a structure similar to that of norepinephrine, is tagged with radioactive iodine (^{123}I or ^{131}I) and used for scintigraphic localization of pheochromocytomas when results of CT scans and MRIs are negative. This tagged compound also is used to localize metastasis from malignant pheochromocytoma.

Laparoscopic adrenalectomy is the most effective treatment for most pheochromocytomas. Preoperative medical therapy is instituted after the biochemical diagnosis is confirmed and before surgical resection. However, no controlled studies have shown which therapy is best. Previously, most patients were treated for 1 to 2 weeks before surgery with a competitive α-adrenergic blocking agent (phenoxybenzamine) at an initial dose of 10 mg once or twice daily, with upward titration based on blood pressure measurements every 2 to 3 days to a maximum of 80 mg/d. Because of its long-lasting effects, phenoxybenzamine contributed to the hypotension commonly observed during the first day after tumor removal. Some centers use short-acting specific α-antagonists, such as prazosin (2-5 mg, three times daily), doxazosin (2-8 mg/d), or terazosin (2-5 mg/d). In patients with tachycardia, β-blockers can be added after α-blockade

is achieved, especially if blood pressure control is not achieved. The goal is to achieve a blood pressure of approximately 120/80 mm Hg. If blood pressure control is still not achieved with α- and β-blockade, other drugs, such as calcium channel blockers (amlodipine or verapamil), can be added as needed. Labetalol, a combined α- and β-blocking agent, also can be used, especially in patients with tachyarrhythmias. Patients with pheochromocytomas who are normotensive also should be treated with α-blockers because these patients often become hypertensive during surgical resection. Nitroprusside is used to control intraoperative hypertension. The anesthesiologist should be aware of the potential for changes in blood pressure during tumor manipulation and the need for volume expansion during and after tumor resection.

The long-term prognosis for patients after resection of a solitary sporadic pheochromocytoma is excellent, although some may have persistent hypertension, and as many as 17% have a recurrence. All patients should have annual follow-up evaluation for at least 10 years with repeat biochemical testing, and those with extra-adrenal lesions or familial disease should be followed clinically with blood pressure monitoring indefinitely and imaging evaluation whenever any change in status occurs. Treatment of malignant pheochromocytoma includes surgical debulking, control of catecholamine-related symptoms with α-blockers and catecholamine synthesis inhibitors, external irradiation, or targeted radiotherapy using ^{131}I-MIBG. Systemic cytotoxic chemotherapy has also been used, although response rates are usually low and short-lived.

KEY POINTS

- The diagnosis of pheochromocytoma relies on the documentation of excessive secretion of catecholamines or their metabolites.

- β-Blockers should not be given to patients suspected of having a pheochromocytoma unless these patients are already being treated with α-adrenergic blocking agents.

- Treatment of pheochromocytoma involves laparoscopic adrenalectomy after appropriate preparation with α-adrenergic blocking agents and control of blood pressure and pulse rate.

Primary Hyperaldosteronism

Primary hyperaldosteronism is a condition characterized by excessive autonomous aldosterone production by the adrenal zona glomerulosa, independent of its physiologic regulator, the renin-angiotensin system. Primary hyperaldosteronism is associated with several pathologic entities, such as solitary aldosterone-producing adrenal adenoma (40%-50%); bilateral adrenal hyperplasia, also known as idiopathic primary hyperaldosteronism (50%-60%); and, more rarely, unilateral hyperplasia or adrenal carcinoma. The main manifestations of primary hyperaldosteronism are hypertension, hypokalemia (although up to 50% of patients can be eukalemic), and metabolic alkalosis. The prevalence of primary hyperaldosteronism in patients with hypertension is variable (1%-5%). Therefore, the diagnosis should be considered in any patient with hypertension, especially hypertension resistant to treatment, associated with spontaneous (unprovoked) hypokalemia (or significant hypokalemia in response to low-dose thiazide treatment), or coexistent with an adrenal incidentaloma.

Evaluation for primary hyperaldosteronism involves the simultaneous measurements of the midmorning ambulatory plasma aldosterone level (typically increased) and plasma renin activity (typically suppressed). In most patients with hyperaldosteronism, the plasma aldosterone level exceeds 15 ng/dL (414 pmol/L), but the plasma renin activity is very low or undetectable. A ratio of plasma aldosterone (measured in ng/dL) to plasma renin activity (measured in ng/mL/h) of greater than 30 has a 90% sensitivity and specificity for the diagnosis of primary hyperaldosteronism; a ratio of 20 to 30 is suggestive of the diagnosis, especially when the plasma aldosterone level is greater than 15 ng/dL (414 pmol/L). Determining the ratio of plasma aldosterone to plasma renin activity is particularly helpful in patients receiving ACE inhibitors, angiotensin receptor blockers, or direct renin inhibitors in whom plasma renin activity is expected to be high and the aldosterone level is usually low (see Figure 6, bottom panel). Testing can be done on random blood samples, even in patients taking antihypertensive medications with the exception of spironolactone and eplerenone, both aldosterone receptor antagonists.

The biochemical diagnosis is confirmed by demonstrating persistent elevation (poor suppressibility) of the plasma aldosterone level in response to a high-sodium load. Sodium chloride can be given orally (2 g three times daily for 3 days) or intravenously (normal saline, 500 mL per hour for 4 hours). During salt loading, plasma aldosterone levels are suppressed to less than 5 ng/dL (138 pmol/L) in healthy persons but remain elevated (often >10 ng/dL [276 pmol/L]) in patients with primary hyperaldosteronism. The decision to pursue salt loading should be made only after at least two plasma aldosterone to plasma renin activity ratios are elevated in the presence of an elevated aldosterone level. It is necessary to ensure that patients are potassium replete before beginning a salt-loading test because increased sodium intake will exacerbate hypokalemia.

Measurement of 24-hour urine aldosterone excretion (typically, <12 micrograms/24 h [33.2 nmol/24h]) during the third day of the salt loading also can confirm the diagnosis, provided adequate salt loading is achieved (as demonstrated by a high urine sodium excretion (greater than 200 meq/24 h [200 mmol/24 h]). After adequate salt loading, a plasma aldosterone level greater than 10 ng/dL (276 pmol/L) is diagnostic of hyperaldosteronism.

After the biochemical diagnosis is confirmed, further studies, such as CT of the adrenal glands, are performed to define the pathologic cause of primary hyperaldosteronism. A solitary adrenal adenoma, which is often 2 cm or less in diameter, is easy to recognize on a CT scan. Bilateral adrenal hyperplasia is characterized by diffuse or focal enlargement of both adrenal glands and is associated with unilateral or bilateral nodules; making this distinction is crucial because of its impact on therapy. However, imaging studies are not always accurate in defining the pathologic entity causing hyperaldosteronism, especially given the high prevalence of adrenal incidentalomas in persons older than 40 years. One definitive approach is to catheterize both adrenal veins and measure plasma aldosterone levels from both sides to determine if aldosterone production is unilateral or bilateral. Because this procedure is technically difficult and can be associated with adverse effects, such as adrenal vein dissection and hemorrhage, it should be used selectively in patients in whom surgery is being considered and performed only at centers with expertise in the procedure.

Referral to an endocrinologist is recommended whenever the biochemical data are not typical because some rare conditions may also present with hypertension, hypokalemia, and metabolic alkalosis but may not be associated with an elevated aldosterone level.

The goals of therapy for hyperaldosteronism are normalization (or at least improvement) of blood pressure, resolution of hypokalemia, and attainment of normal aldosterone levels and effects. The last goal is especially important because aldosterone can have adverse effects over and above its influence on blood pressure or the potassium level. Although laparoscopic surgical resection of a solitary aldosterone-secreting adrenal adenoma is usually recommended, especially in young patients, medical therapy also can be an effective alternative approach when it includes an aldosterone receptor blocker (either spironolactone or eplerenone). After removal of the aldosterone-producing adrenal adenoma, potassium levels become normal in greater than 90% of patients; blood pressure normalizes in two thirds of patients, and its control improves in the remaining third.

The treatment of choice for primary hyperaldosteronism caused by bilateral adrenal hyperplasia is medical therapy with either spironolactone or eplerenone. Spironolactone (50-300 mg/d) is often effective in controlling hypertension and hypokalemia. Besides being an aldosterone antagonist that blocks the aldosterone receptor, spironolactone also blocks the androgen receptor and can cause gynecomastia, mastodynia, impotence, and diminished libido in men and menstrual irregularities in women. Eplerenone (25-100 mg/d) is a more selective aldosterone receptor blocker and has fewer of these adverse events. Some medically treated patients with adrenal adenomas and bilateral adrenal hyperplasia require treatment with amiloride to attain eukalemia; a low-dose thiazide diuretic (12.5-25 mg/d) also can be added to reverse hypervolemia. Patients should be followed indefinitely with monitoring of blood pressure, kidney function, and potassium levels. In premenopausal women, aldosterone antagonists are known to be teratogenic in the male fetus and thus must be avoided unless prevention of pregnancy is secured.

KEY POINTS

- Testing for primary hyperaldosteronism includes measuring simultaneous midmorning ambulatory plasma aldosterone levels and plasma renin activity; a ratio of the former over the latter greater than 20 is suggestive of the diagnosis.

- The biochemical diagnosis of primary hyperaldosteronism is confirmed by demonstrating persistent elevation (poor suppressibility) of the plasma aldosterone level in response to a high salt load.

- Primary hyperaldosteronism caused by a solitary aldosterone-secreting adenoma is best treated by adrenalectomy, whereas disease caused by bilateral adrenal hyperplasia is managed medically by using a nonselective (spironolactone) or a more selective (eplerenone) aldosterone blocking agent.

Adrenocortical Cancer

Adrenocortical cancer is a rare malignancy. As many as 60% of patients with this cancer have symptoms of hormone (cortisol) excess, whereas others have mechanical symptoms related to rapid tumor growth (abdominal fullness, nausea, and back pain) and a few have an incidentally discovered adrenal mass. Given the variable clinical presentation of this entity, diagnosis often requires integration of the clinical, biochemical, and imaging data discussed in previous sections. Most adrenocortical cancers produce multiple corticosteroids, including biologically inactive precursors. The imaging characteristics of adrenocortical cancer include a large mass with irregular borders or shape, occasional calcification, high attenuation (high Hounsfield units) on CT, and delay in contrast medium washout.

The treatment of adrenocortical cancer depends on the extent of disease at presentation. Surgical removal after appropriate biochemical assessment remains the best option, especially in patients with early disease. Even after apparent complete resection, adjuvant therapy with mitotane, a known adrenal cytotoxic drug, may be beneficial. Treatment with mitotane is recommended for patients with persistent disease and others with known metastases and is associated with objective remissions in approximately 25% of patients. The main limiting factors of mitotane use are the associated adverse events, including nausea, vomiting, lethargy, and other neurologic symptoms. Experience with other cytotoxic chemotherapy is limited, but this treatment usually has been ineffective. A poorer prognosis is associated with advanced stages of the disease, the presence of metastasis at diagnosis, an older age, and cortisol hypersecretion by the tumor. In patients without clinically evident disease after initial surgery, the median survival rate is 60% at 5 years. This rate is 20% to 25% for those with metastatic disease. Newer studies suggest that mitotane use may improve future survival, even after apparent complete tumor resection.

KEY POINTS

- The manifestations of adrenocortical cancer include hormone (cortisol) excess and mechanical symptoms due to a rapidly growing mass.

- Surgical resection is the best therapeutic option for adrenocortical cancer followed by use of the cytotoxic drug mitotane.

Reproductive Disorders

Basic Concepts and Common Features

The hypothalamic-pituitary-gonadal axes of men and women share many features. Gonadotropin-releasing hormone (GnRH) is released in a pulsatile manner from the hypothalamus. When released, GnRH stimulates the gonadotropic cells in the anterior pituitary gland to secrete follicle-stimulating hormone (FSH) and luteinizing hormone (LH). FSH and LH stimulate spermatogenesis and testosterone production in the testes and follicular development and estrogen production in the ovaries. Testosterone and estrogen decrease the release of GnRH, FSH, and LH through negative feedback inhibition on the hypothalamus and pituitary gland. Feedback inhibition of FSH is also controlled by inhibin B, a protein product of ovarian granulosa cells and testicular Sertoli cells.

Physiology of Male Reproduction

The testes are composed of seminiferous tubules, Leydig cells, and Sertoli cells. Leydig cells are responsible for testosterone production by LH stimulation, and Sertoli cells are responsible for spermatogenesis by FSH stimulation and testosterone. Testosterone is secreted in a diurnal pattern, with the highest levels achieved in the morning, and can be metabolized to dihydrotestosterone in some tissues, such as the prostate, and to estrogen in other tissues, such as fat. The male reproductive axis is shown in **Figure 11**.

Only 2% of testosterone is free testosterone, 44% is bound to sex hormone–binding globulin (SHBG), and the remaining 54% is bound to albumin. Testosterone's binding affinity for SHBG is much greater than for albumin. As a result, testosterone freely disassociates from albumin. Bioavailable testosterone is approximately the amount of free testosterone plus albumin-bound testosterone. A morning total testosterone level has long been considered the most

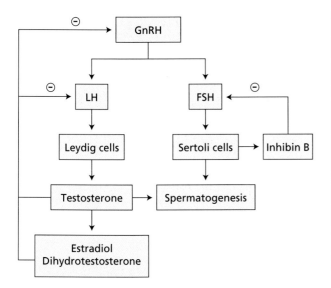

FIGURE 11. Male reproductive axis. Pulses of GnRH elicit pulses of LH and FSH. FSH acts on Sertoli cells, which assist sperm maturation and make inhibin B, the major negative regulator of basal FSH production. The Leydig cells make testosterone, which feeds back to inhibit GnRH and LH release. Some testosterone is irreversibly converted to dihydrotestosterone or estradiol, which are both more potent than testosterone in suppressing GnRH, LH, and FSH. FSH = follicle-stimulating hormone; GnRH = gonadotropin-releasing hormone; LH = luteinizing hormone; – (circled) = negative feedback.

accurate measure of a patient's androgen status except when SHBG is increased (as in the aging man) or decreased (as in obesity). In these circumstances, a serum free testosterone measurement by equilibrium dialysis or a calculated serum free testosterone level is a better measure of a patient's androgen status. Similarly, because of alterations in binding proteins in acutely ill patients, a testosterone measurement should not be obtained because it can lead to an erroneous diagnosis of testosterone deficiency.

Primary Hypogonadism

Primary hypogonadism is due to testicular failure and is defined as a low testosterone level with elevated LH and FSH levels. Primary hypogonadism can have congenital or acquired causes. The most common congenital cause is Klinefelter syndrome (XXY karyotype). Acquired causes include exposure to certain chemotherapy agents, pelvic irradiation, mumps orchitis, trauma, and testicular torsion.

Secondary Hypogonadism

Caused by a hypothalamic or pituitary defect, secondary hypogonadism is defined as a low testosterone level with simultaneously low or inappropriately normal LH and FSH levels. Secondary hypogonadism also can be due to congenital or acquired causes. Idiopathic hypogonadotropic hypogonadism, with anosmia (Kallmann syndrome) or without anosmia, is an example of congenital secondary hypogonadism. Acquired causes include hyperprolactinemia,

functioning or nonfunctioning pituitary adenomas or other sellar masses, chronic opiate use, corticosteroids (exogenous use or excessive endogenous), and infiltrative diseases (such as hemochromatosis).

Androgen Deficiency in the Aging Male

Testosterone levels gradually decrease with age. The degree of decline in the testosterone level is highly variable, and many men will never become hypogonadal. The cause of this decline appears to be multifactorial, with changes in the hypothalamic-pituitary axis and Leydig cell function being the major causes.

Diagnosis and Evaluation of Male Hypogonadism

Symptoms of hypogonadism include low libido, erectile dysfunction, fatigue, and decreased muscle strength. However, these symptoms are common in the general male population and are nonspecific for hypogonadism. More specific signs and symptoms include gynecomastia, decrease in testicular size, and absence of morning erections. Laboratory testing is necessary to make a diagnosis. The best initial test is a morning (8 AM) measurement of the serum total testosterone level. If this level is normal (>350 ng/dL [12 nmol/L]), then hypogonadism is excluded. If abnormal (<200 ng/dL [6.9 nmol/L]), a second confirmatory morning measurement of the total testosterone level should be obtained, according to Endocrine Society guidelines. If the total testosterone level is more equivocal (200-350 ng/dL [6.9-12 nmol/L]) or if an SHBG abnormality is likely in the patient being evaluated, then a serum free testosterone level by equilibrium dialysis or a calculated serum free testosterone level can determine whether hypogonadism is truly present.

When hypogonadism is confirmed, the next step is to determine whether the patient has primary or secondary hypogonadism by measuring LH and FSH levels. Primary hypogonadism is indicated by supranormal LH and FSH levels. In patients with confirmed primary hypogonadism, no clear history of a testicular insult (such as chemotherapy or radiation therapy), and a consistent clinical picture, then a karyotype should be performed to exclude Klinefelter syndrome. If secondary hypogonadism is confirmed by inappropriately normal or low LH and FSH levels, measurement of the serum prolactin level to evaluate for hyperprolactinemia and iron saturation level (transferrin saturation and ferritin levels) to exclude hemochromatosis should be performed to assess for the possible cause. In addition, the presence of any additional pituitary hormone deficiencies should be assessed. An MRI of the pituitary gland should be ordered to exclude hypothalamic or pituitary masses as the cause of decreased gonadotropin production and secretion if any symptoms consistent with mass effect are present, including headaches, visual field changes, a serum total testosterone level less than 150 ng/dL (5.2 nmol/L), an increased prolactin level, or any additional hormonal deficiencies. **Figure 12** shows an algorithm for evaluating hypogonadism.

- Hypogonadism is best diagnosed after two early morning (8 AM) measurements show a decreased total testosterone level.

- After hypogonadism is diagnosed, luteinizing hormone (LH) and follicle-stimulating hormone (FSH) levels should be measured to determine whether the cause is primary (elevated LH and FSH levels) or secondary (low or inappropriately normal LH and FSH levels).

- If primary hypogonadism is confirmed in a patient with no history of a testicular insult and a consistent clinical picture, a karyotype is recommended to exclude Klinefelter syndrome; if secondary hypogonadism is confirmed, the cause should be determined by measurement of prolactin and iron saturation (transferrin saturation and ferritin) levels, evaluation of anterior pituitary function, and (possibly) a pituitary MRI.

Testosterone Replacement Therapy

Various testosterone preparations are available for treatment of male hypogonadism. Transdermal and intramuscular routes of administration are the most widely used.

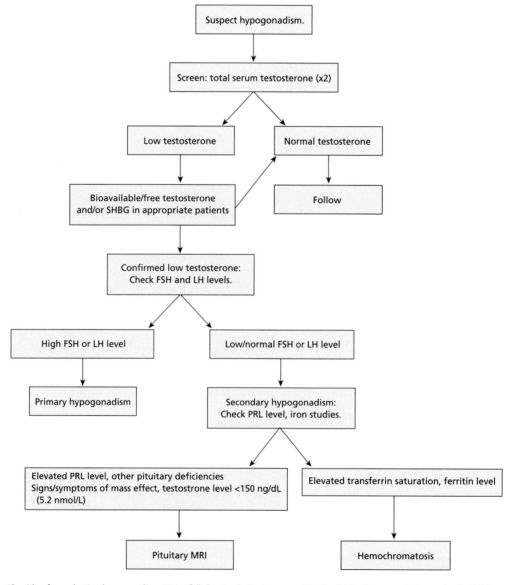

FIGURE 12. Algorithm for evaluating hypogonadism. FSH = follicle-stimulating hormone; LH = luteinizing hormone; PRL = prolactin; SHBG = sex hormone–binding globulin; ×2 = two separate measurements.

In the 1950s, intramuscular testosterone preparations became available. Current preparations include testosterone enanthate and testosterone cypionate, which are administered every 2 to 4 weeks. Advantages to these preparations include their low cost and dosing flexibility. The disadvantage is the large fluctuation in testosterone level after each injection, which can cause fluctuations in mood, energy, libido, and erectile function.

In the 1980s, transdermal preparations that were applied to the scrotum became available. Current transdermal preparations include nongenital patches. Those with an alcohol base often cause skin irritability, and those without an alcohol base can have poor skin adherence, especially in patients who are physically active.

Another testosterone preparation is a buccal tablet applied twice daily. Adverse effects include gum irritation and a bitter taste.

The most popular testosterone preparations currently are hydroalcoholic gels. Advantages to these preparations are the steady level of testosterone provided within 30 minutes of administration and the invisibility of the gel. Disadvantages include the need for daily use, cost, and possible exposure to and absorption by others who come in contact with the patient or his replacement therapy.

Patients receiving testosterone replacement therapy require monitoring of testosterone levels at 3 to 6 months after initiation and annually thereafter, with a goal testosterone level in the midnormal range. For patients receiving intramuscular testosterone preparations, the testosterone level should be checked at the midpoint between scheduled injections. For patients using transdermal preparations, testosterone levels can be checked at any time.

Some of the adverse effects of testosterone replacement—increased hematocrit, worsened sleep apnea, benign prostatic hyperplasia, dyslipidemia, and possibly increased risk of prostate cancer—also need careful monitoring. The Endocrine Society has released clinical guidelines for monitoring these adverse effects (**Table 26**). Recently, long-term adverse cardiovascular effects have been described with testosterone use, which further emphasize the danger of

overdiagnosing hypogonadism or overprescribing testosterone replacement therapy.

KEY POINTS

- Advantages of using a hydroalcoholic gel for testosterone replacement therapy are the steady level of testosterone provided within 30 minutes of administration and the invisibility of the gel; disadvantages include the need for daily use, the cost, and the risk of exposure to and absorption by others who come in contact with the patient.

- After a patient begins testosterone replacement therapy, careful monitoring of testosterone levels and other parameters should occur to assess for adverse effects of treatment, such as increased hematocrit, worsened sleep apnea, benign prostatic hyperplasia, and dyslipidemia.

Anabolic Steroid Abuse in Men

Androgen abuse is common among elite and professional athletes and in young men. The exogenous androgens used for this purpose can suppress endogenous gonadotropins and, therefore, testicular testosterone production. Commonly abused androgens include injectable testosterone esters, oral alkylated testosterone preparations, human chorionic gonadotropin (HCG) injections, aromatase inhibitors, dehydroepiandrosterone (DHEA), and androstenedione supplements.

Physical examination findings may include excessive muscular bulk, acne, gynecomastia, and decreased testicular volume. Low sperm counts also may be present with exogenous androgen use. Androgen abuse can result in hypogonadism and infertility, which occasionally are irreversible. Additional adverse side effects include a low HDL cholesterol level, hepatotoxicity, erythrocytosis, and psychiatric disorders.

Male Infertility

The single best test to assess male fertility is semen analysis. The patient should abstain from sexual activity for 48 to 72 hours to ensure an adequate sample. If semen analysis

TABLE 26. Endocrine Society Clinical Guidelines for Monitoring Adverse Effects of Testosterone Replacement Therapy

Parameter	Recommended Screening Schedule	Alerts
Hematocrit	Value obtained at baseline and then at 3 months and 6 months after therapy initiation, followed by yearly measurements	Value >54%
PSA level	For patients >40 years of age with a baseline value >0.6 ng/mL (0.6 µg/L), DRE and PSA level (determined at 3 and 6 months after therapy initiation followed by regular screening)	Increase >1.4 ng/mL (1.4 µg/L) in 1 y or >0.4 ng/mL (0.4 µg/L) after 6 months of use; abnormal results on DRE; AUA prostate symptoms score/IPSS >19

AUA = American Urological Association; DRE = digital rectal examination; IPSS = International Prostate Symptom Score; µg = microgram(s); PSA = prostate-specific antigen.

Data from Bhasin S, Cunningham GR, Hayes FJ, et al. Testosterone therapy in men with androgen deficiency syndromes: an Endocrine Society Clinical Practice Guideline. J Clin Endocrinol Metab. 2010;95(6):2550. [PMID: 20525905]

results are abnormal, the test should be repeated. If confirmed as abnormal, then a referral to a reproductive endocrinologist or urologist is warranted to determine the best treatment plan.

Gynecomastia

Gynecomastia is a benign but abnormal growth of breast tissue in male patients resulting from an imbalance of testosterone and estrogen, which leads to an increased estrogen-to-testosterone ratio. Causes of this imbalance include medications (such as spironolactone, cimetidine, calcium channel blockers, and ACE inhibitors), liver disease, kidney disease, male hypogonadism, testicular cancer, hyperthyroidism, adrenal tumors, HCG-secreting tumors, and androgen insensitivity syndrome. When this imbalance occurs in the neonatal period and adolescence, gynecomastia is often physiologic, resolving spontaneously most of the time.

Gynecomastia is confirmed on physical examination by the detection of subareolar glandular tissue and should be differentiated from lipomastia, or accumulation of fat in the breast. If gynecomastia is present, a careful evaluation to detect secondary causes, such as chronic illnesses, hyperthyroidism, medications, and drug abuse, is required. The initial laboratory evaluation includes obtaining serum levels of total testosterone, estradiol, HCG, LH, and thyroid-stimulating hormone (TSH). If either primary or secondary hypogonadism is diagnosed, then an evaluation to determine the cause is indicated. If the HCG level is elevated, testicular ultrasonography should be performed first. If the ultrasound is negative for any neoplasm, then chest and abdominal imaging is appropriate to detect malignancy. If the estradiol level is elevated, testicular ultrasonography is performed first; if no mass is detected, adrenal CT or MRI is performed to evaluate for an adrenal mass. If this imaging is negative, the cause is likely to be idiopathic or due to elevated peripheral aromatase activity. If both LH and testosterone levels are elevated and if the rest of the hormonal evaluation is unremarkable, androgen insensitivity syndrome is the likely diagnosis.

Physiology of Female Reproduction

Normal function of the menstrual cycle requires careful coordination of inhibition and stimulation between the hormones of the hypothalamic (GnRH)–pituitary (FSH, LH)–ovarian (estradiol and progesterone) axis. The GnRH pulse frequency varies across the menstrual cycle to promote follicular development and ovulation (**Figure 13**). The FSH level increases slightly in the early follicular phase of the menstrual cycle, which begins with the onset of menstrual bleeding (day 1). This increase leads to recruitment of ovarian follicles, an increase in estradiol (which stimulates endometrial proliferation), and induction of LH receptors in the ovaries. Estradiol exerts acute positive feedback on the pituitary gland, eliciting an LH surge. This LH surge results in ovulation and initiates the luteal phase of the menstrual cycle. Additionally, LH stimulates theca cell androgen production. Androgens are aromatized to estrogen in the granulosa cells by FSH. After the LH surge, the corpus luteum secretes estradiol and progesterone. The declining progesterone levels lead to menstrual bleeding unless conception has occurred.

An average normal menstrual cycle is 28 to 35 days in length. The luteal phase length is constant and usually is 14 days. The follicular phase varies in length from 14 to 21 days, but relatively little variation characterizes follicular phase length in healthy adult women age 20 to 40 years. More cycle length variation occurs in the first 5 years of menstruation, and a decrease in follicular phase length occurs during perimenopause. Menstrual cycles less than 25 days or greater than 35 days are likely anovulatory.

Primary Amenorrhea

Primary amenorrhea is defined as the lack of menses by age 16 years accompanied by a normal body hair pattern and

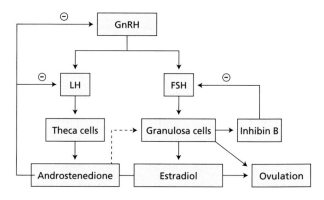

FIGURE 13. Female reproductive axis. As in the male reproductive axis, pulses of GnRH drive LH and FSH production. LH acts on theca cells to stimulate androgen (principally androstenedione) production. Androstenedione is metabolized to estradiol in granulosa cells. FSH acts on granulosa cells to enhance follicle maturation. Granulosa cells produce inhibin B as a feedback regulator of FSH production. FSH = follicle-stimulating hormone; GnRH = gonadotropin-releasing hormone; LH = luteinizing hormone; – (circled) = negative feedback.

normal breast development. Pregnancy must be ruled out in all patients with primary amenorrhea. Approximately 50% of patients with primary amenorrhea have a chromosomal abnormality, such as gonadal dysgenesis, and approximately 15% have an anatomic abnormality of the uterus, vagina, or cervix. Primary ovarian insufficiency due to Turner syndrome, a syndrome characterized by short stature and the loss of a portion or all of one X chromosome, is one of the most common causes of primary amenorrhea. The diagnosis of Turner syndrome can be made on the basis of a karyotype. Diagnosing Turner syndrome is critical because affected patients have a higher incidence of cardiovascular disease, metabolic syndrome, and thyroid dysfunction and should be evaluated annually as adults for these entities.

KEY POINT

- One of the most common causes of primary amenorrhea is primary ovarian insufficiency due to Turner syndrome, which is diagnosed by a karyotype.

Secondary Amenorrhea

Secondary amenorrhea is defined as the absence of a menstrual cycle for three cycles or 6 months in previously menstruating women. Pregnancy is the most common cause of secondary amenorrhea.

Uterine or outflow tract disorders (especially Asherman syndrome), although rare, also must always be considered as a possible cause. Asherman syndrome is due to endometrial scarring after a uterine procedure (usually, repeated dilation and curettage) and should be considered in any woman with amenorrhea and past exposure to uterine instrumentation. The classic presentation is amenorrhea with ovulatory or premenstrual symptoms. After pregnancy is excluded, approximately 40% of secondary amenorrhea will be due to ovarian causes, most commonly polycystic ovary syndrome (PCOS). Additional causes of secondary amenorrhea include hypothalamic amenorrhea, hyperprolactinemia, thyroid disease, and primary ovarian insufficiency.

Functional hypothalamic amenorrhea affects 3% of women between age 18 and 40 years and is a diagnosis of exclusion. Risk factors for this condition include a low body weight and fat percentage, rapid and substantial weight loss, eating disorders, excessive exercise, severe emotional stress, severe nutritional deficiencies, and chronic or acute illness. FSH and LH levels are inappropriately low or normal in this low-estrogen disorder, but FSH is frequently higher than LH. Recovery of menses occurs in 30% to 100% of patients, depending on the cause, with stress and weight loss exhibiting the best prognoses.

Hyperprolactinemia causes secondary amenorrhea through direct inhibition of GnRH secretion. Both hypothyroidism and hyperthyroidism also cause secondary amenorrhea. Hypothyroidism results in increased levels of thyrotropin-releasing hormone through negative feedback, and this hormone, in turn, stimulates prolactin secretion. Hyperthyroidism can cause rapid weight loss, which is known to cause functional hypothalamic amenorrhea.

Primary ovarian insufficiency is defined as amenorrhea before age 40 years in the setting of two elevated FSH levels. Possible secondary causes include Turner syndrome, a fragile X premutation carrier status, autoimmune oophoritis, and the effects of chemotherapy or radiation therapy.

Diagnosis and Evaluation of Amenorrhea

The initial evaluation of amenorrhea includes a thorough history and physical examination and measurement of serum HCG, prolactin, FSH, and TSH levels to assess for pregnancy, hyperprolactinemia, primary ovarian insufficiency, and thyroid disease, respectively. A pelvic ultrasound is required in all patients with primary amenorrhea. A pituitary MRI also is required in these patients if primary ovarian insufficiency is excluded as a cause and in patients with secondary amenorrhea that is hypothalamic in nature but has no clear cause to exclude a pituitary or hypothalamic tumor.

If the prolactin level is elevated, then an evaluation for causes of hyperprolactinemia is necessary, including a review of the patient's medications, thyroid status, and kidney function and, possibly, imaging of the pituitary gland to evaluate for pituitary adenoma. If the FSH level is elevated on two separate measurements, then the diagnosis of primary ovarian insufficiency is made. Patients with these findings also should have a karyotype to evaluate for Turner syndrome and should be tested for the fragile X mutation; a careful review of systems is necessary to assess for autoimmune disease. If the patient has thyroid dysfunction, then treatment of the underlying disorder should result in resumption of menses.

If results of the laboratory tests are normal, the next step is to assess estrogen sufficiency with a progesterone challenge test. Estradiol levels can be variable in amenorrhea of differing causes, but results of a progesterone challenge test will clearly delineate between an estrogen-deficient state (no bleeding) and an estrogen-sufficient state (withdrawal bleeding). If the patient is producing estrogen, she will have withdrawal bleeding within 1 week of completing a course of progesterone. In this case, the patient is not estrogen deficient, and PCOS (or a similar diagnosis) should be considered. If no withdrawal bleeding occurs after the progesterone challenge, then the patient has a low-estrogen state, and hypothalamic amenorrhea is the diagnosis. If no clear cause of the hypothalamic amenorrhea is present, then a pituitary MRI should be ordered to rule out a pituitary adenoma.

KEY POINT

- In a patient with amenorrhea and normal results on initial laboratory studies, the next step in evaluation is a progesterone challenge test.

Hirsutism and Polycystic Ovary Syndrome

Hirsutism is defined as an excess in terminal hair growth in women in androgen-dependent areas of the body. A patient's familial hair pattern and ethnic background should be taken into account when assessing for hirsutism. When hirsutism is present, then the patient must be assessed for virilization, which is commonly due to an ovarian or adrenal tumor. Signs and symptoms of virilization include a deepening of voice, severe acne, clitoromegaly, a decrease in breast size, and male-pattern balding. Other concerning features are rapid onset and progressive hirsutism over a short period of time (such as 1 year) or hirsutism that develops after age 30 years.

Recommended laboratory tests for moderate to severe hirsutism or virilization include measurement of the plasma DHEA sulfate level and serum levels of TSH, prolactin, total testosterone, and follicular phase 17-hydroxyprogesterone to exclude thyroid disease, hyperprolactinemia, ovarian and adrenal tumors, and late-onset congenital adrenal hyperplasia. If the serum total testosterone level is greater than 200 ng/dL (6.9 nmol/L), then a pelvic ultrasound and adrenal CT are necessary to exclude an ovarian or adrenal neoplasm; if the plasma DHEA sulfate level is greater than 700 micrograms/mL (1890 micromoles/L), then an adrenal CT is necessary to exclude an adrenal cortisol-secreting and/or androgen-secreting neoplasm. Most cases of hirsutism have benign causes, with PCOS being the most common.

PCOS is one of the most common endocrine disorders in young women, with a prevalence of approximately 7%. In 1990, the National Institutes of Health defined PCOS as occurring in women who have oligomenorrhea and clinical or biochemical evidence of hyperandrogenism when other endocrine disorders are excluded. In 2003, the American Society for Reproductive Medicine and the European Society of Human Reproduction established new, still debated diagnostic criteria (Rotterdam criteria) stating that two of the following three findings must be present to establish a diagnosis of PCOS: (1) oligo-ovulation or anovulation, (2) clinical or biochemical evidence of hyperandrogenism, and (3) polycystic ovarian morphology on an ultrasound when other endocrine disorders are excluded.

The primary clinical manifestations of PCOS are menstrual irregularity (oligomenorrhea or amenorrhea), ovulatory dysfunction with resultant infertility, insulin resistance, and hyperandrogenism. Oligo-ovulation or anovulation can result in endometrial hyperplasia and/or infertility. Hyperandrogenism presents as hirsutism, acne, or androgenic alopecia. Most patients with PCOS also have insulin resistance, and studies have shown an increased incidence of metabolic syndrome, obesity, impaired glucose tolerance, and frank type 2 diabetes mellitus. Both obese and lean women with PCOS have evidence of insulin resistance, which suggests that this finding is intrinsic to the disorder. Improvement in insulin resistance with weight loss or the use of metformin is associated with a decrease in serum androgen

levels. In fact, patients treated with metformin have not only improved insulin sensitivity and androgen levels, but also improved ovulatory rates with increased pregnancy rates. These data strongly suggest that the insulin resistance of PCOS plays a role in the oligomenorrhea and hyperandrogenism seen in this disorder. More recent studies also have shown frequent associations between the insulin resistance of PCOS and both fatty liver disease and sleep apnea.

Treatment of the clinical manifestations of PCOS depends on which symptom(s) is(are) most problematic to the patient. Weight loss and exercise are mainstays of therapy for all patients with PCOS and have been shown to lessen the severity of clinical manifestations of the disorder. If a patient's major concern is hyperandrogenism, then oral contraceptive therapy is the best choice. Spironolactone may be added after 6 months if acne and hirsutism are still cosmetically bothersome to the patient. Additional treatments for hirsutism include waxing, electrolysis, laser therapy, and topical eflornithine. For the menstrual irregularities associated with PCOS, oral estrogen-progesterone contraceptives are effective and provide endometrial protection. If a patient has a contraindication to oral contraceptives or does not wish to take them, cyclical progesterone can be given to induce withdrawal bleeding. The insulin resistance of PCOS is treated with diet and exercise. Metformin also can be used, especially if acanthosis nigricans or impaired glucose tolerance is present. Infertility in PCOS is usually treated with diet, exercise, clomiphene, or metformin, depending on the patient's age, degree of insulin resistance, and personal preference.

KEY POINTS

- A woman with acute onset of rapidly progressive hirsutism should be assessed for signs of virilization (deepening of the voice, acne, clitoromegaly, decrease in breast size, and male-pattern balding) because of the risk of an androgen-secreting ovarian or adrenal tumor.

- Polycystic ovary syndrome, which is characterized by menstrual irregularities and hyperandrogenism, is associated with insulin resistance and an increased risk of metabolic syndrome, impaired glucose tolerance, and type 2 diabetes mellitus.

- Oral contraceptives are effective in treating the oligomenorrhea of polycystic ovary syndrome (PCOS) and provide endometrial protection; the insulin resistance and obesity of PCOS are best treated with weight loss and exercise, but use of metformin also should be considered.

Anabolic Steroid Abuse in Women

Some women abuse anabolic steroids to enhance their athletic performance or physique. Adverse effects include hirsutism, acne, deepening of the voice, decreased breast size, and clitoromegaly. Withdrawal of androgens does not result in severe hypogonadism, as it does in men. Symptoms of hyperandrogenism with a normal or low testosterone level may be a clue of androgen abuse.

Female Infertility

Infertility is defined as the inability to conceive in 1 year with regular unprotected sexual intercourse. If the female partner is older than 35 years, then infertility is defined as the inability to conceive within 6 months. Infertility evaluation for women includes a careful menstrual history and proper evaluation of oligomenorrhea, if present. Measuring serum TSH and prolactin levels is appropriate to exclude thyroid disease and hyperprolactinemia because even mild abnormalities in thyroid function or prolactin levels can result in infertility. If results of initial testing are normal, then referral to a reproductive endocrinologist is indicated. Further evaluation will typically include a semen analysis of the male partner, confirmation of ovulatory function with measurement of a midluteal progesterone level, ovarian reserve testing by measuring a serum FSH level on day 3 of the menstrual cycle, and hysterosalpingography performed sometime between days 6 and 10 of the menstrual cycle to evaluate for any uterine or tubal abnormalities. If no abnormalities are found, closely monitored therapy with clomiphene or gonadotropins may be initiated.

KEY POINT

- Measuring the serum thyroid-stimulating hormone and prolactin levels is appropriate to exclude thyroid disease and hyperprolactinemia in a woman with infertility; if results of initial testing are normal, then referral to a reproductive endocrinologist for further evaluation and treatment is appropriate.

Calcium and Bone Disorders

Calcium Homeostasis

Precise regulation of calcium homeostasis in the body is critical. Calcium is the main mineral component of the skeleton and plays major roles in neuronal transmission, muscle contraction, and blood clotting; it also is an important intracellular messenger regulating numerous processes throughout the body. The normal range for the total serum calcium level is 9.0 to 10.5 mg/dL (2.2-2.6 mmol/L); 50% to 60% of this calcium is bound to plasma proteins or complexed with anions, and the remaining ionized calcium controls physiologic actions. The normal level of ionized calcium is maintained in a very narrow range (4.4-5.2 mg/dL [1.1-1.3 mmol/L]).

The body regulates serum calcium by controlling its entry through the intestine, its exit through the kidney, and its storage in bone (**Figure 14**). These processes are regulated by parathyroid hormone (PTH) and 1,25-dihydroxyvitamin D. 1,25-Dihydroxyvitamin D is made when exposure of the skin to ultraviolet light triggers conversion of 7-dehydrocholesterol to vitamin D_3 or cholecalciferol. Cholecalciferol also is supplied by dietary sources or nutritional supplements, such as vitamin D_2 (ergocalciferol), a plant steroid. In the liver, vitamins D_2 and D_3 are hydroxylated to 25-hydroxyvitamin D, the storage form of vitamin D, which in turn is hydroxylated in the kidney to the active form, 1,25-dihydroxyvitamin D. PTH and 1,25-dihydroxyvitamin D maintain tight control of the plasma ionized calcium level.

The plasma ionized calcium level is monitored by a parathyroid cell membrane calcium-sensing receptor (CSR).

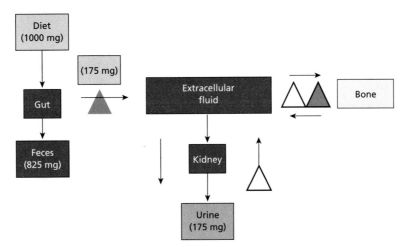

FIGURE 14. Regulation of calcium homeostasis. The flow of calcium through the body (net daily calcium flux) in a hypothetical healthy person with a typical dietary calcium intake of 1000 mg/d is shown. In this example, 175 mg is absorbed by the gut and enters the extracellular fluid compartment (plasma and interstitial fluid). The remaining 825 mg is lost in feces. After filtration of plasma by the kidney, most of the calcium is reclaimed from the filtrate, and in this example, 175 mg is released in urine to maintain net zero change in total body calcium. Processes regulated by parathyroid hormone are indicated by white triangles, and those regulated by 1,25-dihydroxyvitamin D are indicated by teal triangles.

As circulating levels of plasma ionized calcium increase, CSR signaling is activated and causes PTH secretion to decrease; when plasma ionized calcium levels are low, PTH secretion increases. PTH activates bone resorption and distal nephron calcium resorption. PTH also stimulates kidney production of 1,25-dihydroxyvitamin D, thereby increasing calcium absorption by the small intestine. If plasma ionized calcium levels increase above the normal range, PTH secretion declines, which leads to greater calcium losses by the kidneys, reduced 1,25-dihydroxyvitamin D production, and decreased calcium absorption by the intestines. Both PTH and 1,25-dihydroxyvitamin D act on bone to facilitate calcium release. Accordingly, the plasma ionized calcium level is maintained in a narrow range, even at the expense of skeletal calcium when necessary.

Hypercalcemia

Clinical Manifestations of Hypercalcemia

Clinical manifestations of hypercalcemia are the same, regardless of its underlying cause. Most persons with mild hypercalcemia (levels > the normal serum calcium level but <12 mg/dL [3.0 mmol/L]) are asymptomatic, although some report mild fatigue, depression, constipation, mild polyuria, mild increase in thirst, or vague changes in cognition. Typical manifestations of hypercalcemia are more common with serum calcium levels of 12 to 14 mg/dL (3.0-3.5 mmol/L) and include anorexia, nausea, abdominal pain, muscle weakness, and depressed mental status. Dehydration caused by polyuria also is common because hypercalciuria decreases the kidneys' ability to concentrate urine. At calcium levels greater than 14 mg/dL (3.5 mmol/L), lethargy, disorientation, and coma may develop. The severity of the symptoms is determined by the severity of the serum calcium elevation, the rate of increase, and the overall health of the affected person.

Patients with primary hyperparathyroidism (and thus, by definition, hypercalcemia) in the setting of multiple endocrine neoplasia (MEN) types 1 and 2 also may have specific manifestations of the other tumors associated with these syndromes. Patients with hypercalcemia due to sarcoidosis may have inflammatory or pulmonary symptoms. Because hypercalcemia of malignancy typically develops only when a substantial tumor burden is present, most patients with this type of hypercalcemia already have symptoms related to an established cancer diagnosis.

KEY POINT

- Typical manifestations of hypercalcemia include anorexia, nausea, abdominal pain, muscle weakness, dehydration, and depressed mental status; symptom severity is determined by the extent of the serum calcium elevation, the rate of increase, and the overall health of the affected person.

Causes and Diagnosis of Hypercalcemia

Identifying the cause of hypercalcemia (**Table 27**) requires a comprehensive history, physical examination, laboratory tests, and, occasionally, imaging studies. Medications, foods, and nutritional supplements should be reviewed. Family history suggesting inherited disorders of calcium metabolism or related conditions should be elicited. In addition to evaluating patients with suspected hypercalcemia for signs of dehydration and depressed mental status, the clinician should identify signs of common causes of hypercalcemia, such as malignancy and granulomatous diseases. Benign parathyroid conditions do not produce a neck mass. Physical evidence of osteoporosis or kidney stones should also be sought. Other findings depend on the type of hypercalcemia involved (see Table 27).

When an elevated serum calcium level is found, factitious hypercalcemia—caused by increased levels of the plasma proteins that bind calcium—must first be excluded in patients at risk for this condition, including those with HIV infection, chronic hepatitis, and multiple myeloma. The ionized calcium level in these patients remains normal.

After hypercalcemia is confirmed, the next step is the simultaneous measurement of serum PTH and serum or plasma ionized calcium levels. In the absence of plasma protein abnormalities, obtaining a total serum calcium level is usually adequate; ionized calcium samples must be drawn under anaerobic conditions and kept on ice for accurate results. With normal parathyroid glands, hypercalcemia will suppress PTH. If the serum calcium level is elevated and the PTH level is high or inappropriately normal, the diagnosis of PTH-mediated hypercalcemia or primary hyperparathyroidism is made (see later discussion) (**Figure 15**). If PTH levels are low, causes of non–PTH-mediated hypercalcemia should be considered (see later discussion). The serum creatinine level also may be acutely elevated in persons with hypercalcemia who are dehydrated or chronically elevated in those with nephrocalcinosis. The serum phosphorus level may be low in hypercalcemia associated with primary hyperparathyroidism, whereas hyperphosphatemia may occur if the cause is vitamin D intoxication. By changing the set point for the CSR, lithium therapy can lead to mild hypercalcemia and mildly elevated PTH levels that mimic primary hyperparathyroidism but do not require intervention.

Parathyroid Hormone–Mediated Hypercalcemia

Description, Evaluation, and Treatment
Primary hyperparathyroidism is the most common cause of hypercalcemia diagnosed in the outpatient setting. The annual incidence of primary hyperparathyroidism in the United States is approximately four per 100,000 persons. The incidence peaks in the fifth to sixth decade of life, with a female-to-male ratio of 3:2. The clinical manifestations of hyperparathyroidism depend on its severity and chronicity. The hypercalcemia of primary hyperparathyroidism often is

TABLE 27. Differential Diagnosis of Hypercalcemia

Parathyroid Hormone Mediated

Primary hyperparathyroidism
  Parathyroid adenoma(s)
  Parathyroid hyperplasia
  Parathyroid carcinoma

Tertiary hyperparathyroidism

Familial hypocalciuric hypercalcemia

Lithium therapy–associated hypercalcemia

Nonparathyroid Hormone Mediated

Malignancy-associated hypercalcemia
  Humoral hypercalcemia of malignancy
    PTH-related protein (squamous cell carcinoma, adenocarcinoma of the breast or ovary, renal cell carcinoma, transitional cell carcinoma, T-cell lymphoma, islet cell neoplasms, myeloma)
    1,25-Dihydroxyvitamin D (B-cell lymphoma)
  Local osteolytic hypercalcemia (myeloma, breast cancer, lymphoma)

Granulomatous diseases (sarcoidosis, tuberculosis)

Endocrinopathies (hyperthyroidism, adrenal insufficiency)

Certain drugs (thiazide diuretics, excessive calcium supplements, vitamin D or A)

Immobilization

Other (increased plasma protein levels from factitious hypercalcemia, acute kidney failure, total parenteral nutrition, or milk alkali syndrome)

PTH = parathyroid hormone.

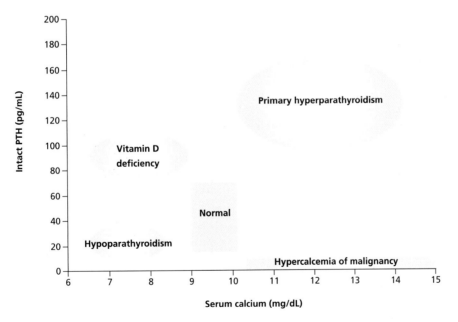

FIGURE 15. Relationship of calcium, PTH, and vitamin D status in normal conditions and in several diseases. PTH = parathyroid hormone.

diagnosed incidentally by routine blood testing before the development of symptoms. This disorder also may be found during the evaluation of osteoporosis or nephrolithiasis. In 75% to 80% of patients with primary hyperparathyroidism, a solitary parathyroid adenoma is present; hyperplasia involving multiple parathyroid glands is found in 15% to 20%, and parathyroid carcinoma is present in less than 1%. Symptoms associated with more severe or prolonged disease include nephrolithiasis, kidney disease due to nephrocalcinosis, fragility fractures, and bone pain.

After the diagnosis of primary hyperparathyroidism is established, additional testing may be necessary to determine whether parathyroidectomy is warranted. Guidelines for surgical intervention in patients with asymptomatic primary hyperparathyroidism were updated at a National Institutes of Health workshop in 2008 (**Table 28**). A parathyroid sestamibi scan or ultrasound may locate the causative adenoma but is not required to diagnose primary hyperparathyroidism.

No current medical therapy is as effective as surgery for primary hyperparathyroidism. A 15-year long-term follow-up study of patients who did not undergo parathyroidectomy showed that one third developed disease progression and most experienced additional bone loss by the study's end. Patients who do not have surgery can be monitored and, in some cases, may benefit from medication. Dietary calcium should not be restricted in these patients, and vitamin D deficiency should be corrected to prevent further elevation of PTH and bone loss. In those with low bone mass, a bisphosphonate will help slow bone loss but will not control hypercalcemia. In patients with symptomatic hypercalcemia who are not surgical candidates or whose causative parathyroid adenoma cannot be localized, the calcimimetic agent cinacalcet can control hypercalcemia. However, this agent has multiple drug interactions and is very expensive, and its long-term safety has not been established, limiting its use to specific clinical situations.

A schedule recommending follow-up testing of persons with primary hyperparathyroidism who do not undergo parathyroidectomy also was developed at the 2008 National Institutes of Health workshop (**Table 29**). Patients who develop criteria for parathyroidectomy should be referred for surgery.

Familial Forms of Hyperparathyroidism
Familial hypocalciuric hypercalcemia (FHH) is a rare autosomal dominant condition caused by inactivating mutations of

TABLE 28. Indications for Surgical Intervention in Patients with Primary Hyperparathyroidism

Increase in serum calcium level ≥1 mg/dL (0.25 mmol/L) above upper limit of normal[a]

Creatinine clearance <60 mL/min (0.06 L/min)[a]

T-score (on DEXA scan) of −2.5 or worse at the lumbar spine, total hip, femoral neck, or distal radius[a]

Age <50 y[a]

Surgery also indicated in patients in whom medical surveillance is neither desired nor possible, including those with significant bone, kidney, gastrointestinal, or neuromuscular symptoms typical of primary hyperparathyroidism

DEXA = dual-energy x-ray absorptiometry.

[a]In otherwise asymptomatic patients.

Adapted from Bilezikian JP, Khan AA, Potts JT Jr; Third International Workshop on the Management of Asymptomatic Primary Hyperthyroidism. Guidelines for the management of asymptomatic primary hyperparathyroidism: summary statement from the Third International Workshop. J Clin Endocrinol Metab. 2009;94(2):336. [PMID: 19193908] Copyright 2009, The Endocrine Society.

TABLE 29. Long-Term Monitoring of Patients with Primary Hyperparathyroidism Who Do Not Undergo Parathyroidectomy

Test	Interval
Serum calcium	Annually
Serum creatinine	Annually
Bone densitometry	Every 1-2 years at three sites (such as the lumbar spine, hip, and distal radius)

Adapted from Bilezikian JP, Khan AA, Potts JT Jr; Third International Workshop on the Management of Asymptomatic Primary Hyperthyroidism. Guidelines for the management of asymptomatic primary hyperparathyroidism: summary statement from the Third International Workshop. J Clin Endocrinol Metab. 2009;94(2):336. [PMID: 19193908] Copyright 2009, The Endocrine Society.

the *CASR* gene. These mutations result in high serum calcium levels and inappropriately normal to mildly elevated serum PTH levels. Patients with FHH have low urine calcium excretion, although this finding may occur in those taking thiazide diuretics, proton pump inhibitors, or lithium. FHH is suspected in patients with a family history of asymptomatic, stable, mild hypercalcemia and in patients whose urine calcium to creatinine clearance ratio is very low (<0.01). The diagnosis of FHH can be made on clinical grounds in a patient with chronic mild hypercalcemia and hypocalciuria, lack of symptoms or sequelae, and a family history of similar findings. FHH can be confirmed with genetic testing for *CASR* gene mutations, although not all mutations have been characterized. FHH is usually a benign condition that requires no intervention but should be recognized to prevent unnecessary parathyroidectomy.

Familial hyperparathyroidism can occur as an isolated entity or as part of the MEN syndromes (types 1 and 2). These syndromes should be considered in all patients with primary hyperparathyroidism, particularly those who are young or have a personal or family history of a related endocrinopathy. Knowing before surgery whether the hyperparathyroidism is familial or not is essential because patients with inherited primary hyperparathyroidism often have multigland parathyroid hyperplasia, and evaluation of all parathyroid glands should occur during surgery. If MEN2 is suspected, pheochromocytoma must be excluded before the patient can safely undergo surgery, and the patient should be evaluated for medullary thyroid cancer.

Nonparathyroid Hormone–Mediated Hypercalcemia

Causes and Diagnosis

If a patient's serum calcium level is elevated and the PTH level is appropriately suppressed to less than normal, then PTH-independent hypercalcemia is likely. A non-PTH disorder is most often responsible for acute hypercalcemia. Cancer is the most common cause of PTH-independent hypercalcemia and the most frequent cause of acute hypercalcemia in a hospitalized patient. When the PTH level is low and the patient does not have a malignancy, diagnostic considerations should include nonmalignant causes, such as vitamin D intoxication or production of 1,25-dihydroxyvitamin D by granulomatous disease (such as sarcoidosis or tuberculosis) (see Table 27).

Malignancy-Associated Hypercalcemia

In malignancy-associated hypercalcemia, the serum calcium elevation is usually moderate or severe, and the PTH level is low (see Figure 15). Evidence of significant dehydration and generalized debility is evident, as are other cancer-related symptoms. In most instances, a cancer diagnosis has already been established.

Humoral hypercalcemia of malignancy (HHM) results from tumor production of a circulating factor that acts on skeletal calcium release, renal calcium handling, or intestinal calcium absorption. Rarely, this disorder can be caused by unregulated production of 1,25-dihydroxyvitamin D (as in B-cell lymphomas) or other mediators that interfere with calcium homeostasis. The most common cause of HHM is PTH-related protein (PTHrP). PTHrP is homologous to PTH, and they share a common receptor. PTHrP and PTH both activate osteoclasts to resorb bone, thereby decreasing calcium excretion and increasing phosphate clearance by the kidneys.

Tumors that cause HHM by secreting PTHrP are typically squamous cell carcinomas (often of the lung), although other tumors (such as breast and renal cell carcinoma) also can be responsible. Tumors produce PTHrP in small amounts. Therefore, HHM typically develops in patients with a large tumor burden and is seldom the presenting feature of a cancer.

Another form of malignancy-associated hypercalcemia is local osteolytic hypercalcemia, which occurs when bony metastases produce factors that activate bone resorption by osteoclasts. The classic tumor associated with this syndrome is multiple myeloma, although other neoplasms (breast cancer, lymphoma) may also be implicated.

KEY POINTS

- If the serum calcium level is elevated and the parathyroid hormone (PTH) level is high or inappropriately normal in a patient with hypercalcemia, the diagnosis is PTH-mediated primary hyperparathyroidism, most often caused by a solitary parathyroid adenoma.

- Tumors that secrete parathyroid hormone–related protein, typically squamous cell carcinomas, are the most common cause of hypercalcemia of malignancy.

Treatment of Acute Hypercalcemia

When the serum calcium level is severely elevated, treatment should include rehydration and increasing urine calcium excretion while simultaneously reducing bone resorption or intestinal calcium absorption, depending on which is the main source of the excess calcium.

Most patients with acute hypercalcemia have volume contraction, which further exacerbates their inability to excrete calcium. Therefore, the first intervention should be intravenous infusion of normal saline. Delivery of sodium and water to the distal nephron will enhance urine calcium excretion. After intravascular volume is replenished, a loop diuretic, such as furosemide, allows additional aggressive saline hydration and may further enhance calcium excretion. However, evidence for the efficacy of furosemide in this setting is lacking.

Nearly all causes of severe hypercalcemia involve increased osteoclast activity, and thus drugs that inhibit bone resorption are useful. The treatment of choice is an intravenous bisphosphonate, such as pamidronate or zoledronate. Zoledronate has greater potency and a longer duration of action than pamidronate. Caution should be exercised with these agents in the setting of kidney dysfunction.

For more rapid resolution of hypercalcemia, subcutaneous injection of calcitonin can be used, either alone or simultaneously with a bisphosphonate. Tachyphylaxis limits the effectiveness of calcitonin to a few days. In severe or refractory hypercalcemia, low-calcium bath hemodialysis may be required. Patients whose kidney function precludes the use of bisphosphonates may respond to off-label use of denosumab, which also reduces osteoclast-mediated bone resorption.

When hypercalcemia results from increased intestinal calcium absorption, as occurs in vitamin D intoxication or granulomatous diseases, glucocorticoid treatment is indicated (for example, prednisone, 10-40 mg/d). Glucocorticoids directly impair intestinal calcium transport and also inhibit kidney or granulomatous 1α-hydroxylase activity, thereby resulting in decreased production of 1,25-dihydroxyvitamin D.

Long-term management should focus on addressing the cause of hypercalcemia. Treatment of the underlying cause may not lead to immediate lowering of the serum calcium level and thus should be coupled with short-term management interventions that should be continued until stabilization is achieved.

KEY POINT

- Treatment of acute hypercalcemia involves administering intravenous fluids, increasing urine calcium excretion, and reducing either bone resorption or intestinal calcium absorption, depending on which is the main source of excess calcium.

Hypocalcemia

Diagnosis and Causes of Hypocalcemia

Hypocalcemia is present when the serum calcium level is less than normal. This diagnosis should be confirmed with repeat measurements and a serum albumin measurement, given that a low plasma calcium-binding protein level can cause a factitious low serum calcium level. The measured serum calcium level should be corrected for a low albumin level by adding 0.8 mg/dL (0.2 mmol/L) of calcium for each 1 g/dL (10 g/L) of albumin that a patient's serum albumin level is less than 4 g/dL (40 g/L). An accurate ionized calcium measurement will circumvent these pitfalls.

Chronic mild to moderate hypocalcemia is usually asymptomatic. However, when the serum calcium level is less than 7.5 to 8.0 mg/dL (1.9-2.0 mmol/L) and the serum albumin level is normal, a patient may develop symptoms of neuromuscular irritability, including tremor, muscle spasms or cramps, or paresthesias. On physical examination, Chvostek sign (contraction of the ipsilateral facial muscles with tapping of the facial nerve) and Trousseau sign (carpopedal spasm

induced by prolonged application of greater-than-systolic pressure by a blood pressure cuff) may be noted. Tetany or seizures may be seen if the serum calcium level becomes severely low. Prolongation of the corrected QT interval and bradycardia may be evident on an electrocardiogram, indicating that the patient is at risk for cardiac arrhythmias.

The cause of hypocalcemia usually is identified by obtaining a careful history (**Table 30**). Dietary calcium and vitamin D intake, inadequate sun exposure, gastrointestinal malabsorption, and alcohol intake should be discussed. Information

TABLE 30. Differential Diagnosis of Hypocalcemia

Condition	Laboratory Findings	Comments
Disorders of vitamin D metabolism (vitamin D deficiency) Lack of sunlight Dermatologic disorders Dietary deficiency Malabsorption Liver disease Kidney disease Vitamin D-dependent rickets, type I (1α-hydroxylase deficiency)	Mild hypocalcemia, hypophosphatemia, elevated PTH level, and decreased 25-hydroxyvitamin D level; decreased 1,25-dihydroxyvitamin D level if kidney disease is present	Vitamin D deficiency widespread among housebound and institutionalized older persons and general medical patients with disorders that predispose to altered vitamin D metabolism
Vitamin D resistance (vitamin D–dependent rickets, type II)	Hypocalcemia, hypophosphatemia, and elevated PTH level; elevated 1,25-dihydroxyvitamin D level when treated with vitamin D	Vitamin D–receptor defect leading to resistance to 1,25-dihydroxyvitamin D
Hypoparathyroidism Postsurgical (most common cause; seen after thyroid, parathyroid, or neck surgery) After external radiation therapy to neck Autoimmune (autoimmune polyglandular syndrome) Congenital (DiGeorge syndrome) Infiltrative (hemochromatosis, sarcoidosis)	Hypocalcemia, hyperphosphatemia, and a low or inappropriately normal PTH level	—
PTH resistance (pseudohypoparathyroidism)	Hypocalcemia, hyperphosphatemia, and elevated PTH level with normal 25-hydroxyvitamin D level	Pseudohypoparathyroidism, type 1a, an autosomal dominant disorder marked by resistance to multiple hormones and Albright hereditary osteodystrophy (short stature, obesity, round facies, brachymetacarpia, and mental deficiency)
Hypomagnesemia Chronic diuretic use Alcoholism Diarrhea Malabsorption Certain drugs (amphotericin B, aminoglycosides, cisplatin)	Hypomagnesemia and hypocalcemia; PTH level potentially low, normal, or high	Hypomagnesemia potentially leading to impaired PTH secretion and PTH resistance, with impaired tissue responsiveness to PTH

(continued on next page)

TABLE 30. Differential Diagnosis of Hypocalcemia (*continued*)

Condition	Laboratory Findings	Comments
Medications Causing altered vitamin D metabolism (phenytoin, phenobarbital, isoniazid, theophylline, rifampin, 5-fluorouracil plus leucovorin) Causing intravascular binding (phosphate, foscarnet, EDTA, citrated blood products) Intravenous bisphosphonates (especially in vitamin D deficiency; contraindicated in hypocalcemia)	Hypocalcemia and low 25-hydroxyvitamin D or 1,25-dihydroxyvitamin D level (with agents that alter vitamin D metabolism)	Hypocalcemia potentially developing rapidly with use of some medications, especially if administered intravenously
Extravascular deposition Pancreatitis Hungry-bone syndrome Rhabdomyolysis Tumor lysis syndrome Osteoblastic metastases	Hypocalcemia and hyper- or hypophosphatemia	In pancreatitis, hypocalcemia from the deposition of calcium in the form of calcium soaps; hyperphosphatemia suggestive of rhabdomyolysis or tumor lysis syndrome with release of phosphate from the bone; hypophosphatemia seen in hungry-bone syndrome or with osteoblastic metastases (of prostate or breast cancer)
Sepsis	Hypocalcemia and low PTH and 1,25-dihydroxyvitamin D levels	Sepsis most likely mediated by the action of inflammatory cytokines on the parathyroid glands, kidneys, and bone
Acute respiratory alkalosis	Normal serum calcium but low ionized calcium levels	Alkalosis leading to increased binding of calcium ions to albumin
Artifactual hypoglycemia with hypoalbuminemia	Low serum calcium and normal ionized calcium levels	Reduced protein binding leading to lower total serum calcium level, with normal ionized fraction

EDTA = ethylenediaminetetraacetic acid; PTH = parathyroid hormone.

about previous head and neck surgery and irradiation should be elicited because these are the most common causes of acquired hypoparathyroidism. The risk for rarer conditions, such as autoimmune disease and iron overload states, also should be determined. Any history of pancreatitis, rhabdomyolysis, tumor lysis syndrome, or ongoing transfusion therapy should be investigated because all are potential causes of hypocalcemia. If the patient's history and physical examination findings do not reveal an obvious reason for the hypocalcemia, simultaneous measurement of PTH and serum calcium levels will determine whether the process is PTH mediated. A low or inappropriately normal PTH level in the setting of a low calcium level indicates hypoparathyroidism. An elevated PTH level is seen in secondary hyperparathyroidism and is an appropriate physiologic response of the parathyroid glands to a low calcium level of any cause. These measurements should be followed by kidney function testing and measurement of magnesium, phosphorus, and 25-hydroxyvitamin D levels (see Figure 15).

Unintentional removal or injury of parathyroid glands during thyroidectomy can result in hypoparathyroidism with hypocalcemia postoperatively. Patients who had severe primary hyperparathyroidism with high bone turnover may experience hungry bone syndrome after parathyroidectomy, which is protracted hypocalcemia with deposition of large quantities of calcium into the unmineralized bone matrix.

Autoimmune destruction or infiltrative diseases, such as hemochromatosis, also may impair parathyroid function. Additionally, congenital absence of the parathyroid glands occurs in DiGeorge syndrome. Functional hypoparathyroidism may result from hypomagnesemia because magnesium is necessary for PTH release and action. Patients with alcoholism can experience this type of hypoparathyroidism and hypocalcemia related to their other nutritional deficiencies. Pseudohypoparathyroidism is caused by inherited PTH resistance, which results in hypocalcemia accompanied by marked elevations of the serum PTH level.

Hypocalcemia may occur in acute pancreatitis, in which fatty acids released through the action of pancreatic enzymes complex with calcium. Hypocalcemia due to the formation of calcium phosphate complexes occurs in severe hyperphosphatemic states, such as kidney failure, rhabdomyolysis, and tumor lysis syndrome. Hypocalcemia may also be seen in patients given multiple erythrocyte transfusions using cells to which calcium chelators have been added. Hypocalcemia due to vitamin D deficiency is typically mild and asymptomatic.

- Hypocalcemia is diagnosed after the serum calcium level is less than normal on repeated measurements, even after correction for hypoalbuminemia, if present.

- If a patient's history and physical examination findings do not clearly indicate a cause of hypocalcemia, then kidney function and parathyroid hormone, magnesium, phosphorus, and vitamin D levels should be checked.

Treatment of Hypocalcemia

In patients with symptoms of marked hypocalcemia, calcium should be delivered by slow continuous intravenous infusion (for example, calcium gluconate as 0.5-1.5 mg elemental calcium/kg/h) to raise the serum calcium level until symptoms are relieved. Concurrently, any deficiency in magnesium or vitamin D should be corrected. Oral calcium should be administered as the intravenous infusion is tapered.

In patients with less severe hypocalcemia, oral administration of calcium should be sufficient. Older persons and those taking proton pump inhibitors may not absorb calcium well, and thus higher dosages may be needed. Vitamin D also should be provided. Recommended daily intake of dietary calcium and vitamin D is provided in **Table 31**. Patients who are vitamin D deficient may require replenishment of their stores before starting a standard daily dose (see later discussion).

In chronic hypoparathyroidism, long-term administration of 1,25-dihydroxyvitamin D is necessary because 1α-hydroxylase will not be active in the kidney in the absence of PTH. A starting dose of 0.25 microgram/d is typical, with titration upward as needed. In patients with hypoparathyroidism, the serum calcium level should be kept at or slightly lower than the lower limit of the normal range (sufficient to relieve symptoms and reverse tetanic signs). Higher serum

calcium levels may exacerbate hypercalciuria, which increases the risk of nephrocalcinosis or kidney stones. Periodic measurement of 24-hour urine calcium excretion is recommended to exclude hypercalciuria.

- In patients with hypoparathyroidism, the serum calcium level should be kept at or slightly less than the lower limit of normal, at a level sufficient to relieve symptoms and reverse tetanic signs; full normalization of this level often results in hypercalciuria, which increases the risk of nephrocalcinosis or kidney stones

Metabolic Bone Disease

Osteoporosis

Epidemiology and Physiology

Osteoporosis is defined as low bone mass involving trabecular bone microarchitecture and connectivity and a thinning of cortical bone, which lead to decreased bone strength and an increased risk of fracture (**Figure 16**). Osteoporosis results from genetic factors and diseases and medications that affect peak bone mass and contribute to the rate of bone loss with aging. Osteoporosis can be diagnosed by measuring bone mineral density (BMD), which reflects the bone calcium content and is a surrogate for bone mass. The World Health Organization (WHO) states that in postmenopausal women and men older than 50 years, osteoporosis is present when the BMD T-score is 2.5 or more standard deviations (SD) less than that of a healthy young adult reference population in whom bone density is at its peak (see later discussion). The presence of a vertebral or hip fracture sustained with low trauma is also diagnostic of osteoporosis. Osteopenia is present in this population when the T-score is 1.1 to 2.4 SDs less than peak bone density.

TABLE 31. U.S. Institute of Medicine 2010 Daily Recommended Intake of Calcium and Vitamin D[a,b]				
Group	Calcium Intake (mg)	Upper Limit of Calcium Intake (mg)	Vitamin D Intake (units)	Upper Limit of Vitamin D Intake (units)
Men and Women (19-50 y, including women who are pregnant and lactating)	1000	2500	600	4000
Men (51-70 y)	1000	2000	600	4000
Women (51-70 y)	1200	2000	600	4000
Men and Women (>70 y)	1200	2000	800	4000

[a]Released November 30, 2010, before U.S. Preventive Services Task Force recent draft statement on vitamin D and calcium supplementation for prevention of cancer and osteoporotic fractures in adults.

[b]For adults age 19 years and older.

Adapted with permission from The National Academies Press, Copyright 2011, National Academy of Sciences. Institute of Medicine of the National Academies. DRIs for Calcium and Vitamin D. 11/30/2011. Available at www.iom.edu/Reports/2010/Dietary-Reference-Intakes-for-Calcium-and-Vitamin-D.aspx. Accessed June 13, 2012.

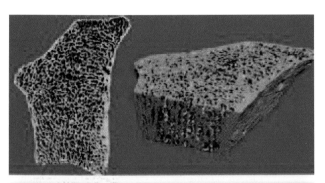

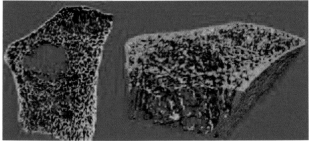

FIGURE 16. Osteoporotic bone. These images are three-dimensional micro-CT images of trabecular bone in the distal radius of a woman with normal bone density (*top*) and a woman with osteoporosis (*bottom*). Note the thinning and loss of trabeculae, which lead to loss of resistance to fracture.

Reprinted from Best Practice and Research in Clinical Endocrinology and Metabolism, 22(5). Griffith JF, Genant HK. Bone mass and architecture determination: state of the art. 752. [PMID: 19028355] Copyright 2008, with permission from Elsevier.

Peak bone mass is achieved in the late 20s or early 30s; after this age, bone density decreases slowly. Because peak bone mass is lower in women than men, women experience higher rates of fracture. The most common sites of fragility fractures are the hips, distal forearms, and vertebrae. The lifetime risk of experiencing any fragility fracture for white women is close to 50%, and for white men is close to 20%. The incidence of hip fracture in women and men at age 65 years is approximately 300 and 150, respectively, per 100,000 person-years. These rates increase to approximately 3000 and 2000, respectively, per 100,000 by age 85 years. Black persons generally have a higher BMD and lower risk for fracture than their white, Hispanic, or Asian counterparts. Hip fracture carries the highest morbidity and mortality of all fractures. Deaths typically occur from associated complications, such as pulmonary embolism and pneumonia. At least one third of patients with hip fracture return to their previous level of functioning, but 20% will require long-term nursing care. Because of the high cost to patients and insurers, preventing hip fracture is a major focus of osteoporosis management.

Bone remodeling occurs continuously in adults. A cycle of bone remodeling begins with the recruitment of bone-resorbing osteoclasts. Osteoblasts are then recruited and fill the resorption pit with new bone matrix. The matrix is then mineralized with hydroxyapatite. Through the process of bone remodeling, the skeleton is constantly rejuvenated and

mineral stores of the skeleton are made available to the body as needed. With advancing age, slightly less bone is formed than was resorbed during each remodeling cycle, which results in the gradual decline in bone mass with aging (see Figure 16). With this decrease in bone mass comes a concomitant increase in fracture risk. The age-related decline in bone mass occurs at a rate of approximately 0.1% to 0.5% per year in both sexes. In women, however, the rate of bone loss accelerates in the perimenopausal period and early menopause because of estrogen deficiency. After this period, a woman may have lost one quarter to one third of her total skeletal mass.

Risk factors for low bone mass and the resultant increased risk of fracture are shown in **Table 32**.

Evaluation

Measurement of bone density is an essential tool to assess fracture risk. Of the available modalities, dual-energy x-ray absorptiometry (DEXA) has the highest accuracy and precision and is most widely used in large clinical trials of osteoporosis medications. In a typical DEXA report, the BMD measurements are converted to T-scores and Z-scores (**Figure 17**). The T-score is the number of SDs the patient's BMD is higher or lower than the mean reference value for young, healthy, sex-matched persons at peak bone density. The Z-score represents the number of SDs the patient's BMD is higher or lower than the mean value for persons of the patient's age and sex. The T-score is used to diagnose osteoporosis and predict fracture risk. The most common sites measured by DEXA are the proximal femur and lumbar spine. In women, each SD less than the peak bone mass represents a loss of 10% to 12% of bone mineral content and corresponds to an approximately 2- to 2.5-fold increase in fracture risk at that site.

The 2010 National Osteoporosis Foundation (NOF) guidelines for osteoporosis screening appear in **Table 33**. DEXA is also appropriate to use in patients with conditions affecting bone mass (such as hyperparathyroidism) and for monitoring patients receiving osteoporosis therapy. When patients begin prescription osteoporosis therapy, their T-scores will improve slightly, but their fracture risk may decline by as much as 30% to 50%. Therefore, in patients receiving therapy for osteoporosis, BMD changes over time, rather than T-scores, should be monitored every 1 to 2 years using the same densitometer.

After the diagnosis of osteoporosis is made, the clinician should consider a selective evaluation for secondary causes of low bone mass if the patient's age and comorbid conditions do not provide an explanation (**Table 34**). A comprehensive history and physical examination can reveal underlying conditions associated with bone loss. The evaluation also should assess the patient for risk factors of low bone mass (see Table 32). Routine blood chemistry studies are reasonable, including a complete blood count and

TABLE 32.	Risk Factors for Low Bone Mass and Fractures

Nonmodifiable Risk Factors

Advanced age

Female sex

First-degree relative with history of hip fracture

Personal history of fragility fracture

Postmenopausal status

White or Asian ancestry

Modifiable Risk Factors

Alcohol abuse

Low body weight

Sedentary lifestyle

Smoking

Conditions

Anorexia nervosa

Chronic kidney disease

Chronic liver disease

COPD

Cushing syndrome

Growth hormone deficiency

Hyperparathyroidism

Hypogonadism

Intestinal malabsorption

Monoclonal gammopathy

Organ transplantation

Rheumatoid arthritis

Thyrotoxicosis

Medications

Carbamazepine

Corticosteroids

Depot medroxyprogesterone acetate

Leuprolide

Phenytoin

Proton pump inhibitors

Causes of Falls

Cognitive decline

Decreased mobility

Impaired neuromuscular function

Low visual acuity

Sedative drug use

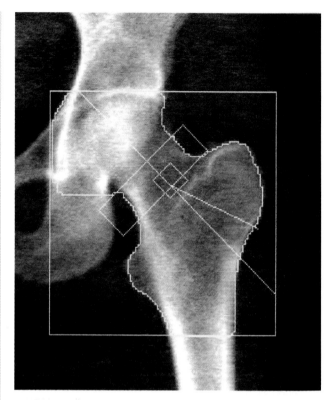

DXA Results Summary:

Region	Area (cm²)	BMC (g)	BMD (g/cm²)	T-Score	Z-Score
Neck	4.75	2.76	0.580	-2.4	-1.7
Troch	7.95	3.58	0.450	-2.5	-2.1
Inter	20.10	14.78	0.735	-2.4	-2.1
Total	**32.80**	**21.11**	**0.644**	**-2.4**	**-2.0**

FIGURE 17. Sample hip dual-energy x-ray absorptiometry report. The scan image of the left hip region shows positioning of the hip, with regions analyzed outlined in yellow. Of particular interest are the total hip (contents of large rectangle) and the femoral neck (contents of small rectangle). The analysis provides the bone mineral density and the patient's results expressed as Z-scores (standard deviations from same-age reference group) and T-scores (standard deviations from young adult reference group at peak bone mass). This patient has osteopenia (T-score of −2.4) in both the femoral neck and total hip. The Z-scores indicate that the bone density is considerably below the age-matched reference range, which raises concern that a condition besides aging has contributed to bone loss. BMC = bone mineral content; BMD = bone mineral density; DXA = dual-energy x-ray absorptiometry; Inter = intertrochanteric space; Troch = greater trochanter.

measurement of serum levels of calcium, phosphorus, electrolytes, creatinine, 25-hydroxyvitamin D, and alkaline phosphatase. Measurement of the serum PTH level is recommended if the serum calcium level is elevated. An elevated PTH level in the setting of a low calcium level and/or low 25-hydroxyvitamin D level indicates secondary hyperparathyroidism, which also can cause bone loss. Subclinical hyperthyroidism should be ruled out by determining the serum thyroid-stimulating hormone level. A 24-hour urine calcium level may reveal calcium malabsorption or excessive

TABLE 33. Guidelines for Osteoporosis Screening

Women age ≥65 y

Men and women age >50 y with fragility or low-trauma fracture

Postmenopausal women age <65 y with one or more of the following risk factors for future fragility fracture: personal history of fracture, secondary cause of low bone mass, low body weight, current smoker, alcohol abuse, or a first-degree family member with a hip fracture

Men and premenopausal women with secondary cause of low bone mass or personal history of low trauma or fragility fracture

Data from National Osteoporosis Foundation. Clinician's Guide to Prevention and Treatment of Osteoporosis. Available at: www.nof.org/sites/default/files/pdfs/NOF_ClinicianGuide2009_v7.pdf, p 13-14. Accessed May 11, 2012.

TABLE 34. Secondary Causes of Low Bone Mass

Endocrine disorders: hyperparathyroidism, osteomalacia, Cushing syndrome, hypogonadism, hyperthyroidism, acromegaly, and diabetes mellitus

Hematopoietic disorders: myeloma, sickle cell disease, thalassemia minor, leukemia, lymphoma, and polycythemia vera

Connective tissue disorders: systemic lupus erythematosus and rheumatoid arthritis

Kidney disease: chronic kidney disease, renal tubular acidosis, and hypercalciuria

Gastrointestinal conditions: malabsorption (gastrectomy, primary biliary cirrhosis, celiac disease, gastric bypass surgery, pancreatic insufficiency, and inflammatory bowel disease)

Exogenous: corticosteroids, proton pump inhibitors, anticonvulsants, heparin, gonadotropin-releasing hormone agonists, depot medroxyprogesterone, chemotherapeutic agents, and excessive alcohol

Genetic: osteogenesis imperfecta, homocystinuria, Marfan syndrome, cystic fibrosis, and hemochromatosis

kidney calcium losses. Testosterone levels should be checked in men who have risk factors or symptoms of hypogonadism, with replacement therapy initiated if indicated. Testing for monoclonal gammopathy in older adults may be appropriate because asymptomatic monoclonal gammopathy may cause bone loss. If no cause is found for the osteoporosis, it is considered idiopathic. Idiopathic osteoporosis is rare in premenopausal women but accounts for approximately 50% of osteoporosis in men of all ages.

Prediction of Fracture Risk

The DEXA T-score allows the prediction of a patient's relative fracture risk. The Fracture Risk Assessment Tool (FRAX) developed by the WHO was designed to predict the absolute fracture risk. Based on data from cohorts around the globe, the FRAX is a Web-based tool (http:www.shef.ac.uk/FRAX/index.jsp)

that incorporates major risk factors and a patient's femoral neck T-score (if available) to calculate an absolute fracture risk over the next 10 years.

FRAX does not include all components of a patient's fracture risk, such as tendency to fall. The effect of osteoporosis drugs on fracture risk as calculated with FRAX is unknown. Nevertheless, the NOF now recommends that FRAX be used as a component of decision-making when deciding which patients with osteopenia may benefit from treatment with antiosteoporotic medications.

Prevention of Osteoporosis and Fracture

First Steps

Lifestyle modifications and adjustment of modifiable risk factors (see Table 32) are the first steps in preventing or treating osteoporosis. Physical therapy evaluation may be appropriate for patients considered at high risk for falls. For frail older patients, medications that may predispose to dizziness should be avoided.

Persons of all ages must consume adequate amounts of both calcium and vitamin D to maintain bone health. Additionally, calcium and vitamin D supplementation has a beneficial effect on postmenopausal bone loss, although not as dramatic as is seen with antiresorptive or anabolic therapies. Recently, the recommended daily allowances of calcium and vitamin D were revised by the U.S. Institute of Medicine (IOM) (see Table 31), and a new vitamin D guideline was provided by the Endocrine Society in 2011. However, controversy exists about the need for higher dosages of calcium and vitamin D supplementation in some populations. In June 2012, the U.S. Preventive Services Task Force (USPSTF) released a draft recommendation statement recommending against supplementation with greater than 1000 mg/d of calcium or with 400 units/d or more of vitamin D for primary prevention of fractures in healthy community-dwelling women who are postmenopausal because of lack of evidence showing safety or efficacy. The USPSTF does, however, recommend vitamin D supplementation for preventing falls in noninstitutionalized older persons.

Antiosteoporosis Pharmacologic Therapy

Osteoporosis is most often prevented or treated with antiresorptive agents (**Table 35**). FDA-approved antiresorptive agents for the treatment of low bone mass include bisphosphonates, selective estrogen receptor modulators, and calcitonin. All of these agents reduce vertebral and nonvertebral (multiple sites, including the hip) fracture rates by 30% to 60% over 2 to 3 years. Only some of the bisphosphonates (and estrogen) have been shown specifically to reduce hip fracture risk. For the prevention of osteoporosis in women, the antiresorptive agents approved by the FDA are alendronate, ibandronate, risedronate, zoledronate, raloxifene, and estrogen.

TABLE 35. FDA-Approved Medications for Osteoporosis and Approved Indications

Medication	Postmenopausal Osteoporosis		Osteoporosis in Men	Corticosteroid-Induced Osteoporosis	
	Prevention	Treatment	Treatment	Prevention	Treatment
Estrogens[a]	Yes	No	No	No	No
Calcitonin[a]	No	Yes[b]	No	No	No
Raloxifene	Yes	Yes	No	No	No
Alendronate[a,c]	Yes	Yes	Yes	No	Yes
Ibandronate[d]	Yes	Yes	No	No	No
Risedronate[a,e]	Yes	Yes	Yes	Yes	Yes
Zoledronate[f]	Yes	Yes	Yes	Yes	Yes
Denosumab[g]	No	Yes	No	No	No
Teriparatide	No	Yes	Yes	No	No

[a]Generic preparation available in the United States.

[b]More than 5 years after menopause.

[c]Oral daily or weekly dosing.

[d]Oral monthly dosing; intravenous dosing every 3 months.

[e]Oral daily, weekly, or monthly dosing.

[f]Intravenous dosing once yearly.

[g]Subcutaneous injection every 6 months.

Bisphosphonates bind to the bone matrix and decrease osteoclast activity, thereby slowing bone resorption while new bone formation and mineralization continue. Alendronate and risedronate have been studied most extensively; over a period of 2 to 3 years, these drugs produce a 6% increase in bone density and a 30% to 50% reduction in fracture risk at both vertebral and nonvertebral sites. Ibandronate reduces the risk of vertebral fracture by as much as 50% after 3 years of therapy but has not been shown in clinical trials to prevent hip fracture. No clear benefit of newer bisphosphonate drugs versus older agents has been demonstrated; the older drugs are available in generic form and may be more cost-effective for long-term therapy (see Table 35). Esophagitis is a risk of oral bisphosphonate therapy, and thus these agents are contraindicated in patients with active esophageal disease or swallowing disorders. Intravenous bisphosphonates are preferred for women with postmenopausal osteoporosis who are unable to take oral bisphosphonates or who desire the convenience of less frequent dosing. However, the costs of these drugs and their administration are significantly greater than those of available oral agents. Intravenous ibandronate is given every 3 months, whereas zoledronate is administered annually. Zoledronate reduces the risk of fracture of the hip and other skeletal sites. An acute-phase reaction (flulike symptoms for several days) is a common adverse effect of zoledronate. Bisphosphonate therapy is not recommended for patients with impaired kidney function (creatinine clearance less than 30-35 mL/min [0.030-0.035 L/min] [normal, 90-140 mL/min {0.09-0.14 L/min}]).

Osteonecrosis of the jaw has been described in patients taking bisphosphonates and is more likely to occur in patients undergoing treatment for cancer who receive frequent doses of intravenous bisphosphonates. The risk of this complication with the dosages used for osteoporosis treatment is estimated at 1 in 10,000. Special care is necessary when patients require dental procedures because extractions may increase the risk of osteonecrosis. Persons with any defect in jaw architecture or with upcoming jaw surgery should not take bisphosphonates. Stopping ongoing therapy for dental procedures is of limited utility because the agents remain in the bone matrix long after discontinuation. Bisphosphonates should be avoided in women of childbearing age. Because of the long biologic half-life of bisphosphonates, a theoretical risk of passage to the fetus exists, even in patients no longer taking them.

Given the persistence of bisphosphonates in the bone matrix, concern exists about adverse effects of prolonged therapy, including an association with atypical femoral fractures. To date, bisphosphonates have not been conclusively proved to be causative. Nevertheless, the FDA issued a Drug Safety Communication in 2010 recommending that patients receiving bisphosphonate therapy be reassessed periodically, particularly after 5 years of use, to determine if treatment remains appropriate. Many experts recommend that after 5 years of therapy, patients be considered for a "drug holiday" lasting 2 years or more. For patients with severe osteoporosis or ongoing fractures, treatment with teriparatide during the bisphosphonate drug holiday should be considered. Persons on drug holiday should be monitored for fracture and evidence of reactivation of bone loss (by BMD testing every 1-2 years); therapy should be restarted if reactivation of bone loss is evident.

Raloxifene, a selective estrogen receptor modulator, is an estrogen agonist in bone but an estrogen antagonist in the breast and uterus. Vertebral fracture risk reduction with raloxifene is comparable to that of estrogen or bisphosphonate therapy. Raloxifene has not been shown, however, to prevent hip fractures. Also, patients treated with raloxifene have a 1.4- to 1.5-fold increased risk of fatal stroke and thromboembolism. Raloxifene is a good choice for women whose bone loss is primarily in the spine, who have a relatively low risk of hip fracture, and who are unable to tolerate oral bisphosphonates. Although generally well tolerated, this drug may exacerbate menopausal hot flushes. Raloxifene is not approved for use in men or premenopausal women.

The beneficial effects of calcitonin are much less pronounced than those of other antiresorptive agents. Calcitonin injections and nasal spray are approved for the treatment of established osteoporosis but not for its prevention. Calcitonin has been shown to prevent primarily vertebral fractures and is generally safe and well tolerated. Because of the availability of other safe and more potent drugs, calcitonin is rarely used for osteoporosis treatment except when other options are lacking.

The use of estrogen to maintain bone health has fallen out of favor because of data from the Women's Health Initiative indicating that estrogen increases the risk of cardiovascular disease and breast cancer. Therefore, estrogen use for osteoporosis prevention should be limited to women who also require its beneficial effects for hot flushes or vaginal dryness.

Denosumab is the newest available antiresorptive agent. This drug is a humanized monoclonal antibody directed against the receptor activator of nuclear factor κB (RANK) ligand, a key signal in activating bone resorption. This leads to decreased osteoclastogenesis. Approved only for women with postmenopausal osteoporosis and a high risk of fracture, denosumab is administered by injection every 6 months. Fracture prevention by denosumab is comparable to that seen with bisphosphonate therapy. Common adverse effects include musculoskeletal pain, hyperlipidemia, and cystitis. An increased risk of infections, particularly skin infections, and osteonecrosis of the jaw also have been reported in association with denosumab use. Denosumab is not appropriate for use in persons who are immunosuppressed or who have hypocalcemia. Given its similar efficacy for fracture prevention as bisphosphonates and its significant risk factor profile and expense, denosumab is not generally used for routine treatment of postmenopausal osteoporosis.

Teriparatide (recombinant human PTH [1-34]) is currently the only available anabolic agent for osteoporosis therapy in the United States and is generally used in patients with severe osteoporosis (T-score ≤−3.5), recurrent fractures, or

continuing bone loss while taking other medications. Although chronic elevation of the serum PTH level results in bone loss, transient spikes have anabolic effects on bone. A daily subcutaneous injection of teriparatide provides a brief increase in the serum PTH level and results in increased BMD. The effects are particularly dramatic in the spine; one study comparing 14 months of teriparatide therapy with alendronate treatment showed that alendronate-treated patients had a 5.6% increase in lumbar spine BMD, whereas teriparatide-treated patients had a 12.2% increase. Teriparatide has a "black box" warning from the FDA concerning a risk of osteosarcoma, which is based on the increased incidence seen in rats. For this reason, the drug is administered for no longer than 2 years, and its use is contraindicated in patients with hyperparathyroidism, Paget disease, unexplained elevation of the alkaline phosphatase level, malignancy involving bone, or a history of radiation therapy. Selection of patients for this costly and potent drug requires care, and consultation with an endocrinologist should be considered.

Simultaneous administration of teriparatide and oral bisphosphonates impairs the anabolic effects of teriparatide and thus is not recommended. When bisphosphonates are used after completion of a course of teriparatide, the increase in BMD due to teriparatide therapy is preserved and followed by additional gain during subsequent bisphosphonate treatment. In clinical practice, many patients being considered for teriparatide therapy have already received long-term bisphosphonate therapy. Whether these patients benefit as much from teriparatide as bisphosphonate-naïve patients do is unclear.

The most comprehensive set of guidelines for identifying patients who will benefit from treatment of low bone mass were updated by the NOF in 2010 (**Table 36**). Follow-up DEXA (using the same machine, if possible) is recommended every 1 to 2 years initially to monitor response to therapy. Stable or improved bone density indicates appropriate response to therapy. Bone loss while receiving

TABLE 36. NOF 2010 Guidelines for Pharmacologic Treatment of Patients with Osteoporosis

Men age >50 y or postmenopausal women with osteoporosis *OR* prior vertebral or hip fracture

Men age >50 y or postmenopausal women with osteopenia *AND* a prior fragility fracture or other medical issues that increase fracture risk

Men and women with osteopenia *AND* a 3% or greater probability of hip fracture or a 20% or greater probability of other major osteoporotic fracture over the next 10 years[a]

NOF = National Osteoporosis Foundation.

[a]Percentages determined by using the U.S.-adapted WHO Fracture Risk Assessment Tool (FRAX) algorithm.

Data from National Osteoporosis Foundation. Clinician's Guide to Prevention and Treatment of Osteoporosis. Available at: www.nof.org/sites/default/files/pdfs/NOF_ClinicianGuide2009_v7.pdf. Accessed July 5, 2012.

therapy should prompt evaluation of medication adherence and unrecognized secondary causes of bone loss (as discussed previously).

- Dual-energy x-ray absorptiometry has the highest accuracy and precision of the modalities available for measuring bone mineral density and assessing fracture risk and is most widely used in large clinical trials of osteoporosis medications.
- Osteoporosis is most often treated with antiresorptive agents, such as bisphosphonates, selective estrogen receptor modulators, and calcitonin; teriparatide is currently the only available anabolic agent for osteoporosis treatment in the United States.

Osteomalacia

In osteomalacia, the bone matrix is normal in quantity but weakened by insufficient mineral content. Osteomalacia in the growing skeleton is termed rickets and is associated with bony deformities, including bowing of the legs. Causes of osteomalacia include deficiencies of calcium, phosphate, or vitamin D, but inhibition of mineralization from any cause may be responsible. These deficiencies may result from nutritional insufficiency, intestinal malabsorption, or abnormalities in vitamin D metabolism due to liver disease, kidney disease (renal tubular acidosis, chronic kidney disease), or antiepileptic drugs. Rarely, osteomalacia occurs because of genetic vitamin D resistance, inherited kidney disorders of phosphate wasting, or oncogenic osteomalacia (a humoral syndrome of increased urine phosphate loss associated with rare tumors of mesenchymal origin). Osteomalacia presents in adults as proximal muscle weakness and diffuse or focal skeletal pain. Osteomalacia also can be asymptomatic, with diagnosis based on clinical evaluation and laboratory and imaging results. Decreased or low-normal levels of calcium and phosphorus are noted, as is an elevated alkaline phosphatase level. Depending on the cause, decreased levels of either 25-hydroxyvitamin D or 1,25-dihydroxyvitamin D may be seen. Plain films may show osteopenia or pseudofractures. When necessary, the diagnosis can be confirmed with a bone biopsy analyzed by an experienced bone pathologist.

The treatment of osteomalacia depends on the pathogenesis of the condition. For patients with dietary insufficiency or malabsorption of vitamin D, high doses of cholecalciferol and calcium (see Table 31) will rapidly correct deficits and heal the bone. An assessment for underlying disorders (such as celiac disease, which may be asymptomatic) should be performed, with other evaluations if indicated. Phosphate-wasting conditions require a different approach, such as phosphate supplementation or localization and removal of any causative tumor.

- For most patients with osteomalacia caused by dietary insufficiency or malabsorption of vitamin D, administration of high doses of cholecalciferol and calcium will rapidly correct deficits and heal the bone.

Vitamin D Deficiency

Guidelines for screening for vitamin D deficiency are lacking, but risk factors include advanced age, dark skin, low sun exposure, and fat malabsorption. Vitamin D deficiency is diagnosed in patients with a low serum 25-hydroxyvitamin D level. The optimal level is currently a matter of debate, with the IOM recommending a level of 20 ng/mL (50 nmol/L) and the Endocrine Society endorsing a level of 30 ng/mL (75 nmol/L). Vitamin D levels are adequate for skeletal health at 20 ng/mL (50 nmol/L), but nonskeletal benefits may require a level of 30 ng/mL (75 nmol/L). The evidence supporting skeletal benefits at a vitamin D level of 20 ng/mL (50 nmol/L) is more robust than is the evidence for the nonskeletal benefits achieved at a level of 30 ng/mL (75 nmol/L). The IOM (see Table 31) and the Endocrine Society recommend the same daily vitamin D dose for each demographic group, but the Endocrine Society cautions that adults may need doses as high as 1500 to 2000 units/d to achieve their recommended serum target level of 30 ng/mL (75 nmol/L) (but see previous discussion of the draft recommendation statement from the USPSTF). For those found to be vitamin D deficient (defined as a 25-hydroxyvitamin D level less than 20 ng/mL [50 nmol/L]), the Endocrine Society recommends a course of ergocalciferol, 50,000 units weekly for 8 weeks, followed by confirmation of a normal serum 25-hydroxyvitamin D level.

Paget Disease of Bone

Clinical Features and Evaluation

Paget disease of bone is a condition in which abnormal osteoclast function leads to accelerated and disordered bone remodeling, which produces highly disorganized and brittle bone microarchitecture in affected areas. This process sometimes leads to deformity of affected bones, increased bone vascularity, nerve impingement syndromes, and a propensity to fracture. Paget disease of bone is commonly seen in older persons and may be familial. The precise cause is unknown, although an inherited or viral origin (or a combination of the two) is suspected. Most persons with Paget disease are asymptomatic, with increased serum alkaline phosphatase levels detected incidentally on blood testing or pathognomonic changes discovered on radiographs. If the disease is severe or extensive, bony deformity and pain result, either from the bony lesions themselves or from complications of the abnormal bone, such as nerve compression, degenerative arthritis or osteosarcoma. The skull may be enlarged, and significant bowing of the long bones of the legs may occur. Skull involvement may cause a sensorineural hearing loss, and bony overgrowth may lead to local impingement on spinal nerve roots with pain or neurologic deficits. Rare complications include high-output heart failure from multiple vascular shunts in bone and transformation to osteosarcoma.

The diagnosis of Paget disease typically is made after finding isolated elevation of the serum alkaline phosphatase level without other evidence of liver disease. A nuclear bone scan is then performed to locate the involved areas (**Figure 18**). Plain radiographs of these areas should be evaluated to exclude metastatic disease and confirm the pagetic findings.

Treatment

Treatment of Paget disease is indicated for patients with bone pain and for patients with involvement of the skull, weight-bearing bones, or joints. The goal of treatment is to decrease pain and reduce risk of pathologic fracture. High-dose antiresorptive agents are given, such as a 2-month course of risedronate, 30 mg/d orally, or a single dose of an injectable bisphosphonate (see previous discussion). Injectable calcitonin is less effective but can be used in patients with impaired kidney function. Disease activity and response to therapy are assessed by serial measurement of alkaline phosphatase levels. The goal of treatment is normalization of the alkaline phosphatase level. Retreatment is indicated if the alkaline phosphatase level (checked every 3 to 6 months) is greater than normal. Patients with skull involvement should also have periodic audiometry to exclude hearing loss.

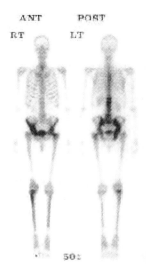

FIGURE 18. Whole-body bone scan images from a patient with Paget disease showing intense tracer uptake in the right proximal tibia, pelvis, left proximal femur and lumbar spine. ANT = anterior; LT = left; POST = posterior; RT = right.

- In Paget disease of bone, disease activity and response to therapy are assessed by serial measurement of the alkaline phosphatase level.

Bibliography

Diabetes Mellitus

ACCORD Study Group, Cushman WC, Evans GW, Byington RP, et al. Effects of intensive blood-pressure control in type 2 diabetes mellitus. N Engl J Med. 2010;362(17):1575-1585. [PMID: 20228401]

Athyros VG, Tziomalos K, Gossios TD, et al; GREACE Study Collaborative Group. Safety and efficacy of long-term statin treatment for cardiovascular events in patients with coronary heart disease and abnormal liver tests in the Greek Atorvastatin and Coronary Heart Disease Evaluation (GREACE) Study: a post-hoc analysis. Lancet. 2010;376(9756):1916-1922. [PMID: 21109302]

Calles-Escandón J, Lovato LC, Simons-Morton DG, et al. Effect of intensive compared with standard glycemia treatment strategies on mortality by baseline subgroup characteristics: the Action to Control Cardiovascular Risk in Diabetes (ACCORD) trial. Diabetes Care. 2010;33(4):721-727. [PMID: 20103550]

Cengiz E, Tamborlane WV, Martin-Fredericksen M, Dziura J, Weinzimer SA. Early pharmacokinetic and pharmacodynamic effects of mixing lispro with glargine insulin: results of glucose clamp studies in youth with type 1 diabetes. Diabetes Care. 2010;33(5):1009-1012. [PMID: 20150302]

International Association of Diabetes and Pregnancy Study Groups Consensus Panel, Metzger BE, Gabbe SJ, Persson B, et al. International Association of Diabetes and Pregnancy Study Groups recommendations on the diagnosis and classification of hyperglycemia in pregnancy. Diabetes Care. 2010;33(3):676-682. [PMID: 20190296]

Juvenile Diabetes Research Foundation Continuous Glucose Monitoring Study Group, Tamborlane WV, Beck RW, Bode BW, et al. Continuous glucose monitoring and intensive treatment of type 1 diabetes. N Engl J Med. 2008;359(14):1464-1476. [PMID: 18779236]

Moghissi ES, Korytkowski MT, DiNardo M, et al; American Association of Clinical Endocrinologists; American Diabetes Association. American Association of Clinical Endocrinologists and American Diabetes Association consensus statement on inpatient glycemic control. Diabetes Care. 2009;32(6):1119-1131. [PMID: 19429873]

O'Kane MJ, Bunting B, Copeland M, Coates VE; ESMON Study Group. Efficacy of self monitoring of blood glucose in patients with newly diagnosed type 2 diabetes (ESMON study): randomised controlled trial. BMJ. 2008;336(7654):1174-1177. [PMID: 18420662]

Poolsup N, Suksomboon N, Rattanasookchit S. Meta-analysis of the benefits of self-monitoring of blood glucose on glycemic control in type 2 diabetes patients: an update. Diabetes Technol Ther. 2009;11(12):775-784. [PMID: 20001678]

Umpierrez GE, Hellman R, Korytkowski MT, et al; Endocrine Society. Management of hyperglycemia in hospitalized patients in non-critical care setting: an Endocrine Society clinical practice guideline. J Clin Endocrinol Metab. 2012;97(1):16-38. [PMID: 22223765]

Zeller M, Danchin N, Simon D, et al; French Registry of Acute ST-Elevation and Non–ST-Elevation Myocardial Infarction Investigators. Impact of type of preadmission sulfonylureas on mortality and cardiovascular outcomes in diabetic patients with acute myocardial infarction. J Clin Endocrinol Metab. 2010;95(11):4993-5002. [PMID: 20702526]

Disorders of the Pituitary Gland

Cook DM, Yuen KC, Biller BM, Kemp SF, Vance ML; American Association of Clinical Endocrinologists. American Association of Clinical Endocrinologists medical guidelines for clinical practice for growth hormone use in growth hormone–deficient adults and transition patients—2009 update. Endocr Pract. 2009;15(Supppl 2):1-29. [PMID: 20228036]

Freda PU, Beckers AM, Katznelson L, et al; Endocrine Society. Pituitary incidentaloma: an Endocrine Society clinical practice guideline. J Clin Endocrinol Metab. 2011;96(4):894-904. [PMID: 21474686]

Laws ER, Jane JA Jr. Neurosurgical approach to treating pituitary adenomas. Growth Horm IGF Res. 2005;15(Suppl A):S36-S41. [PMID: 16039890]

Loh JA, Verbalis JG. Disorders of water and salt metabolism associated with pituitary disease. Endocrinol Metab Clin North Am. 2008;37(1):213-234. [PMID: 18226738]

Melmed S, Casanueva FF, Hoffman AR, et al; Endocrine Society. Diagnosis and treatment of hyperprolactinemia: an Endocrine Society clinical practice guideline. J Clin Endocrinol Metab. 2011;96(2):273-288. [PMID: 21296991]

Melmed S, Colao A, Barkan A, et al; Acromegaly Consensus Group. Guidelines for acromegaly management: an update. J Clin Endocrinol Metab. 2009;94(5):1509-1517. [PMID: 19208732]

Molitch ME. Prolactinomas and pregnancy. Clin Endocrinol (Oxf). 2010;73(2):147-148. [PMID: 20550542]

Sheehan JP, Pouratian N, Steiner L, Laws ER, Vance ML. Gamma Knife surgery for pituitary adenomas: factors related to radiological and endocrine outcomes. J Neurosurg. 2011;114(2):303-309. [PMID: 20540596]

Toogood AA, Stewart PM. Hypopituitarism: clinical features, diagnosis, and management. Endocrinol Metab Clin North Am. 2008;37(1):235-261. [PMID: 18226739]

Disorders of the Thyroid Gland

American Thyroid Association (ATA) Guidelines Taskforce on Thyroid Nodules and Differentiated Thyroid Cancer, Cooper DS, Doherty GM, Haugen BR, et al. Revised American Thyroid Association management guidelines for patients with thyroid nodules and differentiated thyroid cancer [errata in Thyroid. 2010;20(6):674-675 and Thyroid. 2010;20(8):942]. Thyroid. 2009;19(11):1167-1214. [PMID: 19860577] Also available at: www.thyroidguidelines.org/revised/taskforce. Accessed June 8, 2012.

American Thyroid Association Guidelines Taskforce, Kloos RT, Eng C, Evans DB, et al. Medullary thyroid cancer: management guidelines of the American Thyroid Association [erratum in Thyroid. 2009;19(11):1295]. Thyroid. 2009;19(6):565-612. [PMID: 19469690] Also available at: http://thyroidguidelines.net/medullary/taskforce. Accessed June 8, 2012.

Bahn RS, Burch HB, Cooper DS, et al; American Thyroid Association; American Association of Clinical Endocrinologists. Hyperthyroidism and other causes of thyrotoxicosis: management guidelines of the American Thyroid Association and American Association of Clinical Endocrinologists. Endocr Pract. 2011;17(3):456-520. [PMID: 21700562] Also available at: http://thyroidguidelines.net/hyperthyroidism. Accessed June 8, 2012.

Cooper DS. Approach to the patient with subclinical hyperthyroidism. J Clin Endocrinol Metab. 2007;92(1):3-9. [PMID: 17209221]

Devdhar M, Ousman YH, Burman KD. Hypothyroidism. Endocrinol Metab Clin North Am. 2007;36(3):595-615. [PMID: 17673121]

Franklyn JA. Subclinical thyroid disorders—consequences and implications for treatment. Ann Endocrinol (Paris). 2007;68(4):229-230. [PMID: 17651685]

Kwaku MP, Burman KD. Myxedema coma. J Intensive Care Med. 2007;22(4):224-231. [PMID: 17712058]

Nayak B, Burman K. Thyrotoxicosis and thyroid storm. Endocrinol Metab Clin North Am. 2006;35(4):663-686. [PMID: 17127140]

Poppe K, Velkeniers B, Glinoer D. Thyroid disease and female reproduction. Clin Endocrinol (Oxf). 2007;66(3):309-321. [PMID: 17302862]

Stagnaro-Green A, Abalovich M, Alexander E, et al; American Thyroid Association Taskforce on Thyroid Disease During Pregnancy and Postpartum. Thyroid. 2011;21(10):1081-1125. [PMID: 21787128]

Surks MI, Boucai L. Age- and race-based serum thyrotropin reference limits. J Clin Endocrinol Metab. 2010;95(2):496-502. [PMID: 19965925]

Surks MI, Ortiz E, Daniels GH, et al. Subclinical thyroid disease: scientific review and guidelines for diagnosis and management. JAMA. 2004;291(2):228-238. [PMID: 14722150]

Wartofsky L. Myxedema coma. Endocrinol Metab Clin North Am. 2006;35(4):687-698. [PMID: 17127141]

Yassa L, Marqusee E, Fawcett R, Alexander EK. Thyroid hormone early adjustment in pregnancy (the THERAPY) trial. J Clin Endocrinol Metab. 2010;95(7):3234-3241. [PMID: 20463094]

Disorders of the Adrenal Glands

Al-Aridi R, Abdelmannan D, Arafah BM. Biochemical diagnosis of adrenal insufficiency: the added value of dehydroepiandrosterone sulfate measurements. Endocr Pract. 2011;17(2):261-270. [PMID: 21134877]

Allolio B, Fassnacht M. Clinical review: adrenocortical carcinoma: clinical update. J Clin Endocrinol Metab. 2006;91(6):2027-2037. [PMID: 16551738]

Arafah BM. Hypothalamic pituitary adrenal function during critical illness: limitations of current assessment methods. J Clin Endocrinol Metab. 2006;91(10):3725-3745. [PMID: 16882746]

Bornstein SR. Predisposing factors for adrenal insufficiency. N Engl J Med. 2009;360(22):2328-2339. [PMID: 19474430]

Funder JW, Carey RM, Fardella C, et al; Endocrine Society. Case detection, diagnosis, and treatment of patients with primary hyperaldosteronism: an Endocrine Society clinical practice guideline. J Clin Endocrinol Metab. 2008;93(9):3266-3281. [PMID: 18552288]

Lenders JW, Eisenhofer G, Mannelli M, Pacak K. Phaeochromocytoma. Lancet. 2005;366(9486):665-675. [PMID: 16112304]

Nieman LK. Approach to the patient with an adrenal incidentaloma. J Clin Endocrinol Metab. 2010;95(9):4106-4113. [PMID: 20823463]

Nieman LK, Biller BM, Findling JW, et al. The diagnosis of Cushing's syndrome: an Endocrine Society clinical practice guideline. J Clin Endocrinol Metab. 2008;93(5):1526-1540. [PMID: 18334580]

Sprung CL, Annane D, Keh D, et al; CORTICUS Study Group. Hydrocortisone therapy for patients with septic shock. N Engl J Med. 2008;358(2):111-124. [PMID: 18184957]

Young WF Jr. Clinical practice. The incidentally discovered adrenal mass. N Engl J Med. 2007;356(6):601-610. [PMID: 17287480]

Reproductive Disorders

Basaria S, Coviello AD, Travison TG, et al. Adverse events associated with testosterone administration. N Engl J Med. 2010;363(2):109-122. [PMID: 20592293]

Bhasin S, Cunningham GR, Hayes FJ, et al; Task Force, Endocrine Society. Testosterone therapy in men with androgen deficiency syndromes: an Endocrine Society clinical practice guideline. J Clin Endocrinol Metab. 2010;95(6):2536-2559. [PMID: 20525905]

Gordon CM. Clinical practice. Functional hypothalamic amenorrhea. N Engl J Med. 2010;363(4):365-371. [PMID: 20660404]

Hoffman LK, Ehrmann DA. Cardiometabolic features of polycystic ovary syndrome. Nat Clin Pract Endocrinol Metab. 2008;4(4):215-222. [PMID: 18250636]

Martin KA, Chang RJ, Ehrmann DA, et al. Evaluation and treatment of hirsutism in premenopausal women: an Endocrine Society clinical practice guideline. J Clin Endocrinol Metab. 2008;93(4):1105-1120. [PMID: 18252793]

Nelson LM. Clinical practice. Primary ovarian insufficiency. N Engl J Med. 2009;360(6):606-614. [PMID: 19196677]

Nestler JE. Metformin for the treatment of the polycystic ovary syndrome. N Engl J Med. 2008;358(1):47-54. [PMID: 18172174]

Qaseem A, Snow V, Denberg TD, et al; Clinical Efficacy Assessment Subcommittee of the American College of Physicians. Hormonal testing and pharmacologic treatment of erectile dysfunction: a clinical practice guideline from the American College of Physicians. Ann Intern Med. 2009;151(9):639-649. [PMID: 19884625]

Rosner W, Vesper H; Endocrine Society; American Association for Clinical Chemistry; American Association of Clinical Endocrinologists; Androgen Excess/PCOS Society; American Society for Bone and Mineral Research; American Society for Reproductive Medicine; American Urological Association; Association of Public Health Laboratories; Laboratory Corporation of America; North American Menopause Society; Pediatric Endocrine Society. Toward excellence in testosterone testing: a consensus statement. J Clin Endocrinol Metab. 2010;95(10):4542-4548. [PMID: 20926540]

Yeap BB. Testosterone and ill-health in aging men. Nat Clin Pract Endocrinol Metab. 2009;5(2):113-121. [PMID: 19165223]

Calcium and Bone Disorders

Bilezikian JP, Khan AA, Potts JT Jr; Third International Workshop on the Management of Asymptomatic Primary Hyperthyroidism. Guidelines for the management of asymptomatic primary hyperparathyroidism: summary statement from the third international workshop. J Clin Endocrinol Metab. 2009;94(2):335-339. [PMID: 19193908]

Body JJ, Gaich GA, Scheele WH, et al. A randomized double-blind trial to compare the efficacy of teriparatide [recombinant human parathyroid hormone (1-34)] with alendronate in postmenopausal women with osteoporosis. J Clin Endocrinol Metab. 2002;87(10):4528-4535. [PMID: 12364430]

Holick, MF. Vitamin D deficiency. New Engl J Med. 2007;357(3):266-281. [PMID: 17634462]

Inzucchi SE. Management of hypercalcemia. Diagnostic workup, therapeutic options for hyperparathyroidism and other common causes. Postgrad Med. 2004;115(5):27-36. [PMID: 15171076]

Khan AA, Bilezikian JP, Kung AW, et al. Alendronate in primary hyperparathyroidism: a double-blind, randomized, placebo-controlled trial. J Clin Endocrinol Metab. 2004;89(7):3319-3325. [PMID: 15240609]

Rittmaster RS, Bolognese M, Ettinger MP, et al. Enhancement of bone mass in osteoporotic women with parathyroid hormone followed by alendronate. J Clin Endocrinol Metab. 2000;85(6):2129-2134. [PMID: 10852440]

Rubin MR, Bilezikian JP, McMahon DJ, et al. The natural history of primary hyperparathyroidism with or without parathyroid surgery after 15 years. J Clin Endocrinol Metab. 2008;93(9):3462-3470. [PMID: 18544625]

Silverberg SJ, Shane E, Jacobs TP, Siris E, Bilezikian JP. A 10-year prospective study of primary hyperparathyroidism with or without parathyroid surgery [erratum in N Engl J Med. 2000;342(2):144]. N Engl J Med. 1999;341(17):1249-1255. [PMID: 10528034]

U.S. Preventive Services Task Force. Vitamin D and Calcium Supplementation to Prevent Cancer and Osteoporotic Fractures in Adults: Draft Recommendation Statement. AHRQ Publication No. 12-05163-EF-2. Available at: www.uspreventiveservicestaskforce.org/draftrec3.htm. Accessed June 13, 2012.

Endocrinology and Metabolism Self-Assessment Test

This self-assessment test contains one-best-answer multiple-choice questions. Please read these directions carefully before answering the questions. Answers, critiques, and bibliographies immediately follow these multiple-choice questions. The American College of Physicians is accredited by the Accreditation Council for Continuing Medical Education (ACCME) to provide continuing medical education for physicians.

The American College of Physicians designates MKSAP 16 Endocrinology and Metabolism for a maximum of 12 *AMA PRA Category 1 Credits*™. Physicians should claim only the credit commensurate with the extent of their participation in the activity.

Earn "Same-Day" CME Credits Online

For the first time, print subscribers can enter their answers online to earn CME credits in 24 hours or less. You can submit your answers using online answer sheets that are provided at mksap.acponline.org, where a record of your MKSAP 16 credits will be available. To earn CME credits, you need to answer all of the questions in a test and earn a score of at least 50% correct (number of correct answers divided by the total number of questions). Take any of the following approaches:

> ➢ Use the printed answer sheet at the back of this book to record your answers. Go to mksap.acponline.org, access the appropriate online answer sheet, transcribe your answers, and submit your test for same-day CME credits. There is no additional fee for this service.

> ➢ Go to mksap.acponline.org, access the appropriate online answer sheet, directly enter your answers, and submit your test for same-day CME credits. There is no additional fee for this service.

> ➢ Pay a $10 processing fee per answer sheet and submit the printed answer sheet at the back of this book by mail or fax, as instructed on the answer sheet. Make sure you calculate your score and fax the answer sheet to 215-351-2799 or mail the answer sheet to Member and Customer Service, American College of Physicians, 190 N. Independence Mall West, Philadelphia, PA 19106-1572, using the courtesy envelope provided in your MKSAP 16 slipcase. You will need your 10-digit order number and 8-digit ACP ID number, which are printed on your packing slip. Please allow 4 to 6 weeks for your score report to be emailed back to you. Be sure to include your email address for a response.

If you do not have a 10-digit order number and 8-digit ACP ID number or if you need help creating a username and password to access the MKSAP 16 online answer sheets, go to mksap.acponline.org or email custserv@acponline.org.

CME credit is available from the publication date of December 31, 2012, until December 31, 2015. You may submit your answer sheets at any time during this period.

Directions

*Each of the numbered items is followed by lettered answers. Select the **ONE** lettered answer that is **BEST** in each case.*

Self-Assessment Test

Item 1

A 62-year-old man is evaluated before having panretinal laser photocoagulation therapy in both eyes. He has an 18-year history of type 2 diabetes mellitus. He also has diabetic neuropathy and hypertension. At his annual retinal eye examination last week, his vision had deteriorated to 20/30 in his right eye and 20/40 in his left eye; new blood vessels are seen growing on the optic discs of both eyes. Medications are metformin, insulin glargine, simvastatin, ramipril, enteric-coated aspirin, and hydrochlorothiazide.

On physical examination, temperature is 36.9 °C (98.4 °F), blood pressure is 147/86 mm Hg, pulse rate is 88/min, and respiration rate is14/min; BMI is 34. Other than the presence of proliferative diabetic retinopathy, physical examination findings are unremarkable.

Which of the following is the most likely outcome of the planned procedure?

(A) Diminished central vision with retention of peripheral vision
(B) Diminished peripheral and night vision with retention of central vision
(C) Improvement of vision (to 20/20) in both eyes
(D) Loss of binocular vision and depth perception

Item 2

A 61-year-old man is evaluated after a CT scan obtained because of right epigastric pain showed a 7-cm right adrenal mass. The patient reports no change in weight or appetite and no history of hypertension, palpitations, headaches, or excess sweating. He takes no medication.

Physical examination shows a man with normal features. Temperature is 36.7 °C (98.1 °F), blood pressure is 122/76 mm Hg, pulse rate is 74/min and regular, and respiration rate is 16/min; BMI is 29. No plethora, muscle wasting, weakness, or ecchymosis is noted.

Results of laboratory studies, including measurement of serum electrolyte, cortisol, and adrenocorticotropic hormone levels and of the 24-hour urine metanephrine level, are normal, as are results of a dexamethasone suppression test.

The previously obtained CT scan shows a 7-cm right adrenal mass with an attenuation factor of 77 Hounsfield units and a normally sized left adrenal gland. No lymphadenopathy or other masses were detected.

Which of the following is the most appropriate management?

(A) Biopsy of the adrenal mass
(B) Right adrenalectomy
(C) Serum aldosterone to plasma renin activity ratio determination
(D) 24-Hour measurement of urine cortisol excretion

Item 3

An 18-year-old woman is evaluated for a 6-month history of amenorrhea. The patient underwent menarche at age 13 years and had normal menstrual cycles until 6 months ago. She reports no hot flushes, night sweats, weight changes, or cold or heat intolerance. She has had no uterine procedures and has no family history of thyroid disease or primary ovarian insufficiency.

On physical examination, vital signs are normal; BMI is 22. No evidence of hirsutism, acne, alopecia, clitoromegaly, or galactorrhea is found.

Results of laboratory studies are normal, including serum follicle-stimulating hormone, human chorionic gonadotropin, prolactin, free thyroxine (T_4), and thyroid-stimulating hormone levels.

Which of the following is the most appropriate next diagnostic step?

(A) Measurement of total testosterone and dehydroepiandrosterone levels
(B) MRI of the pituitary gland
(C) Pelvic ultrasonography
(D) Progesterone challenge testing

Item 4

A 28-year-old woman is evaluated for a 1-year history of a nonpainful swelling in her neck. Her health has been otherwise excellent, with no weight loss, nervousness, or excessive tiredness. She is interested in becoming pregnant. Her mother and maternal grandmother have thyroid disease treated with levothyroxine.

On physical examination, blood pressure is 130/80 mm Hg, pulse rate is 94/min and regular, and respiration rate is 16/min; BMI is 27. Her thyroid gland is minimally enlarged bilaterally and feels firm. No specific nodules or cervical lymphadenopathy is palpated. Results of cardiac, pulmonary, abdominal, and extremity examinations are normal.

Laboratory studies:

Thyroid-stimulating hormone (TSH)	6.5 µU/mL (6.5 mU/L)
Thyroxine (T_4), free	1.2 ng/dL (15 pmol/L)
Triiodothyronine (T_3), free	4.0 ng/L (6.1 pmol/L)
Thyroid peroxidase antibodies	640 units/L (normal, <20 units/L)

Which of the following is the most appropriate next step in management?

(A) Fine-needle aspiration biopsy of the thyroid gland
(B) Levothyroxine therapy
(C) Repeat TSH measurement in 6 weeks
(D) Thyroid scan

Item 5

A 47-year-old man is evaluated in the emergency department for a 2-week history of a worsening productive cough associated with fever and night sweats. The patient has advanced HIV infection and has lost 8.2 kg (18.0 lb) since his last outpatient visit 3 months ago. He stopped taking all medications, including antiretroviral therapy, 4 months ago.

On physical examination, temperature is 38.2 °C (100.8 °F), blood pressure is 130/78 mm Hg, and pulse rate is 98/min; BMI is 17. The patient appears cachectic and is diaphoretic. Findings on a chest radiograph are consistent with miliary tuberculosis, and he is admitted to an isolation room.

Results of laboratory studies obtained 1 day after admission show a serum calcium level of 10.8 mg/dL (2.7 mmol/L), an albumin level of 2.4 g/dL (24 g/L), and a serum phosphorus level of 4.8 mg/dL (1.55 mmol/L). A serum parathyroid hormone (PTH) level obtained 2 days after admission is 9 pg/mL (9 ng/L).

Which of the following is the most likely underlying mechanism of this patient's hypercalcemia?

(A) Dehydration
(B) Excessive 1,25-dihydroxyvitamin D production
(C) Excessive parathyroid hormone release
(D) Presence of PTH-related protein

Item 6

A 67-year-old woman is evaluated for a 2-day history of severe muscle weakness. The patient experienced significant weight gain and developed hypertension and type 2 diabetes mellitus 2 years ago. She also reports developing muscle weakness of the lower extremities 6 month ago. Her diabetes is only partially controlled by metformin; her blood glucose measurements at home are usually greater than 250 mg/dL (13.9 mmol/L). Other medications are hydrochlorothiazide, lisinopril, amlodipine, and metoprolol.

Physical examination shows a woman who appears chronically ill. Blood pressure is 154/92 mm Hg, and other vital signs are normal; BMI is 40. Skin examination is notable for facial hirsutism. Central obesity, mild proximal muscle weakness, and 2+ peripheral edema are noted.

Results of laboratory studies show a serum creatinine level of 1.3 mg/dL (115 µmol/L), a plasma glucose level of 144 mg/dL (8.0 mmol/L), and a serum potassium level of 2.9 meq/L (2.9 mmol/L).

Which of the following tests should be performed to reveal the cause of her diabetes?

(A) Adrenal CT
(B) C-peptide measurement
(C) Glutamic acid decarboxylase antibody titer
(D) Pancreatic MRI
(E) 24-Hour urine free cortisol excretion

Item 7

A 26-year-old woman is evaluated for hyperprolactinemia after recent follow-up laboratory studies showed a serum prolactin level of 55 ng/mL (55 µg/L). Mild hyperprolactinemia (serum prolactin level of 35 ng/mL [35 µg/L]) was detected 6 years ago during an evaluation for irregular menstrual cycles; an MRI performed at that time showed a pituitary microadenoma. She was treated with a dopamine agonist, and subsequent serum prolactin measurements have shown normal levels until the most recent measurement. The patient underwent menarche at age 13 years and has had irregular menstrual cycles since that time, with multiple missed cycles. She has never been pregnant. Her family history is unremarkable, and she takes no medication.

On physical examination, blood pressure is 108/70 mm Hg, pulse rate is 82/min, and respiration rate is 12/min; BMI is 25. The patient has a normal distribution of body weight. Breast development is normal, but breast tenderness is noted on examination. No galactorrhea, acne, hirsutism, or striae are present.

Laboratory studies confirm a serum prolactin level of 55 ng/mL (55 µg/L) and show a thyroid-stimulating hormone level of 1.2 µU/mL (1.2 mU/L).

Which of the following is the most appropriate next diagnostic test?

(A) Pregnancy test
(B) Random serum growth hormone measurement
(C) Serum cortisol measurement
(D) Visual field testing

Item 8

A 28-year-old woman is reevaluated for worsening eye symptoms. The patient has a 6-month history of Graves disease. Methimazole was initiated but then discontinued when the patient became neutropenic (absolute neutrophil count, 500/µL [0.5×10^9/L]). Although treatment with methimazole abated her symptoms of thyrotoxicosis and normalized results of her thyroid function tests, her eye symptoms have progressed to severe discomfort (burning and itching) in both eyes and diplopia when she looks upward and laterally.

On physical examination, temperature is 37.2 °C (99.0 °F), blood pressure is 130/70 mm Hg, pulse rate is 90/min, and respiration rate is 16/min; BMI is 23. Examination of the thyroid gland shows an enlarged smooth gland without nodules. Examination of the eyes shows significant bilateral chemosis and erythema. Bilateral moderate proptosis and right lid and globe lag are noted. Visual acuity is normal.

Laboratory studies:

Thyroid-stimulating hormone	<0.01 µU/mL (0.01 mU/L)
Thyroxine (T_4), free	2.4 ng/dL (31 pmol/L)
Triiodothyronine (T_3)	230 ng/dL (3.5 nmol/L)
Thyroid-stimulating immunoglobins	340% (normal, <110%)

An MRI of the orbits shows bilateral proptosis and increased size of the extraocular muscles, especially the right inferior rectus muscle. Increased retro-orbital fat is seen, and the optic nerves appear normal

Which of the following is the most appropriate treatment for this patient's hyperthyroidism?

(A) Oral iodine solution
(B) Propylthiouracil
(C) Radioactive iodine therapy
(D) Thyroidectomy

Item 9

A 29-year-old woman is evaluated for recent-onset polyuria. The patient also has a 6-month history of fatigue, decreased energy, nausea, dry skin, and amenorrhea. She had pulmonary sarcoidosis 10 years ago that was successfully treated with a 2-year course of glucocorticoids and has not had any symptoms until now. She currently takes no medication and has no pertinent family history.

On physical examination, vital signs are normal; BMI is 24. Findings from examination of the heart, lungs, and thyroid gland are normal. Skin color and texture are normal, with no areas of hyperpigmentation. Diminished axillary and pubic hair and delayed relaxation of the deep tendon reflexes are noted.

Laboratory studies:

Electrolytes	
Sodium	146 meq/L (146 mmol/L)
Potassium	4.0 meq/L (4.0 mmol/L)
Chloride	96 meq/L (96 mmol/L)
Bicarbonate	28 meq/L (28 mmol/L)
Pregnancy test	Negative
Adrenocorticotropic hormone	12 pg/mL (3 pmol/L)
Cortisol (9 AM)	(Normal, 5-25 µg/dL [138-690 nmol/L])
Baseline	4.5 µg/dL (124 nmol/L)
After cosyntropin stimulation	13 µg/dL (359 nmol/L)
Follicle-stimulating hormone	3 mU/mL (3 units/L)
Luteinizing hormone	2 mU/mL (2 units/L)
Thyroid-stimulating hormone	0.5 µU/mL (0.5 mU/L)
Thyroxine (T_4), free	0.6 ng/dL (8 pmol/L)

A chest radiograph has normal findings.

Which of the following is the most appropriate diagnostic test to perform next?

(A) CT of the adrenal glands
(B) Lung biopsy
(C) Pituitary MRI
(D) Thyroid scan

Item 10

A 54-year-old woman comes to the office for advice regarding maintaining bone health. She has no history of fracture. The patient recently had a lumpectomy and radiation therapy to treat breast cancer, is currently taking tamoxifen, and will begin taking an aromatase inhibitor in 2 months. She underwent menopause at age 52 years and has persistent hot flushes. Her risk factors for osteoporosis include a slim body habitus and a mother who had a hip fracture at age 67 years.

Physical examination findings, including vital signs, are normal. BMI is 20.

Results of routine laboratory studies are normal.

A dual-energy x-ray absorptiometry scan shows T-scores of −2.1 in the lumbar spine, −2.3 in the femoral neck, and −1.9 in the total hip. Her Fracture Risk Assessment Tool (FRAX) score indicates a 22% risk of major osteoporotic fracture and a 2.4% risk of hip fracture over the next 10 years. Optimal calcium and vitamin D supplementation is recommended, and she is encouraged to begin weight-bearing exercise as tolerated.

Which of the following pharmacologic agents can be started in this patient?

(A) Alendronate
(B) Denosumab
(C) Estrogen
(D) Raloxifene
(E) Teriparatide

Item 11

A 15-year-old girl is evaluated for excessive urination and thirst. She has been drinking almost 5 liters (169 ounces) of fluid daily for the past 2 months. The patient's mother has type 2 diabetes mellitus.

On physical examination, vital signs are normal; BMI is 35. Results of general medical and neurologic examinations are unremarkable. She is not dehydrated, and no ketones are detected on her breath.

Laboratory studies:

Hemoglobin A_{1c}	8.7%
Glucose, random	324 mg/dL (18.0 mmol/L)
Electrolytes	Normal
Urine ketones	Absent

In addition to treating the patient's hyperglycemia, which of the following is the most appropriate next step in management?

(A) Measure fasting plasma C-peptide level
(B) Measure fasting plasma insulin level
(C) Measure stimulated plasma C-peptide level
(D) Obtain islet cell and glutamic acid decarboxylase antibody titers

Item 12

A 29-year-old man is evaluated for possible infertility. He and his wife have been trying to conceive for 2 years. His wife had a full anatomic evaluation with normal results. The patient reports normal libido and erectile function and had normal puberty. Family history is unremarkable. He takes no medication.

On physical examination, vital signs are normal; BMI is 22. Visual field examination findings and testicular volume are normal, as is hair distribution. All other physical examination findings are unremarkable.

Which of the following is the most appropriate next diagnostic test?

(A) Luteinizing and follicle-stimulating hormone measurements
(B) Semen analysis
(C) Testicular ultrasonography
(D) Total testosterone measurement

Item 13

A 27-year-old woman is evaluated during the fourth week of an uneventful pregnancy. She has a 3-year history of primary hypothyroidism due to Hashimoto thyroiditis that is treated with levothyroxine, 125 μg/d. She also takes prenatal vitamins and iron sulfate.

On physical examination, temperature is 37.1 °C (98.8 °F), blood pressure is 128/80 mm Hg, pulse rate is 95/min, and respiration rate is 18/min and regular; BMI is 25. She has a mild fine hand tremor. Lung, cardiac, and skin examination findings are normal. The thyroid gland is smooth and slightly enlarged without a bruit or nodules.

Laboratory studies show a serum thyroid-stimulating hormone level of 4.2 μU/mL (4.2 mU/L) and a serum free thyroxine (T_4) level of 1.6 ng/dL (21 pmol/L).

Which of the following is the most appropriate management?

(A) Increase the levothyroxine dosage by 10% now
(B) Increase the levothyroxine dosage by 30% now
(C) Repeat thyroid function tests in 5 weeks
(D) Repeat thyroid function tests in the second trimester

Item 14

A 67-year-old man is evaluated in the emergency department for an explosive headache and blurred vision that began 4 hours ago. He reports a 3-month history of fatigue, weight gain (total, 4.5 kg [10 lb]), and erectile dysfunction. The patient has a 2-year history of atrial fibrillation treated with warfarin and metoprolol.

Physical examination reveals a pale man who appears uncomfortable. Blood pressure is 88/56 mm Hg, pulse rate is 88/min, and respiration rate is 18/min. Visual field examination reveals bitemporal hemianopia. Except for the finding of neck stiffness, the remainder of the physical examination is unremarkable.

Results of laboratory studies are notable for a serum sodium level of 128 meq/L (128 mmol/L).

A noncontrast CT scan shows a heterogeneous sellar mass with suprasellar extension and bowing of the optic chiasm.

In addition to neurosurgical consultation, which of the following is the most appropriate initial management?

(A) Glucocorticoid administration
(B) Insulin tolerance test
(C) Lumbar puncture
(D) Serum prolactin measurement

Item 15

A 62-year-old woman is evaluated for a 1-week history of fatigue, lethargy, constipation, and nocturnal polyuria and polydipsia. The patient has advanced breast cancer, which has metastasized to her liver. Conventional therapy is no longer helpful, and she is scheduled to see her oncologist to discuss the next steps in her cancer management.

Physical examination shows a pale and somnolent woman. Blood pressure is 98/65 mm Hg and resting pulse rate is 103/min. Cardiopulmonary examination findings are normal. The mucous membranes are dry. The liver edge is palpated 3 cm below the right costal margin.

Laboratory studies:

Blood urea nitrogen	37 mg/dL (13.2 mmol/L)
Calcium	15.7 mg/dL (3.9 mmol/L)
Creatinine	1.4 mg/dL (124 μmol/L)
Sodium	151 meq/L (151 mmol/L)

A bone scan shows metastatic disease to the liver.

Which of the following is the most appropriate immediate next step in treating this patient?

(A) An intravenous bisphosphonate
(B) Intravenous furosemide
(C) Intravenous glucocorticoids
(D) Intravenous normal saline

Item 16

A 59-year-old woman is evaluated for muscle cramps and difficult-to-control hypertension. The patient reports no headaches or unexplained sweating. She started taking hydrochlorothiazide 20 months ago when hypertension was diagnosed but changed her medication after developing hypokalemia (serum potassium level, 1.9 meq/L [1.9 mmol/L]). Subsequent addition of lisinopril, atenolol, amlodipine, and potassium chloride has resulted in no improvement in blood pressure control.

Physical examination reveals a woman with normal features. Temperature is 36.5 °C (97.7 °F), blood pressure is 186/102 mm Hg with no orthostatic changes, pulse rate is 66/min with no orthostatic changes, and respiration rate is 16/min; BMI is 29. Results of examination of the lungs, heart, and thyroid gland are normal.

Laboratory studies:

Electrolytes	
Sodium	143 meq/L (143 mmol/L)
Potassium	2.9 meq/L (2.9 mmol/L)
Chloride	96 meq/L (96 mmol/L)
Bicarbonate	33 meq/L (33 mmol/L)

Which of the following is the most appropriate next diagnostic test?

(A) CT of the abdomen
(B) Dexamethasone suppression test
(C) Measurement of plasma catecholamine levels
(D) Serum aldosterone to plasma renin activity ratio determination
(E) 24-Hour measurement of urine free cortisol excretion

Item 17

A 58-year old woman is evaluated for a 3-week history of fatigue and weight loss. The patient has no significant medical history and takes no prescription medication, but she does take a daily over-the-counter multivitamin and a calcium supplement. She has a 50-pack-year smoking history.

Physical examination reveals a lethargic, ill-appearing woman. Temperature is 37.3 °C (99.1 °F), blood pressure is 136/78 mm Hg, pulse rate is 95/min, and respiration rate is 12/min. Other physical examination findings are unremarkable.

Laboratory studies:

Hemoglobin	8.3 g/dL (83 g/L)
Albumin	4.6 g/dL (46 g/L)
Blood urea nitrogen	43 mg/dL (15.4 mmol/L)
Calcium	14.5 mg/dL (3.6 mmol/L)
Creatinine	2.4 mg/dL (212 µmol/L)
Sodium	145 meq/L (145 mmol/L)

A chest radiograph shows a 5-cm mass in the right lower lobe of the lung but is otherwise unremarkable.

Which of the following is the most likely cause of her hypercalcemia?

(A) Malignancy
(B) Primary hyperparathyroidism
(C) Sarcoidosis
(D) Vitamin D intoxication

Item 18

A 42-year-old man is evaluated for a 6-month history of painful and enlarged breasts. The patient had normal puberty and has no relevant personal or family medical history. He takes no medication.

On physical examination, vital signs are normal; BMI is 25. Examination of the chest shows symmetric tender gynecomastia. Testicular volume is normal, no abdominal or testicular masses are palpated, and no lymphadenopathy is noted.

Laboratory studies show a serum human chorionic gonadotropin level of 2 mU/mL (2 units/L) (normal, <5 mU/mL [5 units/L]), a luteinizing hormone level of 5 mU/mL (5 units/L), and a total testosterone level of 400 ng/dL (14 nmol/L).

Which of the following is the most appropriate next diagnostic test?

(A) Adrenal CT
(B) Breast ultrasonography
(C) Estradiol level determination
(D) Karyotype
(E) Testicular ultrasonography

Item 19

A 33-year-old woman is evaluated after having three episodes of severe hypoglycemia, each resulting in a visit to the emergency department, in the past month. Two of the episodes occurred while she was asleep, and the most recent one happened midafternoon yesterday. The patient has a 19-year history of type 1 diabetes mellitus and has been trying to lower her hemoglobin A_{1c} level to less than 7.0% before she tries to get pregnant. She states that she no longer experiences any warning symptoms before she becomes hypoglycemic. The patient had an episode of diabetic ketoacidosis in her teens. She has mild background diabetic retinopathy, some numbness in her feet from peripheral neuropathy, and occasional orthostatic hypotension. She eats a healthy diet, counts carbohydrates, and adjusts her preprandial insulin intake. Medications are insulin glargine, 24 units at bedtime, and insulin glulisine, 6 to 10 units before breakfast, lunch, and dinner, depending on her planned carbohydrate intake and preprandial blood glucose level.

On physical examinations, vital signs are normal; BMI is 30.

Results of laboratory studies show a hemoglobin A_{1c} value of 6.6% and no evidence of microalbuminuria.

Which of the following is the most appropriate treatment for this patient?

(A) Increased carbohydrate intake at meals
(B) Insulin dose reductions
(C) α-Lipoic acid
(D) Preprandial pramlintide
(E) Substitution of insulin detemir for insulin glargine

Item 20

A 40-year-old man is evaluated after the incidental discovery of a small nodule in the right lobe of the thyroid gland on a CT scan obtained because of chest pain. The patient reports feeling well now, with no nervousness, palpitations, neck discomfort, or dysphagia. His mother has papillary thyroid cancer that was diagnosed in her 30s.

Physical examination shows a healthy-appearing, alert man. Vital signs are normal; BMI is 28. Lung, heart, and abdominal examination findings are normal. On neck examination, the thyroid gland is barely palpable, with no nodes or cervical lymphadenopathy.

Laboratory studies show a thyroid-stimulating hormone level of 1.5 µU/mL (1.5 mU/L).

A Doppler ultrasound of the thyroid gland shows a right-lobe 6-mm hypoechoic nodule with microcalcifications, blurred nodule margins, and increased central vascularity. No enlarged cervical lymph nodes are present on either side.

Which of the following is the most appropriate management?

(A) Fine-needle aspiration biopsy
(B) Repeat thyroid ultrasonography in 3 months
(C) Right thyroid lobectomy
(D) Thyroid MRI

Item 21

A 27-year-old man is evaluated for a 7-month history of loss of strength and progressive fatigue and a decreased sense of well being. The patient sustained a severe traumatic brain injury in an automobile collision 16 months ago. He has had no excessive urination, cold intolerance, constipation, or loss of libido or other symptoms of sexual dysfunction. His only medication is a daily multivitamin.

On physical examination, vital signs are normal; BMI is 30. Increased abdominal girth is noted. All other findings, including those from a neurologic examination, are normal.

Laboratory studies:

Complete blood count	Normal
Basic metabolic panel	Normal
Testosterone (8 AM)	980 ng/dL (34 nmol/L)
Thyroid-stimulating hormone	2.0 µU/mL (2.0 mU/L)
Thyroxine (T_4), free	1.4 ng/dL (18 pmol/L)

Which of the following is the most appropriate next diagnostic test?

(A) Fasting growth hormone measurement
(B) Glucose tolerance test
(C) Gonadotropin-releasing hormone test
(D) Insulin-like growth factor 1 measurement

Item 22

A 66-year-old woman comes to the office for management of osteoporosis discovered on a screening dual-energy x-ray absorptiometry (DEXA) scan. The patient has no personal history of fractures and no family history of parathyroid disease or low bone mineral density. She has hypertension treated with lisinopril but takes no other medications or supplements.

On physical examination, vital signs are normal; BMI is 22. Dentition is good. Other than mild kyphosis, physical examination findings are unremarkable.

Laboratory studies:

Albumin	4.0 g/dL (40 g/L)
Calcium	8.7 mg/dL (2.2 mmol/L)
Creatinine	0.7 mg/dL (61.9 µmol/L)
Phosphorus	2.9 mg/dL (0.94 mmol/L)
Parathyroid hormone	176 pg/mL (176 ng/L)

The DEXA scan showed T-scores of −2.1 in the lumbar spine, −3.0 in the femoral neck, and −2.5 in the total hip. Radiographs of the lateral spine show no compression fractures.

Which of the following is the most appropriate next step in management?

(A) Measurement of 1,25-dihydroxyvitamin D level
(B) Measurement of 25-hydroxyvitamin D level
(C) Parathyroidectomy
(D) Repeat DEXA scan in 1 year

Item 23

A 46-year-old woman is evaluated after undergoing a total thyroidectomy 6 weeks ago for metastatic (stage III) papillary thyroid cancer. A 4.5-cm left papillary thyroid cancer was removed. Metastatic disease was identified in a single cervical lymph node (level III). The patient has been taking levothyroxine since the surgery.

On physical examination, blood pressure is 130/70 mm Hg, pulse rate is 88/min and regular, and respiration rate is 16/min and regular. Examination of the neck shows a well-healing incision without palpable masses or lymphadenopathy. The lungs are clear to auscultation, and no murmurs, enlargement, or other abnormalities are seen on cardiac examination. No Chvostek sign is elicited.

Laboratory studies show a serum thyroid-stimulating hormone level of 0.1 µU/mL (0.1 mU/L), an undetectable serum thyroglobulin level (<0.5 ng/mL [0.5 µg/L] [normal, 1.6-59.9 ng/mL {1.6-59.9 µg/L}]), and no thyroglobulin antibodies.

Which of the following is the most appropriate next step in treatment?

(A) Chemotherapy with doxorubicin
(B) External-beam radiation therapy
(C) Radioactive iodine therapy
(D) Observation

Item 24

A 48-year-old man is evaluated during a routine examination. He has a 6-year history of hypertension treated with amlodipine and atenolol and is currently asymptomatic. His father had a myocardial infarction at age 50 years, and his mother developed type 2 diabetes mellitus at age 64 years.

On physical examination, blood pressure is 138/89 mm Hg, pulse rate is 76/min, and respiration rate is 18/min; BMI is 33. Central obesity is noted, but all other findings are unremarkable.

Results of laboratory studies show a hemoglobin A_{1c} level of 6.6% and a fasting plasma glucose level of 114 mg/dL (6.3 mmol/L)

Which of the following diagnostic tests should be performed next?

(A) Oral glucose tolerance test
(B) Repeat measurement of fasting plasma glucose level
(C) Repeat measurement of hemoglobin A_{1c} value
(D) No additional testing

Item 25

A 49-year-old woman is evaluated for a 1-week history of excessive fatigue and nausea. She has a history of hypertension, colon cancer, and unexplained anorexia. She was treated with megestrol, 320 mg/d, for almost a year before running out of her medications 2 weeks ago. She has had no palpitations, headaches, or unexplained sweating. Other medications are metoprolol and hydrochlorothiazide.

On physical examination, temperature is 36.5 °C (97.7 °F), blood pressure is 108/78 mm Hg with no orthostatic changes, pulse rate is 86/min with no orthostatic changes, and respiration rate is 16/min; BMI is 31. Results of examination of the lungs, heart, and thyroid gland are normal. A plethoric rounded face and central obesity with supraclavicular and posterior cervical fat pads are noted.

Laboratory studies:

Electrolytes	
Sodium	133 meq/L (133 mmol/L)
Potassium	3.9 meq/L (3.9 mmol/L)
Chloride	98 meq/L (98 mmol/L)
Bicarbonate	29 meq/L (29 mmol/L)
Adrenocorticotropic hormone	8 pg/mL (2 pmol/L)
Cortisol (9 AM)	2.7 µg/dL (75 nmol/L) (normal, 5-25 µg/dL [138-690 nmol/L])

Which of the following is the most appropriate management?

(A) CT of the adrenal glands
(B) Dexamethasone suppression test
(C) Fludrocortisone
(D) Oral hydrocortisone

Item 26

A 42-year-old man is evaluated for infertility. He and his wife have been trying to conceive for 1 year. They have a 4-year-old child conceived without problems. The patient reports a slightly decreased libido that he attributes to increased stress at work. Puberty was normal. He has osteoarthritis of the hands. Family history is unremarkable. His only medication is ibuprofen as needed.

On physical examination, vital signs are normal; BMI is 24. Testicular volume is decreased bilaterally. Visual field and thyroid examination findings are normal. No gynecomastia is noted.

Laboratory studies:

Alanine aminotransferase	48 units/L
Aspartate aminotransferase	25 units/L
Follicle-stimulating hormone	2 mU/mL (2 units/L)
Luteinizing hormone	2 mU/mL (2 units/L)
Prolactin	12 ng/mL (12 µg/L)
Testosterone, total (8 AM)	
Initial measurement	200 ng/dL (6.9 nmol/L)
Repeat measurement	190 ng/dL (6.5 nmol/L)
Thyroid-stimulating hormone	1.2 µU/mL (1.2 mU/L)
Thyroxine (T$_4$), free	1.2 ng/dL (15 pmol/L)

An MRI of the pituitary gland is normal.

Which of the following is the most appropriate next diagnostic test?

(A) Ferritin and iron saturation measurement
(B) Free testosterone measurement
(C) Karyotyping
(D) Testicular ultrasonography

Item 27

A 29-year-old woman is evaluated for a 2-day history of fever, cough, nasal congestion, myalgia, and fatigue. Addison disease was diagnosed 3 months ago. Medications are hydrocortisone (10 mg at 8 AM, 5 mg at noon, and 5 mg at 6 PM) and fludrocortisone (0.05 mg/d). She has been able to take her medications as scheduled and fluids as needed.

On physical examination, temperature is 38.2 °C (100.8 °F), blood pressure is 102/68 mm Hg without orthostatic changes, pulse rate is 88/min without orthostatic changes, and respiration rate is 21/min; BMI is 31. Erythema is noted in the posterior pharynx, and bilateral small cervical lymph nodes are present. The rest of the physical examination is unremarkable.

Which of the following is the most appropriate treatment?

(A) Hospital admission for intravenous fluids and glucocorticoid therapy
(B) Increased fludrocortisone dose
(C) Increased hydrocortisone dose for 3 days
(D) Symptomatic treatment for upper respiratory tract infection only

Item 28

A 55-year-old man is evaluated for anxiety, heat intolerance, and weight loss (2.3 kg [5 lb]) over the past 6 weeks. The patient also reports decreased visual acuity. He has no neck discomfort. He takes no medication.

Physical examination reveals a nervous man. Blood pressure is 150/70 mm Hg, pulse rate is 110/min and regular, and respiration rate is 16/min; BMI is 27. Other than tachycardia, the cardiopulmonary examination is unremarkable. Eye examination findings are normal. The thyroid gland is enlarged, smooth, and without bruits or nodules. The skin is warm. A bilateral hand tremor is noted. No pretibial myxedema is seen.

Laboratory studies:

Thyroid-stimulating hormone	1.5 µU/mL (0.5 mU/L)
Thyroxine (T$_4$), free	2.4 ng/dL (31 pmol/L)
Triiodothyronine (T$_3$)	220 ng/dL (3.4 nmol/L)
Thyroid-stimulating hormone–receptor and thyroid peroxidase antibodies	Negative

Radioactive iodine (^{123}I) uptake by the thyroid gland at 24 hours is 55% (normal, 10%-30%). A thyroid scan shows homogenous distribution.

Which of the following is the most appropriate next step in management?

(A) Methimazole
(B) Pituitary MRI
(C) Propylthiouracil
(D) Radioactive iodine therapy
(E) Thyroidectomy

Item 29

A 53-year-old man is evaluated after a pheochromocytoma is diagnosed on the basis of a 6-month history of hypertension and a 9-month history of recurrent palpitations, sweating, headaches, and weight loss (total, 4.5 kg [10 lb]) despite a good appetite. Medications are amlodipine, 10 mg/d; hydrochlorothiazide, 25 mg/d; and lisinopril.

Physical examination shows an anxious-looking man. Temperature is 36.5 °C (97.7 °F), blood pressure is 158/96 mm Hg without orthostatic changes, pulse rate is 102/min without orthostatic changes, and respiration rate is 16/min; BMI is 28.

Findings from examination of the lung, heart, and thyroid gland are normal. A mild resting tremor is noted in the upper extremities, but no myopathy or muscle weakness is detected.

Laboratory studies:

Glucose, fasting	150 mg/dL (8.3 mmol/L)
Metanephrine, free	160 pg/mL (0.8 nmol/L) (normal, 12-61 pg/mL [0.1-0.3 nmol/L])
Normetanephrine, free	740 pg/mL (4.1 nmol/L) (normal, 18-112 pg/mL [0.1-0.6 nmol/L])
Thyroid-stimulating hormone	1.2 µU/mL (1.2 mU/L)
Urine	
Creatinine	1100 mg/24 h
Epinephrine	220 µg/24 h (1201 nmol/24 h) (normal, 0-20 µg/24 h [0-109 nmol/24 h])
Metanephrine	0.85 mg/24 h (4.3 mmol/24 h)
Norepinephrine	2350 µg/24 h (13,889 nmol/24 h) (normal, 15-80 µg/24 h [89-473 nmol/24 h])
Normetanephrine	4550 µg/24 h (28,843 nmol/24 h) (normal, 128-484 µg/24 h [699-2643 nmol/24 h])
Vanillylmandelic acid	14 mg/24 h (71 µmol/24 h)

An electrocardiogram shows sinus tachycardia. A CT scan reveals a 3.5-cm left adrenal mass with an attenuation factor of 33 Hounsfield units.

Which of the following is the most appropriate initial management?

(A) Angiotensin receptor blocker therapy
(B) α-Blocker therapy
(C) β-Blocker therapy
(D) Surgery
(E) Observation

Item 30

A 78-year-old woman is evaluated for a 1-week history of diffuse constant headaches only occasionally relieved by acetaminophen. The patient has a history of hypertension and impaired fasting glucose, both of which are controlled with diet and exercise. She is up-to-date with preventive health screening.

Physical examination findings, including vital signs and results of neurologic evaluation, are normal.

Results of laboratory studies show a persistently elevated alkaline phosphatase level of 272 units/L; fractionation of the alkaline phosphatase shows an elevation in the bone isoform level. Other routine laboratory studies, including a complete blood count, are normal.

A bone scan shows uptake in the calvarium, left clavicle, two right ribs, and left acetabulum.

Which of the following is the most appropriate next step in management?

(A) Audiology testing
(B) Bone biopsy
(C) Plain radiographs
(D) Serum collagen type 1 cross-linked C-telopeptide (CTX) measurement
(E) Serum protein electrophoresis

Item 31

A 33-year old woman is evaluated for a 3-week history of fatigue, excessive sweating, and occasional headache on awakening. The patient has had type 1 diabetes mellitus since age 18 years. Her blood glucose log for the past 2 weeks shows fasting blood glucose levels ranging between 125 and 146 mg/dL (6.9-8.1 mmol/L) (average, 135 mg/dL [7.5 mmol/L]) and an average predinner level of 176 mg/dL (9.8 mmol/L). She does not check her level at other times during the day but occasionally experiences hypoglycemic symptoms around lunchtime, especially if she does not eat enough. She lives alone and usually exercises 1 hour each evening. Her diabetes regimen is premixed 70/30 insulin (neutral protamine Hagedorn [NPH] insulin/regular insulin) before breakfast and before dinner.

Physical examination shows a slim but well-appearing woman. Temperature is 36.6 °C (97.9 °F), blood pressure is 104/63 mm Hg, pulse rate is 66/min, and respiration rate is 14/min; BMI is 18. Other physical examination findings are unremarkable.

Results of laboratory studies show a hemoglobin A_{1c} value of 5.7% (estimated average plasma glucose level, 120 mg/dL [6.7 mmol/L]).

Which of the following is the most likely cause of her symptoms?

(A) Dawn phenomenon
(B) Nocturnal hypoglycemia

(C) Sleep apnea

(D) Somogyi phenomenon

Item 32

A 23-year-old woman is evaluated for a 3-month history of amenorrhea and galactorrhea. Her father has a history of recurrent kidney stones, and her brother has peptic ulcer disease.

On physical examination, vital signs are normal; BMI is 23. An expressible clear white nipple discharge is present bilaterally. All other examination findings are normal, including those from a visual field examination.

Laboratory studies:

Calcium	12 mg/dL (3.0 mmol/L)
Creatinine	0.7 mg/dL (61.9 µmol/L)
Parathyroid hormone	178 pg/mL (178 ng/L)
Prolactin	78 ng/mL (78 µg/L)
Thyroid-stimulating hormone	1.5 µU/mL (1.5 mU/L)

An MRI of the brain shows a 7-mm microadenoma of the pituitary gland.

Which of the following is the most likely diagnosis?

(A) Autoimmune polyglandular syndrome type 1

(B) Hashimoto thyroiditis

(C) Multiple endocrine neoplasia type 1 (MEN1)

(D) MEN2

Item 33

A 46-year-old man is evaluated for a 1-year history of low libido and erectile dysfunction. He underwent normal puberty and has two teenaged children. The patient has a history of hypertension. His only medication is chlorthalidone.

On physical examination, temperature is normal, blood pressure is 125/72 mm Hg, and pulse rate is 80/min; BMI is 42. No gynecomastia is present, and testicular volume is normal. A normal male distribution of body hair is noted.

Results of laboratory studies show a serum follicle-stimulating hormone level of 5 mU/mL (5 units/L), a serum luteinizing hormone level of 4 mU/mL (4 units/L), and a serum total testosterone level of 210 ng/dL (7 nmol/L); the serum thyroid-stimulating hormone and prolactin levels are normal.

Which of the following is the most appropriate next diagnostic test?

(A) Free testosterone assessment

(B) Karyotyping

(C) Pituitary MRI

(D) Sperm count

Item 34

A 35-year-old woman is evaluated for a nodule on the right side of her neck that she first noticed 2 weeks ago. The patient also reports recent flushing, diaphoresis, palpitations,

and headaches. She has a history of hypertension treated with hydrochlorothiazide.

On physical examination, blood pressure is 145/95 mm Hg, pulse rate is 100/min and regular, and respiration rate is 16/min. Results of heart, lung, and abdominal examinations are normal. Examination of the thyroid gland shows a 2-cm firm right-sided nodule; all other thyroid findings are normal.

Results of laboratory studies show a serum calcium level of 10.8 mg/dL (2.7 mmol/L) and a thyroid-stimulating hormone (TSH) level of 2.0 µU/mL (2.0 mU/L).

An ultrasound of the thyroid gland shows a 2- × 2-cm solid right-sided nodule with no evidence of lymphadenopathy. Results of a fine-needle aspiration biopsy of the nodule show numerous plasmacytoid-appearing cells staining positive for calcitonin that are consistent with medullary thyroid cancer.

Which of the following is the most appropriate next step in management?

(A) Administer radioactive iodine

(B) Measure plasma free metanephrine and normetanephrine levels

(C) Perform a total lobectomy

(D) Suppress TSH secretion with levothyroxine

Item 35

A 34-year-old woman comes to the office for a routine follow-up evaluation. She has an 18-year history of type 1 diabetes mellitus. Her glycemic control has been poor, with hemoglobin A_{1c} values typically ranging from 8.0% to 10.0%; her most recent hemoglobin A_{1c} value obtained 6 months ago was 8.2%. The patient wants to get her diabetes under better control before conceiving. Her current diabetic regimen is neutral protamine Hagedorn (NPH) insulin at bedtime and before breakfast and insulin lispro before each meal. She takes 1 unit of insulin lispro for every 20 grams of carbohydrate in the meal, plus 1 unit for every 50 mg/dL (2.8 mmol/L) that her premeal blood glucose level is above 120 mg/dL (6.7 mmol/L). For the past 3 months, she has been eating a healthy, high-carbohydrate, high-fiber, and low–glycemic index diet, with consistent amounts of carbohydrate at each meal. Mean blood glucose levels derived from her current blood glucose log are shown; the preprandial (Pre) breakfast levels are fasting, and the postprandial (Post) levels are 2 hours after eating.

Glucose values:

Time	Pre (mg/dL [mmol/L])	Post (mg/dL [mmol/L])	Other (mg/dL [mmol/L])
Breakfast	124 (6.9)	197 (10.9)	—
Lunch	118 (6.5)	236 (13.1)	—
Dinner	121 (6.7)	264 (14.7)	—
Bedtime			
11 PM	—	—	131 (7.3)
3 AM	—	—	122 (6.8)

On physical examination, temperature is normal, blood pressure is 126/73 mm Hg, and pulse rate is 76/min; BMI is 18. All other physical examination findings are unremarkable.

Which of the following modifications to her treatment regimen is most appropriate?

(A) Add pramlintide before each meal
(B) Change the insulin lispro to regular insulin
(C) Change the NPH insulin to insulin glargine
(D) Decrease mealtime carbohydrate intake
(E) Increase the premeal insulin lispro dosage

Item 36

A 43-year-old man is evaluated in the hospital for perioral paresthesias and severe cramping of both hands. He had a total thyroidectomy yesterday because of papillary thyroid cancer. The surgery went well, and no involved lymph nodes were found.

On physical examination, vital signs are normal. Cardiopulmonary and abdominal examinations are unremarkable. Results of muscle strength testing are normal. Although the patient reports cramps, no tetany is detected.

Results of laboratory studies show a serum calcium level of 4.1 mg/dL (1.0 mmol/L), a serum magnesium level of 1.7 mg/dL (0.70 mmol/L), and a serum phosphorus level of 4.7 mg/dL (1.52 mmol/L); kidney function is normal.

A resting electrocardiogram is normal.

Which of the following is the most appropriate immediate treatment for this patient?

(A) Calcitriol
(B) Calcium
(C) Magnesium
(D) Teriparatide

Item 37

A 56-year-old man comes to the office for a follow-up evaluation. Three weeks ago, the patient had surgery to repair a bleeding duodenal ulcer. During his 7-day hospitalization, he was given six units of packed red blood cells. He was discharged 2 weeks ago with instructions to take omeprazole. The patient has a 12-year history of type 2 diabetes mellitus, and his hemoglobin A_{1c} values have ranged from 8.5% to 9.0% for the past 5 years. Since hospital discharge, his blood glucose levels have ranged from 140 to 160 mg/dL (7.8-8.9 mmol/L). He has a 40-pack-year smoking history but has not smoked since the surgery. Although work was increasingly stressful before ulcer repair, he says he has been feeling more relaxed since discharge and has been eating healthier foods. Medications are metformin, glyburide, simvastatin, and omeprazole.

On physical examination, temperature is 36.9 °C (98.4 °F), blood pressure is 142/83 mm Hg, pulse rate is 82/min, and respiration rate is 14/min; BMI is 34. Other physical examination findings are unremarkable.

Results of laboratory studies show a hematocrit of 43% and a hemoglobin A_{1c} value of 6.2% (estimated average plasma glucose level, 130 mg/dL [7.2 mmol/L]).

Which of the following best explains the reduction in his hemoglobin A_{1c} value?

(A) Blood transfusions
(B) Healthier diet
(C) Omeprazole interference with the hemoglobin A_{1c} assay
(D) Smoking cessation

Item 38

A 56-year-old man is evaluated for the gradual onset of low libido and erectile dysfunction over a 3-year period. The patient has a history of hypertension, depression, and chronic pancreatitis. He no longer drinks alcohol. Family history is unremarkable. Medications are lisinopril, methadone, and citalopram.

Physical examination reveals a thin man. Temperature is normal, blood pressure is 132/88 mm Hg, pulse rate is 72/min, and respiration rate is 10/min; BMI is 22. Visual field and thyroid examination findings are normal. The patient has a normal male distribution of body hair, and no gynecomastia or acne is noted. The testes are small and soft.

Results of laboratory studies show a serum follicle-stimulating hormone level of 1.2 mU/mL (1.2 units/L), a serum luteinizing hormone level of 1.1 mU/mL (1.1 units/L), and a serum total testosterone level of 125 ng/dL (4 nmol/L). The serum thyroid-stimulating hormone and prolactin levels are normal, as are results of iron studies.

An MRI of the pituitary gland is normal.

Which of the following is the most likely cause of this patient's hypogonadism?

(A) Anabolic steroid abuse
(B) Citalopram
(C) Lisinopril
(D) Methadone

Item 39

A 29-year-old woman is evaluated for a 3-month history of fatigue, nausea, poor appetite, and salt craving; she has lost 6 kg (13.2 lb) in this period. She has a 5-year history of hypothyroidism treated with levothyroxine and a family history of thyroid disease, scleroderma, and premature gray hair.

Physical examination shows a woman with evenly tanned skin, including non–sun-exposed skin. Temperature is 36.9 °C (98.4 °F), blood pressure is 82/64 mm Hg supine and 72/50 mm Hg sitting, pulse rate is 102/min supine and 124/min sitting, and respiration rate is 16/min; BMI is 23. Results of heart, lung, and thyroid gland examinations are normal. Hyperpigmentation of the gum line is noted. No muscle weakness is detected.

Laboratory studies:

Electrolytes	
Sodium	126 meq/L (126 mmol/L)
Potassium	5.7 meq/L (5.7 mmol/L)
Chloride	101 meq/L (101 mmol/L)

Bicarbonate	22 meq/L (22 mmol/L)
Thyroid-stimulating hormone	6.2 µU/mL (6.2 mU/L)
Adrenocorticotropic hormone (ACTH) (1 PM)	234 pg/mL (51 pmol/L)
Cortisol, random (1 PM)	2.5 µg/dL (69 nmol/L)
Dehydroepiandrosterone sulfate	0.2 µg/mL (0.54 µmol/L)

Which of the following is the most appropriate management?

(A) Hydrocortisone

(B) Increased levothyroxine dosage

(C) Morning (9 AM) measurement of serum cortisol and ACTH levels

(D) MRI of the pituitary gland

Item 40

A 29-year-old woman is evaluated for a 1-week history of new-onset severe headache and progressive fatigue, dizziness, weakness, arthralgia, and nausea. The patient is at 28 weeks' gestation (gravida 2, para 1). Before pregnancy, she had normal menses and no difficulty conceiving. She has a history of Hashimoto thyroiditis. Medications are levothyroxine and a multivitamin.

On physical examination, she is pale and appears ill. Blood pressure is 96/50 mm Hg, pulse rate is 90/min, and respiration rate is 14/min. Vision is normal. No evidence of Cushing syndrome or acromegaly is noted.

A noncontrast brain MRI obtained to evaluate her headache symptoms reveals a symmetric and homogeneous sellar mass measuring 15 mm in diameter with extension to the chiasm without compression. No cavernous sinus invasion is noted.

Laboratory studies:

Adrenocorticotropic hormone	<5 pg/mL (1 pmol/L)
Cortisol (8:00 AM)	7.9 µg/dL (218 nmol/L) (normal, 5-25 µg/dL [138-690 nmol/L])
Prolactin	55 ng/mL (55 µg/L)
Thyroid-stimulating hormone	1.9 µU/mL (1.9 mU/L)
Thyroxine (T_4), free	1.3 ng/dL (17 pmol/L)

Which of the following is the most likely diagnosis?

(A) Craniopharyngioma

(B) Lymphocytic hypophysitis

(C) Prolactinoma

(D) Sheehan syndrome

Item 41

A 48-year-old woman is evaluated after laboratory study results show a hemoglobin A_{1c} value of 8.5% (estimated average plasma glucose level of 197 mg/dL [10.9 mmol/L]). The patient has type 2 diabetes mellitus. Her blood glucose logs indicate an average fasting and preprandial blood glucose level of 132 mg/dL (7.3 mmol/L) for the past 3 months. She also has a history of iron deficiency anemia secondary to menorrhagia and has recently started iron replacement therapy. Other medications are neutral protamine Hagedorn (NPH) insulin at bedtime and metformin three times daily with meals.

On physical examination, temperature is 36.9 °C (98.4 °F), blood pressure is 127/78 mm Hg, pulse rate is 77/min, and respiration rate is 14/min; BMI is 26. All other findings from the physical examination are unremarkable.

Results of laboratory studies are normal except for a repeat hemoglobin A_{1c} value of 8.5% and a fasting plasma glucose level of 130 mg/dL (7.2 mmol/L); a blood glucose level obtained simultaneously on the patient's glucose monitor is 134 mg/dL (7.4 mmol/L).

Which of the following best explains the discrepancy between her average blood glucose levels as measured on the glucose monitor and her hemoglobin A_{1c} values?

(A) Inaccurate glucose monitor

(B) Iron therapy

(C) Nocturnal hypoglycemia

(D) Postprandial hyperglycemia

Item 42

A 57-year-old man develops tingling and numbness around his mouth and cramping in his feet and hands 8 hours after removal of a single enlarged parathyroid gland during minimally invasive surgery. He experienced some postoperative pain and is still hospitalized. The patient has a history of primary hyperparathyroidism and kidney stones. His only medication is a multivitamin.

On physical examination, vital signs are normal. A positive Chvostek sign and Trousseau phenomenon are noted, as is a spontaneous carpopedal spasm. The remainder of the examination is unremarkable.

Laboratory studies:

Albumin	3.9 g/dL (39 g/L)
Calcium	
Before surgery	11.6 mg/dL (2.9 mmol/L)
After surgery	7.2 mg/dL (1.8 mmol/L)
Creatinine	1.3 mg/dL (115 µmol/L)
Phosphorus	1.9 mg/dL (0.61 mmol/L)
Parathyroid hormone	
Before surgery	Elevated
After surgery	Normal
25-Hydroxyvitamin D	32 ng/mL (80 nmol/L)

Which of the following is the most likely cause of this patient's hypocalcemia?

(A) Chronic kidney disease

(B) Dilutional hypocalcemia

(C) Hungry bone syndrome

(D) Hyperventilation

Item 43

An 18-year-old woman is evaluated for a lump in her neck that she first noticed several weeks ago. She is in otherwise excellent health and has no history of radiation exposure or other medical issues. She has no family history of thyroid nodules or thyroid cancer and takes no medication.

On physical examination, vital signs are normal; BMI is 21. Examination of the thyroid gland shows a firm left-sided thyroid nodule that moves when she swallows. The rest of the gland is not palpable, with no cervical lymphadenopathy.

Laboratory studies show a thyroid-stimulating hormone level of 1.0 µU/mL (1.0 mU/L). Results of a complete blood count and comprehensive metabolic profile are normal.

A thyroid ultrasound shows a 2- × 2-cm solid hypo-echoic left-sided thyroid nodule with increased intranodular vascular flow. Results of the fine-needle aspiration (FNA) biopsy are consistent with a follicular neoplasm.

Which of the following is the most appropriate next step in management?

(A) Levothyroxine suppression
(B) Radioactive iodine therapy
(C) Repeat FNA biopsy of the nodule in 6 months
(D) Thyroid lobectomy

Item 44

A 28-year-old woman is evaluated for a 5-month history of amenorrhea. She formerly had normal menses. The patient reports eating a healthy diet and having increased stress at work; she does not exercise. Personal and family medical history is unremarkable. She takes no medication.

On physical examination, temperature is 36.8 °C (98.2 °F), blood pressure is 110/70 mm Hg, pulse rate is 60/min, and respiration rate is 10/min; BMI is 23. Results of visual field, thyroid, and pelvic examinations are normal. Skin examination reveals mild facial acne. No galactorrhea is noted.

Laboratory studies show a serum follicle-stimulating hormone level of 4 mU/mL (4 units/L), a serum prolactin level of 14 ng/mL (14 µg/L), and a serum thyroid-stimulating hormone level of 1.3 µU/mL (1.3 mU/L). Human chorionic gonadotropin testing has negative results, and a progesterone challenge test produces no withdrawal bleeding.

A pituitary MRI is normal.

Which of the following is the most likely cause of this patient's amenorrhea?

(A) Functional hypothalamic amenorrhea
(B) Polycystic ovary syndrome
(C) Primary ovarian insufficiency
(D) Subclinical hypothyroidism

Item 45

A 56-year-old man comes to the office for a follow-up evaluation. Since receiving a diagnosis of type 2 diabetes mellitus 6 months ago, he has been eating a low-fat, high-fiber, high-carbohydrate diet and walking for 20 minutes at night. The patient has never smoked and drinks no alcohol. He originally took metformin to treat his diabetes but stopped because of persistent diarrhea. Current medications are glyburide and ramipril.

On physical examination, temperature is 36.8 °C (98.2 °F), blood pressure is 129/76 mm Hg, pulse rate is 76/min, and respiration rate is 15/min; BMI is 22. Other physical examination findings are normal.

Laboratory studies:

Alanine aminotransferase	102 units/L
Aspartate aminotransferase	96 units/L
Cholesterol	
Total	264 mg/dL (6.83 mmol/L)
LDL	157 mg/dL (4.07 mmol/L)
HDL	42 mg/dL (1.09 mmol/L)
Glucose, fasting	196 mg/dL (10.9 mmol/L)
Hemoglobin A_{1c}	9.8%
Iron studies	Normal
Triglycerides	437 mg/dL (4.94 mmol/L)
Hepatitis virus studies	Negative

Bedtime neutral protamine Hagedorn (NPH) insulin is initiated.

Which of the following is the most appropriate treatment of his hyperlipidemia?

(A) Begin a fibrate now
(B) Begin a statin now
(C) Begin a statin after results of liver chemistry studies normalize
(D) Begin nicotinic acid (niacin) now
(E) Begin either a fibrate or nicotinic acid after results of liver chemistry studies normalize

Item 46

A 58-year-old man is evaluated for a 1-week history of headache that started after he sustained minor head trauma with no loss of consciousness in a motor vehicle collision. A CT scan obtained in the emergency department revealed a sellar mass. The patient has a 2-year history of mild sexual dysfunction but no other symptoms. He takes no medication.

On physical examination, blood pressure is 126/78 mm Hg and pulse rate is 64/min; BMI is 32. Normal secondary sexual characteristics are noted, and no gynecomastia is present. Other examination findings also are normal.

Laboratory studies show normal insulin-like growth factor 1 and morning cortisol levels

An MRI shows a 1.7-cm sellar mass with suprasellar extension but no chiasmal compression.

In addition to assessing adrenal and thyroid function, which of the following is the most appropriate next diagnostic step?

(A) Dexamethasone suppression test
(B) Growth hormone stimulation test
(C) Serum prolactin measurement
(D) Serum sodium and urine osmolality measurements

Item 47

A 57-year-old woman returns to the office to discuss her laboratory results after a recent routine physical examination. She has hypertension treated with lisinopril but is otherwise healthy and takes no vitamins or supplements. At her previous evaluation, blood pressure was 129/84 mm Hg, pulse rate was 86/min, and BMI was 26; all other physical examination findings were normal.

Previous laboratory studies:

Albumin	3.8 g/dL (38 g/L)
Calcium	10.6 mg/dL (2.7 mmol/L)
Creatinine	0.9 mg/dL (79.6 µmol/L)
Parathyroid hormone	61 pg/mL (61 ng/L)

She has no history of fractures, kidney stones, or bone pain but recalls that her brother was evaluated for an elevated serum calcium level several years ago; she says he is currently healthy and has not required any treatment or surgery.

Which of the following is the most appropriate next test in this patient's evaluation?

(A) Measurement of the serum prolactin level
(B) Measurement of the serum 25-hydroxyvitamin D level
(C) Measurement of the urine calcium and urine creatinine levels
(D) Parathyroid sestamibi scan

Item 48

A 64-year-old woman is evaluated in the intensive care unit for persistent hypotension secondary to pyelonephritis-related gram-negative sepsis. The patient was admitted to the hospital 2 days ago and has received appropriate fluid and vasopressor resuscitation and antibiotic therapy. She is no longer receiving vasopressors.

Physical examination reveals a pale woman. Temperature is 37.9 °C (100.2 °F), blood pressure is 92/64 mm Hg supine, pulse rate is 102/min supine, and respiration rate is 16/min. The remaining physical examination findings are unremarkable.

Laboratory studies:

Albumin	2.1 g/dL (21 g/L)
Electrolytes	
Sodium	139 meq/L (139 mmol/L)
Potassium	3.6 meq/L (3.6 mmol/L)
Chloride	109 meq/L (109 mmol/L)
Bicarbonate	23 meq/L (23 mmol/L)
Cortisol, random	15 µg/dL (414 nmol/L)

Which of the following is the most appropriate management?

(A) Continuation of current therapy
(B) Cosyntropin stimulation test
(C) Morning (9 AM) measurement of serum cortisol level
(D) Stress doses of hydrocortisone

Item 49

A 62-year-old woman is admitted to the hospital in a coma. Her daughter says that her mother has had progressive lethargy, malaise, disorientation, and ataxia over the past 2 days. The patient received radioactive iodine therapy 10 years ago for an overactive thyroid gland and has hypertension. She does not drink alcohol or smoke. Medications are levothyroxine and hydrochlorothiazide, although the daughter reports that her mother is only intermittently adherent to her medication regimen.

Physical examination shows an ill-appearing woman who is comatose and not responding to verbal commands. Temperature is 35.9 °C (96.6 °F), blood pressure is 105/65 mm Hg, pulse rate is 75/min, and respiration rate is 10/min. Cardiac examination shows a grade 2/6 holosystolic murmur at the left lower sternal border. Lung examination reveals dependent crackles, but findings are otherwise normal. The thyroid gland is not palpable, and no cervical lymphadenopathy is noted. The skin is dry and cold, and the face, lips, and hands are mildly edematous. Abdominal examination findings are normal.

Laboratory studies:

Leukocyte count	20,000/µL (20 × 10⁹/L), with 80% neutrophils
Electrolytes	
Sodium	132 meq/L (132 mmol/L)
Potassium	3.5 meq/L (3.5 mmol/L)
Chloride	103 meq/L (103 mmol/L)
Bicarbonate	26 meq/L (26 mmol/L)
Glucose	45 mg/dL (2.5 mmol/L)
pH	7.30
Thyroid-stimulating hormone	140 µU/mL (140 mU/L)
Thyroxine (T$_4$), free	0.2 ng/dL (3 pmol/L)
Triiodothyronine (T$_3$)	<20 ng/dL (0.3 nmol/L)

A serum cortisol level is pending.

A chest radiograph shows mild bibasilar infiltrates and an enlarged heart. A CT scan of the head without contrast is normal.

Which of the following is the most appropriate initial treatment of this patient?

(A) Intravenous levothyroxine
(B) Intravenous levothyroxine and hydrocortisone
(C) Intravenous liothyronine
(D) Intravenous liothyronine and hydrocortisone

Item 50

A 47-year-old man is evaluated for a 5-year history of sexual dysfunction and a 3-month history of headache. He reports low libido and erectile dysfunction. Personal and family medical histories are unremarkable. The patient takes no medication.

On physical examination, vital signs are normal; BMI is 24. Funduscopic, visual field, and cranial nerve examination findings are normal. Testes are small and descended bilaterally. No testicular mass is palpated.

Laboratory studies:

Comprehensive metabolic profile	Normal
Follicle-stimulating hormone	2 mU/mL (2 units/L)
Luteinizing hormone	1.3 mU/mL (1.3 units/L)
Prolactin	78 ng/mL (78 µg/L)
Thyroid-stimulating hormone	2.1 µU/mL (2.1 mU/L)
Total testosterone	132 ng/dL (4.6 nmol/L)

Which of the following is the most appropriate initial management?

(A) Cabergoline therapy
(B) Pituitary MRI
(C) Testicular ultrasonography
(D) Testosterone therapy

Item 51

A 35-year-old man is evaluated for a 2-month history of low libido. The patient had a normal puberty. Family history is unremarkable. He drinks two beers per week and takes no medication.

On physical examination, vital signs are normal; BMI is 23. Visual field examination findings are normal, as is testicular size. No gynecomastia is noted.

Laboratory studies:

Follicle-stimulating hormone	6 mU/mL (6 units/L)
Luteinizing hormone	5 mU/mL (5 units/L)
Thyroid-stimulating hormone	2.5 µU/mL (2.5 mU/L)
Total testosterone (4 PM)	200 ng/dL (7 nmol/L)

Which of the following is the most appropriate next diagnostic test?

(A) Measurement of serum ferritin and iron saturation levels
(B) Morning serum free testosterone measurement
(C) Morning serum total testosterone measurement
(D) Testicular ultrasonography

Item 52

A 24-year-old woman is evaluated for a 1-week history of neck discomfort that radiates to the jaw, palpitations, a fast heart rate, anxiety, and fever. The patient reports having a sore throat 4 weeks ago that resolved after a few days. She has no other symptoms and no personal history of thyroid or endocrine disorders. Her only medication is an oral contraceptive.

Physical examination shows an anxious-appearing woman. Temperature is 37.5 °C (99.5 °F), blood pressure is 140/60 mm Hg, pulse rate is 110/min, and respiration rate is 16/min; BMI is 23. Cardiopulmonary examination reveals tachycardia, but other findings are normal. The thyroid gland is slightly enlarged and tender with no nodules. No thyroid bruit is heard, and no cervical lymphadenopathy is palpated. No eye findings or pretibial myxedema is noted. The patient has a fine bilateral hand tremor.

Laboratory studies:

Erythrocyte sedimentation rate	45 mm/h
Thyroid-stimulating hormone	<0.01 µU/mL (0.01 mU/L)
Thyroxine (T_4), free	4.1 ng/dL (53 pmol/L)
Triiodothyronine (T_3)	300 ng/dL (4.6 nmol/L)

A Doppler thyroid ultrasound shows an enlarged thyroid gland with heterogeneous echotexture without cervical lymphadenopathy; no significant vascular flow is evident.

Which of the following is the most appropriate next step in management?

(A) Bilateral fine-needle aspiration biopsy
(B) Methimazole
(C) Serum thyroglobulin measurement
(D) 24-Hour radioactive iodine uptake test

Item 53

An 82-year-old woman is evaluated for the recent development of frequent episodes of confusion and forgetfulness. She has a 6-year history of type 2 diabetes mellitus and a 5-year history of heart failure. Medications are glyburide, furosemide, lisinopril, and potassium supplements.

On physical examination, temperature is normal, blood pressure is 142/77 mm Hg, pulse rate is 87/min, and respiration rate is 16/min; BMI is 20. All other physical examination findings are unremarkable, including those from a mental status examination.

Laboratory studies show a serum creatinine level of 1.3 mg/dL (115 µmol/L) and a hemoglobin A_{1c} value of 6.2%.

Which of the following is the most appropriate immediate next step in management?

(A) Discontinue glyburide
(B) Start glipizide
(C) Start metformin
(D) Start premixed 70/30 insulin (neutral protamine Hagedorn [NPH] insulin/regular insulin)

Item 54

A 58-year-old woman is evaluated during a routine physical examination. She reports no headache, heartburn, breast discomfort, change in energy or mood, or bone pain. The patient has osteoarthritis and a history of a distal tibia fracture sustained 1 year ago when she tripped while walking. She has never had kidney stones and has no family history of endocrinopathies, kidney stones, or bone disease. Medications are ibuprofen as needed and a daily multivitamin.

Physical examination finding, including vital signs, are unremarkable.

Laboratory findings:

Albumin	4.1 g/dL (41 g/L)
Blood urea nitrogen	20 mg/L (7.1 mmol/L)
Calcium	11.1 mg/dL (2.8 mmol/L)

Creatinine	0.7 mg/dL (61.9 µmol/L)
Estimated glomerular filtration rate	65 mL/min/1.73 m²
Parathyroid hormone	63 pg/mL (63 ng/L)

A dual-energy x-ray absorptiometry scan shows T-scores of −1.8 in the lumbar spine, −2.0 in the total hip, −2.2 in the femoral neck, and −2.2 in the distal radius.

Which of the following is the most appropriate next step in managing this patient's disease?

(A) Bisphosphonate therapy

(B) Bone scan

(C) Parathyroidectomy

(D) Parathyroid hormone–related protein measurement

(E) Repeat serum calcium measurement in 1 year

Item 55

A 72-year-old man is hospitalized for treatment of community-acquired pneumonia. Despite 4 days of treatment with intravenous fluids and antibiotics appropriate for the bacteria cultured from sputum and blood, he remains febrile with mild tachycardia. The patient subsequently develops mild hypotension and is transferred to the intensive care unit. Results of two subsequent blood cultures are negative for bacteria. Medical history is significant for hypertension treated with amlodipine and recurrent osteoarthritis treated with intra-articular injections of triamcinolone several times a year; his last injection occurred 3 months ago.

Physical examination shows a pale and anxious man. Temperature is 38.0 °C (100.4 °F), blood pressure is 110/68 mm Hg supine and 102/64 mm Hg sitting, pulse rate is 102/min supine and 124/min sitting, and respiration rate is 21/min; BMI is 33. Lung examination reveals crackles and egophony in the right lower lobe area. Other physical examination findings are unremarkable.

Laboratory studies:

Albumin	2.7 g/dL (27 g/L)
Electrolytes	
Sodium	139 meq/L (139 mmol/L)
Potassium	3.6 meq/L (3.6 mmol/L)
Chloride	109 meq/L (109 mmol/L)
Bicarbonate	23 meq/L (23 mmol/L)
Cortisol, random	9.5 µg/dL (262 nmol/L)
Thyroid-stimulating hormone	Normal

Which of the following is the most appropriate next step in management?

(A) Adrenocorticotropic hormone stimulation test

(B) Hydrocortisone

(C) Pseudomonal antibiotic coverage

(D) Vasopressor support

Item 56

An 88-year-old man is evaluated during a routine physical examination. He reports moderate fatigue but has no other symptoms, such as nervousness, weight gain or loss, joint discomfort, constipation, palpitations, or dyspnea. The patient has a history of hypertension. Medications are daily lisinopril and daily low-dose aspirin.

Physical examination shows an alert and oriented older man. Blood pressure is 140/85 mm Hg; all other vital signs are normal. Cardiac examination shows a grade 1/6 crescendo-decrescendo systolic murmur, and pulmonary examination findings are normal. The thyroid gland is not palpable; no cervical lymphadenopathy is noted. Results of examination of the extremities, including pulses, are normal.

Laboratory studies:

Complete blood count	Normal
Comprehensive metabolic profile	Normal
Thyroid function tests (repeated and confirmed)	
Thyroid-stimulating hormone	6.8 µU/mL (6.8 mU/L)
Thyroxine (T₄), free	1.1 ng/dL (14 pmol/L)
Thyroid peroxidase antibody titer	Normal

Which of the following is the most appropriate management?

(A) Levothyroxine

(B) Liothyronine

(C) Radioactive iodine test

(D) Observation

Item 57

A 38-year-old woman reports a 3-month history of increasing fatigue and weight gain. She underwent transsphenoidal surgery 4 years ago to remove a nonfunctioning pituitary macroadenoma, followed 4 months later by radiation therapy because of residual tumor. She started taking hydrocortisone 14 months ago after adrenal insufficiency was diagnosed. The patient developed amenorrhea 1 year ago and began taking an oral contraceptive. Medications are hydrocortisone, norethindrone with ethinyl estradiol, and a multivitamin.

On physical examination, blood pressure is 102/68 mm Hg, pulse rate is 64/min, and respiration rate is 12/min. Mild periorbital edema is noted. The skin is pale.

Laboratory studies:

Hemoglobin	Normal
Sodium	134 meq/L (134 mmol/L)
Prolactin	22 ng/mL (22 µg/L)
Thyroid-stimulating hormone	1.1 µU/mL (1.1 mU/L)

Which of the following is the most appropriate next diagnostic test?

(A) Morning serum cortisol measurement

(B) Serum free thyroxine (T₄) measurement

(C) Serum growth hormone measurement

(D) Serum luteinizing hormone measurement

Item 58

A 40-year-old woman is evaluated in the emergency department at 1 AM for a 7-hour history of gradually worsening generalized abdominal pain, hyperventilation, and lethargy. Her husband reports difficulty awakening her on several occasions since onset of symptoms, both during the evening and at night. The patient has a 3-day history of nausea and anorexia. She has a 22-year history of type 1 diabetes mellitus treated with insulin. Because she has been unable to eat or drink for the past 3 days, she has reduced her dosage of basal insulin by half and taken no premeal rapid-acting insulin during this period. Her only other medical problem is hypertriglyceridemia. Medications before coming to the emergency department were insulin glargine, prandial insulin glulisine, gemfibrozil, niacin, and daily fish oil.

Physical examination shows a lethargic but arousable woman. Temperature is 96.8 °C (36.0 °F), blood pressure is 105/70 mm Hg, pulse rate is 118/min, and respiration rate is 28/min; BMI is 36. Deep sighing respirations are noted, but the chest is clear to auscultation. She has a sweet smell on her breath. Abdominal examination reveals generalized abdominal tenderness with guarding but no rebound tenderness. Bowel sounds are heard in all four quadrants.

Laboratory studies:

Hemoglobin	14.7 g/dL (147 g/L)
Leukocyte count	23,000/µL (23 × 10⁹/L), with 90% polymorphonuclear leukocytes
Electrolytes	
Sodium	149 meq/L (149 mmol/L)
Potassium	5.1 meq/L (5.1 mmol/L)
Chloride	92 meq/L (92 mmol/L)
Bicarbonate	4 meq/L (4 mmol/L)
Glucose, fasting	615 mg/dL (34.1 mmol/L)
Amylase	1168 units/L
Urinalysis	4+ glucose, 4+ ketones, no bacteria or leukocytes

A chest radiograph is normal.

Besides administering intravenous fluids and insulin, which of the following is the most appropriate management?

(A) Abdominal CT
(B) Endoscopic retrograde cholangiopancreatography
(C) Imipenem
(D) Laparotomy
(E) Serial abdominal examinations

Item 59

A 55-year-old man is reevaluated during a follow-up examination for a wrist fracture and anemia. The patient is otherwise asymptomatic. He was treated in the emergency department 2 weeks ago after he slipped in his driveway and sustained a right wrist fracture; mild iron deficiency anemia was detected at that time. He had normal results of a routine screening colonoscopy 5 years ago. Since his emergency department evaluation, 3 stool samples have been negative for occult blood. He takes no medication.

On physical examination, vital signs are normal; BMI is 19. Other than a cast on his right wrist, all other findings are normal.

Hemoglobin level is 11.9 g/dL (119 g/L), and 25-hydroxyvitamin D level is 17 ng/mL (42 nmol/L). Results of a comprehensive metabolic profile and urinalysis are normal.

A dual-energy x-ray absorptiometry (DEXA) scan shows T-scores of −1.6 in the lumbar spine, −2.2 in the femoral neck, and −1.9 in the total hip.

Which of the following is the most appropriate next step in management?

(A) Begin alendronate
(B) Begin teriparatide
(C) Repeat DEXA scan in 1 year
(D) Screen for celiac disease

Item 60

A 66-year-old woman is evaluated in the emergency department for sudden onset of bilateral flank pain, hypotension, nausea, fatigue, and dizziness. The patient had knee replacement surgery 2 weeks ago and has been taking warfarin for prevention of deep venous thrombosis and oxycodone for pain.

On physical examination, temperature is 38.3 °C (100.9 °F), blood pressure is 98/66 mm Hg supine and 84/60 mm Hg sitting, pulse rate is 102/min supine and 122/min sitting, and respiration rate is 16/min; BMI is 29. Bilateral flank tenderness and dry mucous membranes are noted. The surgical wound is clean.

Laboratory studies:

Hematocrit	21% (34% 5 days ago)
INR	5.5
Leukocyte count	6500/µL (6.5 × 10⁹/L)
Creatinine	1.0 mg/dL (88.4 µmol/L)
Electrolytes	
Sodium	129 meq/L (129 mmol/L)
Potassium	5.4 meq/L (5.4 mmol/L)
Chloride	95 meq/L (95 mmol/L)
Bicarbonate	24 meq/L (24 mmol/L)
Glucose, random	89 mg/dL (4.9 mmol/L)

Which of the following is the most likely cause of her symptoms?

(A) Adrenal hemorrhage
(B) Gastrointestinal bleeding
(C) Narcotic overdose
(D) Septic shock

Item 61

An 82-year-old man is intubated and admitted to the intensive care unit (ICU) for sepsis and hypotension from community-acquired pneumonia. According to his wife, the patient had coronary artery bypass graft surgery 2 years ago and has had intermittent atrial fibrillation since that time that is treated with amiodarone, 200 mg/d. He has no history of thyroid abnormalities. Other medications administered in the ICU are vasopressors, ceftriaxone, and azithromycin.

Physical examination shows a sedated, ill-appearing older man who is intubated and cannot respond to questions. Temperature is 37.8 °C (100.0 °F), blood pressure is 90/50 mm Hg (with vasopressors), pulse rate is 110/min and irregular, and respiration rate is 18/min while intubated; BMI is 30. Cardiac examination reveals an irregular rate without murmurs, rubs, or gallops. Examination of the lungs reveals bibasilar crackles and rhonchi. The thyroid gland is not palpable. No cervical lymphadenopathy is noted. No bowel sounds are heard on abdominal examination. The extremities show 2+ peripheral edema. A few scattered ecchymoses are present on the skin.

Laboratory studies:

Cortisol, random	28 µg/dL (773 nmol/L)
Thyroid antibodies	Pending
Thyroid-stimulating hormone (TSH)	16 µU/mL (16 mU/L)
Thyroxine (T$_4$), free	0.6 ng/dL (8 pmol/L)
Triiodothyronine (T$_3$)	45 ng/dL (0.7 nmol/L)

An electrocardiogram shows tachycardia and atrial fibrillation, and a chest radiograph shows bibasilar infiltrates.

Which of the following is the most likely underlying endocrine disorder in this patient?

(A) Adrenal insufficiency
(B) Euthyroid sick syndrome
(C) Hypothyroidism
(D) TSH-secreting pituitary tumor

Item 62

A 32-year-old woman is evaluated for increased hair growth on the face and chest and a 3-month history of irregular menses. She has a 5-year history of hypothyroidism. Her only medication is levothyroxine.

On physical examination, temperature is 37.0 °C (98.6 °F), blood pressure is 110/72 mm Hg, and pulse rate is 80/min; BMI is 26. Terminal hair growth of the upper lip, chin, sides of the face, and middle of the chest is noted. No acanthosis nigricans or galactorrhea is detected. Palpation of the abdomen reveals no masses. Pelvic examination reveals clitoromegaly.

Laboratory studies:

Dehydroepiandrosterone sulfate	2.78 µg/mL (7.5 µmol/L)
Prolactin	17 ng/mL (17 µg/L)
Total testosterone	279 ng/dL (9.7 nmol/L)
Thyroid-stimulating hormone	1.5 µU/mL (1.5 mU/L)

Which of the following is the most appropriate next diagnostic test?

(A) Adrenal CT
(B) Free testosterone measurement
(C) Pituitary MRI
(D) Transvaginal ultrasonography

Item 63

A 62-year-old man is admitted to the hospital for a right hip replacement. The patient has a 36-year history of type 1 diabetes mellitus. He also has proliferative diabetic retinopathy treated previously with laser therapy and peripheral and autonomic neuropathy. Before admission, the patient's diabetes was treated with premixed 70/30 insulin (neutral protamine Hagedorn [NPH] insulin/regular insulin); he took 18 units of this preparation before breakfast and 12 units before his evening meal. His most recent hemoglobin A$_{1c}$ value indicated good glycemic control.

On physical examination, temperature is normal, blood pressure is 138/79 mm Hg, pulse rate is 88/min, and respiration rate is 16/min; BMI is 22. Other physical examination findings are consistent with the previously established diagnoses of diabetic retinopathy with laser scars, autonomic neuropathy, and osteoarthritis of the right hip.

Which of the following is the most appropriate insulin therapy after surgery?

(A) Insulin glargine once daily and insulin aspart before each meal
(B) Intravenous insulin infusion
(C) Previous schedule of 70/30 insulin
(D) Sliding scale insulin schedule with regular insulin given whenever the blood glucose level is 150 mg/dL (8.3 mmol/L) or greater
(E) Subcutaneous insulin infusion

Item 64

A 33-year-old woman is evaluated for a 5-month history of amenorrhea and a 3-month history of galactorrhea. The patient says her menstrual cycles were normal before onset of amenorrhea. She takes no medication.

On physical examination, vital signs are normal. Visual field findings are normal. Bilateral galactorrhea is noted.

Results of laboratory studies show a serum luteinizing hormone level of 2 mU/mL (2 units/L), a prolactin level of 965 ng/mL (965 µg/L), and a free thyroxine level of 1.1 ng/dL (14 pmol/L). A serum β-human chorionic gonadotropin measurement is normal.

An MRI shows a 1.5-cm sellar mass with suprasellar extension that impinges on the optic chiasm.

Which of the following is the most appropriate initial treatment?

(A) Dopamine agonist therapy
(B) Oral contraceptive
(C) Radiation therapy
(D) Transsphenoidal surgical resection

Item 65

A 72-year-old woman is evaluated in the emergency department for loss of consciousness. Her son, who brought her in, says she seemed confused and agitated when he spoke to her on the telephone less than 2 hours ago. The patient has an 8-year history of type 2 diabetes mellitus. She had strict glycemic control (average hemoglobin A$_{1c}$ level, 6.2%) until last month when she had an infected ulcer between the third and fourth toes of the right foot that resulted in amputation of the middle toe 1 week ago. According to her son, she has been depressed while recovering at home and is not eating or drinking much. Medications are glyburide, cephalexin, and ibuprofen as needed.

On physical examination, temperature is 37.9 °C (100.2 °F), blood pressure is 162/96 mm Hg, pulse rate is 112/min, and respiration rate is 21/min; BMI is 19. The patient remains unconscious and is unresponsive to noxious stimuli. Dense left hemiplegia, warmth, and profuse sweating are noted. No inguinal lymphadenopathy is observed. The right middle toe amputation is healing well without redness, discharge, or swelling. No ankle edema is noted.

Which of the following is the most appropriate next step in management?

(A) Addition of vancomycin and ceftriaxone to the antibiotic regimen
(B) Fingerstick measurement of the blood glucose level
(C) Intravenous infusion of recombinant tissue plasminogen activator
(D) Noncontrast CT of the head

Item 66

A 71-year-old woman is evaluated for a 3-month history of occasional hoarseness and intermittent difficulty swallowing. The patient has a 10-year history of a multinodular goiter. Results of previous fine-needle aspiration biopsies, including one 6 months ago, have been negative for cancer, showing only bland-appearing follicular cells, colloid, and macrophages. She is otherwise healthy and takes no medication.

Physical examination reveals a vigorous woman. Vital signs are normal. The patient's face is slightly flushed and becomes more flushed when she raises her arms. Examination of the neck shows an enlarged thyroid gland that contains several firm but not hard nodules. The gland moves easily with swallowing. All other physical examination findings are normal, with no evidence of thyrotoxicosis.

Results of laboratory studies show a serum thyroid-stimulating hormone level of 0.51 µU/mL (0.51 mU/L) and free thyroxine (T$_4$) level of 1.6 ng/dL (21 pmol/L).

Radioactive iodine uptake is 28%. A thyroid scan reveals multiple patchy areas of either increased or decreased uptake.

A CT scan without contrast shows a large multinodular goiter, with substernal extension and extrinsic moderate compression of the trachea on the right, and a patent airway.

Which of the following is the most appropriate treatment?

(A) External-beam radiation to the neck
(B) Levothyroxine
(C) Methimazole
(D) Thyroidectomy

Item 67

A 42-year-old man is evaluated for a 6-day history of severe burning and stabbing pain in both feet that is worse in the toes. The pain is more severe at night, is aggravated when the bed sheets touch his skin, and is partially relieved when he walks or massages his feet. The patient has an 8-year history of poorly controlled type 1 diabetes mellitus and a 2-year history of hypertension. He was hospitalized briefly 2 weeks ago for treatment of pneumonia and diabetic ketoacidosis. His fasting blood glucose levels have been in the range of 150 to 200 mg/dL (8.3-11.1 mmol/L) since hospital discharge. He does not drink alcohol or smoke. Medications are insulin glargine, insulin glulisine, and lisinopril.

On physical examination, vital signs are normal; BMI is 22. Both feet and ankles are exquisitely sensitive to touch and temperature, especially on the tips of the toes. Pulses are easily palpated in both feet. No fasciculations, muscle weakness, foot ulcers, or foot deformities are noted. Monofilament testing reveals insensate feet bilaterally. Ankle reflexes are absent bilaterally.

Results of laboratory studies show a hemoglobin A$_{1c}$ value of 9.2%.

In addition to improving glycemic control, which of the following is the most appropriate next step in management?

(A) Desipramine
(B) Fluoxetine
(C) Nerve conduction studies
(D) Oxycodone
(E) Sural nerve biopsy

Item 68

A 78-year-old woman is evaluated for a rapidly enlarging neck mass that has been present for 4 weeks and is associated with neck discomfort, dysphagia, and hoarseness. The patient has had Hashimoto thyroiditis and hypothyroidism since age 24 years and has been taking levothyroxine since that time.

Physical examination reveals an older woman in severe distress. Temperature is 39.4 °C (102.9 °F), blood pressure is 145/75 mm Hg, pulse rate is 110/min, and respiration rate is 16/min; BMI is 23. Pulmonary examination reveals dyspnea with bilateral basilar rhonchi, and cardiac examination shows tachycardia without a murmur. The thyroid gland is enlarged and firm without nodules. Facial plethora and distended bilateral cervical neck veins are noted. The patient is hoarse. Bilateral cervical lymphadenopathy is palpated. Although neurologically intact, she finds it difficult to concentrate when asked questions.

A thyroid ultrasound shows an enlarged thyroid gland with heterogeneous echotexture but no specific nodularity and multiple bilateral cervical lymph nodes measuring 1 to 3 cm in diameter.

Which of the following is the most likely diagnosis?

(A) Bleeding into the thyroid gland
(B) Medullary thyroid cancer
(C) Papillary thyroid cancer
(D) Primary thyroid lymphoma

Item 69

A 33-year-old woman is evaluated for a 2-week history of progressive fatigue, dizziness, anorexia, and arthralgia in multiple joints. Six weeks ago, the patient (gravida 2, para 2) had a difficult labor and delivery requiring multiple blood transfusions; her pregnancy had been uneventful. She subsequently was unable to lactate and has had no menses. Her only medication is a daily multivitamin.

Physical examination reveals a pale, thin woman. Temperature is 37.1 °C (98.7 °F), blood pressure is 88/50 mm Hg, pulse rate is 88/min, and respiration rate is 16/min; BMI is 19. Visual field examination findings are normal. No galactorrhea is noted.

Laboratory studies:

Sodium	129 meq/L (129 mmol/L)
Adrenocorticotropic hormone	5 pg/mL (1 pmol/L)
Cortisol (8:00 AM)	2.4 µg/dL (66 nmol/L) (normal, 5-25 µg/dL [138-690 nmol/L])
Follicle-stimulating hormone	1.1 mU/mL (1.1 units/L)
Prolactin	1.3 ng/mL (1.3 µg/L)
Thyroid-stimulating hormone	1.3 µU/mL (1.3 mU/L)

Results of a pituitary MRI are pending.

Which of the following is the most appropriate initial treatment?

(A) Arginine vasopressin replacement therapy
(B) Hydrocortisone
(C) Hypertonic saline
(D) Levothyroxine

Item 70

An 18-year-old woman is evaluated for syncope. She has had three episodes in the past month that resolved after she drank fruit juice with sugar. She has a history of depression treated with citalopram and occasional insomnia treated with zolpidem as needed. Her mother has type 2 diabetes mellitus treated with neutral protamine Hagedorn (NPH) insulin and glyburide.

Several minutes into her evaluation, the patient becomes confused and agitated with tachycardia and profuse sweating. A blood specimen is drawn, and intravenous glucose is administered to resolve her symptoms.

Physical examination shows a pale, thin woman. Vital signs are normal, and other physical examination findings are unremarkable.

Laboratory studies:

C-peptide	0.4 ng/mL (0.13 nmol/L) (normal range, 0.5-2.5 ng/mL [0.16-0.82 nmol/L])
Glucose, fasting	34 mg/dL (1.9 mmol/L)
Insulin	26 µU/mL (187.6 pmol/L) (normal range, 2-20 µU/mL [14.4-144.3 pmol/L])
Sulfonylurea screen	Negative

Which of the following is the most appropriate next step in management?

(A) Abdominal CT
(B) Abdominal octreotide scanning
(C) Gastric emptying study
(D) Psychiatric evaluation

Item 71

A 66-year-old woman is evaluated after a right adrenal mass is found on a CT scan of the abdomen obtained for evaluation of severe abdominal pain, which has since resolved. She has no history of hypertension or diabetes mellitus and has noted no palpitations, headaches, sweating, or weight changes.

On physical examination, temperature is 36.6 °C (97.9 °F), blood pressure is 140/84 mm Hg, pulse rate is 78/min, and respiration rate is 16/min; BMI is 29. The skin is normal, as is the distribution of supraclavicular and posterior cervical fat pads. All other physical examination findings, including those from a neurologic examination, are normal.

Laboratory studies:

Creatinine	1.0 mg/dL (88.4 µmol/L)
Electrolytes	
Sodium	139 meq/L (139 mmol/L)
Potassium	4.1 meq/L (4.1 mmol/L)
Chloride	97 meq/L (97 mmol/L)
Bicarbonate	29 meq/L (29 mmol/L)
Glucose, random	89 mg/dL (4.9 mmol/L)
Cortisol (9 AM)	(Normal, 5-25 µg/dL [138-690 nmol/L])
Baseline	13.8 µg/dL (381 nmol/L)
After 1 mg dexamethasone the night before	1.1 µg/dL (30 nmol/L)
Dehydroepiandrosterone sulfate	0.2 µg/mL (0.54 µmol/L)
Urine metanephrine and normetanephrine	Normal

The previously obtained CT scan shows a right adrenal mass that measures 2.5 cm in its longest dimension and has an attenuation of 9 Hounsfield units.

Which of the following is the most appropriate management?

(A) Metaiodobenzylguanidine (MIBG) scan
(B) MRI
(C) Repeat testing in 6 to 12 months
(D) Right adrenalectomy

Item 72

A 62-year-old man is evaluated in the emergency department for recent onset of fever and severe abdominal pain. He also reports a history of anxiety, frequent palpitations, difficulty concentrating, dyspnea, diarrhea, nausea, vomiting, and weight loss (total, 9.1 kg [20 lb]) over the past few months. He has had no neck discomfort. An abdominal CT

CONT.

scan with iodine contrast obtained several weeks ago when he first experienced abdominal pain was normal. The patient also has a 6-month history of Graves disease treated with methimazole. He takes no other medication.

Physical examination shows an anxious and agitated man. Temperature is 38.9 °C (102.0 °F), blood pressure is 160/90 mm Hg, pulse rate is 130/min and regular, and respiration rate is 22/min. Cardiac examination shows a grade 2/6 holosystolic murmur, and crackles are heard on lung examination. Eye examination shows no acute inflammatory findings. Findings from an examination of the pharynx are normal. The thyroid gland is firm and enlarged bilaterally with no specific nodules palpated. A thyroid bruit is heard. No cervical lymphadenopathy is noted. The skin is warm and moist. Abdominal examination reveals a palpable liver 2 cm below the right costal margin. Examination of the extremities shows 2+ peripheral leg edema. Neurologic examination reveals that the patient is oriented to place but not time, giving the incorrect answer when asked for the year.

Results of laboratory serum studies show a thyroid-stimulating hormone level of less than 0.01 µU/mL (0.01 mU/L), a free thyroxine (T_4) level of 8.2 ng/dL (106 pmol/L), and a triiodothyronine (T_3) level of 650 ng/dL (10 nmol/L).

Which of the following is the most likely diagnosis?

(A) Euthyroid sick syndrome
(B) Myxedema coma
(C) Subacute thyroiditis
(D) Thyroid storm

Item 73

A 31-year-old woman is evaluated during a postpartum examination 6 months after giving birth to her first child. The patient was obese before becoming pregnant, developed gestational diabetes mellitus during pregnancy, and was able to maintain her weight and glucose level within the target range throughout her pregnancy with diet alone. Her infant weighed 4139 grams (146 ounces) at birth.

This patient's infant is at increased risk for which of the following disorders?

(A) Childhood obesity
(B) Maturity-onset diabetes of the young
(C) Type 1A diabetes mellitus
(D) Type 1B diabetes mellitus

Item 74

A 44-year-old man is evaluated for a 2-year history of headache and 1-year history of diabetes mellitus and hypertension. His glove and shoe sizes have increased several times over the past 3 years, and he reports painful knees and hips. The patient also has sleep apnea and carpal tunnel syndrome. Medications are metformin and lisinopril.

On physical examination, blood pressure is 152/92 mm Hg, pulse rate is 82/min, and respiration rate is 16/min. Coarse facial features, frontal bossing, accentuated nasolabial folds, a large tongue, and thick hands and feet are noted.

Which of the following is the most appropriate next diagnostic test?

(A) MRI of the pituitary gland
(B) Random serum growth hormone measurement
(C) Serum insulin-like growth factor 1 measurement
(D) Serum prolactin measurement

Item 75

A 67-year-old man is admitted to the hospital after being found unresponsive and intoxicated at home. Family members report that he has a history of hypertension treated with atenolol and a history of alcoholism. He lives alone and has been resistant to assistance with meals and chores. He takes no other medication.

On physical examination, the patient is lethargic but arousable and smells strongly of alcohol. Vital signs are normal except for a pulse rate of 105/min. Mucous membranes are dry. No pain is elicited on abdominal examination. Chvostek sign and Trousseau phenomenon are noted.

After an electrocardiogram shows tachycardia (heart rate to 105/min) and a prolonged corrected QT interval (0.49 s), the patient is given intravenous fluids with added thiamine and folate. A calcium infusion is initiated.

Laboratory studies (before administration of thiamine, folate, and calcium):

Amylase	110 units/L
Blood urea nitrogen	33 mg/L (11.8 mmol/L)
Creatinine	1.4 mg/dL (124 µmol/L)
Ethanol	249 mg/dL (0.25 g/dL) (normal, <1.0 mg/dL [0.001 g/dL])
Ionized calcium	2.9 mg/dL (0.7 mmol/L) (normal, 3.8-5.3 mg/dL [1.0-1.3 mmol/L])
Phosphorus	2.1 mg/dL (0.68 mmol/L)

In addition to the interventions already underway, measurement of which of the following serum levels is the most appropriate next diagnostic test?

(A) Calcitonin
(B) 1,25-Dihydroxyvitamin D
(C) Magnesium
(D) Parathyroid hormone

Item 76

A 32-year-old man is evaluated for significant blood glucose elevations associated with exercise. The patient has a 22-year history of type 1 diabetes mellitus. He reports that after a recent 6 AM five-mile run, his blood glucose level was 386 mg/dL (21.4 mmol/L); the level was 297 mg/dL (16.5 mmol/L) just before the run and 215 mg/dL (11.9 mmol/L) at bedtime the night before. He took no insulin and ate no food in the morning before his run. During the run, he felt slow and fatigued but was significantly better after drinking water and giving himself insulin. The patient had one episode of diabetic ketoacidosis 15 years ago. Medications are insulin detemir, 16 units/d in the morning, and insulin lispro, 4 to 6 units before each meal, depending on his preprandial blood glucose level and expected carbohydrate intake.

Physical examination findings, including vital signs, are normal.

Which of the following is the most likely cause of his postexercise hyperglycemia?

(A) Excess nocturnal carbohydrate intake
(B) Gastroparesis
(C) Inadequate insulin replacement
(D) Nocturnal hypoglycemia

Item 77

An 18-year-old woman is evaluated for amenorrhea. The patient underwent menarche at age 12 years and has never had any subsequent menses. She has no medical history of note. Family history is remarkable only for hypothyroidism. She takes no medication.

On physical examination vital signs are normal; BMI is 22 (height, 147.3 cm [58.0 in]; weight, 48.6 kg [107.0 lb]). Visual field, thyroid, and pelvic examination findings are normal.

Results of laboratory studies show an initial serum follicle-stimulating hormone level of 53 mU/mL (53 units/L) and a subsequent level of 62 mU/mL (62 units/L) on repeat testing. Serum thyroid-stimulating hormone, human chorionic gonadotropin, and prolactin levels are normal.

Which of the following is the most appropriate next diagnostic test?

(A) Karyotyping
(B) Pelvic ultrasonography
(C) Progesterone challenge test
(D) Serum estradiol measurement

Item 78

A 23-year-old woman is evaluated for a 2-week history of nervousness, palpitations, nausea, vomiting, and weight loss. She is 3 weeks pregnant and says she was previously in excellent health. The patient takes a daily prenatal multivitamin but no other prescription medication, iodine supplement, or other over-the-counter medication.

On physical examination, blood pressure is 130/70 mm Hg, pulse rate is 110/min and regular, and respiration rate is 16/min; BMI is 22. Results of cardiac and lung examinations are normal. Eye examination findings also are normal. Examination of the thyroid gland shows a significantly enlarged gland with a soft bruit but no nodules. No neck tenderness is detected. Abdominal examination reveals a 2-cm patch of vitiligo. A fine bilateral hand tremor and warm, moist skin are noted. No evidence of pretibial myxedema is seen.

Laboratory studies:

Complete blood count	Normal
Comprehensive metabolic profile	Normal
Thyroid-stimulating hormone	<0.01 µU/mL (0.01 mU/L)
Thyroxine (T_4), free	4.0 ng/dL (52 pmol/L)
Triiodothyronine (T_3), free	6 ng/L (9.2 pmol/L)
Human chorionic gonadotropin	Positive
Thyroid peroxidase antibodies	40 units/L (normal, <20 units/L)
Thyroid-stimulating antibodies	140% (normal, <130%)

A thyroid ultrasound shows an enlarged thyroid gland without nodules.

Which of the following is the most appropriate initial treatment?

(A) Methimazole
(B) Propylthiouracil
(C) Thyroidectomy
(D) Reassurance

Item 79

A 21-year-old man comes to the office for a follow-up evaluation. He has a 12-year history of type 1 diabetes mellitus and a recent hemoglobin A_{1c} value of 8.2%. Two days ago, he was brought to the emergency department after having a seizure at 3 AM in his dormitory. Earlier that day, he ate a hearty dinner, played basketball with friends for 3 hours, and then had three beers at a local microbrewery. His glucose monitor showed a blood glucose level of 163 mg/dL (9.0 mmol/L) before he went to bed at 11 PM. His initial plasma glucose level in the emergency department was 28 mg/dL (1.6 mmol/L). He was given intravenous glucose and recovered fully. His only medications are insulin detemir before breakfast and dinner and insulin aspart before all meals.

Physical examination shows a fit, muscular young man. Vital signs are normal; BMI is 19. All other physical examination findings are normal.

Laboratory studies show a hemoglobin A_{1c} value of 8.2%.

Which of the following is the most appropriate advice related to evening exercise to give this patient?

(A) Avoid evening exercise
(B) If alcohol is consumed, drink only light beer
(C) Eat complex carbohydrates at bedtime
(D) Omit the evening dose of insulin detemir and insulin aspart

Item 80

A 38-year-old man is evaluated for a 4-month history of progressive fatigue, cold intolerance, weight gain (total, 5.5 kg [12.0 lb]), occasional headaches, and loss of libido. He has no polydipsia or polyuria.

Physical examination reveals a pale, tired-looking man. Blood pressure is 102/78 mm Hg, pulse rate is 58/min, and respiration rate is 12/min. Deep tendon reflexes have a prolonged relaxation phase. All other examination findings are noncontributory.

Laboratory studies:

Cortisol (8 AM)	7 µg/dL (193 nmol/L) (normal, 5-25 µg/dL [138-690 nmol/L])
Insulin-like growth factor 1	80 ng/mL (80 µg/L) (normal range 101-270 ng/mL [101-270 µg/L])
Testosterone, total	112 ng/dL (3.9 nmol/L)
Thyroid-stimulating hormone	1.1 µU/mL (1.1 mU/L)
Thyroxine, free	0.4 ng/dL (5 pmol/L)

An MRI shows a 1.1-cm sellar mass that fills the sella, with no supra- or parasellar extension.

Levothyroxine is initiated.

Which of the following hormones must be administered simultaneously with levothyroxine?

(A) Glucocorticoid
(B) Growth hormone
(C) Testosterone
(D) Vasopressin

Item 81

A 38-year-old man is evaluated for a mass in his right neck that he first noticed 2 weeks ago while shaving. The patient also reports experiencing a pressure sensation when swallowing solid foods for the past year and daily diarrhea for the past 2 months. His personal medical history is unremarkable. His younger brother has nephrolithiasis, and his father died of a hypertensive crisis and cardiac arrest at age 62 years while undergoing anesthesia induction to repair a hip fracture.

On physical examination, vital signs are normal. A mass is palpated in the right lobe of the thyroid gland. No cervical lymphadenopathy is palpable.

Results of laboratory studies show a serum calcium level of 10.6 mg/dL (2.7 mmol/L) and a thyroid-stimulating hormone level of 1.9 µU/mL (1.9 mU/L).

A chest radiograph is normal. A thyroid ultrasound confirms a 1.4-cm mass in the right lobe of the thyroid gland.

Which of the following is the most likely diagnosis?

(A) Benign familial hypocalciuric hypercalcemia
(B) Multiple endocrine neoplasia type 2
(C) Parathyroid cancer
(D) Sarcoidosis

Item 82

A 25-year-old woman is evaluated for a 2-year history of increasing hair growth on the upper lip, chin, and sides of the face. She underwent menarche at age 12 years and has had irregular menses and some atypical hair growth since

that time. She has no other medical problems and takes no medication.

On physical examination, temperature is normal, blood pressure is 128/70 mm Hg, pulse rate is 70/min, and respiration rate is 10/min; BMI is 27. Thyroid examination findings are normal. Mild acanthosis nigricans of the axillae and neck and terminal hair growth on the chin, upper lip, and sides of the face are noted. No evidence of abdominal or pelvic masses, clitoromegaly, or galactorrhea is detected.

Laboratory studies:

Glucose, fasting	85 mg/dL (4.7 mmol/L)
Dehydroepiandrosterone sulfate	1.8 µg/mL (4.9 µmol/L)
Follicle-stimulating hormone (day 3 of menstrual cycle)	6 mU/mL (6 units/L)
17-Hydroxyprogesterone	100 ng/dL (3 nmol/L) (normal, <200 ng/dL [6 nmol/L])
Prolactin	17 ng/mL (17 µg/L)
Thyroid-stimulating hormone	2.1 µU/mL (2.1 mU/L)
Total testosterone	98 ng/dL (3.4 nmol/L)

Which of the following is the most appropriate treatment for her hirsutism?

(A) Bromocriptine
(B) Dexamethasone
(C) Estrogen-progesterone oral contraceptive
(D) Metformin
(E) Spironolactone

Item 83

A 52-year-old man is seen for follow-up evaluation 12 weeks after undergoing transsphenoidal surgery to treat acromegaly associated with a 2.3-cm pituitary adenoma that had invaded the cavernous sinus. He reports continuing headache and bilateral pain in the hip, knee, and elbows. The patient has a history of type 2 diabetes mellitus, sleep apnea, and hypertension. Medications are metformin, lisinopril, metoprolol, and ibuprofen as needed.

On physical examination, blood pressure is 148/92 mm Hg and pulse rate is 88/min. Frontal bossing, prominent nasolabial folds, a large tongue, and thickened hands and feet are noted.

Laboratory study results show that the serum insulin-like growth factor 1 (IGF-1) level, which was 1030 ng/mL (1030 µg/L) (normal for age, 87-238 ng/mL [87-238 µg/L]) before surgery, is still elevated at 780 ng/mL (780 µg/L).

Which of the following is the most appropriate next step in treatment?

(A) Bromocriptine
(B) Octreotide
(C) Repeat transsphenoidal surgery
(D) Observation

Item 84

A 52-year-old man is evaluated for recent onset of fatigue and muscle weakness. The patient further reports nocturia and polyuria over the past 4 weeks and a 6-kg (13.2-lb) weight loss over the past 2 months. He has COPD and a 55-pack-year smoking history. His only medication is an albuterol inhaler.

On physical examination, temperature is 36.7 °C (98.1 °F), blood pressure is 188/102 mm Hg, pulse rate is 96/min, and respiration rate is 22/min; BMI is 23. Temporal muscle wasting and proximal muscle wasting and weakness are noted in the upper and lower extremities. Hyperpigmented mucous membranes are noted. A view of the patient's toenail beds is shown.

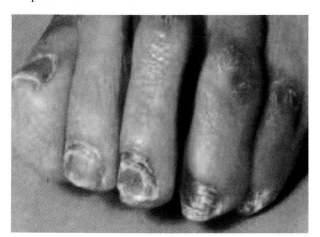

Laboratory studies:

Creatinine	0.8 mg/dL (70.7 µmol/L)
Electrolytes	
Sodium	145 meq/L (145 mmol/L)
Potassium	2.4 meq/L (2.4 mmol/L)
Chloride	101 meq/L (101 mmol/L)
Bicarbonate	33 meq/L (33 mmol/L)
Glucose, random	312 mg/dL (17.3 mmol/L)
Adrenocorticotropic hormone (ACTH)	243 pg/mL (53 pmol/L)
Urine	
Cortisol, free	460 µg/24 h (1268 nmol/24 h)
Potassium, spot test	45 meq/L (45 mmol/L) (normal, 17-164 meq/L [17-164 mmol/L])

Which of the following is the most likely cause of this patient's findings?

(A) Adrenal adenoma

(B) Adrenal carcinoma

(C) Ectopic ACTH secretion

(D) Pituitary adenoma

Answers and Critiques

Item 1   Answer: B

Educational Objective: Predict the results of laser photocoagulation therapy for diabetic retinopathy.

This patient will most likely have diminished peripheral and night vision but retained central vision after photocoagulation. Panretinal laser photocoagulation delivers several thousand small burns to the periphery of the retina, which results in the avascular scarring and shriveling of new vessels shown.

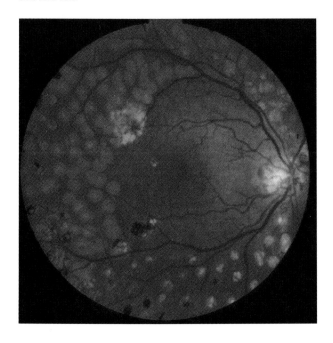

As a result, more retinal blood flow is available for the central part of the retina, which helps retain central vision. However, this procedure also causes deterioration of peripheral vision, which often is most noticeable at night.

This patient's overall visual acuity is unlikely to improve but should not get significantly worse, unless the proliferative retinopathy progresses.

Because central vision remains intact, neither binocular vision nor depth perception will be affected.

> **KEY POINT**
> - Panretinal laser photocoagulation therapy for diabetic retinopathy typically results in retained central vision but poorer peripheral and night vision.

Bibliography
Cheung N, Mitchell P, Wong TY. Diabetic retinopathy. Lancet. 2010;376(9735):124-136. [PMID: 20580421]

Item 2   Answer: B

Educational Objective: Manage an adrenal incidentaloma.

This patient should undergo right adrenalectomy. The increasing use of imaging studies has revealed many previously unrecognized, often asymptomatic adrenal masses (adrenal incidentalomas) in 2% to 3% of the scanned population older than 50 years and in up to 7% of those older than 70 years. Adrenal masses in younger patients are more clinically significant. The evaluation of adrenal masses should address the origin and nature of the mass (primary versus metastatic, benign versus malignant). For a primary tumor, whether it is functioning or not must be determined. Nearly 10% of all adrenal incidentalomas are functioning, although most do not have overt clinical manifestations. He has an incidental but large adrenal mass without any clinical or biochemical features to suggest excessive adrenocortical hormone or catecholamine secretion. The size of the mass (7 cm) and its high CT attenuation (77 Hounsfield units) are suggestive of malignancy. The risk of primary or metastatic cancer is nearly 2% for tumors less than 4 cm in diameter but increases to 25% for tumors 6 cm or larger. For masses 6 cm or larger, surgical removal of the mass is the most appropriate management option.

A biopsy of the adrenal mass is not indicated in this patient because a negative result may be a false-negative, and a positive result only confirms the need to surgically remove the mass.

In the absence of hypertension, hypokalemia, or clinical features suggestive of hypercortisolism, the possibility of hyperaldosteronism or Cushing syndrome is remote. Therefore, neither determining the serum aldosterone to plasma renin activity ratio nor measuring the 24-hour excretion of urine cortisol is likely to be useful.

> **KEY POINT**
> - An adrenal incidentaloma that is 6 cm in size or larger and has a high CT attenuation value has a high likelihood of being malignant; surgical removal of the mass is thus the most appropriate management.

Bibliography
Nieman LK. Approach to the patient with an adrenal incidentaloma. J Clin Endocrinol Metab. 2010;95(9):4106-4113. [PMID: 20823463]

Item 3   Answer: D

Educational Objective: Evaluate secondary amenorrhea.

Progesterone challenge testing is the most appropriate next diagnostic step in this patient. By definition, secondary amenorrhea is the absence of menses for 3 or more consecutive months in a woman who previously has menstruated. Oligomenorrhea (irregular and infrequent menses) is much more common than complete amenorrhea, but the diagnostic considerations are similar. To check for primary ovarian insufficiency and other common endocrinologic causes of amenorrhea, initial laboratory studies should include measurement of the follicle-stimulating hormone (FSH), prolactin, thyroxine (T_4), and thyroid-stimulating hormone levels. Serum FSH values greater than 35 milliunits/mL (35 units/L) are consistent with primary ovarian insufficiency, and values of 20 to 35 milliunits/mL (20-35 units/L) suggest a low ovarian reserve. Her laboratory evaluation has excluded pregnancy, thyroid disease, hyperprolactinemia, and primary ovarian insufficiency. Therefore, the next step is to determine whether she is making adequate estrogen, which the progesterone challenge test can help determine. If withdrawal bleeding occurs, then the patient is producing enough estrogen. If no withdrawal bleeding occurs, then the patient is in a low-estrogen state, and a hypothalamic or pituitary cause is most likely responsible, given her normal FSH level.

Measurement of her total testosterone and dehydroepiandrosterone levels is not indicated at this time because she has no clinical evidence of hyperandrogenism, such as hirsutism or the presence of virilization (voice deepening, clitoral enlargement).

An MRI of the pituitary gland also is not indicated at this time because her prolactin and FSH levels are normal.

Asherman syndrome due to endometrial scarring should be considered as the cause of secondary amenorrhea in any woman who previously had dilation and curettage or a uterine infection. The patient had normal menses until amenorrhea began and has no history of uterine procedures. Therefore, an anatomic abnormality is less likely, and pelvic ultrasonography is not needed.

KEY POINT

- In a patient with secondary amenorrhea and normal findings of screening laboratory studies, the cornerstone of further evaluation is a progesterone withdrawal challenge.

Bibliography

Practice Committee of American Society for Reproductive Medicine. Current evaluation of amenorrhea. Fertil Steril. 2008;90(5 Suppl):S219-S225. [PMID: 19007635]

Item 4   Answer: B

Educational Objective: Manage subclinical hypothyroidism in a woman with multiple risk factors.

This patient should begin receiving levothyroxine therapy because she is at high risk for overt hypothyroidism, given her positive family history, positive thyroid peroxidase antibody assay, small goiter, and desire to become pregnant. Currently, she has subclinical hypothyroidism, which is defined by the presence of an elevated serum thyroid-stimulating hormone

(TSH) level with concomitant thyroxine (T_4) and triiodothyronine (T_3) levels in the reference range. Patients typically have mild or no symptoms of hypothyroidism. The potential causes of subclinical hypothyroidism are the same as for overt hypothyroidism. Evidence suggests that patients with subclinical hypothyroidism also have mild elevations in total cholesterol, LDL cholesterol, and even C-reactive protein levels, and some recent meta-analyses have shown an increased risk for atherosclerosis and cardiac events. However, no data support treatment with levothyroxine to reverse or improve outcomes for these risks. Consensus does exist for treatment of patients with serum TSH levels greater than 10 microunits/mL (10 milliunits/L). Additionally, many advocate a lower threshold for instituting levothyroxine therapy in patients (such as this patient) with anti–thyroid peroxidase antibodies, a strong family history of thyroid disease, a goiter, or pregnancy.

Avoiding hypothyroidism during pregnancy is imperative because overt hypothyroidism has been associated with low birth weight, increased risk of miscarriage, premature birth, and fetal loss. The optimal TSH normal range in a woman desirous of becoming pregnant is 0.5 to 2.5 microunits/mL (0.5-2.5 milliunits/L).

A fine-needle aspiration biopsy of the thyroid gland should be reserved for the evaluation of a thyroid nodule and thus is not indicated in this patient.

Given her high risk of progression to overt hypothyroidism and the potential risk to the fetus should she become pregnant, waiting 6 weeks and then repeating the TSH measurement is not an appropriate choice in this patient.

This patient does not have an indication for a thyroid scan. Physical examination revealed no palpable nodules on or tenderness in the thyroid gland. A thyroid scan would add little to her evaluation and would result in unnecessary radiation exposure.

KEY POINT

- Patients with subclinical hypothyroidism should be treated with levothyroxine if they are at high risk for progression to overt hypothyroidism (thyroid-stimulating hormone level greater than 10 microunits/mL [10 milliunits/L], positive family history, goiter, presence of anti–thyroid peroxidase antibodies, or desire to become pregnant).

Bibliography

Lazarus JH. The continuing saga of postpartum thyroiditis. J Clin Endocrinol Metab. 2011;96(3):614-616. [PMID: 21378224]

Item 5   Answer: B

Educational Objective: Diagnose tuberculosis-induced hypercalcemia.

The patient has disseminated tuberculosis with hypercalcemia due to excessive production of 1,25-dihydroxyvitamin D by the tuberculous granulomas. The granulomas of tuberculosis (and other granulomatous diseases, such as sarcoidosis, Crohn disease, and leprosy) are composed of macrophages that possess the 1α-hydroxylase enzyme needed to convert 25-hydroxyvitamin D to its active form, 1,25-dihydroxyvitamin D. The serum parathyroid hormone level is less than normal, which is an appropriate response to the elevated serum calcium level.

Dehydration might worsen hypercalcemia, but dehydration alone would not explain this patient's suppressed serum parathyroid hormone (PTH) level.

The low serum PTH level argues against excessive PTH release and thus excludes a parathyroid adenoma as the cause of the hypercalcemia. In addition, primary hyperparathyroidism typically is associated with a low serum phosphorus level, which makes hyperparathyroidism an unlikely cause of this patient's hypercalcemia.

Humoral hypercalcemia of malignancy results from the systemic effect of a circulating factor produced by neoplastic cells. The hormone most commonly responsible for this syndrome is PTH-related protein (PTHrP). This protein shares significant homology with PTH. PTHrP has most, if not all, of the metabolic effects of PTH, including osteoclast activation, increased renal tubular calcium reabsorption, and increased clearance of phosphorus by the kidneys. Because tumors that produce PTHrP (squamous cell carcinoma; lung, head, and neck cancer; lymphoma) do so in small quantities, patients who have associated hypercalcemia at presentation usually have an extensive tumor burden. Therefore, it is unusual for hypercalcemia to be the presenting feature of cancer. Additionally, the patient's tuberculosis is a more likely cause of his hypercalcemia.

KEY POINT

- **Hypercalcemia can be caused by the production of 1,25-dihydroxyvitamin D by granulomatous disease.**

Bibliography

Sharma OP. Hypercalcemia in granulomatous disorders: a clinical review. Curr Opin Pulm Med. 2000;6(5):442-447. [PMID: 10958237]

Item 6   Answer: E

Educational Objective: Diagnose Cushing syndrome as a secondary cause of diabetes.

Measurement of the 24-hour excretion of urine free cortisol is the most appropriate next test in this patient to determine the cause of her diabetes mellitus. Various secondary causes of diabetes exist, most involving other endocrinopathies, effects of medications, pancreatic diseases, or genetic conditions. Cushing syndrome is one of these secondary causes of diabetes. The most common cause of Cushing syndrome is corticosteroid therapy, followed by the secretion of adrenocorticotropic hormone (ACTH) by a pituitary adenoma (Cushing disease) and the hyperfunctioning of an adrenocortical adenoma. In this

patient, the combination of diabetes, hypertension, central obesity, hypokalemia, proximal muscle weakness, and edema strongly suggests the presence of Cushing syndrome. The diagnosis can be confirmed by several tests, including measurement of 24-hour excretion of urine free cortisol, an overnight dexamethasone suppression test, or a midnight salivary cortisol measurement.

Adrenal CT is appropriate after Cushing syndrome is diagnosed, especially when it is non–ACTH dependent, to identify the type of adrenal condition responsible. This test would be premature in this patient in whom the diagnosis has not been confirmed.

Residual beta-cell function can be assessed by measuring the C-peptide level, which is often high-normal in early type 2 diabetes because of insulin resistance. Similarly, measuring the glutamic acid decarboxylase antibody titer is useful to confirm the presence of autoimmune (type 1) diabetes when no other evidence exists. However, the C-peptide level will not indicate the cause of diabetes in this patient, and measuring the glutamic acid decarboxylase level also is unlikely to be helpful because she does not have type 1 diabetes.

Pancreatic imaging could be considered when signs and symptoms (such as abdominal or back pain, jaundice, or chronic diarrhea) suggest that an underlying pancreatic disorder is the cause of diabetes. This patient has none of these signs or symptoms, and thus a pancreatic MRI is unlikely to be revealing.

KEY POINT

- **Cushing syndrome is a likely cause of diabetes mellitus in a patient with hypertension, central obesity, and hypokalemia.**

Bibliography

Reimondo G, Pia A, Allasino B, et al. Screening of Cushing's syndrome in adult patients with newly diagnosed diabetes mellitus. Clin Endocrinol (Oxf). 2007;67(2):225-229. [PMID: 17547690]

Item 7   Answer: A

Educational Objective: Evaluate hyperprolactinemia.

A pregnancy test is the most appropriate next test in this woman whose serum prolactin level has again increased. Although she has a history of prolactinemia and associated oligomenorrhea, it is important first to ensure that she is not currently pregnant. Prolactin levels increase during pregnancy. Therefore, an increasing prolactin level in a woman of child-bearing age should not automatically be interpreted as evidence of prolactinemia until pregnancy is excluded as a cause.

Measurement of the growth hormone (GH) level is not useful in the assessment of a woman with amenorrhea or oligomenorrhea unless acromegaly is a possible diagnosis. Even in that setting, however, a random GH value is not useful because of the pulsatile nature of GH secretion.

Clinical features of acromegaly include prognathism; enlargement of the nose, lips, and tongue; frontal bossing; dental malocclusion; increased spacing between the teeth; sleep apnea; enlargement of the hands and feet; arthritis of the hips and knees; carpal tunnel syndrome; oily skin; and skin tags. Prolactin is coproduced with GH in approximately 40% of patients with acromegaly. Some of these patients also may have amenorrhea or galactorrhea. Other than amenorrhea, this patient has no signs or symptoms of acromegaly.

Measuring this patient's serum cortisol level is unlikely to be useful because she has no evidence of Cushing syndrome. Common symptoms of Cushing syndrome include muscle weakness, ecchymosis, hypokalemia, unexplained osteoporosis, new-onset hypertension, and diabetes mellitus but not hyperprolactinemia. However, menstrual irregularities are common in Cushing syndrome.

In patients with compression of the optic chiasm, the most common symptom is diminished vision in the temporal fields. Visual field testing is inappropriate unless a finding suggests a pituitary tumor with evidence of compression of the optic chiasm.

KEY POINT

- **In a woman with a modestly elevated serum prolactin level, pregnancy must first be excluded as a cause before a diagnosis of hyperprolactinemia is made.**

Bibliography

Kreitschmann-Andermahr I, Poll EM, Reineke A, et al. Growth hormone deficient patients after traumatic brain injury—baseline characteristics and benefits after growth hormone replacement—an analysis of the German KIMS database. Growth Horm IGF Res. 2008;18(6):472-478. [PMID: 18829359]

Item 8   Answer: D

Educational Objective: Treat Graves ophthalmopathy.

This patient should undergo thyroidectomy. Clinically significant ophthalmopathy occurs in approximately 5% to 10% of patients with Graves disease. Ophthalmopathy severity varies from mild to severe and may involve lid changes, proptosis or exophthalmos, and inflammatory eye changes, such as chemosis, conjunctival injection, periorbital edema, or iritis. Extraocular muscle involvement can result in double vision, whereas optic nerve compression can result in reduced visual acuity and even blindness. The precise pathophysiology of Graves ophthalmopathy is not well understood. A primary management focus in Graves ophthalmopathy is to establish a euthyroid state because persistent hypothyroidism or hyperthyroidism exacerbates disease activity. The medical treatment for ophthalmopathy includes local measures followed by a trial of corticosteroids. In patients with Graves disease, thyroid surgery usually is reserved for those with a severe allergy or intolerance

to iodine or antithyroid drugs, large or obstructive goiters, or ophthalmopathy.

Oral iodine solution may decrease levels on thyroid function testing for approximately 1 to 2 weeks in some patients, but a patient such as this one who is not taking any thiourea medication that blocks thyroid hormone synthesis may have worsening hyperthyroidism, especially after the initial 1 to 2 weeks.

The use of propylthiouracil also is not appropriate because the patient already has had a severe adverse reaction to methimazole, and the likelihood of a similar or worse reaction to propylthiouracil is high.

Radioactive iodine treatment has been associated with worsening of Graves ophthalmopathy, at least transiently. Therefore, its use as treatment of hyperthyroidism in patients with severe Graves ophthalmopathy is not recommended.

Attempts to modulate the immune response (with the monoclonal antibody rituximab, for example) have had mixed results and at present are still experimental.

KEY POINT

- **In patients with Graves ophthalmopathy, treatment includes establishing normal thyroid function, local measures, prednisone, and thyroidectomy.**

Bibliography

Bahn RS. Graves' ophthalmopathy. N Engl J Med. 2010;362(8):726-738. [PMID: 20181974]

Item 9   Answer: C

Educational Objective: Diagnose central adrenal insufficiency.

This patient with a history of pulmonary sarcoidosis should next have a pituitary MRI. She has symptoms highly suggestive of adrenal insufficiency, hypothyroidism, and hypogonadism. The biochemical findings suggest a central cause of these disorders. Her partial response to cosyntropin stimulation is consistent with partial loss of adrenocorticotropic hormone (ACTH) secretion, or central adrenal insufficiency. The hypothyroidism is also central in origin because it is associated with an inappropriately normal serum thyroid-stimulating hormone level. The polyuria and hypernatremia suggest the development of diabetes insipidus in this patient. These abnormalities are most likely caused by involvement of the hypothalamus and pituitary stalk by sarcoidosis, which led to her biochemical pituitary findings and to central diabetes insipidus, which caused her hypernatremia. Other causes that should be considered are a pituitary adenoma and any other sellar or parasellar mass. A gadolinium-enhanced MRI of the pituitary gland should be performed to exclude these causes and assess for evidence of involvement of these structures with sarcoidosis. However, definitive diagnosis requires biopsy evidence of a noncaseating granuloma in the involved areas. Hypothalamic-pituitary involvement occurs in less than 10% of patients with sarcoidosis and may be difficult to diagnose because patchy involvement of the hypothalamus and pituitary stalk may lead to various combinations of anterior and posterior pituitary hormone deficiencies.

Adrenal CT is not indicated because the cause of the adrenal insufficiency is clearly central ACTH deficiency and not a primary adrenal disease.

In the absence of pulmonary symptoms, a lung biopsy is not needed in this patient. Even if the lung biopsy were positive, imaging is still necessary to address the concerns raised about a possible anatomic abnormality in the sellar region that would explain the loss of pituitary hormone secretion.

Because the hypothyroidism is this patient is central in origin, a thyroid scan measuring radioactive iodine uptake is not indicated.

KEY POINT

- In a patient with symptoms and biochemical findings highly suggestive of central adrenal insufficiency, a pituitary MRI is appropriate to exclude other possible causes, such as a pituitary adenoma or any other sellar or perisellar mass.

Bibliography

Toogood AA, Stewart PM. Hypopituitarism: clinical features, diagnosis, and management. Endocrinol Metab Clin North Am. 2008;37(1):235-261. [PMID: 18226739]

Item 10   Answer: A

Educational Objective: Treat a woman with low bone mass.

The most appropriate medication for this patient is alendronate. She has osteopenia, and her major osteoporotic fracture risk by the Fracture Risk Assessment Tool (FRAX) is in a range for which the National Osteoporosis Foundation (NOF) guidelines favor treatment with antiosteoporotic therapy. The NOF recommends antiosteoporotic therapy for persons whose risk of major osteoporotic fracture over the next 10 years is 20% or greater or whose risk of hip fracture over the next 10 years is 3% or greater. Given her current FRAX score and the expectation that she will lose bone mass more rapidly after an aromatase inhibitor is started, it is reasonable to initiate therapy with alendronate now. Alendronate is approved for both osteoporosis prevention and treatment by the FDA.

Denosumab, a monoclonal antibody that inhibits osteoclast formation, is reserved for patients with a high risk of fracture, including those with multiple risk factors for fracture or a history of previous fractures. This patient does not fulfill these criteria.

Estrogen is contradicted in this patient with a new diagnosis of breast cancer.

Raloxifene, a selective estrogen receptor modulator, is also approved for osteoporosis prevention by the FDA. However, vasomotor symptoms are highly associated with its use, and it may not be well tolerated in a patient already experiencing significant hot flushes.

Teriparatide, or recombinant human parathyroid hormone (1-34), is an anabolic agent that increases bone density and decreases fracture risk. However, teriparatide carries a "black box" warning because of an increased risk of osteosarcoma and is contraindicated in this patient because of her history of radiation therapy, which increases the risk of osteosarcoma. Teriparatide is also contraindicated in persons with malignancy involving bone, Paget disease, or existing hyperparathyroidism or hypercalcemia.

KEY POINT

- In a patient with osteopenia and a history of radiation therapy, alendronate is the most appropriate drug to use for osteoporosis prevention.

Bibliography

Lecart MP, Reginster JY. Current options for the management of postmenopausal osteoporosis. Expert Opin Pharmacother. 2011;12(16):2533-2552. [PMID: 21916810]

Item 11   Answer: D

Educational Objective: Differentiate type 1 from type 2 diabetes mellitus.

This patient's blood should be checked for pancreatic autoantibodies, such as islet cell antibodies (ICAs) and glutamic acid decarboxylase antibodies (GADAs). Although she is obese and has a mother with type 2 diabetes mellitus, she may actually have type 1 diabetes presenting at an earlier stage of the disease process (when she still has significant endogenous insulin secretion) because of her obesity and insulin resistance. In young patients with probable diabetes, the distinction between type 1 and type 2 diabetes should be made as soon as possible. If ICAs and GADAs are found in her blood, she has type 1 diabetes and should begin receiving insulin immediately. Insulin treatment in type 1 diabetes helps preserve endogenous insulin secretion for a longer period of time, which makes it easier to achieve excellent glycemic control without hypoglycemia. If testing does not show these antibodies in her blood, she has type 2 diabetes and should be treated with lifestyle modifications and, possibly, metformin.

Checking this patient's plasma C-peptide level (whether fasting or stimulated) or fasting plasma insulin level will not help distinguish type 1 from type 2 diabetes. A person who is obese and has hyperglycemia but no ketonuria or acidosis is clearly making sufficient endogenous insulin at the moment. Therefore, this patient's plasma C-peptide and insulin levels will both be high, no matter what type of diabetes she has.

- In young patients with probable diabetes mellitus, the distinction between type 1 and type 2 diabetes should be made as soon as possible by checking for the presence of pancreatic autoantibodies, which indicate type 1 disease.

Bibliography

Effect of intensive therapy on residual beta-cell function in patients with type 1 diabetes in the diabetes control and complications trial. A randomized, controlled trial. The Diabetes Control and Complications Trial Research Group. Ann Intern Med. 1998;128(7):517-523. [PMID: 9518395]

Item 12   Answer: B

Educational Objective: Diagnose male infertility.

Semen analysis is the single best test to assess male infertility. The patient should abstain from sexual activity for 48 to 72 hours to have an adequate sample. If semen analysis results are abnormal, the test should be repeated.

Measurement of serum gonadotropin and testosterone levels is not appropriate in the initial evaluation of infertility. If the semen analysis results are abnormal, then luteinizing hormone, follicle-stimulating hormone, and total testosterone studies would be ordered to assess Leydig and Sertoli cell function.

Testicular ultrasonography is not performed in the evaluation of infertility unless an abnormality is detected on testicular examination.

KEY POINT

- Semen analysis is the single best test to assess male infertility.

Bibliography

Cooper TG, Noonan E, von Eckardstein S, et al. World Health Organization reference values for human semen characteristics. Hum Reprod Update. 2010;16(3):231-245. [PMID: 19934213]

Item 13   Answer: B

Educational Objective: Manage hypothyroidism during pregnancy.

This patient's levothyroxine dosage should be increased by 30% now, and the thyroid function tests should be repeated in 2 to 4 weeks. Pregnancy is known to increase levothyroxine requirements in most patients receiving thyroid replacement therapy, and this expected increase should be anticipated by increasing her levothyroxine dosage. The levothyroxine dosage is typically increased in the first (and sometimes in the second) trimester of pregnancy, with a possible total increase of 30% to 50%. During the first trimester, the goal thyroid-stimulating hormone (TSH) level is less than 2.5 microunits/mL (2.5 milliunits/L) because first trimester serum TSH levels between approximately 0.1 and 2.5 microunits/mL (0.1-2.5 milliunits/L)

are associated with fewer maternal and fetal complications. In contrast, the upper range of normal for nonpregnant patients is approximately 4.5 to 5.0 microunits/mL (4.5-5.0 milliunits/L). In pregnant women with hypothyroidism, thyroid function testing should be frequent, preferably every 4 weeks, to protect the health of mother and fetus and to avoid pregnancy complications. When serum TSH values are inappropriately elevated, the dosage of levothyroxine is increased, and free thyroxine (T_4) and TSH levels are monitored every 2 to 4 weeks. The fetus is largely dependent on transplacental transfer of maternal thyroid hormones during the first 12 weeks of gestation. The presence of maternal subclinical or overt hypothyroidism may be associated with subsequent fetal neurocognitive impairment, increased risk of premature birth, low birth weight, increased miscarriage rate, and even an increased risk of fetal death.

Continuing the current levothyroxine dosage is inappropriate in this patient because her TSH level is already too high (4.2 microunits/mL [4.2 milliunits/L]). TSH levels generally should be 0.1 to 2.5 microunits/mL (0.1-2.5 milliunits/L) in the first trimester, 0.2 to 3.0 microunits/mL (0.2-3.0 milliunits/L) in the second, and 0.3 to 3.0 microunits/mL (0.3-3.0 milliunits/L) in the third.

KEY POINT

- Early in pregnancy, levothyroxine requirements are increased in most patients with hypothyroidism by 30% to 50%.

Bibliography

Yassa L, Marqusee E, Fawcett R, Alexander EK. Thyroid hormone early adjustment in pregnancy (the THERAPY) trial. J Clin Endocrinol Metab. 2010;95(7):3234-3241. [PMID: 20463094]

Item 14   Answer: A

Educational Objective: Manage pituitary tumor apoplexy.

This patient with pituitary tumor apoplexy should receive glucocorticoids in addition to undergoing surgical removal of his tumor. His history of fatigue, weight gain, and erectile dysfunction and laboratory finding of hyponatremia suggest panhypopituitarism, and his acute headache and neck stiffness are consistent with hemorrhage. Pituitary tumor apoplexy usually occurs in the setting of a preexisting pituitary adenoma, and thus a neuroimaging scan was appropriately obtained to confirm the diagnosis and show the pituitary anatomy. He also has evidence of bitemporal hemianopia caused by optic chiasmal compression by the mass. The anticoagulant taken by this patient may have predisposed him to hemorrhage.

Pituitary tumor apoplexy is generally a neurosurgical emergency. On occasion, hemorrhagic infarction of a pituitary adenoma may be less urgent, especially in the absence of associated mass effects, and can be managed with conservative follow-up monitoring. In the setting of local mass effects and severe headache, however, neurosurgical decompression of the pituitary gland is necessary. Urgent glucocorticoid administration is often required because of acute adrenocorticotropic hormone deficiency. The leading cause of mortality with pituitary tumor apoplexy is adrenal insufficiency.

An insulin tolerance test usually is performed to rule out both adrenal insufficiency and growth hormone deficiency, and a serum prolactin level typically is obtained after a diagnosis of pituitary adenoma is made to exclude prolactinoma. Because this patient's disorder is a neurosurgical emergency, these tests are inappropriate before the apoplexy is addressed.

A lumbar puncture is useful in patients with suspected meningitis or in whom subarachnoid hemorrhage is suspected despite a negative imaging study. However, the imaging study already provides an explanation for the stiff neck and headache, and a lumbar puncture is not only inappropriate but contraindicated in a patient with pituitary tumor apoplexy.

> **KEY POINT**
>
> • In addition to neurosurgical decompression of the pituitary gland, urgent glucocorticoid administration is often necessary in patients with pituitary tumor apoplexy because of acute adrenocorticotropic hormone deficiency.

Bibliography

Sibal L, Ball SG, Connolly V, et al. Pituitary apoplexy: a review of clinical presentation, management and outcome in 45 cases. Pituitary. 2004;7(3):157-163. [PMID: 16010459]

Item 15   Answer: D
Educational Objective: Treat hypercalcemia.

This patient should be hydrated with normal (0.9%) saline as the next step in her treatment. She has severe symptomatic hypercalcemia in the setting of advanced metastatic breast cancer. The history of polyuria and polydipsia and the physical examination findings of tachycardia and dry mucous membranes suggest significant dehydration, which is confirmed by the elevated blood urea nitrogen and creatinine levels. High calcium levels impair the ability of the nephron to concentrate urine, which results in inappropriate water loss from the kidney. Therefore, the most appropriate next step in this patient's treatment is to restore euvolemia and begin to lower the serum calcium level by saline diuresis. Normalization of intravascular volume with saline will improve delivery of calcium to the renal tubule and aid in excretion of calcium. As the kidneys excrete excess sodium from the saline, excretion of calcium will follow.

Hypercalcemia of malignancy may be due to local osteolytic hypercalcemia or to humoral hypercalcemia of malignancy, in which a tumor that does not involve the skeleton secretes a circulating factor that activates bone resorption.

In this patient, the liver metastases are likely secreting parathyroid hormone–related protein. Control of the tumor with chemotherapy may help the patient's hypercalcemia in the long-run.

Bisphosphonate therapy may be needed if the patient remains hypercalcemic after rehydration, and intravenous furosemide may be appropriate after the patient is adequately hydrated to maintain euvolemia. Glucocorticoid therapy could be considered if bisphosphonate treatment does not adequately lower the serum calcium level. However, none of these treatments should be attempted before the patient is rehydrated with normal saline.

> **KEY POINT**
>
> • In patients with acute hypercalcemia, normalization of intravascular volume with saline will improve delivery of calcium to the renal tubule and aid in excretion of calcium.

Bibliography

Stewart, AF. Clinical practice. Hypercalcemia associated with cancer. N Engl J Med. 2005;352(4):373-379. [PMID: 15673803]

Item 16   Answer: D
Educational Objective: Diagnose hyperaldosteronism.

This patient should have her serum aldosterone to plasma renin activity ratio determined. She has biochemical features indicative of excessive mineralocorticoid secretion. Although several potential mineralocorticoids could be responsible for her symptoms, excessive aldosterone is the most likely cause. Hypertension and hypokalemia are two of the main manifestations of primary hyperaldosteronism. Increases in other mineralocorticoids are seen with unusually excessive cortisol secretion (Cushing syndrome), in which the mineralocorticoid activity of cortisol becomes prominent, and in congenital adrenal hyperplasia due to an enzyme deficiency. This patient's normal findings (except for blood pressure) on physical examination make the first possibility unlikely, and her less than 2-year history of hypertension makes a congenital enzyme deficiency also unlikely. The best screening test for hyperaldosteronism is the determination of the ratio of serum aldosterone to plasma renin activity. The expected findings include an elevated serum aldosterone level and suppressed plasma renin activity. Screening tests can be performed on random blood samples, even in patients taking antihypertensive medications (except the aldosterone receptor antagonists spironolactone and eplerenone). Confirmation of the biochemical diagnosis involves showing persistent elevation (poor suppressibility) of serum aldosterone in response to a high salt load.

Imaging studies are inappropriate before a clear biochemical diagnosis is established. Therefore, CT of the abdomen is premature at this time.

This patient did not exhibit any signs or symptoms that would warrant investigating the possibility of Cushing syndrome. Therefore, neither a dexamethasone suppression test nor a 24-hour measurement of urine free cortisol excretion is likely to be useful.

Nothing in the patient's history or clinical examination findings suggests the possibility of pheochromocytoma. Therefore, measurement of the plasma catecholamine levels is inappropriate as the next diagnostic test.

KEY POINT

- **The best screening test for hyperaldosteronism is the determination of the ratio of serum aldosterone to plasma renin activity.**

Bibliography

Funder JW, Carey RM, Fardella C, et al; Endocrine Society. Case detection, diagnosis, and treatment of patients with primary aldosteronism: an Endocrine Society clinical practice guideline. J Clin Endocrinol Metab. 2008;93(9):3266-3281. [PMID: 18552288]

Item 17   Answer: A

Educational Objective: Diagnose humoral hypercalcemia of malignancy.

This patient has severe hypercalcemia in the setting of a lung mass. This scenario is highly suggestive of humoral hypercalcemia of malignancy (HHM), which results from tumor production of a circulating factor, parathyroid hormone (PTH)–related protein (PTHrP), that acts on skeletal calcium release, calcium handling by the kidney, and intestinal calcium absorption. Tumors that cause HHM by secreting PTHrP are typically squamous cell carcinomas (often of the lung). Rarely, this disorder can be caused by unregulated production of 1,25-dihydroxyvitamin D (as in B-cell lymphomas) or other mediators that interfere with calcium homeostasis. Although PTHrP assays are now available commercially, results may not be available for up to 10 days. Because endogenous PTH secretion is suppressed in the setting of hypercalcemia, a low PTH level provides indirect but strong evidence of the nature of this patient's hypercalcemia. Because HHM results in a fairly rapid rise in the serum calcium level, patients tend to be more symptomatic than patients with hypercalcemia from other, more chronic causes.

Primary hyperparathyroidism is the most common cause of hypercalcemia in the outpatient setting and typically presents at an asymptomatic stage. This disorder is usually due to a benign parathyroid adenoma and not to a lung mass.

Hypercalcemia is frequently associated with sarcoidosis, with 30% to 50% of patients with the disease demonstrating some degree of abnormal calcium metabolism. However, this patient has no history or physical examination findings suggestive of sarcoidosis, and her lung mass would be an atypical manifestation of primary pulmonary sarcoidosis.

The patient takes a daily multivitamin and calcium supplement in over-the-counter dosages. The recommended daily allowance of vitamin D is 600 units. Although the point at which toxicity occurs is not clear, the Institute of Medicine's recommended tolerable intake of vitamin D is 4000 units daily, although substantially greater amounts are usually needed for clinically significant hypervitaminosis to occur. It is unlikely that the amount of vitamin D in her daily multivitamin is enough to cause acute toxicity and hypercalcemia.

KEY POINT

- **Humoral hypercalcemia of malignancy results from tumor production of a circulating factor (parathyroid hormone–related protein [PTHrP]) that acts on skeletal calcium release, calcium handling by the kidney, or intestinal calcium absorption and often involves squamous cell carcinomas of the lung.**

Bibliography

Clines GA. Mechanisms and treatment of hypercalcemia of malignancy. Curr Opin Endocrinol Diabetes Obes. 2011;18(6):339-346. [PMID: 21897221]

Item 18   Answer: C

Educational Objective: Diagnose the cause of gynecomastia.

An estradiol level should be obtained in this patient. Gynecomastia, or the abnormal growth of large mammary glands in men causing breast enlargement, results from an imbalance in the testosterone-to-estrogen ratio in men. This imbalance can be due to either a low testosterone level or an elevated estradiol level. Because the total testosterone level is normal in this patient, an estradiol level must be obtained to check for any elevation.

Adrenal CT is inappropriate in the evaluation of gynecomastia unless the estradiol level is elevated. If the estradiol level is elevated, testicular ultrasonography still should be ordered before adrenal CT to exclude a testicular neoplasm. If the testicular ultrasound shows no neoplasms, then an adrenal CT scan should be ordered to exclude an adrenal neoplasm.

In the evaluation of gynecomastia, breast ultrasonography should be obtained only if uncertainty exists about whether the patient has gynecomastia or lipomastia or if malignancy is a concern (for example, with an asymmetric growth, a breast mass, or unilateral disease). Because these possibilities do not pertain to this patient, breast ultrasonography is not necessary.

A karyotype is not appropriate in this patient. He has normal luteinizing hormone (LH) and testosterone levels. If his LH level were elevated and his testosterone level were decreased, then a karyotype would be indicated to exclude Klinefelter syndrome as a cause of the gynecomastia and hypogonadism.

Testicular ultrasonography is only ordered when the serum estradiol level is elevated to exclude a testicular neoplasm. If the testicular ultrasound is normal, then chest CT might be indicated to exclude a β-human chorionic gonadotropin–secreting mediastinal tumor, which is a rare tumor.

- **Gynecomastia results from an imbalance in the testosterone-to-estrogen ratio in men.**

Bibliography
Braunstein GD. Clinical practice. Gynecomastia. N Engl J Med. 2007;357(12):1229-1237. [PMID: 17881754]

Item 19   Answer: B
Educational Objective: Treat hypoglycemic unawareness.

This patient's dosages of both long-acting and rapid-acting insulin should be decreased by approximately 20%. Hypoglycemia is the major rate-limiting factor in attempting tight glycemic control, especially in patients with type 1 diabetes mellitus. For 48 to 72 hours after a severe episode of hypoglycemia, the body's ability to mount an adrenergic response is blunted, as is the strength of the counterregulatory response. This increases the likelihood of a second severe episode of hypoglycemia that will not be easily recognized (hypoglycemic unawareness), and thus a vicious cycle develops. The best treatment is to reduce the dosage of insulin and scrupulously monitor the blood glucose level for 1 week so that it does not become less than 100 mg/dL (5.6 mmol/L). This intervention allows the brain to reset its adrenergic responses.

Increasing her carbohydrate intake at meals is inappropriate because of her currently healthy diet, her anticipated pregnancy, and the potential for weight gain.

Although α-lipoic acid has shown some efficacy in management of painful diabetic neuropathy, it would have no effect on her hypoglycemic unawareness.

A preprandial injection of pramlintide, a synthetic long-acting analogue of the hormone amylin, is sometimes used in the management of type 1 diabetes to slow down stomach emptying, suppress glucagon secretion, and promote satiety. In this patient, however, pramlintide might actually increase the risk of hypoglycemia.

Switching from insulin glargine to insulin detemir without reducing the dose of insulin is unlikely to be helpful in stopping or reducing this patient's hypoglycemic episodes.

- **Hypoglycemia is the major rate-limiting factor in attempting tight glycemic control, especially in patients with type 1 diabetes mellitus.**

Bibliography
Cryer PE. The barrier of hypoglycemia in diabetes. Diabetes. 2008;57(12):3169-3176. [PMID: 19033403]

Item 20   Answer: A
Educational Objective: Evaluate thyroid nodules with fine-needle aspiration biopsy.

This patient should have a fine-needle aspiration (FNA) biopsy of the thyroid nodule. Most thyroid nodules are benign; only approximately 5% to 15% are malignant. An FNA biopsy is the most accurate method to determine whether a nodule is benign or malignant. FNA biopsy is an outpatient procedure that allows cytologic categorization of the cells within a nodule as benign, suspicious for malignancy, follicular neoplasm, or papillary thyroid cancer. FNA biopsy is also the most sensitive and specific method to help diagnose the cause of a thyroid nodule.

Because thyroid nodules are extremely common, with an estimated 30% to 50% of healthy persons likely to have a thyroid nodule on thyroid ultrasound, guidelines have been developed by the American Thyroid Association to maximize the effectiveness of thyroid FNA biopsy in diagnosing malignancy in a cost-effective manner. These guidelines take into account personal history and risk factors, family history, and ultrasound characteristics of the nodule to help predict the likelihood of malignancy and the need for thyroid FNA biopsy. The recommended nodule size threshold for performing a thyroid FNA biopsy is at least 5 mm in a patient at high risk of thyroid cancer who also has worrisome sonographic characteristics. This patient has a first-degree relative with papillary thyroid cancer. In addition, the thyroid Doppler ultrasound showed a hypoechoic nodule with microcalcifications, blurred nodule margins, and increased central vascularity.

Close monitoring with repeat thyroid ultrasonography in 3 or 6 months is inappropriate management in this patient with significant risk factors and suspicious features on the current ultrasound that should prompt an FNA biopsy.

Thyroid lobectomy is generally appropriate treatment for cancerous thyroid nodules that are less than 1 cm in diameter but is premature in this patient in whom a diagnosis of malignancy has not been established.

MRI has limited utility in evaluating thyroid nodules. Generally less helpful than Doppler ultrasonography in characterizing intrathyroid nodules, MRI may be helpful in detecting local extension of thyroid malignancies or spread into the mediastinum or retro-thyroid regions, if suspected.

- **A fine-needle aspiration biopsy is the most accurate way to determine if a thyroid nodule is benign or malignant.**

Bibliography
American Thyroid Association (ATA) Guidelines Taskforce on Thyroid Nodules and Differentiated Thyroid Cancer; Cooper DS, Doherty GM, Haugen BR, et al. Revised American Thyroid Association management guidelines for patients with thyroid nodules and differentiated thyroid cancer [errata in Thyroid. 2010;20(6):674-675; and Thyroid. 2010;20(8):942]. Thyroid. 2009;19(11):1167-1214. [PMID: 1986057]

Item 21   Answer: D
Educational Objective: Diagnose growth hormone deficiency.

This patient should have his insulin-like growth factor 1 (IGF-1) level measured because he is at risk for growth hormone (GH) deficiency. Up to 40% of patients with a history of traumatic brain injury, particularly when severe, are found subsequently to have hypopituitarism. The most common anterior pituitary hormone disorder after traumatic brain injury is GH deficiency. Acquired GH deficiency in adults is characterized by a change in body composition (increase in central adiposity and reduction in lean skeletal muscle mass), reduction in quality of life, and decrease in bone mineral density. Increased cardiovascular risk also may be present. This patient has had progressive reduction in lean body mass, an increase in central adiposity, and progressive deterioration in his daily performance and quality of life, all of which suggest GH deficiency. In such patients, administration of GH replacement therapy may lead to an increase in muscle mass and quality of life and a reduction in central obesity.

The initial screening test for GH deficiency is measurement of the IGF-1 level. If the IGF-1 value is low, then further testing with a stimulation test to measure GH reserve should be performed to confirm a diagnosis of GH deficiency.

Measurement of the patient's fasting GH level is unlikely to be useful because GH levels are pulsatile and undetectable for much of the day in most patients. Therefore, this test is unlikely to detect GH deficiency.

A glucose tolerance test will not be useful in this patient. The nonsuppressibility of GH during a glucose tolerance test is used to diagnose GH excess in acromegaly, not GH deficiency.

A gonadotropin-releasing hormone test is used to assess luteinizing hormone and follicle-stimulating hormone reserves in the setting of hypogonadotropic hypogonadism. Although this patient has some of the symptoms of male hypogonadism (fatigue and loss of muscle strength), he does not have the anemia, poor libido, or erectile dysfunction commonly associated with the disorder. More importantly, his 8 AM serum testosterone measurement excludes the diagnosis of hypogonadism, which makes a gonadotropin-releasing hormone test unnecessary.

KEY POINT
- **The most common anterior pituitary hormone disorder after traumatic brain injury is growth hormone deficiency, which can be suggested by a decreased serum insulin-like growth factor 1 level and is confirmed by a stimulation test measuring GH reserve.**

Bibliography
Kreitschmann-Andermahr I, Poll EM, Reineke A, et al. Growth hormone deficient patients after traumatic brain injury—baseline characteristics and benefits after growth hormone replacement—an analysis of the German KIMS database. Growth Horm IGF Res. 2008;18(6):472-478. [PMID: 18829359]

Item 22   Answer: B
Educational Objective: Diagnose vitamin D deficiency.

This patient's serum 25-hydroxyvitamin D level should be measured. Results of her recent bone mineral density screening showed osteoporosis of the hip, and laboratory studies showed a high parathyroid hormone (PTH) level in the setting of low serum calcium and phosphorus levels. These findings collectively suggest secondary hyperparathyroidism. In this patient with normal kidney function, secondary hyperparathyroidism is likely due to vitamin D deficiency, a common problem in older adults. Therefore, screening her for vitamin D deficiency by measuring the 25-hydroxyvitamin D level would be the most appropriate next step.

A measurement of the 25-hydroxyvitamin D level is more informative in most patients with hypocalcemia than a measurement of the 1,25-dihydroxyvitamin D level because vitamin D deficiency causes hypocalcemia and stimulates PTH secretion, which in turn stimulates conversion of 25-hydroxyvitamin D to 1,25-dihydroxyvitamin D in the kidneys. Therefore, this patient's serum 1,25-dihydroxyvitamin D level may be normal in the setting of vitamin D deficiency and is not useful to check in this setting.

Parathyroidectomy also would be inappropriate in this patient because the elevation in the PTH level is an appropriate physiologic response to the low calcium (and presumed low vitamin D) level.

Repeat dual-energy x-ray absorptiometry testing in 1 year should not be recommended because this patient already has indications for medical management of her osteoporosis after the high PTH and low calcium levels have been evaluated and treated.

KEY POINT
- **Measurement of the serum 25-hydroxyvitamin D level is an appropriate initial step in the evaluation of hypocalcemia, an elevated parathyroid hormone level, and osteoporosis.**

Bibliography
Holick MF, Binkley NC, Bischoff-Ferrari HA, et al; Endocrine Society. Evaluation, treatment, and prevention of vitamin D deficiency: an Endocrine Society clinical practice guideline [erratum in J Clin Endocrinol Metab. 2011;96(12):3908]. J Clin Endocrinol Metab. 2011;96(7):1911-1930. [PMID: 21646368]

Item 23   Answer: C
Educational Objective: Treat stage III thyroid cancer with radioactive iodine therapy.

The patient should receive radioactive iodine therapy. She has stage III thyroid cancer because her excised malignant thyroid nodule is greater than 4 cm with cervical lymph node involvement (T3N1MX). The American Thyroid Association Guidelines indicate that a patient older than 45 years who has had a total thyroidectomy for a papillary thyroid cancer greater than 4 cm should receive radioactive iodine (^{131}I) because this treatment will decrease the risk of recurrence and death. Decreasing the risk of recurrence is critical because relapsing disease develops in approximately 12% of patients who have no evidence of disease after primary therapy.

Tumors that are not treatable with the combination of surgery, levothyroxine therapy, and repeat doses of ^{131}I are treated with external-beam radiation therapy or chemotherapy (with traditional cytotoxic drugs, such as doxorubicin), but the response to these therapies is poor. This patient has not failed to benefit from first-line therapy, and thus treatment with external-beam radiation or chemotherapy is not yet indicated.

Observation is inadequate postsurgical therapy in this patient who underwent removal of a papillary thyroid cancer greater than 4 cm and a malignant lymph node. Radioactive iodine therapy is needed to decrease the progression of local disease and potentially increase survival in this patient with stage III disease.

KEY POINT

- **Large papillary thyroid cancer (>4 cm) is treated with thyroidectomy and then with radioactive iodine to decrease the risk of recurrence and death.**

Bibliography

American Thyroid Association (ATA) Guidelines Taskforce on Thyroid Nodules and Differentiated Thyroid Cancer; Cooper DS, Doherty GM, Haugen BR, et al. Revised American Thyroid Association management guidelines for patients with thyroid nodules and differentiated thyroid cancer [errata in Thyroid. 2010;20(6):674-675; and Thyroid. 2010;20(8):942]. Thyroid. 2009;19(11):1167-1214. [PMID: 19860577]

Item 24   Answer: C
Educational Objective: Diagnose type 2 diabetes mellitus.

This patient is at high risk for diabetes mellitus and should have his hemoglobin A_{1c} value remeasured. He has a family history of type 2 diabetes and coronary artery disease, is obese, and has hypertension. According to the American Diabetes Association, in the absence of unequivocal symptomatic hyperglycemia, the diagnosis of diabetes must be confirmed on a subsequent day by repeating the same test suggestive of diabetes (in this patient, the hemoglobin A_{1c} measurement). If results of two different diagnostic tests are available and both are diagnostic for diabetes, additional testing is not needed. Although this patient's hemoglobin A_{1c} value is diagnostic of diabetes, his fasting serum glucose level is only in the range of impaired fasting glucose. Because this patient had two different tests

with discordant results, the test that is diagnostic of diabetes (the hemoglobin A_{1c} measurement) should be repeated to confirm the diagnosis.

In this patient without any hyperglycemic symptoms, remeasuring his hemoglobin A_{1c} level is a much simpler and less burdensome way of confirming the diagnosis of diabetes than performing an oral glucose tolerance test.

Because results of measurement of the hemoglobin A_{1c} value and fasting plasma glucose level were discordant, not performing any additional testing is inappropriate.

KEY POINT

- **If results of two different diagnostic tests for diabetes mellitus are discordant, the test that is diagnostic of diabetes should be repeated.**

Bibliography

American Diabetes Association. Standards of medical care in diabetes—2011. Diabetes Care. 2011;34(Suppl 1):S11-S61. [PMID: 21193625]

Item 25   Answer: D
Educational Objective: Manage adrenal insufficiency.

This patient should be treated with oral hydrocortisone. She has clinical and biochemical features of glucocorticoid deficiency 2 weeks after discontinuing megestrol, which she used continuously for 1 year. Megestrol is a progestational agent with strong glucocorticoid activity that is commonly used in patients with anorexia of different causes because it is a potent appetite stimulant. Because of this potent glucocorticoid activity, chronic use of megestrol (and other agents with similar activity) leads to suppression of the hypothalamic-pituitary-adrenal axis. With the suppression of the axis, a sudden discontinuation of the drug leads to symptoms and signs of adrenal insufficiency. This patient's physical examination findings of a plethoric rounded face and central obesity with supraclavicular and posterior cervical fat pads are consistent with prolonged exposure to exogenous agents with glucocorticoid activity, as are her low serum cortisol and plasma adrenocorticotropic hormone levels. Treatment with hydrocortisone for several weeks is necessary to reactivate the axis. The advantages of hydrocortisone are that it is identical to the natural product, has a short half life, and can be tightly titrated easily.

Because adrenal insufficiency that is central in origin indicates a cause other than intrinsic adrenal disease, obtaining a CT scan of the adrenal glands is unwarranted in this patient.

The dexamethasone suppression test is helpful when investigating conditions associated with hypercortisolemia, such as Cushing syndrome. In this patient with a low serum cortisol level and symptomatic adrenal insufficiency, the dexamethasone suppression test is of no value.

Because the patient has central adrenal insufficiency, mineralocorticoid secretion by the adrenal glands is maintained and fludrocortisone therapy is unnecessary.

KEY POINT

- Chronic use of megestrol and similar drugs with strong glucocorticoid activity leads to suppression of the hypothalamic-pituitary-adrenal axis, and sudden discontinuation of these drugs can result in symptoms and signs of adrenal insufficiency.

Bibliography

Leinung MC, Liporace R, Miller CH. Induction of adrenal suppression by megestrol acetate in patients with AIDS. Ann Intern Med. 1995;122(11):843-845. [PMID: 7741369]

Item 26   Answer: A

Educational Objective: Diagnose the cause of secondary hypogonadism.

This patient should have iron saturation studies to determine a possible cause of his central hypogonadism, which is indicated by the low serum testosterone, follicle-stimulating hormone, and luteinizing hormone levels. The evaluation of secondary hypogonadism includes the exclusion of hyperprolactinemia and hemochromatosis as possible causes. This patient's serum prolactin level is normal, but hemochromatosis has not yet been excluded as a cause. His history of osteoarthritis is consistent with a diagnosis of hemochromatosis, as is his slightly elevated alanine aminotransferase level.

Measuring the free testosterone level is not appropriate because this patient does not have any history or physical examination findings suggestive of abnormal sex hormone–binding globulin levels, such as obesity, insulin resistance (for example, type 2 diabetes mellitus), or older age. If he had any of these findings, his total serum testosterone levels would be suspect, and the amount of free testosterone would be a better indicator of hypogonadism.

Karyotyping and testicular ultrasonography are not useful tests in the evaluation of secondary hypogonadism. A karyotype is useful in patients with primary hypogonadism and increased gonadotropin levels to exclude Klinefelter syndrome.

KEY POINT

- The evaluation of secondary hypogonadism includes the exclusion of hyperprolactinemia and hemochromatosis as possible causes.

Bibliography

Bhasin S, Cunningham GR, Hayes FJ, et al; Task Force, Endocrine Society. Testosterone therapy in men with androgen deficiency syndromes: an Endocrine Society clinical practice guideline. J Clin Endocrinol Metab. 2010;95(6):2536-2559. [PMID: 20525905]

Item 27   Answer: C

Educational Objective: Adjust hydrocortisone therapy during a minor illness.

This woman should increase her dose of hydrocortisone approximately threefold for 3 days. This patient with Addison disease (primary adrenal insufficiency) has an upper respiratory tract infection. She has continued to take adequate amounts of fluids and her medications as scheduled. Except for findings related to an upper respiratory tract infection, vital signs and other physical examination findings are normal. What she has not done is adjust her hydrocortisone dose during her intercurrent illness. This step in necessary to minimize the possibility of adrenal crisis. Educating patients about the need to adjust (increase) their dose of hydrocortisone with even minor intercurrent illnesses is crucial in the successful management of adrenal insufficiency.

Because this patient is not hypotensive and is able to take fluids and her medications orally, hospitalization for intravenous administration of fluids and glucocorticoids is unnecessary.

In patients with adrenal insufficiency, fludrocortisone is typically given as mineralocorticoid therapy. The additional glucocorticoid (hydrocortisone) therapy that this patient requires because of her intercurrent illness also will result in additional mineralocorticoid activity. Therefore, adjusting mineralocorticoid dosages during intercurrent medical illnesses is unnecessary.

Symptomatic treatment of her upper respiratory tract infection without adjustment of her hydrocortisone dosage is inappropriate and likely to lead to prolongation and worsening of her symptoms of adrenal insufficiency

KEY POINT

- Adjusting (increasing) the dosage of hydrocortisone with even minor intercurrent illnesses is crucial to avoid adrenal crisis in patients with adrenal insufficiency.

Bibliography

Chakera AJ, Vaidya B. Addison disease in adults: diagnosis and management. Am J Med. 2010;123(5):409-413. [PMID: 20399314]

Item 28   Answer: B

Educational Objective: Diagnose a thyroid-stimulating hormone–secreting pituitary tumor.

This patient should have a pituitary MRI. He has symptoms, clinical examination findings, and laboratory study results that are consistent with hyperthyroidism. The elevated radioactive iodine (^{123}I) uptake excludes subacute or silent thyroiditis. However, he also has a detectable serum thyroid-stimulating hormone (TSH) level. The serum TSH level is typically undetectable (<0.01 microunits/mL [0.01 milliunits/L]) in all patients with thyrotoxicosis due to

Graves disease, a toxic multinodular goiter, or a solitary autonomous thyroid nodule. Thyrotoxicosis with an inappropriately elevated TSH level may be associated with a TSH-secreting pituitary tumor, antibodies that interfere in the serum TSH assay, or laboratory error. The latter two causes, however, are not associated with the clinical and biochemical evidence of hyperthyroidism seen in this patient. Therefore, the most likely diagnosis in this patient is a TSH-secreting pituitary tumor. These tumors secrete TSH that stimulates the thyroid gland to secondarily release thyroxine (T_4) and triiodothyronine (T_3). The serum TSH level in patients with a TSH-secreting pituitary tumor may be detectable (inappropriately normal, detectable, or even elevated) in the setting of elevated T_4 and T_3 levels. The diagnosis should be confirmed with a pituitary MRI, and a full evaluation of pituitary function should be performed because other pituitary hormones may be secreted in excess or be deficient. The primary therapy is neurosurgical resection of the tumor.

For residual disease after surgery, medical therapy with a somatostatin analogue is highly effective in lowering the TSH level and controlling hyperthyroidism in as many as 80% of patients with TSH-secreting tumors. However, radioactive iodine, methimazole, and propylthiouracil have no role.

Because the tumor involves the pituitary gland and not the thyroid gland, thyroidectomy is inappropriate management.

KEY POINT

- A pituitary MRI can confirm the presence of a thyroid-stimulating hormone–secreting pituitary tumor.

Bibliography
Bahn Chair RS, Burch HB, Cooper DS, et al; American Thyroid Association; American Association of Clinical Endocrinologists. Hyperthyroidism and other causes of thyrotoxicosis: management guidelines of the American Thyroid Association and American Association of Clinical Endocrinologists [erratum in Thyroid. 2011;21(10):1169]. Thyroid. 2011;21(6):593-646. [PMID: 21510801]

Item 29   Answer: B
Educational Objective: Treat pheochromocytoma with α-blocker therapy.

This patient should receive α-blocker therapy as initial treatment of his condition. He has classic clinical features of a pheochromocytoma (hypertension, palpitations, sweating, and headaches). The diagnosis is confirmed biochemically by the extreme elevation in plasma metanephrine and normetanephrine levels and 24-hour excretion of urine catecholamines (norepinephrine and epinephrine) and their metabolites (metanephrine, normetanephrine, and vanillylmandelic acid). Anatomically, these findings are associated with an adrenal mass. Although eventual laparoscopic surgical resection of the tumor is necessary, intraoperative and postoperative morbidities should first be minimized by controlling blood pressure and providing adequate α-blockade with preoperative medical therapy. Most patients with a pheochromocytoma previously were treated with the long-acting competitive α-adrenergic blocking agent phenoxybenzamine for several weeks before surgery, but this drug contributed to the hypotension commonly observed during the first day after tumor removal. More recent data show the effectiveness of short-acting specific α-antagonists, such as prazosin, doxazosin, or terazosin, without this adverse effect.

This patient most likely has a pheochromocytoma and is currently being treated with an ACE inhibitor. Adding an angiotensin receptor blocker to his antihypertensive regimen offers no additional therapeutic benefit over that achieved by ACE inhibition because it will not address the pathophysiologic basis of this secondary form of hypertension.

β-Blockers should never be used in patients with suspected or confirmed pheochromocytomas until after they are first treated with α-blockers.

Surgery is the definitive treatment for patients with a pheochromocytoma but should not be performed before therapy with α-blockers.

Although this patient currently seems stable, treatment of this type of tumor cannot be delayed indefinitely because patients can have provoked or unprovoked sudden cardiac episodes that can be fatal. Observation is thus inappropriate as initial treatment.

KEY POINT

- In patients with a biochemically confirmed diagnosis of pheochromocytoma, α-blockade should be instituted before surgery.

Bibliography
Pacak K. Preoperative management of the pheochromocytoma patient. J Clin Endcrinol Metab. 2007;92(11):4069-4079. [PMID: 17989126]

Item 30   Answer: C
Educational Objective: Diagnose Paget disease of bone.

Plain radiographs of the areas showing increased activity on the bone scan should be obtained in this patient. The increased activity may represent Paget disease of bone (osteitis deformans), a focal abnormality of bone metabolism leading to an accelerated rate of bone remodeling that results in disorganized bone matrix and compromise of bone integrity. The diagnosis of Paget disease of bone is best confirmed by plain radiographs of the areas of increased uptake seen on bone scan. Pagetic lesions will show characteristic coarsened bony trabeculae, which are pathognomonic for the disease.

Paget disease of bone may cause a range of clinical symptoms, including bone pain, traumatic and pathologic fractures, skeletal deformities, and cranial nerve impairment due to nerve impingement because of bony overgrowth. Hearing loss related to impairment of cranial nerve VIII is common in Paget disease of bone. Audiology testing to document the patient's baseline hearing status for comparison with future studies should be performed after the diagnosis of Paget disease of bone is confirmed, but not before.

Also part of the differential diagnosis of the bony lesions seen on bone scan is metastatic disease, particularly in an older patient. If plain radiographs do not confirm a diagnosis of Paget disease of bone or show findings consistent with metastatic disease, a bone biopsy can be considered.

Serum collagen type 1 cross-linked C-telopeptide (CTX) measurement may be helpful in monitoring the response of Paget disease to therapy but would not distinguish Paget disease from metastatic lesions.

Serum protein electrophoresis would help diagnose multiple myeloma but would not help distinguish Paget disease from metastases, which is the appropriate goal of the next step in this patient's evaluation.

KEY POINT

- Plain radiographs of pagetic lesions will show characteristic coarsened bony trabeculae, which will confirm the diagnosis of Paget disease of bone.

Bibliography

Josse RG, Hanley DA, Kendler D, Ste Marie LG, Adachi JD, Brown J. Diagnosis and treatment of Paget's disease of bone. Clin Invest Med. 2007;30(5):E210-E223. [PMID: 17892763]

Item 31   Answer: B
Educational Objective: Identify nocturnal hypoglycemia.

This patient's symptoms are most likely caused by nocturnal hypoglycemia. Her hemoglobin A_{1c} value is lower than what her blood glucose log averages suggest. Frequent episodes of significant hypoglycemia for several hours each night would explain this discrepancy. The 70/30 insulin she takes twice daily gives a single large peak 6 to 8 hours after taking it. This patient exercises every evening, which means that her muscles will continue to remove glucose from her blood to replenish their glycogen stores for several hours afterward. This occurrence could cause her blood glucose to decrease to very low levels while she sleeps. Given the duration of her diabetes mellitus, the appropriate adrenergic counterregulatory response may be adequately blunted to not cause her to awaken from sleep but can lead to fatigue, sweating, and headache when she awakens.

The dawn phenomenon is defined as an elevation in blood glucose levels during the early morning hours (4 AM-8 AM) that is thought to be related to the increased physiologic release of cortisol and growth hormone that occur during this time period. The dawn phenomenon is typically

identified by persistent significant elevations of morning blood glucose levels, which were not seen in this patient.

Although sleep apnea may be a cause of fatigue and early morning headache, it is more often seen in obese patients with type 2 diabetes who have an associated high hemoglobin A_{1c} value.

The "Somogyi phenomenon" is a phrase used to describe the theoretical concept that the lower the blood glucose level decreases during the night, the higher it increases the next morning because of increasingly severe rebound hyperglycemia. This idea, however attractive on a theoretical level, has been disproven as a cause of fasting hyperglycemia.

KEY POINT

- Frequent nocturnal hypoglycemia may cause morning fatigue, sweating, and headache in patients with type 1 diabetes mellitus.

Bibliography

Juvenile Diabetes Research Foundation Continuous Glucose Monitoring Study Group. Prolonged nocturnal hypoglycemia is common during 12 months of continuous glucose monitoring in children and adults with type 1 diabetes. Diabetes Care. 2010;33(5):1004-1008. [PMID: 20200306]

Item 32   Answer: C
Educational Objective: Diagnose multiple endocrine neoplasia type 1.

This patient most likely has multiple endocrine neoplasia type 1 (MEN1), which is characterized by tumors of the pituitary gland, the parathyroid glands, and the pancreas (the three "P"s). She has hyperprolactinemia and a pituitary adenoma, the size of which (<1 cm) suggests a microprolactinoma. Additionally, she has primary hyperparathyroidism and a family history that suggests the presence of MEN1 in her kindred. Her father's history of kidney stones suggests that he also has hyperparathyroidism as a result of MEN1, and her brother's history of peptic ulcer disease suggests the presence of a gastrin-secreting pancreatic neuroendocrine tumor in the setting of MEN1. In MEN1, primary hyperparathyroidism most often reflects parathyroid hyperplasia rather than an adenoma. The mutation in the menin gene was most likely inherited in an autosomal dominant fashion in this family.

Autoimmune polyglandular syndrome type 1 is an inherited autosomal recessive disorder characterized by chronic mucocutaneous candidiasis, autoimmune hypoparathyroidism, and adrenal insufficiency. This patient has hyperparathyroidism, not hypoparathyroidism, and thus is unlikely to have autoimmune polyglandular syndrome type 1.

This patient's thyroid-stimulating hormone level is normal, which makes the diagnosis of Hashimoto thyroiditis unlikely.

MEN2 is characterized by primary parathyroid hyperplasia, pheochromocytoma, and medullary thyroid cancer. Although this patient has evidence of primary hyperparathyroidism, she does not have a consistent family history or clinical symptoms or signs of the other components of the genetic abnormality suggestive of this diagnosis.

KEY POINT

- Multiple endocrine neoplasia type 1 is characterized by tumors of the pituitary gland, the parathyroid glands, and the pancreas (the three "P"s).

Bibliography

Brandi ML, Gagel RF, Angeli A, et al. Guidelines for diagnosis and therapy of MEN type 1 and type 2. J Clin Endocrinol Metab. 2001;86(12):5658-5671. [PMID: 11739416]

Item 33   Answer: A
Educational Objective: Diagnose hypogonadism in patients with obesity.

A free testosterone assessment, preferably one using equilibrium dialysis, is the most appropriate diagnostic test to determine whether this patient truly has hypogonadism. A random serum testosterone level greater than 350 ng/dL (12 nmol/L) excludes hypogonadism. Values consistently less than 200 ng/dL (6.9 nmol/L) almost always confirm hypogonadism, but values in the 200 to 350 ng/dL (6.9-12 nmol/L) range are equivocal. Unless the total testosterone level is markedly reduced and the patient has a known pituitary or gonadal pathologic abnormality, a screening testosterone value of 350 ng/dL (12 nmol/L) or lower requires confirmation by a second measurement that includes determination of the free testosterone level. Of note, obesity can cause a decrease in sex hormone–binding globulin levels. Therefore, the free testosterone level can be normal, even when the total testosterone level appears decreased. If the free testosterone level is normal, then hypogonadism is excluded and another etiology of this patient's erectile dysfunction, such as medications, must be explored.

A karyotype is not appropriate in this patient in whom hypogonadism has not been diagnosed and who has normal follicle-stimulating hormone and luteinizing hormone levels, which exclude primary hypogonadism. A karyotype is useful in patients diagnosed with primary hypogonadism to exclude Klinefelter syndrome.

A pituitary MRI is not indicated at this time because the diagnosis of secondary hypogonadism has not been confirmed.

A sperm count is not indicated in this patient because a sperm count will not reliably indicate whether a patient has hypogonadism. Men with low sperm counts can have normal testosterone levels, and men with slightly decreased testosterone levels can have normal sperm counts. In addition, this patient is not seeking fertility at this time.

KEY POINT

- In male patients with obesity, hypogonadism is best diagnosed by a free testosterone assessment because the total testosterone level may be affected by a decrease in the sex hormone–binding globulin level.

Bibliography

Traish AM, Miner MM, Morgentaler A, Zitzmann M. Testosterone deficiency. Am J Med. 2011;124(7):578-587. [PMID: 21683825]

Item 34   Answer: B
Educational Objective: Manage medullary thyroid cancer.

Measurement of the plasma free metanephrine and normetanephrine levels is the most appropriate initial step in management in this patient with a thyroid nodule. She has a history of hypertension, elevated serum calcium and calcitonin levels, and multiple plasmacytoid-appearing cells on fine-needle aspiration (FNA) biopsy of the nodule. These findings are suggestive of medullary thyroid cancer. Although sporadic in greater than 80% of affected patients, medullary thyroid cancer may be associated with multiple endocrine neoplasia type 2A (MEN2A), MEN2B, or familial non-MEN. The MEN2A and MEN2B syndromes are characterized by medullary thyroid cancer and pheochromocytoma. Therefore, the presence of pheochromocytoma must be excluded.

Radioactive iodine is not taken up by parafollicular cells (C cells) and, therefore, is not an appropriate treatment in patients with medullary thyroid cancer.

Because nearly 30% of patients with sporadic medullary thyroid cancer and 100% of patients with inherited medullary thyroid cancer have bilateral disease, total thyroidectomy, not thyroid lobectomy, is always the preferred surgical treatment. After initial surgery, all patients should receive levothyroxine to prevent hypothyroidism.

The administration of levothyroxine without surgery to suppress thyroid-stimulating hormone (TSH) secretion is not indicated because C-cells are not TSH responsive.

KEY POINT

- Although sporadic in greater than 80% of affected patients, medullary thyroid cancer also may be associated with multiple endocrine neoplasia type 2A (MEN2A), MEN2B, or familial non-MEN.

Bibliography

American Thyroid Association Guidelines Task Force; Kloos RT, Eng C, Evans DB, et al. Medullary thyroid cancer: management guidelines of the American Thyroid Association [erratum in Thyroid. 2009;19(11):1295]. Thyroid. 2009;19(6):565-612. [PMID: 19469690]

Item 35 — Answer: E
Educational Objective: Treat type 1 diabetes mellitus.

This patient's preprandial insulin lispro dose should be changed to 1 unit for every 10 grams of carbohydrate to be consumed. She recently has made several healthy changes to her diabetic regimen and lifestyle that have resulted in close-to-ideal fasting and preprandial glucose levels, but her 2-hour postprandial levels are still too high. Changing her insulin lispro dose from 1 unit to cover each 20 grams of carbohydrate to 1 unit to cover every 10 grams of carbohydrate will give her a larger spike of rapid-acting insulin in the first 2 hours after each meal and should lower her postprandial blood glucose levels. This change should result in a lower hemoglobin A_{1c} value after a few months.

Although adding an injection of pramlintide before meals might improve her postprandial blood glucose level, optimization of her current diabetic regimen is likely to successfully control her blood glucoses without introducing an additional and expensive treatment.

Changing from insulin lispro to regular insulin would not improve her blood glucose levels 2 hours after her meals but might cause hypoglycemia 4 to 6 hours after meals.

Changing from neutral protamine Hagedorn (NPH) insulin to insulin glargine would provide no benefit because her fasting and preprandial glucose levels are already at goal, and she is not experiencing nocturnal hypoglycemia. Additionally, insulin glargine is approximately four times more expensive than NPH insulin.

The patient is already somewhat underweight, is planning to get pregnant, and is eating a healthy diet. Therefore, restricting her carbohydrate intake is not appropriate and might lead to hypoglycemia.

KEY POINT
- Evaluating and managing postprandial blood glucose levels can help optimize insulin therapy in patients with type 1 diabetes mellitus.

Bibliography
Singh SR, Ahmad F, Lal A, Yu C, Bai Z, Bennett H. Efficacy and safety of insulin analogues for the management of diabetes mellitus: a meta-analysis. CMAJ. 2009;180(4):385-397. [PMID: 19221352]

Item 36 — Answer: B
Educational Objective: Treat hypoparathyroidism occurring after thyroidectomy.

Calcium is most likely to diminish the acute symptoms in this patient who recently underwent thyroidectomy. Complications of thyroidectomy include the inadvertent removal of or injury to the parathyroid glands. If a substantial amount of parathyroid tissue is not left in vivo, hypoparathyroidism accompanied by hypocalcemia will result postoperatively.

Symptoms are primarily neuromuscular, such as paresthesias and muscle cramps, and tend to be prominent in patients who experience a rapid drop in their serum calcium level after surgery. This patient requires an emergent rapid increase in his serum calcium level, which is best accomplished by oral calcium (carbonate or citrate) supplementation. Intravenous calcium more rapidly increases the serum calcium level and may be indicated in patients with very low (<7.5 mg/dL [1.9 mmol/L]) calcium levels or more significant clinical findings associated with the hypocalcemia, such as severe musculoskeletal weakness, tetany, or electrocardiographic conduction abnormalities. Ultimately, this patient most likely will require more prolonged calcium therapy, depending on the degree of his hypoparathyroidism after surgery.

Although this patient also may require chronic vitamin D supplementation to maintain his serum calcium levels, this would not be an initial intervention in a symptomatic individual with hypocalcemia. Calcitriol (1,25-dihydroxyvitamin D) should be used because the lack of parathyroid hormone (PTH) will diminish the endogenous conversion of 25-hydroxyvitamin D to the more potent 1,25-dihydroxyvitamin D. However, calcitriol by itself will not effectively increase serum calcium levels until several days have elapsed.

Patients with hypomagnesemia may have hypocalcemia that is refractory to correction until the low magnesium levels are repleted. This patient has no evidence of significant hypomagnesemia.

Teriparatide, a recombinant form of PTH, currently is used in the treatment of advanced osteoporosis. Although it holds promise as a potential therapy for chronic hypoparathyroidism, its safety and long-term effectiveness for this use have not been established, and it does not have FDA approval for treatment of acute hypoparathyroidism.

KEY POINT
- In most patients with hypoparathyroidism and hypocalcemia, oral calcium is appropriate emergent therapy because it is rapidly absorbed and will increase the serum calcium level within minutes.

Bibliography
Khan MI, Waguespack SG, Hu MI. Medical management of postsurgical hypoparathyroidism [erratum in: Endocr Pract. 2011;17(6):967]. Endocr Pract. 2011;17(Suppl 1):18-25. [PMID: 21134871]

Item 37 — Answer: A
Educational Objective: Interpret hemoglobin A_{1c} values in a patient with a recent blood transfusion.

The six units of packed red blood cells that this patient received while hospitalized most likely are responsible for his low hemoglobin A_{1c} value. In patients receiving hemodialysis, those with hemolytic anemia or certain hemoglobinopathies, or those with recent blood transfusions, hemoglobin A_{1c} values may be falsely lowered because of the presence of erythrocytes less than 120 days old in the sample. In this patient, not enough time has elapsed since the blood was transfused for the erythrocytes to become glycosylated and reflect a true hemoglobin A_{1c} level.

Although eating a healthier diet might lower his blood glucose levels over the next few months, not enough time has passed for this lifestyle intervention to affect his hemoglobin A_{1c} value so profoundly. His blood glucose log shows premeal values of 140 to 160 mg/dL (7.8-8.9 mmol/L), which means that postprandial values are likely to be even higher and not compatible with a hemoglobin A_{1c} value of 6.2%.

Omeprazole does not interfere with hemoglobin A_{1c} assays and thus is not responsible for his dramatically lower value.

Cessation of cigarette smoking, although an inherently positive lifestyle change, will not affect the hemoglobin A_{1c} level.

KEY POINT

- Hemoglobin A_{1c} values may be falsely lowered in patients who have received recent blood transfusions.

Bibliography

Spencer DH, Grossman BJ, Scott MG. Red cell transfusion decreases hemoglobin A1c in patients with diabetes. Clin Chem. 2011;57(2):344-346. [PMID: 21059826]

Item 38   Answer: D

Educational Objective: Diagnose opiate-induced secondary hypogonadism.

This patient's use of methadone is most likely responsible for his symptoms. Chronic opiate use is an acquired cause of secondary hypogonadism. The mechanism of opiate-induced hypogonadism is thought to be central hypogonadism, with downregulation of gonadotropin-releasing hormone and subsequently luteinizing hormone (LH) and follicle-stimulating hormone (FSH). This, in turn results in decreased testosterone production.

Active or anabolic steroid abuse can decrease patients' endogenous LH, FSH, and testosterone levels. However, these patients typically seek medical attention because of infertility, usually do not have low libido, are very muscular, and may have significant pustular acne. This patient has low libido, is thin (not muscular), and has no acne, all of which make anabolic steroid abuse very unlikely.

Low libido is an adverse effect of citalopram, but the drug should not cause low testosterone levels and thus is not the cause of this patient's symptoms.

Lisinopril has not been associated with low libido or erectile dysfunction and thus also is unlikely to be the cause of this patient's symptoms.

KEY POINT

- The mechanism of opiate-induced hypogonadism is thought to be central hypogonadism, with downregulation of gonadotropin-releasing hormone and subsequently luteinizing hormone and follicle-stimulating hormone, which results in decreased testosterone production.

Bibliography

Bliesener N, Albrecht S, Schwager A, Weckbecker K, Lichtermann D, Kingmüller D. Plasma testosterone and sexual function in men receiving buprenorphine maintenance for opioid dependence. J Clin Endocrinol Metab. 2005;90(1):203-206. [PMID: 15483091]

Item 39   Answer: A

Educational Objective: Manage newly diagnosed adrenal insufficiency.

Hydrocortisone therapy is most appropriate for management of this patient's disorder. She has the classic clinical (fatigue, nausea, weight loss, salt craving) and biochemical (hyponatremia, hyperkalemia, and low cortisol and high adrenocorticotropic hormone [ACTH] levels) features of primary adrenal insufficiency. The laboratory study results also suggest decreased production of mineralocorticoids (hyponatremia and hyperkalemia) and adrenal androgens (low serum dehydroepiandrosterone sulfate level). Although the random serum cortisol level is within the accepted range for the afternoon, it is inappropriately low for the degree of hypotension experienced by this patient—especially because hypotension is a strong stimulus for ACTH and cortisol release. The plasma ACTH level, which was measured at the same time as the serum cortisol level, is extremely elevated and indicates primary adrenal failure. Therefore, all three classes of corticosteroids produced by the adrenal cortex (glucocorticoids, mineralocorticoids, and adrenal androgens) are diminished, which suggests the diagnosis of primary adrenal insufficiency. The disorder is most likely autoimmune in nature, given the patient's family history, and is best treated with hydrocortisone.

Although the serum thyroid-stimulating hormone level is minimally elevated, this patient has newly diagnosed primary adrenal insufficiency that should be addressed before any adjustment in the levothyroxine dosage is made. Increasing the levothyroxine dosage before starting glucocorticoids could accelerate the metabolic clearance of endogenously secreted cortisol and potentially worsen symptoms of adrenal insufficiency.

The abnormalities in this patient's laboratory results are quite clear and associated with clinical symptoms. Therefore, repeat testing of her serum cortisol and plasma ACTH levels at 9 AM is unnecessary.

The increased plasma ACTH level is a physiologic response to the reduction in cortisol and excludes pituitary insufficiency as the cause of the patient's hypocortisolism. An MRI of the pituitary gland is thus not indicated.

KEY POINT

- The diagnosis of primary adrenal insufficiency is suggested when all three classes of corticosteroids produced by the adrenal cortex are diminished.

Bibliography

Chakera AJ, Vaidya B. Addison disease in adults: diagnosis and management. Am J Med. 2010;123(5):409-413. [PMID: 20399314]

Item 40   Answer: B

Educational Objective: Diagnose lymphocytic hypophysitis.

This patient most likely has lymphocytic hypophysitis, an uncommon autoimmune disorder characterized by symmetric enlargement of the sellar contents. Lymphocytic hypophysitis is usually detected during pregnancy or in the postpartum period. Antipituitary antibodies can be detected in patients with this disorder, but these antibodies are not routinely clinically measured. Lymphocytic hypophysitis is a rare cause of hypopituitarism and can be associated with central adrenal insufficiency, as seen in this patient. Adrenocorticotropic hormone deficiency is a common finding in lymphocytic hypophysitis and is a major cause of morbidity and mortality in patients with the disorder. This patient should be treated with glucocorticoid replacement therapy and observation of the mass, which often decreases in size over time. If visual field defects develop, surgery may be necessary.

Craniopharyngioma is a rare, irregular, mixed solid-cystic lesion, often with calcifications, seen in persons of this patient's age that often is associated with panhypopituitarism and diabetes insipidus. The radiographic findings and signs and symptoms in this patient are inconsistent with craniopharyngioma.

Although prolactinomas may enlarge during pregnancy, the serum prolactin level is generally greater than 500 ng/mL (500 micrograms/L), with lesions greater than 10 mm in size (macroadenomas). Given the size of her pituitary lesion, one would expect her serum prolactin level to be much higher than measured. The hyperprolactinemia in this patient most likely reflects her recent gravid state because serum prolactin levels increase throughout pregnancy. The increased size of the normal pituitary gland during pregnancy does not result in associated clinical signs or symptoms of hypopituitarism and will not cause local mass effects.

Sheehan syndrome is defined as pituitary infarction or hemorrhage in the setting of a complicated delivery and thus is not the diagnosis in this patient.

KEY POINT

- Adrenocorticotropic hormone deficiency is a common finding in lymphocytic hypophysitis and is a major cause of morbidity and mortality.

Bibliography

Molitch ME, Gillam MP. Lymphocytic hypophysitis. Horm Res. 2007;68(Suppl 5):145-150. [PMID: 18174733]

Item 41   Answer: D

Educational Objective: Interpret hemoglobin A_{1c} results.

The discrepancy in this patient's glucose monitor readings and hemoglobin A_{1c} values is most likely due to postprandial hyperglycemia. She tests her blood glucose level only in a fasting state and before each meal and does not obtain postprandial or other measurements. Although her records indicate an average level that is close to the target of 130 mg/dL (7.2 mmol/L), her blood glucose level may actually exceed 200 mg/dL (11.1 mmol/L) for several hours after meals. These periods of hyperglycemia will contribute to her elevated hemoglobin A_{1c} value. The hemoglobin A_{1c} level represents the average of her fasting, preprandial, postprandial, nocturnal, and other blood glucose levels during the past 3 months.

Although blood glucose monitors occasionally may produce inaccurate readings, this occurrence is extremely rare and also is unlikely in this patient because the simultaneous laboratory plasma glucose level and glucose monitor reading are within 10% of each other.

Hemoglobin A_{1c} levels vary directly with erythrocyte survival. Levels are falsely high when erythrocyte survival is prolonged (decreased erythrocyte turnover), as occurs in patients with untreated iron, vitamin B_{12}, or folate deficiency anemia. Conversely, hemoglobin A_{1c} levels may be falsely low in patients with the shorter erythrocyte survival associated with rapid cell turnover, as occurs in patients with hemolytic anemia; those being treated for iron, folate, or vitamin B_{12} deficiency; and those being treated with erythropoietin. This patient's history of recent iron deficiency anemia treated with iron is likely to falsely lower, not elevate, her hemoglobin A_{1c} level.

If the patient were having prolonged periods of nocturnal hypoglycemia, she would have a lower-than-expected hemoglobin A_{1c} value.

KEY POINT

- Average glucose monitor readings that do not include postprandial blood glucose levels are likely to differ from average plasma glucose levels derived from hemoglobin A_{1c} values.

Bibliography

Nathan DM, Kuenen J, Borg R, Zheng H, Schoenfeld D, Heine RJ; A1c-Derived Average Glucose Study Group. Translating the A1C assay into estimated average glucose values [erratum in Diabetes Care. 2009;32(1):207]. Diabetes Care. 2008; 31(8):1473-1478. [PMID: 18540046]

Item 42   Answer: C

Educational Objective: Diagnose hypocalcemia due to hungry bone syndrome.

This patient's hypocalcemia is most likely caused by hungry bone syndrome. He has developed hypocalcemia after surgery to correct primary hyperparathyroidism. After parathyroidectomy, patients may experience hungry bone syndrome, in which the unmineralized bone matrix produced during the period of hyperparathyroidism begins to mineralize after the parathyroid level becomes more normal. This results in low serum calcium and phosphorus levels because these minerals are consumed by the bone in the process of mineralization.

Secondary hyperparathyroidism and bone disease affect almost all patients with chronic kidney disease (CKD). Hyperphosphatemia, hypocalcemia, and deficiency of 1,25-dihydroxyvitamin D stimulate parathyroid hormone (PTH) secretion. In patients with stage 2 and stage 3 CKD, increased PTH secretion helps maintain the serum calcium level through increased mobilization of calcium from bone and decreased urine calcium excretion. Patients with stage 3 CKD have transient postprandial hypocalcemia and hyperphosphatemia, both of which contribute to the increase in the PTH level that precedes onset of the sustained hyperphosphatemia characteristic of stage 4 and stage 5 CKD. Although this patient's kidney function is mildly impaired, the dysfunction is not serious enough to cause this severe hypocalcemia, and CKD is not consistent with the measured normal PTH level.

Dilutional hypocalcemia can result from excessive intravenous fluid administration. This patient had minimally invasive surgery and would not have required a large amount of hydration.

Alkalosis due to hyperventilation can cause a decrease in the ionized calcium level because of a shift in calcium ions to the intracellular compartment. However, alkalosis does not affect the total serum calcium level.

KEY POINT

- After parathyroidectomy, patients may experience hungry bone syndrome, in which the unmineralized bone matrix produced during the period of hyperparathyroidism begins to mineralize after the parathyroid level becomes more normal.

Bibliography
Mittendorf EA, Merlino JI, McHenry CR. Post-parathyroidectomy hypocalcemia: incidence, risk factors, and management. Am Surg. 2004;70(2):114-119. [PMID: 15011912]

Item 43   Answer: D
Educational Objective: Manage a thyroid nodule.

This patient should undergo thyroid lobectomy. According to several guidelines, biopsy of any nodule greater than 1 cm in diameter is reasonable, and biopsy of smaller nodules should be considered in patients with risk factors, such as a history of radiation exposure, a family history of thyroid cancer, cervical lymphadenopathy, or worrisome ultrasound characteristics. Therefore, it was appropriate to perform a fine-needle aspiration (FNA) biopsy in this 18-year-old

woman with a 2-cm hypoechoic nodule that also has increased intranodular vascularity, regardless of whether she has a personal or family history of thyroid cancer. Results were consistent with a follicular neoplasm, which has an approximately 15% to 30% chance of harboring cancer. Unlike papillary thyroid cancer, follicular thyroid cancer cannot be diagnosed on the basis of an FNA biopsy because it is difficult to differentiate a malignant from a benign adenoma. Therefore, follicular neoplasms require pathologic examination of a surgical specimen to diagnose or exclude malignancy. Either a thyroid lobectomy or total thyroidectomy is typically recommended for these nodules to allow for complete histologic evaluation.

Thyroid hormone suppression therapy with levothyroxine is frequently used in the treatment of differentiated thyroid cancers to minimize thyroid-stimulating hormone stimulation of tumor growth. However, its use in benign nodules is controversial, and using thyroid suppression therapy in this patient who does not yet have a clear diagnosis would be inappropriate.

Because the patient does not yet have a definitive diagnosis of thyroid cancer, treatment with radioactive iodine is not appropriate. Treatment with radioactive iodine is appropriate after malignancy is established.

Because results of FNA biopsy in this patient already suggest the possibility of malignancy, repeating the study in 6 months would be inappropriate. In any case, a repeat FNA biopsy would not obviate the need for a surgical specimen for a definitive diagnosis.

KEY POINT

- Thyroid lobectomy or total thyroidectomy is typically recommended for thyroid nodules with evidence of a follicular neoplasm.

Bibliography
American Thyroid Association (ATA) Guidelines Taskforce on Thyroid Nodules and Differentiated Thyroid Cancer; Cooper DS, Doherty GM, Haugen BR, et al. Revised American Thyroid Association management guidelines for patients with thyroid nodules and differentiated thyroid cancer [errata in Thyroid. 2010;20(6):674-675; and Thyroid. 2010;20(8):942]. Thyroid. 2009;19(11):1167-1214. [PMID: 19860577]

Item 44   Answer: A
Educational Objective: Diagnose functional hypothalamic amenorrhea.

Functional hypothalamic amenorrhea is the most likely diagnosis in this patient. Hypothalamic amenorrhea may result from several causes, including a tumor or infiltrative lesion, such as a lymphoma or sarcoidosis. More commonly, hypothalamic amenorrhea is functional and due to stress, excessive loss of body weight, excessive exercise, or some combination thereof and is a diagnosis of exclusion. This patient's findings of a low follicle-stimulating hormone (FSH) level and normal thyroid-stimulating hormone

(TSH) and prolactin levels; negative human chorionic gonadotropin test results; and no withdrawal bleeding after a progesterone challenge test all suggest hypothalamic amenorrhea. The pituitary MRI excludes a tumor or infiltrative lesion. The increased stress at work is the likely cause of her functional hypothalamic amenorrhea.

Polycystic ovary syndrome (PCOS) is unlikely because the patient has no evidence of significant hyperandrogenism; only mild facial acne is detected on physical examination. In addition, the progesterone challenge test resulted in no withdrawal bleeding, which indicates that she has low estrogen levels. Patients with PCOS typically have adequate estrogen levels but anovulatory cycles; a progesterone challenge test will produce withdrawal bleeding in these patients.

Primary ovarian insufficiency is not the diagnosis because the patient's FSH level is normal. In women with primary ovarian insufficiency, FSH levels are elevated (in the menopausal range).

Subclinical hypothyroidism is unlikely in this patient because her TSH level is normal, which indicates that she is euthyroid.

KEY POINT

- Functional hypothalamic amenorrhea is a diagnosis of exclusion characterized by a low estrogen state, psychological or physical stress, normal or low follicle-stimulating hormone levels, and negative results on progesterone challenge testing.

Bibliography

Gordon CM. Clinical practice. Functional hypothalamic amenorrhea. N Engl J Med. 2010;363(4):365-371. [PMID: 20660404]

Item 45　　Answer: B

Educational Objective: Treat a patient who has diabetes mellitus, hyperlipidemia, and nonalcoholic fatty liver disease with a statin.

In addition to neutral protamine Hagedorn (NPH) insulin at bedtime, a statin should be added now to this patient's diabetes regimen. He has poorly controlled type 2 diabetes mellitus, and thus adding a bedtime basal insulin to his sulfonylurea is a reasonable step to improve his fasting plasma glucose level and hemoglobin A_{1c} value. His liver chemistry studies show moderately elevated aminotransferase levels, but he has no other evidence of liver disease. This makes the diagnosis of nonalcoholic fatty liver disease most likely. In light of his diabetes and significant hypercholesterolemia, the addition of a statin is likely to be beneficial. Patients with nonalcoholic fatty liver disease are not necessarily at a higher risk of adverse outcomes from statin therapy than patients without the disease, and thus statins are a treatment option in these patients. In a study of 437 patients whose liver chemistry

levels were up to three times the upper limit of normal, treatment with atorvastatin resulted in a threefold reduction in cardiovascular events (10% versus 30% in the nontreatment group) and a greater reduction in liver chemistry levels compared with patients not receiving a statin during 3 years of follow-up evaluation.

Fibrates are most effective for reducing the triglyceride level and have little impact on the LDL cholesterol level, the primary lipid target in this patient.

Starting the statin should not be delayed until after his glycemic control has improved or his liver chemistry tests normalize.

Nicotinic acid can lower the LDL cholesterol level and increase the HDL cholesterol level. Its use is typically limited by its adverse effects. Nicotinic acid can cause elevation of glucose and liver chemistry levels and may cause severe hepatocellular damage. Nicotinic acid would be relatively contraindicated in this patient with probable nonalcoholic fatty liver disease.

KEY POINT

- Statins are a viable treatment option in patients with diabetes mellitus, hyperlipidemia, and nonalcoholic fatty liver disease.

Bibliography

Athyros VG, Tziomalos K, Gossios TD, et al; GREACE Study Collaborative Group. Safety and efficacy of long-term statin treatment for cardiovascular events in patients with coronary heart disease and abnormal liver tests in the Greek Atorvastatin and Coronary Heart Disease Evaluation (GREACE) Study: a post-hoc analysis. Lancet. 2010;376(9756):1916-1922. [PMID: 21109302]

Item 46　　Answer: C

Educational Objective: Manage a sellar mass.

In this patient with an incidental sellar mass, measuring the serum prolactin level should be part of the initial evaluation. The approach to a sellar mass includes assessment for hormone hypersecretion, including evaluation for acromegaly, Cushing syndrome, and a prolactinoma. The absence of clinical findings suggestive of acromegaly or Cushing syndrome and the normal insulin-like growth factor 1 (IGF-1) and morning cortisol levels in this patient suggest a nonfunctioning pituitary macroadenoma. However, prolactin-secreting pituitary adenomas are common, and a serum prolactin level should be obtained to evaluate for this possibility. A male patient can have a prolactinoma without gynecomastia or galactorrhea. Testosterone deficiency with associated diminished libido and erectile dysfunction may be present in the setting of hyperprolactinemia. If a prolactinoma is diagnosed, a dopamine agonist is administered to reduce both the serum prolactin level and the tumor size. Further assessment includes evaluation for hypopituitarism.

A dexamethasone suppression test can help localize the tumor source in a patient with adrenocorticotropic hormone–dependent Cushing syndrome. Because this patient does not have Cushing syndrome, this test is not indicated.

A growth hormone stimulation test can be used to evaluate for possible growth hormone deficiency, but measuring the IGF-1 level is typically the initial screening test because IGF-1 is a marker for endogenous growth hormone levels. This patient has a normal IGF-1 level.

Measurement of the serum sodium and urine osmolality levels evaluates deficiency in antidiuretic hormone (ADH) secretion, which occurs in the hypothalamic region and posterior pituitary gland. Deficiencies of ADH secretion are rarely associated with either functional or nonfunctioning pituitary adenomas, although they may be a result of surgical intervention to treat an adenoma.

KEY POINT

- In a patient with an incidental sellar mass, measuring the serum prolactin level should be part of the initial management.

Bibliography

Freda PU, Beckers AM, Katznelson L, et al; Endocrine Society. Pituitary incidentaloma: an Endocrine Society clinical practice guideline. J Clin Endocrinol Metab. 2011;96(4):894-904. [PMID: 21474686]

Item 47   Answer: C
Educational Objective: Diagnose benign familial hypocalciuric hypercalcemia.

The patient should have her urine levels of calcium and creatinine measured so that the urine calcium-to-creatinine clearance ratio can be calculated. A ratio less than 0.01 would suggest benign familial hypocalciuric hypercalcemia (FHH). Although this low ratio also is seen in as many as one third of patients with primary hyperparathyroidism, this patient has none of the expected complications of primary hyperparathyroidism and has a brother with a similar history. Confirmation of the diagnosis of FHH is often possible by genetic testing for mutations in the *CASR* gene.

Measurement of the serum prolactin level could be considered if multiple endocrine neoplasia type 1 (MEN1) was in the differential diagnosis. However, this patient has no history of other tumors, which makes MEN1 an unlikely diagnosis.

Measurement of the serum 25-hydroxyvitamin D level is unlikely to help in the evaluation of a patient with a high serum calcium level and high-normal parathyroid hormone (PTH) level. The typical pattern seen in vitamin D deficiency is a high PTH level and a normal or mildly low serum calcium level.

A parathyroid sestamibi scan is inappropriate at this point in the patient's evaluation because it is a localization study meant to be performed on patients already deemed appropriate for parathyroidectomy.

KEY POINT

- Benign familial hypocalciuric hypercalcemia is likely in the setting of a mild elevation of the serum calcium level with a high-normal or mildly elevated serum parathyroid hormone level and a family member with similar findings.

Bibliography

Christensen SE, Nissen PH, Vestergaard P, Mosekilde L. Familial hypocalciuric hypercalcaemia: a review. Curr Opin Endocrinol Diabetes Obes. 2011;18(6):359-370. [PMID: 21986511]

Item 48   Answer: A

Educational Objective: Evaluate adrenal function during critical illness.

This patient should continue her current therapy of antibiotics and intravenous fluids. In the setting of a critically ill patient with sepsis and hypotension, the diagnosis of adrenal insufficiency is a possibility. Available assays for measuring the serum cortisol level determine the total (protein-bound and free) hormone level. The physiologic effects of cortisol are determined by the free (or unbound) fraction of the hormone pool. Patients with hypoproteinemia have lower serum total cortisol levels but may have normal serum free cortisol levels. The latter situation becomes clinically relevant in critically ill patients with hypoproteinemia, such as this patient.

A random serum cortisol level greater than 12 micrograms/dL (331 nmol/L) in a critically ill patient who has hypoproteinemia (albumin level <2.5 g/dL [25 g/L]) makes the diagnosis of adrenal insufficiency unlikely. The most appropriate management is to order no additional studies and add no new treatment but instead continue the current therapy of antibiotics and intravenous fluids.

The diagnosis of adrenal insufficiency typically relies on demonstrating a low basal serum cortisol level that does not increase appropriately after stimulation with the adrenocorticotropic hormone analogue cosyntropin. Because the adrenal glands are constantly stimulated by stressful events, such as sepsis, obtaining a cosyntropin stimulation test is unlikely to be of value in this setting.

In most healthy persons, the serum cortisol level is highest in the morning. A low morning serum cortisol measurement is compatible with adrenal insufficiency but is neither sufficiently sensitive nor specific to be diagnostic. Additionally, critically ill patients have maximally stimulated cortisol production throughout the day. Therefore, a morning serum cortisol level will not be significantly different from a random serum cortisol level and is not indicated in this patient.

Because the diagnosis of adrenal insufficiency is unlikely in this patient, the use of hydrocortisone is unnecessary.

KEY POINT

- A random serum cortisol level greater than 12 micrograms/dL (331 nmol/L) in a critically ill patient with hypoproteinemia (albumin level <2.5 g/dL [25 g/L]) makes the diagnosis of adrenal insufficiency unlikely and treatment with hydrocortisone unnecessary.

Bibliography

Arafah BM. Hypothalamic pituitary adrenal function during critical illness: limitations of current assessment methods. J Clin Endocrinol Metab. 2006;91(10):3725-3745. [PMID: 16882746]

Item 49   Answer: B
Educational Objective: Treat myxedema coma.

This patient's symptoms and signs strongly suggest myxedema coma, which should be treated with intravenous levothyroxine and hydrocortisone. Patients with myxedema coma frequently are nonresponsive or poorly responsive and have hypotension, hypoglycemia, bradycardia, and hypothermia. Myxedema coma is considered a medical emergency, and appropriate supportive measures (treatment of possible sepsis and pneumonia, ventilation, and assessment and treatment of cardiac issues) are very important. No consensus exists about the most efficacious thyroid hormone replacement regimen to use for myxedema coma. Intravenous levothyroxine has traditionally been administered, with an initial bolus of 200 to 500 micrograms followed by daily doses between 50 and 100 micrograms until transition to oral administration is feasible. These relatively high doses of levothyroxine are recommended to replenish the depleted tissue stores of thyroid hormone. However, they may be associated with cardiac irregularities and should be used cautiously, especially in patients with known or suspected cardiac disorders (which this patient does not have).

Thyroid hormone replacement therapy by itself may not be sufficient treatment. Patients with secondary hypothyroidism may have a degree of hypopituitarism that can lead to secondary adrenal insufficiency. Patients with myxedema coma should be checked for possible adrenal insufficiency and treated with a stress-dose glucocorticoid, such as hydrocortisone, until adrenal insufficiency is excluded and appropriate adrenal function confirmed.

Supplementation with liothyronine (oral or intravenous) has been proposed but is controversial, especially because a definitive benefit of this therapy has not been shown. If liothyronine is used, it should be administered cautiously in lower doses and in combination with levothyroxine. All underlying precipitating conditions also must be addressed.

KEY POINT

- Intravenous levothyroxine and a glucocorticoid (such as hydrocortisone) is appropriate initial treatment of a patient in myxedema coma.

Bibliography

Kwaku MP, Burman KD. Myxedema coma. J Intensive Care Med. 2007;22(4):224-231. [PMID: 17712058]

Item 50   Answer: B
Educational Objective: Manage hyperprolactinemia.

A pituitary MRI should be performed in this patient to evaluate for a sellar mass. He has hypogonadotropic hypogonadism, which is the likely basis of his sexual dysfunction. His hyperprolactinemia is most likely contributing to the hypogonadism. Before treatment can begin, the cause of the hyperprolactinemia must be determined. This patient has no other disorders (such as hypothyroidism, liver disease, or kidney failure) and takes no medication that could result in hyperprolactinemia. Therefore, MRI is necessary to exclude either a prolactinoma or another sellar mass.

Cabergoline, a dopamine agonist, eventually may be necessary for management of the hyperprolactinemia. However, the cause of the hyperprolactinemia first must be determined.

A testicular ultrasound has no role in managing this patient's disorder. His hypogonadism is most likely due to a central cause (low testosterone and low gonadotropin levels), and he has no palpable mass on testicular examination.

Testosterone therapy would not be indicated in this patient because the cause of his secondary hypogonadism still must be elucidated. If the cause is a pituitary adenoma, then treatment with a dopamine agonist may be sufficient to reverse the hypogonadism.

KEY POINT

- In patients with hypogonadotropic hypogonadism and hyperprolactinemia not caused by another disorder or a medication, a pituitary MRI is appropriate to evaluate for a sellar mass.

Bibliography

Melmed S, Casanueva FF, Hoffman AR, et al; Endocrine Society. Diagnosis and treatment of hyperprolactinemia: an Endocrine Society clinical practice guideline. J Clin Endocrinol Metab. 2011;96(2):273-288. [PMID: 21296991]

Item 51   Answer: C
Educational Objective: Diagnose male hypogonadism.

Obtaining a morning serum total testosterone level is the most appropriate next diagnostic test. According to Endocrine Society guidelines, an initial morning measurement of a patient's total testosterone level should be performed in assessing for hypogonadism; if results are abnormal, a second confirmatory morning measurement should be obtained before testing for secondary causes is begun. This recommendation is based on numerous studies showing that variability in testosterone levels from day to day or diurnally is common, with morning total testosterone levels being the most accurate in indicating a patient's androgen status.

Iron studies to exclude hemochromatosis as a cause of central hypogonadism are not indicated in this patient because a diagnosis of hypogonadism has not been confirmed.

Many free testosterone assays are grossly inaccurate and thus are not currently recommended to diagnose hypogonadism unless the assay measures free testosterone by equilibrium dialysis. Additionally, this patient has no risk factors for altered sex hormone–binding globulin levels (obesity and older age), which would make a total testosterone level less reliable. Therefore, he has no need of a free testosterone assessment.

Testicular ultrasonography is not indicated for the diagnosis of hypogonadism. A testicular examination is adequate for assessing testicular volume.

KEY POINT

- In evaluating a male patient for hypogonadism, a morning measurement of the total testosterone level is the most appropriate initial step.

Bibliography

Bhasin S, Cunningham GR, Hayes FJ, et al; Task Force, Endocrine Society. Testosterone therapy in men with androgen deficiency syndromes: an Endocrine Society clinical practice guideline. J Clin Endocrinol Metab. 2010;95(6):2536-2559. [PMID: 20525905]

Item 52   Answer: D

Educational Objective: Diagnose subacute thyroiditis.

This patient should have a 24-hour radioactive iodine uptake (RAIU) test. She most likely has subacute thyroiditis, a form of destructive thyroiditis, given her neck discomfort, history of a transient possible viral infection 4 weeks ago, fever, elevated erythrocyte sedimentation rate (ESR), and biochemical findings (elevated serum free thyroxine [T_4] and triiodothyronine [T_3] levels and low serum thyroid-stimulating hormone level). The RAIU test measures thyroid gland iodine uptake over a timed period, usually 24 hours. In patients with destructive thyroiditis (or exposure to exogenous thyroid hormones), results of the RAIU test will be less than normal (<5% at 24 hours). In contrast to destructive thyroiditis, Graves disease will show an elevated (or sometimes normal) RAIU, which indicates endogenous excess synthesis and production of thyroid hormones.

Fine-needle aspiration biopsy can be useful in the evaluation of thyroid nodules, which this patient does not have.

Antithyroid agents, such as methimazole or propylthiouracil, have no role in the treatment of destructive thyroiditis because endogenous production of thyroid hormones is very low. Although many patients can be treated expectantly with only β-blocker therapy, prednisone is indicated in patients with significant hormone elevation or pain.

Measurement of the serum thyroglobulin level can help distinguish exogenous levothyroxine ingestion from subacute thyroiditis. However, this patient's history and laboratory findings (tender thyromegaly, fever, elevated ESR) are not compatible with exogenous levothyroxine use.

KEY POINT

- In patients with destructive thyroiditis, results of the 24-hour radioactive iodine uptake test will be less than normal (<5% at 24 hours).

Bibliography

Pearce EN, Farwell AP, Braverman LE. Thyroiditis [erratum in N Engl J Med. 2003;349(6):620]. N Engl J Med. 2003;348(26):2646-2655. [PMID: 12826640]

Item 53   Answer: A

Educational Objective: Manage hypoglycemia in a patient taking a sulfonylurea.

This patient should stop taking glyburide immediately. She has impaired kidney function and heart failure, both of which significantly impair her ability to clear glyburide and glyburide metabolites from her body. The biologic half-life of glyburide is thus prolonged. Because of this long half-life and the degree of this patient's kidney impairment (estimated glomerular filtration rate <50 mL/min/1.73 m^2), merely decreasing her glyburide dosage is insufficient to reliably decrease blood drug levels and prevent the return of hypoglycemia. A hemoglobin A_{1c} value of 6.2% is dangerously low in an older patient with diabetes mellitus and has most likely resulted in frequent episodes of hypoglycemia. These episodes, in turn, have caused her recent episodes of confusion and forgetfulness. Because it may take several days after discontinuation for the glyburide to decrease to undetectable levels, evaluating her plasma glucose level in two weeks would be appropriate as a next step in management.

Although glipizide is safer and has a shorter half-life than glyburide, it also accumulates in patients with chronic kidney disease. More importantly, no hypoglycemic agent (glipizide, metformin, or insulin) should be given to this patient until glyburide is completely cleared from her body, which would completely end the cycle of recurrent hypoglycemic episodes.

KEY POINT

- Sulfonylureas with long half-lives, such as glyburide, should not be used in older patients with type 2 diabetes mellitus and impaired kidney function or heart failure.

Bibliography

Greco D, Pisciotta M, Gambina F, Maggio F. Severe hypoglycaemia leading to hospital admission in type 2 diabetic patients aged 80 years or older. Exp Clin Endocrinol Diabetes. 2010;118(4):215-219. [PMID: 20072965]

Item 54   Answer: C

Educational Objective: Manage primary hyper-parathyroidism.

This patient should undergo a parathyroidectomy. She has hypercalcemia and a high-normal parathyroid hormone (PTH) level, a pattern consistent with primary hyperparathyroidism. Although the PTH level is not above the normal range, it is inappropriately high in light of her significant hypercalcemia. Although many patients with hyperparathyroidism may be appropriately observed closely or treated nonsurgically if they are asymptomatic, symptomatic hypercalcemia (for example, with nephrolithiasis and cardiac arrhythmias) is an indication for parathyroidectomy. Additional indications for surgery are a serum calcium level greater than 1.0 mg/dL (0.3 mmol/L) more than the normal range, a creatinine clearance less than 60 mL/min (0.06 L/min) (normal, 90-140 mL/min [0.09-0.14 L/min]), bone density T-scores less than −2.5 in any area, a previous fragility fracture, and age less than 50 years, regardless of symptoms.

This patient's primary indication for parathyroidectomy is the history of a fragility fracture (a fracture sustained in a fall from a standing height). Although her dual-energy x-ray absorptiometry scan does not show osteoporosis, the history of fragility fracture portends an elevated risk of future fracture. The goal of surgery will be to prevent additional bone loss, fragility fractures, or other possible complications of primary hyperparathyroidism.

Bisphosphonate therapy could be attempted if this patient refused surgery but is not as effective as surgery.

A bone scan might be helpful to evaluate for cancer with bony metastases but would not be useful in this patient with a benign parathyroid condition.

PTH-related protein (PTHrP) secretion is commonly associated with certain malignancies. However, measurement of the PTHrP level is unnecessary in this patient whose hypercalcemia is clearly caused by primary hyperparathyroidism and not by malignancy.

Repeating the serum calcium measurement in 1 year would be appropriate for a patient with primary hyperparathyroidism who did not have indications for surgery now.

KEY POINT

- In a patient with primary hyperparathyroidism and a history of a fragility fracture, parathyroidectomy is the most appropriate management.

Bibliography

Bilezikian JP, Khan AA, Potts JT Jr; Third International Workshop on the Management of Asymptomatic Primary Hyperthyroidism. Guidelines for the management of asymptomatic primary hyperparathyroidism: summary statement from the Third International Workshop. J Clin Endocrinol Metab. 2009;94(2):335-339. [PMID: 19193908]

Item 55   Answer: B

Educational Objective: Manage adrenal function during critical illness.

This patient should be treated with stress doses of hydrocortisone as the next step in management. His pneumonia was treated appropriately with intravenous fluids and antibiotics. However, despite optimal therapy, he continues to do poorly. Although his persistent illness could indicate progression into sepsis and septic shock, it is more likely that his poor response to therapy is the result of adrenal insufficiency. The repeated injections of triamcinolone most likely have suppressed his endogenous pituitary-adrenal axis and put him at increased risk for adrenal insufficiency. The timing of the symptoms is crucial in that they occurred 3 months after the last triamcinolone injection. Although the measured serum cortisol level is within the normal range, it is inappropriately low (even for a serum albumin level of 2.7 g/dL [27 g/L]) for the degree of stress (including hypotension) that he is experiencing. If the plasma adrenocorticotropic hormone (ACTH) level had been measured, it would have been inappropriately low or low-normal as a result of chronic suppression by previous glucocorticoid administration. This subnormal response to hypotension and stress is commonly observed in patients with central adrenal insufficiency.

The most appropriate management, therefore, is to treat this patient with stress doses of hydrocortisone. Glucocorticoid deficiency is associated with increased morbidity and mortality in critically ill patients. When the diagnosis is highly suspected, especially in the proper clinical setting (including previous exposure to glucocorticoids), treatment should be instituted immediately, even if the diagnosis cannot be firmly established in a timely manner.

In a stable patient, an ACTH stimulation test would be an appropriate study to assess for adrenal suppression caused by exogenous glucocorticoids. However, in a patient with likely adrenal insufficiency and vasomotor instability, immediate treatment is indicated before further study.

Although the patient is at risk for a hospital-acquired infection, possibly with a pseudomonal infection, even adequate antibiotic treatment may not be successful without treating his possible adrenal insufficiency.

Continued therapy with intravenous fluids and antibiotics is appropriate, although adding vasopressors without addressing his potential underlying adrenal suppression is not adequate therapy.

KEY POINT

- In a critically ill patient at high risk for adrenal insufficiency, the most appropriate management is treatment with stress doses of hydrocortisone.

Bibliography

Arafah BM. Hypothalamic pituitary adrenal function during critical illness: limitations of current assessment methods. J Clin Endocrinol Metab. 2006;91(10):3725-3745. [PMID: 16882746]

Item 56   Answer: D

Educational Objective: Interpret thyroid function studies in an older patient.

This patient should be monitored for evidence of hypothyroidism and should receive no pharmacologic therapy at present. In older persons with abnormal results on thyroid function testing, such as are seen in this patient, the tests should be repeated several times over a period of months to ensure the stability and accuracy of the results. The normal thyroid-stimulating hormone (TSH) range for most ambulatory outpatients is 0.5-5.0 microunits/mL (0.5-5.0 milliunits/L). However, the normal range is different during pregnancy and in patients older than 80 years. Several studies have shown that an elevated serum TSH level in older patients is not associated with detrimental medical outcomes (such as depressive symptoms and impaired cognitive function) but, in fact, is associated with a lower mortality rate. Although the precise numbers are somewhat controversial, the normal reference range most likely is approximately 1 to 7 microunits/mL (1-7 milliunits/L). It is now recognized that older patients generally should not be given levothyroxine solely for an elevated TSH level. A full consideration of the patient and the clinical context is necessary.

This patient is basically asymptomatic (except for mild fatigue) and in good health. His thyroid peroxidase antibody level and clinical examination findings are basically normal and thus support the concept that he does not require exogenous levothyroxine.

Most evidence to date has shown no clinical advantage of liothyronine over levothyroxine in patients requiring thyroid replacement therapy. Additionally, liothyronine and other triiodothyronine (T_3) preparations have a short half-life and have been associated with acute spikes in serum T_3 levels, which are of particular concern in older adult patients or patients with cardiac abnormalities.

A radioactive iodine test is not useful in establishing the diagnosis of hypothyroidism and thus is inappropriate in this patient.

KEY POINT

- Older patients generally should not be given levothyroxine solely for an elevated thyroid-stimulating hormone level.

Bibliography

Gussekloo J, van Exel E, de Craen AJ, Meinders AE, Frölich M, Westendorp RG. Thyroid status, disability and cognitive function, and survival in old age. JAMA. 2004;292(21):2591-2599. [PMID: 15572717]

Item 57   Answer: B

Educational Objective: Diagnose central hypothyroidism after pituitary irradiation.

This patient most likely has central hypothyroidism and should have her serum free thyroxine (T_4) level measured. Her hypopituitarism is a result of the radiation therapy she received as part of her treatment of a pituitary adenoma. Her symptoms are typical of hypothyroidism, and the signs and symptoms of central hypothyroidism are similar to those of primary hypothyroidism. However, the biochemical diagnosis of central hypothyroidism is established differently because patients may have either a low-normal to overtly low serum thyroid-stimulating hormone (TSH) level. Therefore, the diagnosis is made based on measurement of a low free T_4 level in association with both a low to low-normal TSH level and clinical symptoms suggestive of hypothyroidism. This patient's mild hyponatremia may be caused by her hypothyroidism and should improve with T_4 replacement. In a patient with central hypothyroidism who takes levothyroxine replacement therapy, the goal should be achievement of a normal free T_4 level because monitoring the TSH value is not useful.

Measuring this patient's morning serum cortisol level is inappropriate management because she is receiving glucocorticoid replacement therapy for adrenal insufficiency, which guarantees that the cortisol level will be low.

A random measurement of the serum growth hormone (GH) level is not useful in the assessment of GH deficiency. A serum insulin-like growth factor 1 level would be useful for assessing GH production.

Measurement of this patient's serum luteinizing hormone level will not be useful because the oral contraceptive agent she is taking will have lowered her gonadotropin levels.

KEY POINT

- The diagnosis of central hypothyroidism is made on the basis of the serum free thyroxine (T_4) level.

Bibliography

Darzy KH, Shalet SM. Hypopituitarism following radiotherapy. Pituitary. 2009;12(1):40-50. [PMID: 18270844]

Item 58   Answer: E

Educational Objective: Manage diabetic ketoacidosis.

This patient should first be admitted to the intensive care unit for administration of intravenous fluids and insulin for management of severe diabetic ketoacidosis (DKA) and subsequently have serial abdominal examinations. She has reduced her insulin intake for the past 2 days while she was not feeling well. The insulin requirement usually is increased while a patient is under the stress imposed by illness. Her serum bicarbonate level is now substantially less than 15 meq/L (15 mmol/L), and she has generalized abdominal pain in the absence of specific intra-abdominal findings on physical examination. These findings are common in DKA, with just under half of patients reporting abdominal pain. Serial abdominal examinations are necessary to determine if her abdominal symptoms improve as her ketoacidosis resolves.

Answers and Critiques

The severity of the abdominal pain is related to the degree of metabolic acidosis. In the absence of localized findings, imaging with CT or other invasive procedures, such as laparotomy or endoscopic retrograde cholangiopancreatography, should be considered only if the patient's abdominal pain does not resolve with correction of the acidosis.

DKA also often causes an elevated leukocyte count, an elevated amylase level, and a less-than-normal temperature, all of which this patient has. However, none of these findings reliably suggests infection, and no obvious source of infection is evident. Imipenem thus should not be started.

> ## KEY POINT
> - Diabetic ketoacidosis can cause generalized abdominal pain, leukocytosis, and hyperamylasemia.

Bibliography

Umpierrez G, Freire AX. Abdominal pain in patients with hyperglycemic crises. J Crit Care. 2002;17(1):63-67. [PMID: 12040551]

Item 59   Answer: D
Educational Objective: Manage secondary osteoporosis.

The most appropriate next step in management is to screen this 55-year-old man for celiac disease as part of the evaluation for secondary causes of his low bone mass and fracture. This patient has a history of fragility fracture (fracture sustained in a fall from a standing height), and his bone density results show osteopenia. In an otherwise healthy 55-year-old man, these findings raise concern for a secondary cause of his low bone mass and fragility fracture. Half of the men with osteoporosis will have an identifiable cause. Therefore, screening guided by history and physical examination findings may include testing for hypogonadism, vitamin D deficiency, primary hyperparathyroidism, calcium malabsorption, and multiple myeloma. Measurement of 24-hour urine calcium excretion while the patient consumes 1000 mg/d of calcium also may be useful. Low values for urine calcium may indicate calcium malabsorption, which can be seen in celiac disease. In light of this patient's low BMI, fragility fracture, and history of iron deficiency anemia, celiac disease is a concern, even if gastrointestinal symptoms are absent.

Initiation of alendronate or teriparatide can be considered after the evaluation for secondary causes is completed. These agents will be more effective once the secondary cause of low bone mass has been corrected.

Repeating the bone density test in 1 year without any intervention now would allow time for additional bone loss to occur and thus would not be the best management.

> ## KEY POINT
> - Low urine calcium excretion in a patient with a fragility fracture may indicate calcium malabsorption.

Bibliography

Bours SP, van Geel TA, Geusens PP, et al. Contributors to secondary osteoporosis and metabolic bone diseases in patients presenting with a clinical fracture. J Clin Endocrinol Metab. 2011;96(5):1360-1367. [PMID: 21411547]

Item 60   Answer: A
Educational Objective: Diagnose the cause of acute adrenal insufficiency.

This patient most likely has an adrenal hemorrhage. Acute adrenal insufficiency can result from hemorrhage (spontaneous, after trauma or anticoagulation), emboli (atrial fibrillation), and sepsis (particularly secondary to meningococcemia). Patients typically have abdominal, back, or flank pain; hypotension; fever; and nausea and vomiting. The diagnosis also is suggested by the laboratory findings of hyponatremia, hyperkalemia, and a low hematocrit. This patient developed flank pain, hypotension, nausea, fatigue, and dizziness 2 weeks after knee replacement surgery, and her physical examination and laboratory findings include orthostatic changes in her blood pressure and pulse, hyponatremia, hyperkalemia, and a low hematocrit. Of note, she has been receiving an anticoagulant since surgery, which most likely caused bleeding. After blood samples are drawn for measurement of cortisol and adrenocorticotropic hormone levels, she should be treated immediately for adrenal insufficiency with hydrocortisone and intravenous fluids. Abdominal CT and additional laboratory testing can be performed at a later stage, if necessary, to confirm the diagnosis.

Although gastrointestinal bleeding could explain the patient's hypotension, fatigue, and anemia, it does not explain the rest of her clinical and electrolyte findings.

Similarly, neither a narcotic overdose nor septic shock explains the sudden onset of flank pain, anemia, hyponatremia, and hyperkalemia.

> ## KEY POINT
> - A decreasing hematocrit, hypotension, hyponatremia, hyperkalemia, and acute onset of abdominal, back, or flank pain suggest adrenal insufficiency secondary to an adrenal hemorrhage.

Bibliography

Bornstein SR. Predisposing factors for adrenal insufficiency. N Engl J Med. 2009;360(22):2328-2339. [PMID: 19474430]

Item 61   Answer: C
Educational Objective: Diagnose hypothyroidism in a critically ill patient.

This patient most likely has hypothyroidism, which is strongly suggested by his exceedingly high serum thyroid-stimulating hormone (TSH) level and his low free thyroxine (T_4) and total triiodothyronine (T_3) levels. Additionally, he has been taking amiodarone, which causes hypothyroidism in approximately 10% of North Americans who take it chronically and hyperthyroidism in approximately 1%. Although the role that this patient's hypothyroidism is playing in his medical condition cannot be determined with certainty, judicious administration of exogenous levothyroxine may help his general metabolism, his ability to respond beneficially to corticosteroids, and his hypotension.

Adrenal insufficiency alone is an unlikely explanation for this patient's laboratory test results and clinical presentation. The patient's random serum cortisol level is not consistent with frank adrenal insufficiency, and his TSH level is elevated. Adrenal insufficiency is rare in critically ill patients but must be considered in those with septic shock, who may develop severe, protracted hypotension that is not responsive to standard therapy. Most of these patients have elevated serum total and free cortisol levels. A recent study showed that hydrocortisone therapy (300 mg/d) given to patients with septic shock did not influence mortality but resulted in a faster reversal of shock. Such therapy is not directed at treating an adrenal dysfunction, but rather at controlling the associated overwhelming inflammatory response.

Nonthyroidal illness can alter the results of thyroid function tests, an effect referred to as euthyroid sick syndrome, which is more common in critically ill patients. The mechanisms by which nonthyroidal illness cause thyroid function test abnormalities are unknown but could relate to the systemic release of multiple cytokines. However, the serum TSH level is not expected to increase to greater than 10 microunits/mL (10 milliunits/L) in a patient with nonthyroidal illness, except perhaps in the recovery phase of a serious illness. This patient is acutely and seriously ill, is not in the recovery phase of a serious illness, and has a TSH level of 16 microunits/mL (16 milliunits/L).

A TSH-secreting pituitary tumor is typically associated with inappropriately elevated serum free T_4 and total T_3 levels; this patient's levels are low.

KEY POINT

- Hypothyroidism is characterized by an elevated thyroid-stimulating hormone level in the setting of low triiodothyronine (T_3) and thyroxine (T_4) levels and is a common side effect of amiodarone therapy.

Bibliography
Adler SM, Wartofsky L. The nonthyroidal illness syndrome. Endocrinol Metab Clin North Am. 2007;36(3):657-672. [PMID: 17673123]

Item 62   Answer: D
Educational Objective: Diagnose hyperandrogenism in a patient with a neoplasm.

The most appropriate next diagnostic test is transvaginal ultrasonography to examine this patient's ovaries. Her history and physical examination findings are consistent with hyperandrogenism. Her total testosterone level is elevated, and her dehydroepiandrosterone sulfate (DHEAS) level is normal. In healthy women, the ovaries and adrenal glands contribute equally to testosterone production. However, a testosterone level greater than 200 ng/dL (6.9 nmol/L) in a woman with rapid onset of hyperandrogenic symptoms (increased hirsutism in a short period of time and clitoromegaly) suggests an ovarian neoplasm, which is best diagnosed with a transvaginal ultrasound.

Dehydroepiandrosterone is produced primarily in the adrenal glands and is sulfated in the adrenal glands, liver, and small intestine to become DHEAS. Levels greater than 7.0 micrograms/mL (18.9 micromoles/L) strongly suggest an adrenal source of androgens. In this patient, whose DHEAS level is only 2.9 micrograms/mL (7.8 micromoles/L), imaging of the adrenals would be the next step only if the transvaginal ultrasound showed no ovarian neoplasm.

A free testosterone measurement is not needed because this patient's history and physical examination findings do not suggest an abnormality in her sex hormone–binding globulin level that would make the total testosterone measurement suspect.

Because elevated androgen levels in women have either an ovarian or an adrenal source, a pituitary MRI would not be useful in this patient.

KEY POINT

- In a woman with rapid onset of hyperandrogenic symptoms, especially if her testosterone level is greater than 200 ng/dL (6.9 nmol/L), an ovarian neoplasm is likely and is best diagnosed with a transvaginal ultrasound.

Bibliography
Martin KA, Chang RJ, Ehrmann DA, et al. Evaluation and treatment of hirsutism in premenopausal women: an Endocrine Society clinical practice guideline. J Clin Endocrinol Metab. 2008;93(4):1105-1120. [PMID: 18252793]

Item 63   Answer: A
Educational Objective: Treat a hospitalized patient who has diabetes mellitus with basal insulin.

This patient should begin receiving insulin glargine (once daily) and insulin aspart (before each meal) after surgery. A patient with long-standing type 1 diabetes mellitus makes no endogenous insulin and needs a flexible insulin regimen that includes half his daily requirements as a basal insulin (such as insulin glargine) and the rest as boluses of rapid-acting insulin (such as insulin aspart) before meals.

CONT.

Neither intravenous nor subcutaneous insulin infusions are necessary in this patient, and both would likely require his transfer to the intensive care unit for safe administration.

Given his unpredictable levels of activity and eating while in the hospital, restoring the patient's previous outpatient dosage of premixed insulin is inappropriate.

A sliding scale that does not include basal insulin and does not begin insulin administration unless the blood glucose level is at or above 150 mg/dL (8.3 mmol/L) will cause wide swings from hyperglycemia to hypoglycemia and thus is inappropriate treatment for this patient.

KEY POINT

- **A sliding scale insulin regimen that includes no basal insulin is inappropriate for a hospitalized patient with diabetes mellitus.**

Bibliography

Queale WS, Seidler AJ, Brancati FL. Glycemic control and sliding scale insulin use in medical inpatients with diabetes mellitus. Arch Intern Med. 1997;157(5):545-552. [PMID: 9066459]

Item 64   Answer: A
Educational Objective: Treat a macroprolactinoma.

This patient has a macroprolactinoma, and administration of a dopamine agonist, such as cabergoline, is indicated as the initial treatment. Hyperprolactinemia can cause galactorrhea, oligomenorrhea, and amenorrhea in premenopausal women; erectile dysfunction in men; and decreased libido, infertility, and osteopenia in both sexes. Large tumors also may cause mass effects, which are often the presenting feature in men and postmenopausal women. This patient has amenorrhea and galactorrhea in the setting of a markedly elevated serum prolactin level. The MRI shows a pituitary mass greater than 1 cm that extends to the optic chiasm. These radiographic findings are consistent with a macroprolactinoma with chiasmal compression. The visual field examination indicates that the mass is not currently compressing the chiasm to the point of visual loss. Dopamine agonists normalize prolactin levels, correct amenorrhea and galactorrhea, and decrease tumor size by more than 50% in 80% to 90% of patients. They are used as first-line therapy, unless visual field loss is significant and progressive. Even with mild visual loss, dopamine agonists are usually used as first-line treatment. Cabergoline is generally more efficacious and better tolerated, although more expensive, than bromocriptine.

An oral contraceptive agent will replace gonadal corticosteroids and lead to menstruation but will not reduce tumor size. Simple replacement of estrogen with oral contraceptives is inappropriate therapy in this patient but may be preferable treatment in women with idiopathic hyperprolactinemia or microprolactinomas who do not desire fertility but are estrogen deficient. Because

prolactinomas have estrogen receptors, tumor growth resulting from estrogen replacement therapy is possible. However, with the dosages routinely used in oral contraceptives, this growth is very uncommon.

Surgery is appropriate only in patients with resistance or intolerance to dopamine agonists, with a primarily cystic tumor, or with acute and unstable deterioration of vision. Radiation therapy, including stereotactic radiosurgery, is used even less commonly for prolactinomas but is indicated for macroprolactinomas that do not respond to either medical or surgical treatment.

KEY POINT

- **In a patient with a macroprolactinoma, administration of a dopamine agonist, such as cabergoline, is indicated as the initial treatment.**

Bibliography

Melmed S, Casanueva FF, Hoffman AR, et al; Endocrine Society. Diagnosis and treatment of hyperprolactinemia: an Endocrine Society clinical practice guideline. J Clin Endocrinol Metab. 2011;96(2):273-288. [PMID: 21296991]

Item 65   Answer: B
Educational Objective: Treat profound hypoglycemia in an older patient.

This patient with probable hypoglycemia should have a fingerstick measurement of her blood glucose level. Older patients who take sulfonylureas with long half-lives can have high drug levels in their blood because of decreased clearance, which results in profound and prolonged hypoglycemia. Hypoglycemia should be suspected in any patient with diabetes who has focal neurologic signs and is sweating. The fact that her average hemoglobin A_{1c} level is well below 7.0% further indicates an increased risk for hypoglycemia. Additionally, the patient has not been eating and drinking adequately since her amputation, which also can contribute to the development of hypoglycemia. Hypoglycemia can cause various neurologic findings, including coma and hemiplegia. The most immediate step is to measure her blood glucose level and, if hypoglycemia is present, treat her with glucose to prevent permanent neurologic disability.

This patient has a slight fever but not enough evidence of septicemia to justify starting empiric antibiotic therapy with vancomycin and ceftriaxone. Additionally, septicemia is unlikely to be the cause of a left hemiplegia.

If the patient does not have hypoglycemia, alternative diagnoses can be considered, including stroke. In patients with stroke, a noncontrast head CT to exclude intracerebral hemorrhage is necessary before the administration of thrombolytic drugs, such as recombinant tissue plasminogen activator. However, hypoglycemia should first be excluded as a diagnosis before a head CT or thrombolytic administration.

- Older patients who take sulfonylureas with long half-lives can develop profound hypoglycemia, which can be reversed by an infusion of glucose.

Bibliography

Chiniwala N, Jabbour S. Management of diabetes mellitus in the elderly. Curr Opin Endocrinol Diabetes Obes. 2011;18(2):148-152. [PMID: 21522002]

Item 66   Answer: D

Educational Objective: Treat a multinodular goiter.

This patient should undergo thyroidectomy. In iodine-sufficient areas of the world, multinodular goiter is an idiopathic condition characterized by both solid and partially cystic thyroid nodules that is more common in older persons. Over time, the goiter generally grows and may require treatment. Fine-needle aspiration biopsy is used to exclude cancer in this generally benign condition and has excluded it in this patient. However, goiter growth can lead to impingement of the goiter on the trachea, esophagus, or recurrent laryngeal nerve and result in dyspnea, stridor, chronic cough, a sensation of fullness or pressure, dysphagia, or hoarseness. Hyperthyroidism also may develop if one (or more) of the nodules becomes autonomous and large enough to produce sufficient thyroid hormone to suppress thyroid-stimulating hormone (TSH) and render the patient thyrotoxic. This patient's recent symptoms are most likely due to impingement. Therefore, thyroid surgery is indicated because the local compressive symptoms are prominent and clinically significant.

No evidence of the effectiveness of external-beam radiation therapy for benign thyroid disease has been shown, which makes the therapy inappropriate in this patient.

Levothyroxine will further suppress the TSH level and may render the patient thyrotoxic. The previous practice of giving patients levothyroxine to shrink thyroid nodules has been abandoned because of its inefficacy and the morbidities associated with iatrogenic thyrotoxicosis.

Methimazole is a thioamide drug used to treat hyperthyroidism. Although this patient has a low-normal TSH level, she is not frankly thyrotoxic. Therefore, treating her with an antithyroid medication is unnecessary and will have no effect on goiter size.

In select circumstances, radioactive iodine (^{131}I) can be used to modestly decrease the size of a multinodular goiter but is not a first-line option in the United States, except in patients with thyrotoxicosis due to autonomous function. In a patient with a suppressed TSH level, this therapy will preferentially address the hyperfunctioning areas and spare those regions not visualized on imaging. As a result, the ultimate effect on goiter size may be unpredictable.

- In patients with impingement of a multinodular goiter on the trachea, esophagus, or recurrent laryngeal nerve, a thyroidectomy is indicated if local compressive symptoms are prominent and clinically significant.

Bibliography

Bahn RS, Castro MR. Approach to the patient with nontoxic multinodular goiter. J Clin Endocrinol Metab. 2011;96(5):1202-1212. [PMID: 21543434]

Item 67   Answer: A

Educational Objective: Treat painful diabetic neuropathy.

This patient should be treated with desipramine. He is experiencing an acute episode of painful diabetic neuropathy that developed after a period of poor glycemic control. This disorder involves acute segmental demyelination in the peripheral sensory nerves. Remyelination and recovery can occur if excellent glycemic control (hemoglobin A_{1c} level <7.0%) is established and maintained for several months. Relief of symptoms often is obtained by administering a low-dose tricyclic antidepressant, such as desipramine; topical application of capsaicin cream is also appropriate.

Fluoxetine and other selective serotonin reuptake inhibitors are ineffective for treating painful diabetic neuropathy and should not be used in this patient.

Nerve conduction studies might show marked slowing of nerve conduction, and a sural nerve biopsy would confirm the presence of segmental demyelination. These diagnostic tests, however, are unnecessary in a patient in whom the diagnosis of acute painful diabetic neuropathy is so likely, given his compatible history and physical examination findings.

Starting a potentially addictive and dangerous drug (such as oxycodone), especially when used for prolonged periods, is inappropriate therapy for a condition that may well be self-limiting.

- Symptoms of painful diabetic neuropathy can be treated with a low-dose tricyclic antidepressant and topical application of capsaicin cream.

Bibliography

Hovaguimian A, Gibbons CH. Clinical approach to the treatment of painful diabetic neuropathy. Ther Adv Endocrinol Metab. 2011;2(1):27-38. [PMID: 21709806]

Item 68   Answer: D

Educational Objective: Diagnose thyroid lymphoma.

This patient most likely has primary thyroid lymphoma. A benign goiter would not grow this rapidly and is unlikely to be associated with local symptoms. Thyroid lymphoma occurs most frequently in older patients who have a history of Hashimoto thyroiditis. Primary thyroid lymphoma typically presents as an enlarging neck mass, often with evidence of local compression of adjacent structures (such as dysphagia, hoarseness, stridor, jugular vein distention, and facial edema) and systemic symptoms ("B" symptoms) of lymphoma (such as fever, weight loss, and night sweats). A thyroid fine-needle aspiration (FNA) biopsy can suggest the diagnosis, but a core-needle or excisional biopsy is often needed to establish the diagnosis of lymphoma. Most primary thyroid lymphomas are mucosa-associated lymphoid tumors and respond to systemic chemotherapy. This patient's distended bilateral cervical neck veins suggest obstruction at the level of the thoracic inlet (that is, the thyroid gland).

Bleeding into the thyroid gland is unlikely because the gland is firm on physical examination, without any evidence of fluctuance, and the thyroid ultrasound shows heterogeneous echotexture rather than a cystic mass. Additionally, the patient has Hashimoto thyroiditis (which can predispose to lymphoma), has no history of neck trauma, and was not taking an anticoagulant medication.

With medullary and papillary thyroid cancers, the thyroid gland most likely would contain specific thyroid nodules. These cancers generally grow relatively slowly.

KEY POINT

- **Thyroid lymphoma occurs most frequently in older patients with a history of Hashimoto thyroiditis and typically presents as an enlarging neck mass, often with local and systemic symptoms.**

Bibliography

Graff-Baker A, Sosa JA, Roman SA. Primary thyroid lymphoma: a review of recent developments in diagnosis and histology-driven treatment. Curr Opin Oncol. 2010;22(1):17-22. [PMID: 19844180]

Item 69   Answer: B

Educational Objective: Manage hypopituitarism associated with Sheehan syndrome.

This patient should receive hydrocortisone as initial treatment. Given her low morning serum cortisol level, this patient has adrenal insufficiency, which makes immediate glucocorticoid therapy with hydrocortisone the most appropriate treatment. Her history and biochemical findings are consistent with hypopituitarism due to Sheehan syndrome, which involves pituitary infarction or hemorrhage in the setting of a complicated delivery, particularly one associated with significant blood loss and hypotension. The patient has no history suggestive of a preexisting pituitary lesion, so the pituitary insult most likely occurred at delivery. Nevertheless, pituitary imaging is appropriate to assess for a sellar mass. The cardinal signs of hypopituitarism

due to Sheehan syndrome are subacute, progressive hypopituitarism; an inability to lactate because of prolactin deficiency; and amenorrhea. Central adrenal insufficiency is the primary cause of mortality in Sheehan syndrome.

Although loss of anterior pituitary hormones is common, the development of diabetes insipidus is rare in Sheehan syndrome. Additionally, the patient's clinical and laboratory findings are not consistent with this diagnosis. Therefore, arginine vasopressin replacement therapy is not indicated.

The hyponatremia in this patient is likely related to the hypopituitarism, and the serum sodium level should normalize with pituitary hormone replacement. The hyponatremia is not severe enough or sufficiently symptomatic to warrant aggressive management with hypertonic saline.

This patient could have central hypothyroidism. If her serum free thyroxine level is low, despite her normal serum thyroid-stimulating hormone level, levothyroxine should be administered. However, thyroid hormone replacement is not urgent because she does not have signs of severe hypothyroidism. Therefore, the diagnosis and management of central hypothyroidism should wait until after her adrenal insufficiency is treated with glucocorticoid replacement therapy.

KEY POINT

- **Patients with Sheehan syndrome and adrenal insufficiency should receive immediate glucocorticoid therapy because central adrenal insufficiency is the primary cause of mortality in Sheehan syndrome.**

Bibliography

Kristjansdottir HL, Bodvarsdottir SP, Sigurjonsdottir HA. Sheehan's syndrome in modern times: a nationwide retrospective study in Iceland. Eur J Endocrinol. 2011;164(3):349-354. [PMID: 21183555]

Item 70   Answer: D

Educational Objective: Manage fasting hypoglycemia in a patient without diabetes mellitus.

This patient should undergo a psychiatric evaluation. In a person without diabetes mellitus who has laboratory-documented hypoglycemia, the finding of an inappropriately high serum insulin level and a suppressed serum C-peptide level suggests that the hypoglycemia is due to an exogenous injection of insulin. Some patients with psychiatric issues (such as a history of depression) engage in the use of hypoglycemic agents prescribed to others, frequently as an attention-seeking behavior. Given her mother's diabetic treatment, she has ready access to both insulin and an oral hypoglycemic agent, and her negative sulfonylurea screen indicates that glyburide is not the causative agent. A psychiatric evaluation is critical in establishing a diagnosis and developing a treatment plan to address her dangerous behavior.

Although abdominal CT is an effective means of detecting the presence of an insulinoma, her laboratory study results are inconsistent with endogenous insulin secretion from an insulinoma. If she had an insulinoma, both serum insulin and C-peptide levels would be inappropriately high in the presence of hypoglycemia.

An octreotide scan may be helpful in detecting and localizing primary and metastatic neuroendocrine tumors. Octreotide scanning is particularly useful in diagnosing specific tumors of neural crest origin, particularly neoplasms that express increased levels of somatostatin receptors, such as carcinoid tumors. This study may also have a role in localizing insulin-secreting tumors that are not visible on usual studies (MRIs or CT scans). However, in this patient with a low suspicion for insulinoma, an octreotide scan would not be an appropriate initial study.

Altered gastric emptying, particularly in persons with surgical changes in the stomach and proximal small bowel (as occur with some forms of bariatric surgery), may cause clinical symptoms consistent with relative hypoglycemia (late dumping syndrome). However, this is rarely associated with clinically significant hypoglycemia in an otherwise healthy person. Without a history of altered gastrointestinal anatomy or an underlying disease that might lead to abnormal gastric function (such as diabetes), a gastric emptying study is not indicated.

KEY POINT

- In a person without diabetes mellitus who has laboratory-documented hypoglycemia, the finding of an inappropriately high serum insulin level and a suppressed C-peptide level suggests that the hypoglycemia is due to an exogenous injection of insulin.

Bibliography

Cryer PE, Axelrod L, Grossman AB, et al; Endocrine Society. Evaluation and management of adult hypoglycemic disorders: an Endocrine Society clinical practice guideline. J Clin Endocrinol Metab. 2009;94(3):709-728. [PMID: 19088155]

Item 71   Answer: C

Educational Objective: Manage an asymptomatic incidental adrenal mass.

This patient should have repeat testing in 6 to 12 months. She has an incidentally discovered 2.5-cm adrenal mass with no clinical or biochemical features indicating excess hormonal secretion of glucocorticoids, mineralocorticoids, or adrenal androgens by the adrenal cortex or of catecholamines by the medulla. Neither the size (<4 cm) nor the imaging characteristics (an attenuation <20 Hounsfield units) of this adrenal mass suggest possible malignancy. Therefore, observation and repeat testing in 6 to 12 months would be the most appropriate management.

Incidentally discovered adrenal masses are a common finding on imaging obtained for other purposes. Routine evaluation is assessment of possible malignancy based on the size of the lesion and other radiographic findings (including shape, homogeneity, attenuation, and contrast washout) and of possible biochemical function. Clinical evidence of a possible functional lesion should be sought, including evidence of hypertension, electrolyte abnormalities, or glucocorticoid excess. In the early stages of their disease, some patients with pheochromocytoma or Cushing syndrome may have no obvious clinical manifestations. Thus, all patients with incidental adrenal masses should be screened for those two entities, and those who also have hypertension should be screened for hyperaldosteronism. Pheochromocytoma usually is evaluated with a 24-hour urine collection of catecholamines and Cushing syndrome with a low-dose dexamethasone suppression test. Screening for hyperaldosteronism involves determining the ratio of serum aldosterone to plasma renin activity.

Because this patient is not hypertensive and has no clinical or biochemical evidence of excess catecholamine secretion, a pheochromocytoma is unlikely. Therefore, a metaiodobenzylguanidine(MIBG) scan is neither warranted nor necessary.

Similarly, obtaining an MRI in this patient who already had a CT scan would offer no additional diagnostic information and thus would be unwarranted.

This asymptomatic patient who has a nonfunctioning 2.5-cm adrenal mass with unremarkable imaging characteristics also has no indications for surgical intervention.

KEY POINT

- Incidentally discovered adrenal masses that are small, are associated with no clinical or biochemical features suggestive of excess hormonal secretion, and have no imaging features suggestive of possible malignancy should be followed with observation and repeat testing in 6 to 12 months.

Bibliography

Nieman LK. Approach to the patient with an adrenal incidentaloma. J Clin Endocrinol Metab. 2010;95(9):4106-4113. [PMID: 20823463]

Item 72   Answer: D

Educational Objective: Diagnose thyroid storm.

This patient most likely is experiencing thyroid storm, which is an exaggerated state of thyrotoxicosis. Although some overlap exists, thyroid storm can be differentiated from other forms of thyrotoxicosis by the presence of temperature elevation, significant tachycardia, heart failure, abdominal discomfort, diarrhea, nausea, vomiting, and (sometimes) jaundice. Neurologically, agitation and disorientation can occur. Serum free thyroxine (T_4) and serum triiodothyronine (T_3) levels are elevated in both thyrotoxicosis and thyroid storm, but generally more so in thyroid storm. Thyroid storm most commonly occurs in patients who have untreated hyperthyroidism or are not adherent to their treatment regimen for the disorder but may be precipitated by surgery, trauma, or administration of radiocontrast agents with significant amounts of iodine. Treatment typically consists of a combination of antithyroid drugs (propylthiouracil or methimazole), iodine solution, high-dose corticosteroids, β-blockers, and (rarely) lithium. Even with aggressive therapy and supportive measures, mortality rates are as high as 15% to 20%.

Euthyroid sick syndrome does not cause these symptoms and signs of hyperthyroidism or these elevations in free T$_4$ and total T$_3$ levels. Furthermore, this patient's history of Graves disease makes euthyroid sick syndrome an unlikely diagnosis.

Myxedema coma is another life-threatening thyroid emergency characterized by the combination of mental status changes, hypothermia, hypoventilation, and hyponatremia in a patient whose clinical picture is consistent with hypothyroidism. This patient's T$_3$ and T$_4$ levels are markedly elevated, which excludes the diagnosis of hypothyroidism, and he is hyperthermic, not hypothermic.

Subacute (de Quervain) thyroiditis entails transient destruction of thyroid tissue, which leads to disruption of follicles and release of preformed thyroid hormone into the circulation that may initially cause hyperthyroidism and eventually may result in hypothyroidism. Subacute thyroiditis is thought to occur after a viral infection and usually involves thyroid tenderness, which this patient does not have. In addition, this patient is critically ill from his hyperthyroidism, which is unusual in subacute thyroiditis.

KEY POINT

- **Thyroid storm can be differentiated from other forms of thyrotoxicosis by the presence of temperature elevation, significant tachycardia, heart failure, abdominal discomfort, diarrhea, nausea, vomiting, and (sometimes) jaundice.**

Bibliography

Nayak B, Burman K. Thyrotoxicosis and thyroid storm. Endocrinol Metab Clin North Am. 2006;35(4):663-686. [PMID: 17127140]

Item 73   Answer: A

Educational Objective: Counsel a woman about the risks of gestational diabetes mellitus.

This patient's infant has an increased risk of childhood obesity. Gestational diabetes mellitus is hyperglycemia occurring during pregnancy and is typically identified in the second trimester. This disorder represents the inability of a woman's beta cells to adequately compensate for the degree of insulin resistance associated with various placenta-derived factors. The diagnosis of gestational diabetes is usually made on the basis of an oral glucose tolerance test, although no consensus exists at this time on the diagnostic thresholds. It has been recently recognized that the

offspring of mothers who have prepregnancy obesity and develop gestational diabetes during pregnancy are at increased risk for childhood obesity. The reason for this is not clear but may involve a combination of genetic factors and maternal imprinting of genes during intrauterine life.

Women with gestational diabetes are likely to develop the disorder during future pregnancies and are at increased risk for type 2 diabetes later in life, with some estimates placing the risk of the latter as high as 50% over 10 years.

Several genetic syndromes that are collectively known as maturity-onset diabetes of the young (MODY) develop early in life (teens to early 20s). The pattern of inheritance is autosomal dominant. Several described subtypes of MODY are associated with specific genetic defects in enzymes or transcription factors affecting beta-cell function but not with gestational diabetes.

Type 1 diabetes mellitus mainly affects lean children, teenagers, and young adults. The disorder is characterized by absolute insulin deficiency from selective autoimmune destruction of insulin-secreting pancreatic beta cells. In type 1A diabetes, one or more autoantibodies directed against the beta cells or their products (such as anti–glutamic acid decarboxylase, anti–islet cell autoantigen 512, and anti-insulin antibodies) usually can be detected. Type 1B diabetes is idiopathic, has no autoimmune markers, and occurs more commonly in persons of Asian or African descent. Neither type 1A nor type 1B diabetes is associated with gestational diabetes.

KEY POINT

- **The offspring of mothers with prepregnancy obesity and gestational diabetes mellitus are at increased risk for childhood obesity.**

Bibliography

Landon MB, Gabbe SG. Gestational diabetes mellitus. Obstet Gynecol. 2011;118(6):1379-1393. [PMID: 22105269]

Item 74   Answer: C

Educational Objective: Diagnose acromegaly.

This patient's historical and clinical findings suggest a diagnosis of acromegaly, and this diagnosis should be confirmed by measurement of the serum insulin-like growth factor 1 (IGF-1) level. Acromegaly is due to hypersecretion of growth hormone (GH) and is most commonly caused by a pituitary adenoma. High GH levels stimulate the liver to produce excess IGF-1, and both GH and IGF-1 circulate in the blood, causing the systemic effects of acromegaly. IGF-1 is an integrated measure of GH secretion, and thus measuring the serum IGF-1 level is the single best test for making the diagnosis of acromegaly. A normal serum IGF-1 level rules out acromegaly.

An MRI can show a pituitary adenoma but cannot diagnose acromegaly. After the diagnosis has been established, however, an MRI is necessary to determine the size and location of the pituitary adenoma.

GH is usually secreted episodically in pulses. Therefore, a single random measurement of the serum GH level is not useful in diagnosing acromegaly. GH hypersecretion is autonomous in acromegaly, and GH levels are not suppressible by hyperglycemia, as they normally would be. An oral glucose tolerance test also can be useful in establishing a diagnosis in a patient in whom the diagnosis of acromegaly is not clear.

Although prolactin often is cosecreted by GH-producing tumors, measuring the serum prolactin level is not useful in making the diagnosis of acromegaly because it is neither sensitive nor specific for the disease.

> **KEY POINT**
> - Insulin-like growth factor 1 (IGF-1) is an integrated measure of growth hormone secretion, and thus measuring the serum IGF-1 level is the single best test for making the diagnosis of acromegaly.

Bibliography

Katznelson L, Atkinson JL, Cook DM, Ezzat SZ, Hamrahian AH, Miller KK; American Association of Clinical Endocrinologists. American Association of Clinical Endocrinologists medical guidelines for clinical practice for the diagnosis and treatment of acromegaly—2011 update. Endocr Pract. 2011;17(Suppl 4):1-44. [PMID: 21846616]

Item 75   Answer: C

Educational Objective: Manage hypocalcemia in a malnourished patient with alcoholism.

This patient should next have his serum magnesium level measured. He has a history of chronic alcohol abuse and serum chemistry results that are notable for hypocalcemia. Evidence of tetany and a corrected QT interval prolongation are indications for aggressive intravenous repletion of calcium. In this patient with alcohol abuse and symptomatic hypocalcemia, hypomagnesemia should be suspected. Hypomagnesemia in the setting of severe hypocalcemia should be treated promptly with intravenous magnesium to help increase serum calcium levels and prevent ventricular arrhythmias. In addition, hypomagnesemia can impair the ability to increase serum calcium levels because low levels of magnesium inhibit parathyroid hormone (PTH) secretion and induce resistance to PTH. Therefore, in addition to increasing the patient's serum calcium level, treatment of his hypomagnesemia is essential to restore normal parathyroid function.

Measurement of the serum calcitonin level is typically not helpful in the assessment of hypocalcemia because calcitonin plays only a minor role in calcium homeostasis in humans.

This patient most likely is vitamin D deficient because of poor nutrition associated with his alcohol abuse.

Measurement of the serum 1,25-dihydroxyvitamin D level is unlikely to provide useful information regarding the exact cause of his hypocalcemia, and, in any case, measurement of the serum 25-hydroxyvitamin D level would be the more appropriate test.

The serum PTH level most likely would be inappropriately low in this patient as a result of his chronic alcohol abuse and hypocalcemia. Measuring this level is thus unnecessary.

> **KEY POINT**
> - Hypomagnesemia in the setting of severe hypocalcemia should be treated promptly with intravenous magnesium to help increase serum calcium levels and prevent ventricular arrhythmias.

Bibliography

Iwasaki Y, Asai M, Yoshida M, Oiso Y, Hashimoto K. Impaired parathyroid hormone response to hypocalcemic stimuli in a patient with hypomagnesemic hypocalcemia. J Endocrinol Invest. 2007;30(6):513-516. [PMID: 17646727]

Item 76   Answer: C

Educational Objective: Diagnose postexercise hyperglycemia.

This patient's significantly increased blood glucose level after running most likely results from baseline hypoinsulinemia exacerbated by the physiologic changes associated with prolonged exercise, such as stimulation of hepatic glucose release. A patient who has had type 1 diabetes mellitus for more than 20 years, including one episode of diabetic ketoacidosis, will be completely insulin deficient. Although long-acting, the treatment effect of insulin detemir does not always last a full 24 hours. The fact that his blood glucose level was 215 mg/dL (11.9 mmol/L) at bedtime the night before his run and was even higher the next morning before exercise suggests that he had low levels of insulin present in his system during the night and before starting his run. This hypoinsulinemia most likely triggered increased hepatic gluconeogenesis. In the absence of sufficient plasma insulin, the glucose could not be absorbed by the muscles and other tissues, and his blood glucose level continued to increase. Appropriate treatment is to adjust his insulin regimen to ensure adequate insulin replacement before running to minimize the expected physiologic changes associated with exercise.

Excess carbohydrate intake in the evening would likely contribute to his noted elevated bedtime and pre-exercise blood-glucose levels but would not independently account for the significant rise in his blood glucose level after exercise.

Although this patient may have some degree of gastroparesis given the duration of his diabetes, this disorder is an unlikely explanation for an increased blood glucose level 12 hours or more since he last ate.

Early morning blood glucose elevations may occur in response to the nocturnal hypoglycemia associated with diabetes therapy. Although this patient had an elevated morning blood glucose level before running, his bedtime measurement also was elevated, and he took no additional insulin beyond his single dose of long-acting insulin the morning before. Therefore, nocturnal hypoglycemia is unlikely to be the cause of this patient's exercise-associated hypoglycemia.

KEY POINT

- **Hypoinsulinemia causes increased hepatic glucose output and decreased peripheral glucose uptake, which results in a higher blood glucose level and, ultimately, a higher hemoglobin A_{1c} value; prolonged exercise, which further stimulates hepatic glucose release, exacerbates this condition.**

Bibliography

Temple MY, Bar-Or O, Riddell MC. The reliability and repeatability of the blood glucose response to prolonged exercise in adolescent boys with IDDM. Diabetes Care. 1995;18(3):326-332. [PMID: 7555475]

Item 77   Answer: A
Educational Objective: Diagnose the cause of primary ovarian insufficiency.

Obtaining a karyotype is the most appropriate next diagnostic test because this patient has primary ovarian insufficiency, and Turner syndrome must be excluded as the cause. Primary ovarian insufficiency can be diagnosed because she has two elevated follicle-stimulating hormone (FSH) levels in the setting of amenorrhea. If evidence of Turner syndrome is found, the associated estrogen deficiency must be treated. Turner syndrome is associated with several cardiovascular malformations, including aortic valve disease, aortic dilation, and aortic coarctation; renal malformations, most commonly horseshoe kidney; and autoimmune disorders, such as thyroid disease. Therefore, cardiac imaging and kidney ultrasonography often are recommended for patients with Turner syndrome. Patients with Turner syndrome with mosaicism may have several years of normal menses before entering menopause. Turner syndrome can be associated with a short stature, stocky build, square chest, and webbed neck. This patient's short stature is the only physical examination finding consistent with Turner syndrome.

Pelvic ultrasonography is unlikely to be useful in this patient. The elevated FSH level indicates that the amenorrhea is due to decreased estradiol production from the ovaries.

A progesterone challenge test is useful when trying to determine whether a patient is in a normal or low estrogen state. Laboratory studies and clinical symptoms already have shown that this patient is in a low estrogen state, and a progesterone challenge test would not provide any additional information.

Measuring this patient's serum estradiol level will not add any additional information because the elevated FSH level indicates a low estrogen state.

KEY POINT

- **In a woman with primary ovarian insufficiency, Turner syndrome must be excluded as the cause by obtaining the patient's karyotype.**

Bibliography

Nelson LM. Clinical practice. Primary ovarian insufficiency. N Engl J Med. 2009;360(6):606-614. [PMID: 19196677]

Item 78   Answer: B
Educational Objective: Treat hyperthyroidism in pregnancy.

This patient should receive propylthiouracil. The symptoms, clinical findings, and presence of vitiligo suggest that she has autoimmune Graves hyperthyroidism and not gestational thyrotoxicosis. The hyperthyroidism is more severe in Graves hyperthyroidism than in gestational thyrotoxicosis and often is associated with a significantly enlarged thyroid gland, as in this patient. Although evidence of ophthalmopathy is lacking, this finding is not uncommon in Graves hyperthyroidism. Her thyroid-stimulating antibody and thyroid peroxidase antibody levels also are elevated, albeit minimally, which is consistent with this diagnosis.

Although mild hyperthyroidism in pregnancy may not require treatment, this patient has significant signs and symptoms and moderately elevated thyroid function test results. Untreated hyperthyroidism is associated with an increased risk of miscarriage, fetal growth retardation, premature delivery, and preeclampsia. The presence of maternal thyroid-stimulating antibodies also places the fetus at increased risk for neonatal hyperthyroidism, which can be life threatening. The most appropriate treatment is an antithyroid drug. A recent consensus conference suggested that propylthiouracil should be used in the first trimester of pregnancy in patients with Graves hyperthyroidism who require treatment and that methimazole be substituted in the second and third trimesters.

Methimazole is associated with an increased risk of fetal abnormalities, such as aplasia cutis and choanal atresia, when used in the first trimester. After fetal organogenesis is complete, methimazole should be used. Methimazole is the antithyroid agent of choice except in the first trimester of pregnancy, in the presence of an allergy to methimazole, or in some cases of thyroid storm. Propylthiouracil is associated with a higher risk of severe hepatotoxicity than methimazole. Close monitoring of pregnant women treated with antithyroid agents is required, as is periodic fetal thyroid ultrasonography.

Thyroidectomy is indicated in patients with a toxic adenoma, a toxic multinodular goiter, or a large malignant thyroid nodule but is not warranted in this patient with Graves hyperthyroidism.

Because of the already cited risks of untreated hyperthyroidism in pregnancy, reassurance is inadequate as initial treatment for this patient.

Bibliography

Bahn Chair RS, Burch HB, Cooper DS, et al; American Thyroid Association; American Association of Clinical Endocrinologists. Hyperthyroidism and other causes of thyrotoxicosis: management guidelines of the American Thyroid Association and American Association of Clinical Endocrinologists [erratum in Thyroid. 2011;21(10):1169]. Thyroid. 2011;21(6):593-646. [PMID: 21510801]

Item 79   Answer: C
Educational Objective: Manage delayed hypoglycemia in a patient with type 1 diabetes mellitus.

This patient should eat complex carbohydrates (at least 45 grams) at bedtime on evenings of vigorous exercise. He developed severe hypoglycemia several hours after playing basketball for 3 hours, drinking, and not eating before bedtime. Vigorous exercise depletes the muscles' glycogen stores. Although his blood glucose level was 163 mg/dL (9.0 mmol/L) just before he went to bed, his muscles continued to extract glucose from the blood for several hours to replenish their glycogen stores. The alcohol in his system inhibited the liver's ability to release glucose into the blood, and thus his plasma glucose level decreased severely while he was asleep. A substantial snack containing complex carbohydrates before bedtime would have been absorbed over several hours and thereby prevented hypoglycemia.

It is neither reasonable nor necessary to advise a fit young man with diabetes to avoid exercising in the evening.

Even light beer contains enough alcohol to inhibit hepatic glucose output. If he is willing to make the change, he should be advised to drink no alcohol on evenings of vigorous exercise.

Although omitting the insulin aspart dose might be reasonable, stopping both forms of insulin would be a poor choice. Doing so would cause his plasma glucose level to increase because of hypoinsulinemia. His plasma glucose level most likely would be extremely high by bedtime and even higher the following morning.

Bibliography

Cryer PE. The barrier of hypoglycemia in diabetes. Diabetes. 2008;57(12):3169-3176. [PMID: 19033403]

Item 80   Answer: A
Educational Objective: Treat hypopituitarism.

Glucocorticoid therapy should be started in this patient to prevent progressive adrenal insufficiency. He has hypopituitarism, given the findings of testosterone deficiency and central hypothyroidism (low serum free thyroxine and inappropriately normal serum thyroid-stimulating hormone levels). The MRI shows a suprasellar mass. Neoplastic lesions, particularly pituitary adenomas, cause hypopituitarism by direct compression of the normal pituitary gland or by disruption of the pituitary stalk. Surgery is the primary mode of therapy for tumors that warrant intervention. This patient's serum cortisol value is low normal, which suggests tenuous adrenal reserve. After thyroid hormone replacement therapy is initiated, accelerated metabolism of endogenous cortisol occurs, with induction of progressive central adrenal insufficiency. In a patient with central hypothyroidism, adrenal reserve should be evaluated; if found to be low-normal or overtly low, a glucocorticoid should be administered.

This patient has both growth hormone deficiency (low serum insulin-like growth factor 1 level) and male hypogonadism (low serum testosterone level). However, these are not as serious as the central hypothyroidism, and hormone replacement for these deficiencies can be initiated at a future time.

The patient does not have signs or symptoms of diabetes insipidus. Therefore, vasopressin replacement is not required.

Bibliography

Grossman AB. Clinical review: The diagnosis and management of central hypoadrenalism. J Clin Endocrinol Metab. 2010;95(11):4855-4863. [PMID: 20719838]

Item 81   Answer: B
Educational Objective: Diagnose familial hyperparathyroidism.

The most likely diagnosis is multiple endocrine neoplasia type 2 (MEN2). The finding of mild hypercalcemia in a young man whose family history includes a brother with kidney stones and a father with an anesthesia-induced hypertensive crisis raises concern for MEN2. The patient likely has hyperparathyroidism, and his neck mass is most likely a medullary thyroid cancer. His history of diarrhea suggests a high serum calcitonin level caused by the medullary thyroid cancer. Undiagnosed pheochromocytoma may have been the cause of his father's death, and the brother may have hyperparathyroidism. Together, these personal and family findings suggest that this patient may belong to a MEN2 kindred. MEN2 is caused by germline transmission of a mutant *RET* proto-oncogene. The MEN2 phenotype can include primary hyperparathyroidism, pheochromocytoma, and medullary thyroid cancer. The hyperparathyroidism of MEN2 is due to benign hyperplasia involving all parathyroid glands.

Benign familial hypocalciuric hypercalcemia is a rare familial condition caused by inactivating mutations of the calcium-sensing receptor, which has a major function in regulating calcium metabolism through parathyroid tissue and renal calcium. The disorder is autosomal dominant with high penetrance. Decreased sensitivity of the calcium-sensing receptor to calcium is typical of this disorder and thus higher calcium levels are required to suppress parathyroid hormone secretion. Fractional excretion of calcium is less than 1%, despite the hypercalcemia, and the PTH level is normal or slightly elevated. The clinical significance of this disease lies mostly in its mistaken diagnosis as hyperparathyroidism. Benign hypocalciuric hypercalcemia does not explain the patient's thyroid mass or the father's probable pheochromocytoma.

Parathyroid cancer may be palpable on physical examination, but hyperplastic parathyroid glands with benign enlargement would not. Additionally, parathyroid cancer would cause more severe hypercalcemia and does not explain the patient's personal history of diarrhea or his family history.

Sarcoidosis causes hypercalcemia by production of 1,25-dihydroxyvitamin D by granulomas. This patient's neck mass and normal chest radiograph are not typical of sarcoidosis.

KEY POINT

- **The finding of mild hypercalcemia in a young patient with a family history of related endocrinopathies raises concern for multiple endocrine neoplasia type 2.**

Bibliography

Moline J, Eng C. Multiple endocrine neoplasia type 2: an overview. Genet Med. 2011;13(9):755-764. [PMID: 21552134]

Item 82   Answer: C

Educational Objective: Manage hirsutism in polycystic ovary syndrome.

This patient should begin taking an oral contraceptive. She has polycystic ovary syndrome (PCOS), as indicated by her irregular menses, her clinical and biochemical hyperandrogenism, and the exclusion of other possible causes. The best initial treatment for hirsutism in this population is an oral contraceptive, which decreases luteinizing hormone release through estrogen's negative feedback, thereby decreasing testosterone production by the ovary, and

increases sex hormone–binding globulin levels, thereby decreasing bioavailable testosterone levels.

Bromocriptine is a dopamine agonist indicated for medical treatment of prolactin-secreting pituitary tumors. This patient exhibits no clinical or biochemical evidence of a prolactinoma that would require treatment with a dopamine agonist.

Dexamethasone is used in the treatment of congenital adrenal hyperplasia. This patient's 17-hydroxyprogesterone level is normal, which suggests that she does not have this disorder.

Although early observational trials suggested that metformin may be effective in treating hirsutism in patients with PCOS, subsequent randomized clinical control trials have had mixed results. Therefore, metformin is not the best first-line treatment for symptoms of hyperandrogenism (such as acne, hirsutism, and alopecia) in women with PCOS.

Spironolactone can be very useful for the treatment of hyperandrogenism in PCOS but is added only if an oral contraceptive does not adequately improve symptoms. Because of the teratogenic effects of spironolactone, it is not given to women without an oral contraceptive pill.

KEY POINT

- **The best initial treatment for hirsutism in women with polycystic ovary syndrome is an oral contraceptive.**

Bibliography

Martin KA, Chang RJ, Ehrmann DA, et al. Evaluation and treatment of hirsutism in premenopausal women: an Endocrine Society clinical practice guideline. J Clin Endocrinol Metab. 2008;93(4):1105-1120. [PMID: 18252793]

Item 83   Answer: B

Educational Objective: Treat acromegaly after transsphenoidal surgery.

The most appropriate next step in treating this patient who has acromegaly is administration of octreotide, a somatostatin analogue. The goals of therapy for acromegaly are to normalize the insulin-like growth factor 1 (IGF-1) and growth hormone (GH) levels, reduce tumor bulk, prevent or decrease the number of comorbidities, and reduce the risk of premature death. Transsphenoidal surgery will normalize biochemical IGF-1 and GH levels in as many as 90% of patients with microadenomas and 40% of patients with macroadenomas. In patients (such as this one) whose IGF-1 and GH levels remain elevated postoperatively, somatostatin analogues are commonly used to normalize levels and shrink any residual pituitary tumor. This patient's comorbidities (sleep apnea, hypertension, type 2 diabetes mellitus, arthropathy, and headache) should continue to be monitored and treated, if needed.

Dopamine agonists generally do not work as well as somatostatin analogues in the treatment of acromegaly, and cabergoline, not bromocriptine, is the most effective dopamine agonist for this purpose.

Although this patient already underwent surgical debulking of his tumor, the continued elevation of his GH and IGF-1 levels indicates that residual disease is present, most likely in the cavernous sinus, which is not surgically accessible. Therefore, repeat surgery is unlikely to be useful.

Clinical observation is inappropriate for this patient with residual active acromegaly, which has associated comorbidities and premature mortality. Therefore, therapy is indicated.

KEY POINT

- In patients with acromegaly whose insulin-like growth factor 1 and growth hormone levels remain elevated after transsphenoidal surgery, somatostatin analogues are commonly used to normalize levels and shrink any residual pituitary tumor.

Bibliography

Katznelson L, Atkinson JL, Cook DM, Ezzat SZ, Hamrahian AH, Miller KK; American Association of Clinical Endocrinologists. American Association of Clinical Endocrinologists medical guidelines for clinical practice for the diagnosis and treatment of acromegaly—2011 update. Endocr Pract. 2011;17(Suppl 4):1-44. [PMID: 21846616]

Item 84   Answer: C

Educational Objective: Diagnose ectopic adrenocorticotropic hormone secretion.

The clinical and biochemical features of this patient with Cushing syndrome (hypercortisolism, melanonychia striata on the toenails) are most likely caused by ectopic adrenocorticotropic hormone (ACTH) secretion by a malignant tumor. Patients with these tumors typically have signs and symptoms of malignancy (weight loss,

cachexia, and temporal muscle wasting) and biochemical features of mineralocorticoid activity. This patient most likely has new-onset type 2 diabetes mellitus (recent-onset polyuria and nocturia, high random glucose levels) and classic features of excess mineralocorticoid activity, including hypertension, metabolic alkalosis, and excessive urine potassium loss. He has no history of gastrointestinal fluid losses. Clinical examination shows features consistent with excessive ACTH secretion (hyperpigmented mucous membranes) and excess amounts of glucocorticoids (proximal muscle wasting and weakness). The patient's history of smoking suggests the possibility of an ACTH-producing lung cancer; approximately half of all cases of ectopic ACTH secretion are due to small-cell lung cancer.

Adrenal adenomas can be associated with hypercortisolism but the features tend to be mild, with hypertension and diabetes the most prominent. Adrenal adenomas are associated with suppressed ACTH levels.

Although adrenal carcinomas may be associated with weight loss, rapid onset of cushingoid features, and findings of hypercortisolism, they also are associated with suppressed, not elevated, levels of ACTH.

The clinical and biochemical features of hypercortisolism observed in this patient are not consistent with those seen in patients with ACTH-secreting pituitary adenomas, which generally are associated with lower ACTH levels and slow onset of cushingoid features.

KEY POINT

- Patients with ectopic adrenocorticotropic hormone (ACTH) production typically have weight loss, rapid onset of Cushing syndrome, temporal muscle wasting, and elevated plasma ACTH levels.

Bibliography

Neiman LK, Biller BM, Findling JW, et al. The diagnosis of Cushing's syndrome: an Endocrine Society Clinical Practice Guideline. J Clin Endocrinol Metab. 2008;93(5): 1526-1540. [PMID: 18334580]

Index

A — NAME AND ADDRESS (Please complete.)

Last Name _____ First Name _____ Middle Initial _____

Address _____

Address cont. _____

City _____ State _____ ZIP Code _____

Country _____

Email address _____

ACP
AMERICAN COLLEGE OF PHYSICIANS
INTERNAL MEDICINE | *Doctors for Adults*

Medical Knowledge Self-Assessment Program® 16

TO EARN *AMA PRA CATEGORY 1 CREDITS*™ YOU MUST:

1. Answer all questions.
2. Score a minimum of 50% correct.

===

TO EARN *FREE* SAME-DAY *AMA PRA CATEGORY 1 CREDITS*™ ONLINE:

1. Answer all of your questions.
2. Go to **mksap.acponline.org** and access the appropriate answer sheet.
3. Transcribe your answers and submit for CME credits.
4. You can also enter your answers directly at **mksap.acponline.org** without first using this answer sheet.

To Submit Your Answer Sheet by Mail or FAX for a $10 Administrative Fee per Answer Sheet:

1. Answer all of your questions and calculate your score.
2. Complete boxes A–F.
3. Complete payment information.
4. Send the answer sheet and payment information to ACP, using the FAX number/address listed below.

B — Order Number

(Use the Order Number on your MKSAP materials packing slip.)

C — ACP ID Number

(Refer to packing slip in your MKSAP materials for your ACP ID Number.)

COMPLETE FORM BELOW ONLY IF YOU SUBMIT BY MAIL OR FAX

Last Name _____ First Name _____ MI _____

Payment Information. Must remit in US funds, drawn on a US bank.

The processing fee for each paper answer sheet is $10.

☐ Check, made payable to ACP, enclosed

Charge to ☐ **VISA** ☐ **MasterCard** ☐ **AMERICAN EXPRESS** ☐ **DISCOVER**

Card Number _____

Expiration Date _____ / _____
               MM   YY

Security code (3 or 4 digit #s) _____

Signature _____

Fax to: 215-351-2799

Questions?
Go to **mskap.acponline.org** or email **custserv@acponline.org**

Mail to:
Member and Customer Service
American College of Physicians
190 N. Independence Mall West
Philadelphia, PA 19106-1572

1 Ⓐ Ⓑ Ⓒ Ⓓ Ⓔ
2 Ⓐ Ⓑ Ⓒ Ⓓ Ⓔ
3 Ⓐ Ⓑ Ⓒ Ⓓ Ⓔ
4 Ⓐ Ⓑ Ⓒ Ⓓ Ⓔ
5 Ⓐ Ⓑ Ⓒ Ⓓ Ⓔ

6 Ⓐ Ⓑ Ⓒ Ⓓ Ⓔ
7 Ⓐ Ⓑ Ⓒ Ⓓ Ⓔ
8 Ⓐ Ⓑ Ⓒ Ⓓ Ⓔ
9 Ⓐ Ⓑ Ⓒ Ⓓ Ⓔ
10 Ⓐ Ⓑ Ⓒ Ⓓ Ⓔ

11 Ⓐ Ⓑ Ⓒ Ⓓ Ⓔ
12 Ⓐ Ⓑ Ⓒ Ⓓ Ⓔ
13 Ⓐ Ⓑ Ⓒ Ⓓ Ⓔ
14 Ⓐ Ⓑ Ⓒ Ⓓ Ⓔ
15 Ⓐ Ⓑ Ⓒ Ⓓ Ⓔ

16 Ⓐ Ⓑ Ⓒ Ⓓ Ⓔ
17 Ⓐ Ⓑ Ⓒ Ⓓ Ⓔ
18 Ⓐ Ⓑ Ⓒ Ⓓ Ⓔ
19 Ⓐ Ⓑ Ⓒ Ⓓ Ⓔ
20 Ⓐ Ⓑ Ⓒ Ⓓ Ⓔ

21 Ⓐ Ⓑ Ⓒ Ⓓ Ⓔ
22 Ⓐ Ⓑ Ⓒ Ⓓ Ⓔ
23 Ⓐ Ⓑ Ⓒ Ⓓ Ⓔ
24 Ⓐ Ⓑ Ⓒ Ⓓ Ⓔ
25 Ⓐ Ⓑ Ⓒ Ⓓ Ⓔ

26 Ⓐ Ⓑ Ⓒ Ⓓ Ⓔ
27 Ⓐ Ⓑ Ⓒ Ⓓ Ⓔ
28 Ⓐ Ⓑ Ⓒ Ⓓ Ⓔ
29 Ⓐ Ⓑ Ⓒ Ⓓ Ⓔ
30 Ⓐ Ⓑ Ⓒ Ⓓ Ⓔ

31 Ⓐ Ⓑ Ⓒ Ⓓ Ⓔ
32 Ⓐ Ⓑ Ⓒ Ⓓ Ⓔ
33 Ⓐ Ⓑ Ⓒ Ⓓ Ⓔ
34 Ⓐ Ⓑ Ⓒ Ⓓ Ⓔ
35 Ⓐ Ⓑ Ⓒ Ⓓ Ⓔ

36 Ⓐ Ⓑ Ⓒ Ⓓ Ⓔ
37 Ⓐ Ⓑ Ⓒ Ⓓ Ⓔ
38 Ⓐ Ⓑ Ⓒ Ⓓ Ⓔ
39 Ⓐ Ⓑ Ⓒ Ⓓ Ⓔ
40 Ⓐ Ⓑ Ⓒ Ⓓ Ⓔ

41 Ⓐ Ⓑ Ⓒ Ⓓ Ⓔ
42 Ⓐ Ⓑ Ⓒ Ⓓ Ⓔ
43 Ⓐ Ⓑ Ⓒ Ⓓ Ⓔ
44 Ⓐ Ⓑ Ⓒ Ⓓ Ⓔ
45 Ⓐ Ⓑ Ⓒ Ⓓ Ⓔ

46 Ⓐ Ⓑ Ⓒ Ⓓ Ⓔ
47 Ⓐ Ⓑ Ⓒ Ⓓ Ⓔ
48 Ⓐ Ⓑ Ⓒ Ⓓ Ⓔ
49 Ⓐ Ⓑ Ⓒ Ⓓ Ⓔ
50 Ⓐ Ⓑ Ⓒ Ⓓ Ⓔ

51 Ⓐ Ⓑ Ⓒ Ⓓ Ⓔ
52 Ⓐ Ⓑ Ⓒ Ⓓ Ⓔ
53 Ⓐ Ⓑ Ⓒ Ⓓ Ⓔ
54 Ⓐ Ⓑ Ⓒ Ⓓ Ⓔ
55 Ⓐ Ⓑ Ⓒ Ⓓ Ⓔ

56 Ⓐ Ⓑ Ⓒ Ⓓ Ⓔ
57 Ⓐ Ⓑ Ⓒ Ⓓ Ⓔ
58 Ⓐ Ⓑ Ⓒ Ⓓ Ⓔ
59 Ⓐ Ⓑ Ⓒ Ⓓ Ⓔ
60 Ⓐ Ⓑ Ⓒ Ⓓ Ⓔ

61 Ⓐ Ⓑ Ⓒ Ⓓ Ⓔ
62 Ⓐ Ⓑ Ⓒ Ⓓ Ⓔ
63 Ⓐ Ⓑ Ⓒ Ⓓ Ⓔ
64 Ⓐ Ⓑ Ⓒ Ⓓ Ⓔ
65 Ⓐ Ⓑ Ⓒ Ⓓ Ⓔ

66 Ⓐ Ⓑ Ⓒ Ⓓ Ⓔ
67 Ⓐ Ⓑ Ⓒ Ⓓ Ⓔ
68 Ⓐ Ⓑ Ⓒ Ⓓ Ⓔ
69 Ⓐ Ⓑ Ⓒ Ⓓ Ⓔ
70 Ⓐ Ⓑ Ⓒ Ⓓ Ⓔ

71 Ⓐ Ⓑ Ⓒ Ⓓ Ⓔ
72 Ⓐ Ⓑ Ⓒ Ⓓ Ⓔ
73 Ⓐ Ⓑ Ⓒ Ⓓ Ⓔ
74 Ⓐ Ⓑ Ⓒ Ⓓ Ⓔ
75 Ⓐ Ⓑ Ⓒ Ⓓ Ⓔ

76 Ⓐ Ⓑ Ⓒ Ⓓ Ⓔ
77 Ⓐ Ⓑ Ⓒ Ⓓ Ⓔ
78 Ⓐ Ⓑ Ⓒ Ⓓ Ⓔ
79 Ⓐ Ⓑ Ⓒ Ⓓ Ⓔ
80 Ⓐ Ⓑ Ⓒ Ⓓ Ⓔ

81 Ⓐ Ⓑ Ⓒ Ⓓ Ⓔ
82 Ⓐ Ⓑ Ⓒ Ⓓ Ⓔ
83 Ⓐ Ⓑ Ⓒ Ⓓ Ⓔ
84 Ⓐ Ⓑ Ⓒ Ⓓ Ⓔ
85 Ⓐ Ⓑ Ⓒ Ⓓ Ⓔ

86 Ⓐ Ⓑ Ⓒ Ⓓ Ⓔ
87 Ⓐ Ⓑ Ⓒ Ⓓ Ⓔ
88 Ⓐ Ⓑ Ⓒ Ⓓ Ⓔ
89 Ⓐ Ⓑ Ⓒ Ⓓ Ⓔ
90 Ⓐ Ⓑ Ⓒ Ⓓ Ⓔ

91 Ⓐ Ⓑ Ⓒ Ⓓ Ⓔ
92 Ⓐ Ⓑ Ⓒ Ⓓ Ⓔ
93 Ⓐ Ⓑ Ⓒ Ⓓ Ⓔ
94 Ⓐ Ⓑ Ⓒ Ⓓ Ⓔ
95 Ⓐ Ⓑ Ⓒ Ⓓ Ⓔ

96 Ⓐ Ⓑ Ⓒ Ⓓ Ⓔ
97 Ⓐ Ⓑ Ⓒ Ⓓ Ⓔ
98 Ⓐ Ⓑ Ⓒ Ⓓ Ⓔ
99 Ⓐ Ⓑ Ⓒ Ⓓ Ⓔ
100 Ⓐ Ⓑ Ⓒ Ⓓ Ⓔ

101 Ⓐ Ⓑ Ⓒ Ⓓ Ⓔ
102 Ⓐ Ⓑ Ⓒ Ⓓ Ⓔ
103 Ⓐ Ⓑ Ⓒ Ⓓ Ⓔ
104 Ⓐ Ⓑ Ⓒ Ⓓ Ⓔ
105 Ⓐ Ⓑ Ⓒ Ⓓ Ⓔ

106 Ⓐ Ⓑ Ⓒ Ⓓ Ⓔ
107 Ⓐ Ⓑ Ⓒ Ⓓ Ⓔ
108 Ⓐ Ⓑ Ⓒ Ⓓ Ⓔ
109 Ⓐ Ⓑ Ⓒ Ⓓ Ⓔ
110 Ⓐ Ⓑ Ⓒ Ⓓ Ⓔ

111 Ⓐ Ⓑ Ⓒ Ⓓ Ⓔ
112 Ⓐ Ⓑ Ⓒ Ⓓ Ⓔ
113 Ⓐ Ⓑ Ⓒ Ⓓ Ⓔ
114 Ⓐ Ⓑ Ⓒ Ⓓ Ⓔ
115 Ⓐ Ⓑ Ⓒ Ⓓ Ⓔ

116 Ⓐ Ⓑ Ⓒ Ⓓ Ⓔ
117 Ⓐ Ⓑ Ⓒ Ⓓ Ⓔ
118 Ⓐ Ⓑ Ⓒ Ⓓ Ⓔ
119 Ⓐ Ⓑ Ⓒ Ⓓ Ⓔ
120 Ⓐ Ⓑ Ⓒ Ⓓ Ⓔ

121 Ⓐ Ⓑ Ⓒ Ⓓ Ⓔ
122 Ⓐ Ⓑ Ⓒ Ⓓ Ⓔ
123 Ⓐ Ⓑ Ⓒ Ⓓ Ⓔ
124 Ⓐ Ⓑ Ⓒ Ⓓ Ⓔ
125 Ⓐ Ⓑ Ⓒ Ⓓ Ⓔ

126 Ⓐ Ⓑ Ⓒ Ⓓ Ⓔ
127 Ⓐ Ⓑ Ⓒ Ⓓ Ⓔ
128 Ⓐ Ⓑ Ⓒ Ⓓ Ⓔ
129 Ⓐ Ⓑ Ⓒ Ⓓ Ⓔ
130 Ⓐ Ⓑ Ⓒ Ⓓ Ⓔ

131 Ⓐ Ⓑ Ⓒ Ⓓ Ⓔ
132 Ⓐ Ⓑ Ⓒ Ⓓ Ⓔ
133 Ⓐ Ⓑ Ⓒ Ⓓ Ⓔ
134 Ⓐ Ⓑ Ⓒ Ⓓ Ⓔ
135 Ⓐ Ⓑ Ⓒ Ⓓ Ⓔ

136 Ⓐ Ⓑ Ⓒ Ⓓ Ⓔ
137 Ⓐ Ⓑ Ⓒ Ⓓ Ⓔ
138 Ⓐ Ⓑ Ⓒ Ⓓ Ⓔ
139 Ⓐ Ⓑ Ⓒ Ⓓ Ⓔ
140 Ⓐ Ⓑ Ⓒ Ⓓ Ⓔ

141 Ⓐ Ⓑ Ⓒ Ⓓ Ⓔ
142 Ⓐ Ⓑ Ⓒ Ⓓ Ⓔ
143 Ⓐ Ⓑ Ⓒ Ⓓ Ⓔ
144 Ⓐ Ⓑ Ⓒ Ⓓ Ⓔ
145 Ⓐ Ⓑ Ⓒ Ⓓ Ⓔ

146 Ⓐ Ⓑ Ⓒ Ⓓ Ⓔ
147 Ⓐ Ⓑ Ⓒ Ⓓ Ⓔ
148 Ⓐ Ⓑ Ⓒ Ⓓ Ⓔ
149 Ⓐ Ⓑ Ⓒ Ⓓ Ⓔ
150 Ⓐ Ⓑ Ⓒ Ⓓ Ⓔ

151 Ⓐ Ⓑ Ⓒ Ⓓ Ⓔ
152 Ⓐ Ⓑ Ⓒ Ⓓ Ⓔ
153 Ⓐ Ⓑ Ⓒ Ⓓ Ⓔ
154 Ⓐ Ⓑ Ⓒ Ⓓ Ⓔ
155 Ⓐ Ⓑ Ⓒ Ⓓ Ⓔ

156 Ⓐ Ⓑ Ⓒ Ⓓ Ⓔ
157 Ⓐ Ⓑ Ⓒ Ⓓ Ⓔ
158 Ⓐ Ⓑ Ⓒ Ⓓ Ⓔ
159 Ⓐ Ⓑ Ⓒ Ⓓ Ⓔ
160 Ⓐ Ⓑ Ⓒ Ⓓ Ⓔ

161 Ⓐ Ⓑ Ⓒ Ⓓ Ⓔ
162 Ⓐ Ⓑ Ⓒ Ⓓ Ⓔ
163 Ⓐ Ⓑ Ⓒ Ⓓ Ⓔ
164 Ⓐ Ⓑ Ⓒ Ⓓ Ⓔ
165 Ⓐ Ⓑ Ⓒ Ⓓ Ⓔ

166 Ⓐ Ⓑ Ⓒ Ⓓ Ⓔ
167 Ⓐ Ⓑ Ⓒ Ⓓ Ⓔ
168 Ⓐ Ⓑ Ⓒ Ⓓ Ⓔ
169 Ⓐ Ⓑ Ⓒ Ⓓ Ⓔ
170 Ⓐ Ⓑ Ⓒ Ⓓ Ⓔ

171 Ⓐ Ⓑ Ⓒ Ⓓ Ⓔ
172 Ⓐ Ⓑ Ⓒ Ⓓ Ⓔ
173 Ⓐ Ⓑ Ⓒ Ⓓ Ⓔ
174 Ⓐ Ⓑ Ⓒ Ⓓ Ⓔ
175 Ⓐ Ⓑ Ⓒ Ⓓ Ⓔ

176 Ⓐ Ⓑ Ⓒ Ⓓ Ⓔ
177 Ⓐ Ⓑ Ⓒ Ⓓ Ⓔ
178 Ⓐ Ⓑ Ⓒ Ⓓ Ⓔ
179 Ⓐ Ⓑ Ⓒ Ⓓ Ⓔ
180 Ⓐ Ⓑ Ⓒ Ⓓ Ⓔ

MK

MKSAP® 16

Medical Knowledge Self-Assessment Program®

Infectious Disease

ACP American College of Physicians®
INTERNAL MEDICINE | Doctors for Adults

Welcome to the Infectious Disease Section of MKSAP 16!

Here, you will find updated information on central nervous system infection, skin and soft tissue infection, community-acquired pneumonia, tick-borne disease, urinary tract infection, *Mycobacterium tuberculosis* and nontuberculous mycobacterial infection, sexually transmitted infection, health care–associated infection, HIV infection, and many other clinical challenges. All of these topics are uniquely focused on the needs of generalists and subspecialists *outside* of infectious disease.

The publication of the 16th edition of Medical Knowledge Self-Assessment Program heralds a significant event, culminating 2 years of effort by dozens of leading subspecialists across the United States. Our authoring committees have strived to help internists succeed in Maintenance of Certification, right up to preparing for the MOC examination, and to get residents ready for the certifying examination. MKSAP 16 also helps you update your medical knowledge and elevates standards of self-learning by allowing you to assess your knowledge with 1,200 all-new multiple-choice questions, including 108 in Infectious Disease.

MKSAP began more than 40 years ago. The American Board of Internal Medicine's examination blueprint and gaps between actual and preferred practices inform creation of the content. The questions, refined through rigorous face-to-face meetings, are among the best in medicine. A psychometric analysis of the items sharpens our educational focus on weaknesses in practice. To meet diverse learning styles, we offer MKSAP 16 online and in downloadable apps for PCs, tablets, laptops, and smartphones. We are also introducing the following:

High-Value Care Recommendations: The Infectious Disease section starts with several recommendations based on the important concept of health care value (balancing clinical benefit with costs and harms) to address the needs of trainees, practicing physicians, and patients. These recommendations are part of a major initiative that has been undertaken by the American College of Physicians, in collaboration with other organizations.

Content for Hospitalists: This material, highlighted in blue and labeled with the familiar hospital icon (◨), directly addresses the learning needs of the increasing number of physicians who work in the hospital setting. MKSAP 16 Digital will allow you to customize quizzes based on hospitalist-only questions to help you prepare for the Hospital Medicine Maintenance of Certification Examination.

We hope you enjoy and benefit from MKSAP 16. Please feel free to send us any comments to mksap_editors@acponline.org or visit us at the MKSAP Resource Site (mksap.acponline.org) to find out how we can help you study, earn CME, accumulate MOC points, and stay up to date. I know I speak on behalf of ACP staff members and our authoring committees when I say we are honored to have attracted your interest and participation.

Sincerely,

Patrick Alguire

Patrick Alguire, MD, FACP
Editor-in-Chief
Senior Vice President
Medical Education Division
American College of Physicians

Infectious Disease

Committee

Allan R. Tunkel, MD, PhD, MACP, Editor[2]
Professor of Medicine
Drexel University College of Medicine
Chair, Department of Medicine
Monmouth Medical Center
Long Branch, New Jersey

Thomas Fekete, MD, FACP, Associate Editor[1]
Professor of Medicine
Chief, Infectious Diseases
Section of Infectious Diseases
Temple University Medical School
Philadelphia, Pennsylvania

Karen C. Bloch, MD, MPH [1]
Assistant Professor
Department of Infectious Disease and Preventive Medicine
Division of Infectious Diseases
Vanderbilt University Medical Center
Nashville, Tennessee

Patricia D. Brown, MD, FACP[1]
Associate Professor of Medicine
Division of Infectious Diseases
Wayne State University School of Medicine
Chief of Medicine
Detroit Receiving Hospital
Detroit, Michigan

Larry M. Bush, MD, FACP[2]
Affiliated Professor of Biomedical Sciences
Charles E. Schmidt College of Medicine
Florida Atlantic University
Boca Raton, Florida
Affiliated Associate Professor of Medicine
University of Miami-Miller School of Medicine
JFK Medical Center
Palm Beach County, Florida

Michael Frank, MD, FACP[1]
Professor of Medicine
Residency Program Director
Vice Chair for Education
Department of Medicine
Medical College of Wisconsin
Milwaukee, Wisconsin

Keith S. Kaye, MD, MPH, FACP[2]
Professor of Medicine

Wayne State University
Corporate Medical Director, Infection Prevention, Epidemiology and Antimicrobial
 Stewardship, Detroit Medical Center
Detroit, Michigan

Fred A. Lopez, MD, FACP[2]
Richard Vial Professor and Vice Chair
Department of Medicine
Louisiana State University Health Sciences Center
New Orleans, Louisiana

Annette C. Reboli, MD, FACP[2]
Founding Vice Dean
Professor of Medicine
Cooper Medical School of Rowan University
Cooper University Hospital
Camden, New Jersey

Editor-in-Chief

Patrick C. Alguire, MD, FACP[1]
Senior Vice President, Medical Education
American College of Physicians
Philadelphia, Pennsylvania

Deputy Editor-in-Chief

Philip A. Masters, MD, FACP[1]
Senior Medical Associate for Content Development
American College of Physicians
Philadelphia, Pennsylvania

Senior Medical Associate for Content Development

Cynthia D. Smith, MD, FACP[2]
American College of Physicians
Philadelphia, Pennsylvania

Infectious Disease Clinical Editor

Mary Jane Barchman, MD, FACP[2]

Infectious Disease Reviewers

Robert D. Arbeit, MD[2]
Richard A. Fatica, MD[1]
Gloria T. Fioravanti, DO, FACP[1]

John D. Goldman, MD, FACP[1]
Duane R. Hospenthal, MD, PhD, FACP[1]
Richard H. Moseley, MD, FACP[1]
Mark E. Pasanen, MD, FACP[1]

Infectious Disease Reviewer Representing the American Society for Clinical Pharmacology & Therapeutics

Kevin Leary, MD, FACP[1]

Infectious Disease ACP Editorial Staff

Margaret Wells[1], Managing Editor
Sean McKinney[1], Director, Self-Assessment Programs
John Haefele[1], Assistant Editor

ACP Principal Staff

Patrick C. Alguire, MD, FACP[1]
Senior Vice President, Medical Education

D. Theresa Kanya, MBA[1]
Vice President, Medical Education

Sean McKinney[1]
Director, Self-Assessment Programs

Margaret Wells[1]
Managing Editor

Valerie Dangovetsky[1]
Program Administrator

Becky Krumm[1]
Senior Staff Editor

Ellen McDonald, PhD[1]
Senior Staff Editor

Katie Idell[1]
Senior Staff Editor

Randy Hendrickson[1]
Production Administrator/Editor

Megan Zborowski[1]
Staff Editor

Linnea Donnarumma[1]
Assistant Editor

John Haefele[1]
Assistant Editor

Developed by the American College of Physicians

---

1. Has no relationships with any entity producing, marketing, re-selling, or distributing health care goods or services consumed by, or used on, patients.

2. Has disclosed relationships with entities producing, marketing, re-selling, or distributing health care goods or services consumed by, or used on, patients. See below.

Conflicts of Interest

The following committee members, reviewers, and ACP staff members have disclosed relationships with commercial companies:

Robert D. Arbeit, MD
Employment
Idera Pharmaceuticals
Stock Options/Holdings
Idera Pharmaceuticals

Mary Jane Barchman, MD, FACP
Speakers Bureau
Novartis

Larry Bush, MD, FACP
Speakers Bureau
Cubist, Sanofi-Pasteur

Keith S. Kaye, MD, MPH, FACP
Speakers Bureau
Cubist, Merck, Pfizer, OrthoMcNeil
Consultantship
Merck, Pfizer, OrthoMcNeil, Forest Pharmaceuticals, Theradoc
Research Grants/Contracts
Merck, Pfizer, Cubist, Sage Products, Inc.

Fred A. Lopez, MD, FACP
Royalties
UpToDate

Annette C. Reboli, MD, FACP
Research Grants/Contracts
Merck, Pfizer, T2 BioSystems, Astellas
Royalties
UpToDate
Other
Pfizer, Merck

Cynthia D. Smith, MD, FACP
Stock Options/Holdings
Merck and Company

Allan R. Tunkel, MD, PhD, MACP
Employment
Food and Drug Administration
Research Grants/Contracts
UpToDate
Other
NIH, Infectious Diseases Society of America

Acknowledgments

The American College of Physicians (ACP) gratefully acknowledges the special contributions to the development and production of the 16th edition of the Medical Knowledge Self-Assessment Program® (MKSAP® 16) made by the following people:

Graphic Services: Michael Ripca (Technical Administrator/Graphic Designer) and Willie-Fetchko Graphic Design (Graphic Designer).

Production/Systems: Dan Hoffmann (Director, Web Services & Systems Development), Neil Kohl (Senior Architect), and Scott Hurd (Senior Systems Analyst/Developer).

MKSAP 16 Digital: Under the direction of Steven Spadt, Vice President, ACP Digital Products & Services, the digital version of MKSAP 16 was developed within the ACP's Digital Product Development Department, led by Brian Sweigard (Director). Other members of the team included Sean O'Donnell (Senior Architect), Dan Barron (Senior Systems Analyst/Developer), Chris Forrest (Senior Software Developer/Design Lead), Jon Laing (Senior Web Application Developer), Brad Lord (Senior Web Developer), John McKnight (Senior Web Developer), and Nate Pershall (Senior Web Developer).

The College also wishes to acknowledge that many other persons, too numerous to mention, have contributed to the production of this program. Without their dedicated efforts, this program would not have been possible.

Introducing the MKSAP Resource Site (mksap.acponline.org)

The MKSAP Resource Site (mksap.acponline.org) is a continually updated site that provides links to MKSAP 16 online answer sheets for print subscribers; access to MKSAP 16 Digital, Board Basics® 3, and MKSAP 16 Updates; the latest details on Continuing Medical Education (CME) and Maintenance of Certification (MOC) in the United States, Canada, and Australia; errata; and other new information.

ABIM Maintenance of Certification

Check the MKSAP Resource Site (mksap.acponline.org) for the latest information on how MKSAP tests can be used to apply to the American Board of Internal Medicine for Maintenance of Certification (MOC) points.

RCPSC Maintenance of Certification

In Canada, MKSAP 16 is an Accredited Self-Assessment Program (Section 3) as defined by the Maintenance of Certification Program of The Royal College of Physicians and Surgeons of Canada (RCPSC) and approved by the Canadian Society of Internal Medicine on December 9, 2011. Approval of Part A sections of MKSAP 16 extends from July 31, 2012, until July 31, 2015. Approval of Part B sections of MKSAP 16 extends from December 31, 2012, to December 31, 2015. Fellows of the Royal College may earn three credits per hour for participating in MKSAP 16 under Section 3. MKSAP 16 will enable Fellows to earn up to 75% of their required 400 credits during the 5-year MOC cycle. A Fellow can achieve this 75% level by earning 100 of the maximum of 174 *AMA PRA Category 1 Credits*™ available in MKSAP 16. MKSAP 16 also meets multiple CanMEDS Roles for RCPSC MOC, including that of Medical Expert, Communicator, Collaborator, Manager, Health Advocate, Scholar, and Professional. For information on how to apply MKSAP 16 CME credits to RCPSC MOC, visit the MKSAP Resource Site at mksap.acponline.org.

The Royal Australasian College of Physicians CPD Program

In Australia, MKSAP 16 is a Category 3 program that may be used by Fellows of The Royal Australasian College of Physicians (RACP) to meet mandatory CPD points. Two CPD credits are awarded for each of the 174 *AMA PRA Category 1 Credits*™ available in MKSAP 16. More information about using MKSAP 16 for this purpose is available at the MKSAP Resource Site at mksap.acponline.org and at www.racp.edu.au. CPD credits earned through MKSAP 16 should be reported at the MyCPD site at www.racp.edu.au/mycpd.

Continuing Medical Education

The American College of Physicians is accredited by the Accreditation Council for Continuing Medical Education (ACCME) to provide continuing medical education for physicians.

The American College of Physicians designates this enduring material, MKSAP 16, for a maximum of 174 *AMA PRA Category 1 Credits*™. Physicians should claim only the credit commensurate with the extent of their participation in the activity.

Up to 16 *AMA PRA Category 1 Credits*™ are available from December 31, 2012, to December 31, 2015, for the MKSAP 16 Infectious Disease section.

Learning Objectives

The learning objectives of MKSAP 16 are to:
- Close gaps between actual care in your practice and preferred standards of care, based on best evidence
- Diagnose disease states that are less common and sometimes overlooked and confusing
- Improve management of comorbid conditions that can complicate patient care
- Determine when to refer patients for surgery or care by subspecialists

- Pass the ABIM Certification Examination
- Pass the ABIM Maintenance of Certification Examination

Target Audience

- General internists and primary care physicians
- Subspecialists who need to remain up-to-date in internal medicine
- Residents preparing for the certifying examination in internal medicine
- Physicians preparing for maintenance of certification in internal medicine (recertification)

Earn "Same-Day" CME Credits Online

For the first time, print subscribers can enter their answers online to earn CME credits in 24 hours or less. You can submit your answers using online answer sheets that are provided at mksap.acponline.org, where a record of your MKSAP 16 credits will be available. To earn CME credits, you need to answer all of the questions in a test and earn a score of at least 50% correct (number of correct answers divided by the total number of questions). Take any of the following approaches:

1. Use the printed answer sheet at the back of this book to record your answers. Go to mksap.acponline.org, access the appropriate online answer sheet, transcribe your answers, and submit your test for same-day CME credits. There is no additional fee for this service.

2. Go to mksap.acponline.org, access the appropriate online answer sheet, directly enter your answers, and submit your test for same-day CME credits. There is no additional fee for this service.

3. Pay a $10 processing fee per answer sheet and submit the printed answer sheet at the back of this book by mail or fax, as instructed on the answer sheet. Make sure you calculate your score and fax the answer sheet to 215-351-2799 or mail the answer sheet to Member and Customer Service, American College of Physicians, 190 N. Independence Mall West, Philadelphia, PA 19106-1572, using the courtesy envelope provided in your MKSAP 16 slipcase. You will need your 10-digit order number and 8-digit ACP ID number, which are printed on your packing slip. Please allow 4 to 6 weeks for your score report to be emailed back to you. Be sure to include your email address for a response.

If you do not have a 10-digit order number and 8-digit ACP ID number or if you need help creating a username and password to access the MKSAP 16 online answer sheets, go to mksap.acponline.org or email custserv@acponline.org.

Permission/Consent for Use of Figures Shown in MKSAP 16 Infectious Disease Multiple-Choice Questions

Figure shown in Self-Assessment Test Item 25 reproduced with permission from the Massachusetts Medical Society. From Baker DJ, Reboli AC. [Images in Clinical Medicine]. N Engl J Med. 1997;998. Copyright © 1997 Massachusetts Medical Society.

Disclosure Policy

It is the policy of the American College of Physicians (ACP) to ensure balance, independence, objectivity, and scientific rigor in all of its educational activities. To this end, and consistent with the policies of the ACP and the Accreditation Council for Continuing Medical Education (ACCME), contributors to all ACP continuing medical education activities are required to disclose all relevant financial relationships with any entity producing, marketing, re-selling, or distributing health care goods or services consumed by, or used on, patients. Contributors are required to use generic names in the discussion of therapeutic options and are required to identify any unapproved, off-label, or investigative use of commercial products or devices. Where a trade name is used, all available trade names for the same product type are also included. If trade-name products manufactured by companies with whom contributors have relationships are discussed, contributors are asked to provide evidence-based citations in support of the discussion. The information is reviewed by the committee responsible for producing this text. If necessary, adjustments to topics or contributors' roles in content development are made to balance the discussion. Further, all readers of this text are asked to evaluate the content for evidence of commercial bias and send any relevant comments to mksap_editors@acponline.org so that future decisions about content and contributors can be made in light of this information.

Resolution of Conflicts

To resolve all conflicts of interest and influences of vested interests, the ACP precluded members of the content-creation committee from deciding on any content issues that involved generic or trade-name products associated with proprietary entities with which these committee members had relationships. In addition, content was based on best evidence and updated clinical care guidelines, when such evidence and guidelines were available. Contributors' disclosure information can be found with the list of contributors' names and those of ACP principal staff listed in the beginning of this book.

Hospital-Based Medicine

For the convenience of subscribers who provide care in hospital settings, content that is specific to the hospital setting has been highlighted in blue. Hospital icons (🏥) highlight where the hospital-only content begins, continues over more than one page, and ends.

Educational Disclaimer

The editors and publisher of MKSAP 16 recognize that the development of new material offers many opportunities for error. Despite our best efforts, some errors may persist in print. Drug dosage schedules are, we believe, accurate and in accordance with current standards. Readers are advised, however, to ensure that the recommended dosages in MKSAP 16 concur with the information provided in the product information material. This is especially important in cases of new, infrequently used, or highly toxic drugs. Application of the information in MKSAP 16 remains the professional responsibility of the practitioner.

The primary purpose of MKSAP 16 is educational. Information presented, as well as publications, technologies, products, and/or services discussed, is intended to inform subscribers about the knowledge, techniques, and experiences of the contributors. A diversity of professional opinion exists, and the views of the contributors are their own and not those of the ACP. Inclusion of any material in the program does not constitute endorsement or recommendation by the ACP. The ACP does not warrant the safety, reliability, accuracy, completeness, or usefulness of and disclaims any and all liability for damages and claims that may result from the use of information, publications, technologies, products, and/or services discussed in this program.

Publisher's Information

Unauthorized Use of This Book Is Against the Law

MKSAP 16 ISBN: 978-1-938245-00-8
(Infectious Disease) ISBN: 978-1-938245-09-1

Printed in the United States of America.

For order information in the U.S. or Canada call 800-523-1546, extension 2600. All other countries call 215-351-2600. Fax inquiries to 215-351-2799 or email to custserv@acponline.org.

Errata and Norm Tables

Errata for MKSAP 16 will be available through the MKSAP Resource Site at mksap.acponline.org as new information becomes known to the editors.

MKSAP 16 Performance Interpretation Guidelines with Norm Tables, available July 31, 2013, will reflect the knowledge of physicians who have completed the self-assessment tests before the program was published. These physicians took the tests without being able to refer to the syllabus, answers, and critiques. For your convenience, the tables are available in a printable PDF file through the MKSAP Resource Site at mksap.acponline.org.

Table of Contents

Infectious Disease High-Value Care Recommendations

The American College of Physicians, in collaboration with multiple other organizations, is embarking on a national initiative to promote awareness about the importance of stewardship of health care resources. The goals are to improve health care outcomes by providing care of proven benefit and reducing costs by avoiding unnecessary and even harmful interventions. The initiative comprises several programs that integrate the important concept of health care value (balancing clinical benefit with costs and harms) for a given intervention into various educational materials to address the needs of trainees, practicing physicians, and patients.

To integrate discussion of high-value, cost-conscious care into MKSAP 16, we have created recommendations based on the medical knowledge content that we feel meet the below definition of high-value care and bring us closer to our goal of improving patient outcomes while conserving finite resources.

High-Value Care Recommendation: A recommendation to choose diagnostic and management strategies for patients in specific clinical situations that balances clinical benefit with cost and harms with the goal of improving patient outcomes.

Below are the High-Value Care Recommendations for the Infectious Disease section of MKSAP 16.

- Do not use latex agglutination tests to identify the cause of bacterial meningitis because results of these tests rarely change treatment.
- Pre-lumbar puncture CT scans are only recommended in patients with a suspected mass lesion; who are immunocompromised; who have a history of central nervous system disease; or who present with new-onset seizures, decreased level of consciousness, focal neurologic deficits, or papilledema.
- The diagnosis of skin infections is typically based on clinical findings, not blood, skin, or biopsy cultures.
- Incision and drainage is the primary therapy for a cutaneous abscess, and possibly, antibiotic treatment, depending on extent and severity of infection.
- Ulcers that are clinically uninfected (that is, without purulence or inflammation) should not be treated with antibiotics.
- Blood cultures, sputum Gram stain and culture, and pneumococcal and *Legionella* urine antigen testing are optional in outpatients with community-acquired pneumonia (see Item 79).

- Once patients with pneumonia are ready to switch to oral therapy, most can be safely discharged without observation (see Item 46).
- Follow-up chest imaging is not indicated in most patients with pneumonia who improve with treatment but should be considered in those who are older than 40 years of age and smokers.
- Serologic testing is not recommended for patients with early Lyme disease because a measurable antibody response may not have had time to develop (see Item 23).
- Serologic testing for Lyme disease should be restricted to patients with clinically suggestive signs or symptoms who either reside in or have traveled to an endemic area.
- Urine culture is usually not needed for patients with an uncomplicated urinary tract infection because results rarely change management.
- Urologic investigation, including CT and/or ultrasonography, should be restricted to those with pyelonephritis who have persistent flank pain or fever after 72 hours of antimicrobial therapy.
- Screening for and treatment of asymptomatic bacteriuria is indicated only in pregnant women and patients undergoing invasive urologic procedures (see Item 85).
- Do not obtain MRIs to follow treatment response of patients with osteomyelitis because results are not very specific and can lead to additional unwarranted therapy.
- Do obtain blood cultures in patients with suspected vertebral osteomyelitis because such culture results are positive in more than 50% of patients and can minimize the extent of the evaluation.
- Do not obtain stool cultures in otherwise healthy patients with diarrhea unless they have had symptoms for longer than 3 days, associated fever, or bloody or mucoid stools because results rarely change management (see Item 48).
- Do not obtain stool cultures in hospitalized patients with diarrhea after they have been in the hospital longer than 3 days.
- Do not send formed stool for *Clostridium difficile* toxin testing because positive results are more likely to reflect colonization than active infection.
- Do not send stool for ova and parasites testing in patients with diarrhea lasting fewer than 7 days.
- HIV viral load testing should only be used to diagnose patients with suspected acute-phase HIV and to monitor the efficacy of antiretroviral treatment.

- When influenza virus infection has been documented in the community, a diagnosis can be established clinically and rapid influenza diagnostic tests are unnecessary.
- Prophylactic or therapeutic antiviral therapy should be avoided in persons at low risk for or with equivocal clinical findings of influenza virus infection (see Item 43).

- Use newer antimicrobial agents only when clearly indicated and when appropriate treatment options are unavailable because they are expensive and need to be reserved for the most serious infections.

Infectious Disease

Central Nervous System Infections

Meningitis

Viral Meningitis

Epidemiology and Cause

The aseptic meningitis syndrome is defined as the presence of clinical and laboratory findings consistent with meningitis in a patient who has normal cerebrospinal fluid (CSF) stains and culture on initial evaluation. Viruses are the major cause, and enteroviruses are diagnosed in 85% to 95% of cases. Approximately 30,000 to 75,000 cases are reported annually in the United States, although the actual number is likely underrepresented. Enteroviral meningitis usually occurs in the summer and fall and is spread by the fecal-oral route. Although enteroviral meningitis occurs most often in infants and children, it is also the most common cause of aseptic meningitis in adults.

Meningitis develops in 10% to 30% of patients infected with mumps virus, although mumps is rare in a highly immunized population. Herpes simplex viruses (HSV) account for 0.5% to 3% of cases of aseptic meningitis and are most often associated with primary genital infection due to herpes simplex

virus type 2 (HSV-2). HSV-2 is also the most common cause of the syndrome of benign recurrent lymphocytic meningitis (previously termed Mollaret meningitis). Although encephalitis is the most common neurologic manifestation of West Nile virus infection (seen in fewer than 1% of patients), aseptic meningitis may also occur.

Diagnosis

Adult patients with enteroviral meningitis usually present with the sudden onset of fever, headache, nuchal rigidity, and photophobia. The duration of illness is usually less than 1 week, and many patients report improvement after diagnostic lumbar puncture. Patients with mumps meningitis usually report fever, vomiting, and headache. Salivary gland enlargement occurs in only 50% of these patients. Patients with the syndrome of benign recurrent lymphocytic meningitis characteristically develop approximately 10 episodes of meningitis lasting 2 to 5 days followed by spontaneous recovery.

CSF findings in patients with viral meningitis are shown in **Table 1**. Viral cultures of CSF are insensitive for diagnosis and are not routinely recommended. Nucleic acid amplification tests, such as polymerase chain reaction (PCR), are both sensitive (86% to 100%) and specific (92% to 100%) for diagnosing enteroviral meningitis. PCR has also been useful for diagnosing HSV-induced meningitis and for associating HSV-2

TABLE 1. Typical CSF Findings in Patients with Viral and Bacterial Meningitis

CSF Parameter	Viral Meningitis[a]	Bacterial Meningitis
Opening pressure	≤250 mm H$_2$O	200-500 mm H$_2$O[b]
Leukocyte count	50-1000/μL (50-1000 × 10^6/L)	1000-5000/μL (1000-5000 × 10^6/L)[c]
Leukocyte differential	Lymphocytes[d]	Neutrophils
Glucose	>45 mg/dL (2.5 mmol/L)	<40 mg/dL (2.2 mmol/L)[e]
Protein	<200 mg/dL (2000 mg/L)	100-500 mg/dL (1000-5000 mg/L)
Gram stain	Negative	Positive in 60%-90%[f,g]
Culture	Negative	Positive in 70%-85%[g]

CSF = cerebrospinal fluid; μL= microliter.

[a]Primarily nonpolio enteroviruses (echoviruses and coxsackieviruses).

[b]Values exceeding 600 mm H$_2$O suggest the presence of cerebral edema, intracranial suppurative foci, or communicating hydrocephalus.

[c]Range may be <100/μL (100 × 10^6/L) to >10,000/μL (10,000 × 10^6/L).

[d]May have neutrophil predominance early in infection, but lymphocyte predominance occurs after the first 6 to 48 hours.

[e]The CSF:plasma glucose ratio is ≤0.40 in most patients.

[f]The likelihood of a positive Gram stain correlates with number of bacteria in the CSF.

[g]The yield of positive results is significantly reduced by prior administration of antimicrobial therapy.

with the presence of benign recurrent lymphocytic meningitis. West Nile virus meningitis is best diagnosed by detection of IgM antibodies in CSF.

Treatment

Treatment of patients with enteroviral meningitis is supportive. Whether antiviral therapy alters the course of mild HSV-2 meningitis is unclear. Antiviral suppressive therapy may be considered in patients with benign recurrent lymphocytic meningitis, although there are no clinical trials to date that support the safety and efficacy of this approach. **H**

KEY POINTS

- Aseptic meningitis syndrome is defined as the presence of clinical and laboratory findings consistent with meningitis in a patient who has normal cerebrospinal fluid stains and culture on initial evaluation.

- Polymerase chain reaction is both sensitive and specific for diagnosing enteroviral meningitis and is also useful for diagnosing aseptic meningitis due to herpes simplex virus.

- Treatment of enteroviral meningitis is supportive.

Bacterial Meningitis

Cause

Streptococcus pneumoniae is the most common cause of bacterial meningitis in the United States. Approximately 70% of patients with *S. pneumoniae* meningitis have otitis media, sinusitis, pneumonia, basilar skull fracture with CSF leak, or are immunocompromised (splenectomy or asplenia, hypogammaglobulinemia, multiple myeloma, alcoholism, chronic liver or kidney disease, malignancy, or HIV infection).

Neisseria meningitidis meningitis most often occurs in children and young adults and in patients with properdin and terminal complement (C5, C6, C7, C8, and perhaps C9) deficiencies. *Listeria monocytogenes* meningitis develops most frequently in neonates, older adults (>50 years of age), and in those who are immunocompromised (diabetes mellitus, liver or kidney disease, collagen vascular disorders, disorders of iron overload, HIV infection, transplant recipients, and patients taking anti–tumor necrosis factor α agents such as infliximab and etanercept), although cases have been reported in patients with no underlying disorders. Outbreaks have been associated with ingestion of contaminated coleslaw, soft cheeses, raw vegetables, alfalfa tablets, cantaloupes, and frankfurters and other processed meats. The incidence of invasive listeriosis has been decreasing, most likely as a result of decreased contamination by *L. monocytogenes* in ready-to-eat foods.

Meningitis due to group B streptococci (*Streptococcus agalactiae*) most commonly occurs in neonates. Because of this risk, the Centers for Disease Control and Prevention (CDC) and the American College of Obstetricians and Gynecologists have established guidelines for the prevention of early-onset disease. These guidelines recommend universal screening of all pregnant women for rectovaginal colonization at 35 to 37 weeks' gestation and the administration of antimicrobial prophylaxis to carriers.

Meningitis caused by gram-negative bacilli (*Escherichia coli*, *Klebsiella* species, *Serratia marcescens*, *Pseudomonas aeruginosa*) may occur following head trauma, after neurosurgical procedures, and after placement of ventricular drains. Older adults, immunocompromised patients, and patients with gram-negative bacteremia or disseminated strongyloidiasis are also at risk for gram-negative meningitis. *Haemophilus influenzae*–induced bacterial meningitis in children or adults suggests the presence of sinusitis, otitis media, epiglottitis, pneumonia, diabetes mellitus, alcoholism, splenectomy or asplenia, head trauma with CSF leak, and immunodeficiencies such as hypogammaglobulinemia.

Recurrent bacterial meningitis accounts for about 1% to 6% of cases of community-acquired meningitis. The most common predisposing conditions in adults are remote head trauma and/or CSF leakage. Immunodeficient disorders such as complement deficiencies, asplenia, and HIV infection may also predispose to recurrent bacterial meningitis.

Health care–associated (nosocomial) bacterial meningitis usually occurs in the setting of head trauma, recent neurosurgery, or placement of external or internal ventricular drains and is usually caused by a different spectrum of pathogens than those causing community-acquired bacterial meningitis. Likely pathogens include staphylococci (*Staphylococcus aureus* and coagulase-negative staphylococci), gram-negative bacilli (*P. aeruginosa*), and *Propionibacterium acnes* (especially in patients with internal ventricular drains).

Epidemiology

The epidemiology of bacterial meningitis in the United States has changed significantly since the introduction of conjugate vaccines (**Table 2**). Since licensure of the 7-valent

TABLE 2. Causes of Bacterial Meningitis in the United States

Pathogen	Percentage of Total Cases		
	1986[a]	1995[b]	2003-2007
Haemophilus influenzae	45	7	7
Neisseria meningitidis	14	25	14
Streptococcus pneumoniae	18	47	58
Streptococcus agalactiae	6	12	18
Listeria monocytogenes	3	8	3

[a]Other bacteria represent 14% of total cases.

[b]Because of rounding, the percentage does not total 100%.

pneumococcal conjugate vaccine for children (covering serotypes 4, 6B, 9V, 14, 18C, 19F, and 23F) in 2000, one study reported that the incidence of pneumococcal meningitis decreased from 1.13 cases per 100,000 population between 1998 and 1999 to 0.79 case per 100,000 population between 2004 and 2005. However, the incidence of meningitis caused by serotypes 19A, 22F, and 35B (not covered by the vaccine) increased during this time. In a recent surveillance study conducted by the CDC in eight states representing 17 million persons of all ages, the incidence of bacterial meningitis declined from 2.0 to 1.38 cases per 100,000 population between 1998 and 1999 and 2006 and 2007; the median age of patients with meningitis increased from 30.3 years to 41.9 years. A 13-valent pneumococcal conjugate vaccine has recently been licensed in the United States, which offers additional protection against serotype 19A, but not serotypes 22F and 35B.

A quadrivalent meningococcal conjugate vaccine that provides coverage against four of the five major meningococcal serogroups (A, C, Y, and W135) was licensed for use in the United States in 2005. Routine single-dose vaccination is recommended for all children and adolescents ages 11 to 18 years, and revaccination is recommended for persons at prolonged increased risk of developing meningococcal disease. This vaccine does not provide coverage against serogroup B meningococci, which are responsible for almost one third of cases of invasive meningococcal infection in the United States. Vaccination against *H. influenzae* type b infection has almost eradicated what was once the most common form of bacterial meningitis. Remaining cases of *H. influenzae* meningitis are usually caused by other serotypes or nontypeable strains.

Diagnosis

Patients with bacterial meningitis usually present with some combination of fever, headache, stiff neck, and signs of cerebral dysfunction (confusion, delirium, or a decreased level of consciousness). Clinical features in patients with health care–associated bacterial meningitis most often include fever and a decreased level of consciousness, although these findings may be difficult to recognize in patients who are sedated, have recently undergone a neurosurgical procedure, or have an underlying disease that may mask the signs and symptoms.

Bacterial meningitis is diagnosed by CSF examination (see Table 1). Use of latex agglutination tests, which detect antigens of common meningeal pathogens, is no longer recommended because of the frequency of false-positive and false-negative results and because antigen testing does not modify the decision as to whether to administer antimicrobial therapy. A rapid immunochromatographic test that detects the C polysaccharide cell wall antigen of all strains of *S. pneumoniae* has an overall sensitivity of 95% to 100% and specificity of 100% for the rapid diagnosis of pneumococcal meningitis, although more studies are needed to demonstrate its

usefulness. PCR has a sensitivity of 92% to 100% and specificity of 100% for diagnosing pneumococcal meningitis. Use of PCR for this indication has not been extensively evaluated, and false-positive results have been reported. However, modifications to the technique may make PCR useful in diagnosing patients with bacterial meningitis, especially when CSF Gram stain and culture are negative.

Management

A management algorithm for patients with suspected bacterial meningitis is shown in **Figure 1**.

When acute bacterial meningitis is suspected, blood cultures and lumbar puncture must be performed immediately because lumbar puncture is needed to determine whether CSF findings are consistent with the clinical manifestations and suspected diagnosis. Emergent lumbar puncture should not be performed, however, in patients whose clinical presentation is consistent with a central nervous system (CNS) mass lesion. A CT scan of the head should be done before lumbar puncture in these patients, as well as in patients who are immunocompromised, have a history of CNS disease, present with new-onset seizures, or have a decreased level of consciousness, focal neurologic deficits, or papilledema. Some experts also suggest delaying lumbar puncture in patients with clinical signs of impending brain herniation because of the risk of precipitating herniation even when CT findings are normal. Clinical signs of impending herniation include deteriorating level of consciousness (especially a Glasgow Coma Scale score of ≤11), brainstem signs (including papillary changes, posturing, or irregular respirations), and a seizure.

Empiric antimicrobial therapy is started immediately for all patients after CSF is obtained by lumbar puncture, and adjunctive dexamethasone is also begun for most adult patients. Recommendations for selecting empiric antimicrobial agents are based on the patient's age and underlying condition (**Table 3, see page 5**). For patients in whom the lumbar puncture is delayed, blood culture specimens are obtained and appropriate adjunctive and empiric antimicrobial therapy is started before the lumbar puncture is performed. For all patients, targeted antimicrobial therapy can be initiated after the presumptive pathogen is identified on CSF Gram stain following lumbar puncture (**Table 4, see page 5**). Once the pathogen is positively identified and in vitro susceptibility is known, the antimicrobial regimen can be modified to provide optimal therapy (**Table 5, see page 6**).

Most adult patients with bacterial meningitis should be started on adjunctive dexamethasone when empiric antimicrobial therapy is begun. Adjunctive corticosteroids have been shown to decrease mortality and negative short-term neurologic sequelae in patients in developed countries, although their efficacy in resource-poor countries with significant prevalence of HIV infection and other comorbid diseases has not been established. Use of adjunctive dexamethasone may also be a concern in patients for whom

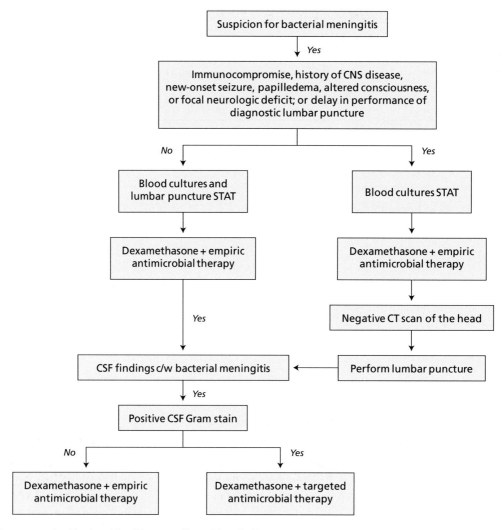

FIGURE 1. Management algorithm for adults with suspected bacterial meningitis.

CNS = central nervous system; c/w = consistent with; CSF = cerebrospinal fluid.

vancomycin is the most appropriate antimicrobial agent, because vancomycin's ability to penetrate the CSF may be reduced when dexamethasone is also administered. However, adjustment of the vancomycin dose to achieve serum trough concentrations of 15 to 20 micrograms/mL may help to overcome this problem. For patients receiving adjunctive dexamethasone and standard antimicrobial therapy with vancomycin and a third-generation cephalosporin (either cefotaxime or ceftriaxone) for treatment of pneumococcal meningitis who do not improve as expected or whose isolate has a cefotaxime or ceftriaxone minimal inhibitory concentration greater than 2.0 micrograms/mL, a repeat lumbar puncture is recommended 36 to 48 hours after initiation of therapy to document CSF sterility.

Outpatient intravenous antimicrobial therapy may be appropriate for selected patients with acute bacterial meningitis because outpatient therapy is associated with decreased costs of hospitalization, decreased risk of hospital-acquired infections, and better quality of life. The following criteria can be used for selecting patients for outpatient intravenous therapy: (1) completion of inpatient therapy for more than 6 days; (2) absence of fever for at least 24 to 48 hours; (3) no significant neurologic dysfunction, focal findings, or seizure activity; (4) clinical stability or improving infection; (5) ability to take fluids by mouth; (6) access to home health nursing for administration of antimicrobial therapy; (7) reliable intravenous line and infusion device (if needed); (8) daily availability of a physician; (9) established plan for physician visits, nurse visits, laboratory monitoring, and emergencies; (10) patient and/or family compliance; and (11) a safe environment with access to a telephone, utilities, food, and a refrigerator. ◧

KEY POINTS

- Approximately 70% of patients with *Streptococcus pneumoniae* meningitis are immunocompromised or have an underlying disorder such as otitis media, sinusitis, or pneumonia.

- Patients with bacterial meningitis may have some combination of fever, headache, stiff neck, and signs of cerebral dysfunction.

- When acute bacterial meningitis is suspected, immediate blood cultures and lumbar puncture must be performed unless lumbar puncture is contraindicated.

- Empiric antimicrobial therapy is started immediately for all patients with suspected bacterial meningitis after lumbar puncture is performed followed by targeted antimicrobial therapy after presumptive identification of the pathogen on cerebrospinal fluid Gram stain.

- Adjunctive dexamethasone should be started immediately for most adult patients with suspected bacterial meningitis who are living in developed countries.

TABLE 4. Recommended Targeted Antimicrobial Therapy for Bacterial Meningitis[a]

Pathogen	Antimicrobial Therapy
Streptococcus pneumoniae[b]	Vancomycin plus a third-generation cephalosporin[c,d]
Neisseria meningitidis	Third-generation cephalosporin[c]
Listeria monocytogenes	Ampicillin or penicillin G[e]
Haemophilus influenzae type b[f]	Third-generation cephalosporin[c]

[a]Based on identification of presumptive pathogen by cerebrospinal fluid Gram stain.

[b]Pending in vitro susceptibility testing, assume that the pneumococcal isolate is highly resistant to penicillin and use combination therapy.

[c]Cefotaxime or ceftriaxone.

[d]Addition of rifampin should be considered.

[e]Addition of an aminoglycoside should be considered.

[f]Pending in vitro susceptibility testing, assume that the pathogen produces β-lactamase.

TABLE 3. Recommended Empiric Antimicrobial Therapy for Suspected Bacterial Meningitis[a]

Community-acquired Meningitis		
Predisposing Factor	**Common Bacterial Pathogens**	**Antimicrobial Therapy**
Age <1 month	*Streptococcus agalactiae, Escherichia coli, Listeria monocytogenes, Klebsiella* species	Ampicillin plus cefotaxime or ampicillin plus an aminoglycoside
Age 1-23 months	*Streptococcus pneumoniae, Haemophilus influenzae, S. agalactiae, Neisseria meningitidis, E. coli*	Vancomycin plus a third-generation cephalosporin[b,c,d]
Age 2-50 years	*S. pneumoniae, N. meningitidis*	Vancomycin plus a third-generation cephalosporin[b,c,d]
Age >50 years	*S. pneumoniae, N. meningitidis, L. monocytogenes,* aerobic gram-negative bacilli	Vancomycin plus ampicillin plus a third-generation cephalosporin[b,c]
Immunocompromised state	*S. pneumoniae, N. meningitidis, L. monocytogenes,* aerobic gram-negative bacilli (including *Pseudomonas aeruginosa*)	Vancomycin plus ampicillin plus either cefepime or meropenem
Health care–associated Meningitis		
Predisposing Factor	**Common Bacterial Pathogens**	**Antimicrobial Therapy**
Basilar skull fracture	*S. pneumoniae, H. influenzae,* group A β-hemolytic streptococci	Vancomycin plus a third-generation cephalosporin[b]
Postneurosurgery or head trauma	*Staphylococcus aureus,* coagulase-negative staphylococci (especially *Staphylococcus epidermidis*), aerobic gram-negative bacilli (including *P. aeruginosa*)	Vancomycin plus either ceftazidime or cefepime or meropenem
Ventricular catheters (external or internal)	*S. aureus,* coagulase-negative staphylococci (especially *S. epidermidis*), aerobic gram-negative bacilli (including *P. aeruginosa*), diphtheroids (including *Propionibacterium acnes*)	Vancomycin plus either ceftazidime or cefepime or meropenem

[a]Based on the patient's age and underlying condition.

[b]Cefotaxime or ceftriaxone.

[c]Some experts would add rifampin if adjunctive dexamethasone is given.

[d]Add ampicillin if the patient has risk factors for or infection with *L. monocytogenes* is suspected.

TABLE 5. Recommended Specific Antimicrobial Therapy for Bacterial Meningitis Based on Pathogen and in vitro Susceptibility Testing

Pathogen/Susceptibilities	Standard Therapy	Alternative Therapies
Streptococcus pneumoniae		
Penicillin MIC ≤0.06 µg/mL	Penicillin G or ampicillin	Third-generation cephalosporin[a]; chloramphenicol
Penicillin MIC ≥0.12 µg/mL		
Cefotaxime or ceftriaxone MIC <1.0 µg/mL	Third-generation cephalosporin[a]	Meropenem; cefepime
Cefotaxime or ceftriaxone MIC ≥1.0 µg/mL	Vancomycin plus a third-generation cephalosporin[a,b]	Moxifloxacin[b,c]
Neisseria meningitidis		
Penicillin MIC <0.1 µg/mL	Penicillin G or ampicillin	Third-generation cephalosporin[a]; chloramphenicol
Penicillin MIC 0.1-1.0 µg/mL	Third-generation cephalosporin[a]	Chloramphenicol; a fluoroquinolone; meropenem
Listeria monocytogenes	Ampicillin or penicillin G[d]	Trimethoprim-sulfamethoxazole
Streptococcus agalactiae	Ampicillin or penicillin G[d]	Third-generation cephalosporin[a]; vancomycin
Haemophilus influenzae		
β-lactamase-negative	Ampicillin	Third-generation cephalosporin[a]; cefepime; aztreonam; chloramphenicol; a fluoroquinolone
β-lactamase-positive	Third-generation cephalosporin[a]	Chloramphenicol; cefepime; aztreonam; a fluoroquinolone
Escherichia coli and other Enterobacteriaceae[e]	Third-generation cephalosporin[a]	Aztreonam; meropenem; a fluoroquinolone; trimethoprim-sulfamethoxazole
Pseudomonas aeruginosa[e]	Ceftazidime[d] or cefepime[d]	Aztreonam[d]; meropenem[d]; ciprofloxacin[d]
Staphylococcus aureus		
Methicillin-sensitive	Nafcillin or oxacillin	Vancomycin; meropenem; linezolid; daptomycin
Methicillin-resistant	Vancomycin[f]	Trimethoprim-sulfamethoxazole; linezolid; daptomycin
Staphylococcus epidermidis	Vancomyin[f]	Linezolid

MIC = minimal inhibitory concentration; µg = micrograms.

[a]Cefotaxime or ceftriaxone.

[b]Addition of rifampin should be considered if the pathogen is sensitive and if the ceftriaxone MIC is >2 micrograms/mL.

[c]Has not been studied in patients with pneumococcal meningitis, but efficacy has been demonstrated in experimental animal models; if used, administering in combination with either a third-generation cephalosporin (cefotaxime or ceftriaxone) or vancomycin should be considered.

[d]Addition of an aminoglycoside should be considered.

[e]Choice of specific antimicrobial therapy should be guided by in vitro susceptibility test results.

[f]Addition of rifampin should be considered.

Focal Central Nervous System Infections

Brain abscess, cranial subdural empyema, and spinal epidural abscess are discussed below.

Brain Abscess

The most common pathogenetic mechanism of brain abscess formation is direct extension from a contiguous focus of infection, most often the middle ear, mastoid cells, or paranasal sinuses (**Table 6**). A second mechanism is

TABLE 6. Predisposing Conditions, Etiologic Agents, and Empiric Antimicrobial Therapy in Patients with Bacterial Brain Abscess

Predisposing Condition	Usual Bacterial Isolates	Empiric Antimicrobial Therapy
Otitis media or mastoiditis	Streptococci (aerobic or anaerobic); *Bacteroides* species; *Prevotella* species; Enterobacteriaceae	Metronidazole plus a third-generation cephalosporin[a]
Sinusitis	Streptococci; *Bacteroides* species; Enterobacteriaceae; *Staphylococcus aureus*; *Haemophilus* species	Metronidazole plus a third-generation cephalosporin[a,b]
Dental sepsis	Mixed *Fusobacterium*, *Prevotella*, and *Bacteroides* species; streptococci	Penicillin plus metronidazole
Penetrating trauma or after neurosurgery	*S. aureus*, streptococci, Enterobacteriaceae, *Clostridium* species	Vancomycin plus a third-generation cephalosporin[a,c]
Lung abscess, empyema, bronchiectasis	*Fusobacterium*, *Actinomyces*, *Bacteroides*, and *Prevotella* species; streptococci; *Nocardia* species	Penicillin plus metronidazole plus a sulfonamide[d]
Endocarditis	*S. aureus*, streptococci	Vancomycin plus gentamicin

[a]Cefotaxime or ceftriaxone; the fourth-generation cephalosporin cefepime may also be used.

[b]Add vancomycin if infection caused by methicillin-resistant *Staphylococcus aureus* is suspected.

[c]Use ceftazidime or cefepime if infection caused by *Pseudomonas aeruginosa* is suspected.

[d]Use trimethoprim-sulfamethoxazole if infection caused by *Nocardia* species is suspected.

hematogenous dissemination from a distant focus of infection; primary sources are chronic pyogenic lung diseases, wound and skin infections, osteomyelitis, pelvic infections, cholecystitis, intraabdominal infections, and infective endocarditis. Patients with congenital heart disease and hereditary hemorrhagic telangiectasia are also at increased risk. Trauma is a third pathogenetic mechanism, occurring secondary to an open cranial fracture with dural breach, as a result of neurosurgery, or after a foreign body injury. The cause of brain abscess is unknown in 10% to 35% of patients.

Most symptoms and signs are related to the size and location of the space-occupying lesion within the brain. Headache is the most common symptom; sudden worsening of the headache may signify rupture of the abscess into the ventricular space and is associated with a high mortality rate. Less than 50% of patients with brain abscess present with the triad of headache, fever, and focal neurologic deficit.

MRI is the diagnostic procedure of choice. Diffusion-weighted MRI can be used to help discriminate between abscess lesions and neoplasms. CT is reserved for patients unable to undergo MRI.

The optimal management of brain abscess requires a multidisciplinary approach. All lesions larger than 2.5 cm should be excised or stereotactically aspirated, and specimens should undergo microbiologic and histopathologic analysis. For abscesses in the early cerebritis stage (that is, the earliest stage of purulent brain infection when there is little or no enhancement on neuroimaging) or when all the abscesses are smaller than 2.5 cm, the largest lesion should be aspirated for diagnosis and microbiologic identification. Following specimen retrieval, it is appropriate to initiate empiric antimicrobial therapy based on the patient's predisposing conditions

and the presumed pathogenesis of brain abscess formation (see Table 6). In patients with significant cerebral edema and mass effect, initiation of corticosteroids is warranted.

Antimicrobial therapy usually lasts 6 to 8 weeks, and parenteral agents are preferred to ensure achievement of adequate tissue levels. Depending on the patient's response clinically and as demonstrated on imaging, this regimen may be followed by prolonged oral antimicrobial therapy if an appropriate agent is available. Shorter courses of therapy (3 to 4 weeks) may be adequate for patients who have undergone complete surgical excision of the brain abscess. Repeat neuroimaging biweekly up to 3 months after completion of therapy is recommended to monitor for re-expansion of the abscess or failure to respond.

KEY POINTS

- To establish the diagnosis and cause of brain abscess, a lesion should be stereotactically aspirated or surgically excised, and specimens should undergo culture and histopathologic analysis.
- In patients with brain abscess, intravenous antimicrobial therapy is usually continued for 6 to 8 weeks, followed by prolonged oral therapy if an appropriate agent is available.

Cranial Subdural Empyema

Paranasal sinusitis is the most common condition (40% to 80% of cases) predisposing to the development of cranial subdural empyema. Bacterial species that are most often isolated include aerobic streptococci, staphylococci, aerobic gram-negative bacilli, and anaerobic streptococci and other anaerobes; polymicrobial infections are common.

CONT.

Cranial subdural empyema can be rapidly progressive in its clinical presentation, with symptoms and signs related to increased intracranial pressure, meningeal irritation, or focal cortical inflammation. Headache is a prominent symptom and becomes generalized as the infection progresses. The diagnostic neuroimaging procedure of choice is MRI, which is preferred to CT because it provides better clarity of morphologic detail; may detect empyemas not seen on CT, such as those located at the base of the brain, along the falx cerebri, or in the posterior fossa; and can differentiate extraaxial empyemas from most sterile effusions and subdural hematomas.

Cranial subdural empyema is a medical and surgical emergency. Given the potential for polymicrobial infection, empiric antimicrobial therapy with vancomycin, metronidazole, and a third- or fourth-generation cephalosporin is warranted. The goals of surgical therapy are to achieve adequate decompression of the brain and evacuate the empyema. The optimal surgical approach is not clearly defined, although craniotomy is most often recommended because it allows wide exposure and better drainage of the empyema, which may be more loculated, tenacious, and extensive than that demonstrated by neuroimaging studies. Retrospective analyses have shown a lower mortality rate in patients with cranial subdural empyema who were treated with craniotomy compared with those who had drainage through craniectomy or burr holes. However, a limited drainage procedure (burr holes) may be preferable in patients with septic shock, those with localized parafalcine collections, and in children with subdural empyema secondary to meningitis.

KEY POINTS

- The clinical presentation of cranial subdural empyema can be rapidly progressive, with symptoms and signs related to increased intracranial pressure, meningeal irritation, or focal cortical inflammation.
- Craniotomy is most often recommended in patients with cranial subdural empyema because it allows wide exposure and better drainage of the empyema compared to more limited procedures.

 Spinal Epidural Abscess

Spinal epidural abscess most often occurs secondary to hematogenous dissemination to the epidural space from foci elsewhere in the body. Therefore, the most common infecting microorganism is *Staphylococcus aureus* (50% to 90% of cases). Gram-negative bacilli and anaerobes may be seen if the infection has a urinary or gastrointestinal source. The clinical presentation progresses through four stages: backache and focal vertebral pain; nerve root pain, manifested by radiculopathy or paresthesias; spinal cord dysfunction; and paraplegia. MRI with gadolinium enhancement is the diagnostic procedure of choice; it can enable visualization of the spinal cord and the epidural space in sagittal and transverse sections and can also identify accompanying osteomyelitis, intramedullary spinal cord lesions, and diskitis.

The principles of therapy for spinal epidural abscess are surgical decompression, drainage of the abscess, and antimicrobial therapy. Empiric antimicrobial therapy should always include an antistaphylococcal agent (usually vancomycin pending organism identification and in vitro susceptibility testing) plus coverage for gram-negative bacilli with agents such as an antipseudomonal cephalosporin or carbapenem, especially for patients with a history of injection drug use or a spinal procedure. Spinal epidural abscess is a surgical emergency requiring surgical drainage with decompression to minimize the likelihood of permanent neurologic sequelae. Antimicrobial therapy alone can be considered in patients who have localized pain and radicular symptoms without long-tract signs; these patients require frequent neurologic examinations and serial MRI studies to demonstrate resolution of the abscess. Emergent surgery is required in patients with increasing neurologic deficit, persistent severe pain, or increasing fever or peripheral leukocyte count. Surgery is not likely to be effective in patients who have experienced complete paralysis for longer than 24 to 36 hours, although some authorities have performed surgery when complete paralysis has lasted less than 72 hours.

KEY POINTS

- The clinical presentation of spinal epidural abscess begins with backache and focal vertebral pain and progresses to nerve root pain, spinal cord dysfunction, and paraplegia.
- The principles of spinal epidural abscess management are surgical decompression, drainage of the abscess, and antimicrobial therapy.
- Antimicrobial therapy alone can be considered in patients with spinal epidural abscess who have localized pain and radicular symptoms without long-tract signs; frequent follow-up neurologic examinations and serial MRI studies to demonstrate abscess resolution are necessary.

Encephalitis

Encephalitis refers to infection of the brain parenchyma with associated neurologic dysfunction. The meninges are also frequently involved, and the terms "encephalitis" and "meningoencephalitis" are used interchangeably. Although more than 100 microorganisms are associated with encephalitis, the most commonly diagnosed causes in the United States are herpes simplex virus and West Nile virus. In more than 50% of patients, however, a cause is not identified despite intensive diagnostic evaluation (**Table 7**).

Clinically, encephalitis is defined by an altered mental status lasting for at least 24 hours. Decreased consciousness may range from mild confusion to coma, and seizures occur in up to 40% of patients. Other common manifestations include hallucinations, ataxia, and cranial neuropathies. Focal neurologic

TABLE 7. Selected Viral Causes of Encephalitis Among Adults in the United States

Cause	Epidemiology	Clinical Features	Diagnosis	Treatment
Eastern equine encephalitis virus	Mosquito-borne infection	Case fatality rate, 50%-70%	Serology	Supportive
Herpes simplex virus-1	Reactivation of latent virus in about two thirds of cases	Temporal lobe seizures, fever	CSF PCR	Acyclovir
Human herpes virus-6	Immunocompromise, particularly bone marrow transplantation	Seizures	CSF PCR	Ganciclovir or foscarnet
JC virus (PML)	AIDS, immunomodulating therapy (natalizumab, rituximab)	Focal neurologic findings, subacute onset	CSF PCR	Decrease immunosuppression, start ART (in patients with AIDS)
Rabies virus	Transmitted by bite of infected animal	Agitation, paresthesias at site of inoculation, hydrophobia, autonomic instability	Serology (serum or CSF), RT-PCR of saliva, immuno-fluorescence staining of nuchal biopsy specimen	Supportive
St. Louis encephalitis virus	Mosquito-borne infection, endemic to United States west of the Mississippi River	Seizures, altered mentation, urinary tract symptoms, SIADH	Serology	Supportive
West Nile virus	Mosquito-borne infection, widely distributed worldwide	Acute flaccid paralysis, parkinsonian symptoms, myoclonus	Serology	Supportive

CSF PCR = cerebrospinal fluid polymerase chain reaction; PML = progressive multifocal leukoencephalopathy; ART = antiretroviral therapy; RT-PCR = reverse transcriptase polymerase chain reaction; SIADH = syndrome of inappropriate antidiuretic hormone secretion.

CONT.

findings may be present when a localized anatomic region of the brain is involved.

Neuroimaging is required to define the location and extent of central nervous system involvement. MRI is more sensitive than CT scanning for this purpose. Lumbar puncture should be performed in all patients without contraindications. The cerebrospinal fluid (CSF) typically exhibits a lymphocytic pleocytosis, although the CSF may be acellular. All patients should be tested for herpes simplex virus. Other serologic studies and molecular testing are based on the season of the year, geographic location, history of exposures, predisposing conditions, and clinical findings (for example, rash). **H**

Herpes Simplex Encephalitis

Herpes simplex encephalitis is the most common cause of endemic encephalitis in the United States, with a predilection for the very young and the elderly. Herpes simplex virus type 1 (HSV-1) accounts for greater than 90% of cases in adults; herpes simplex virus type 2 (HSV-2) causes the remaining cases. More than two thirds of infections are due to reactivation of latent HSV-1 virus rather than to primary infection. Even with antiviral therapy, the mortality rate for herpes simplex encephalitis ranges from 15% to 30%, and neuropsychiatric sequelae are common.

 Most patients present within a week of onset of symptoms, most commonly alterations in mental status and fever.

Orolabial herpetic lesions are present in less than 10% of patients. Because the virus most often infects the temporal lobes, partial complex seizures may occur. Without treatment, infection progresses to bilateral temporal lobe hemorrhagic necrosis, resulting in severe neurologic impairment or death.

Results of routine laboratory studies are nonspecific. CSF pleocytosis is generally present, with a lymphocytic predominance. However, the CSF leukocyte count is normal (0-5/microliter [$0\text{-}5 \times 10^6$/L]) in approximately 5% of patients. Neuroimaging findings that localize inflammation to one or both temporal lobes are strongly suggestive of this diagnosis (**Figure 2**). MRI is superior to CT scanning for identifying early infection when radiographic abnormalities may be subtle. An electroencephalogram may show characteristic periodic lateralizing epileptiform discharges localizing to the temporal lobes.

Microbiologic diagnosis requires detection of HSV in the CSF or brain tissue. HSV polymerase chain reaction (PCR) of CSF has a sensitivity of greater than 95% and specificity approaching 100% for diagnosis. False-negative HSV PCR results may occur early in the course of infection. In most patients, HSV PCR results remain positive for more than 7 days after antiviral therapy is begun. Because CSF viral culture is insensitive and HSV serologic studies are nonspecific, these tests are not indicated for diagnosis.

Intravenous acyclovir is the treatment of choice for herpes simplex encephalitis. Because delay in initiating treatment

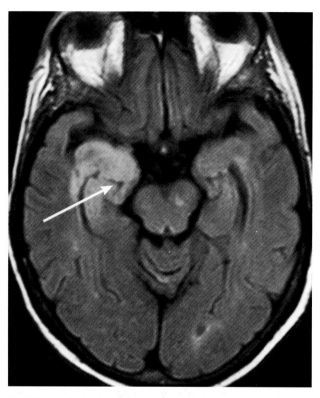

FIGURE 2. Brain MRI exhibiting right temporal lobe enhancement (arrow) in a patient with herpes simplex encephalitis.

CONT.

is associated with adverse neurologic outcomes or death, beginning empiric acyclovir before HSV PCR results are available is recommended. A positive HSV PCR result is diagnostic, and intravenous acyclovir is continued for 14 to 21 days. Oral antivirals such as valacyclovir have poor CSF penetration and result in subtherapeutic levels, mandating continuation of intravenous therapy for the entire treatment course. In patients with a low clinical suspicion for herpes simplex encephalitis, acyclovir may be discontinued when HSV PCR results are negative. Patients with an initially negative HSV PCR in whom there is a strong clinical suspicion for herpes simplex encephalitis should undergo repeat HSV PCR on a second CSF sample 3 to 7 days after the initial lumbar puncture or be treated with a full course of acyclovir. **H**

KEY POINTS

- Herpes simplex virus polymerase chain reaction of cerebrospinal fluid is diagnostic of herpes simplex encephalitis and should be performed in all patients with suspected infection.
- Intravenous acyclovir is the treatment of choice for patients with herpes simplex encephalitis.

West Nile Virus Encephalitis

West Nile virus encephalitis, first detected in the United States in 1999, has become an important cause of epidemic encephalitis nationally, although the regional incidence varies considerably from year to year. The virus is spread by the bite of an infected *Culex* mosquito, with the peak incidence in the late summer and early fall.

West Nile virus encephalitis is asymptomatic in 80% of **H** patients. Symptomatic infections include West Nile fever, occurring in 20% of patients, and West Nile neuroinvasive disease (WNND), occurring in less than 1% of patients, with adults over 50 years of age being disproportionately affected. Patients with West Nile fever develop a self-limited febrile illness associated with fatigue, rash, headache, anorexia, back pain, and myalgia. Clinical manifestations of WNND include meningitis, encephalitis, and myelitis, either alone or as overlapping findings. An objective finding of focal weakness is an important clue to diagnosing WNND. In the most severe cases, this manifests as acute flaccid paralysis and may lead to diaphragmatic involvement with respiratory failure similar to poliomyelitis. Other neurologic findings suggestive of WNND include extrapyramidal signs, which may mimic the tremors and bradykinesia of Parkinson disease. Rash may be present but is more common with West Nile fever than with WNND. Standard laboratory studies in WNND typically reveal a lymphocyte-predominant CSF pleocytosis, although in contrast to most viral encephalitides, neutrophils constitute a substantial proportion of the differential count. MRI of the brain is often normal or shows nonspecific abnormalities. Bilateral enhancement of the thalamus and basal ganglia on T2-weighted MRI images has been reported in a subset of patients with WNND.

Detection of West Nile virus IgM antibody in the CSF of symptomatic patients is diagnostic of WNND. The antibody is reliably detected within 9 days of onset of fever and often persists for more than 1 year. Serologic cross-reactivity with other flaviviruses (for example, St. Louis encephalitis virus, Japanese encephalitis virus, dengue virus, yellow fever virus) may cause false-positive West Nile virus IgM antibody results following recent infection with or immunization against one of these viruses. Nucleic acid amplification techniques are insensitive in diagnosing WNND because of the very brief period of viremia occurring in WNND.

Treatment of West Nile virus infection is supportive, although ongoing studies are evaluating the role of immunotherapy. There are no commercially available human vaccines against this virus. Prevention involves minimizing the risk of transmission from infected mosquitoes. **H**

KEY POINTS

- Clinical manifestations of West Nile neuroinvasive disease include meningitis, encephalitis, and myelitis, either alone or in combination; an objective finding of focal weakness is characteristic.
- The diagnosis of West Nile neuroinvasive disease is established by detection of West Nile virus IgM antibody in the CSF of symptomatic patients.
- Treatment of West Nile virus infection is supportive.

Prion Diseases of the Central Nervous System

Introduction

Prions are novel pathogens composed of transmissible proteins that lack associated genetic material and cause five recognized clinical syndromes in humans (**Table 8**). Creutzfeldt-Jakob disease and variant Creutzfeldt-Jakob disease occur most often. Common features of all prion diseases include progressive neurologic impairment, the absence of inflammatory cerebrospinal fluid (CSF) findings, and the presence of spongiform changes on neuropathologic examination. There are currently no treatments available for these conditions, which are invariably fatal.

Creutzfeldt-Jakob Disease

Creutzfeldt-Jakob disease (CJD) is classified as sporadic (sCJD), familial (fCJD), iatrogenic (iCJD), and variant (vCJD). The most common form is sCJD (85% of cases), followed by fCJD (10% to 15% of cases); iCJD and vCJD each account for approximately 1% of cases.

sCJD typically affects older adults with onset between 50 and 70 years of age. Patients may present with psychiatric manifestations, cognitive decline, or motor dysfunction. Extrapyramidal signs are present in approximately 65% of patients. Myoclonus and rapidly progressive dementia are hallmarks of this disease (**Table 9**). The median survival after symptom onset is 5 months.

The diagnosis of sCJD is challenging because routine laboratory testing is unrevealing. The CSF is typically acellular, although the total protein level may be elevated. Detection of elevated levels of 14-3-3 protein, a specific neuronal protein, in the cerebrospinal fluid may be an indirect marker of sCJD, but this test has low sensitivity and specificity and is only available through the National Prion Disease Pathology Surveillance Center (www.cjdsurveillance.com). The electroencephalogram may show a characteristic periodic sharp wave pattern in the later stages of disease. MRI is a useful diagnostic tool, with findings of areas of focal cortical hyperintensity on diffusion-weighted imaging or fluid-attenuated inversion recovery (FLAIR) sequences predictive of infection. Neural tissue evaluation demonstrating spongiform changes and histopathologic staining for prion protein (PrPsc) confirm the diagnosis, but results are rarely available pre-mortem.

In general, invasive neurosurgical procedures for patients with suspected prion disease are discouraged because of the potential for contamination of surgical instruments and exposure of health care workers to infectious tissues. If necessary, disposable instruments or those able to be specially sterilized

TABLE 9.	World Health Organization Criteria for Probable Sporadic Creutzfeldt-Jakob Disease (All Four Criteria Must Be Met)

1. Progressive dementia

2. Clinical signs (requires at least two of the following with duration <2 years):
   a. Myoclonus
   b. Pyramidal or extrapyramidal dysfunction
   c. Visual or cerebellar disturbance
   d. Akinetic mutism

3. Laboratory or EEG findings (at least one of the following):
   a. Characteristic EEG findings (1- to 2-Hz periodic sharp waves)
   b. Cerebrospinal fluid positive for 14-3-3 protein

4. No alternative diagnosis identified by routine investigation

EEG = electroencephalogram.

TABLE 8. Classification of Prion Diseases				
Disease	**Epidemiology**	**Pathophysiology**	**Clinical Findings**	**Time to Death**
Kuru	Papua New Guinea (Fore tribe)	Exposure to human brain tissue by cannibalism	Tremors, ataxia, movement disorders, dementia	<2 years
Gerstmann-Sträussler-Scheinker syndrome	Inherited, autosomal dominant	*PRNP* gene mutation	Progressive cerebellar degeneration with dementia	<5 years
Fatal familial insomnia	Inherited	*PRNP* gene mutation	Insomnia, myoclonus, autonomic dysfunction, endocrinopathy (dementia rare)	<1 year
Sporadic Creutzfeldt-Jakob disease	Mean age of onset, 65 years	Spontaneous mutation of host protein to form prion protein PrPsc	Rapidly progressive dementia, myoclonus, extrapyramidal signs	<6 months
Variant Creutzfeldt-Jakob disease	Most cases identified in the United Kingdom and Europe. Mean age of onset, 29 years	Dietary consumption of meat contaminated with brain tissue from animals with bovine spongiform encephalopathy	Paresthesias, psychiatric symptoms, delayed onset of dementia	~1 year

should be used; involvement by infection prevention practitioners is essential. Similarly, harvesting tissues from patients with suspected spongiform encephalopathy should be avoided.

Variant Creutzfeldt-Jakob Disease

In the late 1990s, a cluster of cases suggestive of sCJD was reported from the United Kingdom. In contrast to patients with sCJD, patients with this disorder were younger, had primarily psychiatric presentations, and had less rapid disease progression. These findings ultimately led to recognition of this outbreak as a unique prion disease, termed vCJD.

Neuropathologic findings unique to vCJD include heavy concentrations of amyloid plaque in the cerebrum and cerebellum that stain for a type of prion protein (PrPsc type 4 pattern) that is not found in other human prion diseases but is described in animals and animal products infected with bovine spongiform encephalopathy. Coupled with epidemiologic data, the consumption of animal protein, particularly beef, during a large-scale epidemic of bovine spongiform encephalopathy supports animal-to-human transmission.

The diagnosis is made by radiographic and neuropathologic examination. Characteristic findings on MRI (pulvinar sign) and identification of the PrPsc protein in tonsillar tissue facilitate pre-mortem diagnosis. Changes in animal feeding and butchering practices have led to sharp decreases in the incidence of vCJD.

KEY POINTS

- Common features of all prion diseases include progressive neurologic impairment, the absence of inflammatory cerebrospinal fluid findings, and the presence of spongiform changes on neuropathologic examination.

- Neural tissue evaluation demonstrating spongiform changes and histopathologic staining for prion protein (PrPsc) confirm the diagnosis of sporadic Creutzfeldt-Jakob disease, but results are rarely available pre-mortem, and invasive neurosurgical procedures pose a risk of secondary transmission.

- Patients with variant Creutzfeldt-Jakob disease have prion protein (PrPsc) that can be identified in tonsillar tissue, allowing pre-mortem confirmatory pathologic diagnosis.

Skin and Soft Tissue Infections

Introduction

The most common microorganisms causing skin infection are streptococci, particularly group A β-hemolytic streptococci (GABHS), and *Staphylococcus aureus*. The presence of lymphangitis and a "peau d'orange" appearance of the skin are more consistent with streptococcal infection, whereas an abscess or drainage from an existing wound or site of previous penetrating trauma suggests *S. aureus* as the likely pathogen.

Erysipelas is a superficial infection involving the upper dermis and is primarily due to infection with GABHS. Tender, warm, intensely erythematous plaques with well-demarcated, indurated borders and associated edema are characteristic findings. Fever is often present. Although erysipelas usually involves the lower extremities, the upper extremities and face also may be affected.

Cellulitis involves the deep dermis and subcutaneous fat tissue. In contrast to erysipelas, cellulitis is characterized by spreading erythema that is not well demarcated (**Figure 3**). As in erysipelas, edema, redness, warmth, fever, and leukocytosis often occur. If furuncles, carbuncles, or abscesses are present, cellulitis is usually due to *S. aureus*. **Table 10** provides additional cellulitis risk factors with microbiologic associations that should be considered in the appropriate clinical situation.

The diagnosis of skin infections is often based on clinical findings because a microbial diagnosis is established in only a few patients. Blood culture results are positive in only about 5% of patients and appear most helpful in those who appear toxic or are immunocompromised. Because of low yield and questionable accuracy, cultures obtained by punch biopsy or needle aspiration of a lesion are not routinely performed. Most cases of diffuse, nontraumatic cellulitis with nondiagnostic culture results are due to β-hemolytic streptococci and typically respond to β-lactam antibiotics. Purulent cellulitis is more suggestive of staphylococcal disease and should be treated empirically with effective therapy against methicillin-resistant *S. aureus* (MRSA) infection. Recommended empiric antimicrobial agents for outpatients with a community-associated (CA)-MRSA skin or soft tissue infection include trimethoprim-sulfamethoxazole, a tetracycline (for example, doxycycline), clindamycin, and linezolid. **H**

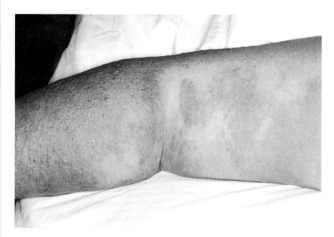

FIGURE 3. Spreading, undemarcated erythema of cellulitis; purulent drainage or exudate may also be present.

TABLE 10. Cellulitis Pathogens Associated with Specific Behaviors/Risk Factors

Pathogen	Risk Factor	Comment
Aeromonas hydrophila	Contact with or participation in recreational sports in freshwater lakes, streams, rivers (including brackish water); contact with leeches	Cellulitis nonspecific in clinical appearance; minor trauma to skin usually leads to inoculation of organism
Vibrio vulnificus, other *Vibrio* species	Contact with salt water or brackish water; contact with drippings from raw seafood	May cause cellulitis through direct inoculation into skin or may be ingested, leading to bacteremia with secondary skin infection. Hallmark is hemorrhagic bullae in area of cellulitis lesion(s)
Erysipelothrix rhusiopathiae	Contact with saltwater marine life (can also infect freshwater fish)	Cellulitis usually involves the hand or arm, and occurs in those handling fish, shellfish, or occasionally, poultry or meat contaminated with bacterium. Causes erysipeloid disease
Pasteurella multocida	Contact primarily with cats	Cellulitis occurs as a result of cat scratch or bite
Capnocytophaga canimorsus	Contact primarily with dogs	Cellulitis and sepsis particularly in patients with hyposplenism
Bacillus anthracis	Target of bioterrorism	Edematous pruritic lesion with central eschar; spore-forming organism
Francisella tularensis	Contact with or bite from infected animal (particularly cats); arthropod bites (particularly ticks)	Ulceroglandular syndrome characterized by ulcerative lesion with central eschar and localized tender lymphadenopathy; constitutional symptoms often present
Mycobacterium marinum	Contact with fresh water or salt water, including fish tanks and swimming pools	Lesion often trauma-associated and often involving upper extremity; papular lesions become ulcerative at site of inoculation; ascending lymphatic spread can be seen ("sporotrichoid" appearance); systemic toxicity usually absent

KEY POINTS

- The presence of lymphangitis and a "peau d'orange" appearance of the skin are more consistent with streptococcal infection, whereas an abscess or drainage from an existing wound or site of previous penetrating trauma is more suggestive of staphylococcal infection.

- The diagnosis of skin infections is often clinical because a microbial diagnosis is established in only a few patients.

Community-Associated Methicillin-Resistant *Staphylococcus aureus*

CA-MRSA is a significant public health problem. Most CA-MRSA isolates contain genes encoding for multiple toxins, including cytotoxins that result in leukocyte destruction and tissue necrosis. CA-MRSA most often causes purulent skin and soft tissue infections (SSTI) and, less commonly, pneumonia. Healthy young persons tend to be infected, and outbreaks occur in athletes, prison inmates, men who have sex with men, children in day care centers, injection drug users, homeless persons, and military personnel, particularly when close contact or crowded conditions exist. CA-MRSA is now the most common identifiable cause of SSTI in patients seen in the emergency department. These genetically distinct CA-MRSA strains are also replacing MRSA strains as causes of infection in hospitals and other health care settings. The emergence of CA-MRSA has affected empiric treatment of SSTI because these new strains have distinct antibiotic susceptibility patterns.

Clinical practice guidelines by the Infectious Diseases Society of America have been published for the management of SSTI in the era of CA-MRSA. Incision and drainage is the primary therapy for a cutaneous abscess. Antibiotic treatment is also recommended when (1) patients are very young or elderly; (2) multiple sites of infection, systemic illness, comorbidities, or immunosuppression is present; (3) infection quickly progresses and is associated with concomitant cellulitis; (4) there is poor response to incision and drainage; or (5) abscesses are in locations where they are difficult to drain, such as the face, genitalia, or hand. Empiric therapy for CA-MRSA is indicated for patients with purulent cellulitis.

Oral antibiotic agents for outpatient treatment of CA-MRSA include clindamycin, trimethoprim-sulfamethoxazole, tetracyclines, and linezolid. However, clindamycin resistance among patients with CA-MRSA should be monitored locally, and some experts recommend avoiding empiric

CONT.

therapy with clindamycin when local resistance rates exceed 10% to 15%. In addition, results of susceptibility testing for clindamycin may be misleading, with treatment failures reported in patients in whom the isolate was shown to be susceptible to clindamycin but resistant to erythromycin. Fluoroquinolones are not recommended because of the concern for development of MRSA resistance during treatment as well as the increased prevalence of resistance already observed in many areas. Only linezolid and clindamycin also provide reliable coverage for β-hemolytic streptococci. When patients require hospitalization for a complicated SSTI, such as deep infection, infected burns and ulcers, and surgical wound infections, surgical debridement and broad-spectrum antibiotics, including those with coverage for MRSA, should be considered. Appropriate antibiotics for empiric MRSA coverage in this setting include vancomycin, daptomycin, telavancin, ceftaroline, and linezolid. **H**

KEY POINTS

- Community-associated methicillin-resistant *Staphylococcus aureus* most often causes purulent skin and soft tissue infection and, less commonly, pneumonia.

- The emergence of community-associated methicillin-resistant *Staphylococcus aureus* has affected empiric treatment of skin and soft tissue infections because these new strains have distinct antibiotic susceptibility patterns.

- Incision and drainage is the primary therapy for a cutaneous abscess in patients with community-associated methicillin-resistant *Staphylococcus aureus* infection, and possibly, depending on the extent and severity of infection, antibiotic treatment.

H Necrotizing Fasciitis

Necrotizing fasciitis is an SSTI that extends beyond the epidermis, dermis, and subcutaneous fat tissues to involve the fascia and, potentially, the underlying muscle. This life-threatening infection is often classified according to its associated microbiologic findings. Type I necrotizing fasciitis is a polymicrobial infection usually encompassing a combination of streptococci, staphylococci, aerobic gram-negative bacilli, and anaerobes such as *Clostridium*, *Bacteroides*, and *Peptostreptococcus* species. One example of type I necrotizing fasciitis is perineal fasciitis, also known as Fournier gangrene. Type II necrotizing fasciitis is a monomicrobial infection typically caused by *Streptococcus pyogenes* ("flesh-eating bacteria"). Other bacteria that can cause a similar infection are *Vibrio vulnificus*, *S. aureus*, and *Streptococcus agalactiae*. *V. vulnificus* is a curved gram-negative rod found in warm coastal waters such as the Gulf of Mexico. Patients who are immunocompromised, especially those with iron overload syndromes such as cirrhosis, are at increased risk for developing

necrotizing fasciitis secondary to *V. vulnificus* after ingestion of raw or undercooked shellfish or after traumatized skin is exposed to contaminated sea water (**Figure 4**). Clostridial myonecrosis, or gas gangrene, is a similarly presenting necrotizing infection that is differentiated by muscle involvement. This infection is usually associated with trauma, recent surgery, or injection drug use and is caused primarily by *Clostridium perfringens*, although other *Clostridium* species have been reported.

Necrotizing fasciitis is often associated with a preexisting skin infection or trauma, including chronic vascular or pressure ulcers (for example, diabetic foot ulcers) and surgical wounds. However, an obvious portal of entry may not be evident. Necrotizing fasciitis usually involves the lower extremities, followed by the upper extremities, but any site can be affected (**Figure 5**).

Cutaneous manifestations may initially include erythematous lesions associated with significant pain and edema. The severity of pain is often disproportionate to the visible skin findings. The lesions may rapidly increase in size and develop a violaceous, bullous, and gangrenous appearance. Palpation of affected areas may demonstrate "woody" induration and crepitus as a result of soft tissue–associated gas. Patients may be toxic, with fever, hypotension, mental status changes, tachycardia, leukocytosis, and laboratory evidence of multi-organ dysfunction. Streptococcal-associated necrotizing fasciitis is associated with toxic shock syndrome in up to 50% of patients. Anesthesia may develop in the affected area as a result of localized nerve necrosis.

Clinical suspicion of necrotizing fasciitis is important in directing early evaluation, including surgical consultation. Evidence of systemic inflammation, including elevations of the total leukocyte count, erythrocyte sedimentation rate, and serum C-reactive protein level, is often present, and the serum creatine kinase level may also be increased. MRI of the

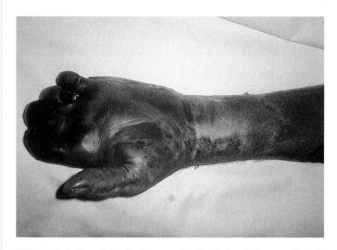

FIGURE 4. Necrotizing fasciitis secondary to *Vibrio vulnificus*, manifested as hemorrhagic bullous lesions.

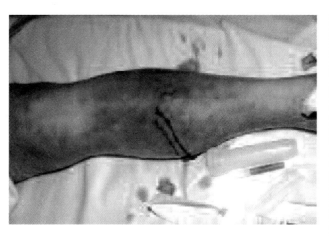

FIGURE 5. Necrotizing fasciitis of the left calf of an elderly patient with peripheral arterial disease.

CONT.

affected area can localize and determine the extent of fascial plane involvement. Blood cultures and staining of wound-associated tissue may be helpful.

Because mortality rates range from 30% to 70% and are increased when surgery is delayed, timely surgical exploration is essential to determine the extent of necrosis and debride all necrotic tissue; sometimes, surgery is pursued when the diagnosis is uncertain. Cultures of infected tissue should be obtained during surgical intervention. Repeat surgical evaluation is pursued in most patients 24 to 36 hours later and continued daily as indicated.

In addition to supportive care and surgery, empiric broad-spectrum antibiotics are appropriate for patients with suspected necrotizing fasciitis. Initial therapy should include coverage for *S. aureus* (including MRSA), streptococci, gram-negative bacilli, and anaerobes. Regimens consisting of an anti-MRSA agent such as vancomycin or daptomycin or linezolid plus (1) piperacillin-tazobactam, (2) cefepime and metronidazole, or (3) a carbapenem (for example, meropenem or imipenem) are reasonable. Clindamycin should be part of the initial regimen when infection due to GABHS or clostridia is suspected. When type II necrotizing fasciitis secondary to GABHS or clostridial myonecrosis is present, combined therapy with both penicillin and clindamycin is indicated. Clindamycin may be beneficial in early treatment because of its ability to suppress toxin production, although 5% or more of streptococci and staphylococci may be resistant to this drug. Antibiotics can be discontinued once surgical debridement is no longer needed and clinical improvement is evident.

Studies regarding use of intravenous immune globulin (IVIG) to treat streptococcal necrotizing fasciitis are conflicting. To date, there are no definitive recommendations for use of IVIG in patients with necrotizing fasciitis, although some experts recommend its use in patients with associated toxic shock or a high risk of death.

- Cutaneous manifestations of necrotizing fasciitis often initially include erythematous lesions associated with significant pain and edema.

- Timely surgical exploration is essential in patients with necrotizing fasciitis to determine the extent of necrosis and debride all necrotic tissue.

- Empiric broad-spectrum antibiotics are appropriate for patients with suspected necrotizing fasciitis.

Toxic Shock Syndrome

Toxic shock syndrome (TSS) is an uncommon, and potentially fatal, infection caused by toxin-producing staphylococci and streptococci. Menstruation-associated staphylococcal TSS was described in the 1980s in women who used tampons. Nonmenstruation-associated staphylococcal TSS occurs in patients with surgical and obstetrical wound infections, sinus infection with nasal packings, osteomyelitis, skin ulcers, burns, and pneumonia and in injection drug users. Clinical features may include chills, malaise, fever, hypotension, erythematous rash, and multi-organ involvement (**Table 11**). Patients may have no localizing signs of infection when systemic toxicity develops.

TABLE 11. Diagnostic Criteria for Staphylococcal Toxic Shock Syndrome

The presence of:
Fever >38.9 °C (102.0 °F)
Systolic blood pressure less than 90 mm Hg
Diffuse macular rash with subsequent desquamation, especially on palms and soles
Involvement of three of the following organ systems:
Gastrointestinal (nausea, vomiting, diarrhea)
Muscular (severe myalgia or fivefold or greater increase in serum creatine kinase level)
Mucous membrane (hyperemia of the vagina, conjunctivae, or pharynx)
Kidney (blood urea nitrogen or serum creatinine level at least twice the upper limit of normal)
Liver (bilirubin, aspartate aminotransferase or alanine aminotransferase concentration twice the upper limit of normal)
Blood (platelet count <100,000/μL [100 × 10⁹/L])
Central nervous system (disorientation without focal neurologic signs)
Negative serologies for Rocky Mountain spotted fever, leptospirosis, and measles; negative cerebrospinal fluid cultures for organisms other than *Staphylococcus aureus*

μL = microliter.

Adapted with permission from Moreillon P, Aue Y-A, Glauser MP. *Staphylococcus aureus.* In: Mandell GL, Dolin R, Bennett JE, eds. Principles and Practice of Infectious Disease. 6th ed. Philadelphia, PA: Churchill Livingstone; 2005:2331. Copyright 2005, Elsevier.

CONT.

Streptococcal TSS can occur secondary to infection with any β-hemolytic streptococcus, although *S. pyogenes* is most common. Most cases occur in the setting of SSTIs, although streptococci may also gain entry through mucous membranes such as in pharyngitis. Surgical procedures, blunt trauma with hematoma and ecchymoses, influenza and varicella infections, and NSAID use have also been associated with this syndrome. A portal of entry may not be evident in about 50% of patients. The diagnostic criteria for streptococcal TSS are found in **Table 12**. Bacteremia is more common and mortality rates are higher in patients with streptococcal TSS than in those with staphylococcal TSS.

Patients with TSS require early supportive therapy and treatment of any underlying infection. Site management may include debridement and removal of foreign bodies. Empiric broad-spectrum antibiotics similar to those given for necrotizing fasciitis should be administered until the pathogen or pathogens are identified. Once culture results are known, antibiotic coverage can be targeted. Because of its ability to inhibit toxin production and modulate production of tumor necrosis factor, clindamycin is also included when either staphylococcal or streptococcal involvement is suspected. IVIG is sometimes recommended for treatment of streptococcal TSS based on observational data that showed better survival in patients treated with IVIG. Hyperbaric oxygen may also be helpful as adjunctive therapy, but more studies are needed before its standard use is recommended.

Secondary transmission of GABHS-induced TSS to close contacts of patients has been reported. Contact isolation precautions should be initiated for patients with suspected or known invasive GABHS-induced disease, including TSS and necrotizing fasciitis, until 24 hours of antibiotic therapy has been completed. Although not routinely recommended, postexposure penicillin-based prophylaxis may be considered for household contacts of patients with invasive GABHS

infection, including those who are older than 65 years of age or have conditions associated with an increased risk of developing invasive infection (for example, diabetes mellitus, cardiac disease, varicella infection, cancer, HIV infection, corticosteroid use, or injection drug use).

KEY POINT

- Patients with toxic shock syndrome require early supportive care, treatment of any underlying infection, possible debridement and removal of foreign bodies, and administration of empiric broad-spectrum antibiotics until microbial identification is made.

Animal Bites

Animal bites are responsible for 1% of all visits to the emergency department in the United States. Approximately 5% to 20% of these bites are infected. Complications include formation of abscesses, soft tissue infection, tenosynovitis, septic arthritis, osteomyelitis, and bacteremia. The animal involved and the location of the bite are important. Dog bites are less likely to become infected than cat bites. Infections after a bite are due to oral flora of the animal and microorganisms present on the skin of the patient. Infections after dog and cat bites are usually due to a mix of aerobic and anaerobic microorganisms. Staphylococci and streptococci are reported in approximately 40% of bite wounds, and anaerobes commonly found in the oral flora of both cats and dogs, including *Bacteroides*, *Porphyromonas*, and *Prevotella* species, are reported in these infections. *Pasteurella* species, particularly *P. multocida*, are gram-negative coccobacilli that are frequently isolated from wounds after cat and dog bites, scratches, or licks. *Capnocytophaga canimorsus* is a gram-negative rod that can cause overwhelming sepsis, most often in patients with asplenia, following a dog or cat bite or scratch.

A thorough history of both the patient and the animal is needed in the evaluation of patients with animal bites. The type of animal involved, the circumstances under which the attack occurred, the timing of the bite, and the health status of the animal are important. The patient's immune status, including tetanus and rabies immunization history, use of immunosuppressive medications, and presence of any immunocompromising disorders, should be determined. Physical examination should identify the location and extent of injury; evidence of necrosis or crush injury; presence of edema, erythema, or purulent discharge; nerve involvement; and range of motion and function. Adequate wound irrigation and debridement are required, and the need for additional tetanus and rabies prophylaxis is determined. Radiographic evaluation is obtained when bone involvement is possible, crepitus is present, or foreign bodies are suspected.

TABLE 12. Diagnostic Criteria for Streptococcal Toxic Shock Syndrome
Definite Case:
Isolation of GABHS from a sterile site
Probable Case:
Isolation of GABHS from a nonsterile site
Hypotension
The presence of two of the following findings:
Kidney (acute kidney insufficiency or failure)
Liver (elevated aminotransferase concentrations)
Skin (erythematous macular rash, soft tissue necrosis)
Blood (coagulopathy, including thrombocytopenia and disseminated intravascular coagulation)
Pulmonary (acute respiratory distress syndrome)
GABHS = group A β-hemolytic streptococci.

Antibiotic prophylaxis should be considered for any immunocompromised patient and for patients who have wounds on the hands or near a joint or bone, moderate or severe wounds at any site, significant crush injuries, or wounds with associated edema. A 3- to 5-day course of amoxicillin-clavulanate is recommended. Patients with a β-lactam allergy may be given a fluoroquinolone or doxycycline or trimethoprim-sulfamethoxazole plus an anti-anaerobic agent such as clindamycin.

Antibiotics are given when wounds are infected. Patients not requiring hospitalization can be treated with the same oral agents used for prophylaxis. Hospitalization is needed for patients with severe or deep infections; nerve, tendon, or crush injuries; or infected hand bites. Intravenous antibiotic regimens may include β-lactam/β-lactamase combinations, cefoxitin, or carbapenems. Patients who are allergic to penicillin can be treated with a fluoroquinolone plus clindamycin. The addition of agents such as vancomycin can be considered in patients with suspected infection caused by MRSA. Therapy is usually required for less than 2 weeks, although longer courses of 3 to 4 weeks for joint infection and at least 4 to 6 weeks for bone infection are appropriate.

Cat-scratch disease is an infection that most often occurs in immunocompetent children and young adults following inoculation of the fastidious gram-negative bacterium *Bartonella henselae* after a cat scratch or bite. A pustule or papule or erythema develops at the site of inoculation several days to 2 weeks after the scratch or bite. Significant tender regional lymphadenopathy, occasionally suppurative, develops 2 to 3 weeks after inoculation in areas that drain the infected site. The lymphadenopathy generally resolves within months, and extranodal disease is rare. The diagnosis is often made clinically, although a laboratory diagnosis is possible through culture, serology, histopathology, or nucleic acid–based testing. Although cat-scratch disease is generally a self-limited infection when antibiotics are not given, some experts recommend a short course of antibiotic therapy, usually with azithromycin.

KEY POINTS

- Dog bites are less likely to become infected than cat bites.
- Following a dog or cat bite, adequate wound irrigation and debridement are required, and the need for tetanus and rabies prophylaxis is determined.
- Antibiotic prophylaxis following a dog or cat bite should be considered for any immunocompromised patient and for patients who have wounds on the hands or near a joint or bone, moderate or severe wounds at any site, significant crush injuries, or wounds with associated edema.
- Antibiotics should be given to all patients with an infected dog or cat bite.

Human Bites

Human bite wounds are categorized as self-inflicted, occlusional, or clenched-fist injuries. Self-inflicted wounds such as paronychia are incidental and result from thumb sucking or nail biting. Occlusional bite wounds result from intentional bites, usually in the setting of a confrontation, and often involve the fingers (in particular the index or middle finger), hand, and other upper extremity locations. Clenched-fist injuries result from a punch to the mouth of another person and commonly cause a traumatic laceration of the third, fourth, or fifth metacarpal head.

Infection caused by human oral flora is typically polymicrobial, including α-hemolytic streptococci, staphylococci, *Haemophilus* species, and *Eikenella corrodens,* as well as anaerobes, many of which produce β-lactamases.

Initial evaluation and management are similar to that for animal bites and should also include evaluation for potentially transmissible pathogens, including those causing HIV infection, herpes simplex virus infection, syphilis, and hepatitis B and C virus infection. Patients who have human bite wounds without evidence of infection should receive prophylactic amoxicillin-clavulanate for 3 to 5 days. Patients with clenched-fist injuries require particular attention because such injuries are prone to deeper infection involving the tendons, joints, and bone. In these patients, radiographic evaluation, consultation with a hand surgeon to determine the need for exploration of the wound, and possibly, hospitalization, are indicated. Broad-spectrum antibiotics with anaerobic coverage such as β-lactam/β-lactamase inhibitors, cefoxitin, or carbapenems can be administered empirically. Vancomycin can be considered for patients with risk factors for MRSA infection.

KEY POINTS

- Patients who have human bite wounds without evidence of infection should receive prophylactic amoxicillin-clavulanate for 3 to 5 days.
- Patients with clenched-fist injuries usually require radiographic evaluation, consultation with a hand surgeon, and possibly, hospitalization.

Diabetic Foot Infections

Foot infections are common in patients with diabetes mellitus because of the neuropathy, vascular insufficiency, and immunodeficiency associated with this disease. Most infections begin after trauma and are categorized as mild, moderate, or severe.

Mild infections are most often caused by staphylococci and streptococci.

Findings include purulence or inflammation (pain, tenderness, warmth, erythema, and induration) and cellulitis that extends no deeper than the superficial soft tissue and spreads 2 cm or less around the ulcer. Systemic findings are absent.

Patients with moderate infections have cellulitis that extends beyond 2 cm around the ulcer, gangrene, lymphangitic spread, deep tissue abscess, or deep tissue spread, including extension to the muscle, joint, tendon, or bone. Systemic findings are absent. Severe infections are limb-threatening and are associated with metabolic instability or systemic toxicity, such as fever, tachycardia, hypotension, kidney insufficiency, mental status changes, and leukocytosis. These more extensive infections are usually polymicrobial, including staphylococci, streptococci, enteric gram-negative bacilli, *Pseudomonas aeruginosa*, and anaerobes.

Ulcers that are clinically uninfected (that is, without purulence or inflammation) should not be treated with antibiotics. In the absence of recent antibiotic use, most patients with mild and many with moderate diabetic foot infections can receive empiric treatment with a short course of oral antibiotics directed against aerobic gram-positive staphylococci and streptococci, similar to skin infections in nondiabetic individuals. Severe limb-threatening infections require surgical evaluation and initial broad-spectrum antibiotic coverage commensurate with the severity of the systemic findings. Definitive antibiotic treatment should be adjusted based on results of cultures obtained from deeper tissue during surgical debridement or by aspiration. Superficial swab cultures are misleading and should be avoided.

Two common problems are usually encountered in patients with significant diabetic foot infections: (1) arterial insufficiency from macrovascular complications of diabetes, and (2) osteomyelitis. An assessment for possible arterial insufficiency (see MKSAP 16 Cardiovascular Medicine) should be undertaken. Evaluation for potential bone infection is more challenging, because bone changes related to neuropathy and Charcot changes (bony abnormalities due to repeated trauma) can mimic osteomyelitis. The role of MRI to identify occult osteomyelitis has not been fully resolved, but the presence of bone infection usually becomes apparent over time, as wound healing is poor or drainage recurs after ulcer closure. Wound care consisting of wound cleansing, debridement, and off-loading of local foot pressure is essential for optimal healing of all diabetic foot wounds and is often best managed with close involvement of podiatrists and wound care specialists.

KEY POINTS

- Diabetic foot ulcers that are clinically uninfected should not be treated with antibiotics.
- Mild and many moderate diabetic foot infections can be treated with a short course of oral antibiotics directed against aerobic gram-positive staphylococci and streptococci.
- Severe diabetic foot infections are limb-threatening and require surgical evaluation and initial broad-spectrum antibiotic coverage commensurate with the severity of the systemic findings.

Community-Acquired Pneumonia

Epidemiology

Community-acquired pneumonia (CAP) is defined as an acute pneumonia occurring in persons who have not been hospitalized recently and are not living in facilities such as nursing homes. Underlying disease such as chronic bronchitis and COPD, cardiovascular disease, and diabetes mellitus increases the risk of CAP. Smokers are at increased risk for invasive pneumococcal infections even if they do not have structural lung disease. Other risk factors include alcoholism and the presence of neurologic diseases that increase the risk of aspiration. With few exceptions (for example, *Legionella* pneumonia due to inhalation of contaminated aerosolized water), CAP is caused by microaspiration of organisms that may colonize the oropharynx, which often occurs during sleep. In contrast, aspiration pneumonia refers to pneumonia that occurs following a large-volume aspiration of gastric contents, which results in a chemical pneumonitis followed by a bacterial infection.

CAP occurs most commonly in elderly patients; 60% of all hospitalizations for pneumonia occur in patients over 65 years of age. Additional risk factors in this age group include cardiopulmonary disease, poor functional status, low weight, and recent weight loss. Pneumonia is the eighth leading cause of death in the United States and the most common cause of death from an infectious disease. The mortality rate for outpatients with CAP is less than 5%; the mortality rate for inpatients is 10% but can be as high as 30% for patients who are admitted to the intensive care unit (ICU).

The cost of caring for patients with CAP is estimated to exceed 17 billion dollars annually. Various aspects of caring for hospitalized patients are considered quality indicators, and hospital performance influences reimbursement to health care institutions by Medicare and other third-party payers. Guidelines are available to direct antibiotic selection in patients with CAP and are discussed later. Numerous studies have shown that use of guideline-concordant antibiotics is associated with decreased mortality rates in hospitalized patients. A marked reduction in 30-day mortality rates in elderly patients with CAP from 1987 to 2005 has recently been reported. Greater use of pneumococcal and influenza vaccination and use of guideline-concordant antibiotics are hypothesized as possible explanations for this reduction, although it has never been shown that pneumococcal vaccination reduces mortality from pneumonia in this population.

KEY POINT

- Community-acquired pneumonia occurs most often in elderly patients; 60% of all hospitalizations for pneumonia are in patients over 65 years of age.

Microbiology

Streptococcus pneumoniae is the most commonly documented pathogen in patients with CAP and the most frequent cause of bacteremic pneumonia acquired in the community. *Haemophilus influenzae* and *Moraxella catarrhalis* are also common pathogens. Other gram-negative organisms are responsible for a small proportion of cases of CAP. Enteric gram-negative bacilli can cause CAP in patients with chronic medical comorbidities, chronic liver disease, and alcoholism. *Klebsiella pneumoniae* is reported in patients with alcoholism. *Pseudomonas aeruginosa* is a potential cause of CAP in patients with chronic underlying structural lung disease (such as bronchiectasis or cystic fibrosis), frequent exacerbations of severe COPD, and a history of long-term corticosteroid therapy, but many such patients have risk factors for health care–associated pneumonia. *Staphylococcus aureus*, including community-associated methicillin-resistant *S. aureus* infection (CA-MRSA), is a less common potential cause of CAP. *S. aureus* should be considered when CAP occurs following influenza, in patients with cavitary pneumonia in whom there are no risk factors for aspiration, in injection drug users, and in patients with a recent history of a CA-MRSA skin and soft tissue infection.

Regardless of antimicrobial susceptibility, CAP due to *S. aureus* is associated with a higher mortality rate and more prolonged length of stay compared with CAP from other causes. *Mycoplasma pneumoniae* and *Chlamydophila pneumoniae* infection are more likely to occur in outpatients with CAP. *Legionella* infection must be considered, especially in cases of severe CAP and in patients with a recent history of travel. *Legionella* infections are more common in the summer and sometimes occur in epidemics when a common-source reservoir aerosolizes bacteria that are inhaled by susceptible patients. Respiratory viruses, including influenza, parainfluenza, respiratory syncytial virus, and adenovirus, may cause CAP. Outbreaks of severe CAP due to adenovirus type 14 have recently been described. Epidemiologic history that should prompt consideration of less common pathogens is outlined in **Table 13**.

KEY POINTS

- *Streptococcus pneumoniae* is the most frequently documented pathogen in patients with community-acquired pneumonia; *Haemophilus influenzae* and *Moraxella catarrhalis* are also common.

- Community-acquired pneumonia due to *Staphylococcus aureus* is associated with higher mortality rates and more prolonged hospitalizations compared with community-acquired pneumonia due to other pathogens.

Diagnosis

The acute onset of cough (especially with purulent sputum production), fever, chills, pleuritic chest pain, and dyspnea is characteristic of pneumonia. The presentation may be much more nonspecific in elderly patients, who may present with confusion or an exacerbation of an underlying chronic cardiopulmonary disease. Tachypnea is the most sensitive finding suggesting pneumonia in this age group.

When obtaining a history in patients with suspected CAP, risk factors for health care–associated pneumonia, such as antibiotic therapy or hospitalization in the preceding 90 days, must be excluded. Any epidemiologic exposures that might suggest the possibility of unusual pathogens must also be determined.

Clinical findings alone are not sufficient to confirm a diagnosis of pneumonia; a chest radiograph should be obtained in all patients. In patients who have a clinical presentation compatible with pneumonia and focal auscultatory findings on chest examination, an initial normal chest radiograph, although uncommon, should not exclude the diagnosis of CAP. A repeat chest radiograph in 24 to 48 hours may show airspace disease.

The role of routine diagnostic testing to determine the microbial cause of CAP is controversial. The Infectious Diseases Society of America/American Thoracic Society (IDSA/ATS) Consensus Guidelines suggest that microbiologic diagnostic testing is optional in outpatients. In patients who are hospitalized but not in the ICU, diagnostic testing is recommended for those in whom outpatient antibiotic therapy was ineffective and for those with cavitary infiltrates, alcoholism, chronic liver disease, functional or anatomic asplenia, severe obstructive or structural lung disease, or leukopenia. The *Legionella* urine antigen test should also be performed in patients with a recent travel history. Diagnostic testing is considered optional in other hospitalized patients.

There is strong consensus that patients with CAP who require ICU admission should have blood cultures, sputum Gram stain and culture (or culture of an endotracheal aspirate in intubated patients), and pneumococcal and *Legionella* urine antigen testing. The sensitivity of the pneumococcal urine antigen test is 70%, with a specificity as high as 96%, and the test has a rapid turnaround time. Although the *Legionella* urine antigen test detects only *L. pneumophila* serogroup 1, this strain is responsible for 85% or more of cases of legionellosis. Reported sensitivity of this test varies from 70% to 90%, with a specificity of 99%.

Blood culture results are positive in 5% to 14% of hospitalized patients with CAP. Obtaining blood culture samples before antibiotic therapy is begun is one of the Medicare quality of care indicators for CAP. Data indicate that obtaining blood cultures is associated with lower mortality rates in patients older than 65 years of age. Patients with a large pleural effusion on presentation (typically defined as an effusion occupying half or more of the hemithorax on an upright chest radiograph or a fluid level of more than 1 cm on lateral decubitus films) should undergo thoracentesis; in addition, these patients should have blood and sputum cultures and pneumococcal and *Legionella* urine antigen tests. Studies to date have not demonstrated a significant

TABLE 13. Possible Microbial Causes of Community-Acquired Pneumonia

Clinical Presentation	Commonly Encountered Pathogens
Aspiration	Gram-negative enteric pathogens, oral anaerobes
Cough >2 weeks with whoop or posttussive vomiting	*Bordetella pertussis*
Lung cavity infiltrates	Community-associated methicillin-resistant *Staphylococcus aureus*, oral anaerobes, endemic fungal pathogens, *Mycobacterium tuberculosis*, atypical mycobacteria

Epidemiology or Risk Factor	Commonly Encountered Pathogens
Alcoholism	*Streptococcus pneumoniae*, oral anaerobes, *Klebsiella pneumoniae*, *Acinetobacter* species, *M. tuberculosis*
COPD and/or smoking	*Haemophilus influenzae*, *Pseudomonas aeruginosa*, *Legionella* species, *S. pneumoniae*, *Moraxella catarrhalis*, *Chlamydophila pneumoniae*
Exposure to bat or bird droppings	*Histoplasma capsulatum*
Exposure to birds	*Chlamydophila psittaci*
Exposure to rabbits	*Francisella tularensis*
Exposure to farm animals or parturient cats	*Coxiella burnetii*
Exposure to rodent excreta	Hantavirus
HIV infection (early)	*S. pneumoniae, H. influenzae, M. tuberculosis*
HIV infection (late)	Those with early HIV infection plus *Pneumocystis jirovecii*, *Cryptococcus, Histoplasma, Aspergillus*, atypical mycobacteria (especially *Mycobacterium kansasii*), *P. aeruginosa*
Hotel or cruise ship stay in previous 2 weeks	*Legionella* species
Travel or residence in southwestern United States	*Coccidioides* species, hantavirus
Travel or residence in Southeast and East Asia	*Burkholderia pseudomallei*
Influenza activity in community	Influenza, *S. pneumoniae, Staphylococcus aureus, H. influenzae*
Injection drug use	*S. aureus*, anaerobes, *M. tuberculosis, S. pneumoniae*
Endobronchial obstruction	Anaerobes, *S. pneumoniae, H. influenzae, S. aureus*
Bronchiectasis or cystic fibrosis	*Burkholderia cepacia, P. aeruginosa, S. aureus*
Bioterrorism	*Bacillus anthracis, Yersinia pestis, Francisella tularensis*

Adapted with permission from Mandell LA, Wunderink RG, Anzueto A, et al; Infectious Diseases Society of America; American Thoracic Society. Infectious Diseases Society of America/American Thoracic Society consensus guidelines on the management of community-acquired pneumonia in adults. Clin Infect Dis. 2007;44 Suppl 2:S27-72. [PMID: 17278083] Copyright 2007, Oxford University Press.

 CONT.

difference between empiric therapy and pathogen-directed therapy, except among patients in the ICU. Pathogen-directed therapy, however, does allow for focusing and reducing antibiotic coverage, which may be associated with fewer adverse effects. Confirming an etiologic diagnosis may be especially helpful when patients fail to respond to antibiotic therapy.

The role of inflammatory biomarkers such as procalcitonin in the diagnosis and management of pneumonia remains investigational. **H**

KEY POINTS

- The acute onset of cough (especially with purulent sputum production), fever, chills, pleuritic chest pain, and dyspnea is characteristic of community-acquired pneumonia.
- The presence of tachypnea is the most sensitive finding suggesting pneumonia in elderly patients.

- Blood cultures, sputum Gram stain and culture, and pneumococcal and *Legionella* urine antigen testing are indicated for patients with community-acquired pneumonia who require admission to an intensive care unit.

Management
Site of Care

Deciding whether to hospitalize a patient for treatment of CAP has a major impact on the cost of care, because the greatest expenditure for treating CAP occurs among hospitalized patients. Studies have shown that most patients with CAP prefer outpatient treatment, if possible.

Several scoring systems are available to help determine mortality risk to guide decisions regarding the need for hospitalization. The CURB-65 score uses five indicators of severity of illness (confusion, blood urea nitrogen level >20 mg/dL (7.14 mmol/L), respiration rate ≥30/min, systolic blood pressure <90 mm Hg or diastolic blood pressure <60 mm Hg, and age ≥65 years). One point is scored for each positive indicator. Patients with a score of 0 or 1 have a low mortality risk and can be considered for outpatient treatment. Those with a score of 2 or more should be hospitalized. Patients with a score of 3 or more should be considered for admission to the ICU. The Pneumonia Severity Index (PSI) assigns patients to one of five mortality risk groups. Patients in PSI risk groups I and II are generally treated as outpatients. Those in risk group III may require brief hospitalization for observation, whereas those in risk groups IV and V generally require hospital admission. The calculation of the PSI score includes 20 different variables and therefore requires access to a decision support tool (http://pda.ahrq.gov/clinic/psi/psicalc.asp).

Studies have shown that both scoring systems perform well in terms of predicting mortality. For predicting the risk of mortality, recent investigation suggests that the negative predictive value of these scoring systems is greater than the positive predictive value. Both the PSI and the CURB-65 scores have been shown to predict the time to clinical stability in hospitalized patients with CAP.

Prediction rules are only one part of clinical decision-making concerning when and whether to hospitalize patients with pneumonia. Some patients with a low mortality risk may still require admission because of inadequate social support, exacerbation of underlying chronic pulmonary or cardiovascular disease, inability to tolerate oral therapy, or other indicators of severity of illness not accounted for in the scoring systems. Pulse oximetry should be performed to document the adequacy of oxygenation in individuals who will be managed as outpatients.

CAP is considered severe when a patient requires initial admission to the ICU or early transfer to the ICU. Ways of identifying patients with severe CAP at the time of presentation are being studied because delayed ICU admission is an independent predictor of in-hospital mortality in such patients, and greater than 50% of ICU deaths due to CAP occurs in patients who were initially admitted to the medical ward. The IDSA/ATS guidelines propose major and minor criteria for admission to the ICU. The major criteria include the need for mechanical ventilation and vasopressor support. The minor criteria incorporate the original ATS minor criteria for severe CAP and the CURB-65 criteria (**Table 14**). It is currently proposed that patients with three or more minor criteria should be admitted to the ICU. These criteria have not undergone extensive prospective validation, although recent investigation has shown that the negative predictive value of the severe CAP minor criteria is greater than 90%.

TABLE 14. IDSA/ATS Minor Criteria for Severe Community-Acquired Pneumonia

Clinical Criteria
Confusion (new-onset disorientation to person, place, or time)
Hypothermia (core temperature <36.0 °C [96.8 °F])
Respiration rate ≥30/min[a]
Hypotension necessitating aggressive fluid resuscitation
Multilobar pulmonary infiltrates

Laboratory Criteria
Arterial Po_2/Fio_2 ratio ≤250[a]
Leukopenia (<4000 cells/μL [4.0 × 10⁹/L])
Thrombocytopenia (<100,000 /μL [10 × 10⁹/L])
Blood urea nitrogen >20 mg/dL (7.1 mmol/L)

μL = microliter; IDSA/ATS = Infectious Diseases Society of America/American Thoracic Society.

[a]A patient who requires noninvasive positive-pressure ventilation should be considered to meet this criterion.

Reprinted with permission from Mandell LA, Wunderink RG, Anzueto A, et al; Infectious Diseases Society of America; American Thoracic Society. Infectious Diseases Society of America/American Thoracic Society consensus guidelines on the management of community-acquired pneumonia in adults. Clin Infect Dis. 2007;44 Suppl 2:S27-72. [PMID: 17278083] Copyright 2007, Oxford University Press.

Antibiotic Therapy

Most patients with CAP are treated empirically. Even if a microbial diagnosis is eventually confirmed, initial antibiotic therapy needs to be chosen based on limited information. The selection of antibiotic therapy depends on the site of care (outpatient, medical ward, or ICU) and the presence of risk factors for certain pathogens.

In outpatients, risk factors for drug-resistant *S. pneumoniae* influence the selection of empiric therapy. These risk factors include age older than 65 years, recent (within the past 3 months) β-lactam therapy, medical comorbidities, immunocompromising conditions and immunosuppressive therapy, alcoholism, and exposure to a child in day care. Recommendations for outpatient antibiotic therapy for CAP are provided in **Table 15**. A treatment duration of 5 to 7 days is appropriate for most outpatients.

TABLE 15. Antibiotic Therapy for Community-Acquired Pneumonia in Outpatients

Risk Factors	Treatment
Previously healthy and no risk factor(s) for drug-resistant *Streptococcus pneumoniae*	Macrolide (azithromycin, clarithromycin, or erythromycin) or doxycycline
Risk factor(s) for drug-resistant *S. pneumoniae* or underlying comorbidities	Respiratory fluoroquinolone (moxifloxacin, gemifloxacin, or levofloxacin) **or** β-lactam[a] plus a macrolide or doxycycline

[a]Amoxicillin, 1 g every 8 hours, or amoxicillin-clavulanate, 2 g every 12 hours (preferred), or cefpodoxime or cefuroxime, 500 mg twice daily (alternative).

CONT.

Recommendations for empiric antibiotic therapy for inpatients (medical ward and ICU) are provided in **Table 16**. The selection of empiric antibiotics for patients with severe CAP is influenced by the presence of risk factors for *P. aeruginosa* and CA-MRSA infection. Antibiotic coverage for possible *P. aeruginosa infection* is appropriate for patients with severe CAP who have a sputum Gram stain that shows gram-negative rods. Empiric antibiotics should include coverage for CA-MRSA in patients with a compatible sputum Gram stain.

For patients with a confirmed microbial cause of CAP, therapy is directed at the isolated pathogen (**Table 17**). Several retrospective studies have suggested that combined β-lactam and macrolide therapy is potentially beneficial in patients with bacteremic pneumococcal pneumonia. Suggested explanations for this benefit include the possibility of coinfection with an atypical pathogen and the anti-inflammatory effect of macrolides, independent of their antimicrobial activity. No prospective clinical trials of combination therapy have been undertaken to date.

The timing of initial empiric antibiotic therapy for hospitalized patients is one of the quality of care indicators by Medicare and other third-party payers. Starting antibiotics within 6 hours of presentation is indicated, based on studies that showed decreased mortality rates among Medicare patients who received antibiotic therapy within 8 hours of presentation and a second analysis that showed decreased mortality rates if antibiotic therapy was begun within 4 hours of presentation. Some experts, however, are concerned that too much emphasis on meeting time criteria for antibiotic administration may increase unnecessary antibiotic use. The IDSA/ATS guidelines simply recommend giving the first dose of antibiotics while the patient is still in the emergency department.

In hospitalized patients, intravenous antibiotic therapy can be changed to oral therapy when criteria for clinical stability are met (temperature ≤37.8 °C [100.0 °F], pulse rate ≤100/min, respiration rate ≤24/min, systolic blood pressure ≥90 mm Hg, arterial oxygen saturation ≥90% or Po_2 ≥ 60 mm Hg [7.9 kPa] on ambient air, ability to tolerate oral intake, and normal mental status). Once patients are ready to switch to oral therapy, they can be safely discharged without observation on oral therapy unless an underlying comorbidity is present requiring continued hospitalization. A 7-day course of therapy (including therapy received during hospitalization) is sufficient for most patients, provided the initial antibiotic was active against the isolated pathogen. More prolonged therapy is required for patients who take longer to become clinically stable, those with cavitary pneumonia, and those with pneumonia due to *S. aureus* or *P. aeruginosa*. Patients with pneumococcal bacteremia do not require a more prolonged course of intravenous antibiotic therapy, although they may take longer to become clinically stable. When indicated, patients should receive pneumococcal and influenza vaccination during their hospitalization for CAP, as vaccination is part of the pneumonia quality of care indicators.

Complications

Failure to improve after initial empiric therapy may be because of misdiagnosis of CAP (for example, cryptogenic organizing pneumonia, vasculitis, pulmonary embolism) or to a resistant pathogen. Patients with persistent fever and those who initially improve and then relapse require evaluation for a

TABLE 16. Empiric Antibiotic Therapy for Community-Acquired Pneumonia in Inpatients	
Inpatient Setting	**Treatment**
Medical ward	β-lactam[a] plus a macrolide or doxycycline; **or** respiratory fluoroquinolone (moxifloxacin, gemifloxacin or levofloxacin)
Intensive care unit	β-lactam[b] plus either azithromycin or a fluoroquinolone[c]; if penicillin-allergic, a respiratory fluoroquinolone[d] plus aztreonam
If risk factor(s) for *Pseudomonas aeruginosa* or gram-negative rods on sputum Gram stain	Antipseudomonal β-lactam with pneumococcal coverage (cefepime, imipenem, meropenem, or piperacillin-tazobactam) plus ciprofloxacin or levofloxacin (750 mg); **or** antipseudomonal β-lactam with pneumococcal coverage plus an aminoglycoside plus azithromycin; **or** antipseudomonal[e] β-lactam with pneumococcal coverage plus an aminoglycoside plus a respiratory fluoroquinolone
If risk factor(s) for CA-MRSA or compatible sputum Gram stain	Add vancomycin or linezolid to β-lactam[b] plus either azithromycin or a fluoroquinolone[c]

CA-MRSA = community-associated methicillin-resistant *Staphylococcus aureus*.

[a]Cefotaxime, ceftriaxone, or ampicillin; ertapenem is an alternative in patients with an increased risk of enteric gram-negative pathogens (not *P. aeruginosa*).

[b]Cefotaxime, ceftriaxone, or ampicillin-sulbactam.

[c]Moxifloxacin, gemifloxacin, ciprofloxacin, or levofloxacin.

[d]Moxifloxacin, gemifloxacin, or levofloxacin.

[e]Aztreonam can be used in a patient with a severe β-lactam allergy.

TABLE 17. Pathogen-Specific Therapy for Community-Acquired Pneumonia

Pathogen	Preferred Therapy	Alternative Therapy
Streptococcus pneumoniae		
Penicillin MIC <2 µg/mL	Penicillin G, amoxicillin	Macrolide, oral[a] or parenteral[b] cephalosporin, doxycycline, respiratory fluoroquinolone[c]
Penicillin MIC ≥2 µg/mL	Cefotaxime, ceftriaxone, respiratory fluoroquinolone[c]	Vancomycin, linezolid, and 3 g/d amoxicillin if penicillin MIC ≤4 µg/mL
Haemophilus influenzae		
β-Lactamase negative	Amoxicillin	Fluoroquinolone, doxycycline, azithromycin, clarithromycin[d]
β-Lactamase positive	Second- or third-generation cephalosporin, amoxicillin-clavulanate	Fluoroquinolone, doxycycline, azithromycin, clarithromycin
Mycoplasma pneumoniae, _Chlamydophila pneumoniae_	Macrolide, tetracycline	Fluoroquinolone
Legionella species	Fluoroquinolone, azithromycin	Doxycycline
Enterobacteriaceae	Use the most appropriate narrow-spectrum agent appropriate for treatment of pneumonia based on susceptibility test results in vitro	
Pseudomonas aeruginosa	Antipseudomonal β-lactam plus aminoglycoside or ciprofloxacin or levofloxacin (based on susceptibility test results in vitro)	Aminoglycoside plus ciprofloxacin or levofloxacin (based on susceptibility test results in vitro)
Staphylococcus aureus		
Methicillin susceptible	Nafcillin	Cefazolin, clindamycin[e]
Methicillin resistant	Vancomycin[f] or linezolid	Trimethoprim-sulfamethoxazole

MIC = minimal inhibitory concentration; µg = micrograms.

[a]Cefpodoxime, cefprozil, cefuroxime, cefdinir, cefditoren.

[b]Cefuroxime, cefotaxime, ceftriaxone.

[c]Levofloxacin, gemifloxacin, moxifloxacin.

[d]Azithromycin is more active in vitro than clarithromycin against _H. influenzae_.

[e]If susceptibility is documented, including disk diffusion test (D-test) if erythromycin resistant.

[f]Consider alternative if vancomycin MIC is ≥2 micrograms/mL.

Adapted with permission from Mandell LA, Wunderink RG, Anzueto A, et al. Infectious Diseases Society of America/American Thoracic Society consensus guidelines on the management of community-acquired pneumonia in adults. Clin Infect Dis. 2007;44(Suppl 2):S27-72. Copyright 2007, Oxford University Press.

possible parapneumonic effusion or empyema. Up to one third of patients hospitalized for the treatment of CAP develop a parapneumonic effusion. Thoracentesis to exclude a complicated parapneumonic effusion or empyema is necessary only if patients fail to respond clinically. Drug fever or a nosocomial infection should be considered in patients who have a persistent fever.

Follow-up

Follow-up chest imaging is not indicated in most patients who improve with treatment. However, a follow-up chest radiograph should be considered to document clearance of pulmonary infiltrates and determine the presence of a possible pulmonary malignancy 6 to 8 weeks after completing treatment for patients who are older than 40 years of age and for smokers. In a recent study, 9.2% of patients hospitalized for pneumonia were diagnosed with a pulmonary malignancy following hospitalization. The median time to diagnosis was 297 days; only 27% were diagnosed within 90 days of admission. Smokers should receive counseling regarding smoking cessation. Such counseling is one of the quality of care indicators for pneumonia. The success of any smoking intervention is modest, but the association of smoking with pneumonia and with progressive lung disease makes this a logical time for counseling.

Outpatients and hospitalized patients who were treated for CAP should generally have a follow-up office visit 10 to

14 days after completing therapy. Hospitalized patients who required more than 3 days to become clinically stable are at increased risk for rehospitalization and death and require early follow-up after initial discharge. Studies have shown that the median time for resolution of respiratory symptoms in patients with CAP is 14 days. However, one third of patients continue to have at least one pneumonia-related symptom at 28 days. Patients who recover from an episode of CAP are at significantly increased risk of dying, although the leading causes of death are comorbidities such as COPD and cardiovascular disease.

KEY POINTS

- Most patients with community-acquired pneumonia are treated empirically; the selection of antibiotic therapy depends on the site of care and the presence of risk factors for certain pathogens.

- In outpatients with community-acquired pneumonia, risk factors for drug-resistant *Streptococcus pneumoniae* influence the selection of empiric antibiotic therapy.

- When indicated, hospitalized patients with community-acquired pneumonia should receive pneumococcal and influenza vaccinations.

- In patients with community-acquired pneumonia, failure to improve after initial empiric therapy may be because of misdiagnosis of community-acquired pneumonia or a resistant pathogen.

Tick-Borne Diseases

Lyme Disease

Lyme disease is the most common arthropod-borne infection in the United States, with 22,561 confirmed cases reported in 2010. The incidence varies geographically, and hyperendemic areas in the northeast and north central United States reflect the geographic density of the vector deer tick, *Ixodes scapularis*, in these areas (**Figure 6**). The causative spirochete is *Borrelia burgdorferi sensu stricto*, which is transmitted to humans following vector tick attachment and feeding. Because the nymphal deer tick is so small, fewer than 50% of infected patients recall a tick attachment. Deer ticks may also serve as vectors for other tick-borne infections (**Table 18**), and coinfection may occur.

Lyme disease has three distinct stages: early localized, early disseminated, and late (**Table 19**). The clinical manifestations of Lyme disease depend on the stage of infection. Early localized Lyme disease typically occurs 1 to 2 weeks following infection. The initial clinical manifestation is erythema migrans (EM), an erythematous skin lesion at the site of tick attachment that is noted in 70% to 80% of patients with confirmed infection (**Figure 7**). Classically, the border of EM expands over several days, and the lesion often develops central clearing, leading to the description of a "target" or "bulls-eye" appearance. Atypical EM may present as a confluent erythematous macule that sometimes has a vesicular or necrotic

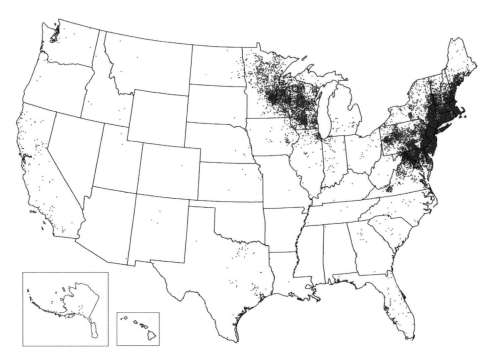

FIGURE 6. Geographic distribution of Lyme disease cases in the United States, 2010.

Courtesy of the Centers for Disease Control and Prevention. Accessed on June 14, 2012, at www.cdc.gov/ncidod/dvbid/lyme/ld_Incidence.htm.

TABLE 18. Selected Human Tick-Borne Diseases in the United States

Disease	Pathogen	Vector	Predominant United States Geographic Distribution
Lyme disease	*Borrelia burgdorferi*	Deer tick	Northeast and north central
Babesiosis	*Babesia microti*	Deer tick	Northeast and north central
Southern tick–associated rash illness	Unknown	Lone Star tick	Southeast, south central, and mid-Atlantic
Human monocytic ehrlichiosis	*Ehrlichia chaffeensis*	Lone Star tick	Southeast, south central, and mid-Atlantic
Human granulocytic anaplasmosis	*Anaplasma phagocytophilum*	Deer tick	Northeast and north central
Rocky Mountain spotted fever	*Rickettsia rickettsii*	Dog tick	Continental

eschar in the center. Secondary cellulitis that develops at the site of tick attachment may also mimic EM.

If early localized Lyme disease is not treated, progression to later stages may occur. Early disseminated Lyme disease is associated with spirochetemia that develops several weeks after the initial infection. Patients frequently present with a febrile illness associated with myalgia, headache, fatigue, and lymphadenopathy. Multiple EM lesions are common at this stage and are found at anatomic sites distinct from the initial

tick attachment. Localized infection associated with early disseminated Lyme disease may involve the heart and central nervous system. Lyme myocarditis is reported in 5% of untreated patients and ranges from asymptomatic first-degree heart block to complete heart block. Conduction abnormalities due to Lyme disease are reversible and respond to antibiotics. Neurologic manifestations of early disseminated Lyme disease include cranial nerve palsy (unilateral or bilateral), aseptic meningitis, and radiculopathy.

TABLE 19. Clinical Presentation and Treatment of Lyme Disease

Clinical Manifestations	Diagnostic Testing	Antibiotic Formulation and Duration (see also Table 20)
Early Localized Stage (Incubation period: 3-30 days)		
EM at site of tick attachment	Visualization of EM	Oral , 14-21 days[a]
Early Disseminated Stage (Incubation period: 3-6 weeks)		
Multiple EM lesions distinct from site of tick attachment	ELISA with confirmatory Western blot	Oral, 14-21 days
Cranial nerve palsy (unilateral or bilateral)	ELISA with confirmatory Western blot	Oral, 14-21 days
Meningitis	ELISA with confirmatory Western blot	IV, 10-28 days
Myocarditis	ELISA with confirmatory Western blot	First-degree heart block, asymptomatic: oral, 14-21 days
		Second-degree AV or complete heart block: IV followed by oral (once patient is stabilized), 14-21 days
Late Stage (Incubation Period: Months to Years)		
Arthritis	ELISA with confirmatory Western blot, PCR of synovial fluid	Oral, 28 days
Recurrent arthritis after treatment	Western blot, PCR of synovial fluid	Oral or IV, 28 days
Encephalopathy or encephalomyelitis	ELISA with confirmatory Western blot, PCR of cerebrospinal fluid (low sensitivity)	IV, 14-28 days
Post-Lyme Disease Syndrome		
Nonspecific headache, arthralgia, fatigue	None	Supportive care; antibiotics not indicated

AV = atrioventricular; ELISA = enzyme-linked immunosorbent assay; EM = erythema migrans; IV = intravenous; PCR = polymerase chain reaction.

[a]Range of 10-21 days if doxycycline is used, 14-21 days for alternative agents.

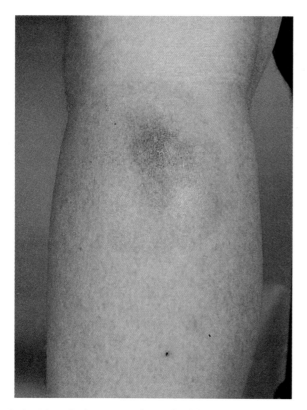

FIGURE 7. Erythema migrans lesion of early localized Lyme disease manifested as "target lesion" with central clearing.

Late-stage Lyme disease occurs in as many as 60% of untreated patients. Lyme arthritis is characterized by migratory monoarticular or oligoarticular inflammation, which often improves spontaneously and then recurs in the same joint or another joint months to years later. The knee is involved in 85% of patients. In the United States, late neurologic complications are rare, and affected patients usually present with an encephalopathy with deficits in cognition and short-term memory.

The diagnosis of early localized Lyme disease is clinical and is based on visualization of the EM skin lesion. Serologic testing is not recommended at this stage, because a measurable antibody response may not have had time to develop. However, laboratory confirmation of infection is required for all later stages of Lyme disease. Detection of antibodies against *B. burgdorferi* using a two-stage approach is recommended. The initial test is an enzyme-linked immunosorbent assay (ELISA), which is sensitive but not sufficiently specific for diagnosis. A positive or equivocal ELISA should therefore be followed by a confirmatory Western blot to detect antibodies directed against specific *B. burgdorferi* epitopes. Interpretation of the Western blot is standardized and is based on the absolute number of positive bands. Testing for IgM antibody to *B. burgdorferi* should be restricted to patients with less than 1 month of symptoms, because an isolated IgM antibody titer in the absence of detectable IgG

antibody after this period likely represents a false-positive test result. Neurologic involvement is supported by cerebrospinal fluid (CSF) pleocytosis and a positive ratio of CSF to serum antibodies or a positive CSF polymerase chain reaction (PCR), although CSF PCR must be considered experimental in the diagnosis of central nervous system Lyme disease.

Serologic testing for Lyme disease should be restricted primarily to patients with clinically suggestive signs or symptoms (other than erythema migrans) who reside in or have traveled to an endemic area. The finding of *B. burgdorferi* antibodies in patients who have nonspecific symptoms of fatigue or myalgia or who are unlikely to have been exposed to a vector tick likely represents a false-positive test result. Serologic testing following a tick bite in an asymptomatic patient is not indicated. Because *B. burgdorferi* antibodies remain positive indefinitely, serial testing is also not recommended.

Treatment recommendations vary and are based on the disease stage and organ involvement (**Table 20**); (see also Table 19). Empiric doxycycline is the recommended treatment of erythema migrans. Post–Lyme disease syndrome, sometimes erroneously called "chronic Lyme disease," presents a particular treatment challenge. This syndrome refers specifically to patients with confirmed Lyme disease, based on stringent clinical and laboratory criteria, who have persistent constitutional symptoms despite appropriate antibiotic treatment. Supportive therapy to ameliorate symptoms is appropriate for these patients, but prolonged durations or repeated courses of antibiotics (oral or intravenous) are ineffectual and strongly discouraged.

KEY POINTS

- The initial clinical manifestation of Lyme disease is erythema migrans, which is an erythematous skin lesion at the site of tick attachment.

- Although serologic studies are not recommended for diagnosing early localized Lyme disease, two-stage laboratory testing (enzyme-linked immunosorbent assay followed by confirmatory Western blot when the initial screening test is positive or equivocal) is required for the diagnosis of all later stages of infection.

- Serologic testing for Lyme disease should be restricted to patients with clinically suggestive signs or symptoms who either reside in or have traveled to an endemic area.

- The finding of *B. burgdorferi* antibodies in patients who have nonspecific symptoms of fatigue or myalgia or who are unlikely to have been exposed to a vector tick likely represents a false-positive test result for Lyme disease.

TABLE 20. Preferred Antibiotic Treatment of Lyme Disease

Antibiotic	Dosage
Oral regimens	
Doxycycline[a]	100 mg twice daily
Amoxicillin	500 mg three times daily
Cefuroxime	500 mg twice daily
Parenteral regimen	
Ceftriaxone	2 g daily

[a]Doxycycline is also active against *Anaplasma phagocytophilum* and is the preferred agent for patients ages 8 years and older who are not pregnant or breast-feeding.

Data from Wormser GP, Dattwyler RJ, Shapiro ED, et al. The clinical assessment, prevention, and treatment of Lyme disease, human granulocytic anaplasmosis, and babesiosis: clinical practice guidelines by the Infectious Diseases Society of America. Clin Infect Dis. 2006;43(9):1089-1134 [PMID: 17029130] Copyright 2006 Oxford University Press. Used with permission.

Babesiosis

Babesiosis is a tick-borne protozoal infection. The geographic distribution of babesiosis due to *Babesia microti*, the most common pathogen, corresponds to that of Lyme disease (see Figure 6) because both infections are transmitted by the same vector tick species. Other *Babesia* species cause clinically similar infections but are endemic to the northwestern and midwestern United States. Person-to-person transmission may occur after transfusion of infected blood products from an asymptomatic donor. Following infection, protozoa persist and replicate inside human erythrocytes. Most infections with *B. microti* are asymptomatic and, when infection is clinically apparent, symptoms range from a self-limited febrile illness to fulminant multiorgan system failure and death.

Patients with mild infection present with fever and findings related to hemolysis, including splenomegaly, hepatomegaly, and jaundice. Asplenic patients tend to have high levels of parasitemia and more severe disease. Other risk factors for more severe disease include older age, HIV infection, and other immunocompromised states. The clinical presentation in patients with severe babesiosis may include profound hemolytic anemia, acute kidney injury, disseminated intravascular coagulation, high-output heart failure, and circulatory collapse.

Laboratory findings reflect the presence of hemolysis and include a macrocytic anemia (due to increased numbers of reticulocytes), increased serum bilirubin level, decreased haptoglobin concentration, and increased serum lactate dehydrogenase level. Thrombocytopenia and elevated serum liver enzyme values are also common.

The preferred method for diagnosing babesiosis is PCR using whole blood specimens, which is more sensitive than direct microscopy. Visualization of intraerythrocytic ring forms on a thin-preparation blood smear is suggestive of babesiosis, but differentiation from falciparum malaria may be difficult if the patient has a compatible travel history for both infections. Serologic testing is not recommended because seroconversion may lag behind onset of clinical symptoms, or conversely, detectable antibodies may reflect a previous asymptomatic infection.

Treatment is indicated for all symptomatic patients with laboratory confirmation of infection as well as for asymptomatic patients with documented persistence of parasites for more than 3 months. Treatment regimens for patients with mild disease include the combination of atovaquone and azithromycin or quinine and clindamycin; the former regimen is better tolerated. Quinine combined with clindamycin is the treatment of choice for severe disease, and exchange transfusion is recommended for patients with greater than 10% parasitemia. Symptoms typically respond rapidly to therapy but may recur in immunocompromised patients.

KEY POINTS

- Babesiosis may be asymptomatic and when clinically apparent ranges from a self-limited febrile illness to fulminant multiorgan system failure and death.

- The preferred method for diagnosing babesiosis is polymerase chain reaction on whole blood specimens, which is more sensitive than direct microscopy.

- Treatment regimens for patients with mild babesiosis include the combination of atovaquone and azithromycin or quinine and clindamycin.

Southern Tick–Associated Rash Illness

Southern tick–associated rash illness (STARI) is clinically indistinguishable from the early localized form of Lyme disease. However, STARI occurs in a geographically distinct distribution in the southeast, mid-Atlantic, and south central United States. Results of testing in patients with STARI will be negative for *B. burgdorferi* infection. The causative agent has not been identified, but the vector appears to be the Lone Star tick, *Amblyomma americanum*.

The primary clinical manifestation of STARI is an EM skin lesion that is often associated with fever, headache, and myalgia. Much like the early localized form of Lyme disease, the diagnosis of STARI is clinical and is based on recognition of the classic EM lesion. Treatment with doxycycline is recommended, although disease progression to later stages has not been reported in untreated patients.

KEY POINTS

- The distinguishing clinical manifestation of Southern tick–associated rash illness is erythema migrans, which is often associated with fever, headache, and myalgia.

- Doxycycline is the recommended treatment for Southern tick–associated rash illness.

Ehrlichiosis and Anaplasmosis

Human monocytic ehrlichiosis (HME) and human granulocytic anaplasmosis (HGA) are clinically similar tick-borne rickettsial diseases that occur in geographically distinct areas of the United States. The different distribution is based on the endemicity of the vector ticks (see Table 18). Both diseases usually occur within 1 to 2 weeks after inoculation and are characterized by a nonfocal febrile illness with frequent headache, myalgia, and fatigue. Skin lesions are described in fewer than 30% of adults with HME and are very uncommon in patients with HGA. The most common skin lesion in patients with HME is a maculopapular rash, but a petechial eruption similar to that seen with Rocky Mountain spotted fever has been described (see Figure 8, discussed below). Meningoencephalitis is also more frequent in patients with HME, occurring in 20% of these patients.

Both HME and HGA are associated with leukopenia (particularly lymphopenia), thrombocytopenia, and elevated serum liver enzyme values. The abnormal liver enzyme findings may lead to the erroneous diagnosis of acute cholecystitis and possible unnecessary surgical intervention. In patients with clinical signs suggestive of meningoencephalitis, the CSF typically shows a lymphocytic pleocytosis with a mildly elevated protein concentration; rarely, CSF findings suggestive of bacterial meningitis have been reported.

The causative agents, *Ehrlichia chaffeensis* and *Anaplasma phagocytophilum*, are trophic for monocytes and neutrophils, respectively. In approximately 20% of patients, the diagnosis is suggested by the presence of intraleukocytic clusters of bacteria (morulae) on a buffy coat stain. Antibodies are seldom detected at the time of acute infection and appear 2 to 4 weeks following clinical illness. Because treatment delay has been associated with increased mortality rates for both HME and HGA, empiric antibiotics should be started when either infection is suspected clinically, followed by laboratory confirmation later if necessary.

Doxycycline, 100 mg twice daily for 7 to 14 days, is used to treat HME and HGA. Symptoms respond to treatment within 24 to 72 hours, and an alternative diagnosis should be considered if defervescence does not occur during this time. **H**

KEY POINTS

- Both human monocytic ehrlichiosis and human granulocytic anaplasmosis are characterized by a nonfocal febrile illness with frequent headache, myalgia, and fatigue.
- Results of serologic testing may be negative in patients with acute human monocytic ehrlichiosis and human granulocytic anaplasmosis infection but may be positive 2 to 4 weeks after development of clinical illness if the diagnosis requires confirmation.
- Treatment of human monocytic ehrlichiosis and human granulocytic anaplasmosis should be initiated when infection is suspected because treatment delays are associated with poorer outcomes.
- Doxycycline is the treatment of choice for both human monocytic ehrlichiosis and human granulocytic anaplasmosis.

Rocky Mountain Spotted Fever **H**

Rocky Mountain spotted fever (RMSF) is a tick-borne rickettsial disease found throughout the contiguous United States. The incubation period following infection ranges from 2 to 14 days. Fever is almost always present and is variably accompanied by headache, myalgia, confusion, and gastrointestinal symptoms. The characteristic finding of RMSF is a petechial rash (**Figure 8**). The rash is ultimately identified in 90% of patients but is present at the onset of fever in only 15%. Initial skin findings are nonblanching macules on the wrists and ankles that progress over days to a petechial skin eruption involving the trunk, extremities, palms, and soles, but sparing the face. Skin lesions do not occur in 10% of patients, and the absence of lesions is a risk factor for an adverse outcome, presumably because of delay in recognizing the infection and initiating treatment.

Laboratory findings in patients with RMSF include thrombocytopenia and elevated serum liver enzyme values. In contrast to ehrlichiosis and anaplasmosis, leukocyte counts tend to be normal. Patients with RMSF meningoencephalitis typically have a lymphocytic pleocytosis.

Serologic testing is generally used for diagnosis. However, seroconversion often lags behind the onset of clinical symptoms. A fourfold rise in antibody titer or seroconversion noted on a convalescent serum sample obtained 2 to 4 weeks after the acute illness is considered diagnostic. Immunohistochemical studies of a skin biopsy specimen showing *Rickettsi rickettsii* may confirm the diagnosis at the time of presentation. Doxycycline should be started empirically whenever RMSF is suspected and should not be withheld or discontinued based on serologic test results. **H**

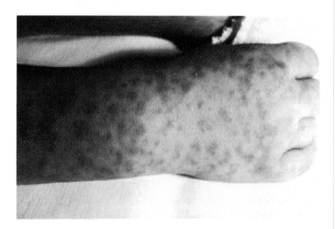

FIGURE 8. Petechial skin lesions associated with Rocky Mountain spotted fever.

Picture courtesy of Centers for Disease Control and Prevention. Accessed on June 14, 2012, at www.cdc.gov/rmsf/symptoms/index.html.

Urinary Tract Infections

Epidemiology and Microbiology

Urinary tract infection (UTI) is defined as inflammation of the uroepithelium that involves the lower urinary tract (cystitis), upper urinary tract (pyelonephritis), or both. In the United States, UTIs account for approximately 100,000 hospital admissions each year at a cost of 1.6 billion dollars annually. UTIs are more common in women than in men, with most occurring between the ages of 16 and 35 years. One in three women will have a UTI by age 24 years, and recurrence rates are reported to be as high as 45%. Bacteremia develops in approximately 2% to 4% of patients with nosocomial UTIs, which is associated with a 13% mortality rate. In addition, increased antimicrobial resistance among causative pathogens is posing management challenges in outpatient and hospital settings.

Escherichia coli, the most common pathogen causing UTIs, is responsible for approximately 85% of cases. In addition, coagulase-negative staphylococci such as *Staphylococcus saprophyticus* may cause approximately 10% of UTIs. Gram-negative bacilli other than *E. coli* account for approximately 5% of UTIs. Gram-negative bacilli such as *Proteus*, *Pseudomonas*, *Klebsiella*, and *Enterobacter* species are frequent pathogens in recurrent UTIs and UTIs associated with structural urinary tract abnormalities. Multiple pathogens may be isolated when structural abnormalities are present.

Multidrug-resistant pathogens are more common in hospitalized patients, kidney transplant recipients, and patients with underlying urologic abnormalities, previous UTIs, recent antibiotic treatment, or immunocompromising conditions. Fungi, such as *Candida* species, are more frequent pathogens in patients with diabetes mellitus or chronic indwelling urinary catheters and those receiving antibiotics.

KEY POINTS

- Urinary tract infections are more common in women than in men; one in three women will have a urinary tract infection by age 24 years.

- *Escherichia coli* is the causative pathogen in 85% of urinary tract infections.

Diagnosis

UTIs are categorized as uncomplicated or complicated. An uncomplicated UTI is an infection occurring in a normal urinary tract and generally responds well to conventional antimicrobial treatment. Complicated UTIs are infections that occur in patients with structural or functional urinary tract abnormalities and are seen most often in infants, older patients, patients with indwelling urinary catheters, and those with renal calculi. Patients with spinal cord injuries, diabetes mellitus, multiple sclerosis, and AIDS are also more likely to develop complicated UTIs. In general, UTIs in pregnant women and men are considered to be complicated. Complicated UTIs may be associated with multidrug-resistant pathogens and require radiographic investigation more often than do uncomplicated UTIs.

Symptoms of UTI vary widely depending on patient age and severity of infection. Symptoms may include dysuria, frequency, nocturia, enuresis, urgency, hematuria, low back pain, suprapubic pain, flank pain, fever, chills, rigors, and in the elderly, new incontinence and altered mental status.

Definitive laboratory diagnosis requires microscopic urinalysis. The presence of 10 or more leukocytes/microliter of unspun urine from a midstream, clean-catch sample indicates significant pyuria and is indicative of a UTI. The presence of hematuria is helpful in the differential diagnosis because this finding is suggestive of a UTI but not of vaginitis or urethritis.

Urine dipsticks for detecting the presence of leukocyte esterase (suggesting pyuria) and nitrite (produced by bacteria in the urine) are clinically convenient and relatively reliable in confirming infection, particularly if both indicators are positive and the patient has signs or symptoms consistent with UTI. However, in clinical circumstances suggestive of UTI, negative or discordant findings cannot exclude infection, and microscopic analysis is warranted.

Urine culture is usually not needed for patients with an uncomplicated UTI because a treatment response to antimicrobial agents will have occurred before the results become available. A urine culture should be obtained in (1) patients with suspected pyelonephritis, a complicated UTI, or recurrent UTIs (not associated with sexual activity); (2) patients for whom routine treatment may not be available (for example, because of allergies); or (3) patients in whom the presence of a resistant organism is strongly suspected. Cultures are recommended for pregnant women with asymptomatic bacteriuria and for all patients before urologic manipulation. The presence of 10^5 or more colony-forming units (CFU) of bacteria/mL of urine from a midstream, clean-catch sample indicates significant bacteriuria and is diagnostic of UTI in most patients. However, in women with acute dysuria and pyuria, a urine culture yielding 10^2 or more CFU of bacteria/mL is diagnostic of UTI. Recovery of mixed bacteria from a single urine culture sample suggests contamination.

Urologic investigation, including CT and/or ultra-sonography, is not necessary for most patients with UTI but is indicated for those with pyelonephritis who have persistent flank pain or fever after 72 hours of antimicrobial therapy to exclude a perinephric or intrarenal abscess. Older men with recurrent UTIs should also undergo urologic investigation to rule out structural defects, including prostatitis.

KEY POINTS

- Uncomplicated urinary tract infections (UTIs) generally respond well to antimicrobial therapy, whereas complicated UTIs are often associated with multi-drug-resistant pathogens in patients with other comorbidities.
- The presence of 10 or more leukocytes/microliter of unspun urine from a midstream, clean-catch sample or a urine dipstick showing leukocyte esterase indicates significant pyuria and is indicative of a urinary tract infection.
- Urine culture is usually not needed for patients with an uncomplicated urinary tract infection because a treatment response to antimicrobial therapy will have occurred before the results become available.

Management

Cystitis in Women

Dysuria is the most frequent manifestation of cystitis in women and usually occurs together with one or more of the following: urgency, frequency, suprapubic pain, and hematuria. Fever is usually absent. The presence of pyuria is sufficient for diagnosing cystitis in young, sexually active, nonpregnant women. A urine culture should be performed if the diagnosis is unclear, the patient is pregnant, or the infection has recurred after treatment

Various antimicrobial agents are available for treating acute uncomplicated cystitis in women (**Table 21**). Fluoroquinolones and β-lactam agents are not recommended as first-line agents; the fluoroquinolones should be considered as alternative agents. Recommended antibiotics for treating cystitis in pregnant patients include amoxicillin and nitrofurantoin.

KEY POINTS

- Dysuria is the most common manifestation of acute cystitis in women, usually accompanied by urgency, frequency, suprapubic pain, or hematuria, but typically not fever.
- Trimethoprim-sulfamethoxazole, nitrofurantoin monohydrate macrocrystals, and fosfomycin are recommended for treating acute uncomplicated cystitis in women.

Recurrent Urinary Tract Infections in Women

Recurrent UTIs often occur in healthy, young, sexually active women who have a normal urinary tract. In some reports, more than 25% of women who experience their first UTI develop a recurrent infection within months. A recurrent UTI is classified as either a relapse or reinfection. A relapse is present if the current infection is caused by the same pathogen as the initial UTI and occurs within 2 weeks of completing the initial therapy. A reinfection is diagnosed if the current infection is caused by a different strain than that causing the initial UTI or if a urine culture sample was sterile between the two episodes of UTI. Most recurrences are reinfections. Risk factors that increase the likelihood for recurrent UTI include biologic (vaginal colonization with uropathogens), genetic (nonsecretor of ABH blood group antigens), and pelvic structure factors; frequency of sexual activity; spermicide use; a new sexual partner; a history of UTIs at or before age 15 years; and a family history of a mother with recurrent UTIs. Among postmenopausal women, risk factors include urinary incontinence, the presence of a cystocele or postvoid urine residual, and a history of UTIs before menopause.

Prevention strategies for recurrent UTIs include avoiding spermicides. Other factors that might decrease risk but have not been demonstrated to do so in controlled studies include postcoital voiding and liberal fluid intake. The role of cranberry juice in prevention remains unclear. Continuous or postcoital antimicrobial prophylaxis may be considered in patients with two or more symptomatic infections within 6 months or three or more episodes within 12 months. Management of these patients may also include early institution of self-treatment based on positive dipstick findings or clinical symptoms of UTI. Intravaginal estrogen cream is an option for postmenopausal women with recurrent UTIs.

TABLE 21. Recommended First-Line Antimicrobial Agents for Acute Uncomplicated Cystitis in Women

Agent	Dose and Duration	Comments
Trimethoprim-sulfamethoxazole	160/800 mg (one double-strength tablet) orally twice daily for 3 days	Avoid if resistance rates to uropathogens are >20% or if used to treat a urinary tract infection in preceding 3 months
Nitrofurantoin monohydrate macrocrystals	100 mg orally twice daily for 5 days	Avoid if pyelonephritis is suspected
Fosfomycin	3 g orally (single dose)	Has lower efficacy compared with some other agents; avoid if pyelonephritis is suspected

A urologic workup is generally not required for recurrent UTIs unless a structural or physiologic abnormality is suspected. Recurrent UTIs due to *Proteus* species may be associated with nephrolithiasis and require additional diagnostic studies. Multiple relapses due to the same pathogenic strain are also an indication for urologic workup.

KEY POINT

- Antimicrobial prophylaxis may be considered if recurrent urinary tract infections develop in women who have two or more symptomatic infections within 6 months or three or more episodes within 12 months.

Acute Pyelonephritis

Pyelonephritis is an inflammation of the renal parenchyma typically resulting from an ascending bladder infection. Clinical manifestations may include flank pain radiating to the groin, fever, chills, nausea, vomiting, and concurrent or antecedent symptoms of a lower UTI.

Empiric antimicrobial therapy should be initiated after a urine culture is obtained. When a patient does not require hospitalization, ciprofloxacin, 500 mg orally twice daily for 7 days, with or without an initial loading dose of ciprofloxacin, 400 mg intravenously, is an appropriate choice in geographic areas where fluoroquinolone resistance rates are less than 10%. In areas where fluoroquinolone resistance rates are higher, an initial single parenteral dose of a long-acting cephalosporin (such as ceftriaxone, 1 g) or a consolidated 24-hour dose of an aminoglycoside is also recommended prior to oral fluoroquinolone therapy. Oral β-lactam agents are less effective than other available agents for the treatment of pyelonephritis.

Patients with pyelonephritis requiring hospitalization should be treated initially with intravenous antimicrobial agents, including a fluoroquinolone (with the exception of moxifloxacin); an aminoglycoside with or without ampicillin; an extended-spectrum cephalosporin or extended-spectrum penicillin with or without an aminoglycoside; or a carbapenem. Choices should be based on local resistance data.

KEY POINTS

- Clinical manifestations of acute pyelonephritis include flank pain radiating to the groin, fever, chills, nausea, vomiting, and concurrent or antecedent symptoms of a lower urinary tract infection.
- In patients with acute pyelonephritis, empiric antimicrobial therapy should be administered after a urine culture is obtained.

Asymptomatic Bacteriuria

Asymptomatic bacteriuria is defined as the presence of specified numbers of bacteria in a urine specimen of an asymptomatic patient. Screening for and treatment of asymptomatic bacteriuria has been shown to be indicated only in pregnant women and men and women undergoing invasive urologic procedures. Screening for bacteriuria in other patient populations is not recommended and should not be a component of routine medical care.

KEY POINT

- Treatment of asymptomatic bacteriuria is recommended only for pregnant women and for men and women undergoing invasive urologic procedures.

Acute Prostatitis

Isolated bladder infection in men is rare. Often, bladder infection and symptoms of UTI are associated with acute bacterial prostatitis. Patients with acute prostatitis often develop a sudden febrile illness with chills, low back pain, or perineal pain accompanied by symptoms of a lower UTI. The diagnosis is based on clinical findings. Digital rectal examination often shows an edematous, tender prostate. Urinalysis often reveals pyuria and bacteriuria. A clean-catch urine culture is recommended to determine the causative pathogen. Enteric gram-negative pathogens are most common. Trimethoprim-sulfamethoxazole is the treatment of choice, and a fluoroquinolone (ciprofloxacin or levofloxacin) is an alternative option. The duration of therapy is typically 4 to 6 weeks.

KEY POINTS

- Clinical manifestations of acute prostatitis include a sudden febrile illness with chills, low back pain, or perineal pain accompanied by symptoms of a lower urinary tract infection.
- Trimethoprim-sulfamethoxazole is the antimicrobial agent of choice for treating acute prostatitis.

Mycobacterium tuberculosis Infection

Introduction

About two billion people worldwide are believed to have latent tuberculosis infection (LTBI), and each year about nine million people develop active disease. Public health approaches to control tuberculosis include primary prevention (isolating and treating patients with active disease and administering bacillus Calmette-Guérin [BCG] vaccine to persons at risk) and secondary prevention (treating patients with LTBI). Despite these measures, about two million people worldwide die of active disease each year. About 25% of those who die are coinfected with HIV.

Epidemiology

The number of new cases of tuberculosis reported yearly in the United States declined by about 58% from 1993 through 2010, when 11,182 cases were reported, representing an all-time low since reporting began in the United States in 1953. However, the percentage of cases in foreign-born persons increased during this period and constituted 60% of all cases in the United States in 2010. The rate of infection in foreign-born persons is 11 times higher than that of persons born in the United States. Eighty percent of all cases of tuberculosis in foreign-born persons living in the United States develop in Hispanics and Asians, and Mexico, the Philippines, India, Vietnam, and China are the top five countries of origin. Racial and ethnic minority groups are also disproportionately affected. In 2010, blacks or African Americans represented 40% of all new reported cases of tuberculosis in U.S.-born persons. Hispanics represent the largest proportion of total cases reported (29%).

KEY POINTS

- In the United States, the number of new cases of tuberculosis reported yearly declined by about 58% from 1993 through 2010.

- The rate of tuberculosis infection in foreign-born persons living in the United States is 11 times higher than that of persons born in the United States.

Pathophysiology

Mycobacterium tuberculosis is an acid-fast bacillus that causes primary tuberculosis infection when airborne respiratory droplets are inhaled and delivered to the terminal airways. Macrophages ingest the mycobacteria, which continue to multiply intracellularly and can potentially spread to other organs through the lymphatics and bloodstream. Most persons remain asymptomatic because their immune system contains the mycobacteria, and the only clues to the presence of infection are new reactivity to the tuberculin skin test (or interferon-γ release assay) or radiographic evidence such as localized scarring of the pulmonary parenchyma and lymph nodes (the Ghon complex). These findings indicate the presence of LTBI, which is not contagious. Progression to active disease can occur after initial infection (primary progressive tuberculosis) or by reactivation of LTBI. Without treatment, about 10% of persons infected with *M. tuberculosis* develop active tuberculosis during their lifetime, and approximately 50% of these persons will develop active disease within the first 2 years after being infected. Impairment of host defenses, such as in patients receiving immunosuppressive agents (corticosteroids or tumor necrosis factor antagonists) or those with HIV infection, diabetes mellitus, chronic kidney disease, malnutrition, and malignancy, increases the risk for primary progressive tuberculosis and reactivation of LTBI.

KEY POINTS

- Progression to active tuberculosis can occur after initial infection (primary progressive tuberculosis) or by reactivation of latent tuberculosis infection.

- Without treatment, about 10% of persons infected with *Mycobacterium tuberculosis* will develop active tuberculosis during their lifetime.

Clinical Manifestations

As noted earlier, patients with LTBI are asymptomatic. Although patients with LTBI do not have systemic manifestations of active tuberculosis, they are at increased risk for future development of active disease. Active disease is characterized by pulmonary and constitutional signs and symptoms (fever, night sweats, cough, chest pain, weight loss, and anorexia) that can develop insidiously. The cough is often chronic and can be nonproductive or productive, bloody, and purulent.

Findings on physical examination are nonspecific and range from normal to subtle to overtly abnormal, depending on the extent of parenchymal and pleural involvement. Immunocompromised patients, including those with HIV infection, often do not have typical signs and symptoms of tuberculosis and are more likely to develop extrapulmonary or disseminated disease. Extrapulmonary disease commonly involves the lymph nodes, bones, joints, and pleura. However, any site, including genitourinary, peritoneal, meningeal, pericardial, and laryngeal tissue, may be involved, and infection at these sites may mimic various other diseases.

KEY POINTS

- Patients with latent tuberculosis infection are asymptomatic.

- Patients with active tuberculosis may have pulmonary and constitutional signs and symptoms that can develop insidiously.

- Immunocompromised patients, including those with HIV infection, often do not have typical signs and symptoms of tuberculosis and are more likely to develop extrapulmonary or disseminated disease.

Diagnostic Testing

Two tests (discussed below) are available to detect LTBI: the Mantoux tuberculin skin test (TST) and interferon-γ release assays (IGRAs). However, neither test is able to distinguish between latent and active infection. Therefore, any individual with a positive test for LTBI should be carefully evaluated for the possibility of active infection.

In patients presenting with clinical findings consistent with active infection, in addition to a thorough history and physical examination, a test for *M. tuberculosis* infection; a chest radiograph; and microbiologic tests, including acid-fast stains and culture of clinical specimens, should be done.

TABLE 22. Interpretation of Tuberculin Skin Test Results

Criteria for Tuberculin Positivity by Risk Group		
≥5 mm Induration	**≥10 mm Induration**	**≥15 mm Induration**
HIV-positive persons Recent contacts of persons with active TB Persons with fibrotic changes on chest radiograph consistent with old TB Patients with organ transplants and other immunosuppressive conditions (receiving the equivalent of ≥15 mg/d of prednisone for >4 weeks)	Recent (<5 years) arrivals from high-prevalence countries Injection drug users Residents or employees of high-risk congregate settings: prisons and jails, nursing homes and other long-term facilities for the elderly, hospitals and other health care facilities, residential facilities for patients with AIDS, homeless shelters Mycobacteriology lab personnel; persons with clinical conditions that put them at high risk for active disease; children aged <4 years or exposed to adults in high-risk categories	All others with no risk factors for TB

TB = tuberculosis infection.

Tuberculin Skin Test

The Mantoux TST involves injecting purified protein derivative intradermally (usually into the volar aspect of the forearm) and assessing the skin response. Measurement of induration (not erythema) is determined 48 to 72 hours later and, when positive, indicates a delayed-type hypersensitivity response. To increase the specificity of the test, criteria for positivity are based on the patient's risk factors for infection with *M. tuberculosis* (**Table 22**). Patients with HIV infection or other serious immunocompromising conditions who are close contacts of persons with active tuberculosis should be treated for LTBI regardless of the results of a TST or IGRA once active disease has been excluded.

Causes of false-negative results of the TST (occurring in at least 20% of persons with known active tuberculosis) include recently acquired tuberculosis infection, age younger than 6 months, overwhelming tuberculosis, recent vaccination with a live virus (for example, measles), recent viral infection (for example, measles, varicella), and anergy. False-positive results can be due to BCG vaccination and infection with nontuberculous mycobacteria. For persons who undergo routine serial testing, a positive TST result is considered an increased induration of 10 mm or more within a 2-year interval. Interpretation of the TST in persons with a history of BCG vaccination is the same as for persons who never received the vaccine (unless BCG vaccination was very recent), although IGRA assays (discussed next) may be preferred for those who were vaccinated with BCG.

Remote exposure to tuberculosis may result in an initially negative TST result that can become positive several weeks later. This "booster effect" represents a true-positive result and is especially helpful in evaluating elderly patients with a remote history of LTBI or differentiating remote exposures from new exposures in patients who undergo serial testing. The booster effect is also more common in patients with a history of BCG vaccination and in those with nontuberculous mycobacterial infections.

Interferon-γ Release Assays

The Centers for Disease Control and Prevention endorses the use of IGRAs in all clinical settings in which the TST is recommended. Two types of IGRAs are increasingly being used. Both indicate sensitization to *M. tuberculosis* by measuring release of interferon-γ in the blood by T cells as a response to *M. tuberculosis*–associated antigens. IGRAs are generally thought to be as sensitive as but more specific than the TST in diagnosing tuberculosis. As with the TST, a more vigorous IGRA response is needed for a low-risk person to be considered infected. Similar to the TST, IGRAs are not recommended for testing individuals who are at low risk for LTBI and development of active disease if infected. The exception is testing individuals who will be at increased risk in the future.

IGRAs are preferred to the TST when persons have received BCG either as treatment for cancer or as a vaccine or when testing persons who often fail to return for a follow-up reading of the TST (for example, injection drug users or homeless persons). Conversely, the TST is preferred when testing children younger than 5 years of age. In this population, some experts have recommended testing with both the TST and an IGRA to increase the specificity of diagnosis. An IGRA or a TST may be used for testing recent contacts of someone with active tuberculosis or for periodic screening of persons who are at risk for occupational exposure (for example, health care workers).

Compared with TST, the initial costs of IGRA testing are higher and laboratory processing is required. However, unlike TST, IGRA testing does not require a follow-up visit and interpretation to complete the testing process. Thus, when deciding which test to use, the costs and availability of both of these tests, as well as patient reliability and convenience, should be considered.

Culture and Other Microbiologic Tests

Bacteriologic evaluation of clinical specimens is recommended when active tuberculosis is suspected. Histopathologic evidence of caseating granulomas is helpful but not diagnostic, and just the presence of acid-fast bacilli (AFB) does not confirm a diagnosis of tuberculosis. Cultures need to be performed for confirmation. Because acid-fast staining characteristics from clinical specimens depend on the concentration of mycobacteria (sensitivity of 45% to 80%), culture should be obtained even when smears for AFB are negative. Routine cultures done on solid media optimized for the growth of mycobacteria are slow: the median time to positivity is 3 to 4 weeks, and some specimens can still grow after 5 weeks. Liquid media techniques that do not rely on the presence of visible colonies but can detect microbial metabolism turn positive within a median time of about 1 week. The Centers for Disease Control and Prevention also recommends performing nucleic acid amplification (NAA) testing on a sputum specimen when the diagnosis of tuberculosis is suspected but not established. The positive predictive value of NAA testing is greater than 95% in patients with AFB-positive smears. Perhaps more importantly, these tests are positive in 50% to 80% of patients with AFB-negative, culture-positive smears. A positive NAA test in a patient with suspected tuberculosis should prompt initiation of treatment regardless of whether the sputum smear is AFB-positive or -negative. NAA tests for tuberculosis have the added advantage of providing results within 2 days. They should not be used when the suspicion for tuberculosis is low, because their positive predictive value is less than 50% in this setting. These tests are also expensive and may not be suitable for low-resource areas.

Bronchoscopy, including bronchoalveolar lavage and biopsy, can be considered in patients who are suspected of having tuberculosis but whose sputum studies are negative. Evaluation of patients with suspected pleural tuberculosis may include biopsy to detect granulomas because the yield from pleural fluid cultures in these patients is low (<25%); pleural biopsy yields granulomas in 75% of cases. Some experts recommend measurement of pleural fluid adenosine deaminase levels to establish the diagnosis of pleural tuberculosis in patients with exudative lymphocytic pleural effusions.

Analysis of cerebrospinal fluid from patients with suspected tuberculous meningitis classically reveals a lymphocytic pleocytosis, decreased glucose levels, and elevated protein levels. However, cerebrospinal fluid stains for AFB are usually negative (positivity generally <25%). Cultures are also negative in up to 25% of patients. Assays for polymerase chain reaction have a high specificity (98%) but an average sensitivity of only about 50% in diagnosing tuberculous meningitis.

Drug susceptibility testing of the initial isolate should be routinely performed.

Radiographic Imaging

Primary progressive tuberculosis may present as localized infiltrates or paratracheal and hilar lymphadenopathy on chest radiographs. Reactivation pulmonary tuberculosis typically appears as fibrocavitary disease in the superior segments of the lower lobes or apical-posterior segments of the upper lobes. Atypical radiographic findings such as miliary patterns, middle and lower lung zone involvement, mediastinal lymphadenopathy, and pleural involvement are especially likely in patients with AIDS. CT scans may be helpful for detecting subtle manifestations of pulmonary tuberculosis that are not seen on plain radiographic films or for evaluating tuberculous involvement in extrapulmonary locations.

KEY POINTS

- Measurement of induration (not erythema) is used to determine a positive or negative response to the tuberculin skin test.
- Remote exposure to tuberculosis may result in an initially negative tuberculin skin test that can become positive several weeks later.
- Interferon-γ release assays are generally as sensitive as but more specific than the tuberculin skin test in diagnosing tuberculosis.
- Patients with suspected active tuberculosis require a tuberculin skin test or interferon-γ release assay; a chest radiograph; and microbiologic tests, including acid-fast stains and culture of clinical specimens.
- When active tuberculosis is suspected, culture should always be obtained, even when smears for acid-fast bacilli are negative.
- Nucleic acid amplification testing on a sputum specimen is recommended when the diagnosis of tuberculosis is suspected but not established.
- Bronchoscopy, including bronchoalveolar lavage and biopsy, can be considered in patients who are suspected of having tuberculosis but whose sputum studies are negative.

Treatment

In patients with evidence of tuberculosis infection as documented by a positive TST or IGRA and in whom active tuberculosis has been excluded, treatment should be initiated for LTBI. Treatment of LTBI usually involves a 9-month course of isoniazid. Because peripheral neuropathy may be associated with isoniazid therapy, concurrent treatment with pyridoxine (vitamin B$_6$) should be considered, particularly in those with an increased risk of neuropathy (diabetes, uremia, alcoholism, HIV infection, malnutrition, seizure disorder, or pregnancy). An alternative therapy is rifampin daily for 4 months. Recently, the Centers for Disease Control and Prevention also included 3 months of directly observed, once-weekly rifapentine and isoniazid combination therapy for treatment of latent tuberculosis.

Active tuberculosis is treated with multiple drugs for at least 6 months and involves an initial treatment phase and a continuation phase. In patients who are not believed to be infected with drug-resistant mycobacteria, the initial phase usually consists of a 2-month course of isoniazid, rifampin, ethambutol, and pyrazinamide. Interruptions in treatment are not uncommon. Treatment guidelines recommend that an interruption of 2 or more weeks during the initial 2-month phase of therapy requires restarting the same regimen from the beginning. The continuation phase generally involves treatment with isoniazid and rifampin for either 4 or 7 months. The 7-month course is given when patients have cavitary pulmonary disease at diagnosis and positive sputum cultures after completing initial therapy. Treatment of extrapulmonary tuberculosis is similar to that of pulmonary disease except for patients with tuberculous meningitis for whom the ideal duration of therapy is unknown; these patients are usually treated for 9 to 12 months. An initial course of adjunctive corticosteroids should be given to patients with tuberculous pericarditis or tuberculous meningitis to decrease the potentially deleterious inflammatory effects of treatment.

Drugs used to treat tuberculosis have a toxicity profile that should be discussed with the patient before therapy is begun (**Table 23**). In addition, drugs such as the rifamycins (including rifampin, rifapentine, and rifabutin) are potent inducers of the cytochrome P-450 hepatic enzyme system, which results in reduced serum concentrations of many drugs, including warfarin. Before treatment is begun, the

TABLE 23. Antituberculous Drugs		
Agent	**Side Effects**	**Notes**
First-Line Medications		
Isoniazid	Rash; liver enzyme elevation; hepatitis; peripheral neuropathy; lupus-like syndrome	Hepatitis risk increases with age and alcohol consumption. Pyridoxine may prevent peripheral neuropathy. Adjust for kidney injury.
Pyrazinamide	Hepatitis; rash; GI upset; hyperuricemia	May make glucose control more difficult in diabetic patients. Adjust for kidney injury.
Rifampin	Hepatitis; rash; GI upset	Contraindicated or should be used with caution when administered with protease inhibitors and non-nucleoside reverse transcriptase inhibitors. Do not administer to patients also taking saquinavir/ritonavir. Colors body fluids orange.
Rifabutin	Rash; hepatitis; thrombocytopenia; severe arthralgia; uveitis; leukopenia	Dose adjustment required if taken with protease inhibitors or non-nucleoside reverse transcriptase inhibitors. Monitor for decreased antiretroviral activity and for rifabutin toxicity.
Rifapentine	Similar to rifampin	Contraindicated in HIV-positive patients (unacceptable rate of failure/relapse).
Ethambutol	Optic neuritis; rash	Baseline and periodic tests of visual acuity and color vision. Patients are advised to call immediately if any change in visual acuity or color vision. Adjust for kidney injury.
Second-Line Medications[a]		
Streptomycin	Auditory, vestibular, and kidney toxicity	Avoid or reduce dose in adults >59 years. Monitor hearing and kidney function tests. Adjust for kidney injury.
Cycloserine	Psychosis; convulsions; depression; headaches; rash; drug interactions	Pyridoxine may decrease CNS side effects. Measure drug serum levels.
Capreomycin	Kidney, vestibular and auditory toxicity	Monitor hearing and kidney function tests. Adjust for kidney injury.
Ethionamide	GI upset; hepatotoxicity; hypersensitivity	May cause hypothyroidism.
Kanamycin and amikacin	Auditory, vestibular, and kidney toxicity	Not approved by the FDA for TB treatment. Monitor vestibular, hearing, and kidney function.
Levofloxacin, moxifloxacin, gatifloxacin	GI upset; dizziness; hypersensitivity; drug interactions	Not approved by the FDA for TB treatment. Should not be used in children.
Para-aminosalicylic acid	GI upset; hypersensitivity; hepatotoxicity	May cause hypothyroidism, especially if used with ethionamide. Measure liver enzymes.

CNS = central nervous system; FDA = U.S. Food and Drug Administration; GI = gastrointestinal; TB = tuberculosis.

[a]Use these drugs in consultation with a clinician experienced in the management of drug-resistant TB.

following studies should be performed: hepatitis B and C virus serologic tests for at-risk patients; platelet count; and measurement of serum aminotransferase, bilirubin, alkaline phosphatase, and creatinine levels. Color vision and visual acuity testing is also needed if ethambutol is to be used.

Directly observed therapy is preferred for patients in whom self-administered treatment cannot be assured because nonadherence can result in ongoing transmission of mycobacteria, drug-resistance, and relapsed infection. Otherwise, at a minimum, patients should undergo a monthly clinical evaluation for documentation of adherence and detection of any adverse medication reactions. In patients receiving first-line antituberculosis medications, routine laboratory tests for monitoring kidney and liver function and platelet count are not needed unless clinically indicated or if abnormalities were documented at baseline.

Treatment durations and recommendations are generally the same for patients with tuberculosis who are coinfected with HIV. Dose adjustments for antiretroviral therapy (ART) and rifamycin agents may be required because of drug interactions. Treatment of tuberculosis in patients with HIV infection should be started at or before the initiation of ART. Early initiation of ART in HIV-infected patients with tuberculosis appears to be most beneficial in those with advanced immunosuppression.

Multidrug-Resistant and Extensively Drug-Resistant Tuberculosis

Resistance to commonly used antituberculosis drugs is increasingly being recognized worldwide. Infection with potentially drug-resistant strains should be suspected in (1) patients who were previously treated for tuberculosis, especially if treatment was inadequate because of patient nonadherence or an inappropriate initial regimen; (2) patients who were infected in countries where high rates of drug resistance are present; (3) adherent patients who are not responding to standard empiric therapy; and (4) close contacts of patients with drug-resistant tuberculosis. Multidrug-resistant (MDR) tuberculosis strains are resistant to at least isoniazid and rifampin. Extensively drug-resistant (XDR) strains are MDR strains that are also resistant to fluoroquinolones and to at least one of the following three second-line injectable drugs: kanamycin, capreomycin, and amikacin. In the United States, 88 cases of primary MDR tuberculosis were reported in 2010; 82% involved foreign-born persons. Between 1993 and 2007, a total of 83 cases of XDR tuberculosis were reported in the United States.

Although the presence of MDR and XDR strains is thought to be associated with higher mortality rates, these strains are potentially curable when use of antituberculosis drugs is directed by comprehensive drug susceptibility testing. The drug regimen for treating MDR and XDR tuberculosis usually includes more medications, and the duration of treatment is much longer. Because of the delay in obtaining results from susceptibility testing, patients may initially receive an ineffective

regimen. Development of more rapid diagnostic studies for susceptibility testing, including automated rapid liquid culture techniques and NAA assays, is needed. Surgery may be required for management of localized drug-resistant pulmonary tuberculosis, particularly XDR strains, when patients do not respond to appropriate medical therapy.

KEY POINTS

- Treatment for latent tuberculosis infection usually involves a 9-month course of isoniazid along with pyridoxine (vitamin B_6).
- Active tuberculosis treatment involves an initial phase (usually a 2-month course of isoniazid, rifampin, ethambutol, and pyrazinamide) and a continuation phase (usually a 4- or 7-month course of isoniazid and rifampin).
- Directly observed therapy is preferred when treating patients with tuberculosis because medication nonadherence can result in transmission of mycobacteria, drug-resistance, and relapsed infection.
- Multidrug-resistant tuberculosis strains are resistant to at least isoniazid and rifampin; extensively drug-resistant strains are also resistant to fluoroquinolones and to at least one of the following: kanamycin, capreomycin, and amikacin.

Prevention

BCG vaccine is derived from an attenuated strain of *Mycobacterium bovis*. Although the vaccine is widely used worldwide, it is not generally administered in the United States. BCG vaccine is most effective for preventing disseminated disease and tuberculous meningitis in children. Its protective effect in adults is variable. BCG vaccine should not be given to immunocompromised patients because it is a live vaccine and may cause disseminated disease.

KEY POINT

- Bacillus Calmette-Guérin vaccine is most effective for preventing disseminated tuberculosis and tuberculous meningitis in children.

Nontuberculous Mycobacterial Infections

The term "nontuberculous mycobacteria (NTM)" refers to a group of environmental mycobacteria that are found in soil and natural and treated water. Most identified species are nonpathogenic. NTM are also found as colonizers of medical equipment and surgical solutions, which may explain nosocomial transmission of pathogenic microorganisms.

NTM infections tend to affect young adults and elderly persons. The most common clinical manifestations are pulmonary,

TABLE 24. Diseases Caused by Common Nontuberculous Mycobacterial Species

Disease	*Mycobacterium* species
Pulmonary disease	M. avium complex, M. kansasii, M. abscessus, M. xenopi, M. malmoense
Lymphadenitis	M. avium complex, M. malmoense, M. scrofulaceum
Skin, soft tissue, and musculoskeletal diseases	M. abscessus, M. chelonae, M. fortuitum, M. marinum, M. ulcerans
Disseminated disease	M. avium complex, M. kansasii, M. abscessus, M. xenopi, M. genavense, M. haemophilum, M. chelonae
Health care–associated infections	M. abscessus, M. chelonae, M. fortuitum

most frequently in patients with advanced HIV infection and less often in patients who are immunocompromised. Whether tumor necrosis factor-α blocking agents also predispose to NTM infection is currently unknown.

The same techniques used in culture of *M. tuberculosis* are used in culture of NTM. Detecting NTM isolated from anatomic sites that are generally thought to be sterile suggests NTM infection. Because a single specific test to differentiate NTM colonization from active infection is not available, diagnostic criteria have been developed to aid in determining which patients require treatment (**Table 25**).

KEY POINTS

- Most infections caused by nontuberculous mycobacteria affect young adults and elderly persons.
- The most common clinical manifestations of nontuberculous mycobacterial infections are pulmonary, lymphatic, cutaneous, soft tissue, and disseminated infections.
- Because a single specific test to differentiate nontuberculous mycobacterial colonization from active infection is not available, diagnostic criteria have been developed to aid in determining which patients require treatment.

Mycobacterium avium Complex Infection

Mycobacterium avium complex (MAC) is the most common cause of NTM lung disease and is acquired by inhaling the

lymphatic, cutaneous, soft tissue, and disseminated infection (**Table 24**). Host defenses, body morphotype, and immune status figure significantly in the clinical manifestations of NTM infection. Structural lung conditions (including COPD, bronchiectasis, cystic fibrosis, and pneumoconiosis) and esophageal motility disorders appear to be associated with NTM lung disease. The presence of a slender body habitus, pectus excavatum, scoliosis, and mitral valve prolapse may also be associated with NTM lung disease, especially in postmenopausal women. Abnormalities in interferon-γ and interleukin-12 pathways also predispose to developing severe NTM infections. Disseminated disease is observed

TABLE 25. Diagnostic Criteria for Nontuberculous Mycobacterial Lung Disease

Criteria	Findings
Clinical and imaging criteria	Evidence of pulmonary symptoms and abnormal chest imaging studies (nodular or cavitary lung lesions on radiographs and high-resolution CT scans), with exclusion of other possible causes
Laboratory (microbiologic) criteria	Positive isolation of NTM from at least two separate sputum samples
	or
	Positive isolation of NTM from at least one bronchoalveolar lavage sample
	or
	Histopathologic demonstration of AFB and/or granulomatous disease with a positive culture for NTM from lung tissue specimen; or histopathologic demonstration of AFB and/or granulomatous disease on lung tissue specimen with a positive culture for NTM from one or more sputum samples or bronchoalveolar lavage sample
Other considerations	The isolation of an unusual NTM species or of an NTM species that is usually a contaminant should prompt consultation with an infectious diseases specialist.
	The suspicion of NTM lung disease that does not fulfill the above diagnostic criteria should prompt follow-up until a definitive diagnosis is made or excluded.
	Whether to treat pulmonary infections due to NTM should be based on the potential benefits and risks for individual patients.

AFB = acid-fast bacilli; NTM = nontuberculous mycobacteria.

Data from Griffith DE, Aksamit T, Brown-Elliott BA, et al; the ATS Mycobacterial Diseases Subcommittee; American Thoracic Society; Infectious Disease Society of America. An official ATS/IDSA statement: diagnosis, treatment, and prevention of nontuberculous mycobacterial diseases. Am J Respir Crit Care Med. 2007;175(4):367-416. [Erratum in: Am J Respir Crit Care Med. 2007;175(7):744-745 (dosage error in article text)]. [PMID: 17277290] aerosolized microorganisms from colonized soil and water. Two distinct presentations of MAC lung infection are common. The first is a fibrocavitary disease (similar to tuberculosis) that often involves the upper lobes, occurs primarily in middle-aged men with a history of smoking or other chronic lung injury, and, if left untreated, progresses rapidly to cavitary lung destruction and respiratory failure. The second type of infection tends to occur in middle-aged or elderly women who have no history of smoking or underlying lung disease (Lady Windermere syndrome). Patients have a chronic cough and nodular infiltrates (nodular bronchiectatic disease) that frequently involve the right middle lobe or lingula. Although this disease generally has an indolent course, some patients may have aggressive disease with fever, weight loss, and progressive respiratory insufficiency.

Other presentations of MAC infection are less common. A hypersensitivity-like pneumonitis, referred to as "hot tub lung," is linked to inhalation of aerosolized household water colonized by MAC. The onset is subacute; patients present with dyspnea, cough, and fever, and resolution occurs following removal of the aerosol. Lymphadenitis, primarily of the head and neck, is the primary presentation of NTM infection in children, and MAC is isolated in about 80% of these patients. Disseminated MAC disease is one of the most common infections in patients with advanced HIV infection, particularly those with CD4 cell counts less than 50/microliter.

Antimicrobial therapy is indicated for most patients in whom MAC is determined to be an invasive pathogen. In vitro susceptibility testing is usually not indicated before therapy is begun. Treatment usually consists of a combination of a macrolide (clarithromycin, azithromycin), ethambutol, and a rifamycin (rifampin, rifabutin). Adding amikacin or streptomycin is recommended for the first 2 to 3 months of therapy for patients with severe or previously treated MAC infection. Surgical intervention may be indicated when disease is predominantly localized to one lung. Adding corticosteroids for treatment of MAC hypersensitivity-like pneumonitis may hasten recovery. Lymphadenitis caused by MAC should be treated with excisional surgery alone.

KEY POINTS

- *Mycobacterium avium* complex most often manifests as a tuberculosis-like infection in middle-aged men with a history of smoking and chronic lung disease and in middle-aged or elderly women with no history of smoking or underlying lung disease.
- Treatment of *Mycobacterium avium* complex infection generally includes a combination of a macrolide (clarithromycin, azithromycin), ethambutol, and a rifamycin (rifampin, rifabutin).

Mycobacterium kansasii

Mycobacterium kansasii is the second most common NTM species causing lung disease. Unlike other NTM species, *M. kansasii* is not normally found in natural environments but is commonly isolated from urban municipal water supplies. A single clinical isolate is therefore unlikely to represent colonization and should be considered diagnostic of disease. Patients with *M. kansasii* lung infection have symptoms and signs suggestive of tuberculosis. Treatment consists of isoniazid, rifampin, and ethambutol given daily for 18 months, and results of sputum cultures must be negative for at least 12 months before therapy is discontinued.

KEY POINTS

- Patients with *Mycobacterium kansasii* lung disease present with symptoms and signs suggestive of tuberculosis.
- Treatment of *Mycobacterium kansasii* lung disease consists of isoniazid, rifampin, and ethambutol.

Rapidly Growing Mycobacteria

Rapidly growing mycobacteria (RGM) are defined by their brief growing period in culture media (within 7 days). They are generally ubiquitous saprophytes that are widely distributed in nature. The three most clinically relevant species are *M. fortuitum*, *M. chelonae*, and *M. abscessus*. RGM have a wide spectrum of clinical manifestations, including pulmonary, skin, soft tissue, and musculoskeletal infections. They are sometimes acquired by direct inoculation such as with cosmetic procedures. Dissemination of RGM is rare and occurs only in patients who are severely immunocompromised. RGM, especially *M. fortuitum* and *M. abscessus*, may also be associated with health care–associated infections, including, but not limited to, surgical site, catheter-related bloodstream, and prosthetic device–related infections. The common factor in these infections is exposure to colonized liquid, usually tap water. Because drug susceptibility varies among the RGM species, in vitro susceptibility testing of all clinically significant RGM isolates is recommended before therapy is begun. Treatment with a multiple antibiotic regimen is required.

KEY POINTS

- Rapidly growing mycobacteria have a wide spectrum of clinical manifestations, including pulmonary, skin, soft tissue, and musculoskeletal infections, and are sometimes acquired by direct inoculation.
- Treatment of infection due to rapidly growing mycobacteria requires in vitro susceptibility testing and combination antibiotic therapy.

Fungal Infections

Systemic Candidiasis

Systemic or invasive candidiasis includes candidemia, disseminated candidiasis, and focal organ involvement. *Candida* bloodstream infection, such as catheter-related candidemia, may initially be the primary disorder but may lead to disseminated or focal organ involvement as a result of hematogenous spread. In disseminated or focal organ involvement, candidemia may be present secondary to the primary infection, but in many circumstances, blood cultures are negative. Although *Candida albicans* is the most common pathogen, identification of non-*albicans* species is increasing. Any *Candida* species that is obtained from a blood culture should never be considered a contaminant but instead should initiate investigation for a cause.

Risk factors for systemic candidiasis include medications (broad-spectrum antibiotics, chemotherapeutic agents, immunosuppressive agents), catheter-related causes (central venous catheters, parenteral nutrition, hemodialysis), and hospitalization (especially a prolonged stay in an intensive care unit). Patients with malignancies, acute kidney injury, neutropenia, and severe acute pancreatitis are at increased risk as are transplant recipients and those recovering from recent surgery.

Clinical Manifestations and Diagnosis

Initial clinical manifestations of systemic candidiasis range from fever, hypotension, and leukocytosis to sepsis syndrome and septic shock, which are indistinguishable from severe bacterial infection. Characteristic eye and skin lesions may be present. Eye lesions are characterized by distinctive white exudates in the retina. Skin lesions are generally painless papules or pustules on an erythematous base. Tissue from the skin lesions contains yeast and can help determine the diagnosis rapidly. Other common sites of dissemination are the kidneys, liver, spleen, and brain. However, microabscesses in all organs have been described. Although *Candida* can infect any organ, the most frequent focal infections are urinary tract infections, peritonitis, bone and joint infections, endophthalmitis, and meningitis. Even though *Candida* is frequently isolated from the sputum, pneumonia from this pathogen is extremely rare. Chronic disseminated candidiasis (also called hepatosplenic candidiasis) occurs in patients with hematologic malignancies who are no longer neutropenic. Clinical manifestations include fever, right upper quadrant abdominal pain, nausea, and vomiting. The gold standard for diagnosing systemic candidiasis is a positive culture from the blood or a normally sterile body fluid or site. A negative culture does not exclude this diagnosis. If organ involvement is suspected, biopsy specimens should be obtained and sent for histopathologic studies and culture. Identification of the specific *Candida* species is important to guide appropriate antifungal therapy.

Treatment

Empiric therapy for suspected candidiasis is similar to that for proven infection. Fluconazole or an echinocandin (caspofungin, anidulafungin, or micafungin) is recommended as initial therapy for most non-neutropenic patients with candidemia. Fluconazole is preferred for patients who are less critically ill. An echinocandin is preferred for patients with moderate to severe illness who recently received an azole. Changing from an echinocandin to fluconazole is indicated if the *Candida* isolate is likely to be susceptible to fluconazole and if the patient is clinically stable. An echinocandin is initially preferred for infection due to *Candida glabrata,* and an oral azole agent may be substituted at a later date. However, fluconazole and voriconazole susceptibility testing is needed before changing to an azole in patients with *C. glabrata* infection. Susceptibility testing may also be indicated for other *Candida* species in which azole resistance is suspected.

Fluconazole is recommended for infection due to *Candida parapsilosis.* Voriconazole is used as step-down oral therapy for infection due to *Candida krusei* or voriconazole-susceptible *C. glabrata.* Treatment of uncomplicated candidemia should be continued for 2 weeks after clearance of the pathogen from the bloodstream and resolution of symptoms.

Removal of intravenous catheters is strongly recommended for non-neutropenic patients with candidemia because catheter removal has been associated with a shorter duration of infection and improved patient outcomes. Candidemia caused by *C. parapsilosis* is almost always catheter-related.

In neutropenic patients with proven *Candida* infection, an echinocandin or voriconazole (if coverage of molds is desired) may be used. Because neutropenic patients may develop candidemia if the pathogen enters the bloodstream from the gastrointestinal tract, the role of catheter removal is less clear. However, if candidemia persists for more than a few days in a neutropenic patient with a catheter, the catheter should be removed. Empiric therapy for suspected invasive candidiasis in neutropenic patients may include a lipid formulation of amphotericin B, an echinocandin, or voriconazole.

Therapy is not usually indicated for patients with asymptomatic cystitis caused by *Candida* species unless the patient is neutropenic or is undergoing a urologic procedure. The treatment of choice for symptomatic cystitis and pyelonephritis is fluconazole.

Treatment for most focal infections is consistent with the recommendations for the treatment of candidemia, except that echinocandins should not be used to treat meningitis or endophthalmitis because of poor penetration.

Aspergillosis and Aspergilloma

Aspergillus species are ubiquitous in the environment. The primary route of acquisition is inhalation of aerosolized spores, and the principal site of disease is the lung. The most common *Aspergillus* species causing infection are *A. fumigatus*, *A. flavus*, *A. niger*, and *A. terreus*, and the most common forms of pulmonary infection are allergic bronchopulmonary aspergillosis, aspergilloma (fungus ball), and invasive aspergillosis.

Allergic bronchopulmonary aspergillosis most often occurs in patients with chronic asthma or cystic fibrosis. Diagnostic criteria include asthma, central bronchiectasis, fleeting pulmonary infiltrates on chest imaging studies, and laboratory studies showing eosinophilia, elevated serum IgE levels, cutaneous reactivity to *Aspergillus* antigens, and the presence of *Aspergillus*-precipitating antibodies. Recommended treatment is administration of oral corticosteroids during an acute phase or exacerbation. Adding the antifungal agent itraconazole has been shown to improve outcomes and have a corticosteroid-sparing effect.

Symptoms of aspergilloma (fungus ball) include cough, hemoptysis, dyspnea, weight loss, fatigue, fever, and chest pain. Hemoptysis can be life-threatening. Radiographic studies show a rounded mass in a preexisting pulmonary cavity or cyst or in areas of devitalized lung. Sputum culture is usually positive for *Aspergillus*. Surgical resection is considered the definitive therapy.

Invasive sinopulmonary aspergillosis and disseminated aspergillosis generally occur in immunocompromised patients. The lung is the most common site of invasive disease. The organism invades blood vessels and causes distal infarction of tissue. Patients may present with fever, cough, chest pain, hemoptysis, and pulmonary infiltrates or nodules on chest radiographs. Wedge-shaped densities resembling infarcts may also be seen on radiographs. CT scans may show a target lesion with a necrotic center surrounded by a ring of hemorrhage (the halo sign). Dissemination may occur to the central nervous system (CNS) and cause a brain abscess or to blood vessels in the heart, gastrointestinal tract, or skin. Diagnosis may be difficult, because *Aspergillus* is a frequent contaminant in sputum.

The diagnosis of invasive aspergillosis is established by tissue biopsy showing *Aspergillus* in histopathologic and culture specimens, especially specimens that were obtained from a normally sterile site. Blood cultures are rarely positive. The galactomannan antigen immunoassay is a useful diagnostic test for detecting fungi in serum, cerebrospinal fluid, and bronchoalveolar lavage fluid, and serial measurements can be used for monitoring therapy. The β-D-glucan assay and polymerase chain reaction are also promising diagnostic tests. Treatment of invasive aspergillosis includes conventional and lipid formulations of amphotericin B, voriconazole, itraconazole, posaconazole, or caspofungin. Voriconazole is superior to conventional amphotericin B for primary therapy. The lipid formulation of amphotericin B, echinocandins, or other triazole agents are indicated for patients who cannot tolerate voriconazole, have contraindications to its use, or have progressive infection. Combination therapy is not routinely recommended. **H**

Mucormycosis

Mucormycosis (formerly zygomycosis) is an acute and rapidly progressive infection that most commonly occurs in patients with hematologic malignancies associated with prolonged neutropenia, other disorders causing prolonged neutropenia or immunosuppression, severe burns or trauma, or poorly controlled diabetes mellitus. Patients taking corticosteroids, cytotoxic agents, or deferoxamine are also at increased risk. Rhinocerebral mucormycosis is the most common presentation; pulmonary, gastrointestinal, cutaneous, and disseminated infections rarely occur. Rhinocerebral mucormycosis is a rapidly fatal infection that spreads from the sinuses retroorbitally and to the CNS. Patients present with headache, epistaxis, and ocular findings, including proptosis, periorbital edema, and decreased vision. Examination of the nose or palate may show black necrotic tissue, which is usually pathognomonic. Pulmonary mucormycosis with thrombosis and infarction most frequently develops in patients with hematologic malignancies. Cutaneous mucormycosis is rare and develops most often in burn and trauma patients or as a result of dissemination from another site. Gastrointestinal mucormycosis is also rare, occurring primarily in patients with gastrointestinal tract abnormalities or severe malnutrition.

CONT. Isolated CNS mucormycosis may result from hematogenous spread and occurs in injection drug users.

The diagnosis of mucormycosis is confirmed by tissue biopsy and culture. Histopathologic studies show characteristic broad, irregular, ribbon-like, aseptate hyphae that exhibit broad right-angle branching. Blood cultures are usually negative. Therapy requires both medical and surgical interventions. High-dose conventional or lipid-based amphotericin B is the antifungal agent of choice. Immediate, aggressive surgical debridement is essential and may have to be repeated.

KEY POINTS

- Rhinocerebral mucormycosis is a rapidly fatal infection; finding black necrotic tissue on examination of the nose or palate is pathognomonic.

- Treatment of mucormycosis requires a combination of high-dose conventional or lipid-based amphotericin B and immediate, aggressive surgical debridement.

Cryptococcosis

Cryptococcosis is an invasive mycosis that occurs worldwide. The lungs are the primary portal of entry for *Cryptococcus* species. Although immunocompetent hosts are generally able to contain the pathogen as a result of cell-mediated immunity, immunocompromised patients are at risk for pulmonary infection that can rapidly disseminate. Disseminated infection most often involves the CNS and causes subacute or chronic meningoencephalitis or meningitis. Headache and alterations in mental status are the most common symptoms. Fever and nuchal rigidity occur less often. Complications include hydrocephalus, encephalitis, brainstem vasculitis, involvement of the optic pathways, and mass lesions (cryptococcomas) of the brain. Other forms of disseminated cryptococcosis include skin, prostate, bone, eye, and urinary tract involvement. Whenever cryptococcosis occurs at a site outside the CNS, a lumbar puncture should be done to determine if CNS infection is also present.

The diagnosis is made initially by histopathologic studies showing cryptococci *or* cryptococcal antigen in serum or cerebrospinal fluid and is confirmed by isolation of cryptococci in culture. Pulmonary cryptococcosis found incidentally in an asymptomatic immunocompetent host may resolve without treatment. However, all patients with CNS cryptococcosis or extrapulmonary disease require therapy. Fluconazole is the antifungal agent of choice for primary cutaneous infection without evidence of dissemination and for isolated mildly symptomatic pulmonary disease. The preferred treatment for disseminated infection, infection in an immunocompromised patient, or cryptococcal meningoencephalitis or meningitis is amphotericin B plus flucytosine, given as induction therapy for 2 weeks; 4 weeks of induction therapy are recommended for non–HIV-infected, nontransplant patients. Consolidation therapy with fluconazole is then administered for at least

8 weeks. Maintenance therapy can be discontinued in HIV-positive patients who are receiving effective antiretroviral therapy, have a CD4 cell count of 100/microliter or greater for 3 or more months, and have been receiving antifungal therapy for at least 1 year. Organ transplant recipients who must remain on high-dose immunosuppressive agents may require lifelong maintenance therapy. An important part of treating patients with CNS cryptococcosis is management of elevated intracranial pressure (for example, frequent lumbar punctures and removal of cerebrospinal fluid) or placement of a ventriculoperitoneal shunt if the patient is receiving appropriate antifungal therapy and other measures to reduce elevated intracranial pressure have failed.

KEY POINTS

- The diagnosis of cryptococcosis is made initially by histopathologic studies showing cryptococci or cryptococcal antigen in tissue, serum, or cerebrospinal fluid and is confirmed by isolation of cryptococci in culture.

- The preferred treatment of disseminated cryptococcosis, cryptococcal infection in an immunocompromised host, or cryptococcal meningoencephalitis or meningitis is amphotericin B plus flucytosine induction therapy followed by fluconazole consolidation therapy.

Blastomycosis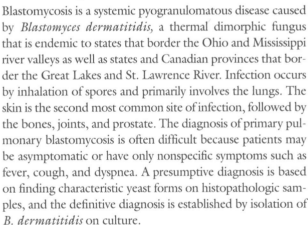

Blastomycosis is a systemic pyogranulomatous disease caused by *Blastomyces dermatitidis,* a thermal dimorphic fungus that is endemic to states that border the Ohio and Mississippi river valleys as well as states and Canadian provinces that border the Great Lakes and St. Lawrence River. Infection occurs by inhalation of spores and primarily involves the lungs. The skin is the second most common site of infection, followed by the bones, joints, and prostate. The diagnosis of primary pulmonary blastomycosis is often difficult because patients may be asymptomatic or have only nonspecific symptoms such as fever, cough, and dyspnea. A presumptive diagnosis is based on finding characteristic yeast forms on histopathologic samples, and the definitive diagnosis is established by isolation of *B. dermatitidis* on culture.

Acute pulmonary blastomycosis may be mild and self-limited in the immunocompetent host and may not require treatment; however, therapy may prevent extrapulmonary dissemination. All immunocompromised patients and all patients with moderate to severe pneumonia or disseminated infection require treatment. Oral itraconazole is the agent of choice for patients with mild to moderate pulmonary blastomycosis and is given for 6 to 12 months. Patients with moderately severe to severe disease should receive a conventional or lipid formulation of amphotericin B for 1 to 2 weeks followed by oral itraconazole for 6 to 12 months.

CONT.

Extrapulmonary blastomycosis can occur in the absence of lung disease. Cutaneous blastomycosis is most common and is frequently a marker for disseminated infection. Mild to moderate disseminated extrapulmonary blastomycosis is treated with oral itraconazole, and moderately severe to severe disease requires a conventional or lipid formulation of amphotericin B. **H**

KEY POINTS

- A presumptive diagnosis of pulmonary blastomycosis is based on the finding of characteristic yeast forms on histopathologic samples, and the definitive diagnosis is established by isolation of *Blastomyces dermatitidis* on culture.
- Patients with mild or moderate pulmonary blastomycosis are treated with oral itraconazole, and those with moderately severe to severe disease should receive a conventional or lipid formulation of amphotericin B followed by oral itraconazole.

Histoplasmosis

Histoplasmosis is caused by *Histoplasma capsulatum*, a thermal dimorphic fungus that is endemic to the midwestern states of the Ohio and Mississippi river valleys. Infection is usually asymptomatic but occasionally causes acute and chronic pulmonary disease, granulomatous mediastinitis, fibrosing mediastinitis, broncolithiasis, pulmonary nodules (histoplasmomas), and acute and chronic disseminated disease. The diagnosis is established by histopathologic studies, antigen determination, and isolation of *H. capsulatum* on culture. Because the sensitivity of these studies differs depending on the extent of infection and the time following exposure, a battery of tests is usually required to confirm the diagnosis.

In most symptomatic patients, disease is mild and resolves without therapy. Therapy is indicated for patients with moderately severe or severe infection, acute diffuse pulmonary involvement, and chronic cavitary pulmonary disease. Treatment should also be considered for patients with mild infection who are immunocompromised or have had symptoms for 4 or more weeks. Itraconazole is the antifungal agent of choice for mild to moderate histoplasmosis, and a conventional or lipid formulation of amphotericin B is used to treat moderately severe to severe infection. **H**

KEY POINTS

- The diagnosis of histoplasmosis is established by histopathologic studies, antigen determination, and isolation of *Histoplasma capsulatum* on culture.
- Itraconazole is the antifungal agent of choice for treating mild to moderate histoplasmosis, and a conventional or lipid formulation of amphotericin B is used to treat moderately severe to severe infection.

Coccidioidomycosis

Coccidioidomycosis is caused by the thermal dimorphic fungi *Coccidioides immitis* and *Coccidioides posadasii,* which are endemic to the deserts of the southwestern United States, parts of Mexico, and Central and South America. Most infections are caused by inhalation of spores and are asymptomatic. Primary infection most frequently presents as community-acquired pneumonia occurring 1 to 3 weeks following exposure. In endemic areas, up to one third of cases of community-acquired pneumonia are caused by *Coccidioides* species. Valley fever is a subacute infection with respiratory symptoms, fever, and erythema nodosum. Extrapulmonary infection most commonly involves the skin, bones, joints, and CNS. The diagnosis is established by isolation of *Coccidioides* species in culture. Serologic tests are useful both for diagnosis and for monitoring the course of therapy and are the preferred method for diagnosing primary coccidioidal infections. Serologic studies are more helpful than culture in establishing the cause of chronic coccidioidal meningitis because cultures of cerebrospinal fluid are frequently negative. Because a negative serologic test does not exclude infection, repeated tests are needed to improve sensitivity.

Treatment is indicated for patients with severe disease or those with an increased risk for disseminated infection. Ketoconazole, fluconazole, and itraconazole are all reasonable treatment options for uncomplicated primary coccidioidal infection. The duration of therapy generally ranges from 3 to 6 months. An amphotericin B–based regimen is indicated for patients with severe coccidioidal pneumonia. Oral fluconazole is the antifungal agent of choice for treatment of meningitis, and therapy should be continued for life because relapses are common after medication is discontinued. However, intrathecal amphotericin B is indicated for patients who fail to respond to azole agents and for women during the first trimester of pregnancy. **H**

KEY POINTS

- Primary coccidioidomycosis most frequently presents as community-acquired pneumonia occurring 1 to 3 weeks following exposure.
- Serologic tests are useful for diagnosing primary coccidioidal infection and monitoring the course of therapy; repeated testing may be needed to improve sensitivity.
- Treatment of uncomplicated primary coccidioidal infection is ketoconazole, fluconazole, or itraconazole for 3 to 6 months.

Sporotrichosis

Infections caused by *Sporothrix schenckii* are usually associated with inoculation of skin from contaminated soil that tends to occur while gardening. A papule appears days to weeks later at the site of inoculation and usually ulcerates. Similar lesions then occur along lymphatic channels proximal to the inoculation site. The diagnosis is established by culture. Itraconazole is the treatment of choice for cutaneous and osteoarticular *S. schenckii* infection.

KEY POINT

• Cutaneous and osteoarticular *Sporothrix schenckii* infections are treated with itraconazole.

Sexually Transmitted Infections

Introduction

Sexually transmitted infections can be categorized as those that cause cervicitis and urethritis (and resultant complications such as pelvic inflammatory disease and epididymitis-orchitis), genital ulcers, and external genital warts. The diagnosis and treatment of sexually transmitted infections are important not only in the care of individual patients but also for preventing transmission of infection to other persons.

Cervicitis and Urethritis

Cervicitis and urethritis are most commonly caused by *Chlamydia trachomatis* and *Neisseria gonorrhoeae*. In women, herpes simplex virus (HSV) may also cause cervicitis. In men, urethritis may be due to HSV, *Trichomonas vaginalis*, and *Mycoplasma genitalium*. *N. gonorrhoeae* and *C. trachomatis* may cause proctitis in both men and women who have receptive anal intercourse.

Women with cervicitis generally present with purulent vaginal discharge. Intermenstrual bleeding (especially after intercourse) and dysuria may also develop. On examination, the vulva and the vaginal mucosa appear normal, but the cervix is inflamed, and mucopurulent discharge may be seen from the endocervical canal. Bleeding may occur when a swab is passed through the cervical os. Men with urethritis present with dysuria and penile discharge. Purulent discharge may be noted at the urethral meatus or expressed by applying gentle pressure with the forefinger on the dorsum of the penis and the thumb on the ventral surface at the base and moving towards the meatus.

Patients with proctitis present with rectal pain, tenesmus, and rectal discharge. Anoscopy reveals erythematous, friable mucosa in the rectal vault. In addition to *N. gonorrhoeae* and *C. trachomatis*, the differential diagnosis of proctitis includes HSV and syphilis.

KEY POINTS

• Cervicitis and urethritis are most commonly caused by *Chlamydia trachomatis* and *Neisseria gonorrhoeae*.

• Women with cervicitis generally present with purulent vaginal discharge; intermenstrual bleeding (especially after intercourse) and dysuria may also develop.

• Men with urethritis present with dysuria and penile discharge.

Chlamydia trachomatis Infection

Risk factors for *C. trachomatis* infection include age 25 years or younger, new or multiple sexual partners, and engaging in unprotected sex. Infection may be asymptomatic. Sequelae of untreated infection in women include pelvic inflammatory disease, ectopic pregnancy, and infertility. Annual screening of sexually active young women (≤25 years of age) and of older women with other risk factors is recommended. Nucleic acid amplification tests are the most sensitive diagnostic modality and may be performed on an endocervical or urethral swab or a urine sample. In patients with documented infection, all sexual partners in the 60 days preceding the onset of symptoms (or the last sexual partner if more than 60 days have elapsed since symptom onset) should be referred for evaluation and treatment.

Treatment of *C. trachomatis* infection is discussed later in this section. Test of cure is recommended only for pregnant women.

KEY POINTS

• Risk factors for *Chlamydia trachomatis* infection include age 25 years or younger, new or multiple sexual partners, and engaging in unprotected sex; sexually active women aged 25 years or younger and older women with risk factors should be screened annually.

• Nucleic acid amplification tests are the most sensitive study to diagnose *Chlamydia trachomatis* infection and may be performed on an endocervical or urethral swab or a urine sample.

Neisseria gonorrhoeae Infection

The highest rates of *N. gonorrhoeae* infection occur in sexually active young women. However, more infections are diagnosed in men because of the high rates of infection in men who have sex with men and the greater ease of diagnosis in male patients. Although visualization of intracellular gram-negative diplococci on a cervical or urethral smear has a high specificity for *N. gonorrhoeae*, the absence of this finding is not sensitive enough to exclude infection. Nucleic acid amplification tests therefore are preferred.

N. gonorrhoeae may cause pharyngeal infection (most cases of which are asymptomatic) and disseminated gonococcal infection (DGI). DGI presents as a febrile arthritis-dermatitis syndrome with migratory polyarthralgia evolving into frank arthritis with or without tenosynovitis that involves one or more joints. *N. gonorrhoeae* infection should be considered in the differential diagnosis of monoarticular septic arthritis in a sexually active patient. Skin lesions occur in 75% of patients with DGI. The classic lesion is characterized by a small number of necrotic vesicopustules on an erythematous base. Blood and synovial fluid cultures are often negative. A high index of clinical suspicion for DGI should prompt the collection of specimens from the cervix or urethra, pharynx, and rectum for culture to make a presumptive diagnosis.

There is a high rate of coinfection with *C. trachomatis* in patients diagnosed with *N. gonorrhoeae*. Consequently, it is recommended that individuals diagnosed with *N. gonorrhoeae* be treated concurrently for both infections.

As described for sexual partners of patients with *C. trachomatis* infection, sexual partners of patients with *N. gonorrhoeae* infection should be referred for evaluation and treatment. Treatment is discussed later in this section.

KEY POINTS

- Patients with *Neisseria gonorrhoeae* infection should also be treated for *Chlamydia trachomatis* infection because of the high rate of coinfection.
- All recent sexual partners of patients with *Neisseria gonorrhoeae* or *Chlamydia trachomatis* infection should be referred for evaluation and treatment of possible infection.

Complications of Cervicitis and Urethritis

Pelvic Inflammatory Disease

Pelvic inflammatory disease (PID) is an ascending infection of the genital tract. Patients may present with endometritis, salpingitis, or both, and PID can be complicated by the development of a tubo-ovarian abscess. PID is considered a polymicrobial infection. *C. trachomatis* and *N. gonorrhoeae* cause most infections; other possible pathogens include enteric gram-negative organisms, organisms that originate from the normal vaginal flora (especially anaerobes), and streptococci. The risk of PID is particularly high in sexually active young women (especially adolescents). The possibility of PID should be considered in women who present with pelvic or lower abdominal pain, particularly if accompanied by vaginal discharge, intermenstrual bleeding, or dyspareunia. The presenting symptoms can be mild. However, a high index of suspicion for PID must be maintained, especially in sexually active young women because unrecognized and untreated infection can lead to fallopian tube scarring and infertility.

The clinical diagnosis of PID is imprecise. PID should be considered in sexually active women who present with lower abdominal or pelvic pain and one or more of the

following findings: cervical motion tenderness, uterine tenderness, or adnexal tenderness. The presence of mucopurulent cervical discharge or numerous leukocytes in a wet mount of vaginal secretions increases the specificity of the diagnosis. Other findings that increase diagnostic specificity include fever (temperature >38.3 °C [100.9 °F]), an increased erythrocyte sedimentation rate or C-reactive protein concentration, and confirmation of infection caused by either *N. gonorrhoeae* or *C. trachomatis*. Patients in whom the diagnosis is suspected should be tested for these two pathogens, although recommended antimicrobial regimens for PID target all possible causative organisms. Many women with PID can be managed as outpatients with oral antibiotic therapy. Hospitalization is recommended for patients with the following criteria: (1) inability to exclude a surgical emergency as the cause of clinical findings; (2) pregnancy; (3) failure to respond to outpatient treatment with oral therapy; (4) inability to tolerate oral therapy; (5) severe signs of systemic toxicity, such as nausea, vomiting, and high fever; or (6) suspected tubo-ovarian abscess.

KEY POINTS

- The risk of pelvic inflammatory disease is particularly high in sexually active young women (especially adolescents).
- Pelvic inflammatory disease should be considered in sexually active women who present with lower abdominal or pelvic pain and one or more of the following findings: cervical motion tenderness, uterine tenderness, or adnexal tenderness.

Epididymitis

Acute epididymitis in sexually active men younger than age 35 years is most frequently due to *C. trachomatis*; *N. gonorrhoeae* also causes epididymitis in this age group. In older men, most infections occur in conjunction with urinary tract infection caused by enteric gram-negative organisms. Urinary obstruction secondary to benign prostatic hyperplasia is a common predisposing factor. Infection due to Enterobacteriaceae should also be considered in men who have sex with men who are the insertive partner in anal intercourse.

Patients with epididymitis present with unilateral pain and tenderness in the epididymis and testis (epididymitis-orchitis). The spermatic cord is enlarged and tender on palpation. The finding of leukocytes (≥10/hpf) on urine microscopic examination or positive leukocyte esterase on urine dipstick is supportive of the diagnosis. Patients with sudden onset of severe testicular pain or those without pyuria should be evaluated for possible testicular torsion. When *N. gonorrhoeae* or *C. trachomatis* infection is suspected, a urethral swab or urine sample should be obtained for nucleic acid amplification testing. Urine culture and susceptibility testing should also be done.

- Patients with epididymitis present with unilateral pain and tenderness in the epididymis and testis (epididymitis-orchitis) and an enlarged and tender spermatic cord.

Treatment

Recommendations for treatment of cervicitis, urethritis, proctitis, and associated complications are listed in **Table 26**. Antibiotic recommendations for the management of infections due to *N. gonorrhoeae* have changed significantly in the past several years because of increasing antimicrobial resistance among *N. gonorrhoeae* isolates in the United States. In 2010, the Centers for Disease Control and Prevention (CDC) recommended administration of ceftriaxone, 250 mg intramuscularly as a single dose, for the treatment of all infections due to *N. gonorrhoeae* because of reports of decreased susceptibility of *N. gonorrhoeae* isolates to cephalosporins and increasing reports of clinical failures with lower doses of ceftriaxone (125 mg). Oral cefixime should be used only if ceftriaxone is unavailable. In addition, all patients treated for *N. gonorrhoeae* should receive azithromycin or doxycycline (azithromycin is preferred) not just because of the high rate of coinfection with *C. trachomatis*, but because of the additional activity of these agents against isolates with decreased susceptibility to cephalosporins.

Cervicitis and urethritis can be treated empirically or based on the results of diagnostic testing. Patients who are seen in the emergency department or urgent care clinic and those who are unlikely to follow up after diagnostic testing

TABLE 26. Treatment of *Chlamydia trachomatis* and *Neisseria gonorrhoeae* Infections and Their Complications

Clinical Syndrome	Preferred Regimen	Alternative Regimen
Cervicitis and urethritis (empiric therapy)	Ceftriaxone, 250 mg IM single dose **plus** azithromycin, 1 g PO single dose	Cefixime, 400 mg PO single dose **plus** doxycycline, 100 mg PO twice daily for 7 days
Chlamydia cervicitis, urethritis, or proctitis	Azithromycin, 1 g PO single dose **or** doxycycline, 100 mg PO twice daily for 7 days	Erythromycin base, 500 mg PO four times daily **or** erythromycin ethylsuccinate, 800 mg PO four times daily **or** levofloxacin, 500 mg PO daily **or** ofloxacin, 300 mg PO twice daily for 7 days
Gonococcal cervicitis, urethritis, or proctitis and pharyngeal infection[a]	Ceftriaxone, 250 mg IM single dose **plus** azithromycin, 1 g PO single dose (preferred) **or** doxycycline, 100 mg PO twice daily for 7 days	Cefixime, 400 mg PO single dose plus azithromycin, 1 g PO single dose (preferred) **or** doxycycline, 100 mg PO twice daily for 7 days; test of cure of *N. gonorrhoeae* 1 week following treatment
Disseminated gonococcal infection	Ceftriaxone, 1 g IM or IV every 24 h	Cefotaxime, 1 g IV every 8 h **or** ceftizoxime, 1 g IV every 8 h
Pelvic inflammatory disease		
Parenteral Therapy	Cefotetan, 2 g every 12 h; **or** cefoxitin, 2 g every 6 h **plus** doxycycline, 100 mg PO or IV every 12 h **or** Clindamycin, 900 mg every 8 h **plus** gentamicin, 2 mg/kg loading dose followed by 1.5 mg/kg every 8 hours or a single daily dose of 3-5 mg/kg/d	Ampicillin-sulbactam, 3 g every 6 h **plus** doxycycline, 100 mg PO or IV every 12 h
Oral/IM Therapy	Ceftriaxone, 250 mg IM single dose **plus** doxycycline, 100 mg PO twice daily for 14 days **with or without** metronidazole, 500 mg PO twice daily for 14 days **or** Cefoxitin, 2 g IM single dose, with probenecid, 1 g PO **plus** doxycycline, 100 mg PO every 12 h for 14 days **with or without** metronidazole, 500 mg PO twice daily for 14 days	
Epididymitis[b]	Ceftriaxone, 250 mg IM single dose **plus** doxycycline, 100 PO twice daily for 10 days	

IM = intramuscularly; IV = intravenously; PO = orally.

[a]Treatment for possible *Chlamydia* infection is recommended for all patients diagnosed with gonorrhea.

[b]The recommended regimen for acute epididymitis likely due to enteric gram-negative organisms is levofloxacin, 500 mg PO daily, or ofloxacin, 300 mg PO twice daily × 10 days.

CONT.

should receive single-dose empiric therapy for both *N. gonorrhoeae* and *C. trachomatis* at the time of diagnosis. Patients diagnosed with any one sexually transmitted infection should be offered testing for other sexually transmitted infections, including HIV. **H**

KEY POINTS

- Ceftriaxone, 250 mg intramuscularly as a single dose, plus azithromycin (preferred) or doxycycline is the currently recommended treatment for *Neisseria gonorrhoeae* infection.
- Patients with cervicitis and urethritis can be treated empirically, or therapy can be based on results of diagnostic testing.
- Patients diagnosed with any one sexually transmitted infection should be offered testing for other sexually transmitted infections, including HIV.

Genital Ulcers

Herpes Simplex Virus Infection

Herpes simplex virus (HSV) is the most common cause of genital ulcer disease in the United States. Up to 50% of primary genital infections are due to HSV-1, whereas recurrent genital and perianal ulcers caused by this virus are generally due to HSV-2. This distinction has clinical implications because subclinical viral shedding and recurrent ulcers are less likely in patients with HSV-1 infections. Although most patients with HSV-2 infection have mild or subclinical disease and have never been diagnosed with genital ulcers, they may still shed virus and serve as a source of transmission to others.

Patients with symptomatic primary infection have multiple genital lesions in various stages of evolution from vesicles to pustules to shallow ulcerations on an erythematous base (see MKSAP 16 Dermatology). Women may present with cervicitis, and both men and women may have urethritis. Patients often have tender inguinal lymphadenopathy and significant systemic symptoms. Patients with recurrent infection present with fewer lesions; many patients may experience a prodrome of burning or pruritus in the genital region before the appearance of ulcers. Systemic symptoms are absent. Atypical clinical presentations, including the presence of linear fissures, are well described.

The initial clinical diagnosis of genital HSV infection should always be confirmed by viral culture or nucleic acid amplification tests such as polymerase chain reaction (PCR). PCR has superior sensitivity. Confirming HSV-1 as the cause of a primary genital infection is particularly important because this information will significantly impact patient counseling regarding risk of transmission and recurrence. Serologic tests that are type specific (can reliably distinguish HSV-1 from HSV-2) can be used for patients with a negative culture or those who present with a history of genital HSV infection that was never confirmed by culture or PCR.

Antiviral medications can reduce symptoms in patients with primary and recurrent HSV infections (**Table 27**). Patients who experience frequent recurrences of genital HSV infection (six or more episodes per year) or those who have less frequent recurrences associated with severe symptoms may be offered long-term suppressive therapy (see Table 27). Because recurrences become less frequent over time, the need for ongoing suppressive therapy should be reviewed periodically. Daily suppressive therapy with valacyclovir has been shown to reduce the risk of transmission between heterosexual partners.

Patients diagnosed with genital HSV infection need to be counseled regarding the chronic nature of their infection and the risk of transmission as a result of asymptomatic viral shedding. Patients should inform sexual partners of their diagnosis, use condoms consistently, and avoid sexual activity when experiencing prodromal symptoms or ulcer outbreaks. Type-specific serologic testing of sexual partners can determine if they are at risk of acquiring infection. Pregnant women with genital HSV infection should inform their obstetrician, and later, their newborn's pediatrician, of their diagnosis.

TABLE 27. Treatment of Herpes Simplex Virus Genital Infections	
Clinical Syndrome	**Recommended Regimen**
Primary infection[a]	Acyclovir, 400 mg three times daily **or** acyclovir, 200 mg five times daily **or** famciclovir, 250 mg three times daily **or** valacyclovir, 1 g twice daily; all regimens for 7-10 days (all regimens to be given orally)
Recurrent infection	Acyclovir, 400 mg three times daily for 5 days **or** acyclovir, 800 mg twice daily for 5 days **or** acyclovir, 800 mg three times daily for 2 days **or** famciclovir, 125 mg twice daily for 5 days **or** famciclovir, 1 g twice daily for 1 day **or** famciclovir, 500 mg once followed by 250 mg twice daily for 2 days **or** valacyclovir, 500 mg twice daily for 3 days **or** valacyclovir, 1 g once daily for 5 days
Suppressive therapy	Acyclovir, 400 mg twice daily **or** famciclovir, 250 mg twice daily **or** valacyclovir, 500 mg daily[b] **or** valacyclovir, 1 g daily

[a]Therapy can be extended if healing is incomplete after 10 days of treatment.

[b]The 500-mg dose of valacyclovir may be less effective than the 1-g dose in patients who have very frequent recurrences (≥10 episodes per year).

- Although most patients with genital herpes simplex virus type 2 infections have mild or subclinical disease and have never been diagnosed with genital ulcers, they may still shed virus and serve as a source of transmission to others.
- The initial clinical diagnosis of genital herpes simplex virus infection should always be confirmed by viral culture or polymerase chain reaction.
- Patients with genital herpes simplex virus infection should be counseled to inform sexual partners of their diagnosis, use condoms consistently, and avoid sexual activity when experiencing prodromal symptoms or ulcer outbreaks.

Syphilis

In the past decade, many urban areas in the United States have reported an increase in the number of cases of syphilis, especially among men who have sex with men. Clinical manifestations are classified according to stage to assist in decisions regarding treatment and follow-up.

Primary syphilis presents as an ulcer (chancre) that appears at the site of inoculation and may occur on the mouth, external genitalia, perianal area, or anal canal. Chancres are usually single, but several lesions can develop. A typical chancre is a painless round lesion with a raised regular border that has a firm induration on palpation. Genital lesions are frequently associated with nontender inguinal lymphadenopathy. The clinical diagnosis of primary syphilis is usually confirmed by serologic testing, although very early treatment may abort the antibody response.

The most common clinical manifestation of secondary syphilis is a generalized rash that is typically nonpruritic and often involves the palms and soles. Lesions may be macular, papular, or pustular. Silvery gray erosions with an erythematous border may be visualized on mucosal surfaces (mucus patches). Patients with secondary syphilis frequently have systemic symptoms.

Patients with positive serologic tests for syphilis but no clinical manifestations of disease have latent infection. If previous positive serologic test results are available and the infection is known to have been present for 1 year or less, patients are classified as having early latent infection. All other patients are classified as having late latent infection or syphilis of unknown duration.

Tertiary syphilis includes neurologic manifestations, ocular manifestations, cardiovascular disease (aortitis), and gummas (which can occur in any organ). Tertiary neurologic manifestations include meningovascular disease and parenchymatous disease. However, patients with neurosyphilis may be asymptomatic. Cerebrospinal fluid (CSF) examination should be performed in patients with neurologic or ophthalmic symptoms or signs, evidence of active tertiary syphilis, and serologic treatment failure.

Penicillin is the treatment of choice for all stages of syphilis, and treatment recommendations are provided in **Table 28**. Serologic testing is performed to document response to therapy. A fourfold (two-dilution) change in titer is considered significant.

Patients with primary and secondary syphilis should have repeat serologic tests at 6 and 12 months after treatment. All patients diagnosed with syphilis should be tested for HIV infection. The sexual partners of patients diagnosed with any stage of syphilis should also be evaluated. Partners

TABLE 28. Treatment of Syphilis		
Stage	**Recommended Regimen**[a]	**Alternative Regimen for Penicillin-Allergic Patients**
Primary and secondary	Benzathine penicillin G, 2.4 million units IM single dose	Doxycycline, 100 mg PO twice daily **or** tetracycline, 500 mg PO four times daily for 14 days
Early latent	Benzathine penicillin G, 2.4 million units IM single dose	Doxycycline, 100 mg PO twice daily **or** tetracycline, 500 mg PO four times daily for 14 days
Late latent or syphilis of unknown duration	Benzathine penicillin G, 2.4 million units IM at 1-week intervals for 3 doses	Doxycycline, 100 mg PO twice daily **or** tetracycline, 500 mg PO four times daily for 28 days
Neurosyphilis	Aqueous crystalline penicillin G, 18-24 million units daily given as 3-4 million units IV every 4 h or by continuous infusion for 10-14 days **or** procaine penicillin, 2.4 million units IM daily **plus** probenecid, 500 mg PO four times daily, both for 10-14 days	Ceftriaxone, 2 g IM **or** IV daily for 10-14 days[b]

IM = intramuscularly; IV = intravenously; PO = orally.

[a]Penicillin is the only effective antimicrobial agent for treatment of syphilis at any stage in pregnancy; therefore, pregnant penicillin-allergic patients should be desensitized and treated with the appropriate penicillin regimen as outlined above.

[b]Limited data are available to support the use of this alternative regimen, and the possibility of cross-reaction in penicillin-allergic patients must be considered.

exposed to a patient with primary, secondary, or early latent syphilis within the previous 3 months should be treated even if serologic test results are negative.

- Primary syphilis presents as an ulcer (chancre) at the site of inoculation; secondary syphilis is characterized by a generalized rash (especially on the palms and soles); and tertiary syphilis is associated with neurologic and ocular manifestations, cardiovascular disease, and gummas.
- Penicillin is the treatment of choice for all stages of syphilis.
- Partners exposed to a patient with primary, secondary, or early latent syphilis within the previous 3 months should also be treated for syphilis, even if serologic test results are negative.

Chancroid

Although chancroid is the most frequent cause of genital ulcer disease worldwide, it is uncommon in the United States where it is most often reported as an outbreak of infections in urban areas that typically occurs in association with trading sex for drugs, particularly crack cocaine.

Chancroid is caused by *Haemophilus ducreyi*. Lesions may be single or multiple and begin as tender, erythematous papules that become pustular and rupture to form a painful ulcer. Patients may have tender, enlarged inguinal lymph nodes that are frequently unilateral and may suppurate and drain.

The CDC recommends that a clinical diagnosis of chancroid be made in patients with all of the following criteria: (1) single or multiple painful genital ulcers, (2) no evidence to support a diagnosis of syphilis, (3) a typical clinical presentation and appearance of the ulcer, and (4) a negative test for the presence of HSV in the ulcer exudate.

Treatment of chancroid is outlined in **Table 29**. Patients must have a repeat evaluation within 1 week of treatment to document improvement. Failure to respond to therapy may indicate that the diagnosis is incorrect, and the patient should be referred to a clinician with expertise in the evaluation and management of genital ulcer disease.

- Chancroid lesions may be single or multiple and begin as tender, erythematous papules that become pustular and rupture to form a painful ulcer.
- Patients treated for chancroid must have a repeat evaluation within 1 week of beginning therapy because failure to document improvement may indicate an incorrect diagnosis.

Lymphogranuloma Venereum

Lymphogranuloma venereum (LGV) is caused by *C. trachomatis* (serovars L1, L2, and L3). Infection is only rarely reported in the United States. LGV presenting as proctitis and proctocolitis (sometimes with isolated perianal ulcers) among men who have sex with men has been recently reported in many countries in Western Europe. Classic LGV presents as a papule or ulcer at the site of inoculation that is painless and resolves without treatment. Painful unilateral inguinal lymphadenopathy then develops and is accompanied by fever and malaise. Lymph nodes may suppurate and drain. Genital specimens or lymph node drainage specimens can be tested for *C. trachomatis* using nucleic acid amplification techniques. Nucleic acid amplification testing can also be used in patients with proctitis, although these tests are not approved by the FDA for rectal specimens. Patients who have a compatible clinical presentation may be treated presumptively (see Table 29).

- Lymphogranuloma venereum typically presents as a papule or ulcer at the site of inoculation that is painless and resolves without treatment.

Genital Warts

Genital warts (condylomata acuminata) are most often due to human papillomavirus (HPV) serotypes 6 and 11, although many other serotypes can cause these lesions. HPV serotypes 16 and 18 are strongly associated with cervical cancer. Perianal warts are common in men who have sex with men and are associated with anal cancer. Warts most commonly are flesh-colored exophytic lesions that appear hyperkeratotic and are often pedunculated. Genital warts are asymptomatic in most persons. Diagnosis can be made based on the clinical appearance of the lesions.

Two HPV vaccines are currently licensed in the United States for the prevention of infection due to HPV serotypes associated with genital warts and cervical cancer. In 2011, the

TABLE 29. Treatment of Chancroid and Lymphogranuloma Venereum	
Clinical Entity	**Recommended Regimen**
Chancroid	Azithromycin, 1 g PO single dose **or** ceftriaxone, 250 mg IM single dose **or** ciprofloxacin, 500 mg PO twice daily for 3 days **or** erythromycin base, 500 mg PO three times daily for 7 days
Lymphogranuloma venereum	Doxycycline, 100 mg PO twice daily for 21 days (preferred) **or** erythromycin base, 500 mg PO four times daily for 21 days (alternative)
IM = intramuscularly; PO = orally.	

CDC's Advisory Committee on Immunization Practices (ACIP) recommended the routine vaccination of males 11 or 12 years old with three doses of the quadrivalent HPV vaccine for protection against HPV and HPV-related conditions and cancers in males. The vaccination of males with HPV may also provide indirect protection of women by reducing transmission of HPV. Catch-up vaccination is recommended for all men aged 19 to 21 years. Men aged 22 to 26 years should be vaccinated if they have underlying immunosuppression (including HIV infection) or if they are men who have sex with men. Women 19 to 26 years of age who were not previously vaccinated should also receive the HPV vaccine.

Treatment is only indicated for patients who have symptomatic lesions or who are concerned about the cosmetic appearance of the warts. However, treatment does not eliminate the possibility of HPV transmission. Patient-applied topical agents and physician-administered treatments are available.

KEY POINTS

- Genital warts most commonly present as asymptomatic, flesh-colored, exophytic lesions that appear hyperkeratotic and are often pedunculated.
- Treatment of genital warts is only indicated for patients who have symptomatic lesions or are concerned about the cosmetic appearance of the warts.

Osteomyelitis

Pathophysiology and Classification

Although normal bone is resistant to infection because it is not exposed to microbes, pathogens may reach the bone through hematogenous spread, direct inoculation following trauma or surgery, or by contiguous spread from colonized or infected adjacent soft tissues. Pathologic hallmarks of acute osteomyelitis include the presence of polymorphonuclear leukocytes, thrombosis of small vessels, and bone necrosis. The subsequent accompanying separated pieces of dead bone are known as the sequestrum. Once the sequestrum has formed and new bone formation has begun, the infection is considered chronic. Lymphocytes, histiocytes, and plasma cells are observed histologically, and sinus tracts and local bone loss are seen clinically.

Hematogenous osteomyelitis is generally a disease of children, but it also accounts for approximately 20% of cases in adults. Unlike in children in whom the most frequent sites of infection are the growing ends or metaphyses of long bones where rapid bone turnover occurs, the vertebral column is the most common location for hematogenous osteomyelitis in adults. The sternoclavicular and sacroiliac bones may be involved, especially in injection drug users. The bacteremic events responsible for hematogenous osteomyelitis may be related to intravascular catheters, distant foci of infection, or

infective endocarditis. Except in patients with endocarditis, the bacteremia is often not apparent. Typically, a single (monomicrobial) bacterial species is responsible for hematogenous osteomyelitic infection. Although most cases are caused by *Staphylococcus aureus,* aerobic gram-negative bacilli cause disease in many patients. *Pseudomonas aeruginosa* and *Salmonella* species are associated with infections in injection drug users and patients with sickle cell disease, respectively.

Osteomyelitis associated with a contiguous focus of infection, vascular insufficiency, or decubitus ulcers may be polymicrobial or monomicrobial, with *S. aureus* as the most common organism. The presence of a foreign body and weak host defenses predispose to infection with less pathogenic organisms. Pathogens found alone or in combination in patients with contiguous osteomyelitis include gram-negative bacilli, enterococci, anaerobes, and fungi.

KEY POINTS

- Although most cases of hematogenous osteomyelitis are caused by *Staphylococcus aureus,* aerobic gram-negative bacilli such as *Pseudomonas aeruginosa* and *Salmonella* species are associated with infections in injection drug users and patients with sickle cell disease, respectively.
- *Staphylococcus aureus* is the most common causative organism of contiguous osteomyelitis, vascular insufficiency, or decubitus ulcers, and infection may be polymicrobial or monomicrobial.

Clinical Manifestations

The clinical manifestations of acute osteomyelitis customarily present subacutely, usually with dull pain from the infected bone. Local erythema, warmth, edema, and palpable tenderness often follow. Pus may spread into joints, presenting as septic arthritis. Fever may or may not be present. Patients with infection of the spine or pelvic joints may have constant pain exacerbated by movement. Chronic pain following the placement of a prosthetic joint or loosening of its components should be considered suspicious for prosthetic joint infection. The clinical features of chronic osteomyelitis are similar to those of acute osteomyelitis, but the presence of a draining sinus tract is somewhat pathognomonic of chronic osteomyelitis.

KEY POINTS

- The clinical manifestations of acute osteomyelitis customarily present subacutely, usually with dull pain from the infected bone, followed by local erythema, warmth, edema, and palpable tenderness; fever may or may not be present.
- The clinical features of chronic osteomyelitis are similar to those of acute osteomyelitis, but the presence of a draining sinus tract is pathognomonic of chronic osteomyelitis.

Diagnosis

Imaging Studies

In patients with osteomyelitis, conventional plain radiographs are limited by their poor sensitivity and specificity. Soft tissue swelling may be an early finding, but osseous abnormalities can take 2 weeks to become visible.

Nuclear imaging modalities include the three-phase bone scan, gallium scanning, and tagged leukocyte scanning. A three-phase bone scan uses a radionuclide tracer (usually technetium-99m) that is injected; γ images of the area of interest are taken at specific times following injection. Osteomyelitis shows enhancement in all three phases, whereas overlying soft tissue infections do not. Gallium-67 has an affinity for acute phase reactants and will accumulate in areas of infection following injection. Tagged leukocyte scanning involves use of a radiotracer to label autologous leukocytes, which are reinjected; they will accumulate at sites of infection or inflammation. All three nuclear imaging studies have high sensitivity (>90%) for osteomyelitis. However, specificity is more variable because these studies tend to be falsely positive in patients with conditions involving inflammation or bone turnover, such as degenerative joint disease, trauma, surgery, or cancer. The specificity of these tests is significantly improved when there is no evidence of another process involving the area of interest as documented by normal plain radiography.

MRI has generally become the preferred imaging technique for diagnosing osteomyelitis. It is readily available, quickly obtained, has a high sensitivity for bone infection, and can help exclude disease in the setting of a negative study. It may show evidence of bone infection within several days of onset, can delineate bone anatomy and changes in the surrounding soft tissues, and tends to be more effective than nuclear imaging in detecting osteomyelitis in specific anatomic locations such as the feet and vertebrae. However, the specificity of MRI is limited because the bone marrow edema changes seen in patients with osteomyelitis may be from other causes and may persist for months after effective therapy. Because follow-up MRIs can be confusing and lead to additional unwarranted therapy, they are generally not necessary. However, if an MRI is obtained, findings that are most worrisome will show new areas of bone involvement.

CT scanning is a reasonable choice when MRI is contraindicated, such as in patients with cardiac pacemakers, defibrillators, metallic artifacts, or kidney failure (gadolinium contraindicated).

Laboratory Studies

Blood tests lack specificity to assist in the initial diagnosis of osteomyelitis. The leukocyte count may not be elevated, but inflammatory markers, such as the erythrocyte sedimentation rate and C-reactive protein level, are generally increased; however, normal values do not exclude the diagnosis. Blood cultures may identify bacteremia in a small fraction of cases (almost all are acute osteomyelitis). In such cases, the infecting organism is likely to be identified. Nevertheless, blood cultures are recommended in all cases of suspected osteomyelitis because identifying a microorganism may eliminate the need for more extensive testing.

Bone Biopsy

Bone biopsy is considered the gold standard for diagnosing osteomyelitis and can be done by open surgical biopsy or needle aspiration. Bone biopsies showing microorganism inflammation and osteonecrosis can corroborate the diagnosis.

With the exception of *S. aureus*, collection of microorganisms isolated from culture specimens of superficial wounds or sinus tracts correlates poorly with deep cultures from bone; therefore, this approach is of limited value. Collection of surface swab cultures should be discouraged because it can misdirect therapy.

KEY POINTS

- In patients with osteomyelitis, conventional plain radiographs are limited by their poor sensitivity and specificity because osseous abnormalities can take 2 weeks to become visible.
- MRI is the preferred imaging modality for detecting osteomyelitis and has reliable sensitivity.
- Bone biopsy can be done in patients with osteomyelitis by open surgical biopsy or needle aspiration and is diagnostic when results demonstrate microorganism inflammation and osteonecrosis.

Treatment

Treatment is initiated once the diagnosis of osteomyelitis is established and the inciting pathogen identified. Successful treatment generally requires a combination of surgical debridement, removal of orthopedic hardware (if present and feasible), and administration of appropriate antibiotics for a prolonged period (see MKSAP 16 Rheumatology). The application of vacuum-assisted closure devices and use of hyperbaric oxygen exposure are adjunctive therapies, which may offer benefit for a selective group of patients. Prognosis depends on factors such as the chronicity of disease, organisms involved, comorbidities, and physiologic state of the infected individual, as well as the ability to remove all infected hardware or prosthetic devices. In patients in whom cure cannot be achieved, chronic suppressive antibiotic treatment is warranted. Similarly, in patients with no systemic or severe local signs of infection and in whom a prosthesis is not loose or in whom surgery is not possible or desired, lifelong oral antimicrobial therapy may be considered in an attempt to suppress the infection and retain usefulness of the total joint replacement.

- Successful treatment of osteomyelitis generally requires a combination of surgical debridement, removal of orthopedic hardware (if present and feasible), and administration of appropriate antibiotics for a prolonged period.
- In patients with osteomyelitis in whom cure cannot be achieved, chronic suppressive antibiotic treatment is warranted.

Evaluation and Management of Diabetes Mellitus–Associated Osteomyelitis

In patients with diabetes mellitus, skin and soft tissue infections and subsequent ulcer formation, particularly on the feet, may progress unrecognized, eventually resulting in contiguous osteomyelitis. Therefore, patients with diabetes must be vigilant to any signs of soft tissue disease and seek evaluation expeditiously, before a potentially limb-threatening condition develops.

Important clinical signs suggestive of a deeper infectious process in patients with diabetic foot ulcers are tenderness, erythema, warmth, and the presence of purulent material in the ulcer or from a sinus tract. Gas in the soft tissues, suggested by crepitus, bullous formation, and skin color changes, may indicate necrotizing fasciitis. Severe ischemia with gangrene may also occur.

Many patients with diabetes and complex foot infection lack classic systemic signs of infection, including fever. In general, ulcers that are greater than 2 cm, are present for 2 weeks or longer, and are characterized by visible bone or a positive probe-to-bone test, are predictive of contiguous osteomyelitis.

The approach to imaging and laboratory studies in patients with diabetes-associated osteomyelitis is the same as that for patients with osteomyelitis; however, the presence of visualized bone or palpation of bone by a sterile, blunt, stainless steel probe in the depth of a foot ulcer should obviate the need for diagnostic imaging.

Combined medical and surgical therapy, wound management, glucose control, and administration of antibiotics are recommended to increase the likelihood for a successful outcome. Debridement and culture before institution of antimicrobial therapy are recommended. Early surgical intervention for debridement and drainage decreases the risk for amputations. Revascularization procedures, if indicated, improve the arterial blood supply, promoting healing and preventing further ischemic necrosis.

Broad-spectrum antimicrobial treatment is usually required as initial therapy owing to the polymicrobial nature of diabetic foot infections. Patients with severe infections or those with suspected or proven osteomyelitis generally require parenteral therapy. Oral antimicrobial therapy may be adequate for patients with milder infections involving pathogens sensitive to agents demonstrating good oral bioavailability. Although not supported by good comparative data, standard treatment regimens include monotherapy or combination therapy with agents possessing good activity against staphylococci, streptococci, aerobic gram-negative bacilli, and anaerobes. Vancomycin combined with an agent active against gram-negative organisms would be appropriate empiric therapy. Advanced-generation cephalosporins (for example, ceftriaxone and cefepime) or fluoroquinolones (for example, ciprofloxacin or levofloxacin), combined with an agent with anaerobic activity, such as metronidazole or clindamycin, are also acceptable choices. In addition, a β-lactam/β-lactamase inhibitor combination drug and a carbapenem agent such as meropenem would provide appropriate coverage. The increasing prevalence of methicillin-resistant *S. aureus* emphasizes the importance of establishing a microbiologic diagnosis. The initial empiric antimicrobial regimen should be narrowed after culture and sensitivity information becomes available, with the understanding that not every isolate from these polymicrobial infections requires treatment. The duration of antimicrobial therapy should be individualized based on the clinical circumstances. Generally, therapy should be given until the wound and the signs of infection have resolved. In patients with osteomyelitis, antimicrobial therapy is usually given for 6 weeks following surgical debridement unless the infected bone has been totally removed, in which case the medication can be stopped once the wound has adequately healed.

- Diabetic foot ulcers that are generally greater than 2 cm, are present for 2 weeks or longer, and are characterized by visible bone or a positive probe-to-bone test are predictive of contiguous osteomyelitis.
- Debridement and culture before institution of antimicrobial therapy are recommended in patients with diabetes mellitus and osteomyelitis.
- In patients with osteomyelitis, antimicrobial therapy is usually given for 6 weeks following surgical debridement unless the infected bone has been totally removed, in which case the medication can be stopped after the wound has adequately healed.

Evaluation and Management of Vertebral Osteomyelitis

Infection of the vertebral bones and contiguous disk space, termed spondylodiskitis, most often occurs as a consequence of bacteremia. The segmental arteries that supply the vertebral column bifurcate, thereby permitting the infecting organism to simultaneously reach two adjacent vertebral bodies, with subsequent bony destruction. The intervertebral disk space becomes secondarily involved by direct invasion from the adjacent bones. Alternatively, these anatomic areas can become infected following spinal surgery or as a rare complication from injection or catheter placement. The lumbar spine is involved most frequently, followed by the thoracic and cervical vertebrae. *S. aureus* (including methicillin-resistant *S. aureus*) is the most commonly involved pathogen, although, coagulase-negative staphylococci may also be a cause of infection in the spine. Gram-negative bacilli, streptococci, *Candida* species, and unusual organisms (for example, *Brucella* species) may also be involved.

Progressively worsening back or neck pain over several weeks without an alternative explanation should prompt an evaluation for possible vertebral osteomyelitis. Tenderness localized over the spinal site of infection is common, and neurologic deficits may occur.

Although fever and elevated leukocyte counts are present in only half of patients, an increased erythrocyte sedimentation rate (often >100 mm/h) and C-reactive protein level are present in more than 80% of patients. Obtaining blood cultures, which are positive in more than 50% of patients, is essential, because isolation of a probable pathogen can minimize the extent of the evaluation and facilitate focused antibiotic therapy.

The lack of sensitivity of plain radiographs limits their utility in patients with vertebral osteomyelitis. MRI offers the best sensitivity, but false-positive scans may occur in patients with uninfected fractures. Radionuclide scans may be helpful diagnostic aids but, with the exception of gallium scans, lack sufficient specificity. A CT-guided percutaneous needle aspiration biopsy and culture are needed to confirm the diagnosis when blood cultures are negative. Even in patients in whom the first sample is nondiagnostic, a second biopsy attempt can help to determine the microbial cause. Ideally, biopsy attempts should be performed before antibiotics are given, but biopsy should not be avoided in patients already receiving therapy.

The mainstay of vertebral osteomyelitis treatment includes prolonged pathogen-directed, or occasionally, empiric parenteral antimicrobial therapy. In patients in whom a pathogen is not isolated, an empiric regimen including a reliable agent aimed at gram-positive cocci, such as vancomycin, with a broad-spectrum antibiotic against gram-negative bacilli, such as cefepime or ceftriaxone, would be reasonable. Oral antimicrobial agents are generally not used for treatment of vertebral osteomyelitis except in specific situations, such as when a fluoroquinolone (ciprofloxacin)-sensitive gram-negative bacillus proves to be the infecting pathogen, or possibly, when long-term chronic antimicrobial suppression is warranted, such as in patients with retained orthopedic hardware.

Antimicrobial therapy is generally given for 6 to 8 weeks, but prolonged therapy may be necessary in patients with extensive or advanced disease. Surgical intervention is rarely required except when it is necessary to stabilize the spine, drain an abscess, or pursue the diagnosis in patients in whom empiric treatment is not effective. H

Follow-up MRI is usually not warranted except for patients in whom improvement is expected but not achieved, when complications develop, or when inflammatory markers remain elevated without explanation.

KEY POINTS

- Progressively worsening back or neck pain over several weeks without an alternative explanation and localized tenderness over the spinal site of infection should prompt an evaluation for possible vertebral osteomyelitis.

- An increased erythrocyte sedimentation rate (often >100 mm/h) and C-reactive protein level are present in more than 80% of patients with vertebral osteomyelitis.

- Obtaining blood cultures, which are positive in more than 50% of patients, is essential in diagnosing patients with vertebral osteomyelitis.

- A CT-guided percutaneous needle aspirate biopsy and culture are needed to confirm the diagnosis of vertebral osteomyelitis when blood cultures are negative.

Fever of Unknown Origin

Introduction

Fever is a complex cytokine-mediated response of the body to many infectious and noninfectious causes. Although the source of fever is often determined by a thorough history, physical examination, and basic laboratory studies, the cause cannot be established in a subgroup of patients who are said to have fever of unknown origin (FUO). FUO is classically defined as an illness that lasts at least 3 weeks in a patient with a temperature greater than 38.3 °C (101.0 °F) on several occasions and whose diagnosis remains uncertain despite having been evaluated in a hospital for at least 1 week.

However, because of improved diagnostic methods, it has been suggested that the classic definition of FUO should be changed, with a particular focus on specific risk groups:

- Classic FUO: temperature higher than 38.0 °C (100.4 °F) for more than 3 weeks and either more than 3 days of hospital investigation or more than two outpatient visits without determination of the cause.

- Health care–associated FUO: temperature higher than 38.0 °C (100.4 °F) for more than 3 days in a hospitalized patient receiving acute care with infection not present or incubating on admission.

CONT.

- Immune-deficient FUO: temperature higher than 38.0 °C (100.4 °F) in a patient in whom the diagnosis remains uncertain after more than 3 days despite appropriate investigation, including at least 48 hours' incubation of microbiologic cultures.
- HIV-related FUO: temperature higher than 38.0 °C (100.4 °F) in a patient with confirmed HIV infection for more than 3 weeks in outpatients or more than 3 days in inpatients.

Causes

Although some FUOs are due to infections, other broad diagnostic categories include noninfectious inflammatory disorders (connective tissue diseases, vasculitis syndromes, and granulomatous diseases), malignancies, and other specific disorders. Historically, infections were considered the most likely cause of fever, followed by noninfectious inflammatory disorders and malignancies. More recently, infections and malignancies have become less commonly associated with FUO, and undetermined causes are increasing in prevalence. However, even with current diagnostic methods, the cause remains undetermined in a significant number of patients.

The patient's age may provide a clue to diagnosis. Infections and malignancies are responsible for most FUOs in adults; however, malignancy is an uncommon cause in children. Noninfectious multisystemic inflammatory disorders (polymyalgia rheumatica, temporal arteritis, and rheumatoid arthritis) are most frequently associated with FUO in older patients.

The duration of fever is also important in diagnosing FUOs. For example, factitious fever and granulomatous diseases should be strongly considered in patients with a history of unexplained fever of more than 6 months.

Immune status should also be considered because this may alter the differential diagnosis of potential causes. The number of immunocompromised persons (transplant recipients and patients receiving cancer therapy) and patients with stable AIDS infection has increased in recent years. In patients with neutropenia and fever, the initial diagnostic consideration should include bacterial infection, particularly because an impaired immune response may change the typical presentation of many infections. Persistent fever may also be due to fungi, including infections caused by *Aspergillus* and *Candida* species. In patients with AIDS and a low CD4 cell count, the most common causes of FUO are infections (particularly mycobacterial infections), followed by malignancies such as non-Hodgkin lymphoma.

In all patients with FUO, the response to empiric antimicrobial therapy may provide a clue as to whether a bacterial infection may be the underlying cause. An initial response with relapse may suggest a localized infection, such as an abscess. No response may be associated with an atypical infection or a noninfectious cause.

Occult abscesses in the kidneys, liver, and spleen may not always have well-defined localizing features, especially in elderly or immunocompromised patients. Blood culture results are not always positive, and other serologic test results may be insensitive in these patients. Similarly, patients with vertebral osteomyelitis may not have localizing symptoms.

Infective endocarditis was once a common cause of FUO. However, modern microbiologic techniques are effective in identifying causative pathogens, including the HACEK organisms (*H*aemophilus aphrophilus, *A*ctinobacillus actinomycetemcomitans, *C*ardiobacterium hominis, *E*ikenella corrodens, and *K*ingella kingae). Exceptions are pathogens associated with culture-negative infective endocarditis, including *Coxiella burnetii*, *Tropheryma whipplei*, and *Brucella*, *Bartonella*, *Chlamydia*, *Histoplasma*, and *Legionella* species. Tuberculosis may not always be suspected as a cause of FUO, particularly in patients without a clear exposure history and without pulmonary symptoms or findings. This is particularly true in immunocompromised patients with atypical clinical manifestations, such as those with extrapulmonary involvement.

Patients with acute HIV infection may present with fever and various other findings. Enzyme-linked immunosorbent assays (ELISA) for HIV can be negative during early infection; a repeat ELISA or a viral load determination may be necessary for diagnosis. Because fever is an integral part of the mononucleosis syndromes, Epstein-Barr virus and cytomegalovirus infections should always be considered. Results of mononucleosis testing may be negative in up to 15% of younger patients, and the presentation of Epstein-Barr virus infection in older adults may differ from that seen in younger individuals. Toxoplasmosis can cause fever and lymphadenopathy, but the acute illness is seldom diagnosed or treated except in the setting of pregnancy.

Neoplastic-associated causes of FUO include lymphoma, posttransplant lymphoproliferative disorders, leukemia, myelodysplastic syndromes, renal cell carcinoma, hepatocellular carcinoma, liver metastases, colon cancer, and atrial myxoma. A clue to cancer-related fever is that patients often appear less toxic and may not be aware of having fever. Noninfectious inflammatory disorders to be considered include systemic lupus erythematosus, cryoglobulinemia, polyarteritis nodosa, and granulomatosis with polyangiitis (also known as Wegener granulomatosis). Adult-onset Still disease should be considered in a patient with arthritis, evanescent rash, fever, neutrophilic leukocytosis, pharyngitis, lymphadenopathy, hepatosplenomegaly, and abnormal liver chemistry test results. Giant cell arteritis should be suspected in patients over 50 years of age who present with jaw claudication, headache, visual disturbances, a significantly elevated erythrocyte sedimentation rate, and polymyalgia rheumatica.

Medications may be associated with FUO. Drug fever may cause rash and eosinophilia and can be diagnosed when fever resolves after discontinuation of the causative agent.

Hereditary periodic fever syndromes are rare but should be considered when fever-free intervals of at least 14 days occur in patients with recurrent FUO. These include hyper-immunoglobulin D syndrome (HIDS), tumor-necrosis factor receptor-1–associated periodic syndrome (TRAPS), Muckle-Wells syndrome, and familial Mediterranean fever.

Familial Mediterranean fever is an autosomal recessive disease occurring in certain ethnic groups, including persons of Jewish, Armenian, Arab, and Turkish descent, and is characterized by serositis, arthritis, chest and abdominal pain, and rarely, a distal lower extremity rash. Patients with the Muckle-Wells syndrome, an autosomal dominant disorder resulting from a defective gene that encodes the cryopyrin protein, exhibit progressive sensorineural hearing loss; episodic urticarial rash, fever, abdominal pain, and arthralgia/arthritis; and possibly, eventual amyloidosis. HIDS, an autosomal recessive disease, presents at a very young age and manifests as recurrent episodes of fever, abdominal pain, diarrhea, lymphadenopathy, maculopapular rash, and joint pain; elevated serum IgD and IgA levels are characteristic. TRAPS is an autosomal dominant syndrome characterized by recurrent presentations of fever; tender, erythematous patches; periorbital edema; conjunctivitis; abdominal pain; arthritis; and testicular pain.

Miscellaneous causes of FUO include subacute thyroiditis or hyperthyroidism, sarcoidosis, pulmonary embolism, retroperitoneal or abdominal hematoma, pheochromocytoma, factitious fever, and habitual hyperthermia.

KEY POINTS

- Fever of unknown origin may be due to infections, noninfectious inflammatory disorders, malignancies, and many other disorders.

- Infections that commonly cause fever of unknown origin include tuberculosis, infective endocarditis, and intra-abdominal and pelvic abscesses.

- Hereditary periodic fever syndromes, such as hyper-immunoglobulin D syndrome, tumor-necrosis factor receptor-1–associated periodic syndrome, Muckle-Wells syndrome, and familial Mediterranean fever, should be considered when fever-free intervals of at least 14 days occur in patients with recurrent fever of unknown origin.

Evaluation

A comprehensive history and thorough physical examination, which should be repeated as the illness evolves, are essential in the evaluation of patients with FUO. The history should determine the presence of immunocompromising conditions or a predisposition to infective endocarditis (including injection drug use and valvular abnormalities), as well as medications, immunizations, hobbies, travel, sexual activity (including a history of sexually transmitted infections), and recent contacts with domestic or farm animals, insects, and ill persons. The physical examination should include pelvic, rectal, and temporal artery evaluation. The presence of rash, lymphadenopathy, cardiac murmurs, hepatosplenomegaly, and arthritic changes can provide valuable clues to the diagnosis.

Initial laboratory studies may include a complete blood count, erythrocyte sedimentation rate, measurement of C-reactive protein, peripheral blood smear, complete metabolic profile with liver chemistry studies, urinalysis with microscopic evaluation, and urine and blood cultures. Further testing should be done based on potential causes as assessed during the history and physical examination and may include an antinuclear antibody assay, measurement of rheumatoid factor, serum and urine protein electrophoresis, and serologic studies for hepatitis, syphilis, HIV, cytomegalovirus, Epstein-Barr virus, and *C. burnetii* (Q fever); tuberculosis testing (skin and interferon-γ release assays) may also be appropriate. Imaging should be directed by the potential cause of the FUO, and extensive studies based solely on the presence of an FUO should not be done. Based on the history and physical examination, a chest radiograph, echocardiogram, and CT scans of the abdomen, chest, and pelvis may be appropriate, depending on clinical considerations. Nuclear imaging studies are considered useful by some clinicians in identifying an inflammatory source of fever when initial imaging studies are normal. Further evaluation, including biopsies, is dictated by results of abnormal tests. Bone marrow examination may be useful in patients with anemia and thrombocytopenia.

Up to 50% of patients with FUO will not have an identified cause despite an extensive evaluation. The prognosis is generally good for these patients because symptoms tend to resolve within months of development. Although empiric antibiotics with or without corticosteroids are often considered, their use should be discouraged if the patient is stable and has no localizing signs.

KEY POINTS

- A comprehensive history and thorough physical examination, which often needs to be repeated as the illness evolves, are essential in the evaluation of a patient with fever of unknown origin.

- Laboratory testing and imaging studies of patients with fever of unknown origin should be directed by the potential cause and findings on history and physical examination.

- Up to 50% of patients with fever of unknown origin will not have an identified cause despite an extensive evaluation.

Primary Immunodeficiencies

Introduction

Although uncommon, primary immunodeficiency syndromes should be considered in patients with frequent, multiple, or prolonged infections caused by certain pathogens such as *Streptococcus pneumoniae*, *Neisseria* species, and *Haemophilus influenzae*. Primary immunodeficiency syndromes are relatively rare and generally manifest in children.

Selective IgA Deficiency

Selective absence of serum and secretory IgA, inherited as an incompletely penetrant autosomal dominant or autosomal recessive trait, is the most common primary immunodeficiency and has a worldwide prevalence of approximately 1 in 300 to 700 persons. IgA is the major immunoglobulin in external secretions (for example, saliva, tears, nasal secretions) and blocks the binding of antigens (pathogens and toxins) to cell receptors. It binds antigens and facilitates their clearance by ciliated epithelium. Most patients with selective IgA deficiency develop few or no recurrent infections, although some have chronic or recurrent respiratory tract infections, atopic disorders, and an increased frequency of autoimmune disorders. Gastrointestinal and urogenital tract infections may also occur. Other immunoglobulin concentrations are usually normal, although an IgG_2 subclass deficiency has been reported in patients with the most morbidity, and IgM concentrations may be abnormal. Serum autoantibodies to IgA are found in up to 40% of patients with recurrent infections. Some patients have severe anaphylactic reactions to administration of intravenous immune globulin or blood products.

Common Variable Immunodeficiency

Common variable immunodeficiency (CVID) occurs in both adults and children. Most patients present before age 30 years. Approximately 1 in 25,000 persons is affected worldwide, and the disorder is more prevalent among those of northern European descent. CVID is caused by impaired B cell differentiation and defective immunoglobulin production. Serum IgG levels are markedly reduced, and serum IgA or IgM levels (or both) are frequently low.

Patients with CVID frequently develop chronic lung diseases, autoimmune disorders, malabsorption, recurrent infections, and lymphoma, and their response to vaccination is poor or absent. Sinopulmonary infections, ear infections, and conjunctivitis are common and are most often caused by pneumococci, *Mycoplasma* species, and *Haemophilus influenzae*. Some patients are also susceptible to infection with enteroviruses, *Candida* species, and *Giardia lamblia*. Septic arthritis and chronic pulmonary diseases (bronchiectasis, restrictive or obstructive lung disease) have also been reported. Gastrointestinal diseases occur in approximately 20% of patients with CVID and include inflammatory bowel disease, sprue-like disorders, and pernicious anemia. Approximately 25% of patients have an autoimmune disorder, such as rheumatoid arthritis or hemolytic anemia and thrombocytopenia. Up to 20% of patients have evidence of granulomatous disease associated with noncaseating granulomas in lymphoid or solid organs.

Patients with CVID usually show impaired responses to vaccines. If CVID is suspected, quantitative serum IgG, IgA, and IgM levels should be measured. If levels are low, antibody response to vaccination should be tested by determining the response to protein- and polysaccharide-based vaccines. Such testing is not needed in patients with very low (<200 mg/dL [2.0 g/L]) or undetectable serum IgG levels because these patients will most likely not respond to vaccines.

Use of immune globulin replacement therapy has reduced the number of recurrent infections in patients with CVID. Prophylactic antibiotics should not be routinely administered to all patients but should be reserved for those with chronic lung disease and those who require oral corticosteroids or immunosuppressive agents for more than 1 month.

Abnormalities in the Complement System

Complement deficiency states may be inherited or acquired. Complement deficiencies predispose to bacterial infections and autoimmune disorders. The frequency of inherited complement deficiencies in the general population is about 0.03%. Most complement deficiencies are inherited as autosomal recessive traits. However, C1 inhibitor deficiency is inherited as an autosomal dominant trait, and properdin deficiency is an X-linked disorder. Deficiencies of C3, factor H, factor I, and properdin are associated with severe recurrent infections caused by encapsulated organisms such as *Streptococcus pneumoniae*. Deficiency of the terminal complement components C5, C6, C7, and C8 increases susceptibility to disseminated neisserial infections (primarily due to meningococci but also to gonococci), which tend to be recurrent and have mild to moderate clinical manifestations. Inherited defects of the alternative complement pathway, including factor D and properdin, are rare. Patients with properdin deficiency are at risk for neisserial infections. Recurrent pneumonia and otitis media have also been reported in these patients. Systemic lupus erythematosus (SLE) is the most common autoimmune disorder in patients with complement deficiencies. Autoimmune disease (most commonly SLE) is more common in those with inherited complement deficiencies, especially those with C1, C4, C2, or C3 deficiency.

When a complement pathway defect is suspected, patients should be tested for total hemolytic complement (CH_{50}). If the serum CH_{50} concentration is very low or undetectable, specific complement components should be measured.

Vaccination is the most effective way to prevent infections in patients with complement deficiencies. All routine vaccinations (especially meningococcal, pneumococcal, and *Haemophilus influenzae* vaccines) should be administered. Conjugate vaccines are preferred to polysaccharide vaccines in these patients.

KEY POINTS

- Patients with common variable immunodeficiency frequently develop chronic lung diseases, autoimmune disorders, malabsorption, recurrent infections, and lymphoma, and their response to vaccination is poor or absent.

- In patients with suspected chronic variable immunodeficiency and low serum immunoglobulin levels, the antibody response to vaccination should be tested to help establish the diagnosis.

- When a complement pathway defect is suspected, patients should be tested for total hemolytic complement (CH_{50}).

- Vaccination is the most effective way to prevent infections in patients with complement deficiency.

Bioterrorism

Introduction

Bioterrorism is defined as the intentional release of bacteria, viruses, or toxins for the purpose of harming or killing civilians.

A bioterrorism attack results in an increased incidence of a disease (epidemic) above its usual rate in a population (endemic), which occurs suddenly and within a relatively confined geographic area (outbreak). Biologic agents that can potentially be used are prioritized into three classes (A, B, and C), based on their ability to cause illness and death, capacity for dissemination, public perception as related to plausible civil disruption, and special needs required for effective public health intervention. Class A agents have the greatest potential for causing a major public health impact associated with a high mortality rate and are discussed in this chapter (**Table 30**).

In general, class B agents (for example, *Coxiella burnetii*, *Brucella* species, *Salmonella* species, *Vibrio cholerae*) are disseminated less easily, result in less morbidity and lower mortality rates, and would be expected to have a lower medical and public health impact. Class C agents include emerging pathogens (for example, Nipah virus, hantavirus) that are currently not believed to have a high risk for use as bioterrorism agents but could have the potential for wide dissemination in the future.

Except for smallpox (eradicated by vaccine), all of the major bioterrorism agents are naturally occurring. Epidemiologic features may help distinguish a bioterrorism attack from a naturally occurring disease. Illness due to bioterrorism is more likely to be associated with suddenness of onset, a large number of cases, increased severity or an uncommon clinical presentation, and an unusual geographic, temporal, or demographic clustering of cases. Syndromic surveillance refers to using health-related data to signal the probability that a case or an outbreak of illness is related to bioterrorism and therefore warrants a further public health response.

TABLE 30. Class A Bioterrorism Agents				
Disease - Agent	**Incubation Period**	**Clinical Features**	**Treatment**	**Prophylaxis**
Anthrax – *Bacillus anthracis*	1 to 60 days	Inhalational (febrile respiratory distress); cutaneous (necrotic eschar); gastrointestinal (distention, peritonitis)	Ciprofloxacin or doxycycline plus 1 or 2 additional agents[a]	Ciprofloxacin or doxycycline
Smallpox virus – variola virus	7 to 17 days	Fever followed by pustular cutaneous rash	Supportive care	Vaccine if exposure was in the past 3 days
Plague – *Yersinia pestis*	1 to 6 days	Fulminant pneumonia and sepsis	Streptomycin or gentamicin	Doxycycline or ciprofloxacin
Botulism – *Clostridium botulinum*	2 hours to 8 days	Cranial nerve palsies and descending flaccid paralysis	Antitoxin and supportive care	Antibotulinum antitoxin
Tularemia – *Francisella tularensis*	3 to 5 days	Fever, respiratory distress, and sepsis	Streptomycin or gentamicin (severe disease); doxycycline or ciprofloxacin (nonsevere disease)	Doxycycline or ciprofloxacin
Viral hemorrhagic fever – various viruses	Variable	Hemorrhage and multiorgan failure	Supportive care	None available

[a]Penicillin, ampicillin, imipenem, meropenem, clindamycin, rifampin, vancomycin, or clarithromycin.

- Bioterrorism is defined as the intentional release of bacteria, viruses, or toxins for the purpose of harming or killing civilians.

- Biologic agents that can potentially be used for bioterrorism are prioritized into three classes (A, B, and C), with class A agents having the greatest potential for causing a major public health impact associated with a high mortality rate.

Anthrax

Anthrax infection is caused by the bacterium *Bacillus anthracis* ("coal" in Greek) to describe the distinctive black eschar associated with cutaneous disease. This gram-positive, "box-car"–shaped, aerobic, nonmotile bacillus is found in soil worldwide, predominantly in agricultural areas (**Figure 9A**). Under favorable environmental conditions, it transforms into 1- to 5-micron spores that may remain viable for decades (**Figure 9B**). Spores may be acquired by inhalation, cutaneous contact, or ingestion. Cutaneous anthrax is most common, but inhalational anthrax is most likely to be lethal. Gastrointestinal anthrax is uncommon in humans.

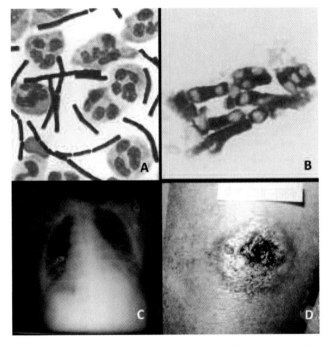

FIGURE 9. *A,* "box-car"–shaped, gram-positive *Bacillus anthracis* bacilli in the cerebrospinal fluid of the index case of inhalational anthrax due to bioterrorism in the United States; *B,* terminal and subterminal spores of *B. anthracis; C,* widened mediastinum on chest radiograph due to hemorrhagic lymphadenopathy in a patient with anthrax; *D,* black eschar lesion of cutaneous anthrax.

Because spores are easily dispersed by aerosolization and infective spores can be sent by mail (for example, the October 2001 occurrence of bioterrorism-related anthrax in the United States), even a single case of inhalational anthrax should raise the possibility of deliberate spread. Inhaled spores are transported to draining mediastinal lymph nodes. After an incubation period of 1 to 6 days (potentially up to 60 days), a prodromal "flu-like" illness characterized by low-grade fever, malaise, fatigue, myalgia, and headache occurs. Cough, dyspnea, and chest pain are rapidly followed by fulminant septic shock and death.

B. anthracis is diagnosed by culture or polymerase chain reaction (PCR) of blood, tissue, or fluid samples. The presence of mediastinal widening on a chest radiograph or CT scan is suggestive of inhalational anthrax in the right clinical setting (**Figure 9C**).

Inhalational anthrax is initially treated with intravenous ciprofloxacin or doxycycline combined with one or two additional antibiotics (see Table 30); total treatment course is 60 days, although oral antibiotics may be substituted for intravenous agents after the first 10 to 14 days. Postexposure prophylaxis with ciprofloxacin or doxycycline should be started as soon as possible following an actual or suspected anthrax attack. Although not licensed by the FDA for this purpose, a cell-free anthrax vaccine is available for postexposure immunization and is administered intramuscularly as a three-dose series in conjunction with the postexposure antibiotic regimen.

Cutaneous anthrax develops on exposed areas of the body after contact with infective spores and may occur even when skin is intact. A small pruritic papule forms at the inoculation site 1 to 7 days after exposure, followed by a vesicle and then an ulcer that evolves into a flat black eschar (**Figure 9D**). Most lesions occur on the head, neck, or extremities. Vesicular fluid and biopsy samples should be sent for culture and PCR, preferably before beginning antibiotic therapy. Unless there is definite evidence that the infection was naturally acquired, a 60-day course of ciprofloxacin or doxycycline is recommended as first-line therapy. Antibiotics do not affect the evolution of skin lesions. However, if cutaneous anthrax is not treated, the mortality rate is estimated to be 10% to 20% because of secondary bacteremic spread.

Gastrointestinal anthrax is uncommon in humans and usually results from the ingestion of undercooked meat contaminated with spores of *B. anthracis* from an infected animal. A high mortality rate (25% to 60%) is reported and is probably the result of late diagnosis and delay in treatment.

Although meningitis or meningoencephalitis may develop in patients with all three forms of anthrax, most central nervous system involvement occurs in patients with inhalational disease. It is often hemorrhagic and may rarely be the presenting manifestation of anthrax. However, the cerebrospinal fluid is not the initial site of infection. Prognosis is extremely poor. **H**

- Because anthrax spores are easily dispersed by aerosolization and infective spores can be sent by mail, even a single case of inhalational anthrax should raise the possibility of a bioterrorism attack.
- Clinical manifestations of inhalational anthrax include low-grade fever, malaise, fatigue, myalgia, headache, cough, dyspnea, and chest pain, which are rapidly followed by fulminant septic shock and death.
- Inhalational anthrax is treated with a 60-day course of ciprofloxacin or doxycycline combined with one or two additional antibiotics.
- Cutaneous anthrax is characterized by a small pruritic papule followed by a vesicle and then an ulcer that evolves into a flat black eschar; most lesions occur on the head, neck, or extremities.

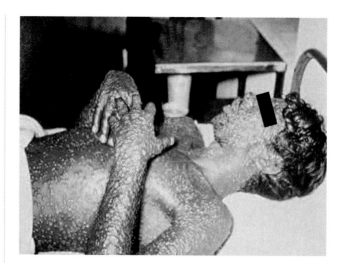

FIGURE 10. Diffuse synchronous skin lesions of smallpox.

Smallpox (Variola)

Smallpox is caused by variola, a selective human-only virus. Although it was once the leading cause of death due to an infectious agent, smallpox has been eradicated worldwide. The virus now exists in only a few laboratory repositories, and routine civilian vaccination against smallpox was suspended in the United States in 1971. The disease is easily acquired, because inhaling only a few virions carried on airborne droplets from an infected patient is sufficient to cause infection. Aerosol infectivity, the high degree of contagion, and widespread susceptibility because of a large nonimmunized population make smallpox a serious bioterrorism threat.

An initially asymptomatic respiratory tract infection and subsequent viremia develop during a 7- to 17-day incubation period. High fever, headache, vomiting, and backache then occur and last for 2 to 4 days, during which time the patient is extremely ill. The rash first appears on the buccal and pharyngeal mucosa and most often spreads to the hands and face and then to the arms, legs, and feet. The centrifugally distributed skin lesions evolve synchronously (same stage of maturation on any one area of the body) from macules to papules to vesicles to pustules and eventually become crusted (**Figure 10**). Patients remain contagious until all scabs and crusts are shed. Blindness due to keratitis or corneal ulceration is a serious complication. The overall mortality rate is about 30%.

Smallpox should be differentiated from varicella (chickenpox) (see Viral Infections), in which the rash starts centrally on the trunk and spreads toward the periphery, although the greatest number of lesions remain concentrated on the trunk (centripetal distribution). Unlike smallpox lesions, varicella lesions show differing stages of maturation on any one area of the body. A much milder form of smallpox, also known as variola minor or alastrim, has a typical febrile prodrome and rash, but is associated with a mortality rate of less than 1%.

The diagnosis of smallpox is primarily clinical, although PCR assays are available. The Centers for Disease Control and Prevention (CDC) provides a useful diagnostic tool (http://emergency.cdc.gov/agent/smallpox/diagnosis/#diagnosis). There is currently no established treatment for smallpox, although the antiviral agent cidofovir may have some therapeutic efficacy. Postexposure vaccination with vaccinia virus should be performed, with attention to its known potential adverse complications. One strategy, referred to as "ring vaccination," targets vaccination of close contacts of patients with smallpox who will be at greatest risk of contracting the disease. When given within 3 days of exposure, this active immunization can prevent or significantly lessen the severity of smallpox symptoms in most people.

- The smallpox rash first appears on the buccal and pharyngeal mucosa and spreads to the hands and face and then to the arms, legs, and feet; lesions evolve synchronously from macules to papules to vesicles to pustules and eventually become crusted.
- There is currently no established treatment for smallpox, although the antiviral agent cidofovir may have some therapeutic efficacy.

Plague

Plague, also known as the "Black Death," has been responsible for several pandemics. The infection is caused by the bacterium *Yersinia pestis*, a gram-negative coccobacillus that generally infects rodents and is transmitted to humans by the bite of an infected flea.

Bubonic plague is characterized by purulent lymphadenitis near the inoculation site and is more common in the naturally occurring zoonotic form of infection. Septicemic plague refers to the syndrome of overwhelming *Y. pestis* bacteremia, which is often characterized by disseminated intravascular coagulation and multiorgan dysfunction usually following primary cutaneous exposure. Primary pneumonic plague is caused by direct inhalation of respiratory droplets from infected humans or animals (particularly domestic cats) or potentially as a result of intentional aerosol release of pathogens. Since primary lung infection and human-to-human spread with *Y. pestis* are extremely rare, a case of pneumonic plague should suggest bioterrorism. Secondary pneumonic plague refers to hematogenous spread of *Y. pestis* to the lungs in patients with untreated bubonic or septicemic disease.

After a short incubation period of 1 to 6 days, patients with pneumonic plague present with sudden fever, chest discomfort, a productive cough, hemoptysis, and radiographic evidence of bronchopneumonia. Sputum Gram stain (and possibly blood smear) may identify gram-negative bacilli demonstrating the classic bipolar staining or "safety pin" shape.

Without rapid treatment, the mortality rate approaches 100%. Streptomycin and gentamicin are the antibiotics of choice, and doxycycline and fluoroquinolones are alternative agents. The antibiotics are continued for 10 days. Respiratory droplet isolation precautions must be instituted for at least 48 hours after starting antibiotic therapy. Postexposure prophylactic antibiotics (doxycycline or a fluoroquinolone for 7 days) should be given to asymptomatic persons known to have been exposed to aerosolized *Y. pestis* or to those who have had close contact with an infected patient. No effective vaccine for prevention of primary pneumonic plague is currently available.

KEY POINTS

- Because primary pneumonic plague is extremely rare, an identified case should suggest the possibility of bioterrorism.
- Patients with pneumonic plague present with sudden fever, chest discomfort, a productive cough, hemoptysis, and radiographic evidence of bronchopneumonia.
- Streptomycin and gentamicin are the antibiotics of choice for treating pneumonic plague.
- Postexposure prophylactic antibiotics (doxycycline or a fluoroquinolone for 7 days) should be given to asymptomatic persons known to have been exposed to aerosolized *Y. pestis* or to those who have had close contact with an infected patient.

Botulism

Botulinum toxin is the most lethal biologic substance known. The toxin is produced by the anaerobic, gram-positive, spore-forming bacillus *Clostridium botulinum*. After the toxin

enters the systemic circulation, it is transported to sites of acetylcholine-mediated neurotransmission. Because the toxin prevents release of acetylcholine, muscular contractions cannot occur and flaccid paralysis results.

Of the seven distinct antigenic forms of botulinum toxin, almost all human cases of botulism have been caused by serotypes A, B, and E. Ingestion of preformed toxin from exposure to home-canned foods or in vivo toxin production after spore germination following ingestion (infant botulism with honey) or wound contamination are the most common forms of botulism illness.

Aerosol-disseminated botulism (lethal inhaled toxin dose, 0.70 to 0.90 micrograms) and foodborne botulism would be the most likely types identified in a bioterrorism attack. Contaminating the water supply with botulinum toxin is believed to be an impractical and unlikely scenario. Clinical manifestations develop within 24 to 72 hours of toxin exposure (possibly more quickly following inhalation) and consist of a classic triad of (1) descending flaccid paralysis with prominent bulbar signs, (2) normal body temperature, and (3) normal mental status. Bulbar signs include the "4 Ds": Diplopia, Dysarthria, Dysphonia, and Dysphagia. Paralysis may progress to involve the respiratory muscles. The differential diagnosis includes the Guillain-Barré syndrome and myasthenia gravis, which are the two disorders that most closely mimic the clinical syndrome of botulism.

The presumptive diagnosis is based on the clinical presentation. Confirmation depends on identifying botulinum toxin from samples of the patient's blood, stool, gastric contents, and wound swabs, as well as from suspected foods. The standard method of identification is a mouse bioassay conducted at the CDC laboratories. Treatment includes supportive care and early administration of an equine-derived trivalent antitoxin available from the CDC through state and local health departments. However, the antitoxin will not reverse existing paralysis.

KEY POINTS

- Clinical manifestations of botulism consist of a classic triad of (1) descending flaccid paralysis with prominent bulbar signs [diplopia, dysarthria, dysphonia, and dysphagia], (2) normal body temperature, and (3) normal mental status.
- Treatment of botulism includes supportive care and the early administration of an equine-derived trivalent antitoxin.

Tularemia

Tularemia is a widespread zoonotic disease caused by a small, fastidious, gram-negative coccobacillus, *Francisella tularensis*. The organism occurs naturally throughout North America and Eurasia and has been isolated from over 250 species of wildlife. Humans become infected via arthropod bites (predominantly ticks), ingestion of contaminated food or water, handling of infectious animal tissue, and inhalation of aerosols. Exposure to very few organisms is sufficient to produce disease. No human-to-human transmission occurs.

Tularemia is characterized by several distinct presentations. A bioterrorism attack would probably involve aerosolized *F. tularensis,* with the principal presentations being pneumonic, typhoidal, septicemic, and potentially, oropharyngeal. Following a usual incubation period of 3 to 5 days, all patients develop the abrupt onset of fever, chills, myalgia, and anorexia. A dry cough is common in all forms of the disease, and a sore throat, abdominal pain, and diarrhea may be present. Relative bradycardia (pulse-temperature dissociation) may be noted.

Patients with pneumonic tularemia from either hematogenous spread or direct inhalation have no or minimal sputum production, substernal tightness, and pleuritic chest pain. Severe respiratory failure may develop. Chest radiograph findings show subsegmental or lobar infiltrates (including ovoid densities) and pleural effusions. Hilar lymphadenopathy is common. All forms of tularemia may spread to various organs and be associated with septic shock.

The diagnosis relies on a high index of clinical suspicion. Samples of blood, tissue, sputum, or fluid aspirates should be collected. Because *F. tularensis* is highly infectious, samples should only be sent to Biosafety Level 3 laboratories, and laboratory personnel must be notified in advance to take necessary precautions. *F. tularensis* does not grow readily on routine culture media, and serologic studies are generally needed to confirm the diagnosis. However, the natural delay in the development of antibody titers makes serologic studies impractical for rapid diagnosis after an intentional release. PCR and immunofluorescence testing may be performed directly on tissue specimens. A granulomatous infiltrate in tissue samples resulting from a cell-mediated immune response to infection with *F. tularensis* may be misdiagnosed as tuberculosis if the granulomas are caseating.

The treatment of choice for pneumonic, septicemic, or typhoidal tularemia is streptomycin or gentamicin for 7 to 14 days. Treatment following a mass exposure or postexposure prophylaxis after intentional release of *F. tularensis* is a 14-day course of doxycycline or ciprofloxacin. Mortality rates may be as high as 30% in untreated patients with pneumonic or typhoidal tularemia. The *F. tularensis* vaccine once approved for laboratory workers is no longer available for use.

KEY POINTS

- Patients with all forms of tularemia experience abrupt-onset fever, chills, myalgia, and anorexia.
- Serologic studies are impractical for rapid diagnosis of tularemia after a bioterrorism attack.
- The treatment of choice for pneumonic, typhoidal, or septicemic tularemia is streptomycin or gentamicin for 7 to 14 days.

Viral Hemorrhagic Fever

Viral hemorrhagic fevers (VHFs) are a group of febrile illnesses caused by RNA viruses from four families (**Table 31**). These viruses are considered likely candidates for use as biologic weapons because of their high infectivity and virulence after low-dose exposure, their capacity for causing significant morbidity and mortality, and the few, if any, treatment options available. The viruses are widely distributed in nature and, with the exception of dengue virus, are both stable and infectious by airborne dissemination.

The pathogenesis of VHF is poorly understood. Because the target organ is the vascular bed, the dominant clinical features are usually due to microvascular damage and changes in vascular permeability. After a variable incubation period of 2 to 21 days, all of the VHF pathogens cause a febrile prodrome, myalgia, and prostration. Early signs of infection often include conjunctival injection, mild hypotension, and petechial hemorrhages. Patients with advanced VHF develop shock and generalized bleeding from the mucous membranes, skin, and gastrointestinal tract, which are frequently accompanied by neurologic, hematopoietic, and pulmonary involvement.

In naturally occurring VHF, an appropriate epidemiologic exposure history would aid in the diagnosis. In a bioterrorism attack, however, deliberate aerosolization would be the most likely route of dissemination and would result in the simultaneous presentation of multiple patients. Specific diagnostic studies are available at the CDC laboratories that detect viral RNA by reverse transcription PCR, presence of viral protein antigens, development of IgM antibodies, or isolation of the virus.

Intensive supportive care is the mainstay of treatment. Potentially effective antiviral agents are limited (for example, ribavirin for Arenaviridae and Bunyaviridae viruses). Because of the potential for person-to-person transmission of some VHF pathogens, such as Ebola virus, appropriate isolation measures

TABLE 31.	Families of Viral Hemorrhagic Fever
Virus Family	**Disease**
Flaviviridae	Yellow fever
	Dengue fever
	Various tick-borne flavivirus hemorrhagic fevers
Filoviridae	Ebola hemorrhagic fever
	Marburg hemorrhagic fever
Arenaviridae	Lassa fever
	Various South American hemorrhagic fevers
Bunyaviridae	Rift Valley fever
	Crimean Congo hemorrhagic fever
	Hantavirus pulmonary syndrome
	Hemorrhagic fever with renal syndrome

CONT.

for individuals with suspected or confirmed VHF include a combination of airborne and contact precautions. **H**

KEY POINTS

- Patients with viral hemorrhagic fever present with a febrile prodrome, myalgia, and prostration.
- Patients with advanced viral hemorrhagic fever experience shock and generalized bleeding from the mucous membranes, skin, and gastrointestinal tract.
- Intensive supportive care is the mainstay of treatment of viral hemorrhagic fever.

Travel Medicine

The practice of travel medicine encompasses both prevention (pre-travel advice about preventable infections, appropriate prophylaxis and immunizations, and behavioral practices to avoid exposure to infective agents) and treatment of returning travelers who have symptoms of infection. The most common travel-associated infections are listed in **Table 32**.

TABLE 32. Common Travel-Associated Infections

Febrile illnesses

Malaria

Dengue fever

Typhoid fever

Rickettsial infection

Yellow fever

Mononucleosis syndrome
(cytomegalovirus and Epstein-Barr virus)

Brucellosis

Travelers' diarrhea

Bacterial agents: *Escherichia coli*, *Campylobacter*, *Salmonella*, and *Shigella* species

Viral agents: rotavirus

Protozoa: *Cryptosporidium*, microsporidia, *Giardia*, and *Isospora* species

Malaria

Malaria is caused by infection with various *Plasmodium* species parasites that are transmitted by the bite of the female *Anopheles* mosquito. Malaria can be prevented by use of bed nets, insect repellents containing about 30% *N,N*-diethyl-3-methylbenzamide (DEET), and adherence to an appropriate chemoprophylaxis regimen. Yet, despite all precautions, infection can occur. The most common symptoms are fever (occurring in characteristic paroxysms of 48- or 72-hour cycles), headache, myalgia, nausea, vomiting, abdominal pain, and diarrhea. Patients found to have hyperparasitemia, defined as 5% to 10% or more of parasitized erythrocytes, may develop more severe signs and symptoms collectively referred to as complicated malaria because of the parasitized erythrocytes' adherence to and sequestration in small blood vessels. Generally more often associated with *Plasmodium falciparum* infection, this form of disease may be characterized by alteration in mentation with seizures, hepatic failure, disseminated intravascular coagulation, brisk intravascular hemolysis, metabolic acidosis, kidney insufficiency, and hypoglycemia. Patients with long-standing infection may present with anemia and splenomegaly. Thrombocytopenia and abnormal liver chemistry test results are also frequent findings.

The diagnosis of malaria relies on examination of peripheral blood smears. In some patients, the precise identification of the malarial species requires laboratory molecular techniques. The characteristics of the different malarial species are summarized in **Table 33**. *P. falciparum*, more so than other malaria species, and *Plasmodium knowlesi* may cause severe and potentially lethal infection.

Plasmodium knowlesi, the recently described species infecting macaque monkeys in Southeast Asia and now also known to infect humans, completes its blood stage cycle every 24 hours. Consequently, very high parasite loads develop, and a potentially severe and fatal infection can occur. On peripheral blood smear examination, *P. knowlesi* mimics *Plasmodium malariae*, with demonstration of all stages of the parasite in the circulation. Owing to the absence of its specific macaque reservoir hosts, this fifth *Plasmodium* species is not encountered in Africa.

TABLE 33. Characteristics of *Plasmodium* species

Characteristics	*P. vivax*	*P. ovale*	*P. malariae*	*P. falciparum*	*P. knowlesi*
Incubation period	10-30 days	10-20 days	15-35 days	8-25 days	Indeterminate
Geographic distribution	Tropical and temperate zones	West Africa and Southeast Asia	Tropical zones	Tropical and temperate zones	South and Southeast Asia
Parasitemia level	Low	Low	Very low	High	Can be high
Risk of disease severity	Low risk	Low risk	Very low risk	High risk	High risk
Disease relapse risk	Yes	Yes	Yes	None	None
Chloroquine resistance	Yes	No	Rare	Yes	No

CONT.

Clues to the diagnosis of falciparum malaria include travel to Africa, early onset of infection after returning from an endemic area, a peripheral blood smear showing a high level of parasitemia invading both young and old erythrocytes, and typically, the presence of thin, often multiple, "ring forms" lining the inner surface of the erythrocytes. Moreover, with *P. falciparum* infection, there is an absence of trophozoites and schizonts, although banana-shaped gametocytes may be detected in the smear.

The risk of exposure to malaria, presence of antimalarial drug resistance in endemic areas, and recommendations for chemoprophylaxis depend on the travel destination. Antimalarial chemoprophylaxis regimens are listed in **Table 34**. Unless travel is absolutely necessary, pregnant women are advised against entering malarial areas of the world. Chloroquine chemoprophylaxis can be safely administered during pregnancy. For travel to areas where chloroquine-resistant malaria is present, mefloquine is recommended for all travelers, although its safety is less well studied.

Information about malaria prophylaxis and treatment is frequently updated in the "Yellow Book" publication from the Centers for Disease Control and Prevention; the 2012 guidelines are now available (http://wwwnc.cdc.gov/travel/yellowbook/2012/chapter-3-infectious-diseases-related-to-travel/malaria.htm).

KEY POINTS

- The most common symptoms of malaria are fever (occurring in characteristic paroxysms of 48- or 72-hour cycles), headache, myalgia, nausea, vomiting, abdominal pain, and diarrhea.
- *Plasmodium falciparum* and *Plasmodium knowlesi* may cause severe and potentially lethal malaria.
- The risk of exposure to malaria, presence of antimalarial drug resistance in endemic areas, and recommendations for chemoprophylaxis depend on the travel destination.

TABLE 34. Antimalarial Chemoprophylaxis Regimens

Drug	Dose	Time of Prophylaxis Initiation	Time of Prophylaxis Discontinuation
For endemic areas with chloroquine-resistant *Plasmodium falciparum*			
Mefloquine	250 mg once weekly	1-2 weeks before travel	4 weeks after returning
Atovaquone/proguanil	250 mg/100 mg once daily	1-2 days before travel	7 days after returning
Doxycycline	100 mg once daily	1-2 days before travel	4 weeks after returning
For endemic areas with chloroquine-sensitive *Plasmodium falciparum*			
Chloroquine	500 mg once weekly	1-2 weeks	4 weeks
Hydroxychloroquine	400 mg once weekly	1-2 weeks	4 weeks
Atovaquone/proguanil	250/100 mg once daily	1-2 days	7 days
Mefloquine	250 mg once weekly	2 weeks	4 weeks
Doxycycline	100 mg once daily	1-2 days	4 weeks
Primaquine[a]	26.3 mg once daily	1-2 days	1 week
For endemic areas with *Plasmodium vivax*			
Primaquine[a]	52.6 mg once daily	1-2 days	1 week
Chloroquine	500 mg once weekly	1-2 days	4 weeks
Hydroxychloroquine	400 mg once weekly	1-2 days	4 weeks
Atovaquone/proguanil	250/100 mg once daily	1-2 days	7 days
Mefloquine	250 mg once weekly	2 weeks	4 weeks
Doxycycline	100 mg once daily	1-2 days	4 weeks
Prophylaxis for relapse due to *Plasmodium vivax* or *Plasmodium ovale*			
Primaquine[a]	52.6 mg once daily	As soon as possible	2 weeks

[a]Contraindicated in persons with severe forms of glucose-6-phosphate dehydrogenase deficiency or methemoglobin reductase deficiency; should not be administered to pregnant women.

Reprinted with permission from Freedman, DO. Clinical practice. Malaria prevention in short-term travelers. N Engl J Med. 2008;359(6):603-612. [PMID: 18687641] Copyright 2008 Massachusetts Medical Society.

Typhoid Fever

Typhoid fever is a potentially life-threatening febrile illness caused by the bacterium *Salmonella enterica* serotype Typhi (formerly *Salmonella typhi*). Nontyphoidal *Salmonella* infection is discussed elsewhere in this syllabus (see Infectious Gastrointestinal Syndromes). Typhoid fever most often occurs in travelers who recently returned from endemic areas and is caused by consumption of water or food contaminated by human feces. Unlike other salmonellae, *S. enterica* serotype Typhi causes disease only in humans. Travelers to South, East, and Southeast Asia are at especially increased risk for infection.

Symptoms include fatigue, fever ("enteric fever" daily for 4 to 8 weeks in untreated patients), headache, cough, anorexia, hepatosplenomegaly, and, at times, a macular rash on the trunk (rose spots) that appears after an incubation period of 6 to 30 days. Diarrhea may be present early and resolve spontaneously. However, many patients with typhoid fever have constipation at diagnosis. Serious complications, such as intestinal hemorrhage or perforation, may occur 2 to 3 weeks after infection develops. Invasion of the gallbladder by typhoid bacilli may result in the long-term typhoid carrier state, especially in patients with gallstones.

The diagnosis of typhoid fever often relies on isolation of the organism in the blood, bone marrow, stool, and/or urine. Serologic studies may also be used. The classic Widal test, which measures anti-O and H antigen titers, has been widely substituted with newer, more sensitive and specific assays developed to detect antibodies to lipopolysaccharide or outer membrane proteins of *S. enterica* serotype *Typhi*. Fluoroquinolones, most often ciprofloxacin, are generally used for empiric therapy. However, because fluoroquinolone resistance is becoming high in South Asia and increasing in other areas, a third-generation cephalosporin (for example, ceftriaxone) is becoming the empiric antibiotic of choice pending in vitro susceptibility testing. Typhoid vaccine is recommended for travelers to areas at risk for infection. Either an oral live-attenuated vaccine or an intramuscular cell-free Vi capsular polysaccharide vaccine may be used. Both vaccines protect approximately 50% to 80% of recipients. 🄷

KEY POINTS

- Symptoms of typhoid fever include fatigue, fever ("enteric fever" daily for 4 to 8 weeks in untreated patients), headache, cough, anorexia, hepatosplenomegaly, and, at times, a macular rash.

- Although fluoroquinolones are frequently used for empiric treatment of typhoid fever, a third-generation cephalosporin is becoming the drug of choice because of increasing fluoroquinolone resistance.

- An oral live-attenuated typhoid vaccine and an intramuscular cell-free Vi capsular polysaccharide typhoid vaccine are available, and both vaccines are equally effective.

Travelers' Diarrhea

Travelers' diarrhea is the most common infection in travelers to developing countries and is estimated to affect 40% to 60% of travelers. It is usually a self-limited condition but may occasionally induce life-threatening volume depletion. This food- and waterborne illness is caused by various pathogens (see Table 32). The risk of transmission may be reduced by appropriate selection of food and water sources. It is advisable to avoid consuming water and drinks and ice made from tap water and to avoid brushing teeth with tap water. It is also prudent to not eat undercooked meats and poultry, unpasteurized dairy products, and fruits that are not peeled just prior to eating. Carbonated drinks and beer and wine are thought to be safe. Water may be purified by adding sodium hypochlorite (2 drops/1.89 L) or tincture of iodine (5 drops/0.95 L) to local water sources or boiling water for 3 minutes before allowing it to cool. Antibiotic prophylaxis for travelers' diarrhea is not recommended for most patients; however, it may be considered for patients with coexisting inflammatory bowel disease. The Infectious Diseases Society of America has published guidelines for the use of oral agents for prophylaxis and for treatment of travelers' diarrhea with a prolonged clinical course (**Table 35**). Bismuth subsalicylate can be used to prevent or treat diarrhea, but excessive doses are required that are inconvenient and can lead to salicylate toxicity. Rifaximin, a nonabsorbed antibiotic, is effective and safe when prescribed at doses of 200 mg, once or twice daily for 2 weeks, particularly when *Escherichia coli* will be the most likely acquired pathogen during travel.

TABLE 35. Treatment and Prophylaxis for Travelers' Diarrhea	
Agent	**Treatment Regimen (oral)**
Bismuth subsalicylate	1 oz every 30 min for 8 doses
Norfloxacin	400 mg twice daily for 3 days
Ciprofloxacin	500 mg twice daily for 3 days
Ofloxacin	200 mg twice daily for 3 days
Levofloxacin	500 mg once daily for 3 days
Azithromycin	1000 mg, single dose
Rifaximin	200 mg three times daily for 3 days
Agent	**Prophylaxis Regimen (oral)**
Bismuth subsalicylate	Two tablets chewed 4 times daily
Norfloxacin	400 mg daily[a]
Ciprofloxacin	500 mg daily[a]
Rifaximin	200 mg once or twice daily[a]

[a]Chemoprophylaxis is recommended for no more than 2 to 3 weeks (the period studied in trials and a period short enough to minimize the risk of antimicrobial-associated adverse effects).

Reprinted with permission from Hill DR, Ericsson CD, Pearson RD, et al; Infectious Diseases Society of America. The practice of travel medicine: guidelines by the Infectious Diseases Society of America. Clin Infect Dis. 2006;43(12):1499-1539. [PMID: 17109284] Copyright 2006 Oxford University Press.

Antimotility agents such as diphenoxylate and loperamide may relieve symptoms but should be given only with antibiotic diarrhea treatment. These agents should not be used when dysenteric disease or bloody diarrhea is present.

KEY POINTS

- Travelers' diarrhea is usually self-limited but may occasionally induce life-threatening volume depletion.

- Antimotility agents such as diphenoxylate and loperamide may relieve symptoms of travelers' diarrhea but should be given only with antibiotic diarrhea treatment and should not be used in patients with dysenteric disease or bloody diarrhea.

Dengue Fever

Dengue fever is caused by four serotypes of viruses belonging to the family Flaviviridae (DENV-1 through DENV-4) and is transmitted by a mosquito vector (*Aedes aegypti*) with prominent diurnal activity. Although dengue fever is becoming ubiquitous in many parts of the world, geographic areas with the highest endemicity include the Caribbean, South and Central America, and Asia.

Infection may be asymptomatic or may cause an acute febrile illness associated with frontal headache, myalgia, and retro-orbital pain, with or without minor spontaneous bleeding manifestations (purpura, melena, conjunctival injection). Because prominent lumbosacral pain is a frequent manifestation, the term "breakbone fever" has been used to describe infection with the dengue virus. Some patients develop a macular or scarlatiniform rash as the fever abates. The rash spares the palms and soles and evolves into areas of petechiae on extensor surfaces. A second febrile period ("saddleback" pattern) may occur. In patients with severe infection, a life-threatening hemorrhagic or shock syndrome may develop that includes liver failure and encephalopathy. This entity appears to be related to previous dengue viral infection, often of a different type. Laboratory findings may include leukopenia, thrombocytopenia, and elevated serum aminotransferase levels.

The diagnosis is often made based on clinical findings and is sometimes confirmed by enzyme-linked immunosorbent assay or reverse transcriptase polymerase chain reaction. Since there is no specific antiviral agent for treatment of dengue fever, therapy is supportive. No effective vaccine is currently available.

KEY POINTS

- Patients with dengue fever may be asymptomatic or may have an acute febrile illness associated with frontal headache, myalgia, and retro-orbital pain, with or without minor spontaneous bleeding manifestations or prominent lumbosacral pain.

- There is no specific antiviral agent for treating dengue fever, and no vaccine is available.

Hepatitis A Virus Infection

Hepatitis A virus (HAV) infection is acquired by ingesting contaminated water or food. Travelers to developing countries should be given HAV vaccine 1 month before going to an endemic area, provided they have not been previously immunized or have not contracted HAV infection in the past. A second booster dose is given 6 to 12 months after the initial vaccination. Serum immune globulin, once widely used for pre-exposure passive protection, is rarely indicated except perhaps for the very young (<12 months), for immunocompromised persons (who are less responsive to HAV vaccine), and for persons who choose not to be vaccinated. If HAV infection does occur, therapy is symptomatic, as no antiviral agent is currently available for treatment.

KEY POINT

- Travelers to areas endemic for hepatitis A virus (HAV) infection should be given HAV vaccine 1 month before departure and a second booster dose 6 to 12 months later.

Rickettsial Infection

Rickettsioses are caused by obligate intracellular gram-negative bacteria that are transmitted by small vectors (fleas, lice, mites, and ticks). *Rickettsia typhi*, which causes endemic or murine typhus, is transmitted by fleas from a rodent reservoir, and *Rickettsia prowazekii*, which causes epidemic or louse-borne typhus, is transmitted by human body lice. Outbreaks of rickettsial infection have been reported during periods of war and natural disasters and are associated with poor hygienic conditions and tick infestation. The clinical presentation is usually vague and includes fever, headache, and malaise, which are often accompanied by a maculopapular, vesicular, or petechial rash. An eschar at the site of the insect bite often develops after infection with *Rickettsia africae* (African tick typhus), *Rickettsia conorii* (Mediterranean spotted fever), and *Orientia tsutsugamushi* (previously *Rickettsia tsutsugamushi* [scrub typhus]). Infection with *R. africae* is a very common cause of fever in travelers to South Africa.

When clinically suspected, the diagnosis may be confirmed by polymerase chain reaction, immunohistochemical analysis of tissue samples, or culture during the acute stage of illness before antibiotic therapy is begun. The treatment of choice is doxycycline. No vaccine or antimicrobial prophylaxis is available. Prevention therefore relies on minimizing exposure to vectors (for example, by use of repellents) when traveling in endemic areas.

KEY POINTS

- The clinical presentation of a rickettsial infection is usually vague and includes fever, headache, and malaise, often accompanied by a maculopapular, vesicular, or petechial rash.

- Doxycycline is the antibiotic of choice for treating rickettsial infections; no vaccine or antimicrobial prophylaxis is available.

Brucellosis

Infection by human pathogenic species of the gram-negative coccobacillus *Brucella* (*B. abortus*, *B. melitensis*, *B. suis*, and *B. canis*) is acquired by ingestion of contaminated milk, by direct inoculation through skin wounds and mucous membranes, or by inhalation after exposure to domestic animals giving birth. Since this is a zoonotic infection with reservoirs in cattle and other animals, travelers usually become infected after consuming unpasteurized milk, other dairy products, or undercooked meat in countries where brucellosis is endemic. The Mediterranean basin, Indian subcontinent, Arabian Peninsula, and parts of Central and South America, Mexico, Asia, and Africa are high-prevalence areas. After a variable incubation period of usually weeks, patients develop fever, myalgia, fatigue, headache, and night sweats. Some patients may develop endocarditis and neuropsychiatric symptoms.

The diagnosis is established by isolating the organism in blood or bone marrow cultures or by specific serologic testing. The treatment of choice for brucellosis is a combination of doxycycline, rifampin, and streptomycin (or gentamicin). Antimicrobial prophylaxis is not recommended. Infection prevention relies on avoiding the ingestion of unpasteurized products or exposure to cattle or other animals in endemic areas. H

KEY POINTS

- Clinical manifestations of brucellosis include fever, myalgia, fatigue, headache, and night sweats and, less often, endocarditis and neuropsychiatric symptoms.
- The treatment of choice for brucellosis is a combination of doxycycline, rifampin, and streptomycin (or gentamicin).

Travel-Associated Fungal Infections

Most pathogenic fungi are endemic to the soil of certain geographic areas (**Table 36**) and are acquired either by inhalation of airborne mycelial organisms or by direct inoculation through cutaneous wounds or abrasions (see Fungal Infections). Although most of these infections are asymptomatic in immunocompetent hosts, immunocompromised patients are at risk of developing serious, often systemic, clinical manifestations. *Histoplasma capsulatum*, a dimorphic fungal organism that is particularly endemic to the southeastern United States, is found in high concentrations in soil contaminated with bird or bat droppings. The infection is acquired through inhalation of the fungus in its mold form.

TABLE 36. Common Travel-Associated Acquired Fungal Infections

Organism	Geographic Distribution
Coccidioides species	Southwest United States
	Mexico
	Central and South America
Histoplasma species	Ohio River Valley
	Mexico
	Central America
Penicillium marneffei	Southeast Asia
	China

Infection due to *Penicillium marneffei* is a rapidly growing problem among HIV-infected or generally immunocompromised persons living in or traveling to Southeast Asia. In this subset of persons, *P. marneffei* infection causes serious systemic manifestations associated with a high mortality rate. Survival depends on early diagnosis and institution of appropriate antifungal therapy, often for life, because of the propensity for relapses.

Since prophylaxis with antimycotic agents is not recommended and vaccines are not available, travelers to endemic areas may decrease their risk of contracting a fungal infection by limiting their exposure to outdoor dust and/or wearing well-fitted dust masks. H

KEY POINTS

- Infection due to *Penicillium marneffei* is a rapidly growing problem among HIV-infected or generally immunocompromised persons living in or traveling to Southeast Asia.
- Since prophylaxis with antimycotic agents is not recommended and vaccines are not available, travelers to endemic areas may decrease their risk of contracting a fungal infection by limiting their exposure to outdoor dust and/or wearing well-fitted dust masks.

Infectious Gastrointestinal Syndromes

Diarrhea is the most common clinical presentation of gastroenteritis but may also be caused by extraintestinal infections (Legionnaires disease, toxic shock syndrome), medications (amoxicillin-clavulanate), or noninfectious diseases (ischemic colitis, inflammatory bowel disease, celiac disease). Noninfectious causes of diarrhea are discussed elsewhere (see MKSAP 16 Gastroenterology and Hepatology).

Classification schema for infectious diarrhea have been developed to maximize judicious testing and aid empiric therapy, recognizing that the yield of stool culture for all patients with diarrhea is low. Infectious diarrhea can be broadly categorized as community acquired (including travelers' diarrhea), health care associated, or persistent (lasting >7 days). Most episodes of diarrhea caused by bacteria and viruses are brief, with symptoms persisting for less than 1 week even in the absence of treatment. Diarrhea in an otherwise healthy person lasting for more than 7 days suggests a parasitic or noninfectious origin.

The diagnostic yield of bacterial stool culture is low (less than 3%); however, identification of a pathogen has important treatment and public health implications and may be useful in identifying and tracking a foodborne outbreak. Because most cases of community-acquired diarrhea are self-limited, stool cultures are not required in all cases; cultures are generally indicated for symptoms lasting longer than 72 hours, particularly in patients with associated fever, tenesmus, or bloody or mucoid stools. Stool cultures are rarely positive if gastrointestinal symptoms have been present for more than 1 week's duration or if diarrhea develops in a hospitalized patient more than 3 days after admission. Routine bacterial stool cultures detect infection with *Salmonella*, *Shigella*, and *Campylobacter* species. Directed testing for Shiga toxin–producing *Escherichia coli* (STEC) may be reflexively performed in some laboratories when stool cultures are ordered. When not done automatically, STEC testing should be performed on all samples with visible or occult blood. Assays for *Clostridium difficile* are indicated for patients with recent antibiotic use, hospitalization, or comorbid disease. A focused history may elucidate epidemiologic features that may further guide diagnostic testing and empiric treatment (**Table 37**).

Infectious diarrhea is frequently transmitted by consumption of infected food products. Although knowing the type of food ingested is rarely useful in identifying a causative agent, the time from ingestion to development of symptoms may be helpful. Onset of gastrointestinal symptoms within 6 hours of ingestion is suggestive of a preformed toxin, such as *Staphylococcus aureus* or *Bacillus cereus* food poisoning, which are associated with nausea and vomiting rather than diarrhea. Symptoms due to most infections caused by ingesting viable bacteria develop 24 to 72 hours following ingestion. Person-to-person transmission can occur by fecal-oral spread and is particularly common for pathogens that cause infection with low inoculums (for example, *Shigella* species) and in preschools or health care settings where fecal soilage leads to environmental contamination.

The physical examination is important to assess the severity of illness but rarely provides clues to the causative organism. In contrast, laboratory findings may suggest specific pathogens. Grossly bloody stools are associated with infection caused by *Escherichia coli* O157:H7 or other

TABLE 37. Epidemiologic and Clinical Features Suggestive of Specific Pathogens in Patients with Diarrhea	
Exposure, Symptom, or Risk Factor	**Pathogen**
Raw or undercooked eggs	*Salmonella*
Reptiles (turtles, snakes, lizards)	*Salmonella*
Puppy or kitten with diarrhea	*Campylobacter*
Travel to developing countries	≤7 days: bacterial (ETEC, EAEC, Enterobacteriaceae); >7 days: parasites
Recent antibiotics or hospitalization	*Clostridium difficile*
Chitterlings (pork intestines)	*Yersinia*
Seafood or seawater exposure	*Vibrio*
Cruise ship	Norovirus
Drinking from untreated natural bodies of water	*Giardia lamblia*
Ingestion of untreated fresh water or contaminated shellfish	*Aeromonas* or *Plesiomonas*
Day care centers	*Shigella*, *G. lamblia*, norovirus, rotavirus
Bloody stools (gross blood or heme-positive)	STEC, *Shigella*, *Salmonella* *Campylobacter*, *Entamoeba*
Mimic of acute appendicitis	*Yersinia*

EAEC = enteroaggregative *Escherichia coli*; ETEC = enterotoxigenic *E. coli*; STEC = Shiga toxin–producing *E. coli*.

STEC. Invasive pathogens such as *Salmonella*, *Shigella*, and *Campylobacter* species may also cause bloody stools. Fecal leukocytes, when present, suggest an invasive pathogen, but the sensitivity of this finding is low.

All patients should be evaluated for evidence of volume depletion, and fluid resuscitation is a cornerstone of treatment. Use of antimotility agents such as loperamide is reserved for patients with mild diarrhea and is discouraged for patients with fever, significant abdominal pain, or bloody stools. Decisions regarding empiric antibiotic therapy must be individualized based on suspicion for a particular pathogen and should be carefully considered because treatment of some types of infectious diarrhea may prolong bacterial shedding or increase the risk for complications (see later discussion of specific causes of diarrhea). Viral infections, noninvasive bacterial infections, and many parasitic infections generally resolve without antimicrobial therapy.

KEY POINTS

- Most episodes of diarrhea caused by bacteria and viruses are brief, with symptoms persisting for less than 1 week; diarrhea in an otherwise healthy person lasting more than 7 days suggests a parasitic or noninfectious origin.

- Onset of gastrointestinal symptoms within 6 hours of ingestion suggests a pre-formed toxin, such as *Staphylococcus aureus* or *Bacillus cereus* food poisoning, whereas symptoms due to most infections caused by ingesting viable bacteria develop 24 to 72 hours following ingestion.

Campylobacter Infection

Several *Campylobacter* species are capable of causing human disease, with *Campylobacter jejuni* most frequently associated with gastroenteritis. *Campylobacter* are normal bowel flora in many animals, including livestock. Foodborne transmission as a result of inadequate cooking or preparation of poultry is the most common route of infection. Diarrhea, fever, and abdominal pain are frequently present, and onset occurs several days after ingestion of bacteria. Grossly bloody stools are noted in fewer than 10% of patients; however, occult blood is found in a significantly higher percentage. Fecal leukocytes are variably present. The diagnosis is established by isolation of bacteria on stool culture. Late complications of *Campylobacter* infection include a reactive arthritis and Guillain-Barré syndrome.

Campylobacter infection typically resolves spontaneously even without antibiotic treatment. Treatment is indicated for patients with severe symptoms (high fever, frequent or bloody stools), or symptoms lasting longer than 7 days. Treatment should also be considered for patients at highest risk for complications, including those at extremes of age and patients who have a comorbid illness or are severely immunocompromised. Fluoroquinolone resistance among *Campylobacter* isolates approaches 20% in the United States and may be higher when infections are acquired during travel abroad. In contrast, most isolates are susceptible to macrolides, and recommended treatment for *Campylobacter* gastroenteritis is azithromycin or erythromycin.

KEY POINTS

- The most frequent symptoms of *Campylobacter* infection are diarrhea, fever, and abdominal pain, with onset several days after ingestion of bacteria.
- Recommended treatment for *Campylobacter* gastroenteritis is azithromycin or erythromycin.

Shigella Infection

There are four species of *Shigella* (*S. dysenteriae, S. boydii, S. flexneri,* and *S. sonnei*), all of which have been associated with diarrheal illness. Because shigellosis can be caused by very low infectious inoculums (<100 organisms), both foodborne and fecal-oral transmission can occur. Outbreaks of shigellosis in day-care centers and residential institutions typically occur through the fecal-oral route of infection.

Shigellosis most frequently presents as dysentery, characterized by bloody or mucoid stools, abdominal cramps, tenesmus, and high fever. The bacteria invade colonic tissue and cause inflammation. Fecal leukocytes are found in many patients. The diagnosis is established by bacterial stool culture. Reactive arthritis has been reported as a rare complication following resolution of infection.

Empiric therapy should be considered for patients with clinical evidence of dysentery pending culture confirmation of infection. Treatment is recommended for all patients with a positive culture for *Shigella* to decrease the duration of bacterial shedding and limit secondary spread of infection, even if symptoms have resolved by the time culture results are available. Most isolates remain susceptible to fluoroquinolones, and treatment with one of these agents for 5 days is recommended.

KEY POINTS

- Shigellosis most frequently presents as dysentery, characterized by bloody or mucoid stools, abdominal cramps, tenesmus, and high fever.
- Treatment with a fluoroquinolone is recommended for all patients with a positive culture for *Shigella*, even if symptoms have resolved by the time culture results are available.

Salmonella Infection

Salmonella infections are caused by several closely related bacteria belonging to a single species, *Salmonella enterica*. Organisms may be further characterized microbiologically by serotype. Isolates are often referred to by the genus and serotype (for example, *Salmonella enteritidis*) rather than the taxonomically correct, but lengthier, designation (*S. enterica* serotype Enteritidis).

Clinically, infections may be broadly categorized as typhoidal (associated with *S. enterica* serotype Typhi or *S. enterica* subtype paratyphi) or nontyphoidal. Although typhoid fever is endemic to developing countries, infection in the United States is usually limited to travelers returning from endemic areas (see Travel Medicine). In contrast, nontyphoidal serotypes of *Salmonella* are common causes of gastroenteritis in the United States. *Salmonella* organisms are most frequently transmitted by consumption of contaminated food, especially undercooked or raw eggs. Contaminated chicken and other meat products, milk, fruits, and vegetables have also caused outbreaks. Approximately 5% of patients develop infection after being exposed to reptiles, including turtles, snakes, and lizards.

Symptomatic disease typically occurs within 72 hours of ingestion and even without treatment resolves in 7 to 10 days in most patients. Clinically, *Salmonella* gastroenteritis is indistinguishable from other forms of invasive diarrhea. Associated symptoms include fever and abdominal pain, with gross or occult blood variably present in stool specimens. The diagnosis is established by bacterial stool culture.

Bacteremia occurs in 5% of patients and may cause endovascular infections, particularly aortitis. This uncommon complication of *Salmonella* infection should be considered in patients with known atherosclerotic vascular disease and persistent bacteremia despite antibiotic therapy; diagnosis is established by abdominal CT scan. Risk factors for salmonellosis include age greater than 65 years, use of agents that decrease stomach acid production (antacids, proton pump inhibitors), or impaired cellular immunity (HIV/AIDS, corticosteroid use, transplant recipients). Patients with sickle cell diseases are also at increased risk for disseminated salmonellosis, and osteomyelitis is a reported complication in these patients.

Several studies have found that antibiotic therapy for *Salmonella* gastroenteritis does not decrease the duration of symptoms and may actually prolong fecal shedding of bacteria. Consequently, treatment is discouraged for patients younger than 50 years of age who have relatively mild disease. Antibiotic therapy is indicated for patients with severe infection who require hospitalization in whom bacteremia or other disseminated infection is a concern. Treatment is also recommended for milder disease in the following groups of patients, who are most susceptible to complications of salmonellosis: (1) patients younger than 6 months or older than 50 years of age; (2) presence of prosthetic heart valves or joints; (3) comorbidities (malignancy, uremia, sickle cell disease); (4) significant atherosclerotic disease (because of risk of infectious arteritis); and (5) impaired cellular immunity.

Antibiotic treatment should be based on individual susceptibility patterns when these are known. Most isolates are susceptible to fluoroquinolones, which offer the advantage of oral dosing and are recommended for empiric therapy. Treatment is continued for 5 to 7 days for patients with severe disease or those at risk for complications due to bacteremia (groups 1 to 4). Treatment should be continued for at least 14 days for patients with cellular immune defects (group 5), in whom relapsing infection is common. The median duration of fecal shedding of bacteria after symptomatic infection is 5 weeks; however, surveillance cultures to document clearance are generally not recommended. Strict attention to hand hygiene should be emphasized to prevent secondary infection by person-to-person transmission.

KEY POINTS

- *Salmonella* gastroenteritis is indistinguishable from other forms of invasive diarrhea.
- Treatment of *Salmonella* gastroenteritis is discouraged for healthy patients younger than 50 years of age who have relatively mild disease.

Escherichia coli Infection

Escherichia coli are considered normal intestinal flora; however, specific strains are associated with various diarrheal syndromes (**Table 38**). Most diarrheagenic *E. coli* strains cause a self-limited and nonspecific gastroenteritis. Routine bacterial stool cultures do not distinguish between normal colonic and diarrheagenic *E. coli*, and diagnostic testing is generally restricted to epidemiologic studies or outbreak investigations. The exception is Shiga toxin–producing *E. coli* (STEC), which causes hemorrhagic gastroenteritis. The first reported outbreak of STEC was associated with ingestion of contaminated hamburger meat, and subsequent investigations have confirmed the role of transmission through ingestion of contaminated food products and water. A large European outbreak of hemorrhagic colitis in 2011 caused by *E. coli* O104:H4 was linked to consumption of raw sprouts. Person-to-person transmission may also occur by fecal-oral contamination and contact with animals at farms or petting zoos.

STEC causes diarrhea by production of Shiga toxin. *E. coli* O157:H7 is the most commonly identified STEC, but other strains, including the newly identified *E. coli* O104:H4, may cause a clinically identical hemorrhagic colitis, characterized by bloody diarrhea and abdominal pain in the absence of fever. Approximately 10% of patients with *E. coli* O157:H7 infection develop hemolytic uremic syndrome associated with kidney failure, hemolysis, and thrombocytopenia. Children are more susceptible than adults to this syndrome.

Routine stool cultures are not useful for isolating STEC. The Centers for Disease Control and Prevention (CDC)

TABLE 38. Diarrheagenic Strains of *Escherichia coli*

Strain	Epidemiology	Clinical Findings
Enteroaggregative *E. coli* (EAEC)	Diarrhea in travelers, young children, and patients with HIV infection	Watery diarrhea, fever typically absent
Enteroinvasive *E. coli* (EIEC)	All ages, primarily in developing countries	Inflammatory diarrhea (dysentery) with fever, abdominal pain
Enteropathogenic *E. coli* (EPEC)	Sporadic, occasionally persistent diarrhea in young children	Nausea, vomiting, malnutrition (when chronic)
Enterotoxigenic *E. coli* (ETEC)	Diarrhea in travelers, foodborne outbreaks	Watery diarrhea, fever typically absent
Shiga-toxin producing *E. coli* (STEC)	Foodborne outbreaks (associated with beef and other contaminated food), person-to-person, and zoonotic transmission	Bloody stools, progression to hemolytic uremic syndrome

recommends that specific testing for *E. coli* O157:H7 be performed automatically by the laboratory on all stool specimens in patients with suspected community-acquired bacterial enteritis. *E. coli* O157:H7 can be cultured on a selective medium such as sorbitol-MacConkey agar. Culture-based techniques do not identify other strains of STEC; however, immunoassays to detect Shiga toxin are available and may have public health implications in identifying non-O157:H7 STEC-associated outbreaks.

Treatment of STEC infection is supportive. Antibiotics do not decrease the duration of symptoms and may increase the risk of developing hemolytic uremic syndrome. Empiric antibiotics should generally be withheld in patients presenting with bloody diarrhea unless there is supporting evidence for a cause other than STEC infection, and antibiotics should be discontinued if cultures confirm *E. coli* O157:H7 infection.

KEY POINTS

- Although most diarrheagenic *Escherichia coli* strains cause a self-limited and nonspecific gastroenteritis, Shiga toxin–producing *E. coli* (STEC) causes hemorrhagic gastroenteritis.
- *Escherichia coli* O157:H7 is the most commonly identified Shiga toxin–producing *E. coli*.
- *Escherichia coli* O157:H7 cannot be cultured on routine media but can be isolated on specialized sorbitol-MacConkey agar.
- Treatment of Shiga toxin–producing *Escherichia coli* infection is supportive.

Yersinia Infection

Yersiniosis refers to infection caused by *Yersinia enterocolitica* or *Y. pseudotuberculosis* but does not include infection caused by *Y. pestis*, the etiologic agent of plague (see Bioterrorism). Yersiniosis typically occurs following ingestion of contaminated food or water. Outbreaks of *Y. enterocolitica* have been traced to consumption of chitterlings (pork intestines). *Yersinia* gastroenteritis is clinically indistinguishable from other forms of inflammatory diarrhea and is most commonly identified in young children. In some cases, diarrhea may be absent with bacteria localizing to lymphoid tissue in Peyer patches and associated mesenteric lymph nodes. This presentation may mimic appendicitis clinically, leading to unnecessary appendectomy. Postinfectious complications occurring in yersiniosis include erythema nodosum and reactive arthritis.

Diagnosis is made by bacterial culture. *Yersinia* organisms grow poorly in routine stool cultures and, even on non-selective media, may be slow growing at normal temperatures. When yersiniosis is suspected, the laboratory should be notified to allow for plating onto specific media and cold-enrichment, which may increase the yield of the culture. Whether antibiotic treatment of infection limited to the gastrointestinal tract is beneficial is unknown, and delays in diagnosis often result in symptom resolution before infection is confirmed by culture. Treatment with fluoroquinolones may be indicated for patients with severe or prolonged symptoms.

Vibrio Infection

Vibrio species is a relatively uncommon cause of gastroenteritis in the United States. Conversely, *V. cholerae* is endemic throughout the developing world and is a significant cause of life-threatening diarrhea related to inadequate sanitation. Imported disease may occur in returning travelers as was the case with the recent cholera epidemic in Haiti following the devastating earthquake in 2010.

V. parahaemolyticus is the most common species causing diarrhea in the United States. The organism is widely distributed in salt water, with human infection associated with ingestion of contaminated seafood, particularly raw shellfish. Most infections are characterized by a relatively mild diarrhea, although this can be variably accompanied by nausea and vomiting, fever, and, occasionally, bloody stools. Infection may be particularly severe in patients with pre-existing liver disease, and this is a risk factor for secondary sepsis. In contrast, *V. vulnificus*, also found in saline environments, tends to cause bloodstream infections following ingestion, with diarrhea an uncommon manifestation.

Diarrhea caused by *Vibrio* species is likely underdiagnosed, because the organism requires specific media for culture from stool. The laboratory should be notified when *Vibrio*-associated diarrhea is suspected based on ingestion of raw or undercooked seafood or travel to a coastal region. Antibiotic treatment is indicated for severe illness, particularly in patients with liver disease. Doxycycline and the fluoroquinolones are both active against these organisms.

Clostridium difficile Infection

Clostridium difficile infection (CDI) is the most common cause of health care–associated diarrhea. Risk factors for CDI include use of antibiotics or chemotherapeutic agents in the 8 weeks preceding infection because this causes alterations in enteric flora that allow bacterial overgrowth and toxin production. Although some studies have identified an epidemiologic association between the use of proton pump inhibitors and CDI, other well-controlled studies have suggested that this may be the result of confounding by underlying severity of illness and duration of hospital stay. Asymptomatic *C. difficile* colonization is common in hospitalized patients, and secondary environmental contamination occurs when fecal continence is impaired. *C. difficile* spores are resistant to many disinfectants, including alcohol-based hand sanitizers,

CONT.

and appropriate infection control measures (gowns, gloves, washing hands with soap and water) are recommended to reduce the risk of person-to-person transmission in the health care setting. In recent years, increasingly severe cases of CDI have been reported throughout North America. These infections may occur without previous antibiotic use or health care exposure and have been attributed to a more virulent strain of *C. difficile* termed NAP1/BI/027.

The hallmark of CDI is watery diarrhea that is frequently associated with fever and abdominal pain or cramps. Diarrhea may be absent in patients with significant ileus or toxic megacolon (maximum colonic diameter greater than 7 cm on radiography), leading to a delay in diagnosis. Grossly bloody stools are rare, although fecal occult blood testing may be positive. A pronounced peripheral leukocytosis is common and is a poor prognostic sign. In one study, 25% of hospitalized patients with a leukocyte count greater than 30,000/microliter (30×10^9/L) had CDI, suggesting that this diagnosis should be considered in all hospitalized patients who develop an unexplained leukemoid reaction.

Diagnosis of CDI requires laboratory confirmation of infection in a patient with diarrhea. Testing formed stools is not recommended because a positive result suggests *C. difficile* colonization that does not require treatment. Similarly, serial testing of stool specimens to document clearance of *C. difficile* is not indicated. When test results obtained on an initial appropriately collected stool sample are negative, the yield of sequential tests is low. Sequential testing should therefore be reserved for patients with ongoing symptoms in the absence of an alternative cause.

Stool culture for *C. difficile* with subsequent cytotoxicity testing is the most sensitive test for CDI. However, this study is time consuming and work intensive and is only done in research laboratories. Most commercial laboratories use an enzyme-linked immunosorbent assay to detect toxins A and

B. The sensitivity of this assay on a single diarrheal stool sample ranges from 63% to 94%. One strategy to improve sensitivity is through a two-step method that uses enzyme immunoassay detection of glutamate dehydrogenase (GDH) as an initial screen, followed by cell cytotoxicity assay or toxigenic culture as the confirmatory test for GDH-positive specimens. Polymerase chain reaction (PCR) testing to detect toxin-producing genes is also commercially available and is a highly sensitive and rapid means of diagnosis. Endoscopic examination showing colonic ulcerations with overlying pseudomembrane formation is suggestive of CDI, but these findings are seen in only 50% of patients.

Recently published treatment guidelines reflect the evolving epidemiology of CDI (**Table 39**), with vancomycin increasingly being preferred for treatment of severe or refractory infections. Both the type of antibiotic and the route of administration are important in ensuring that adequate drug levels are present at the luminal site of infection. Enteral administration of metronidazole is preferred except when significant ileus prevents transit of the drug, in which case intravenous administration is indicated. Vancomycin remains in the colonic lumen with minimal systemic absorption. Intravenous vancomycin does not penetrate into the colon and is therefore ineffective for treating CDI. When beginning antibiotic treatment of CDI, any other nonessential systemic antibiotics that may promote colonic overgrowth of *C. difficile* should be discontinued. Despite appropriate initial treatment, CDI recurs in approximately 20% of patients. The role of ancillary therapy (for example, rifampin, cholestyramine, probiotic agents) or alternative agents (for example, nitazoxanide, rifaximin) for treating recurrent infections has not been established. Fidaxomicin has recently been approved by the FDA for treatment of mild to moderate CDI and appears to be as effective as vancomycin but is associated with a lower

TABLE 39. Treatment Recommendations for *Clostridium difficile* Infection		
Presentation	**Severity**	**Antibiotic Regimen**
Initial episode	Mild to moderate	Metronidazole, 500 mg orally every 8 hours for 10-14 days
Initial episode	Severe	Vancomycin, 125 mg orally every 6 hours for 10-14 days
Initial episode	Severe with multiorgan system failure or hypotension	Vancomycin, 500 mg orally or by nasogastric tube every 6 hours for 10-14 days **plus** metronidazole, 500 mg intravenously every 8 hours for 10-14 days
Initial episode	Severe with ileus or toxic megacolon	Same as for severe infection with multiorgan system failure with the addition of vancomycin by rectal tube
First recurrence		Treatment regimen based on severity, as in initial episode
Second recurrence		Vancomycin taper: vancomycin, 125 mg orally four times daily for 10-14 days, then 125 mg orally twice daily for 7 days, then 125 mg orally daily for 7 days, then 125 mg orally every 2 to 3 days for 2-8 weeks

Adapted with permission from Cohen SH, Gerding DN, Johnson S, et al; Society for Healthcare Epidemiology of America; Infectious Diseases Society of America. Clinical practice guidelines for Clostridium difficile infection in adults: 2010 update by the society for healthcare epidemiology of America (SHEA) and the infectious diseases society of America (IDSA). Infect Control Hosp Epidemiol. 2010;31(5):431-455. [PMID: 20307191] Copyright 2010 The University of Chicago Press.

CONT.

relapse rate; it is very expensive, and its role as initial therapy or for treatment of relapsing disease has not yet been defined. H

Viral Gastroenteritis

Viral gastroenteritis remains a significant cause of death among young children in developing countries. Although viral infections are the leading cause of gastroenteritis in the United States, they typically result in a relatively mild, self-limited illness. The two most common causes of viral gastroenteritis are rotavirus, which occurs almost exclusively in children under the age of 5 years, and noroviruses. Large outbreaks of gastroenteritis due to noroviruses have been documented in health care institutions, schools, cruise ships, and other settings where many people are housed in close proximity. Noroviruses are almost ideally suited for person-to-person transmission, as illness occurs with ingestion of fewer than 100 viral particles and fecal shedding of several million viral copies continues for prolonged periods following resolution of symptoms. In addition to fecal-oral transmission, infection can occur by ingestion of contaminated food or water, environmental contamination, or airborne inhalation of the virus.

Norovirus infection causes the abrupt onset of nausea, vomiting, and diarrhea, either singly or in combination, with fever noted in at least 50% of patients. The stool is typically watery without blood or leukocytes. Symptoms develop within 48 hours of infection and typically resolve after 72 hours, although findings may persist for longer periods in elderly or immunocompromised patients. Laboratory diagnosis is not routinely done because of the self-limited nature of the infection but may be important for public health investigations. If laboratory studies are indicated, PCR may be diagnostic. Antiviral agents are not available, and treatment, even in patients with severe infection, is supportive.

Parasitic Infections

Parasitic infection should be considered as a potential cause for diarrhea lasting for more than 7 days. In the United States, *Blastocystis* species are the most common parasites detected microscopically; however, whether this parasite is pathogenic is controversial. Reports have suggested resolution of gastrointestinal symptoms following treatment with metronidazole or other antimicrobial agents, but whether this is due to eradication of *Blastocystis* organisms or to treatment of other undiagnosed pathogens is unknown. Most authorities recommend reserving treatment only for patients with diarrhea lasting longer than 7 days in whom other infectious or noninfectious causes have been excluded. *Giardia lamblia* and *Cryptosporidium parvum* are the most commonly identified parasitic agents definitively known to cause diarrhea in the United States. Amebiasis is relatively uncommon in the United States but can cause hemorrhagic colitis in travelers and may occur several years after return from an endemic area.

Giardia Infection

G. lamblia is an environmental protozoal parasite that exists in fresh water sources throughout the United States and abroad. Cysts enter natural water supplies through excretion in animal feces, and ingestion of untreated water from contaminated streams or rivers is the major route of human infection. Hikers, campers, and outdoor enthusiasts are at highest risk of infection. Less commonly, infection is transmitted person-to-person by fecal-oral contamination.

Infection is asymptomatic in more than 50% of patients, and the protozoa clear spontaneously. In the remaining patients, symptoms typically occur 1 to 2 weeks after infection and include watery, foul-smelling diarrhea; bloating; flatulence; and belching. Significant weight loss is common because of anorexia and malabsorption, but fever is distinctly unusual. Gastrointestinal symptoms can persist for several weeks to months in the absence of treatment. Patients with hypogammaglobulinemia are at increased risk of developing severe or chronic infection.

Giardiasis can be diagnosed by examination of stool specimens for ova and parasites. Because protozoa may be shed sporadically in stool, examination of at least three specimens is suggested. Antigen testing of stool using immunoassays is more sensitive than microscopy for the diagnosis of *Giardia*, and is the preferred diagnostic test. Treatment is indicated for all symptomatic patients. First-line therapy is metronidazole for 7 to 10 days. Other active agents include tinidazole, nitazoxanide, mebendazole, and albendazole. Lactose intolerance is common following giardiasis and may persist for several weeks after completion of antibiotic therapy.

Cryptosporidium Infection

Cryptosporidium species, including *Cryptosporidium parvum*, are ubiquitous protozoal water parasites and have been responsible for large infectious outbreaks associated with contamination of municipal water supplies. Cryptosporidiosis is often asymptomatic, and infection in healthy persons is characterized by a relatively mild and self-limited diarrheal illness. In contrast, infection in patients with AIDS may result in prolonged diarrhea associated with significant weight loss and wasting. Patients with advanced HIV infection and low CD4 cell counts may also develop infection of the biliary tree causing acalculous cholecystitis

Cryptosporidia are not detected on routine examination of stool specimens for ova and parasites, but protozoa can be visualized with partial acid-fast staining of stools. Serologic assays directed against antigens in the stool have increased sensitivity compared with microscopic examination. Treatment in immunocompetent patients is often unnecessary, as cryptosporidiosis typically resolves spontaneously. Nitazoxanide may hasten resolution of symptoms in patients with severe infection. Treatment is challenging in patients with HIV infection because symptoms are often refractory to nitazoxanide and other antimicrobial agents. Reconstitution of cellular immunity may be curative in these patients, and optimization of antiretroviral therapy is indicated. Repletion of fluid losses and nutritional supplementation are important ancillary treatments.

Amebiasis

Amebiasis refers to infection with the protozoa *Entamoeba histolytica*, which is spread primarily through ingestion of contaminated food or water. Therefore, infection is more frequent in developing countries where sanitation may be suboptimal or in institutional settings owing to environmental contamination. Most infections are subclinical, with asymptomatic shedding of cysts over prolonged periods. In a minority of patients, invasive disease causes an inflammatory colitis characterized by bloody stools. Invasive disease is more common at the extremes of age and in immunocompromised patients. Amebic liver abscess is a well-described complication occurring when trophozoites enter the portal vein circulation and may occur in the absence of colitis.

Definitive diagnosis is established by stool antigen detection of *E. histolytica*. Serologic tests may support the diagnosis, particularly in patients with amebic liver abscess, because stool tests may be negative when disease is localized to the liver. Microscopy can identify trophozoites and cysts, but fecal shedding may be intermittent. *E. histolytica* is morphologically indistinguishable from other nonpathogenic entamoebae, potentially leading to misdiagnosis. Treatment of symptomatic patients is with metronidazole, followed by a luminally active agent such as paromomycin or iodoquinol to eradicate intestinal reservoirs. Asymptomatic patients with

confirmed *E. histolytica* in stool should also receive a luminal amebicide.

KEY POINTS

- Signs and symptoms of giardiasis include watery, foul-smelling diarrhea; bloating; flatulence; belching; and often significant weight loss; however, fever is distinctly uncommon.

- First-line treatment of giardiasis is metronidazole for 7 to 10 days.

- Cryptosporidiosis is often asymptomatic in healthy persons or causes a relatively mild and self-limited diarrheal illness; infection in patients with advanced HIV infection may be associated with severe diarrhea, weight loss, and wasting.

- Although treatment of cryptosporidiosis in immunocompetent patients is often unnecessary, nitazoxanide may hasten resolution of symptoms in patients with severe infection.

- Amebiasis (*Entamoeba histolytica* infection) is spread primarily through ingestion of contaminated food or water and occurs more frequently in developing countries where sanitation may be suboptimal or in institutional settings owing to environmental contamination.

Infections in Transplant Recipients

Introduction

Transplantation of solid organs or hematopoietic stem cells continues to become more common as both the indications and the range of acceptable candidates increase. Advances in surgical techniques have reduced the rate of postoperative infections, and better immunosuppressive regimens have reduced the incidence of acute rejection. Despite these advances, infection remains common after transplantation and is responsible for up to 50% of deaths in solid-organ transplant recipients.

Antirejection Drugs in Transplant Recipients

A classification of the most commonly used agents to prevent or treat rejection in solid-organ transplant recipients is shown in **Table 40**. Different classes, and to some extent, even different agents within a class, have different risks for infectious complications. Most transplant centers use a three-drug regimen consisting of prednisone, a calcineurin inhibitor, and an antimetabolite (usually mycophenolate mofetil). Regimens that minimize use of corticosteroids are associated with

TABLE 40.	Immunosuppressive Agents Used in Transplant Recipients
Class	**Agents**
Corticosteroids	Prednisone, others
Cytotoxic agents (DNA synthesis inhibitors, antimetabolites)	Mycophenolate mofetil
	Azathioprine
	Methotrexate
	Cyclophosphamide
Calcineurin pathway inhibitors	Cyclosporine
	Tacrolimus
mTOR inhibitors	Sirolimus (rapamycin)
	Everolimus
Lymphocyte-depleting antibodies	
Polyclonal	Antithymocyte globulins
Monoclonal	Muromonab (anti-CD3 antibody)
	Basiliximab (anti-IL-2 receptor)
	Daclizumab (anti-IL-2 receptor)
	Rituximab (anti-CD20 antibody)
	Alemtuzumab (anti-CD52 antibody)

IL-2 = interleukin 2; mTOR = mammalian target of rapamycin.

reduced rates of *Pneumocystis jirovecii* and other fungal infections. Cyclosporine-based regimens are associated with reduced rates of infections compared with regimens that utilize high doses of cytotoxic agents.

Immunosuppression prior to allogeneic hematopoietic stem cell transplantation (HSCT) involves a conditioning regimen of whole-body irradiation and myeloablative high-dose chemotherapy. Posttransplant treatment, including treatment of graft-versus-host disease (GVHD), may include corticosteroids, cytotoxic agents, and/or antilymphocyte antibodies. The lymphocyte-depleting agents are primarily used for early induction therapy or for treatment of acute rejection or GVHD and can have a prolonged effect that lasts for months. However, lymphocyte depletion, especially of T cells, is associated with an increased risk for infection with cytomegalovirus (CMV), polyoma BK virus, *P. jirovecii* and other fungi and for development of Epstein-Barr virus (EBV)–associated posttransplant lymphoproliferative disease (PTLD).

Many of the immunosuppressive agents have significant drug interactions that must be considered before starting any agent. Overlapping toxicities must also be considered, especially nephrotoxicity, cytopenias, and a prolonged QT interval. Interactions affecting drug metabolism and levels are also common. Important examples are the interactions of cyclosporine, tacrolimus, and sirolimus with macrolide antibiotics and with azole antifungal agents, which result in increased levels of one or both drugs.

KEY POINTS

- Most transplant centers use a three-drug regimen consisting of prednisone, a calcineurin inhibitor, and an antimetabolite (usually mycophenolate mofetil) to prevent or treat rejection in solid-organ transplant recipients.

- Immunosuppression prior to allogeneic hematopoietic stem cell transplantation involves a conditioning regimen of whole-body irradiation and myeloablative high-dose chemotherapy; posttransplant treatment may include corticosteroids, cytotoxic agents, and/or antilymphocyte antibodies.

- Many of the immunosuppressive agents have significant drug interactions that must be considered before starting any new drug in transplant recipients.

Posttransplantation Infections
Timeline and Type of Transplant

The risk for infections after transplantation depends on a number of factors, including the organ transplanted, immunosuppressive regimen used, development of rejection or GVHD and the treatment used, characteristics of both donor and recipient, and time since transplantation. Because some pathogens can be transmitted in the transplanted organ, donors are usually screened for active bacterial or fungal infections, various viruses (CMV, EBV, hepatitis B and C viruses, HIV), and tuberculosis.

CONT.

In the early period (first month after solid-organ transplantation), patients are at risk for surgical site and wound infections, which are usually bacterial, as well as for other nosocomial infections, such as central line infections, pneumonia, and *Clostridium difficile* infection. Specific sites of likely bacterial infection are related in part to the organ transplanted (for example, urinary tract infection in kidney transplant recipients).

In the middle period (after 1 month), the consequences of immunosuppression on cell-mediated immunity predominate, and CMV reactivation and infection are common. Other viruses can also reactivate and cause disease during this period, including EBV, polyoma BK virus, and hepatitis B and C viruses. Infections with intracellular bacteria such as *Legionella* species and with opportunistic pathogens such as *P. jirovecii* and other fungi may also occur.

In the late period (more than a few months posttransplantation), depletion of cell-mediated immunity continues at a reduced level, and opportunistic infections are less common. CMV infection may still occur, particularly in patients requiring more intense immunosuppression, and EBV-associated PTLD may develop. Polyomavirus infections more commonly present in this time period. Certain bacterial infections (such as *Listeria* and *Nocardia* infections) and fungal infections also become relatively more frequent, as do severe episodes of community-acquired infections.

The relationship between risk for different infections and time period after HSCT is depicted in **Figure 11**. Risk for

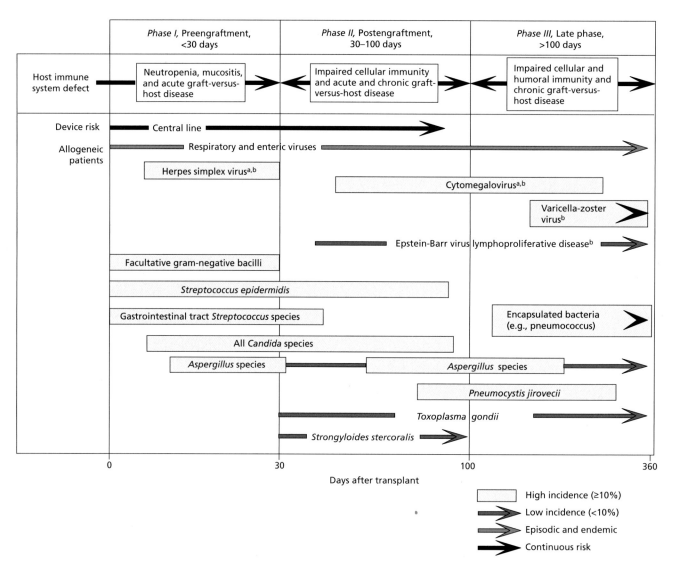

FIGURE 11. Phases of opportunistic infections in allogeneic hematopoietic stem cell transplant recipients. a = without standard prophylaxis; b = primarily among persons who are seropositive before transplant.

Reprinted with permission from CDC, Infectious Disease Society of America, and the American Society of Blood and Marrow Transplantation. Centers for Disease Control and Prevention. Guidelines for preventing opportunistic infections among hematopoietic stem cell transplant recipients. Recommendations of CDC, the Infectious Disease Society of America, and the American Society of Blood and Marrow Transplantation. Cytotherapy. 2001;3(1):41-54. [PMID: 12028843] infection is affected by the recipient's underlying disease, how well matched the donor and recipient are, and the presence of GVHD and consequent need for immunosuppression. Risk for infection following HSCT differs from that after solid-organ transplantation because of the profound neutropenia that follows HSCT, which increases the risk for bacterial and invasive fungal infections. **H**

KEY POINTS

- The risk for infection after transplantation depends on the organ transplanted, immunosuppressive regimen used, development of rejection or graft-versus-host disease and the treatment used, characteristics of both donor and recipient, and time since transplantation.

- The risk for infection after hematopoietic stem cell transplantation (HSCT) differs from that following solid-organ transplantation because of the profound neutropenia that follows HSCT, which increases the risk for bacterial and invasive fungal infections.

Specific Posttransplantation Infections
Viral Infections

CMV is the most important viral infection that occurs after transplantation. Reactivation and disease are most likely in CMV seronegative recipients of an organ from a seropositive donor. Onset usually occurs between 2 weeks and 4 months posttransplant, but may occur later because of prophylaxis. Reactivation is more likely to occur in the transplanted organ, and this may affect the clinical presentation. Patients may have a nonspecific febrile illness, often with leukopenia or thrombocytopenia. CMV can also cause a pneumonitis associated with high mortality rates or gastrointestinal tract or liver disease, including colitis, esophagitis, and hepatitis. As opposed to CMV infection in patients with AIDS, retinitis or central nervous system infection is rare in transplant recipients.

The most important consequence of EBV infection is B-lymphocyte proliferation leading to PTLD, which is more common following solid-organ transplantation than after HSCT. Patients usually present with fever and an extranodal mass or lymphadenopathy. Polyoma BK virus may cause nephropathy and ureteral strictures in kidney transplant recipients and may cause hemorrhagic cystitis in HSCT recipients. Hepatitis B and C may recur, especially after liver transplantation.

Bacterial Infections

Bacterial infections are common in the early period after transplantation, although prophylaxis has reduced this risk. The site of infection after solid-organ transplantation is often related to the surgical site and the transplanted organ. Examples are cholangitis and peritonitis after liver transplantation and pneumonia after lung transplantation. Pathogens include gram-negative bacilli (such as *Escherichia coli* and *Klebsiella* species) and staphylococci. Multidrug-resistant organisms, including *Pseudomonas aeruginosa* and

methicillin-resistant *Staphylococcus aureus*, are common, and organisms "carried over" from pretransplantation colonization (such as *Burkholderia cepacia* in patients receiving a lung transplant for cystic fibrosis) may cause infection.

The early period after HSCT is characterized by infections due to bacteria that are typically associated with neutropenia, including gram-negative bacilli and streptococci. During the late period after HSCT, an increase in infection by encapsulated organisms such as *Streptococcus pneumoniae* occurs. Because antibiotic regimens are likely to be given after any type of transplantation, *Clostridium difficile* infection must be considered in a patient presenting with diarrhea, fever, or leukocytosis.

Legionella infection tends to cause a severe, rapidly progressive, multilobar pneumonia in transplant recipients. *Listeria monocytogenes* causes bacteremia and meningoencephalitis, which may include cranial nerve and brainstem involvement manifesting as rhombencephalitis. Patients with *Nocardia* infection usually present with lung nodules, but dissemination occurs in about 25% of these patients and most often leads to brain abscesses. Tuberculosis usually occurs as reactivation disease in the first year after transplantation. Although tuberculosis may cause classic fever, cough, and focal lung lesions, about 50% of patients will have disseminated or extrapulmonary disease and may present with only sweats and weight loss.

Fungal Infections

Aspergillus species is the most common cause of invasive fungal infection after transplantation, especially following lung transplantation and during the neutropenic phase after HSCT. Invasive aspergillosis involves the lungs more often than the sinuses, and patients typically present with fever and possibly dry cough and chest pain. Dissemination to the brain is most common and is characterized by headache, focal deficits, and/or mental status changes. Non-*Aspergillus* molds, including the agents of mucormycosis, are increasingly being seen, including *Mucor* species and *Rhizopus* species, and have presentations indistinguishable from invasive aspergillosis.

Invasive *Candida* infections are common after transplantation, especially following liver transplantation and HSCT (particularly during the neutropenic phase). Fluconazole prophylaxis has reduced the overall incidence of these infections, but has also shifted the distribution of isolates to drug-resistant *Candida albicans* and *Candida glabrata*. Mucocutaneous infections, such as thrush and esophagitis, more commonly develop later after transplantation in patients who require ongoing immunosuppression.

Cryptococcus neoformans infection may develop in the late period after solid-organ transplantation but is uncommon following HSCT. Most patients have a subacute onset of fever, headache, and mental status changes (the latter two findings suggesting meningitis). Histoplasmosis and coccidioidomycosis can occur late after solid-organ transplantation in the Midwest and Southwest United States, respectively, but are rare following HSCT. Patients present with fever and respiratory signs and symptoms and possibly localized signs related to dissemination.

The incidence of *Pneumocystis* pneumonia after transplantation has been reduced significantly as a result of prophylaxis with trimethoprim-sulfamethoxazole and is usually a mid- to late-period posttransplantation opportunistic infection. Compared with *Pneumocystis* pneumonia in AIDS patients, pneumonia in transplant recipients has a more acute onset and is a more rapidly progressive illness.

Protozoa and Helminths

Toxoplasma gondii can reactivate after transplantation and usually causes central nervous system disease presenting as fever, headache, and focal neurologic changes. Imaging studies of the brain show multiple ring-enhancing lesions. Cardiac toxoplasmosis is a special problem in heart transplant recipients and may be caused by an infected transplanted heart.

Infection with *Strongyloides stercoralis* is more common in tropical and subtropical areas and can persist for many years in a subclinical state. Immunosuppression can then result in a hyperinfection syndrome; migration of *S. stercoralis* organisms in the lung and gastrointestinal tract can be associated with bacterial seeding, resulting in pneumonia and gram-negative bacteremia associated with a high mortality rate.

KEY POINTS

- The most common viral infections in transplant recipients are caused by cytomegalovirus, Epstein-Barr virus, polyoma BK virus, and hepatitis B and C viruses.
- Bacterial infections are common in the early period after transplantation, although prophylaxis has reduced this risk.
- Multidrug-resistant organisms, including *Pseudomonas* species and methicillin-resistant *Staphylococcus aureus*, are common in transplant recipients.
- *Aspergillus* species is the most common cause of invasive fungal infection in transplant recipients, especially following lung transplantation and during the neutropenic phase after hematopoietic stem cell transplantation.
- *Toxoplasma gondii* infection following transplantation can cause central nervous system disease and cardiac toxoplasmosis.

Prevention of Infections in Transplant Recipients

Prevention of infections after transplantation relies on reducing exposures and administering prophylactic agents and immunizations. Prophylactic antibiotics are usually given

after solid-organ transplantation and HSCT. Prophylaxis reduces the incidence of postoperative infections after solid-organ transplantation and may include fluconazole for *Candida* prophylaxis, especially for liver transplant recipients. During the neutropenic phase after HSCT, bacterial prophylaxis with a fluoroquinolone is usually given along with fluconazole or another antifungal agent.

Considerable attention has been given to reducing CMV disease after transplantation. True prophylaxis requires giving an agent broadly to every recipient at risk, whereas preemptive therapy targets those who show signs of early infection (such as a positive polymerase chain reaction) before development of disease. Both approaches are used for prevention, and the preferred agent is intravenous ganciclovir or oral valganciclovir, administered for the first 3 to 4 months after transplantation.

Trimethoprim-sulfamethoxazole is used to prevent *Pneumocystis* pneumonia and also provides activity against some gram-negative bacteria and *Listeria*, *Nocardia*, and *Toxoplasma* species. It is often continued for 12 months or more. Patients with latent tuberculosis infection should be given preventive isoniazid, preferably before transplantation. Antiviral therapy can be given to reduce recurrence of hepatitis B virus infection after liver transplantation.

Recommendations for immunizations in transplant recipients are shown in **Table 41**. Generally, solid-organ transplant recipients receive all vaccinations before transplantation, and HSCT recipients are revaccinated after immune system reconstitution. Because of the risk due to immunosuppression, live attenuated vaccines are usually contraindicated after solid-organ transplantation or HSCT.

KEY POINTS

- Prophylactic antibiotics are usually given after solid-organ transplantation and hematopoietic stem cell transplantation.
- Solid-organ transplant recipients generally receive all recommended vaccinations before transplantation, and hematopoietic stem cell transplant recipients are revaccinated after immune system reconstitution.

Hospital-Acquired Infections

Epidemiology

Nosocomial, or hospital-acquired infections (HAIs), are one of the 10 leading causes of death and the most common complication in hospitalized patients in the United States. HAIs are defined as infections that develop after 48 hours of hospitalization, with no evidence that the infection was present or incubating at the time of admission. Between 5% and 10% of patients admitted to acute care hospitals (approximately 2 million patients per year) acquire one or more HAIs, resulting in

TABLE 41. Immunization Recommendations for Adult Transplant Recipients

Immunization	SOT Recipients	HSCT Recipients[a]
Pneumococcal	Polysaccharide vaccine pretransplant; repeat at 5 years	Conjugate vaccine, three to four doses starting 3-6 months posttransplant
Influenza (inactivated only)	Annually	Annually
Tetanus, diphtheria, and acellular pertussis (Tdap)	Complete series pretransplant, including Tdap booster	Tdap, three doses starting 6-12 months posttransplant
Measles-mumps-rubella	Contraindicated after transplantation	One dose 24 months posttransplant, only if no GVHD or immunosuppression
Inactivated polio	Complete series pretransplant	Three doses starting 6-12 months posttransplant
Haemophilus influenzae type b	No recommendations	Three doses starting 6-12 months posttransplant
Meningococcal	As per general recommendations	As per general recommendations
Hepatitis A virus	Complete series pretransplant if not already immune	As per general recommendations
Hepatitis B virus	Complete series pretransplant if not already immune	Three doses starting 6-12 months posttransplant if otherwise indicated
Varicella -zoster virus	Varicella pretransplant if not already immune; zoster pretransplant if meets general recommendations; both are contraindicated posttransplant	Not recommended; absolutely contraindicated before 24 months and in presence of GVHD or immunosuppression
Human papillomavirus	As per general recommendations; give pretransplant	As per general recommendations

GVHD = graft-versus-host disease; HSCT = hematopoietic stem cell transplantation; SOT = solid-organ transplantation.

[a]For multiple-dose immunizations, the period between doses is generally 1 to 2 months.

90,000 deaths and accounting for costs of 4.5 to 6.5 billion dollars annually.

Health care–associated infections have a more expansive definition. These include HAIs as well as infections in patients who were recently hospitalized, attend infusion centers, or reside in long-term-care facilities. This chapter will focus only on HAIs.

Health care organizations, professional associations, government and accrediting agencies, and third-party payers have all developed initiatives related to the prevention or reduction of HAIs. In 2008, the Centers for Medicare and Medicaid Services stopped reimbursing hospitals for some costs associated with certain HAIs, and this policy will be broadened in the near future. Hospitals are required to report their rates of HAIs to selected organizations and sometimes to the general public. Although prevention of infections primarily focuses on patient safety, prevention may also potentially reduce hospital costs and enhance institutions' reputations.

Prevention

Preventing HAIs requires a multifaceted and multidisciplinary approach. A stable infection control infrastructure is of paramount importance. One of the most important components of HAI prevention is hand hygiene compliance. Hand hygiene, enacted before and after patient contact, consists of hand washing with soap and water for at least 15 to 30 seconds; alcohol-based hand disinfectants are acceptable alternatives to soap and water. Standardization of cleaning practices and immunization of health care workers are additional measures. Many successful HAI prevention initiatives involve "bundles" of processes. Often, the individual impact of each component of a bundle on HAIs is not clearly defined, but when all components of the "entire" bundle are practiced together, infection rates decrease.

KEY POINTS

- Hospital-acquired infections are defined as infections that develop after 48 hours of hospitalization, with no evidence that the infection was present or incubating at the time of admission.

- Hospital-acquired infections are one of the 10 leading causes of death and the most common complication in hospitalized patients in the United States.

- Hand hygiene is the single most important measure to prevent hospital-acquired infections.

Catheter-Associated Urinary Tract Infections

Catheter-associated urinary tract infection (CAUTI) is defined as a UTI occurring in a catheterized patient and accounts for more than 97% of UTIs acquired in the hospital. CAUTI is the most common type of HAI, with an average of 16.8 cases per 1000 catheter days.

Risk factors for CAUTI are listed in **Table 42**.

Diagnosis

The diagnosis of CAUTI is challenging. In patients with indwelling urethral, indwelling suprapubic, or intermittent catheterization, CAUTI is defined by the presence of symptoms or signs compatible with UTI with no other identified source of infection, along with 10^3 or more colony-forming units (cfu)/mL of one or more bacterial species in a single catheter urine specimen or in a midstream voided urine specimen from a patient whose catheter had been removed within the previous 48 hours. Symptoms and signs of a UTI may include new-onset or worsening fever, rigors, altered mental status, malaise or lethargy with no other identified cause, flank pain, costovertebral angle tenderness, acute hematuria, pelvic discomfort, and, in those whose catheters have been removed, dysuria, urgent or frequent urination, or suprapubic pain or tenderness. Because pyuria is not a reliable indicator of a UTI in a catheterized patient, systemic symptoms of infection may be the only indicators, especially in patients who have spinal cord injuries or who cannot provide a reliable history.

Treatment

Before initiating treatment for presumed CAUTI, a urine specimen for culture should be obtained to guide therapy and to account for the wide spectrum of potential organisms and the increased likelihood of antimicrobial resistance. If the catheter cannot be discontinued and has been in place for more than 2 weeks, the urine culture specimen should be obtained from a freshly placed catheter. The duration of treatment is 7 days for patients in whom symptoms resolve promptly and 10 to 14 days for those in whom response is delayed, regardless of whether the catheter remains in place.

Prevention

Measures and interventions to prevent CAUTI are shown in **Table 43**. Factors that have no role in the prevention of CAUTI include (1) screening for asymptomatic bacteriuria in catheterized patients; (2) treatment of asymptomatic bacteriuria, except in pregnant women and before invasive urologic procedures; (3) catheter irrigation; (4) routine changes of catheters; and (5) cleaning the meatal area with antiseptics before or during catheterization. The effect of using catheters coated with antiseptics (silver alloy or antibiotic) on the incidence of CAUTI remains unclear. Studies have demonstrated that antiseptic-coated catheters decrease the incidence

TABLE 42. Risk Factors for Catheter-Associated Urinary Tract Infection

Unmodifiable Risk Factors

Female sex

Age >50 years

Presence of a rapidly fatal underlying illness

Presence of diabetes mellitus

Serum creatinine >2.0 mg/dL (176.8 μmol/L) at time of catheterization

Modifiable Risk Factors

Prolonged duration of catheterization

Nonadherence to appropriate catheter care

Catheter insertion after day 6 of hospitalization

Catheter insertion performed outside the operating room

μmol = micromoles.

TABLE 43. Prevention of Catheter-Associated Urinary Tract Infection

Period	Preventive Measures
Prior to catheterization	Avoid catheterization whenever possible
	Use condom catheters or intermittent catheterization whenever possible
At time of catheter insertion	Adhere to hand hygiene practices by health care workers
	Use proper aseptic techniques when inserting the catheter
	Use smaller catheters to decrease urethral trauma
After catheter insertion	Promote early catheter removal whenever possible
	Secure the catheter
	Maintain a closed drainage system
	Avoid unnecessary system disconnections
	Use aseptic technique when handling the catheter, including for sample collection
	Maintain unobstructed urine flow
	Empty the collecting bag regularly, using a separate collecting container for each patient
	Keep the collecting bag below the level of the bladder

CONT.
of asymptomatic bacteriuria but do not significantly reduce the risk for symptomatic UTI. Antiseptic-coated catheters cost more than standard urinary catheters. In the absence of new evidence demonstrating their efficacy, they should not be used as a primary modality for preventing CAUTI. **H**

KEY POINTS

- Catheter-acquired urinary tract infection is the most common type of hospital-acquired infection.
- Pyuria is not a reliable indicator of a urinary tract infection in a catheterized patient.
- Antiseptic-coated catheters should not be used as a primary modality for preventing catheter-acquired urinary tract infection.

H Surgical Site Infections

Surgical site infections (SSIs) are diagnosed when the following two criteria are met: (1) infection occurs within 30 days after an operative procedure and (2) infection involves either the skin or soft tissue (incisional SSI) or an organ/space that was operated on or manipulated during the surgical procedure (organ/space SSI). Incisional SSIs are further classified as superficial (involving only the skin and/or subcutaneous tissue) and deep (involving the soft tissue). Primary incisional infections are those that develop in the primary surgical incision; secondary incisional infections are those that develop in the secondary incision in patients who have had surgery with more than one incision (for example, the donor site [leg] in coronary artery bypass surgery). In organ/space SSI, any part of the body can be involved, excluding the skin incision, fascia, or muscle layers. If an implant is placed during surgery, SSI can occur up to 1 year postoperatively. Implant infections are not associated with a superficial incisional SSI and should always be considered to be deep incisional or organ/space infections.

SSIs occur in 2% to 5% of patients undergoing surgery in the United States each year and account for 300,000 to 500,000 infections annually. *Staphylococcus aureus* is the most common cause, accounting for approximately 20% to 37% of SSIs. Methicillin-resistant *S. aureus* (MRSA) is a leading cause of SSIs in some tertiary care and community hospitals. SSIs lead to increased duration of hospitalization (>1 week of additional postoperative hospital days), a 2- to 11-fold increased risk of death for infected patients, and increased health care costs ($3000 to $29,000 per patient and approximately 10 billion dollars annually for the U.S. health care system). Risk factors for SSI are shown in **Table 44**.

Diagnosis

SSI typically manifests during the second or third postoperative week, although it can occur much later if an implant was placed during surgery. Diagnosis of superficial incisional SSI is typically based on signs and symptoms, including purulent drainage, pain, tenderness, redness, or heat. Patients with

TABLE 44. Risk Factors for Surgical Site Infection

Period	Risk Factors
Preoperative	Modifiable factors: obesity, tobacco use, use of immunosuppressants, length of preoperative hospitalization
	Unmodifiable factors: age, diabetes mellitus
Perioperative	Wound class, length of surgery, shaving of hair, hypoxia, hypothermia
Postoperative	Hyperglycemia, substandard wound care, blood transfusion

deep incisional SSI or organ/space SSI are typically more symptomatic than patients with superficial SSI owing to inflammation or abscess involving an organ or soft tissues. Frequently, cultures obtained during incision and drainage or debridement are positive.

Cultures should be obtained whenever deep incisional or organ/space SSI is suspected. Optimal cultures are taken from the deepest layer involved and should be obtained under controlled conditions such as in the operating room or by needle aspiration. Superficial swab cultures are potentially misleading and have a specificity of less than 30%. If necessary for evaluation of possible SSI, advanced imaging (CT or MRI) is more reliable than plain radiographs for diagnosing SSI.

The diagnosis of SSI in a patient with an implant or prosthetic joint can be challenging. Radiographic findings are usually nonspecific, and clinical signs and symptoms may be subtle. Multiple cultures should be obtained from deep infected tissues surrounding the prosthetic joint. Sonication, the use of ultrasound to agitate and dislodge bacteria from a removed and infected implant, is another method used to increase the yield of cultures to establish an accurate microbiologic diagnosis; however, because of the complexities associated with this technique, it is not practiced routinely in many laboratories (see MKSAP 16 Rheumatology for further discussion of Prosthetic Joint Infections).

Treatment

Surgical opening of the incision with debridement and removal of necrotic tissue is the most important aspect of treatment of deep incisional and organ/space SSIs. Antimicrobial therapy is an important adjunct. The type of debridement and duration of postoperative antimicrobial therapy depend on the anatomic site of infection, the invasiveness of the SSI, and whether foreign material was implanted or fully removed.

Prevention

The major measures to prevent SSIs are listed in **Table 45**. Checklists have played an important role in decreasing SSI rates, because they help to ensure compliance with multiple infection control measures. The impact of preoperative nasal

TABLE 45. Prevention of Surgical Site Infection

Preoperative Preventive Measures	Comments
Control/eliminate modifiable risk factors	Including uncontrolled diabetes mellitus or hyperglycemia, obesity, tobacco use, use of immunosuppressive agents, and length of preoperative hospitalization
Provide antibiotic prophylaxis	Administer 30 to 60 min before incision (60-120 min before incision for vancomycin and the fluoroquinolones)
	Maintain therapeutic antibiotic levels until wound closure, even if additional doses are needed intraoperatively
	Do not give prophylactic antibiotics for longer than 24 h after surgery

Perioperative Preventive Measures	Comments
Avoid shaving of hair	If necessary, clipping is preferred
Use chlorhexidine-based surgical preparation	May be superior to povidone iodine–based antiseptics
Minimize traffic in and out of operating room	None
Administer supplemental oxygen	Still controversial (most experience in procedures involving colorectal surgery)
Use checklists to improve compliance with preventive processes	None

Postoperative Preventive Measures	Comments
Optimize glucose control	Maintaining plasma glucose levels below 200 mg/dL (11.1 mmol/L) for 48 h postoperatively is recommended
Monitor and report risk-adjusted SSI rates to surgeons	None

SSI = surgical site infection.

decolonization of *S. aureus* on risk for SSI is controversial. The results of controlled clinical trials have been mixed, with the most convincing evidence in cardiothoracic surgery in the setting of preoperative nasal decolonization combined with chlorhexidine bathing. Based on current evidence, if nasal decolonization of *S. aureus* is performed, it should be conducted in conjunction with chlorhexidine bathing.

KEY POINTS

- Surgical site infections are diagnosed when infection occurs within 30 days after an operative procedure and involves the skin/soft tissue or an organ/space that underwent surgery or was manipulated during the procedure.

- *Staphylococcus aureus* is the most common cause of surgical site infections.

- Radiographic findings in patients with surgical site infections who have an implant or prosthetic joint are usually nonspecific, and clinical signs and symptoms may be subtle.

Central Line–Associated Bloodstream Infections

Central line–associated bloodstream infection (CLABSI) is a bloodstream infection originating from a central line without another recognizable focus of infection. Catheter-related bloodstream infection (CRBSI) is a type of CLABSI in which cultures of the catheter tip grow the same organism found in blood culture specimens. In the United States, 80,000 episodes of CLABSI occur in intensive care units (ICUs) each year and are attributed with causing 28,000 deaths annually. The epidemiology of CLABSI outside the intensive care unit is less well studied, but rates are lower. Independent risk factors for CLABSI are shown in **Table 46**.

Diagnosis

CLABSI should be highly suspected in patients who do not have an obvious source of infection from a site other than the central line and in whom the same pathogen is isolated from a peripheral blood culture specimen and from either a blood culture specimen obtained by aspirating blood through the central line or a culture of the catheter tip. It is important to recognize that central venous catheter tips are often colonized with bacteria in the absence of clinical infection. Thus, a positive culture of a central venous catheter performed as part of a routine screening protocol in the absence of positive blood cultures or signs of infection does not require treatment. Blood cultures (at least two sets) should be obtained from different anatomic sites (at least one peripheral site). A threefold greater colony count from the culture drawn through a catheter compared with a peripheral blood culture is a strong predictor for CLABSI. "Time to positivity" is the time between blood culture incubation and growth detection. When blood cultures are drawn from a central line and from

TABLE 46. Independent Risk Factors for Central Line–Associated Bloodstream Infection

Period	Risk Factors
Before central line insertion	Premature birth
	Neutropenia
	Prolonged hospitalization
During central line insertion	Catheterization in a site other than the subclavian vein[a]
	Substandard catheter care
	Heavy microbial colonization of the skin at the insertion site
After central line insertion	Prolonged duration of catheterization
	Total parenteral nutrition delivered through the catheter
	Heavy microbial colonization of the catheter hub

[a]Femoral vein placement is associated with greatest infection risk, and internal jugular vein placement with the second greatest infection risk.

Note: Female sex and subclavian vein insertion site were independently associated with decreased risk for infection.

a peripheral site within 30 minutes of one another, if the central line culture turns positive at least 2 hours before growth is reported on the peripheral culture, a central line infection is strongly supported. The semiquantitative roll-plate method for culturing the distal tip of a central venous catheter is a validated method for detecting catheter colonization and contributes diagnostic information when the same pathogen is recovered from both the catheter tip and the blood culture specimen. Typically, blood cultures should become negative once an infected central line is removed and appropriate therapy is administered. If bacteremia persists, a diagnostic workup for a deeper source of infection is appropriate.

Treatment

Removal of the central line is the most important intervention in treating CLABSI and is especially important when the pathogen is *S. aureus*, *Pseudomonas aeruginosa*, or *Candida* species. If salvage of a central line is attempted, use of an antibiotic lock is an optional adjunct to administration of systemic antibiotics.

Prevention

Early CLABSI occurs in the first 5 to 7 days following central line insertion and is typically caused by pathogens introduced during insertion. Late CLABSI occurs 5 to 7 days or more after insertion and is generally caused by pathogens introduced during catheter use or care. Methods to prevent early CLABSI mostly relate to improving catheter insertion techniques. Hand hygiene, basic aseptic techniques, and full

barrier precautions are mandatory. In adults, the femoral vein should be avoided for venous access whenever possible, and use of chlorhexidine-based antiseptics (in preference to iodines or alcohol) for skin preparation is advocated. Once a catheter is inserted, it should be removed as soon as the indication for placement has resolved. Appropriate disinfection before and after accessing any part of the catheter helps prevent late CLABSI. Antiseptic sponge products are effective in preventing CLABSI and should be changed every 5 to 7 days or sooner if they become soiled. If a gauze dressing is used, the insertion site should be inspected, prepped again, and dressed every 48 hours using sterile technique, and dressings should be replaced when they become damp, loosened, or soiled. If a transparent dressing is used, the dressing should be changed every 7 days or sooner if it becomes non-intact. Whenever central line dressings are changed, the insertion site and catheter hub should be disinfected with a chlorhexidine-based antiseptic. In patients with central lines in place, especially patients in the ICU, daily bathing with chlorhexidine body wash has been shown to reduce the risk for CLABSI. Intravenous administration sets should be replaced every 96 hours. Hemodialysis catheter insertion sites may be treated with povidone-iodine ointment or polymyxin ointment whenever the dialysis catheter is accessed as long as these antiseptics do not interfere with the catheter material (based on the manufacturer's recommendations).

Use of antiseptic- or antimicrobial-coated or impregnated central venous catheters for adult patients has been shown to reduce rates of CLABSI, although there is a lack of consensus about the cost-benefit ratio of their use. However, their use is recommended if the CLABSI rate is not decreasing in centers after successful implementation of a comprehensive strategy to reduce CLABSI rates. Use of antibiotic or alcohol locks as prophylaxis, systemic antimicrobial prophylaxis, and routine replacement of central lines are not recommended, although the use of an antibiotic lock solution can be considered in patients with long-term catheters who have a history of multiple CRBSIs despite maximal adherence to aseptic technique.

The Institute for Healthcare Improvement launched a campaign in 2004 introducing a bundle of evidence-based interventions for reducing CLABSI. The bundle includes a checklist that lists the following processes associated with reduced risk for CLABSI: (1) hand hygiene prior to line insertion, (2) use of maximal barrier precautions, (3) use of chlorhexidine skin antiseptic, and (4) optimal catheter site selection (preferring the subclavian site and avoiding the femoral site). Subsequent additions to this bundle include use of daily chlorhexidine-based body washes, use of prepackaged central line insertion kits, and daily review of central line necessity. Increased education of staff regarding use of central line bundles, checklists, and central line kits or carts has been shown to significantly reduce rates of CLABSI. For example, rates in the United States decreased in 2008-2009 compared with those in 2001. H

- Primary hospital-acquired bloodstream infection comprises both central line–associated bloodstream infection and catheter-related bloodstream infection and is defined as an infection originating from a central line without another recognizable focus of infection.

- Removal of the central line is the most important intervention in treating central line–associated bloodstream infection and is especially important when the pathogen is *Staphylococcus aureus*, *Pseudomonas aeruginosa*, or *Candida* species.

- Using a "bundle" of evidence-based interventions for preventing central line–associated bloodstream infections has been shown to significantly reduce infection rates.

TABLE 47. Risk Factors for Hospital-Acquired Pneumonia and Ventilator-Associated Pneumonia

Risk Factors	Variables
Comorbid conditions, exposures, and events	Advanced age
	Altered mental status
	Underlying chronic lung disease
	Rapidly or ultimately fatal disease
	Neurologic disease
	Trauma
	Previous antibiotic use
	Abdominal or thoracic surgery
	Mechanical ventilation
	Recent large-volume aspiration
	Nasogastric intubation
Medications	H_2 blockers
	Corticosteroids

Hospital-Acquired Pneumonia and Ventilator-Associated Pneumonia

Hospital-acquired pneumonia (HAP) is defined as a pneumonia that occurs 48 hours or more after hospital admission and was not incubating at the time of admission. Ventilator-associated pneumonia (VAP) is a subset of HAP and refers to pneumonia that develops more than 48 to 72 hours after mechanical ventilation was begun.

HAP is the second leading cause of hospital-acquired infection after catheter-associated urinary tract infection and is a common cause of infection in the ICU. Most cases of HAP in the ICU are due to VAP. The frequency of HAP is reportedly higher in certain patient populations, such as the elderly, newborns, and adult ICU patients. In one multinational study, HAP was the single most common type of infection. More than 50% of the antibiotics prescribed in the ICU are for the treatment of HAP, and HAP increases hospital stays by an average of 7 to 9 days per patient and increases health care costs by more than $40,000 per patient. The crude mortality rate may be as high as 70%. Multiple risk factors for HAP and VAP have been identified (**Table 47**). Mechanical ventilation is the single strongest independent risk factor for HAP; the incidence of pneumonia is 6- to 20-fold greater in ventilated than nonventilated patients. Re-intubation is an additional risk factor for VAP.

Diagnosis

Diagnosis of HAP and VAP is challenging. The two primary approaches to diagnosing these infections are through clinical and radiographic findings and bacteriologic test results. HAP should be suspected in patients with a new or progressive pulmonary infiltrate on chest radiograph with clinical findings suggesting infection (new onset of fever, purulent sputum, leukocytosis, and decreased oxygenation). When fever, leukocytosis, purulent sputum, and a positive lower respiratory tract culture are present without a new lung infiltrate, the diagnosis of nosocomial tracheobronchitis should be considered. Tracheobronchitis may mimic many of the clinical signs and symptoms of HAP and may respond to antibiotics. Bacterial colonization of the lower respiratory tract is common in intubated patients, and a positive culture does not necessarily indicate clinical infection. Additional components of diagnosing VAP include (1) obtaining blood cultures, (2) performing a diagnostic thoracentesis if a significant pleural effusion is present (or if a patient has a pleural effusion and appears toxic) to rule out empyema or a complicated parapneumonic effusion, and (3) obtaining lower respiratory tract samples for culture, ideally before antibiotics are initiated or changed.

Samples of lower respiratory tract secretions should be obtained from all patients with suspected HAP and should be ideally collected before antibiotic therapy is initiated or changed. Samples can include an endotracheal aspirate, bronchoalveolar lavage sample, or protected specimen brush sample.

Treatment

Delay in initiating appropriate antimicrobial therapy for HAP is associated with adverse outcomes. That some patients are at risk for HAP caused by multidrug-resistant organisms (see following discussion) should be considered when empiric therapy is selected. Risk factors for multidrug-resistant organisms include recent use of antibiotics, current hospitalization of 5 days or more, immunosuppression, and recent health care–associated exposures. If the presence of multidrug-resistant organisms is suspected, broad-spectrum antibiotic coverage for both gram-positive and gram-negative organisms (including MRSA and *P. aeruginosa*) should be prescribed as guided by the local hospital antibiogram. Antifungal and antiviral agents are not routinely prescribed.

CONT.

"De-escalation," or narrowing of empiric antimicrobial coverage once culture results are available and the patient has stabilized (typically on hospital day 3 or 4), is another important component of treating HAP. Treatment for 8 days is sufficient for patients with VAP, as long as empiric therapy was effective and patients do not have pneumonia due to *Pseudomonas* species or *Acinetobacter* species. The four important components of treating HAP and VAP are to (1) treat early, (2) administer empiric broad-spectrum antimicrobial agents, (3) de-escalate antimicrobial coverage when appropriate, and (4) consider short-duration therapy (8 days) whenever feasible.

Prevention

The most effective way to prevent VAP is to avoid unnecessary mechanical ventilation. Use of noninvasive ventilation techniques whenever possible and aggressive weaning efforts for patients who do require mechanical ventilation are advocated. Adherence to an evidence-based VAP-prevention "bundle" of interventions is recommended, which includes (1) keeping the head of the bed elevated at greater than 30 degrees, (2) daily assessments of readiness to wean, and (3) use of chlorhexidine mouth care. Respiratory equipment has been associated with outbreaks of VAP, and equipment should be disinfected or sterilized according to published guidelines. Continuous intermittent subglottic suctioning has been demonstrated to reduce the risk for VAP. The data regarding use of endotracheal tubes coated with antiseptics in preventing VAP are promising, but coated tubes are not currently recommended by guidelines. Selective use of oral and digestive decontamination has been demonstrated to be an effective preventive intervention in Europe but not in the United States, where the prevalence of antibiotic-resistant pathogens is higher.

KEY POINTS

- Hospital-acquired pneumonia is defined as a pneumonia that occurs 48 hours or more after hospital admission that was not incubating at the time of admission.
- Ventilator-associated pneumonia is defined as pneumonia that develops more than 48 to 72 hours after beginning mechanical ventilation.
- Mechanical ventilation is the single strongest independent risk factor for development of hospital-acquired pneumonia and ventilator-associated pneumonia.
- The four important components for treating hospital-acquired pneumonia and ventilator-associated pneumonia are to (1) treat early, (2) administer empiric broad-spectrum antimicrobial agents, (3) de-escalate antimicrobial coverage when appropriate, and (4) consider short-duration therapy (8 days) whenever feasible.

Hospital-Acquired Infections Caused by Multidrug-Resistant Organisms

Hospital-acquired infections (HAIs) are commonly caused by multidrug-resistant organisms. Examples of gram-positive multidrug-resistant organisms include MRSA and vancomycin-resistant enterococci. The vast majority of HAIs caused by MRSA are due to hospital-acquired MRSA, although community-associated MRSA has also been implicated. Frequently encountered gram-negative multidrug-resistant organisms include extended-spectrum β-lactamase (ESBL)–producing Enterobacteriaceae, carbapenem-resistant Enterobacteriaceae, *Acinetobacter baumannii*, and multidrug-resistant strains of *P. aeruginosa*.

The prevalence of multidrug-resistant organisms as causative pathogens for HAIs is continually increasing. Infections caused by multidrug-resistant organisms are associated with worse outcomes compared with infections caused by drug-susceptible strains of the same species. Multidrug-resistant infections were historically acquired only in nosocomial settings but are now being encountered in long-term care facilities (for example, nursing homes) and in patients without any contact with health care environments. Although the development of multidrug resistance is complex, its rapid expansion and increasing clinical significance highlight the need for diligent stewardship in using antibiotics in all settings.

Treatment of HAIs caused by multidrug-resistant organisms is frequently complicated by delays in beginning effective antimicrobial therapy. Treatment principles include the following:

1. MRSA infection is often treated with vancomycin. However, if the minimal inhibitory concentration to vancomycin is elevated (≥2 micrograms/mL) and the patient is not clinically responding to therapy, other agents may be considered, such as linezolid or clindamycin for pneumonia and daptomycin for bloodstream infections.

2. Linezolid and daptomycin are generally used to treat invasive infections due to vancomycin-resistant enterococci. However, if ampicillin is active against the causative organism, it should be used as the preferred therapeutic agent.

3. Carbapenems are the antibiotics of choice for invasive infections such as bacteremia caused by ESBL-producing pathogens. Group 1 carbapenems (for example, ertapenem) can be used to treat these infections as long as they are not caused by *Pseudomonas* or *Acinetobacter* species. Fluoroquinolones are also a therapeutic option if the pathogen is susceptible. Cephalosporins and penicillins, including cefepime and β-lactam/β-lactamase combinations, should not be used.

4. Therapeutic options for infections caused by carbapenem-resistant Enterobacteriaceae are limited. Polymyxins, tigecycline, and sometimes, aminoglycosides are often the only

CONT.

available active antimicrobial agents. Tigecycline monotherapy should not be used when bacteremia is suspected.

5. Some strains of non-fermenter, multidrug-resistant gram-negative organisms, such as *A. baumannii* and *P. aeruginosa*, may only be susceptible to polymyxins. *A. baumannii* sometimes retains susceptibility to tigecycline and/or minocycline. Minocycline, if active against the *A. baumannii* strain being treated, is preferred over tigecycline for treatment of urinary tract infection because it achieves higher urinary concentrations.

6. The role of polymyxin-based combination therapy (vs. monotherapy) for multidrug-resistant organisms such as *Acinetobacter* species, *P. aeruginosa*, and carbapenem-resistant Enterobacteriaceae remains uncertain as does the role of aerosolized colistin for treatment of ventilator-associated pneumonia.

Although contact precautions are effective measures to prevent nosocomial spread of multidrug-resistant organisms, their success depends on the compliance of health care workers. Cohort units with dedicated staff are an additional measure to control spread of these organisms. Communication between hospitals and surrounding long-term care facilities can help to identify suspected and known carriers of multidrug-resistant organisms at the time of hospital admission. A surveillance system to monitor rates of multidrug-resistant infections is an important component of hospital infection control. **H**

KEY POINTS

- The prevalence of multidrug-resistant organisms as causative pathogens for hospital-acquired infections is continually increasing.

- Treatment of hospital-acquired infections caused by multidrug-resistant organisms is frequently complicated by delays in beginning effective antimicrobial therapy.

- Although contact precautions are effective measures to prevent nosocomial spread of multidrug-resistant organisms, their success depends on the compliance of health care workers.

Infective Endocarditis Prevention

Background

Infective endocarditis is the net result of the several separate events. Damage to the heart valve or other surface can serve as a nidus for a thrombus composed of platelets, fibrin, and microbes. Turbulent blood flow contributes to this process as does foreign material, including prosthetic valves and pacemakers.

The intensity of bacteremia in the setting of infective endocarditis is variable. Spontaneous bacteremia can occur, but even minor trauma such as that associated with toothbrushing or interventions that manipulate the teeth and periodontal tissues, oropharynx, or gastrointestinal, urologic, and gynecologic tracts can elicit brief periods of bacteremia. Even though numerous bacteria may transiently enter the bloodstream, the risk for infective endocarditis is higher with bacteria such as streptococci, staphylococci, and enterococci, in which specific mediators of bacterial adherence are present (see MKSAP 16 Cardiovascular Medicine for discussion of Infective Endocarditis diagnosis and treatment).

KEY POINT

- Even though numerous bacteria may transiently enter the bloodstream, the risk for infective endocarditis is higher with bacteria such as streptococci, staphylococci, and enterococci, in which specific mediators of bacterial adherence are present.

Rationale

Interventions to prevent infective endocarditis have included correction of predisposing conditions, reduction of skin and oropharyngeal bacterial colonization, and elimination of the point of entry for potential pathogens. Administration of systemic antimicrobial agents, given before invasive procedures associated with transient bacteremia containing organisms causing infective endocarditis, has received the greatest attention as a preventive strategy. The American Heart Association (AHA) infective endocarditis prophylaxis recommendations, which were revised in 2007, acknowledge that this infection is much more likely to result from regular exposure to random bacteremia associated with daily activities than from bacteremia caused by a dental, gastrointestinal, genitourinary, or gynecologic tract procedure. It is likely that the risk of antibiotic-associated adverse events exceeds the benefit, if any, from prophylactic antibiotic therapy in these settings; therefore, the recommended indications for prophylaxis have been narrowed significantly relative to prior guidelines. These changes and their rationale will need to be discussed with patients, particularly low-risk patients who had previously received prophylaxis for dental procedures and are accustomed to this practice.

The AHA currently recommends prophylaxis for patients **H** with cardiac conditions with the highest risk for adverse outcome from infective endocarditis rather than prophylaxis for those with an increased lifetime risk for this infection. Infective endocarditis prophylaxis is recommended for patients with (1) a prosthetic cardiac valve; (2) a previous episode of infective endocarditis; (3) congenital heart disease characterized by unrepaired cyanotic congenital heart disease, including palliative shunts and conduits; a completely repaired congenital heart defect with prosthetic material or device during the first 6 months after the procedure; and repaired congenital heart disease with residual defects; or (4) for cardiac transplantation recipients in whom cardiac valvulopathy develops. **H**

- Infective endocarditis is now thought to be much more likely to result from regular exposure to random bacteremia associated with daily activities than from bacteremia caused by a dental, gastrointestinal, genitourinary, or gynecologic tract procedure.

- The risk for antibiotic-associated adverse events exceeds the benefit, if any, from infective endocarditis prophylaxis.

- The American Heart Association currently recommends infective endocarditis prophylaxis for patients with a prosthetic cardiac valve, a history of infective endocarditis, certain types of congenital heart disease, or those who are cardiac transplantation recipients in whom cardiac valvulopathy develops.

Recommended Prophylactic Regimens

In patients who meet current AHA infective endocarditis criteria, a single dose of a prophylactic antimicrobial agent should be given 30 to 60 minutes before all dental procedures involving manipulation of gingival tissue, the periapical region of teeth, or perforation of the oral mucosa in those patients with cardiac conditions discussed previously. If the antimicrobial agent is inadvertently not administered before the procedure, the medication may be given up to 2 hours after the procedure. **Table 48** lists the preferred antimicrobial regimens for use before a dental procedure.

Although a link between invasive respiratory tract procedures and infective endocarditis has never been demonstrated, antimicrobial prophylaxis (see Table 48) may be considered for patients with the cardiac conditions discussed previously who undergo an invasive respiratory tract procedure. Infective endocarditis prophylaxis is not recommended for patients who undergo genitourinary or gastrointestinal procedures, including upper endoscopy or colonoscopy with or without biopsy.

Appropriate treatment for patients with bacteriuria is recommended to prevent wound infection or infection from genitourinary tract procedures. In patients at risk for infective endocarditis who are about to undergo a surgical procedure that involves infected skin and/or related tissues, it is recommended that the treatment regimen for the infection have adequate activity against staphylococci and β-hemolytic streptococci, because these organisms have a greater propensity to cause infective endocarditis. **H**

- In patients who meet current American Heart Association infective endocarditis criteria, a single dose of a prophylactic antimicrobial agent should be given 30 to 60 minutes before all dental procedures involving manipulation of gingival tissue, the periapical region of teeth, or perforation of the oral mucosa.

- In patients who meet current American Heart Association infective endocarditis criteria, if the antibiotic dose is inadvertently not administered before the procedure, the medication may be given up to 2 hours after the procedure.

TABLE 48. Prophylactic Regimens for Infective Endocarditis Before a Dental Procedure

Situation	Agent[a]	Adults	Children
Oral	Amoxicillin	2 g	50 mg/kg
Unable to take oral medication	Ampicillin	2 g IM or IV	50 mg/kg IM or IV
	or		
	Cefazolin or ceftriaxone	1 g IM or IV	50 mg/kg IM or IV
Allergic to penicillin or ampicillin – oral	Cephalexin	2 g	50 mg/kg
	or		
	Clindamycin	600 mg	20 mg/kg
	or		
	Azithromycin or clarithromycin	500 mg	15 mg/kg
Allergic to penicillin or ampicillin and unable to take oral medication	Cefazolin or ceftriaxone	1 g IM or IV	50 mg/kg IM or IV
	or		
	Clindamycin	600 mg IM or IV	20 mg/kg IM or IV

IM = intramuscular; IV = intravenous.

[a]Regimen consists of a single dose 30 to 60 minutes before the dental procedure, or, if inadvertently not administered, drug may be given up to 2 hours after the procedure.

Adapted from Wilson W, Taubert KA, Gewitz M, et al; American Heart Association. Prevention of infective endocarditis: guidelines from the American Heart Association: a guideline from the American Heart Association Rheumatic Fever, Endocarditis and Kawasaki Disease Committee, Council on Cardiovascular Disease in the Young, and the Council on Clinical Cardiology, Council on Cardiovascular Surgery and Anesthesia, and the Quality of Care and Outcomes Research Interdisciplinary Working Group. J Am Dent Assoc. 2008;139 Suppl:3S-24S. [PMID: 18167394]. Copyright 2008 American Dental Association.

HIV/AIDS

Epidemiology and Prevention

In the United States in 2009, one million persons were estimated to be infected with HIV, with about one third unaware of their diagnosis. The infrastructure for testing and early treatment is established in most developed countries and in many developing countries, but failure to seek testing and financial and other barriers to treatment still exist. Untested and untreated persons may be responsible for ongoing viral spread.

HIV is spread through sexual contact, contaminated blood such as from injection drug use or occupational exposure, or perinatally; barrier precautions, including condoms, can decrease the risk for sexually transmitted infection. In addition, in 2012, the FDA approved the drug emtricitabine/tenofovir disoproxil fumarate for pre-exposure prophylaxis against HIV infection in uninfected individuals who are at high risk of HIV infection and who may engage in sexual activity with HIV-infected partners. The drug is contraindicated for pre-exposure prophylaxis in persons with unknown or positive HIV status.

Postexposure prophylaxis, which can significantly lower the risk of infection if initiated early enough, is standard after occupational exposure and is becoming more accepted following sexual or other exposures. Pre-exposure prophylaxis has been found to be effective in reducing the risk of acquiring HIV infection; however, the merits of taking indefinite antiretroviral therapy are controversial (see Management of the Pregnant Patient with HIV Infection for discussion of perinatal HIV prevention).

KEY POINTS

- HIV is spread through sexual contact, contaminated blood, or perinatally; barrier precautions, including condoms, can decrease the risk for infection.
- Postexposure HIV prophylaxis can significantly lower the risk of infection if initiated early enough and is standard procedure after occupational exposure.

Pathophysiology and Natural History

HIV is a retrovirus that primarily infects CD4 cells, including T-helper lymphocytes, which replicate and integrate into the host cell genome. Infection leads to destruction of these cells and, eventually, to immune system compromise, predisposing to opportunistic infections and AIDS.

Acute Retroviral Syndrome

Up to 90% of persons who become infected with HIV experience an acute symptomatic illness within 2 to 4 weeks of infection, although an accurate diagnosis is not established in most patients during this time. Symptoms typically last 2 to 3 weeks and may range from a simple febrile illness to a full-blown, mononucleosis-like syndrome (**Table 49**). Because of the lack of immune response in early infection, virus levels tend to be very high, resulting in high levels of infectivity during this period. Patients presenting with the acute retroviral syndrome are usually in the "window period," during which time seroconversion of the disease has not yet occurred and results of HIV antibody testing are negative. However, viral-specific tests, such as those for nucleic acid, are usually positive at quite high levels during this time frame and can be used to establish the diagnosis. Symptoms of acute HIV infection resolve with or without treatment, and most acute infections are undiagnosed. The benefit of beginning antiretroviral therapy during acute infection has not been proved but is suggested by theoretical considerations and retrospective data.

Chronic HIV infection

After acute retroviral syndrome, a period of years of asymptomatic, but still active, infection occurs, during which depletion of CD4 T-lymphocytes progresses. Patients may develop symptoms of chronic HIV infection during this period (**Table 50**). Before progression to AIDS (see Opportunistic Infections), patients may experience common infections that do not qualify as opportunistic infections but are more prolonged or severe in the context of HIV infection. Examples include recurrent or refractory vaginal candidiasis, severe oral or genital herpes simplex virus infection, pneumococcal pneumonia, and herpes zoster virus infection.

AIDS

A diagnosis of AIDS is established with development of certain AIDS-indicator opportunistic infections or malignancies (see Opportunistic Infections) or when the CD4 cell count decreases to less than 200/microliter.

TABLE 49. Signs and Symptoms of the Acute Retroviral Syndrome (Primary HIV Infection)

Sign/Symptom	Frequency (%)
Fever	96
Lymphadenopathy	74
Pharyngitis	70
Rash	70
Myalgia/arthralgia	54
Diarrhea	32
Headache	32
Nausea/vomiting	27
Hepatosplenomegaly	14
Weight loss	13
Thrush	12
Neurologic symptoms	12

TABLE 50. Signs and Symptoms of Chronic HIV Infection

Lymphadenopathy

Fevers, night sweats

Fatigue

Weight loss

Chronic diarrhea

Seborrheic dermatitis, psoriasis, tinea, onychomycosis

Oral aphthous ulcers, oral hairy leukoplakia, gingivitis/periodontitis

Peripheral neuropathy

Leukopenia, anemia, thrombocytopenia

Nephropathy

KEY POINTS

- Up to 90% of persons who become infected with HIV experience an acute symptomatic illness within 2 to 4 weeks of infection, although an accurate diagnosis is not established in most patients during this time.

- Symptoms of acute retroviral syndrome typically last 2 to 3 weeks and may range from a simple febrile illness to a full-blown, mononucleosis-like syndrome.

- An AIDS diagnosis is established when certain AIDS-indicator opportunistic infections or malignancies develop or when the CD4 cell count falls below 200/microliter.

Screening and Diagnosis

Because previous testing guidelines excluded many undiagnosed persons with HIV infection, the Centers for Disease Control and Prevention (CDC) released new HIV testing recommendations in 2006, significantly widening the scope of testing and encouraging reduction of barriers to widespread testing. Most, but not all, states have since revised or repealed laws requiring written consent for HIV testing, consistent with the CDC's recommendations for adoption of "opt-out" screening (the patient is informed and testing proceeds unless the patient declines). All adolescents and adults aged 13 to 64 years are recommended to undergo testing at least once unless the prevalence in the specific population is less than 0.1%. In addition, the American College of Physicians has issued a guidance statement recommending that this age range be expanded to include persons through age 75 years because of increased rates of infection in this population. Persons at high risk for HIV infection (injection drug users and their sex partners, persons who exchange sex for money or drugs, sex partners of those with HIV infection, men who have sex with men, and persons and their sex partners who have had more than one sex partner since their last HIV test) should undergo repeat testing at least annually. The guidelines reinforce the importance of HIV screening in all pregnant women as early as possible in pregnancy to implement measures to minimize perinatal transmission. In addition, in 2012, the FDA approved an at-home, rapid HIV screening test. The self-administered test uses swabs of oral fluids from the upper and lower gums to identify HIV antibodies, and results are available within 20 to 40 minutes. Physicians should advise patients that a positive test result requires confirmatory testing in the office. Moreover, because HIV antibodies may not appear during the window period (see Acute Retroviral System, discussed previously) patients with negative home test results should undergo repeat testing within 3 months.

The diagnosis of HIV infection is established by a two-stage serologic testing process. The initial test is an enzyme immunoassay (EIA). A negative EIA is generally considered adequate to exclude infection except during the acute phase following primary infection (the window period) before seroconversion occurs and when serologic testing, including Western blot assay, may be falsely negative. In these patients, EIA testing should be repeated 6 to 12 weeks later when seroconversion is established. If an acute diagnosis is necessary during the window period, a specific viral test such as the quantitative RNA polymerase chain reaction assay may be useful; in acute infection, the viral load is usually very high (often >100,000 copies/mL). However, use of a viral load study for routine diagnosis or in situations other than during the acute phase of infection is discouraged because of decreased sensitivity and specificity of the test at lower viral loads and the significant cost relative to EIA. In a patient with a positive EIA, the test should be repeated. Repeatedly positive EIA results are confirmed by Western blot assay. Combination testing with EIA followed by Western blot assay has a sensitivity of 99.5% and specificity of 99.99%. Rapid HIV tests are now available in kits that can be used in the clinical setting. These are EIA tests, and positive results require standard follow-up confirmatory testing. Because the EIA requires confirmatory testing, it is never appropriate to tell patients they have HIV infection based on results of any EIA alone before the Western blot results are known.

A negative Western blot assay indicates a false-positive EIA result. An indeterminate Western blot assay indicates the presence of antibody bands to certain viral antigens, but results are insufficient to establish the diagnosis of HIV infection. This may occur during the "window period" of acute infection when patients are just beginning to develop antibodies to HIV. Repeatedly indeterminate Western blot results usually indicate a cross-reacting antibody caused by infections or immunologic diseases other than HIV infection. Indications for HIV testing are shown in **Table 51**.

KEY POINTS

- All persons aged 13 to 64 years are recommended to undergo HIV testing at least once unless the prevalence in the specific population is less than 0.1%.

- Persons likely to be at high risk for HIV infection should undergo repeat HIV testing at least annually.

- The diagnosis of HIV infection is established by a two-stage serologic testing process consisting of enzyme immunoassay (EIA) followed by Western blot assay confirmatory testing of positive EIA results.
- Standard HIV testing may be unreliable in early infection, and repeat testing or other tests such as quantitative RNA polymerase chain reaction assay can help to establish the diagnosis.

Initiation of Care

Initial Evaluation and Laboratory Testing

Initial evaluation of the newly diagnosed patient with HIV infection includes a complete history, including social and sexual history, and physical examination with attention to signs and symptoms of opportunistic infections and other complications. Counseling on HIV transmission and prevention is also appropriate.

Laboratory tests indicated for patients with newly diagnosed HIV infection are shown in **Table 52**. Baseline testing assesses the patient's hematologic and metabolic status and assesses for coinfections that would need to be addressed.

Baseline viral resistance testing is now recommended for all newly diagnosed patients with HIV infection to guide the choice of antiretroviral therapy (See Drug Resistance Testing). The CD4 T-lymphocyte cell count (CD4 cell count) and quantitative measurement of HIV RNA (viral

TABLE 51. Indications for HIV Testing
Symptoms/signs of acute retroviral syndrome
Symptoms/signs of chronic HIV infection
Opportunistic infection
Severe, recurrent, or persistent infection that does not qualify as opportunistic
Presence of tuberculosis, HBV infection, HCV infection, other sexually transmitted infections, hemophilia
History of at-risk behavior (multiple sex partners, men who have sex with men, injection drug use) or sexual partner of someone who engages in at-risk behavior
Persons aged 13-64 years, unless in population areas with low (<0.1%) prevalence
Known or suspected HIV exposure
Victim of sexual assault
Patient request
All pregnant women
Child born to mother infected with HIV
Occupational exposure to blood/body fluid (both source patient and exposed worker)
Blood/semen/organ donor
HBV = hepatitis B virus; HCV = hepatitis C virus.

TABLE 52. Laboratory Testing as Part of the Evaluation of HIV Infection
Repeat HIV antibody testing if no documentation
Viral resistance testing at baseline and for treatment failure
Quantitative HIV RNA assay (viral load)
T-cell subsets (CD4 cell count)
Complete blood count with differential
Chemistries, including kidney function and fasting plasma glucose
Liver chemistry studies/liver enzymes
Fasting serum lipid profile
Tuberculin skin test or interferon-γ release assay for tuberculosis exposure
Serologic testing for hepatitis A, B, and C virus infection
Serologic testing for syphilis; testing for other sexually transmitted infections
Pap test
Toxoplasma serology
Varicella and cytomegalovirus serologies in high-risk individuals

load) are the most important tests for monitoring disease stage and effectiveness of treatment. The baseline CD4 cell count may be important in deciding when to initiate antiretroviral therapy. Follow-up monitoring of the viral load is critical in assessing the adequacy of the therapeutic regimen. Repeat testing of CD4 cell count, viral load, complete blood count, and kidney and liver function should be performed whenever HIV regimens are begun or modified, 2 to 8 weeks after therapy is changed, and every 3 to 6 months in patients whose regimens remain stable.

Immunizations and Prophylaxis for Opportunistic Infections

Because of their increased risk for pneumococcal pneumonia and other invasive pneumococcal diseases, all patients with HIV infection should receive pneumococcal polysaccharide vaccine immunization. Three doses of the hepatitis B virus (HBV) vaccine are indicated in patients who are not already immune to or infected with HBV. Annual influenza vaccination is appropriate, and recommendations for tetanus, diphtheria, and acellular pertussis; hepatitis A virus; human papillomavirus; and meningococcal vaccines are the same as those for the general population. Live virus vaccines, such as the measles-mumps-rubella and varicella-zoster vaccines, are not appropriate in patients with HIV infection, although studies evaluating the safety and effectiveness of the zoster vaccine in individuals with HIV infection with high CD4 cell counts are ongoing.

Indications and preferred agents for primary prophylaxis of opportunistic HIV/AIDS infections are shown in

Table 53. It is important to exclude active infection with *Mycobacterium avium* complex clinically and with negative blood cultures, because the single agent selected as prophylaxis would not be effective treatment for the active infection, and resistance could emerge, making the active infection even more difficult to treat. Similarly, it is important to exclude active tuberculosis with tuberculin skin testing or the interferon-γ release assay to determine whether prophylactic treatment or treatment for active disease is necessary.

KEY POINTS

- A thorough history, including social and sexual history, and physical examination with attention to signs and symptoms of opportunistic infections and other complications, as well as counseling on HIV transmission and prevention, are appropriate in patients with newly diagnosed HIV.

- Baseline viral resistance testing is now recommended for all newly diagnosed patients with HIV infection to guide the choice of antiretroviral therapy.

- The CD4 T-lymphocyte cell count and quantitative measurement of HIV RNA viral load are the most important tests for monitoring disease stage and effectiveness of treatment.

- All patients with HIV infection should receive pneumococcal polysaccharide vaccine immunization; hepatitis B virus vaccine (if not already immune to or infected by); annual influenza vaccination; and vaccines for tetanus, diphtheria, and acellular/pertussis; hepatitis A; human papillomavirus; and meningococcal vaccines as indicated in the general population.

- In patients with HIV infection, it is important to exclude active infection with *Mycobacterium avium* complex clinically and with negative blood cultures and active tuberculosis with tuberculin skin testing or the interferon-γ release assay to determine whether prophylactic treatment or treatment for active disease is necessary.

Complications of HIV Infection in the Antiretroviral Therapy Era

The development of medication regimens that effectively lower HIV viral loads to undetectable levels has transformed HIV infection from a uniformly fatal illness into a manageable chronic disease. However, as opportunistic infections and AIDS-related malignancies occur less frequently, other complications of HIV have increased in importance. These medication regimens have been referred to as highly active antiretroviral therapy (HAART), a term that initially was used to differentiate more aggressive, usually multiple-drug therapy, from single- or double-drug therapy that was once the standard approach. Currently, combination therapy is used routinely, and the distinction between antiretroviral therapy (ART) and HAART is less meaningful. Consequently, the term ART will be used in the discussion of HIV therapy in this section.

Metabolic Disorders

Metabolic changes in patients with HIV infection can be caused by antiretroviral medications or the infection itself. HIV infection is associated with decreased total, HDL, and LDL serum cholesterol levels and increased serum triglyceride levels. ART tends to reverse some of these changes: total and LDL cholesterol increase, but HDL cholesterol remains decreased and triglycerides remain elevated. Some antiretroviral agents, including many protease inhibitors, are particularly associated with hyperlipidemia. Atorvastatin has been shown to be effective in treating hyperlipidemia in patients with HIV infection; however, because of interactions with the protease inhibitor ritonavir, atorvastatin should be started at a lower dose in these patients.

Insulin resistance may also develop or worsen with treatment of HIV infection. Measurement of fasting lipids and fasting glucose or hemoglobin A_{1c} levels is appropriate after initiation of or a change in antiretroviral regimens and requires periodic follow-up during therapy.

Changes in lipids may be accompanied by lipodystrophy as well as changes in body fat distribution, including truncal and visceral fat accumulation and loss of subcutaneous fat in the face and extremities. This peripheral

TABLE 53. Prophylaxis for Opportunistic Infections in HIV/AIDS

Opportunistic Infection	Indication	Preferred Drug
Pneumocystis jirovecii	CD4 cell count <200/µL	TMP/SMX, double-strength tablet once daily or three times weekly
Toxoplasmosis	CD4 cell count <100/µL and positive serology	TMP/SMX, double-strength tablet once daily
Mycobacterium avium complex	CD4 cell count <50/µL	Azithromycin, 1200 mg/week
Tuberculosis	TST >5 mm or positive IGRA	INH, 300 mg/d for 9 months

IGRA = interferon-γ release assay; INH = isoniazid; TMP/SMX = trimethoprim-sulfamethoxazole; TST = tuberculin skin test; µL = microliter.

lipoatrophy may be reduced with avoidance of the thymidine analogue reverse transcriptase inhibitors (RTIs) (stavudine and zidovudine).

Mitochondrial toxicity leading to lactic acidosis, which can be fatal if not recognized early, has decreased with replacement of stavudine, didanosine, and zidovudine with lamivudine or emtricitabine and tenofovir in most regimens.

Osteopenia and osteoporosis may also be increased in patients with HIV infection; bone densitometry screening is not recommended for all patients but should be considered for those older than 50 years or with other risk factors.

HIV can also lead to chronic kidney disease through development of HIV-associated nephropathy. HIV-associated nephropathy, when diagnosed early, can be reversed with treatment of HIV. Patients in whom HIV-associated nephropathy progresses may require kidney dialysis or transplantation.

Liver disease is also increasing in patients with HIV infection, partly because of the high prevalence of coinfection with HBV or hepatitis C virus (HCV). Patients with HIV infection with chronic HBV infection requiring treatment should be given a multidrug regimen with agents active against both HBV and HIV infection. Patients co-infected with HIV and HCV have an increased risk for progression to chronic liver disease and cirrhosis.

KEY POINT

- Metabolic disorders, including hyperlipidemia, insulin resistance, body fat distribution changes, chronic kidney or liver disease and cirrhosis, and osteopenia and osteoporosis, are associated with HIV infection and HIV treatment.

Cardiovascular Disease

An increased risk for cardiovascular disease is associated not only with the use of some antiretroviral agents but also with HIV infection itself. The SMART study, which randomized subjects with CD4 cell counts greater than 350/microliter to continuous ART versus CD4 cell count–guided treatment interruptions, found that patients in the treatment-interruptions arm not only had more infectious complications (as expected), but they also experienced more cardiovascular disease end points and death, which led to early termination of the study. These results suggest that any increased cardiovascular risk caused by the metabolic side effects of treatment is more than offset by the risk from uncontrolled HIV infection, at least in those patients with CD4 cell counts less than 350/microliter. This increased risk is thought to be related to ongoing chronic inflammation, contributing to increased atherosclerosis. Chronic care of patients with HIV infection requires attention to modifiable cardiovascular risk factors, such as smoking, hyperlipidemia, hypertension, and diabetes.

KEY POINTS

- Any increased cardiovascular risk caused by the metabolic side effects of HIV treatment is more than offset by the risk from uncontrolled HIV infection.

- Chronic care of patients with HIV infection requires attention to modifiable cardiovascular risk factors, such as smoking, hyperlipidemia, hypertension, and diabetes mellitus.

Immune Reconstitution Inflammatory Syndrome

With the initiation of ART, viral load levels fall sharply, CD4 cell counts increase, and immune responses improve. In the presence of an opportunistic infection, which may not have been clinically recognized previously, this reconstitution of the immune response can lead to dramatic inflammatory responses as the newly revived immune system reacts to high burdens of antigens. This inflammatory presentation of infections is called immune reconstitution inflammatory syndrome (IRIS) and usually occurs a few weeks to a few months after initiation of ART. IRIS occurs with various opportunistic infections but most commonly in patients with mycobacterial infections, such as tuberculosis or *M. avium* complex, or disseminated fungal infections. Continuation of treatment is appropriate in patients with IRIS, but concomitant corticosteroids may be required to moderate excessive inflammation.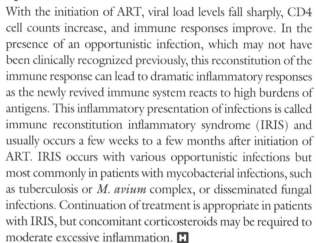

KEY POINTS

- Immune reconstitution inflammatory syndrome can occur after initiation of antiretroviral therapy as a dramatic inflammatory response to a previously clinically unrecognized opportunistic infection when the newly revived immune system reacts to high burdens of antigens.

- Continuation of treatment is appropriate in patients with immune reconstitution inflammatory syndrome, but concomitant corticosteroids may be required to moderate excessive inflammation.

Opportunistic Infections

Most opportunistic infections are unlikely to occur in patients with a CD4 cell count higher than 200/microliter, which is why this is the threshold value used to define AIDS.

Oral candidiasis (thrush) may occur in patients with CD4 cell counts greater than 200/microliter, especially in those with other risk factors, such as history of use of inhaled corticosteroids or broad-spectrum antibiotics, but extension to esophageal candidiasis occurs more often in patients with AIDS. Diagnosis is usually based on findings of visual inspection showing characteristic whitish plaques on the oral mucosa. Treatment of oral candidiasis includes topical agents such as clotrimazole troches. Dysphagia or other swallowing symptoms in patients with visible thrush suggest esophageal

CONT.

candidiasis, which requires treatment with a systemic agent such as fluconazole.

Cryptococcal infection starts in the lung but rarely presents until it is disseminated, most commonly to the meninges or skin. Cryptococcal meningitis may occur in patients with higher CD4 cell counts but occurs more typically in those with counts less than 100/microliter. It has a subacute or chronic presentation, characterized by headaches and changes in mental status, and systemic symptoms such as fever, sweats, and weight loss. Focal neurologic deficits usually involve cranial nerves. Diagnosis is established by culture or cryptococcal antigen testing on cerebrospinal fluid or serum. Treatment consists of induction therapy with amphotericin B deoxycholate or the lipid formulation of amphotericin B, combined with flucytosine, followed by consolidation therapy with fluconazole. Attention to increased intracranial pressure is crucial to reduce the risk for mortality and neurologic sequelae such as blindness. Even with effective treatment, there is significantly increased risk of early mortality in patients with disseminated cryptococcal disease.

Pneumocystis jirovecii pneumonia occurs in patients with CD4 cell counts less than 200/microliter and usually presents subacutely with dyspnea, dry cough, and fever. The chest radiograph typically shows diffuse bilateral interstitial or alveolar infiltrates, and diagnosis can be confirmed by identification of stains of the organism in sputum or bronchoalveolar lavage fluid. The preferred treatment is high-dose trimethoprim-sulfamethoxazole. The patient may worsen clinically following initiation of appropriate treatment, and corticosteroids should be used as adjunctive therapy in those with an arterial Po_2 of less than 70 mm Hg (9.3 kPa) while breathing ambient air or an alveolar-arterial oxygen gradient of greater than 35 mm Hg.

Toxoplasma gondii is a protozoan transmitted through the ingestion of undercooked meat or contact with cat feces. Toxoplasmosis primarily causes encephalitis in patients with CD4 cell counts less than 100/microliter. The illness is characterized by fever, headache, focal neurologic deficits, and, possibly, seizures. Contrast-enhanced CT of the head or MRI of the brain usually shows multiple ring-enhancing lesions. MRI is the imaging modality of choice because it has higher sensitivity and can better differentiate toxoplasmosis from other infections and central nervous system lymphoma. Treatment is typically empiric (pyrimethamine plus sulfadiazine or pyrimethamine plus clindamycin, or alternatively, trimethoprim-sulfamethoxazole), with clinical and radiologic responses occurring within 1 to 2 weeks.

The most common mycobacterial diseases in AIDS are tuberculosis and disseminated *M. avium* complex infection. Unlike in HIV-negative individuals, the presentation of tuberculosis in patients with AIDS is more likely to be extrapulmonary or associated with atypical chest radiographic findings without upper lobe cavitary lesions. Treatment of tuberculosis in patients with AIDS is complicated by drug interactions with antiretroviral agents and usually requires the use of reduced doses of rifabutin instead of rifampin. Disseminated *M. avium* complex infection usually is characterized by CD4 cell counts less than 50/microliter and fever, sweats, weight loss, lymphadenopathy, hepatosplenomegaly, and cytopenia. Specific mycobacterial blood cultures are usually positive. Treatment consists of a macrolide-based (clarithromycin or azithromycin) multidrug regimen.

Patients with cytomegalovirus (CMV) infection usually have CD4 cell counts less than 50/microliter. Gastrointestinal involvement is most commonly characterized by ulcers in the esophagus or colon, although CMV infection may occur anywhere in the gastrointestinal tract. CMV may infect the central nervous system, causing encephalitis or polyradiculitis. Prior to ART, the most common and significant presentation of CMV was CMV retinitis. The incidence of this illness has decreased significantly and is currently limited to patients with advanced immunosuppression who have not responded to ART. Patients with CMV retinitis may initially present with only floaters, but their condition will progress to blindness. Urgent ophthalmologic evaluation and initiation of ganciclovir, valganciclovir, or foscarnet therapy are necessary in patients with suspected CMV retinitis.

Molluscum contagiosum, caused by a poxvirus, is characterized by dome-shaped papules with central umbilication, most commonly occurring on the face and neck; these papules usually resolve with initiation of ART (**Figure 12**).

Bacillary angiomatosis is the most common manifestation of *Bartonella* infection in patients with AIDS and is characterized by skin lesions that may be confused with Kaposi sarcoma. Kaposi sarcoma presents with red, purple, or brown macules,

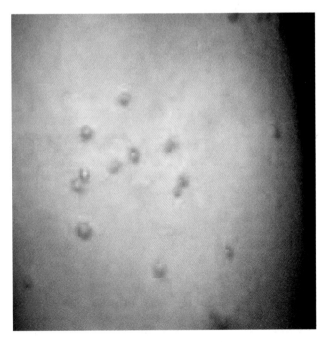

FIGURE 12. The dome-shaped papules with central umbilication of molluscum contagiosum.

CONT.

papules, plaques, or nodules on the skin or mucous membranes and is now known to be caused by a human herpesvirus (HHV-8). It occurs primarily in men who have sex with men and is rare in other HIV risk groups (**Figure 13**). ⊞

KEY POINTS

- Dysphagia or other swallowing symptoms in patients with HIV infection and visible oral thrush are suggestive of esophageal candidiasis, which requires treatment with a systemic agent such as fluconazole.

- Disseminated cryptococcal infection is characterized by headaches and neurologic deficits with changes in mental status, cranial nerve involvement, and systemic symptoms such as fever, sweats, and weight loss.

- Increased intracranial pressure in patients with disseminated cryptococcus can cause death and neurologic sequelae such as blindness.

- *Pneumocystis jirovecii* pneumonia occurs in patients with CD4 cell counts less than 200/microliter.

- Toxoplasmosis primarily causes encephalitis in patients with CD4 cell counts less than 100/microliter and is characterized by fever, headache, focal neurologic deficits, and possibly, seizures.

- The presentation of tuberculosis in patients with AIDS, unlike in HIV-negative individuals, is more likely to be extrapulmonary or associated with atypical chest radiographic findings without upper lobe cavitary lesions.

- Patients with cytomegalovirus disease usually have CD4 cell counts less than 50/microliter and retinitis or gastrointestinal involvement.

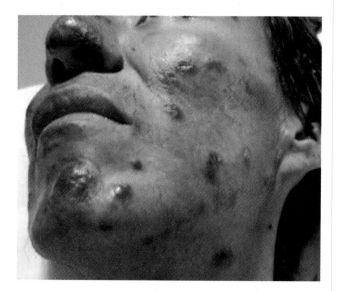

FIGURE 13. The lesions of Kaposi sarcoma, characterized by red, purple, or brown macules, papules, plaques, or nodules on the skin or mucous membranes.

Management of HIV Infection

The management of HIV infection continues to evolve rapidly. The U.S. Department of Health and Human Services (DHHS) and the National Institutes of Health regularly update guidelines on management of HIV infection, including the use of antiretroviral agents, prevention and treatment of opportunistic infections, and HIV testing and prophylaxis. The most recent guidelines are available at the AIDS info Web site (www.aidsinfo.nih.gov).

When to Initiate Treatment

Because the benefits of treating HIV earlier have been demonstrated, and the treatment regimens have become less complex and better tolerated, indications for when to begin ART have expanded. Current indications for initiation of ART, according to the DHHS guidelines, are listed in **Table 54**. In addition, the International AIDS Society U.S.A. Panel recommends treatment of those with active HCV coinfection and those who are at high risk for or have active cardiovascular disease, regardless of CD4 cell count. Whether to initiate treatment in all patients with HIV infection, even those with a CD4 cell count greater than 500/microliter, is an area of considerable controversy. A large NIH-sponsored prospective randomized controlled trial with clinical end points (the START study) is ongoing to address this question.

KEY POINT

- Antiretroviral therapy is recommended for patients with active hepatitis B or C virus coinfection, high risk for or active cardiovascular disease, a history of AIDS-defining opportunistic infection or malignancy, symptomatic HIV infection, a CD4 cell count <500 cells/microliter, HIV-associated nephropathy, or pregnancy.

TABLE 54. Indications for Initiation of Antiretroviral Therapy in HIV Infection

History of AIDS-defining opportunistic infection or malignancy[a]
Symptomatic HIV infection
CD4 cell count <500/µL
Presence of HIV-associated nephropathy
Active coinfection with hepatitis B or C virus
Pregnancy, to prevent perinatal transmission

µL = microliter.

[a]AIDS-defining illnesses include esophageal or pulmonary candidiasis; invasive cervical cancer; extrapulmonary coccidioidomycosis, cryptococcosis, or histoplasmosis; chronic intestinal cryptosporidiosis or isosporiasis; cytomegalovirus retinitis or infection other than liver, spleen, or lymph nodes; herpes simplex virus infection (chronic ulcers, bronchitis, pneumonitis, esophagitis); HIV encephalopathy; Kaposi sarcoma; lymphoma (Burkitt, immunoblastic, primary brain); lymphoid interstitial pneumonia; *Mycobacterium tuberculosis* at any site; extrapulmonary *Mycobacterium avium* complex or *Mycobacterium kansasii*; *Pneumocystis jirovecii* infection; progressive multifocal leukoencephalopathy; recurrent *Salmonella* bacteremia; toxoplasmosis of brain; HIV wasting syndrome; or recurrent bacterial pneumonia.

Antiretroviral Regimens

The objective of HIV treatment is to fully suppress viral replication to prevent the development of viral drug resistance, resulting in a rapid and progressive decrease of viral load levels within the first few weeks of treatment, and, within a few months of treatment, undetectable viral load levels that remain undetectable during therapy. Adhering to such a regimen requires a level of commitment often difficult for patients to maintain. Consequently, clinicians must discuss adherence with patients before initiation of therapy and at every follow-up visit. Maximal suppression of the virus generally requires the use of at least three drugs from at least two different classes. See **Table 55** for a list of agents currently in use in the United States.

The current preferred initial regimen in patients without viral drug resistance combines two nucleoside analogue RTIs (tenofovir and emtricitabine) with a nonnucleoside RTI (efavirenz), available as a once-daily, combination single pill. The use of a combination pill improves adherence and effectiveness. However, efavirenz should not be used in women who are or may become pregnant because of its association with neural tube defects (see Management of Pregnant Patients with HIV Infection). Other preferred regimens for patients who cannot take efavirenz use the same nucleoside "backbone," consisting of tenofovir and emtricitabine, with an integrase inhibitor (raltegravir) or a protease inhibitor (atazanavir or darunavir) as the third drug rather than efavirenz. Protease inhibitors are almost always given with a small dose of ritonavir, which is used to boost the drug levels of protease inhibitors, rather than as an antiretroviral agent itself. Ritonavir, even at small doses, has potent actions on multiple pathways of drug metabolism, including inhibition of the cytochrome P-450 enzyme system responsible for metabolism of many drugs. The use of ritonavir allows smaller and less frequent dosing of the regimen's other protease inhibitor, yet results in more steady and reliable drug levels, improving tolerability and effectiveness. Other drug interactions in patients with HIV infection are also common. For example, atazanavir should not be given with proton pump inhibitors, and protease inhibitors should not be given with lovastatin or simvastatin.

TABLE 55. Antiretroviral Agents Available in the United States to Treat HIV Infection

Class	Agents[a]
Nucleoside analogue RTIs	Abacavir
	Didanosine
	Emtricitabine
	Lamivudine
	Stavudine
	Tenofovir
	Zidovudine
Nonnucleoside RTIs	Efavirenz
	Etravirine
	Nevirapine
	Rilpivirine
Protease inhibitors	Atazanavir
	Darunavir
	Fosamprenavir
	Indinavir
	Lopinavir
	Nelfinavir
	Ritonavir
	Saquinavir
	Tipranavir
Entry inhibitors	Enfuvirtide
	Maraviroc
Integrase inhibitor	Raltegravir

[a]Some agents are also available as components of combination medications.

RTIs = reverse transcriptase inhibitors.

KEY POINTS

- Clinicians must discuss the importance of adherence with their patients with HIV infection before initiation of antiretroviral drug therapy and at every follow-up visit.

- Maximal suppression of HIV generally requires the use of at least three drugs from at least two different classes.

- The current preferred initial HIV antiretroviral regimen in patients without viral drug resistance combines two nucleoside analogue reverse transcriptase inhibitors with a nonnucleoside reverse transcriptase inhibitor in a once-daily, combination single pill.

- Protease inhibitors are almost always given with a small dose of ritonavir, which is used to boost the drug levels of protease inhibitors rather than as an antiretroviral agent itself.

Resistance Testing

Baseline testing of a patient's HIV isolate for antiretroviral resistance should be performed to guide the choice of agents, because previous infection with a resistant virus may have occurred. Resistance testing is also appropriate in the setting of treatment failure as evidenced by suboptimally controlled viral loads (lack of decreased or suppressed viral load, or previously undetectable viral loads that have become detectable on repeated testing). Generally, about 500 copies of virus/mL of blood are required for resistance testing to be adequately performed. Testing for treatment failure should be done while the patient is still receiving therapy, because false-negative results may occur with removal of the selective pressure provided by the drugs.

- Resistance testing of a patient's HIV isolate should be performed to guide the choice of agents at baseline and in treatment failure as evidenced by suboptimally controlled viral loads.

- Testing for treatment failure should be done while the patient is still receiving therapy.

Management of Pregnant Patients with HIV Infection

HIV testing for all pregnant women is appropriate. About one in four neonates born to women with HIV infection will acquire HIV infection perinatally if antiretroviral therapy is not given. Appropriate antiretroviral therapy can reduce the risk of HIV transmission to the newborn to less than 2%. Because HIV infection can be transmitted through breast milk, mothers with HIV infection should not breastfeed their infants if an alternative method is available. The preferred antiretroviral regimen in pregnancy is zidovudine, lamivudine, and lopinavir/ritonavir; efavirenz is teratogenic and should not be given in pregnancy. Indications for antiretroviral therapy in women after delivery are the same as those for the nonpregnant adult.

- HIV testing for all pregnant women is appropriate.

- In pregnant women with HIV infection, appropriate antiretroviral therapy can reduce the risk of HIV transmission to the newborn to less than 2%.

- The preferred antiretroviral regimen in pregnancy is zidovudine, lamivudine, and lopinavir/ritonavir; efavirenz is teratogenic and should not be given in pregnancy.

Viral Infections

Influenza Viruses

Overview

Influenza virus infection is a highly contagious, acute, febrile respiratory illness that causes outbreaks annually and is responsible for approximately 36,000 deaths annually. Influenza A, B, and C viruses are human pathogens, although influenza C infection is rare. Influenza A viruses infect a wide range of hosts and are classified into subtypes based on their surface proteins, hemagglutinin and neuraminidase. Influenza virus variants result from frequent minor antigenic changes (drifts) caused by point mutations and recombination events that occur during viral replication. Major changes in the surface glycoproteins are referred to as antigenic shifts. Antigenic shifts are associated with epidemics and pandemics of influenza A virus infection, whereas antigenic drifts are associated with more localized outbreaks. Antigenic shifts only occur among influenza A viruses. New influenza A virus subtypes can cause a pandemic when they bring about illness in humans, are transmitted efficiently from human to human, and when little or no preexisting immunity is present among humans. In the spring of 2009, infection of humans with a novel influenza A virus (H1N1) was identified, and this virus caused a worldwide pandemic. Outbreaks caused by influenza B viruses are generally less severe than those caused by influenza A viruses; however, it is impossible to clinically differentiate between influenza A and B virus infection.

Outbreaks of influenza have a seasonal distribution and occur almost exclusively during the winter months in the Northern and Southern Hemispheres. In tropical regions, influenza occurs throughout the year. Although influenza viruses can cause disease among persons in any age group, rates of infection are highest among children. Serious illness and death are highest among children younger than 2 years and adults older than 65 years and those who have medical conditions that confer risk for complications. Seasonal influenza is estimated to cause approximately 36,000 deaths annually.

- New influenza A virus subtypes can cause a pandemic when they cause illness in humans, are transmitted efficiently from human to human, and when there is little or no preexisting immunity present among humans.

- Outbreaks caused by influenza B viruses are generally less severe than those caused by influenza A virus; however, it is impossible to clinically differentiate between influenza A and B virus infection.

Clinical Features and Evaluation

Typical symptoms of influenza in adults are fever, headache, myalgia, nonproductive cough, sore throat, and nasal discharge. Gastrointestinal symptoms may occur in children. The incubation period is 1 to 4 days.

The most common complication of influenza is pneumonia, occurring in patients with underlying chronic illnesses. Primary viral pneumonia, secondary bacterial pneumonia, or both may occur. The most common bacterial pathogens are *Streptococcus pneumoniae, Staphylococcus aureus,* and *Haemophilus influenzae.* Other less common influenza complications include myocarditis, pericarditis, myositis, rhabdomyolysis, encephalitis, aseptic meningitis, transverse myelitis, and Guillain-Barré syndrome.

When influenza has been documented in the community, a clinical diagnosis can be made based on signs and symptoms. The standard laboratory study used to confirm influenza virus infection is reverse transcriptase polymerase chain reaction or viral culture. Rapid influenza diagnostic tests are immunoassays that can identify the presence of influenza A and B viral nucleoprotein antigens in respiratory secretions and display results qualitatively as positive or negative. Several rapid influenza diagnostic tests are commercially available, and results are generally available within 15 minutes or less. Rapid influenza diagnostic tests are helpful in confirming disease if positive. However, because they have limited sensitivity, negative results do not exclude the diagnosis, and other studies are indicated if confirmation is necessary. However, these tests are useful for public health purposes in detecting influenza virus outbreaks and guiding decisions about implementation of prevention and control measures.

KEY POINTS

- Typical symptoms of influenza in adults are fever, headache, myalgia, nonproductive cough, sore throat, and nasal discharge; the incubation period is 1 to 4 days.

- The most common complication of influenza is pneumonia, occurring in patients with underlying chronic illnesses.

- When influenza has been documented in the community, a clinical diagnosis can be made based on signs and symptoms.

Management

Influenza vaccination is the most effective method for preventing influenza infection and its complications. Two types of influenza vaccine are available: trivalent inactivated influenza vaccine and live intranasal influenza vaccine. The trivalent inactivated influenza vaccine can be used in persons older than 6 months, including healthy persons, those with chronic medical conditions, and pregnant women. Live intranasal influenza vaccine is administered as a nasal spray. It can be used for healthy persons aged 2 to 49 years who are not pregnant or immunocompromised. In 2010, the Centers for Disease Control and Prevention's (CDC's) Advisory Committee on Immunization Practices (ACIP) began recommending annual influenza vaccination for all persons older than 6 months.

Antiviral medications with activity against influenza viruses are an important adjunct to influenza vaccination in preventing and treating influenza. Two FDA-approved influenza antiviral medications, oseltamivir and zanamivir, were recommended for use as influenza treatment and chemoprophylaxis in the United States during the 2011-2012 influenza season. These agents are neuraminidase inhibitors and are active against influenza A and B viruses. Because of high rates of adamantane resistance in the United States, the CDC-ACIP advised against the use of amantadine and rimantadine for the treatment or chemoprophylaxis of influenza A virus infection. Because resistance patterns may change rapidly, treatment recommendations should be reviewed each year.

Treatment is indicated for hospitalized patients; those with severe, complicated, or progressive illness; and those at high risk for influenza complications. However, prophylactic or therapeutic treatment in individuals at low risk or those with equivocal clinical findings of influenza infection should be avoided. When indicated, treatment should be started within the first 2 days of symptom onset and may reduce the duration of illness and decrease the risk for serious complications. Prompt initiation of treatment without awaiting confirmation of laboratory studies is recommended. For pregnant women and patients with severe or progressive illness, antiviral treatment started within 3 to 4 days of symptom onset may still be beneficial. ◨

KEY POINTS

- All persons older than 6 months are now recommended to receive annual influenza vaccination.

- Antiviral treatment of influenza is indicated for hospitalized patients; those with severe, complicated, or progressive illness; or those at high risk for influenza complications.

- When indicated, antiviral treatment of influenza should be started within the first 2 days of symptom onset and may reduce the duration of illness and decrease the risk for serious complications.

Herpes Simplex Viruses

Overview

Herpes simplex virus (HSV) infection can occur at any skin location. Lesions on abraded skin or the fingers (herpetic whitlow) were once common among health care workers before improvements in hand hygiene and the use of gloves emerged. Recurrent HSV-1 keratitis is a primary cause of corneal blindness in industrialized nations and is characterized by dendritic ulcers, which are detected by fluorescein staining.

HSV is the most common cause of sporadic encephalitis ◨ in the United States. HSV encephalitis begins unilaterally in the temporal lobe and then spreads contralaterally, causing hemorrhagic necrosis. Manifestations include personality and behavioral changes, headache, fever, decreased consciousness, and abnormal speech. Focal seizures may also occur. Focal lesions are usually disclosed on imaging studies. Examination of the cerebrospinal fluid reveals pleocytosis and sometimes the presence of erythrocytes; the glucose level is usually normal. Cerebrospinal fluid testing for HSV DNA by polymerase chain reaction is appropriate. Prompt treatment is required as soon as the diagnosis is suspected. In patients who are immunocompromised, HSV may cause pneumonia, aseptic meningitis, esophagitis, colitis, hepatitis, or disseminated cutaneous disease. Oral and genital lesions may be particularly extensive. ◨

The clinical manifestations, evaluation, and diagnosis of herpes simplex virus infection and herpes zoster virus infection are discussed in MKSAP 16 Dermatology and the Sexually Transmitted Infection section.

- Clinical manifestations of herpes simplex encephalitis include personality and behavioral changes, headache, fever, decreased consciousness, and abnormal speech.

Management

Acyclovir, valacyclovir, and famciclovir are efficacious for treating mucocutaneous and visceral HSV infection, preventing HSV reactivation in immunocompromised hosts, and preventing symptomatic reactivation of recurrent genital herpes. Consideration of suppressive therapy is warranted for patients with a history of frequent (more than six per year) recurrences or severe recurrences of genital HSV or who are immunocompromised.

For patients with HSV encephalitis and other serious life-threatening infections or for those who cannot tolerate oral therapy, intravenous acyclovir is the treatment of choice. Topical agents, such as trifluorothymidine, vidarabine, and cidofovir, are available for treating HSV ocular infections. Topical corticosteroids are contraindicated in patients in whom HSV is known or suspected to be the cause of an ocular infection.

Patients with resistance to acyclovir, which is more common in those who are severely immunocompromised, are treated with foscarnet or cidofovir. Valacyclovir, in high doses, has been associated (rarely) with thrombotic thrombocytopenic purpura after extended use in patients with AIDS.

KEY POINTS

- Acyclovir, valacyclovir, and famciclovir are efficacious for treating mucocutaneous and visceral herpes simplex virus (HSV) infection, preventing HSV reactivation in immunocompromised hosts, and preventing symptomatic reactivation of recurrent genital herpes.

- For herpes simplex virus encephalitis and other serious life-threatening infections or in the setting of intolerance to oral therapy, intravenous acyclovir is the treatment of choice.

- Topical corticosteroids are contraindicated in patients in whom herpes simplex virus is known or suspected to be the cause of an ocular infection.

Varicella-Zoster Virus

Overview

Varicella-zoster virus, a herpesvirus, causes two distinct forms of clinical disease: varicella (chickenpox) infection and herpes zoster (shingles).

Varicella represents the primary infection with varicella-zoster virus and is a highly contagious disease characterized by a generalized vesicular rash (**Figure 14**). It is characterized by a vesicular eruption that spreads from the face and extremities toward the trunk (centripetally). Several stages of lesions, including macules, papules, vesicles, pustules, and scabbed

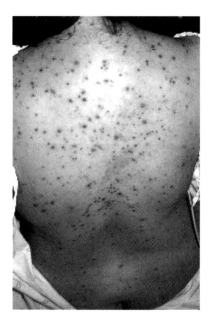

FIGURE 14. Varicella (chickenpox) rash is a vesicular eruption in which several stages of lesions (macules, papules, vesicles, pustules, and scabbed lesions) may be present simultaneously.

lesions, may be present simultaneously. Systemic symptoms are more pronounced in adults. Varicella can be more severe and disseminate in patients who are immunocompromised and in pregnant women. Complications may include secondary bacterial infections of the skin, including invasive streptococcal superinfection; pneumonia; encephalitis; optic neuritis; transverse myelitis; and Guillain-Barré syndrome.

Varicella is usually diagnosed clinically based on its characteristic appearance and history of exposure, although viral culture and immunohistochemical tests can be done.

Herpes zoster virus infection represents reactivation of prior infection with varicella-zoster virus and generally manifests as a vesicular rash in a dermatomal distribution. It should be considered in patients with pain along an affected dermatome, followed in 2 to 3 days by the typical diagnostic vesicular eruption (**Figure 15**).

KEY POINTS

- Varicella represents primary infection with varicella-zoster virus and is characterized by a vesicular eruption that spreads centripetally and encompasses several stages of lesions, including macules, papules, vesicles, pustules, and scabbed lesions, simultaneously.

- Herpes zoster is a reactivation of prior varicella-zoster virus infection and typically results in a vesicular rash in a dermatomal distribution.

Management

Varicella vaccine is highly effective and is recommended for routine vaccination in children between 12 to 15 months of

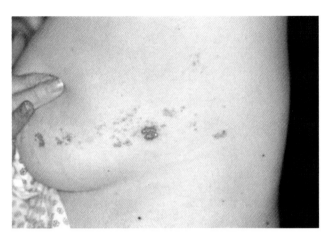

FIGURE 15. Pink to red papules and vesicles in a unilateral dermatomal distribution characteristic of herpes zoster virus infection.

age, with a second dose given at 4 to 6 years of age. In patients 13 years or older who have not been immunized or have no evidence of immunity, two doses of vaccine should be given 4 to 8 weeks apart; a second ("catch-up") dose should also be given to patients older than 13 who previously received only one dose of vaccine as a child.

Varicella-zoster immune globulin, if it can be procured, or varicella-zoster immune globulin product (VariZIG), is useful in preventing and lessening symptomatic varicella after a significant exposure in high-risk patients, such as those who are immunocompromised, have a negative or unknown history of chickenpox, and have not been vaccinated against varicella-zoster virus infection. It is also recommended for pregnant women who are seronegative for varicella-zoster virus infection and who have had significant exposure to the virus as well as for newborn infants of mothers who had varicella less than 5 days before delivery or 48 hours postpartum.

Herpes zoster vaccine is indicated for the prevention of herpes zoster infection in persons aged 60 years or older. It has been found to reduce the incidence of herpes zoster infection and decrease the incidence and severity of postherpetic neuralgia.

Acyclovir is approved for the treatment of varicella and herpes zoster virus infection. This agent reduces the duration of lesion formation and number of new lesions and decreases systemic symptoms in normal hosts. Treatment is recommended for adolescents, adults, and those at high risk for complications. Treatment should be initiated within 24 hours of onset of lesions.

Acyclovir, valacyclovir, and famciclovir are approved oral agents for the treatment of herpes zoster. Valacyclovir and famciclovir have better oral bioavailability than acyclovir and are better for hastening healing of skin lesions and reducing the risk for postherpetic neuralgia. Concomitant administration of corticosteroids with antiviral therapy for herpes zoster virus infection remains controversial.

KEY POINTS

- Varicella vaccine is recommended for routine vaccination in children between 12 and 15 months of age, with a second dose recommended at 4 to 6 years of age.
- Herpes zoster vaccine is indicated for the prevention of herpes zoster in persons aged 60 years or older.
- In patients with varicella-zoster virus infection, acyclovir shortens the duration of lesion formation, reduces the number of new lesions, and diminishes systemic symptoms and is recommended for adolescents, adults, and those at high risk for complications.

New Topics in Anti-infective Therapy

Introduction

Several newer antimicrobial agents have been licensed over the past decade that have improved the options for treatment of various infections caused by gram-positive and gram-negative bacteria. Their introduction is particularly important because antimicrobial resistance to many currently used antibiotics is becoming increasingly widespread. However, these new antibiotics are extremely expensive, and the risk of inappropriate use or overuse of these drugs could lead to low-value care and further resistance, potentially making treatment of many common infections problematic. Consequently, these medications should be used only when clearly indicated and when other appropriate treatment options are not available.

Emergence of resistant microorganisms has also led to a reexamination of older, well-known, and economical antibiotics that have retained activity against certain resistant pathogens. Indications are increasingly being recognized for these familiar agents in the treatment of infections involving organisms that are resistant to many currently used antibiotics.

KEY POINTS

- Several newer antimicrobial agents have improved the options for treatment of various gram-positive and gram-negative infections, but these agents should be used only when clearly indicated and when other appropriate treatment options are unavailable.
- Indications are increasingly being recognized for older, well-known agents in the treatment of infections with organisms that are resistant to many currently used antibiotics.

Newer Antibacterial Drugs
Lipopeptides and Glycolipopeptides

Daptomycin is a lipopeptide with bactericidal activity against gram-positive aerobic organisms, including methicillin-resistant

CONT.

Staphylococcus aureus (MRSA) and vancomycin-resistant enterococci (VRE) (**Table 56**). Daptomycin retains activity against many strains of *S. aureus* that have elevated minimal inhibitory concentrations (MICs) to vancomycin (≥2 micrograms/mL). Daptomycin is indicated for the treatment of complicated skin and soft tissue infections involving staphylococci, streptococci, and *Enterococcus faecalis*. Daptomycin is also an important agent in the treatment of bloodstream infections, including right-sided endocarditis caused by sensitive staphylococci (including MRSA) that are nonresponsive to vancomycin, particularly when the MIC to vancomycin is 2 micrograms/mL or higher. Daptomycin is not effective in

the treatment of pneumonia because it is inactivated by pulmonary surfactant. An important side effect of daptomycin is rhabdomyolysis; serum creatine kinase levels should be monitored weekly in patients receiving daptomycin, with discontinuation of treatment in patients whose creatine kinase level is elevated more than five times the upper limit of normal. Serious eosinophilic pneumonia developing during daptomycin treatment that has regressed on discontinuation of daptomycin has also been noted.

Telavancin is a glycolipopeptide with activity against gram-positive aerobic bacteria, including MRSA (see Table 56). Telavancin has lower MICs to *S. aureus* than vancomycin as

Agent	Route	Dose for Patients with Normal Kidney and/or Liver Function	Relative Cost	Adverse Events	Issues/ Limitations	FDA Indications
Ceftaroline	IV	600 mg every 12 h	$$	Similar to other cephalosporins; generally well tolerated	No clinical experience for MRSA outside of skin infections; limited activity against gram-negative bacilli	Community-acquired bacterial pneumonia except that caused by MRSA; acute bacterial skin and skin structure infections
Daptomycin	IV	6 mg/kg/d	$$$	Well tolerated; creatine kinase elevations	Inactivated by pulmonary surfactant; optimal dose still unknown	Complicated skin and skin structure infections; *S. aureus* bloodstream infections (bacteremia), including those with right-sided infective endocarditis, caused by methicillin-susceptible and methicillin-resistant isolates
Doripenem	IV	500 mg every 8 h	$$	Similar to other carbapenems, but lower risk for seizures	CNS penetration not well defined	Complicated intraabdominal infections; complicated urinary tract infections, including pyelonephritis
Linezolid	IV, PO	600 mg every 12 h	$$$	Thrombocytopenia; neuropathies	Toxicities may limit duration of therapy; selective serotonin reuptake inhibitor (SSRI) interaction	Vancomycin-resistant *Enterococcus faecium* infections, including cases with concurrent bacteremia; nosocomial pneumonia; complicated skin and skin structure infections, including diabetic foot infections without concomitant osteomyelitis; uncomplicated skin and skin structure infections; community-acquired pneumonia
Telavancin	IV	10 mg/kg/d	$$$	Nephrotoxicity	Significant interaction with coagulation tests; optimal doses unknown in patients with kidney dysfunction	Complicated skin and skin structure infections
Tigecycline	IV	100 mg x 1; 50 mg every 12 h	$$$	Nausea/vomiting; pancreatitis	Low serum concentrations	Complicated skin and soft tissue infection; complicated intraabdominal infection; community-acquired bacterial pneumonia

IV = intravenous; MRSA = methicillin-resistant *Staphylococcus aureus*; CNS = central nervous system; PO = orally.

CONT.

well as a longer half-life than that of vancomycin, which allows for a simpler dosing regimen. Telavancin can cause nephrotoxicity; patients receiving this agent require monitoring of kidney function. Telavancin is FDA approved for the treatment of skin and soft tissue infections.

Oxazolidinones

Linezolid is an oxazolidinone agent with bacteriostatic activity against gram-positive aerobic bacteria, including MRSA and VRE (see Table 56). Major uses for linezolid are oral therapy for indicated MRSA infections (see Table 56) and intravenous or oral therapy for pneumonia. The high penetration of linezolid into respiratory secretions contributes to its efficacy in the treatment of pneumonia. Urinary concentrations are also high, facilitating bactericidal concentrations against enterococci. An important side effect of linezolid is myelosuppression, notably thrombocytopenia, with an incidence as high as 10% with long-term use. Patients treated with linezolid should receive weekly complete blood counts. Long courses of linezolid therapy are associated with mitochondrial toxicity, including potentially irreversible peripheral or optic neuropathy.

β-Lactam Antibiotics

Ceftaroline is an advanced-generation cephalosporin with activity against gram-positive aerobic bacteria, including MRSA, and some gram-negative aerobic bacteria, including nonextended-spectrum β-lactamase–producing Enterobacteriaceae. Ceftaroline is not considered effective against strains of *Pseudomonas aeruginosa* and *Acinetobacter baumannii*. This drug is approved for the treatment of skin and soft tissue infections, including those caused by MRSA, and community-acquired pneumonia, except for pneumonia caused by MRSA because ceftaroline's efficacy against MRSA pneumonia has not been studied in clinical trials.

Doripenem is a group 2 carbapenem with in vitro activity similar to that of imipenem and meropenem except that doripenem is more active against *P. aeruginosa* than imipenem and meropenem. Although doripenem may still retain activity against strains of *P. aeruginosa* that are resistant to other carbapenems, the true clinical efficacy of this finding is unclear. This agent is approved for the treatment of complicated intraabdominal and urinary tract infections and also is used to treat health care–associated infections such as hospital-acquired and ventilator-associated pneumonia. No seizure events directly attributable to doripenem have been reported.

Glycylcyclines

Tigecycline is a glycylcycline agent with bacteriostatic activity against aerobic gram-positive bacteria (including MRSA and VRE), gram-negative bacteria (including carbapenem-resistant Enterobacteriaceae [CRE] and *A. baumannii*, but not *P. aeruginosa*), and some anaerobes. It is approved for the treatment of complicated skin and skin structure infections, complicated intraabdominal infections, and community-acquired pneumonia. Tigecycline does not attain high serum concentrations and should not be used for treating bacteremia. Nor does it achieve adequate urine concentrations; consequently, it is not indicated for treating urinary tract infections. An important treatment niche for this agent is possible management of patients with highly resistant gram-negative organisms. Resistance to tigecycline may occur in patients receiving this agent, and treatment failures have been reported. Nausea and vomiting are the most common side effects; cases of pancreatitis have also been reported. H

KEY POINTS

- Daptomycin is indicated for complicated skin and soft tissue infections involving staphylococci, streptococci, and *Enterococcus faecalis*.

- Telavancin is active against gram-positive aerobic bacteria, including methicillin-resistant *Staphylococcus aureus*.

- Telavancin has a lower minimal inhibitory concentration to *Staphylococcus aureus* than vancomycin and a longer half-life than that of vancomycin, allowing for a simpler dosing regimen.

- Major uses for linezolid are oral therapy for methicillin-resistant *Staphylococcus aureus* infections and intravenous or oral therapy for pneumonia.

- Linezolid causes myelosuppression, notably thrombocytopenia, with an incidence as high as 10% with long-term use; patients receiving linezolid require weekly complete blood counts.

- Ceftaroline is approved for treating skin and soft tissue infections, including those caused by methicillin-resistant *Staphylococcus aureus* (MRSA), and community-acquired pneumonia, except for pneumonia caused by MRSA.

- Doripenem is approved for complicated intraabdominal and urinary tract infections and also is used to treat health care–associated infections.

New Uses for Older Antimicrobial Agents

Trimethoprim-sulfamethoxazole

Trimethoprim-sulfamethoxazole (TMP-SMX) is a combination antimicrobial agent that is bactericidal against many pathogens (**Table 57**). TMP-SMX is used as a primary therapeutic agent against *Stenotrophomonas maltophilia* and *Pneumocystic (carinii) jirovecii*. TMP-SMX has retained excellent activity against MRSA, is orally bioavailable, and is an important agent in the treatment of skin and soft tissue infections caused by community-associated MRSA. The role of TMP-SMX in treating bacteremia or pneumonia remains unclear. Limitations of this drug include allergy (including Stevens-Johnson syndrome), hyperkalemia, and possible kidney toxicity.

TABLE 57. Older Antimicrobial Agents for New Indications

Drug	Route	Dosage[a]	Daily cost	Adverse Events	Issues/Limitations	Emerging Uses
Colistin	IV	5 mg/kg/d	$$	Nephrotoxicity; neurotoxicity	Pharmacologic properties poorly defined; significant unknowns on dosing	Treatment of multidrug-resistant gram-negative bacilli
Fosfomycin	PO, IV	3 g x 1 PO; 1-16 g/d IV	PO: $$; IV: unavailable	Gastrointestinal	Only available orally in United States; systemic experience limited to combination therapy	Urinary tract infection due to VRE or multidrug-resistant gram-negative (e.g., ESBL-producing organism or CRE)
Trimethoprim-sulfamethoxazole	IV, PO	5 mg/kg every 12 h (dose based on TMP component)	IV: $$; PO: $	Hypersensitivity; hyperkalemia	Limited data in ESKAPE pathogens; shortage of IV formulation	Skin and soft tissue infection from MRSA

IV = intravenous; PO = oral; ESBL – extended-spectrum β-lactamase; CRE – carbapenem-resistant Enterobacteriaceae; MRSA = methicillin-resistant *Staphylococcus aureus*; VRE = vancomycin-resistant enterococci; TMP = trimethoprim-sulfamethoxazole; ESKAPE = *Enterococcus faecium, Staphylococcus aureus, Klebsiella pneumoniae, Acinetobacter baumannii, Pseudomonas aeruginosa,* and *Enterobacter* species.

[a]Refers to the dosage for patients with normal kidney and/or liver function.

Polymyxins

Colistin (polymyxin E) and polymyxin B are the two commercially available polymyxin antimicrobial agents (see Table 57) with bactericidal activity against many strains of gram-negative bacilli, including *P. aeruginosa, A. baumannii,* and the Enterobacteriaceae. Polymyxins are important in the treatment of gram-negative bacilli that are resistant to all other antimicrobials, including CRE, *P. aeruginosa,* and *A. baumannii.* Colistin, which is administered in the form of its prodrug, colistimethate sodium, has become the most commonly used form of polymyxin for parenteral administration and has also been used as nebulization therapy for pneumonia in patients with cystic fibrosis and pneumonia caused by multidrug-resistant gram-negative organisms as well as for intrathecal or intraventricular therapy in patients with meningitis caused by resistant strains of *A. baumannii.* Given concerns of risk for prescribing errors in the United States, colistin dosing is based on milligrams of colistin base activity (CBA). Limitations of colistin include nephrotoxicity and neurotoxicity.

Fosfomycin

Fosfomycin is a phosphonic acid derivative with bactericidal activity against many gram-positive and gram-negative organisms, including MRSA, VRE, and multidrug-resistant gram-negative organisms (see Table 57). Only the oral formulation is available in the United States, although it is not widely available, and attainable serum concentrations are low. An important use of this agent is in the treatment of lower urinary tract infection (cystitis). Fosfomycin can be especially useful in patients with allergies to multiple antibiotics because it is not cross-allergenic with any other agent.

Aminoglycosides

Aminoglycosides are bactericidal antimicrobials that are primarily used as companion drugs to broaden activity or provide synergy against treatment of gram-negative bacilli or to provide synergistic activity against gram-positive bacteria. However, these agents have retained activity against some multidrug-resistant strains of gram-negative bacilli, including *A. baumannii, P. aeruginosa,* and CRE, and have become important agents of last resort in the treatment of infections caused by these bacteria. Once-daily dosing of these agents is becoming the preferred mode of administration for treatment of infection caused by gram-negative bacilli. The major limitations of the aminoglycosides are nephrotoxicity and ototoxicity (vestibular and cochlear).

Rifamycins

Rifampin is a rifamycin that has retained activity against many strains of MRSA and is often used in combination with other agents for the treatment of infections caused by MRSA and coagulase-negative staphylococci, especially in patients who also have infection associated with indwelling foreign bodies. A major limitation of rifampin is its potential to induce hepatic microsomal enzymes, causing multiple drug-drug interactions. Rifampin should not be used as monotherapy for the treatment of bacterial infection because of the rapid emergence of resistance. Rifaximin is a nonabsorbable rifamycin derivative that has been useful in the treatment and prophylaxis of travelers' diarrhea. It has also shown benefit in the management of hepatic encephalopathy. ⊞

- Trimethoprim-sulfamethoxazole is used as a primary agent against *Stenotrophomonas maltophilia* and *Pneumocystis jirovecii*, and it has retained excellent activity against methicillin-resistant *Staphylococcus aureus* (MRSA), is orally bioavailable, and is important in treating skin and soft tissue infections caused by community-associated MRSA.

- Polymyxins are important in the treatment of gram-negative bacilli that are resistant to all other antimicrobials, including carbapenem-resistant Enterobacteriaceae, *Pseudomonas aeruginosa*, and *Acinetobacter baumannii*.

- Fosfomycin is active against many gram-positive and gram-negative organisms, including methicillin-resistant *Staphylococcus aureus*, vancomycin-resistant enterococci, and multidrug resistant gram-negative organisms.

- Aminoglycosides have retained activity against some multidrug-resistant strains of gram-negative bacilli, including *Acinetobacter baumannii*, *Pseudomonas aeruginosa*, and carbapenem-resistant Enterobacteriaceae.

- Once-daily dosing of aminoglycosides is becoming the preferred mode of administration for treatment of infection caused by gram-negative bacilli.

- Rifampin has retained activity against many strains of methicillin-resistant *Staphylococcus aureus* (MRSA) and is often used in conjunction with other agents to treat infections caused by MRSA and coagulase-negative staphylococci, especially in patients who also have infection associated with indwelling foreign bodies.

- Rifampin should not be used as monotherapy for the treatment of bacterial infection because of the rapid emergence of resistance.

Antimicrobial Stewardship

Antimicrobial stewardship focuses on optimizing antimicrobial therapy through appropriate empiric therapy, narrowing the spectrum of coverage once clinical data become available, and shortening the duration of therapy whenever possible. Once a specific organism is isolated and its sensitivities to available antibiotics known, it is beneficial to focus or "de-escalate" therapy to avoid the selection of organisms resistant to currently effective broad-spectrum antibiotics. Important goals of stewardship are to limit the emergence of antimicrobial resistance and reduce inappropriate antimicrobial usage.

Core members of the stewardship team include an infectious diseases physician, an infectious diseases pharmacist (or professionals with interest and experience in antimicrobial therapeutics), a health care epidemiologist, a clinical microbiologist, and an information systems specialist. Support from hospital administration to provide the necessary infrastructure and involvement of quality assurance and patient safety programs are important to the success of antimicrobial stewardship programs.

- Important goals of antimicrobial stewardship are to limit the emergence of antimicrobial resistance and reduce inappropriate antimicrobial usage.

Outpatient Antimicrobial Therapy

Outpatient antimicrobial therapy (OPAT) encompasses intravenous, intramuscular, and subcutaneous antimicrobial therapy administered without hospitalization. OPAT can be delivered at home or in other nonhospital settings. Patients receiving OPAT should be clinically stable. OPAT requires teamwork among a physician, nurse, pharmacist, and case manager. Creation of a schedule of visits and periodic laboratory monitoring are also required. The home situation should include family/caregiver support, transportation, availability of emergency services (if needed), telephone, running water, and refrigeration. Conditions commonly treated with OPAT include skin and soft tissue infections, osteomyelitis, and bacteremia. It is preferable to use agents for OPAT that are dosed infrequently, such as ceftriaxone or vancomycin, and the first dose of therapy should be administered in a supervised setting. OPAT can be delivered through peripheral short catheters, peripherally inserted central catheters, and tunneled or nontunneled central catheters.

- Outpatient antimicrobial therapy encompasses intravenous, intramuscular, and subcutaneous antimicrobial therapy administered without hospitalization, and it can be delivered at home or in other nonhospital settings.

- Patients for whom outpatient antimicrobial therapy is being considered require a home situation with family/caregiver support, transportation, availability of emergency services, telephone, running water, and refrigeration.

- It is preferable to use agents for outpatient antimicrobial therapy that are dosed infrequently, such as ceftriaxone or vancomycin, and the first dose should be administered in a supervised setting.

Hyperbaric Oxygen

Hyperbaric oxygen is sometimes used to promote wound healing. Data are limited regarding use of this modality for treatment of acute, life-threatening soft tissue infections, although the recognized infectious diseases for which hyperbaric oxygen is used include clostridial gangrene, necrotizing fasciitis, and refractory osteomyelitis.

Hyperbaric oxygen is also sometimes used to treat chronic nonhealing ulcers. Some studies have reported decreased amputation rates associated with use of hyperbaric oxygen. Hyperbaric oxygen might be used as adjunctive therapy for severe diabetic foot infections or nonhealing infections despite appropriate antimicrobial and surgical therapy.

Absolute contraindications to hyperbaric oxygen therapy include untreated pneumothorax and recent chemotherapy with doxorubicin or cisplatin. The most common adverse effect is barotrauma to the middle ear, cranial sinuses, or the teeth; oxygen toxicity is a rare complication.

KEY POINTS

- In patients with chronic, nonhealing ulcers, decreased amputation rates have been reported with use of hyperbaric oxygen.
- Absolute contraindications to hyperbaric oxygen therapy include untreated pneumothorax and recent chemotherapy with doxorubicin or cisplatin.

Bibliography

Central Nervous System Infections

Bloch KC, Glaser C. Diagnostic approaches for patients with suspected encephalitis. Curr Infect Dis Rep. 2007;9(4):315-322. [PMID: 17618552]

Boström A, Oertel M, Ryang Y, et al. Treatment strategies and outcome in patients with non-tuberculous spinal epidural abscess—a review of 46 cases. Minim Invasive Neurosurg. 2008;51(1):36-42. [PMID: 18306130]

Brouwer MC, McIntyre P, de Gans J, Prasad K, van de Beek D. Corticosteroids for acute bacterial meningitis. Cochrane Database Syst Rev. 2010;9:CD004405. [PMID: 20824838]

Brouwer MC, Tunkel AR, van de Beek D. Epidemiology, diagnosis, and antimicrobial treatment of acute bacterial meningitis. Clin Microbiol Rev. 2010;23:467-492. [PMID: 20610819]

Carpenter J, Stapleton S, Holliman R. Retrospective analysis of 49 cases of brain abscess and review of the literature. Eur J Clin Microbiol Infect Dis. 2007;26(1):1-11. [PMID: 17180609]

Centers for Disease Control and Prevention (CDC). Licensure of a 13-valent pneumococcal conjugate vaccine (PCV13) and recommendations for use among children – Advisory Committee on Immunization Practices (ACIP), 2010. MMWR Morb Mortal Wkly Rep. 2010;59(9):258-261. [PMID: 20224542]

Darouiche RO. Spinal epidural abscess. N Engl J Med. 2006;355(19):2012-2020. [PMID: 17093252]

Glaser CA, Honarmand S, Anderson LJ, et al. Beyond viruses: clinical profiles and etiologies associated with encephalitis. Clin Infect Dis. 2006;43(12):1565-1577. [PMID: 17109290]

Hsu HE, Shutt KA, Moore MR, et al. Effect of pneumococcal conjugate vaccine on pneumococcal meningitis. N Engl J Med. 2009;360(3):244-256. [PMID: 19144940]

Ihekwaba UK, Kudesia G, Mckendrick MW. Clinical features of viral meningitis in adults: significant differences in cerebrospinal fluid findings among herpes simplex virus, varicella zoster virus, and enterovirus infections. Clin Infect Dis. 2008;47(6):783-789. [PMID: 18680414]

Lee TH, Chang WN, Su TM, et al. Clinical features and predictive factors of intraventricular rupture in patients who have bacterial brain abscess. J Neurol Neurosurg Psychiatry. 2007;78(3):303-309. [PMID: 17012340]

Lu CH, Chang WN, Lui CC. Strategies for the management of bacterial brain abscess. J Clin Neurosci. 2006;13(10):979-985. [PMID: 17056261]

Mailles A, Stahl JP; Steering Committee and Investigators Group. Infectious encephalitis in france in 2007: a national prospective study. Clin Infect Dis 2009;49(12):1838-1847. [PMID: 19929384]

Murray KO, Walker C, Gould E. The virology, epidemiology, and clinical impact of West Nile virus: a decade of advancements in research since its introduction into the Western Hemisphere. Epidemiol Infect. 2011;139(6):1-11. [PMID: 21342610]

Nathoo N, Nadvi SS, Gouws E, van Dellen JR. Craniotomy improves outcome for cranial subdural empyema: computed tomography–cra experience with 699 patients. Neurosurgery. 2001;49(4):872-878. [PMID: 11564248]

Osborn MK, Steinberg JP. Subdural empyema and other suppurative complications of paranasal sinusitis. Lancet Infect Dis. 2007;7(1):62-67. [PMID: 17182345]

Sendi P, Bregenzer T, Zimmerli W. Spinal epidural abscess in clinical practice. QJM. 2008;101(1):1-12. [PMID: 17982180]

Tebruegge M, Curtis N. Epidemiology, etiology, pathogenesis, and diagnosis or recurrent bacterial meningitis. Clin Microbiol Rev. 2008;21(3):519-537. [PMID: 18625686]

Thigpen MC, Whitney CG, Messonnier N, et al; Emerging Infections Program Network. Bacterial meningitis in the United States, 1998-2007. N Engl J Med. 2011;364(21):2016-2025. [PMID: 21612470]

Tunkel AR, Glaser CA, Bloch KC, et al; Infectious Diseases Society of America. The management of encephalitis: clinical practice guidelines by the Infectious Diseases Society of America. Clin Infect Dis. 2008;47(3):303-327. [PMID: 18582201]

Tunkel AR, Hartman BJ, Kaplan SL, et al. Practice guidelines for the management of bacterial meningitis. Clin Infect Dis. 2004;39(9):1267-1284. [PMID: 15494903]

van de Beek D, Drake JM, Tunkel AR. Nosocomial bacterial meningitis. N Engl J Med. 2010;362(2):146-154. [PMID: 20071704]

Werno AM, Murdoch DR. Medical microbiology: laboratory diagnosis of invasive pneumococcal disease. Clin Infect Dis. 2008;46(6):926-932. [PMID: 18260752]

Prion Diseases of the Central Nervous System

Holman RC, Belay ED, Christensen KY, et al. Human prion diseases in the United States. PLoS One. 2010;5(1):e8521. [PMID: 20049325]

Rosenbloom MH, Atri A. The evaluation of rapidly progressive dementia. Neurologist. 2011;17(2):67-74. [PMID: 21364356]

Ryou C. Prions and prion diseases: fundamentals and mechanistic details. J Microbiol Biotechnol. 2007;17(7):1059-1070. [PMID: 18051314]

Skin and Soft Tissue Infections

Anaya DA, Pellinger EP. Necrotizing soft tissue infection: diagnosis and management. Clin Infect Dis. 2007;44(5):705-710. [PMID: 17278065]

Björnsdóttir S, Gottfredsson M, Thórisdóttir AS, et al. Risk factors for acute cellulitis of the lower limb: a prospective case-control study. Clin Infect Dis. 2005;41(10):1416-1422. [PMID: 16231251]

Lipsky BA, Berendt AR, Cornia PB, et al. 2012 Infectious Diseases Society of America clinical practice guideline for the diagnosis and treatment of diabetic foot infections. Clin Infect Dis. 2012;54(12):132-173. [PMID: 22619242]

Liu C, Bayer A, Cosgrove SE, et al; Infectious Diseases Society of America. Clinical practice guidelines by the Infectious Diseases Society of America for the treatment of methicillin-resistant Staphylococcus aureus infections in adults and children. Clin Infect Dis. 2011;52(3):e18-55. Epub 2011 Jan 4. [PMID: 21208910]

Semel JD, Goldin H. Association of athlete's foot with cellulitis of the lower extremities: diagnostic value of bacterial cultures of ipsilateral interdigital space samples. Clin Infect Dis. 1996;23(5):1162–1164. [PMID: 8922818]

Stevens DL, Bisno AL, Chambers HF, et al; Infectious Diseases Society of America. Practice guidelines for the diagnosis and management of skin and soft tissue infections. Clin Infect Dis. 2005;41(10):1373-1406. [PMID: 16231249]

Stevens DL, Eron LL. Cellulitis and soft-tissue infections. Ann Intern Med. 2009;150(1):ITC11. [PMID: 19124814]

Wong CH, Khin LW, Heng KS, Tan KC, Low CO. The LRINEC (Laboratory Risk Indicator for Necrotizing Fasciitis) score: a tool for distinguishing necrotizing fasciitis from other soft tissue infections. Crit Care Med. 2004;32(7):1535-1541. [PMID: 15241098]

Community-Acquired Pneumonia

Chalmers JD, Singanayagam A, Akram AR, et al. Severity assessment tools for predicting mortality in hospitalized patients with community-acquired pneumonia. Systematic review and meta-analysis. Thorax. 2010;65(10):878-883. [PMID: 20729231]

Christ-Crane, Opal SM. Clinical review: the role of biomarkers in the diagnosis and management of community-acquired pneumonia. Crit Care. 2010;14(1):203. [PMID: 20236471]

Jackson ML, Nelson JC, Jackson LA. Risk factors for community-acquired pneumonia in immunocompetent seniors. J Am Geriatr Soc. 2009;57(5):822-828. [PMID: 19453307]

Lewis PF, Schmidt MA, Lu X, et al. A community-based outbreak of severe respiratory illness caused by human adenovirus serotype 14. J Infect Dis. 2009;199(10):1427-1434. [PMID: 19351259]

Mandell LA, Wunderink RG, Anzueto A, et al; Infectious Diseases Society of America; American Thoracic Society. Infectious Diseases Society of America/American Thoracic Society consensus guidelines on the management of community-acquired pneumonia in adults. Clin Infect Dis. 2007;(44)(suppl 2):S27-72. [PMID: 17278083]

Mortensen EM, Copeland LA, Pugh MJ, et al. Diagnosis of pulmonary malignancy after hospitalization for pneumonia. Am J Med. 2010;123(1):66-71. [PMID: 20102994]

Niederman N. In the clinic. Community-acquired pneumonia. Ann Intern Med. 2009;151(7):ITC4-2-ITC4-14; quiz ITC4-16. [PMID: 19805767]

Restrepo MI, Mortensen EM, Rello J, Brody J, Anzueto A. late admission to the ICU in patients with severe community-acquired pneumonia is associated with higher mortality. Chest. 2010;137(3):552-557. [PMID: 19880910]

Ruhnke GW, Coca-Perraillon M, Kitch BT, Cutler DM. Marked reduction in 30-day mortality among elderly patients with community-acquired pneumonia. Am J Med. 2011;124(2):171-178.e1. [PMID: 21295197]

Waterer GW, Rello J, Wunderink RG. Management of community-acquired pneumonia in adults. Am J Respir Crit Care Med. 2011;183(2):157-164. [PMID: 20693379]

Tick-Borne Diseases

Chapman AS, Bakken JS, Folk SM, et al; Tickborne Rickettsial Diseases Working Group; CDC. Diagnosis and management of tickborne rickettsial diseases: Rocky Mountain spotted fever, ehrlichiosis, and anaplasmosi—United States: a practical guide for physicians and other health-care and public health professionals. MMWR Recomm Rep. 2006;55(RR-4):1-27. [PMID: 16572105]

Halperin JJ, Shapiro ED, Logigian E, et al; Quality Standards Subcommittee of the American Academy of Neurology. Practice parameter: treatment of nervous system Lyme disease (an evidence-based review): report of the Quality Standards Subcommittee of the American Academy of Neurology. Neurology. 2007;69(1):91-102. [PMID: 17522387]

Ismail N, Bloch KC, McBride JW. Human ehrlichiosis and anaplasmosis. Clin Lab Med. 2010;30(1):261-292. [PMID: 20513551]

Murray TS, Shapiro ED. Lyme disease. Clin Lab Med. 2010;30(1):311-328. [PMID: 20513553]

O'Connell S. Lyme borreliosis: current issues in diagnosis and management. Curr Opin Infect Dis. 2010;23(3):231-235. [PMID: 20407371]

Stanek G, Wormser GP, Gray J, Strle F. Lyme borreliosis. Lancet. 2012;379(9814):461-473. [PMID: 21903253]

Wormser GP, Dattwyler RJ, Shapiro ED, et al. The clinical assessment, treatment, and prevention of lyme disease, human granulocytic anaplasmosis, and babesiosis: clinical practice guidelines by the Infectious Diseases Society of America. Clin Infect Dis. 2006;43(9):1089-1134. [PMID: 17029130]

Urinary Tract Infections

Dielubanza EJ, Schaeffer AJ. Urinary tract infections in women. Med Clin North Am. 2011;95(1):27-41. [PMID: 21095409]

Foxman B. The epidemiology of urinary tract infection. Nat Rev Urol. 2010;7(12):653-660. [PMID: 21139641]

Gupta K, Hooton TM, Naber KG, et al; Infectious Diseases Society of America; European Society for Microbiology and Infectious Diseases. International clinical practice guidelines for the treatment of acute uncomplicated cystitis and pyelonephritis in women: A 2010 update by the Infectious Diseases Society of America and the European Society for Microbiology and Infectious Diseases. Clin Infect Dis. 2011;52(5):e103-120. [PMID: 21292654]

Nicolle LE, Bradley S, Colgan R, Rice JC, Schaeffer A, Hooton TM; Infectious Diseases Society of America; American Society of Nephrology; American Geriatric Society. Infectious Diseases Society of America guidelines for the diagnosis and treatment of asymptomatic bacteriuria in adults. Clin Infect Dis. 2005;40(5):643-654. [PMID: 15714408]

Mycobacterium tuberculosis **Infection**

American Thoracic Society; CDC; Infectious Diseases Society of America. Treatment of tuberculosis. MMWR Recomm Rep. 2003;52(RR-11):1-77. [PMID: 12836625]

Blanc F-X, Sok T, Laureillard D, et al; CAMELIA (ANRS 1295–CIPRA KH001) Study Team. Earlier versus later start of antiretroviral therapy in HIV-infected adults with tuberculosis. N Engl J Med. 2011;365(16):1471-1481. [PMID: 22010913]

Caminero JA, Sotgiu G, Zumla A, Migliori GB. Best drug treatment for multidrug-resistant and extensively drug-resistant tuberculosis. Lancet Infect Dis. 2010;10(9):621-629. [PMID: 20797644]

Centers for Disease Control and Prevention (CDC). Recommendations for use of an isoniazid-rifapentine regimen with direct observation to treat latent Mycobacterium tuberculosis infection. MMWR Morb Mortal Wkly Rep. 2011;60(48):1650-1653. [PMID: 22157884]

Centers for Disease Control and Prevention (CDC). Reported tuberculosis in the United States, 2010. Atlanta, GA: U.S. Department of Health and Human Services, CDC, October 2011.

Centers for Disease Control and Prevention (CDC). Updated guidelines for the use of nucleic acid amplification tests in the diagnosis of tuberculosis. MMWR Morb Mortal Wkly Rep. 2009;58(01):7-10. [PMID: 19145221]

Diagnostic Standards and Classification of Tuberculosis in Adults and Children. This official statement of the American Thoracic Society and the Centers for Disease Control and Prevention was adopted by the ATS Board of Directors, July 1999. This statement was endorsed by the Council of the Infectious Disease Society of America, September 1999. Am J Respir Crit Care Med. 2000;161(4 pt 1):1376-1395. [PMID: 10764337]

Mazurek GH, Jereb J, Vernon A, LoBue P, Goldberg S, Castro K; IGRA Expert Committee; Centers for Disease Control and Prevention (CDC). Updated guidelines for using Interferon Gamma Release Assays to detect Mycobacterium tuberculosis infection - United States, 2010. MMWR Recomm Rep. 2010;59(RR-5):1-25. [PMID: 20577159]

Bibliography

Nontuberculous Mycobacterial Infections

Griffith DE, Aksamit T, Brown-Elliot BA, et al; ATS Mycobacterial Diseases Subcommittee; American Thoracic Society; Infectious Disease Society of America. An official ATS/IDSA statement: diagnosis, treatment, and prevention of nontuberculous mycobacterial diseases. Am J Respir Crit Care Med. 2007;175(4):367-416. [PMID: 17277290]

Jarzembowski JA, Young MB. Nontuberculous mycobacterial infections. Arch Pathol Lab Med. 2008:132(8):1333-1341. [PMID: 18684037]

Piersimoni C, Scarparo C. Pulmonary infections associated with nontuberculous mycobacteria in immunocompetent patients. Lancet Infect Dis. 2008;8(5):323-334. [PMID: 18471777]

Tortoli E. Clinical manifestations of nontuberculous mycobacteria infections. Clin Microbiol Infect. 2009;15(10):906-910. [PMID: 19845702]

Fungal Infections

Billie J. New non-culture-based methods for the diagnosis of invasive candidiasis. Curr Opin Crit Care. 2010;16(5):460-464. [PMID: 20736833]

Chen SC, Playford EG, Sorrell TC. Antifungal therapy in invasive fungal infections. Curr Opin Pharmacol. 2010;10(5):522-530. Epub 2010 Jul 2. [PMID: 20598943]

Kauffman CA. Histoplasmosis. Clin Chest Med. 2009;30(2):217-225. [PMID: 19375629]

Pappas PG, Kauffman CA, Andes D, et al; Infectious Diseases Society of America. Clinical practice guidelines for the management of candidiasis: 2009 update by the Infectious Diseases Society of America. Clin Infect Dis. 2009;48(5):503-535. [PMID: 19191635]

Perfect JR, Dismukes WE, Dromer F, et al. Clinical practice guidelines for the management of cryptococcal disease: 2010 update by the Infectious Diseases Society of America. Clin Infect Dis. 2010;50(3):291-322. [PMID: 20047480]

Smith JA, Kauffman CA. Blastomycosis. Proc Am Thorac Soc. 2010;7(3):173-180. [PMID: 20463245]

Spellberg B, Ibrahim AS. Recent advances in the treatment of mucormycosis. Curr Infect Dis Rep. 2010;12(6):423-429. [PMID: 21308550]

Thursky KA, Playford EG, Seymour JF, et al. Recommendations for the treatment of established fungal infections. Intern Med J. 2008;38(6b):496-520. [PMID: 18588522]

Vyas KS, Bariola JR, Bradsher RW Jr. Treatment of endemic mycoses. Expert Rev Respir Med. 2010;4(1):85-95. [PMID: 20387295]

Walsh TJ, Anaissie EJ, Denning DW, et al; Infectious Diseases Society of America. Clin Infect Dis. 2008;46(3):327-360. [PMID: 18177225]

Sexually Transmitted Infections

Martin-Iguacel R, Llibre JM, Nielsen H, et al. Lymphogranuloma venereum proctocolitis: a silent endemic disease in men who have sex with men in industrialized countries. Eur J Clin Microbiol Infect Dis. 2010;29(8):917-925. [PMID: 20509036]

U.S. Preventive Services Task Force. Screening for chlamydial infection: U.S. Preventive Services Task Force recommendation statement. Ann Intern Med. 2007;147(2):128-134. [PMID: 17576996]

Wilson JF. In the clinic. Vaginitis and cervicitis. Ann Intern Med. 2009;151(5):ITC3-1-ITC3-15 [PMID: 19721016]

Workowski KA, Berman S; Centers for Disease Control and Prevention (CDC). Sexually transmitted diseases treatment guidelines, 2010. MMWR Recomm Rep. 2010;59(RR 1-12):1-110. [Erratum in MMWR Recomm Rep. 2011;60(1):18]. [PMID: 21160459]

Osteomyelitis

Conterno LO, da Silva Filho CR. Antibiotics for treating chronic osteomyelitis in adults. Cochrane Database Syst Rev. 2009;(3):CDO4439. [PMID: 19588358]

Lew DP, Waldvogel FA. Osteomyelitis. N Engl J Med. 1997;336(14):999-1007. [PMID: 9077380]

Pineda C, Vargas A, Rodriguez AV. Imaging of osteomyelitis: current concepts. Infec Dis Clin North Am. 2006;20(4):789-825. [PMID: 17118291]

Powlson AS, Coll AP. The treatment of diabetic foot infections. J Antimicrob Chemother. 2010;65(suppl 3):iii3-9. [PMID: 20876626]

Rao N, Lipsky BA. Optimizing antimicrobial therapy in diabetic foot infections. Drugs. 2007;67(2):195-214. [PMID: 17284084]

Zimmerli W. Clinical practice. Vertebral osteomyelitis. N Engl J Med. 2010;362(11):1022-1029. [PMID: 20237348]

Fever of Unknown Origin

Bleeker-Rovers CP, Vos FJ, de Kleijn EM, et al. A prospective multicenter study on fever of unknown origin: the yield of a structured diagnostic protocol. Medicine (Baltimore). 2007;86(1):26-38. [PMID: 17220753]

Hot A, Jaisson I, Girard C, et al. Yield of bone marrow examination in diagnosing the source of fever of unknown origin. Arch Intern Med. 2009;169(21):2018-2023. [PMID: 19933965]

Mourad O, Palda V, Detsky AS. A comprehensive evidence-based approach to fever of unknown origin. Arch Intern Med. 2003;163(5):545-551. [PMID: 12622601]

Vanderschueren S, Knockaert D, Adriaenssens T, et al. From prolonged febrile illness to fever of unknown origin: the challenge continues. Arch Intern Med. 2003;163(9):1033-1041. [PMID: 12742800]

Primary Immunodeficiencies

Maarschalk-Ellerbroek LJ, Hoepelman IM, Ellerbroek PM. Immunoglobulin treatment in primary antibody deficiency. Int J Antimicrob Agents. 2011;37(5):396-404. [PMID: 21276714]

Morimoto Y, Routes JM. Immunodeficiency overview. Prim Care. 2008;35(1):159-173. [PMID: 18206723]

Nelson KS, Lewis DB. Adult-onset presentations of genetic immunodeficiencies: genes can throw slow curves. Curr Opin Infect Dis. 2010;23(4):359-364. [PMID: 20581672]

Notarangelo LD. Primary immunodeficiencies. J Allergy Clin Immunol. 2010;125(2)(suppl 2):S182-194. Epub 2009 Dec 29. [PMID: 20042228]

Oliveira JB, Fleisher TA. Laboratory evaluation of primary immunodeficiencies. J Allergy Clin Immunol. 2010;125(2)(suppl 2):S297-S305. Epub 2009 Dec 29. [PMID: 20042230]

Park MA, Li JT, Hagan JB, Maddox DE, Abraham RS. Common variable immunodeficiency: a new look at an old disease. Lancet. 2008;372(9637):489-502. [PMID: 18692715]

Ram S. Lewis LA, Rice PA. Infections of people with complement deficiencies and patients who have undergone splenectomy. Clin Microbiol Rev. 2010;23(4):740-780. [PMID: 20930072]

Wood P, UK Primary Immunodeficiency Network. Clin Med. 2009;9(6):595-599. [PMID: 20095309]

Yel L. Selective IgA deficiency. J Clin Immunol. 2010;30(1):10-16. Epub 2010 Jan 26. [PMID: 20101521]

Bioterrorism

Arnon S, Schecter R, Inglesby TV, et al; Working Group on Civilian Biodefense. Botulinum toxin as a biological weapon: medical and public health management. JAMA. 2001;285(8):1059-1070. [PMID: 11209178]

Bartlett JG, Inglesby TV, Boria L. Management of anthrax. Clin Infect Dis. 2002;35(7):851-858. [PMID: 12228822]

Borchardt SM, Ritger KA, Dworkin MS. Categorization, prioritization, and surveillance of potential bioterrorism agents. Infect Dis Clin North Am. 2006;20(2):213-225, vii-viii. [PMID: 16762736]

Boria L, Inglesby TV, Peters CJ, et al; Working Group on Civilian Biodefense. Hemorrhagic Fever Viruses as Biological Weapons: medical and public health management. JAMA. 2002;287(18):2391-2405. [PMID: 11988060]

Breman JG, Henderson DA. Diagnosis and management of smallpox. N Engl J Med. 2002;346(17):1300-1308. [PMID: 11923491]

Bush LM, Abrams BH, Beall A, Johnson CC. Index case of fatal inhalational anthrax due to bioterrorism in the United States. N Engl J Med. 2001;345(22):1607-1610. [PMID: 11704685]

Dennis DT, Inglesby TV, Henderson DA, et al; Working Group on Civilian Biodefense. Tularemia as a biological weapon: medical and public health management. JAMA. 2001;285(21):2763-2773. [PMID: 11386933]

Inglesby TV, Dennis DT, Henderson DA, et al; Working Group on Civilian Biodefense. Plague as a biological weapon: medical and public health management. JAMA. 2000;283(17):2281-2290. [PMID: 10807389]

Inglesby TV, O'Toole T, Henderson DA, et al; Working Group on Civilian Biodefense. Anthrax as a biological weapon, 2002: updated recommendations for management. JAMA. 2002;287(17):2236-2252. [PMID: 11980524]

Travel Medicine

Ariza J, Bosilkovski M, Cascio A, et al; International Society of Chemotherapy; Institute of Continuing Medical Education of Ioannina. Perspectives for the treatment of brucellosis in the 21st century: the Ioannina recommendations. PLoS Med. 2007;4(12):e317. [PMID: 18162038]

Cao C, Liang L, Wang W, et al. Common reservoirs for Penicillium marneffei infection in humans and rodents, China. Emerg Infect Dis. 2011;17(2):209-214. [PMID: 21291590]

Centers for Disease Control and Prevention (CDC). Acinetobacter baumannii infections among patients at military medical facilities treating injured U.S. service members, 2002-2004. MMWR Morb Mortal Wkly Rep. 2004;53(45);1063-1066. [PMID: 15549020]

Cetron MS, Marfin AA, Julian KG, et al. Yellow Fever vaccine. Recommendations of the Advisory Committee on Immunization Practices (ACIP), 2002. MMWR Recomm Rep. 2002;51(RR-17):1-11; quiz CE1-4. [PMID: 12437192]

Galgiani JN, Ampel NM, Blair JE, et al; Infectious Diseases Society of America. Coccidioidomycosis. Clin Infect Dis. 2005;41(9):1217-1223. [PMID: 16206093]

Hill DR, Baird JK, Parise ME, Lewis LS, Ryan ET, Magill AJ. Primaquine: report from CDC expert meeting on malaria chemoprophylaxis I. Am J Trop Med Hyg. 2006;75(3):402-415. [PMID: 16968913]

Hill DR, Ericsson CD, Pearson RD et al; Infectious Diseases Society of America. The Practice of Travel Medicine: Guidelines by the Infectious Diseases Society of America. Clin Infect Dis. 2006;43(12):1499-1539. [PMID: 17109284]

Parola P, Paddock CD, Raoult D. Tick-borne rickettsioses around the world: emerging diseases challenging old concepts. Clin Microbiol Rev. 2005;18(4):719-756. [PMID: 16223955]

Steinberg EB, Bishop R, Haber P, et al. Typhoid fever in travelers: who should be targeted for prevention? Clin Infect Dis. 2004;39(2):186-191. [PMID: 15307027]

Teixeira MG, Barreto ML. Diagnosis and management of dengue. BJM. 2009;339:b4338. [PMID: 19923152]

Infectious Gastrointestinal Syndromes

Buchholz U, Bernard H, Werber D, et al. German outbreak of Escherichia coli O104:H4 associated with sprouts. N Engl J Med. 2011;365(19)1763-1770. [PMID: 22029753]

Cabada MM, White AC Jr. Treatment of cryptosporidiosis: do we know what we think we know? Curr Opin Infect Dis. 2010;23(5):494-499. [PMID: 20689422]

Cohen SH, Gerding DN, Johnson S, et al; Society for Healthcare Epidemiology of America; Infectious Diseases Society of America. Clinical practice guidelines for Clostridium difficile infection in adults: 2010 update by the society for healthcare epidemiology of America

(SHEA) and the infectious diseases society of America (IDSA). Infect Control Hosp Epidemiol. 2010;31(5):431-455. [PMID: 20307191]

Division of Viral Diseases, National Center for Immunization and Respiratory Diseases, Centers for Disease Control and Prevention. Updated norovirus outbreak management and disease prevention guidelines. MMWR Recomm Rep. 2011;60(RR-3):1-18. [PMID: 21368741]

Guerrent RL, Van Gilder T, Steiner TS, et al; Infectious Diseases Society of America. Practice guidelines for the management of infectious diarrhea. Clin Infect Dis. 2001;32(3):331-351. [PMID: 11170940]

Kelly CP, LaMont JT. Clostridium difficile—more difficult than ever. N Engl J Med. 2008;359(18):1932-1940. [PMID: 18971494]

Kent AJ, Banks MR. Pharmacological management of diarrhea. Gastroenterol Clin North Am. 2010;39(3):495-507. [PMID: 20951914]

Loo VG, Poirier L, Miller MA, et al. A predominantly clonal multi-institutional outbreak of Clostridium difficile-associated diarrhea with high morbidity and mortality. N Engl J Med. 2005;353(23):2442-2449. [PMID: 16322602]

Louis TJ, Miller MA, Mullane KM, et al; OPT-80-003 Clinical Study Group. Fidaxomicin versus vancomycin for Clostridium difficile infection. N Engl J Med. 2011;364(5):422-431. [PMID: 21288078]

Orth D, Grif K, Zimmerhackl LB, Würzner R. Prevention and treatment of enterohemorrhagic Escherichia coli infections in humans. Expert Rev Anti Infect Ther. 2008;6(1):101-108. [PMID: 18251667]

Tan KS, Mirza H, Teo JD, Wu B, Macary PA. Current views on the clinical relevance of Blastocystis spp. Curr Infect Dis Rep. 2010;12(1):28-35. [PMID: 21308496]

Valdez Y, Ferreira RB, Finlay BB. Molecular mechanisms of Salmonella virulence and host resistance. Curr Top Microbiol Immunol. 2009;337:93-127. [PMID: 19812981]

Infections in Transplant Recipients

Avery RK. Infectious disease following kidney transplant: core curriculum 2010. Am J Kidney Dis. 2010;55(4):755-771. [PMID: 20338466]

Eid AJ, Razonable RR. New developments in the management of cytomegalovirus infection after solid organ transplantation. Drugs. 2010;70(8):965-981. [PMID: 20481654]

Nishi SPE, Valentine VG, Duncan S. Emerging bacterial, fungal, and viral respiratory infections in transplantation. Infect Dis Clin North Am. 2010;24(3):541-555. [PMID: 20674791]

Nucci M, Anaissie E. Fungal infections in hematopoietic stem cell transplantation and solid-organ transplantation—focus on aspergillosis. Clin Chest Med. 2009;30(2):295-306, vii. [PMID: 19375636]

AST Infectious Diseases Community of Practice. The American Society of Transplantation Infectious Diseases Guidelines, Second Edition. Am J Transplant. 2009;9(suppl 4):S1-S281.

Tomblyn M, Chiller T, Einsele H, et al; Center for International Blood and Marrow Research; National Marrow Donor program; European Blood and MarrowTransplant Group; American Society of Blood and Marrow Transplantation; Canadian Blood and Marrow Transplant Group; Infectious Diseases Society of America; Society for Healthcare Epidemiology of America; Association of Medical Microbiology and Infectious Disease Canada; Centers for Disease Control and Prevention. Guidelines for preventing infectious complications among hematopoietic cell transplantation recipients: a global perspective. Biol Blood Marrow Transplant. 2009;15(10):1143-1238. [PMID: 19747629]

Hospital-Acquired Infections

American Thoracic Society, Infectious Diseases Society of America. Guidelines for the management of adults with hospital-acquired, ventilator-associated, and healthcare-associated pneumonia. Am J Respir Crit Care Med. 2005;171(4):388-416. [PMID: 15699079]

Anderson DJ. Surgical site infections. Infect Dis Clin North Am. 2011;25(1):135-153. [PMID: 21315998]

Boucher HW, Talbot GH, Bradley JS, et al. Bad bugs, no drugs: no ESKAPE! An update from the Infectious Diseases Society of America. Clin Infect Dis. 2009;48(1):1-12. [PMID: 19035777]

Burke JP. Infection control - a problem for patient safety. N Engl J Med. 2003;348(7):651-656. [PMID: 12584377]

Chenoweth CE, Saint S. Urinary tract infections. Infect Dis Clin North Am. 2011;25(1):103-115. [PMID: 21315996]

Hidron AI, Edwards JR, Patel J, et al; National Healthcare Safety Network Team; Participating National Healthcare Safety Network Facilities. NHSN annual update: antimicrobial-resistant pathogens associated with healthcare-associated infections: annual summary of data reported to the National Healthcare Safety Network at the Centers for Disease Control and Prevention, 2006-2007. Infect Control Hosp Epidemiol. 2008;29(11):996-1011. [PMID: 18947320]

Hooton TM, Bradley SF, Cardenas DD, et al; Infectious Diseases Society of America. Diagnosis, prevention, and treatment of catheter-associated urinary tract infection in adults: 2009 International Clinical Practice Guidelines from the Infectious Diseases Society of America. Clin Infect Dis. 2010;50(5):625-663. [PMID: 20175247]

Horan TC, Andrus M, Dudeck MA. CDC/NHSN surveillance definition of health care-associated infection and criteria for specific types of infections in the acute care setting. Am J Infect Control. 2008;36(5):309-332. [PMID: 18538699]

Lin MY, Hota B, Khan YM, et al; CDC Prevention Epicenter Program. Quality of traditional surveillance for public reporting of nosocomial bloodstream infection rates. JAMA. 2010;304(18):2035-2041. [PMID: 21063013]

Mermel LA, Allon M, Bouza E, et al. Clinical practice guidelines for the diagnosis and management of intravascular catheter-related infection: 2009 Update by the Infectious Diseases Society of America. Clin Infect Dis. 2009;49(1):1-45. [PMID: 19489710]

O'Grady NP, Alexander M, Burns LA, et al; Healthcare Infection Control Practices Advisory Committee (HICPAC) (Appendix 1). Summary of recommendations: Guidelines for the Prevention of Intravascular Catheter-related Infections. Clin Infect Dis. 2011;52(9):1087-1099. [PMID: 21467014]

Weber DJ, Rutala WA. Central line-associated bloodstream infections: prevention and management. Infect Dis Clin North Am. 2011;25(1):77-102. [PMID: 21315995]

Yokoe DS, Mermel LA, Anderson DJ, et al. A compendium of strategies to prevent healthcare-associated infections in acute care hospitals. Infect Control Hosp Epidemiol. 2008;29(suppl 1):S12-S21. [PMID: 18840084]

Infective Endocarditis Prevention

Gould FK, Elliott TS, Foweraker J, et al; Working Party of the British Society for Antimicrobial Chemotherapy. Guidelines for the prevention of endocarditis: report of the Working Party of the British Society for Antimicrobial Chemotherapy. J Antimicrob Chemother. 2006;57(6):1035-1042. [PMID: 16624872]

Wilson W, Taubert KA, Gewitz M, et al; American Heart Association. Prevention of infective endocarditis: guidelines from the American Heart Association: a guideline from the American Heart Association Rheumatic Fever, Endocarditis, and Kawasaki Disease Committee, Council on Cardiovascular Disease in the Young, and the Council on Clinical Cardiology, Council on Cardiovascular Surgery and Anesthesia, and the Quality of Care and Outcomes Research Interdisciplinary Working Group. Circulation. 2007;116(15):1736-1754. [PMID: 17446442]

HIV/AIDS

Aberg JA, Kaplan JE, Libman H, et al; HIV Medicine Association of the Infectious Diseases Society of America. Primary care guidelines for the management of persons infected with human immunodeficiency virus: 2009 update by the HIV Medicine Association of the Infectious Diseases Society of America. Clin Infect Dis. 2009;49(5):651-681. [PMID: 19640227]

Branson BM, Handsfield HH, Lampe MA, et al; Centers for Disease Control and Prevention (CDC). Revised recommendations for HIV testing of adults, adolescents, and pregnant women in health-care settings. MMWR Recomm Rep. 2006;55(RR-14):1-17. [PMID: 16988643]

Cohen MS, Gay CL, Busch MP, Hecht FM. The detection of acute HIV infection. J Infect Dis. 2010;202(suppl 2):S270-S277. [PMID: 20846033]

Farrugia PM, Lucariello R, Coppola, JT. Human immunodeficiency virus and atherosclerosis. Cardiol Rev. 2009;17(5):211-215. [PMID: 19690471]

Feinberg, J. Management of newly diagnosed HIV infection. Ann Intern Med. 2011;155(7):ITC41. [PMID: 21969353]

Kaplan JE, Benson C, Holmes KH, Brooks JT, Pau A, Masur H; Centers for Disease Control and Prevention (CDC); National Institutes of Health; HIV Medicine Association of the Infectious Diseases Society of America. Guidelines for prevention and treatment of opportunistic infections in HIV-infected adults and adolescents: recommendations from the CDC, National Institutes of Health, and the HIV Medicine Association of the Infectious Diseases Society of America. MMWR Recomm Rep. 2009;58(RR-4):1-207. [PMID: 19357635]

Landovitz RJ, Currier JS. Postexposure prophylaxis for HIV infection. N Engl J Med. 2009;361(18):1768-1775. [PMID: 19864675]

Panel on Antiretroviral Guidelines for Adults and Adolescents. Guidelines for the use of antiretroviral agents in HIV-1-infected adults and adolescents. Department of Health and Human Services. January 10, 2011;1-166. Available at www.aidsinfo.nih.gov/ContentFiles/AdultandAdolescentGL.pdf. Accessed July 9, 2012.

Panel on Treatment of HIV-Infected Pregnant Women and Prevention of Perinatal Transmission. Recommendations for use of antiretroviral drugs in pregnant HIV-1-infected women for maternal health and interventions to reduce perinatal HIV transmission in the United States. May 24, 2010;1-117. Available at www.aidsinfo.nih.gov/ContentFiles/PerinatalGL.pdf. Accessed July 9, 2012.

Qaseem A, Snow V, Shekelle P et al. and the Clinical Efficacy Assessment Subcommittee, American College of Physicians. Screening for HIV in health care settings: a guidance statement from the American College of Physicians and HIV Medicine Association. Ann Intern Med. 2009 Jan 20;150(2):125-31. Epub 2008 Nov 30. PubMed [PMID: 19047022]

Taylor S, Jayasuriya A, Smit E. Using HIV resistance tests in clinical practice. J Antimicrob Chemother. 2009;64(2):218-222. [PMID: 19535382]

Thompson MA, Aberg JA, Cahn P, et al; International AIDS Society-USA. Antiretroviral treatment of adult HIV infection: 2010 recommendations of the International AIDS Society-USA Panel. JAMA. 2010;304(3):321-333. [PMID: 20639566]

Viral Infections

Bond D, Mooney J. A literature review regarding the management of varicella-zoster virus. Musculoskeletal Care. 2010;8(2):118-122. [PMID: 20301227]

Cernik C, Gallina K, Brodell RT. The treatment of herpes simplex infections: an evidence-based review. Arch Intern Med. 2008;168(11):1137-1144. [PMID: 18541820]

Fiore AE, Bridges CB, Cox NJ. Seasonal influenza vaccines. Curr Top Microbiol Immunol. 2009;333:43-82. [PMID: 19768400]

Fiore AE, Fry A, Shay D, Gubareva L, Bresee JS, Uyeki TM; Centers for Disease Control and Prevention (CDC). Antiviral agents for the treatment and chemoprophylaxis of influenz — recommendations of the Advisory Committee on Immunization Practices (ACIP). MMWR Recomm Rep. 2011;60(1):1-24. [PMID: 21248682]

Jefferson T, Jones M, Doshi P, Del Mar C, Dooley L, Foxlee R. Neuraminidase inhibitors for preventing and treating influenza in healthy adults. Cochrane Database Syst Rev. 2010;(2):CD001265. [PMID: 20166059]

Mubareka S, Leung V, Aoki FY, Vinh DC. Famciclovir: a focus on efficacy and safety. Expert Opin Drug Saf. 2010;9(4):643-658. [PMID: 20429777]

Oxman MN. Zoster vaccine: current status and future prospects. Clin Infect Dis. 2010;51(2):197-213. [PMID: 20550454]

Strasfeld L, Chou S. Antiviral drug resistance: mechanisms and clinical implications. Infect Dis Clin North Am. 2010;24(3):809-833. [PMID: 20674805]

Vigil KJ, Chemaly RF. Valacyclovir: approved and off-label uses for the treatment of herpes virus infections in immunocompetent and immunocompromised adults. Expert Opin Pharmacother. 2010;11(11):1901-1913. [PMID: 20536295]

Whitley RJ, Volpi A, McKendrick M, Wijck A, Oaklander AL. Management of herpes zoster and post-herpetic neuralgia now and in the future. J Clin Virol. 2010;48(suppl 1):S20-S28. [PMID: 20510264]

New Topics in Anti-infective Therapy

Chen LF, Kaye D. Current use for old antibacterial agents: polymyxins, rifamycins, and aminoglycosides. Infect Dis Clin North Am. 2009;23(4):1053-1075, x. [PMID: 19909897]

Dellit TH, Owens RC, McGowan JE Jr, et al; Infectious Diseases Society of America; Society for Healthcare Epidemiology of America. Infectious Diseases Society of America and the Society for Healthcare Epidemiology of America guidelines for developing an institutional program to enhance antimicrobial stewardship. Clin Infect Dis. 2007;44(2):159-177. [PMID: 17173212]

Eskes A, Ubbink DT, Lubbers M, Lucas C, Vermeulen H. Hyperbaric oxygen therapy for treating acute surgical and traumatic wounds. Cochrane Database Syst Rev. 2010;(10):CD008059. [PMID: 20927771]

Lipsky BA, Berendt AR, Deery HG, et al; Infectious Diseases Society of America. Diagnosis and treatment of diabetic foot infections. Plast Reconstr Surg. 2006;117(7 suppl):212S-238S. [PMID: 16799390]

Pogue JM, Marchaim D, Kaye D, Kaye KS. Re-visiting "older" antibiotics in the era of multi-drug resistance. Pharmacotherapy. 2011;31(9):912-921. [PMID: 21923592]

Tice AD, Rehm SJ, Dalovisio JR, et al; IDSA. Practice guidelines for outpatient parenteral antimicrobial therapy. IDSA guidelines. Clin Infect Dis. 2004;38(12):1651-1672. [PMID: 15227610]

Infectious Disease Self-Assessment Test

This self-assessment test contains one-best-answer multiple-choice questions. Please read these directions carefully before answering the questions. Answers, critiques, and bibliographies immediately follow these multiple-choice questions. The American College of Physicians is accredited by the Accreditation Council for Continuing Medical Education (ACCME) to provide continuing medical education for physicians.

The American College of Physicians designates MKSAP 16 Infectious Disease for a maximum of 16 *AMA PRA Category 1 Credits*™. Physicians should claim only the credit commensurate with the extent of their participation in the activity.

Earn "Same-Day" CME Credits Online

For the first time, print subscribers can enter their answers online to earn CME credits in 24 hours or less. You can submit your answers using online answer sheets that are provided at mksap.acponline.org, where a record of your MKSAP 16 credits will be available. To earn CME credits, you need to answer all of the questions in a test and earn a score of at least 50% correct (number of correct answers divided by the total number of questions). Take any of the following approaches:

➢ Use the printed answer sheet at the back of this book to record your answers. Go to mksap.acponline.org, access the appropriate online answer sheet, transcribe your answers, and submit your test for same-day CME credits. There is no additional fee for this service.

➢ Go to mksap.acponline.org, access the appropriate online answer sheet, directly enter your answers, and submit your test for same-day CME credits. There is no additional fee for this service.

➢ Pay a $10 processing fee per answer sheet and submit the printed answer sheet at the back of this book by mail or fax, as instructed on the answer sheet. Make sure you calculate your score and fax the answer sheet to 215-351-2799 or mail the answer sheet to Member and Customer Service, American College of Physicians, 190 N. Independence Mall West, Philadelphia, PA 19106-1572, using the courtesy envelope provided in your MKSAP 16 slipcase. You will need your 10-digit order number and 8-digit ACP ID number, which are printed on your packing slip. Please allow 4 to 6 weeks for your score report to be emailed back to you. Be sure to include your email address for a response.

If you do not have a 10-digit order number and 8-digit ACP ID number or if you need help creating a username and password to access the MKSAP 16 online answer sheets, go to mksap.acponline.org or email custserv@acponline.org.

CME credit is available from the publication date of December 31, 2012, until December 31, 2015. You may submit your answer sheets at any time during this period.

Directions

*Each of the numbered items is followed by lettered answers. Select the **ONE** lettered answer that is **BEST** in each case.*

Item 1

An 18-year-old woman is evaluated 4 weeks following hospitalization for her second episode of pneumococcal pneumonia in 18 months. She received the pneumococcal vaccine 20 months ago. The patient was also diagnosed with giardiasis 2 years ago. She also has a history of asthma. Her mother has selective IgA deficiency, and her brother has lymphoma. Her review of systems is negative for findings associated with autoimmune disorders, including systemic lupus erythematosus.

On physical examination, vital signs are normal. Faint crackles are heard at the posterior left lung base.

Laboratory studies show a hemoglobin level of 8.6 g/dL (86 g/L), a mean corpuscular volume of 120 fL, and a leukocyte count of 6800/μL (6.8 × 10⁹/L) with a normal differential. HIV serology results are negative.

Which of the following is most likely to establish the diagnosis?

(A) Check response to pneumococcal and tetanus vaccines
(B) Measure CD4 cell count
(C) Measure serum IgG, IgM, and IgA levels
(D) Measure total hemolytic complement level

Item 2

A 33-year-old man is evaluated after learning that a person living in his home was recently found to have active tuberculosis. The patient has no acute symptoms. He was recently diagnosed with HIV infection, and his CD4 cell count is 250/μL. He is a U.S. citizen and has no history of incarceration, homelessness, or travel to areas with an increased prevalence of tuberculosis. He takes no medications but had been planning to begin antiretroviral therapy at his next office visit.

On physical examination, vital signs are normal. The remainder of the examination, including cardiopulmonary findings, is normal.

A tuberculin skin test induces 0 mm of induration. A chest radiograph is normal.

Which of the following is the most appropriate next step in the management of this patient?

(A) Begin isoniazid and pyridoxine
(B) Begin isoniazid, rifampin, pyrazinamide, pyridoxine, and ethambutol
(C) Begin rifampin and pyrazinamide
(D) No additional evaluation or therapy is needed

Item 3

A 64-year-old woman is hospitalized for a 2-day history of fever and chills and a 1-day history of hypotension and dyspnea. Medical history is significant for adenocarcinoma of the colon diagnosed 3 weeks ago for which she had a partial colectomy. Her course was complicated by the development of a polymicrobial intra-abdominal abscess. After drainage of the abscess, she received hyperalimentation through a central line catheter and ceftriaxone and metronidazole for 7 days.

On physical examination, temperature is 39.0 °C (102.2 °F), blood pressure is 90/60 mm Hg, pulse rate is 120/min, and respiration rate is 20/min. There are erythema and purulent drainage at the site of a right subclavian central venous catheter. The rest of the examination is normal.

Laboratory studies indicate a leukocyte count of 16,000/μL (16 × 10⁹/L). Serum creatinine level is 3.6 mg/dL (318.2 μmol/L) compared with a value of 1.2 mg/dL (106.1 μmol/L) at admission. Two sets of blood cultures obtained 2 days ago are growing yeast.

In addition to central venous catheter removal, which of the following is the most appropriate treatment option for this patient?

(A) Caspofungin
(B) Conventional amphotericin B
(C) Fluconazole
(D) Liposomal amphotericin B
(E) Voriconazole

Item 4

A 42-year-old man is evaluated for recurrent diarrhea. Four weeks ago, the patient was diagnosed with a mild *Clostridium difficile* infection and treated with a 14-day course of metronidazole, 500 mg orally every 8 hours, with resolution of his symptoms. He currently takes no medications.

One week after his last dose of metronidazole, he again develops recurrent watery stools without fever or other symptoms. There is no visible blood or mucus in the stools.

Physical examination findings are noncontributory.

Results of laboratory studies show a leukocyte count of 10,400/μL (10.4 × 10⁹/L) and a normal serum creatinine level. A stool sample tests positive for occult blood, and results of a repeat stool assay are again positive for *C. difficile* toxin.

Which of the following is the most appropriate treatment at this time?

(A) Oral metronidazole for 14 days
(B) Oral metronidazole taper over 42 days
(C) Oral vancomycin for 14 days
(D) Oral vancomycin plus parenteral metronidazole for 14 days
(E) Oral vancomycin taper over 42 days

Item 5

A 28-year-old woman is evaluated for a 2-day history of painful genital lesions accompanied by dysuria, generalized myalgia, malaise, and fever. She is sexually active.

On physical examination, temperature is 37.8 °C (100.0 °F), and the remaining vital signs are normal. Examination of the genital area discloses painful vesicular lesions on an erythematous base.

Which of the following is the most appropriate treatment?

(A) Acyclovir
(B) Benzathine penicillin G
(C) Ceftriaxone and azithromycin
(D) Fluconazole

Item 6

A 35-year-old man is evaluated in the emergency department for a 6-day history of fever, headache, malaise, myalgia, dry cough, shortness of breath, and vague chest pain. He recently returned from filming a documentary on hibernating Indiana bats in the caves of Ohio. Medical history is noncontributory.

On physical examination, temperature is 38.3 °C (100.9 °F). Pulmonary examination discloses a few bilateral wheezes. The remainder of the examination, including vital signs, is normal.

The hemoglobin level is 10.5 g/dL (105 g/L), and the leukocyte count is 8000/µL (8.0 × 10⁹/L) with 53% neutrophils, 35% lymphocytes, and 12% monocytes. HIV serologic testing is negative.

The chest radiograph shows hilar lymphadenopathy and interstitial infiltrates.

The preliminary blood and sputum cultures are negative for organisms.

Which of the following is the most likely diagnosis?

(A) Blastomycosis
(B) Coccidioidomycosis
(C) Cryptococcosis
(D) Histoplasmosis

Item 7

An 82-year-old woman is evaluated for a 3-week history of pain in the right knee. She underwent right knee arthroplasty 3 years ago. Ten months following her arthroplasty, she developed a methicillin-resistant *Staphylococcus aureus* (MRSA) infection that required removal of the prosthetic joint and a new total knee arthroplasty as well as 6 weeks of vancomycin and rifampin antimicrobial therapy.

On physical examination, vital signs are normal. Examination of the knee joint and surrounding tissues is unremarkable.

Leukocyte-tagged nuclear imaging studies demonstrate focal uptake at the proximal tibia, and radiographic findings are consistent with sequestrum formation at the same anatomic location.

Culture of the joint fluid reveals MRSA sensitive to vancomycin, daptomycin, linezolid, trimethoprim-sulfamethoxazole, tetracycline, and rifampin.

The patient refuses to undergo any further surgical procedures.

Which of the following is the most appropriate management of this patient?

(A) Lifelong oral rifampin
(B) Lifelong oral trimethoprim-sulfamethoxazole
(C) Six weeks of parenteral vancomycin and oral rifampin
(D) Symptomatic treatment

Item 8

A 47-year-old woman is evaluated in the emergency department for abdominal pain and diarrhea. The diarrhea began 3 days ago as semi-formed stools, but in the last 24 hours, the patient has noted streaks of bright red blood in the stools. She has abdominal cramps that are unrelated to bowel movements but no fever. Five days before her symptoms developed, the patient attended a cookout where she ate potato salad, coleslaw, and a hamburger. Two other guests have also developed a diarrheal illness.

On physical examination, temperature and blood pressure are normal; the pulse rate is 115/min. Abdominal examination discloses hyperactive bowel sounds with diffuse tenderness to palpation. Remaining physical examination findings are noncontributory.

Results of laboratory studies show a leukocyte count of 17,400/µL (17.4 × 10⁹/L) and a serum creatinine level of 1.0 mg/dL (88.4 µmol/L). A stool sample shows gross blood.

Which of the following pathogens is most likely causing this patient's current illness?

(A) *Bacillus cereus*
(B) *Campylobacter jejuni*
(C) Shiga toxin–producing *Escherichia coli*
(D) *Staphylococcus aureus*
(E) *Yersinia enterocolitica*

Item 9

A 33-year-old woman is evaluated for a 2-day history of diarrhea. She describes the stools as mucoid but without visible blood. Bowel movements are associated with mild abdominal cramping. She has no nausea or vomiting. The patient works with infants in a day care center, and several children have recently had a diarrheal illness.

On physical examination, temperature is 37.8 °C (100.0 °F); other vital signs are normal. Abdominal examination discloses normal bowel sounds and diffuse mild tenderness to palpation.

A stool sample shows no gross blood, but results of guaiac testing and a test for fecal leukocytes are positive.

The patient is advised to increase fluid intake and take over-the-counter antipyretic agents for fever. No antibiotics are prescribed. Two days later, a stool culture is reported to be growing *Shigella sonnei*. The patient is contacted and reports that her diarrhea and fever have both resolved and that she wishes to return to work.

Which of the following is the most appropriate treatment at this time?

(A) Azithromycin

(B) Ciprofloxacin

(C) Metronidazole

(D) No treatment is needed

Item 10

A 52-year-old man is admitted to the hospital with fatigue and fever of 3 days' duration. He is a health care worker and has a bicuspid aortic valve. He takes no medications.

Blood cultures are obtained at the time of admission, and he is started on empiric vancomycin for possible endocarditis.

On hospital day 2, his initial blood cultures become positive for gram-positive cocci in clusters, and on hospital day 3, his blood cultures grow methicillin-resistant *Staphylococcus aureus*. Susceptibility to vancomycin is intermediate (MIC = 4 μg/mL).

On hospital day 4, the patient continues to appear ill. Temperature is 38.6 °C (101.5 °F), blood pressure is 105/65 mm Hg, and pulse rate is 110/min. On cardiopulmonary examination, the lungs are clear, and a grade 2/6 systolic ejection murmur is heard at the right upper sternal border, but there is no evidence of heart failure or septic emboli.

Which of the following is the most appropriate management?

(A) Discontinue vancomycin and begin daptomycin

(B) Discontinue vancomycin and begin linezolid

(C) Discontinue vancomycin and begin trimethoprim-sulfamethoxazole

(D) Increase vancomycin dose

Item 11

An 18-year-old woman is evaluated for a 5-day history of a thick yellow vaginal discharge that is occasionally tinged with blood, especially after intercourse. She has no dyspareunia or abdominal pain. She has been sexually active with a single male partner for the past 3 months and uses oral contraceptives. Her partner has no symptoms.

On physical examination, temperature is 37.2 °C (98.9 °F), blood pressure is 105/65 mm Hg, pulse rate is 70/min, and respiration rate is 10/min. A pelvic examination reveals no abnormalities of the vulva or vaginal mucosa. The cervix is inflamed, and copious mucopurulent secretions are noted. No cervical motion tenderness, uterine tenderness, adnexal tenderness, or masses are identified on bimanual examination.

A wet mount of vaginal secretions shows numerous leukocytes, with a pH of 5.5. The whiff test is negative. There are no trichomonads or clue cells. A urine pregnancy test is negative.

Which of the following is the most appropriate treatment?

(A) Oral cefixime

(B) Oral ciprofloxacin and oral azithromycin

(C) Parenteral ceftriaxone and oral azithromycin

(D) Parenteral cefoxitin and oral doxycycline

Item 12

A 63-year-old man undergoes annual screening for tuberculosis. The patient is a physician, and this screening is required for maintaining his hospital appointment. His medical history is significant for bladder cancer diagnosed 1 year ago that was treated with bacillus Calmette-Guérin. There is no current evidence of active bladder cancer on follow-up cystoscopy, and he has no respiratory or systemic symptoms.

On physical examination, vital signs are normal. The remaining physical examination findings, including cardiopulmonary examination, are normal.

Which of the following is the most appropriate next step in management?

(A) Chest radiograph

(B) Interferon-γ release assay

(C) Tuberculin skin test

(D) Two-step tuberculin skin testing

Item 13

A 28-year-old woman is evaluated in the emergency department for an injury to the hand sustained after punching another woman in the mouth 5 hours ago. She is allergic to penicillin, which causes hives, facial edema, and wheezing. All immunizations are current, including tetanus toxoid, diphtheria toxoid, and acellular pertussis vaccine administered 4 years ago.

On physical examination, temperature is normal, blood pressure is 125/70 mm Hg, pulse rate is 75/min, and respiration rate is 14/min. The dorsum of the left hand has several tiny punctures with minimal erythema and tenderness. There is no purulence or other evidence of infection, and no underlying tissue is visible.

Results of a urine pregnancy test are negative. Radiographs of the left hand show no fracture, foreign body, or gas.

Which of the following is the most appropriate management?

(A) Cephalexin

(B) Clindamycin and moxifloxacin

(C) Tetanus immunization

(D) Trimethoprim-sulfamethoxazole

(E) Observation

Item 14

A 20-year-old man is evaluated following exposure to a relative who was found to have an active varicella-zoster infection that developed about 2 days after their contact. The patient was recently diagnosed with acute myeloid leukemia and completed one cycle of induction therapy with standard-dose cytarabine and daunorubicin. He does not recall having had chickenpox as a child and has never received a varicella vaccine.

On physical examination, temperature is normal, blood pressure is 110/70 mm Hg, pulse rate is 70/min, and respiration rate is 12/min. There is no skin rash.

The leukocyte count is 600/µL (0.6×10^9/L), and the absolute neutrophil count is 200/µL. Testing for varicella antibody is negative.

Which of the following is the most appropriate management of this patient?

(A) Acyclovir
(B) Varicella vaccine
(C) Varicella-zoster immune globulin product
(D) No treatment

Item 15

A 73-year-old woman is evaluated for a 2-day history of fatigue, fever, nausea, and vomiting but no localizing symptoms. She is otherwise healthy.

On physical examination, she appears ill. Temperature is 39.8 °C (103.6 °F), blood pressure is 125/75 mm Hg, pulse rate is 115/min, and respiration rate is 15/min. Cardiopulmonary and abdominal examinations are unremarkable.

Laboratory studies indicate a leukocyte count of 17,500/µL (17.5×10^9/L) with 85% neutrophils. A urinalysis demonstrates more than 50 leukocytes/hpf and is positive for leukocyte esterase. Gram-negative rods are seen on microscopic examination. A chest radiograph is normal.

She is admitted to the hospital and treated with aggressive intravenous fluid therapy and empiric piperacillin-tazobactam. On hospital day 2, her urine and blood cultures become positive for *Escherichia coli* susceptible to piperacillin-tazobactam, imipenem, ciprofloxacin, ampicillin, and nitrofurantoin.

Which of the following is the most appropriate management?

(A) Continue piperacillin-tazobactam
(B) Discontinue piperacillin-tazobactam and begin ampicillin
(C) Discontinue piperacillin-tazobactam and begin ciprofloxacin
(D) Discontinue piperacillin-tazobactam and begin imipenem
(E) Discontinue piperacillin-tazobactam and begin nitrofurantoin

Item 16

A 55-year-old man is evaluated in the emergency department after experiencing fever and chills yesterday evening and bilateral arm pain and a rash on the upper extremities upon awakening this morning. The patient ate raw oysters from the Gulf Coast 3 nights ago. He was recently diagnosed with hemochromatosis.

On physical examination, the patient is ill appearing. Temperature is 39.1 °C (102.4 °F), blood pressure is 85/50 mm Hg, pulse rate is 130/min, and respiration rate is 28/min. Skin findings of the upper extremity are shown.

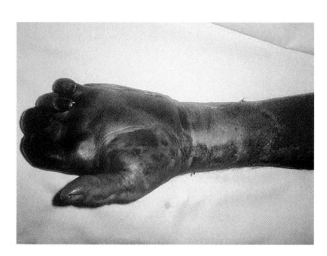

Cardiopulmonary examination findings are normal. On abdominal examination, there is shifting dullness and no guarding or rebound. No signs of meningeal irritation are present.

Laboratory studies:

Leukocyte count	28,000/µL (28×10^9/L) with 93% neutrophils, 6% lymphocytes, and 1% monocytes
Ferritin	1000 ng/mL (1000 µg/L)
Albumin	2.3 g/dL (23 g/L)
Aspartate aminotransferase	145 units/L
Alanine aminotransferase	100 units/L

The peripheral blood smear is normal.

Which of the following pathogens is most likely causing this patient's current findings?

(A) *Babesia microti*
(B) *Capnocytophaga canimorsus*
(C) *Rickettsia rickettsii*
(D) *Vibrio vulnificus*

Item 17

A 23-year-old man was admitted to a hospital 2 days ago with a 3-day history of fever, severe headache and backache, vomiting, and sores in the back of his throat. The patient is a soldier. Yesterday, he developed spots on his hands and face, and today, the spots have spread to his arms and trunk, and he has developed a papular rash on his face and hands; all of the lesions are now at the same stage of development. The patient's nurse, a 28-year-old woman, did not use any personal protective equipment during her first 2 days of his care.

Which of the following interventions is most appropriate for the nurse?

(A) Acyclovir
(B) Cidofovir
(C) Smallpox vaccine
(D) Varicella vaccine
(E) No intervention is required

Item 18

A 45-year-old woman is evaluated for nausea, anorexia, and fatigue. She had a kidney transplant 7 months ago and has been doing well since then, with normal blood pressure, a normal serum creatinine level, and an at-goal tacrolimus level on routine follow-up last month. Medications are tacrolimus, mycophenolate mofetil, and prednisone. She reports that 5 days ago, she also began taking some leftover clarithromycin that she had at home because she thought she was getting a sinus infection.

On physical examination, temperature is 37.2 °C (99.0 °F), blood pressure is 142/90 mm Hg, pulse rate is 104/min, and respiration rate is 20/min. Cardiopulmonary examination is normal. The abdomen is soft and nontender. The surgical site of the transplanted kidney is well healed.

Laboratory studies indicate a blood urea nitrogen level of 51 mg/dL (18.2 mmol/L) and a serum creatinine level of 3.7 mg/dL (327.1 µmol/L).

Dipstick and microscopic urinalysis are normal.

Which of the following is the most likely cause of this patient's acute kidney injury?

(A) Clarithromycin-induced interstitial nephritis
(B) Mycophenolate mofetil toxicity
(C) Organ rejection
(D) Tacrolimus toxicity

Item 19

A 32-year-old man is admitted to the hospital with a 5-day history of fever, chills, and myalgia. The patient works as a wildlife biologist. Most of his time is spent outdoors in rural areas. He removed an attached tick from his right leg 3 weeks ago but recalls no rash.

On physical examination, temperature is 38.8 °C (101.8 °F), and pulse rate is 115/min. The patient is oriented and conversant. There is no nuchal rigidity. Neurologic examination is notable for right lower extremity weakness, with 2/5 strength with foot dorsiflexion and plantar flexion, 2/5 strength with knee flexion and extension, and 3/5 strength with hip flexion. Right knee and ankle deep tendon reflexes are absent but are intact on the left side. Sensation is preserved. Remaining physical examination findings are unremarkable.

Laboratory studies, including a complete blood count with differential and metabolic panel, are normal. A CT scan of the head without contrast is normal. Lumbar puncture is performed. The cerebrospinal fluid (CSF) leukocyte count is 227/µL (227×10^6/L), with 45% neutrophils. The CSF protein level is 75 mg/dL (750 mg/L). A Gram-stained CSF specimen is negative.

Which of the following CSF diagnostic studies should be performed next?

(A) Cytomegalovirus polymerase chain reaction (PCR)
(B) PCR for *Ehrlichia* species
(C) PCR for *Borrelia burgdorferi* species
(D) West Nile virus IgM antibody assay

Item 20

A 59-year-old woman is evaluated for a dry cough with moderate exertional dyspnea, which has remained stable in intensity over the past 7 months. The onset of her respiratory symptoms does not correlate with any unusual exposures. She has intermittently been treated with oral antibiotics for outpatient pneumonia without a change in her symptoms. She has no systemic signs or symptoms and otherwise feels well. Medical history is unremarkable. She does not smoke. She has lived most of her adult life in the southeastern United States. She currently takes no medications.

On physical examination, vital signs are normal. Pulmonary auscultation reveals scattered rhonchi. The remainder of the examination, including cardiac examination, is normal.

A CT scan of the lungs demonstrates scattered nodular infiltrates, mostly confined to the right middle and bilateral upper lobes.

Normal respiratory flora grow from a sputum culture, and although the smear for acid-fast bacilli is negative, the culture eventually grows *Mycobacterium avium* complex by DNA gene-probe testing.

Which of the following is the most appropriate next step in management?

(A) Bronchoalveolar lavage
(B) Clarithromycin, ethambutol, and rifampin
(C) Repeat sputum acid-fast bacilli smear and culture
(D) Video-assisted thorascopic lung biopsy
(E) Observation

Item 21

A 40-year-old woman is admitted to the hospital for headaches, fever, and sweats of 3 weeks' duration as well as diplopia and increased somnolence that began yesterday. She was diagnosed with HIV infection 2 months ago with a CD4 cell count of 166/µL and an HIV RNA viral load of 66,923 copies/mL, and she immediately began taking antiretroviral therapy. She had been tolerating her medications and felt well until her current symptoms started. Medications are tenofovir, emtricitabine, efavirenz, and trimethoprim-sulfamethoxazole.

On physical examination, temperature is 38.2 °C (100.8 °F), blood pressure is 154/96 mm Hg, pulse rate is 64/min, and respiration rate is 18/min. She is awake but drowsy and is oriented to person and place but not time. The left eye cannot move laterally with leftward gaze. The rest of the neurologic examination is unremarkable.

CT scan of the head shows mildly increased ventricle size and mild cerebral atrophy, which is confirmed by MRI of the brain. Lumbar puncture is performed.

Cerebrospinal fluid analysis:

Leukocyte count	122/µL (122 × 10⁶/L) with 18% polymorphonuclear cells and 82% mononuclear cells
Glucose	62 mg/dL (3.4 mmol/L)
Protein	433 mg/dL (4330 mg/L)

The CD4 cell count is 251/µL, and the HIV RNA viral load is 675 copies/mL.

Infection with which of the following is the most likely cause of this patient's clinical presentation?

(A) *Cryptococcus neoformans*
(B) Cytomegalovirus
(C) *Histoplasma capsulatum*
(D) *Toxoplasma gondii*

 Item 22

An 18-year-old woman is evaluated in the emergency department for a 2-day history of fever, headache, vomiting, and photosensitivity. She noted painful ulcers on the vulva 10 days ago. Her boyfriend has had penile ulcers. Medical history is otherwise unremarkable.

On physical examination, temperature is 38.5 °C (101.3 °F), blood pressure is 100/60 mm Hg, pulse rate is 110/min, and respiration rate is 14/min. Nuchal rigidity is noted. The eyes appear normal. She has no oral or skin lesions. There are a few shallow ulcers on the vulva. There are no changes in sensorium. Neurologic examination is nonfocal.

Cerebrospinal fluid (CSF) analysis:

Leukocyte count	200/µL (200 × 10⁶/L) with 90% lymphocytes
Erythrocyte count	10/µL (10 × 10⁶/L)
Glucose	60 mg/dL (3.3 mmol/L)

Plasma glucose level is 100 mg/dL (5.6 mmol/L). A Gram stain of the CSF is negative.

Which of the following is the most likely diagnosis?

(A) Acute bacterial meningitis
(B) Acute retroviral syndrome
(C) Behçet disease
(D) Herpes simplex virus–induced aseptic meningitis

Item 23

A 22-year-old man is evaluated for a skin eruption on his leg. The patient lives in Virginia and is active outdoors. One week ago, he found a black tick on his lower leg, which his roommate removed with a tweezers. Yesterday he developed diffuse myalgia, neck stiffness, and fatigue. These symptoms have persisted, and today he notes erythema at the site of the previously attached tick.

On physical examination, temperature is 38.1 °C (100.6 °F); other vital signs are normal. There is no nuchal rigidity. Skin findings are shown.

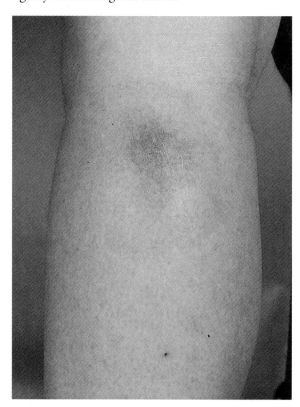

Which of the following is the most appropriate initial management?

(A) *Borrelia burgdorferi* polymerase chain reaction on skin biopsy specimen
(B) Empiric intravenous ceftriaxone
(C) Empiric oral doxycycline
(D) Serologic testing for Lyme disease

Item 24

A 35-year-old woman is evaluated for a 1-day history of fever, headache, myalgia, arthralgia, and neck stiffness. The patient is sexually active. She had a similar episode 2 years ago, at which time results of cerebrospinal fluid (CSF) analysis showed lymphocytic meningitis. All culture results were negative, and her symptoms resolved over the next 3 days.

On physical examination, temperature is 38.3 °C (101.0 °F), blood pressure is 110/70 mm Hg, pulse rate is 90/min, and respiration rate is 12/min. There are no oral or genital ulcers. There is mild neck stiffness. Remaining physical examination findings, including mental status evaluation and complete neurologic examination, are normal. Funduscopic examination is normal.

Examination of the CSF shows a leukocyte count of 90/µL (90 × 10⁶/L) with 95% lymphocytes, a glucose level of 68 mg/dL (3.8 mmol/L), and a protein level of 70 mg/dL (700 mg/L). A Gram-stained CSF specimen is negative.

Which of the following diagnostic studies will most likely establish the cause of this patient's meningitis?

(A) CSF cytology
(B) CSF IgM assay for West Nile virus
(C) CSF polymerase chain reaction for herpes simplex virus type 2
(D) MRI of the brain

Item 25

A 42-year-old man is admitted to the hospital for a 2-week history of headache and fever and a 1-week history of skin lesions. He was diagnosed with AIDS 5 years ago. He has not taken antiretroviral therapy for the past year. His only current medication is trimethoprim-sulfamethoxazole.

On physical examination, temperature is 38.0 °C (100.4 °F). Skin findings are shown.

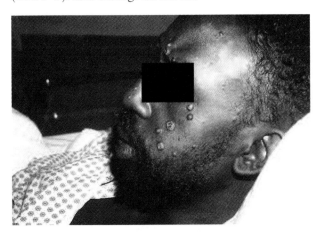

The remainder of the physical examination is normal.

Results of the serum cryptococcal antigen assay are positive at a titer of 1:1024. Blood cultures from admission are growing budding yeast. Cerebrospinal fluid (CSF) opening pressure is 220 mm H₂0. CSF cryptococcal antigen and culture results are pending. A Gram stain of the CSF is negative.

Cerebrospinal fluid analysis:
Leukocyte count   2/µL (2.0 × 10⁶/L)
Erythrocyte count   10/µL (10 × 10⁶/L)
Protein   70 mg/dL (700 mg/L)
Glucose   70 mg/dL (3.9 mmol/L)

The plasma glucose level is 100 mg/dL (5.6 mmol/L).
A CT scan of the head is normal.

Which of the following is the most appropriate initial treatment?

(A) Conventional amphotericin B and flucytosine
(B) Caspofungin
(C) Fluconazole
(D) Itraconazole

Item 26

A 23-year-old woman is evaluated for a 5-day history of yellow vaginal discharge accompanied by lower abdominal pain and dyspareunia. The remainder of the medical history is noncontributory.

On physical examination, temperature is 38.0 °C (100.4 °F), blood pressure is 110/60 mm Hg, pulse rate is 90/min, and respiration rate is 12/min. The cervix appears inflamed, with a small amount of mucopurulent discharge. There is no cervical motion tenderness, but there is tenderness to palpation of the uterus on bimanual examination. No adnexal tenderness or masses are noted.

A serum pregnancy test is negative.

Which of the following is the most appropriate treatment?

(A) Intravenous clindamycin and gentamicin for 7 days
(B) Oral ciprofloxacin and metronidazole for 14 days
(C) Single-dose intramuscular ceftriaxone and oral doxycycline for 14 days
(D) Single-dose intramuscular ceftriaxone and single-dose oral azithromycin

Item 27

A 31-year-old woman is evaluated for recurrent episodes of genital symptoms that consist of itching, irritation, and burning in the vulvar area without vaginal discharge. The patient has experienced two similar episodes over the past 3 years, but she has never noticed any lesions in the genital region. She has had six lifetime sexual partners.

On physical examination, vital signs are normal. An examination of the external genitalia reveals a linear fissure between the labia minora and the labia majora on the left. A pelvic examination is normal.

HIV and syphilis screening are performed.

Which of the following is the most appropriate next diagnostic test to perform?

(A) Herpes simplex virus polymerase chain reaction
(B) Serology for *Chlamydia trachomatis* serovars L1, L2, and L3
(C) Tzanck smear
(D) Wet mount with potassium hydroxide

Item 28

A 22-year-old man is evaluated for a painless penile lesion first noted 3 days ago. He has no fever or other symptoms. He has had three male sexual partners in the past 6 months and uses condoms inconsistently. He undergoes HIV testing every year, and his most recent results 7 months ago were negative.

On physical examination, vital signs are normal. Skin findings on the shaft of the penis are shown.

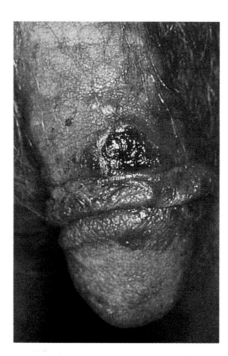

There is no evidence of penile discharge or other genital lesions. He has no other skin or oral lesions. Shotty, nontender inguinal lymphadenopathy is noted.

Which of the following is the most likely diagnosis?

(A) Chancroid
(B) Herpes simplex virus infection
(C) Human papillomavirus infection
(D) Syphilis

Item 29

A 24-year-old man is admitted to the hospital with a 4-day history of fever, malaise, and arthralgia of the elbows, wrists, and knees. Two days ago, he developed progressive pain and swelling of the right knee. He also has a rash on his right arm.

On physical examination, temperature is 38.2 °C (100.8 °F), blood pressure is 110/60 mm Hg, pulse rate is 95/min, and respiration rate is 12/min. There is evidence of tenosynovitis of the left wrist. The right knee is swollen and warm, with significant effusion. The rash on his arm is shown (see top of right-hand column).

Blood cultures are obtained, and an arthrocentesis of the right knee is performed. The synovial fluid leukocyte count is 60,000/μL (60 × 10^9/L) with 90% polymorphonuclear neutrophils. The Gram stain is negative.

Which of the following is the most appropriate diagnostic test to perform next?

(A) Antinuclear antibody and rheumatoid factor assays
(B) Biopsy and culture of a skin lesion

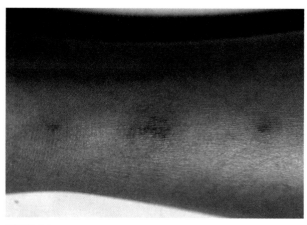

ITEM 29

(C) HLA B27 testing
(D) Nucleic acid amplification urine test for *Neisseria gonorrhoeae*

Item 30

A 35-year-old man is evaluated for a 2-week history of nonproductive cough and fever. He has a 20-year history of asthma. Three weeks ago, he visited friends in Indiana. He has no dyspnea, hemoptysis, or worsening of his baseline asthma symptoms. His only medication is an albuterol inhaler as needed.

On physical examination, temperature is 38.0 °C (100.4 °F), blood pressure is 130/70 mm Hg, pulse rate is 88/min, and respiration rate is 16/min. Crackles are heard in both lungs.

Laboratory studies show a normal leukocyte count and serum creatinine level.

Chest radiograph reveals patchy pulmonary infiltrates with mild hilar lymphadenopathy.

Which of the following is the most appropriate management?

(A) Lipid amphotericin B
(B) Fluconazole
(C) Itraconazole
(D) No treatment

Item 31

A 46-year-old man is admitted to the hospital with a ruptured gallbladder requiring emergent open cholecystectomy.

An indwelling urinary catheter is inserted prior to surgery, and a drain is left in his upper right abdominal quadrant.

The patient is stabilized and transferred to the surgical intensive care unit.

In addition to removing the urinary catheter at the first possible moment, which of the following will decrease this patient's risk of catheter-associated urinary tract infection?

(A) Daily cleansing of the meatal area of the catheter with antiseptics

(B) Maintenance of urine-collecting bag below the level of the bladder

(C) Routine catheter change every 5 days

(D) Treatment of asymptomatic bacteriuria

(E) Use of antiseptic-coated urinary catheters

Item 32

A 46-year-old man with quadriplegia is evaluated for fever and increased muscle spasticity. He self-catheterizes intermittently four times daily because of chronic bladder dysfunction, although an indwelling urinary catheter was placed 2 weeks ago because of difficulty with self-catheterization.

On physical examination, the temperature is 38.9 °C (102.0 °F). The remainder of the examination is consistent with the diagnosis of quadriplegia. An indwelling bladder catheter is in place.

A urinalysis and culture are obtained.

Which of the following is required to establish the diagnosis of catheter-associated urinary tract infection in this patient?

(A) Grossly cloudy urine

(B) Positive urine dipstick for leukocyte esterase

(C) Positive urine Gram stain

(D) Urine culture with more than 10^3 colony-forming units/mL

Item 33

A 29-year-old man is evaluated for newly diagnosed HIV infection. He has no symptoms and is willing to start combination antiretroviral therapy if necessary. He has no other medical problems and takes no medications.

Physical examination is normal.

The complete blood count, serum chemistries, and liver enzymes are normal. CD4 cell count is 424/μL. HIV RNA viral load is 21,317 copies/mL. HIV resistance testing is negative for mutations. A hepatitis B virus surface antibody assay, serologic testing for syphilis, and a hepatitis C virus antibody assay are negative.

In addition to periodic follow-up monitoring, which of the following is the most appropriate management of this patient's HIV infection?

(A) Begin combination antiretroviral therapy now

(B) Withhold treatment until CD4 cell count falls below 350/μL

(C) Withhold treatment until HIV RNA viral load exceeds 55,000 copies/mL

(D) Withhold treatment until symptoms develop

Item 34

A 26-year-old man is evaluated for a 3-day history of fever, myalgia, dry cough, and malaise. He has no known drug allergies, and the remainder of the medical history is noncontributory.

On physical examination, temperature is 38.3 °C (100.9 °F), blood pressure is 125/75 mm Hg, pulse rate is 95/min, and respiration rate is 16/min. Oxygen saturation is 100% with the patient breathing ambient air. Crackles are heard in the left lung base.

Chest radiograph shows left lower lobe airspace disease.

Which of the following oral agents is the most appropriate treatment?

(A) Amoxicillin

(B) Azithromycin

(C) Cefuroxime

(D) Ciprofloxacin

Item 35

A 25-year-old woman is evaluated for a 1-week history of cough and fever, painful nodules on the extensor surfaces of the arms and the legs, and arthralgia of the knees and ankles. Her symptoms developed 3 weeks after she vacationed in the Arizona desert.

On physical examination, temperature is 39.0 °C (102.2 °F), blood pressure is 100/60 mm Hg, pulse rate is 110/min, and respiration rate is 18/min. Crackles and egophony are heard in the posterior left lower lung field. There is no evidence of joint effusions. Findings of the skin examination of the lower extremities are shown.

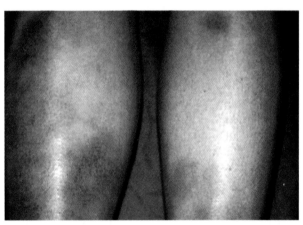

Laboratory studies indicate an erythrocyte sedimentation rate of 70 mm/h and a normal complete blood count.

A chest radiograph reveals a dense infiltrate of the left lower lobe and left hilar lymphadenopathy. Gram stains of sputum are negative.

Which of the following is the most likely diagnosis?

(A) Blastomycosis

(B) Coccidioidomycosis

(C) Histoplasmosis

(D) Sporotrichosis

Item 36

A 22-year-old woman is evaluated for a 1-day history of dysuria and urinary urgency and frequency. She had an episode of cystitis 2 years ago. The patient has a sulfa allergy.

On physical examination, temperature is normal, blood pressure is 110/60 mm Hg, pulse rate is 60/min, and respiration rate is 14/min. There is mild suprapubic tenderness, but no flank tenderness. The remainder of the examination is normal.

Urine dipstick analysis shows 3+ leukocyte esterase. A pregnancy test is negative.

Treatment with which of the following antibiotics is most appropriate?

(A) Amoxicillin
(B) Fosfomycin
(C) Levofloxacin
(D) Nitrofurantoin

Item 37

A 30-year-old man is admitted to the hospital with a 1-month history of fever, night sweats, cough, weight loss, and chest pain. The patient is homeless. A diagnosis of pericardial tamponade is established.

Pericardiocentesis is performed, following which there is no recurrence of a significant pericardial effusion. Microbiologic examination of pericardial fluid identifies *Mycobacterium tuberculosis*.

In addition to four-drug antituberculous therapy, which of the following is the most appropriate next treatment?

(A) Indomethacin and colchicine
(B) Pericardial window
(C) Prednisone
(D) Surgical pericardiectomy

Item 38

A 21-year-old man undergoes evaluation in the intensive care unit (ICU) before surgical intervention scheduled for tomorrow. He was admitted to the surgical ICU 17 days ago for multiple gunshot wounds. He is mechanically ventilated and had a central line catheter placed in the right femoral vein. *Acinetobacter baumannii* has been isolated from blood cultures drawn from the central line catheter, sputum, and one of the abdominal drains. The patient shares the room with one additional patient, who is also mechanically ventilated.

Which of the following is most likely to reduce spread of this patient's *Acinetobacter* infection to his roommate?

(A) Clean the patients' room with bleach
(B) Ensure strict staff adherence to hand hygiene practices
(C) Give prophylactic antimicrobial agents active against *Acinetobacter* species to the roommate
(D) Replace source patient's central line catheter, endotracheal tube, and abdominal drain with new devices

Item 39

A 59-year-old woman is evaluated for a 1-week history of increasing pain of the right foot. She recalls stepping on a nail about 1 month before her symptoms began. The patient has a 5-year history of heart failure secondary to idiopathic dilated cardiomyopathy. She has an implantable cardioverter-defibrillator, and her current medications are carvedilol, lisinopril, furosemide, and spironolactone.

On physical examination, vital signs are normal. Examination of the foot reveals tenderness and warmth directly below the proximal fifth metatarsal bone.

A radiograph of the right foot is normal.

Which of the following is the most appropriate next step to establish the diagnosis?

(A) CT scan
(B) Gallium scan
(C) MRI
(D) Three-phase bone scan

Item 40

A 54-year-old man is evaluated in the emergency department for a 2-week history of fever and chills occurring every 1 to 2 days. He also has a significant headache, muscle pain, and intermittent diarrhea. The patient is an archeology professor who returned 2 weeks ago from a 6-week "dig" in Thailand in Southeast Asia. He received pre-travel prophylactic vaccinations, including combined hepatitis A and B virus vaccines, as well as yellow fever, typhoid, and Japanese encephalitis vaccines. In addition, he completed a regimen of mefloquine for malaria chemoprophylaxis.

On physical examination, he appears ill but is awake and alert. Temperature is 39.4 °C (102.9 °F), blood pressure is 100/62 mm Hg, pulse rate is 118/min, and respiration rate is 20/min. Cardiopulmonary examination is unremarkable. There is mild splenomegaly.

A complete blood count indicates a leukocyte count of 8900/µL (8.9×10^9/L), a platelet count of 82,000/µL (82×10^9/L), and a hemoglobin level of 10 g/dL (100 g/L). He also has a mildly increased serum indirect bilirubin level and elevated serum alanine and aspartate aminotransferase levels. A peripheral blood smear is shown.

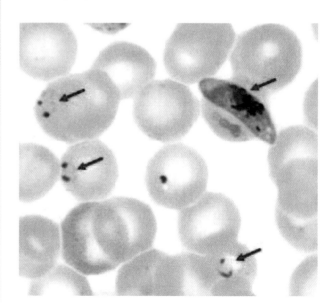

Against which of the following malaria species should treatment be initiated in this patient?

(A) *Plasmodium falciparum*
(B) *Plasmodium malariae*
(C) *Plasmodium ovale*
(D) *Plasmodium vivax*

Item 41

A 25-year-old woman undergoes evaluation. Treatment for active pulmonary tuberculosis was initiated 6 weeks ago. The mycobacteria were susceptible to all first-line antituberculous agents, and a 2-month course of isoniazid, rifampin, ethambutol, and pyrazinamide was prescribed as initial therapy. However, the patient was lost to follow-up for 3 weeks, during which time she discontinued all medications.

On physical examination, temperature is 37.7 °C (99.9 °F), blood pressure is 110/70 mm Hg, pulse rate is 90/min, and respiration rate is 18/min. The remainder of her physical examination is normal.

Which of the following is the most appropriate management?

(A) Continue the same treatment to complete the planned total number of doses, provided all doses are completed within 3 months
(B) Repeat sputum smear for acid-fast bacilli; if results are negative, treatment can be considered complete
(C) Restart different treatment with at least two new drugs to which the mycobacteria were originally susceptible
(D) Restart the same treatment from the beginning

Item 42

A 70-year-old man is evaluated for a 6-month history of hyperkeratotic skin lesions. The patient lives in Michigan. He is otherwise healthy.

On physical examination, temperature is normal, blood pressure is 150/78 mm Hg, pulse rate is 80/min, and respiration rate is 14/min. The lungs are clear.

A representative skin lesion on the face is shown.

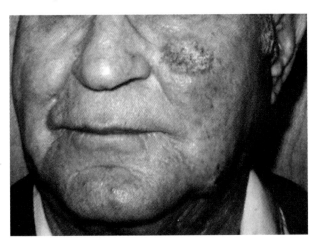

Skin biopsy shows a pyogranulomatous broad-based budding yeast. Chest radiograph

Which of the following is the most appropriate treatment of this patient?

(A) Amphotericin B
(B) Fluconazole
(C) Itraconazole
(D) Surgical excision

Item 43

A 42-year-old woman is evaluated for a 4-day history of mild fever, headache, myalgia, nonproductive cough, and sore throat. There is a confirmed influenza A (H1N1) outbreak in the local community. She has no other medical illnesses.

On physical examination, temperature is 38.2 °C (100.8 °F), blood pressure is 130/70 mm Hg, pulse rate is 88/min, and respiration rate is 14/min. She does not appear ill. There is diffuse muscle tenderness to palpation. The lungs are clear. The abdomen is soft and nontender.

Laboratory studies show a leukocyte count of 5600/μL (5.6×10^9/L) and a serum creatinine level of 1.0 mg/dL (88.4 μmol/L).

Which of the following is the most appropriate treatment?

(A) Amantadine
(B) Oseltamivir
(C) Rimantadine
(D) Zanamivir
(E) No treatment

Item 44

A 53-year-old man is evaluated for a 2-day history of swelling and pain of the right knee. Active tuberculosis was recently diagnosed, and the patient has been treated with isoniazid, rifampin, and pyrazinamide for the past 7 weeks. Ethambutol, which was also started 7 weeks ago, had to be discontinued 1 week ago after the patient experienced decreased visual acuity ascribed to optic neuritis. Mycobacteria are fully susceptible to all first-line antituberculous agents. His medical history also includes hypertension for which he takes amlodipine.

On physical examination, vital signs are normal. The right knee is warm, erythematous, and swollen, and he has difficulty bearing weight on this leg because of intense pain. Range of motion of the knee is restricted and elicits pain.

A serum uric acid level obtained today is 10.5 mg/dL (0.62 mmol/L). A complete blood count reveals a leukocyte count of 14,700/μL (14.7×10^9/L) with 87% polymorphonuclear cells and 13% lymphocytes. An arthrocentesis of the right knee is performed and reveals a synovial fluid leukocyte count of 30,000/μL (30×10^9/L) (90% polymorphonuclear cells, 10% lymphocytes). Gram stain is negative, but polarized light microscopy reveals intra- and extracellular monosodium urate crystals.

Which of the following is most likely responsible for this patient's clinical findings?

(A) Amlodipine
(B) Isoniazid
(C) Pyrazinamide
(D) Rifampin

Item 45

A 52-year-old man is admitted to the intensive care unit with fever and hypotension. He sustained a burn injury 1 year ago with involvement of approximately 20% of his skin surface area. Since his injury, he has been hospitalized frequently for skin grafting procedures, most recently 1 week ago involving the anterior left thigh. At the site of his latest skin graft, he has developed purulent drainage over the past 24 hours. The patient takes no medications, including antibiotics.

On physical examination, temperature is 38.8 °C (101.8 °F), blood pressure is 95/50 mm Hg, and the pulse rate is 115/min. Cardiopulmonary examination is unremarkable. He has multiple well-healed skin graft sites except for his recent graft site on the anterior left thigh, which shows an area of devitalized skin with eschar formation and peripheral erythema and drainage of a moderate amount of pus.

Empiric vancomycin is initiated.

Two sets of blood cultures obtained at the onset of fever on admission are positive for *Pseudomonas aeruginosa*. Empiric vancomycin and cefepime are initiated. Antibiotic sensitivity studies show that the organism is pan-resistant to all antimicrobial agents to which it was tested, including all β-lactam antimicrobial agents, carbapenems, fluoroquinolones, and aminoglycosides.

Which of the following is the most appropriate antibiotic treatment for this patient?

(A) Intravenous colistin
(B) Intravenous minocycline
(C) Intravenous rifampin
(D) Intravenous tigecycline

Item 46

A 47-year-old man is admitted to the hospital with community-acquired pneumonia. He has hypertension and a 25-pack-year smoking history. His only current medication is chlorthalidone.

On physical examination, the patient is in mild respiratory distress. Temperature is 40.1 °C (104.2 °F), blood pressure is 145/85 mm Hg, pulse rate is 130/min, and respiration rate is 16/min. Oxygen saturation is 89% with the patient breathing ambient air. Pulmonary examination demonstrates dullness to percussion with bronchial breath sounds localized to the right lung base.

A chest radiograph shows right lower lobe consolidation without significant pleural effusion. Intravenous ceftriaxone and azithromycin are initiated. On the second hospital day, blood cultures obtained on admission are positive

for gram-positive cocci in pairs and chains. The ceftriaxone is continued and the azithromycin is stopped.

On the morning of hospital day 3, the patient is feeling better, has been afebrile for the past 12 hours, and is eating and drinking well. The blood culture isolate is identified as *Streptococcus pneumoniae* susceptible to penicillin. Temperature is 37.0 °C (98.6 °F), blood pressure is 140/80 mm Hg, pulse rate is 88/min, and respiration rate is 16/min. Oxygen saturation is 97% with the patient breathing ambient air.

Which of the following is the most appropriate management?

(A) Discharge on oral levofloxacin to complete 7 days of therapy
(B) Discharge on oral amoxicillin to complete 14 days of therapy
(C) Discharge on oral amoxicillin to complete 7 days of therapy
(D) Switch to oral amoxicillin and discharge tomorrow, if stable

Item 47

A 56-year-old man is evaluated in the emergency department for a 3-day history of fever, myalgia, dyspnea, and mid-anterior chest discomfort. He works at a local airport as an airplane mechanic where small aircraft are used for crop-dusting nearby fields. The remainder of the medical history is unremarkable.

On physical examination, temperature is 38.7 °C (101.7 °F), blood pressure is 94/60 mm Hg, pulse rate is 115/min, and respiration rate is 24/min. The patient appears confused. The skin is cool and mottled. No rash is present. Pulmonary examination discloses diminished breath sounds bilaterally at the lung bases. Other than distant heart sounds and tachycardia, the cardiac examination is normal. There are no focal neurologic findings.

A chest radiograph is shown.

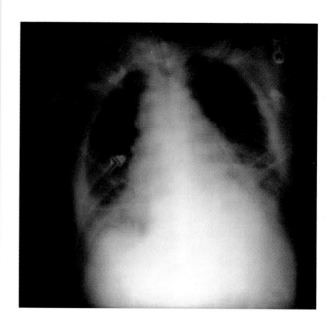

CONT.

Which of the following is the most likely infectious agent?

(A) *Bacillus anthracis*
(B) *Erysipelothrix rhusiopathiae*
(C) *Listeria monocytogenes*
(D) *Nocardia* species

Item 48

A 55-year-old man undergoes follow-up evaluation for treatment of *Blastocystis* infection. Ten days ago, the patient went to a walk-in clinic because of diarrhea. Probable viral gastroenteritis was diagnosed, and loperamide was prescribed. Stool studies were performed at that time. Cultures for bacteria were negative, but a microscopic examination for ova and parasites showed *Blastocystis* species. He was contacted by the clinic and told to seek further medical attention because of his stool studies.

Diarrhea resolved within 24 hours of starting loperamide, and the patient is currently asymptomatic. He takes no medications.

On physical examination today, vital signs are normal. There is no abdominal tenderness.

Which of the following is the most appropriate intervention at this time?

(A) Begin ciprofloxacin
(B) Begin metronidazole
(C) Repeat stool examination for ova and parasites
(D) No additional evaluation or treatment is indicated

Item 49

A 62-year-old man is admitted to the hospital with confusion. His wife reports that he is a truck driver, but he has been unable to work for the past 3 weeks because he can no longer follow map directions. Yesterday, she found him putting his clothes in the dishwasher rather than the washing machine. The patient has insomnia and fatigue but no headache, photophobia, stiff neck, fever, or other localizing symptoms or signs. He has never traveled outside the United States.

On physical examination, vital signs are normal. He appears disheveled and is conversant but slow to respond to questions. Myoclonic movements of the upper extremities are noted at rest. Remaining physical examination findings are unremarkable.

Results of a complete blood count and metabolic panel are normal. Urine culture findings are negative. Lumbar puncture is performed. The cerebrospinal fluid (CSF) leukocyte count is 2/μL (2.0 × 10⁶/L). CSF protein and glucose levels are normal.

MRI of the brain shows atrophy appropriate for his age, but no focal lesions.

Which of the following is the most likely diagnosis?

(A) Cryptococcal meningitis
(B) Neurosyphilis
(C) Sporadic Creutzfeldt-Jakob disease
(D) Tuberculous meningitis

Item 50

A 48-year-old woman is admitted to the hospital with a 1-week history of nasal congestion, rhinorrhea, dry cough, fever, chills, and myalgia. She was beginning to feel better until 48 hours ago when she developed a recurrence of fever and chills, a cough productive of blood-streaked yellow sputum, and right-sided pleuritic chest pain. She has had no recent hospitalizations. Medical history is significant for type 2 diabetes mellitus. She has no history of tobacco, alcohol, or recreational drug use. Current medications are metformin and glipizide.

On physical examination, temperature is 39.0 °C (102.2 °F), blood pressure is 100/50 mm Hg, pulse rate is 110/min, and respiration rate is 24/min. Crackles are heard over the right lateral chest with egophony and increased fremitus.

Laboratory studies indicate a leukocyte count of 20,000/μL (20 × 10⁹/L), a blood urea nitrogen level of 28 mg/dL (10.0 mmol/L), and a serum creatinine level of 1.3 mg/dL (114.9 μmol/L). Chest radiograph shows right middle lobe airspace disease with a small area of cavitation and blunting of the right costophrenic angle.

Which of the following is the most appropriate empiric treatment of this patient?

(A) Aztreonam
(B) Ceftriaxone and azithromycin
(C) Ceftriaxone, azithromycin, and vancomycin
(D) Moxifloxacin

Item 51

A 35-year-old man is evaluated in the emergency department in April for symptoms of diplopia and difficulty swallowing food and water of 24 hours' duration; his wife is being evaluated in the emergency department for similar symptoms. The patient and his wife returned to their home in Connecticut 2 days ago from a 7-day Caribbean cruise during which they went snorkeling, ate pork at an island barbeque, and hiked in a forest. Review of systems is otherwise negative.

On physical examination, vital signs are normal. The patient is alert and oriented. He has dysphonia and dysarthria, obvious bilateral ocular palsies, an absent gag reflex, and symmetric upper extremity motor weakness without any objective sensory abnormalities. The remainder of the examination is unremarkable.

Which of the following is the most likely diagnosis?

(A) Botulism
(B) Guillain-Barré syndrome
(C) Paralytic shellfish poisoning
(D) Tick paralysis

Item 52

A 33-year-old woman is evaluated for a 5-week history of whitish spots in the mouth and the back of the throat and discomfort with swallowing solid foods. This is her first episode of these symptoms. She has had no mouth pain, trouble ingesting liquids or pills, nausea, vomiting, diarrhea, fever, chills, sweats, or skin problems. She has a 3-year history of HIV infection and also has moderately severe asthma, which is now well controlled with inhaled medications that were recently prescribed. Her medications are tenofovir, emtricitabine, raltegravir, and inhaled fluticasone and salmeterol.

On physical examination, her vital signs are normal. Whitish plaques are seen on the palate and posterior pharynx. The remainder of the physical examination is normal.

Her last CD4 cell count was 458/μL. The HIV RNA viral load is undetectable.

Which of the following is the most appropriate management of this patient?

(A) Clotrimazole troches
(B) Fluticasone cessation
(C) Intravenous amphotericin B
(D) Nystatin swish-and-swallow
(E) Oral fluconazole

Item 53

A 74-year-old man is evaluated in the emergency department for a 3-day history of fever and chills as well as confusion. He has a 5-week history of a nonhealing ulcer on the plantar surface of his left foot. He has diabetes mellitus, hypertension, and peripheral vascular disease for which he takes metformin, glyburide, lisinopril, chlorthalidone, and aspirin. He has no known medication allergies.

On physical examination, temperature is 39.0 °C (102.2 °F), blood pressure is 92/60 mm Hg, pulse rate is 108/min, and respiration rate is 18/min. He appears ill and is slow to respond. Examination of the left foot discloses a 3.5 × 2.5-cm ulcer with surrounding erythema and warmth. A foul odor and edema and tenderness involving the entire foot are noted. Pedal pulses are absent. The underlying bone is detected with a metal probe.

Laboratory studies indicate a leukocyte count of 21,500/μL (21.5 × 10⁹/L) with 18% band forms. Serum electrolyte levels and kidney function tests are normal.

A radiograph of the left foot reveals soft tissue swelling with erosion of the cortex at the head of the metatarsal bone beneath the site of the ulceration.

Which of the following is the most appropriate empiric antimicrobial regimen?

(A) Aztreonam and metronidazole
(B) Cefazolin and metronidazole
(C) Clindamycin and gentamicin
(D) Vancomycin and meropenem

Item 54

A 25-year-old woman who is 12 weeks pregnant is found to be HIV positive during a routine pregnancy evaluation. She is asymptomatic. Her medical history is unremarkable, and her only medication is a prenatal vitamin.

On physical examination, vital signs are normal. No lymphadenopathy, thrush, or skin lesions are noted. The remainder of the examination is normal.

Hemoglobin is 11 g/dL (110 g/L). HIV antibody testing is positive by enzyme immunoassay and confirmed by Western blot analysis. CD4 cell count is 865/μL, and HIV RNA viral load is 510 copies/mL. Rapid plasma reagin and hepatitis B serologies are negative. HIV genotyping shows no resistance mutations. The remaining laboratory studies are unremarkable.

Which of the following is the most appropriate management?

(A) Begin antiretroviral therapy at the onset of labor
(B) Begin tenofovir, emtricitabine, and efavirenz now
(C) Begin zidovudine, lamivudine, and lopinavir-ritonavir now
(D) Repeat CD4 cell count and treat if 500/μL or lower

Item 55

A 19-year-old man is evaluated for a sore throat, daily fever, frontal headache, myalgia, and arthralgia of 5 days' duration. He also has severe discomfort in the lower spine and a rash on his trunk and extremities. He returned from a 7-day trip to the Caribbean 8 days ago. The remainder of the history is noncontributory.

On physical examination, temperature is 38.3 °C (100.9 °F), blood pressure is 104/72 mm Hg, pulse rate is 102/min, and respiration rate is 16/min. His posterior pharynx is notably injected but without exudate. He has a maculopapular rash on his chest, arms, and legs that spares the palms and soles. There is no palpable lymphadenopathy. The remainder of the examination, including cardiopulmonary and abdominal examinations, is normal.

Laboratory studies:
Leukocyte count	3100/μL (3.1 x 10⁹/L)
Platelet count	85,500/μL (85.5 x 10⁹/L)
Hemoglobin	13.9 g/dL (139 g/L)
Alanine aminotransferase	114 units/L
Aspartate aminotransferase	154 units/L
Total bilirubin	1.2 mg/dL (20.5 μmol/L)

Which of the following is the most likely diagnosis?

(A) Dengue fever
(B) Leptospirosis
(C) Malaria
(D) Syphilis
(E) Yellow fever

Item 56

A 24-year-old man is evaluated for an increasingly painful boil on his back that has been present for 3 days and has increased in size. The patient has had similar lesions on his back and chest previously, but these were smaller and spontaneously drained and resolved without requiring medical attention. The remainder of the medical history is noncontributory.

On physical examination, vital signs are normal, and the patient is not ill appearing. Examination of the back discloses a 7-cm fluctuant, tender, oval-shaped lesion, with surrounding erythema extending 3 cm from the edge of the lesion. The remainder of the physical examination is normal.

An aspirate of the lesion reveals purulent material, a Gram stain of which demonstrates many leukocytes and many gram-positive cocci in clusters. A culture is sent for processing. Incision and drainage of the lesion produces approximately 5 mL of pus.

Which of the following is the most appropriate antibiotic treatment for this patient?

(A) Amoxicillin-clavulanate

(B) Azithromycin

(C) Moxifloxacin

(D) Rifampin

(E) Trimethoprim-sulfamethoxazole

Item 57

A 23-year-old man undergoes preliminary evaluation. He has just been admitted to a detoxification center because of injection drug use.

On physical examination, temperature is 36.8 °C (98.2 °F), blood pressure is 125/75 mm Hg, pulse rate is 90/min, and respiration rate is 18/min. Findings of physical examination demonstrate evidence of injection drug use on the bilateral upper extremities but are otherwise normal.

Tuberculin skin testing induces 6 mm of induration. The patient has not had previous tuberculin skin tests. Results of a serologic test for HIV infection are negative.

Which of the following is the most appropriate next step in the management of this patient?

(A) Chest radiograph

(B) Isoniazid

(C) Isoniazid, rifampin, pyrazinamide, and ethambutol

(D) No additional therapy or evaluation

Item 58

A 44-year-old woman is evaluated for a 1-week history of low-grade fever, fatigue, and body aches. She had a kidney transplant 5 months ago; at the time of transplantation, she was seropositive for Epstein-Barr virus and seronegative for cytomegalovirus with a seropositive donor. Her recent course has been uncomplicated with no episodes of rejection. She completed cytomegalovirus prophylaxis with valganciclovir last month. Medications are tacrolimus, mycophenolate mofetil, prednisone, and trimethoprim-sulfamethoxazole.

On physical examination, temperature is 37.8 °C (100.0 °F), blood pressure is 136/88 mm Hg, pulse rate is 96/min, and respiration rate is 16/min. There is no lymphadenopathy. The transplant surgical wound site is without erythema or drainage. Cardiopulmonary examination is normal. The abdomen is soft and nontender.

Laboratory studies:

Hematocrit	33%
Leukocyte count	3200/μL (3.2×10^9/L)
Platelet count	112,000/μL (112×10^9/L)
Alkaline phosphatase	155 units/L
Alanine aminotransferase	52 units/L
Aspartate aminotransferase	48 units/L
Bilirubin	0.6 mg/dL (10.3 μmol/L)
Blood urea nitrogen	18 mg/dL (6.4 mmol/L)
Creatinine	1.1 mg/dL (97.2 μmol/L)

Microscopic urinalysis is unremarkable. The chest radiograph is normal.

Infection with which of the following is the most likely diagnosis?

(A) Cytomegalovirus

(B) Epstein-Barr virus

(C) *Listeria monocytogenes*

(D) Polyoma BK virus

Item 59

A 70-year-old man is evaluated in the emergency department for a 1-day history of fever and altered mental status. Medical history is significant for coronary artery disease and hypertension treated with hydrochlorothiazide, aspirin, lisinopril, and atenolol.

On physical examination, temperature is 38.3 °C (101.0 °F), blood pressure is 98/58 mm Hg, pulse rate is 100/min, and respiration rate is 20/min. The patient is confused and oriented only to person. He is unable to answer any questions. His neck is supple, and neurologic examination findings are nonfocal. He has no rash.

A CT scan of the head without contrast reveals evidence of mild cerebral edema.

Lumbar puncture is performed. Opening pressure is 300 mm H_2O. Cerebrospinal fluid (CSF) analysis demonstrates a leukocyte count of 1200/μL (1200×10^6/L) with 60% neutrophils and 40% lymphocytes, a glucose level of 30 mg/dL (1.7 mmol/L), and a protein level of 350 mg/dL (3500 mg/L). A Gram-stained CSF specimen is negative.

Dexamethasone followed by vancomycin, ampicillin, and ceftriaxone are begun in the emergency department, and the patient is admitted to the hospital. The next day, his clinical condition is unchanged.

Which of the following is the most appropriate management at this time?

(A) Add rifampin

(B) Continue current management

(C) Place an external ventricular drain

(D) Repeat the CSF analysis

Item 60

A 68-year-old woman is admitted to the intensive care unit with severe community-acquired pneumonia complicated by hypercapnic respiratory failure. Medical history is significant for COPD, with several exacerbations occurring in the past 6 months that were successfully managed with prednisone in the outpatient setting. She also has a 60-pack-year smoking history. Medications are prednisone, albuterol, fluticasone-salmeterol, and tiotropium.

The patient is intubated and placed on mechanical ventilation. On physical examination, temperature is 37.8 °C (100.0 °F), blood pressure is 160/100 mm Hg, pulse rate is 115/min, and respiration rate is 22/min. There are diminished breath sounds throughout the lung fields, with scattered rhonchi, wheezing, and marked prolongation of the expiratory phase.

A chest radiograph shows hyperinflation, with flattening of the diaphragms and right lower lobe consolidation with air bronchograms.

Results of a Gram stain and culture of the endotracheal aspirate show numerous polymorphonuclear cells, few epithelial cells, and moderate gram-negative rods.

Which of the following is the most appropriate initial treatment?

(A) Aztreonam and azithromycin
(B) Cefepime, tobramycin, and azithromycin
(C) Cefotaxime and azithromycin
(D) Cefotaxime, azithromycin, and levofloxacin

Item 61

A 57-year-old woman is admitted to the hospital with a 2-day history of fever and confusion. Medical history is significant for hypertension treated with metoprolol.

On physical examination, temperature is 39.0 °C (102.2 °F); other vital signs are normal. The patient is alert but lethargic and answers questions with one-word responses. She is oriented to person only. Passive flexion of the neck elicits mild nuchal rigidity. Remaining physical examination findings are unremarkable.

Lumbar puncture is performed. Opening pressure is 21 mm H$_2$O. The cerebrospinal fluid (CSF) leukocyte count is 147/microliter (147×10^6/L) with 77% lymphocytes. CSF glucose and protein levels are normal. An MRI of the brain is normal.

Treatment with empiric acyclovir, 10 mg/kg intravenously every 8 hours, is initiated. By hospital day 3, the patient's fever has resolved and her mental status has normalized. Results of a CSF herpes simplex virus (HSV) polymerase chain reaction (PCR) performed at admission are negative.

Which of the following is the most appropriate management of this patient's acyclovir therapy?

(A) Change intravenous acyclovir to oral acyclovir to complete a 14-day course
(B) Continue intravenous acyclovir pending results of repeat HSV PCR
(C) Continue intravenous acyclovir to complete a 14-day course
(D) Discontinue intravenous acyclovir

Item 62

A 35-year-old man is evaluated in the emergency department for redness and pus that developed near a scratch on his left forearm.

On physical examination, temperature is 37.4 °C (99.4 °F), blood pressure is 140/80 mm Hg, pulse rate is 80/min, and respiration rate is 14/min. A 3 × 2-cm erythematous, warm patch is present over the left forearm with some associated purulent exudate but no fluctuance, drainable abscess, or lymphadenopathy.

Laboratory studies indicate a leukocyte count of 10,000/µL (10×10^9/L) with 70% neutrophils and 30% lymphocytes.

Which of the following is the most appropriate outpatient therapy?

(A) Amoxicillin
(B) Cephalexin
(C) Dicloxacillin
(D) Trimethoprim-sulfamethoxazole

Item 63

A 25-year-old man is evaluated for a 2-week history of purulent drainage from a small opening in a previously healed right lower extremity wound; this was preceded by about 10 days of tenderness and redness at the wound site. Six months ago, the patient had a motorcycle accident in which he sustained an open comminuted fracture of the proximal tibia. Management consisted of surgical debridement and lavage followed by open reduction and internal fixation with a metal plate and screws as well as empiric antibiotic therapy. Culture results during and after surgery were negative.

On physical examination, the patient appears well. Temperature is 37.2 °C (98.9 °F), blood pressure is 120/75 mm Hg, and respiration rate is 12/min. There is a well-healed surgical incision overlying the right tibia except for a 2-mm opening at the distal margin with minimal surrounding erythema and slight purulent drainage. The remainder of the examination is normal.

Swab samples obtained from the wound are sent to the microbiology laboratory for aerobic and anaerobic culture and sensitivity testing. *Proteus mirabilis* and an enterococcal species are isolated from the culture, both susceptible to all antibiotics tested.

Which of the following is the most appropriate next step in management?

(A) Bone biopsy cultures
(B) Intravenous ampicillin-sulbactam
(C) Oral ciprofloxacin and amoxicillin
(D) Technetium 99m–labeled bone scan

Item 64

A 28-year-old man is admitted to the hospital for 3 weeks of increasing dyspnea on exertion, dry cough, pleuritic chest pain, and fever. The patient has been in a monogamous relationship with a male partner for the past 3 years but had multiple partners of both sexes previously.

On physical examination, temperature is 38.6 °C (101.5 °F), blood pressure is 110/66 mm Hg, pulse rate is 112/min, and respiration rate is 24/min. The oropharynx demonstrates scattered white plaques. Lung auscultation discloses diffuse crackles bilaterally. The remainder of the examination is normal.

Arterial blood gas levels with the patient breathing ambient air show a pH of 7.48, P_{CO_2} of 30 mm Hg (4.0 kPa), and P_{O_2} of 62 mm Hg (8.2 kPa). A rapid HIV test is positive. Sputum Gram stain shows few neutrophils, pseudohyphae, and mixed bacteria. A chest radiograph shows bilateral diffuse reticular infiltrates.

Which of the following is the most likely diagnosis?

(A) Cytomegalovirus pneumonia
(B) *Mycobacterium avium* complex infection
(C) *Pneumocystis jirovecii* pneumonia
(D) Pulmonary candidiasis

Item 65

A 40-year-old man is admitted to the emergency department with a 1-day history of headache and epistaxis. He has had type 1 diabetes mellitus requiring insulin for 30 years and two episodes of ketoacidosis in the past year.

On physical examination, temperature is 36.0 °C (96.8 °F), blood pressure is 100/70 mm Hg, pulse rate is 120/min, and respiration rate is 22/min. There is mild proptosis of the right eye with periorbital edema and a black eschar on the inferior turbinate of the right nostril. Skin examination shows no other lesions. The remainder of the examination is normal.

Laboratory studies are consistent with diabetic ketoacidosis. Blood cultures are negative. A chest radiograph is normal.

CT of the head reveals mild proptosis of the right eye and right ethmoid and maxillary sinusitis with bony erosion. Intravenous amphotericin B is instituted.

In addition to treatment of this patient's diabetic ketoacidosis and institution of antifungal therapy, which of the following is the most important next step in treatment?

(A) Add piperacillin-tazobactam
(B) Add posaconazole
(C) Administer hyperbaric oxygen treatment
(D) Perform surgical debridement

Item 66

A 35-year-old man is evaluated in the emergency department following the acute onset of bilateral lower extremity paralysis. The patient has a history of injection drug use. He was well until 5 days ago, when he developed severe pain in the middle of his back that was not relieved by topical heat or ibuprofen. Today, he was unable to walk and was brought to the hospital by ambulance.

On physical examination, temperature is 37.8 °C (100.0 °F), blood pressure is 120/74 mm Hg, pulse rate is 98/min, and respiration rate is 14/min. Neurologic examination findings show 0/5 motor strength in both lower extremities and absent sensation below the level of the umbilicus.

Emergent MRI of the spine reveals evidence of osteomyelitis involving the lower half of the T10 vertebral body and the upper half of the T11 vertebral body, diskitis at the T10-T11 disk space, and an epidural mass compressing the spinal cord.

Blood cultures are obtained.

Which of the following is the most appropriate next step in management?

(A) Antimicrobial therapy
(B) CT-guided bone biopsy
(C) Emergent radiation therapy
(D) Emergent surgical decompression

Item 67

A 64-year-old woman is hospitalized for a 24-hour history of diffuse erythroderma, nausea, vomiting, and a rapidly progressive left lower leg soft tissue infection associated with fever, tachycardia, and hypotension.

An emergent MRI of the left lower leg is compatible with superficial fascial necrosis. Empiric broad-spectrum antibiotics are initiated, and emergent surgical débridement and fasciotomy are performed.

Gram stain reveals gram-positive cocci in short chains ultimately identified as *Streptococcus pyogenes*.

Which of the following precautions is most appropriate for this patient to prevent spread of this organism?

(A) Airborne precautions
(B) Contact precautions
(C) Droplet precautions
(D) Standard precautions only

Item 68

A 35-year-old man is evaluated during a routine follow-up visit. He was diagnosed with HIV infection 2 years ago. He started combination antiretroviral therapy with tenofovir, emtricitabine, and efavirenz and within 4 months had an undetectable HIV RNA viral load and a normal CD4 cell count. The patient has been adherent to his medication regimen. He is presently asymptomatic, feeling well, and having no problems with his medications.

The physical examination is normal.

Laboratory studies show an HIV RNA viral load of 275 copies/mL, with repeated results indicating 710 copies/mL. The CD4 cell count is normal. The remaining laboratory tests, including complete blood count, serum chemistries, and liver enzymes, are normal.

Which of the following is the most appropriate next step in the management of this patient?

(A) Continue present medication regimen and follow up in 4 weeks

(B) Discontinue present medication regimen and perform resistance testing in 1 week

(C) Discontinue present medication regimen and repeat CD4 cell count and HIV RNA viral load in 4 weeks

(D) Perform viral resistance testing and continue present medication regimen pending results

Item 69

A 20-year-old man is evaluated for a scratch on his right arm from a pet kitten that occurred 3 weeks ago. The patient now has a skin lesion at the inoculation site and painful swelling in the ipsilateral axillary area. He is also experiencing malaise. Medical history is unremarkable.

On physical examination, temperature is 37.2 °C (99.0 °F), blood pressure is 120/80 mm Hg, pulse rate is 80/min, and respiration rate is 14/min. A red papule is present on the biceps area of the right arm, and tender right axillary lymphadenopathy with overlying erythema is noted. The remainder of the examination is normal.

Laboratory studies indicate a leukocyte count of 11,500/µL (11.5×10^9/L) with 83% neutrophils and 17% lymphocytes and a normal metabolic panel.

Which of the following is the most appropriate treatment?

(A) Azithromycin

(B) Dicloxacillin

(C) Itraconazole

(D) Linezolid

Item 70

A 72-year-old man is evaluated for fatigue and weakness of 8 months' duration. The patient is a retired businessman who is an avid gardener and recalls many tick attachments over the past several years. He lives in Texas but has traveled extensively throughout the United States.

The patient was seen in a walk-in clinic 1 week ago and had laboratory testing for Lyme disease. An enzyme-linked immunosorbent assay for *Borrelia burgdorferi* was positive. A Western blot assay was negative for IgG antibodies and positive for IgM antibodies.

On physical examination today, vital signs are normal. Remaining physical examination findings are unremarkable.

An electrocardiogram is normal.

Which of the following is the most appropriate management?

(A) Initiate additional evaluation for fatigue and weakness

(B) Repeat serologic testing for *Borrelia burgdorferi* in 1 month

(C) Treat with ceftriaxone

(D) Treat with doxycycline

Item 71

A 32-year-old woman is evaluated for a 2-day history of dysuria and urinary urgency and frequency and a 1-day history of fever. She has had no nausea or vomiting.

On physical examination, temperature is 38.5 °C (101.3 °F), blood pressure is 120/70 mm Hg, pulse rate is 90/min, and respiration rate is 12/min. There is right flank tenderness on palpation.

A urinalysis shows more than 20 leukocytes/hpf and 4+ bacteria. A pregnancy test is negative.

In addition to obtaining a urine culture, which of the following is the most appropriate empiric treatment?

(A) Ampicillin

(B) Ciprofloxacin

(C) Nitrofurantoin

(D) Trimethoprim-sulfamethoxazole

Item 72

A 55-year-old man undergoes follow-up evaluation for worsened cholesterol levels. He has a history of multidrug-resistant HIV infection, but he has been responding well to his current antiretroviral regimen for the past 6 months. The patient follows a healthy diet and exercise regimen. He currently smokes cigarettes and has no family history of premature coronary artery disease. Medications are tenofovir, emtricitabine, raltegravir, and ritonavir-boosted darunavir.

Physical examination is unremarkable.

Laboratory studies:

Alanine aminotransferase	26 units/L
Aspartate aminotransferase	34 units/L
Cholesterol	
Total	264 mg/dL (6.8 mmol/L)
LDL	170 mg/dL (4.4 mmol/L)
HDL	46 mg/dL (1.2 mmol/L)
Triglycerides	240 mg/dL (2.7 mmol/L)

Which of the following is the most appropriate management?

(A) Encourage strict dietary lipid restriction and recheck lipid panel in 6 months

(B) Start atorvastatin

(C) Start fenofibrate

(D) Start simvastatin

Item 73

A 55-year-old man is evaluated for a 2-day history of fever, headache, and confusion. Medical history is significant for type 2 diabetes mellitus treated with metformin. The patient has no known drug allergies.

On physical examination, temperature is 39.2 °C (102.6 °F), blood pressure is 100/60 mm Hg, pulse rate is 118/min, and respiration rate is 24/min. He is confused but responds to vigorous stimulation. There are no rashes. Neurologic examination findings are nonfocal.

Laboratory studies show a leukocyte count of 22,000/µL (22×10^9/L) with 40% band forms.

CONT.

A CT scan of the head without contrast is normal.

Lumbar puncture is performed. Cerebrospinal fluid (CSF) leukocyte count is 1500/μL (1500 × 10⁶/L) with 95% neutrophils, glucose level is 26 mg/dL (1.4 mmol/L), and protein level is 200 mg/dL (2000 mg/L). A CSF Gram stain is shown.

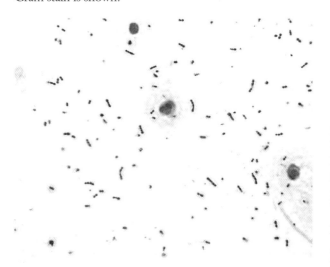

In addition to adjunctive dexamethasone, which of the following antimicrobial regimens should be initiated at this time?

(A) Ampicillin and ceftriaxone
(B) Ceftriaxone
(C) Levofloxacin
(D) Vancomycin and ceftriaxone
(E) Vancomycin and gentamicin

Item 74

A 27-year-old man is hospitalized for fatigue, fever, and chills that developed 48 hours ago after his return from a camping trip in New Mexico. On the day of admission, he developed shortness of breath, pleuritic chest pain, and a productive cough with blood-streaked sputum. His medical history is otherwise unremarkable, and he takes no medications.

On physical examination, he is in moderate respiratory distress. Temperature is 38.6 °C (101.5 °F), blood pressure is 110/65 mm Hg, and pulse rate is 110/min. Oxygen saturation with the patient breathing ambient air is 85%. Cardiopulmonary examination discloses diffuse crackles bilaterally and tachycardia. The remainder of the physical examination is normal.

Laboratory studies indicate a leukocyte count of 17,500/μL (17.5 × 10⁹/L) with 75% band forms and normal serum electrolyte levels and kidney and liver chemistry results. A chest radiograph shows diffuse infiltrates bilaterally.

Microscopic examination of the blood obtained on admission reveals gram-negative bipolar-staining bacilli.

Which of the following is the most likely infectious agent?

(A) *Legionella pneumophila*
(B) *Pseudomonas aeruginosa*

(C) *Salmonella enteritidis*
(D) *Yersinia pestis*

Item 75

A 22-year-old woman is evaluated for an 8-day history of escalating fever, abdominal pain, headache, sore throat, dry cough, and initial constipation followed by frequent loose, watery stools. She returned 2 weeks ago from rural India where she spent the month of July. In preparation for travel, she took atovaquone-proguanil for malaria prophylaxis and had ciprofloxacin in the event of a diarrheal illness. Two weeks before her trip, she received a tetanus, diphtheria, and acellular pertussis vaccination and live oral vaccine for typhoid fever. She has received a complete hepatitis A and B virus vaccine series. She is otherwise healthy and takes no medications.

On physical examination, temperature is 39.5 °C (103.1 °F), blood pressure is 106/72 mm Hg, pulse rate is 64/min, and respiration rate is 16/min. She has a faint salmon-colored maculopapular rash on the trunk. Cardiopulmonary examination is normal. Splenomegaly but no palpable tenderness is noted on abdominal examination.

Laboratory studies:

Hemoglobin	10.5 g/dL (105 g/L)
Leukocyte count	3150/μL (3.15 × 10⁹/L) with 55% neutrophils, 42% lymphocytes, and 3% monocytes
Platelet count	106,000/μL (106 x 10⁹/L)
Alanine aminotransferase	167 units/L
Aspartate aminotransferase	98 units/L
Total bilirubin	2.4 mg/dL (41.0 μmol/L)
Sodium	130 meq/L (130 mmol/L)

Which of the following is the most likely diagnosis?

(A) Brucellosis
(B) Leishmaniasis
(C) Malaria
(D) Typhoid fever

Item 76

A 42-year-old man is evaluated in the emergency department for a 3-day history of dyspnea and dizziness. He is training for a marathon and initially attributed his symptoms to overexertion and dehydration. Despite refraining from training and increasing his fluid intake, his symptoms have persisted. He has no chest pain, fever, or cough. Medical history is unremarkable. The patient is a college professor in Rhode Island. He has not noted any tick attachments or antecedent rash.

On physical examination, he appears well. Temperature is normal, blood pressure is 100/60 mm Hg, and pulse rate is 35/min. Other than bradycardia, the remaining physical examination findings are unremarkable.

Results of initial laboratory studies show a normal complete blood count, metabolic panel, and cardiac enzyme

CONT.

measurements. The admission electrocardiographic rhythm strip is shown.

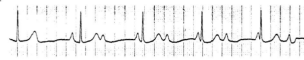

Serologic testing for *Borrelia burgdorferi* is performed. Both the initial enzyme-linked immunosorbent assay and a confirmatory Western blot assay are positive.

Which of the following is the most appropriate initial treatment?

(A) Intravenous ceftriaxone
(B) Oral cefuroxime
(C) Oral doxycycline
(D) Placement of a permanent pacemaker
(E) Observation

Item 77

A 25-year-old woman is evaluated for redness that developed over her right leg at the site of a mosquito bite. She is otherwise healthy and takes no medications.

On physical examination, temperature is 37.2 °C (99.0 °F), blood pressure is 120/70 mm Hg, pulse rate is 70/min, and respiration rate is 14/min. There is an erythematous 3 × 3-cm patch on the right thigh. The area is warm to the touch with no evidence of purulence, fluctuance, crepitus, or lymphadenopathy.

Which of the following is the most appropriate empiric outpatient therapy?

(A) Cephalexin
(B) Doxycycline
(C) Fluconazole
(D) Metronidazole
(E) Trimethoprim-sulfamethoxazole

Item 78

A 46-year-old woman is evaluated before undergoing a dental cleaning procedure involving deep scaling. She has a history of mitral valve prolapse without regurgitation and also had methicillin-resistant *Staphylococcus aureus* (MRSA) aortic valve endocarditis 10 years ago treated successfully with antibiotics. The patient notes an allergy to penicillin characterized by hypotension, hives, and wheezing. The remainder of the history is noncontributory.

On physical examination, vital signs are normal. Cardiopulmonary examination discloses a late systolic click. The remainder of the examination is normal.

Which of the following is the most appropriate prophylactic regimen for this patient before her dental procedure?

(A) Amoxicillin
(B) Cephalexin
(C) Clindamycin

(D) Vancomycin
(E) No prophylaxis

Item 79

A 36-year-old man is admitted to the emergency department for a 1-week history of fever, chills, and cough productive of yellow sputum and a 2-day history of progressive dyspnea.

The patient experiences progressive respiratory distress in the emergency department and is intubated and placed on mechanical ventilation. Two sets of blood cultures are obtained, and empiric antibiotic therapy is begun.

On physical examination, temperature is 38.8 °C (101.8 °F), blood pressure is 85/50 mm Hg, pulse rate is 130/min, and respiration rate is 28/min. BMI is 28. Bronchial breath sounds are heard over the left and right lower lung fields.

Laboratory studies indicate a hemoglobin level of 10.7 g/dL (107 g/L), a leukocyte count of 4000/µL (4.0 × 10^9/L), and a platelet count of 97,000/µL (97 × 10^9/L).

A chest radiograph shows findings consistent with consolidation in the left and right lower lobes and patchy airspace opacity in the right middle lobe.

In addition to Gram stain and culture of an endotracheal aspirate, which of the following is the most appropriate next step in the evaluation?

(A) Bronchoscopy with quantitative cultures
(B) *Legionella* and *Streptococcus pneumoniae* urine antigen assays
(C) *Legionella* serologic testing
(D) No further testing

Item 80

A 65-year-old man is evaluated for a 1-day history of left arm and left leg weakness. His wife has also noted some asymmetry of his face. Medical history is significant for hypertension and type 2 diabetes mellitus. Medications are lisinopril and metformin.

On physical examination, temperature is 37.2 °C (99.0 °F), blood pressure is 170/100 mm Hg, pulse rate is 90/min, and respiration rate is 14/min. Neurologic examination findings include a central cranial nerve VII palsy on the left, 2/5 motor strength of the left upper extremity, and 4/5 motor strength of the left lower extremity. There are no sensory deficits. Hyperreflexia of the left arm and leg is noted, and the left plantar response is positive.

Laboratory studies indicate a normal complete blood count and serum chemistry studies, including liver chemistry studies and kidney function tests.

MRI of the brain with contrast shows a 3-cm ring-enhancing lesion in the right parietal region with surrounding edema and a midline shift to the left.

Which of the following diagnostic studies should be performed next?

(A) Stereotactic CT-guided aspiration of the lesion
(B) CT scan of the chest, abdomen, and pelvis
(C) Lumbar puncture
(D) Whole-body PET scan

Item 81

A 61-year-old man undergoes preoperative evaluation before coronary artery bypass surgery and aortic valve replacement surgery, both scheduled for tomorrow. He has been hospitalized in the cardiac intensive care unit (ICU) for 4 days after collapsing and experiencing cardiogenic shock. He was intubated in the field with a standard, non-silver-coated endotracheal tube and placed on mechanical ventilation in the ICU. He is being treated with both paralytic and sedating medications, in addition to a proton pump inhibitor and intravenous nitroglycerin.

On physical examination, the patient's condition has stabilized and he is afebrile. No attempts are made to wean him from the ventilator because of his impending surgery and his heart condition.

Which of the following is the most appropriate measure to prevent ventilator-associated pneumonia in this patient?

(A) Bathe patient daily in chlorhexidine
(B) Begin preoperative antimicrobial prophylaxis immediately and continue until extubation
(C) Maintain the head of bed above a 30° angle
(D) Perform tracheotomy and remove endotracheal tube
(E) Replace endotracheal tube with a silver-coated endotracheal tube

Item 82

A 55-year-old woman is evaluated for a 1-day history of diarrhea. She has had four liquid stools in the past 24 hours without visible mucus or blood. The patient does not have fever, nausea, vomiting, abdominal pain, or cramping. She returned yesterday from a 2-week trip to Guatemala, where she traveled to rural areas, swam in a local river, and brushed her teeth with tap water.

On physical examination, she is thin and in no acute distress. Vital signs, including temperature, are normal. She has no rash. Her mucous membranes are moist. Bowel sounds are mildly hyperactive, but no focal abdominal tenderness or peritoneal signs are present. Rectal examination is nontender with heme-negative brown stool in the vault.

Which of the following stool studies should be done next?

(A) Culture for bacteria
(B) Culture for viruses
(C) Examination for ova and parasites
(D) Testing for fecal leukocytes
(E) No diagnostic testing is indicated

Item 83

A 26-year-old man is admitted to the emergency department with a 3-day history of dysuria with yellow urethral discharge.

On physical examination, temperature is 37.3 °C (99.1 °F), blood pressure is 120/70 mm Hg, pulse rate is 82/min, and respiration rate is 12/min. There are purulent secretions noted at the urethral meatus. No tenderness of the epididymis, spermatic cords, or testes is noted.

A Gram stain of the urethral discharge is shown.

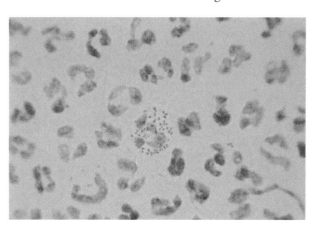

Which of the following is the most appropriate treatment?

(A) Azithromycin
(B) Cefoxitin
(C) Ceftriaxone and azithromycin
(D) Ciprofloxacin and azithromycin

Item 84

A 30-year-old woman is evaluated in the emergency department for a right lower extremity skin infection. She works in a nursing facility where she experienced a minor laceration of the right shin 3 days ago. She initially applied a topical sterile dressing but developed purulent drainage from her wound with increasing surrounding tenderness and a fever over the past 24 hours.

On physical examination, temperature is 38.5 °C (101.3 °F), blood pressure is 125/75 mm Hg, pulse rate is 90/min, and respiration rate is 18/min. An area of purulent cellulitis measuring approximately 4 × 5 cm is present over the right lower extremity surrounding a 1.5-cm laceration. There is no fluctuance. Cardiopulmonary examination is normal. No costovertebral angle tenderness or signs of meningeal irritation are present.

Laboratory studies indicate a leukocyte count of 14,000/µL (14 × 10⁹/L) with 90% neutrophils and 10% lymphocytes. Urinalysis is normal. A radiograph of the right lower extremity shows only soft tissue swelling.

Which of the following β-lactam antibiotics is most appropriate for treatment of this infection?

(A) Ceftaroline
(B) Ceftriaxone
(C) Meropenem
(D) Oxacillin

Item 85

A 65-year-old man undergoes a routine examination. He feels well. He has a history of hypertension treated with lisinopril. The remainder of the history is noncontributory.

On physical examination, temperature is 37.2 °C (99.0 °F), blood pressure is 124/84 mm Hg, pulse rate is 86/min, and respiration rate is 22/min. Physical examination is notable for a soft, nontender enlarged prostate without nodules.

As part of a health insurance evaluation, urinalysis and culture are performed. Urinalysis shows 1+ protein and trace leukocyte esterase, and the urine culture grows more than 10^5 colony-forming units of *Escherichia coli* susceptible to ciprofloxacin and trimethoprim-sulfamethoxazole.

Which of the following is the most appropriate management?

(A) Ciprofloxacin
(B) Kidney ultrasound
(C) Repeat urinalysis and urine culture
(D) Trimethoprim-sulfamethoxazole
(E) No further evaluation or treatment necessary

Item 86

A 25-year-old woman is evaluated in the emergency department for anaphylaxis following a transfusion of packed red blood cells after trauma resulting from a motor vehicle collision 3 weeks ago. She was diagnosed with systemic lupus erythematosus after a pregnancy 2 years ago. She has a history of eczema since childhood as well as a history of recurrent sinopulmonary and urinary tract infections. Six months ago, she was diagnosed with chronic, unexplained diarrhea.

On physical examination, temperature is 37.5 °C (99.5 °F), blood pressure is 112/60 mm Hg, pulse rate is 80/min, and respiration rate is 14/min. The skin is pruritic and red with poorly demarcated, eczematous, crusted, papulovesicular plaques and excoriations located in the antecubital and popliteal fossae. The remainder of her physical examination is normal.

Laboratory studies show a leukocyte count of 8000/μL (8.0×10^9/L).

A chest radiograph is normal.

Which of the following is the most likely diagnosis?

(A) C1-inhibitor deficiency
(B) Terminal complement deficiency
(C) Properdin deficiency
(D) Selective IgA deficiency

Item 87

A 56-year-old woman is evaluated in the emergency department in May for a 2-day history of fever, myalgia, and headache. She works as a horse trainer on a farm in Oklahoma and recalls removing at least three ticks from her skin in the past 2 weeks.

On physical examination, the patient appears ill. Temperature is 39.3 °C (102.7 °F); other vital signs are normal. There is no nuchal rigidity, lymphadenopathy, or rash. Remaining physical examination findings are nonfocal.

Laboratory studies:

Leukocyte count	14,600/μL (14.6×10^9/L) with 87% neutrophils
Platelet count	136,000/μL (136×10^9/L)
Alanine aminotransferase	177 units/L
Aspartate aminotransferase	211 units/L
Alkaline phosphatase	114 units/L
Creatinine	1.4 mg/dL (123.7 μmol/L)

Serologic testing *for Rickettsia rickettsii*, *Anaplasma phagocytophilum*, and *Ehrlichia chaffeensis* is performed.

Which of the following is the most appropriate next step in the management of this patient?

(A) Begin empiric amoxicillin
(B) Begin empiric doxycycline
(C) Withhold antibiotics unless a petechial skin rash develops
(D) Withhold antibiotics while awaiting serologic results

Item 88

A 28-year-old woman who is 3 months pregnant undergoes evaluation in September. She is a nurse and works at a local hospital. There is an influenza A virus outbreak in the community, and she wants to prevent infection during her pregnancy.

On physical examination, temperature is 36.5 °C (97.7 °F), blood pressure is 110/70 mm Hg, pulse rate is 88/min, and respiration rate is 14/min. The remainder of the examination is normal.

Which of the following is the most appropriate influenza virus prophylaxis for this patient?

(A) Amantadine
(B) Live attenuated intranasal influenza vaccine
(C) Oseltamivir
(D) Trivalent inactivated influenza vaccine

Item 89

A 22-year-old man is evaluated for a 1-day history of fever, rash, and abdominal pain. He has a 5-year history of recurrent episodes of these symptoms plus occasional joint pain in the knee or hip that resolves spontaneously after several days.

On physical examination, temperature is 38.6 °C (101.5 °F), blood pressure is 120/70 mm Hg, pulse rate is 70/min, and respiration rate is 14/min. A sharply demarcated, tender, raised, erythematous, warm rash is present over the dorsa of both feet and both anterior legs that extends approximately 10 cm in diameter. There is no inguinal lymphadenopathy or fluctuance, ulcer, or purulence. Abdominal examination discloses normal bowel sounds and minimal tenderness to palpation. Distal pulses are normal.

Laboratory studies indicate a leukocyte count of 13,000/μL (13×10^9/L) with 80% neutrophils, 17% lymphocytes, and 3% monocytes and a platelet count of 400,000/μL (400×10^9/L).

Which of the following is the most likely diagnosis?

(A) Erythromelalgia
(B) Familial Mediterranean fever
(C) Staphylococcal cellulitis
(D) Sweet syndrome

Item 90

A 32-year-old woman who is 41 weeks pregnant is admitted to the hospital for an elective cesarean delivery. The woman is a known carrier of group B *Streptococcus* as evidenced by a vaginal/rectal surveillance culture obtained at gestational week 36. She has gestational diabetes that has been well controlled throughout pregnancy with diet only. She also has a 10-pack-year smoking history and continues to smoke approximately 5 cigarettes daily. Her only medication is a daily prenatal vitamin.

Physical examination, including vital signs, is normal.

Which of the following is the most appropriate measure for preventing surgical site infection in this patient?

(A) Decolonization of group B *Streptococcus* vaginal/rectal carriage before surgery
(B) Prophylactic antibiotics for 72 hours after incision
(C) Shaving of the surgical field
(D) Surgical antimicrobial prophylaxis 30 to 60 minutes before initial incision

Item 91

A 32-year-old man undergoes follow-up evaluation for recurrent genital herpes simplex virus infection. His most recent outbreak was the third episode within 8 months and consisted of painful vesicles on the penile shaft and perianal area. The lesions resolved after acyclovir therapy, which is consistent with his response to treatment of previous episodes. He was diagnosed with HIV infection 10 years ago and discontinued antiretroviral therapy (ART) 1 year ago because of adverse effects. His last CD4 cell count was 30/µL. His only medication is trimethoprim-sulfamethoxazole.

On physical examination, temperature is normal, blood pressure is 130/70 mm Hg, pulse rate is 80/min, and respiration rate is 14/min. He presently has no active lesions.

In addition to encouraging this patient to restart his antiretroviral therapy, which of the following is the most appropriate therapy to prevent symptomatic genital herpes simplex virus reactivation?

(A) Acyclovir
(B) Cidofovir
(C) Foscarnet
(D) Valganciclovir

Item 92

A 50-year-old woman is admitted to the emergency department for a 2-day history of fever and chills, dyspnea, hemoptysis, and left-sided pleuritic chest pain. She underwent allogeneic hematopoietic stem cell transplantation for myelodysplastic syndrome 6 months ago; until 2 days ago she had been doing well. Her medications are trimethoprim-sulfamethoxazole, acyclovir, prednisone, and cyclosporine.

On physical examination, temperature is 39.3 °C (102.7 °F), blood pressure is 110/68 mm Hg, pulse rate is 122/min, and respiration rate is 24/min. Dullness to percussion, crackles, and egophony are heard at the left lung base. The remainder of the examination is normal.

Laboratory studies show a leukocyte count of 4400/µL (4.4×10^9/L), a platelet count of 155,000/µL (155×10^9/L), and a hematocrit of 30%.

Chest radiograph shows a dense infiltrate in the left lower lobe.

Infection with which of the following is the most likely diagnosis?

(A) *Candida krusei*
(B) Cytomegalovirus
(C) *Pneumocystis jirovecii*
(D) *Streptococcus pneumoniae*

Item 93

A 27-year-old man is evaluated in the emergency department for a 2-day history of fever, weakness, and dark-colored urine. The patient returned yesterday from a 2-week camping trip to Cape Cod, Massachusetts. While there, he developed a target-shaped lesion on his thigh. He was evaluated at a walk-in clinic, where early-stage Lyme disease was diagnosed. He is currently on day 10 of a 14-day course of doxycycline.

On physical examination, temperature is 38.5 °C (101.3 °F), blood pressure is 122/66 mm Hg, and pulse rate is 118/min. The previously noted lesion on the thigh has resolved. He is jaundiced. The liver is tender and is palpable 5 cm below the costophrenic margin.

Laboratory studies:

Hemoglobin	8.4 g/dL (84 g/L)
Reticulocyte count	10%
Leukocyte count	12,600/µL (12.6×10^9/L)
Platelet count	110,000/µL (110×10^9/L)
Lactate dehydrogenase	675 units/L
Total bilirubin	8.3 mg/dL (145.3 µmol/L)

Which of the following pathogens is most likely causing this patient's current findings?

(A) *Anaplasma phagocytophilum*
(B) *Babesia microti*
(C) *Borrelia burgdorferi*
(D) *Rickettsia rickettsii*
(E) West Nile virus

Item 94

A 58-year-old man is admitted to the emergency department with a 2-day history of fever, chills, cough, progressively worsening dyspnea, and left-sided pleuritic chest pain. He has no other medical problems and takes no medications.

Pneumonia is diagnosed, and two sets of blood cultures and a urine sample for pneumococcal and *Legionella* antigens are obtained. Treatment with cefotaxime and azithromycin is begun. The patient is admitted to the medical ward.

On physical examination, temperature is 38.2 °C (100.8 °F), blood pressure is 130/80 mm Hg, pulse rate is 115/min, and respiration rate is 28/min. Oxygen saturation is 87% with the patient breathing ambient air. Markedly diminished breath sounds are heard in the left lung base with dullness to percussion.

Chest radiograph shows consolidation of the left lower lobe and lingula with a pleural effusion to the midpoint of the left hemithorax on upright images.

Which of the following is the most appropriate management of this patient?

(A) Add metronidazole to ceftriaxone and azithromycin
(B) Change antimicrobial therapy to cefepime and vancomycin
(C) Diagnostic ultrasound-guided thoracentesis if no improvement within 24 to 48 hours
(D) Immediate ultrasound-guided thoracentesis

Item 95

A 33-year-old woman undergoes routine evaluation. She feels well but inquires about HIV screening because she has had several lifetime partners, but within monogamous relationships and always using condoms. She has had no known sex partners with HIV infection and reports that none of her partners were known injection drug users or men who have sex with men. She has no history of sexually transmitted infections, has never been pregnant, and is sexually active only with her husband of 8 years. Her husband is healthy but has never been tested for HIV infection. Her only medication is an oral contraceptive.

Physical examination is normal.

Which of the following is the most appropriate next step in the management of this patient?

(A) HIV antibody enzyme immunoassay
(B) HIV antibody Western blot assay
(C) HIV nucleic acid amplification test
(D) No testing indicated

Item 96

A 36-year-old woman is evaluated for fever and headache 7 days after undergoing a craniotomy for removal of a mass lesion in her right frontal lobe. Pathologic examination demonstrated a malignant astrocytoma. The patient had been doing well before development of the current symptoms.

On physical examination, temperature is 38.9 °C (102.0 °F); other vital signs are normal. Her neck is stiff. The remaining physical examination findings are normal.

Laboratory studies show a leukocyte count of 9600/µL (9.6 × 10⁹/L) with a normal differential.

MRI of the brain reveals postoperative changes but only minimal cerebral edema in the area of the surgery. Lumbar puncture is performed.

Cerebrospinal fluid analysis:
Leukocyte count	450/µL (450 × 10⁶/L)
Erythrocyte count	100/µL (100 × 10⁶/L)
Glucose	45 mg/dL (2.5 mmol/L)
Protein	500 mg/dL (5000 mg/L)
Gram stain	Negative

In addition to vancomycin, which of the following empiric antimicrobial agents should be administered now?

(A) Ceftriaxone
(B) Gentamicin
(C) Meropenem
(D) Metronidazole
(E) Trimethoprim-sulfamethoxazole

Item 97

A 70-year-old woman undergoes evaluation. She will be traveling to Mexico for vacation, visiting several Mexican villages with accommodations at local inns. In preparation for her travel, she has received the full hepatitis A vaccine series and has been instructed on protection against mosquitoes and other biting insects. She is current with all age-appropriate recommended vaccinations. Medical history is significant for intermittent flares of inflammatory bowel disease for which she takes 5-aminosalicylic acid. She is otherwise healthy and takes no other medications.

Physical examination, including vital signs, is normal.

Because of her underlying gastrointestinal condition, the patient is concerned about developing a diarrheal illness during her travel.

Which of the following will be most helpful in reducing this patient's risk for travelers' diarrhea?

(A) Avoidance of tap water
(B) Prophylactic bismuth subsalicylate
(C) Prophylactic *Lactobacillus* probiotic
(D) Prophylactic loperamide
(E) Prophylactic rifaximin

Item 98

A 22-year-old man is evaluated for diarrhea and weight loss. The patient has a 3-week history of foul-smelling, large-volume, watery stools associated with abdominal bloating. There is no visible blood or mucus in the stools. He reports a 4.5-kg (10-lb) weight loss, which he attributes to a poor appetite. One month before symptoms developed, he took a 2-week hiking trip along the Appalachian Trail, where he slept in primitive camp sites without running water. His girlfriend, who accompanied him on the trip, is well.

On physical examination, the patient appears thin but is in no acute distress. Vital signs are normal. Abdominal examination discloses high-pitched, increased bowel sounds and diffuse tenderness to palpation, without peritoneal signs.

Results of a stool examination are negative for occult blood and fecal leukocytes.

Which of the following stool studies is most likely to be diagnostic?

(A) Stool assay for *Giardia* antigen
(B) Stool culture for bacteria
(C) Stool examination for ova and parasites
(D) Stool sample for modified acid-fast staining for *Cryptosporidium*

Item 99

A 19-year-old man is evaluated in the emergency department for a 10-day history of fever, cervical lymphadenopathy, malaise and fatigue, sore throat, headache, and nausea, but no vomiting, diarrhea, abdominal pain, nasal congestion, or cough. He had a rash a few days ago that has resolved. He is sexually active with both men and women and does not use condoms.

On physical examination, temperature is 38.1 °C (100.6 °F), blood pressure is 110/88 mm Hg, pulse rate is 96/min, and respiration rate is 16/min. He appears uncomfortable but is not in distress. Significant lymphadenopathy is noted in the cervical, axillary, and inguinal regions. The oropharynx is erythematous with mildly enlarged tonsils but no exudate. Sclerae and conjunctivae are clear, and the skin is without rash. The remainder of the examination, including cardiac, joint, abdominal, and genital findings, is unremarkable.

Results of the heterophile antibody test, rapid streptococcal antigen test, HIV enzyme immunoassay, and rapid plasma reagin test are negative.

Which of the following is the most appropriate diagnostic test to perform next?

(A) CD4 cell count
(B) HIV nucleic acid amplification test
(C) HIV Western blot assay
(D) Repeat HIV enzyme immunoassay

Item 100

A 32-year-old woman who is 5 months pregnant undergoes evaluation before international travel. The patient is a photojournalist, and in 3 weeks, she will be traveling to a rural area in Kenya, Africa, on assignment for 10 days. The patient takes a prenatal vitamin.

Physical examination, including vital signs, is normal. The patient is given advice on mosquito bite avoidance and insect repellent (DEET).

Which of the following is the most appropriate malaria chemoprophylaxis of this patient?

(A) Atovaquone-proguanil
(B) Chloroquine
(C) Doxycycline
(D) Mefloquine

Item 101

A 36-year-old man who was admitted to the intensive care unit for treatment of multiple traumatic injuries sustained in a motor vehicle accident is diagnosed with ventilator-associated pneumonia.

On physical examination, temperature is 38.3 °C (101.0 °F), blood pressure is 130/88 mm Hg, pulse rate is 108/min, and respiration rate is 22/min. Breath sounds reveal bilateral basilar crackles. The remainder of the physical examination, consistent with his history of multiple trauma-related injuries, is otherwise noncontributory.

A chest radiograph reveals bilateral lower lobe infiltrates. A quantitative bronchoalveolar lavage culture grows methicillin-resistant *Staphylococcus aureus* with susceptibilities to vancomycin, daptomycin, linezolid, rifampin, and tigecycline. Two sets of blood cultures are negative.

Vancomycin is initiated, and on hospital day 3, the patient develops an urticarial rash. The patient's clinical status has remained unchanged.

In addition to discontinuing vancomycin, which of the following is the most appropriate treatment?

(A) Daptomycin
(B) Linezolid
(C) Rifampin
(D) Tigecycline

Item 102

A 60-year-old man is evaluated in the emergency department for swelling and erythema of the right leg with associated fever.

On physical examination, temperature is 38.1 °C (100.6 °F), blood pressure is 135/85 mm Hg, pulse rate is 99/min, and respiration rate is 16/min. BMI is 28. An area of cellulitis measuring 4 × 3 cm is present on the distal right lower extremity with associated tenderness, warmth, and edema but without necrosis, purulent exudate, fluctuance, or lymphadenopathy. Tinea pedis infection is found between several toes of both feet. The remainder of the physical examination is normal.

Laboratory studies indicate a leukocyte count of 12,000/μL (12×10^9/L) with 80% neutrophils, 18% lymphocytes, and 2% monocytes. A metabolic panel is normal. Topical clotrimazole is prescribed for the tinea pedis infection.

The patient refuses hospital admission.

Which of the following is the most appropriate outpatient therapy?

(A) Clindamycin
(B) Doxycycline
(C) Rifampin
(D) Trimethoprim-sulfamethoxazole

Item 103

A 68-year-old man is admitted to the emergency department for a 3-day history of cough and increasing dyspnea. He was previously healthy and takes no medications.

On physical examination, temperature is 38.6 °C (101.5 °F), blood pressure is 145/90 mm Hg, pulse rate is 100/min, and respiration rate is 30/min. Oxygen saturation is 95% with the patient breathing ambient air. There are crackles in the right lower posterior lung field. The remainder of the physical examination is normal.

Laboratory studies:

Hemoglobin	12.2 g/dL (122 g/L)
Leukocyte count	10,700/µL (10.7 × 10⁹/L)
Platelet count	210,000/µL (210 × 10⁹/L)
Blood urea nitrogen	25 mg/dL (8.9 mmol/L)
Creatinine	1.0 mg/dL (88.4 µmol/L)
Glucose	110 mg/dL (6.1 mmol/L)
Electrolytes	Normal

Chest radiograph shows right lower lobe airspace disease.

Results of blood cultures, sputum Gram stain, and pneumococcal urine antigen assays are pending.

Which of the following is the most appropriate management of this patient?

(A) Administer a single dose of empiric intravenous antibiotic therapy and discharge on oral antibiotic therapy

(B) Begin empiric antibiotic therapy and admit to the intensive care unit

(C) Begin empiric antibiotic therapy and admit to the medical ward

(D) Discharge and prescribe oral antibiotic therapy

Item 104

A 30-year-old man is evaluated for a 3-month history of fever, night sweats, and headache. The patient has a history of injection drug use and is currently incarcerated.

On physical examination, temperature is 38.3 °C (101.0 °F), blood pressure is 110/65 mm Hg, pulse rate is 95/min, and respiration rate is 20/min. He is oriented but lethargic. Cardiopulmonary and neurologic examinations are normal.

The leukocyte count is 15,000/µL (15 × 10⁹/L) with 70% neutrophils, 20% lymphocytes, and 10% monocytes, and the serum albumin level is 2.3 g/dL (23 g/L). The remaining metabolic panel and results of urinalysis are normal.

Lumbar puncture is performed. Opening pressure is 250 mm H₂O. Cerebrospinal fluid (CSF) examination shows a cell count of 400/µL (400 × 10⁶/L) with 95% lymphocytes, a protein level of 200 mg/dL (2000 mg/L), and a glucose level of 20 mg/dL (1.1 mmol/L). CSF polymerase chain reaction is positive for *Mycobacterium tuberculosis*, and CSF culture grows *M. tuberculosis*. Blood culture specimens show no growth. A CT scan of the head reveals basilar meningeal enhancement.

Treatment with isoniazid, rifampin, pyrazinamide, and ethambutol and corticosteroids is begun. Mycobacteria are fully susceptible to all four antituberculous agents.

Which of the following is the most appropriate treatment duration?

(A) 4 to 6 months
(B) 9 to 12 months
(C) 15 to 18 months
(D) 24 months

Item 105

A 29-year-old man is evaluated in the hospital 2 weeks after allogeneic hematopoietic stem cell transplantation for acute myeloid leukemia. He has had a dry cough and persistent fever for 3 days despite taking antibiotic agents. The patient and donor were both seropositive for cytomegalovirus. His medications are imipenem, ciprofloxacin, vancomycin, acyclovir, and fluconazole.

On physical examination, temperature is 38.5 °C (101.3 °F), blood pressure is 122/74 mm Hg, pulse rate is 98/min, and respiration rate is 18/min. Skin examination shows some petechiae but no lesions or rash. Cardiopulmonary and abdominal examinations are normal. The intravenous catheter site is without erythema or drainage.

Laboratory studies show a hematocrit of 24%, a leukocyte count of 100/µL (0.10 × 10⁹/L), and a platelet count of 15,000/µL (15 × 10⁹/L). Chest radiograph discloses scattered opacities. A noncontrast CT scan of the chest demonstrates nodular infiltrates without cavitation.

Which of the following is the most likely infectious cause of this patient's fever?

(A) *Aspergillus*
(B) Cytomegalovirus
(C) Mucormycosis (zygomycosis)
(D) *Pneumocystis jirovecii*

Item 106

A 26-year-old woman undergoes follow-up evaluation after completing an appropriate antibiotic course for a urinary tract infection (UTI) diagnosed 3 days ago; she is currently asymptomatic. She has had five similar episodes in the past year, the symptoms for all of which began after sexual intercourse and responded well to antibiotic treatment. She has increased her fluid intake and routinely voids after sexual intercourse. She is sexually active with one partner and does not use spermicides. Her only form of birth control is an intrauterine device, which has been in place for 6 months. She is otherwise healthy, with no medical problems and no history of sexually transmitted infections. She currently takes no medications.

Physical examination, including vital signs, is normal.

Which of the following is the most appropriate next step to reduce this patient's risk for UTIs?

(A) Chronic suppressive therapy with trimethoprim-sulfamethoxazole

(B) Drinking cranberry juice

(C) Postcoital antimicrobial prophylaxis

(D) Removal of intrauterine device

(E) Using a spermicide prior to intercourse

Item 107

A 28-year-old man undergoes follow-up evaluation and review of his most recent routine laboratory studies. He has asymptomatic HIV infection and is adherent to his antiretroviral therapy regimen. He has had two sexual partners within the past 6 months. Although he has communicated his HIV status to both partners, he still has not used condoms consistently. His only medication is efavirenz-emtricitabine-tenofovir. He has no medication allergies.

Physical examination is normal with the exception of shotty axillary and inguinal lymphadenopathy, unchanged from previous examinations. His neurologic examination is normal.

A comprehensive metabolic profile is normal. The CD4 cell count is 680 cells/µL, HIV RNA viral load is undetectable, and the serum rapid plasma reagin titer is 1:16 compared with negative results 6 months ago. Results of serum fluorescent treponemal antibody absorption testing are positive.

Which of the following is the most appropriate treatment?

(A) Aqueous crystalline penicillin G intravenously for 10 days

(B) Intramuscular benzathine penicillin G weekly for three doses

(C) Oral doxycycline for 14 days

(D) Single-dose intramuscular benzathine penicillin G

Item 108

A 27-year-old woman is evaluated for a 2-day history of fever, hemoptysis, and chest pain. She was recently diagnosed with acute myeloid leukemia and completed her last course of chemotherapy 2 weeks ago. Her course has been complicated by profound neutropenia, thrombocytopenia, and fever that initially resolved after treatment with cefepime and vancomycin.

On physical examination, temperature is 38.9 °C (102.0 °F), blood pressure is 110/70 mm Hg, pulse rate is 100/min, and respiration rate is 20/min. A friction rub is heard at the left posterior lung base.

Laboratory studies indicate a leukocyte count of 100/µL (0.10×10^9/L). Serum galactomannan antigen immunoassay results are positive, consistent with a diagnosis of invasive pulmonary aspergillosis.

A chest radiograph shows a pleural-based nodular density at the left lung base.

A CT scan of the chest is shown.

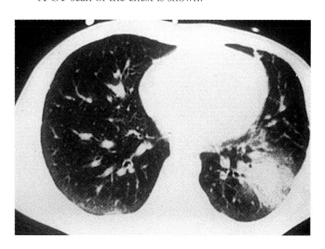

Which of the following is the most appropriate treatment?

(A) Itraconazole

(B) Liposomal amphotericin B

(C) Micafungin

(D) Voriconazole

Answers and Critiques

Item 1   Answer: C

Educational Objective: Diagnose common variable immunodeficiency.

Serum levels of IgG, IgA, and IgM should be measured. There is a high probability that this patient has common variable immunodeficiency (CVID). The onset is usually between 15 and 25 years of age, and a history of recurrent respiratory tract infections with encapsulated organisms such as *Streptococcus pneumoniae* and *Haemophilus influenzae* is common; giardiasis can also occur. Patients with CVID have a higher incidence of autoimmune disorders, particularly autoimmune hemolytic anemia and thrombocytopenia, pernicious anemia, and rheumatoid arthritis, as well as disorders of the gastrointestinal tract leading to diarrhea and malabsorption. This patient's anemia and high mean corpuscular volume are suggestive of vitamin B_{12} deficiency. There is a familial predisposition to selective IgA deficiency and malignancies. A higher incidence of CVID exists in those of northern European ancestry.

If serum IgG and IgA or IgM levels are low, the antibody response to protein- and polysaccharide-based vaccines should then be assessed. If IgG levels are very low (<200 mg/dL [2.0 g/L]) or undetectable, assessment of vaccine response is not necessary because antibody levels are predictably absent. Therefore, the first step in the evaluation of patients with suspected CVID is measurement of serum immunoglobulin levels.

A low CD4 cell count may occur in patients with CVID; however, measurement of the CD4 cell count would not contribute to the diagnosis. Involvement of cellular immunity in CVID is variable. T-cell numbers, including CD4 cells or T-cell function, can be normal in nearly 50% of patients.

Total hemolytic complement should be checked whenever a complement deficiency is suspected. A low total hemolytic complement level is seen with classical and terminal complement pathway deficiencies. Complement deficiencies involving the early components of the complement system are associated with autoimmune disorders, most specifically systemic lupus erythematosus. These patients may experience recurrent infections caused by encapsulated organisms such as *Streptococcus pneumoniae* or disseminated neisserial infections. Deficiencies in the terminal components of the complement system are associated with recurrent neisserial infections including meningitis and disseminated gonorrheal infection. The patient's clinical presentation is most compatible with CVID, not deficiencies in the early or terminal complement system.

> **KEY POINT**
>
> - Patients with common variable immunodeficiency frequently develop sinopulmonary infections, autoimmune disorders, malabsorption, and lymphoma, and their response to vaccination is poor.

Bibliography

Chapel H, Cunningham-Rundles C. Update in understanding common variable immunodeficiency disorders (CVIDs) and the management of patients with these conditions. Br J Haematol. 2009;145(6):709-727. [PMID: 19344423]

Item 2   Answer: A

Educational Objective: Manage an immunocompromised patient who has been exposed to a close contact with active tuberculosis.

Isoniazid and pyridoxine should be started for treatment of latent tuberculosis infection (LTBI). This patient has HIV infection and was recently exposed to a close contact with active tuberculosis. Patients with HIV infection or other serious immunocompromising conditions who are close contacts of persons with active tuberculosis should be treated for LTBI regardless of the results of a tuberculin skin test or interferon-γ release assay (IGRA) once active disease has been excluded. This patient is asymptomatic and has a normal chest radiograph, which exclude active disease. Patients with LTBI are typically treated with a 9-month regimen of isoniazid. Pyridoxine may also be given to certain patients at risk for developing peripheral neuropathy secondary to isoniazid. These include patients with HIV infection, diabetes mellitus, uremia, alcoholism, malnutrition, and seizure disorders, as well as pregnant women. In this patient, the tuberculin skin test or IGRA should be repeated 8 to 10 weeks after the most recent exposure. If results are still negative, isoniazid and pyridoxine can be discontinued. However, some experts recommend a complete course of treatment for LTBI in patients with HIV infection, who may not be able to mount a positive tuberculin skin test or IGRA response because of anergy.

Isoniazid, rifampin, pyrazinamide, pyridoxine, and ethambutol are used to treat active tuberculosis. This patient is asymptomatic and has a normal chest radiograph, making active disease highly unlikely.

The use of rifampin and pyrazinamide for treatment of LTBI is not recommended by the Centers for Disease Control and Prevention and the American Thoracic Society because of associated hepatic toxicity, which results in increased rates of hospitalization and death.

This patient with HIV infection and a recent exposure to a close contact with active tuberculosis requires treatment for latent tuberculosis infection, regardless of the results of a tuberculin skin test or IGRA; providing no further evaluation or treatment would not be appropriate.

KEY POINT

- Regardless of their response to a tuberculin skin test or interferon-γ release assay, patients with HIV infection who have had a known recent exposure to a close contact with active tuberculosis should receive treatment for latent tuberculosis infection after active disease has been excluded.

Bibliography

National Tuberculosis Controllers Association; Centers for Disease Control and Prevention (CDC). Guidelines for the investigation of contacts of persons with infectious tuberculosis: Recommendations from the National Tuberculosis Controllers Association and CDC. MMWR Recomm Rep. 2005;54(RR-15):1-47. [PMID: 16357823]

Item 3   Answer: A
Educational Objective: Treat life-threatening candidemia.

This patient should be treated with caspofungin. She has fungemia, which is most likely caused by *Candida* species. The most likely source is the central venous catheter, the site of which shows obvious signs of infection including erythema and purulent drainage. She has multiple risk factors for candidemia, including exposure to broad-spectrum antibiotics and having received parenteral nutrition via a central venous catheter. In addition to catheter removal, it is essential that antifungal therapy be instituted promptly. Because she is severely ill, the therapy of choice is an echinocandin agent. The Infectious Diseases Society of America guidelines do not distinguish among the echinocandins; therefore, any of them (caspofungin, anidulafungin, or micafungin) would be appropriate.

Amphotericin B or a lipid formulation of amphotericin B is an alternative choice if there is intolerance to or limited availability of other antifungal agents. This patient has kidney failure, which would be exacerbated by either formulation of amphotericin B.

Fluconazole is recommended for patients who are less critically ill than this patient and who have had no recent exposure to azole antifungal agents. When this patient becomes clinically stable, she can be transitioned from receiving an echinocandin to fluconazole if the isolate is likely to be susceptible to fluconazole.

Voriconazole is effective for the treatment of candidemia, but it offers little advantage over fluconazole and is recommended as step-down oral therapy for selected patients with candidiasis caused by *Candida krusei* or voriconazole-susceptible *Candida glabrata*.

KEY POINT

- Antifungal therapy with an echinocandin agent (caspofungin, anidulafungin, or micafungin) is the treatment of choice for critically ill patients with candidemia.

Bibliography

Pappas PG, Kauffman CA, Andes D, et al; Infectious Diseases Society of America. Clinical practice guidelines for the management of candidiasis: 2009 update by the Infectious Diseases Society of America. Clin Infect Dis. 2009;48(5):503-535. [PMID: 19191635]

Item 4   Answer: A
Educational Objective: Treat recurrent mild to moderate *Clostridium difficile* infection.

This patient has recurrent mild to moderate *Clostridium difficile* infection (CDI) and requires a repeat course of oral metronidazole for 14 days. The most appropriate treatment regimen for both the initial episode and the first recurrence of CDI is determined by the severity of the illness. Severe CDI is characterized by leukocytosis, defined as a leukocyte count greater than 15,000/microliter (15×10^9/L), and a significant decrease in kidney function, defined as an increase in the serum creatinine level greater than 1.5 times the baseline level. Patients without clinical or laboratory findings consistent with severe disease are at low risk for complications, and the recommended treatment is metronidazole for 10 to 14 days. Despite appropriate initial therapy, CDI recurs in approximately 20% of patients. The choice of therapy for the first recurrence does not decrease the probability of a second recurrence, and treatment is determined by the severity of illness in the same way as for the initial presentation.

Prolonged courses of metronidazole, such as a taper over 42 days, are not recommended because neurotoxicity can develop.

Oral vancomycin for 10 to 14 days is indicated for patients meeting the criteria for severe CDI, which this patient does not have.

Combination therapy with oral vancomycin and parenteral metronidazole is reserved for patients in whom enteral antimicrobial agents may not reach the distal colon, such as those with ileus or megacolon.

Patients who have a second recurrence of CDI of any degree of severity should be treated with a prolonged vancomycin taper over 4 to 8 weeks.

KEY POINT

- In patients with *Clostridium difficile* infection, the most appropriate treatment regimen for both the initial episode and the first recurrence is determined by the severity of the illness.

Bibliography

Cohen SH, Gerding DN, Johnson S, et al; Society for Healthcare Epidemiology of America; Infectious Diseases Society of America.

Clinical practice guidelines for Clostridium difficile infection in adults: 2010 update by the Society for Healthcare Epidemiology of America (SHEA) and the Infectious Diseases Society of America (IDSA). Infect Control Hosp Epidemiol. 2010;31(5):431-455. [PMID: 20307191]

Item 5   Answer: A

Educational Objective: Treat primary genital herpes simplex virus infection.

The most appropriate treatment is acyclovir. This patient's clinical examination findings are consistent with herpes simplex virus (HSV) infection. Because she has several lesions accompanied by systemic symptoms (malaise, fever), she most likely has a primary infection. Both HSV-1 and HSV-2 can cause primary genital infection; the incidence of primary infection from HSV-1 has increased in recent years. HSV-1 genital infections are less likely to be associated with recurrences and subclinical viral shedding. Although the clinical presentation is consistent with HSV infection, the diagnosis should be confirmed by viral culture or polymerase chain reaction testing; direct fluorescence antibody testing is a much less sensitive diagnostic modality. Pending the results of diagnostic testing, the patient should begin receiving antiviral therapy to reduce the severity and duration of symptoms. Acyclovir, valacyclovir, and famciclovir are all recommended for the treatment of primary HSV infections; acyclovir is available generically and therefore is the least-expensive treatment option. Valacyclovir has the advantage of twice-daily dosing compared with thrice-daily dosing of acyclovir or famciclovir. Regardless of the regimen chosen, the patient should be treated for 7 to 10 days. Patients with newly diagnosed genital HSV infection must be counseled regarding the risks of recurrence and transmission. Women and men with genital HSV infection should be educated regarding the risk of neonatal infection. Chronic therapy with valacyclovir has been shown to reduce the risk of transmission of infection to sexual partners.

Benzathine penicillin G is the appropriate treatment choice for primary syphilis. Syphilis is characterized by chancres, which are usually single painless lesions with a clean base (unless secondarily infected), although multiple lesions can also occur.

Ceftriaxone plus azithromycin is appropriate treatment for mucopurulent cervicitis. HSV infection can cause cervicitis, but the presentation would be characterized by ulcerative lesions on the cervix.

Single-dose fluconazole is the appropriate treatment for candidal vaginitis, which may include fissures and excoriations from pruritus, but ulcerative lesions would not be typical.

KEY POINT

- Pending the results of diagnostic testing, patients with suspected primary herpes simplex virus infection should begin receiving empiric antiviral therapy with acyclovir, valacyclovir, or famciclovir to reduce the severity and duration of symptoms.

Bibliography

Workowski KA, Berman S; Centers for Disease Control and Prevention (CDC). Sexually transmitted diseases treatment guidelines, 2010. MMWR Recomm Rep. 2010;59(RR-12):1-110. [PMID: 21160459]

Item 6   Answer: D

Educational Objective: Diagnose acute pulmonary histoplasmosis.

This patient's recent travel history and clinical symptoms are most consistent with acute pulmonary histoplasmosis (also known as "Ohio Valley fever"). *Histoplasma capsulatum*, a dimorphic fungal organism that is particularly endemic to the southeastern United States, is found in high concentrations in soil contaminated with bird or bat droppings. The infection is acquired through inhalation of the fungus in its mold form. Although most acute infections are asymptomatic, some persons develop a flu-like syndrome (fever, myalgia, malaise) and pulmonary symptoms (dyspnea, cough, chest discomfort). In a few patients, histoplasmosis may become disseminated, causing bone marrow involvement and pancytopenia, as well as involvement of the meninges, adrenal glands, and other organs. Persons who have a weakened immune system such as from AIDS or immunosuppressive therapy for autoimmune conditions, neoplasms, or transplantation are at higher risk for disseminated histoplasmosis. This patient's travel history and symptoms are suspicious for histoplasmosis, and diagnosis may be confirmed by laboratory testing.

Symptoms caused by acute infection with *Blastomyces dermatitidis*, which is also a dimorphic fungus, are very similar to those caused by *H. capsulatum*. In addition, the endemic geographic distribution of *Blastomyces* and *Histoplasma* overlap. However, acute pulmonary blastomycosis is rarely associated with hilar lymphadenopathy, a common finding in acute pulmonary histoplasmosis. Furthermore, acute blastomycosis is more often associated with exposure to soil containing decaying vegetation and wood products, not bat caves.

This patient's clinical-epidemiologic scenario is not consistent with that of acute pulmonary coccidioidomycosis because *Coccidioides immitis* is endemic to the southwestern United States (Arizona, New Mexico, California, and west Texas).

Infection caused by *Cryptococcus neoformans* typically affects immunocompromised persons and most often causes localized pulmonary lesions.

- *Histoplasma capsulatum* is a dimorphic fungal organism endemic to the southeastern United States; is found in soil contaminated with bird or bat droppings; and is characterized by a flu-like syndrome and dyspnea, cough, and chest discomfort.

Bibliography

Dylewski J. Acute pulmonary histoplasmosis. CMAJ. 2011;183(14): E1090. [PMID: 21810958]

Item 7   Answer: B

Educational Objective: Manage a patient with a prosthetic joint infection.

The most appropriate management of this patient who has requested no further surgery is to retain her prosthesis and administer lifelong therapy with trimethoprim-sulfamethoxazole. This patient most likely has chronic osteomyelitis in her tibia with a chronically infected prosthetic joint. Ideally, removal of all the hardware and debridement of the necrotic bone tissue, followed by a prolonged course of a pathogen-directed parenteral or oral antimicrobial treatment regimen, would occur. However, the patient has refused a surgical management option. In patients with no systemic or severe local signs of infection and in whom the prosthesis is not loose or in whom surgery is not possible or desired, lifelong oral antimicrobial therapy may be considered in an attempt to suppress the infection and retain usefulness of the total joint replacement. The success of this treatment modality partly depends on the relative virulence of the causative microorganism and its sensitivity to an orally absorbed antimicrobial drug. Assuming no known allergies to sulfa-containing medications, trimethoprim-sulfamethoxazole would be an acceptable choice.

The use of rifampin alone in treating methicillin-resistant *Staphylococcus aureus* infections often leads to the development of organism resistance to this drug and is not recommended.

Repeating an antimicrobial regimen to eradicate this chronic bone-joint infection with retained hardware would unnecessarily expose the patient to the risks associated with lengthy parenteral antimicrobial treatment and would provide only a minimal chance of eradication of the infectious process.

Careful observation with symptomatic relief but no antimicrobial treatment would confer a risk for local extension of the septic process and possible systemic spread of the infection.

- In patients with prosthetic joint infection with no systemic or severe local signs of infection and in whom the prosthesis is not loose or surgery is not possible or desired, lifelong oral antimicrobial therapy may be considered to suppress the infection and retain usefulness of the total joint replacement.

Bibliography

Cobo J, Del Pozo JL. Prosthetic joint infection: diagnosis and management. Expert Rev Anti Infect Ther. 2011;9(9):787-802. [PMID: 21905787]

Item 8   Answer: C

Educational Objective: Identify infectious causes of hemorrhagic colitis.

The most likely pathogen is Shiga toxin–producing *Escherichia coli* (STEC). The presence of visible blood in the stool is diagnostic of hemorrhagic colitis, and the STEC strain *E. coli* O157:H7 is the most common cause of this condition in the United States. Both *E. coli* O157:H7 and the newly described *E. coli* O104:H4 (which caused a large outbreak of hemorrhagic gastroenteritis in Europe in 2011) induce vascular damage by producing a Shiga toxin. Gross blood is found in stool samples in more than 60% of patients with *E. coli* O157:H7 infection, and a history of visible blood in the stool can be elicited in more than 90% of patients. STEC organisms are typically foodborne pathogens, and clusters or outbreaks of disease may develop in persons who have eaten contaminated foods. Other clinical findings suggestive of STEC infection include abdominal tenderness and leukocytosis. Fever is relatively uncommon and develops in only one third of patients.

Bacillus cereus and *Staphylococcus aureus* are both associated with foodborne gastrointestinal disease caused by a preformed toxin. Therefore, symptoms occur less than 24 hours after ingestion rather than after several days as in STEC infection and are characterized by nausea and vomiting rather than by diarrhea.

Campylobacter jejuni and *Yersinia enterocolitica* also cause foodborne gastroenteritis, but grossly bloody stools are uncommon, and fever occurs in most patients.

- **The presence of visible blood in the stool is diagnostic of hemorrhagic colitis, which in the United States is most often caused by Shiga toxin–producing *Escherichia coli*.**

Bibliography

Guerrant RL, Van Gilder T, Steiner TS, et al; Infectious Diseases Society of America. Practice guidelines for the management of infectious diarrhea. Clin Infect Dis. 2001;32(3):331-351. [PMID: 11170940]

Item 9   Answer: B

Educational Objective: Treat shigellosis.

This patient has shigellosis, and even though her symptoms have resolved, she requires treatment with ciprofloxacin. *Shigella* organisms are extremely infectious even at a low inoculum, and outbreaks of disease in day care settings and nursing homes are well described. The spectrum of clinical disease ranges from a mild, self-limited gastrointestinal illness to dysentery associated with bloody diarrhea and fever. While culture results are pending, empiric therapy with ciprofloxacin is indicated for patients with severe symptoms who have a high clinical suspicion for shigellosis and also for those with milder disease such as the elderly, immunocompromised, and those working in food services and child care centers because treatment shortens the duration of fever, diarrhea, and shedding of the organism by about 48 hours. Otherwise, in patients with milder symptoms, obtaining culture results before beginning treatment is a reasonable approach. However, once a microbiologic diagnosis is established, treatment is generally indicated even if the illness has resolved to hasten clearance of fecal shedding of bacteria and reduce the risk of secondary spread to other persons. Use of a fluoroquinolone is appropriate because most *Shigella* organisms have not developed resistance to these agents. Treatment is usually for 3 days in immunocompetent individuals; conversion of stools to negative generally requires at least 48 hours of antibiotic treatment, and patients at high risk of spreading the disease should avoid exposure during that period.

Azithromycin is the recommended empiric therapy for *Campylobacter* infection because of the high rates of fluoroquinolone resistance in these organisms.

Metronidazole is not active against aerobic bacteria and is not effective therapy for *Shigella* infection.

KEY POINT

- In a patient with shigellosis confirmed by microbiologic diagnosis, ciprofloxacin is indicated to hasten clearance of fecal shedding of bacteria and reduce the risk of secondary spread to other persons even if the illness has resolved.

Bibliography

Guerrant RL, Van Gilder T, Steiner TS, et al; Infectious Diseases Society of America. Practice guidelines for the management of infectious diarrhea. Clin Infect Dis. 2001;32(3):331-351. [PMID: 11170940]

Item 10   Answer: A

Educational Objective: Manage a patient with bloodstream infection due to vancomycin-intermediate methicillin-resistant *Staphylococcus aureus*.

In this patient, vancomycin should be discontinued and daptomycin should be initiated. The causative pathogen is a vancomycin-intermediate *Staphylococcus aureus* (VISA), which has a minimal inhibitory concentration (MIC) of 4 micrograms/mL to vancomycin. Although vancomycin is a reasonable initial choice for empiric therapy for treating a possible methicillin-resistant *S. aureus* (MRSA) bloodstream infection, daptomycin is recommended as an alternative to vancomycin for treatment of bloodstream infection caused by vancomycin-intermediate *S. aureus*, particularly in patients treated with vancomycin who do not appear to be responding to treatment. Daptomycin is a bactericidal agent, which has been studied extensively for treatment of bloodstream infections due to *S. aureus*, including MRSA. Daptomycin retains activity against many strains of *S. aureus* with elevated MICs to vancomycin ($\geq$2 micrograms/mL).

Linezolid has activity against *S. aureus* but is not indicated for the treatment of bloodstream infection.

Recently, trimethoprim-sulfamethoxazole has been used more frequently for treatment of MRSA skin infection, but it is not recommended as a primary agent for the treatment of bloodstream infection.

Because of the intermediate sensitivity of the identified organism to vancomycin, optimal pharmacodynamic targets may not be possible by increasing the vancomycin dose. To avoid treatment-related toxicity, the use of an alternative agent is preferred versus increasing the vancomycin dose.

KEY POINT

- Daptomycin is recommended for treatment of bloodstream infections caused by methicillin-resistant *Staphylococcus aureus* when the minimal inhibitory concentration to vancomycin is more than 2 micrograms/mL.

Bibliography

Liu C, Bayer A, Cosgrove SE, et al. Clinical practice guidelines by the Infectious Diseases Society of America for the treatment of methicillin-resistant *Staphylococcus aureus* infections in adults and children: executive summary. Clin Infect Dis. 2011;52(3):285-292. [PMID: 21217178]

Item 11   Answer: C

Educational Objective: Treat cervicitis.

The most appropriate treatment is ceftriaxone plus azithromycin. The findings on pelvic examination confirm that the patient's vaginal discharge is due to mucopurulent cervicitis, which is most commonly caused by *Neisseria gonorrhoeae* and *Chlamydia trachomatis* infection. The presence of leukocytes, an elevated pH level, and a negative whiff test are consistent with this diagnosis. The patient should be treated with a single-dose regimen that will provide coverage against the two most common pathogens. The preferred treatment of cervicitis is ceftriaxone, 250 mg intramuscularly in a single dose, plus azithromycin, 1 g orally in a single dose. Ceftriaxone provides coverage against *N. gonorrhoeae*, and azithromycin has activity against *C. trachomatis*. Reports of decreased susceptibility to cephalosporins have led to the recommendation that all infections (cervicitis, urethritis, pharyngitis, and proctitis) be treated with a 250-mg dose, rather than a 125-mg dose of ceftriaxone, as was recommended previously.

Cefixime is an alternative to ceftriaxone for the management of cervicitis or urethritis (although parenteral therapy with ceftriaxone is preferred); however, all patients should also be treated for possible chlamydial disease with a single dose of azithromycin or 7 days of doxycycline.

Fluoroquinolones such as ciprofloxacin are no longer recommended for treatment of the gonorrheal component of cervicitis because of the emergence of resistance to these agents.

The combination of cefoxitin (or cefotetan) plus doxycycline would be appropriate therapy for a patient with pelvic inflammatory disease. However, the absence of uterine, adnexal, and cervical motion tenderness in this patient makes such a diagnosis unlikely.

KEY POINT

- **The preferred treatment of cervicitis is ceftriaxone, 250 mg intramuscularly in a single dose, plus azithromycin, 1 g orally in a single dose.**

Bibliography

Centers for Disease Control and Prevention (CDC). Cephalosporin susceptibility among Neisseria gonorrhoeae isolates—United States, 2000-2010. MMWR Morb Mortal Wkly Rep. 2011;60(26):873-877. [PMID: 21734634]

Item 12   Answer: B

Educational Objective: Evaluate for *Mycobacterium tuberculosis* infection in a patient who received bacillus Calmette-Guérin cancer therapy.

In this physician who has a history of bladder cancer treated with bacillus Calmette-Guérin (BCG), tuberculosis screening using an interferon-γ release assay (IGRA) is preferred. Either an IGRA or a tuberculin skin test (TST) can be used to diagnose tuberculosis, although neither can distinguish between latent tuberculosis infection and active disease. However, an IGRA is preferred for two groups of patients: those who have received BCG as a vaccine or as cancer therapy and those who are unlikely to return for interpretation of the TST. Conversely, the TST is preferred for testing children who are younger than 5 years of age.

If the IGRA result is positive, active disease should be excluded by determining whether associated signs and symptoms are present (fever, chills, night sweats, weight loss, cough), obtaining a chest radiograph, and possibly obtaining microbiologic examination of sputum (or other involved fluids or tissues) when appropriate. When active disease has been ruled out, a diagnosis of latent tuberculosis infection is made.

A two-step tuberculin test is sometimes done in patients who will be undergoing serial testing (such as a physician) to establish a baseline result for future testing. This is particularly useful in individuals with a remote exposure to tuberculin antigens (BCG, previous infection, or atypical mycobacterial infection) because their immune response to these antigens may have waned. The initial test "boosts" the immune response, possibly improving the reliability of the subsequent test. However, this test would not be desirable in this patient with recent BCG treatment.

KEY POINT

- **The interferon-γ release assay is preferred over the tuberculin skin test for tuberculosis screening when patients have received bacillus Calmette-Guérin either as a vaccine or as cancer therapy.**

Bibliography

Mazurek GH, Jereb J, Vernon A, et al; IGRA Expert Committee; Centers for Disease Control and Prevention (CDC). Updated guidelines for using interferon gamma release assays to detect Mycobacterium tuberculosis infection - United States, 2010. MMWR Recomm Rep. 2010;59(RR-5):1-25. [PMID: 20577159]

Item 13   Answer: B

Educational Objective: Manage a patient with a clenched-fist injury who is allergic to penicillin.

The most appropriate treatment is clindamycin and moxifloxacin. This patient, who is allergic to penicillin, has a clenched-fist injury to the left hand and requires immediate prophylaxis with clindamycin and moxifloxacin. Clenched-fist injuries result unintentionally when a person punches the mouth of another person. Initial evaluation and management are similar to that for human and animal bites. Patients with clenched-fist injuries are at increased risk for infection involving deep structures, including tendons, joints, and bones. The Infectious Diseases Society of America practice guidelines for skin and soft tissue infections recommend that all patients with human bite wounds should receive prompt prophylaxis. Infection is caused by human oral flora and typically involves a mixture of aerobic organisms, including α-hemolytic streptococci, staphylococci, *Haemophilus* species, and *Eikenella corrodens*, and anaerobic organisms, many of which produce β-lactamases. Although amoxicillin-clavulanate is an oral agent that provides such coverage, it should not be given to a patient with a history of a hypersensitivity reaction to penicillin. Instead, the combination of clindamycin and moxifloxacin provides the polymicrobial coverage needed for human bite wound–associated prophylaxis in patients with a type 1 β-lactam allergy. Moxifloxacin is effective against *E. corrodens*, and clindamycin is active against anaerobes, staphylococci, and streptococci. Clindamycin is a pregnancy risk category B drug and moxifloxacin a category C (risk cannot be ruled out) drug.

Cephalexin is active against streptococci and staphylococci but not *E. corrodens* and gram-negative anaerobes. This agent also should not be given to a patient who has an IgE-mediated penicillin allergy.

This patient does not require tetanus immunization because she was vaccinated 4 years ago, and the vaccine is effective for 10 years.

Trimethoprim-sulfamethoxazole, which can be given to patients who are allergic to penicillin, provides good coverage for aerobic bacteria but has limited activity against anaerobes. Adding an anaerobic antimicrobial agent such as metronidazole to trimethoprim-sulfamethoxazole would provide adequate coverage.

Observation is inappropriate because patients with clenched-fist injuries are at high risk for developing an infection and require immediate antimicrobial prophylaxis.

KEY POINT

- **The combination of clindamycin and moxifloxacin is the recommended antimicrobial prophylactic regimen for a patient with a clenched-fist injury who is allergic to penicillin.**

Bibliography

Stevens DL, Bisno AL, Chambers HF, et al; Infectious Diseases Society of America. Practice guidelines for the diagnosis and management of skin and soft tissue infections. Clin Infect Dis. 2005;41(10):1373-1406. [PMID: 16231249]

Item 14   Answer: C

Educational Objective: Prevent varicella infection in a patient with leukemia.

This patient should receive varicella-zoster immune globulin (VZIG) if it can be procured. He is severely immunocompromised and at high risk for serious complications of varicella virus infection. However, the production of VZIG has been discontinued by the manufacturer, and an investigational varicella-zoster immune globulin product (VariZIG™) is available under a compassionate-use protocol. If a VZIG product cannot be obtained, the Centers for Disease Control and Prevention suggest the use of intravenous immune globulin. Susceptible persons who are immunocompromised or pregnant should receive a VZIG product or intravenous immune globulin within 96 hours of exposure, and this patient should be treated because his exposure was within this time frame. Patients who receive a VZIG preparation should be monitored for development of varicella for 28 days after exposure because the immune globulin may prolong the incubation period.

Treating immunocompromised persons with acyclovir for postexposure prophylaxis of varicella virus has not been studied; however, treatment of active varicella infection in this immunocompromised host is indicated.

The varicella vaccine is a live virus vaccine and is contraindicated for use in immunocompromised patients. However, because of the infection's association with high morbidity and the excellent efficacy of the vaccine, the vaccine is used in selected groups of immunocompromised persons such as those with leukemia who are in remission. Nonetheless, the varicella vaccine would not be an option for this patient with active leukemia under treatment.

Withholding treatment is not appropriate because the varicella virus causes significant morbidity and mortality in immunocompromised hosts.

KEY POINT

- **Varicella-zoster immune globulin (VZIG) or investigational VZIG (VariZIG™) or intravenous immune globulin (if a VZIG product is unavailable) should be used in immunocompromised or pregnant persons within 96 hours of exposure to the varicella virus to prevent infection.**

Bibliography

Fisher JP, Bate J, Hambleton S. Preventing varicella in children with malignancies: what is the evidence? Curr Opin Infect Dis. 2011;24(3):203-211. [PMID: 21455062]

Item 15   Answer: B

Educational Objective: Understand the goals of antimicrobial stewardship and de-escalation of empiric antimicrobial therapy in the clinical setting.

In this patient, piperacillin-tazobactam should be discontinued and ampicillin begun. The primary reason for this recommendation is to reduce the likelihood of induction of resistance to broad-spectrum antibiotics used in empiric therapy. The early use of aggressive antibiotic treatment is widely accepted for critically ill patients before confirmation of a specific diagnosis. In this patient, treatment with a broad-spectrum antibiotic with activity against the likely infecting organism identified in the urine by the presence of gram-negative rods was indicated. However, once a specific organism is isolated and its sensitivities to available antibiotics known, it is beneficial to focus or "de-escalate" therapy to avoid the selection of organisms resistant to currently effective broad-spectrum antibiotics. Willingness to de-escalate therapy can be challenging in a patient who has responded well to broad-spectrum antibiotic coverage. However, failure to curtail excess antibiotic use is an ecologic hazard for the patient and the medical unit as a whole. Ampicillin is a narrow-spectrum agent with activity against this infectious pathogen and is a good choice for de-escalation.

Nitrofurantoin is also a narrow-spectrum agent but is not significantly absorbed into the bloodstream and thus would not be an appropriate therapeutic choice for bloodstream infection.

Piperacillin-tazobactam, imipenem, and ciprofloxacin are each active against this infectious pathogen but provide unnecessarily broad-spectrum coverage, which can promote the emergence of antimicrobial resistance.

Eh

Answers and Critiques

Answers and Critiques

KEY POINT

- Antimicrobial stewardship is a growing quality-based movement focused on optimizing antimicrobial prescribing and limiting unnecessary prescribing.

Bibliography

Dellit TH, Owens RC, McGowan JE Jr, et al. Infectious Diseases Society of America; Society for Healthcare Epidemiology of America. Infectious Diseases Society of America and the Society for Healthcare Epidemiology of America guidelines for developing an institutional program to enhance antimicrobial stewardship. Clin Infect Dis. 2007;44(2):159-177. [PMID: 17173212]

Item 16   Answer: D

Educational Objective: Diagnose *Vibrio vulnificus*–associated necrotizing fasciitis.

This patient most likely has necrotizing fasciitis secondary to *Vibrio vulnificus* infection. He has hemochromatosis with evidence of portal hypertension (ascites). *V. vulnificus* infection should always be considered in a patient with liver disease who presents with sepsis and cutaneous manifestations of hemorrhagic bullae after possible exposure to this waterborne, gram-negative rod. Increased iron availability has been shown to enhance the virulence and growth of *V. vulnificus*, which perhaps explains why patients with hemochromatosis are more likely to develop infection in addition to their having the decreased opsonization and serum bactericidal activity found in patients with liver disease. Septicemia occurs after ingestion of raw or undercooked shellfish, usually oysters. Patients may also develop wound-associated *V. vulnificus* infection when the pathogen is inoculated through traumatized skin. This organism thrives in warm brackish or salt water, such as the Gulf of Mexico, and most infections occur during the summer months, when seawater temperatures facilitate its growth.

Babesia microti is the pathogen responsible for babesiosis, a tick-associated infection that occurs in the coastal northeastern and upper midwestern United States. Flu-like symptoms develop about 1 week after tick exposure, and the diagnosis is typically established by evaluation of a peripheral blood smear that shows intraerythrocytic parasites. Rash is not a typical feature of babesiosis. Patients with decreased splenic function are more likely to develop serious complications.

Capnocytophaga canimorsus is a gram-negative rod that can cause cellulitis and overwhelming sepsis in patients with decreased splenic function who have been bitten by a dog or cat.

Rickettsia rickettsii is a tick-associated pathogen responsible for Rocky Mountain spotted fever (RMSF). Although liver chemistry studies can be abnormal in patients with both RMSF and *V. vulnificus* infection, the rash in RMSF characteristically begins on the palms, soles, wrists, and ankles before moving centripetally to involve the trunk. The rash is initially maculopapular but eventually becomes petechial. Aseptic meningitis may also develop. RMSF is unlikely in this patient with hemorrhagic bullae.

KEY POINT

- Patients with liver disease are at increased risk for developing necrotizing fasciitis secondary to *Vibrio vulnificus* infection after eating raw or undercooked shellfish or following exposure of traumatized skin to contaminated sea water.

Bibliography

Bross MH, Soch K, Morales R, Mitchell RB. Vibrio vulnificus infection: diagnosis and treatment. Am Fam Physician. 2007;76(4):539-544. [PMID: 17853628]

Item 17   Answer: C

Educational Objective: Manage a health care provider with exposure to suspected smallpox.

The most appropriate intervention for this patient's nurse is smallpox vaccine. This patient most likely has active smallpox (variola) infection, to which his nurse has likely experienced unprotected respiratory exposure. Smallpox infection is initially asymptomatic, with respiratory tract infection and viremia occurring during a 7- to 17-day incubation period. High fever, headache, vomiting, and backache follow, lasting 2 to 4 days. The smallpox rash first appears on the buccal and pharyngeal mucosa and most often spreads to the hands and face before spreading to the trunk, arms, legs, and feet. The centrifugally distributed skin lesions evolve synchronously (same stage of maturation on any one area of the body) from macules to papules to vesicles to pustules and eventually become crusted. Patients remain contagious until all scabs and crusts are shed. Presumably, the soldier's infection was acquired through exposure to an intentional spread of smallpox virus through an act of bioterrorism because smallpox was eradicated in 1979, and no known naturally occurring case has been reported in more than 3 decades. Vaccination with the live virus preparation, vaccinia, made from a distinct and separate related pox virus, provides immunity to smallpox. When given within 3 days of exposure, this active vaccine can prevent or significantly lessen the severity of smallpox symptoms in most people and is indicated in all exposed persons.

Chickenpox is the viral exanthem infection most likely to be confused with smallpox. The varicella-zoster virus infection differs from smallpox in the former's centripetal mode of rash distribution, which is most concentrated on the torso, with fewest lesions on the hands and feet, as well as the presence of various stages of lesions (papules, vesicles, and crusts) existing simultaneously. Acyclovir is not an appropriate prophylactic agent for either chickenpox or smallpox.

Cidofovir, an intravenous antiviral agent demonstrating in vitro antiviral activity against the smallpox virus, may theoretically be clinically useful in the event of a widespread smallpox outbreak or to treat severe vaccine-related reactions; however, it currently is not indicated to prevent or treat smallpox.

Considering the patient's signs and symptoms and potential occupational exposure to smallpox through an act of bioterrorism, providing no intervention to his nurse, who was exposed to this patient within the past few days, would not be prudent.

KEY POINT

- Vaccination with the live virus preparation, vaccinia, provides immunity to smallpox, and, when given within 3 days of exposure, can prevent or significantly lessen the severity of smallpox symptoms in most people.

Bibliography

Guharoy R, Panzik R, Noviasky JA, et al. Smallpox: clinical features, prevention, and management. Ann Pharmacother. 2004;38(3):440-447. [PMID: 14755066]

Item 18   Answer: D

Educational Objective: Diagnose tacrolimus nephrotoxicity in a patient following kidney transplantation.

This patient has tacrolimus toxicity resulting in acute kidney injury. The most common manifestation of tacrolimus nephrotoxicity is an acute increase in the serum creatinine and blood urea nitrogen levels; other manifestations of nephropathy include tubular disorders and a hemolytic-uremic syndrome. Patients may also have hypertension, neurotoxicity, and metabolic abnormalities, including hyperglycemia, hyperkalemia, and hypomagnesemia. Many of the immunosuppressive agents are associated with significant drug interactions. Interactions affecting drug metabolism occur when cyclosporine, tacrolimus, or sirolimus is combined with macrolide antibiotics or azole antifungal agents, the interaction of which results in increased levels of one or both drugs. Tacrolimus metabolism by hepatic cytochrome P-450 enzymes is significantly inhibited by the macrolide antibiotic clarithromycin, and the interaction between these two agents leads to several-fold increases in tacrolimus levels, resulting in toxicity. If a macrolide antibiotic must be used in a transplant recipient, azithromycin, which is not a significant inhibitor of the cytochrome P-450 enzyme system, should be chosen.

The most common side effects of mycophenolate mofetil are gastrointestinal (nausea, diarrhea, and cramping) and bone marrow suppression but not acute kidney injury. Antibiotics have no effect on mycophenolate mofetil drug levels.

Acute interstitial nephritis is most commonly caused by a hypersensitivity reaction to a medication and may manifest as fever, rash, and eosinophilia. Urine findings may include leukocyte casts, eosinophils, and a urine protein-creatinine ratio usually less than 2.5 mg/mg. There are no findings to suggest acute interstitial nephritis in this patient, and clarithromycin is an exceedingly rare cause of drug-induced interstitial nephritis.

Organ rejection could cause acute kidney injury; however, this patient's condition has been stable, with no medical problems for 7 months following transplantation. Therefore, her current symptoms and findings are more likely attributable to toxicity from a known drug interaction between clarithromycin and tacrolimus than rejection.

KEY POINT

- Drug toxicity can occur when cyclosporine, tacrolimus, or sirolimus is combined with macrolide antibiotics or azole antifungal agents.

Bibliography

Spriet I, Meersseman W, de Hoon J, von Winckelmann S, Wilmer A, Willems L. Mini-series: II. Clinical aspects. Clinically relevant CYP450-mediated drug interactions in the ICU. Intensive Care Med. 2009;35(4):603-612. [PMID: 19132344]

Item 19   Answer: D

Educational Objective: Diagnose West Nile virus myelitis.

This patient presents with the acute onset of asymmetric flaccid paralysis consistent with West Nile virus (WNV) myelitis, and a WNV IgM antibody assay should be performed to confirm the diagnosis. WNV has been identified as an important cause of encephalitis throughout the continental United States. Birds are the main reservoir of this virus in nature. Several species of mosquitoes can acquire the virus after biting a bird with high-level viremia and transmit the infection to humans. A poliomyelitis-like syndrome has been described in as many as 12% of patients with WNV neuroinvasive disease. Neuromuscular symptoms range in severity from mild unilateral weakness to quadriplegia with respiratory failure. WNV myelitis may occur in isolation or may be part of an overlap syndrome with encephalitis or meningitis. WNV IgM antibody is detectable in the cerebrospinal fluid (CSF) in greater than 90% of patients with WNV neuroinvasive disease at the time of presentation. Because WNV viremia is of brief duration, CSF viral cultures are positive in less than 10% of patients, and results of WNV polymerase chain reaction are positive in less than 60% of patients.

Cytomegalovirus may cause a polyradiculopathy, but this occurs almost exclusively in patients with advanced HIV infection and is characterized by sensory loss and urinary retention.

Although ehrlichiosis may cause a febrile illness that is variably associated with meningoencephalitis, this infection is not associated with focal paralysis.

Neurologic manifestations of *Borrelia burgdorferi*, the causative agent of Lyme disease, typically occur more than a month after infection. Early disseminated Lyme disease may present as aseptic meningitis, cranial neuropathy, or

CONT.

radiculopathy. Encephalopathy or encephalomyelitis has been reported in late disease.

> **KEY POINT**
> - West Nile virus (WNV) IgM antibody is detectable in the cerebrospinal fluid in greater than 90% of patients with WNV neuroinvasive disease at the time of presentation.

Bibliography

Sejvar JJ, Bode AV, Marfin AA, et al. West Nile virus-associated flaccid paralysis. Emerg Infect Dis. 2005;11(7):1021-1027. [PMID: 16022775]

Item 20   Answer: C

Educational Objective: Diagnose *Mycobacterium avium* complex lung disease.

This patient requires a repeat acid-fast bacilli smear and culture before treatment is initiated. Nontuberculous mycobacteria (NTM), also referred to as atypical mycobacteria, when acting as invasive pathogens most often involve the lungs. Because NTM species are readily recovered from the environment (especially tap water and soil), when they are isolated from nonsterile human sites, results must be interpreted within the context of the patient's clinical syndrome to avoid treating for colonization alone. *Mycobacterium avium* complex (MAC) is the most frequently recognized NTM causing pulmonary disease and develops after inhalation of the organism. Although the classic presentation of pulmonary MAC disease is a subacute to chronic illness occurring in persons with a history of underlying pulmonary disease, MAC has also been increasingly recognized in middle-aged to elderly women with no preexisting lung disease. The more indolent clinical course in this latter group of patients consists mainly of chronic cough. Systemic symptoms are generally absent. Discrete pulmonary nodules best visualized on CT scan of the lungs are very commonly found.

Because of the significant frequency of positive sputum cultures for MAC in persons without active disease, it is often difficult to differentiate colonization from actual active lung disease. The isolation of MAC from a single sputum culture has a low predictive value and therefore is not proof of infection with NTM. To avoid unnecessary, lengthy, multidrug antimicrobial therapy, clinicians can follow specific diagnostic criteria to define a clinical case of MAC lung disease. Along with her symptoms and chest CT scan abnormalities, this patient would require a second positive MAC sputum culture obtained through a routine sputum culture, a bronchial wash or lavage, or a histopathologic specimen for a diagnosis to be established. Because the patient is clinically stable, isolating the organism from a second sputum sample would be the least-invasive and lowest-risk method for confirming the diagnosis. If a repeat culture were negative for MAC, then more aggressive interventions, such as bronchoalveolar lavage or lung biopsy, to

assess for the presence of the infection or other potential causes of her symptoms would be indicated.

Initiating treatment before confirming the diagnosis would be premature.

Instituting no further evaluation would not be prudent given the potential significance of her clinical symptoms and radiographic findings.

> **KEY POINT**
> - *Mycobacteria avium* complex infection occurs frequently in middle-aged to elderly women with no preexisting lung disease and most often consists of chronic cough, the absence of systemic symptoms, and discrete pulmonary nodules commonly located in the middle lobe or lingular areas and best visualized by CT.

Bibliography

Kasperbauer SH, Daley CL. Diagnosis and treatment of infections due to Mycobacterium avium complex. Semin Respir Crit Care Med. 2008;29(5):569-576. [PMID: 18810690]

Item 21   Answer: A

Educational Objective: Diagnose cryptococcal meningitis in a patient with HIV infection and immune reconstitution inflammatory syndrome.

The most likely diagnosis is *Cryptococcus neoformans* infection. This patient with AIDS has developed symptoms of meningitis after initiation of antiretroviral treatment, which is consistent with immune reconstitution inflammatory syndrome (IRIS), most likely from cryptococcal meningitis. With the initiation of combination antiretroviral therapy, viral load levels decrease sharply, CD4 cell counts increase, and immune responses improve. In the presence of an opportunistic infection, which may not have been clinically recognized previously, this process can lead to dramatic inflammatory responses as the newly revived immune system reacts to high burdens of antigens. IRIS usually occurs a few weeks to a few months after initiation of antiretrovirals in the setting of various opportunistic infections, most commonly mycobacterial or disseminated fungal infections, including cryptococcal meningitis. This patient's prolonged duration of symptoms, including headache, mental status changes, and cranial nerve involvement, are typical of cryptococcal meningitis as are the lumbar puncture results showing evidence of inflammation. Fungal cultures of cerebrospinal fluid may eventually grow the organism, but results of cryptococcal serum or cerebrospinal fluid antigen testing will be available more quickly and have a sensitivity of more than 95%. Acute treatment consists of intravenous amphotericin B followed by long-term oral fluconazole, with special attention to management of increased intracranial pressure.

Cytomegalovirus infection can cause encephalitis, but it is much less common, especially in patients with CD4 cell counts greater than 100/microliter; the MRI would also likely show periventricular involvement.

Histoplasmosis is caused by *Histoplasma capsulatum*, a thermal dimorphic fungus endemic to the midwestern states of the Ohio and Mississippi river valleys. Patients may have acute or chronic pulmonary disease, and immunocompromised patients, especially, may present with disseminated disease. Central nervous system involvement can occur, but usually as part of obvious dissemination including pulmonary disease, which is not consistent with this patient's presentation.

Toxoplasmosis can cause encephalitis in patients with AIDS, usually in those with CD4 cell counts less than 100/microliter and headache, mental status changes, and focal deficits. But the MRI findings in affected patients would show the characteristic multiple ring-enhancing lesions of the toxoplasmic abscesses, which are not present in this patient.

> **KEY POINT**
>
> - In patients with HIV infection, immune reconstitution inflammatory syndrome can occur a few weeks to a few months after initiation of antiretroviral therapy and results in a dramatic inflammatory response to opportunistic infections.

Bibliography

Letendre SL, Ellis RJ, Everall I, Ances B, Bharti A, McCutchan JA. Neurologic complications of HIV disease and their treatment. Top HIV Med. 2009;17(2):46-56. [PMID: 19401607]

Item 22   Answer: D

Educational Objective: Diagnose aseptic meningitis caused by herpes simplex virus type 2 infection.

This patient's clinical illness and cerebrospinal fluid (CSF) findings are most consistent with aseptic meningitis caused by herpes simplex virus (HSV). Aseptic meningitis is defined as meningeal inflammation without a known bacterial or fungal cause. Most cases are caused by viruses, although aseptic meningitis may also be associated with difficult-to-identify infectious agents, inflammation triggered by medications, malignancy, and other systemic inflammatory conditions. Although HSV-1 is typically associated with encephalitis, overt viral meningitis is much more common with HSV-2. The genital lesions of HSV-2 usually precede or accompany the onset of meningitis.

Typical CSF findings of acute bacterial meningitis include a leukocyte count of 1000 to 5000/microliter (1000 to 5000 × 10⁶/L), a predominance of neutrophils, a glucose level of less than or equal to 40 mg/dL (2.2 mmol/L), a CSF-to-plasma glucose ratio of less than or equal to 0.4, and Gram stain positivity of 60% to 90%.

The differential diagnosis of HSV aseptic meningitis includes illnesses with concurrent genital or perineal ulcerations and central nervous system involvement, such as

other viral causes, Behçet disease, porphyria, collagen vascular diseases, and inflammatory bowel disease. Patients with Behçet disease have recurrent painful oral and genital aphthous ulcerations, skin lesions, and uveitis; this disease is relatively rare in the United States. Neurologic manifestations are seen in up to 25% of patients. When Behçet disease causes aseptic meningitis, the level of pleocytosis is usually less than 100 cells/microliter. Additionally, the lack of history or findings of other manifestations of this uncommon condition makes this an unlikely diagnosis.

Acute retroviral infection may present with a syndrome characterized by fatigue, fever, pharyngitis, and lymphadenopathy. A small percentage of patients may have central nervous system involvement, including meningitis. The rash associated with acute HIV infection tends to be a diffuse, maculopapular eruption across the chest, back, face, and upper extremities; it may affect the palms and soles and is generally not painful or pruritic. Although it should be considered that this patient is at risk for acute HIV infection, her presentation is less consistent with this diagnosis.

> **KEY POINT**
>
> - Aseptic meningitis is commonly associated with genital infection from herpes simplex virus 2 and is characterized by recurrent episodes of fever, headache, vomiting, and photosensitivity.

Bibliography

Davis LE. Acute and recurrent viral meningitis. Curr Treat Options Neurol. 2008;10(3):168-177. [PMID: 18579020]

Item 23   Answer: C

Educational Objective: Manage a patient with an erythema migrans skin lesion.

The skin lesion shown is consistent with erythema migrans, and oral doxycycline should be started immediately. Erythema migrans may be due to either early localized Lyme disease or Southern tick–associated rash illness. Although these two infections are caused by specific tick vectors with relatively distinct geographic distributions, both ticks are endemic to Virginia. Geographic location is therefore of little value in differentiating between these two syndromes in this patient. However, empiric doxycycline is the recommended treatment for erythema migrans regardless of the cause. Treatment should be given based on the clinical finding of an expansile, target-like skin lesion, particularly at the site of a known tick attachment.

Borrelia burgdorferi polymerase chain reaction testing is not indicated. Although *B. burgdorferi* may be amplified from erythema migrans skin biopsy specimens if the diagnosis is uncertain, this study is generally not needed because the presence of the characteristic erythema migrans rash, such as is seen in this patient, dictates treatment.

Intravenous ceftriaxone is reserved for patients with cardiac or neurologic manifestations of disseminated Lyme disease.

Serologic testing for *B. burgdorferi* is not recommended because false-negative antibody assay results may occur in patients with early localized Lyme disease and would be negative in patients with Southern tick–associated rash illness.

KEY POINT

- Empiric oral doxycycline is the recommended treatment for erythema migrans regardless of the cause.

Bibliography

Stonehouse A, Studdiford JS, Henry CA. An update on the diagnosis and treatment of early Lyme disease: "focusing on the bull's eye, you may miss the mark". J Emerg Med. 2010;39(5):e147-151. [PMID: 17945460]

Item 24   Answer: C

Educational Objective: Diagnose herpes simplex virus type 2–induced benign recurrent lymphocytic meningitis.

This patient most likely has benign recurrent lymphocytic meningitis, and the most appropriate study to confirm the diagnosis is cerebrospinal fluid (CSF) polymerase chain reaction for herpes simplex virus type 2 (HSV-2). Benign recurrent lymphocytic meningitis, formerly known as Mollaret meningitis, is most often caused by HSV-2, although some cases have been associated with HSV-1 and Epstein-Barr virus. Patients usually experience 2 to 3 to at least 10 episodes of meningitis (most often characterized by headache, fever, and stiff neck) that last for 2 to 5 days and are followed by spontaneous recovery. About 50% of patients may also have transient neurologic manifestations, such as seizures, hallucinations, diplopia, cranial nerve palsies, or an altered level of consciousness. Disease occurs in patients without symptoms or signs of genital or cutaneous infection. Nucleic acid amplification tests, such as CSF polymerase chain reaction to detect the DNA of HSV-2, will establish the diagnosis. Patients usually recover without therapy; it is not clear whether antiviral agents alter the course of mild infection.

Given the recurrent nature of this patient's illness, it is unlikely to be caused by a malignancy. Cytologic studies are therefore unnecessary at this time. Cytology may reveal Mollaret cells, which are large atypical monocytes, but they are not seen in all cases, and their presence does not establish the etiologic diagnosis.

The recurrent episodes that this patient has experienced also make West Nile virus infection unlikely.

MRI of the brain would be appropriate if the patient had the clinical presentation of encephalitis (fever, hemicranial headache, language and behavioral abnormalities, memory impairment, cranial nerve deficits, and seizures), which is most often caused by HSV-1 rather than HSV-2.

KEY POINT

- Herpes simplex virus type 2 is the most common cause of benign recurrent lymphocytic meningitis, and the diagnosis is established by cerebrospinal fluid polymerase chain reaction.

Bibliography

Shalabi M, Whitley RJ. Recurrent benign lymphocytic meningitis. Clin Infect Dis. 2006;43(9):1194-1197. [PMID: 17029141]

Item 25   Answer: A

Educational Objective: Treat cryptococcal meningitis in a patient with AIDS.

This patient should be treated with conventional amphotericin B and flucytosine. He has AIDS and disseminated cryptococcosis, including cryptococcal meningitis. Headache and alterations in mental status are the most common symptoms. The skin lesions, which are molluscum-like, are characteristic of disseminated cryptococcosis. The cerebrospinal fluid (CSF) profile, including the paucity of leukocytes, is consistent with cryptococcal meningitis in the setting of AIDS. Control of CSF pressure is crucial to a successful outcome in patients with cryptococcal meningoencephalitis. If the CSF pressure is greater than or equal to 250 mm H_2O and there are symptoms of increased intracranial pressure, the pressure should be relieved by CSF drainage. The treatment of cryptococcal meningoencephalitis in HIV-infected patients consists of three stages: (1) induction, (2) consolidation, and (3) maintenance (suppression). The induction therapy of choice in patients with normal kidney function is conventional amphotericin B plus flucytosine for at least 2 weeks. The 2-week induction course is followed by oral fluconazole for a minimum of 8 weeks. Lipid formulations of amphotericin B are reserved for those with or predisposed to kidney dysfunction.

Echinocandins such as caspofungin have no role in the treatment of cryptococcal meningoencephalitis because they lack activity against cryptococci and have poor penetration into the CSF.

Other regimens for induction therapy in patients with cryptococcal meningoencephalitis include amphotericin B plus fluconazole, high-dose fluconazole plus flucytosine, high-dose fluconazole alone, and itraconazole alone, although itraconazole is discouraged because of poor penetration into the CSF.

KEY POINT

- Conventional amphotericin B plus flucytosine is the preferred treatment for cryptococcal meningitis in a patient with AIDS.

Bibliography

Perfect JR, Dismukes WE, Dromer F, et al. Clinical practice guidelines for the management of cryptococcal diseases: 2010 update by the Infectious Diseases Society of America. Clin Infect Dis. 2010;50(3):291-322. [PMID: 20047480]

Item 26   Answer: C

Educational Objective: Treat pelvic inflammatory disease in an outpatient.

This patient has pelvic inflammatory disease (PID) and requires a single dose of parenteral ceftriaxone followed by 14 days of oral doxycycline. This regimen may be given with or without oral metronidazole. The patient has evidence of cervicitis; however, the presence of uterine tenderness should prompt a diagnosis of PID. The clinical diagnosis of PID is imprecise. Because of the potential serious sequelae of untreated PID, including tubal scarring that can lead to infertility, ectopic pregnancy, and chronic pelvic pain syndromes, an approach using a very low threshold for diagnosis is recommended. The Centers for Disease Control and Prevention (CDC) guidelines recommend that women who present with abdominal or pelvic pain and have cervical motion tenderness, adnexal tenderness, or uterine tenderness be treated for PID. This infection is always considered to be polymicrobial. Antimicrobial regimens for PID must include coverage for *Neisseria gonorrhoeae*, *Chlamydia trachomatis*, aerobic gram-negative rods, and anaerobes that may be found in the vaginal flora. Early follow up (within 72 hours) must be arranged, and hospitalization is required for patients who do not respond to treatment with oral therapy or who cannot take oral therapy owing to nausea and vomiting. Male partners of women with PID who have had sexual contact in the past 60 days should be referred for evaluation and treatment.

The combination of clindamycin and gentamicin is an acceptable parenteral treatment for PID. However, this patient does not have signs of systemic toxicity, so outpatient treatment is appropriate.

Ciprofloxacin can no longer be used for the treatment of infections that may be due to *N. gonorrhoeae* because of increasing fluoroquinolone resistance.

Single-dose intramuscular ceftriaxone plus single-dose oral azithromycin is appropriate management for cervicitis, but single-dose therapy would not be sufficient for the treatment of PID.

KEY POINT

- **Women with abdominal or pelvic pain and cervical motion tenderness, adnexal tenderness, or uterine tenderness who can tolerate outpatient therapy should be treated for pelvic inflammatory disease, with single-dose intramuscular ceftriaxone and oral doxycycline for 14 days.**

Bibliography

Workowski KA, Berman S; Centers for Disease Control and Prevention (CDC). Sexually transmitted diseases treatment guidelines, 2010. MMWR Recomm Rep. 2010;59(RR-12):1-110. [PMID: 21160459]

Item 27   Answer: A

Educational Objective: Diagnose genital herpes simplex virus infection.

The most appropriate diagnostic test to perform next is herpes simplex virus (HSV) polymerase chain reaction (PCR) assay of the fissure. The patient has a history of recurrent genital symptoms consisting of itching and burning, which is a very characteristic prodrome of recurrent genital HSV infection. Although the patient reports no history of genital lesions, serologic surveys have shown that most patients with serologic evidence of HSV-2 infection do not have a history of symptomatic genital ulcer disease. The presence of a fissure is well described as an atypical presentation of genital HSV-2 infection. PCR is the most sensitive diagnostic methodology for confirming that the lesion is due to HSV; alternatively, a viral culture can be obtained. Viral cultures are less expensive than HSV PCR but are less sensitive.

Lymphogranuloma venereum (LGV) is a genital ulcer disease caused by the L1, L2, and L3 serovars of *Chlamydia trachomatis*. Classic LGV presents as a painless papule or ulcer at the site of inoculation that resolves without treatment and is followed by painful unilateral inguinal lymphadenopathy accompanied by fever and malaise. This patient's symptoms are not compatible with LGV, and serologic testing for this infection is not indicated.

A Tzanck smear for HSV is limited by low sensitivity and specificity and is only helpful when results are positive.

Patients with candidal vulvovaginitis may have vaginal pruritus and burning associated with fissures, but evidence of vaginal discharge and small erythematous papular lesions (satellite lesions) should be visible, peripheral to the involved area. Consequently, wet mount of vaginal secretions with the addition of potassium hydroxide is not necessary.

KEY POINT

- **Polymerase chain reaction is the most sensitive and specific diagnostic test for confirming a diagnosis of herpes simplex virus infection.**

Bibliography

Van Wagoner NJ, Hook EW 3rd. Herpes diagnostic tests and their use. Curr Infect Dis Rep. 2012;14(2):175-184. [PMID: 22311664]

Item 28   Answer: D

Educational Objective: Diagnose primary syphilis.

This patient's clinical presentation and examination findings are most consistent with a syphilitic chancre. Chancres are most frequently single lesions, but multiple lesions can occur, and the lesions are generally painless. The ulcer's border is raised and has a firm, cartilaginous consistency. The incidence of primary and secondary syphilis in the United States has increased among certain populations, especially young men who have sex with men, particularly those who are members of racial and ethnic minorities. A recent epidemiologic study from New York City found that men who have sex with men are at a 140-fold higher risk of newly diagnosed syphilis compared with heterosexual men. Factors such as drug use and the perception that unprotected oral sex is "safer" than anal intercourse are believed to be contributing to this increase. Because the methodology needed to demonstrate *Treponema pallidum* organisms in clinical specimens is not available in most settings, the clinical diagnosis can be confirmed by serologic testing; however, the serum rapid plasma reagin titer is frequently negative in primary syphilis. This patient should be offered HIV testing, screening for gonorrhea and chlamydia infection, and risk reduction counseling. In addition to syphilis, the differential diagnosis of genital ulcer disease includes chancroid and herpes simplex virus infection. Bacterial secondary infection of traumatic genital lesions can also have the appearance of an ulcer.

Chancroid causes single or multiple painful ulcers with a ragged border; the ulcer's base has a granulomatous appearance, frequently with a purulent exudate. This patient does not have chancroid.

Herpes simplex virus infection generally presents with multiple painful ulcers that were initially vesicular on an erythematous base.

Human papillomavirus infection causes genital warts, not ulcerative lesions.

KEY POINT

- Syphilitic chancres are most frequently single, painless lesions, with a raised border and a firm cartilaginous consistency; multiple lesions can also occur.

Bibliography

Su JR, Beltrami JF, Zaidi AA, Weinstock HS. Primary and secondary syphilis among black and Hispanic men who have sex with men: case report data from 27 States. Ann Intern Med. 2011;155(3):145-151. [PMID: 21810707]

Item 29   Answer: D

Educational Objective: Diagnose disseminated gonococcal infection.

The most appropriate next step in diagnosis is a nucleic acid amplification urine test for *Neisseria gonorrhoeae*. This is a noninvasive, sensitive test for diagnosing gonorrhea in men that provides rapid results (within hours) and can help guide therapy pending return of blood and synovial fluid culture results. Mucosal cultures, including of the throat, anus, urethra, or cervix, may also be helpful in establishing the diagnosis because they tend to have a higher diagnostic yield than blood and synovial fluid cultures in patients with disseminated gonococcal infection (DGI).

Although this young patient may have an autoimmune inflammatory arthritis such as systemic lupus erythematosus

or rheumatoid arthritis, he has evidence of an arthritis-dermatitis syndrome and should be evaluated for DGI. In contrast to nongonococcal septic arthritis, patients with DGI present with migratory joint symptoms and often have involvement of several joints with tenosynovitis rather than involvement of just a single joint. Asymmetric joint involvement helps distinguish DGI from autoimmune disease–associated polyarthritis, which is typically symmetric. Skin lesions are found in more than 75% of patients with DGI but may be few in number; consequently, a careful examination of the skin must be performed. Lesions are most likely to be found on the extremities. The classic lesion is characterized by a small number of necrotic vesicopustules on an erythematous base. Organisms are rarely cultured from the skin lesions of DGI, although they may be demonstrated through nucleic acid amplification techniques.

The prevalence of HLA B27 in patients with reactive arthritis is only 50%; consequently, HLA B27 testing is not very useful in establishing a diagnosis. In addition, reactive arthritis tends to present as a symmetric oligoarthritis, and this patient's arthritis is asymmetric. The associated rash, keratoderma blennorrhagica, consists of hyperkeratotic lesions on the palms and soles, which are not present in this patient. Patients with reactive arthritis may also have conjunctivitis, urethritis, oral ulcers, and circinate balanitis.

KEY POINT

- To confirm a presumptive diagnosis of disseminated gonococcal infection, in addition to blood and synovial fluid cultures, specimens should be obtained from mucosal surfaces, including the throat, anus, and urethra, or cervix, which can be tested via nucleic acid amplification tests or culture.

Bibliography

García-De La Torre I, Nava-Zavala A. Gonococcal and nongonococcal arthritis. Rheum Dis Clin North Am. 2009;35(1):63-73. [PMID: 19480997]

Item 30   Answer: D

Educational Objective: Manage mild pneumonia caused by *Histoplasma capsulatum* in a healthy host.

This patient has mild pulmonary histoplasmosis, which is self-limiting and requires no treatment in a healthy host. In those who become ill, the incubation period is 7 to 21 days, and most have symptoms by day 14. Histoplasmosis is common in states bordering the Ohio river valley and the lower Mississippi river. Infection may be asymptomatic, but the diagnosis should be considered in any patient with pulmonary and systemic symptoms following potential exposure in a geographically endemic area. In most symptomatic patients, disease is mild and resolves without therapy within 1 month. In a few patients, particularly those with immunocompromise (such as HIV infection) or other concurrent illnesses, severe pneumonia with respiratory failure may result. Histoplasmosis may also cause chronic infection, including pulmonary and mediastinal masses, cavitary lesions, central nervous system involvement, pericarditis, and arthritis and arthralgia. Antifungal treatment is indicated for severe or moderately severe acute pulmonary, chronic pulmonary, disseminated, and central nervous system histoplasmosis or for those patients whose symptoms do not improve within 1 month. Evidence of effectiveness, however, is lacking to support this recommendation.

If treatment is indicated for acute pulmonary histoplasmosis, the treatment of choice is itraconazole. Lipid formulations of amphotericin B are indicated for more severe forms of pulmonary histoplasmosis. Fluconazole has been used for treatment of histoplasmosis, but it is less effective than itraconazole. Fluconazole resistance has also been noted in some patients who have not responded to therapy.

KEY POINT

- **Mild forms of histoplasmosis do not require treatment, whereas more severe forms may be treated with amphotericin B or one of the newer triazole antifungal agents.**

Bibliography

Wheat LJ, Freifeld AG, Kleiman MB, et al; Infectious Diseases Society of America. Clinical practice guidelines for the management of patients with histoplasmosis: 2007 update by the Infectious Diseases Society of America. Clin Infect Dis. 2007;45(7):807-825. [PMID: 17806045]

Item 31   Answer: B

Educational Objective: Prevent catheter-associated urinary tract infection.

This patient's urine-collecting bag should be maintained below the level of the bladder to avoid catheter-associated urinary tract infection (CAUTI). The most effective way to prevent UTIs is to decrease catheter use. Devices should be used for specific indications. Examples include (1) to diagnose pathologic findings in the lower urinary tract or the cause of urinary retention, (2) to monitor fluid status in acutely ill patients when this directly impacts medical treatment, and (3) to manage patients with stage 3 or 4 pressure ulcers on the buttocks. However, urinary catheters often are used for convenience, which significantly increases the risk of UTIs. If the catheter is needed, measures are required to decrease the risk of bacteriuria and subsequent infection. These include hand washing, using an aseptic technique and sterile equipment for catheter insertion and care, securing the catheter properly, and maintaining unobstructed urine flow and closed sterile drainage. Finally, to prevent the backflow of stagnating, contaminated urine, it is important to keep the collecting bag below the level of the bladder at all times.

There is no proven preventive benefit associated with cleansing the meatal area of the catheter with antiseptics.

Although removing the catheter at the first possible opportunity is an important measure in preventing CAUTI, routine exchange of urinary catheters is not necessary or effective.

Screening and treatment of asymptomatic bacteriuria does not improve patient outcomes in nonpregnant patients and does not prevent CAUTI.

Using antiseptic-coated catheters has not yet been demonstrated to significantly affect the incidence of CAUTI, although it significantly reduces colonization rates and colonization densities of urinary catheters.

KEY POINT

- **Maintaining the urine-collecting bag below the level of the bladder is an established measure for preventing catheter-associated urinary tract infections.**

Bibliography

Chenoweth CE, Saint S. Urinary Tract Infections. Infect Dis Clin North Am. 2011;25(1):103-115. [PMID: 21315996]

Item 32   Answer: D

Educational Objective: Diagnose catheter-associated urinary tract infection.

A urine culture demonstrating more than 10^3 colony-forming units (CFU)/mL will establish the diagnosis of catheter-associated urinary tract infection (CAUTI). CAUTI can be difficult to diagnose, and it may be difficult to distinguish colonization in a patient with a bladder catheter from true infection. The Infectious Diseases Society of American (IDSA) has suggested criteria to aid in the diagnosis of CAUTI. In patients with indwelling urethral, indwelling suprapubic, or intermittent catheterization, CAUTI is defined by the presence of symptoms or signs compatible with UTI with no other identified source of infection and 10^3 or more CFU/mL of one or more bacterial species in a single catheter urine specimen. Signs and symptoms compatible with CAUTI include new-onset or worsening of fever, rigors, altered mental status, malaise, or lethargy with no other identified cause; flank pain; costovertebral angle tenderness; acute hematuria; and pelvic discomfort. In patients with spinal cord injury, increased spasticity, autonomic dysreflexia, or sense of unease are also compatible with CAUTI.

The cloudiness of the urine or detection of organisms on urine Gram stain is not adequate for establishing a diagnosis of CAUTI. Cloudy appearance of urine is not diagnostic of UTI and is not part of the IDSA UTI definition.

The presence of positive leukocyte esterase on a dipstick urinalysis is consistent with the presence of leukocytes in the urine. Although the absence of evidence of leukocytes in the urine has a high negative predictive value for UTI, in a patient with an indwelling catheter in which colonization and concentration of normal urinary contents may occur, the presence of urinary leukocytes is not sufficient to make a diagnosis of CAUTI.

> **KEY POINT**
>
> - Catheter-associated urinary tract infection is defined by the presence of symptoms or signs compatible with urinary tract infection with no other identified source of infection and 10^3 or more colony-forming units/mL of one or more bacterial species in a single catheter urine specimen.

Bibliography

Hooton TM, Bradley SF, Cardenas DD, et al; Infectious Diseases Society of America. Diagnosis, prevention, and treatment of catheter-associated urinary tract infection in adults: 2009 International Clinical Practice Guidelines from the Infectious Diseases Society of America. Clin Infect Dis. 2010;50(5):625-663. [PMID: 20175247]

Item 33   Answer: A
Educational Objective: Manage newly diagnosed HIV infection.

The most appropriate management is treatment with tenofovir, emtricitabine, and efavirenz now. Because of the benefits associated with earlier initiation of combination antiretroviral therapy and the diminished complexity of and greater tolerance to these regimens, indications for when to begin therapy have expanded. The Department of Health and Human Services 2011 guidelines recommend initiation of antiretroviral therapy for patients with a history of an AIDS-defining opportunistic infection or malignancy, the presence of symptoms, a CD4 cell count less than 500/microliter, HIV-associated nephropathy, active co-infection with hepatitis B virus infection, and pregnancy (to prevent perinatal transmission). In addition, the International AIDS Society–USA Panel recommends treatment of those with active hepatitis C virus co-infection and those who are at high risk for or have active cardiovascular disease, regardless of CD4 cell count. Whether to start treatment in all patients with HIV infection is controversial and remains under investigation as of this writing.

Based on accumulating data from cohort studies showing better outcomes in those patients who initiate treatment earlier, recent guidelines have raised the CD4 cell count threshold from 350/microliter to 500/microliter, below which antiretroviral treatment should be started.

Because the CD4 cell count is a better indicator of risk for progression and disease than is HIV RNA viral load, recent guidelines have removed viral load levels as an indicator of need for initiation of antiretroviral therapy.

Because this patient's CD4 cell count is less than 500/microliter, he should initiate HIV treatment regardless of whether symptoms are present.

> **KEY POINT**
>
> - Initiating combination antiretroviral therapy is appropriate in patients with HIV infection and a CD4 cell count less than 500/microliter, regardless of whether symptoms are present.

Bibliography

Panel on Antiretroviral Guidelines for Adults and Adolescents. Guidelines for the use of antiretroviral agents in HIV-1-infected adults and adolescents. Department of Health and Human Services. October 14, 2011;1-167. Available at: www.aidsinfo.nih.gov/ContentFiles/AdultandAdolescentGL.pdf. Accessed December 20, 2011.

Item 34   Answer: B
Educational Objective: Treat community-acquired pneumonia in an outpatient.

This patient should be treated with azithromycin. His clinical presentation and radiographic findings are consistent with community-acquired pneumonia (CAP). In outpatients, risk factors for drug-resistant *Streptococcus pneumoniae* infection influence the selection of empiric therapy. These risk factors include age greater than 65 years, recent (within the past 3 months) β-lactam therapy, medical comorbidities, immunocompromising conditions and immunosuppressive therapy, alcoholism, and exposure to a child in day care. This patient is a young, healthy man with no risk factors for drug-resistant *S. pneumoniae* infection; therefore, treatment with a macrolide agent, such as azithromycin, will provide adequate coverage for the likely pathogens, including drug-sensitive *S. pneumoniae*, *Haemophilus influenzae*, *Mycoplasma*, and *Chlamydophila* species.

Amoxicillin would not provide coverage for the atypical pathogens such as *Mycoplasma* or *Chlamydophila* and would not cover all *H. influenzae* strains because an increasing number of strains are β-lactamase producing. Although very few studies exist on the microbiology of CAP in outpatients, *Mycoplasma* and *Chlamydophila* more likely cause pneumonia in ambulatory patients. High-dose amoxicillin combined with a macrolide is an alternative for patients with risk factors for drug-resistant *S. pneumoniae* infection.

Cefuroxime will provide coverage for drug-sensitive *S. pneumoniae* and *H. influenzae* but not for atypical pathogens. A respiratory fluoroquinolone such as moxifloxacin or levofloxacin provides appropriate coverage for the likely pathogens associated with CAP but is unnecessarily broad for this indication. A respiratory fluoroquinolone would be appropriate if this patient had risk factors for infection with drug-resistant *S. pneumoniae*.

Ciprofloxacin has very poor activity against *S. pneumoniae* and should never be used as empiric therapy for CAP.

KEY POINT

- In previously healthy patients with pneumonia but no risk factors for drug-resistant *Streptococcus pneumoniae* infection, treatment with a macrolide agent, such as azithromycin, will provide adequate coverage for the likely pathogens.

Bibliography

Mandell LA, Wunderink RG, Anzueto A, et al; Infectious Diseases Society of America; American Thoracic Society. Infectious Diseases Society of America/American Thoracic Society consensus guidelines on the management of community-acquired pneumonia in adults. Clin Infect Dis. 2007;44(suppl 2):S27-72. [PMID: 17278083]

Item 35   Answer: B

Educational Objective: Diagnose acute coccidioidomycosis.

This patient has the acute form of coccidioidomycosis infection. Coccidioidomycosis is endemic to the desert regions of the southwestern United States and to Central and South America. It is estimated that only half of patients infected acutely come to medical attention. Those who do frequently present with what is known as "valley fever," a subacute respiratory illness with systemic symptoms, such as fever and fatigue, which persist for weeks to months. Some symptomatic patients also note joint symptoms, a presentation frequently described as "desert rheumatism." Erythema nodosum (painful nodules on the extensor surfaces of the extremities) is also a common manifestation of acute coccidioidomycosis infection. Although uncommon in immunocompetent persons, complicated disease may occur, particularly in those with impaired cell-mediated immunity. Persons of American Indian, African, or Filipino descent are also more likely to develop serious infection. Routine laboratory findings are usually normal except for an increased erythrocyte sedimentation rate. Because the manifestations of early coccidioidal infections are nonspecific, epidemiologic clues are important when deciding to perform specific laboratory testing. The incubation period is 1 to 3 weeks. Culture is the most sensitive means of establishing the diagnosis, but identification of spherules by direct examination is more rapid. Serologic studies are also available for diagnosing coccidioidomycosis infection.

Although blastomycosis and histoplasmosis can also cause pneumonia and erythema nodosum, blastomycosis is endemic to the Mississippi river and Ohio river basins and around the Great Lakes. The diagnosis may be confirmed by the appearance of characteristic broad-based budding organisms in sputum or tissue samples by potassium hydroxide (KOH) preparation or cytohistologic methods. Histoplasmosis is also endemic to the states bordering the Ohio river valley and the lower Mississippi River. It does not produce spherules, and the yeast forms seen in clinical specimens are relatively small.

Sporotrichosis is a very rare cause of pneumonia and very rarely has been associated with erythema nodosum. Symptoms and signs of pulmonary sporotrichosis include productive cough, lung nodules and cavitations, fibrosis, and hilar lymphadenopathy. It is a chronic disease with slow progression. It does not form spherules.

KEY POINT

- Coccidioidomycosis is a common pulmonary fungal infection endemic to the desert regions of the southwestern United States and to Central and South America, is frequently asymptomatic, and may present with a subclinical pulmonary infection, systemic symptoms, joint pain, and erythema nodosum.

Bibliography

Ampel NM. New perspectives on coccidioidomycosis. Proc Am Thorac Soc. 2010;7(3):181-185. [PMID: 20463246]

Item 36   Answer: D

Educational Objective: Manage acute, uncomplicated cystitis in a woman.

This patient has acute, uncomplicated cystitis, and she should be given nitrofurantoin for 5 days. Nitrofurantoin is a first-line agent for uncomplicated cystitis owing to its efficacy, current minimal resistance, and minimal propensity to select drug-resistant organisms. A 3-day regimen of nitrofurantoin is not as effective as a 3-day regimen of trimethoprim-sulfamethoxazole or fluoroquinolone agents. Nitrofurantoin should not be used if early pyelonephritis is suspected. If the patient had not been allergic to sulfa drugs, a 3-day course of trimethoprim-sulfamethoxazole would have been appropriate if local resistance rates of urinary tract pathogens did not exceed 20% or if the infecting organism was known to be susceptible.

Amoxicillin or ampicillin should not be used unless the infecting organism is known to be susceptible because of the relatively high frequency of *Escherichia coli* species resistant to these agents among patients with community-acquired urinary tract infections.

Fosfomycin is another alternative first-line agent for uncomplicated cystitis if it is available, but it has inferior efficacy compared with other short-course, first-line agents. It should not be used if early pyelonephritis is suspected.

Fluoroquinolone agents, such as levofloxacin, are alternatives for patients who are allergic to or intolerant of first-line agents or live in areas where resistance to trimethoprim-sulfamethoxazole is higher than 20%. Fluoroquinolones are highly effective agents, and 3-day regimens are equivalent in efficacy to longer treatment courses. They should be reserved for more serious infections than acute cystitis.

- Nitrofurantoin or trimethoprim-sulfamethoxazole is the preferred management strategy for acute, uncomplicated cystitis in nonpregnant young women.

Bibliography

Gupta K, Hooton TM, Naber KG, et al; Infectious Diseases Society of America; European Society for Microbiology and Infectious Diseases. International clinical practice guidelines for the treatment of acute uncomplicated cystitis and pyelonephritis in women: a 2010 update by the Infectious Diseases Society of America and the European Society for Microbiology and Infectious Diseases. Clin Infect Dis. 2011;52(5):e103-120. [PMID: 21292654]

Item 37   Answer: C

Educational Objective: Treat tuberculous pericarditis.

The most appropriate treatment at this time is prednisone. This patient has tuberculous pericarditis resulting in cardiac tamponade and requiring pericardiocentesis. In addition to antituberculous therapy for at least 6 months, consensus guidelines of the American Thoracic Society, Centers for Disease Control and Prevention, and the Infectious Diseases Society of America recommend use of adjunctive corticosteroid therapy. Specifically, adults with tuberculous pericarditis should receive prednisone for the first 11 weeks of therapy. The following doses and duration of prednisone are recommended: 60 mg/d for 4 weeks, then 30 mg/d for 4 weeks, then 15 mg/d for 2 weeks, and finally 5 mg/d for the last week. The use of corticosteroids appears to be associated with improved survival and decreased need for pericardiectomy.

NSAIDs, such as indomethacin, and colchicine can be considered for patients with acute idiopathic or viral pericarditis. These agents are helpful in resolving acute inflammation and symptoms and in preventing recurrences. However, this patient has known tuberculous pericarditis, and the role of NSAIDs and colchicine in the treatment of this disorder in lieu of prednisone is not supported by current guidelines.

At this point, the patient has no indications for more invasive treatment of his tamponade, including pericardial window or pericardiectomy, and he is likely to respond to antituberculous therapy. Indications for more invasive treatment include recurrent pericardial effusions, loculated effusion, or diagnostic need for pericardial biopsy.

- In addition to rifampin, isoniazid, pyrazinamide, and ethambutol therapy, adjunctive corticosteroids are recommended for the treatment of patients with tuberculous pericarditis.

Bibliography

American Thoracic Society, CDC, Infectious Diseases Society of America. Treatment of tuberculosis. MMWR Recomm Rep. 2003;52(RR-11):1-77. [PMID: 12836625]

Item 38   Answer: B

Educational Objective: Prevent transmission of hospital-acquired infection.

Hand hygiene is the single most important measure to prevent infections, including from multidrug-resistant organisms. Hand hygiene, enacted before and after patient contact, consists of hand washing with soap and water for at least 15 to 30 seconds; alcohol-based hand disinfectants are acceptable alternatives to soap and water. In addition to hand hygiene, standard precautions include the use of barrier protection, including wearing gloves and personal protective equipment for the mouth, nose, and eyes; appropriate handling of patient care equipment and instruments/devices (avoiding exposure to skin and using appropriate cleaning techniques); and proper handling, transporting, and processing of used/contaminated linen.

Bleach has an important role in cleaning the rooms of patients with *Clostridium difficile* infection but has not proved helpful in controlling patient-to-patient transmission of infection with *Acinetobacter baumannii*.

Prophylactically treating the roommate for *Acinetobacter* infection is not nearly as effective or safe as proper hand hygiene. Furthermore, improper use of antibiotics in this fashion is likely to quickly lead to antibiotic resistance.

Removing the contaminated catheters and drains from a source patient has not been demonstrated to reduce the risk for spread of pathogens to other patients.

- Hand hygiene is the single most important measure to prevent spread of hospital-acquired infections.

Bibliography

Burke JP. Infection control - a problem for patient safety. N Engl J Med. 2003;348(7):651-656. [PMID: 12584377]

Item 39   Answer: A

Educational Objective: Evaluate a patient with osteomyelitis.

The next study that should be performed is a CT scan of the foot. The clinical hallmarks of acute osteomyelitis are local pain and fever, particularly in patients with acute hematogenous osteomyelitis, but these symptoms may be absent in patients with chronic and contiguous osteomyelitis.

Given the limitations of physical examination findings in the diagnosis of osteomyelitis, radiologic studies are frequently used. In patients in whom radiographic results are negative but clinical suspicion for osteomyelitis remains high, MRI is indicated. MRI scans show changes of acute osteomyelitis within days of infection and are superior to and more sensitive (90%) and specific (80%) than plain films and CT scans; can detect soft tissue abscesses and epidural, paravertebral, or psoas abscesses possibly requiring surgical drainage; and can delineate anatomy before surgery. Nonetheless, false-positive MRI results may occur in patients with noninfectious conditions such as fractures, tumors, and healed osteomyelitis. In patients with a pacemaker or metal hardware precluding MRI or in those in whom MRI results are inconclusive, CT scans or (if metal hardware is likely to impair CT imaging) nuclear studies may be used instead of MRI. CT reveals excellent anatomic imaging details, and it is the imaging study of choice for patients with osteomyelitis when MRI cannot be obtained.

Nuclear imaging studies can reliably detect the presence of inflammation related to acute infection. However, such visualized abnormalities, which may be caused by bone turnover or inflammation, can also be from other noninfectious causes, including trauma, neoplasm, and degenerative joint disease. Gallium scanning, once a gold standard for cancer diagnosis, may still be used to visualize inflammation and chronic infections, partly because gallium binds to the membranes of neutrophils recruited to a site of infection. However, leukocyte-labeled nuclear scans have almost entirely replaced this imaging technique. Except in the setting of diminished blood flow to the affected area, a negative three-phase bone scan confers a high negative predictive value for osteomyelitis.

KEY POINT

- CT scan is the imaging study of choice for suspected osteomyelitis when MRI cannot be performed.

Bibliography

Chihara S, Segreti J. Osteomyelitis. Dis Mon. 2010;56(1):5-31. [PMID: 19995624]

Item 40   Answer: A

Educational Objective: Diagnose a returning traveler with malaria.

The most likely malaria species against which treatment should be directed is *Plasmodium falciparum*. Malaria should be considered the most likely cause of fever in any traveler returning from a malaria-endemic area of the world. After Africa, Asia is the geographic destination with the highest risk of imported malaria. *P. falciparum* causes most malaria cases diagnosed in the United States following travel. Although mostly all cases occur in travelers who did not take any chemoprophylaxis or who were not adherent to it, infection can still be contracted despite compliance with all medical and preventive measures. In this instance, the patient spent time in Thailand, one of the rare malaria-infested zones where mefloquine-resistant *P. falciparum* has been reported.

There are no pathognomonic clinical signs or symptoms of malaria. In general, the signs and symptoms of uncomplicated malaria are nonspecific and infrequently occur before 1 to 4 weeks after return from travel. Fever, present in 100% of patients, may have a recurring cyclical pattern every 48 or 72 hours, varying according to the specific *Plasmodium* species and corresponding to the synchrony of organism replication. However, classic periodic malarial fever is most often absent in imported cases. Other common symptoms include myalgia, headache, and gastrointestinal discomfort. The degree of anemia depends on the duration of disease and degree of parasitemia. Although leukocyte counts may be variable, thrombocytopenia is present in greater than 50% of patients. Kidney impairment may also occur, the pathogenesis of which likely relates to hemolysis and erythrocyte sequestration within the kidney circulation. The term "blackwater fever" is given to the very dark urine secondary to significant hemoglobinuria sometimes observed in patients with severe *falciparum* malaria. Moreover, overwhelming disease may occur in patients who have anatomic or functional asplenia. The standard for malaria diagnosis is the Giemsa-stained blood smear by light microscopy. *P. falciparum* can involve erythrocytes of any size and are characterized by ring forms, some of which may be multiple, positioned along the periphery of the erythrocyte against the inner surface of its membrane. Classic "banana-shaped" gametocytes, if detected, can help to distinguish *falciparum* malaria species from the other potential *Plasmodium* species.

Infection with *Plasmodium malariae* should be considered if the paroxysms of fever occur every 72 hours and when the parasitized erythrocytes demonstrate the characteristic band form trophozoite, neither of which is consistent with this patient's clinical scenario.

Infection with *Plasmodium ovale* and *Plasmodium vivax* may show trophozoite and schizont forms on the peripheral blood smear with Schüffner dots inside of enlarged erythrocytes, inconsistent with this patient's peripheral blood smear findings.

KEY POINT

- A diagnosis of malaria should be considered in the differential diagnosis of travelers returning from malaria-endemic areas who present with fever and a peripheral smear indicating *Plasmodium* organisms in the erythrocytes.

Bibliography

Taylor SM, Molyneux ME, Simel DL, et al. Does this patient have malaria? JAMA. 2010;304(18):2048-2056. [PMID: 21057136]

Item 41   Answer: D

Educational Objective: Manage a patient with active tuberculosis who has discontinued her medications.

This patient's therapy for active tuberculosis should be restarted from the beginning. She is infected with a strain of *Mycobacterium tuberculosis* that is sensitive to all first-line antituberculous agents, but she interrupted her initial 2-month phase of treatment. Interruptions in treatment are not uncommon. Decisions regarding subsequent therapy are based on the duration of treatment and when the medications were discontinued. Consensus guidelines recommend that an interruption of 2 or more weeks during the initial 2-month phase of therapy requires restarting the same regimen from the beginning.

When the lapse is less than 2 weeks, recommendations are that the initial regimen should be continued until the planned total number of doses is taken, provided that all doses are taken within 3 months.

Regardless of whether results of a sputum smear are negative for acid-fast bacilli, the recommended treatment regimen for a pulmonary infection caused by a fully susceptible strain of *M. tuberculosis* includes an initial 2-month phase followed by a continuation phase of at least 4 months' duration.

Because all of this patient's medications were discontinued at the same time, there is no indication that the strain of tuberculosis has developed resistance; therefore, there is no need to restart a different treatment regimen.

KEY POINT

- **When a patient with active tuberculosis being treated with initial-phase antituberculous agents discontinues treatment for 2 weeks or longer, the same antituberculous regimen should be restarted from the beginning.**

Bibliography

American Thoracic Society; CDC; Infectious Diseases Society of America. Treatment of tuberculosis. MMWR Recomm Rep. 2003;52(RR-11):1-77. [PMID: 12836625]

Item 42   Answer: C

Educational Objective: Treat mild disseminated extrapulmonary blastomycosis in a healthy host.

This patient, who is a healthy host, has mild disseminated extrapulmonary blastomycosis and should be treated with oral itraconazole for 6 to 12 months or until all signs and symptoms of the disease have abated. Up to 40% of those infected with blastomycosis develop extrapulmonary infection, which is usually cutaneous (most commonly), genitourinary, osteoarticular, or central nervous system (CNS) disease. Two types of cutaneous lesions (verrucous and ulcerative) occur frequently in the absence of clinically active pulmonary disease and are the most common extrapulmonary manifestation of blastomycosis. Verrucous lesions usually are found on exposed skin. Over time, lesions may undergo central clearing, scar formation, and depigmentation. Both verrucous and ulcerative lesions may occur in the same patient. Definitive diagnosis requires growth of the organism in culture. A presumptive diagnosis is made by visualizing the characteristic yeast with broad-based buds in pus, secretions, or tissue. Because of toxicity, conventional amphotericin B and amphotericin B lipid formulations are reserved for patients with moderately severe to severe pulmonary, disseminated, and CNS

blastomycosis, whereas itraconazole is the drug of choice for the treatment of non–life-threatening, non–CNS blastomycosis. Itraconazole drug levels should be measured during the first month of treatment in patients with disseminated or pulmonary blastomycosis.

Fluconazole has a very limited role in the treatment of blastomycosis. Results from one study using low to standard doses were disappointing, whereas higher doses were more efficacious.

Because the response to antifungal therapy is very good, there is no role for surgical excision of skin lesions caused by blastomycosis.

KEY POINT

- **Mild to moderate disseminated extrapulmonary blastomycosis can be effectively treated with oral itraconazole.**

Bibliography

Chapman SW, Dismukes WE, Proia LA, et al; Infectious Diseases Society of America. Clinical practice guidelines for the management of blastomycosis: 2008 update by the Infectious Diseases Society of America. Clin Infect Dis. 2008;46(12):1801-1812. [PMID: 18462107]

Item 43   Answer: E

Educational Objective: Manage influenza virus infection during an outbreak in the community.

This patient has classic symptoms of influenza occurring during a confirmed outbreak of influenza A (H1N1) virus infection in the community. She has mild illness and is otherwise healthy; therefore, she does not need treatment with an antiviral medication. The Advisory Committee on Immunization Practices (ACIP) recommends early antiviral treatment of suspected or confirmed influenza for hospitalized patients; those with severe, complicated, or progressive illness; and those at high risk for influenza complications. Other high-risk medical conditions include cardiovascular disease (except isolated hypertension), active cancer, chronic kidney disease, chronic liver disease, hemoglobinopathies, immunocompromise (including HIV disease), and neurologic diseases that impair handling of respiratory secretions. When treatment is indicated, it should be started within the first 2 days of symptom onset to reduce the duration of illness and decrease the risk for serious complications. Oseltamivir or zanamivir is indicated for those with influenza A (H1N1), influenza A (H3N2), or influenza B virus infection or for those in whom the influenza virus type or influenza A virus subtype is unknown. Oseltamivir and zanamivir differ in pharmacokinetics, safety profile, route of administration, approved age groups, and recommended dosages. Zanamivir is administered by an inhaler device and is not recommended for persons with underlying airways disease such as asthma or COPD.

Amantadine and rimantadine are related antiviral medications in the adamantane class that are active against influenza A viruses but not influenza B viruses. In recent years, widespread adamantane resistance among influenza A (H3N2 and H1N1) strains has been noted. These agents are not recommended for antiviral treatment or chemoprophylaxis of currently circulating influenza A strains.

KEY POINT

- Antiviral therapy is not indicated for mild influenza in healthy persons.

Bibliography

Fiore AE, Fry A, Shay D, Gubareva L, Bresee JS, Uyeki TM; Centers for Disease Control and Prevention (CDC). Antiviral agents for the treatment and chemoprophylaxis of influenza —- recommendations of the Advisory Committee on Immunization Practices (ACIP). MMWR Recomm Rep. 2011;60(1):1-24. [PMID: 21248682]

Item 44   Answer: C

Educational Objective: Understand the potential side effects associated with first-line drugs used to treat tuberculosis.

Pyrazinamide is most likely responsible for causing an acute attack of gout in this patient who is being treated for active tuberculosis. Pyrazinamide can cause hyperuricemia and gout by inhibiting renal tubular excretion of uric acid. Other potential side effects include hepatitis, rash, and gastrointestinal upset. Pyrazinamide is contraindicated for use in patients with active gout and should be used with caution in those with a known history of chronic gout.

Amlodipine is commonly associated with nausea, flushing, palpitations, dizziness, peripheral edema, and muscle pain; however, it does not increase uric acid levels, and its use is not contraindicated in patients with gout.

Side effects of isoniazid use include hepatitis, rash, peripheral neuropathy, and a lupus-like syndrome, but not hyperuricemia.

Rifampin can cause rash, hepatitis, gastrointestinal upset, and orange-coloring of body fluids. Of note, rifampin enhances kidney excretion of uric acid.

KEY POINT

- Pyrazinamide use is associated with hyper-uricemia, which can result in gouty arthritis.

Bibliography

American Thoracic Society; CDC; Infectious Diseases Society of America. Treatment of tuberculosis. MMWR Recomm Rep. 2003;52(RR-11):1-77 [PMID: 12836625]

Item 45   Answer: A

Educational Objective: Treat extensively drug-resistant *Pseudomonas aeruginosa.*

This patient requires treatment with intravenous colistin. Extensively drug-resistant *Pseudomonas aeruginosa* is a treatment challenge. This organism frequently colonizes

clinical settings, such as intensive care units, and is the most common cause of widely resistant gram-negative health care–acquired pneumonia. Patients with burns also appear to be particularly susceptible to pseudomonal infection, which confers a poor prognosis, even with aggressive treatment. This resistance pattern and susceptibility in this patient make selection of adequate antibiotic therapy difficult. Colistin (polymyxin E) is an older antimicrobial agent that historically was used infrequently owing to high rates of nephrotoxicity. Recently, colistin has been used more frequently because it is one of the few agents with reliable activity against resistant gram-negative bacilli, such as extensively drug-resistant *P. aeruginosa*, and it is the only agent of the options listed that that is effective in this setting and achieves adequate systemic drug levels.

Minocycline and rifampin, which are older antimicrobial agents, lack reliable pseudomonal activity and are therefore inappropriate for use in this situation.

Tigecycline, a newer glycylcycline agent, has no pseudomonal activity.

KEY POINT

- Colistin is one of the only available options for treatment of extensively drug-resistant *Pseudomonas aeruginosa* infection.

Bibliography

Pogue JM, Marchaim D, Kaye D, Kaye DS. Revisiting "older" antimicrobials in the era of multidrug resistance. Pharmacotherapy. 2011;31(9):912-921. [PMID: 21923592]

Item 46   Answer: C

Educational Objective: Manage a hospitalized patient with bacteremic pneumococcal pneumonia.

This patient with bacteremic pneumococcal pneumonia should be discharged on oral amoxicillin to complete 7 days of therapy. His physical examination findings on hospital day 3 (afebrile, pulse rate ≤100/min, respiration rate ≤24/min, and systolic blood pressure ≥90 mm Hg) plus normal oxygen saturation while breathing ambient air indicate that he is clinically stable and should be considered for discharge. In addition, patients considered stable for discharge should have a normal (or baseline) mental status and be able to tolerate oral therapy. The presence of pneumococcal bacteremia does not warrant a more prolonged course of intravenous therapy. Once patients are clinically stable, they are at very low risk for subsequent clinical deterioration and can be safely discharged from the hospital.

Levofloxacin would provide unnecessarily broad-spectrum coverage for this patient's penicillin-susceptible pneumonia, and levofloxacin would be a more expensive treatment option.

Seven days of therapy is sufficient for treatment of community-acquired pneumonia in most patients, especially those who have a prompt clinical response to treatment, even in the setting of bacteremic infection. A 14-day

CONT.

treatment regimen would be unnecessarily long for this patient.

Studies have shown that continued observation after switching from intravenous to oral therapy is not necessary.

KEY POINT

- **Hospitalized patients with bacteremic community-acquired pneumonia who respond promptly to therapy do not require a more prolonged course of intravenous therapy and can be discharged home on oral medication when they are clinically stable.**

Bibliography

Weinstein MP, Klugman KP, Jones RN. Rationale for revised penicillin susceptibility breakpoints versus Streptococcus pneumoniae: coping with antimicrobial susceptibility in an era of resistance. Clin Infect Dis. 2009;48(11):1596-1600. [PMID: 19400744]

Item 47   Answer: A

Educational Objective: Diagnose anthrax infection.

The most likely infectious agent is *Bacillus anthracis*. This patient most likely has inhalational anthrax, a form of disease previously diagnosed only in persons having potential occupational exposure to this bacillus. The spores of *B. anthracis* lie dormant in soil. Disease may follow infection with spores acquired through cutaneous contact, ingestion, or inhalation. The rapid development of a septic state following a nonspecific prodromal flu-like syndrome is characteristic of inhalational anthrax. Although anthrax does not generally manifest as pneumonitis, migration of inhaled spores to the mediastinal lymph nodes leads to tissue destruction and hemorrhage, resulting in the classic widening of the mediastinum and occasional bloody pleural effusions demonstrated on chest radiograph or CT imaging. The diagnosis is confirmed by isolation of the organism (commonly from blood cultures with inhalational disease) or by detection of its presence in tissue or fluid through polymerase chain reaction testing.

Erysipelothrix rhusiopathiae, another infrequently encountered gram-positive bacillus recognized as a pathogen in animals and a colonizer in fish, is most commonly associated with human infection in persons with occupational exposure to contaminated meat or fish. Most infections are cutaneous; the rarely occurring invasive form develops primarily as infective endocarditis.

Although *Listeria monocytogenes* is often acquired through ingestion of contaminated foods or unpasteurized milk products, severe disease most often occurs in the very young, elderly, or those who have an underlying state of immunocompromise. Generally, *L. monocytogenes* presents as a diarrheal illness, but it may lead to sepsis and central nervous system involvement. This patient's constellation of signs and symptoms is not consistent with *L. monocytogenes*.

Nocardia infections can manifest as cutaneous, lymphocutaneous, pulmonary, or central nervous system disease. Nodular and cavitary lesions are predominantly observed when the lungs are involved. Bacteremia with this weakly staining gram-positive bacillus is rare.

KEY POINT

- **The rapid development of a septic state following a nonspecific prodromal flu-like syndrome and widening of the mediastinum is characteristic of inhalational anthrax.**

Bibliography

Inglesby TV, O'Toole T, Henderson DA, et al. Anthrax as a biologic weapon, 2002: updated recommendations for management. JAMA. 2002;287(17):2236-2252. [PMID: 11980524]

Item 48   Answer: D

Educational Objective: Manage a patient with stool samples containing *Blastocystis* species.

Asymptomatic patients in whom *Blastocystis* species are found in stool samples do not require therapy or additional studies to document eradication of the organisms. *Blastocystis* species are protozoal parasites that are frequently found in human stool samples submitted for microscopic examination. However, their clinical significance is uncertain. Epidemiologic studies have found no significant difference in the prevalence of *Blastocystis* species in stool samples of patients with diarrheal illnesses compared with asymptomatic control patients. Fecal carriage may persist for many months in the absence of symptoms. Studies evaluating treatment of symptomatic patients have provided conflicting reports regarding resolution of gastrointestinal symptoms. Most authorities recommend reserving treatment only for patients with diarrhea lasting longer than 7 days in whom other infectious or noninfectious causes have been excluded.

Ciprofloxacin is not active against *Blastocystis* species.

Treatment regimens reported to be effective against *Blastocystis* species include metronidazole, trimethoprim-sulfamethoxazole, and nitazoxanide. Controversy exists as to whether resolution of symptoms with one of these agents is attributable to eradication of *Blastocystis* organisms or to treatment of another undiagnosed pathogen.

There is controversy regarding obtaining stool studies in patients with diarrhea. Clinically meaningful results occur in an estimated 2% to 6% of stool cultures, and most episodes of mild to moderate diarrhea are self-limited. Additionally, positive culture results may be difficult to interpret, particularly in patients whose symptoms have resolved. Thus, for cases of mild to moderate diarrhea, symptomatic treatment for 48 to 72 hours is reasonable before cultures are obtained, whereas immediate studies are generally recommended for patients with severe symptoms, significant comorbidities, the immunosuppressed, and those with public contact (such as food preparers or child

Answers and Critiques

care workers) who may require negative stool studies to return to work.

KEY POINT

- Asymptomatic patients in whom *Blastocystis* species are found in stool samples do not require therapy or additional studies to document eradication of the organisms.

Bibliography

Tan KS, Mirza H, Teo JD, Wu B, Macary PA. Current Views on the Clinical Relevance of Blastocystis spp. Curr Infect Dis Rep. 2010;12(1):28-35. [PMID: 21308496]

Item 49   Answer: C

Educational Objective: Diagnose sporadic Creutzfeldt-Jakob disease.

This patient most likely has sporadic Creutzfeldt-Jakob disease (sCJD). All forms of CJD are associated with the accumulation of the prion protein in neural tissue, spongiform brain pathology without inflammation, normal cerebrospinal fluid (CSF), relentless symptomatic progression, and no specific treatment. The findings of rapidly progressive dementia and myoclonus, together with his age, bland CSF findings, and a nondiagnostic neuroimaging study, are most consistent with sCJD. The definitive diagnosis of sCJD requires visualization of spongiform changes on pathologic examination of brain tissue. Supportive findings include evidence of 1- to 2-Hz periodic sharp waves on an electroencephalogram or the presence of the 14-3-3 protein in a CSF sample, although the latter finding is nonspecific.

Cryptococcal and *Mycobacterium tuberculosis* infections of the central nervous system cause a subacute to chronic meningitis associated with CSF pleocytosis, headache, fever, and meningeal signs. Myoclonus is not a feature of these infections.

Tertiary neurosyphilis may cause dementia. However, this typically progresses over months to years rather than weeks and is associated with CSF pleocytosis.

KEY POINT

- Sporadic Creutzfeldt-Jakob disease is characterized by rapidly progressive dementia and myoclonus, bland cerebrospinal fluid findings, and nondiagnostic neuroimaging studies, but the definitive diagnosis requires finding spongiform changes on pathologic examination of brain tissue.

Bibliography

Gao C, Shi Q, Tian C, et al. The epidemiological, clinical, and laboratory features of sporadic Creutzfeldt-Jakob disease patients in China: surveillance data from 2006 to 2010. PLoS One. 2011;6(8):e24231. [PMID: 21904617]

Item 50   Answer: C

Educational Objective: Treat a patient with suspected community-associated methicillin-resistant *Staphylococcus aureus* pneumonia.

The most appropriate empiric treatment is ceftriaxone, azithromycin, and vancomycin. The patient has no risk factors for health care–associated pneumonia; therefore, initial empiric antibiotic therapy would include ceftriaxone (or cefotaxime) and azithromycin (or doxycycline) to provide coverage for the most common community-acquired pneumonia (CAP) pathogens, *Streptococcus pneumoniae*, *Haemophilus influenzae*, and the atypical pathogens. However, the presence of a cavitary infiltrate warrants consideration of additional pathogens. In this patient with no risk factors for aspiration pneumonia, involvement of *Staphylococcus aureus*, including possible community-associated methicillin-resistant *S. aureus* (CA-MRSA) infection, is a consideration. CA-MRSA pneumonia can occur following an influenza-like illness; the classic history is a viral syndrome that seems to be improving and then suddenly worsens. *S. aureus* is responsible for less than 10% of cases of CAP; however, the risk increases when pneumonia occurs after influenza infection. Because this patient with a cavitary infiltrate and influenza-like prodrome may have *S. aureus* infection, initial empiric antibiotics should include coverage for CA-MRSA. Consequently, vancomycin should be added to ceftriaxone and azithromycin.

Aztreonam provides coverage only for aerobic gram-negative rods. Although gram-negative pathogens can cause necrotizing pneumonia, initial empiric coverage should not be limited to only gram-negative organisms.

Moxifloxacin does not provide adequate coverage for CA-MRSA.

KEY POINT

- Community-associated methicillin-resistant *Staphylococcus aureus* pneumonia can occur following an influenza-like illness and requires initial empiric antibiotics with ceftriaxone or cefotaxime and azithromycin or doxycycline plus vancomycin.

Bibliography

Taneja C, Haque N, Oster G, et al. Clinical and economic outcomes in patients with community-acquired Staphylococcus aureus pneumonia. J Hosp Med. 2010;5(9):528-534. [PMID: 20734457]

Item 51   Answer: A

Educational Objective: Diagnose botulism.

The most likely diagnosis is botulism. Ingestion of preformed toxin from exposure to home-canned foods, or in vivo toxin production after spore germination following ingestion (infant botulism with honey) or wound contamination, are the most common forms of botulism.

CONT.

Distinguishing naturally occurring foodborne botulism from botulism contracted through deliberate contamination of foods with botulinum toxin may be difficult. Both modes of exposure would likely present within 1 to 5 days of toxin ingestion with a classic triad of symmetric, descending flaccid paralysis with prominent bulbar palsies; normal body temperature; and a clear sensorium. Bulbar signs include the "4 Ds": Diplopia, Dysarthria, Dysphonia, and Dysphagia. Respiratory dysfunction may result from upper airway obstruction or diaphragmatic weakness. A diagnosis can be confirmed by detection of toxin in serum, stool, gastric aspirate, or suspect foods. Treatment is mainly supportive and consists of passive immunization using trivalent equine antitoxin (A, B, and E) and close monitoring of the respiratory status. Antibiotics would be indicated only in patients with complications, such as nosocomial infections.

Guillain-Barré syndrome can clinically mimic botulism because it is characterized by oculomotor dysfunction; however, this condition is usually associated with a history of antecedent infection (gastroenteritis from *Campylobacter* infection), ascending paralysis, and paresthesias. This constellation of symptoms and findings is not consistent with that of this patient.

Paralytic shellfish poisoning is characterized by a history of ingestion of any type of filter-feeding molluscan shellfish (for example, clams, oysters, scallops, or mussels) in which a specific neurotoxin (saxitoxin) produced by microscopic algae has accumulated, particularly in temperate and tropical locations. Symptoms may begin a few minutes to hours after ingestion and commonly include tingling of the lips and tongue that progresses to paresthesias of the digits of the hands and feet, with loss of control of the arms and legs. Depending on the quantity of toxin ingested, muscles of the thorax and abdomen may become paralyzed, resulting in respiratory difficulties

Tick paralysis, associated with *Dermacentor* ticks and most often encountered in the United States Pacific Northwest, also produces an ascending paralysis, predominantly affecting proximal large muscles. This patient's recent travel itinerary and physical examination findings are not consistent with tick paralysis.

KEY POINT

- Botulism presents with a classic triad of symmetric, descending flaccid paralysis with prominent bulbar palsies (diplopia, dysarthria, dysphonia, and dysphagia); normal body temperature; and a clear sensorium.

Bibliography

Cherington M. Botulism: update and review. Semin Neurol. 2004;24(2):155-163. [PMID: 15257512]

Item 52   Answer: E

Educational Objective: Manage a patient with esophageal candidiasis.

This patient should be treated with oral fluconazole. She has evidence of oral candidiasis (thrush), with typical white plaques on visual inspection and symptoms of dysphagia indicating esophageal involvement. Although oral candidiasis has been typically associated with advanced immunosuppression in patients with HIV (CD4 cell counts <200/microliter), it may occur with higher CD4 cell counts in the setting of other risk factors, such as inhaled corticosteroids or broad-spectrum antibiotics.

Although isolated oral disease can be treated with topical agents such as nystatin or clotrimazole, this patient's swallowing symptoms suggest concurrent esophageal disease. Esophageal candidiasis requires systemic therapy such as fluconazole, which can be administered orally as long as the patient can swallow pills.

Although this patient's inhaled corticosteroids may have predisposed her to oral candidiasis, the most appropriate management is to treat the candidal disease and not to discontinue the inhaled corticosteroids, which are an important part of the successful management of her asthma.

This patient has no history of previous treatment with fluconazole and is therefore unlikely to have fluconazole-resistant *Candida*.

Amphotericin B is an intravenous treatment, is associated with increased toxicity, and is not as convenient as oral therapy; consequently, it is not warranted as initial treatment of esophageal candidiasis.

KEY POINT

- Oral candidiasis with esophageal involvement is characterized by whitish plaques on the oral mucosa and difficulty swallowing; treatment with a systemic agent such as fluconazole is required.

Bibliography

Kaplan JE, Benson C, Holmes KH, Brooks JT, Pau A, Masur H; Centers for Disease Control and Prevention (CDC); National Institutes of Health; HIV Medicine Association of the Infectious Diseases Society of America. Guidelines for prevention and treatment of opportunistic infections in HIV-infected adults and adolescents: recommendations from CDC, the National Institutes of Health, and the HIV Medicine Association of the Infectious Diseases Society of America. MMWR Recomm Rep. 2009;58(RR-4):1-207. [PMID: 19357635]

Item 53   Answer: D

Educational Objective: Empirically treat diabetes mellitus–associated osteomyelitis.

The most appropriate empiric treatment of this patient is vancomycin and meropenem. This patient is experiencing a septic syndrome and limb-threatening foot infection.

Limb-threatening infections are characterized by extensive spreading cellulitis, extending far beyond the wound or ulcer, with systemic illness and possible sepsis with ulcers extending deep into the subcutaneous tissue, as well as tissue ischemia. Limb-threatening infections are polymicrobial, including staphylococci, streptococci, enteric gram-negative rods, *Pseudomonas aeruginosa*, and anaerobes. Ideally, a biopsy of the affected bone and deep soft tissues should be attempted before empiric antimicrobial therapy is initiated. However, in the setting of sepsis and a limb-threatening infection in a patient with diabetes mellitus, antimicrobial therapy using agents directed at suspected pathogens should urgently be administered. Surgical debridement will also be required. Patients with severe infections should receive parenteral therapy. Pending the results of microbiologic cultures, vancomycin and meropenem would be an appropriate combination of agents, predictably supplying broad coverage against the potential pathogens of concern.

Because they are not active against gram-positive cocci, aztreonam and metronidazole would not provide coverage against streptococci and staphylococci. Although metronidazole has excellent activity against anaerobic gram-negative bacilli, the narrow spectrum of activity of cefazolin versus many gram-negative bacilli, as well as its inactivity against methicillin-resistant strains, may be inadequate.

Because of clindamycin's methicillin-resistant activity, this agent cannot reliably treat serious infections potentially involving staphylococci.

The use of gentamicin or other aminoglycosides to provide coverage against aerobic gram-negative bacilli in empiric antibiotic regimens for treatment of complex diabetic foot infections is not currently recommended because of the narrow toxicity-to-benefit ratio with such use. In addition, aminoglycosides may exhibit diminished antimicrobial activity in a necrotic, anaerobic environment.

KEY POINT

- In the setting of sepsis and a limb-threatening infection in a patient with diabetes mellitus, antimicrobial therapy with agents directed at suspected pathogens should urgently be administered.

Bibliography

Powlson AS, Coll AP. The treatment of diabetic foot infections. J Antimicrob Chemother. 2010;65(suppl 3):iii3-9. [PMID: 20876626]

Item 54   Answer: C

Educational Objective: Manage HIV infection in pregnancy.

The most appropriate management of this pregnant patient is immediate institution of antiretroviral therapy with zidovudine, lamivudine, and lopinavir-ritonavir. About one in four neonates born to women with HIV infection will acquire HIV infection perinatally if antiretroviral therapy is not given. Appropriate antiretroviral therapy can reduce the risk of HIV transmission to the newborn to less than 2%. This patient should receive antiretroviral therapy now, regardless of CD4 cell count, viral load, or presence or absence of symptoms.

Although about two thirds of perinatal HIV transmission occurs during delivery, one third occurs in utero; consequently, antiretroviral therapy should be started now and not withheld until the onset of labor to maximally reduce chances of perinatal transmission.

Efavirenz is contraindicated in women who are or who may be pregnant because of the risk for teratogenicity.

Withholding treatment until there is a decrease in CD4 cell count or onset of HIV symptoms would not be appropriate because all pregnant women with HIV infection should receive antiretroviral therapy to reduce the likelihood for perinatal transmission.

KEY POINT

- In pregnant women with HIV infection, antiretroviral therapy with zidovudine, lamivudine, and lopinavir-ritonavir can reduce the risk of HIV transmission to the newborn to less than 2% and should be given regardless of CD4 cell count, viral load, or presence or absence of HIV symptoms.

Bibliography

Panel on Treatment of HIV-Infected Pregnant Women and Prevention of Perinatal Transmission. Recommendations for use of antiretroviral drugs in pregnant HIV-1-infected women for maternal health and interventions to reduce perinatal HIV transmission in the United States. September 14, 2011;1-207. Available at: www.aidsinfo.nih.gov/ContentFiles/PerinatalGL.pdf. Accessed December 20, 2011.

Item 55   Answer: A

Educational Objective: Diagnose dengue fever.

Dengue fever, a flavivirus infection transmitted by the bite of the *Aedes aegypti* mosquito, is the most prevalent mosquito-borne viral illness in the world. Dengue is endemic to many parts of the world, especially Southeast Asia and tropical geographic areas. A significant rise in the incidence of dengue has occurred recently in the Caribbean islands and Latin America, resulting from the reestablishment of the *A. aegypti* vector in these areas. On several occasions, domestically acquired (autochthonous) cases in the United States, generally limited to the southern states, have been reported. Classic manifestations in symptomatic persons present after an incubation period of 4 to 7 days. Typically, patients experience abrupt fever with chills, severe frontal headache, retro-orbital pain, and musculoskeletal pain, characteristically severe in the lumbar spine, earning dengue the name "break-bone fever." A nonspecific macular or maculopapular rash, sparing the palms and soles, often

Answers and Critiques

develops within 3 to 4 days of onset of illness, tending to coincide with the resolution of fever. Referred to as a "saddle-back" pattern, a second episode of fever and symptoms may occur in some patients. Abnormal laboratory findings include leukopenia, neutropenia, thrombocytopenia, and mildly elevated liver aminotransferase concentrations, with the serum aspartate aminotransferase level often higher than the serum alanine aminotransferase level. The febrile illness may be followed by a prolonged episode of fatigue. Full recovery is expected in all infected persons. The diagnosis of dengue fever remains mainly clinical. During the early phase of illness, real-time reverse transcriptase polymerase chain reaction can be useful in detecting virus in the blood. However, acute and convalescent serologic testing is commonly used to confirm a diagnosis in returning travelers. Treatment of dengue fever involves symptomatic relief. Currently, no vaccine is clinically available to protect against infection.

Leptospirosis, caused by infection with pathogenic spirochetes belonging to the genus *Leptospira,* is endemic throughout the world. Infection occurs through direct or indirect contact with urine or tissues of infected animals, most often rodents and other small mammals. In most infected patients, a self-limited illness characterized by high fever, myalgia, abdominal pain, and conjunctival suffusion occurs, with a rash developing infrequently.

Malaria does not cause a rash and is not endemic to the Caribbean islands except for the Dominican Republic and Haiti.

Yellow fever, another flavivirus infection contracted through the bite of the *A. aegypti* mosquito, occurs mostly in areas of sub-Saharan Africa and South America, but is not endemic to the Caribbean islands.

KEY POINT

- Classic manifestations of dengue infection in symptomatic persons include fever with chills, severe frontal headache, retro-orbital pain, and musculoskeletal pain that is characteristically severe in the lumbar spine, as well as a nonspecific macular or maculopapular rash sparing the palms and soles.

Bibliography
Ross TM. Dengue virus. Clin Lab Med. 2010;30(1):149-160. [PMID: 20513545]

Item 56   Answer: E

Educational Objective: Treat a community-associated methicillin-resistant *Staphylococcus aureus* skin infection.

Trimethoprim-sulfamethoxazole (TMP-SMX) is an older antibiotic drug that has been used with increasing frequency for treatment of skin and soft tissue infections caused by community-associated methicillin-resistant

Staphylococcus aureus (CA-MRSA), and it has retained excellent activity against most strains of CA-MRSA. This patient presents with a cutaneous abscess that is larger than 5 cm with purulent drainage and associated cellulitis. A Gram stain of the lesion aspirate is suggestive of *S. aureus,* which is consistent with CA-MRSA infection. Treatment with TMP-SMX is appropriate empiric therapy after drainage of the lesion. Limitations of TMP-SMX include sulfa allergy (including Stevens-Johnson syndrome), hyperkalemia, and possible kidney toxicity. Therapy may be further directed once culture and sensitivity results have returned.

Amoxicillin-clavulanate is an expanded spectrum β-lactam antimicrobial agent, but it is not active against MRSA.

Azithromycin, a macrolide, has poor activity against MRSA and should not be used for empiric treatment of CA-MRSA.

Moxifloxacin, a fluoroquinolone, has increased activity against *S. aureus* compared with other fluoroquinolones, but resistance to this agent has emerged among CA-MRSA strains; consequently, moxifloxacin is not a good empiric choice.

Rifampin has activity against some strains of MRSA but should not be used as a single agent for treatment of infection because of the risk for rapid emergence of resistance.

KEY POINT

- Trimethoprim-sulfamethoxazole is a first-line choice for treatment of skin and soft tissue infection due to suspected or confirmed community-associated methicillin-resistant *Staphylococcus aureus.*

Bibliography
Liu C, Bayer A, Cosgrove SE, et al. Clinical practice guidelines by the Infectious Diseases Society of America for the treatment of methicillin-resistant Staphylococcus aureus infections in adults and children: executive summary. Clin Infect Dis. 2011;52(3):285-292. [PMID: 21217178]

Item 57   Answer: D

Educational Objective: Interpret a tuberculin skin test reaction in a patient who uses injection drugs.

No additional evaluation or treatment is indicated for a person who uses injection drugs and has a tuberculin skin test reaction of less than 10 mm of induration.

Certain high-risk groups require a chest radiograph to exclude active tuberculosis when their tuberculin skin test reaction is greater than or equal to 5 mm. These groups include recent contacts of patients with active tuberculosis, patients with HIV infection, persons with fibrotic changes on prior chest radiographs consistent with old healed tuberculosis, and organ transplant recipients and patients with other immunocompromising conditions. High-risk persons who require a chest radiograph when their tuberculin skin test reaction is greater than or equal to 10 mm include injection drug users; persons from countries with a high prevalence of tuberculosis who immigrated to the United States less than 5 years ago; employees or residents of high-risk congregate settings such as prisons, nursing homes, hospitals, or homeless shelters; mycobacteriology laboratory workers; patients with clinical conditions that put them at increased risk for active tuberculosis (for example, chronic kidney disease; diabetes mellitus; silicosis; lymphoproliferative disorders; cancer of the neck, head, or lung; gastrectomy or jejunoileal bypass and weight loss of ≥10% from ideal body weight); children who are younger than 4 years of age; and adolescents, children, and infants who are exposed to adults in high-risk categories. Asymptomatic persons in either of these two groups who have a chest radiograph that is normal or is inconsistent with active tuberculosis should receive treatment for latent tuberculosis infection because they are at increased risk for tuberculosis. Treatment will substantially reduce the risk that latent tuberculosis will progress to active disease. Treatment of latent tuberculosis typically consists of isoniazid for 9 months unless there is strong suspicion of infection with isoniazid-resistant mycobacteria (for example, exposure to a person with known isoniazid-resistant tuberculosis). In this situation, rifampin for 4 months is a reasonable alternative. Recently, the Centers for Disease Control and Prevention also included 3 months of directly observed, once-weekly rifapentine and isoniazid combination therapy for treatment of latent tuberculosis.

Four-drug therapy with isoniazid, rifampin, pyrazinamide, and ethambutol is used to treat active tuberculosis. There is no evidence that the asymptomatic person described here has active tuberculosis.

KEY POINT

- A tuberculin skin test reaction of less than 10 mm in a person who uses injection drugs requires no additional evaluation or treatment.

Bibliography
American Thoracic Society. Targeted tuberculin testing and treatment of latent tuberculosis infection. MMWR Recomm Rep. 2000;49(RR-6):1-51. [PMID: 10881762]

Item 58   Answer: A
Educational Objective: Diagnose cytomegalovirus infection after kidney transplantation.

This patient has cytomegalovirus (CMV) infection and disease presenting as the CMV syndrome, which typically occurs in the first few months after transplantation. Typical findings include fever, cytopenias, and hepatitis and may include pneumonitis or colitis. The onset of CMV in this patient was delayed by the prophylaxis given for the first few months following transplantation. The periods following solid organ transplant during which opportunistic infections can occur are the early period (within the first month after

transplantation), the middle period (the first few months after transplantation), and the late period (more than a few months after transplantation). This patient is at higher risk for CMV infection because she was a seronegative recipient of an organ from a seropositive donor. Testing for CMV viremia should be performed, and treatment with intravenous ganciclovir or oral valganciclovir should be started.

This patient is also at risk for Epstein-Barr virus reactivation and disease, and this would be the appropriate time frame (5 months posttransplantation) for this infection to occur; however, in transplant recipients, this infection usually presents with lymphadenopathy as Epstein-Barr virus–associated posttransplant lymphoproliferative disease. Lymphadenopathy is absent in this patient.

Listeria monocytogenes infection may occur during this posttransplantation time frame but more often causes meningoencephalitis with headache and mental status changes or neurologic deficits, which this patient does not have.

Polyoma BK virus infection is a late complication of transplantation. Kidney transplant recipients with BK virus infection may develop BK-related nephropathy, organ rejection, or ureteral strictures. Transplant recipients with BK-related nephropathy have decoy cells in the urine (cells with intranuclear inclusions), evidence of which is absent in this patient.

KEY POINT

- Cytomegalovirus infection typically occurs in the first few months after solid organ transplantation (the middle period); is characterized by fever, malaise, leukopenia, and thrombocytopenia; and may involve the lungs or gastrointestinal tract.

Bibliography
De Keyzer K, Van Laecke S, Peeters P, Vanholder R. Human cytomegalovirus and kidney transplantation: a clinician's update. Am J Kidney Dis. 2011;58(1):118-126. [PMID: 21684438]

Item 59   Answer: B

Educational Objective: Manage bacterial meningitis.

Continuation of current management is indicated for this patient with acute bacterial meningitis. *Streptococcus pneumoniae* and *Listeria monocytogenes* are the most likely causative pathogens in this age group. The recommended empiric antimicrobial regimen is the combination of vancomycin, ampicillin, and a third-generation cephalosporin (either cefotaxime or ceftriaxone) pending culture results and in vitro susceptibility testing of the isolated pathogen. Because this patient may possibly have pneumococcal meningitis, he received adjunctive dexamethasone, which can attenuate release of bacterial virulence components as a result of antimicrobial-induced lysis. Administration of dexamethasone may limit some of the pathophysiologic consequences of bacterial meningitis (including subarachnoid

CONT.

space inflammation, cerebral edema, and increased intracranial pressure). Although adjunctive dexamethasone has been shown to reduce the likelihood of adverse outcomes and death in adults with pneumococcal meningitis, it should be given concomitant with or just before the first dose of an antimicrobial agent to achieve these benefits.

Adding rifampin can be considered in patients with resistant pneumococcal meningitis when in vitro testing demonstrates that the organism is susceptible to this agent.

Placement of an external ventricular drain is only appropriate for treatment of hydrocephalus, which was not seen on this patient's neuroimaging studies.

Repeating the cerebrospinal fluid analysis is indicated for patients who have not improved after 36 to 48 hours of appropriate therapy, especially for patients with pneumococcal meningitis who are also being treated with adjunctive dexamethasone.

KEY POINT

- Recommended empiric therapy for bacterial meningitis is the combination of vancomycin, ampicillin, and a third-generation cephalosporin (cefotaxime or ceftriaxone), with adjunctive dexamethasone for suspected or proven pneumococcal meningitis concomitant with or just prior to the first dose of antimicrobial therapy.

Bibliography

Brouwer MC, McIntyre P, de Gans J, et al. Corticosteroids for acute bacterial meningitis. Cochrane Database Syst Rev. 2010;(9):CD004405. [PMID: 20824838]

 Item 60   Answer: B

Educational Objective: Treat *Pseudomonas aeruginosa* pneumonia.

The most appropriate treatment is cefepime, tobramycin, and azithromycin. This patient has severe community-acquired pneumonia (CAP) and risk factors for *Pseudomonas aeruginosa* infection given her underlying frequent exacerbations of severe COPD and long-term corticosteroid therapy. In addition, her sputum Gram stain reveals gram-negative rods. Consequently, antibiotic therapy should include coverage for possible *P. aeruginosa* until further information is obtained from the sputum culture. Because of increasing antimicrobial resistance among gram-negative pathogens, empiric coverage for possible *P. aeruginosa* infection should include an antipseudomonal β-lactam agent with pneumococcal coverage (cefepime, imipenem, meropenem, or piperacillin-tazobactam) plus ciprofloxacin or levofloxacin; or an antipseudomonal β-lactam agent with pneumococcal coverage plus an aminoglycoside plus azithromycin; or an antipseudomonal β-lactam with pneumococcal coverage plus an aminoglycoside plus a respiratory fluoroquinolone.

Aztreonam is an alternative antipseudomonal agent that can be used for patients with severe β-lactam allergy

and would require combination with a second agent with antipseudomonal activity, as described above.

Neither cefotaxime plus azithromycin nor the combination of cefotaxime, azithromycin, and levofloxacin would provide adequate coverage against possible infection with *P. aeruginosa* in this critically ill patient.

KEY POINT

- Because of increasing antimicrobial resistance among gram-negative pathogens, empiric coverage for critically ill patients with possible *Pseudomonas aeruginosa* infection should include two antipseudomonal agents.

Bibliography

Mandell LA, Wunderink RG, Anzueto A, et al. Infectious Diseases Society of America/American Thoracic Society consensus guidelines on the management of community-acquired pneumonia in adults. Clin Infect Dis. 2007;44(suppl 2):S27-72. [PMID: 17278083]

Item 61   Answer: D

Educational Objective: Manage a patient with meningoencephalitis.

Because this patient has a low probability for herpes simplex encephalitis, intravenous acyclovir should be discontinued. The patient presents with meningoencephalitis, defined as an altered mental status lasting at least 24 hours that is variably associated with fever, seizures, pleocytosis, and abnormal neuroimaging studies. Herpes simplex encephalitis is the most common cause of sporadic encephalitis in the United States and one of the few treatable causes of encephalitis. It is classically associated with localized infection of the temporal lobe; however, atypical presentations have been described. Treatment guidelines recommend initiation of empiric acyclovir in all patients with encephalitis pending diagnostic testing for HSV. HSV polymerase chain reaction (PCR) of cerebrospinal fluid (CSF) has a sensitivity of 95% and a specificity of 98% for the diagnosis of herpes simplex encephalitis. Given the excellent performance characteristics of this assay, it is appropriate to discontinue acyclovir in a patient with a low probability for herpes simplex encephalitis.

Oral formulations of acyclovir and valacyclovir do not achieve therapeutic CSF levels, which precludes treatment of encephalitis with these agents in patients with presumed or confirmed herpes simplex encephalitis.

False-negative HSV PCR results may occur very early in the course of infection. However, more than 90% of patients with herpes simplex encephalitis have abnormalities on MRI of the brain. Consequently, in patients with MRI studies confirming temporal lobe inflammation, acyclovir should be continued pending repeat testing on a second CSF sample obtained 2 to 4 days later. However, this patient has a normal MRI and a negative HSV PCR, which effectively excludes the diagnosis of herpes simplex encephalitis; a second HSV PCR is not needed. A positive

NT.

HSV PCR result is diagnostic of herpes simplex encephalitis. Therefore, only patients with positive results should continue to receive intravenous acyclovir for 14 to 21 days.

KEY POINT

- In patients with a low clinical suspicion for herpes simplex encephalitis, empiric acyclovir therapy may be discontinued when herpes simplex virus polymerase chain reaction results are negative.

Bibliography

Tunkel AR, Glaser CA, Bloch KC, et al; Infectious Diseases Society of America. The management of encephalitis: clinical practice guidelines by the Infectious Diseases Society of America. Clin Infect Dis. 2008;47(3):303-327. [PMID: 18582201]

Item 62   Answer: D

Educational Objective: Treat a patient with purulent cellulitis.

This patient has purulent cellulitis (cellulitis associated with purulent drainage or an exudate but without a drainable abscess), and outpatient treatment with trimethoprim-sulfamethoxazole should be initiated. This infection is most likely caused by community-associated methicillin-resistant *Staphylococcus aureus* (CA-MRSA). Novel CA-MRSA strains have emerged across the United States. These strains are distinct from hospital-associated or health care–associated MRSA strains, have different virulence factors, and often have different antimicrobial susceptibility patterns. Initial cases of skin and soft tissue infections, including cellulitis with or without abscesses, occurred in children, student and professional athletes, prisoners, men who have sex with men, and American Indians. CA-MRSA strains continue to spread throughout the community and beyond these initially defined subpopulations, and now many patients do not have identifiable risk factors. Recommended empiric antimicrobial agents for outpatients with a CA-MRSA skin or soft tissue infection include trimethoprim-sulfamethoxazole, a tetracycline (for example, doxycycline), clindamycin, and linezolid.

Amoxicillin, cephalexin, and dicloxacillin are β-lactam agents with activity against β-hemolytic streptococci but not CA-MRSA. These agents are indicated for treatment of patients with nonpurulent cellulitis.

KEY POINT

- Recommended empiric antibiotic agents for outpatients with purulent cellulitis caused by community-associated methicillin-resistant *Staphylococcus aureus* include trimethoprim-sulfamethoxazole, a tetracycline (for example, doxycycline), clindamycin, and linezolid.

Bibliography

Liu C, Bayer A, Cosgrove SE, et al; Infectious Diseases Society of America. Clinical practice guidelines by the Infectious Diseases Society of America for the treatment of methicillin-resistant

Staphylococcus aureus infections in adults and children. Clin Infect Dis. 2011;52(3):e18-55. Epub 2011 Jan 4. [PMID: 21208910]

Item 63   Answer: A

Educational Objective: Manage a patient with osteomyelitis.

The most appropriate next step in management is deep bone biopsy culture before antimicrobial therapy is begun. The development of a draining sinus tract from the wound above a bone that underwent surgical instrumentation is highly suspicious for underlying contiguous osteomyelitis. The patient's current condition is presumably related to his initial open trauma or surgery 6 months ago. Microbiologic isolates from cultures obtained from a wound or draining sinus tract generally do not reliably correlate with the pathogen in the infected bone with the occasional exception of *Staphylococcus aureus*. Owing to limited utility and the possibility for providing misinformation, the use of microbiologic isolates from the culture of wounds or draining sinus tracts to guide therapy, such as treatment with ampicillin-sulbactam against the organisms identified from a wound swab in this patient, is discouraged. Instead, identification of the causative pathogen(s) is best attempted by bone biopsy performed surgically or percutaneously with radiographic guidance. Once the causative organism is recovered, treatment (usually consisting of at least 6 weeks of parenteral antimicrobial therapy) can be initiated. Debridement of necrotic material is often necessary, and, if feasible, removal the metallic hardware is performed to optimize the chances of microbiologic eradication and clinical success.

Prolonged oral ciprofloxacin has proved to be an effective therapy for bone biopsy culture–proven osteomyelitis involving susceptible gram-negative bacilli. However, oral amoxicillin would not be an adequate choice for treating the rare circumstance of enterococcal osteomyelitis.

A three-phase technetium-99m-labeled bone scan is a very sensitive imaging modality for detecting the presence of suspected osteomyelitis. However, this study lacks specificity and would be expected to be abnormal owing to the patient's recent surgery and, therefore, could not reliably confirm a diagnosis of bone infection.

KEY POINT

- In patients with suspected osteomyelitis, the microbiologic isolates from cultures obtained from a wound or draining sinus tract generally do not reliably correlate with the pathogen in the infected bone with the occasional exception of *Staphylococcus aureus*.

Bibliography

Zuluaga AF, Wilson G, Saldarriaga JG, et al. Etiologic diagnosis of chronic osteomyelitis: a prospective study. Arch Intern Med. 2006;166(1):95-100. [PMID: 16401816]

Item 64   Answer: C

Educational Objective: Diagnose *Pneumocystis* pneumonia in a patient with AIDS.

The most likely diagnosis is *Pneumocystis jirovecii* pneumonia. This patient with known HIV risk factors and a reactive rapid HIV test very likely has HIV infection, although confirmation with Western blot testing still must be performed. He is most likely presenting with *Pneumocystis* pneumonia (PCP) caused by *Pneumocystis jirovecii*. His subacute presentation with dry cough and dyspnea and chest radiograph findings of diffuse interstitial disease constitute the typical presentation of PCP in patients with AIDS, which is also the most common opportunistic infection in patients not taking *Pneumocystis* prophylaxis. Bronchoscopy with lavage can be done with special stains to confirm the diagnosis. Because this patient's arterial PO_2 level is less than 70 mm Hg (9.3 kPa), treatment would include corticosteroids plus trimethoprim-sulfamethoxazole.

Although it can cause pneumonia in transplant recipients, cytomegalovirus (CMV) is an unusual cause of pneumonia in patients with AIDS. In such patients, CMV is more likely to present as retinitis or gastrointestinal disease, with CD4 cell counts less than 50/microliter.

Mycobacterium avium complex usually causes disseminated disease in patients with AIDS and CD4 cell counts less than 50/microliter who present with systemic symptoms, such as fevers, sweats, weight loss, and involvement of the liver, spleen, and lymph nodes, not as pulmonary disease.

Candida is generally a very rare cause of pulmonary infection, even in immunocompromised hosts. The presence of pseudohyphae in this patient's sputum is most likely a result of his oral candidiasis as demonstrated by his examination findings and is not evidence of pulmonary involvement.

KEY POINT

- **In patients with AIDS, *Pneumocystis* pneumonia is the most common opportunistic infection in patients not taking *Pneumocystis* prophylaxis and is typically characterized by a subacute presentation with dry cough and dyspnea and chest radiograph findings of diffuse interstitial disease.**

Bibliography

Carmona EM, Limper AH. Update on the diagnosis and treatment of Pneumocystis pneumonia. Ther Adv Respir Dis. 2011;5(1):41-59. [PMID: 20736243]

Item 65   Answer: D

Educational Objective: Treat mucormycosis (previously zygomycosis) in a patient with diabetic ketoacidosis.

Based on his clinical scenario and physical examination findings, this patient most likely has rhino-orbital mucormycosis (previously zygomycosis) and requires emergency surgical debridement and intravenous amphotericin B. Because of a recent change in taxonomy, the class name Zygomycetes has been replaced, and, therefore, the term "zygomycosis" is no longer appropriate. Classic manifestations of mucormycosis are sinusitis, rhino-orbital infection, and rhinocerebral infection. Following inhalation of spores, infection is initially localized to the nasal turbinates and sinuses. Infection can progress rapidly to the orbit or brain. Prompt administration of intravenous amphotericin B and aggressive surgical debridement are essential in cases of suspected mucormycosis given the high mortality rate (25% to 62%) associated with this disorder.

Piperacillin-tazobactam is a broad-spectrum β-lactam/β-lactamase inhibitor combination that is used to treat polymicrobial bacterial infections. It does not possess antifungal activity and, therefore, would not be appropriate as the next important step in managing a life-threatening fungal infection.

Oral posaconazole is a broad-spectrum azole antifungal agent that has in vitro activity against mucormycoses. This agent may have a role in step-down therapy for patients who have responded to amphotericin B or as salvage therapy for patients who have not responded to first-line treatment, but it would not be appropriate first-line treatment in this patient.

The efficacy of hyperbaric oxygen treatment of mucormycosis has not been definitively demonstrated in clinical trials. Hyperbaric oxygen is not a first-line treatment and should not be considered in this patient.

KEY POINT

- **Successful management of mucormycosis (previously zygomycosis) hinges on prompt administration of appropriate antifungal therapy coupled with aggressive surgical debridement.**

Bibliography

Sun HY, Singh N. Mucormycosis: its contemporary face and management strategies. Lancet Infect Dis. 2011;11(4):301-311. [PMID: 21453871]

Item 66   Answer: D

Educational Objective: Manage a patient with an epidural abscess and neurologic deficits.

This patient most likely has an epidural abscess complicated by spinal cord compression and requires emergent surgical decompression. This procedure should be performed in patients presenting within 24 to 36 hours of developing complete paralysis to minimize the likelihood of permanent neurologic sequelae.

Empiric antimicrobial therapy should be administered intraoperatively once appropriate culture specimens are obtained. Medical therapy alone can be considered for patients who have only localized pain and/or radicular symptoms, but these patients require careful observation with frequent neurologic examinations and MRI studies to demonstrate resolution of the abscess.

CT-guided bone biopsy might yield positive culture results but would not treat this patient's neurologic compromise.

Emergent radiation therapy should not be administered for a bacterial abscess or before a definitive diagnosis is established. In addition, malignancy is not likely in this patient based on his initial MRI findings.

KEY POINT

- Patients with an epidural abscess and complete paralysis lasting less than 24 to 36 hours should undergo emergent surgical decompression.

Bibliography

Darouiche RO. Spinal epidural abscess. N Engl J Med. 2006;355(19):2012-2020. [PMID: 17093252]

Item 67   Answer: B

Educational Objective: Initiate appropriate infection control measures in a patient with invasive disease secondary to *Streptococcus pyogenes* infection.

To prevent dissemination of infection resulting from this patient's group A β-hemolytic streptococcal (*Streptococcus pyogenes*) (GABHS) necrotizing fasciitis and toxic shock syndrome (TSS), contact precautions must be instituted. Once *S. pyogenes* is confirmed as the cause of infection, parenteral clindamycin and penicillin are recommended. Secondary transmission of GABHS-induced TSS to close contacts of patients has been reported. Contact isolation precautions should be initiated for patients with suspected or known invasive GABHS-induced disease, including TSS and necrotizing fasciitis, until they have completed 24 hours of antibiotic therapy. Gloves and gowns should be worn by anyone entering the room. Postexposure penicillin-based prophylaxis may be considered for high-risk household contacts of patients with invasive GABHS infection, including those who are older than 65 years of age or have conditions associated with an increased risk of developing invasive infection (for example, diabetes mellitus, cardiac disease, varicella infection, cancer, HIV infection, corticosteroid use, or injection drug use).

Airborne precautions are recommended for patients infected with microorganisms such as rubella virus and *Mycobacterium tuberculosis*, which are transmitted by airborne droplet nuclei less than 5 micrometers in size. Organisms causing avian influenza, varicella, disseminated zoster, severe acute respiratory syndrome, smallpox, and the agents of viral hemorrhagic fever require airborne and contact precautions. Airborne precautions include placing patients in an isolation room with high-efficiency particulate air filtration and negative pressure. Visitors to the room should wear appropriate respiratory protective gear when entering as should patients during transport out of the room. Persons who are not immune to measles or varicella infection should not enter the room.

Droplet precautions are used for protection against microorganisms transmitted by respiratory droplets greater than 5 micrometers in size. These droplets can usually be transmitted to susceptible recipient mucosal surfaces over short distances measuring less than 3 to 10 feet. Examples of other pathogens and diseases requiring institution of droplet isolation precautions include *Neisseria meningitidis*, pneumonic plague, diphtheria, *Haemophilus influenzae* type b, *Bordetella pertussis*, influenza, mumps, rubella, and parvovirus B19.

Standard precautions are used with all patients and include protecting breaks in the skin or mucous membranes from possible pathogenic exposures, hand washing before and after patient contact, wearing gloves when contacting blood or bodily fluids, hand washing after glove removal, and wearing a mask and eye protection when needed to decrease risk for splash- or aerosol-associated exposures. However, using only standard precautions in this patient with GABHS infection would provide inadequate protection.

KEY POINT

- Infection control management of patients with suspected or known invasive disease caused by group A β-hemolytic streptococci, including toxic shock syndrome and necrotizing fasciitis, consists of contact precautions until completion of 24 hours of antibiotic therapy.

Bibliography

Siegel JD, Rhinehart E, Jackson M, Chiarello L; Health Care Infection Control Practices Advisory Committee. 2007 Guideline for Isolation Precautions: Preventing Transmission of Infectious Agents in Health Care Settings. Am J Infect Control. 2007;35(10 suppl 2):S65-164. [PMID: 18068815]

Item 68   Answer: D

Educational Objective: Manage HIV treatment failure.

The patient should undergo viral resistance testing while continuing his present medication regimen, with a treatment change based on resistance testing results. Resistance testing is appropriate in the setting of treatment failure as evidenced by suboptimally controlled HIV RNA viral loads (lack of suppressed viral loads or previously undetectable viral loads that have become detectable on repeated testing). This patient is adherent to his antiretroviral therapy, and his previously undetectable viral load is now repeatedly detectable, indicating treatment failure. Resistance testing should be performed to guide the selection of a new treatment regimen. The present regimen should be continued to sustain partial suppression of the virus pending results of resistance testing. A new regimen can be instituted once resistance testing results become available.

Continuing the same therapeutic regimen in this patient with demonstrated treatment failure would lead to development of further resistance, higher virus levels, and an eventual decline in CD4 cell count.

Resistance testing should be done while the patient continues the current regimen. Discontinuing the regimen would allow a significant increase in viral load. Resistance testing done while the patient is not receiving therapy may be unreliable without the selective pressure of the medications to maintain the presence of mutations in the predominant virus population.

This patient requires antiretroviral therapy and has been tolerating it well. The Strategies for Management of AntiRetroviral Treatment (SMART) study showed that for such patients, therapy should be maintained and a drug holiday avoided because it is associated with increased complications and mortality.

KEY POINT

• **In patients with HIV infection, resistance testing is appropriate in the setting of treatment failure as evidenced by suboptimally controlled viral loads (lack of suppressed viral loads or previously undetectable viral loads that have become detectable on repeated testing).**

Bibliography

Taylor S, Jayasuriya A, Smit E. Using HIV resistance tests in clinical practice. J Antimicrob Chemother. 2009;64(2):218-222. [PMID: 19535382]

Item 69   Answer: A
Educational Objective: Treat cat-scratch disease.

This patient has cat-scratch disease, and treatment with azithromycin is recommended. Cat-scratch disease most often occurs in immunocompetent children and young adults and is caused by inoculation of the fastidious gram-negative bacterium *Bartonella henselae* after the scratch or bite of a kitten or cat. A pustule or papule or erythema develops at the site of inoculation several days to 2 weeks after the injury. Significant tender regional lymphadenopathy develops 2 to 3 weeks after inoculation in areas that drain the infected site. These lymph nodes suppurate in a small number of patients. Lymphadenopathy generally resolves within months, and extranodal disease is rare. *B. henselae* infection also should be considered in the differential diagnosis of fever of unknown origin. Although cat-scratch disease is usually a self-limited illness, some experts recommend a short course of treatment with azithromycin. Other agents that can be used include doxycycline, rifampin, clarithromycin, trimethoprim-sulfamethoxazole, and ciprofloxacin.

Linezolid and dicloxacillin are used primarily to treat gram-positive bacteria such as staphylococci and streptococci and are not effective against gram-negative organisms such as *B. henselae*.

Lymphocutaneous sporotrichosis is the most common form of sporotrichosis caused by the fungus *Sporothrix*

schenckii. Following cutaneous inoculation, typically of the hand or forearm, a papule or nodule with overlying erythema develops and may ulcerate. Similar lesions develop along lymphatic channels proximal to the draining lymph nodes. Itraconazole is the preferred treatment. This patient does not have findings consistent with sporotrichosis, and treatment with itraconazole is not indicated.

KEY POINT

• **Azithromycin is an effective antibiotic agent for treatment of cat-scratch disease.**

Bibliography

Stevens DL, Bisno AL, Chambers HF, et al; Infectious Diseases Society of America. Practice guidelines for the diagnosis and management of skin and soft tissue infections. Clin Infect Dis. 2005;41(10):1373-1406. [PMID: 16231249]

Item 70   Answer: A
Educational Objective: Interpret serologic testing for *Borrelia burgdorferi* infection.

This patient requires additional evaluation for fatigue and weakness. He has vague constitutional symptoms of several months' duration that are nonfocal, nonspecific, and not suggestive of Lyme disease. Investigation for other possible causes is therefore indicated.

Despite this patient's low clinical suspicion for Lyme disease, serologic testing was performed. This is a common problem when patients are searching for answers for nonspecific, troublesome symptoms. The recommended diagnostic strategy is two-stage serologic testing for the presence of antibodies to *Borrelia burgdorferi*. The initial screening test is an immunofluorescent assay or enzyme-linked immunosorbent assay, both of which are exquisitely sensitive but nonspecific. If the initial test is equivocal or positive, as it was in this patient, a confirmatory Western blot assay is performed. Standardized criteria are available for interpretation of Western blot IgG and IgM antibody assays based on the number of positive bands. Interpretation of a positive IgM antibody result with a negative IgG antibody result requires clinical correlation. If symptoms are present for less than 1 month, findings may represent delayed seroconversion following acute infection, and repeat testing at a later date is recommended to confirm the diagnosis. However, when symptoms have been present for more than 1 month, particularly when the symptoms are nonspecific (as they are in this patient), a positive IgM antibody result in the absence of IgG antibodies most likely represents a false-positive test result, and no additional testing for Lyme disease is needed.

Because the patient requires further evaluation and is very unlikely to have Lyme disease, treatment of this infection with either ceftriaxone or doxycycline is not indicated.

- Patients with nonspecific symptoms, such as fatigue, myalgia, or arthralgia, with a low pretest probability for Lyme disease, should not be tested for this disease.

Bibliography

Centers for Disease Control and Prevention (CDC). Recommendations for test performance and interpretation from the Second National Conference on Serologic Diagnosis of Lyme Disease. MMWR Morb Mortal Wkly Rep. 1995;11;44(31):590-591. [PMID: 7623762]

Item 71   Answer: B
Educational Objective: Treat pyelonephritis in a young woman in an outpatient setting.

This patient has signs and symptoms consistent with mild pyelonephritis, and because she does not require hospitalization, the optimal management is to obtain a urine culture and start a 7-day course of oral ciprofloxacin, with or without an initial loading dose of ciprofloxacin, 400 mg intravenously. Optimal treatment of acute, uncomplicated pyelonephritis depends on the severity of illness and local resistance patterns as well as host factors such as allergies. Therapy with fluoroquinolone antibiotics is indicated when the prevalence of resistance of community uropathogens to this class of medications does not exceed 10%. If the prevalence of fluoroquinolone resistance is greater than 10%, a single dose of a long-acting intravenous agent such as ceftriaxone or an aminoglycoside should be administered.

Ampicillin would not be appropriate because oral β-lactam agents are less effective than other antibiotics for treating pyelonephritis, and resistance rates are high.

Nitrofurantoin should not be used to treat pyelonephritis because it does not achieve adequate levels in renal tissue.

In a study comparing a 7-day regimen of oral ciprofloxacin with a 14-day regimen of trimethoprim-sulfamethoxazole for women with mild to moderate pyelonephritis, ciprofloxacin had significantly higher clinical and microbiologic cure rates. Trimethoprim-sulfamethoxazole would be appropriate if the pathogen was known to be susceptible.

KEY POINT

- Standard outpatient management of mild pyelonephritis in women who are not pregnant is an oral fluoroquinolone, such as ciprofloxacin, for 7 days.

Bibliography

Gupta K, Hooton TM, Naber KG, et al; Infectious Diseases Society of America; European Society for Microbiology and Infectious Diseases. International clinical practice guidelines for the treatment of acute uncomplicated cystitis and pyelonephritis in women: a 2010 update by the Infectious Diseases Society of America and the European Society for Microbiology and Infectious Diseases. Clin Infect Dis. 2011;52(5):e103-e120. [PMID: 21292654]

Item 72   Answer: B
Educational Objective: Manage hyperlipidemia in a patient with HIV infection.

The most appropriate management of this patient is initiation of atorvastatin. Metabolic changes in patients with HIV infection can be caused by antiretroviral medications or the infection itself. HIV infection is associated with decreased total, HDL, and LDL cholesterol levels and increased triglyceride levels. Treatment with antiretroviral therapy tends to reverse some of these changes: total and LDL cholesterol increase, but HDL cholesterol remains decreased and triglycerides remain elevated. Some antiretroviral agents, including many protease inhibitors, are particularly associated with hyperlipidemia. This patient's LDL cholesterol level is still higher than goal (130 mg/dL [4.1 mmol/L]) despite diet and exercise. Treatment with a statin is therefore indicated. Atorvastatin has been shown to be effective in treating hyperlipidemia in patients with HIV infection; because of interactions with the protease inhibitor ritonavir, atorvastatin should be started at a lower dose.

This patient has a relatively healthy lifestyle except for smoking, and additional therapeutic changes would likely not have an adequately positive effect on his lipids given their current levels.

Reduction in LDL cholesterol, not triglycerides, is the primary goal of this patient's therapy, and a statin is a better choice than a fibrate for reducing LDL cholesterol levels.

Simvastatin is contraindicated in patients taking HIV protease inhibitors because of cytochrome P-450 drug metabolism interactions, which would raise simvastatin concentrations to dangerous levels.

KEY POINT

- Atorvastatin is effective for treating hyperlipidemia in patients with HIV infection and should be started at a lower dose in patients taking protease inhibitors to avoid drug interactions.

Bibliography

Farrugia PM, Lucariello R, Coppola JT. Human immunodeficiency virus and atherosclerosis. Cardiol Rev. 2009;17(5):211-215. [PMID: 19690471]

Item 73   Answer: D
Educational Objective: Treat a patient with pneumococcal meningitis.

Vancomycin and ceftriaxone are indicated for this patient, who most likely has acute bacterial meningitis. Cerebrospinal fluid analysis was consistent with this diagnosis, and Gram stain revealed gram-positive diplococci, suggesting that *Streptococcus pneumoniae* is the bacterial pathogen. Pending in vitro susceptibility testing of the isolated organism, the patient should be presumed to have pneumococcal meningitis caused by a pathogen that is resistant to penicillin G. The combination of vancomycin and a third-generation cephalosporin (either ceftriaxone or cefotaxime) is therefore recommended because these agents have been shown to be synergistic in killing resistant pneumococci in experimental animal models of pneumococcal meningitis. Once results of in vitro susceptibility testing are available, antimicrobial therapy can be modified for optimal treatment.

Levofloxacin has not been studied in patients with bacterial meningitis, and the other antimicrobial combinations have not shown efficacy in the treatment of pneumococcal meningitis caused by highly penicillin-resistant strains.

KEY POINT

- **The recommended empiric therapy for pneumococcal meningitis is vancomycin plus a third-generation cephalosporin (either ceftriaxone or cefotaxime).**

Bibliography

Brouwer MC, Tunkel AR, van de Beek D. Epidemiology, diagnosis, and antimicrobial treatment of acute bacterial meningitis. Clin Microbiol Rev. 2010;23(3):467-492. [PMID: 20610819]

Item 74   Answer: D

Educational Objective: Diagnose *Yersinia pestis* infection.

The most likely infectious agent is *Yersinia pestis*, the causative agent of plague. *Y. pestis* is endemic to the southwestern United States where the population of reservoir rodents is dense, with transmission usually by flea bite. The bipolar staining Gram-negative bacillus giving the appearance of a closed "safety pin" is virtually pathognomonic for *Y. pestis*.

Plague typically consists of three clinical syndromes: (1) pneumonic plague, occurring with inhalation of bacteria; (2) bubonic plague, characterized by purulent lymphadenitis near the inoculation site (more common in the naturally occurring zoonotic form of infection); and (3) septicemic plague, a septic presentation that can arise from either of the other syndromes. Bubonic plague, with systemic symptoms associated with an intensely painful, swollen group of lymph nodes (bubo), is the most common form and represents 85% of all cases. Pneumonic plague is the most fulminant and lethal form of the disease, occurring primarily through direct inhalation of infectious respiratory droplets from infected animals or people or from intentional aerosol release as an act of bioterrorism. The pneumonic form of disease is virtually 100% fatal if treatment is not administered within 24 hours. Based on ease of access, the potential lethality of the aerosolized form, lack of preventive measures, and rapidity of clinical progression, the Centers for Disease Control and Prevention have designated *Y. pestis* a Category A bioterrorism agent.

Legionella infection (Legionnaires disease) generally requires the inhalation of an infectious aerosol of *Legionella pneumophila* from a contaminated water source. Although frequently associated with systemic symptoms and abnormal laboratory findings, pneumonia is the primary clinical manifestation of infection following a few days of a nonspecific prodromal illness. *L. pneumophila* is a gram-negative bacillus and is difficult to isolate from cultures of sputum or blood; the presence of gram-negative, bipolar bacilli in the blood is not consistent with Legionnaires disease.

Community-acquired pneumonia involving *Pseudomonas aeruginosa* is quite uncommon in young immunocompetent hosts without underlying lung disease.

Gastroenteritis is the most common presentation of *Salmonella enteritidis*, with nontyphoidal strains only rarely causing pleuropulmonary infections.

KEY POINT

- **Plague typically consists of three clinical syndromes: (1) pneumonic plague, occurring with inhalation of bacteria (most likely bioterrorism scenario); (2) bubonic plague, characterized by purulent lymphadenitis near the inoculation site; and (3) septicemic plague, a septic presentation arising from either of the other syndromes.**

Bibliography

Prentice MB, Rahalison L. Plague. Lancet. 2007;369(9568):1196-1207. [PMID: 17416264]

Item 75   Answer: D

Educational Objective: Diagnose typhoid fever in a returning traveler.

This patient most likely has typhoid fever. Most cases are diagnosed in returning international travelers. Typhoid fever may develop following the ingestion of *Salmonella enterica* serotype Typhi, or occasionally, *S. enterica* subtype paratyphi organisms. The incubation period for *S. typhi* infection ranges from 1 to 4 weeks.

The clinical presentation of typhoid fever is typically a rising fever, with temperatures as high as 40.0 °C (104.0 °F), accompanied by relative bradycardia and significant abdominal pain, almost always accompanied by constipation. Diarrhea may be present initially, but more often develops later as the disease progresses. Approximately one third of patients develop salmon-colored, blanching, 1- to 4-cm maculopapules on the trunk. A distended and tender abdomen with splenomegaly is often present. Laboratory abnormalities include anemia, leukopenia, thrombocytopenia, and elevations in serum bilirubin and aminotransferase levels. Hyponatremia is common. The diagnosis is mainly clinical and is established by isolation of *S. typhi* or *S. paratyphi* from blood, bone marrow, stool, or skin. Two vaccines are available for protection against infection with *S. typhi*, although neither is completely effective.

Brucellosis is a worldwide zoonotic infection. The clinical manifestations are generally chronic in nature and often include fever, bone and joint symptoms, and neurologic and neuropsychiatric symptoms frequently accompanied by severe weakness and malaise. Rash is not typically associated with this infection.

Leishmaniasis is a protozoal disease transmitted to humans through the bite of a female sandfly. Patients with visceral leishmaniasis present with weight loss, fever, hepatosplenomegaly, pancytopenia, and hypergammaglobulinemia. The incubation period is typically several months after time of exposure in an endemic area.

Malaria is often characterized by a cyclic pattern of fever without prominent gastrointestinal symptoms or rash.

KEY POINT

- Typhoid fever should be considered in patients returning from endemic areas who present with a rash, rising fever, abdominal pain, and constipation possibly followed by diarrhea.

Bibliography
Meltzer E, Schwartz E. Enteric fever: a travel medicine oriented view. Curr Opin Infect Dis. 2010;23(5):432-437. [PMID: 20613510]

Item 76   Answer: A
Educational Objective: Treat Lyme myocarditis.

Intravenous ceftriaxone is the most appropriate therapy for this patient, who has complete heart block with serologic testing indicating *Borrelia burgdorferi* infection, consistent with Lyme myocarditis. The most common cardiac manifestation of early disseminated Lyme disease is disturbance of the atrioventricular conduction system, ranging from asymptomatic first-degree heart block to third-degree (complete) heart block. For patients with second- or third-degree heart block, intravenous ceftriaxone is recommended. In addition, symptomatic patients or those with second- or third-degree heart block should be hospitalized for cardiac monitoring during treatment.

Asymptomatic patients with first-degree heart block may be treated as outpatients with an oral regimen such as cefuroxime or doxycycline.

Although placement of a temporary pacemaker may be required for symptomatic patients, the conduction abnormalities are reversible, and use of a permanent pacemaker is not indicated.

Observation is not appropriate because antibiotic treatment should be initiated immediately.

KEY POINT

- Intravenous ceftriaxone is the recommended therapy for patients with Lyme myocarditis associated with second- or third-degree heart block.

Bibliography
Wormser GP, Dattwyler RJ, Shapiro ED, et al. The clinical assessment, treatment, and prevention of lyme disease, human granulocytic anaplasmosis, and babesiosis: clinical practice guidelines by the Infectious Diseases Society of America. Clin Infect Dis. 2006;43(9):1089-1134. [PMID: 17029130]

Item 77   Answer: A
Educational Objective: Treat nonpurulent cellulitis.

This patient has nonpurulent cellulitis that is most likely caused by β-hemolytic streptococci, and empiric outpatient treatment with a β-lactam agent such as cephalexin or dicloxacillin is recommended. Cellulitis is a bacterial skin infection involving the dermis and subcutaneous tissues. This infection is most frequently associated with dermatologic conditions involving breaks in the skin, such as eczema, tinea pedis, or chronic skin ulcers, and conditions leading to chronic lymphedema, such as mastectomy and lymph node dissections or saphenous vein grafts used in bypass surgery. Cellulitis should be suspected in patients with the acute onset of spreading erythema, edema, pain or tenderness, and warmth. Fever, although common, is not uniformly present. Patients with severe disease may have associated systemic toxicity. The most common pathogens are *Staphylococcus aureus* and the β-hemolytic streptococci, especially group A β-hemolytic streptococci (GABHS). GABHS is most often associated with nonpurulent cellulitis, whereas *S. aureus* may cause concomitant abscesses, furuncles, carbuncles, and bullous impetigo.

Doxycycline and trimethoprim-sulfamethoxazole have activity against community-associated methicillin-resistant *S. aureus* but are not reliably effective against β-hemolytic streptococci.

Fluconazole is an antifungal agent. Fungi do not usually cause cellulitis in young, healthy persons, but fungal infection should be considered in immunocompromised patients.

Metronidazole is an antimicrobial agent used to treat some anaerobic bacterial and protozoal infections. Although metronidazole is active against some microaerophilic bacteria, it is not effective for treatment of β-hemolytic streptococci.

KEY POINT

- Outpatients with nonpurulent cellulitis should be treated empirically with a β-lactam agent such as cephalexin or dicloxacillin that is active against β-hemolytic streptococci.

Bibliography
Gunderson CG. Cellulitis: definition, etiology, and clinical features. Am J Med. 2011;124(12):1113-1122. [PMID: 22014791]

Item 78   Answer: C
Educational Objective: Manage a patient with a history of infective endocarditis before a dental procedure.

This patient with a history of infective endocarditis requires antimicrobial prophylaxis with clindamycin before her dental procedure. The American Heart Association (AHA) infective endocarditis guidelines, revised in 2007, now recommend that only patients with cardiac conditions associated with the highest risk of adverse outcome from endocarditis receive antimicrobial prophylaxis before undergoing a dental procedure involving manipulation of gingival tissue or the periapical region of teeth or perforation of the oral mucosa. These conditions include the presence of a prosthetic cardiac valve, history of infective endocarditis, unrepaired cyanotic congenital heart disease, congenital heart disease repair with prosthetic material or device for the first 6 months after intervention, presence of palliative shunts and conduits, and cardiac valvulopathy in cardiac transplant recipients. The suggested antibiotic prophylactic regimens before dental procedures for patients with these indications are agents directed against viridans group streptococci, administered as a single dose 30 to 60 minutes before the procedure. Clindamycin, azithromycin, or clarithromycin would be appropriate choices for this patient, who experienced anaphylaxis after receiving penicillin.

Amoxicillin and cephalosporins such as cephalexin should not be used in patients with a history of anaphylaxis after receiving penicillin.

Vancomycin is not required because, despite this patient's history of methicillin-resistant *Staphylococcus aureus* endocarditis, this previous infection does not influence the antibiotic choice for prophylactic endocarditis treatment.

According to the AHA guidelines, a history of infective endocarditis is one of the indications for infective endocarditis prophylaxis before a dental procedure involving gingival manipulation; consequently, providing no prophylaxis to this patient would not be appropriate.

KEY POINT

- The indications for infective endocarditis antimicrobial prophylaxis for patients who will undergo a dental procedure involving manipulation of gingival tissue or the periapical region of teeth or perforation of the oral mucosa are (1) the presence of a prosthetic cardiac valve, (2) a history of infective endocarditis, (3) unrepaired cyanotic congenital heart disease, (4) congenital heart disease repair with prosthetic material or device for the first 6 months after intervention, (5) presence of palliative shunts and conduits, and (6) cardiac valvulopathy in cardiac transplant recipients.

Bibliography

Wilson W, Taubert KA, Gewitz M, et al. American Heart Association Rheumatic Fever, Endocarditis, and Kawasaki Disease Committee; American Heart Association Council on Cardiovascular Disease in the Young; American Heart Association Council on Clinical Cardiology; American Heart Association Council on Cardiovascular Surgery and Anesthesia; Quality of Care and Outcomes Research Interdisciplinary Working Group. Prevention of infective endocarditis. Guidelines from the American Heart Association. A guideline from the American Heart Association Rheumatic Cardiovascular Disease in the Young, and the Council on Clinical Cardiology, Council on Cardiovascular Surgery and Anesthesia, and the Quality of Care and Outcomes Research Interdisciplinary Working Group. Circulation. 2007;116(15):1736-1754. [PMID: 17446442]

Item 79   Answer: B

Educational Objective: Diagnose severe community-acquired pneumonia.

This patient requires *Legionella* and *Streptococcus pneumoniae* urine antigen assays. The role of routine diagnostic testing to determine the microbial cause of community-acquired pneumonia (CAP) is controversial. The Infectious Diseases Society of America/American Thoracic Society (IDSA/ATS) consensus guidelines suggest that diagnostic testing in outpatients, except for pulse oximetry, is optional. However, this hospitalized patient has severe CAP, defined as CAP in a patient necessitating admission to an intensive care unit or transfer to an intensive care unit within 24 hours of admission. Blood cultures, *Legionella* and *Streptococcus pneumoniae* urine antigen assays, and endotracheal aspirate for Gram stain and culture are recommended for hospitalized patients with severe CAP.

Bronchoscopy with quantitative culture can be used as a diagnostic tool in the evaluation of patients with pneumonia. When bronchoscopy was compared with evaluation using clinical features suggesting pneumonia and endotracheal aspirate for Gram stain and qualitative culture in patients with ventilator-associated pneumonia, clinical outcomes for the two approaches were equivalent. However, bronchoscopy with quantitative culture has not been prospectively studied for the management of patients with severe CAP.

Serology for atypical pathogens such as *Legionella* species is not recommended because convalescent titers would need to be obtained 6 to 8 weeks after initial testing to establish a diagnosis.

This hospitalized patient has severe CAP; consequently, providing no further evaluation would not be appropriate.

KEY POINT

- Blood cultures, *Legionella* and *Streptococcus pneumoniae* urine antigen assays, and endotracheal aspirate for Gram stain and culture are recommended for hospitalized patients with severe community-acquired pneumonia.

Bibliography

Niederman N. In the clinic. Community-acquired pneumonia. Ann Intern Med. 2009;151(7):ITC4-2-ITC4-14; quiz ITC4-16. [PMID: 19805767]

Item 80   Answer: A

Educational Objective: Diagnose a suspected brain abscess.

This patient most likely has a brain abscess, and stereotactic CT-guided aspiration of the lesion should be done next. The diagnosis of brain abscess should be considered in patients with a central nervous system mass lesion. Most of the symptoms and signs relate to the size and location of the abscess. Less than 50% of patients with a bacterial brain abscess present with the triad of headache, fever, and focal neurologic deficits. Although the most common predisposing conditions are a result of hematogenous spread or a contiguous focus of infection, 10% to 35% of brain abscesses are cryptogenic. Suspected abscesses that are greater than 2.5 cm in diameter on neuroimaging studies should be excised or aspirated under CT guidance. The specimens should then be sent for microbiologic examination (including stains and culture for bacteria, nocardia, mycobacteria, and fungi) and for histopathologic examination (including special stains for identification of these organisms). Although other causes may account for this patient's mass lesion, including a neoplasm, a definitive diagnosis should be established rather than assuming that this is a malignant lesion.

Lumbar puncture is not indicated for patients with central nervous system mass lesions because of the potential complication of brain herniation.

Whole-body PET scanning or CT scanning of the chest, abdomen, and pelvis might be useful in localizing an unknown infectious or malignant focus but would not be performed before definitively diagnosing the primary central nervous system lesion, which may reveal significant information that would further guide the diagnostic evaluation and appropriate treatment.

KEY POINT

- **In patients with a central nervous system mass lesion, a definitive diagnosis, such as brain abscess, should be determined rather than assuming that the lesion is malignant.**

Bibliography

Lu CH, Chang WN, Liu CC. Strategies for the management of bacterial brain abscess. J Clin Neurosci. 2006;13(10):979-985. [PMID: 1705626]

Item 81   Answer: C

Educational Objective: Prevent ventilator-associated pneumonia.

The head of this patient's bed should be maintained above an angle of 30°. Ventilator-associated pneumonia (VAP) is a subset of hospital-acquired pneumonia (HAP) and refers to pneumonia that develops more than 48 to 72 hours after mechanical ventilation is begun. As in the prevention of central line–associated bloodstream infections (CLABSI), using and implementing a prevention "bundle" is a successful method for reducing the rate of VAP in a facility. A VAP prevention bundle of interventions includes: (1) maintaining the head of the patient's bed above a 30° angle, (2) daily assessments of the patient's readiness to wean from the ventilator, and (3) chlorhexidine mouth washes.

Use of chlorhexidine-based antiseptic to bathe hospitalized patients in intensive care units is a common practice. The benefit of chlorhexidine bathing has been studied relative to CLABSI prevention and spread of multidrug-resistant organisms such as *Acinetobacter baumannii*. However, controlled data pertaining to the specific role of chlorhexidine-based bathing on VAP prevention are still lacking.

Prolonged durations of perioperative surgical prophylactic antimicrobial agents have not been demonstrated to reduce the risk for VAP.

Performing early tracheotomy has not been clearly demonstrated as a method for reducing VAP.

The data regarding the role of antiseptic-coated endotracheal tubes in VAP prevention are promising, but silver-coated endotracheal tubes are not currently formally recommended for VAP prevention. In clinical studies, patients were initially intubated with silver-coated endotracheal tubes; however, the effect on VAP prevention of extubating patients and then re-intubating them with silver-coated endotracheal tubes has not been studied.

KEY POINT

- **In patients receiving mechanical ventilation, maintaining the head of the bed above a 30° angle helps reduce the risk for ventilator-associated pneumonia.**

Bibliography

American Thoracic Society; Infectious Diseases Society of America. Guidelines for the management of adults with hospital-acquired, ventilator-associated, and healthcare-associated pneumonia. Am J Respir Crit Care Med. 2005;171(4):388-416. [PMID: 15699079]

Item 82   Answer: E

Educational Objective: Diagnose travelers' diarrhea.

No additional diagnostic testing is indicated. This patient has travelers' diarrhea, which is an extremely common illness among visitors to developing countries, especially following ingestion of unprocessed water or raw fruits and vegetables. Travelers' diarrhea may be caused by several different pathogens. The most common pathogen is enterotoxigenic *Escherichia coli* (ETEC), which typically causes a self-limited, relatively mild diarrheal illness that can be treated symptomatically without the need for diagnostic testing.

Routine stool cultures cannot differentiate ETEC from *E. coli* organisms that are part of the normal fecal flora. However, stool cultures for bacteria should be obtained in patients with diarrhea lasting longer than 72 hours, particularly if associated with fever, tenesmus, or blood in the stool.

Stool cultures for viruses are rarely indicated for other than epidemiologic investigation because results are not useful for guiding therapy.

Symptoms lasting longer than 7 days may indicate a parasitic intestinal infection, and examination of the stool for ova and parasites is the recommended initial diagnostic test.

The presence of fecal leukocytes is suggestive of an inflammatory bacterial diarrhea; however, positive results also may be characteristic of other conditions. In this patient, who is at low risk for inflammatory diarrhea, this test would not be cost-effective because, regardless of the results, it would be unlikely to change management.

KEY POINT

- **The most common pathogen responsible for travelers' diarrhea is enterotoxigenic *Escherichia coli*, which typically causes a self-limited, relatively mild diarrheal illness that can be treated symptomatically and warrants no diagnostic testing.**

Bibliography

Hill DR, Ericsson CD, Pearson RD, et al; Infectious Diseases Society of America. The practice of travel medicine: Guidelines by the Infectious Diseases Society of America. Clin Infect Dis. 2006;43(12):1499-1539. [PMID: 17109284]

Item 83   Answer: C
Educational Objective: Treat a patient with gonococcal urethritis.

The most appropriate treatment is ceftriaxone and azithromycin. This patient presents with symptoms and signs consistent with urethritis, including laboratory findings indicating intracellular gram-negative diplococci visualized on a Gram stain of urethral discharge. If available, Gram stain results are extremely useful in the evaluation of men with symptomatic gonococcal urethritis because more than 95% of patients have this finding. Ceftriaxone is the preferred treatment option. Patients with gonococcal urethritis (or cervicitis) should also be treated for possible chlamydial infection because the risk of coinfection is high. Consequently, a single dose of azithromycin plus ceftriaxone should be given to this patient.

A high (2-g) dose of azithromycin may be sufficient for treating infection with *Neisseria gonorrhoeae* and also *Chlamydia trachomatis* but is limited by the high frequency of gastrointestinal side effects, increasing resistance, and expense associated with such use.

Cefoxitin has activity against penicillinase-producing *N. gonorrhoeae* but would not be effective in a single dose without the simultaneous administration of probenecid. In addition, it would fail to cover possible coinfection with *C. trachomatis*.

The combination of ciprofloxacin and azithromycin would not be adequate therapy for this patient. Strains of gonorrhea have become increasingly resistant to fluoroquinolones in recent years; consequently, fluoroquinolones such as ciprofloxacin are no longer recommended for treatment of these infections.

KEY POINT

- **Patients with gonococcal urethritis (or cervicitis) should also be treated for possible coinfection with chlamydial infection with ceftriaxone plus a single dose of azithromycin.**

Bibliography

Workowski KA, Berman S; Centers for Disease Control and Prevention (CDC). Sexually transmitted diseases treatment guidelines, 2010. MMWR Recomm Rep. 2010;59(RR-12):1-110. [PMID: 21160459]

Item 84   Answer: A
Educational Objective: Treat possible methicillin-resistant *Staphylococcus aureus* infection in a patient with purulent cellulitis.

Empiric ceftaroline is the most appropriate β-lactam antibiotic for this patient with purulent cellulitis presumably caused by methicillin-resistant *Staphylococcus aureus* (MRSA). Development of MRSA requires the acquisition of a *mec* gene, which encodes for penicillin-binding protein 2a in the bacterial membrane. Drug resistance develops because of the low affinity of penicillin-binding protein 2a for β-lactam agents. MRSA organisms are resistant to oxacillin, nafcillin, and dicloxacillin, as well as to carbapenems (including meropenem) and monobactam antibiotics. All cephalosporins, including ceftriaxone, are also inactive against MRSA, except ceftaroline, a new fifth-generation cephalosporin approved by the FDA for treating skin infections and community-acquired bacterial pneumonia. Ceftaroline, unlike other β-lactam agents, has a high affinity for penicillin-binding protein 2a. This drug also has activity against staphylococci and streptococci as well as some gram-negative organisms (including *Haemophilus influenzae*) and Enterobacteriaceae (including *Klebsiella* species and *Escherichia coli*). Ceftaroline is administered intravenously and requires dose adjustment based on kidney function.

KEY POINT

- **Ceftaroline is a new β-lactam antibiotic with significant activity against methicillin-resistant *Staphylococcus aureus* and other aerobic and anaerobic gram-positive organisms and aerobic gram-negative bacteria, and it can be used for complicated soft tissue infections and community-acquired pneumonia.**

Bibliography

Saravolatz LD, Stein GE, Johnson LB. Ceftaroline: A novel cephalosporin with activity against methicillin-resistant Staphylococcus aureus. Clin Infect Dis. 2011;52(9):1156-1163. [PMID: 21467022]

Item 85   Answer: E

Educational Objective: Manage a patient with asymptomatic bacteriuria.

Asymptomatic bacteriuria in the elderly does not require treatment. The prevalence of asymptomatic bacteriuria is higher among women than men and occurs more commonly in pregnant patients, patients with diabetes, and the elderly. Asymptomatic bacteriuria becomes more common among men at age 65 years or older. In asymptomatic men, asymptomatic bacteriuria is defined as a single, clean-catch, voided urine specimen with one bacterial species isolated in a quantitative count of 10^5 or more colony-forming units/mL. Evidence has shown that treating asymptomatic bacteriuria in elderly patients has no effect on the incidence of symptomatic urinary tract infections, prevalence of bacteriuria, or survival. Screening or treatment of asymptomatic bacteruria is not indicated in nonpregnant women or patients with diabetes, spinal cord injuries, or with chronic indwelling urinary catheters. Treatment of these populations puts the patients at risk for drug side effects and increases the probability of antibiotic resistance. Treating asymptomatic bacteriuria is appropriate in pregnancy and before invasive urologic procedures.

Ciprofloxacin and trimethoprim-sulfamethoxazole are both appropriate choices for treating symptomatic urinary tract infection, which is not required in this patient.

Medical evaluation, such as kidney ultrasonography, is not indicated for asymptomatic bacteriuria.

Repeating a urinalysis and urine culture will likely provide similar results and will not help in managing this patient.

KEY POINT

- Except for pregnancy and prior to invasive urologic procedures, treatment of asymptomatic bacteriuria is not indicated.

Bibliography
Matthews SJ, Lancaster JW. Urinary Tract Infections in the elderly population. Am J Geriatr Pharmacother. 2011;9(5):286-309. [PMID: 21840265]

Item 86   Answer: D

Educational Objective: Diagnose selective IgA deficiency.

Selective IgA deficiency is the most likely diagnosis in this patient. Although most patients with selective IgA deficiency are asymptomatic, some have chronic or recurrent respiratory tract infections, atopic disorders (such as eczema), or a high incidence of autoimmune diseases, such as rheumatoid arthritis or systemic lupus erythematosus. Gastrointestinal and urinary tract infections may occur as well as severe anaphylactic reactions after intravenous administration of blood products or immune globulin preparations. Patients with undetectable serum levels of IgA may form antibodies directed against IgA, which rarely can be responsible for transfusion reactions.

C1-inhibitor deficiency is an autosomal dominant disorder associated with hereditary angioedema. Most patients have a family history of angioedema, and the condition often presents as recurrent episodes of subcutaneous edema, unexplained episodes of abdominal pain, or laryngeal edema. A single episode of angioedema following an erythrocyte transfusion is most compatible with selective IgA deficiency, not C1-inhibitor deficiency.

Terminal complement deficiency (C5-C9) is inherited as an autosomal co-dominant disorder and is associated with susceptibility to systemic neisserial infections, especially meningococcal disease.

Inherited defects of properdin are rare. Those with this deficiency are at risk for recurrent infection with *Neisseria meningitidis*, not anaphylaxis.

KEY POINT

- **Most patients with selective IgA deficiency are at risk for severe anaphylactic reactions after intravenous administration of blood products or immune globulin preparations.**

Bibliography
Yel L. Selective IgA deficiency. J Clin Immunol. 2010;30(1):10-16. [PMID: 20101521]

Item 87   Answer: B

Educational Objective: Manage tick-borne rickettsial infection.

Doxycycline should be started now. This patient presents with a febrile illness in the spring and a history of tick exposure, raising concern for a tick-borne infection. Results of serologic testing for any of the tick-borne rickettsial pathogens are often negative during the acute phase of the illness. Molecular testing for *Ehrlichia* and *Anaplasma* spp. by whole blood polymerase chain reaction is more sensitive during the acute phase but may be negative if the patient has received prior antibiotics. If one of these diseases is suspected based on epidemiologic and clinical data, empiric treatment should be initiated immediately without awaiting laboratory confirmation because a delay in therapy is associated with a significant increase in morbidity.

Human granulocytic anaplasmosis (HGA, caused by *Anaplasma phagocytophilum*), human monocytic ehrlichiosis (HME, caused by *Ehrlichia chaffeensis*), and Rocky Mountain spotted fever (RMSF, caused by *Rickettsia rickettsii*) present as nonfocal febrile illnesses that are variably associated with cytopenias and increased serum liver enzyme values. Clinically, these three syndromes are difficult to differentiate from each other, although a petechial skin eruption is seen in up to 85% of patients with RMSF but in many fewer adults with HME or HGA. The characteristic rash in RMSF begins as blanching erythematous macules around the wrists and ankles; lesions spread centripetally and become petechial. The rash is found in only 15% of patients on presentation but appears in most patients by day 4. The absence of the rash presents a diagnostic challenge because of the nonspecific nature of the presentation, but treatment should be initiated regardless of the absence of skin lesions if there is clinical concern for a tick-borne rickettsial infection.

The tick vector for HGA is the same species of tick that causes Lyme disease and is endemic to the northeastern United States and the Great Lakes region. In contrast, the tick vector for HME is distributed throughout the south central United States, and RMSF is found throughout the continental United States.

Doxycycline is the antibiotic of choice for treatment of these tick-borne illnesses; β-lactam antibiotics such as amoxicillin are not effective against these infections.

KEY POINT

- **Because results of serologic testing for any of the tick-borne rickettsial pathogens are often negative during the acute phase of the illness, empiric treatment with doxycycline should be initiated immediately if one of these diseases is suspected based on epidemiologic and clinical data.**

Bibliography

Chapman AS, Bakken JS, Folk SM, et al; Tickborne Rickettsial Diseases Working Group; CDC. Diagnosis and management of tickborne rickettsial diseases: Rocky Mountain spotted fever, ehrlichiosis, and anaplasmosis—United States: a practical guide for physicians and other health-care and public health professionals. MMWR Recomm Rep. 2006;55(RR-4):1-27. [PMID: 16572105]

Item 88   Answer: D

Educational Objective: Prevent influenza virus infection in a pregnant woman.

This patient should receive trivalent inactivated influenza vaccine. Pregnant women are at higher risk for complications from seasonal influenza viruses, and severe disease has been reported during pandemics. Vaccination is the best way to prevent influenza. Ideally, vaccination with the trivalent inactivated influenza vaccine is indicated in pregnant women whose last two trimesters coincide with influenza season, but it can be administered at any time, regardless of trimester of pregnancy. The influenza vaccine should not be given to persons with anaphylactic hypersensitivity to eggs or to those with a history of Guillain-Barré syndrome, both of which are rare.

Chemoprophylaxis with antiviral medications is not a substitute for influenza vaccination when influenza vaccine is available. Oseltamivir, zanamivir, and the adamantanes (amantadine and rimantadine) are efficacious in the prevention of influenza after exposure to a household member or other close contact with confirmed influenza. Emergence

of resistance has become an issue that now limits the use of the adamantanes. Antiviral therapy should be considered for those who are at higher risk for complications but who have not been vaccinated and have family or other close contacts in whom influenza virus infection is suspected or confirmed. An alternative to chemoprophylaxis is to start early therapy at the onset of signs or symptoms. Before instituting pre-exposure chemoprophylaxis, it is important to consider that adverse effects associated with long-term use are uncertain and prolonged use of antiviral agents may lead to resistance. The neuraminidase inhibitors and the adamantanes are pregnancy category C agents, which means that data from clinical studies are not adequate to assess the safety of these medications for pregnant women. Pregnant women with confirmed or suspected influenza should receive antiviral treatment, and pregnancy is not a contraindication to oseltamivir or zanamivir use.

The live attenuated intranasal influenza vaccine is contraindicated in pregnancy as well as in patients with chronic metabolic diseases, diabetes mellitus, kidney dysfunction, hemoglobinopathies, immunosuppression, and chronic diseases that can compromise respiratory function or the handling of respiratory secretions.

KEY POINT

- **Vaccination with the trivalent inactivated influenza vaccine is the most effective method for preventing influenza infection and its complications in healthy persons, those with chronic medical conditions, and pregnant women.**

Bibliography

Yudin MH. Optimizing knowledge of antiviral medications for prophylaxis and treatment of influenza during pregnancy. Expert Rev Respir Med. 2011;5(4):495-501. [PMID: 21859269]

Item 89   Answer: B

Educational Objective: Diagnose familial Mediterranean fever.

This patient most likely has familial Mediterranean fever (FMF), which occurs in ethnic groups originating in the Mediterranean basin. Symptoms of this autosomal recessive disorder typically develop in patients before the age of 20 years and are characterized by acute, self-limited episodes of fever associated with abdominal, chest, or joint pain caused by serosal inflammation. Cutaneous manifestations of FMF mimic erysipelas and usually develop over a distal lower extremity (most often unilaterally but occasionally bilaterally). A neutrophilic leukocytosis is characteristic. Elevated levels of acute phase reactants, including the erythrocyte sedimentation rate and C-reactive protein level, are also common. The genetic association, as well as the episodic presentation of acute, self-limited episodes with concomitant skin abnormalities, distinguishes cutaneous manifestations caused by FMF from those caused by bacterial skin and soft tissue infections. The preferred treatment is colchicine.

Erythromelalgia typically manifests as paroxysmal bilateral erythema of the extremities with associated warmth and burning pain. This condition is often precipitated by warmer external temperatures and febrile episodes and is aggravated by the dependent position. The episodic presentation, inciting factors, and bilateral extremity distribution are helpful in distinguishing erythromelalgia from skin and soft tissue infections. Serosal inflammation is not a feature of this disease.

Staphylococcal cellulitis is less likely because of the bilateral symmetric distribution of this patient's skin findings and the absence of purulence and lymphadenopathy. His history of previous episodes that resolved without antibiotic treatment makes staphylococcal cellulitis unlikely.

Sweet syndrome, or acute febrile neutrophilic dermatitis, most commonly affects middle-aged women after an upper respiratory tract infection. Sweet syndrome may be idiopathic or may be associated with an underlying condition. Patients with Sweet syndrome present with the abrupt onset of fever, arthralgia, myalgia, and cutaneous lesions. Individual lesions are tender, nonpruritic, brightly erythematous, well-demarcated papules and plaques that appear on the neck, upper trunk, and typically, upper extremities. This patient's skin lesions are not consistent with those of Sweet syndrome. In addition, Sweet syndrome is not typically associated with abdominal pain, and it does not typically remit after several days.

KEY POINT

- **Familial Mediterranean fever is a hereditary periodic fever syndrome that is characterized by serosal inflammation in the chest, abdomen, or joints and an erysipelas-like rash.**

Bibliography

Falagas ME, Vergidis PI. Narrative reviews: Diseases that masquerade as infectious cellulitis. Ann Intern Med. 2005;142(1):47-55. [PMID: 15630108]

Item 90　　Answer:　D

Educational Objective: Prevent surgical site infection in a pregnant woman.

This patient should receive antimicrobial prophylaxis 30 to 60 minutes before surgery with therapeutic levels maintained throughout surgery. There are several measures that help to prevent surgical site infections (SSIs). Antibiotic prophylaxis should be administered 30 to 60 minutes before surgical incision; vancomycin and the fluoroquinolones can be administered 60 to 120 minutes before incision. If the procedure is prolonged, it is important to repeat the dosage to maintain therapeutic levels throughout the procedure depending on the agent's half-life. Preoperative measures to prevent SSIs include control or elimination of modifiable risk factors (for example, uncontrolled

diabetes mellitus or hyperglycemia, obesity, tobacco use, use of immunosuppressive agents, length of preoperative hospitalization) and antibiotic prophylaxis. Perioperative measures to prevent SSIs are to avoid shaving of hair, provide aggressive glucose control, use chlorhexidine-based surgical preparation, minimize traffic into and out of the operating room, administer supplemental oxygen, and use checklists to improve compliance with preventive processes.

Decolonization of group B *Streptococcus* vaginal/rectal carriage is important for prevention of early-onset neonatal group B streptococcal disease but has no role in the prevention of SSIs.

Antimicrobial prophylaxis should be stopped promptly after the procedure ends, within 24 hours following incision. Continuing antibiotics beyond this period is not recommended.

Shaving of hair prior to surgery is a risk factor for, not a protective factor against, SSIs.

KEY POINT

- **To minimize the risk for surgical site infection, antimicrobial prophylaxis should be administered 30 to 60 minutes before surgical incision, with therapeutic levels maintained throughout the procedure.**

Bibliography

Anderson DJ. Surgical site infections. Infect Dis Clin North Am. 2011;25(1):135-153. [PMID: 21315998]

Item 91　　Answer:　A

Educational Objective: Treat recurrent genital herpes simplex virus infection in a patient with AIDS.

The most appropriate treatment is acyclovir. This severely immunocompromised patient with AIDS and a very low CD4 cell count presents with recurrent genital and perianal herpes simplex virus infection. The lesions have resolved, and the suppressive treatment of choice is acyclovir. Chronic suppressive antiviral therapy prevents outbreaks of genital herpes and is warranted in immunocompromised hosts or those with frequent (>6 episodes per year) or severe recurrences. He should be encouraged to re-initiate antiretroviral therapy because immune reconstitution will also reduce recurrent episodes of herpes simplex virus infection.

Cidofovir and foscarnet are intravenous preparations reserved for treatment of acyclovir-resistant herpesvirus infections. Cidofovir is also available as an ointment, which can hasten healing of acyclovir-resistant lesions; however, cidofovir can also cause mucocutaneous ulcers. The intravenous form can cause rash, neutropenia, and kidney failure. Foscarnet can also cause serious adverse effects, including kidney insufficiency, nausea, paresthesias, and seizures.

Valganciclovir is the prodrug of ganciclovir. It has broad-spectrum activity against herpesviruses. It is currently approved for treatment, suppression, and prevention of cytomegalovirus infections. Its principal toxicity is myelosuppression.

KEY POINT

- Acyclovir is efficacious for treating genital herpes simplex virus infection and preventing symptomatic reactivation in immunocompromised hosts.

Bibliography

Cernik C, Gallina K, Brodell RT. The treatment of herpes simplex infections: an evidence-based review. Arch Intern Med. 2008;168(11):1137-1144. [PMID: 18541820]

Item 92   Answer: D

Educational Objective: Diagnose *Streptococcus pneumoniae* infection after transplantation.

This patient with fever, chills, cough, and pleuritic chest pain most likely has *Streptococcus pneumoniae* infection. The periods following hematopoietic stem cell transplantation (HSCT) during which opportunistic infections can occur are the pre-engraftment phase (>30 days after transplantation), the postengraftment phase (30 to 100 days after transplantation), and the late phase (>100 days after transplantation). This patient underwent HSCT 6 months ago, and this late posttransplantation time frame is associated with a high risk for infection with encapsulated bacterial organisms such as *S. pneumoniae*. Consequently, immunization with a full series of conjugated pneumococcal vaccines is indicated, beginning 3 to 6 months after transplantation.

Candida (no matter which species) is a very rare cause of pneumonia, even in immunocompromised patients.

Cytomegalovirus infection frequently occurs after the first month of transplantation but occurs less commonly 6 to 12 months after transplantation. Also, cytomegalovirus pneumonia would more likely cause diffuse interstitial infiltrates rather than lobar consolidation as demonstrated on this patient's chest radiograph.

Pneumocystis pneumonia may occur in patients following HSCT, but this patient is taking trimethoprim-sulfamethoxazole, which is very effective as prophylaxis against *Pneumocystis jirovecii*. In addition, *Pneumocystis* pneumonia would be less likely to have a lobar presentation.

KEY POINT

- In the late posttransplantation phase (more than a few months after transplantation), hematopoietic stem cell transplant recipients are at high risk for infection with encapsulated organisms such as *Streptococcus pneumoniae*.

Bibliography

Wingard JR, Hsu J, Hiemenz JW. Hematopoietic stem cell transplantation: an overview of infection risks and epidemiology. Infect Dis Clin North Am. 2010;24(2):257-272. [PMID: 20466269]

Item 93   Answer: B

Educational Objective: Diagnose babesiosis.

The most likely pathogen is *Babesia microti*. This patient has a febrile illness associated with clinical and laboratory evidence of hemolysis following a camping trip in New England. This presentation is highly suggestive of babesiosis, a tick-borne protozoal infection caused by *B. microti*. The vector tick is *Ixodes scapularis*, the same arthropod that transmits Lyme disease (caused by *Borrelia burgdorferi*) and human granulocytic anaplasmosis (caused by *Anaplasma phagocytophilum*). Consequently, coinfection with more than one of these tick-borne pathogens may develop. Although all three pathogens may cause a febrile illness, only *B. microti* results in significant hemolysis because of multiplication of the organisms within erythrocytes.

Because Lyme disease, human granulocytic anaplasmosis, and Rocky Mountain spotted fever (RMSF) (caused by *Rickettsia rickettsii*) are all treated with doxycycline, the onset of new symptoms in a patient taking this antibiotic would support development of another infection, such as babesiosis. This patient is unlikely to have RMSF because it is not associated with hemolysis but is often associated with a rash. The characteristic rash of RMSF begins as blanching erythematous macules around the wrists and ankles, progressing to petechiae. The rash is found in only 15% of patients on presentation but appears in 85% to 90% of patients by day 4. RMSF is more common in the southeastern and south central United States.

West Nile virus may cause a febrile illness that is variably associated with fever and central nervous system manifestations but is not associated with hemolysis. West Nile virus is usually transmitted by mosquitoes and is not a tick-borne disease.

KEY POINT

- Because the same vector tick carries pathogens responsible for babesiosis, Lyme disease, and human granulocytic anaplasmosis, coinfection among these three entities may occur; however, only babesiosis causes hemolysis.

Bibliography

Wormser GP, Dattwyler RJ, Shapiro ED, et al. The clinical assessment, treatment, and prevention of lyme disease, human granulocytic anaplasmosis, and babesiosis: clinical practice guidelines by the Infectious Diseases Society of America. Clin Infect Dis. 2006;43(9):1089-1134. [PMID: 17029130]

Item 94   Answer: D

Educational Objective: Manage a parapneumonic effusion.

This patient requires immediate ultrasound-guided thoracentesis. Patients such as this with community-acquired pneumonia (CAP) and a large associated pleural effusion (typically defined as an effusion occupying half or more of the hemithorax on an upright chest radiograph or a fluid level of more than 1 cm on lateral decubitus films) should undergo prompt thoracentesis as part of the initial evaluation to confirm the microbial cause of the pneumonia and exclude a complicated parapneumonic effusion or empyema. Delay in the diagnosis of a complicated pleural effusion or empyema may result in a loculated effusion, often necessitating more invasive management, such as video-assisted thoracoscopic surgery or open thoracotomy.

The presence of a pleural effusion does not affect the selection of empiric antibiotic therapy; consequently, adding metronidazole or changing therapy from cefotaxime and azithromycin to cefepime and vancomycin would be unnecessary.

Pleural effusions can occur in 20% to 40% of hospitalized patients with CAP. A small pleural effusion that develops during treatment does not require thoracentesis as long as the patient is responding appropriately to antibiotic treatment.

KEY POINT

- Patients with community-acquired pneumonia and a large associated pleural effusion should undergo prompt thoracentesis to confirm the microbial cause of the pneumonia and exclude a complicated parapneumonic effusion or empyema.

Bibliography
Colice GL, Curtis A, Deslauriers J, et al. Medical and surgical treatment of parapneumonic effusions: an evidence-based guideline. Chest. 2000;118(4):1158-1171. [PMID: 11035692]

Item 95   Answer: A

Educational Objective: Screen for HIV infection.

The first step in the management of this patient is screening by HIV antibody enzyme immunoassay (EIA). Although this patient has no symptoms or significant risk factors for HIV infection, she has asked about receiving HIV screening. The Centers for Disease Control and Prevention (CDC) now recommend HIV screening for all persons between the ages of 13 and 64 years at least once and that those with risk factors undergo annual testing. In addition, the American College of Physicians has issued a guidance statement recommending that this age range be expanded to include patients through age 75 years because of increased rates of infection in this population. HIV antibody EIA is the appropriate first test when screening for HIV infection, and when combined with a Western blot if the EIA is positive, has 99% sensitivity and specificity for the diagnosis of HIV infection.

The Western blot assay is the confirmatory test for HIV infection and should only be used to confirm that a

reactive EIA is a true positive and not a false-positive result. It should not be used as the initial step in screening.

This patient has no symptoms of acute HIV infection; consequently, there is no concern she may be in the "window period" of acute HIV infection, during which false-negative antibody testing results can occur that require HIV nucleic acid amplification testing to establish a diagnosis. In addition, HIV nucleic acid amplification testing is less sensitive and specific than standard HIV antibody EIA screening followed by Western blot confirmatory testing.

Initiating no testing for this patient, who has never had HIV screening and who has specifically requested it, would not be the most appropriate management.

KEY POINT

- All persons between the ages of 13 and 75 years should be tested for HIV infection at least once, and those with risk factors should undergo annual testing.

Bibliography
Branson BM, Handsfield HH, Lampe MA, et al. ; Centers for Disease Control and Prevention (CDC). Revised recommendations for HIV testing of adults, adolescents, and pregnant women in health-care settings. MMWR Recomm Rep. 2006;55(RR-14):1-17; quiz CE1-4. [PMID: 16988643]

Item 96   Answer: C

Educational Objective: Treat a patient with bacterial meningitis following neurosurgery.

In addition to vancomycin, meropenem is the most appropriate antimicrobial agent for this patient, who has most likely developed bacterial meningitis following a neurosurgical procedure. The most common pathogens that cause meningitis in this setting are gram-positive organisms (such as *Staphylococcus aureus* and coagulase-negative staphylococci) and gram-negative bacilli. Based on the possibility of staphylococcal meningitis, including that caused by methicillin-resistant strains, vancomycin should be included in the empiric therapeutic regimen. Multiple gram-negative bacilli must also be considered, including *Pseudomonas aeruginosa* and *Acinetobacter* species. Of the possible choices listed, meropenem is the best agent to treat the most likely gram-negative bacilli in a patient with nosocomial meningitis.

Ceftriaxone and trimethoprim-sulfamethoxazole are not active against *P. aeruginosa.*

Although gentamicin has activity against many gram-negative bacilli, it does not achieve adequate cerebrospinal fluid concentrations after parenteral administration to treat gram-negative meningitis.

Metronidazole is only active against anaerobic bacteria.

- Empiric therapy for patients with nosocomial meningitis should include vancomycin plus an agent that penetrates well into cerebrospinal fluid and has in vitro activity against gram-negative bacilli, including *Pseudomonas aeruginosa* and *Acinetobacter* species.

Bibliography

van de Beek D, Drake JM, Tunkel AR. Nosocomial bacterial meningitis. N Engl J Med. 2010;362(2):146-154. [PMID: 20071704]

Item 97 — Answer: E

Educational Objective: Prevent travelers' diarrhea in a patient with inflammatory bowel disease.

This patient should be given prophylactic rifaximin to reduce her risk for travelers' diarrhea. Travelers' diarrhea is the most common illness in persons visiting developing countries, with an overall incidence of about 20% to 60%. The risk of acquiring this condition correlates directly with the geographic region visited. The highest risk is associated with travel to Mexico, South and Central America, Asia, and countries in Africa other than South Africa. Travelers' diarrhea is defined as the occurrence of three or more unformed stools per day with abdominal pain or cramps, nausea or vomiting, bloody stools, or fever. Diarrhea is usually self-limited, generally lasting 1 to 4 days, although in some patients, symptoms persist longer. Bacteria such as enterotoxigenic *Escherichia coli* cause most episodes of travelers' diarrhea. Other causative bacterial organisms include *Salmonella, Shigella, Campylobacter, Aeromonas,* and *Vibrio* species. Protozoan pathogens are isolated in less than 10% of patients. Travelers' diarrhea caused by viral diseases is uncommon, but in certain circumstances such as on cruise ships, it may be caused by norovirus infection. No definitive microbiologic agent is identified in about 30% of patients.

Reducing the risk for travelers' diarrhea involves multiple modalities. The use of prophylactic antibiotics has proved effective but is not recommended for the average traveler owing to potential side effects. Antibiotics may be warranted in some instances, such as this patient whose inflammatory bowel disease could be greatly exacerbated by an episode of travelers' diarrhea, and others with immunocompromising illnesses and chronic diseases that could be exacerbated in the setting of dehydration or electrolyte imbalance. Historically, the fluoroquinolone class of antibiotics has been used to treat travelers' diarrhea, although the development of fluoroquinolone resistance has led to increased interest in alternative agents. Rifaximin, a nonabsorbed antibiotic, is effective and safe when prescribed at doses of 200 mg, once or twice daily for 2 weeks, particularly when *E. coli* will be the most likely acquired pathogen during travel.

Although it may seem logical that avoiding tap water that is potentially contaminated with diarrhea-producing microorganisms would decrease the risk for travelers' diarrhea, this practice has only been shown to confer a small benefit. Nonetheless, instituting water purification techniques, such as boiling tap water for 3 minutes and then cooling it to room temperature, are highly recommended.

Taking bismuth subsalicylate at the high dose required to diminish the incidence of travelers' diarrhea is not convenient and could lead to salicylate toxicity.

The effectiveness of probiotics in reducing the risk for travelers' diarrhea remains uncertain, with results varying depending on the preparation studied.

The use of antimotility medications, such as loperamide or diphenoxylate, to prevent travelers' diarrhea has not been shown to be effective as a prophylactic intervention.

- Although travelers' diarrhea is self-limited and generally requires no prophylactic medication, antibiotics are indicated in patients whose conditions could be exacerbated by an episode of travelers' diarrhea, such as inflammatory bowel disease, immunocompromising illnesses, and chronic diseases such as cardiac disease.

Bibliography

DuPont HL, Ericsson CD, Farthing MJ, et al. Expert review of the evidence for prevention of travelers' diarrhea. J Travel Med. 2009;16(3):149-160. [PMID: 19538575]

Item 98 — Answer: A

Educational Objective: Diagnose giardiasis.

The study most likely to establish a diagnosis is a stool assay for *Giardia* antigen. This patient's clinical presentation of a prolonged gastrointestinal illness characterized by watery diarrhea and weight loss and his history of camping in the preceding month are strongly suggestive of infection with *Giardia lamblia*. This parasitic infection is typically transmitted by ingestion of *Giardia* cysts found in natural bodies of water. Giardiasis can be prevented by boiling or filtering water or by iodine treatment. Most infections are asymptomatic. Symptomatic infection often involves the small bowel and is characterized by large-volume liquid stools and bloating or belching. Although fever is rare, weight loss due to anorexia and malabsorption is an almost universal finding. A monoclonal antibody assay that detects *Giardia* antigen directly on a stool sample is recommended for diagnosis.

Stool cultures for bacteria have a low yield in diagnosing a diarrheal illness lasting more than 7 to 10 days and, in addition, would not be useful in this patient who has a protozoal infection.

Although giardiasis may be diagnosed by microscopic examination for ova and parasites identifying *Giardia* trophozoites or cysts, the intermittent shedding of these organisms makes this a less sensitive test than the *Giardia* antigen assay. In situations in which antigen testing is not readily available, examination of three stool specimens for ova and parasites may be diagnostic.

Modified acid-fast staining of a stool sample is needed to visualize *Cryptosporidium*, *Isospora*, and *Cyclospora* organisms but is not indicated for the diagnosis of *Giardia*.

KEY POINT

- The most sensitive test for diagnosing giardiasis is a stool assay for *Giardia* antigen.

Bibliography

Pawlowski SW, Warren CA, Guerrant R. Diagnosis and treatment of acute or persistent diarrhea. Gastroenterology. 2009;136(6):1874-1886. [PMID: 19457416]

Item 99   Answer: B

Educational Objective: Diagnose the acute retroviral syndrome.

The most appropriate next diagnostic test is an HIV nucleic acid amplification test. This patient's medical history and timing of symptoms are typical of acute HIV infection. Although his symptoms could also represent infectious mononucleosis or syphilis, preliminary results for those conditions are negative. Most persons in whom HIV infection develops experience an acute symptomatic illness within 2 to 4 weeks of infection. Symptoms typically last for a few weeks and range from a simple febrile illness to a full-blown mononucleosis-like syndrome. Because patients lack an immune response during this period, virus levels tend to be very high, resulting in high levels of infectivity. Symptoms of acute HIV infection resolve with or without treatment, and most acute infections are undiagnosed. Patients presenting with symptomatic acute HIV infection (the acute retroviral syndrome) are usually in the "window period," which may extend for 3 to 6 weeks, during which time seroconversion of the disease has not yet occurred and results of HIV antibody testing are negative. However, viral-specific tests, such as those for nucleic acid, are usually positive at quite high levels during this time frame and can be used to establish the diagnosis.

Measurement of CD4 cell counts is neither sensitive nor specific for HIV infection and should be performed only after the diagnosis of HIV is already established. The CD4 cell count can be normal in HIV infection, and conversely, can be depressed from many other conditions that can present similarly to acute HIV infection.

During the window period of acute HIV infection, antibody testing is unreliable. Therefore, antibody-based testing, whether by repeat enzyme immunoassay or Western blot, would not be useful.

KEY POINT

- Most persons in whom HIV infection develops experience an acute symptomatic illness within 2 to 4 weeks of infection, with symptoms ranging from a simple febrile illness to a mononucleosis-like syndrome.

Bibliography

Cohen MS, Gay CL, Busch MP, Hecht FM. The detection of acute HIV infection. J Infect Dis. 2010;202(suppl 2):S270-S277. [PMID: 20846033]

Item 100   Answer: D

Educational Objective: Prevent malaria in a pregnant patient.

This patient should receive chemoprophylaxis with mefloquine. Because malaria in a pregnant woman can be very deleterious to both the mother and the fetus, it is advisable that travel to malaria-endemic areas be delayed until after delivery of the fetus. However, when pregnant travelers cannot or will not defer travel, chemoprophylaxis with mefloquine during the second and third trimesters of pregnancy has been found to be safe and is the recommended drug for travel to areas of the world where chloroquine-resistant malaria is found. Safety data on the use of this medication during the first trimester are less available.

Owing to the predominance of chloroquine-resistant *Plasmodium falciparum* species in Africa, chemoprophylaxis with chloroquine would be inadequate, even though this drug has been deemed safe during pregnancy.

Doxycycline, although active against all malaria species, including chloroquine resistant-strains, should not be used during pregnancy. Potential adverse effects of doxycycline to the fetus include inhibition of bone growth, dysplasia, and dental discoloration.

Atovaquone-proguanil, a preferred agent for preventing malaria in chloroquine-resistant zones, is not recommended for prophylaxis in pregnant women owing to insufficient data.

KEY POINT

- Chemoprophylaxis with mefloquine during the second and third trimesters of pregnancy is safe and recommended for pregnant travelers who cannot defer travel to areas of the world where chloroquine-resistant malaria is found.

Bibliography

Schlagenhauf P, Petersen E. Malaria chemoprophylaxis: strategies for risk groups. Clin Microbiol Rev. 2008;21(3):466-472. [PMID: 18625682]

Item 101   Answer: B

Educational Objective: Treat a patient with ventilator-associated, methicillin-resistant *Staphylococcus aureus* pneumonia.

This patient requires discontinuation of vancomycin and initiation of intravenous linezolid. Linezolid is an oxazolidinone drug with bacteriostatic activity against gram-positive aerobic bacteria, including methicillin-resistant *Staphylococcus aureus* (MRSA) and vancomycin-resistant enterococci, and it has performed well in randomized controlled trials compared with vancomycin. The pharmacokinetics of linezolid in the lung are favorable, and it is an excellent alternative to vancomycin for treatment of MRSA. An important side effect of linezolid is myelosuppression, notably thrombocytopenia. Weekly complete blood counts should be obtained in patients treated with linezolid.

Daptomycin is effective in treating staphylococcal bacteremia and right-sided infective endocarditis in addition to skin and skin structure infections. It is equally effective for methicillin-susceptible *Staphylococcus aureus* (MSSA) and MRSA infections. Although daptomycin is no more effective than β-lactams for treating MSSA infections, it may be a useful alternative to vancomycin for treating MRSA infections in patients with fluctuating kidney function or in patients who require a relatively high (≥2 micrograms/mL) vancomycin minimal inhibitory concentration (MIC). Daptomycin is bound by surfactant, and it is not effective in the treatment of pneumonia.

Rifampin often has good in vitro activity against *S. aureus* but should not be used as a single agent because resistance to this agent can emerge rapidly.

Tigecycline is indicated for the treatment of community-acquired pneumonia but not for hospital-acquired (or ventilator-associated) pneumonia. An FDA warning reported increased mortality rates among patients treated with tigecycline in randomized controlled trials of patients with hospital-acquired pneumonia. Consequently, tigecycline should not be used for treatment of ventilator-associated pneumonia unless there are no alternative therapies.

KEY POINT

- Linezolid is an FDA-approved option for treating methicillin-resistant *Staphylococcus aureus* pneumonia, including ventilator-associated pneumonia, as well as vancomycin-resistant enterococci.

Bibliography
Liu C, Bayer A, Cosgrove SE, et al. Clinical practice guidelines by the Infectious Diseases Society of America for the treatment of methicillin-resistant Staphylococcus aureus infections in adults and children: executive summary. Clin Infect Dis. 2011;52(3):285-292. [PMID: 21217178]

Item 102   Answer: A

Educational Objective: Treat a patient with nonpurulent cellulitis with systemic symptoms.

This patient has nonpurulent cellulitis with associated fever and leukocytosis and should be treated with clindamycin to provide coverage for both β-hemolytic streptococci and community-associated methicillin-resistant *Staphylococcus aureus* (CA-MRSA). Although β-hemolytic streptococci are most likely causing his infection, coverage for CA-MRSA is also recommended by some experts because of the patient's associated systemic symptoms. Known risk factors for lower-extremity cellulitis include tinea pedis, onychomycosis, chronic leg ulcerations, varicose veins of the leg, phlebitis, obesity, type 2 diabetes mellitus, and heart failure. Treatment of this patient's tinea pedis is an appropriate intervention to prevent recurrent cellulitis.

Doxycycline and trimethoprim-sulfamethoxazole are active against CA-MRSA but do not provide reliable coverage for β-hemolytic streptococci. If either of these agents is used, a β-lactam agent such as amoxicillin should be added to provide coverage for β-hemolytic streptococci.

Although rifampin is active against staphylococci and streptococci, it should never be used as monotherapy because of the development of resistance. Only limited data are available to recommend the use of rifampin as an adjunctive agent for treatment of skin and soft tissue infections.

KEY POINT

- In an outpatient with nonpurulent cellulitis and associated systemic symptoms, treatment with clindamycin is recommended to provide activity against both β-hemolytic streptococci and community-associated methicillin-resistant *Staphylococcus aureus*.

Bibliography
Liu C, Bayer A, Cosgrove SE, Daum RS, et al; Infectious Diseases Society of America. Clinical practice guidelines by the Infectious Diseases Society of America for the treatment of methicillin-resistant Staphylococcus aureus infections in adults and children. Clin Infect Dis. 2011;52(3):e18-55. Epub 2011 Jan 4. [PMID: 21208910]

Item 103   Answer: C

Educational Objective: Choose the appropriate site of care for a patient with community-acquired pneumonia.

The patient needs to be started on empiric antibiotic treatment for community-acquired pneumonia (CAP) and admitted to the medical ward. Rules that predict mortality risk can be used to guide site-of-care decisions in patients with CAP. The CURB-65 score estimates mortality risk based on the following indicators: confusion, blood urea nitrogen level greater than 19.6 mg/dL (7.0 mmol/L), respiration rate 30/min or more, systolic blood pressure less than 90 mm Hg or diastolic blood pressure 60 mm Hg or less, and age 65 years or older. One point is scored for each positive indicator. Patients with a score of 0 or 1 have a low mortality risk and can be considered for outpatient treatment. Those with a score of 2 or more should be hospitalized. Patients with a score of 3 or more should be considered for admission to the intensive care unit (ICU). This patient's CURB-65 score is 3, and his predicted mortality risk is 17%; hospitalization is generally recommended for persons with scores of 2 or higher.

Discharging this patient on oral antibiotic therapy after empiric treatment with intravenous antibiotic therapy would not be appropriate because, in addition to empiric antibiotic therapy, this patient requires hospitalization.

Admission to the ICU should be considered in patients with CURB-65 scores of 3 or higher. To help further define the population of patients who would benefit from admission to the ICU, the Infectious Diseases Society of America/American Thoracic Society (IDSA/ATS) consensus guidelines for the management of community-acquired pneumonia have proposed major and minor criteria for ICU admission. Major criteria include the need for vasopressor support or mechanical ventilation. Minor criteria include confusion, hypothermia, respiration rate of 30/min or more (or the need for noninvasive positive-pressure ventilation), hypotension requiring aggressive fluid resuscitation, multilobar infiltrates, arterial PO_2/FIO_2 ratio of 250 or less, leukopenia, thrombocytopenia, and blood urea nitrogen level of greater than 20 mg/dL (7.1 mmol/L). This patient has two minor criteria; ICU admission should be considered in patients with three or more minor criteria.

Because the patient's CURB-65 score predicts a significant mortality risk, outpatient therapy would not be appropriate.

KEY POINT

- In patients with community-acquired pneumonia, the CURB-65 score assigns one point for each positive indicator (confusion, blood urea nitrogen level >19.6 mg/dL [7.0 mmol/L], respiration rate ≥30/min, systolic blood pressure <90 mm Hg or diastolic blood pressure ≤60 mm Hg, and age ≥65 years), with a score of 0 or 1 indicating consideration for outpatient management, and a score of 2 or more indicating the need for hospitalization.

Bibliography

Mandell LA, Wunderink RG, Anzueto A, et al. Infectious Diseases Society of America; American Thoracic Society. Infectious Diseases Society of America/American Thoracic Society consensus guidelines on the management of community-acquired pneumonia in adults. Clin Infect Dis. 2007;44(suppl 2):S27-72. [PMID: 17278083]

Item 104   Answer: B

Educational Objective: Treat a patient with tuberculous meningitis.

This patient has tuberculous meningitis and requires treatment for 9 to 12 months. He has several characteristic features of this infection, including headache, fever, and lethargy. Results of lumbar puncture show an increased opening pressure and a cerebrospinal fluid (CSF) lymphocytic pleocytosis, an elevated CSF protein level, and a decreased CSF glucose level. A CT scan shows basilar meningeal involvement (hydrocephalus may be seen also).

In general, the recommendations for treatment of extrapulmonary tuberculosis are the same as those for treatment of pulmonary disease. For most patients with extrapulmonary tuberculosis caused by strains that are fully susceptible to all drugs, the recommended treatment duration is 6 to 9 months. This includes a 2-month initial phase of isoniazid, rifampin, pyrazinamide, and ethambutol followed by a continuation phase of isoniazid and rifampin for 4 or 7 months. The 7-month continuation phase is recommended when pyrazinamide cannot be administered during the initial phase. However, treatment of tuberculous meningitis is an exception to these recommendations. The American Thoracic Society, Centers for Disease Control and Prevention, and the Infectious Diseases Society of America consensus guidelines recommend that patients with tuberculous meningitis be treated for 9 to 12 months rather than the standard 6 to 9 months. Adjunctive corticosteroids are also recommended. Serial lumbar punctures should be considered to assess the response of the CSF cell count and protein and glucose levels to therapy.

Four months of therapy is inappropriate because at least 6 months of treatment is recommended for patients with any form of extrapulmonary tuberculosis.

Therapeutic durations longer than 9 to 12 months are recommended for patients with various patterns of multidrug-resistant tuberculosis.

KEY POINT

- The recommended duration of antituberculous treatment in patients with tuberculous meningitis is 9 to 12 months.

Bibliography

American Thoracic Society; CDC; Infectious Diseases Society of America. Treatment of tuberculosis. MMWR Recomm Rep. 2003;52(RR-11):1-77. [PMID: 12836625]

Item 105   Answer: A

Educational Objective: Diagnose invasive aspergillosis after transplantation.

This patient has aspergillosis. *Aspergillus* species is the most common cause of invasive fungal infection after transplantation, especially following lung transplantation and during

CONT.

the neutropenic phase after hematopoietic stem cell transplantation (HSCT). Invasive aspergillosis involves the lungs more often than the sinuses, and patients typically have fever, and possibly, dry cough or hemoptysis, and chest pain. Dissemination to the brain may be characterized by headache, focal deficits, or mental status changes. This patient's risk factors for invasive fungal disease include profound neutropenia of prolonged duration, persistent fever while receiving broad-spectrum antibacterial coverage, and pulmonary nodules. The treatment of choice is voriconazole. This patient has been taking fluconazole prophylaxis, which provides coverage for most *Candida* species but not for *Aspergillus* species.

Cytomegalovirus (CMV) pneumonia is less likely to occur in the first few weeks after HSCT (pre-engraftment phase) than in the period after the first few weeks through the first few months following transplantation (postengraftment phase). CMV infection would also be unlikely to cause pulmonary nodules on imaging.

Mucormycosis (zygomycosis) is a rapidly progressive fungal infection that most commonly occurs in patients with hematologic malignancies or other disorders associated with prolonged neutropenia or immunosuppression, severe burns or trauma, or diabetic ketoacidosis. Corticosteroids, cytotoxic agents, or deferoxamine also confers an increased risk. Rhinocerebral or pulmonary involvement occurs most commonly. Invasive aspergillosis is much more commonly associated with early fungal infections following stem cell transplantation than is mucormycosis.

Pneumocystis jirovecii infection is less likely to occur in the acute setting immediately following transplantation. The chest radiograph typically shows bilateral interstitial infiltrates, but rarely, findings can vary from a normal radiograph to consolidation, cysts, nodules, pleural effusions, or a pneumothorax.

KEY POINT

- Invasive aspergillosis is a common fungal infection following transplantation (especially of the lung and during the neutropenic phase after hematopoietic stem cell transplantation) and may be characterized by fever, dry cough, or hemoptysis.

Bibliography
Asano-Mori Y. Fungal infections after hematopoietic stem cell transplantation. Int J Hematol. 2010;91(4):576-587. [PMID: 20432074]

Item 106   Answer: C

Educational Objective: Manage postcoital urinary tract infection.

The most appropriate next step in preventing recurrent urinary tract infections (UTIs) in this patient is postcoital ciprofloxacin. Recurrent UTIs in young, sexually active women are more commonly a reinfection rather than

relapse and are often associated with sexual intercourse. Consequently, a detailed sexual history should be obtained from female patients with a presentation such as that in this patient. Symptoms of UTI are often related to the use of spermicidal agents because spermicides decrease the number of healthy vaginal lactobacilli and predispose women to UTIs. However, this patient does not use spermicidal agents. The recommended prophylaxis against recurrent UTI is liberal fluid intake and postcoital voiding. Although these recommendations are not evidenced-based, they are unlikely to be harmful. If UTIs continue to occur despite these measures as they have in this patient, prophylaxis with a postcoital antibiotic such as ciprofloxacin is appropriate.

Chronic suppressive antibiotic therapy can be an effective method for preventing postcoital UTI, but patients may have difficulty adhering to this regimen, and it is associated with increased costs, resistance, and candidal superinfections.

Randomized clinical trials have not demonstrated that drinking cranberry juice reduces the incidence of recurrent UTI, including postcoital UTI.

Removal of this patient's intrauterine device (IUD) is not warranted because IUDs are not associated with UTIs.

Adding a spermicide is likely to increase, not decrease, this patient's incidence of UTI.

KEY POINT

- Antibiotic prophylaxis following intercourse is appropriate for preventing recurrent postcoital urinary tract infections in women.

Bibliography
Dielubanza EJ, Schaeffer AJ. Urinary tract infections in women. Med Clin North Am. 2011;95(1):27-41. [PMID: 21095409]

Item 107   Answer: D

Educational Objective: Treat early-latent syphilis.

The Centers for Disease Control and Prevention (CDC) recommends a single dose of intramuscular benzathine penicillin G for the treatment of primary, secondary, and early-latent syphilis. This regimen is appropriate for individuals with coexisting HIV infection as well.

This asymptomatic patient who has serologic evidence of syphilis now but had negative serologic results for syphilis 6 months ago has early-latent syphilis. Recent epidemiologic data have shown that the rates of syphilis and other sexually transmitted infections (STIs) are increasing among men who have sex with men, especially among younger men, those in urban areas (particularly members of racial and ethnic minorities), and men who use drugs during sex. Periodic screening for STIs in persons at risk is an important part of HIV primary care. This patient should receive counseling regarding STI risk reduction and should be encouraged to refer his sexual partners for evaluation. Persons exposed to sexual partners diagnosed with primary, secondary, or early-latent syphilis within the preceding 90 days should be treated, regardless of serologic results. Individuals exposed to sexual partners with syphilis more than 90 days before a diagnosis was established should receive treatment if there is any concern regarding whether they will undergo follow-up serologic testing.

The recommended treatment for late-latent syphilis, which is defined as syphilis of more than 1 year in duration or syphilis of unknown duration, consists of three doses of intramuscular benzathine penicillin G.

Aqueous crystalline intravenous penicillin G is the treatment of choice for patients with neurosyphilis, but this patient does not have evidence of central nervous system involvement. The need for cerebrospinal fluid (CSF) examination in all patients with HIV infection and syphilis is controversial. CSF abnormalities suggestive of neurosyphilis are more likely in individuals with rapid plasma reagin titers of 1:32 or higher and those with CD4 cell counts of 350 cells/microliter or less; however, the CDC guidelines do not recommend routine CSF examination in patients with HIV infection who do not have neurologic symptoms.

Doxycycline is an alternative treatment in patients who are allergic to penicillin. This patient does not have a penicillin allergy.

KEY POINT

- The Centers for Disease Control and Prevention recommends a single dose of intramuscular benzathine penicillin G for the treatment of primary, secondary, and early-latent syphilis.

Bibliography

Workowski KA, Berman S; Centers for Disease Control and Prevention (CDC). Sexually transmitted diseases treatment guidelines, 2010. MMWR Recomm Rep. 2010;59(RR-12):1-110. [PMID: 21160459]

Item 108   Answer: D

Educational Objective: Treat invasive pulmonary aspergillosis in a patient with leukemia.

This patient should be treated with voriconazole. She has probable invasive pulmonary aspergillosis, for which acute leukemia with profound and prolonged neutropenia is a risk factor. She has classic symptoms and signs of an angioinvasive fungal infection, including fever, cough, chest pain, hemoptysis, and pulmonary nodules on chest radiograph. In addition, her CT scan demonstrates evidence of the "halo sign," which is an area of low attenuation surrounding a nodule, reflecting hemorrhage into the tissue surrounding the fungus. The halo sign is not diagnostic of aspergillosis and may occur in infection caused by other angioinvasive fungi. Evidence from a large randomized controlled trial supports voriconazole as the treatment of choice in patients with invasive aspergillosis. Standard procedures for establishing a definitive diagnosis of pulmonary aspergillosis are bronchoalveolar lavage with or without biopsy, transthoracic percutaneous needle aspiration, or video-assisted thoracoscopic biopsy. The galactomannan antigen immunoassay is an important non–culture-based method of diagnosing invasive aspergillosis. It has good sensitivity in detecting invasive aspergillosis in patients with hematologic malignancy. When combined with early use of CT, the serum galactomannan antigen immunoassay permits early treatment with antifungal therapy.

Liposomal amphotericin B may be considered an alternative primary therapy for some patients. Amphotericin B formulations, itraconazole, posaconazole, and echinocandin agents such as caspofungin and micafungin are appropriate as salvage therapy in patients who are refractory to, or intolerant of, voriconazole.

KEY POINT

- Voriconazole is the drug of choice for immunocompromised patients with invasive pulmonary aspergillosis.

Bibliography

Walsh TJ, Anaissie EJ, Denning DW, et al; Infectious Diseases Society of America. Treatment of aspergillosis: clinical guidelines of the Infectious Diseases Society of America. Clin Infect Dis. 2008;46(3):327-360. [PMID: 18177225]

Index

Cephalosporins
  for bacterial meningitis, Q59
  for typhoid fever, 63
Cerebritis, in brain abscess, 7
Cerebrospinal fluid analysis
  in bacterial meningitis, 1t, 3
  in Creutzfeldt-Jakob disease, 11
  in cryptococcosis, 41
  in herpes simplex encephalitis, 9, 10
  in herpes simplex virus infections, 95
  in syphilis, 47
  in tuberculosis, 34
  in viral meningitis, 1, 1t
  in West Nile virus, 10
Cervicitis, 43
  complications of, 44
  in genital herpes simplex infections, 46
  gonococcal, 45t
  treatment of, 45–46, 45t, Q11
Chancres, syphilitic, 47, 48, Q28
Chancroid, 48, 48t
Charcot changes, in diabetic foot infections, 18
Chest pain, in anthrax, 57, 58
Chickenpox. *See* Varicella
Children
  cat-scratch disease in, 17
  hematogenous osteomyelitis in, 49
  influenza in, 94
  primary immunodeficiencies in, 55
  tuberculin skin testing in, 33
  viral gastroenteritis in, 71
Chlamydia infections, fever of unknown origin in, 53
Chlamydia trachomatis infections, 43, 44
  treatment of, 45–45, 45t
Chlamydophila pneumoniae infections, 19
Chlorhexidine, 81
Chloroquine, as malaria prophylaxis, 62, 62t
  Plasmodium resistance to, 61t, Q100
Cholecystitis, acalculous, 72
Chronic kidney disease, in HIV/AIDS, 90
Cidofovir
  for acyclovir-resistant herpesvirus infections, Q91
  for smallpox, 58
Ciprofloxacin
  for pyelonephritis, 31, Q71
  for shigellosis, Q9
  for travelers' diarrhea, 63t
Cisplatin, as contraindication to hyperbaric oxygen therapy, 102
Clarithromycin
  as infective endocarditis prophylaxis, 85t
  for *Mycobacterium avium* complex treatment, 38
Clenched-fist injuries, antibiotic treatment for, Q13
Clindamycin
  for babesiosis, 27
  for clenched fist injuries, Q13
  for nonpurulent cellulitis, Q102
  for purulent cellulitis, Q62
  for toxic shock syndrome, 16
Clindamycin resistance, in methicillin-resistant *Staphylococcus aureus* pneumonia, 13–14
Clostridium botulinum, as botulism causal agent, 56t, 59
Clostridium difficile infections
  diarrhea in, 69–71, 70t
  in transplant recipients, 74, 75
  treatment of, 70–71, 70t, Q4
Clostridium infections, necrotizing fasciitis in, 14
Clostridium perfringens infections, necrotizing fasciitis in, 14
Coccidioides. See Coccidioidomycosis
Coccidioidomycosis, 42, 65, 65t
  acute, Q35
  in transplant recipients, 75–76
Colistin base activity (CBA), 100
Colistin, 100, 100t, Q45
Colitis, hemorrhagic, 68, Q8
Colony-forming units (CFUs), of bacteria in urine, 29, Q32
Coma, in encephalitis, 8
Common variable immunodeficiency (CVID), 55, Q1
Complement deficiencies, 55–56
Computed tomography, of osteomyelitis, 50, Q39
Condylomata acuminata, 48–49
C1 inhibitor deficiency, 55
Constipation, in typhoid fever, Q75

Contact precautions, for
Corticosteroids
  for allergic bronchopulmonary aspergillosis, 40
  in combination with herpes zoster antiviral therapy, 97
  topical, contraindication in herpes simplex virus infections, 96
  for tuberculous pericarditis, Q37
  use in transplant recipients, 72, 73t
Cough
  in anthrax, 57, 58
  in aspergillomas, 40
  in aspergillosis, 75, Q105
  in community-acquired pneumonia, 19, 20
  in histoplasmosis, Q6
  in influenza, 94
  in *Mycobacterium avium* complex infections
  in *Pneumocystis jirovecii* infections, Q64
  in pneumonic plague, 59
  in typhoid fever, 63
Coxiella burnetii, as bioterrorism agent, 53, 56
Cranial nerve palsy, in Lyme disease, 25, 25t
Craniotomy, for subdural empyema, 8
C-reactive protein
  in necrotizing fasciitis, 14
  in osteomyelitis, 50
  in vertebral osteomyelitis, 52
Creutzfeldt-Jakob disease, 11–12, 11t
  sporadic, 11t, Q49
  variant, 11t, 12
Cryptococcosis, 41
  disseminated, in HIV/AIDS, 91, 92
Cryptosporidiosis, 72
CURB-65 score, for community-acquired pneumonia, 20–21, Q103
Cycloserine, for tuberculosis, 35t
Cyclosporine, drug interactions of, 73, Q18
Cystitis
  diagnosis of, 30
  in women, 30, Q36
Cytomegalovirus infections
  fever of unknown origin in, 53
  in HIV/AIDS, 91, 92
  in transplant donors, screening for, 73
  in transplant recipients, 73, 74, 75, Q58
    prevention of, 76
  in travelers, 61t
Cytotoxins A and B, in *Clostridium difficile* infections, 71

Daptomycin, 97–98, 98t, Q10
Darunavir, 93, 93t
Dementia, in Creutzfeldt-Jakob disease, 11, Q49
Dengue fever/virus, 60, 61t, 64, Q55
Dental procedures, infective endocarditis prophylaxis before, 85, 85t, Q78
Dental sepsis, brain abscess in, 7t
Dexamethasone, for bacterial meningitis, 3–4, Q59
Diabetes mellitus
  foot infections in, 17–18, 51
  osteomyelitis in, 51, Q53
  urinary tract infections in, 29
Diarrhea, 66
  bloody, 64
  in HIV/AIDS, 87t
  infectious (bacterial or viral), 65–72
    in *Campylobacter* infections, 66, 66t, 67
    clinical features of, 66, 66t
    in *Clostridium difficile* infections, 69–71
    epidemiology of, 66t
    in *Escherichia coli* infections, 66, 66t
    in giardiasis, 66t, 71, Q98
    in malaria, 61, 62
    in salmonellosis, 66, 66t
    in shigellosis, 66, 66t, 67, Q9
    transmission of, 66
    in *Vibrio* infections, 66t
    in viral gastroenteritis, 71
    in yersiniosis, 66t
  noninfectious causes of, 65
  in parasitic infections, 66, 71–72
  travelers', 61t, 63–64, 63t, Q82, Q97
Dicloxacillin, for cellulitis, Q77
Diphenoxylate, for traveler's diarrhea, 64
Disseminated gonococcal infection, 43–44, 45t, Q29
Disseminated intravascular coagulation, in septicemic plague, 58–59

A — NAME AND ADDRESS (Please complete.)

Last Name _____ First Name _____ Middle Initial _____

Address _____

Address cont. _____

City _____ State _____ ZIP Code _____

Country _____

Email address _____

ACP
AMERICAN COLLEGE OF PHYSICIANS
INTERNAL MEDICINE | *Doctors for Adults*

Medical Knowledge Self-Assessment Program® 16

TO EARN *AMA PRA CATEGORY 1 CREDITS*™ YOU MUST:

1. Answer all questions.
2. Score a minimum of 50% correct.

- -

TO EARN *FREE* SAME-DAY *AMA PRA CATEGORY 1 CREDITS*™ ONLINE:

1. Answer all of your questions.
2. Go to **mksap.acponline.org** and access the appropriate answer sheet.
3. Transcribe your answers and submit for CME credits.
4. You can also enter your answers directly at **mksap.acponline.org** without first using this answer sheet.

To Submit Your Answer Sheet by Mail or FAX for a $10 Administrative Fee per Answer Sheet:

1. Answer all of your questions and calculate your score.
2. Complete boxes A–F.
3. Complete payment information.
4. Send the answer sheet and payment information to ACP, using the FAX number/address listed below.

B — Order Number

(Use the Order Number on your MKSAP materials packing slip.)

C — ACP ID Number

(Refer to packing slip in your MKSAP materials for your ACP ID Number.)

COMPLETE FORM BELOW ONLY IF YOU SUBMIT BY MAIL OR FAX

Last Name | First Name | MI

Payment Information. Must remit in US funds, drawn on a US bank.

The processing fee for each paper answer sheet is $10.

☐ Check, made payable to ACP, enclosed

Charge to ☐ **VISA** ☐ **MasterCard** ☐ **AMERICAN EXPRESS** ☐ **DISCOVER**

Card Number _____

Expiration Date _____ / _____   Security code (3 or 4 digit #s) _____
                   MM   YY

Signature _____

Fax to: 215-351-2799

Questions?
Go to **mksap.acponline.org** or email **custserv@acponline.org**

Mail to:
Member and Customer Service
American College of Physicians
190 N. Independence Mall West
Philadelphia, PA 19106-1572

1 Ⓐ Ⓑ Ⓒ Ⓓ Ⓔ
2 Ⓐ Ⓑ Ⓒ Ⓓ Ⓔ
3 Ⓐ Ⓑ Ⓒ Ⓓ Ⓔ
4 Ⓐ Ⓑ Ⓒ Ⓓ Ⓔ
5 Ⓐ Ⓑ Ⓒ Ⓓ Ⓔ

6 Ⓐ Ⓑ Ⓒ Ⓓ Ⓔ
7 Ⓐ Ⓑ Ⓒ Ⓓ Ⓔ
8 Ⓐ Ⓑ Ⓒ Ⓓ Ⓔ
9 Ⓐ Ⓑ Ⓒ Ⓓ Ⓔ
10 Ⓐ Ⓑ Ⓒ Ⓓ Ⓔ

11 Ⓐ Ⓑ Ⓒ Ⓓ Ⓔ
12 Ⓐ Ⓑ Ⓒ Ⓓ Ⓔ
13 Ⓐ Ⓑ Ⓒ Ⓓ Ⓔ
14 Ⓐ Ⓑ Ⓒ Ⓓ Ⓔ
15 Ⓐ Ⓑ Ⓒ Ⓓ Ⓔ

16 Ⓐ Ⓑ Ⓒ Ⓓ Ⓔ
17 Ⓐ Ⓑ Ⓒ Ⓓ Ⓔ
18 Ⓐ Ⓑ Ⓒ Ⓓ Ⓔ
19 Ⓐ Ⓑ Ⓒ Ⓓ Ⓔ
20 Ⓐ Ⓑ Ⓒ Ⓓ Ⓔ

21 Ⓐ Ⓑ Ⓒ Ⓓ Ⓔ
22 Ⓐ Ⓑ Ⓒ Ⓓ Ⓔ
23 Ⓐ Ⓑ Ⓒ Ⓓ Ⓔ
24 Ⓐ Ⓑ Ⓒ Ⓓ Ⓔ
25 Ⓐ Ⓑ Ⓒ Ⓓ Ⓔ

26 Ⓐ Ⓑ Ⓒ Ⓓ Ⓔ
27 Ⓐ Ⓑ Ⓒ Ⓓ Ⓔ
28 Ⓐ Ⓑ Ⓒ Ⓓ Ⓔ
29 Ⓐ Ⓑ Ⓒ Ⓓ Ⓔ
30 Ⓐ Ⓑ Ⓒ Ⓓ Ⓔ

31 Ⓐ Ⓑ Ⓒ Ⓓ Ⓔ
32 Ⓐ Ⓑ Ⓒ Ⓓ Ⓔ
33 Ⓐ Ⓑ Ⓒ Ⓓ Ⓔ
34 Ⓐ Ⓑ Ⓒ Ⓓ Ⓔ
35 Ⓐ Ⓑ Ⓒ Ⓓ Ⓔ

36 Ⓐ Ⓑ Ⓒ Ⓓ Ⓔ
37 Ⓐ Ⓑ Ⓒ Ⓓ Ⓔ
38 Ⓐ Ⓑ Ⓒ Ⓓ Ⓔ
39 Ⓐ Ⓑ Ⓒ Ⓓ Ⓔ
40 Ⓐ Ⓑ Ⓒ Ⓓ Ⓔ

41 Ⓐ Ⓑ Ⓒ Ⓓ Ⓔ
42 Ⓐ Ⓑ Ⓒ Ⓓ Ⓔ
43 Ⓐ Ⓑ Ⓒ Ⓓ Ⓔ
44 Ⓐ Ⓑ Ⓒ Ⓓ Ⓔ
45 Ⓐ Ⓑ Ⓒ Ⓓ Ⓔ

46 Ⓐ Ⓑ Ⓒ Ⓓ Ⓔ
47 Ⓐ Ⓑ Ⓒ Ⓓ Ⓔ
48 Ⓐ Ⓑ Ⓒ Ⓓ Ⓔ
49 Ⓐ Ⓑ Ⓒ Ⓓ Ⓔ
50 Ⓐ Ⓑ Ⓒ Ⓓ Ⓔ

51 Ⓐ Ⓑ Ⓒ Ⓓ Ⓔ
52 Ⓐ Ⓑ Ⓒ Ⓓ Ⓔ
53 Ⓐ Ⓑ Ⓒ Ⓓ Ⓔ
54 Ⓐ Ⓑ Ⓒ Ⓓ Ⓔ
55 Ⓐ Ⓑ Ⓒ Ⓓ Ⓔ

56 Ⓐ Ⓑ Ⓒ Ⓓ Ⓔ
57 Ⓐ Ⓑ Ⓒ Ⓓ Ⓔ
58 Ⓐ Ⓑ Ⓒ Ⓓ Ⓔ
59 Ⓐ Ⓑ Ⓒ Ⓓ Ⓔ
60 Ⓐ Ⓑ Ⓒ Ⓓ Ⓔ

61 Ⓐ Ⓑ Ⓒ Ⓓ Ⓔ
62 Ⓐ Ⓑ Ⓒ Ⓓ Ⓔ
63 Ⓐ Ⓑ Ⓒ Ⓓ Ⓔ
64 Ⓐ Ⓑ Ⓒ Ⓓ Ⓔ
65 Ⓐ Ⓑ Ⓒ Ⓓ Ⓔ

66 Ⓐ Ⓑ Ⓒ Ⓓ Ⓔ
67 Ⓐ Ⓑ Ⓒ Ⓓ Ⓔ
68 Ⓐ Ⓑ Ⓒ Ⓓ Ⓔ
69 Ⓐ Ⓑ Ⓒ Ⓓ Ⓔ
70 Ⓐ Ⓑ Ⓒ Ⓓ Ⓔ

71 Ⓐ Ⓑ Ⓒ Ⓓ Ⓔ
72 Ⓐ Ⓑ Ⓒ Ⓓ Ⓔ
73 Ⓐ Ⓑ Ⓒ Ⓓ Ⓔ
74 Ⓐ Ⓑ Ⓒ Ⓓ Ⓔ
75 Ⓐ Ⓑ Ⓒ Ⓓ Ⓔ

76 Ⓐ Ⓑ Ⓒ Ⓓ Ⓔ
77 Ⓐ Ⓑ Ⓒ Ⓓ Ⓔ
78 Ⓐ Ⓑ Ⓒ Ⓓ Ⓔ
79 Ⓐ Ⓑ Ⓒ Ⓓ Ⓔ
80 Ⓐ Ⓑ Ⓒ Ⓓ Ⓔ

81 Ⓐ Ⓑ Ⓒ Ⓓ Ⓔ
82 Ⓐ Ⓑ Ⓒ Ⓓ Ⓔ
83 Ⓐ Ⓑ Ⓒ Ⓓ Ⓔ
84 Ⓐ Ⓑ Ⓒ Ⓓ Ⓔ
85 Ⓐ Ⓑ Ⓒ Ⓓ Ⓔ

86 Ⓐ Ⓑ Ⓒ Ⓓ Ⓔ
87 Ⓐ Ⓑ Ⓒ Ⓓ Ⓔ
88 Ⓐ Ⓑ Ⓒ Ⓓ Ⓔ
89 Ⓐ Ⓑ Ⓒ Ⓓ Ⓔ
90 Ⓐ Ⓑ Ⓒ Ⓓ Ⓔ

91 Ⓐ Ⓑ Ⓒ Ⓓ Ⓔ
92 Ⓐ Ⓑ Ⓒ Ⓓ Ⓔ
93 Ⓐ Ⓑ Ⓒ Ⓓ Ⓔ
94 Ⓐ Ⓑ Ⓒ Ⓓ Ⓔ
95 Ⓐ Ⓑ Ⓒ Ⓓ Ⓔ

96 Ⓐ Ⓑ Ⓒ Ⓓ Ⓔ
97 Ⓐ Ⓑ Ⓒ Ⓓ Ⓔ
98 Ⓐ Ⓑ Ⓒ Ⓓ Ⓔ
99 Ⓐ Ⓑ Ⓒ Ⓓ Ⓔ
100 Ⓐ Ⓑ Ⓒ Ⓓ Ⓔ

101 Ⓐ Ⓑ Ⓒ Ⓓ Ⓔ
102 Ⓐ Ⓑ Ⓒ Ⓓ Ⓔ
103 Ⓐ Ⓑ Ⓒ Ⓓ Ⓔ
104 Ⓐ Ⓑ Ⓒ Ⓓ Ⓔ
105 Ⓐ Ⓑ Ⓒ Ⓓ Ⓔ

106 Ⓐ Ⓑ Ⓒ Ⓓ Ⓔ
107 Ⓐ Ⓑ Ⓒ Ⓓ Ⓔ
108 Ⓐ Ⓑ Ⓒ Ⓓ Ⓔ
109 Ⓐ Ⓑ Ⓒ Ⓓ Ⓔ
110 Ⓐ Ⓑ Ⓒ Ⓓ Ⓔ

111 Ⓐ Ⓑ Ⓒ Ⓓ Ⓔ
112 Ⓐ Ⓑ Ⓒ Ⓓ Ⓔ
113 Ⓐ Ⓑ Ⓒ Ⓓ Ⓔ
114 Ⓐ Ⓑ Ⓒ Ⓓ Ⓔ
115 Ⓐ Ⓑ Ⓒ Ⓓ Ⓔ

116 Ⓐ Ⓑ Ⓒ Ⓓ Ⓔ
117 Ⓐ Ⓑ Ⓒ Ⓓ Ⓔ
118 Ⓐ Ⓑ Ⓒ Ⓓ Ⓔ
119 Ⓐ Ⓑ Ⓒ Ⓓ Ⓔ
120 Ⓐ Ⓑ Ⓒ Ⓓ Ⓔ

121 Ⓐ Ⓑ Ⓒ Ⓓ Ⓔ
122 Ⓐ Ⓑ Ⓒ Ⓓ Ⓔ
123 Ⓐ Ⓑ Ⓒ Ⓓ Ⓔ
124 Ⓐ Ⓑ Ⓒ Ⓓ Ⓔ
125 Ⓐ Ⓑ Ⓒ Ⓓ Ⓔ

126 Ⓐ Ⓑ Ⓒ Ⓓ Ⓔ
127 Ⓐ Ⓑ Ⓒ Ⓓ Ⓔ
128 Ⓐ Ⓑ Ⓒ Ⓓ Ⓔ
129 Ⓐ Ⓑ Ⓒ Ⓓ Ⓔ
130 Ⓐ Ⓑ Ⓒ Ⓓ Ⓔ

131 Ⓐ Ⓑ Ⓒ Ⓓ Ⓔ
132 Ⓐ Ⓑ Ⓒ Ⓓ Ⓔ
133 Ⓐ Ⓑ Ⓒ Ⓓ Ⓔ
134 Ⓐ Ⓑ Ⓒ Ⓓ Ⓔ
135 Ⓐ Ⓑ Ⓒ Ⓓ Ⓔ

136 Ⓐ Ⓑ Ⓒ Ⓓ Ⓔ
137 Ⓐ Ⓑ Ⓒ Ⓓ Ⓔ
138 Ⓐ Ⓑ Ⓒ Ⓓ Ⓔ
139 Ⓐ Ⓑ Ⓒ Ⓓ Ⓔ
140 Ⓐ Ⓑ Ⓒ Ⓓ Ⓔ

141 Ⓐ Ⓑ Ⓒ Ⓓ Ⓔ
142 Ⓐ Ⓑ Ⓒ Ⓓ Ⓔ
143 Ⓐ Ⓑ Ⓒ Ⓓ Ⓔ
144 Ⓐ Ⓑ Ⓒ Ⓓ Ⓔ
145 Ⓐ Ⓑ Ⓒ Ⓓ Ⓔ

146 Ⓐ Ⓑ Ⓒ Ⓓ Ⓔ
147 Ⓐ Ⓑ Ⓒ Ⓓ Ⓔ
148 Ⓐ Ⓑ Ⓒ Ⓓ Ⓔ
149 Ⓐ Ⓑ Ⓒ Ⓓ Ⓔ
150 Ⓐ Ⓑ Ⓒ Ⓓ Ⓔ

151 Ⓐ Ⓑ Ⓒ Ⓓ Ⓔ
152 Ⓐ Ⓑ Ⓒ Ⓓ Ⓔ
153 Ⓐ Ⓑ Ⓒ Ⓓ Ⓔ
154 Ⓐ Ⓑ Ⓒ Ⓓ Ⓔ
155 Ⓐ Ⓑ Ⓒ Ⓓ Ⓔ

156 Ⓐ Ⓑ Ⓒ Ⓓ Ⓔ
157 Ⓐ Ⓑ Ⓒ Ⓓ Ⓔ
158 Ⓐ Ⓑ Ⓒ Ⓓ Ⓔ
159 Ⓐ Ⓑ Ⓒ Ⓓ Ⓔ
160 Ⓐ Ⓑ Ⓒ Ⓓ Ⓔ

161 Ⓐ Ⓑ Ⓒ Ⓓ Ⓔ
162 Ⓐ Ⓑ Ⓒ Ⓓ Ⓔ
163 Ⓐ Ⓑ Ⓒ Ⓓ Ⓔ
164 Ⓐ Ⓑ Ⓒ Ⓓ Ⓔ
165 Ⓐ Ⓑ Ⓒ Ⓓ Ⓔ

166 Ⓐ Ⓑ Ⓒ Ⓓ Ⓔ
167 Ⓐ Ⓑ Ⓒ Ⓓ Ⓔ
168 Ⓐ Ⓑ Ⓒ Ⓓ Ⓔ
169 Ⓐ Ⓑ Ⓒ Ⓓ Ⓔ
170 Ⓐ Ⓑ Ⓒ Ⓓ Ⓔ

171 Ⓐ Ⓑ Ⓒ Ⓓ Ⓔ
172 Ⓐ Ⓑ Ⓒ Ⓓ Ⓔ
173 Ⓐ Ⓑ Ⓒ Ⓓ Ⓔ
174 Ⓐ Ⓑ Ⓒ Ⓓ Ⓔ
175 Ⓐ Ⓑ Ⓒ Ⓓ Ⓔ

176 Ⓐ Ⓑ Ⓒ Ⓓ Ⓔ
177 Ⓐ Ⓑ Ⓒ Ⓓ Ⓔ
178 Ⓐ Ⓑ Ⓒ Ⓓ Ⓔ
179 Ⓐ Ⓑ Ⓒ Ⓓ Ⓔ
180 Ⓐ Ⓑ Ⓒ Ⓓ Ⓔ

MKSAP® 16

Medical Knowledge Self-Assessment Program®

Cumulative Index

Cumulative Index

Editor-in-Chief

Patrick C. Alguire, MD, FACP[1]
Senior Vice President, Medical Education
American College of Physicians
Philadelphia, Pennsylvania

Deputy Editor-in-Chief

Philip A. Masters, MD, FACP[1]
Senior Medical Associate for Content Development
American College of Physicians
Philadelphia, Pennsylvania

Senior Medical Associate for Content Development

Cynthia D. Smith, MD, FACP[2]
American College of Physicians
Philadelphia, Pennsylvania

Associate Editors

Virginia U. Collier, MD, MACP[2]
Hugh R. Sharp, Jr. Chair of Medicine
Christiana Care Health System
Newark, Delaware
Professor of Medicine
Jefferson Medical College of Thomas Jefferson University
Philadelphia, Pennsylvania

Richard S. Eisenstaedt, MD, FACP[1]
Professor of Medicine
Temple University School of Medicine
Chair, Department of Medicine
Abington Memorial Hospital
Abington, Pennsylvania

Jack Ende, MD, MACP[1]
Professor of Medicine
University of Pennsylvania
Chief, Department of Medicine
Penn Presbyterian Medical Center
Philadelphia, Pennsylvania

Thomas Fekete, MD, FACP[1]
Professor of Medicine
Section of Infectious Diseases

Temple University Medical School
Philadelphia, Pennsylvania

Howard H. Weitz, MD, FACP[1]
Professor of Medicine
Director, Jefferson Heart Institute
Director, Division of Cardiology
Jefferson Medical College of Thomas Jefferson University
Philadelphia, Pennsylvania

ACP Principal Staff

Patrick C. Alguire, MD, FACP[1]
Senior Vice President, Medical Education

D. Theresa Kanya, MBA[1]
Vice President, Medical Education

Sean McKinney[1]
Director, Self-Assessment Programs

Margaret Wells[1]
Managing Editor

Valerie Dangovetsky[1]
Program Administrator

Becky Krumm[1]
Senior Staff Editor

Ellen McDonald, PhD[1]
Senior Staff Editor

Katie Idell[1]
Senior Staff Editor

Randy Hendrickson[1]
Production Administrator/Editor

Megan Zborowski[1]
Staff Editor

Linnea Donnarumma[1]
Assistant Editor

John Haefele[1]
Assistant Editor

Developed by the American College of Physicians

Conflicts of Interest

The following committee members, reviewers, and ACP staff members have disclosed relationships with commercial companies:

Virginia U. Collier, MD, MACP
Stock Options/Holdings
Celgene, Pfizer, Merck, Schering-Plough, Abbott, Johnson and Johnson, Medtronic, McKesson, Amgen

Cynthia D. Smith, MD, FACP
Stock Options/Holdings
Merck and Company

Acknowledgments

The American College of Physicians (ACP) gratefully acknowledges the special contributions to the development and production of the 16th edition of the Medical Knowledge Self-Assessment Program® (MKSAP® 16) made by the following people:

Graphic Services: Michael Ripca (Technical Administrator/Graphic Designer) and Willie-Fetchko Graphic Design (Graphic Designer).

Production/Systems: Dan Hoffmann (Director, Web Services & Systems Development), Neil Kohl (Senior Architect), and Scott Hurd (Senior Systems Analyst/Developer).

MKSAP 16 Digital: Under the direction of Steven Spadt, Vice President, ACP Digital Products & Services, the digital version of MKSAP 16 was developed within the ACP's Digital Product Development Department, led by Brian Sweigard (Director). Other members of the team included Sean O'Donnell (Senior Architect), Dan Barron (Senior Systems Analyst/Developer), Chris Forrest (Senior Software Developer/Design Lead), Jon Laing (Senior Web Application Developer), Brad Lord (Senior Web Developer), John McKnight (Senior Web Developer), and Nate Pershall (Senior Web Developer).

The College also wishes to acknowledge that many other persons, too numerous to mention, have contributed to the production of this program. Without their dedicated efforts, this program would not have been possible.

Introducing the MKSAP Resource Site (mksap.acponline.org)

The MKSAP Resource Site (mksap.acponline.org) is a continually updated site that provides links to MKSAP 16 online answer sheets for print subscribers; access to MKSAP 16 Digital, Board Basics® 3, and MKSAP 16 Updates; the latest details on Continuing Medical Education (CME) and Maintenance of Certification (MOC) in the United States, Canada, and Australia; errata; and other new information.

ABIM Maintenance of Certification

Check the MKSAP Resource Site (mksap.acponline.org) for the latest information on how MKSAP tests can be used to apply to the American Board of Internal Medicine for MOC points.

RCPSC Maintenance of Certification

In Canada, MKSAP 16 is an Accredited Self-Assessment Program (Section 3) as defined by the Maintenance of Certification Program of The Royal College of Physicians and Surgeons of Canada (RCPSC) and approved by the Canadian Society of Internal Medicine on December 9, 2011. Approval of Part A sections of MKSAP 16 extends from July 31, 2012, until July 31, 2015. Approval of Part B sections of MKSAP 16 extends from December 31, 2012, to December 31, 2015. Fellows of the Royal College may earn three credits per hour for participating in MKSAP 16 under Section 3. MKSAP 16 will enable Fellows to earn up to 75% of their required 400 credits during the 5-year MOC cycle. A Fellow can achieve this 75% level by earning 100 of the maximum of 174 *AMA PRA Category 1 Credits*™ available in MKSAP 16. MKSAP 16 also meets multiple CanMEDS Roles for RCPSC MOC, including that of Medical Expert, Communicator, Collaborator, Manager, Health Advocate, Scholar, and Professional. For information on how to apply MKSAP 16 CME credits to RCPSC MOC, visit the MKSAP Resource Site at mksap.acponline.org.

The Royal Australasian College of Physicians CPD Program

In Australia, MKSAP 16 is a Category 3 program that may be used by Fellows of The Royal Australasian College of Physicians (RACP) to meet mandatory CPD points. Two CPD credits are awarded for each of the 174 *AMA PRA Category 1 Credits*™ available in MKSAP 16. More information about using MKSAP 16 for this purpose is available at the MKSAP Resource Site at mksap.acponline.org and at www.racp.edu.au. CPD credits earned through MKSAP 16 should be reported at the MyCPD site at www.racp.edu.au/mycpd.

Continuing Medical Education

The American College of Physicians is accredited by the Accreditation Council for Continuing Medical Education (ACCME) to provide continuing medical education for physicians.

The American College of Physicians designates this enduring material, MKSAP 16, for a maximum of 174 *AMA PRA Category 1 Credits*™. Physicians should claim only the credit commensurate with the extent of their participation in the activity.

Learning Objectives

The learning objectives of MKSAP 16 are to:

- Close gaps between actual care in your practice and preferred standards of care, based on best evidence
- Diagnose disease states that are less common and sometimes overlooked and confusing
- Improve management of comorbid conditions that can complicate patient care
- Determine when to refer patients for surgery or care by subspecialists
- Pass the ABIM Certification Examination
- Pass the ABIM Maintenance of Certification Examination

Target Audience

- General internists and primary care physicians
- Subspecialists who need to remain up-to-date in internal medicine
- Residents preparing for the certifying examination in internal medicine
- Physicians preparing for maintenance of certification in internal medicine (recertification)

Earn 'Same-Day' CME Credits Online

For the first time, print subscribers can enter their answers online to earn CME credits in 24 hours or less. You can submit your answers using online answer sheets that are provided at mksap.acponline.org, where a record of your MKSAP 16 credits will be available. To earn CME credits, you need to answer all of the questions in a test and earn a score of at least 50% correct. (Number of correct answers divided by the total number of questions.) Take any of the following approaches:

1. Use the printed answer sheet at the back of this book to record your answers. Go to mksap.acponline.org, access the appropriate online answer sheet, transcribe your answers, and submit your test for same-day CME credits. There is no additional fee for this service.

2. Go to mksap.acponline.org, access the appropriate online answer sheet, directly enter your answers, and submit your test for same-day CME credits. There is no additional fee for this service.

3. Pay a $10 processing fee per answer sheet and submit the printed answer sheet at the back of this book by mail or fax, as instructed on the answer sheet. Make sure you calculate your score and fax the answer sheet to 215-351-2799 or mail the answer sheet to Member and Customer Service, American College of Physicians, 190 N. Independence Mall West, Philadelphia, PA 19106-1572, using the courtesy envelope provided in your MKSAP 16 slipcase. You will need your 10-digit order number and 8-digit ACP ID number, which are

printed on your packing slip. Please allow four to six weeks for your score report to be emailed back to you. Be sure to include your email address for a response.

If you do not have a 10-digit order number and 8-digit ACP ID number or if you need help creating a username and password to access the MKSAP 16 online answer sheets, go to mksap.acponline.org or email custserv@acponline.org.

Disclosure Policy

It is the policy of the American College of Physicians (ACP) to ensure balance, independence, objectivity, and scientific rigor in all of its educational activities. To this end, and consistent with the policies of the ACP and the Accreditation Council for Continuing Medical Education (ACCME), contributors to all ACP continuing medical education activities are required to disclose all relevant financial relationships with any entity producing, marketing, re-selling, or distributing health care goods or services consumed by, or used on, patients. Contributors are required to use generic names in the discussion of therapeutic options and are required to identify any unapproved, off-label, or investigative use of commercial products or devices. Where a trade name is used, all available trade names for the same product type are also included. If trade-name products manufactured by companies with whom contributors have relationships are discussed, contributors are asked to provide evidence-based citations in support of the discussion. The information is reviewed by the committee responsible for producing this text. If necessary, adjustments to topics or contributors' roles in content development are made to balance the discussion. Further, all readers of this text are asked to evaluate the content for evidence of commercial bias and send any relevant comments to mksap_editors@acponline.org so that future decisions about content and contributors can be made in light of this information.

Resolution of Conflicts

To resolve all conflicts of interest and influences of vested interests, the ACP precluded members of the content-creation committee from deciding on any content issues that involved generic or trade-name products associated with proprietary entities with which these committee members had relationships. In addition, content was based on best evidence and updated clinical care guidelines, when such evidence and guidelines were available. Contributors' disclosure information can be found with the list of contributors' names and those of ACP principal staff listed in the beginning of this book.

Educational Disclaimer

The editors and publisher of MKSAP 16 recognize that the development of new material offers many opportunities for error. Despite our best efforts, some errors may persist in print. Drug dosage schedules are, we believe, accurate and in accordance with current standards. Readers are advised, however, to ensure that the recommended dosages in MKSAP 16 concur with the information provided in the product information material. This is especially important in cases of new, infrequently used, or highly toxic drugs. Application of the information in MKSAP 16 remains the professional responsibility of the practitioner.

The primary purpose of MKSAP 16 is educational. Information presented, as well as publications, technologies, products, and/or services discussed, is intended to inform subscribers about the knowledge, techniques, and experiences of the contributors. A diversity of professional opinion exists, and the views of the contributors are their own and not those of the ACP. Inclusion of any material in the program does not constitute endorsement or recommendation by the ACP. The ACP does not warrant the safety, reliability, accuracy, completeness, or usefulness of and disclaims any and all liability for damages and claims that may result from the use of information, publications, technologies, products, and/or services discussed in this program.

Publisher's Information

Unauthorized Use of This Book Is Against the Law

MKSAP 16 ISBN: 978-1-938245-00-8

Printed in the United States of America.

For order information in the U.S. or Canada call 800-523-1546, extension 2600. All other countries call 215-351-2600. Fax inquiries to 215-351-2799 or email to cust-serv@acponline.org.

Errata and Norm Tables

Errata for MKSAP 16 will be available through the MKSAP Resource Site at mksap.acponline.org as new information becomes known to the editors.

MKSAP 16 Performance Interpretation Guidelines with Norm Tables, available July 31, 2013, will reflect the knowledge of physicians who have completed the self-assessment tests before the program was published. These physicians took the tests without being able to refer to the syllabus, answers, and critiques. For your convenience, the tables will be made available in a printable PDF file at the MKSAP Resource Site at mksap.acponline.org.

Interpretation Key

Each of the 11 books of MKSAP 16 is page-numbered individually beginning with number 1. Each entry of the cumulative index consists of the page number on which a particular term appears, followed, in parentheses, by a code designating the particular book. For example, in the index entry:

Amoxicillin

    for *H. pylori* infection, 15(GA), 16t(GA)

    for infective endocarditis prophylaxis, 8(ID)

15(GA) refers to page 15 of the Gastroenterology and Hepatology syllabus;

16t(GA) refers to a table on page 16 of the Gastroenterology and Hepatology syllabus; and

8(ID) refers to page 8 of the Infectious Disease syllabus

The codes for the books are as follows:

CV = Cardiovascular Medicine
DM = Dermatology
EN = Endocrinology and Metabolism
GA = Gastroenterology and Hepatology
GIM = General Internal Medicine
HO = Hematology and Oncology
ID = Infectious Disease
NP = Nephrology
NR = Neurology
PM = Pulmonary and Critical Care Medicine
RM = Rheumatology

Cumulative Index

Cumulative Index

MKSAP® 16

Medical Knowledge Self-Assessment Program®

General Internal Medicine

Welcome to the General Internal Medicine section of MKSAP 16!

Here, you will find updated information on routine care of the healthy patient; patient safety; professionalism and ethics; palliative care; chronic pain; acute and chronic cough; chronic fatigue; musculoskeletal pain; dyslipidemia; obesity; men's and women's health; eye, ear, nose, mouth, and throat disorders; mental and behavioral health; geriatric medicine; perioperative medicine; and many other clinical challenges. All of these topics are uniquely focused on the needs of both generalists and those who practice subspecialty internal medicine.

The publication of the 16th edition of Medical Knowledge Self-Assessment Program heralds a significant event, culminating 2 years of effort by dozens of leading subspecialists across the United States. Our authoring committees have strived to help internists succeed in Maintenance of Certification, right up to preparing for the MOC examination, and to get residents ready for the certifying examination. MKSAP 16 also helps you update your medical knowledge and elevates standards of self-learning by allowing you to assess your knowledge with 1,200 all-new multiple-choice questions, including 168 in General Internal Medicine.

MKSAP began more than 40 years ago. The American Board of Internal Medicine's examination blueprint and gaps between actual and preferred practices inform creation of the content. The questions, refined through rigorous face-to-face meetings, are among the best in medicine. A psychometric analysis of the items sharpens our educational focus on weaknesses in practice. To meet diverse learning styles, we offer MKSAP 16 online and in downloadable apps for PCs, tablets, laptops, and smartphones. We are also introducing the following:

High-Value Care Recommendations: The General Internal Medicine section starts with several recommendations based on the important concept of health care value (balancing clinical benefit with costs and harms) to address the needs of trainees, practicing physicians, and patients. These recommendations are part of a major initiative that has been undertaken by the American College of Physicians, in collaboration with other organizations.

Content for Hospitalists: This material, highlighted in blue and labeled with the familiar hospital icon (⬛), directly addresses the learning needs of the increasing number of physicians who work in the hospital setting. MKSAP 16 Digital will allow you to customize quizzes based on hospitalist-only questions to help you prepare for the Hospital Medicine Maintenance of Certification Examination.

We hope you enjoy and benefit from MKSAP 16. Please feel free to send us any comments to mksap_editors@acponline.org or visit us at the MKSAP Resource Site (mksap.acponline.org) to find out how we can help you study, earn CME, accumulate MOC points, and stay up to date. I know I speak on behalf of ACP staff members and our authoring committees when I say we are honored to have attracted your interest and participation.

Sincerely,

Patrick Alguire, MD, FACP
Editor-in-Chief
Senior Vice President
Medical Education Division
American College of Physicians

General Internal Medicine

Committee

Gary H. Tabas, MD, FACP, Editor[1]
Professor of Medicine
Division of General Internal Medicine
Department of Medicine
University of Pittsburgh School of Medicine
University of Pittsburgh Medical Center Presbyterian—Shadyside
Pittsburgh, Pennsylvania

Jack Ende, MD, MACP, Associate Editor[1]
Professor of Medicine
University of Pennsylvania
Chief, Department of Medicine
Penn Presbyterian Medical Center
Philadelphia, Pennsylvania

Paul B. Aronowitz, MD, FACP[1]
Adjunct Associate Professor of Medicine
Dartmouth Medical School
Associate Professor of Clinical Medicine
University of California, San Francisco
Program Director
Internal Medicine Residency Program
California Pacific Medical Center
San Francisco, California

Rosemarie L. Conigliaro, MD, FACP[1]
Professor of Medicine
Senior Assistant Dean for Curriculum
University of Kentucky College of Medicine
Lexington, Kentucky

Rosanne Granieri, MD, FACP[1]
Professor of Medicine
Division of General Internal Medicine
Department of Medicine
University of Pittsburgh School of Medicine
Pittsburgh, Pennsylvania

Eric H. Green, MD, MSc, FACP[1]
Associate Professor of Clinical Medicine
Drexel University College of Medicine
Philadelphia, Pennsylvania
Associate Program Director
Internal Medicine Residency Program
Mercy Catholic Medical Center
Darby, Pennsylvania

Scott Herrle, MD, MS[1]
Assistant Professor of Medicine
University of Pittsburgh School of Medicine
VA Pittsburgh Healthcare System
Pittsburgh, Pennsylvania

Christopher L. Knight, MD, FACP[2]
Associate Professor
Department of Medicine
University of Washington
Seattle, Washington

Megan McNamara, MD, MSc[1]
Assistant Professor of Medicine
Director of Student Assessment, Program Evaluation, and the Center for the Advancement of Medical Learning
Case Western Reserve University School of Medicine
Cleveland, Ohio

Mohan Nadkarni, MD, FACP[1]
Professor of Medicine
Chief, Section of General Internal Medicine
University of Virginia Health System
Charlottesville, Virginia

Consulting Contributor

P. Preston Reynolds, MD, PhD, FACP[1]
Professor of Medicine
Division of General Medicine, Geriatrics and Palliative Care
Center for Biomedical Ethics and Humanities
University of Virginia Health System
Charlottesville, Virginia

Editor-in-Chief

Patrick C. Alguire, MD, FACP[1]
Senior Vice President, Medical Education
American College of Physicians
Philadelphia, Pennsylvania

Deputy Editor-in-Chief

Philip A. Masters, MD, FACP[1]
Senior Medical Associate for Content Development
American College of Physicians
Philadelphia, Pennsylvania

Senior Medical Associate for Content Development

Cynthia D. Smith, MD, FACP[2]
American College of Physicians
Philadelphia, Pennsylvania

General Internal Medicine Clinical Editor

Michele Heisler, MD[1]

General Internal Medicine Reviewers

Stewart Babbott, MD, FACP[1]
Elizabeth A. Cerceo, MD, FACP[1]
John K. Chamberlain, MD, MACP[1]
Timi Edeki, MD[2]
Douglas Einstadter, MD, MPH, FACP[1]
Stephanie L. Elkins, MD[2]
Richard M. Hoffman, MD, MPH, FACP[2]
Medha Munshi, MD[2]
Asher Tulsky, MD, FACP[1]
Peter H. Wiernik, MD, FACP[2]

General Internal Medicine Reviewers Representing the American Society for Clinical Pharmacology & Therapeutics

John Thomas Callaghan, MD, PhD[2]
Anne N. Nafziger, MD, FACP[2]

General Internal Medicine ACP Editorial Staff

Becky Krumm[1], Senior Staff Editor
Sean McKinney[1], Director, Self-Assessment Programs
Margaret Wells[1], Managing Editor
John Haefele[1], Assistant Editor

ACP Principal Staff

Patrick C. Alguire, MD, FACP[1]
Senior Vice President, Medical Education

D. Theresa Kanya, MBA[1]
Vice President, Medical Education

Sean McKinney[1]
Director, Self-Assessment Programs

Margaret Wells[1]
Managing Editor

Valerie Dangovetsky[1]
Program Administrator

Becky Krumm[1]
Senior Staff Editor

Ellen McDonald, PhD[1]
Senior Staff Editor

Katie Idell[1]
Senior Staff Editor

Randy Hendrickson[1]
Production Administrator/Editor

Megan Zborowski[1]
Staff Editor

Linnea Donnarumma[1]
Assistant Editor

John Haefele[1]
Assistant Editor

Developed by the American College of Physicians

---

1. Has no relationships with any entity producing, marketing, re-selling, or distributing health care goods or services consumed by, or used on, patients.

2. Has disclosed relationships with entities producing, marketing, re-selling, or distributing health care goods or services consumed by, or used on, patients. See below.

Conflicts of Interest

The following committee members, reviewers, and ACP staff members have disclosed relationships with commercial companies:

John Thomas Callaghan, MD
Employment
Eli Lilly & Co. (Retiree)
Stock Options/Holdings
Eli Lilly, Abbott, Isis
Consultantship
Marcadia, Biogen Idec

Timi Edeki, MD
Employment
AstraZeneca
Stock Options/Holdings
Abbott Laboratories

Stephanie L. Elkins, MD
Speakers Bureau
Celgene, Cephalon Oncology, GlaxoSmithKline

Richard M. Hoffman, MD, MPH, FACP
Employment
Foundation for Informed Medical Decision Making
Research Grants/Contracts
NIH
Royalties
UpToDate

Christopher L. Knight, MD, FACP
Royalties
Oakstone Medical Publishing

Medha Munshi, MD
Consultantship
Novartis (spouse), Celgene (spouse), Millenium (spouse)

Anne N. Nafziger, MD, FACP
Consultantship
Bertino Consulting

Cynthia D. Smith, MD, FACP
Stock Options/Holdings
Merck and Company

Peter H. Wiernik, MD, FACP
Honoraria
Celgene

Acknowledgments

The American College of Physicians (ACP) gratefully acknowledges the special contributions to the development and production of the 16th edition of the Medical Knowledge Self-Assessment Program® (MKSAP® 16) made by the following people:

Graphic Services: Michael Ripca (Technical Administrator/Graphic Designer) and Willie-Fetchko Graphic Design (Graphic Designer).

Production/Systems: Dan Hoffmann (Director, Web Services & Systems Development), Neil Kohl (Senior Architect), and Scott Hurd (Senior Systems Analyst/Developer).

MKSAP 16 Digital: Under the direction of Steven Spadt, Vice President, ACP Digital Products & Services, the digital version of MKSAP 16 was developed within the ACP's Digital Product Development Department, led by Brian Sweigard (Director). Other members of the team included Sean O'Donnell (Senior Architect), Dan Barron (Senior Systems Analyst/Developer), Chris Forrest (Senior Software Developer/Design Lead), Jon Laing (Senior Web Application Developer), Brad Lord (Senior Web Developer), John McKnight (Senior Web Developer), and Nate Pershall (Senior Web Developer).

The College also wishes to acknowledge that many other persons, too numerous to mention, have contributed to the production of this program. Without their dedicated efforts, this program would not have been possible.

Introducing the MKSAP Resource Site (mksap.acponline.org)

The MKSAP Resource Site (mksap.acponline.org) is a continually updated site that provides links to MKSAP 16 online answer sheets for print subscribers; access to MKSAP 16 Digital, Board Basics® 3, and MKSAP 16 Updates; the latest details on Continuing Medical Education (CME) and Maintenance of Certification (MOC) in the United States, Canada, and Australia; errata; and other new information.

ABIM Maintenance of Certification

Check the MKSAP Resource Site (mksap.acponline.org) for the latest information on how MKSAP tests can be used to apply to the American Board of Internal Medicine for Maintenance of Certification (MOC) points.

RCPSC Maintenance of Certification

In Canada, MKSAP 16 is an Accredited Self-Assessment Program (Section 3) as defined by the Maintenance of Certification Program of The Royal College of Physicians and Surgeons of Canada (RCPSC) and approved by the Canadian Society of Internal Medicine on December 9, 2011. Approval of Part A sections of MKSAP 16 extends from July 31, 2012, until July 31, 2015. Approval of Part B sections of MKSAP 16 extends from December 31, 2012, to December 31, 2015. Fellows of the Royal College may earn three credits per hour for participating in MKSAP 16 under Section 3. MKSAP 16 will enable Fellows to earn up to 75% of their required 400 credits during the 5-year MOC cycle. A Fellow can achieve this 75% level by earning 100 of the maximum of 174 *AMA PRA Category 1 Credits*™ available in MKSAP 16. MKSAP 16 also meets multiple CanMEDS Roles for RCPSC MOC, including that of Medical Expert, Communicator, Collaborator, Manager, Health Advocate, Scholar, and Professional. For information on how to apply MKSAP 16 CME credits to RCPSC MOC, visit the MKSAP Resource Site at mksap.acponline.org.

The Royal Australasian College of Physicians CPD Program

In Australia, MKSAP 16 is a Category 3 program that may be used by Fellows of The Royal Australasian College of Physicians (RACP) to meet mandatory CPD points. Two CPD credits are awarded for each of the 174 *AMA PRA Category 1 Credits*™ available in MKSAP 16. More information about using MKSAP 16 for this purpose is available at the MKSAP Resource Site at mksap.acponline.org and at www.racp.edu.au. CPD credits earned through MKSAP 16 should be reported at the MyCPD site at www.racp.edu.au/mycpd.

Continuing Medical Education

The American College of Physicians is accredited by the Accreditation Council for Continuing Medical Education

(ACCME) to provide continuing medical education for physicians.

The American College of Physicians designates this enduring material, MKSAP 16, for a maximum of 174 *AMA PRA Category 1 Credits™*. Physicians should claim only the credit commensurate with the extent of their participation in the activity.

Up to 24 *AMA PRA Category 1 Credits™* are available from December 31, 2012, to December 31, 2015, for the MKSAP 16 General Internal Medicine section.

Learning Objectives

The learning objectives of MKSAP 16 are to:
- Close gaps between actual care in your practice and preferred standards of care, based on best evidence
- Diagnose disease states that are less common and sometimes overlooked and confusing
- Improve management of comorbid conditions that can complicate patient care
- Determine when to refer patients for surgery or care by subspecialists
- Pass the ABIM Certification Examination
- Pass the ABIM Maintenance of Certification Examination

Target Audience

- General internists and primary care physicians
- Subspecialists who need to remain up-to-date in internal medicine
- Residents preparing for the certifying examination in internal medicine
- Physicians preparing for maintenance of certification in internal medicine (recertification)

Earn "Same-Day" CME Credits Online

For the first time, print subscribers can enter their answers online to earn CME credits in 24 hours or less. You can submit your answers using online answer sheets that are provided at mksap.acponline.org, where a record of your MKSAP 16 credits will be available. To earn CME credits, you need to answer all of the questions in a test and earn a score of at least 50% correct (number of correct answers divided by the total number of questions). Take any of the following approaches:

1. Use the printed answer sheet at the back of this book to record your answers. Go to mksap.acponline.org, access the appropriate online answer sheet, transcribe your answers, and submit your test for same-day CME credits. There is no additional fee for this service.

2. Go to mksap.acponline.org, access the appropriate online answer sheet, directly enter your answers, and submit your test for same-day CME credits. There is no additional fee for this service.

3. Pay a $10 processing fee per answer sheet and submit the printed answer sheet at the back of this book by mail or fax, as instructed on the answer sheet. Make sure you calculate your score and fax the answer sheet to 215-351-2799 or mail the answer sheet to Member and Customer Service, American College of Physicians, 190 N. Independence Mall West, Philadelphia, PA 19106-1572, using the courtesy envelope provided in your MKSAP 16 slipcase. You will need your 10-digit order number and 8-digit ACP ID number, which are printed on your packing slip. Please allow 4 to 6 weeks for your score report to be emailed back to you. Be sure to include your email address for a response.

If you do not have a 10-digit order number and 8-digit ACP ID number or if you need help creating a username and password to access the MKSAP 16 online answer sheets, go to mksap.acponline.org or email custserv@acponline.org.

Permission/Consent for Use of Figures Shown in MKSAP 16 General Internal Medicine Multiple-Choice Questions

The figures shown in Self-Assessment Test Item 29, Item 148, and Item 61 appear courtesy of Edward A. Jaeger, MD, Jefferson Medical College, Wills Eye Institute, Philadelphia, PA. The figure shown in Self-Assessment Test Item 163 is reprinted with permission from Physicians' Information and Education Resource (ACP PIER). Philadelphia, PA: American College of Physicians.

Disclosure Policy

It is the policy of the American College of Physicians (ACP) to ensure balance, independence, objectivity, and scientific rigor in all of its educational activities. To this end, and consistent with the policies of the ACP and the Accreditation Council for Continuing Medical Education (ACCME), contributors to all ACP continuing medical education activities are required to disclose all relevant financial relationships with any entity producing, marketing, re-selling, or distributing health care goods or services consumed by, or used on, patients. Contributors are required to use generic names in the discussion of therapeutic options and are required to identify any unapproved, off-label, or investigative use of commercial products or devices. Where a trade name is used, all available trade names for the same product type are also included. If trade-name products manufactured by companies with whom contributors have relationships are discussed, contributors are asked to provide evidence-based citations in support of the discussion. The information is reviewed by the committee responsible for producing this text. If necessary, adjustments to topics or contributors' roles in content development are made to balance the discussion. Further, all readers of this text are asked to evaluate the content for evidence of commercial bias and send any relevant comments to mksap_editors@acponline.org so that future decisions about content and contributors can be made in light of this information.

Resolution of Conflicts

To resolve all conflicts of interest and influences of vested interests, the ACP precluded members of the content-creation committee from deciding on any content issues that involved generic or trade-name products associated with proprietary entities with which these committee members had relationships. In addition, content was based on best evidence and updated clinical care guidelines, when such evidence and guidelines were available. Contributors' disclosure information can be found with the list of contributors' names and those of ACP principal staff listed in the beginning of this book.

Hospital-Based Medicine

For the convenience of subscribers who provide care in hospital settings, content that is specific to the hospital setting has been highlighted in blue. Hospital icons (🏥) highlight where the hospital-only content begins, continues over more than one page, and ends.

Educational Disclaimer

The editors and publisher of MKSAP 16 recognize that the development of new material offers many opportunities for error. Despite our best efforts, some errors may persist in print. Drug dosage schedules are, we believe, accurate and in accordance with current standards. Readers are advised, however, to ensure that the recommended dosages in MKSAP 16 concur with the information provided in the product information material. This is especially important in cases of new, infrequently used, or highly toxic drugs. Application of the information in MKSAP 16 remains the professional responsibility of the practitioner.

The primary purpose of MKSAP 16 is educational. Information presented, as well as publications, technologies, products, and/or services discussed, is intended to inform subscribers about the knowledge, techniques, and experiences of the contributors. A diversity of professional opinion exists, and the views of the contributors are their own and not those of the ACP. Inclusion of any material in the program does not constitute endorsement or recommendation by the ACP. The ACP does not warrant the safety, reliability, accuracy, completeness, or usefulness of and disclaims any and all liability for damages and claims that may result from the use of information, publications, technologies, products, and/or services discussed in this program.

Publisher's Information

Unauthorized Use of This Book Is Against the Law

Errata and Norm Tables

Errata for MKSAP 16 will be available through the MKSAP Resource Site at mksap.acponline.org as new information becomes known to the editors.

MKSAP 16 Performance Interpretation Guidelines with Norm Tables, available July 31, 2013, will reflect the knowledge of physicians who have completed the self-assessment tests before the program was published. These physicians took the tests without being able to refer to the syllabus, answers, and critiques. For your convenience, the tables are available in a printable PDF file through the MKSAP Resource Site at mksap.acponline.org.

Table of Contents

General Internal Medicine High-Value Care Recommendations

The American College of Physicians, in collaboration with multiple other organizations, is embarking on a national initiative to promote awareness about the importance of stewardship of health care resources. The goals are to improve health care outcomes by providing care of proven benefit and reducing costs by avoiding unnecessary and even harmful interventions. The initiative comprises several programs that integrate the important concept of health care value (balancing clinical benefit with costs and harms) for a given intervention into various educational materials to address the needs of trainees, practicing physicians, and patients.

To integrate discussion of high-value, cost-conscious care into MKSAP 16, we have created recommendations based on the medical knowledge content that we feel meet the below definition of high-value care and bring us closer to our goal of improving patient outcomes while conserving finite resources.

High-Value Care Recommendation: A recommendation to choose diagnostic and management strategies for patients in specific clinical situations that balances clinical benefit with cost and harms with the goal of improving patient outcomes.

Below are the High-Value Care Recommendations for the General Internal Medicine section of MKSAP 16.

- The value of the periodic health examination for healthy, asymptomatic adults is debatable and there is no consensus interval.
- The U.S. Preventive Services Task Force recommends against screening for the following conditions: carotid artery stenosis, COPD, hereditary hemochromatosis, and peripheral arterial disease.
- According to the U.S. Preventive Services Task Force, screening for coronary artery disease is not recommended in low-risk persons, and the evidence for screening high-risk persons is inconclusive, as is the evidence for screening using nontraditional risk factors, such as high-sensitivity C-reactive protein, homocysteine level, Lp(a) lipoprotein level, ankle-brachial index, carotid intima-media thickness, and coronary artery calcium score.
- The U.S. Preventive Services Task Force recommends against routine screening for hepatitis C virus infection in the general population.
- The U.S. Preventive Services Task Force recommends against screening for asymptomatic bacteriuria in men and nonpregnant women.
- Evidence for the benefits of screening mammography is lacking for women age 75 years and older.

- The American Cancer Society does not recommend using MRI for breast cancer screening in average-risk women and finds the evidence regarding breast self-examination to be insufficient.
- Owing to poor specificity, cervical cancer screening with human papillomavirus (HPV) DNA testing alone is not recommended, although clinicians can consider using HPV DNA testing along with cervical cytology in women age 30 years and older to help guide further investigation and decrease the frequency of testing (see Item 34).
- Owing to limitations of currently available screening tests and unclear benefits of screening, prostate cancer screening remains controversial (see Item 49).
- The American College of Physicians and the American Academy of Family Physicians both recommend that clinicians have individualized discussions with their patients regarding obtaining prostate-specific antigen (PSA) measurements and support obtaining PSA levels after such discussions in patients 50 years and older who have life expectancies of at least 10 years (see Item 49).
- Palliative care consultation programs are associated with significant hospital cost savings, with an adjusted net savings of $1696 in direct costs for patients discharged alive from the hospital and $4908 net savings for patients dying in the hospital as compared with patients who receive usual care (see Item 76).
- Evidence suggests that more aggressive care at the end of life—whether prolonged hospitalization, intensive care unit admission, or performance of procedures—does not improve either quality or duration of life (see Item 89).
- Feeding tubes are not recommended for terminal cancer.
- There is no specific role for diagnostic testing in the assessment and management of chronic noncancer pain because abnormalities that are identified may not be the source of the patient's pain (see Item 117).
- Routine antibiotic treatment of uncomplicated upper respiratory tract infections and acute bronchitis in nonelderly immunocompetent patients is not recommended (see Item 13).
- Patients with chronic fatigue for longer than 1 month rarely have abnormalities on either physical or laboratory evaluation; testing should thus be judicious and performed only when clearly indicated (see Item 7).
- Patients with chronic fatigue syndrome should have regular follow-up to monitor their symptoms, for support and validation, and to avoid unnecessary diagnostic and treatment interventions.

- Tests with the lowest likelihood of affecting diagnosis or management of syncope include head CT scan, carotid Doppler ultrasonography, electroencephalography, and cardiac enzyme levels; these studies may be indicated if symptoms point to specific etiologies but otherwise should be omitted from the work-up (see Item 86 and Item 156).
- Neurocardiogenic and orthostatic syncope both are generally benign in nature and do not require hospitalization (see Item 86).
- Patients with nonspecific low back pain and no symptoms or signs to suggest systemic illness should not routinely receive additional diagnostic testing (see Item 91).
- Mechanical neck pain outside of the setting of acute trauma rarely requires imaging, although plain films can be helpful in patients older than 50 years to exclude malignancy and to assess for osteoarthritic changes (see Item 37).
- A repeat lipid screening interval of 5 years is considered appropriate in low-risk patients, with a shorter interval in those with borderline results and a longer interval in those with consistently normal results.
- Several nontraditional risk factors may be related to cardiovascular outcomes, including levels of Lp(a) lipoprotein, small LDL particles, HDL subspecies, apolipoproteins B and A-1, and the total cholesterol/HDL cholesterol ratio; however, the U.S. Preventive Services Task Force and updated National Cholesterol Education Program Adult Treatment Panel III (ATP III) guidelines do not recommend measuring or treating any of these risk factors when managing lipid levels (see Item 66).
- The benefits of statin therapy are generally class specific, and there is no compelling evidence that newer agents are more effective than established statin medications, which may be more cost effective.
- Because the risk of significant liver or muscle damage is very low in patients on statin therapy, routine follow-up testing is not indicated and should be performed based on the development of symptoms or other clinical findings while on therapy (see Item 158).
- Cardiovascular primary prevention with statin therapy in older patients (ages 65-80 years) is controversial.
- Because many episodes of erectile dysfunction are transient, an extensive laboratory evaluation is not mandatory at presentation without symptoms or findings suggestive of an underlying systemic disorder or before implementing lifestyle modification or counseling therapy.
- In adult men, asymptomatic hydroceles and varicoceles can usually be diagnosed clinically and generally do not require advanced imaging or treatment.
- Intrauterine devices (IUDs) combine the highest contraceptive efficacy (typical failure rate <1%) with the lowest cost.

- Initial evaluation of women with dysmenorrhea includes a thorough history, with particular attention to sexual activity and risks for abuse or infection; unless pelvic pathology is suspected (previous radiation, trauma, infection, foreign body), treatment may be initiated without further evaluation (see Item 131).
- There is no role for antibiotic eye drops in the treatment of viral conjunctivitis (see Item 11).
- Treatment of allergic conjunctivitis includes oral antihistamines, topical antihistamines, and artificial tears; antibiotic treatment is not indicated.
- Imaging of the central nervous system is not considered part of a routine evaluation for bilateral hearing loss.
- For the diagnosis of sinusitis, imaging is rarely necessary in an average-risk patient; however, it should be considered in immunocompromised patients at risk for unusual organisms, such as fungal or pseudomonal sinusitis (see Item 107).
- Empiric antibiotic treatment for acute pharyngitis not based on a clinical decision tool (such as the Centor criteria) should be discouraged (see Item 161).
- In the management of epistaxis, unless the patient has severe bleeding or has an associated systemic disease, laboratory studies and imaging are usually not necessary (see Item 4).
- In patients with dental infections without cellulitis or systemic symptoms, antibiotic therapy is not necessary if dental intervention can be performed within several days.
- Visualizing a hemorrhoid or other source of rectal bleeding in a low-risk patient younger than 40 years without other symptoms to suggest inflammatory bowel disease or colon cancer may spare the patient further endoscopic evaluation (see Item 48).
- When a somatoform disorder is suspected, laboratory and other testing should be ordered logically to evaluate plausible medical diagnoses; extensive and elaborate testing to explore unsupported or very unlikely diagnoses should be avoided (see Item 85).
- Frequent, routine review to verify need for medication and appropriate dosing is an important aspect of optimal geriatric care (see Item 46).
- Interventions to prevent pressure ulcers are much more cost effective than the prolonged and intensive efforts required for treatment of existing ulcers (see Item 24).
- Comprehensive batteries of laboratory testing, chest radiographs, and electrocardiograms should not be routinely performed in the preoperative setting without specific indication as they may result in further testing, delay surgery, and add expense, and such testing rarely influences perioperative care (see Item 8).
- Preoperative tests should be based on known or suspected comorbidities and should only be ordered when a result will alter management (see Item 8).

- Comprehensive preoperative testing has not been shown to be helpful in cataract surgery and is not endorsed by any major specialty society or payor.
- Preoperative pulmonary function testing should be reserved for patients with unexplained dyspnea (see Item 47).
- Laboratory testing for underlying bleeding disorders and anemia should be reserved for patients in whom there is a reasonable probability of an abnormal test and is not required as a routine component of preoperative evaluation (see Item 8).
- Blood transfusion is reserved for patients with symptomatic anemia, a preoperative hemoglobin concentration below 6 g/dL, postoperative hemoglobin concentration below 7 g/dL, or patients with symptomatic cardiovascular disease and hemoglobin concentrations between 6 and 10 g/dL.

General Internal Medicine

Interpretation of the Medical Literature

Study Design

Threats to Validity

Investigators attempt to infer validity, or "truth," by comparing two groups of people in a well-designed study. Many factors can threaten a study's validity, including errors in measurement, data collection, selection of subjects, or analysis. *Internal validity* refers to the degree to which the investigators' conclusions (usually implying cause and effect) are supported by the study. *External validity* refers to the generalizability of the study. There is always some error in any research study. Error is typically shown in scientific publications by way of a confidence interval (CI), typically the 95% confidence interval, which signifies that the investigators can be 95% certain that the value derived from a study truly lies within that interval. If the CI is wide, the point estimate is said to have less certainty, or precision; this is often due to small sample size. A small sample size can also decrease the *power* of a study. Power is the probability of detecting a difference between two groups when a true difference exists. Random error due to chance alone can sometimes result in uneven distribution of patient characteristics, affecting study results. When error is not random, but is applied differentially to one group, it is called *bias.* Bias can occur in selection of patients, measurement, and analysis. Selection bias occurs when patients chosen for a study group have characteristics that can affect the results of the study. Bias can be minimized using carefully constructed research protocols that ensure that the comparison groups are selected, measured, and analyzed in the same way.

Another major challenge in interpreting studies is confounding. A confounder is a third factor that influences both exposure (treatment) and outcome. For example, the false conclusion that smokeless tobacco in the form of snuff poses a greater risk for developing coronary artery disease (CAD) than cigarette smoking could occur because being male (the confounder, which is associated with CAD) is more likely among snuff users than among cigarette smokers. A failure to recognize the presence of a confounder distorts the cause-effect relationship. Confounding can be minimized by using a randomized study design or with statistical techniques if randomization is not possible.

Experimental Studies

In an experimental study, patient selection, treatment, and analysis are determined from the outset to minimize error and bias. In addition, many experimental studies blind patients, treating physicians, and investigators to which treatment a patient is receiving in order to reduce bias, because knowledge of which treatment a patient receives can affect patient reporting and investigator assessment of outcomes. To minimize bias associated with measurement, assessors of clinical outcomes are typically blinded even if patients and treating physicians cannot be blinded.

Various types of study designs are compared in **Table 1**. In a randomized controlled trial (RCT), randomization is performed in an effort to distribute all potential prognostic factors equally across both the experimental and the control groups, minimizing confounding and bias. Although historically, most RCTs compared a new intervention with a placebo, RCTs can also compare a new therapy with an existing one. The objective of these trials, which are often used when the new therapy is less costly or easier to use, is typically to prove that the new therapy is "noninferior" to accepted therapies. These studies require careful attention to the power of the study; studies with small numbers of patients can mask a true difference.

Well-designed RCTs typically have a high degree of precision and internal validity. However, RCTs are typically conducted on patients with a narrow spectrum of disease and use treatment protocols that may be difficult to implement outside of a research setting. Therefore, many RCTs lack generalizability.

Two other experimental study designs are used when randomization of individual patients is unfeasible or unethical (for example, evaluating a new patient safety initiative). In a quasi-experimental study design, data can be compared in the same group of patients both before and after an intervention. In cluster-randomized studies, groups of patients are randomized, rather than individual patients.

Observational Studies

In an observational study, the investigator has no role in assigning individuals to interventions, but rather compares the effects of exposures or treatments among two or more observed groups. By their very nature, observational studies are more susceptible to bias and confounding than experimental studies. Strengths of observational studies, however, include their ability to include a broader spectrum of disease (and diseases or exposures that are rare) and that treatments

TABLE 1. Types of Study Designs

Study Design	Description	Strengths	Weaknesses	Key Threats to Validity
Experimental Studies				
Randomized controlled trial (RCT)	Patients receive one of two interventions, often one being a placebo	Strongest design for determining causation	Expensive, time-consuming, not practical for many clinical situations Limited follow-up duration Limited number of outcomes that can be assessed Limited generalizability	If randomization is ineffective If data are not analyzed according to initially assigned group If key individuals are aware of group assignment (not blinded) If follow-up is incomplete
Cluster-randomized trial	Patients grouped by clusters (e.g., nursing unit) rather than assigned randomly	Same as for RCTs Can be used if randomization of patients is not ethical or feasible	Same as for RCTs Challenging to analyze	Same as for RCTs If analysis does not account for clustering
Quasi-experimental design	Review of data collected before and after an intervention	Can be used if randomization of patients is not ethical or feasible	Patients not randomized	If no adjustment for possible confounding
Observational Studies				
Cohort study	Studies outcomes of groups using observed assignment	Able to detect associations, but these are not always cause-effect relationships Able to study multiple outcomes over a long period of time Large sample size	Requires complicated statistical techniques to minimize confounding Prospective designs can be expensive and take many years before results are available	Selection bias in cohort Bias in measurement of exposures and outcomes If important confounders not accounted for
Case-control study	Compares past exposures in patients with and without disease	Useful for rare diseases or exposures Inexpensive	High risk for bias High risk for confounding Cannot assess incidence/prevalence	Selection bias, especially in controls Measurement bias, especially recall bias

are administered in a "real-world" environment. Two types of observational studies are cohort studies and case-control studies. A cohort study compares the outcomes of groups with and without exposures or treatments not initiated by the investigator; for example, rates of lung cancer between smokers and nonsmokers. Cohorts are compared by following them forward in time (prospectively) or by looking backward in time (retrospectively); prospective design minimizes recall bias (inaccurate recall of past events).

A case-control study retrospectively compares the experience of patients who have a disease with those who do not have the disease. For example, patients with and without lung cancer can be compared with respect to their exposure to asbestos. Case-control studies are particularly useful to study rare diseases or diseases that occur many years after specific exposures. These studies are highly susceptible to

bias, especially recall bias, as patients with disease may be more likely to remember previous exposures. Careful attention is needed in both measurement of exposures and selection of controls.

Other observational study designs are limited in their ability to establish causality but may be useful as relatively inexpensive means of generating hypotheses for future research or for determining estimates of prevalence of a disease. A cross-sectional study assesses for both exposure and disease at the same time point (rather than prospectively or retrospectively). A case series is a report of clinical outcomes in a group of patients; the absence of a control group prevents any conclusions about the effectiveness of the treatment. Epidemiologic studies compare outcomes, in aggregate, of two different populations (countries, socioeconomic groups). These studies are potentially subject to the *ecologic fallacy*, erroneously assuming that population-level associations imply individual-level associations.

Other Study Designs

Systematic reviews summarize existing experimental or observational studies in a rigorous way. Systematic reviews are characterized by a focused clinical question, exhaustive review of the published literature, a systematic protocol for selecting articles and abstracting data (often utilizing independent reviewers), qualitative or quantitative combination of the results, and narrative summary of strengths and limitations of the analysis. Systematic reviews that quantitatively combine data are called meta-analyses. The strength of systematic reviews lies in combining the data from many small studies to minimize the impact of random error. Potential weaknesses, in addition to the weaknesses of the composite studies, include study identification and selection variability in the design of the included studies.

In general, meta-analyses are considered the highest quality sources of evidence, followed (in descending order) by qualitative systematic reviews, RCTs, cohort studies, and case-control studies. Within each category, however, quality may vary, so a well-designed prospective cohort study may be superior to a small RCT with a high rate of drop-out.

Comparative effectiveness research (CER) is intended to produce evidence that can help patients, physicians, and policy makers better understand the effectiveness, benefits, and harms of treatments or procedures. CER employs systematic reviews as well as new clinical trials to determine effectiveness in routine clinical practice.

KEY POINTS

- Internal validity refers to the degree to which the investigators' conclusions are supported by the study; external validity refers to the generalizability of the study.
- Bias occurs when systematic differences between groups affect the outcome of a study.
- Meta-analyses are considered the highest quality sources of evidence, followed (in descending order) by qualitative systematic reviews, RCTs, cohort studies, and case-control studies.

Statistical Analysis

Published studies of therapies typically express results in either relative or absolute terms (**Table 2**). Relative comparisons, such as relative risk, odds ratio, and hazard ratio, compare the ratio between rates of events (such as death or hospitalizations) in two groups. Absolute comparisons, such as absolute risk differences, express absolute differences in rates of disease or events in two groups. Relative risk differences may exaggerate the impact of an intervention, especially for relatively uncommon outcomes. For example, an intervention that reduces the rate of a disease from 20% to 10% and an intervention that reduces it from 2% to 1% each have a relative risk reduction (RRR) of 50%. However, the absolute risk reduction (ARR) for the first case is 10%, whereas the ARR for the second is 1%. The effect size, a measure of the general impact of an intervention, is best characterized by the number needed to treat (NNT), which is number of patients needed to receive a

TABLE 2. Common Terms Used in the Interpretation of the Medical Literature for Therapeutics			
Term	**Definition**	**Calculation**	**Notes**
Absolute risk (AR)	The probability of an event occurring in a group during a specified time period	AR = patients with event in group / total patients in group	Also known as *event rate*; can be for benefits or harms. Often, an experimental event rate (EER) is compared with a control event rate (CER)
Relative risk (RR)	The ratio of the probability of developing a disease with a risk factor present to the probability of developing the disease without the risk factor present	RR = EER / CER	Used in cohort studies and randomized controlled trials Any two ARs can be substituted for EER and CER
Absolute risk reduction (ARR)	The difference in rates of events between experimental group (EER) and control group (CER)	ARR = | EER − CER |	Any two ARs can be substituted for EER and CER
Relative risk reduction (RRR)	The ratio of absolute risk reduction to the event rate among controls	RRR = | EER − CER | / CER	Any two ARs can be substituted for EER and CER
Number needed to treat (NNT)	Number of patients needed to receive a treatment for one additional patient to benefit	NNT = 1 / ARR	A good estimate of the effect size
Number needed to harm (NNH)	Number of patients needed to receive a treatment for one additional patient to be harmed	NNH = 1 / ARI	ARI = absolute risk increase and equals | EER − CER | when the event is an unfavorable outcome (e.g., drug side effect)

treatment for one additional patient to be expected to benefit from the intervention. NNT is the reciprocal of the ARR. In the example above, the NNT in the first case is 10 (1/0.10) and in the second case, 100 (1/0.01). Number needed to harm (NNH) is the reciprocal of the absolute risk increase (ARI), and reflects the number of patients that would need to be treated to expect one of them to be harmed by the intervention. Defining risk in absolute terms and calculating the NNT/NNH is the best way to understand the magnitude of difference in the sample (effect size).

A *P* value allows the reader to assess how likely any difference seen is due to chance alone. For example, a *P* value of less than 0.05 (corresponding to a less than 1 in 20 chance of getting the results found in the trial assuming there is no difference between the treatments) is often accepted as a cut-off for statistically significant results. *P* values are related to both the degree of difference found between groups and the number of patients in a study, so studies with many patients often produce highly statistically significant results. However, it is important to recognize that differences found to be statistically significant in large trials may not be clinically important. For example, a large study could find a statistically significant decrease in an event rate from 0.2% in the control group to 0.1% in the treatment group. However, the ARR would be 0.1%, yielding a NNT of 1000.

Many measures are used to define the properties of diagnostic tests (**Table 3**), including sensitivity, specificity, and predictive value. Understanding these characteristics for a given test is essential in knowing how effective and helpful a study will be in the diagnostic process. For example, the sensitivity is an indicator of the ability of a test to detect a disease if it is present, and the specificity reflects how effectively a test can exclude illness in a patient without the disease. Both sensitivity and specificity are properties of the test itself and do not vary with the prevalence of disease. The predictive value of a test, however, does vary according to the prevalence of the disease. For example, consider a test with 90% sensitivity and 90% specificity. In a population in which 80% of people have the disease (prevalence of 80%), positive test results will be true positives 97% of the time (positive predictive value [PPV]); however, negative test results will be true negatives only 69% of the time (negative predictive value [NPV]). Conversely, if only 8% of the population has the disease (prevalence of 8%), the PPV of the test is 44% and the NPV is 99%.

The Bayes theorem uses sensitivity, specificity, and the pretest probability of a disease to calculate the posttest probability of the disease. The likelihood ratio (LR) is the ratio of the probability of a particular test result (positive or negative) among patients with a disease to the probability of that same result among patients without the disease. The pretest odds of a disease multiplied by the LR equals the posttest odds of the disease. The posttest odds can be converted to a percentage to yield the more commonly used posttest probability.

KEY POINTS

- Defining risk in absolute terms and calculating number needed to treat/harm is the best way to understand the magnitude of difference in the sample (effect size).

- The positive predictive value of a test increases with increasing prevalence of the disease being tested for, whereas the negative predictive value increases with *decreasing* prevalence of the disease.

Sources of Evidence

The Cochrane collection offers a single source for systematic reviews (www.mrw.interscience.wiley.com/cochrane/); PubMed's clinical queries page offers assistance for common clinical searches (www.ncbi.nlm.nih.gov/pubmed/clinical), including searches for systematic reviews and other clinical study categories; and PubMed (www.ncbi.nlm.nih.gov/pubmed/) can be used for more comprehensive searches. Textbooks and review articles typically offer "predigested" evidence on a clinical topic, although they lack the formal rigor of a systematic review. Guidelines, in contrast, allow groups of experts to synthesize and interpret available evidence. The authors grade their recommendations based on the quality of the evidence reviewed. As guidelines are evidence-supported expert opinion, there are often differences between guidelines put out by different organizations. These differences may reflect the unconscious biases of the authors and sponsoring organization. The American College of Physicians (ACP) publishes clinical practice guidelines, guidance statements, and best practice advice based on reviews of available evidence (www.acponline.org/clinical_information/guidelines). A useful compilation of guidelines is also available at www.guidelines.gov. Critical evaluation tools and evidence-based medicine (EBM) calculators are available at www.cebm.net. Other EBM resources include ACP's PIER (http://pier.acponline.org), ACP Journal Club (www.acpjc.org), ACP JournalWise (www.journalwise.org), and Clinical Evidence (http://clinicalevidence.bmj.com).

Routine Care of the Healthy Patient

Important Health Care Initiatives and Trends

Many recent national initiatives attempt to improve quality and safety of patient care, standardize practice patterns, provide more transparency about hospital outcomes, and nudge heterogeneous health care systems into the electronic age (**Table 4**). In a health care system with many stakeholders with varying and sometimes conflicting goals, there is an

TABLE 3.	Common Terms Used in the Interpretation of the Medical Literature for Diagnostic Tests		
Term	**Definition**	**Calculation**	**Notes**
Prevalence (Prev)	Proportion of patients with disease in the population	Prev = (TP + FN) / (TP + FP + FN + TN)	
Sensitivity (Sn)	Proportion of patients with disease who have a positive test	Sn = TP / (TP + FN)	
Specificity (Sp)	Proportion of patients without disease who have a negative test	Sp = TN / (FP + TN)	
Positive predictive value (PPV)	Proportion of patients with a positive test who have disease	PPV = TP / (TP + FP)	Increases with *increasing* prevalence
Negative predictive value (NPV)	Proportion of patients with a negative test who do not have disease	NPV = TN / (TN + FN)	Increases with *decreasing* prevalence
Positive likelihood ratio (LR+)	The likelihood that a positive test result would be expected in a patient with the disease that a positive test result would be expected in a patient without a disease	LR+ = Sn / (1 − Sp)	
Negative likelihood ratio (LR−)	The likelihood that a negative test result would be expected in a patient with the disease compared with the likelihood that a negative test result would be expected in a patient without a disease	LR− = (1 − Sn) / Sp	
Pretest odds	The odds that a patient has the disease before the test is performed	Pretest odds = $\dfrac{\text{pretest probability}}{1 - \text{pretest probability}}$	
Posttest odds	The odds that a patient has the disease after a test is performed	Posttest odds = pretest odds × LR	LR+ is used if result of test is positive; LR− is used if result of test is negative. A nomogram is available to calculate posttest probability using pretest probability and LR without having to convert pretest probability to odds (see www.cebm.net/index.aspx?o=1043)
Pretest probability	Proportion of patients with the disease before a test is performed	Pretest probability can be estimated from population prevalence, clinical risk calculators, or clinical experience if no evidence-based tools exist	
Posttest probability	Proportion of patients with the disease after a test is performed	Posttest probability = $\dfrac{\text{posttest odds}}{1 + \text{posttest odds}}$	

FN = false negative; FP = false positive; TN = true negative; TP = true positive.

increasing drive to stress value—health outcomes achieved per dollar spent—for the patient above all else.

Value in health care is defined by the outcomes achieved rather than by the volumes of procedures performed or services rendered. To determine value, the measurement of processes and their improvement is trumped by the measurement of clinical outcomes and the economic costs of attaining those outcomes. This measurement can be complex. For example, measurement of the outcome of care of a patient with cardiovascular disease should include the costs of treating comorbidities or contributory risk factors, such as hypertension, hyperlipidemia, and obesity, as well as the costs associated with potential adverse effects of treatments.

Frail elderly persons with limited life expectancies should have different outcome measures than younger adults. For example, seeking to achieve a hemoglobin A_{1c} level below 7% in an 80-year-old woman with multiple comorbidities who is recently diagnosed with diabetes mellitus would have less value (in terms of improved clinical outcomes, potential adverse effects, and economic costs) than achieving that clinical target in a young adult recently diagnosed with diabetes.

TABLE 4. Important Health Care Initiatives, Organizations, and Terms

Term	Definition	Additional Resources
Diabetes Recognition Program (DRP)	A voluntary NCQA program designed to provide clinicians with tools to support the delivery and recognition of consistent high quality care in diabetes	www.ncqa.org/tabid/139/Default.aspx
Electronic Health Record (EHR) incentive program	Medicare program to provide incentive payments to physicians and hospitals that demonstrate meaningful use of certified EHR technology	www.cms.gov/ehrincentiveprograms
Healthcare Effectiveness Data and Information Set (HEDIS)	Measures that are widely used across health systems (e.g., β-blocker use after myocardial infarction or breast cancer screening)	www.ncqa.org/tabid/187/default.aspx
Hospital Compare	U.S. Health and Human Services (HHS) Web site that compares Medicare data between hospitals	hospitalcompare.hhs.gov
Physician Quality Reporting System (PQRS [formerly PQRI])	The 2006 Tax Relief and Health Care Act required the establishment of a physician quality reporting system, including an incentive payment for eligible professionals who satisfactorily report data on quality measures for covered professional services furnished to Medicare beneficiaries	www.cms.gov/pqri
National Committee for Quality Assurance (NCQA)	Not-for-profit organization dedicated to improving health care quality	www.ncqa.org/tabid/675/Default.aspx
Accountable care organization (ACO)	A formally organized entity comprising physicians (primary care, specialists, subspecialists) and other health service professionals that is responsible through contracts with payers for providing a broad set of health care services to a specific population of people. A key goal of the ACO structure is to control growth of health care costs while maintaining or improving quality of care.	www.acponline.org/ppvl/policies/aco.pdf
Concierge medicine	Relationship between a patient and a physician in which the patient pays an annual fee for increased access to that physician	www.physiciansnews.com/business/204.kalogredis.html
Electronic prescribing	Computer-based electronic generation, transmission, and filling of a prescription, taking the place of paper and faxed prescriptions	www.ama-assn.org/ama/pub/physician-resources/health-informationtechnology/health-it-basics/eprescribing.page
Patient-centered medical home (PCMH)	Team-based model of care led by primary care physician providing continuous, coordinated care for the patient	www.acponline.org/running_practice/pcmh/
Pay for performance (P4P)	Payment to providers of health care based upon quality of care rather than just services provided	www.ahrq.gov/qual/pay4per.htm

In practice, many quality performance measures assess compliance with care processes rather than the outcomes of those processes. For example, all of the more than 70 Healthcare Effectiveness Data and Information Set (HEDIS) measures updated by the National Committee for Quality Assurance (NCQA) each year are process measures. None are outcome measurements. This method of quality improvement attempts to standardize the provision of care by different providers (for example, measurement of hemoglobin A_{1c} in patients with diabetes) but rarely measures the actual outcomes of that care (for example, risk of microvascular or macrovascular disease in diabetes). Performance measures stressing value will emphasize outcomes and the costs to achieve those outcomes more heavily than the processes utilized in care. Practicing physicians will need to be vigilant for the types of metrics by which they are measured, both responding to and influencing the development of specific process and outcome care measures.

Screening

Screening, which typically refers to the identification of a condition in the asymptomatic state, should be reserved for common conditions, with well-understood natural histories, that have significant negative consequences on society and for which early detection provides clinical benefits. Early detection and treatment of the condition should lead to increased survival or improved quality of life compared with identification at a later, symptomatic stage. The screening test needs to be acceptable to persons available for screening and should possess adequate sensitivity and specificity such that the frequency of false-positive and false-negative results is minimized.

Evaluating the effectiveness of screening tests in reducing morbidity and mortality is best accomplished with randomized controlled trials. Three types of bias are commonly observed in such studies. *Lead-time bias* occurs when a screening test leads to earlier identification of a condition, and an apparent improvement in 5-year survival, but does not actually result in improved mortality. *Length bias* occurs when the variable rate of progression of a disease is not accounted for. For example, a patient with a prolonged asymptomatic phase (for example, a slowly progressing cancer) has a greater likelihood of being identified in a screening study than a patient with a more rapidly progressing cancer. This results in an apparent—but not actual—survival benefit. *Overdiagnosis* in screening refers to the identification of cancers that are not destined to progress, thereby inflating survival statistics.

Balancing the benefits of screening with the potential to identify inaccurate or insignificant findings that lead to additional low yield, high cost, and low value testing; increased patient anxiety; and possible harm to patients requires an understanding of specific screening tests and their appropriate use. The American College of Physicians (ACP) has developed a number of clinical practice guidelines, guidance statements, and best practice statements to help understand the optimal use of specific screening tests. The U.S. Preventive Services Task Force (USPSTF) has systematically reviewed the available evidence and published evidence-based recommendations on screening for a wide range of conditions (www.uspreventiveservicestaskforce .org/recommendations.htm). **Table 5** summarizes these recommendations (see Geriatric Medicine for preventive care measures specific to the geriatric patient). A Web-based and mobile application for use at the point of care to individualize screening recommendations from the USPSTF is available (http://epss.ahrq.gov/PDA/index.jsp). Other organizations also publish focused guidelines for proper use of screening tests, and multiple clinical calculators and risk assessment tools are available to assess the need for specific screening tests.

TABLE 5.	Summary of USPSTF Screening Recommendations
Condition	**Recommendation**
Depression	All adults, when appropriate support system available
Alcohol misuse	All adults
Obesity	All adults
Hypertension	All adults
Lipid disorders	All men ≥35 years of age; consider in men 20-35 years of age with increased cardiovascular risk. Women ≥45 years of age with increased cardiovascular risk; consider in women 20-45 years of age with increased cardiovascular risk.
Diabetes mellitus	All adults with sustained blood pressure >135/80 mm Hg
Osteoporosis	Women ≥65 years of age; any other woman whose fracture risk is ≥ that of a 65-year old white woman without additional risk factors.
Abdominal aortic aneurysm	One-time screening in all men 65-75 years of age who have ever smoked
HIV infection	All persons at increased risk of HIV infection
Hepatitis B virus infection	All pregnant women at the first prenatal visit
Chlamydial infection	All women ≤24 years of age who are sexually active; all women >24 years of age who are at increased risk of infection.
Gonorrhea	Sexually active women who are at increased risk of infection
Asymptomatic bacteriuria	Pregnant women at 12-16 weeks' gestation or at the first prenatal visit, whichever comes first.
Syphilis	High-risk persons and pregnant women
Breast cancer	Biennial screening mammography for average-risk women 50-74 years of age; initiation of screening between 40 and 49 years of age should be individualized.
Cervical cancer	Screen with Pap smear: initiate no sooner than 21 years of age; test every 3 years thereafter or, for women aged 30-65 years who want to lengthen the duration of screening, every 5 years if combined with HPV testing. Screening is not indicated in women following hysterectomy and without previous high-risk Pap smears. Screening may be discontinued at age 65 years in non–high-risk women with no recent abnormal Pap smears.
Colon cancer	All adults 50-75 years of age (see MKSAP 16 Gastroenterology and Hepatology)

HPV = human papillomavirus; USPSTF = U.S. Preventive Services Task Force.

Screening During the History and Physical Examination

The USPSTF recommends screening adults for depression when appropriate supports are available for accurate diagnosis, treatment, and follow up. There is little evidence to support one screening method over another, although evidence suggests that asking two questions ("Over the past 2 weeks, have you felt down, depressed, or hopeless?" and "Over the past 2 weeks, have you felt little interest or pleasure in doing things?") will detect almost all cases of significant depression and may be as effective as longer instruments. There is also evidence that asking only one question, "Have you felt sad or depressed much of the time during the past year?" is also effective. A positive response to any of these questions requires additional assessment to determine diagnosis and treatment.

Several organizations, including the USPSTF, the American Medical Association, the American Society of Addiction Medicine, and the Canadian Task Force on Preventive Health Care recommend screening and performing behavioral counseling interventions to reduce alcohol misuse by adults. The USPSTF recommends that all adults be asked about tobacco use. Although the USPSTF concludes that there is insufficient evidence to recommend screening for illicit substance use, they also conclude that there is little evidence of harms associated with either screening or subsequent behavioral interventions. Screening for alcohol misuse, smoking, and drug use is discussed further in Lifestyle Risk Factors.

Owing to the increasing rate of obesity in our society, the USPSTF recommends screening all adults for obesity and, for those determined to be obese, to offer intensive counseling and behavioral interventions to promote sustained weight loss.

The USPSTF recommends screening all adults age 18 years and older for hypertension but concludes that evidence is lacking regarding the optimal interval of screening. The Seventh Report of the Joint National Committee on Prevention, Detection, Evaluation, and Treatment of High Blood Pressure (JNC 7) recommends screening every 2 years for those with blood pressures of less than 120/80 mm Hg and every year for those with systolic blood pressures of 120 to 139 mm Hg and diastolic blood pressures of 80 to 89 mm Hg. According to JNC 7 guidelines, the mean of two or more seated clinic measurements should be used to make the diagnosis of hypertension. A recent study confirms the importance of using multiple measurements to make the diagnosis of hypertension and the potential error in using only one measurement.

Because of insufficient evidence, the USPSTF does not recommend for or against screening for glaucoma in adults or for either visual acuity or dementia in older adults. There was also insufficient evidence for the USPSTF to recommend for or against screening for family and intimate partner violence among children, women, and older adults.

Periodic Health Examination

Although most Americans view the periodic health examination as essential to high quality care, the value of the periodic health examination for healthy, asymptomatic adults is debatable and there is no consensus interval. At the very least, it appears that the periodic health examination improves the delivery of some preventive services and reduces patient worry. Executive periodic physical examinations, frequently performed on behalf of many corporations, remain controversial without clear evidence of benefit.

Specific Screening Tests

The USPSTF strongly recommends screening for dyslipidemia in certain populations based on age, sex, and cardiovascular risk factors (see Table 5). The National Cholesterol Education Program's Adult Treatment Program III recommends obtaining a fasting lipid profile once every 5 years in all adults over the age of 20 years with a normal initial lipid profile (see Dyslipidemia for specific lipid values).

The USPSTF recommends screening for type 2 diabetes in asymptomatic adults with a sustained blood pressure of greater than 135/80 mm Hg. In contrast, the American Diabetes Association recommends screening all adults age 45 years and older without risk factors and all adults with a BMI of equal to or greater than 25 who have one or more of the following risk factors: gestational diabetes, hypertension, hyperlipidemia, and family history of type 2 diabetes in a first-degree relative. Appropriate screening tests include a fasting plasma glucose level, hemoglobin A_{1c} level, or a 2-h, 75-g oral glucose tolerance test. The USPSTF concludes that there is insufficient evidence regarding screening for gestational diabetes.

The USPSTF recommends screening for osteoporosis in all women age 65 years or older and also in younger women with an elevated fracture risk. Although the USPSTF concludes that evidence is insufficient to recommend screening in men, ACP practice guidelines from 2008 recommend screening those men who are at increased risk. The USPSTF currently has no guidelines regarding screening for vitamin D deficiency.

According to the USPSTF, screening for abdominal aortic aneurysm (AAA) should be performed with abdominal ultrasonography on a one-time basis in all men between the ages of 65 and 75 years who have ever smoked (defined as 100 lifetime cigarettes). They make no recommendation for or against screening men who have never smoked and recommend against routine screening for AAA in women regardless of smoking history.

The USPSTF recommends against screening for the following conditions: carotid artery stenosis, COPD, hereditary hemochromatosis, and peripheral arterial disease. Screening for coronary artery disease is not recommended in low-risk persons, and the evidence for screening high-risk persons is inconclusive, as is the evidence for screening using nontraditional risk factors, such as high-sensitivity C-reactive protein level, homocysteine level, Lp(a) lipoprotein level, ankle-brachial index, carotid intima-media thickness, and coronary artery calcium score. Owing to insufficient evidence, the USPSTF does not recommend for or against screening for thyroid disease.

Screening for Infectious Diseases

The Centers for Disease Control and Prevention (CDC) recommend that all persons between the ages of 13 and 64 years be screened for HIV infection, whereas the USPSTF recommends screening only persons at increased risk of infection. In addition, the USPSTF recommends that all pregnant women be screened for HIV infection.

The USPSTF strongly recommends screening for hepatitis B virus infection in all pregnant women at their first prenatal visit but otherwise recommends against routine screening.

The USPSTF recommends against routine screening for hepatitis C virus infection in the general population and found insufficient evidence to recommend for or against screening in persons at increased risk. The CDC recommends screening persons at increased risk of infection (history of illicit injection drug use, history of receiving clotting factors before 1987 or blood products or organs before 1992, or on chronic hemodialysis at any time). Additionally, the CDC recommends one-time testing for baby boomers (born 1945-1965) regardless of risk factors, followed by a brief screening for alcohol use in those identified as having hepatitis C virus infection.

The USPSTF recommends screening for chlamydial infection in all women 24 years of age or younger who are sexually active and all women older than 24 years who are at increased risk of infection (history of sexually transmitted infection [STI], new or multiple sexual partners, inconsistent condom use, or exchanging sex for drugs or money). There is insufficient evidence to recommend for or against chlamydial infection screening in men.

According to the USPSTF, screening for gonorrhea infection should be limited to sexually active women who are at increased risk of infection (same risk factors as for chlamydial infection). The task force recommends against screening low-risk men and women and states that there is insufficient evidence for screening in all other groups.

Although the USPSTF recommends against screening for asymptomatic bacteriuria in men and nonpregnant women, it supports screening with urine culture for pregnant women at 12 to 16 weeks' gestation or at the first prenatal visit, whichever comes first. Syphilis screening is recommended in all high-risk persons and in all pregnant women but not in other persons.

Cancer Screening Tests

Breast Cancer Screening

Age is the most important risk factor for women developing breast cancer. A woman's individual risk of developing breast cancer can be determined using the breast cancer risk assessment tool (www.cancer.gov/bcrisktool), which is based on the Gail model.

Mammography, the most widely used method of screening for breast cancer, is the only available breast cancer screening modality that has been shown to reduce mortality, with the strongest evidence for its use being in average-risk women between the ages of 50 and 69 years. Screening mammography may be less effective for average-risk women between the ages of 40 and 49 years owing to the lower incidence of breast cancer and lower accuracy of mammography in this age group. Whereas two randomized controlled trials have demonstrated the benefits of screening mammography in average-risk women between the ages of 70 and 74 years, evidence for the benefits of screening mammography is lacking for women age 75 years and older.

The optimal frequency of mammography screening is unclear for all age groups. For average-risk women, the USPSTF recommends performing biennial screening mammography for women ages 50 to 74 years. This approach yields a median breast cancer reduction of 16.5% compared with no screening (number needed to invite [NNI] to screening to prevent one breast cancer death = 1339, ages 50-59 years; NNI = 377, ages 60-69 years). In contrast, the USPSTF states that initiation of screening between the ages of 40 and 49 years (NNI = 1904) should be individualized, taking into account both the patient's risk and the testing characteristics of mammography. The ACP provides similar recommendations for women in their 40s. A recent study supports these recommendations, finding that mammography performed every 2 years was effective in women with relatively high breast density or who possess additional risk factors for developing breast cancer. The American Cancer Society (ACS), American Medical Association, American College of Obstetricians and Gynecologists (ACOG), and the National Comprehensive Cancer Network (NCCN) all recommend beginning annual mammography at the age of 40 years. The ACS does not recommend using MRI for breast cancer screening in average-risk women and finds the evidence regarding breast self-examination to be insufficient. No mention is made of what age to stop annual screening mammography in the ACOG, ACS, or NCCN guidelines.

Women who are either *BRCA1* or *BRCA2* mutation carriers have a high risk of developing breast cancer by the age of 70 years (65% and 45%, respectively). Despite most patients having a family history of breast cancer, less than 10% of all women with breast cancer have an inherited genetic mutation. Features of the family history that should raise concern for an inherited syndrome include having multiple affected family members, young age at time of diagnosis, and the presence of multiple primary tumors. The USPSTF and NCCN both recommend referral to a geneticist if concern exists for an inherited syndrome. The ACS recommends screening with annual MRI alternating every

6 months with annual mammography for women with a greater than 25% lifetime risk of developing breast cancer beginning at the age of 30 years and continuing as long as the woman is in good health.

Based on the results of the Study of Tamoxifen and Raloxifene (STAR) trial, which demonstrated a 50% reduction in the incidence of hormone receptor–invasive breast cancer with the use of these agents, postmenopausal women with a ≥1.66 risk of developing breast cancer over the next 5 years based on the Gail model should be offered a 5-year course of either tamoxifen or raloxifene.

Cervical and Anal Cancer Screening
Screening with conventional cervical cytology (Pap smear) results in a 95% decrease in mortality from cervical cancer. **Table 6** summarizes the recommendations from major professional organizations. Owing to poor specificity, screening with human papillomavirus (HPV) DNA testing alone is not recommended, although clinicians can consider using HPV DNA testing along with cervical cytology in women age 30 years and older to help guide further investigation and decrease the frequency of testing.

If cervical cytology is interpreted as unsatisfactory, the test should be immediately repeated. When interpreted as atypical squamous cells of undetermined significance, acceptable options include referring for colposcopy, obtaining HPV DNA testing and then referring for colposcopy if positive, or repeating the Pap smear in 6 to 12 months. With any other abnormal result, the patient should be referred for colposcopy.

Although some experts recommend anal cytologic screening for anal cancer in high-risk persons (persons who practice receptive anal intercourse, have known anal HPV infection, or who have HIV infection), the USPSTF, ACS, and the CDC do not currently recommend such screening.

Prostate Cancer Screening
Owing to limitations of currently available screening tests and unclear benefits of screening, prostate cancer screening remains controversial. The two most commonly used methods of screening for prostate cancer include prostate-specific antigen (PSA) measurement and digital rectal examination (DRE), with the former being more sensitive.

The USPSTF has concluded that the harms of screening for prostate cancer outweigh the benefits in men of any age regardless of risk factors. In contrast, the ACS and American Urological Association (AUA) recommend offering both PSA measurement and DRE to men on an annual basis beginning at the age of 50 years. The ACP and American Academy of Family Physicians (AAFP) both recommend that clinicians have individualized discussions with their patients regarding obtaining PSA measurements and support obtaining PSA levels after such discussions in patients 50 years and older who have life expectancies of at least 10 years. Men should be informed about the gaps in the evidence and should be assisted in considering their personal preferences before deciding whether or not to be tested. The presence of benign prostatic hyperplasia symptoms should not increase the propensity to screen for prostate cancer with PSA testing.

Additional Cancer Screening Tests
The USPSTF recommends against routine screening for bladder, ovarian, and pancreatic cancers. The USPSTF concludes that the evidence is insufficient to recommend for or against screening for skin and oral cancer. The USPSTF recommends that fair-skinned persons aged 10 to 24 years be counseled about reducing their exposure to ultraviolet radiation to reduce the risk of skin cancer. Colon cancer screening is discussed in depth in MKSAP 16 Gastroenterology and Hepatology.

TABLE 6. Recommendations for Cervical Cancer Screening from Major Professional Organizations			
Professional Organization	**Age to Initiate Screening**	**Screening Interval**	**Age to Discontinue Screening**
American Cancer Society	21 y	Ages 21-29 y: cytology alone every 3 y Ages 30-65 y: cytology alone every 3 y, or cytology with HPV co-testing every 5 y	65 y if no recent abnormal Pap smears and no risk factors
U.S. Preventive Services Task Force	21 y	Every 3 y, or every 5 y with HPV co-testing for women ages 30-65 y	65 y if no recent abnormal Pap smears and no risk factors
American College of Obstetrics and Gynecology	21 y	Ages 21-29 y: cytology alone every 2 y Ages 30-65 y: cytology alone every 3 y if three consecutive Pap smears have been negative and no risk factors	65-70 y if three or more consecutive negative Pap smears, including no abnormal Pap smears within the past 10 years, and no risk factors

NOTE: Risk factors for cervical cancer: history of in utero diethylstilbestrol exposure, immunocompromise, HIV positivity.

HPV = human papillomavirus.

KEY POINTS

- The U.S. Preventive Services Task Force recommends periodic screening for alcohol misuse, smoking, obesity, and hypertension in all adults and for hyperlipidemia, osteoporosis (women), and abdominal aortic aneurysm (men, one-time screening) based on age and risk factors.
- The U.S. Preventive Services Task Force recommends pregnant women be screened for HIV infection, hepatitis B virus infection, syphilis, and asymptomatic bacteriuria.
- The U.S. Preventive Services Task Force recommends screening persons at increased risk for sexually transmitted infections for HIV infection, hepatitis C virus infection, chlamydial infection (women), and gonorrhea infection (women).
- The U.S. Preventive Services Task Force recommends periodic screening for breast cancer (women ≥50 years of age), cervical cancer, and colon cancer (50-75 years of age).

Family History and Genetic Testing

Taking a Family History

Family history has an important role in the practice of medicine; it can motivate behavior change, help prevent or predict disease, and improve health outcomes. As many common diseases have genetic contributions, obtaining a family history may identify patients who would benefit from genetic testing. For the clinician, the details of the family history help establish the risk (or pretest probability) of genetically associated disease in an individual patient, and forms the basis upon which clinical decisions regarding the need for additional testing may be made.

The definition of *family* may differ among patients, so clarification may be necessary. The accuracy of the information obtained may vary based on the method by which it is obtained (for example, through standardized form, computer, or in person) as well as on patient characteristics.

Key elements of a family history include number of relatives affected by a condition, relationship degree, gender, age at onset, ethnicity, and lineage (maternal or paternal). Additional demographic and environmental data may be needed, as these may modify risk. Available evidence suggests that patients are better at reporting information on first-degree relatives and are more accurate in reporting the absence than the presence of diseases. Older persons report more accurate family histories than younger persons; women and persons with higher educational levels report more information.

Barriers to obtaining an accurate family history include patient understanding, lack of available knowledge about family medical issues, desire to hide or protect, anxiety about subsequent testing or procedures, and fear of psychological harm. Provider barriers include limited clinic time, lack of tools to analyze and interpret data, and lack of understanding of the implications of the data, especially regarding necessity of further genetic testing.

Caveats to Genetic Testing

The advent of greater availability to the public of genetic tests through direct-to-consumer marketing of personal DNA analysis is likely to have an effect on the process of genetic testing and counseling. Current recommendations support the concept that knowledge of one's DNA is only one component of a complex process. As demand for genetic knowledge increases, primary care providers may be asked to weigh in on issues for which they were not specifically trained. The American College of Medical Genetics recommends that a knowledgeable health care provider be involved in the process of ordering and interpreting genetic tests, that the patient be informed about what the test can actually reveal, and that attention be paid to privacy issues as well as the potential psychological impact of knowing that one is a carrier of a genetic disease.

Specific components of genetic testing should include the following: ethical considerations, including patient autonomy regarding the decision to test and the amount of information the patient wishes to know (the right "not to know"); legal considerations, including informed consent and confidentiality; and issues of potential genetic discrimination by the employment or insurance sectors. In addition, religious and cultural considerations may come into play. Patients should be made aware that not all genetic testing and counseling is covered by insurance plans. Finally, providers may be faced with family members who do not wish to disclose information to others who may be affected, thus creating an ethical conflict for the provider.

Referral for Genetic Counseling

Controversy exists as to whether primary care providers have the training to provide adequate genetic counseling. However, the supply of trained genetic specialists may currently be inadequate for providing all recommended genetic counseling services. Different types of genetic tests require different levels of genetic counseling. In more routine testing, in which adequate physician training and patient education materials are available (for example, routine prenatal testing for α-fetoprotein and markers for inborn errors of metabolism), referral may not be necessary. Recommendations for referral for genetic counseling include situations in which patients, families, or providers require assistance in interpreting family and medical histories to assess chance of disease and whether genetic testing is an option, and to promote informed choices about further actions based on risk.

Specific indications for genetic testing include the following: to diagnose a condition in a person with signs and symptoms of a disease; to assess risk status for a family member who may be an asymptomatic carrier or at risk to develop a disease (for example, muscular dystrophy, cystic fibrosis, Huntington disease); concerns about cancer risk based on family history; an abnormal prenatal or newborn screening test that may indicate increased risk of a genetic disorder; concern about risk to a future pregnancy because of family history, maternal age, or a previous abnormal pregnancy outcome; maternal exposure to teratogens; or an ethnic background suggesting an increased risk for a genetic disease (for example, sickle cell disease, thalassemia, Tay-Sachs disease, or Fanconi anemia).

The genetic counseling process includes a complete genetic pedigree, usually of three generations; risk assessment; review of medical records; physical examination of the patient and/or relatives; laboratory testing as appropriate; a discussion of options and potential courses of action; and a thorough explanation of the potential consequences of the genetic testing process. Genetic counselors may also recommend to test or not to test and must always provide posttest counseling.

KEY POINT

- Recommendations regarding genetic testing include that a knowledgeable health care provider be involved in the process of ordering and interpreting genetic tests, that the patient be informed about what the test can actually reveal, and that attention be paid to privacy issues as well as the potential psychological impact of knowing that one is a carrier of a genetic disease.

Immunization

Immunization is a cornerstone of both pediatric and adult preventive care and a major component of public health policy. Vaccination, or the administration of live, attenuated virus or inactivated virus proteins, can protect a person from acquiring, having complications from, or dying of an infection. Vaccination also reduces transmission and spread of a disease in the population at large, thereby helping even unvaccinated persons. More than 24 different vaccines are currently available for clinical use. Recommendations for their use are updated frequently by the CDC's Advisory Committee on Immunization Practices (ACIP). Current recommendations are available at www.cdc.gov/vaccines/pubs/ACIP-list.htm. Although a few vaccinations are recommended for all adults, most are limited to persons of a specific age group or with certain comorbid illnesses (**Table 7**).

A comprehensive approach to vaccination requires information about previous vaccination as well as current health and comorbid conditions. Many recommendations have changed over time, and adults may need "catch-up" vaccinations. Clinicians should pay particular attention to previous vaccination for pertussis, pneumococcal disease, human papillomavirus, and herpes zoster, as recommendations regarding these vaccinations are newer or have recently changed. Unfortunately, patients may not remember previous vaccinations, and documentation of childhood vaccination may be difficult to obtain. Patient self-report should only be considered valid for influenza and pneumococcal vaccination. For all other vaccines, clinicians should either revaccinate for age-appropriate diseases or obtain serology to document immunity viruses.

TABLE 7. Summary of Recommendations for Vaccines for Adults[a]		
Vaccine	**Type**	**Indications**
Influenza	Live, attenuated or inactivated	All adults
Tetanus, diphtheria, pertussis (Td, Tdap)	Inactivated	All adults. Booster every 10 y. One-time Tdap for all (see text)
Varicella	Live, attenuated	Persons born after 1980, HCWs, persons with ↑ risk of disseminated varicella without documented vaccination or immunity.
Herpes zoster	Live, attenuated	Adults ≥60 y
Pneumococcal disease	Inactivated	Adults ≥65 y; adults 19-64 y with risk factors (see Table 8)
Human papillomavirus	Inactivated	Females 11-26 y; males 11-21 y (permitted 21-26 y)
Measles, mumps, rubella	Live, attenuated	Adults born after 1957 without documented vaccination or immunity. One dose usually sufficient; second dose indicated in HCWs, international travelers, college students, and post-exposure.
Meningococcal disease	Inactivated	Adolescents; persons living in dormitories; persons with HIV or asplenia
Hepatitis A	Inactivated	Travelers to endemic areas, men who have sex with men, users of illicit drugs, persons with chronic liver disease.
Hepatitis B	Inactivated	Adults with increased risk of transmission, morbidity, or exposure (see Table 9)

HCW = health care worker.

[a]Full recommendations are available at www.cdc.gov/vaccines/pubs/ACIP-list.htm.

Vaccines with live, attenuated virus are generally contraindicated in patients with immunodeficiency, although most patients with HIV infection with a CD4 cell count above 200/microliter can receive these vaccines. Inactivated vaccines typically are contraindicated only when the patient has had an allergic reaction to the vaccine. In order to achieve a sustained immunologic response, most immunizations require a series of vaccinations. Manufacturer's guidelines for vaccines indicate the minimum interval between vaccinations, and good immunologic response is typically seen if longer intervals are used. Thus, in patients whose vaccination series was interrupted (for example, a patient who received only two of three injections in a series), the clinician can resume a vaccination series where it was interrupted. Restarting a vaccination sequence is rarely, if ever, required. Although most vaccines should not be given to a patient with a serious acute illness, a patient with mild or moderate disease (such as upper respiratory tract infection), even if associated with fever, can be vaccinated. Multiple vaccines can be given at the same time, although each should be administered at a different site.

Vaccinations Recommended for All Adults

Influenza
Influenza is a respiratory virus that spreads seasonally, with peak activity typically in the fall and winter. Because of antigenic drift, a different strain typically circulates each year, and immunity to the previous year's influenza (vaccine-induced or natural) is not protective of future infection. Vaccination has been shown to reduce incidence, morbidity, and mortality from influenza, and is thought to provide a public health benefit by reducing community spread of influenza. Two types of vaccination are used: a live, attenuated vaccine and an inactivated vaccine. Each is developed during the spring based on projections of the most likely strains to be responsible for the following winter's infections. The live, attenuated vaccine is administered as a single intranasal infusion and is approved for nonpregnant persons from 2 years to 49 years of age without medical conditions that predispose to influenza or its complications (see below). The inactivated vaccine is given as a single intramuscular injection and is approved for adults of any age. Both types are contraindicated in patients with a history of Guillain-Barré syndrome after influenza or severe egg allergy (for example, anaphylaxis), as the vaccine is produced in chicken eggs. Patients without a history of severe egg allergy can be vaccinated, although some patients should be observed for 30 minutes after inoculation. The inactivated vaccine often produces local reaction at the vaccine site and may induce a brief period of myalgia and low-grade fever. The live, attenuated vaccine frequently has side effects of rhinorrhea, headache, and cough. Between 10% and 78% of recipients of either vaccine will have a mild adverse effect.

Influenza vaccination is currently recommended for all adults, although in a time of scarcity, patients more likely to become infected by or develop serious complications from influenza should be prioritized. This includes patients older than 50 years and those younger than 50 years who have cardiovascular disease, pulmonary disease, or immunodeficiency. In addition, health care workers should be prioritized. Vaccination can start whenever the vaccine is available; mass vaccination events should be planned starting in the fall. Clinicians should continue offering vaccination until influenza activity fades in their community, typically in March or April.

Each season, vaccines contain influenza A (including H1N1) and influenza B.

Tetanus, Diphtheria, and Pertussis
Primary vaccination for tetanus and diphtheria (Td) with a three-shot series in childhood followed by booster vaccination every 10 years is highly effective in preventing these diseases. The incidence of adult pertussis has been rising, likely due in part to a declining immunity among adults. Therefore, all adults 19 years and older who have not received a dose of Tdap (tetanus and diphtheria combined with acellular pertussis) should be administered a dose regardless of the interval since their last tetanus and diphtheria toxoid–containing vaccine (although it may also be given in place of a scheduled decennial Td booster). Because recent data suggest that the actual burden of pertussis in persons older than 65 years may be at least 100 times greater than previously reported, pertussis vaccination with at least one dose of Tdap is particularly important in this patient population. Postpartum women, health care workers, and adults who have close contact with infants younger than 12 months (such as child-care workers and grandparents) should also receive a one-time booster of Tdap regardless of the timing of their last Td booster. As this is a relatively recent update, many adults currently coming due for their Td booster should more appropriately receive Tdap.

Vaccinations Recommended for Some Adults

Varicella and Herpes Zoster
The primary focus of varicella immunization is in pediatric care, and childhood vaccination has been recommended since 1996. Persons born before 1980 in the United States are considered likely to have immunity resulting from childhood exposure. Persons born after 1980, health care workers, and those born before 1980 who have a high risk for disseminated varicella should receive a two-dose varicella vaccination series unless they have serologic evidence of varicella immunity or physician-documented evidence of either varicella or varicella vaccination. Patient or parent self-report is not considered reliable. Childhood recommendations changed in 2007 from a single to a two-step varicella vaccination, and some persons may need a single catch-up immunization.

Because the varicella vaccine is a live, attenuated vaccine, vaccination should be done with caution in immunocompromised patients. Pregnant women should not be vaccinated. Women who become pregnant within 1 month of vaccination should be counseled that there is a low risk of birth defects.

A more concentrated version of the live attenuated virus is used for immunization again herpes zoster. In clinical trials, vaccinated patients had a much lower rate of both herpes zoster and postherpetic neuralgia. All adults aged 60 years and older should be vaccinated unless vaccination is contraindicated because of immunodeficiency, regardless of whether they have experienced previous episodes of zoster.

Pneumococcal Disease

Immunization with the 23-valent pneumococcal polysaccharide vaccine decreases the risk of invasive pneumococcal disease. A single dose is recommended for all persons aged 65 years or older and those 19 to 64 years with specific risk factors (**Table 8**); these risk factors were broadened in 2010 to include smokers and persons with asthma. Revaccination after 5 years is recommended in patients who have asplenia or immunocompromise, including kidney failure. Patients vaccinated before age 65 years should receive a booster at 65 years, or 5 years after their initial vaccination if they were initially vaccinated between the ages of 60 and 64 years. There is no current recommendation for additional boosters and no recommendation for a booster for those vaccinated after age 65 years. A 13-valent pneumococcal conjugate vaccine is also available. The ACIP has approved its use in patients 19 years of age and older with immunocompromising conditions, defined as

functional or anatomic asplenia, HIV infection, cancer, advanced kidney disease, or other immunocompromising conditions; however, the recommended dosing regimen for these patients is not yet available. Although it is also FDA-approved for use in persons 50 years of age and older, the ACIP has not yet made a recommendation for its routine use in this patient population as an alternative to the polysaccharide vaccine.

Human Papillomavirus

Human papillomavirus (HPV) is the most common STI in the United States, and exposure to certain serotypes can lead to genital warts and cervical cancer. Vaccination against the most pathogenic serotypes has been shown to reduce infection with HPV as well as the development of precancerous cervical lesions and genital warts. The vaccine is an inactivated vaccine and is licensed for males and females between the ages of 9 and 26 years. Vaccination is recommended for all girls and boys starting at age 11 or 12 years. The CDC recommends catch-up vaccination of women to age 26 years and men to age 21 years but permits vaccination of men up to age 26 years. Both a bivalent and quadrivalent vaccine exist; both are licensed and recommended for females, but only the quadrivalent vaccine is recommended for males. Ideally, vaccination should begin before a person has sexual intercourse, but vaccination is still indicated in individuals who have had

TABLE 8. Indications for Pneumococcal Polysaccharide Vaccination in Adults 19 to 64 Years of Age[a]		
Patient Category	**Specific Indications**	**Dosing Interval**
Immunocompetent patients[b]	Chronic cardiovascular disease (including hypertension)	Single vaccination; single booster at age 65 y or 5 y after initial vaccination, whichever is later
	Chronic pulmonary disease (including asthma and COPD)	
	Diabetes mellitus	
	Chronic liver disease (including cirrhosis)	
	Alcoholism	
	Cigarette smoking	
	Cerebrospinal fluid leak	
	Cochlear implant	
Immunocompromised patients[c]	HIV infection	Two doses separated by 5 y
	Chronic kidney disease or nephrotic syndrome	
	Malignancy (leukemia, lymphoma, generalized malignancy)	
	Use of immunosuppressive treatment (corticosteroids, antirejection medication, radiation therapy)	
	Multiple myeloma	
	Congenital or acquired immunodeficiency	
Patients with asplenia[c]	Functional asplenia (sickle cell disease, other hemoglobinopathies)	Two doses separated by 5 y
	Anatomic asplenia (congenital, surgical, others)	

[a]Vaccination recommended for all adults aged 65 years or older.

[b]A 13-valent pneumococcal conjugate vaccine has been FDA approved for use in patients 50 years of age and older, although the ACIP has not made a recommendation for routine use in this patient population.

[c]A 13-valent pneumococcal conjugate vaccine has been approved by the ACIP for use in patients 19 years of age and older with immunocompromising conditions, defined as functional or anatomic asplenia, HIV infection, cancer, advanced kidney disease, or other immunocompromising conditions; however, the recommended dosing regimen for these patients is not yet available.

intercourse or even have evidence of HPV infection, as immunization can prevent infection with other serotypes. The vaccine is administered as a series of three injections.

Measles, Mumps, and Rubella

Measles, mumps, and rubella have been nearly eliminated in the United States after the introduction of universal childhood vaccination. Adults born before 1957 are considered immune to these diseases. Younger adults without either a documented history of immunization or documented immunity should receive a single dose of measles, mumps, and rubella (MMR) vaccine; this is especially important in women of reproductive age. Health care workers, persons exposed to measles or mumps, international travelers, and students in post-secondary education should receive a second vaccination. MMR is a live, attenuated vaccine that is contraindicated in severe immunodeficiency and pregnancy.

Meningococcal Disease

Vaccination against meningococcus is primarily recommended for adolescents. Unvaccinated adults living in college dormitories or who are in the military should receive a single dose, whereas those with asplenia, complement deficiencies, or HIV infection should receive two doses. Patients with asplenia and those with complement deficiencies should receive boosters every 5 years.

Hepatitis A

Universal vaccination of children against hepatitis A is currently recommended by the ACIP. As hepatitis A epidemics are typically spread by children, this strategy provides a combination of both individual and "herd" immunity and has decreased the extent of hepatitis A outbreaks among adults. Currently, hepatitis A vaccination is recommended for adults with increased likelihood of exposure, including travelers to endemic areas, men who have sex with men, and users of illicit drugs (both injected and noninjected drugs). Hepatitis A vaccination is also recommended for adults with chronic liver disease. The vaccination is not recommended for patients with chronic hepatitis B or C without evidence of liver dysfunction. Immunization typically consists of two injections separated by at least 6 months.

Hepatitis B

Hepatitis B is a vaccine-preventable disease with potential serious complications, and universal vaccination of children is currently recommended. In adults, vaccination is recommended for unvaccinated persons with increased risk of exposure from a sexual, percutaneous, or mucosal source; those planning travel to an endemic area; those with increased risk for morbidity; and any other person who requests vaccination (**Table 9**). Several vaccination strategies exist, all requiring at least three injections.

Special Considerations for Health Care Workers

Health care workers have additional vaccination requirements, both because of their potential exposures to disease and their ability to act as a vector to spread diseases to or between patients. All health care workers should be vaccinated against or have serologic evidence of immunity to hepatitis B, varicella, measles, mumps, and rubella; most employers routinely request or provide pre-employment screening and/or vaccination. In addition, health care workers should receive a one-time Tdap vaccination. Annual influenza vaccination is also recommended for all health care workers, and there have been efforts by some states to require these vaccinations.

TABLE 9. Indications for Adult Hepatitis B Vaccination	
Patient Category	**Specific Indications**
Increased risk of sexual transmission	More than one sex partners/6 months
	Men who have sex with men
	Evaluation or treatment for sexually transmitted infection
	Sex partner of a patient with hepatitis B
Increased risk of percutaneous or mucosal transmission	Current or recent injection drug user
	Close contact of a person with hepatitis B
	Resident or staff of long-term facility for developmentally disabled
	Health care worker or public-safety worker who may be exposed to blood or blood-contaminated fluids
	End-stage kidney disease
Increased risk of morbidity	HIV infection
	Chronic liver disease
	Diabetes mellitus (type 1 or 2) in ages 19-59 y (and at clinician's discretion for age ≥60 y)
Others	Travelers to countries with endemic hepatitis B
	Anyone who requests hepatitis B vaccination

- Annual influenza vaccination is recommended for all adults without contraindications.

- Herpes zoster vaccination is recommended for all adults older than 60 years without contraindications.

- Pneumococcal polysaccharide vaccination is recommended for all adults aged 65 years or older; younger persons who should receive the vaccine include those with specific risk factors, including smokers and those with asthma.

- All health care workers should be vaccinated against or have serologic evidence of immunity to hepatitis B, varicella, measles, mumps, and rubella, receive a one-time Tdap vaccination, and receive an annual influenza vaccination.

Lifestyle Risk Factors

Behavioral Counseling

Motivational interviewing describes a patient-centered counseling process whereby the provider engages the patient in behavior change and allows the patient to direct many aspects of the change process, exploring how behavior changes relate to their key goals and values. Many studies attest to the success of motivational interviewing for addressing dietary and lifestyle changes, substance abuse, and other behaviors known to be detrimental to patients' health. Many providers give patients information and advice in an effort to convince them to change behavior. In contrast, motivational interviewing uses patient-identified issues to initiate and continue the change process. Classic motivational interviewing teaches that patients may be ambivalent about making behavioral changes, and that the purpose of motivational interviewing is to encourage patients themselves to identify and voice reasons for making behavioral changes.

Components of motivational interviewing include using open-ended questions; inviting patients to consider how and why they might change behavior; eliciting patients' understanding of the problem or process and what they feel might be barriers to and facilitators of change; providing information and support; and accepting their current level of commitment to change. Key features of motivational interviewing are that the patient chooses the agenda, the provider is not in "control" and does not tell the patient what he or she should do, and the provider assesses the patient's sense of the importance of issues for him or her and level of confidence in making changes, which are usually small and incremental.

Motivational interviewing is one form of a *brief intervention*, which consists of delivering clear, concise advice designed to increase patients' awareness of an unhealthy behavior and its negative consequences. Brief interventions usually involve one or two counseling sessions of 10 to 30 minutes each, usually following a positive screen for unhealthy behaviors. Sessions as short as 5 minutes, referred to as *brief advice*, may also be effective. Brief interventions can easily be administered in a busy office setting, an emergency department, or other urgent-care or community-based settings. One framework for administering a brief intervention is the FRAMES (Feedback, Responsibility, Advice, Menu, Empathy, Self-efficacy) model, whereby clinicians provide *feedback* on risks, with an emphasis on the patient's *responsibility* to change behavior; clear *advice*, with a *menu* of change options; support and *empathy*; and facilitate the patient's *self-efficacy*. Brief interventions may be delivered by physicians, nurses, health educators, counselors, or via printed or computer-based information. Follow-up is critical to assess patient progress.

Diet and Physical Activity

Despite a large body of literature attesting to the benefits of counseling interventions for increasing physical activity, few studies have been performed in the primary care setting. Most studies that have demonstrated a benefit relied on specially trained health educators or nurses, counselors or psychologists, dietitians or nutritionists, or exercise instructors or physiologists; very few involved primary care providers.

A recent systematic review showed that medium- to high-intensity dietary behavioral counseling, with or without physical activity counseling, resulted in small but statistically significant improvements in adiposity, blood pressure, and cholesterol level, as well as moderate to large changes in self-reported dietary and physical activity behaviors. The evidence for changes in physiologic outcomes was strongest for high-intensity counseling interventions. Benefits beyond 1 year are limited and require continued high-intensity interventions, defined as frequent (monthly) contacts in person, by phone, or by e-mail. Several advisory groups recommend 150 minutes of leisure-time physical activity per week, usually broken into five 30-minute sessions weekly. Several national organizations recommend seeing a physician before embarking on an exercise program only if there is a history of heart disease or hypertension, musculoskeletal disorder, or if symptoms such as chest pain or dizziness have been experienced when trying to exercise in the past.

- Key features of motivational interviewing are that the patient chooses the agenda, the provider is not in "control" and does not tell the patient what he or she should do, and the provider assesses the patient's sense of the importance of issues for him or her and level of confidence in making changes, which are usually small and incremental.

- Physician evaluation before embarking on an exercise program is recommended only if there is a history of heart disease or hypertension, musculoskeletal disorder, or if symptoms such as chest pain or dizziness have been experienced when trying to exercise in the past.

Substance Use Disorders

Tobacco

Smoking is a leading cause of illness and death in the United States. Smoking is no longer viewed as a habit but as a chronic disease, and scientifically validated treatments are available for tobacco use and dependence. Thus, tobacco use assessment should be performed for all patients. Brief advice from a physician has been shown to increase tobacco cessation rates. Despite the availability of several FDA-approved medications for smoking cessation, the proportion of smokers who make quit attempts has increased very little, and many smokers who do attempt to quit do not take advantage of these new treatment options. In addition, innovative and more effective counseling strategies are needed, especially in adolescents and young adults.

Current recommendations are that all clinicians assess tobacco use at every visit, given the likely need for repeated quit attempts and the importance of reinforcing positive behaviors. Clinicians should encourage every patient to make a quit attempt and counsel the patient appropriately. One simple approach for use in the clinical setting is the 5 A's (Ask, Advise, Assess, Assist, and Arrange), wherein the clinician *asks* patients about their smoking status at every visit, *advises* them to quit, *assesses* their willingness/readiness to quit at this time, *assists* them with a quit plan, and *arranges* for follow-up. For smokers not ready to quit, motivational interviewing, with emphasis on nonconfrontational strategies and discussion of patient choices, has shown higher cessation rates than use of brief advice or usual care. High-intensity counseling (greater time and number of sessions) is more effective than low-intensity strategies; for clinicians with limited time, recommendations are to use adjunctive telephone counseling, as every state in the United States has telephone counseling quit line services. In addition, counseling that addresses practical problem-solving skills and social support has been shown to be more effective.

Combining counseling with medication use is more effective than either intervention alone. In addition, combinations of nicotine replacement therapy (available as nicotine gum, inhaler, lozenge, nasal spray, and patch) with bupropion have been shown to be more effective than either alone. Varenicline has been demonstrated to be more effective than bupropion, and combinations of varenicline with various nicotine replacement therapies have showed cessation rates higher than nicotine replacement or bupropion alone. Precautions for bupropion include contraindication in patients on monoamine oxidase inhibitors or with seizure or eating disorders; varenicline must be used with caution in patients with kidney impairment or on dialysis, and in patients with cardiovascular disorders; both drugs must be used with caution in patients with serious psychiatric illness, as they may cause neuropsychiatric symptoms such as personality changes, vivid dreams, or suicidal ideation. The specific method or medication chosen is less critical than that a cessation plan is agreed upon and arranged. The various options offer alternatives for patients with contraindications, side effects, or who have relapsed with one type of treatment.

Hospitalization provides a unique counseling opportunity for patients with smoking-related diseases, especially cardiovascular disease. Smoking cessation counseling that begins during hospitalization and continues after discharge increases the odds of long-term abstinence. The Joint Commission (formerly JCAHO) has instituted an accreditation requirement to provide tobacco cessation interventions for patients hospitalized for acute myocardial infarction, heart failure, and pneumonia. ◨

Alcohol

Alcohol misuse includes "risky" or "hazardous" and "harmful" drinking patterns. *Hazardous drinking* is a pattern of alcohol consumption that increases the risk of harmful consequences. *Harmful drinking* refers to alcohol consumption resulting in negative psychological, physical, and social effects but without meeting criteria for dependence. *Alcohol dependence* is a cluster of behavioral, cognitive, and physiologic phenomena that may develop after repeated alcohol use, which includes a strong desire to consume alcohol, impaired control over its use, persistent drinking despite harmful consequences, increased tolerance, and physical withdrawal when use is discontinued. A standard alcoholic beverage is considered to be one 16-ounce beer, one 5-ounce glass of wine, or one shot (1.5 ounces) of spirits.

The USPSTF recommends screening and counseling for all adults for alcohol use and abuse, identifying quantity and frequency of drinking, adverse consequences, and patterns of use. The Alcohol Use Disorders Identification Test (AUDIT) is the most studied screening tool for detecting alcohol-related problems in primary care settings. It consists of ten questions and is easy to administer; a three-question version (the AUDIT-C) is more sensitive but less specific than the ten-question AUDIT (www.hepatitis.va.gov/provider/tools/audit-c.asp). The four-item CAGE questionnaire may also be used. (Have you ever felt you should Cut down on your drinking? Have people Annoyed you by criticizing your drinking? Have you ever felt bad or Guilty about your drinking? Have you ever had a drink first thing in the morning to steady your nerves or get rid of a hangover [Eye-opener]?) With a cutoff of two positive answers, the CAGE questionnaire is 77% to 95% sensitive and 79% to 97% specific for detecting alcohol abuse or dependence in primary care settings and indicates that further assessment is warranted. The AUDIT is more sensitive than the CAGE questionnaire in identifying hazardous drinking and alcohol dependence, whereas the CAGE is easier to deliver in a primary care setting. The TWEAK test, designed specifically for pregnant women, identifies a lower level of alcohol use, as any amount of alcohol may be considered hazardous to the fetus. Clinicians should choose a screening test appropriate to their practice, and provide counseling and intervention when patients screen positive.

Effective interventions for alcohol-use disorders include counseling regarding appropriate amounts and negative consequences, and agreeing on goals for reducing alcohol intake. Sessions may be performed by the provider or other members of the health care team and are most effective when combined with other assistance such as Alcoholics Anonymous or specialty referral. Frequent follow-up and reassessment are important.

No guidelines clearly delineate how often alcohol screening should be performed; however, all adults should be screened and all women who are pregnant or contemplating pregnancy should be advised of the known ill effects of alcohol on the fetus. Patients with a history of alcohol or other substance abuse are at higher risk for alcohol abuse or relapse and should be screened frequently. The effects of screening adolescents are not known.

Drugs

Unlike alcohol use, all illicit drug use may be considered harmful as any use carries a risk for health and legal ramifications, even amounts and patterns of use that do not meet criteria for drug dependence. Patients with drug abuse are more likely to experience anxiety, depression, psychosis, chronic back and other pain disorders, peptic ulcer disease, headache, chronic lung disease (usually from associated tobacco use), and alcohol-related illnesses, such as pancreatitis, hepatitis, and gastritis. Additional risks associated with illicit drug use include unsafe sexual practices, STIs, and intravenous injection–associated complications.

Prevalence of drug use (illicit and prescription) is much lower than for alcohol and depends on the clinical setting. Several screening instruments have been validated for drug use in the primary care setting. The Alcohol Smoking and Substance Involvement Screening Test (ASSIST) may be used for tobacco, alcohol, marijuana, cocaine, stimulants, sedatives, opioids, and several other agents. It has excellent sensitivity and specificity but is considered too long for use in the primary care setting. The 10-item Drug Abuse Screening Test (DAST-10) is similar to the AUDIT and used for assessing drug use. A single-item screening question, "How many times in the past year have you used an illegal drug or used prescription medications for nonmedical reasons?" was 100% sensitive and 74% specific in a single urban primary care practice for the detection of a current drug use disorder, similar to the longer DAST-10, and may be more appropriate in a busy primary care setting with time constraints. Currently no practice guidelines exist for screening patients for unhealthy drug use.

Once patients have been identified as using drugs, the same interventional techniques (brief interventions, motivational interviewing) may be used for counseling, although data are limited regarding outcomes of these interventions.

Challenges unique to this population include the high likelihood of drug dependence and polysubstance use; the legal ramifications of illicit drug use, and, in the case of prescription drug use, the distinction between appropriate and inappropriate use.

KEY POINTS

- All patients who smoke should be offered cessation assistance, including counseling and medical therapy.
- Smoking cessation counseling that begins during hospitalization and continues after discharge increases the odds of long-term abstinence.

Sexual Behavior

All sexually active adolescents are considered at increased risk for STIs, including chlamydial infection, hepatitis B and C, HIV, HPV, and herpes simplex virus. Adults considered at increased risk include those with multiple sexual partners, a current or previous (in the past year) STI, and all non-monogamous sexually active partners in communities with high rates of STIs. The USPSTF recommends that providers take a sexual history and perform risk assessment during periodic and other health-related visits, particularly in high-risk patients.

Once risk and behavioral factors have been identified, targeted counseling should be provided. Counseling issues may include numbers of partners, partner selection, what constitutes consensual sexual behavior, proper use of condoms and other contraceptives, and appropriate vaccines (HPV, hepatitis). Current USPSTF recommendations are to provide high-intensity counseling targeted to sexually active adolescents and adults at risk for STIs. "High-intensity" counseling refers to a single 4-hour session or a minimum of three 1-hour sessions, with longer duration or counseling up to 16 hours or 10 sessions; this intensity is unlikely to be achieved in the primary care setting. Evidence exists, however, that as little as one or two 20-minute sessions in a primary care office are effective for reducing STIs. Recommendations regarding counseling for low-risk adults and non–sexually active adolescents are lacking.

Domestic Violence

Domestic violence, which refers to intimate partner violence as well as child and elder abuse, is defined as intentional controlling or violent behavior by a person in an intimate relationship with the victim. Risk factors for intimate partner violence include low socioeconomic status, young age, psychiatric illness, alcohol or substance abuse, separated or divorced status, and history of childhood sexual or physical abuse. Risk factors specific for elder abuse include increasing age, non-white race, functional impairment, cognitive disability, low self-esteem, and lack of social support. Victims of domestic violence have a high rate of disability and somatic symptoms, such as chronic pain, headache, and abdominal pain, as well as vaginal and urinary tract infections, STIs, and depression. Providers are often unaware that their patients are victims of domestic violence, despite its pervasiveness in clinical practice. Domestic violence is associated with high-risk behaviors such as substance abuse and risky sexual behavior, eating disorders, and limited access to health care.

Recommendations for screening for domestic violence vary, as there is no gold standard screening test. However, a 2012 USPSTF systematic review concluded that screening instruments can accurately identify women experiencing intimate partner violence, and that screening may improve health outcomes in this population. Studies suggest that women (who constitute the majority of victims) are comfortable with questions from their health care providers regarding abuse. Patients with repeated traumas, even minor, should be asked about abuse. However, many providers may not feel comfortable asking, nor be versed in further counseling strategies and legal issues if their patient is a domestic violence victim. Health care providers' primary responsibilities are to assist with health, assess for safety, and maintain a supportive relationship. Improved health outcomes have been shown even if victims remain in the abusive relationship when their providers have given validation, support, empathy, and non-judgmental, patient-centered discussions about available options and services. Many domestic violence victims are helped by the acknowledgment that violence is unacceptable, that they do have choices, and that they may proceed at their own pace.

KEY POINT

- Health care providers' primary responsibilities in caring for a patient who may be a victim of domestic violence are to assist with health, assess for safety, and maintain a supportive relationship.

Patient Safety

Introduction

Overall, patients in the United States receive only approximately 50% of recommended preventive care measures, while unnecessary procedures and tests continue to be performed, partially owing to payment systems that incentivize quantity over quality as well as to a culture that tends to demand more testing rather than less. The harms to patients from such excessive testing are being increasingly recognized and documented, such as recent reports of harm from radiation exposure from excessive imaging.

Principles of Patient Safety

In the report *To Err is Human: Building a Safer Health System*, the Institute of Medicine defined safety as "freedom

from accidental injury." Since publication of this report in 2000, the patient safety movement has evolved to focus on systems of care and the potential to do harm to patients inherent in the structure of those systems. Emphasis is placed on creating systems of care that have built-in safety nets for avoiding patient harm. The construction of these systems has relied on the concept of the "Swiss cheese model" of medical errors (**Figure 1**). In this model, bad outcomes result when errors occur at several layers in the system. Efforts to improve patient safety also encourage the growth and discussion of patient safety, wherein participants feel they can openly discuss and address medical errors or concerns that an error may occur if the system is not changed.

Quality Improvement Models

Most health care quality improvement programs utilize the Model for Improvement, which emphasizes methods with specific and measurable results. The key to quality improvement using this model is to establish what is to be accomplished with a change, clarify how the results of a change will be measured, and determine what changes will be made that will lead to improvement. These changes are tested and implemented using the Plan-Do-Study-Act (PDSA) cycle (**Figure 2**).

Several important quality improvement models have gained popularity in the United States over the past decade. One is the "lean thinking" model developed by Toyota, which aims to optimize efficiency, value, and safety on a continuous basis. Other systems sometimes utilized are Six Sigma and the Malcolm Baldrige Model for Performance Excellence. Six Sigma is a disciplined, data-driven approach for identifying and removing the causes of defects (errors) and minimizing variability in patient care processes (aiming for six standard deviations between the mean and the "customer's" specification limit). A Six Sigma process is one in which there are only 3.4 errors per million events. For example, in

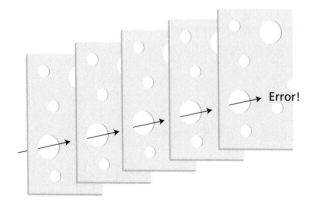

FIGURE 1. "Swiss cheese" model of error.

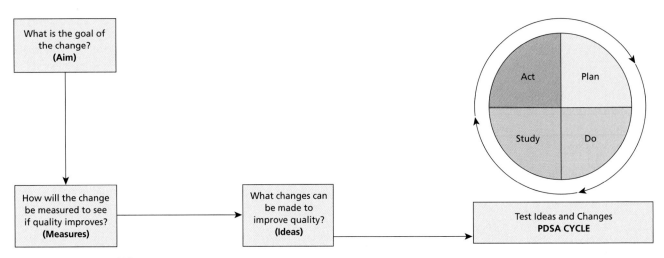

FIGURE 2. PDSA Model for Improvement.

assessing prescribing errors, 99.99966% of prescriptions would have no errors. The Baldrige model focuses on seven components: leadership, strategic planning, student and stakeholder focus, information and analysis, faculty and staff focus, educational and support process management, and organizational performance results.

Measurement of Quality Improvement

Quality improvement measurement began in 1996, when the Joint Commission (formerly JCAHO) implemented the ORYX initiative, a national program for the measurement of hospital quality. This movement gathered momentum in 2004, when the Joint Commission began requiring the collection and reporting of core measure sets (myocardial infarction, congestive heart failure, pneumonia, and pregnancy). A set of quality indicators have been developed to measure health care quality that make use of readily available hospital inpatient and outpatient administrative data. For example, prevention quality indicators identify numbers of hospital admissions that evidence suggests could have been avoided through access to high-quality outpatient care. Inpatient quality indicators assess quality of care inside hospitals as well as across geographic areas, including inpatient mortality for medical conditions and surgical procedures. Patient safety indicators measure potentially avoidable complications and iatrogenic events.

Sources of Error

Diagnostic Errors

A diagnostic error is defined as a diagnosis that is missed, delayed, or wrong; this error may or may not result in harm. Misdiagnosis-related harm is preventable harm resulting from a diagnostic error. Despite the fact that 40,000 to 80,000 deaths result from misdiagnosis annually in the United States

and that tort claims for diagnostic errors are twice as common as claims for medication errors, the science of diagnostic errors is in its infancy. Approximately 40% of malpractice payments in 2003 were related to diagnostic errors, with average payouts of $300,000/claim. The lack of attention to this important area is largely because of the complexity of most diagnostic errors. Diagnostic errors tend to result from a faulty cognitive approach (for example, settling on a diagnosis too soon or not re-examining new information adequately) or from systems-based issues (for example, communication breakdown or failure to obtain important data in a timely way). Suggestions to help avoid diagnostic errors are provided in **Table 10**.

Medication Errors

Between 500,000 and 1.5 million preventable adverse drug events occur each year in the United States, with an estimated 1 medication error daily for each hospitalized patient. Common medication errors by individual physicians include failure to recognize drug interactions among prescribed medications or to adjust dosing to account for impaired kidney or liver function or other conditions requiring dosing adjustments. The focus of efforts to reduce medication errors has been on computerized order entry, banning of abbreviations causing medication errors, bar code implementation in pharmacies, and medication reconciliation at the time of hospital admission and discharge.

Transitions of Care

Transitions of care between the inpatient and outpatient settings present unique challenges in patient safety. Forty percent of discharged patients will have pending studies of which patients and outpatient physicians are not aware despite the need for action on them. One in five patients discharged from the hospital will suffer an adverse event related to medical

TABLE 10. Twelve Tips for Avoiding Diagnostic Errors

Technique	Comments
(1) Understand heuristics[a]	*Availability heuristic:* Diagnosing based upon what is most easily available in the physician's mind (e.g., because of a patient recently seen) rather than what is most probable
	Anchoring heuristic: Settling on a diagnosis early in the diagnostic process despite data that refute the diagnosis or support another (premature closure)
	Representativeness heuristic: Application of pattern recognition (a patient's presentation fits a "typical" case, therefore it must be that case)
(2) Utilize "diagnostic timeouts"	Taking time to periodically review a case based on data but without assuming that the diagnosis is that which was previously reached
(3) Practice "worst-case scenario medicine"	Consider the most life-threatening diagnoses first: • Lessens chance of missing these diagnoses • Does not mandate testing for them, however
(4) Use systematic approach to common problems	For example, anatomic approach to abdominal pain beginning from exterior to interior
(5) Ask why	For example, when a patient presents with diabetic ketoacidosis or a COPD exacerbation, ask what prompted this acute exacerbation of a chronic condition
(6) Utilize the clinical examination	Decreases reliance on a single test and decreases chance of premature closure
(7) Use Bayesian theory	Utilize pre- and posttest probabilities • Helps avert premature closure based on a single test result
(8) Acknowledge the effect of the patient	How does the patient make the physician feel? • Physicians may avoid making bad diagnoses in patients they identify with • Physicians may discount important data in patients with whom they have difficult encounters
(9) Look for clinical findings that do not fit the diagnosis	Encourages a comprehensive approach and incorporates healthy skepticism
(10) Consider "zebras"	Resist temptation to lock onto common diagnoses at risk of missing the uncommon
(11) Slow down and reflect	Difficult to do in most health care systems, which stress the economy of "getting it right the first time"
(12) Admit mistakes	Awareness of one's own fallibility may lead to fewer diagnostic errors later

[a]Heuristics are shortcuts in reasoning used in discovery, learning, or problem solving.

Based on Trowbridge RL. Twelve tips for teaching avoidance of diagnostic errors. Med Teach. 2008;30(5):496-500. [PMID: 18576188]

CONT.

management within 3 weeks of hospital discharge, 66% of which are related to medications. Fourteen percent of elderly patients with medication discrepancies between prescribed outpatient and discharge medications are rehospitalized within 30 days, compared with 6% of those without medication discrepancies. Timely follow-up with a primary care physician after hospital discharge, particularly within 1 month, leads to lower rates of rehospitalization.

The key components of good transitions of care include effective hospitalist–to–primary care physician communication both during hospitalization and at the time of discharge (hand-off), pre-discharge patient education, medication reconciliation, and timely post-hospitalization follow-up. Despite the importance of the discharge summary, it often fails to arrive to the primary care physician in a timely fashion and frequently does not convey important information about diagnosis, medications, test results, follow-up plans, or

pending studies. The quality of discharge summaries is improved with the use of standardized content (**Table 11**).

Medication reconciliation can be arduous and time-consuming. Information gathered at the time of hospitalization should include that provided by the patient, caregivers, primary care providers, and, when necessary, prescription information from the patient's outpatient pharmacy. This information should be entered on a standardized form or electronic record in the patient's medical chart. This form can then be compared with medications prescribed throughout the hospitalization and at the time of discharge. Medication reconciliation is a dynamic process that should occur throughout the hospital stay as new information is obtained or medications are altered or discontinued. Patients should receive a list of medications at the time of discharge and be informed of previous medications which have been discontinued or changed (and the reason for the change). When

TABLE 11. Suggested Content of a Standardized Discharge Summary

Dates of admission and discharge

Reason for hospitalization

Discharge diagnosis

Significant findings from admission work-up:

• History and physical examination

• Laboratory studies

• Imaging studies

• Other tests

Procedures performed

Results of procedures and significant testing

Condition at discharge

Discharge medications and reasons for any changes from admission medications

Follow-up issues

Pending studies and laboratory tests

Counseling provided to patient and family

Follow-up appointments/plans

H CONT. medication reconciliation efforts are led by pharmacists, the rate of adverse drug events at 30 days is 1% versus 11% in control patients. **H**

KEY POINTS

• Common medication errors include failure to recognize drug interactions among prescribed medications or to adjust dosing to account for impaired kidney or liver function.

• Medication reconciliation should occur throughout the hospital stay; patients should receive a list of medications at the time of discharge.

• Timely follow-up with a primary care physician after hospital discharge (≤1 month) leads to lower rates of rehospitalization.

Health Information Technology and Patient Safety

Health information technology comes in three general forms: computerized physician order entry (CPOE), electronic health record (EHR), and clinical decision support. Each of these technologies can be used in an inpatient or outpatient environment and can improve patient safety. Health information technology systems should allow information sharing and integration across the continuum of care.

CPOE refers to the direct entry of orders (for example, prescriptions, radiology) into a computer interface by a physician. CPOE eliminates medication error related to physician handwriting, ensuring that the medication, dose, and directions are exactly what is requested. CPOE improves efficiency by eliminating delays between order entry and order receipt.

A patient's EHR comprises a collection of clinical data (notes, reports) in a computerized format. The EHR should allow multiple users, including specialists, primary care physicians, and the patient, to maintain an accurate, dynamic health record.

Clinical decision support refers to the use of these technologies to supplement a practitioner's clinical reasoning. For example, a CPOE system can warn the ordering clinician about drug interactions, need for renal dosing, or potential contraindications to studies. An EHR interface can prompt physicians to order needed medications, screening tests, or chronic disease management.

Health information technology is not a panacea. The potential for new errors is present in all systems; for example, CPOE can allow multiple physicians to enter potentially conflicting orders simultaneously. Poorly designed systems can introduce even more errors.

National Patient Safety Goals

Each year, the Joint Commission publishes national patient safety guidelines (www.jointcommission.org/standards _information/npsgs.aspx). These guidelines span the continuum of care, including acute care hospitals, ambulatory practices, nursing homes, and free-standing surgical centers, although not every standard is applicable at every site. The goals are focused on those that have the highest impact for both quality and patient safety. Each goal provides specific objectives and metrics. For example, under the goal *Improve accuracy of patient identification* are objectives such as "Use at least two patient identifiers when providing care, treatment, and services." The Joint Commission also includes measurable elements of performance such as "Label containers used for blood and other specimens in the presence of the patient." These safety goals provide a frame for interdisciplinary collaboration around quality and safety and can provide concrete objectives and criteria for quality improvement projects.

Professionalism and Ethics

Professionalism

In exchange for the authority to train, license, certify, and credential physicians, the medical profession has an obligation to society to ensure that physicians uphold ethical and professional behaviors, including maintenance of clinical competence and the fulfillment of clinical and hospital responsibilities in a timely manner. This obligation requires that physicians honestly assess their knowledge and skills and pursue learning where gaps exist. It also creates the expectation that physicians will disclose errors to patients and others and perform duties and meet standards established by local medical and hospital staffs.

In the routine delivery of patient care, physicians must model exemplary interactions with trainees and colleagues, both physician and nonphysician. Teamwork and collaboration, with mutual respect and recognition of one another's contributions to the health care team, are fundamental in today's health care environment and fundamental to demonstrating professionalism with trainees.

As part of their contract with society, physicians must also advance the public good, which requires they serve as judicious stewards of public resources. The Charter on Medical Professionalism comprises three principles and ten commitments (**Table 12**). Three commitments link

professionalism with the public's health: the commitment to improving quality of care, the commitment to improving access to care, and the commitment to a just distribution of finite resources.

Together, these commitments create an expectation that every physician advocate for and work to ensure that all persons have access to quality health care, and that medical care is delivered equitably across racial, ethnic, religious, and socioeconomic groups. A commitment to social justice requires physicians to guard the health of the public by eliminating unsafe and low-value services that generate expenses for care with potential harm and little to no benefit to the patient. The American College of Physicians' High-Value, Cost-Conscious Care initiative strives to promote this commitment by helping physicians assess the value and the costs of specific interventions.

TABLE 12. Principles and Commitments of Professionalism	
Principle or Commitment	**Comment**
Fundamental Principle	
Primacy of patient welfare	Altruism is a central trust factor in the physician-patient relationship. Market forces, societal pressures, and administrative exigencies must not compromise this principle.
Patient autonomy	Patients' decisions about their care must be paramount, as long as those decisions are in keeping with ethical practice and do not lead to demands for inappropriate care.
Social justice	Physicians should work actively to eliminate discrimination in health care, whether based on race, gender, socioeconomic status, ethnicity, religion, or any other social category.
Professional Commitment	
Competence	Physicians must be committed to lifelong learning and to maintaining the medical knowledge and clinical and team skills necessary for the provision of quality care.
Honesty with patients	Obtain informed consent for treatment or research. Report and analyze medical errors in order to maintain trust, improve care, and provide appropriate compensation to injured parties.
Patient confidentiality	Privacy of information is essential to patient trust and even more pressing with electronic medical records.
Appropriate patient relations	Given the inherent vulnerability and dependency of patients, physicians should never exploit patients for any sexual advantage, personal financial gain, or other private purpose.
Improve quality of care	Work collaboratively with other professionals to reduce medical errors, increase patient safety, minimize overuse of health care resources, and optimize the outcomes of care.
Improve access to care	Work to eliminate barriers to access based on education, laws, finances, geography, and social discrimination. Equity requires the promotion of public health and preventive medicine, as well as public advocacy, without concern for the self-interest of the physician or the profession.
Just distribution of resources	Work with other physicians, hospitals, and payers to develop guidelines for cost-effective care. Providing unnecessary services not only exposes one's patients to avoidable harm and expense but also diminishes the resources available for others.
Scientific knowledge	Uphold scientific standards, promote research, create new knowledge, and ensure its appropriate use.
Manage conflicts of interest	Medical professionals and their organizations have many opportunities to compromise their professional responsibilities by pursuing private gain or personal advantage. Such compromises are especially threatening with for-profit industries, including medical equipment manufacturers, insurance companies, and pharmaceutical firms. Physicians have an obligation to recognize, disclose to the general public, and deal with conflicts of interest that arise.
Professional responsibilities	Undergo self-assessment and external scrutiny of all aspects of one's performance. Participate in the processes of self-regulation, including remediation and discipline of members who have failed to meet professional standards.

Adapted with permission from ABIM Foundation. American Board of Internal Medicine; ACP-ASIM Foundation. American College of Physicians-American Society of Internal Medicine; European Federation of Internal Medicine. Medical professionalism in the new millennium: a physician charter. Ann Intern Med. 2002;136(3):243-246. [PMID: 11827500] Copyright 2002, American College of Physicians.

KEY POINT

- Physicians have a responsibility to guard the health of the public by eliminating unsafe and low-value services that generate expenses for care with potential harm and little to no benefit to the patient.

Decision-Making and Informed Consent

Decision-making is at the core of medicine. A common source of ethical challenges in practice is that while the authority for decision-making rests with the patient, the knowledge needed for informed decision-making is often in the hands of the clinician.

Informed Consent

Informed consent requires that the patient understand the nature of the decision being made or intervention being proposed, alternative options to the proposed intervention or decision, and the risks and benefits of each of the various alternatives. To obtain informed consent, the clinician explains the options and their risks and benefits to the patient and makes a recommendation if there is a preferred course of action. In addition, the clinician must assess the patient's understanding of the options and verify the patient's final decision. Although clinicians should make a recommendation if they feel that a particular choice is the most medically appropriate, they must not coerce or entice the patient into making that choice.

The greater the complexity of the decision, the greater the importance of detailed informed consent. Complexity can be characterized by three domains: the potential effect on the patient; the consensus within the medical community as to the appropriate action; and the number and uncertainty of possible outcomes. By convention, most invasive procedures such as surgery require written informed consent, which should reflect the outcome of the conversation described above. However, other complex decisions may also benefit from the principles of informed decision-making, even if an explicit signed consent document is not required. For example, deciding whether to obtain a screening mammography in a woman younger than 50 years is a complex decision by the criteria above, and the principles of informed consent apply even if one does not obtain a specific signed consent for the test in question. In a study of outpatient practices, it was shown that fewer than 10% of all clinical decisions made met standards for informed decision-making, and fewer than 1% of complex decisions were considered fully informed.

Assessing Decision-Making Capacity

The core components of decisional capacity are understanding the situation at hand, understanding the risks and benefits of the decision being made, and the ability to communicate a decision. Assessing understanding can be challenging,

particularly in patients with underlying mental health disorders or cognitive deficits. A diagnosis of dementia or a mental illness does not necessarily mean that a patient is incapable of making health care decisions. The clinician must assess whether or not the patient's decision appears consistent with his or her values and goals of care. If it does, it can probably be accepted as valid. A decision that seems inconsistent is a prompt to further explore the patient's beliefs, values, and comprehension of the situation and the decision. A given decision does not have to be rational, however, nor need it reflect what most people would do in that situation. Patients who are able to understand the consequences may refuse life-saving therapy, even for reasons that may be difficult to understand, such as religious preferences, community beliefs, or other values. The decisional capacity of these patients should only be questioned if they are acting in a way that is inconsistent with their personal beliefs or those of their community.

Advance Directives and Surrogate Decision-Making

When patients lack the capacity to make a decision on their own, they may have provided guidance in the form of an advance directive. Advance directives fall into two broad categories: instructive directives and proxy directives. Advance directive documents may include both components, for example, a living will (instructive) and durable power of attorney for health care (proxy).

Instructive directives provide guidance about what the patient would want to have done in certain situations. These may be straightforward, such as a request not to receive cardiopulmonary resuscitation. They may also be complicated, such as instructions for what specific life-sustaining treatment the patient may or may not want if they are unable to communicate their wishes (for example, in a persistent vegetative state). Instructive directives are subject to interpretation, as they cannot capture all the nuances of a given clinical situation. Many U.S. states have legal guidelines and forms that address the scope of advance directives, but unfortunately the legal forms may be difficult for patients to read and understand.

Proxy directives designate a surrogate decision maker (also known as a durable power of attorney for health care). Ideally, before incapacity occurs, the patient will have designated a surrogate to make health care decisions. If not, the clinician must try to identify the legal next of kin who is empowered to act as a surrogate decision maker. This is typically determined by state law in the United States. Most jurisdictions also have a mechanism to appoint a legal guardian in situations in which the patient is incapable of making health care decisions and there is no designated surrogate or next of kin.

The role of the surrogate is to strive to make decisions based on what the patient would have wanted in that situation (the ethics concept of *substituted judgment*). A living will or instructive directive can help inform the surrogate's decisions. If the surrogate has no knowledge of what the patient would have wanted, either because this was never discussed or because the surrogate did not know the patient well, a secondary standard would be to make decisions the surrogate considers to be in the patient's best interest. If the surrogate's decisions seem inconsistent with the patient's values or previous directives, the clinician should proceed with extreme caution. Ethics consultations are helpful in reconciling conflicts.

KEY POINT

- The core components of decisional capacity are understanding the situation at hand, understanding the risks and benefits of the decision being made, and the ability to communicate a decision.

Withholding or Withdrawing Treatment

Although a primary goal of care is usually to sustain life, there are circumstances under which life-sustaining treatment should be withheld or withdrawn. The emotional implications may differ whether one withholds care (never starts a treatment) or withdraws care (stops a treatment previously started), but the two are equivalent from the standpoint of medical ethics.

The two most common reasons to withhold or withdraw treatment are that the patient or the surrogate has decided that the patient no longer wishes to receive such treatment, or that life-sustaining treatment no longer offers benefit to the patient. If the patient has decided that he or she no longer wishes treatment, the decision to withhold or withdraw is usually straightforward. In most cases, it is reasonable to continue efforts at relief of symptoms and discomfort, while stopping invasive or uncomfortable treatments that serve only to sustain life. In some circumstances, clinicians may disagree with the patient's decision to withhold or withdraw treatment, particularly if they feel that the patient's death is not imminent or inevitable. However, there is ample legal and ethical precedent for competent patients to refuse care. Unless the patient is a minor or lacks decisional capacity, the clinician should abide by the patient's wishes.

A scenario in which life-sustaining treatment no longer offers benefit to the patient who wants it can be more challenging. Although one is on solid ethical ground denying futile treatment, the precise definition of futility can be quite difficult. A treatment is futile either when it has a very low probability of producing any benefit whatsoever (quantitative futility), or when the amount or quality of benefit produced is so small as to be trivial (qualitative futility). If the physician feels that a specific intervention is unlikely to produce an outcome that the patient would find to be meaningfully beneficial, the intervention is likely futile. Although physicians have no ethical obligation to provide futile treatments, even if the

patient wants them, they may need to request ethical and legal consultations in such cases.

Populations that have historically faced discrimination by the health care system and may have greater mistrust of health care providers' intentions, such as blacks in the United States, are more likely to request aggressive end-of-life treatment. Physicians need to be sensitive to such cultural and historical factors that may shape patients' and their families' attitudes about end-of-life care.

KEY POINT

- Competent patients may refuse care even if the clinician believes that the patient's death is not imminent or inevitable; unless the patient is a minor or lacks decisional capacity, the clinician should abide by the patient's wishes.

Physician-Assisted Suicide and Euthanasia

The issue of when it is appropriate to provide a treatment that may hasten the death of a dying patient is a heavily debated area of medical ethics. Most agree by virtue of the principle of double effect that it is ethically permissible to give a terminally ill patient a treatment that may hasten death when the primary intent is therapeutic. A common example is high doses of opiate analgesics used to relieve pain or dyspnea in a patient who is dying.

The practice of prescribing medications or interventions with the primary intent of hastening a patient's death (physician aid in dying, physician-assisted suicide) remains intensely controversial. Although the American Medical Association and the American College of Physicians have both taken positions against the practice, it is legal in some states under specific circumstances.

Active administration of a drug to cause death (active euthanasia) is illegal in all states, regardless of consent. All requests for a hastened death should be carefully evaluated and responded to with empathy and compassion, regardless of the physician's ethical position on the specifics of the request.

KEY POINTS

- A terminally ill patient may be given a treatment that may hasten death when the primary intent is to provide therapy for another condition.
- Active administration of a drug with the intent to cause death is illegal in all states, regardless of consent.

Confidentiality

Implicit in the physician-patient relationship is a commitment to confidentiality. Information disclosed by a patient to a physician should not be disclosed to anyone not directly involved in the patient's care (and therefore bound by a similar requirement for confidentiality). Patients may specify other persons, such as friends or family members, with whom they wish the physician to share information, but in the absence of specific permission, the physician should not disclose anything.

Confidentiality is not absolute, however. Situations in which there is an established risk of patients harming themselves or others may require the clinician to disclose confidential information. If the clinician believes that the patient poses a serious risk of harm to a specific person, he or she has a duty to warn that person. This is usually best handled with the assistance of law enforcement authorities, and it is also often helpful to get legal advice, if available. Another situation in which confidentiality may be sacrificed for the public welfare is for reportable communicable diseases, which are usually determined by local jurisdictions and public health departments.

Constraints on decisional capacity also have implications for confidentiality. If the patient is unable to make an important medical decision, then the person who is making that decision for him or her is entitled to be fully informed as to the aspects of the patient's condition that pertain to the decision. In the case of minor children, parents usually have a legal right to be informed about the child's condition, and the physician has an obligation to disclose any suspicion of abuse. Both ethics and law regarding confidentiality can be complicated for adolescents. Some U.S. states have laws specifically protecting adolescent confidentiality for certain medical issues such as reproductive health. When interviewing adolescents, the physician should perform at least some of the interview without the parents present and explicitly discuss with the patient what will and what will not be confidential, informed by an awareness of applicable local law.

KEY POINTS

- A physician may be required to disclose confidential information if the patient poses a serious risk of harm to self or others or has a reportable communicable disease.

- If a patient is unable to make an important medical decision, the person who is making that decision for him or her is entitled to be fully informed as to the aspects of the patient's condition that pertain to the decision.

Conflicts of Interest

The fiduciary nature of the physician-patient relationship dictates that the physician place the interests of the patient above his or her own. There are, however, numerous opportunities for conflicts of interest. A common area of conflict with the physician's own interests is that of financial relationships. At the most basic level, physician payment structures can generate conflicts of interest. In fee-for-service systems such as those prevalent in the United States, physician compensation often increases with the number and complexity of services provided. Moreover, if the physician has a financial interest in facilities used for diagnosis or treatment, he or she has an incentive to provide additional diagnostic or therapeutic services, or to provide those services in a manner that increases compensation (for example, intravenous instead of subcutaneous or oral medication administration). Although these relationships are regulated by federal law in the United States, regulation has not eliminated them or the associated financial incentives.

The relationships between physicians and companies in the health care industry that profit from physician decisions have also come under increasing scrutiny. The manufacturers of prescription drugs and medical devices devote considerable funds to marketing their products, using both direct and indirect approaches to influence physician behavior. A considerable amount of medical research is funded by companies that stand to gain from the results, which has led to concerns about bias in the content or publication of research papers. In addition, concern has been raised regarding whether experts whose research is heavily funded by industry can make impartial decisions when serving on panels to draft clinical practice guidelines. Many physicians also benefit indirectly from industry funding for continuing medical education programs. Both industry and accrediting organizations have developed standards to help manage these relationships. The Institute of Medicine has published recommendations for controlling conflicts of interest (**Table 13**).

Medical Error Disclosure

Research shows that patients expect disclosure of harmful medical errors. The National Quality Forum endorsed guidelines in 2006 that included three key components of error disclosure:

- Provide facts about the event (including an analysis of system failure, if available)

- Express regret for the unanticipated outcome

- Give a formal apology if the unanticipated outcome was caused by error or system failure

Apologizing for errors can be particularly difficult owing to concern that an apology or admission of responsibility may cause problems in subsequent malpractice litigation. A majority of U.S. states now have laws that offer at least limited protection for apologies or expressions of regret. Caution is indicated, however; whereas apologizing for errors is both ethically and interpersonally desirable, it is reasonable to obtain additional counsel on the legal implications.

TABLE 13. A Selection of Institute of Medicine Recommendations for Individual Physicians to Control Conflicts of Interest
Forgo all gifts or items of material value from pharmaceutical, medical device, and biotechnology companies, accepting only payment at fair market value for a legitimate service in specified situations.
Do not make educational presentations or publish scientific articles that are controlled by industry or contain substantial portions written by someone who is not identified as an author or who is not properly acknowledged.
Do not meet with pharmaceutical and medical device sales representatives except by documented appointment and at the physician's express invitation.
Do not accept drug samples except in certain situations for patients who lack financial access to medications.
Until institutions change their policies, physicians and trainees should voluntarily adopt these recommendations as standards for their own conduct.

Adapted with permission from Steinbrook R. Controlling conflict of interest—proposals from the Institute of Medicine. New Engl J Med. 2009;360(21):2160-2163. [PMID: 19403898] Copyright 2009, Massachusetts Medical Society.

Sexual Contact between Physician and Patient

The inherent asymmetry of power and trust in the physician-patient relationship makes it ethically unacceptable to maintain a sexual relationship with a patient, even if the patient initiates sexual contact.

Sexual relationships with former patients are also concerning. The greater the depth and duration of the previous professional physician-patient relationship, the more caution is needed. Relationships with patients whom the physician was treating for a mental health disorder are particularly problematic and may result in civil liability or professional disciplinary action in some jurisdictions, regardless of patient consent or the time elapsed since terminating the physician-patient relationship. In general, a physician considering a sexual relationship with a former patient is advised to solicit the opinions of legal counsel or an ethicist before proceeding with the relationship.

The Impaired Physician and Colleague Responsibility

Members of the medical profession have an obligation to protect the welfare of patients, which includes taking action when a colleague puts patients at risk. Many states have mandatory reporting statutes that require a physician to report to appropriate authorities when a colleague continues to practice despite his or her inability to do so safely because of impairment from substance use or illness.

In a 2009 survey, the majority of respondents endorsed a duty to report, but of the 17% who had direct knowledge of an impaired colleague, only two-thirds actually reported him or her to the relevant authority. Beliefs that someone else was taking care of the problem or that nothing would happen were the most common reasons for failure to report. Common signs of physician impairment at work are shown in **Table 14**.

All U.S. states now have physician health programs (PHPs) that allow for anonymous reporting of impaired

TABLE 14. Signs of Physician Impairment in the Work Setting
Late to appointments; increased absences; unknown whereabouts
Unusual rounding times, either very early or very late
Increase in patient complaints
Increased secrecy
Decrease in quality of care; careless medical decisions
Incorrect charting or writing of prescriptions
Decrease in productivity or efficiency
Increased conflicts with colleagues
Increased irritability and aggression
Smell of alcohol; overt intoxication; needle marks
Erratic job history

Adapted with permission from Ross S. Identifying an Impaired Physician. Virtual Mentor. December 2003, Volume 5, Number 12. Accessed at http://virtualmentor.ama-assn.org/2003/12/cprl1-0312.html. 22 December 2011. The viewpoints expressed in Virtual Mentor are those of the authors and do not necessarily reflect the views and policies of the AMA. Copyright 2003, American Medical Association.

physicians, and many states stipulate those licensed to practice by the state must report impaired colleagues. Once the PHP is notified of a possibly impaired physician, assessment, treatment, and monitoring can be arranged. If a physician voluntarily participates in the PHP's treatment and monitoring program, the PHP will often advocate for him or her with the state medical board, resulting in mitigation or even avoidance of formal disciplinary action as long as the physician remains in compliance.

Palliative Care

Introduction

The primary focus of palliative care is to relieve patient suffering and to improve the quality of patients' lives and those of their caregivers. Palliative care involves a multifaceted approach that includes clarifying goals of treatment, managing symptoms, mobilizing resources to optimize care and social support, and integrating care across settings—whether home, nursing home, or hospital. Despite its widespread availability, palliative care continues to be underutilized. Much of the resistance to initiating palliative care stems from the traditional care dichotomy between "doing everything" versus providing comfort care—a dichotomy that often fails to focus on relieving suffering and improving quality of care.

Palliative care is often thought of as end-of-life care only, but palliative care addresses pain, suffering, and quality of life across all stages of treatment and does not exclude life-prolonging treatment and rehabilitation. *Nonhospice* palliative care may be offered along with curative or life-prolonging therapies for patients with complex, life-threatening disorders. *Hospice* palliative care is offered when patients reach their final weeks or months of life, when the likely harm of life-prolonging or curative therapies exceeds benefit, and these therapies are discontinued. Hospice services can be provided in a patient's home, in specialized hospice units in hospitals, or in community-based facilities, depending on patients' and their family's individual needs and preferences.

Emerging data for concurrent palliative care intervention in the treatment of cancer strongly suggest that patients using palliative care services have higher scores for quality of life and mood than those undergoing cancer treatment alone. In a study of 151 patients with newly diagnosed metastatic non–small cell lung cancer randomly assigned to standard oncologic therapy alone versus early palliative care with standard oncologic therapy, patients in the palliative care group had a mean survival of 11.6 months as compared with 8.9 months in the group not provided early palliative care. The intervention group also experienced less depression and better quality of life.

Palliative care consultation programs are also associated with significant hospital cost savings, with an adjusted net savings of $1696 in direct costs for patients discharged alive from the hospital and $4908 net savings for patients dying in the hospital as compared with patients who receive usual care.

KEY POINT

- Palliative care addresses pain, suffering, and quality of life across all stages of treatment and does not exclude life-prolonging treatment and rehabilitation.

Deciding When Hospice Palliative Care Is Indicated

Approximately 30% of Medicare's expenditures occur in patients' last year of life. Evidence suggests that more aggressive care at the end of life—whether prolonged hospitalization, intensive care unit admission, or performance of procedures—does not improve either quality or duration of life. The problem with estimating when the last year of life has arrived is that patients do not progress in identical patterns.

Prognostication can be even more difficult when a patient does not have cancer (**Figure 3**). In patients with cancer, the clinical course frequently ends with an obvious decline in the final weeks or months of disease. Patients with organ failure often have gradual decline with serious exacerbations followed by improvement; it can be very challenging to predict timing of death in these patients. A third group of patients are those with frailty, sometimes with concomitant dementia. These patients have long, slow declines but without discrete exacerbations of disease.

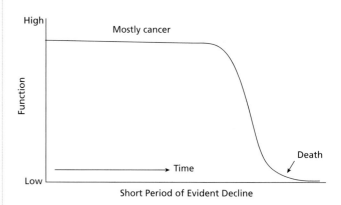

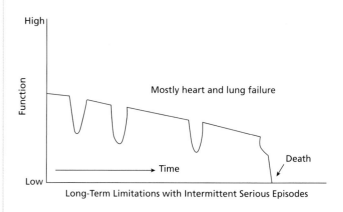

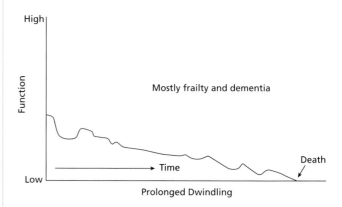

FIGURE 3. Trajectories of late-life illness.

Recent evidence suggests that minority patients receive more intensive care at the end of life than they would if they were more adequately communicated with regarding advance care planning, prognosis, and treatment alternatives, such as nonhospice or hospice palliative care. The National Comprehensive Cancer Network has recommended that patients be screened for palliative care needs at initial presentation with cancer as well as at subsequent visits, and that palliative care services be available to all patients with cancer.

KEY POINT

- More aggressive care at the end of life does not improve either quality or duration of life.

Assessment and Communication

The cornerstone of both hospice and nonhospice palliative care is communication with patients, families, and caregivers. The first step in this communication is to establish goals of care in a patient-centered, open-ended format. Adequate time needs to be allotted to ensure that these discussions provide the opportunity for actively listening to the patient and key care providers (rather than being physician-centered—oriented toward efficiency and completing the task). The initial meeting or meetings should emphasize discovery of what the patient knows and understands regarding the diagnosis and prognosis. This discussion should allow opportunity to clarify how much the patient actually wants to know and should respect the diverse ways in which patients and their families process information about life-altering or life-threatening medical conditions. Medical jargon should be avoided and medical information conveyed succinctly and empathetically. Several meetings may be necessary to allow further processing of information and preparation of more questions by the patient or family members. As issues are addressed and worked through, a plan should be presented in a clear and succinct manner. Next steps should be outlined and, when necessary, carefully reiterated.

KEY POINT

- The first step in communication with patients, families, and caregivers regarding palliative care is to establish goals of care in a patient-centered, open-ended format.

Symptom Management

Symptoms common in patients with cancer and other life-threatening illnesses are myriad. Numerous symptom assessment instruments have been validated in the medical literature. The Edmonton Symptom Assessment Scale is a brief survey that asks patients to rate several symptoms on a scale (pain, dyspnea, fatigue, nausea, depression, anxiety, drowsiness, appetite, sense of well being) and also allows them to add one additional symptom and rate it. These symptoms may occur because of the underlying disease or secondary to treatments for symptoms of the disease.

Pain

Undertreated patient pain is a major problem in both the inpatient and outpatient settings. Assessment of pain can be difficult, particularly in patients with dementia, delirium, or somnolence caused by medications being used to treat pain.

Strong evidence from randomized trials supports treating cancer-related pain with NSAIDs, opioids, and radiation therapy; evidence regarding the use of bisphosphonates for cancer pain is less convincing. There is a lack of studies providing strong evidence on effective ways to treat pain in advanced heart failure or dementia. Opioid use in the treatment of noncancer pain continues to be controversial.

The World Health Organization analgesic ladder provides a stepwise approach to the management of pain (**Figure 4**). Pain management in palliative care, as with other conditions, should begin with nonopioid analgesia, including acetaminophen and NSAIDs (see Common Symptoms, Chronic Noncancer Pain). Adjuvant pain medications are used to treat pain symptoms that respond poorly to analgesic agents, such as neuropathic or bony

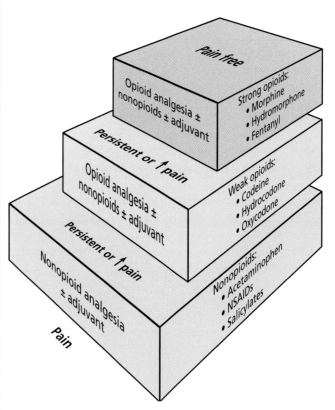

FIGURE 4. World Health Organization analgesic ladder.

CONT.

metastatic pain. Examples of these medications include anticonvulsants, corticosteroids, and antidepressants. Corticosteroids are useful for treating spinal cord compression or brain metastases, but data are lacking in support of their use in other cancer-related pain. Benzodiazepines should generally be avoided as they may actually worsen pain and also cause confusion and agitation in patients who are elderly or have dementia.

Various opioid analgesics are listed in **Table 15**. A weaker opioid analgesic (such as oxycodone) can be added at any point along the World Health Organization ladder. If pain persists or worsens, stronger opioid analgesia should be started. The usual starting dose of short-acting morphine is 5 to 15 mg orally in opiate-naïve patients and the elderly or 1 to 5 mg intravenously. Shorter-acting morphine can be used for breakthrough pain but should be changed to long-acting morphine if a patient develops persistent pain throughout the day or beyond 24 hours of treatment with shorter-acting opioids. A starting dosage of long-acting morphine is usually 30% to 50% of a patient's total average 24-hour usage. This dosage is increased every 3 to 4 days. Analgesia dosage for breakthrough pain should be 10% to 20% of the total daily opioid dose or 25% to 30% of the single standing dose. Analgesia should be gradually increased, with the firm goal of controlling pain. Beliefs about "maximum" dosages do not usually apply.

Although many health care providers worry about respiratory depression as a side effect of morphine, respiratory depression occurs rarely in patients who are actively in pain. In the elderly, however, it is generally best to start at the lower range. Hydromorphone is a semisynthetic opioid agonist that is similar to morphine but has a more favorable pharmacokinetic profile. Fentanyl is more expensive but can be administered as a lollipop, transdermally, or intravenously. Methadone, a long-acting opioid, has an unpredictable half-life and has been reported to cause QT interval prolongation and arrhythmias. It should be used with caution, with monitoring of the QT interval. Meperidine should be avoided because it can cause seizures, especially in the setting of kidney failure, as well as confusion and mood alterations. A fentanyl transdermal patch is an excellent alternative to decrease frequency of dosing but is substantially more expensive than long-acting morphine and takes up to 24 hours to take effect, making dose adjustment slightly more complicated.

When using opioids, it is important to be sensitive to patient concerns about addiction, as these concerns may present an obstacle to attaining adequate pain control. It is extremely rare for patients to become addicted to opioids in the acute hospital setting and rare to become addicted when being treated in the setting of cancer-related pain. Occasionally, opioid use may result in opioid-induced hyperalgesia. This is a poorly understood phenomenon whereby increased dosages of opioids exacerbate pain rather than

relieve it. Other important side effects of morphine include xerostomia, constipation, sedation, myoclonus, urinary hesitancy, nausea, and itching.

Constipation

Constipation is common in cancer patients, particularly in the elderly. It is defined as fewer than three bowel movements per week, the subjective sensation of incomplete bowel movements, or difficult passage of stool. It is important to obtain a history about a patient's premorbid bowel habits in order to establish a baseline. Forty percent to 95% of cancer patients suffer from constipation, and 95% of patients on opioids report constipation. Opioids cause constipation by binding to the μ receptor in the bowel, diminishing intestinal activity and reducing intestinal secretions. Constipation is also exacerbated by decreased activity and, toward the end of life, by reduced mobility and access to the toilet. Other contributing factors in cancer patients include hypercalcemia and bowel obstruction (from primary or metastatic disease or treatment-related adhesions).

A bowel regimen should be prescribed for any patient starting opioid analgesic agents and should include both a stool softener and a laxative. "Rescue laxatives," such as lactulose, magnesium citrate, or enemas, may be needed if the patient fails to have at least three bowel movements weekly or reports symptoms of constipation on a standard bowel regimen. ⊞

Some data indicate that opioid rotation can improve constipation. Three studies have showed reduced reliance on laxatives when oral morphine was switched to a fentanyl transdermal patch.

Fatigue

Fatigue, the subjective feeling of physical, emotional, or mental exhaustion, is one of the most common and distressing symptoms related to cancer and cancer treatment. In contrast to fatigue in a healthy person, fatigue in a cancer patient is not relieved by rest. It affects 60% to 90% of patients with cancer and up to 96% of patients undergoing radiation or chemotherapy. Notably, as cancer progresses, fatigue worsens. Fatigue can also be an early harbinger of recurrent cancer.

Treatment of fatigue in cancer and other end-stage illnesses, such as heart failure and COPD, begins with education of the patient and family members about modes of energy conservation and distraction. Various modalities have been evaluated in reducing cancer-related fatigue, including biofeedback and exercise programs, but the small patient populations in these studies make it difficult to establish firm evidence-based recommendations about interventions. However, given the low morbidity of such treatments, it is reasonable to try an exercise or rehabilitation program.

TABLE 15. Common Noninjected Narcotics Used in Palliative Care for Chronic Pain

Agent	Drug:Morphine Potency Ratio[a]	Form	Starting Dose	Onset	Duration	Comments
Morphine	—	Immediate release	10 mg q 3-4 h	30 min	4 h	Tablet, solution, and rectal suppository
		Controlled/ sustained release[b]	15-30 mg q 12 h	2-4 h	12 h	Tablets, ranging from 15-200 mg
Oxycodone	2:1	Immediate release	2.5-5 mg q 6 h	10-15 min	3-6 h	Tablet and solution form
		Extended release[b]	10 mg q 12 h	1 h	12 h	Tablets 60 mg or higher for use only in opioid-tolerant patients.
Fentanyl	4:1[c]	Immediate release	200-µg lozenge: may repeat once in 15 min, then q 6 h 100-µg buccal tablet: may repeat once in 30 min, then q 4 h	5-15 min	4-8 h	Not recommended for opioid-naïve patients. Transmucosal lozenge or buccal tablet should be used only in patients who are already receiving narcotics and are opioid tolerant. Limit to 4 or fewer daily—additional doses mark need for adjustment of basal pain medication.
		Extended release	25-µg patch q 72 h	12-24 h	72 h	Not recommended for opioid-naive patients. Patients should be on at least 60 mg oral morphine equivalents/d before starting. Dose should not be adjusted upward based on supplemental opiate need for 3 days after initial placement or 6 days after subsequent dose changes. 17 hours are required for 50% decrease in fentanyl levels after removal.
Codeine	1:3-8 (variable)	Immediate release	30-60 mg q 4-6 h	30-60 min	4-6 h	Tablet and liquid, usually taken with adjunct analgesics due to weak strength. Variable efficacy due to differences in metabolism to morphine with CYP2D6 enzyme.
Hydromorphone	4:1	Immediate release	2-4 mg q 3-6 h	15-30 min	4-5 h	Also available as liquid, rectal suppository. Dose adjustment required with kidney failure.
		Extended release	8-64 mg q 24 h	1-2 h	24 h	For use in opioid-tolerant patients only. Dose adjustment required with kidney failure.
Hydrocodone	1:1	Immediate release	5-15 mg q 3-8 h	30-60 min	4-8 h	Available as combination product with adjunct analgesics.

q = every; µg = microgram.

[a]A ratio of 2:1 indicates that the medication is twice as powerful as an equivalent mg strength of morphine. No fixed conversion ratio is likely to be satisfactory in all patients, especially patients receiving large opioid doses.

[b]Divide cumulative daily dose of short-acting narcotic into two divided doses of the longer-acting narcotic.

[c]The fentanyl comparison is a µg-to-mg conversion.

Dyspnea

Dyspnea is a common and troubling symptom for patients with cancer as well as advanced COPD and heart failure. Up to 70% of cancer patients suffer from dyspnea in the last 6 weeks of life, and for 30%, it is rated as moderate to severe in intensity. Strong evidence supports the use of β-agonists, morphine, pulmonary rehabilitation, and oxygen for symptom relief in COPD. Although opioids are frequently used in cancer-related dyspnea, evidence is weak for their use in this situation. However, options are limited in treating cancer-related dyspnea, and opioid use is standard of care. Morphine use in cancer-related dyspnea is prescribed the same way it is used in cancer pain. Benzodiazepines are also sometimes used to treat cancer-related dyspnea but have not been well studied. Oxygen may also be used in treating cancer-related dyspnea, but evidence for functional improvement is lacking.

Nausea

Chronic nausea, defined as nausea lasting longer than 1 week, affects up to 60% of cancer patients in the last 6 months of life regardless of whether they receive chemotherapy. Metoclopramide is a dopamine agonist with prokinetic activity through the cholinergic system. It has a short half-life but can be given intravenously, subcutaneously, or orally and results in symptomatic improvement in 50% of patients. Serotonin antagonists (ondansetron) are effective for chemotherapy-related nausea but are expensive and unproven in the chronic palliative care setting. Dronabinol is a cannabinoid that is effective in chemotherapy-related nausea and AIDS-related wasting, but it has not been well studied for chronic palliative care patients. It may cause somnolence, confusion or euphoria. Dexamethasone has been increasingly used for palliative care as an antiemetic. A trial of 2 to 4 mg intravenously can be tried for patients not responding to other antiemetic agents.

Anorexia and Nutrition

Loss of appetite can be one of the most disturbing symptoms for patients and their providers. Reassurance often needs to be provided, and advance directives regarding feeding tubes should ideally be clarified in advance of the anorexia that occurs at the end of life. Feeding tubes are controversial and probably do not confer a survival advantage to cancer patients unless used as a temporizing measure in the treatment of head and neck or gastrointestinal cancers. Feeding tubes are not recommended for terminal cancer. Two classes of drugs have been shown to improve appetite in patients with cancer but do not provide a survival advantage. Progestational agents, such as megestrol, improve appetite and weight gain. Side effects include thromboembolism, impotence, edema, and vaginal bleeding. Corticosteroids have also been found to improve appetite in patients with cancer, but the proper dosing regimen has not been established.

Depression

Depression is a common symptom in patients approaching the end of life. Tricyclic antidepressants and selective serotonin reuptake inhibitors have been found to be equally effective, provided treatment duration is 6 weeks or longer. Randomized controlled trials have also found consistent efficacy in nonpharmacologic interventions, such as psychotherapy, education, and individual and group support.

Delirium

Delirium is common at the end of life and can be caused by advanced medical conditions, the medications being used to palliate symptoms, or a combination of both. Family members frequently need to be reassured that delirium is common. Opioid analgesia can be reduced provided pain remains controlled. If opioid dosage cannot be reduced owing to pain or dyspnea, haloperidol can be given at a dose of 0.5 to 1 mg intramuscularly. Additional sedative agents (such as benzodiazepines) may be required but can further exacerbate delirium in patients who are elderly or have dementia.

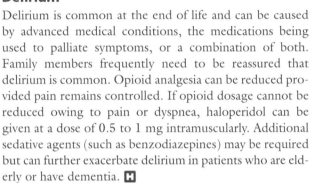

KEY POINTS

- Respiratory depression as a side effect of morphine occurs rarely in patients who are actively in pain.
- A bowel regimen should be prescribed for any patient starting opioid analgesic agents.

Bereavement and Grief

Although providing psychosocial, spiritual, and bereavement support for patients and their families is considered an essential part of hospice palliative care, effective ways to do this are not well demonstrated in the medical literature. Approximately 15% of bereaved survivors in the U.S. experience complicated grief, defined as grief persisting more than 6 months after a death. Its chief symptom is a yearning for a loved one so intense that it incapacitates all other desires. Many interventions have been studied, but thus far, none have shown results adequate to provide evidence-based guidance in this area. It is important, however, for physicians to be sensitive to the needs of bereaved survivors given the depth of despair for which they are at risk.

Common Symptoms

Overview

Common symptoms generally fall into a few major categories, including pain, upper respiratory, neurologic, dermatologic, musculoskeletal, and psychological. Common symptoms account for more than half of visits to the general internist. Most symptoms improve within 2 weeks, but up to 25% of these common symptoms become recurrent or chronic. Patients may present with symptoms as the primary reason for a visit or as a secondary concern during an appointment for follow-up of chronic medical conditions. Symptoms for which no demonstrable pathology is found are designated as somatic. Up to one third of symptoms presented in primary care visits have no demonstrable cause. Some patients may feel uncomfortable discussing sensitive or difficult issues, and talking about a common symptom may feel more acceptable to them. Examples of these hidden agendas include concerns about sexual dysfunction, sexually transmitted infection, incontinence, and depression or other psychological issues. Asking patients if they have other concerns during the visit can often uncover these issues. Depression, anxiety, or somatization should be considered in patients presenting with multiple symptoms in different parts of the body.

Clinical decision rules (CDRs) aid in the diagnosis and management of many common symptoms. Examples of CDRs include the Centor score to diagnose group A streptococcal pharyngitis and the Ottawa ankle rule to determine which patients with ankle injuries require imaging. There is a growing literature regarding the evidence-based approach to evaluating and managing many common symptoms; for example, the Rational Clinical Examination series published by the Journal of the American Medical Association.

Chronic Noncancer Pain

Chronic pain is defined as persistent pain of sufficient duration and intensity to have a significant impact on a patient's quality of life, functional status, and well-being. Pain may be considered chronic if it persists for longer than the anticipated healing time, although various time frames have been proposed (persistence of pain for more than 6 weeks, 3 months, or 6 months). Chronic noncancer pain (CNCP) affects as many as 50 million Americans and is associated with many conditions encountered in primary care, including fibromyalgia, postherpetic neuralgia, diabetic neuropathy, and osteoarthritis. CNCP exacts a significant personal and economic burden, with costs estimated at $85 billion annually as a result of job loss, missed work days, and medical visits. (Cancer pain is discussed in Palliative Care).

Assessment

CNCP may affect many aspects of a patient's life, and guidelines from the Institute for Clinical Systems Improvement emphasize that an initial assessment should evaluate each patient's pain within the context of his or her psychological state and beliefs, family supports, and social and work environments. Physicians should first obtain information about pain location, character, intensity, duration, relieving and exacerbating factors, and previous treatments. Patients should be questioned regarding the impact of pain on their activity level, ability to work, mood, sleep, and relationships with others. The patient's symptoms and goals for treatment need to be explored in a thorough, patient-centered manner. The Brief Pain Inventory (BPI), a patient-completed questionnaire, is a standardized tool for obtaining information about a patient's pain symptoms efficiently. Screening for depression and anxiety, as well as substance abuse, is essential, since these diagnoses may significantly affect treatment options. A history of physical, verbal, or sexual abuse has been associated with chronic pain syndromes, and providers should carefully assess for current or previous threats to a patient's well-being and safety. **Table 16** lists the key elements of the CNCP assessment, as well as suggested strategies for obtaining this information.

All patients with CNCP should receive a complete physical examination, with special attention to the musculoskeletal and nervous systems. Muscle strength and tone should be assessed, joints inspected for signs of effusion or erythema, and trigger points identified. Testing of sensation is essential for diagnosing absent or abnormal sensory states, such as allodynia (pain with stimuli that are usually not painful) or hyperalgesia (increased sensitivity to pain).

There is no specific role for diagnostic testing in the assessment and management of CNCP, as abnormalities that are identified may not be the source of the patient's pain. Tests for certain conditions may be considered, such as an MRI for evaluating back pain if conditions such as spinal stenosis or herniated disk disease are suspected. Similarly, nerve conduction studies may be helpful in select patients if the diagnosis or etiology of neuropathy is uncertain.

Based on findings from the history and physical examination, a patient's pain should be classified into one of five types: neuropathic pain, muscle pain, inflammatory pain, mechanical/compressive pain, and mixed (**Table 17**). This classification is helpful for choosing mechanism-specific treatment options that are most likely to alleviate the pain. Before initiating treatment, providers should assess for common behavioral, social, or systems barriers that may prevent a patient from experiencing functional improvement, irrespective of the treatment plan. Behavioral barriers include low motivation, unrealistic expectations, poor adherence, chemical dependency, and passivity. Social barriers include time constraints, lack of social support, cultural and language barriers, and financial issues. Systems barriers include formulary and coverage restrictions and difficulty accessing behavioral health care. Identifying these barriers can help providers develop a realistic expectation of what can be accomplished in management of a patient's pain. Patients involved in litigation may display limited response to treatment.

TABLE 16. Key Elements in the Assessment of the Patient with Chronic Noncancer Pain

Key Element	Notes[a]
General Assessment	
Pain location, intensity, quality, onset, relieving and exacerbating factors	The Brief Pain Inventory, Chronic Pain Grade, and Neuropathic Pain Scale are all helpful for assessing multiple aspects of a patient's pain.
Functional status	The Physical Functional Ability Questionnaire (FAQ 5) is brief and easy to complete.
Mental health disorders (depression, anxiety, substance abuse)	The Patient Health Questionnaire (PHQ-9) screens for major depressive disorder. The CAGE Questionnaire is a brief screen for alcohol use disorders (see Routine Care of the Healthy Patient).
Verbal, physical, or sexual abuse	Sensitivity and empathy are essential when eliciting this information.
Assessment for Opioid Therapy	
Risk stratification for initiating therapy	The Screener and Opioid Assessment for Patients with Pain (SOAPP) and Opioid Risk Tool (ORT) are patient-completed. The Diagnosis, Intractability, Risk, and Efficacy (DIRE) tool is provider-completed.
Follow-up	The 6 A's are a useful framework for follow-up visits: Analgesia, Activities of daily living, Adverse events, Aberrant behavior, Assessment, Action plan.

[a]Several tools are available for assessments; listed scales are examples.

TABLE 17. Classification of Chronic Pain Mechanisms and Recommended Pharmacologic Therapies

Mechanism of Pain	Description	Examples	Medications
Neuropathic	Burning, shooting, stabbing	Diabetic peripheral neuropathy, postherpetic neuralgia, fibromyalgia[a], multiple sclerosis, trigeminal neuralgia	*Systemic:* gabapentin, pregabalin, TCAs, duloxetine, venlafaxine, tramadol, opioids, carbamazepine *Local:* topical lidocaine 5% patch, capsaicin
Muscle	Tender trigger points. Pain often involves the neck, shoulders, arms, low back, hips, lower extremities	Myofascial pain syndrome, fibromyalgia[a]	TCAs, milnacipran (for fibromyalgia)
Inflammatory	Involved joints are warm, erythematous, and swollen	Rheumatoid arthritis and other inflammatory arthropathies	DMARDs, NSAIDs, TCAs
Mechanical/compressive	Aggravated by activity, relieved by rest	Back pain, neck pain, musculoskeletal pain	NSAIDs, acetaminophen, TCAs, duloxetine

DMARD = disease-modifying antirheumatic drug; TCA = tricyclic antidepressant.

[a]Fibromyalgia pain may be both neuropathic and muscular in origin.

Management

General Principles

The goal of CNCP treatment is to improve function and quality of life in the context of pain that may be ongoing. A comprehensive treatment plan may include physical rehabilitation, cognitive-behavioral therapy (CBT), management of comorbid psychiatric conditions, complementary and alternative therapy, and pharmacologic therapies. A graded exercise program will help to improve functional status, and machine muscle strengthening, aerobic low-impact exercises, and flexion/extension exercises are equally beneficial. "Passive" modalities (transcutaneous electrical nerve stimulation [TENS], massage, and ultrasound) should only be used in the context of an active exercise program; massage therapy may be particularly beneficial for patients with low back pain, fibromyalgia, and knee osteoarthritis. All patients should be taught self-management strategies that can improve pain, such as ice and heat therapy.

CBT techniques include biofeedback, mindfulness-based stress reduction, imagery, and hypnosis, and have been shown to have small but positive effects on pain, disability, and mood. Depression and CNCP are frequently coexistent, and simultaneous treatment should be initiated if the depression is mild to moderate in severity. In contrast, psychiatric therapy is the initial focus of treatment in the setting of severe major depressive disorder and CNCP, as untreated patients will not be able to actively work toward achieving rehabilitation and treatment goals.

Acupuncture has been studied for various CNCP syndromes. The limited evidence for effectiveness for neck pain does not appear to be clinically significant. The improvement with acupuncture in chronic back pain, osteoarthritic knee pain, and fibromyalgia has not been demonstrated to be superior to sham acupuncture. Recent studies have shown that manipulative therapy, when included as part of an interdisciplinary treatment program, can reduce chronic pain. Herbal medications should be used cautiously because of the risk for drug interactions and adverse effects. Feverfew and willow bark appear to be effective for treating headaches and back pain, respectively, but little evidence supports the use of glucosamine, chondroitin, dimethylsulfoxide, or devil's claw.

Nonopioid Medical Therapies

Although medication is not the sole focus of the treatment plan, it is a useful adjunct to care for many patients with CNCP. The World Health Organization analgesic ladder (see Palliative Care), although developed for the palliative care setting, is widely used in the management of CNCP. Pharmacologic pain management should begin with nonopioid agents, such as acetaminophen, NSAIDs, and the selective cyclooxygenase-2 (COX-2) inhibitor celecoxib. Adjuvant therapies include antidepressants, anticonvulsants, muscle relaxants, and topical medications. Tramadol is a unique analgesic that activates μ-opioid receptors and also inhibits serotonin reuptake. It is effective for the treatment of moderate to severe chronic pain, but may increase the risk for suicide in certain patients; moreover, tramadol may be abused or subject to criminal diversion. Caution is necessary when initiating tramadol in patients who are taking serotonin reuptake inhibitors, as cotreatment can increase the risk for serotonin syndrome.

Factors to consider when selecting a medication include the type of pain being treated, side effects, drug interactions, and patient comorbidities. Medications that are appropriate for each type of pain are listed in Table 17.

Acetaminophen is generally safe but should not exceed 4 g/d and should be avoided or used cautiously in patients with liver disease. NSAIDs are reasonable alternatives or supplements to acetaminophen, especially if pain is associated with inflammation. NSAIDs and COX-2 inhibitors should be used cautiously, as they can increase the risk of gastritis, kidney dysfunction, and adverse cardiovascular outcomes. In older patients, the risk for adverse reactions is increased, and the American Geriatrics Society recommends acetaminophen, rather than NSAIDs, as first-line therapy. Older patients who

are treated with an NSAID should also be prescribed a proton pump inhibitor to reduce gastric toxicity; this should be considered in any patient on long-term NSAIDs. Contraindications to NSAID therapy include current peptic ulcer disease, chronic kidney disease, and heart failure. For patients with high cardiovascular risk, naproxen may be a safer choice than diclofenac or ibuprofen. Diclofenac has been associated with increased cardiovascular risk as compared with other NSAIDs, and ibuprofen interferes with the antiplatelet effects of aspirin.

Adjuvant therapies such as gabapentin and pregabalin are efficacious for the treatment of neuropathic pain and have few drug interactions. According to a Cochrane systematic review, pregabalin dosed at 600 mg/d provided substantial pain relief for postherpetic neuralgia, diabetic neuropathy, and fibromyalgia (number needed to treat = 3.9, 5.0, and 11.0, respectively), but treatment-associated dizziness and somnolence were common. Tricyclic antidepressants (TCAs) can be effective for fibromyalgia and other central sensitization pain syndromes, but may produce significant adverse reactions, including constipation, dry mouth, conduction abnormalities, and urinary retention; their use should be avoided in the elderly. Duloxetine, a norepinephrine transporter (NET) inhibitor that has been approved for the treatment of fibromyalgia and diabetic neuropathy, and tramadol both also inhibit serotonin uptake, making them effective for neuropathic pain. In patients with postherpetic neuralgia and diabetic neuropathy, combination therapy with gabapentin and nortriptyline, as compared with monotherapy with each agent, produces better pain relief with fewer adverse reactions.

Opioid Therapy

Opioid therapy should be reserved for patients with moderate to severe neuropathic pain that has been unresponsive to other pharmacologic therapy. It is typically not beneficial in patients with inflammatory or mechanical/compressive pain. The significant side effects associated with opioid therapy (constipation, fatigue, nausea), as well as the attendant risks for abuse and addiction, make appropriate patient selection essential. The most important risk factors for aberrant drug-taking behaviors are a personal or family history of drug or alcohol abuse, age younger than 45 years, and a history of psychiatric disease. Other risk factors include female sex, cigarette smoking, preadolescent sexual abuse (in women), previous legal problems, history of motor vehicle accidents, and poor family support. The DIRE score (Diagnosis, Intractability, Risk, and Efficacy) is a physician-completed risk-stratification tool that can be helpful for determining which patients are most suitable for opioid therapy; higher scores (that is, a more severe diagnosis, clearly intractable pain, lower psychosocial risk, no chemical dependence history, and higher efficacy of opioids already used) predict greater success with treatment. The DIRE score can be accessed at www .icsi.org/pain__chronic__assessment_and_management_of _14399/pain__chronic__assessment_and_management_of __guideline_.html (Appendix E). Table 16 lists additional tools that may be helpful for assessing risk.

Patients who are selected for opioid therapy should have a thorough understanding of its risks and benefits. The patient and the physician should work together to develop an opioid management plan, or pain contract, that outlines agreed-upon goals and rules of treatment. (An example is available in the chronic pain guideline linked to above, Appendix F.) Typically, pain contracts include stipulations that pain medications will not be sought elsewhere, that the patient will abstain from illicit drugs, will keep clinic appointments as scheduled, and will obtain randomly scheduled urine toxicology screens. A copy of this signed document can be given to the patient and reviewed periodically at follow-up visits to ensure that treatment expectations are being met.

Medication selection should be influenced by the severity and frequency of pain; long-acting opioids, which maintain more consistent drug levels, are preferred for the treatment of CNCP. Physicians should be cautious when initiating methadone, which can cause QT-interval prolongation, hypotension, and cardiac arrhythmias. An electrocardiogram should be obtained at baseline, after 30 days of treatment, and annually thereafter. Methadone should be started at low doses and gradually increased to effective doses. Although methadone requires regular monitoring of QT intervals, it can be effective when other opioids are not. In addition, methadone lacks the euphoric effects of morphine and other opioids that can contribute to dose escalation and potential abuse.

Careful monitoring of patients treated with opioid therapy is essential, and clinicians can use the "6 A's" as a framework for assessment during follow-up visits. Patients should be queried about the effectiveness of *Analgesia*, the benefit of therapy on their *Activities of daily living*, *Adverse events* associated with treatment, and *Aberrant behaviors* suggesting drug abuse; providers should also *Assess mood* and review the *Action (treatment) plan*. Clues to aberrant drug-taking behaviors include multiple episodes of prescription loss, repeated requests for dose increases or early refills, drug requests by name, missed appointments, repeatedly seeking prescriptions from other clinicians, not following through with other components of the treatment plan, and aggressive complaining about needing more of the drug. Random urine drug testing, which is recommended for all patients on opioid therapy, may be conducted more frequently if patients exhibit any of these behaviors. When interpreting the results of urine drug testing, providers should consider the possibility of false-positive and false-negative tests, and correlate results clinically (that is, a specific type of urine testing is required for hydrocodone).

Patients should be seen monthly for the first 3 months after opioid therapy is initiated; once a stable regimen is achieved, visits may occur every 3 to 6 months. More frequent visits, with possible therapy restructuring or discontinuation of opioid therapy, should occur if there is evidence of drug abuse or misuse, significant side effects, or lack of functional improvement. Patients on high doses of opioid therapy should also be seen more frequently, as a recent retrospective cohort study suggests that such patients are at higher risk for medically serious or fatal overdose. That study found that patients prescribed 100 mg/d of opioid medication were nine times more likely to have an overdose than patients prescribed 20 mg/d or less. Patients prescribed 50 mg/d to 99 mg/d were at four times the risk of those on lower doses.

KEY POINTS

- Before initiating treatment for chronic noncancer pain, providers should assess for common behavioral, social, or systems barriers that may prevent a patient from experiencing functional improvement.

- All patients with chronic noncancer pain should be taught self-management strategies that can improve pain.

- Pharmacologic management of chronic pain should start with acetaminophen, NSAIDs, and adjuvant pain therapies.

- Opioid therapy should be reserved for patients with chronic moderate to severe neuropathic pain that has been unresponsive to other treatments.

Cough

Cough is one of the most common symptoms for which patients seek medical attention from either a primary care physician or a pulmonologist. In addition, it has significant impact on health care expenditures. According to the American College of Chest Physicians, up to 30,000,000 physician visits annually are for cough-related symptoms, and billions of dollars are spent on medication for symptomatic relief.

A cough is triggered by chemical or mechanical stimulation of cough receptors. These receptors are located in the upper and lower respiratory tracts as well as in the stomach, gastroesophageal junction, diaphragm, esophagus, pericardium, and ears. The knowledge of the location of cough receptors and the chemical and mechanical triggers of the cough reflex contributes to understanding the differential diagnosis. Recent guidelines suggest an empiric and integrative approach to the management of cough based on duration of cough.

Acute Cough

Acute cough is a cough that is present for less than 3 weeks. Upper respiratory tract infections (rhinosinusitis, pharyngitis) and acute bronchitis are the most common causes. Other considerations include exacerbations of COPD, pneumonia, allergic rhinitis, left ventricular failure, asthma, medications, and aspiration.

Rhinosinusitis (the common cold) and acute bronchitis are most commonly caused by viruses (influenza A and B, parainfluenza, coronavirus, rhinovirus, and respiratory syncytial virus). Nonviral causes include *Mycoplasma pneumoniae*, *Chlamydophila pneumoniae*, and *Bordetella pertussis* (whooping cough). Fever may or, more likely, may not be present. Cough with purulent sputum is not a reliable indicator of a bacterial infection. In acute bronchitis, the cough generally lasts more than 5 days and, although most resolve in 3 weeks, bronchial hyperreactivity can lead to persistence of cough for up to 8 weeks.

The incidence of pertussis has increased over the past two decades. If suspected, culture via nasopharyngeal aspirate or swab and macrolide antibiotic treatment are indicated.

Routine antibiotic treatment of uncomplicated upper respiratory tract infections and acute bronchitis in nonelderly immunocompetent patients is not recommended. Despite recommendations to avoid antibiotics in most patients, antibiotic overuse is common. Up to 60% of patients who present with upper respiratory tract infection symptoms or acute bronchitis are given antibiotics. Patient satisfaction with care for acute bronchitis depends primarily on physician-patient communication rather than on antibiotic prescription.

Lower respiratory tract infection or pneumonia can present with cough, but these infections generally are accompanied by fever, constitutional symptoms, pleuritic chest pain, and abnormalities on pulmonary examination. In patients with such findings and moderate to severe symptoms, a chest radiograph should be obtained. Influenza should be considered in any patient during the appropriate season who presents with cough, fever, myalgia, and headache.

Approximately 15% of patients on an ACE inhibitor develop cough. The cough usually begins within 1 week of starting therapy, although in some patients it may be delayed. The medication should be discontinued. Cough generally abates within 1 to 4 weeks. Since this is a class-specific effect, rechallenge with a different ACE inhibitor is not recommended. An angiotensin receptor blocker can be substituted for an ACE inhibitor as these medications generally do not cause cough.

Treatment of the patient with acute cough is based on primary diagnosis and is mainly supportive. For patients with the common cold, first-generation antihistamines, decongestants, inhaled ipratropium bromide, cromolyn sodium, and naproxen are helpful in decreasing sneezing and rhinorrhea. Newer-generation nonsedating antihistamines are ineffective. A review of 17 trials in adults concluded that centrally acting (codeine, dextromethorphan) or peripherally acting (moguisteine, benzonatate) antitussive therapy results in little, if any, improvement in cough associated with upper respiratory tract infection. The American College of Chest Physicians does not recommend their use. β_2-agonists should not be used unless cough is accompanied by wheezing.

Subacute and Chronic Cough

Subacute cough, a cough of 3 to 8 weeks' duration, is most commonly postinfectious. If an infectious origin is unlikely, upper airway cough syndrome (UACS, previously called postnasal drip syndrome), asthma, pertussis, acid reflux, or acute exacerbation of primary lung disease should be considered. Chronic cough is defined as the persistence of cough for longer than 8 weeks. The most common causes are UACS, asthma, nonasthmatic eosinophilic bronchitis (NAEB), and gastroesophageal reflux disease (GERD). In several case series, UACS, asthma, and GERD accounted for 90% of patients with chronic cough (excluding those with cough related to smoking or ACE inhibitors). Other, less common, causes are chronic bronchitis, bronchiectasis, lung cancer, aspiration, irritation of the external auditory canal, and psychogenic. There are often multiple causes for a case of chronic cough.

The medical history and physical examination may suggest a potential cause or causes, but neither is reliable for definitively ruling in or ruling out specific disease. Patients with chronic cough, especially smokers, should undergo chest radiography. If the chest radiograph is normal, the physician should consider UACS, asthma, NAEB, and GERD and begin a stepwise, sequential approach for evaluation and treatment (**Figure 5**). The definitive diagnosis may be known only after successful individual or joint empiric treatment.

The use of a systematic algorithmic approach in the immunocompetent patient with chronic cough can lead to successful outcomes in more than 90% of patients. In general, unless symptoms point to a specific diagnosis or there is a definitive finding on chest radiograph, empiric therapy for UACS for 2 to 3 weeks is started first. If there is no response, evaluation and treatment for asthma, NAEB, and GERD should ensue. All patients with chronic cough who smoke should receive smoking cessation counseling.

Specific therapy for each diagnosis should be optimized. For patients with UACS, first-generation antihistamines and decongestants remain first-line therapy. Patients with cough-variant asthma may demonstrate reversible airflow obstruction or airway hyperreactivity with bronchoprovocation testing.

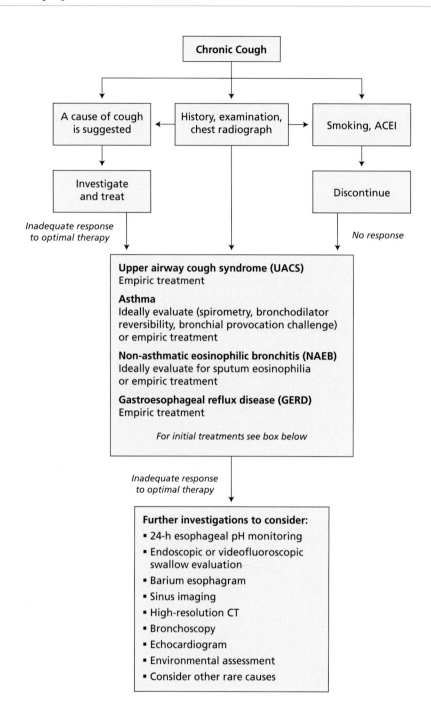

FIGURE 5. Evaluation of chronic cough. ACEI = angiotensin-converting enzyme inhibitor; LTRA = leukotriene receptor antagonist.

However, as bronchoprovocation testing may yield false-positive results, asthma should be diagnosed as a cause of chronic cough only if symptoms abate after 2 to 4 weeks of standard antiasthmatic therapy with an inhaled bronchodilator and inhaled corticosteroids. NAEB is diagnosed in patients who have sputum eosinophilia but are without airway hyperreactivity. These patients are treated with inhaled corticosteroids. GERD may be diagnosed in patients with typical symptoms or in those who fit a typical clinical profile and in whom near-complete or complete resolution of symptoms occurs with antireflux treatment. Typical heartburn symptoms may be present in only 60% patients with chronic cough caused by GERD. Although 24-hour pH monitoring may be helpful in the evaluation of patients with suspected GERD, empiric treatment can be initiated before testing. Effective treatment modalities include dietary and lifestyle modification and acid suppressive therapy with proton pump inhibitors for 1 to 3 months (see MKSAP 16 Gastroenterology and Hepatology).

When disease-based specific therapy fails, cough suppressants may be helpful. Unlike in treatment of acute cough, some clinical trials suggest that centrally acting narcotic (morphine or codeine) or nonnarcotic (dextromethorphan) medications may be effective in the treatment of chronic cough. Peripherally acting antitussives may also be beneficial. As with any long-term medication, risks and benefits need to be considered.

Cough in the Immunocompromised Patient

In addition to being at risk for the common community-acquired infections seen in the immunocompetent host, the immunocompromised patient is at risk for various opportunistic infections that may present with cough, such as tuberculosis, *Pneumocystis jirovecii* pneumonia, and aspergillosis. The degree and duration of immunosuppression, along with whether the primary impairment is in humoral or cell-mediated immunity, can assist in determining the more likely causes. Definitive work-up is indicated in immunocompromised patients with cough. Empiric antibiotic therapy should be initiated while diagnostic testing is used. Treatment can be modified based on subsequent microbiologic test results.

Hemoptysis

Hemoptysis is defined as coughing up any amount of blood from the lower respiratory tract. Hemoptysis must be distinguished from hematemesis or nasopharyngeal bleeding. Massive hemoptysis (>200 mL/d) can be life-threatening. The most common causes of hemoptysis are infection (airway inflammation) and malignancy. Other sources include the tracheobronchial tree (bronchitis, bronchiectasis, tumor), pulmonary parenchyma (abscess; pneumonia, including tuberculosis; Goodpasture syndrome, granulomatosis with polyangiitis [also known as Wegener granulomatosis]), and pulmonary vasculature (arteriovenous malformation, pulmonary

embolism, mitral stenosis, left-sided heart failure). All patients with hemoptysis should undergo chest radiography and, if indicated, chest CT or bronchoscopy.

KEY POINTS

- Routine antibiotic treatment of uncomplicated upper respiratory tract infections and acute bronchitis in nonelderly immunocompetent patients is not recommended.
- Neither centrally acting nor peripherally acting antitussive agents have demonstrated improvement in acute cough associated with upper respiratory tract infection.

Chronic Fatigue and Chronic Fatigue Syndrome

Fatigue is a common symptom in primary care, occurring in a fifth to a quarter of patients. Fatigue is difficult to define and quantify and is often viewed as a minor problem. Chronic fatigue is variably defined as lasting longer than 30 days or longer than 3 months, with a resulting inability to perform desired activities. Chronic fatigue may be secondary to various diseases, including malignancy; autoimmune and endocrine disorders; neurologic diseases (multiple sclerosis, Parkinson disease); chronic kidney, lung, heart, or liver disease; HIV infection; substance abuse; medication side effects; and heavy metal poisoning.

Chronic fatigue syndrome (CFS) is a distinct entity of fatigue that persists for 6 months or more. Diagnostic criteria developed for research purposes have been applied widely in the clinical setting. The International CFS Study Group definition includes medically unexplained fatigue of longer than 6 months' duration after clinical evaluation, with four or more of the following symptoms: subjective memory impairment, sore throat, tender lymph nodes, muscle or joint pain, headache, unrefreshing sleep, and postexertional malaise lasting longer than 24 hours; exclusion criteria include the presence of substance abuse, an eating disorder, an underlying psychiatric disorder, dementia, or severe obesity (BMI ≥ 45). Chronic fatigue of longer than 6 months' duration that does not meet criteria for CFS is designated idiopathic chronic fatigue.

Diagnosis and Evaluation of Chronic Fatigue

There are no specific recommendations regarding diagnostic evaluation for chronic fatigue. Patients with fatigue greater than1 month rarely have abnormalities on either physical or laboratory evaluation; testing should thus be judicious and performed only when clearly indicated. The degree of functional limitation of patients with fatigue is often underestimated by health care providers, resulting in inadequate or incomplete attention and treatment.

Historical elements associated with CFS include unrefreshing sleep, subjective memory impairment, and substantial curtailment in previous level of functioning. CFS has been associated with various conditions, including post–viral infection (parvovirus B19), childhood trauma, and preexisting psychiatric disorders; many associations have not been reproduced in other studies, or are only seen in small numbers of patients, and thus cannot be clearly attributed as causes of CFS.

Physical examination in patients with chronic fatigue is usually normal and performed with the intent to exclude other possible organic causes. Findings of fever, lymphadenopathy, and muscle wasting warrant further evaluation for organic causes and should not be attributed to CFS. Selected laboratory or other diagnostic studies may help identify the cause of chronic fatigue or rule out treatable causes.

Management of Chronic Fatigue and Chronic Fatigue Syndrome

Management of CFS is challenging and requires a comprehensive strategy tailored to the patient's individual goals and needs. Providers must consider the risks of over-investigation, including reinforcement of the patient's belief that a treatable organic cause may be found, the potential hazards of testing itself, and false-positive findings, as well as time and cost issues. Treatment is directed at the underlying illness, if identified; nonspecific therapies include counseling, exercise, and possibly medications. Nonpharmacologic therapy includes lifestyle modification, sleep hygiene, and graded activity; selected patients may benefit from referral for CBT, physical rehabilitation, or psychiatric management. One goal should be to prevent further deterioration in functional ability, which may be accomplished with supportive management and by limiting largely ineffective treatments, such as corticosteroids and immunotherapy. Patients with comorbid depression should be offered antidepressant therapy, but no specific class of medications is recommended specifically for CFS. The limited number of small randomized controlled trials (RCTs) do not provide conclusive evidence for the effectiveness of dietary supplements and herbal remedies for CFS.

Patients with CFS should have regular follow-up to monitor their symptoms, for support and validation, and to avoid unnecessary diagnostic and treatment interventions. Prognosis is variable and related primarily to severity and degree of impairment. In studies, patients with less impairment or fatigue of shorter duration were more likely to recover, although functional outcome is often not reported or standardized, thus limiting the definition of recovery. Other predictors of poor outcome include self-reported poor health and coexisting somatic or mental health disorders.

KEY POINTS

- Fever, lymphadenopathy, or muscle wasting in a patient with chronic fatigue warrants further evaluation for organic causes and should not be attributed to chronic fatigue syndrome.
- Treatment of chronic fatigue syndrome is largely nonpharmacologic and includes lifestyle modification, sleep hygiene, graded activity, and cognitive-behavioral therapy.
- Patients with chronic fatigue syndrome should have regular follow-up to monitor their symptoms, for support and validation, and to avoid unnecessary diagnostic and treatment interventions.

Dizziness

Dizziness is a frustrating and acutely debilitating symptom for many patients. It is more common in women, and prevalence in the elderly may be as high as 37%. Patients with dizziness are at increased risk for falls and nursing home placement. Although most causes of dizziness have a benign course, they may be associated with life-threatening consequences, including stroke and death.

The evaluation of dizziness is challenging and without universally accepted guidelines. The history and physical examination are the most effective diagnostic tools and are used to classify dizziness into four categories: (1) vertigo, (2) presyncope, (3) dysequilibrium, and (4) other causes. The history and physical examination can also help to distinguish peripheral or otologic disease from central disease. Although categorization is attractive, it is not always possible, especially in the elderly. Up to one half of geriatric patients with dizziness have multiple causes in more than one category. Nonetheless, this schema forms the current best framework for diagnosis, evaluation, and management.

In general, key elements of the history include timing of symptoms, duration, provocative or palliative measures, and risk factors for atherosclerotic disease. All patients should have orthostatic vital signs taken and undergo thorough cardiac and neurologic examinations. Routine laboratory testing is not helpful.

Vertigo

Vertigo is the illusion of movement, either personal or environmental, caused by unilateral or asymmetric disruption of peripheral or central vestibular structures. It is typically, but not always, rotational. In studies that examined dizziness in primary care, specialty, or emergency settings, vertigo was the most common type, present in approximately half of patients. It may be accompanied by severe nausea, vomiting, nystagmus, and postural instability. Central causes of vertigo include vascular disease and stroke, mass lesions of the brainstem and cerebellum, multiple sclerosis, migraine, and seizures.

Peripheral causes of vertigo include benign paroxysmal positional vertigo (BPPV), vestibular neuronitis, and Meniere disease. Less common peripheral causes include aminoglycoside toxicity, herpes zoster, otitis media, and perilymph fistulas.

Diagnosing the cause of vertigo is critical because targeted, disease-specific treatment can improve symptoms and prognosis. The duration of symptoms can guide the differential diagnosis (**Table 18**), and results from the Dix-Hallpike maneuver can distinguish central from peripheral disease (**Table 19**). In the Dix-Hallpike maneuver, the patient is instructed to sit upright, turn the head 45 degrees, and keep both eyes open during the entire maneuver. The examiner supports the head and, while instructing the patient to lie down, rapidly places the head below the level of the examining table. The examiner notes nystagmus and subjective symptoms. The test is repeated with the head turned to the opposite side.

Peripheral Vertigo

Clinical Presentation
The most common cause of vertigo is BPPV. Patients with BPPV classically report recurrent, intense, and brief episodes of vertigo (1 minute or less) with a rapid change in head position, such as turning the head while driving or turning over in bed. Auditory or associated neurologic symptoms are absent. BPPV is caused by movement of otoliths or other debris in the semicircular canals (most commonly the posterior semicircular canal) induced by head movement. This leads to perturbation of sensory receptors in the vestibular labyrinth. Recurrences are common, reported to be 18% at 1 year and 30% at 3 years.

Vestibular neuronitis is acute in onset (hours) and is frequently associated with a viral infection that affects the vestibular portion of the eighth cranial nerve. Nausea and vomiting are common; no brainstem symptoms are present (distinguishing it from central vertigo). Hearing usually is not affected, but if it is, the term labyrinthitis is used. Symptoms can be very severe, and although symptoms usually peak during the first 24 hours and resolve within 7 days, full recovery may take longer. Residual dizziness can last for months.

Meniere disease, also known as idiopathic endolymphatic hydrops, is characterized by the classic triad of vertigo, unilateral low frequency hearing loss, and tinnitus, occasionally associated with aural fullness. Endolymphatic hydrops refers to a condition of increased hydraulic pressure in the inner ear endolymphatic system leading to these symptoms. In Meniere disease, the cause of the increased pressure is not known. Vertigo may be the first presenting sign. The diagnosis may be secured only after repeated attacks of vertigo with associated hearing loss.

Treatment
BPPV can be treated by the Epley maneuver (**Figure 6**), which can be curative. This maneuver attempts to move the debris floating in the semicircular canal to a position where it can exit into the utricular cavity. An evidence-based review of all major studies analyzing repositioning procedures concluded that this therapy is beneficial. In one study, 61% of the treated group had complete resolution of symptoms at 4 weeks compared with 20% in the control (sham-treated) group. The number needed to treat was 2.4. Medications generally are ineffective in BPPV.

For other causes of vertigo, particularly vestibular neuronitis, treatment options are generally limited to symptom relief. Vestibular suppressants and antiemetic drugs (antihistamines, benzodiazepines, and phenothiazines) are the three major drug

TABLE 18. Duration of Vertigo and Suggested Causes

Duration of Vertigo	Underlying Cause
Seconds	Benign paroxysmal positional vertigo
Minutes to hours	Transient ischemic attack
	Meniere disease
	Perilymph fistula
	Migraine
Days	Acute vestibular neuronitis/labyrinthitis
	Ischemia/stroke
	Migraine
	Multiple sclerosis
Weeks	Psychogenic

TABLE 19. Interpretation of Dix-Hallpike Maneuver Findings in Evaluation of Vertigo

Characteristic	Peripheral Disease	Central Disease
Latency of nystagmus	2-40 s	No latency
Duration of nystagmus	<1 min	>1 min
Severity of symptoms	Severe	Less severe
Habituation	Yes	No
Fatigability	Yes	No
Direction of nystagmus	Horizontal, with rotational component; never vertical	Can be vertical, horizontal, or torsional; may change with position

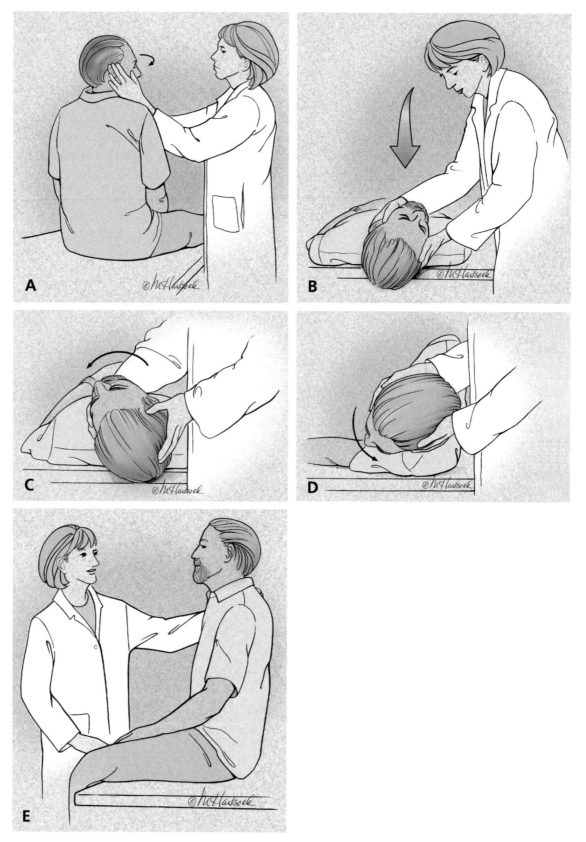

FIGURE 6. Epley maneuver for relieving benign paroxysmal positional vertigo. The patient sits on the examination table, with eyes open and head turned 45 degrees to the right (*A*). The physician supports the patient's head as the patient lies back quickly from a sitting to supine position, ending with the head hanging 20 degrees off the end of the examination table and still turned to the right (*B*). The physician turns the patient's head 90 degrees to the left side. The patient remains in this position for 30 seconds (*C*). The physician turns the patient's head an additional 90 degrees to the left while the patient rotates his or her body 90 degrees in the same direction. The patient remains in this position for 30 seconds (*D*). The patient sits up on the left side of the examination table (*E*). The procedure may be repeated on either side until the patient experiences relief of symptoms.

classes that may modify the intensity of symptoms. The most common drugs are centrally active antihistamine anticholinergic medications. These medications have been shown to reduce symptom severity. Benzodiazepines act centrally to suppress vestibular responses. Phenothiazine antiemetics are useful when nausea and vomiting accompany vertigo. Side effects of all of these medications include sedation. Some experts advocate corticosteroid therapy, but robust outcome data are lacking. Data for calcium channel blockers, betahistine, corticosteroids and ginger root are either weak or conflicting. Medications are recommended only for short periods (24-48 hours). More prolonged use may suppress vestibular feedback and central compensation mechanisms, leading to prolongation of symptoms.

Referral to a trained therapist for vestibular rehabilitation (VR) is helpful for peripheral vertigo, especially if initiated early. In a review of 27 moderate- to high-quality trials enrolling community-dwelling adults, VR proved to be effective. Compared with control groups, VR led to improvement in symptoms, walking, balance, vision, and activities of daily living. Exercises include learning to bring on symptoms to desensitize the vestibular system, learning to coordinate head and eye movements, and improving balance and walking skills.

Although caffeine restriction, salt restriction, and diuretic therapy have been advocated for Meniere disease, a recent review concluded that there is insufficient high-quality evidence to recommend these interventions. Similarly, there are no strong data for corticosteroids or immunosuppressive therapy.

Central Vertigo
Ischemia, infarction, and hemorrhage of the brainstem or cerebellum are life-threatening causes of vertigo. Patients at risk are those with hypertension, tobacco use, hyperlipidemia, diabetes mellitus, atrial fibrillation, and preexisting atherosclerotic vascular disease. Up to one quarter of patients with risk factors for stroke who present with severe vertigo or nystagmus or who are unable to stand without support have infarction of the inferior cerebellum.

The distinction between vertigo due to vascular disease and vertigo due to vestibular neuronitis is critical. Neurologic symptoms are absent in patients with vestibular neuronitis. However, patients with vertigo due to brainstem ischemia, infarction, or hemorrhage may demonstrate diplopia, dysarthria, dysphagia, and focal numbness or weakness. Those with cerebellar disease may present with gait abnormalities and headache. MRI of the brain with angiography is the preferred diagnostic test. Patients with brainstem or cerebellar disease require immediate medical or neurosurgical intervention.

Presyncope
Presyncope is the sensation of near loss of consciousness. The main cause is a global and temporary decrease in cerebral perfusion owing to cardiovascular disease (ischemia, arrhythmia, valvular heart disease), hypotension, carbon monoxide poisoning, anemia, or vasovagal reaction (see Syncope, below).

Dysequilibrium
Dysequilibrium is defined as imbalance or unsteadiness while standing or walking, without the sensation originating in the head. It is relieved with sitting or recumbency. Dysequilibrium is caused by defective sensory input (vision, vestibular), impaired proprioception or motor function, generalized weakness, Parkinson disease, joint pain, or anxiety or other psychiatric disorders. Medications can be contributing factors. A multidisciplinary approach to treatment is frequently indicated. The plan may include physical therapy, assistance devices for ambulation, audiometry testing, vision testing, and medication reconciliation.

Nonspecific Dizziness
Vague signs of dizziness, lightheadedness, or "wooziness" comprise the last and typically most frustrating category of dizziness. Although frequently attributed to psychiatric disorders, especially anxiety and depression, there may be overlap with other categories. Other specific causes include hypoglycemia, hyperglycemia, electrolyte abnormalities, thyroid disorders, anemia, and multiple classes of medications.

KEY POINTS
- All patients being evaluated for dizziness should have orthostatic vital signs taken and undergo thorough cardiac and neurologic examinations; routine laboratory testing is not helpful.
- Benign paroxysmal positional vertigo (BPPV) can be treated by the Epley maneuver, which attempts to move the debris floating in the semicircular canal to a position where it can exit into the utricular cavity; medications generally are ineffective for BPPV.
- Patients with vertigo accompanied by diplopia, dysarthria, dysphagia, focal numbness, gait abnormalities, or headache may have brainstem or cerebellar disease requiring immediate medical or neurosurgical intervention.

Insomnia
Insomnia is defined as any difficulty with sleep initiation, duration, consolidation, or quality that occurs despite adequate opportunity for sleep (in contradistinction to sleep deprivation) and results in daytime sleepiness or other adverse effects on daytime activities. It can be primary or secondary, the latter being more common. Causes include underlying medical problems such as chronic pain, depression, GERD, and obstructive sleep apnea. Insomnia also may be secondary to a poor sleep environment, medications, or other substances. It can be acute (transient) or chronic (occurring at least three times weekly for at least 1 month). Insomnia is sometimes defined as initial (difficulty falling asleep), middle (awakenings during the night), and terminal (early morning awakening).

Insomnia is more common in women, the elderly, patients with comorbid medical problems, shift workers, and persons of lower socioeconomic status. Patients with chronic insomnia are more likely to use health resources, be absent or late to work, and be involved in motor vehicle collisions, and they have an increased risk of suicide, depression, anxiety, and substance abuse. As many as 50% of patients identify some aspect of sleep disorder; clinicians should consider screening for insomnia by asking every patient about their sleep.

Evaluation of Insomnia

Several sleep questionnaires exist for use in patients in whom a sleep problem has been identified. Alternatively, physicians can ask about key components of the problem, including characterization of the sleep disturbance (duration, frequency, severity, progression), precipitating factors, past problems, and previous treatments and response. A thorough sleep history includes patterns of sleep and wakefulness (time to bed, time to sleep, number of awakenings), nocturnal symptoms, pre-sleep and sleep environment, and daytime activities. Interviewing a bed partner may provide additional information. A formal sleep diary may also be used. Important questions include information about medication and other substance use, especially over-the-counter (OTC) medications, caffeine, and alcohol.

Physical examination should assess for obesity, body habitus consistent with obstructive sleep apnea (enlarged tongue or tonsils, increased neck circumference), thyroid dysfunction, heart failure, and neurologic disease. Mental status examination should focus on mood and level of alertness. Laboratory and other diagnostic evaluations should be performed judiciously. An overnight polysomnography may be indicated if obstructive sleep apnea or other primary sleep disturbance (for example, restless legs syndrome or periodic limb movements of sleep) is strongly suspected, or in patients refractory to initial therapy.

Management of Insomnia

Therapy for insomnia is directed at treating any underlying cause or associated comorbid conditions. Pain, esophageal reflux, heart failure, and obstructive sleep apnea should be treated as appropriate. Nonpharmacologic interventions are preferred, especially in the elderly and in those with chronic insomnia.

Sleep hygiene refers to behavioral and environmental factors that affect sleep. Improving sleep hygiene is an important component of insomnia management; alone, however, this is often insufficient to treat chronic insomnia. Components of sleep hygiene include maintenance of a stable bedtime and awakening time, appropriate exposure to light during daytime and darkness during nighttime, avoidance of stimulants and exercise after 6 PM, use of the bed for sleeping and sex only, a maximum of 8 hours in bed, adjusting the bed and room comfort level, and relaxation strategies before bedtime.

CBT has been to shown to be more effective for both primary and secondary insomnia than drug therapy. Several sessions weekly are required over a several-week period. Adjunct medications may be used with CBT initially, but long-term studies indicate that CBT alone is best for maintenance therapy. Other, less common, treatments include sleep restriction, biofeedback, and relaxation techniques.

The decision to initiate pharmacologic treatment should take into account the patient's response to other therapies, patient preferences, treatment goals, comorbid conditions, medication interactions, adverse effects, and cost. Initial recommendations are for short- and intermediate-acting benzodiazepine γ-aminobutyric acid (GABA)-receptor agonists, nonbenzodiazepine GABA-receptor agonists, and type A melatonin-receptor agonists (**Table 20**). Nonbenzodiazepine GABA-receptor agonists are preferred over other sedating agents, including sedating antidepressants, owing to their lack of effect on sleep architecture and their superior safety profile. With benzodiazepines, caution is warranted regarding dependence and tolerance, as well as side effects of daytime sedation and psychomotor impairment. They should not be used in patients with a history of drug or alcohol abuse. Nonbenzodiazepine GABA-receptor agonists, such as zolpidem and zaleplon, have fewer adverse effects, mostly owing to their shorter half-life. Adverse effects of these agents include nausea, vertigo, nightmares, disorientation, and agitation. Zolpidem is associated with cases of somnambulism, such as nocturnal eating, driving, and walking. Data are limited regarding hypnotic agents for long-term therapy. The FDA recommends that treatment be limited to 1 month, and sleep specialists do not recommend long-term therapy. Small studies have show effectiveness for zolpidem for up to 8 weeks and for eszopiclone for up to 6 months.

Other sedative-hypnotic agents (chloral hydrate, barbiturates), gabapentin, and antipsychotic medications are not recommended for use for primary insomnia. Antidepressant medications are recommended for use only when insomnia is one of the manifestations of an underlying depressive disorder. Use of tricyclic antidepressants is discouraged owing to their significant side effect profile; antidepressants that are most efficacious for use in insomnia are low-dose trazodone or mirtazapine. Antihistamines are often used to treat insomnia, especially diphenhydramine, owing to its OTC availability and inclusion in OTC products marketed specifically for sleep. Because these drugs antagonize central H_1 receptors, their side-effect profile is significant and is predominantly anticholinergic with carryover sedation and should be avoided for chronic insomnia. Diphenhydramine has a long half-life and is an inhibitor of CYP2D6 drug metabolism. Thus, with its anticholinergic profile, it is a particularly bad choice for elderly patients, especially those with mild cognitive impairment or Alzheimer disease or who are exposed to polypharmacy. OTC melatonin is available, and in this form is a nonspecific agonist of melatonin receptors. It may be helpful for short-term use for jet lag and other circadian rhythm disorders; however, its effectiveness compared with specific melatonin receptor agonists available

TABLE 20. Drug Treatment of Primary Insomnia

Agent, Dosage	Half-Life (hour)	Side Effects
Benzodiazepines		Daytime sedation, dizziness, anterograde amnesia, falls, rebound insomnia
Estazolam, 1-2 mg	10-24	
Flurazepam, 15-30 mg	2-3	
Quazepam, 7.5-30 mg	40	
Temazepam, 7.5-30 mg	8-15	
Triazolam, 0.125-0.5 mg	2-5	
Nonbenzodiazepine sedative – hypnotic agents		Daytime sedation, dizziness, anterograde amnesia, falls, rebound insomnia
Zolpidem, 5-10 mg	3	
Zaleplon, 5-10 mg	1	
Eszopiclone, 2-3 mg	5-7	Unpleasant taste, dry mouth, drowsiness, dizziness
Melatonin-receptor agonist		
Ramelteon, 8 mg	2-5	Drowsiness, dizziness, increased serum prolactin levels

Adapted with permission from Wilson JF. In the clinic. Insomnia. Ann Intern Med. 2008;148(1):ITC13-1-ITC13-16. [PMID: 18166757] Copyright 2008, American College of Physicians.

by prescription for acute and chronic insomnia is not known. Many patients drink alcohol to help with sleep; although alcohol may help in falling asleep, it interferes with sleep architecture and often causes sleep disruption in the latter half of the night. Dopaminergic agents may be helpful for patients with insomnia associated with restless legs syndrome (see MKSAP 16 Neurology).

Referral to a sleep specialist is indicated if the etiology of insomnia remains unclear, if daytime functioning is impaired, if the insomnia is refractory to therapy, or if the patient requests it. Consultation may also be helpful for patients with restless legs syndrome or other primary sleep disorders, such as narcolepsy. Pulmonary, otolaryngology, or dental referral may be helpful for patients with obstructive sleep apnea or if specific upper airway anatomic abnormalities are suspected. Psychiatric referral is helpful for patients with concurrent psychiatric disorders, patients requiring high doses of medications for treatment, patients with insomnia refractory to treatment, or patients requiring tapering or titration of medications or combinations of medications.

KEY POINTS

- The first-line treatment of insomnia is improving sleep hygiene; additional options include cognitive-behavioral therapy and medications.
- Short- and intermediate-acting benzodiazepine γ-aminobutyric acid (GABA)-receptor agonists, nonbenzodiazepine GABA-receptor agonists, and melatonin-receptor agonists are all effective in the treatment of insomnia, but have different risks of long-term dependence and tolerance as well as side effects.

- Antihistamines such as diphenhydramine have a long half-life, have significant anticholinergic side effects, and often have carry-over sedation; they are a poor choice for treating insomnia in the elderly.

Syncope

Syncope is defined as the transient loss of consciousness with loss of postural tone and spontaneous recovery, resulting from global cerebral hypoperfusion. Loss of consciousness distinguishes syncope from pseudosyncopal events, such as drop attacks and simple falls, and global cerebral hypoperfusion distinguishes syncope from other causes of loss of consciousness, such as seizure and stroke. The loss of consciousness of syncope is usually less than 1 minute, with complete restoration of orientation and function at the time of recovery.

Neurocardiogenic Syncope

Neurocardiogenic syncope, the most common type, is predominantly a clinical diagnosis. Vasovagal neurocardiogenic syncope (the common "faint") results from a reflex withdrawal of sympathetic tone accompanied by an increase in vagal tone, precipitating a drop in blood pressure and heart rate. Without the surge in vagal tone, bradycardia is absent; this variant is called vasodepressor syncope. Patients with neurocardiogenic syncope often experience a prodromal phase, usually longer than 10 seconds, characterized by palpitations, nausea, blurred vision, warmth, diaphoresis, or lightheadedness, although these symptoms are less common in the elderly. Provoking factors include prolonged standing, postural change, hot environments, emotional distress, and preload-reducing situations (dehydration, use of diuretics or vasodilators). The first episode usually occurs at a young age, and recurrences are common. Variants of neurocardiogenic syncope that are specifically situational include cough, sneeze, defecation, swallow, micturition, laughter, post-exercise, and post-prandial syncope. Carotid sinus syncope occurs after mechanical manipulation of the carotid sinuses, altering sympathetic and parasympathetic tone; it may be reproduced by carotid sinus massage and is more common in the elderly, in men, and in those with underlying structural heart disease.

Orthostatic Hypotension

Orthostatic hypotension is characterized by an abnormal drop in blood pressure with standing (greater than 20 mm Hg systolic or 10 mm Hg diastolic). Since orthostatic changes may be "initial" (immediate), "classic" (within 3 minutes), or delayed, syncope may occur immediately (0-3 minutes) or be delayed (up to 30 minutes). Orthostatic syncope is more common in the elderly; in those taking vasoactive drugs, diuretics, or alcohol; and in the setting of volume depletion or autonomic failure, such as primary or idiopathic autonomic neuropathy. It may occur in association with Parkinson disease, diabetes, amyloidosis, Shy-Drager syndrome, and lower motor neuron injuries. Patients commonly have symptoms of dizziness, weakness, and fatigue, both before and after the event.

A unique variant of orthostatic intolerance is postural orthostatic tachycardia syndrome, usually seen in young women and related to inadequate venous return with significant tachycardia; patients may experience symptoms of lightheadedness and palpitations, but not syncope.

Cardiac Causes of Syncope

Cardiac diseases account for the remaining causes of true syncope and predominate in the elderly. Arrhythmias are the most common and the most worrisome causes of syncope and include bradycardias (sinus and atrioventricular node dysfunction) as well as tachyarrhythmias (supraventricular and ventricular; atrial tachyarrhythmias rarely cause syncope). Patients with an arrhythmogenic cause of syncope usually have had only one or two episodes, with less than 5 seconds of warning symptoms before each episode. Patients often have underlying structural heart disease as a contributing cause. A prolonged QT interval may result in arrhythmia causing syncope and can be drug-related (see MKSAP 16 Cardiovascular Medicine). Clues to arrhythmia include brief or absent prodrome, palpitations immediately preceding the episode, and syncope occurring in the supine position. (An exception is ventricular tachycardia, which usually has a warning prodrome of more than 5 seconds and associated diaphoresis).

Other cardiac causes resulting in inadequate cardiac output and subsequent cerebral hypoperfusion include valvular heart disease, cardiac tumors, pericardial disease, and cardiomyopathy. Clues to structural heart disease include relationship to exercise or exertion, sensitivity to volume status, and association with medications. Cardiac ischemia, pulmonary embolism, and aortic dissection are unusual causes of syncope and rarely occur without other symptoms.

Diagnostic Evaluation of Syncope

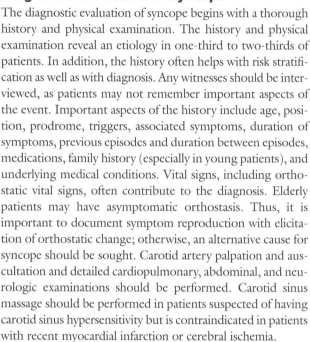

The diagnostic evaluation of syncope begins with a thorough history and physical examination. The history and physical examination reveal an etiology in one-third to two-thirds of patients. In addition, the history often helps with risk stratification as well as with diagnosis. Any witnesses should be interviewed, as patients may not remember important aspects of the event. Important aspects of the history include age, position, prodrome, triggers, associated symptoms, duration of symptoms, previous episodes and duration between episodes, medications, family history (especially in young patients), and underlying medical conditions. Vital signs, including orthostatic vital signs, often contribute to the diagnosis. Elderly patients may have asymptomatic orthostasis. Thus, it is important to document symptom reproduction with elicitation of orthostatic change; otherwise, an alternative cause for syncope should be sought. Carotid artery palpation and auscultation and detailed cardiopulmonary, abdominal, and neurologic examinations should be performed. Carotid sinus massage should be performed in patients suspected of having carotid sinus hypersensitivity but is contraindicated in patients with recent myocardial infarction or cerebral ischemia.

Despite its low diagnostic yield, a 12-lead electrocardiogram (ECG) remains the first and most widely recommended test to perform in patients being evaluated for syncope, partly owing to its noninvasive nature, availability, and low cost. Although this test is relatively insensitive for finding a specific cause of syncope, its specificity is high, and an abnormal ECG is used to identify and stratify patients for additional testing.

The remainder of the evaluation should be directed by the unique circumstances of the patient's event. Guidelines for syncope generally do not dictate the degree of detail considered necessary for further testing. Echocardiography is recommended in patients suspected of having structural heart disease. If an arrhythmia is suspected, documentation of the arrhythmia is indicated either by inpatient telemetry or ambulatory monitoring (see MKSAP 16 Cardiovascular Medicine). No specific routine laboratory studies are recommended, although women of reproductive age warrant a pregnancy test. Tests with the lowest likelihood of affecting diagnosis or management include head CT scan, carotid Doppler ultrasonography, electroencephalography, and measurement of cardiac enzyme levels; these studies may be indicated if symptoms point to specific etiologies but otherwise should be omitted from the work-up. Recommendations to not routinely perform cardiac enzyme testing are supported by evidence that patients with cardiac ischemia almost always present with chest pain or ECG changes. Neurologic studies

CONT.

have only been shown to be useful in patients with new neurologic findings on initial evaluation. Tilt-table testing should be reserved for patients with suspected neurocardiogenic syncope not confirmed by history and physical examination, for those with recurrent syncopal episodes, and for patients suspected of having arrhythmogenic syncope or who have a high risk profile for cardiovascular events in whom previous testing has not been revealing.

Risk Stratification and Management of Syncope

Several risk scores have been developed and validated in order to identify patients with syncope at high risk of adverse events. Causes of syncope vary according to the clinical setting in which the evaluation was conducted (office versus emergency department), and a significant number of patients (40%-50%) never present for evaluation; this number is higher in younger persons. Risk stratification thus is subject to patient population and setting. None of the current risk assessment tools is widely accepted in emergency practice.

Neurocardiogenic and orthostatic syncope both are generally benign in nature and do not require hospitalization. An exception is an elderly patient in whom a secondary cause of orthostasis is suspected or in whom recurrent episodes carry risk for harm from trauma. For neurocardiogenic causes, management may consist of patient education with specific instructions on abortive and preventive strategies. These isometric counter-pressure maneuvers include leg crossing, hand-grip, squatting, and muscle tensing. β-Blockers are no longer indicated in vasovagal syncope.

Orthostatic hypotension is associated with a two-fold increase in mortality from underlying causes; these should be treated appropriately. For benign orthostatic causes, treatment consists of the maneuvers listed above, as well as positional changes, maintenance of adequate fluid intake, compression stockings, and possibly midodrine or fludrocortisone if indicated (frequent episodes with subsequent risk of trauma; syncope during high-risk or competitive activities, such as in pilots or athletes). These patients have an excellent prognosis and no increase in mortality. Patients with carotid sinus hypersensitivity benefit from insertion of a dual-chamber permanent pacemaker.

Cardiac causes of syncope carry a high mortality in all age groups; 6-month mortality is greater than 10% and is related to the underlying cause, not the syncope itself. Although younger patients are more likely to have benign causes of syncope, patients with suspected cardiac causes warrant further inpatient evaluation regardless of age. High-risk patients requiring immediate in-hospital telemetry are those with exertional or supine syncope, palpitations before the event, a family history of sudden death, nonsustained ventricular tachycardia, and abnormal ECG findings (conduction abnormalities, bradycardia). Other indications for hospitalization include chest pain, heart failure, syncope without warning

signs, hemorrhage, suspected or known heart disease, and frequent recurrent episodes.

KEY POINTS

- Tests in the evaluation of syncope with the lowest likelihood of affecting diagnosis or management include head CT scan, carotid Doppler ultrasonography, electroencephalography, and measurement of cardiac enzyme levels; these studies should not be performed in the absence of symptoms pointing to specific etiologies.

- Indications for hospitalization in patients with syncope include chest pain, heart failure, syncope without warning signs, hemorrhage, suspected or known heart disease, and frequent recurrent episodes.

- High-risk patients with syncope requiring immediate in-hospital telemetry are those with exertional or supine syncope, palpitations before the event, a family history of sudden death, nonsustained ventricular tachycardia, or abnormal electrocardiographic findings.

Chest Pain

Chest pain accounts for 2% of all outpatient visits to primary care physicians and 5.5 million visits to emergency departments in the United States annually. It is the most common symptom in persons 50 to 64 years of age presenting for emergency care. Approximately 3 million patients are hospitalized each year for further evaluation and treatment. Although a few patients presenting with chest pain have true medical emergencies or require inpatient care, prompt and accurate diagnosis is nonetheless essential. The physician must not only distinguish ischemic from nonischemic chest pain but also distinguish emergent causes of chest pain from nonemergent ones. Misdiagnosis can be catastrophic for the patient and a source of a malpractice claim against the physician.

The most likely cause of chest pain varies according to patient characteristics and the presentation setting. In the outpatient setting, musculoskeletal causes are the most common, accounting for approximately 40% of cases, followed by gastrointestinal disease (19%). In the emergency department, acute coronary syndromes are more common, accounting for up to 13% of patient visits.

Differential Diagnosis

The differential diagnosis of chest pain largely consists of cardiac, pulmonary, gastrointestinal, and musculoskeletal disease. Dermatologic disease (herpes zoster affecting thoracic dermatomes) and psychiatric conditions (anxiety, panic attack) also can result in chest pain. Whereas most causes of chest pain can be evaluated and treated in a nonurgent fashion, others, such as acute coronary syndromes,

CONT.

aortic dissection, tension pneumothorax, and pulmonary embolism, require rapid triage for definitive diagnosis and intervention.

Cardiac Causes of Chest Pain

Cardiac causes of chest pain include ischemia (acute coronary syndromes, stable angina), aortic dissection, myocarditis, pericarditis, and aortic stenosis. A standard diagnostic approach is to distinguish ischemic chest pain from nonischemic causes as the first step. Characterization of the chest pain is helpful, as pain descriptors provided by the patient can increase or decrease the likelihood of ischemia. (Assessment of pretest probability of ischemic heart disease based on age, sex, and description of the pain is discussed in MKSAP 16 Cardiovascular Medicine.) In a meta-analysis describing the value and limitations of the chest pain history in the evaluation of patients with suspected acute myocardial infarction, radiation to the right arm or shoulder and radiation to both arms or shoulders had the highest positive likelihood ratios (LR+) of 4.7 and 4.1, respectively. Other pain descriptors that increase the likelihood of acute myocardial infarction are pain associated with exertion (LR+ 2.4), radiation to the left arm (LR+ 2.3), diaphoresis (LR+ 2.0), nausea or vomiting (LR+ 1.9), and pain that is pressure-like (LR+ 1.3). Descriptors that decrease the likelihood of acute myocardial infarction include pleuritic pain (LR+ 0.2); pain described as either positional, sharp, or reproducible with palpation (LR+ 0.3); and pain that is either inframammary in location or not associated with exertion (LR+ 0.8). In one study of 48 patients, no patient with sharp or stabbing pain that was positional, pleuritic, or reproducible with palpation and who had no history of angina or myocardial infarction was diagnosed with acute myocardial infarction at discharge. There is no predictable association between acute myocardial infarction and relief of chest pain with nitroglycerin. A high index of suspicion is necessary in women, the elderly, and patients with diabetes, as they may not present with classic symptoms.

Patients presenting with acute chest pain can be stratified into high, intermediate, or low risk of having an acute coronary syndrome based on information easily available in the office setting, including pain descriptors, history of heart disease, cardiac risk factors, and 12-lead ECG (**Table 21**). The ECG can be diagnostic (new ST-segment elevation or depression, T-wave inversion in multiple leads). In some patients, however, the ECG is normal or near-normal even in the presence of acute ischemia, and serial evaluations may be necessary.

Several more detailed prediction tools and algorithms have been published in an attempt to guide further evaluation and therapy and minimize unnecessary testing. These tools,

TABLE 21. Likelihood that Signs and Symptoms Represent an Acute Coronary Syndrome Secondary to CAD

	High Likelihood	Intermediate Likelihood	Low Likelihood
Feature	Any of the following:	Absence of high-likelihood features and presence of any of the following:	Absence of high- or intermediate-likelihood features but may have:
History	Chest or left arm pain or discomfort as chief symptom reproducing prior documented angina Known history of CAD, including MI	Chest or left arm pain or discomfort as chief symptom Age >70 y Male sex Diabetes mellitus	Probable ischemic symptoms in absence of any of the intermediate-likelihood characteristics Recent cocaine use
Physical examination	Transient MR murmur, hypotension, diaphoresis, pulmonary edema, or crackles	Extracardiac vascular disease	Chest discomfort reproduced by palpation
ECG	New, or presumably new, transient ST-segment deviation (1 mm or greater) or T-wave inversion in multiple precordial leads	Fixed Q waves ST-segment depression 0.5 to 1 mm or T-wave inversion greater than 1 mm	T-wave flattening or inversion less than 1 mm in leads with dominant R waves Normal ECG
Cardiac markers	Elevated serum cardiac troponin I, troponin T, or creatine kinase MB	Normal	Normal

CAD = coronary artery disease; ECG = electrocardiogram; MI = myocardial infarction; MR = mitral regurgitation.

CONT.
utilizing history, physical examination, ECG, and cardiac bio-markers (creatine kinase MB, troponin), are predominantly used in emergency departments.

Aortic dissection is characterized by sudden and severe pain at onset, often with a tearing, splitting, or ripping quality that radiates to the back. Asymmetric intensity of peripheral pulses (pulse deficit) is a strong predictor (LR+ 5.7), and the chest radiograph may demonstrate a widened mediastinum. These classic features are often absent, however, and an acute aortic condition must be considered in any patient with severe thoracic pain. Pericarditis and myocarditis usually present with pleuritic chest pain. The pain in pericarditis is unaffected by exercise, worsens with recumbency, and is relieved with sitting forward. A pericardial rub may be present. Classic ECG findings are diffuse ST-segment elevation and PR-segment depression. Aortic stenosis may cause exertional chest pain, which may be accompanied by syncope, dyspnea, and other signs of heart failure.

Pulmonary Causes of Chest Pain

Pulmonary causes of chest pain include pulmonary embolism, pneumothorax, pleuritis, pneumonia, pulmonary hypertension, and other parenchymal lesions. In general, the pain with pulmonary embolism, pneumothorax, pleuritis, and pneumonia is pleuritic in nature and accompanied by dyspnea.

With pulmonary embolism, pain may be accompanied by cough, wheezing, hemoptysis, tachypnea, and tachycardia. Risk factors include immobilization, recent surgery, paresis, history of deep venous thrombosis, malignancy, obesity, tobacco use, and estrogen therapy. The diagnosis is made by ventilation-perfusion scan, chest CT angiography, or pulmonary artery angiography (see MKSAP 16 Pulmonary and Critical Care Medicine). In low-probability scenarios, a negative D-dimer test can be helpful in ruling out thromboembolism.

Pneumothorax can be primary (spontaneous) or secondary. Rupture of a subpleural bleb underlies a spontaneous pneumothorax, and lifetime recurrence rates are up to 50%. Secondary pneumothorax occurs in patients with underlying pulmonary disease such as COPD, cystic fibrosis, or tuberculosis. Physical examination demonstrates decreased chest expansion, decreased breath sounds, and hyperresonance to percussion, all on the affected side. Diagnosis is made by chest radiograph. Tension pneumothorax, heralded by hypotension and tracheal deviation to the unaffected side, is a medical emergency.

Pulmonary hypertension includes pulmonary arterial hypertension and pulmonary hypertension secondary to other conditions, including heart, lung, and thromboembolic disease. The chest pain associated with pulmonary hypertension is not pleuritic but usually is accompanied by exertional dyspnea and fatigue. In most patients, the pain is due to ischemia from either subendocardial hypoperfusion or compression of coronary arteries by enlarged pulmonary arteries. On physical examination, jugular venous pressure is often elevated, there may be a parasternal heave, the S_2 heart sound is widely split, and the P_2 (pulmonic valve) component of S_2 is loud.

Gastrointestinal Causes of Chest Pain

The most common gastrointestinal cause of chest pain is GERD. Although often described as burning, it can mimic angina and be relieved by nitroglycerin. It generally is worsened with bending over or recumbency and relieved with antacids, H_2 blockers, or proton pump inhibitors. Other, less common, gastrointestinal causes of chest pain include cholecystitis, cholangitis, esophageal spasm, peptic ulcer disease, and pancreatitis.

Musculoskeletal Causes of Chest Pain

Musculoskeletal chest pain is common, especially in women. Etiologies include costochondritis, osteoarthritis, and muscle strain. The pain is sharp, occasionally pleuritic, worsened or reproduced with movement or palpation, and relieved with NSAIDs. It may last for weeks. Pain that worsens with movement can raise concern for ischemia, and a careful history is essential. Imaging is usually not indicated or helpful.

Chest Pain and Decision to Hospitalize

The decision to hospitalize a patient with chest pain is challenging. The goal is to identify patients with life-threatening disease who require immediate attention while minimizing unnecessary work-up and treatment in others. A rapid clinical determination of the likelihood of an acute coronary syndrome (see Table 21) is the essential first task for the physician and should guide the decision. In addition, the physician should consider the likelihood of short-term adverse outcomes (death, nonfatal myocardial infarction) in patients with an acute coronary syndrome. Patients suspected of having an acute coronary syndrome should be admitted. Low-risk patients can be further stratified with stress testing.

The use of formal risk scores (TIMI, GRACE, PURSUIT) can be useful in further risk stratification and management. While some centers utilize chest pain evaluation units (CPEUs) to streamline evaluation and limit unnecessary coronary care unit admissions, the true cost-effectiveness of these units is unknown.

Despite a comprehensive history, physical examination, and ECG, approximately 2% of patients with an acute coronary syndrome are missed in the emergency department. Women younger than 55 years old and those who are nonwhite, those who report dyspnea as a chief symptom, or those who have normal ECGs are more likely to be discharged. In one study, the risk-adjusted mortality ratio for those not hospitalized compared with those who were was 1.9 (95% CI, 0.7-5.2).

Patients with pneumothorax, pulmonary embolism, and pericarditis are generally hospitalized for further care.

CONT.

Aortic dissection and tension pneumothorax always require admission. **H**

KEY POINTS

- Characteristics of chest pain that increase the likelihood of ischemia include radiation of pain to either or both arms or shoulders; pain associated with exertion, diaphoresis, or nausea or vomiting; and pain that is pressure-like.

- Characteristics of chest pain with a lower likelihood of ischemia include pleuritic pain; pain that is positional, sharp, or reproducible with palpation; pain that is not associated with exertion; and pain that is inframammary in location.

- There is no predictable association between acute myocardial infarction and relief of chest pain with nitroglycerin.

- An acute aortic condition must be considered in any patient with severe thoracic pain.

Edema

Excess fluid accumulation in the interstitial space leads to edema. Such fluid accumulation results from increased capillary hydrostatic pressure, increased capillary permeability, or decreased plasma oncotic pressure, as well as from retention of sodium and water by the kidneys. Lymphedema, a type of nonpitting edema due to extravasation of high–protein content lymphatic fluid, is caused by congenital lymphatic disease or damage to the lymphatic vessels from surgery, radiation, obstruction, or recurrent cellulitis.

The differential diagnosis of the patient with edema is broad but can be narrowed by history and physical examination. Causes of bilateral edema include heart failure, nephrotic syndrome, cirrhosis, hypoproteinemia, constrictive pericarditis, chronic venous insufficiency, lymphedema, and medications (including minoxidil, nifedipine, amlodipine, thiazolidinediones, NSAIDs, and fludrocortisone). If central venous pressure is elevated, cardiac disease or pulmonary hypertension is likely; if normal, other causes should be considered. The most common causes of unilateral leg edema are deep venous thrombosis, cellulitis, and malignant lymphedema.

The management of edema involves identifying and reversing the underlying disorder. Diuretics should be used carefully, especially in patients whose sodium retention is secondary to a reduction in cardiac output. In these patients, diuretics may further reduce intravascular volume. In patients with chronic venous insufficiency (stasis edema) or lymphedema, diuretic therapy should be avoided because fluid mobilization from the interstitial to the vascular space does not predictably occur. Sodium restriction, leg elevation, and compressive stockings can be helpful.

KEY POINT

- In patients with chronic venous insufficiency or lymphedema, diuretic therapy should be avoided because fluid mobilization from the interstitial to the vascular space does not predictably occur.

Musculoskeletal Pain

Acute Low Back Pain

Diagnosis and Evaluation

The prognosis for acute musculoskeletal low back pain is excellent. More than 70% of patients presenting to primary care clinics recover completely, and fewer than 10% seek ongoing care after 3 months. Because of this, initial diagnostic evaluation of acute low back pain should focus on identifying patients at risk for nonmusculoskeletal causes, such as malignancy, infection, or underlying systemic illness. Particular attention should be paid to diagnosis of conditions that require urgent evaluations (tumor, infection, rapidly progressive neurologic symptoms, cauda equina syndrome) and those for which specific treatments may be more effective than symptomatic therapy (rheumatologic diseases, compression fractures).

Psychosocial factors are more useful than the physical examination in predicting the course of recovery in acute back pain. Presence of depression, passive coping strategies, job dissatisfaction, higher disability levels, disputed compensation claims, and somatization all may predict poorer outcomes. In patients with risk factors for ongoing pain, quantitative assessment of the patient's pain and function can be valuable.

History

Age is the most useful screening factor in low back pain. Cancer, compression fractures, and spinal stenosis are all significantly more likely in older patients. Age older than 50 years has a 75% to 90% sensitivity and 60% to 70% specificity for these three diagnoses. Spondyloarthropathies almost always present before the age of 40 years, but this finding is very nonspecific (sensitivity 100%, specificity 7%). Other important factors in the history are shown in **Table 22**.

Neurologic history and physical examination should focus on differentiating disk herniation and accompanying sciatica (unilateral sharp or burning pain radiating down the back or side of the leg, usually to the foot or ankle) from lesions that compress the central spinal cord (cauda equina syndrome). Key findings associated with central spinal cord compression include bowel and bladder dysfunction (particularly urinary retention or incontinence), diminished sensation over the perineum, bilateral or multilevel neurologic deficits, and rapidly progressive neurologic deficits.

TABLE 22. History Features and Suggested Diagnoses in Low Back Pain

Suggested Diagnosis	History Feature
Cancer	Unexplained weight loss
	Failure to improve after 1 month
	No relief with bed rest
Infection	Fever
	Injection drug abuse
	Urinary tract infection
	Skin infection
Inflammatory/rheumatologic condition	Presence of morning stiffness
	Pain not relieved when supine
	Pain persisting for >3 months
	Gradual onset
	Involvement of other joints
Nerve root irritation (radiculopathy)	Sciatica
	Increased pain with cough, sneeze, or Valsalva maneuver
Spinal stenosis	Severe leg pain
	No pain when seated
	Pseudoclaudication
Compression fracture	Trauma
	Corticosteroid use
	Osteoporosis
Cauda equina syndrome	Bowel or bladder dysfunction
	Saddle sensory loss
	Rapidly progressive neurologic deficits

Physical Examination

Clinicians should inspect for scoliosis and kyphosis, noting any erythema or edema that suggests underlying infection or inflammation. Skin findings (for example, psoriasis) that may suggest an underlying inflammatory arthritis should also be noted. Palpation and percussion of the back can help differentiate vertebral tenderness from pain originating in the paraspinous soft tissues. The presence of vertebral tenderness should increase suspicion of compression fracture or infection. The straight-leg raise test (reproduction of pain extending below the knee with 10 degrees to 60 degrees of leg elevation), weakness and diminished reflexes at the ankles, and sensory loss in the feet are all associated with disk herniation. The crossed straight-leg raise test (lifting the unaffected side causing pain in the opposite leg) is less sensitive but more specific than performing the straight-leg raise test on the affected side. The quality of pain is not important

in the straight-leg raise tests; what matters is that the pain radiates below the knee.

Lumbar spinal stenosis is more common in patients older than 65 years and is anecdotally associated with increased pain when walking and relief when sitting, often called neurogenic claudication or pseudoclaudication. Evidence regarding the diagnostic value of neurogenic claudication is limited, however, and the available data suggest a poor positive likelihood ratio. An abnormal Romberg test or a wide-based gait in the presence of pain suggesting spinal stenosis are specific but not sensitive findings.

Further Diagnostic Testing

Patients with nonspecific low back pain and no symptoms or signs to suggest systemic illness should not routinely receive additional diagnostic testing. The American College of Physicians recommends that diagnostic imaging for low back pain be obtained in patients acutely only if they have evidence of a severe progressive neurologic deficit or signs or symptoms suggestive of a serious or specific underlying condition. There is no evidence to suggest an optimal imaging strategy for such patients if pain persists beyond 1 to 2 months, although plain radiography may be reasonable in this circumstance. For patients with a history that suggests malignancy or fracture, plain radiography is recommended for initial imaging. Complete blood count and erythrocyte sedimentation rate can also be helpful in evaluating patients for infection or evidence of systemic illness. In patients with rapidly progressive neurologic symptoms (but not stable mild neurologic symptoms), cauda equina syndrome, or suspicion for epidural abscess or osteomyelitis, MRI is the preferred modality because of better visualization of soft tissues and the spinal canal. If MRI is not feasible, CT myelography is a viable alternative. Noncontrast CT is useful for detecting sacroiliitis and is a reasonable diagnostic study in patients in whom an inflammatory spondyloarthropathy is suspected.

Patients whose symptoms specifically suggest radiculopathy or spinal stenosis should not receive additional imaging unless they have an inadequate response to noninvasive management and are considering surgery or epidural corticosteroid injection. For patients who are considering an invasive intervention, MRI is usually the initial study of choice. Asymptomatic herniated disks are common findings on MRI, so disk herniations that do not cause nerve root impingement or correlate anatomically with the patient's symptoms should be approached with suspicion.

Treatment

Because the overall prognosis for acute musculoskeletal low back pain is excellent, therapeutic interventions should focus on mitigating symptoms and maintaining function while the patient recovers. Most patients without sciatica show substantial improvement within 2 weeks. Patients with sciatica may be slower to improve, but three quarters of patients are substantially better after 3 months. Pain from spinal stenosis is less likely to improve, although even with this condition, some fluctuation is common.

Nonpharmacologic Treatment

Patients should be encouraged to maintain their daily activities as best they can. Bed rest has been shown in several trials to decrease functional recovery and increase pain in patients both with and without sciatica. Spinal manipulation therapy has been shown to be associated with modest benefits in treatment of acute low back pain, comparable to conventional therapy. Most randomized trials of manipulation involved 2 to 3 weeks of therapy; there is no evidence to suggest that long-term manipulation is any more helpful. Massage and yoga have been shown to be helpful in small studies. The improvement seen with acupuncture in chronic back pain is not superior to sham acupuncture. Supervised exercise therapy and physical therapy have not been shown to be effective early in the course of low back pain, but are helpful in patients whose pain persists for more than 4 weeks and to prevent recurrences.

Pharmacologic Treatment

First-line pharmacotherapy for most patients with acute low back pain includes acetaminophen and NSAIDs. NSAIDs should be used with caution in patients at increased risk for nephrotoxicity (older patients and patients with diabetes mellitus, heart failure, or preexisting kidney disease) or gastrointestinal ulcer. Concurrent treatment with a proton pump inhibitor or misoprostol or use of a cyclooxegenase-2 (COX-2) selective NSAID reduces risk of ulcers in patients at high risk and is specifically recommended for patients older than 75 years. Some patients may also be at increased risk of hypertension and cardiovascular events when using NSAIDs, although different drugs have shown these effects to varying degrees in observational studies. When NSAIDs are used, the lowest effective dose should be used for the shortest possible period, especially in older patients and those with comorbidities that put them at risk for complications. Acetaminophen has fewer adverse effects, but doses should be limited to a maximum of 4 g/d to reduce the risk of hepatotoxicity, although even this dose may be linked to hepatotoxicity in patients with moderate to high alcohol use.

Opioid analgesics or tramadol may be helpful in patients with acute low back pain for whom NSAIDs or acetaminophen do not provide adequate relief. Although reasonably safe for short-term use in modest doses, opioids should be used with caution in elderly patients and patients with chronic mechanical low back pain and used only with extreme caution or avoided altogether in patients with a history of addiction or substance abuse.

There are several drugs with diverse mechanisms of action that are collectively referred to as skeletal muscle relaxants. Evidence suggests these drugs may have some modest benefit in pain relief in acute low back pain. All can cause dizziness and sedation, however, and should be used with caution in older patients.

Interventional and Surgical Treatment

Many injection therapies have been tried in the management of low back pain. Epidural corticosteroid injections may provide short-term relief in patients with disk herniations causing radiculopathy, but evidence is mixed and long-term outcomes are unchanged. Facet joint injections, trigger point injections, and prolotherapy lack compelling supportive evidence; American Pain Society guidelines recommend against their use.

Surgery has clearly shown benefit only in patients with disk herniation causing persistent radiculopathy, patients with painful spinal stenosis, and patients with cauda equina syndrome. For patients with radiculopathy, diskectomy and microdiskectomy show improved outcomes at 6 to 12 weeks compared with nonsurgical therapy, although both surgical and nonsurgical groups tend to continue to improve with time, and differences in outcomes diminish over 1 to 2 years. In spinal stenosis, decompressive laminectomy shows moderate benefits compared with nonsurgical therapy for the first 1 to 2 years, again with diminishing effects in long-term follow-up.

Cauda equina syndrome is considered an emergency because of the risk of rapid, irreversible loss of neurologic function and because of its association with urgent underlying conditions, such as neoplasia or infection. Management typically involves prompt surgical decompression of the affected area of the spinal cord.

For patients with neither radiculopathy nor spinal stenosis, the value of surgery is questionable. Available evidence is of moderate quality and suggests that outcomes from surgery are similar to those of nonsurgical therapy. When benefit has been shown in clinical trials, it is limited to a narrow group of patients with more than 1 year of moderately severe pain and disability and without serious medical or psychiatric comorbidities.

KEY POINTS

- Patients with nonspecific low back pain and no symptoms or signs to suggest systemic illness should not routinely receive additional diagnostic testing.
- Most patients with acute low back pain improve within 3 months with conservative therapy.

Neck Pain

Diagnosis and Evaluation

Neck pain typically arises from three broad categories of conditions: mechanical neck pain arising from muscles, joints, and associated tissues; neurogenic neck pain arising from a cervical nerve root to the spinal cord; and neck pain associated with systemic disease. Initial approach to the history and physical examination should aim to differentiate these categories.

Mechanical neck pain is typically an aching pain localized to the neck, although it may be referred up toward the head or down toward the shoulder girdle. The history may include injury (for example, whiplash or acute strain) or unaccustomed activity, suggesting an overuse syndrome. Physical examination often reveals decreased range of motion, tenderness over soft tissues, and pain caused or exacerbated by flexion or extension of the neck.

Neurogenic pain is typically burning and often radiates to the shoulder or down the arm. Patients may have dermatomal numbness or muscle weakness in the distribution of a cervical nerve root. Involvement of multiple spinal levels, spasticity, hyperreflexia, gait abnormality, or leg weakness all suggest central spinal cord compression.

Patients with underlying systemic illnesses frequently have symptoms suggesting the underlying problem. These may include fever, weight loss, joint pain or arthritis elsewhere, symptoms of polymyalgia rheumatica (headache, visual changes, shoulder and hip girdle pain), or history of immunosuppression, cancer, or injection drug use. Anterior neck pain is an unusual presentation of cervical spine disease and should lead the clinician to suspect other anatomic structures as possible sources of pain. Physical examination should be directed toward identifying underlying systemic illness based on symptoms and risk factors.

Imaging studies should be directed based on suspicions raised during history and physical examination. Mechanical neck pain outside of the setting of acute trauma rarely requires imaging, although plain films can be helpful in patients older than 50 years to exclude malignancy and to assess for osteoarthritic changes. Patients with weakness, hyporeflexia, or symptoms or signs of spinal cord involvement should be evaluated with MRI or CT myelography. Patients with symptoms or signs of systemic illness and a suspected anatomic abnormality in the neck (tumor, abscess, pathologic fracture, or disease of anterior neck structures) should have imaging directed at the suspected underlying cause.

Blood tests are not routinely needed for evaluation of patients with neck pain, but should be ordered as appropriate to exclude or confirm underlying systemic illness. Erythrocyte sedimentation rate, C-reactive protein, and complete blood count can be useful in evaluating for infection or inflammatory conditions.

Treatment

Most patients with neck pain recover with conservative therapy. For patients with mechanical neck pain, mobilization and a gentle home exercise program have been shown to be beneficial. For patients with cervical radiculopathy, the role of either hard or soft cervical collars is unclear, and acupuncture does not appear to offer clinically significant benefit. As in low back pain, acetaminophen and NSAIDs are first-line pharmacotherapy for most patients with acute neck pain. Opioids and skeletal muscle relaxants should be reserved for patients with a poor response to acetaminophen and NSAIDs or who are having difficulty sleeping (in which case sedation is a desirable effect). Patients with neurogenic neck pain may find additional benefit from medications targeting neuropathic pain (see Common Symptoms, Chronic Noncancer Pain, Management).

Interventional therapy is not beneficial for patients with mechanical neck pain. Epidural corticosteroid injection may be beneficial in patients with stable radiculopathy that fails to respond to conservative therapy. Surgery is clearly indicated in patients with progressive neurologic symptoms that stem from a defined anatomic abnormality. The role of surgery in patients with chronic neck pain without progressive neurologic deficits is controversial; limited data suggest faster short-term pain relief but no long-term difference compared with conservative management.

KEY POINTS

- Mechanical neck pain outside of the setting of acute trauma rarely requires imaging, although plain films can be helpful in patients older than 50 years to exclude malignancy and to assess for osteoarthritic changes.

- Most patients with neck pain recover with conservative therapy.

Shoulder Pain

Diagnosis and Evaluation

Important historical features to elicit in the evaluation of shoulder pain include location, severity, chronicity, circumstances of onset, history of trauma, and associated symptoms. Shoulder pain may arise from structures of the shoulder (intrinsic disorders) or may be referred from other sites (extrinsic disorders). Pain with movement of the shoulder along with stiffness, locking, catching, and instability all suggest an intrinsic disorder, whereas a normal shoulder examination or the presence of constitutional symptoms and respiratory or gastrointestinal symptoms suggests an extrinsic or systemic etiology. Neck pain, decreased range of motion of the neck, paresthesias, and pain that radiates down the arm past the elbow suggest cervical spine disease. Pain that worsens with intake of food raises the possibility of pain referred from a gallbladder disorder. Discomfort with physical (non-shoulder) exertion should raise concern for cardiac ischemia. Other extrinsic causes of shoulder pain include pneumonia, apical lung masses, and diaphragmatic irritation due to a variety of causes.

Examination of the shoulder should include inspection, palpation, range-of-motion testing (both passive and active), and provocative maneuvers. It is important to begin by fully exposing both shoulders and examining for any asymmetry or muscle wasting. Palpation should include the acromioclavicular (AC) joint, bicipital groove, all bony structures, and the cervical spine. Pain that is only present with active but not passive range-of-motion testing suggests an extraarticular condition; pain with both active and passive range-of-motion testing suggests an intraarticular condition. Pain that occurs between 60 and 120 degrees of abduction suggests a rotator cuff impingement syndrome, whereas pain with more than 120 degrees of abduction favors AC joint pathology.

Many provocative tests are commonly performed in the assessment of shoulder pain (**Table 23**). The Apley scratch test can be used to assess range of motion. The Neer (**Figure 7**) and Hawkins (**Figure 8**) tests are both useful for diagnosing rotator cuff impingement. The Yergason test (**Figure 9**) is used to assess inflammation of the long head of the biceps and lesions of the glenoid labrum. The apprehension test (**Figure 10**) assesses anterior glenohumeral instability.

Rotator Cuff Disorders

Rotator cuff tendinitis (inflammation of the rotator cuff tendons) can result from repetitive overhead motions, shoulder instability, or trauma. The supraspinatus tendon is most commonly affected and is sometimes accompanied by tendinitis of the long head of the biceps muscle.

Impingement syndrome results from compression of the rotator cuff between the inferior surface of the acromion and the superior surface of the humeral head. Impingement

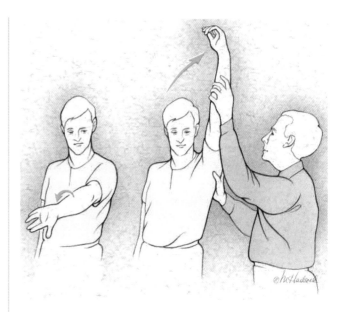

FIGURE 7. Neer test. The examiner applies forced flexion to the affected arm while the arm is fully pronated. This test is considered positive if pain is elicited and suggests either rotator cuff tendinitis or subacromial impingement.

© Maria Hartsock, CMI. Reprinted from Woodward TW, Best TW. The painful shoulder: part I. Clinical evaluation. Am Fam Physician. 2000;61(10):3079-3088. [PMID: 10839557]

symptoms are worse with abduction of the arm, as the space between the acromion and humeral head is smallest with this movement. Impingement can be caused by spurs on the

TABLE 23. Tests Used in Shoulder Evaluation and Significance of Positive Finding		
Test	**Maneuver**	**Diagnosis Suggested by Positive Result**
Apley scratch test	Patient touches superior and inferior aspects of opposite scapula	Loss of range of motion: rotator cuff problem
Neer test	Forced flexion of pronated arm	Subacromial impingement (89% sensitivity; 31% specificity)
Hawkins test	Forward flexion of the shoulder to 90 degrees and internal rotation	Supraspinatus tendon impingement (92% sensitivity; 25% specificity)
Drop-arm test	Attempted slow lowering of arm to waist	Rotator cuff tear
Cross-arm test	Forward elevation to 90 degrees and active adduction	Acromioclavicular joint arthritis
Spurling test	Spine extended with head rotated to affected shoulder while axially loaded	Cervical nerve root disorder
Apprehension test	Anterior pressure on the humerus with external rotation	Anterior glenohumeral instability
Relocation test	Posterior force on humerus while externally rotating the arm	Anterior glenohumeral instability
Sulcus sign	Pulling downward on elbow or wrist	Inferior glenohumeral instability
Yergason test	Elbow flexed to 90 degrees with forearm pronated	Biceps tendon instability or tendinitis
Speed maneuver	Elbow flexed 20 to 30 degrees and forearm supinated	Biceps tendon instability or tendinitis
"Clunk" sign	Rotation of loaded shoulder from extension to forward flexion	Labral disorder

Reprinted with permission from The Painful Shoulder: Part I. Clinical Evaluation., May 15, 2000, Vol 61, No 10, American Family Physician Copyright © 2000 American Academy of Family Physicians. All Rights Reserved.

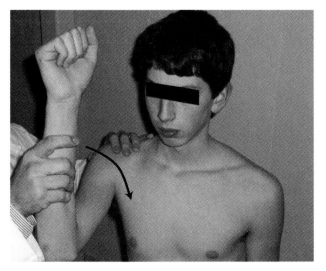

FIGURE 8. Hawkins test for shoulder impingement. The patient holds the arm extended anteriorly at 90 degrees with the forearm bent to 90 degrees (at 12 o'clock), as if holding a shield. The scapula should be stabilized by the examiner. The arm is then internally rotated to cross in front of the body. A positive test elicits pain in the shoulder.

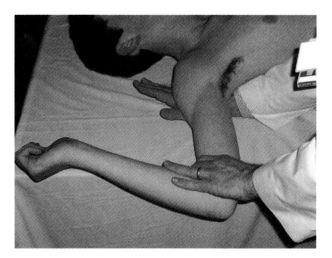

FIGURE 10. Apprehension test. The patient is placed supine on a table. With the arm abducted at 90 degrees and the forearm flexed, the examiner stands at the bedside facing the patient and places one hand under the affected shoulder. With the other hand, gentle pressure is placed on the forearm. Pain or apprehension constitutes a positive test.

acromion, calcification of the coracoacromial ligament, or superior migration of the humeral head during abduction. If left untreated, impingement may lead to a full-thickness rotator cuff tear.

Patients with either rotator cuff tendinitis or impingement have pain located over the lateral deltoid that is present with abduction and internal rotation of the arm. Nighttime symptoms are common. Examination reveals pain with

abduction between 60 degrees and 120 degrees. Pain may be elicited with deep palpation of the lateral deltoid inferior to the acromion process. Both the Neer and Hawkins tests are sensitive but less specific for diagnosing impingement syndrome.

Weakness and loss of function should raise concern for a rotator cuff tear. Examination findings include supraspinatus weakness, weakness with external rotation, evidence of impingement, and a positive drop-arm test. When the diagnosis is not clear or if concern exists for a rotator cuff tear, imaging of the shoulder should be obtained. MRI is the preferred imaging modality (>90% sensitivity), although ultrasonography, in experienced hands, is also an option.

Management of rotator cuff disease is multifaceted. Initially, management includes rest, modification of activities, and NSAIDs to help reduce inflammation and provide pain relief. Subacromial corticosteroid injection has been shown to improve pain for up to 9 months. Physical therapy focused on strengthening the rotator cuff muscles using low-resistance exercises may be beneficial in stabilizing the head of the humerus and reducing impingement. Partial-thickness tears can be managed similar to tendinitis. Full-thickness tears may require surgical intervention depending on other patient characteristics (such as age, type of daily activities, or profession).

Adhesive Capsulitis

Adhesive capsulitis (frozen shoulder) is caused by thickening of the capsule surrounding the glenohumeral joint. It is associated with diabetes, Parkinson disease, stroke, previous trauma, and hypothyroidism but may be idiopathic, particularly in the elderly. It can also occur in the setting of a shoulder or arm injury with concomitant restriction in movement

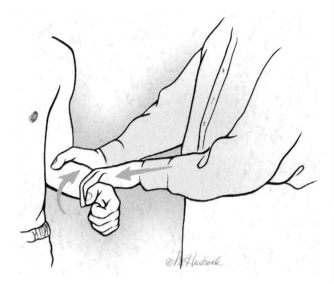

FIGURE 9. The Yergason test consists of resisted supination with the arm at the patient's side and the elbow at 90 degrees of flexion. The test is positive if shoulder pain is elicited.

© Maria Hartsock, CMI. Reprinted from Woodward TW, Best TW. The painful shoulder: part I. Clinical evaluation. Am Fam Physician. 2000;61(10):3079-3088. [PMID: 10839557]

of the shoulder by the patient. Pain is characteristically slow in onset and is located near the insertion of the deltoid muscle. Patients often avoid lying on the affected side. On examination, there is loss of both active and passive range of motion. Radiographic findings are usually absent.

Initial treatment consists of physical therapy and medication with NSAIDs. Subacromial corticosteroid injection (and intra-articular corticosteroids for refractory cases) is most useful in patients with concurrent rotator cuff pathology. Recovery is typically prolonged (up to 2 years). Consideration for surgical intervention is reserved for those in whom conservative therapy has failed.

Acromioclavicular Joint Degeneration

AC joint degeneration typically results from trauma (in younger patients) or osteoarthritis (in older patients). Bilateral involvement should raise concern for rheumatoid arthritis. On examination, there is pain on palpation of the AC joint. Palpable osteophytes may be present. Pain characteristically occurs with shoulder adduction and abduction above 120 degrees. Plain radiography, if obtained, reveals degenerative changes. Therapy consists of NSAIDs and possibly intra-articular corticosteroid injections. Exercises focused on improving scapular retraction may be beneficial. If these therapies fail, surgical referral is warranted.

> **KEY POINTS**
>
> - Management of rotator cuff disease includes rest, activity modification, and anti-inflammatory therapy; after resolution of symptoms, an exercise program to strengthen the rotator cuff muscles should be initiated.
> - Management of adhesive capsulitis consists of physical therapy and oral anti-inflammatory agents; recovery is typically prolonged.

Elbow Pain

Diagnosis and Evaluation

One should begin by obtaining a complete description of the patient's pain. Examination of the elbow includes inspection, palpation, range-of-motion testing, and special tests (see individual conditions below). The neck, shoulder, and wrist should also be examined, as pain can be referred to the elbow from each of these sites.

Epicondylitis

Lateral epicondylitis (tennis elbow) is caused by overuse of the wrist extensor muscles and is most commonly observed in nonathletes, such as computer users who use a mouse. The pain is located laterally, characteristically radiates down the forearm to the dorsal hand, and worsens with activity and at night. On examination, there is tenderness to palpation where the extensor muscles attach to the lateral epicondyle. Pain increases with forced extension of the wrist.

Medial epicondylitis (golfer's elbow) is characterized by pain in the medial elbow and proximal forearm that occurs with activities that require wrist flexion. On examination, there is tenderness to palpation from the medial epicondyle to the pronator teres and flexor carpi radialis muscles. Pain increases with wrist flexion and resisted forearm supination.

Rest, avoidance of activities that worsen pain, stretching, and resistance exercises constitute initial therapy. Corticosteroid injection and oral NSAIDs may provide short-term (but not long-term) relief of symptoms when other measures fail. Surgery may be required for refractory cases.

Olecranon Bursitis

Olecranon bursitis, characterized by painful swelling of the posterior elbow, can result from repetitive trauma, inflammation (gout, rheumatoid arthritis), or infection. On examination, there is localized swelling posterior to the olecranon process without limitation of range of motion of the elbow. When pain, inflammation, or fever is present, fluid should be aspirated for Gram stain, culture, and crystal analysis to rule out septic bursitis and to evaluate for gout. Treatment options include NSAIDs and corticosteroid injection (once infection has been ruled out). Chronic effusions may require surgical intervention.

Ulnar Nerve Entrapment

Entrapment of the ulnar nerve at the elbow (cubital tunnel syndrome) commonly manifests with pain in the elbow with flexion that radiates to the hand accompanied by paresthesias and sensory loss involving the fourth and fifth fingers (**Figure 11**). Weakness is a late finding. Treatment consists of splinting, NSAIDs, and surgical decompression when severe.

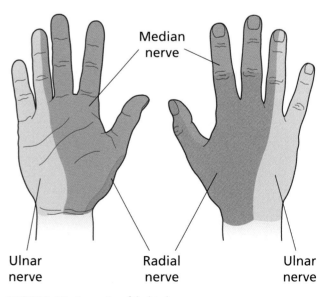

FIGURE 11. Innervation of the hand.

Wrist and Hand Pain

Indications for Imaging

Radiographs (posteroanterior, posteroanterior oblique, and lateral views) should be obtained in all patients with wrist or hand pain with both a history of trauma and localized tenderness to palpation to exclude fracture. Radiographs are also helpful in patients with suspected osteoarthritis.

Carpal Tunnel Syndrome

Carpel tunnel syndrome is caused by compression of the median nerve at the level of the wrist. Risk factors include female sex, obesity, pregnancy, diabetes, hypothyroidism, connective tissue disorders, and rheumatoid arthritis.

The most common clinical presentation is of pain and paresthesias in the distribution of the median nerve (see Figure 11). Patients may also report paresthesias involving all five fingers. Pain is usually worse at night and may radiate into the proximal arm. If left untreated, thenar muscle atrophy may occur. Symptoms may be unilateral or bilateral, with bilateral symptoms occurring in up to 65% of patients at the time of presentation.

The most useful history and examination findings in diagnosing carpal tunnel syndrome are use of a hand symptom diagram, thumb abduction and opposition weakness, and hypalgesia in the territory of the median nerve. The Phalen maneuver and Tinel sign are frequently used but have poor test characteristics. Nerve conduction studies are widely considered to be the diagnostic standard for carpal tunnel syndrome (sensitivity >85%, specificity >95%) and are helpful to obtain when the diagnosis is uncertain.

First-line therapies include avoidance of repetitive motions involving the wrist and hand and nocturnal splinting of the wrist at a neutral angle. Corticosteroid injection of the carpal tunnel appears to provide short-term benefit in patients with mild to moderate disease. A 2-week course of oral corticosteroids appears to be effective on at least a short-term basis. NSAIDs, diuretics, and pyridoxine have all been used, but evidence of their efficacy is lacking.

Surgery is indicated in patients with at least moderately severe disease with persistent symptoms (6 or more months), severe motor impairment, and nerve conduction studies that confirm the diagnosis.

Other Causes of Wrist and Hand Pain

Fracture should be suspected when there is a history of direct trauma and localized tenderness to palpation on examination. Distal radius and scaphoid fractures most commonly result from a fall on an outstretched hand. If clinical suspicion for a scaphoid fracture is high, treatment should not be delayed even if radiographs are normal, as lack of treatment can lead to avascular necrosis. Hamate fractures can result from direct trauma or from repetitive trauma, such as from swinging a golf club or baseball bat.

De Quervain tenosynovitis is caused by inflammation of the abductor pollicis longus and extensor pollicis brevis tendons in the thumb. It is usually associated with repetitive use of the thumb but can also be associated with other conditions, including pregnancy, rheumatoid arthritis, and calcium apatite deposition disease. The typical presentation is of pain on the radial aspect of the wrist that occurs when the thumb is used to pinch or grasp. Examination findings include localized tenderness over the distal portion of the radial styloid process and pain with resisted thumb abduction and extension. Patients also report pain with the Finkelstein test, in which the patient is asked to make a fist over the fully flexed thumb and then to ulnar deviate the hand. This test is positive when pain is present on the radial side of the thumb. Acute therapy consists of applying ice and taping or splinting the thumb to prevent movement. Persistence of symptoms may require injection with a corticosteroid and local anesthetic or use of a short-arm cast with thumb spica. Surgery should be considered in patients with persistent symptoms after a repeat injection.

Ganglion cysts, swellings that overlie either joints or tendons typically on the dorsal surface, arise as a result of chronic irritation of the wrist. If the cyst is not painful, no intervention is required. Treatment options for painful cysts include surgical resection or injection with either a crystalline corticosteroid (preceded by aspiration of the contents) or with hyaluronic acid (followed by aspiration).

Osteoarthritis of the hand is common, often involving the first carpometacarpal joint and the proximal and distal interphalangeal joints. Osteoarthritis of the wrist (radiocarpal arthritis) is uncommon and is almost always post-traumatic. Clinical manifestations of osteoarthritis of the hands and wrists include decreased range of motion, pain that worsens with activity and improves with rest, and swelling. Onset is usually insidious. On examination, one may note bony enlargement of the involved joints. A combination of pharmacologic and nonpharmacologic treatments, individualized to the patient, is recommended. It is important to educate patients about joint protection and refer to physical therapy or provide instructions on hand exercises. Application of heat and ultrasound have been found to be helpful. For mild to moderate pain and when only a few joints are affected, local or topical treatments (topical NSAIDs, capsaicin) are often more effective than systemic treatments.

KEY POINTS

- Radiographs should be obtained in all patients with wrist or hand pain with both a history of trauma and localized tenderness to palpation.

- First-line therapies for carpal tunnel syndrome include avoidance of repetitive motions involving the wrist and hand and nocturnal splinting of the wrist at a neutral angle.

- If clinical suspicion for a scaphoid fracture is high, treatment should not be delayed even if radiographs are normal.

Hip Pain

Diagnosis and Evaluation

Because hip pain can have nonmusculoskeletal causes, it is essential to inquire about symptoms related to the gastrointestinal, gynecologic, and genitourinary systems. On examination, one should observe gait, inspect both the affected and unaffected hips, palpate the sacroiliac joints and bony structures of the hip, including the greater trochanter, and assess range of motion. The FABER test (**Figure 12**) is used to assess Flexion, ABduction, and External Rotation of the hip. It is essential to also perform abdominal, genital, back, and knee examinations, as pain can be referred to the hip from each of these sites. Neurologic and vascular examination of the lower extremities also may help to reveal a cause.

Radiography should be obtained in all patients presenting with acute hip pain to evaluate for fracture. MRI is helpful to evaluate for fracture when radiography is negative but clinical suspicion is high and also to evaluate for avascular necrosis, infection, and tumor, if concern exists.

Specific Causes of Hip Pain

The location of the pain helps to focus the broad differential diagnosis. Anterior (groin) pain is most often caused by osteoarthritis of the hip. The pain is usually chronic, insidious in onset, and worsens with activity. Early morning stiffness may also be present but usually improves with activity. Examination is usually remarkable for decreased and painful internal rotation. Pain may also be produced by logrolling (rocking thigh back and forth with both hands while the patient is supine). When anterior hip pain is acute in onset, the differential diagnosis includes osteonecrosis (most

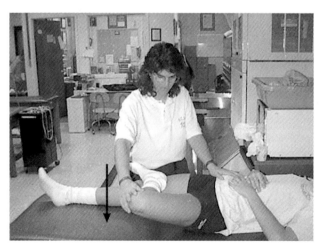

FIGURE 12. The FABER test assesses Flexion, ABduction, and External Rotation of the hip. With the leg in a figure-four position, the normal leg should attain a parallel plane with the table. Gentle downward pressure on the knee in this position simultaneously places stress on the ipsilateral sacroiliac joint.

common in the setting of corticosteroid or excessive alcohol use), fracture (suspect when trauma is present), septic arthritis, and acute synovitis. The examination findings for each of these conditions are similar to those seen with osteoarthritis. An extra-articular cause of anterior hip pain should be suspected when hip range of motion is normal and when pain is not elicited by movement of the hip. Extra-articular causes include inguinal hernia, lower abdominal pathology, and lumbar disk disease at the L1 level.

Lateral hip pain is most often caused by trochanteric bursitis, usually resulting from gait abnormalities. Patients with trochanteric bursitis report pain when lying on the affected side in the area of greater trochanter. On examination, there is point tenderness to palpation approximately 2.5 cm (1 in) posterior and superior to the greater trochanter. Treatment consists of correction of the underlying etiology, heat, stretching, and corticosteroid injection. Another cause of lateral hip pain is entrapment of the lateral femoral cutaneous nerve (meralgia paresthetica), frequently presenting as an oval-shaped area of burning, numbness, or tingling on the distal lateral thigh. Lumbar disk disease at the L4-L5 level may also present with pain in the region of the lateral hip and thigh.

Posterior hip pain can result from sacroiliitis, lumbosacral disk disease, and, rarely, pathology affecting the hip joint. Sacroiliac pathology can lead to pain referred to the gluteal region and is characterized by tenderness to palpation of the sacroiliac joint. Spinal disease often causes pain accompanied by paresthesias and back pain. Piriformis syndrome is caused by compression of the sciatic nerve by the piriformis muscle, leading to pain in the buttocks and the distribution of the sciatic nerve. Piriformis syndrome should be considered when sciatica is present without clear evidence of lumbosacral disk disease.

KEY POINT

- In the evaluation of hip pain, it is essential to perform abdominal, genital, back, and knee examinations, as pain can be referred to the hip from each of these sites.

Knee Pain

Diagnosis and Evaluation

Determining the chronicity of pain helps to focus the broad differential diagnosis. The most common cause of chronic knee pain is osteoarthritis. The presence of multijoint involvement along with systemic symptoms raises concern for an inflammatory condition, such as rheumatoid arthritis. The differential diagnosis for acute knee pain includes trauma, overuse, spontaneous meniscal tear, infection, crystalline disease, and inflammatory arthritis. Septic arthritis must be treated without delay.

On examination, both knees should be fully exposed, and the affected knee compared with the unaffected knee. Any asymmetry or swelling should be noted, as should any erythema, ecchymoses, or muscle atrophy. The presence of swelling, especially if the pain is acute and the overlying skin is erythematous, should be considered an indication to perform arthrocentesis to evaluate for both septic arthritis and a crystalline disorder.

All knee structures should be palpated, and range of motion should be evaluated. The integrity of the anterior cruciate ligament can be assessed by performing the anterior drawer and Lachman tests (**Figure 13**). The posterior drawer test is used to assess the posterior cruciate ligament; with the knee at 90 degrees of flexion and the hip at 45 degrees of flexion, posterior force is applied to the proximal tibia and both the extent of movement and the firmness of the endpoint are assessed. A varus stress test assesses the integrity of the lateral collateral ligament, and a valgus stress test assesses the integrity

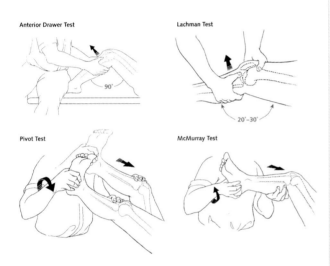

FIGURE 13. Tests for assessing integrity of knee ligaments and injury to knee menisci. (*Top left*) Anterior drawer test (anterior cruciate ligament): Place patient supine, flex the hip to 45 degrees and the knee to 90 degrees. Sit on the dorsum of the foot, wrap your hands around the hamstrings (ensuring that these muscles are relaxed), then pull and push the proximal part of the leg, testing the movement of the tibia on the femur. Do these maneuvers in three positions of tibial rotation: neutral, 30 degrees externally, and 30 degrees internally rotated. A normal test result is no more than 6 to 8 mm of laxity. (*Top right*) Lachman test (anterior cruciate ligament): Place patient supine on examining table, leg at the examiner's side, slightly externally rotated and flexed (20-30 degrees). Stabilize the femur with one hand and apply pressure to the back of the knee with the other hand with the thumb of the hand exerting pressure placed on the joint line. A positive test result is movement of the knee with a soft or mushy end point. (*Bottom left*) Pivot test (anterior cruciate ligament): Fully extend the knee, rotate the foot internally. Apply a valgus stress while progressively flexing the knee, watching and feeling for translation of the tibia on the femur. (*Bottom right*) McMurray test (meniscus): Flex the hip and knee maximally. Apply a valgus (abduction) force to the knee while externally rotating the foot and passively extending the knee. An audible or palpable snap during extension suggests a tear of the medial meniscus. For the lateral meniscus, apply a varus (adduction) stress during internal rotation of the foot and passive extension of the knee.

of the medial collateral ligament (**Figure 14**). The McMurray test (see Figure 13) can be used to detect medial and lateral meniscal injuries, but its low sensitivity increases the likelihood of false-negative results. The medial-lateral grind test is considered the most sensitive (69%) and specific (86%) test for assessing the intactness of the menisci. It is performed with the patient in the supine position. The examiner places the patient's calf in one hand and places the thumb and index finger of the opposite hand over the joint line and then applies varus and valgus stresses to the tibia during both extension and flexion. The test is considered to be positive when the examiner detects a grinding sensation over the joint line with these maneuvers.

Radiographs should be obtained if there is a history of trauma. MRI is useful if concern exists for ligamentous or meniscal injury.

Degenerative Joint Disease

Osteoarthritis most commonly involves the medial compartment of the knee. Pain typically worsens with use and improves with rest. Although morning stiffness may be present, it usually resolves with activity and there are no systemic symptoms. Examination may reveal joint line tenderness, decreased range of motion, crepitus, effusion, and palpable bony changes. Radiographs may aid in determining severity (see MKSAP 16 Rheumatology).

Trauma

Ligamentous injuries of the knee are common. Injury to the anterior cruciate ligament frequently occurs when the patient plants one foot and quickly turns in the opposite direction. Often, a "pop" is heard, swelling quickly develops, and the patient is not able to complete the activity that was being performed when the injury occurred. Medial collateral ligament injuries occur when the knee experiences a valgus force, and lateral collateral ligament injuries occur when the knee experiences a varus force. Medial collateral ligament injuries are much more common than lateral collateral ligament injuries. Meniscal injuries occur with sudden twisting motions of the knee, although "spontaneous" meniscal tears without evidence of significant trauma may occur, primarily in older patients owing to chronic degeneration of the meniscus. Although painful, the patient is able to immediately bear weight. Swelling may occur.

Appropriate treatment of knee trauma is highly dependent on the nature and extent of injury, the degree of dysfunction, and the overall medical status of the patient. Many traumatic knee injuries may be managed without surgical intervention; orthopedic input may be helpful in establishing an optimal therapeutic approach.

Patellofemoral Pain Syndrome

Patellofemoral pain syndrome, an overuse syndrome, typically manifests as anterior knee pain that is worse with prolonged sitting and with walking up and down stairs. It is commonly

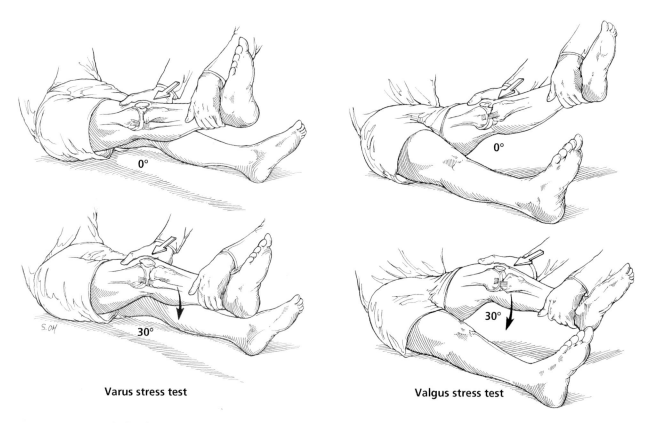

Varus stress test   **Valgus stress test**

FIGURE 14. Varus and valgus forces applied to knee.

seen in runners but also occurs in nonrunners, and it affects women more than men. On examination, the pain may be reproduced by applying pressure to the surface of the patella (patellofemoral compression test) with the knee in extension and moving the patella laterally or medially. Radiographs are unnecessary as the diagnosis is clinical.

Treatment can be divided into acute (first week) and recovery phases. Treatment during the acute phase focuses on pain control and consists of activity modification, short-term use of NSAIDs, and other conservative measures, such as icing. Treatment during the recovery phase should consist of a rehabilitation program that focuses on strengthening the hip abductor and quadriceps muscles and stretching, although there is no single accepted program.

Bursitis

Pes anserine bursitis manifests as pain located near the antero-medial aspect of the proximal tibia and is most commonly caused by overuse or direct trauma. On examination, tenderness is elicited at the level of the tibial tuberosity (approximately 4 cm [1.5 in] below the level of the medial joint line). Swelling may be present at the insertion of the medial hamstring muscles. Treatment consists of avoiding squatting and limiting repetitive bending and direct pressure on the bursa. Placing a pillow between the legs at night and avoiding

crossing the legs may be helpful, as may the application of ice. Oral NSAIDs have limited usefulness owing to the lack of penetration to the bursal space.

Prepatellar bursitis, inflammation of the bursa lying between the patella and the overlying skin, frequently results from repeated trauma ("housemaid's knee") but can also be caused by infection or gout. Patients with prepatellar bursitis present with pain in the anterior aspect of the knee. Erythema, swelling, and tenderness to palpation may be observed near the lower pole of the patella. Treatment consists of rest and avoidance of kneeling.

Iliotibial Band Syndrome

Iliotibial band syndrome presents as lateral knee pain that is worse with walking up or down steps. It is caused by friction between the iliotibial band and the lateral femoral condyle and is frequently seen in runners and cyclists. Tenderness is present at the lateral femoral epicondyle (approximately 3 cm [1.2 in] proximal to the joint line). A Noble test is performed by having the patient, in the supine position, repeatedly flex and extend the knee with the clinician's thumb placed over the lateral femoral epicondyle. A positive Noble test reproduces the patient's pain.

Treatment is conservative and typically consists of rest, stretching, NSAIDs, and addressing contributing factors (such as running).

Baker Cyst

Patients with a popliteal (Baker) cyst report the insidious onset of posterior knee pain and may also note a sense of posterior fullness. It can represent either a true cyst or may be an extension of an intra-articular knee effusion. Examination reveals palpable fullness in the posteromedial knee. Treatment is usually aimed at the underlying condition but may require aspiration and, in a small number of patients, surgical resection.

KEY POINT

- The medial-lateral grind test is the most sensitive and specific test for assessing the intactness of the menisci.

Ankle and Foot Pain

Ankle Sprains

Ankle sprains usually involve a combination of plantar flexion and inversion leading to damage to the lateral ligaments. The anterior talofibular ligament is the most commonly injured. Patients with ankle sprains initially present with pain, swelling, and diminished proprioception. Although typically a self-limited condition, residual symptoms, including pain, instability, and stiffness, are common and may persist for years. Ankle sprains can be graded by severity: ligamentous stretching with no instability and mild pain (grade I); partial ligamentous tear with moderate tenderness to palpation and pain with ambulation (grade II); and complete ligamentous tear with instability, severe pain, and inability to ambulate (grade III).

Evaluation should begin with a determination of the circumstances under which the ankle was injured and whether the ankle was inverted or everted. The inability to bear weight immediately after injury suggests a possible fracture or a more serious sprain. A popping sound when the injury occurred suggests ligament rupture.

Examination should include inspection, palpation, range-of-motion testing, assessment of weightbearing status, and focused testing of the ankle. Palpation should include the bony structures of the ankle and the entire length of the tibia and fibula. The Achilles tendon should also be palpated along its entire course. Specific tests allow for assessment of the integrity of the structures of the ankle. Compression of the fibula and tibia at the midcalf ("squeeze test") should be performed, as pain with this maneuver in the area of the distal tibia and fibular syndesmosis indicates a syndesmosis sprain ("high ankle sprain"). The talar tilt test, used to assess the calcaneofibular ligament, is performed by holding the distal end of the tibia and fibula in one hand while using the other hand to invert the ankle. It is considered positive if the tilt is 5% to 10% greater on the affected side as compared with the unaffected side. The Ottawa ankle and foot rules are a highly sensitive tool to help the clinician determine when it is appropriate to obtain radiographic studies in patients presenting with a history of trauma (**Figure 15**).

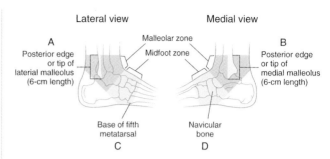

FIGURE 15. Ottawa ankle and foot rules. An ankle radiographic series is indicated if a patient has pain in the malleolar zone and any of these findings: bone tenderness at *A*, bone tenderness at *B*, or inability to bear weight immediately and in the emergency department (or physician's office). A foot radiographic series is indicated if a patient has pain in the midfoot zone and any of these findings: bone tenderness at *C*, bone tenderness at *D*, or inability to bear weight immediately and in the emergency department (or physician's office).

Reproduced with permission from Davis MF, Davis PF, Ross DS. ACP Expert Guide to Sports Medicine. Philadelphia, PA: American College of Physicians, 2005:404. Copyright 2005, American College of Physicians.

Early management of uncomplicated ankle sprains (grade I) includes controlling swelling with ice, compression, and elevation. NSAIDs can be used to help with pain control and to reduce inflammation. Range-of-motion exercises should be started promptly. Further rehabilitation, including proprioceptive training, is essential to prevent chronic instability. Management of grade II sprains is similar but may require limiting weightbearing in addition to stabilization during recovery. Grade III sprains may require surgical intervention given the presence of complete tearing and loss of ankle stability, particularly with failure to respond to more conservative therapies.

Hind Foot Pain

Plantar fasciitis, the most common cause of heel pain, is characterized by intense, sharp pain in the heel with the first steps after long periods of inactivity (such as in the morning or after resting) and initially improves with walking but subsequently worsens. Risk factors include pes planus, running, occupations requiring prolonged standing, and obesity. Examination is notable for tenderness to palpation at the anteromedial aspect of the heel. Radiographs have limited utility but frequently reveal heel spurs and can help to rule out stress fractures of the calcaneus. Cornerstones of therapy include weight loss when appropriate, exercises that stretch the plantar fascia and calf, appropriate footwear, activity modification, and analgesics. Orthotics or night splints may be helpful for some patients. Corticosteroid injections appear to provide short-term improvement in symptoms, although long-term efficacy has not been established. Most cases (>80%) resolve within a year of onset of symptoms, regardless of therapy.

Achilles tendinopathy is caused by recurrent microtrauma and can be either acute or chronic. Acute Achilles tendon pain most commonly results from an abrupt increase in activity level whereas chronic pain (lasting >3 months) results from poor mechanics (pes planus, pes cavus, limb length discrepancy) and improper footwear. Risk factors include male sex, increasing age, history of fluoroquinolone or corticosteroid use, and obesity. Treatment includes avoidance of potentially aggravating activities, using a heel lift, and a 7- to 10-day course of NSAIDs.

Rupture of the Achilles tendon commonly occurs when the patient is pushing off with the foot. Patients may hear a popping sound and usually experience severe pain at the time of injury, although up to one-third of patients do not experience pain. On examination, clinicians can perform the Thompson test (sensitivity, 96%; specificity, 93%) by squeezing the patient's calf while the patient kneels with the feet hanging over the edge of the examining table. Absence of resultant plantar flexion supports the presence of an Achilles tendon rupture. Diagnostic ultrasound can be obtained when the diagnosis is in question. Partial Achilles tendon rupture can be managed similarly to chronic Achilles tendinopathy; surgical intervention is required for complete tendon rupture.

Midfoot Pain

Tarsal tunnel syndrome is due to compression of the tibial nerve at the level of the ankle and is typically manifested as pain and paresthesias in the midfoot. The most common cause of tarsal tunnel syndrome is from scar tissue or loose bony or cartilaginous fragments from fracture of the calcaneus, medial malleolus, or talus. Symptoms also commonly occur in the heel and toes and are worse at night and with prolonged standing. Examination findings can include the presence of a Tinel sign posterior to the medial malleolus (an electric shot sensation upon percussion of the posterior tibial nerve) and sensory loss on the plantar surface of the foot. If severe, atrophy of the intrinsic muscles of the foot may result. Treatment options include NSAIDS, orthotics, and modifications to footwear.

Although uncommon, stress fractures involving the bones of the midfoot can affect runners.

Forefoot Pain

In hallux valgus deformity (bunion), the first toe deviates laterally, and a bony deformity develops on the medial aspect of the first metatarsophalangeal (MTP) joint. This is typically accompanied by the inflammation of a bursa on the medial aspect of the first MTP joint, especially with tight-fitting shoes. Treatment is usually conservative and includes NSAIDs and accommodating footwear. When these interventions fail, orthotics, bracing, and surgical intervention may be required.

Morton neuroma, a common cause of metatarsalgia, results in burning pain in the space between the third and fourth toes or, less commonly, between the second and third toes. It results from entrapment of one of the common digital nerves. Pain is usually worse with standing and is most common in women who wear high heels. On examination,

there is tenderness to palpation of the affected interdigital space. Treatment consists of avoiding high heels and wearing cushioning under the forefoot. NSAIDs are not usually helpful, but corticosteroid injection is helpful in select patients.

KEY POINT

- The Ottawa ankle and foot rules are highly sensitive for ruling out fracture.

Dyslipidemia

Screening

The U.S. Preventive Services Task Force (USPSTF) strongly recommends initiating screening in men at age 35 years, and in women who are at increased risk of cardiovascular disease at age 45 years; screening may also be considered in both men and women beginning at age 20 years who have increased cardiovascular risk. A repeat screening interval of 5 years is considered appropriate in low-risk individuals, with a shorter interval in those with borderline results, and a longer interval in patients with consistently normal testing. The National Cholesterol Education Program Adult Treatment Panel III (ATP III) guidelines recommend initiating screening for lipid disorders at the age of 20 years for all adults, with screening at 5-year intervals for low-risk individuals. More frequent measurements are required for persons with multiple risk factors or in those with zero or one cardiovascular risk factors and an LDL cholesterol level only slightly lower than the goal level. The preferred screening test is a fasting lipoprotein profile including measurements of total cholesterol, HDL cholesterol, and triglycerides in order to calculate the LDL cholesterol level. (LDL cholesterol = total cholesterol − HDL cholesterol − [triglycerides ÷ 5]) The ATP III classification of lipid levels is shown in **Table 24**.

KEY POINTS

- The U.S. Preventive Services Task Force strongly recommends initiating lipid screening in men at age 35 years and in women who are at increased cardiovascular risk at age 45 years, and possibly earlier in both men and women at increased risk for cardiovascular disease.
- The National Cholesterol Education Program Adult Treatment Panel III recommends initiating lipid screening in all adults at age 20 years.

Evaluation of Lipid Levels

LDL Cholesterol

LDL cholesterol comprises 60% to 70% of serum cholesterol and is the most atherogenic of the lipoproteins. Cholesterol treatment guidelines focus on reducing LDL cholesterol as

TABLE 24. Adult Treatment Panel III Classification of Lipid Levels (mg/dL)

LDL Cholesterol—Primary Target of Therapy

<100 mg/dL (2.59 mmol/L)	Optimal
100-129 mg/dL (2.59-3.34 mmol/L)	Near optimal/above optimal
130-159 mg/dL (3.36-4.11 mmol/L)	Borderline high
160-189 mg/dL (4.14-4.89 mmol/L)	High
≥190 mg/dL (4.92 mmol/L)	Very high

Total Cholesterol

<200 mg/dL (5.18 mmol/L)	Desirable
200-239 mg/dL (5.18-6.19 mmol/L)	Borderline high
≥240 mg/dL (6.21 mmol/L)	High

HDL Cholesterol

<40 mg/dL (1.03 mmol/L)	Low
≥60 mg/dL (1.55 mmol/L)	High

Reprinted from ATP III Guidelines At-A-Glance Quick Desk Reference. National Heart, Lung, and Blood Institute. NIH Publication 01-3305. May 2001. Accessed August 8, 2011, at www.nhlbi.nih.gov/guidelines/cholesterol/atglance.pdf.

the primary target of therapy. LDL cholesterol levels have been linked to new and recurrent coronary heart disease (CHD) in numerous trials; higher levels of LDL cholesterol are associated with a greater cardiovascular risk, and a 1% reduction in LDL cholesterol reduces risk by 1%. As outlined in the ATP III guidelines, a patient's goal LDL cholesterol level is determined by counting the number of cardiac risk factors and assessing the short-term risk for an acute coronary syndrome (**Table 25**). For patients without diabetes or

CHD, the risk for a cardiovascular event over the next 10 years may be estimated using the Framingham risk calculator (http://hp2010.nhlbihin.net/atpiii/calculator.asp?usertype=prof). Patients are thus stratified into three different cardiac risk categories (<10%, 10%-20%, >20% risk over 10 years) and treatment goals vary accordingly. Certain medications and medical conditions can cause abnormal LDL cholesterol levels, including diabetes, hypothyroidism, and kidney disease. Suggestive history and physical examination findings should prompt evaluation for these disorders before initiating LDL cholesterol–lowering therapy.

Triglycerides

Elevated triglyceride levels reflect the presence of atherogenic VLDL remnants and are a marker for low HDL cholesterol levels, increased insulin resistance, and other components of the metabolic syndrome. It is controversial whether serum triglyceride levels themselves are an independent predictor of cardiac risk. However, as triglyceride-rich VLDL remnants have been associated with cardiovascular disease, the ATP III guidelines designate non-HDL cholesterol, which comprises LDL cholesterol together with VLDL cholesterol, as a secondary target for lipid-lowering therapy when triglyceride levels are greater than 200 mg/dL (2.26 mmol/L). The goal for non-HDL cholesterol (total cholesterol – HDL cholesterol) is 30 mg/dL (0.34 mmol/L) higher than the goal for LDL cholesterol.

The American Heart Association (AHA) suggests that the "optimal" triglyceride level is less than 100 mg/dL (1.13 mmol/L), but studies have not shown benefit for using medication to reach this target. Because lifestyle factors, including physical inactivity and a high-carbohydrate diet, have been

TABLE 25. Adult Treatment Panel III Recommendations for LDL Cholesterol Level Management

Risk Category	LDL Cholesterol Goal	Initiate TLC	Consider Drug Therapy[a]
High risk: CHD or CHD equivalents[b] (10-year risk >20%)	<100 mg/dL (2.59 mmol/L) (optional goal: <70 mg/dL [1.81 mmol/L])[c]	≥100 mg/dL (2.59 mmol/L)	≥130 mg/dL (3.37 mmol/L) 100 to 129 mg/dL (2.59 to 3.34 mmol/L): drug optional[d]
Moderately high risk: ≥2 risk factors (10-year risk 10% to 20%)	<130 mg/dL (3.37 mmol/L)	≥130 mg/dL (3.37 mmol/L)	≥130 mg/dL (3.37 mmol/L)
Moderate risk: ≥2 risk factors (10-year risk <10%)	<130 mg/dL (3.37 mmol/L)	≥130 mg/dL (3.37 mmol/L)	≥160 mg/dL (4.14 mmol/L)
Lower risk: 0 to 1 risk factor	<160 mg/dL (4.14 mmol/L)	≥160 mg/dL (4.14 mmol/L)	≥190 mg/dL (4.92 mmol/L); 160 to 189 mg/dL (4.14 to 4.90 mmol/L): drug optional

CHD = coronary heart disease; TLC = therapeutic lifestyle changes.

[a]When LDL cholesterol–lowering drug therapy is employed, intensity of therapy should be sufficient to achieve at least a 30% to 40% reduction in LDL cholesterol levels.

[b]CHD risk equivalents include peripheral arterial disease, abdominal aortic aneurysm, carotid artery disease, transient ischemic attacks or stroke of carotid origin or 50% obstruction of a carotid artery, diabetes, and 10-year risk for CHD ≥20%.

[c]ATP III Update 2004: Implications of recent clinical trials for the ATP III Guidelines. Available at www.nhlbi.nih.gov/guidelines/cholesterol/atp3upd04.htm.

[d]If a high-risk person has high triglyceride or low HDL cholesterol levels, combining a fibrate or nicotinic acid with an LDL cholesterol–lowering drug can be considered.

Data from the National Heart Lung and Blood Institute. National Cholesterol Education Program. Third Report of the Expert Panel on Detection, Evaluation, and Treatment of High Blood Cholesterol in Adults (Adult Treatment Panel III): Executive Summary. www.nhlbi.nih.gov/guidelines/cholesterol/atp_iii.htm. Published May 2001. Accessed July 14, 2009.

linked to elevated triglyceride levels, weight loss, exercise, and decreased consumption of carbohydrates and fructose are recommended for patients with borderline (150-199 mg/dL [1.69-2.24 mmol/L]) and high (200-499 mg/dL [2.26-5.63 mmol/L]) triglyceride levels. In accordance with ATP III guidelines, pharmacotherapy is recommended if the non-HDL cholesterol level is above goal, or if triglyceride levels are greater than 500 mg/dL (5.65 mmol/L), because of the increased risk for pancreatitis. Additionally, treating chronic diseases (diabetes, obesity, kidney disease) or eliminating medications that are associated with high triglyceride levels (corticosteroids, protease inhibitors, β-blockers, estrogens) may be beneficial.

HDL Cholesterol

HDL cholesterol makes up about 20% to 30% of serum cholesterol, and low levels have been linked to increased mortality from cardiovascular disease; a 1% decrease in serum HDL cholesterol level is associated with a 2% to 3% increase in cardiovascular risk. Reflecting this inverse relationship, the presence of a high HDL cholesterol level, defined as greater than 60 mg/dL (1.55 mmol/L), subtracts one risk factor when counting risk factors for LDL cholesterol treatment goals. Although HDL cholesterol level is the lipid risk factor most tightly correlated with cardiovascular risk, this may be related in part to the close association among low HDL cholesterol, small, dense LDL particles, and high triglyceride levels. Thus, the updated ATP III guidelines do not designate HDL cholesterol level as a specific target for lipid-lowering therapy. Causes of low HDL cholesterol level include elevated triglyceride levels, obesity, physical inactivity, smoking, high carbohydrate diets, type 2 diabetes, β-blockers, anabolic steroid use, progestational medications, and genetic factors.

Nonstandard Lipid Risk Factors

Several nontraditional risk factors may be related to cardiovascular outcomes, including levels of Lp(a) lipoprotein, small LDL particles, HDL subspecies, apolipoproteins B and A-1, and the total cholesterol/HDL cholesterol ratio. However, the USPSTF and updated ATP III guidelines do not recommend measuring or treating any of these risk factors when managing lipid levels.

Management of Dyslipidemias

Therapeutic Lifestyle Changes

Therapeutic lifestyle changes are the cornerstone of lipid-lowering therapy, and the ATP III guidelines recommend them for all patients with abnormal lipid levels. Saturated fat intake should be reduced to less than 7% of total calories (about 19 g of saturated fat for a 2500-calorie diet) and dietary cholesterol consumption decreased to less than 200 mg/d. Incorporating these changes alone into a standard Western diet can reduce LDL cholesterol levels by 9% to 12%; combining these changes with exercise can result in an LDL cholesterol reduction of up to 15%. Referral to a nutrition professional is also helpful. If goal LDL cholesterol levels are not reached after 6 weeks, the addition of 2 g/d of dietary plant sterols and stanols, found in certain fortified margarines and spreads, can enhance LDL cholesterol lowering by approximately 10%. Similarly, intake of viscous fiber, found in oatmeal, fruits, legumes, and certain vegetables, results in a modest LDL cholesterol reduction.

Drug Therapy

Providers should consider initiating drug therapy in patients who have not achieved LDL cholesterol goals after 3 months of therapeutic lifestyle changes, and simultaneously with lifestyle changes in patients with CHD or CHD risk equivalents who are unlikely to achieve LDL cholesterol goals with dietary therapy alone. The ATP III guidelines for LDL cholesterol goals and treatment strategies are listed in Table 25. Several medications are effective for reducing LDL cholesterol (**Table 26**).

Statins are considered first-line therapy, as they are the most effective for LDL cholesterol lowering and also reduce the risk for CHD outcomes in both primary and secondary prevention. Additionally, statins have been shown to reduce markers of inflammation, including high-sensitivity C-reactive protein levels, and this effect may contribute to their clinical benefits. Several studies have shown that statins reduce total mortality by 20% to 30% in patients with established CHD disease, but a recent meta-analysis of statin treatment for primary prevention in high-risk patients (which included data from the JUPITER trial) failed to show a mortality benefit. The updated ATP III guidelines recommend a goal LDL cholesterol level of less than 100 mg/dL (2.59 mmol/L) in high-risk patients and an optional goal of less than 70 mg/dL (1.81 mmol/L) in very high-risk patients, such as those with established cardiovascular disease plus diabetes.

Physicians should consider potencies, drug interactions, and metabolism when choosing among the currently available statins. The benefits of statin therapy are generally class specific, and there is no compelling evidence that newer agents are more effective than established statin medications, which may be more cost effective. The ATP III guidelines recommend titrating the statin dose to reduce LDL cholesterol levels by 30% to 40%; each doubling of the statin dose reduces LDL cholesterol level by a mean of approximately 6%. However, higher doses of statins are associated with an increased risk for myopathy. The FDA has recently recommended that an 80-mg dosage of simvastatin be prescribed only to those who have been tolerating it well for 12 months or more. Other risk factors for statin-induced myopathy include increased age, multiple medical problems, female sex, and cotreatment with certain medications. Inhibitors of the cytochrome P-450 3A4 (CYP3A4) isoenzyme, including cyclosporine, amiodarone, fibrates, and protease inhibitors,

TABLE 26. Medications for Treating Abnormal Lipid Levels

Agent	Changes in Lipid Values	Evidence	Notes
Statins	LDL cholesterol ↓ 18%-55% HDL cholesterol ↑ 5%-15% TGs ↓ 7%-30%	Reduced CHD in 1° and 2° prevention. Mortality benefit in 2° prevention.	Most effective agents for reducing LDL cholesterol. See Table 27 for adverse effects. Higher doses increase risk for adverse events. Contraindicated in pregnancy.
Bile acid sequestrants	LDL cholesterol ↓ 15%-30% HDL cholesterol ↑ 3%-5% No effect or possible ↑ in TGs	Reduced CHD in 1° prevention.	Avoid in patients with high TGs (>200 mg/dL [2.26 mmol/L]). Constipation, abdominal pain, and nausea are common side effects, but are seen less frequently with colesevelam.
Fibrates	LDL cholesterol ↓ 5%-20% (↑ in patients with elevated TGs) HDL cholesterol ↑ 10%-35% TGs ↓ 20%-50%	Reduced CHD in 1° and 2° prevention.	Most effective agents for reducing TGs, but may raise LDL cholesterol. Combination therapy with statins reduces overall cholesterol profile but may increase risk for myopathy. Avoid in patients with gallstones or kidney disease.
Nicotinic acid	LDL cholesterol ↓ 5%-25% HDL cholesterol ↑ 15%-35% TGs ↓ 20%-50%	Reduced CHD and atherosclerotic progression in 2° prevention.	Most effective agent for increasing HDL cholesterol. Flushing is common, but may be less frequent with sustained-release formulations or with prior administration of aspirin. Other adverse events include hepatotoxicity, gout, and hyperglycemia.
Ezetimibe	LDL cholesterol ↓ 18%	No evidence for cardiovascular benefit in 1° or 2° prevention.	Can reduce LDL cholesterol by an additional 19% when added to statin therapy. May be associated with myopathy.
Omega-3 fatty acids	TGs ↓ 30%-50%	Mixed evidence for reduction of CHD in 2° prevention.	Used as an alternative to fibrates or nicotinic acid for lowering TGs. Therapeutic doses range from 3-12 g/d.

1° = primary; 2° = secondary; CHD = coronary heart disease; TG = triglycerides.

should be used cautiously or not at all in patients taking CYP3A substrates, such as simvastatin, lovastatin, and atorvastatin. In contrast, pravastatin is metabolized renally, and fluvastatin and rosuvastatin are metabolized by CYP2C9, potentially making these better choices in patients treated with multiple medications. Additional adverse events associated with statin use and potential management strategies are listed in **Table 27**. Patients should be monitored for adverse events by obtaining serum creatine kinase and aminotransferase levels before initiating statin therapy. Because the risk of significant liver or muscle damage is very low, routine follow-up testing is not indicated and should be performed based on the development of symptoms or other clinical findings while on therapy.

Critics of the ATP III "treat to target" approach, outlined above, note that many patients do not achieve target LDL cholesterol levels, possibly because of the complexity of the treatment guidelines and the potential adverse effects associated with high-dose statins. A recent decision analysis compared the "treat to target" approach with a "tailored" approach, which eliminates the process of adjusting statin dosing according to achieved LDL cholesterol levels, and instead uses a fixed dose of statin based on the calculated 5-year cardiovascular risk. In this analysis, both approaches would treat similar numbers of patients with statins, but the tailored treatment approach prevented more cardiac morbidity and mortality.

Bile acid sequestrants are most effective when used in combination with statins, but may be used as monotherapy in patients who are considering pregnancy or need only modest LDL cholesterol reduction. Ezetimibe monotherapy can reduce LDL cholesterol by 18%, but evidence of improvement in cardiovascular outcomes with this medication is lacking; it may be considered in patients who are intolerant of statin therapy.

Combination Drug Therapy

Combination drug therapy may be required to achieve LDL cholesterol goals in select patients. Bile acid sequestrants are particularly effective at lowering LDL cholesterol when combined with statins and can produce an additional 12% to 16% LDL cholesterol reduction. This combination is efficacious with low to moderate doses of statins, and should be considered early in therapy for patients with very high LDL cholesterol levels and in patients who may not tolerate high doses of statins. If combined statin-sequestrant therapy is unsuccessful at achieving the target LDL cholesterol level, nicotinic acid may be added as a third agent.

TABLE 27. Major Adverse Events Associated with Statin Use

Adverse Event	Definition	Incidence	Management strategy
Myalgia	Muscle ache or weakness *without* an increase in CK	5%-10%	Investigate for other causes of muscle pain, including vitamin D deficiency, thyroid disease, fibromyalgia, medications, exercise, and strenuous work. Follow symptoms and CK levels weekly; discontinue statin or decrease dose if symptoms worsen or CK levels increase. Once symptoms resolve and CK levels return to baseline, consider use of a statin or alternative LDL cholesterol–lowering medications associated with less risk for myopathy: fluvastatin, rosuvastatin, pravastatin, ezetimibe, bile acid sequestrants. Consider supplementation with coenzyme Q10.
Myositis	Muscle ache or weakness *with* an increase in CK less than 10× ULN	NA	Same as for myalgia.
Rhabdomyolysis	Muscle ache or weakness *with* an increase in CK > 10× ULN and creatinine elevation, accompanied by myoglobinuria	0.09%	Discontinue statin therapy immediately. Monitor symptoms and CK levels. Statin may be restarted, preferably at a lower dose, once symptoms resolve completely and CK levels normalize.
Elevated aminotransferases	Incidental asymptomatic elevation of serum aminotransferase levels to less than 3× ULN with no associated histopathologic changes	3%	Continue statin therapy. Elevation is typically transient and occurs during the first 12 weeks of therapy. Recheck liver chemistry tests only if clinically indicated.
Hepatotoxicity	Alanine aminotransferase > 3× ULN with total bilirubin levels > 2× ULN	1%	Discontinue statin therapy and recheck liver chemistry test results. If liver chemistry test results normalize, consider rechallenge with the same statin at a lower dose or a different statin. If liver chemistry test results remain elevated, continue to withhold statin, screen for underlying liver disease, and consider drug interactions.

CK = creatine kinase; NA = not available; ULN = upper limit of normal.

Statins and fibrates can be used together cautiously to target both LDL and non-HDL cholesterol goals. Gemfibrozil raises the serum concentrations of statins by twofold or more, thereby increasing the risk for myopathy; fenofibrate is thus preferred for combination therapy.

The ARBITER 6-HALTS study compared the effectiveness of niacin or ezetimibe, when added to statin therapy, for reducing carotid intima-media thickness and altering lipid levels. HDL cholesterol levels in the niacin group increased by 18%, and LDL cholesterol levels in the ezetimibe group decreased by 19%; an improvement in carotid intima-media thickness was noted only for the niacin group. In two recent trials, combination treatment with simvastatin and fenofibrate (the ACCORD-Lipid trial) and simvastatin and niacin (the AIM-High trial) as compared with simvastatin monotherapy did not reduce cardiovascular risk.

Management of Hypertriglyceridemia

Lifestyle changes are the primary therapy for treatment of hypertriglyceridemia, and patients should be encouraged to lose weight, exercise regularly, and restrict alcohol use and excessive carbohydrate intake. In patients with above-goal LDL cholesterol and triglyceride levels, treatment with a statin, which reduces triglycerides by 20% to 40%, is first-line therapy. Patients with hypertriglyceridemia and elevated non-HDL cholesterol (≥30 mg/dL [0.77 mmol/L] above LDL cholesterol goal) and normal LDL cholesterol levels may be treated with nicotinic acid or a fibrate initially according to ATP III guidelines. Nicotinic acid reduces triglyceride levels by 30% to 50% and increases HDL cholesterol levels by 20% to 30% and may be the most efficacious monotherapy in patients with elevated non-HDL cholesterol levels. Fibrates are also effective for reducing triglycerides and increasing HDL cholesterol levels (changes of 40%-60% and 15%-25%, respectively), but they can raise LDL cholesterol levels by up to 30%. Thus, fibrate monotherapy may be ineffective for achieving non-HDL cholesterol goals. Therapeutic doses of eicosapentaenoic acid (3 to 9 g/d), which is found in fish oil supplements, can lower triglyceride levels by up to 50%, and may be an alternative to nicotinic acid or fibrate therapy. Evidence is lacking, however, that treatment with fish oil supplementation reduces mortality or cardiovascular events. In a recent randomized controlled trial among patients with established cardiovascular disease, investigators failed to show a reduction in cardiovascular events with low-dose daily supplementation of marine fatty acids, including eicosapentaenoic acid and docosahexaenoic acid.

Management of Low HDL Cholesterol

Low levels of HDL cholesterol are associated with increased cardiac risk, and treatment with medications that increase HDL cholesterol levels, such as nicotinic acid and fibrates, have been shown to reduce cardiovascular outcomes in several large studies. However, this effect may be mediated by treatment modification of the lipoprotein derangements that are associated with low HDL cholesterol levels, including small, dense LDL particles and elevated triglycerides. Thus, evidence of a direct relationship between raising HDL cholesterol levels and decreased cardiac risk is lacking.

In patients with CHD or CHD risk equivalents, treatment of abnormal LDL cholesterol levels should be the primary target of therapy. Once the goal LDL cholesterol level has been achieved, the addition of nicotinic acid or a fibrate may raise HDL cholesterol levels. In the VA-HIT trial, patients with established cardiovascular disease, low LDL cholesterol levels, and low HDL cholesterol levels were treated with gemfibrozil for 5 years. Gemfibrozil increased HDL cholesterol and decreased triglyceride levels, and this was associated with a 22% reduction in cardiovascular events.

Therapeutic lifestyle changes are the primary therapy for patients with low cardiac risk and abnormal HDL cholesterol levels. Weight reduction and increased physical activity can increase HDL cholesterol levels by up to 30%; smoking cessation can also increase HDL cholesterol slightly. There is no clear evidence, however, that initiating drug therapy to raise HDL cholesterol levels in low-risk patients is beneficial. Moreover, a trial attempting to raise HDL cholesterol levels using the cholesteryl-ester transfer protein inhibitor torcetrapib was terminated early because of excess deaths in the torcetrapib group.

KEY POINTS

- Therapeutic lifestyle changes are the cornerstone of lipid-lowering therapy and are recommended for all patients with abnormal lipid levels.

- Lipid-lowering drug therapy should be considered in patients who have not achieved LDL cholesterol goals after 3 months of therapeutic lifestyle changes, and simultaneously with lifestyle changes in patients with coronary heart disease or risk equivalents who are unlikely to achieve LDL cholesterol goals with dietary therapy alone.

- Baseline serum creatine kinase and aminotransferase levels should be obtained before initiating statin therapy; routine follow-up testing is not indicated.

Metabolic Syndrome

Epidemiology and Pathophysiology

The metabolic syndrome consists of a group of risk factors for cardiovascular disease and type 2 diabetes. Various criteria exist for making this diagnosis; the ATP III criteria are presented in **Table 28**. The designation of metabolic syndrome as a "syndrome" remains controversial. Some experts in the fields of diabetes, dyslipidemia, and obesity feel that focusing on interventions aimed at improving the individual constituents of the metabolic syndrome are more important than lumping those metabolic abnormalities into a syndrome. Others, however, feel that grouping the risk factors into a syndrome creates a lower threshold for education and intervention and that attaching a name may also help motivate patients to exercise, consume healthier diets, and lose weight.

The epidemic of obesity and insulin resistance in the United States has led to a sharply rising prevalence of metabolic syndrome, from an estimated 50 million cases in 1990 to 64 million by the year 2000. Metabolic syndrome is associated with a 7-fold increased risk for the future development of type 2 diabetes. It is also associated with a 2-fold increase in cardiovascular events and a 1.5-fold increase in all-cause mortality. The cardiovascular risk is present before the development of diabetes.

The clinical features and cardiovascular risks associated with this syndrome appear to be related to the dysregulation of adipose tissue. Cytokines secreted by adipose cells lead to a proinflammatory state believed to accelerate atherosclerosis, plaque rupture, and atherothrombosis. Insulin-like growth factor is also believed to play a role in metabolic syndrome and increased cardiovascular risk.

Management of Metabolic Syndrome

The "ABCDE" approach has been advocated as a reasonable approach to management of metabolic syndrome (**Table 29**).

TABLE 28. Criteria for Metabolic Syndrome

Any Three of the Following:	
Risk Factor	**Defining Level**
Abdominal obesity (waist circumference)	>40 in (>102 cm) in men; >35 in (>88 cm) in women
Triglyceride level[a]	≥150 mg/dL (1.70 mmol/L)
HDL cholesterol	<40 mg/dL (1.04 mmol/L) in men; <50 mg/dL (1.30 mmol/L) in women
Blood pressure	≥130/≥85 mm Hg
Fasting glucose	≥110 mg/dL (6.11 mmol/L)

[a]Triglyceride level ≥150 mg/dL (1.70 mmol/L) as a single factor correlates highly with presence of metabolic syndrome.

Data from the National Heart Lung and Blood Institute. National Cholesterol Education Program. Third Report of the Expert Panel on Detection, Evaluation, and Treatment of High Blood Cholesterol in Adults (Adult Treatment Panel III): Executive Summary. www.nhlbi.nih.gov/guidelines/cholesterol/atp_iii.htm. Published May 2001. Accessed July 14, 2009.

TABLE 29. "ABCDE" Approach to Management of Metabolic Syndrome

A	Assessment, aspirin	Diagnose metabolic syndrome, calculate Framingham risk score
		Begin aspirin if ≥6% 10-year Framingham risk
B	Blood pressure control	Goal <130/80 mm Hg if intermediate Framingham risk (≥ 6% 10-year risk)
C	Cholesterol management	LDL cholesterol: Statin therapy preferred; LDL cholesterol goal <100 mg/dL (2.59 mmol/L) for high-risk patients, <130 mg/dL (3.36 mmol/L) for intermediate-risk patients (per ATP III guidelines; see Table 25)
		Non-HDL cholesterol: Statin intensification and fenofibrate therapy; non-HDL cholesterol goal <130 mg/dL (3.36 mmol/L) for high-risk patients, <160 mg/dL (4.14 mmol/L) for intermediate-risk patients (per ATP III guidelines)
		Niacin for increasing HDL cholesterol controversial
D	Diabetes prevention, diet	Intensive lifestyle modification
		Metformin when indicated
		Weight loss
		Low glycemic diet
		Consider Mediterranean diet
E	Exercise	Daily vigorous activity
		Recommend use of pedometer; goal >10,000 steps/d

ATP III = National Cholesterol Education Program Adult Treatment Panel III.

Adapted with permission from Blaha MJ, Bansal S, Rouf R, Golden SH, Blumenthal RS, Defilippis AP. A practical "ABCDE" approach to the metabolic syndrome. Mayo Clin Proc. 2008;83(8):932-941. [PMID: 18674478] Copyright 2008, Elsevier.

The first step is assessment and diagnosis of metabolic syndrome. The Framingham risk calculator can then be used to calculate the patient's 10-year risk of myocardial infarction or death due to cardiovascular disease. As patients with metabolic syndrome are at increased risk of thrombosis owing to increased platelet aggregation, aspirin (81 mg/d) should be started in patients with intermediate or high Framingham risk (without contraindications to aspirin) to decrease platelet aggregation. The use of aspirin in low-risk patients is controversial owing to conflicting results in various studies.

Data are not clear about target blood pressures in metabolic syndrome, but some authors suggest a goal blood pressure of below 130/80 mm Hg in patients with intermediate or high Framingham 10-year risk. Owing to mounting evidence that β-blockers and thiazide diuretics worsen glucose tolerance, the American Heart Association and others have removed these drugs as recommended first-line agents to treat blood pressure that is above goal in patients with metabolic syndrome. ACE inhibitors and angiotensin receptor blockers to treat high blood pressure may be better choices in these patients because they have consistently been shown to improve glycemic control.

Although LDL cholesterol is not considered in diagnosing the metabolic syndrome, it is considered to be the principal lipoprotein determinant of atherosclerosis. It is generally recommended that in intermediate- and high-risk patients, statins be used. Fibrate therapy should be instituted in intermediate- and high-risk patients with metabolic syndrome and elevated triglyceride levels.

Lifestyle modification, increased physical activity, weight loss, and diet should be emphasized in all metabolic syndrome interventions. Weight loss reduces oxidative stress and improves all of the components of metabolic syndrome. A diet with a high glycemic load leads to more insulin resistance; therefore, a low-glycemic diet should be emphasized. Cardiac and respiratory fitness is associated with increased insulin sensitivity, decreased incidence of metabolic syndrome and decreased cardiovascular mortality.

KEY POINT

- Aspirin should be started in patients with metabolic syndrome without contraindications who have an intermediate or high Framingham cardiovascular risk.

Dyslipidemia Management in Older Patients

Older patients (ages 65-80 years) with established cardiovascular disease derive similar benefit as younger patients from statin therapy and tolerate these medications well. Primary prevention with statins in this age group, however, is controversial. Cardiovascular risk factor assessment may be less reliable in older patients, and older age confers an increased risk for statin-associated myopathy. Thus, risks and benefits of primary prevention with statin therapy must be weighed carefully in this age group.

- Risks and benefits of primary prevention with statin therapy must be weighed carefully in older patients, as cardiovascular risk factor assessment is less reliable and adverse effects are more frequent in this age group.

Dyslipidemia Management and Stroke Prevention

The American Heart Association (AHA) guidelines on stroke prevention highlight the importance of lipid-lowering therapy. For prevention of recurrent transient ischemic attack or stroke in patients with a history of CHD or elevated cholesterol levels, treatment should be aimed at lipid lowering according to ATP III guidelines. Lipid lowering for secondary stroke prevention in patients *without* a history of cardiac disease should aim for an LDL cholesterol level below 70 mg/dL (1.81 mmol/L) or an LDL cholesterol reduction of at least 50%. Secondary stroke prevention may also include treatment with niacin or gemfibrozil to increase low HDL cholesterol levels.

Aspirin as an Adjunct to Dyslipidemia Management

Aspirin reduces cardiovascular risk by irreversibly inhibiting platelets by inactivating cyclooxygenase-1, thus blocking the formation of thromboxane A_2. Although well established for the secondary prevention of cardiovascular disease, the USPSTF recommends against the routine use of aspirin in primary prevention in men aged 44 years and younger as well as in women aged 54 years and younger. Because the risk of first myocardial infarction is reduced by aspirin use in men ages 45 to 79 years, they recommend its use if the harm of gastrointestinal bleeding does not outweigh the benefit. Calculating Framingham risk scores can be used to help determine CHD risk in this patient population. Similarly, in women ages 55 to 79 years treated with aspirin, there is a statistically significant decreased risk of ischemic stroke but not a decrease in cardiovascular death or myocardial infarction. Again, the USPSTF recommends weighing the potential harm (gastrointestinal bleeding) against the benefit. The data are unclear regarding harm versus benefit of aspirin in men and women older than 80 years. **Table 30** shows the 10-year CHD risk levels for men and stroke risk for women at which the benefit of aspirin exceeds harms. The USPSTF emphasizes an individualized approach based on shared decision-making between physicians and patients.

The optimal dose of aspirin for primary prevention is unclear, as dosages used in studies have varied from 50 mg/d to 1500 mg/d. Given no evidence of improved outcomes and the increased risk of bleeding with higher doses, the USPSTF recommends the use of 75 mg/d aspirin when indicated for this purpose.

The risk of gastrointestinal bleeding increases with age. A history of peptic ulcer disease increases the risk of serious bleeding 2 to 3 fold. Other risk factors for serious gastrointestinal bleeding include male sex (twice the risk of women) and NSAID therapy (4 times the risk compared with aspirin alone).

- The U.S. Preventive Services Task Force recommends aspirin in men ages 45-79 years for primary prevention of cardiovascular disease and in women ages 55-79 years for primary prevention of stroke if the bleeding risks do not outweigh benefit.

Obesity

Definition and Epidemiology

Nearly 34% of adults and 17% of children in the United States are obese, defined as a BMI of 30 or greater. These are double and triple the rates, respectively, of a quarter century ago, and these numbers continue to rise. The highest rates are in black women (50%) and Hispanic women (43%). The Institute of Medicine identifies obesity as an "emerging priority area" for national action.

TABLE 30. CHD Risk Levels at Which Cardiovascular Disease Events Prevented is Closely Balanced to Serious Bleeding Events in Patients Taking Aspirin for Primary Prevention

Men		Women	
Age	10-Year CHD Risk, %	Age	10-Year Stroke Risk, %
45–59 y	≥4	55–59 y	≥3
60–69 y	≥9	60–69 y	≥8
70–79 y	≥12	70–79 y	≥11

CHD = coronary heart disease.

Reprinted from US Preventive Services Task Force. Aspirin for the prevention of cardiovascular disease: U.S. Preventive Services Task Force recommendation statement. Ann Intern Med. 2009;150(6):396-404. [PMID: 19293072]

In adults, obesity is defined by BMI (body mass divided by the square of the height), and online BMI calculators are widely available (www.nhlbisupport.com/bmi/). Categories of obesity and overweight based on BMI proposed by the World Health Organization and National Institutes of Health (NIH) are listed in **Table 31**, along with the most recent prevalence estimates for U.S. men and women.

Obese and overweight persons are at increased risk for heart disease, hypertension, dyslipidemia, type 2 diabetes mellitus, stroke, osteoarthritis, sleep apnea, gallbladder disease, certain cancers (endometrial, breast, colon), and overall mortality. These risks increase progressively with rising BMI. Obesity also is associated with reduced quality of life, societal discrimination, and increased health care costs. It is estimated that obesity added $147 billion to health care costs in 2008. In persons aged 65 years and older, obesity is associated with impaired physical functioning, including difficulty with activities of daily living.

Screening and Evaluation

The NIH and the U.S. Preventive Services Task Force (USPSTF) recommend screening all adults for obesity. The USPSTF recommends screening by calculating the BMI. The NIH recommends screening both with BMI and waist circumference measurement. Waist circumference is measured with a measuring tape placed around the abdomen at the level of the iliac crest. Central adiposity (waist circumference in men >102 cm [40 in]; in women >88 cm [35 in]) is associated with an increased risk for type 2 diabetes, dyslipidemia, hypertension, and heart disease, not only in obese persons, but also in those who are overweight.

The assessment of the obese patient begins with the history and physical examination. The history should specifically elicit chronology of weight gain, family history of obesity, medications that can promote weight gain (**Table 32**), exercise, eating patterns, and symptoms and risk factors for cardiovascular disease. The general physical examination of the obese patient can

TABLE 32. Medications That Cause Weight Gain

Drug Category	Medications
Atypical antipsychotic agents	Clozapine, olanzapine, quetiapine, risperidone
Antidiabetic drugs	Sulfonylureas, thiazolidinediones, insulin
Corticosteroids	Glucocorticoids (e.g., prednisone)
Tricyclic antidepressants	Amitriptyline, imipramine, doxepin
Selective serotonin reuptake inhibitors	Paroxetine
Anticonvulsant agents	Valproic acid, carbamazepine
β-Blockers	Propranolol, atenolol, metoprolol

be challenging owing to excessive intervening adipose tissue, and formal instruction in specific maneuvers in the physical examination receives limited attention in standard textbooks. However, practical suggestions to augment accuracy of the examination have been published (http://jama.jamanetwork.com/article.aspx?doi=10.1001/jama.2010.1950).

Assessment for comorbidities associated with obesity should be considered. The USPSTF does not recommend specific laboratory tests based on the presence of obesity alone, but the American Diabetes Association (ADA) recommends screening for diabetes in patients with a BMI of 25 or greater who have other risk factors for diabetes. Although the major cause of obesity is imbalance between caloric intake and energy expenditure, physicians should consider less common causes, including hypothyroidism and Cushing syndrome.

KEY POINTS

- All adults should be screened for obesity using BMI calculation.
- Central adiposity is associated with an increased risk for type 2 diabetes, dyslipidemia, hypertension, and heart disease in both overweight and obese persons.

TABLE 31. Classification of Obesity

Category	Adult BMI	2007-2008 U.S. Prevalence of Obesity[a]	
		Men ≥20 y (%)	Women ≥20 y (%)
Underweight	<18.5		
Normal weight	18.5-24.9		
Overweight	25.0-29.9	30	29
Obese	≥30.0	32	36
Obesity class I	30.0-34.9	21	18
Obesity class II	35.0-39.9	7	11
Obesity class III	≥40.0	4	7
Summary (obese plus overweight)	≥25.0	62	65

[a]Data from U.S. Health and Human Services Centers for Disease Control and Prevention. Health United States, 2010. Available at www.cdc.gov/nchs/data/hus/hus10.pdf. Accessed January 4, 2012.

Treatment

After the initial assessment of the obese patient, the physician should determine the patient's level of motivation for weight loss, and an individualized treatment plan should follow. Success can be enhanced by a combined team of health professionals, including a dietitian, a behavioral therapist, and an exercise therapist. Adherence to strategies that decrease caloric input and increase energy expenditure will result in weight loss. A combined approach of diet and physical activity is likely to be more successful than an individual one, but strategies that focus on decreasing caloric input are more successful than those that only focus on energy expenditure. The goal is to achieve a reduction in body weight of 10% at a rate of 0.5 to 1 kg (1-2 lb) per week during a 6-month period. This degree of weight loss will reduce the risk of many medical complications of obesity. In addition to lifestyle modification (behavioral changes, exercise, and diet), medication and surgery have become increasingly popular options. The overall management of the obese patient is presented in **Figure 16**.

KEY POINT

- A recommended weight loss goal is a reduction in body weight of 10% at a rate of 0.5 to 1 kg (1-2 lb) per week during a 6-month period.

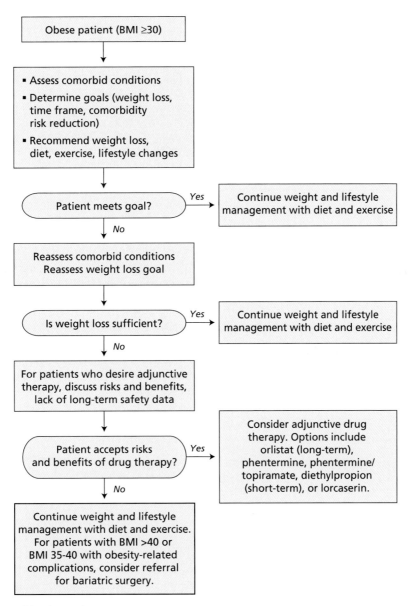

FIGURE 16. Management of the obese patient.

Lifestyle Modification

The USPSTF recommends that clinicians offer all obese patients intensive counseling and behavioral interventions. This includes counseling in diet and exercise. Lifestyle modification has been shown to be the most effective intervention to prevent type 2 diabetes, and the ADA recommends lifestyle modification for diabetes prevention.

Behavioral Therapy

Behavioral therapy focuses the patient's attention on his or her personal maladaptive eating patterns and assists the patient to control or modify food intake, increase exercise, and avoid stimuli that trigger eating. Behavioral therapy is best when accomplished by a therapist trained in this technique and in combination with other modalities but can be initiated by the primary care physician. Principles of behavioral therapy using motivational interviewing are discussed in Routine Care of the Healthy Patient. In a systematic evidence review for the USPSTF on the effectiveness of primary care–relevant treatment for obesity in adults, 21 studies that used behavioral interventions resulted in a weight loss of 1.5 to 5.0 kg (3.3-11 lb) at 12 to 18 months, compared with little or no weight loss in the control groups. Behavioral therapy is time intensive, and regain of weight is common. However, in a recent randomized controlled trial of patients who successfully completed an initial behavioral weight loss program, monthly brief personal contact follow-up was associated with sustained weight loss. The use of technology-based interventions (Web-based interactive interventions) provided early but transient benefit.

Exercise

Exercise as monotherapy is likely not adequate for significant weight loss. In a 12-month study of moderate to vigorous exercise for 1 hour daily, 6 days per week, women lost only 1.4 kg (3.1 lb) and men lost 1.8 kg (4 lb). However, exercise at a level of walking 60 to 90 minutes per day is effective in maintaining weight that is lost and, therefore, is a useful adjunct to any weight loss program. Exercise has other health benefits, including improving cardiovascular health and decreasing waist circumference.

Consistent Dietary Caloric Restriction

Consistent dietary caloric restriction leads to successful weight loss. Obese patients can lose approximately 0.45 kg (1 lb) weekly by decreasing their intake by 500 to 1000 kcal/d below what is needed to maintain current weight. Total calories should not be restricted to less than 800 kcal/d as "very-low-calorie" diets are no more effective than low-calorie diets for successful long-term weight loss and have higher adverse consequences. No one diet has consistently been shown to be superior to others when long-term outcomes are measured. A meta-analysis comparing low-fat to low-carbohydrate diets found that whereas weight loss was better in the short term for the low-carbohydrate diet, there was no difference at 1 year. A randomized trial comparing outcomes of an intensive behavioral intervention combined with either a low-fat or a low-protein diet resulted in an 11% weight loss at 1 year and a 7% weight loss in 2 years in both groups. The low-carbohydrate diet group demonstrated a 23% increase in HDL cholesterol levels at 2 years. Exercise can enhance weight loss, especially when begun during the early phases, but caloric restriction is the key aspect to continued loss of weight. Recent evidence suggests that inadequate sleep (<7-9 hours) also compromises the success rates of typical dietary interventions.

KEY POINTS

- All obese patients should be offered intensive counseling and behavioral interventions to encourage weight loss, including counseling in diet and exercise.
- No one diet has been demonstrated superior to others in achieving long-term weight loss.

Pharmacologic Therapy

With the rising prevalence of obesity, drug therapy has emerged as an attractive option for weight loss in obese patients, especially when lifestyle modification is ineffective. However, both short-term and long-term safety and efficacy may limit use in many patients. Current FDA-approved options for drug therapy in the United States include sympathomimetic drugs that suppress appetite (phentermine, diethylpropion) and drugs that alter fat absorption (orlistat). Several appetite suppressant medications, including sibutramine, have been removed from the market over the years owing to safety concerns.

Sympathomimetic drugs are approved only for short-term use as an adjunct to other weight loss programs. Although studies have documented weight loss with continuous and intermittent use (net loss, 3.6 kg [7.9 lb]), most users regain weight upon discontinuation. Significant increases in blood pressure and arrhythmias can occur with phentermine; caution is indicated in patients with hypertension and cardiovascular disease. However, in a recent study of low-dose, controlled-release phentermine plus topiramate combined with office-based lifestyle intervention, modest weight loss was achieved (8.1 kg [17.8 lb] at 56 weeks compared with 1.4 kg [3.1 lb] in the placebo group). Significant improvement was noted in waist circumference, blood pressure, and lipid levels in the treatment group. Combination phentermine/topiramate has been FDA-approved for the treatment of obesity.

Orlistat, now available over-the-counter, is a lipase inhibitor that leads to fat malabsorption. In a recent meta-analysis on the pharmacologic treatment of obesity, the mean weight loss in patients treated with orlistat was 2.9 kg (6.4 lb) at 12 months. Secondary benefits included reductions in LDL cholesterol level and blood pressure and, in patients with diabetes, improvement in glycemic control. Approximately 15%

to 30% of patients experience gastrointestinal side effects (flatus, abdominal cramps, fecal incontinence, oily spottage), especially while consuming high-fat diets. Orlistat has not been associated with serious cardiovascular side effects. However, a recently completed review by the FDA noted rare reports of severe liver injury with orlistat. Malabsorption of fat-soluble vitamins A, D, and E has been reported, and vitamin supplementation is advisable while taking the medication.

In 2012, lorcaserin, a brain serotonin 2C receptor agonist, was FDA approved for adults with BMI greater than 30 or greater than 27 with obesity-related complications. In conjunction with a reduced-calorie diet and exercise counseling, lorcaserin was associated with an average weight loss of 3% at 1 year. Lorcaserin should be used with caution in patients who are on medications that increase serotonin levels. It has not been studied in patients with significant valvular heart disease.

KEY POINT

- Pharmacologic options for weight loss include orlistat for long-term use, the appetite suppressants phentermine and diethylpropion for short-term use, and lorcaserin.

Surgery

For class II or III obese patients (BMI ≥35) in whom diet, exercise, and/or medication have failed, especially those with significant obesity-related comorbidities, weight loss surgery should be considered. The NIH Consensus Development Conference Statement suggested the following criteria for considering a patient for bariatric surgery:

1. Patients should be well-informed, motivated, able to participate in treatment and long-term follow-up, and have acceptable operative risks.
2. Patients should have a BMI that exceeds 40.
3. Patients with a BMI between 35 and 40 with obesity-related comorbidities, such as severe sleep apnea, diabetes, or severe joint disease, should be considered.
4. Patients should be evaluated by a multidisciplinary team with medical, surgical, psychiatric, and nutritional expertise.

Surgical therapies involve restriction of stomach size and malabsorption of ingested calories as their mechanisms of action. According to worldwide survey data, the most common procedures are Roux-en-Y gastric bypass (65.1%), laparoscopic adjustable band procedures (24%), vertical banded gastroplasties (5.4%), and biliopancreatic diversion (4.8%) (**Figure 17**). The laparoscopic adjustable band procedure is increasing in popularity among patients and physicians, although the weight loss with this procedure, and restrictive surgeries in general, is less robust compared with gastric bypass. The two most common procedures are compared in **Table 33**.

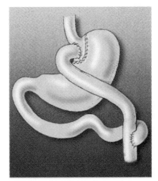

Roux-en-Y gastric bypass

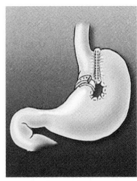

Vertical banded gastroplasty

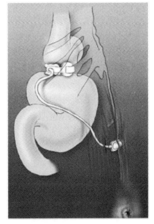

Adjustable gastric band

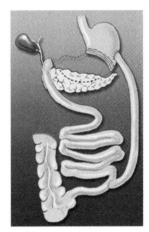

Biliopancreatic diversion with duodenal switch

FIGURE 17. Surgical procedures for obesity.

Reprinted with permission from Maggard MA, Shugarman LR, Suttorp M, et al. Meta-analysis: surgical treatment of obesity. Ann Intern Med. 2005;142(7):547-559. [PMID: 15809466] Copyright 2005, American College of Physicians.

Randomized controlled and cohort studies comparing bariatric surgery with nonsurgical interventions have found that surgery results in more dramatic and sustained weight loss and leads to improvement in obesity-related comorbidities. In a meta-analysis comprising 16,944 patients with a mean BMI of 47 (range 32-69) who underwent some type of bariatric procedure, the average weight loss at 12 months was 43.46 kg (95.6 lb) for Roux-en-Y gastric bypass, 32.16 kg (70.8 lb) for vertical band gastroplasty, 30.19 kg (66.4 lb) for adjustable gastric banding, and 51.93 kg (114.2 lb) for biliopancreatic diversion. Diabetes resolved in 76.8% of patients, hypertension resolved in 61.7%, obstructive sleep apnea resolved in 85.7%, and hyperlipidemia improved in 70%. Another meta-analysis reached similar conclusions. In a large retrospective cohort study, all-cause mortality decreased by 40% in the surgery group compared with the control group at a mean follow-up of 7.1 years. However, in a recent subset of obese, high-risk, primarily male patients, bariatric surgery was not significantly associated with survival during a mean of

TABLE 33.	Comparison of Commonly Used Bariatric Procedures	
Characteristic	Laparoscopic Adjustable Gastric Banding	Roux-en-Y Gastric Bypass
Mechanism of weight loss	Restrictive	Restrictive and malabsorptive
Technique	Adjustable silicone ring is placed around the top part of the stomach, creating a 15-30 mL pouch.	7-10 mL gastric pouch is separated from the rest of the stomach and connected to the small intestine, bypassing the rest of the stomach and duodenum.
Dietary program	<800 kcal/d for 18-36 months; 1000-1200 kcal/d thereafter.	<800 kcal/d for 12-18 months; 1000-1200 kcal/d thereafter in three small, high-protein meals per day.
	Certain foods can get "stuck" (rice, bread, meats, nuts), causing pain and vomiting.	Avoid sugar and fats to prevent "dumping syndrome."
Hospital length of stay	<1 day	3-4 days
Weight loss at 12 months	30.19 kg (66.4 lb)	43.46 kg (95.6 lb)
30-day mortality	0.1%	0.5%
Incidence of postoperative complications	10%	15%
Nonoperative complications	Nausea, vomiting, reflux	Cholelithiasis, nutritional deficiencies (vitamin B_{12}, other B vitamins, iron, calcium, folic acid, vitamin D; rare: magnesium, copper, zinc, vitamin A, vitamin C)

6.7 years of follow-up. Some studies document short-term improvements in quality of life.

Bariatric surgery carries procedure-specific short-term and long-term risks. Surgical mortality rates are low (<1%) and appear to be reduced with the laparoscopic approach and with surgeons who perform a high volume of the procedures. Complications of bariatric surgery are discussed in MKSAP 16 Gastroenterology and Hepatology. Long-term multidisciplinary follow-up of the patient after bariatric surgery is essential. An average of 20% to 25% of lost weight is regained in 10 years. Dietary counseling, increased physical activity (at least 150 minutes weekly), and behavioral modification are recommended. For patients who have undergone a Roux-en-Y procedure, recent guidelines suggest twice yearly monitoring of vitamin D, calcium, phosphorus, parathyroid hormone, and alkaline phosphatase levels. To assess nutritional deficiencies after a malabsorptive procedure, ferritin, vitamin B_{12}, folate, vitamin D, and calcium levels should be assessed every 6 months for the first 2 years and annually thereafter. Bone mineral density testing is recommended yearly until stable.

KEY POINT

- Bariatric surgery may be considered for patients with a BMI above 40 or with a BMI above 35 with obesity-related complications.

Men's Health

Male Sexual Dysfunction

Male sexual dysfunction is common and causes significant distress. Many men, however, hesitate to bring such symptoms to the attention of their health care providers. Sexual dysfunction can be categorized as either erectile dysfunction (ED), ejaculatory dysfunction, or decreased libido.

Erectile Dysfunction

ED, the most common form of sexual dysfunction in men, is the inability to maintain an erection sufficient for satisfactory sexual performance. Up to one in three men experience ED at some point in their lives.

Risk Factors

The prevalence of ED increases with age, with up to 30% of men older than 70 years being affected. Obese men have close to a two-fold greater risk of developing ED than men of normal weight. Risk is similarly increased in men who smoke cigarettes compared with nonsmokers. Other modifiable risk factors include sedentary lifestyle and use of a variety of substances, including alcohol, barbiturates, cocaine, heroin, marijuana, and methamphetamines. Not only do ED and cardiovascular disease share many risk factors (diabetes mellitus, hyperlipidemia, and hypertension), ED is itself a cardiac risk factor that independently predicts mortality and confers a risk similar to that of moderate smoking. Hormonal disorders associated with ED include hypogonadism, hypothyroidism, and hyperprolactinemia. The risk of ED increases with a history of previous pelvic irradiation, surgery (including, but not limited to, prostate surgeries), or trauma. Neurologic conditions associated with an increased risk of ED include dementia, multiple sclerosis, prior cerebrovascular accident, and quadri- or paraplegia.

ED is a common side effect of medications. Up to one-quarter of all cases of ED are thought to be due to medications. **Table 34** provides a list of medications commonly associated

TABLE 34. Medications Commonly Associated with Erectile Dysfunction

Antidepressants
  Monoamine oxidase inhibitors
  Selective serotonin reuptake inhibitors
  Tricyclic antidepressants

Benzodiazepines

Opioids

Anticonvulsants
  Phenytoin
  Phenobarbital

Antihypertensives
  α-Blockers
  β-Blockers
  Calcium channel blockers
  Clonidine
  Spironolactone
  Thiazide diuretics

5α-Reductase inhibitors
  Dutasteride
  Finasteride

with ED. Various psychiatric conditions are associated with ED, including anxiety, depression, and prior sexual abuse. Relationship discord and stress can also lead to ED.

Diagnosis and Evaluation

The initial evaluation of a man reporting ED consists of obtaining medical, psychosocial, and sexual histories in addition to performing a focused physical examination and a limited laboratory investigation. During the medical history, it is important to first obtain an accurate description of what the patient is experiencing, as some patients confuse premature ejaculation with ED. Clinicians should seek to determine the presence or absence of medical conditions, medications, and other risk factors associated with ED. A psychosocial history should be performed with the purpose of identifying any underlying psychological conditions that may be contributory. Sexual history includes libido (loss is seen with androgen deficiency, depression, and as a side effect of medication use); ability to achieve and maintain erections, including circumstances (the sudden onset of the loss of ability to achieve an erection suggests a psychogenic origin but can also occur following radical prostatectomy and after trauma); ability to achieve orgasm, including quality and timing (if situational, suggests psychogenic origin); and penile curvature (its presence, along with penile pain, suggests Peyronie disease); and presence of early morning erections (presence suggests intact corpus cavernosae blood flow and intact neurogenic reflexes). The severity of ED symptoms can be assessed using the International Index of Erectile Function–5 (IIEF-5), a validated, five-item questionnaire (available at www.hiv.va.gov/provider/manual-primary-care/urology-tool2.asp). It is also

important to inquire about lifestyle factors and the sexual function of the patient's partners.

During the physical examination, the patient's BMI, blood pressure, and heart rate should be determined. A genital, digital rectal, and screening neurologic examination in addition to an assessment of lower extremity pulses and secondary sexual characteristics should also be performed. Because many episodes of ED are transient, an extensive laboratory evaluation is not mandatory at presentation without symptoms or findings suggestive of an underlying systemic disorder or before implementing lifestyle modification or counseling therapy. If indicated for suspected abnormalities or persistent symptoms, a reasonable initial laboratory investigation consists of obtaining a fasting serum glucose level, lipid panel, thyroid-stimulating hormone level, and early morning total testosterone level. Additional laboratory tests should only be obtained on the basis of findings in the history and physical examination.

Treatment

The first step in successfully treating ED is to attempt to identify an underlying etiology. If possible, treatment should be directed toward the underlying condition. Regardless of etiology, first-line therapies for ED consist of both lifestyle modifications and pharmacotherapy with phosphodiesterase type 5 (PDE-5) inhibitors. In one study, nearly one third of obese men had improved ED symptoms simply by exercising regularly and losing weight. Attempts should therefore be made to lower the patient's BMI below 30. Patients should be counseled to stop smoking and consideration should be given to stopping (if possible) any medications that are associated with ED. Psychosexual therapy performed by a sex therapist has been found to improve ED in 40% to 80% of patients.

PDE-5 inhibitors function by increasing cyclic guanosine monophosphate (cGMP) levels, which leads to smooth muscle relaxation and engorgement. Improvement in ED appears to be dose related for both sildenafil (up to 50 mg) and vardenafil (all doses) but not tadalafil. All PDE-5 inhibitors improve erections and sexual intercourse success compared with placebo and possess approximately equivalent efficacy. The efficacy of PDE-5 inhibitors is further improved when combined with other ED therapies such as psychotherapy and attempts at weight loss. Because ED shares many risk factors with atherosclerotic disease and itself is an independent risk factor, an assessment of the patient's cardiovascular risk should be made before prescribing a PDE-5 inhibitor. This can be accomplished using guidelines established by the Second Princeton Consensus Conference (**Table 35**).

PDE-5 inhibitors are generally well tolerated. Headache, the most common side effect, occurs in approximately 10% of patients. Dizziness, dyspepsia, flushing, rhinitis, syncope, and visual disturbances occur less commonly. Nonarteritic anterior optic neuropathy, although

TABLE 35. Second Princeton Consensus Conference Guidelines for Treatment of Erectile Dysfunction in Patients with Cardiovascular Disease or Cardiac Risk Factors

Risk Level	Treatment Recommendation
Low risk	
Asymptomatic and <3 major cardiac risk factors[a]	Can initiate or resume sexual activity or treat for ED with PDE-5 inhibitor (if not using nitrates)
Controlled hypertension	
Mild stable angina	
Post successful coronary revascularization	
MI (>6-8 weeks before)	
Mild valvular disease	
Left ventricular dysfunction (NYHA functional class I)	
Intermediate/indeterminate risk	
Asymptomatic and ≥3 major cardiac risk factors[a]	Further cardiac evaluation (stress test or cardiology consultation) and restratification before resumption of sexual activity or treatment for ED
Moderate stable angina	
Recent MI (2-6 weeks)	
Left ventricular dysfunction (ejection fraction <40%) or heart failure (NYHA class II)	
Noncardiac atherosclerotic disease (clinically evident PAD, history of stroke/TIA)	
High risk	
Unstable or refractory angina	Defer sexual activity or ED treatment until cardiac condition is stabilized and reassessed
Uncontrolled hypertension	
Moderate to severe heart failure (NYHA class III-IV)	
Recent MI (<2 weeks)	
High-risk arrhythmia	
Obstructive hypertrophic cardiomyopathy	
Moderate to severe valvular disease (particularly aortic stenosis)	

ED = erectile dysfunction; MI = myocardial infarction; NYHA = New York Heart Association; PAD = peripheral arterial disease; PDE = phosphodiesterase; TIA = transient ischemic attack.

[a]Major cardiac risk factors are: age, hypertension, diabetes mellitus, smoking, dyslipidemia, sedentary lifestyle, family history of premature coronary artery disease. (Male sex is excluded.)

Recommendations from Kostis JB, Jackson G, Rosen R, et al. Sexual dysfunction and cardiac risk (the Second Princeton Consensus Conference). Am J Cardiol. 2005;96(2):313-321. [PMID: 16018863]

extremely rare, has been documented and is caused by crossover inhibition of PDE-6 receptors. The use of PDE-5 inhibitors is contraindicated in patients taking nitrates owing to the potential for profound hypotension. Caution should be exercised when using PDE-5 inhibitors in patients concomitantly taking drugs that inhibit the cytochrome P-450 3A4 pathway, such as protease inhibitors, erythromycin, and ketoconazole. A comprehensive list of interacting medications can be accessed at http://medicine.iupui.edu/clinpharm/ddis/ClinicalTable.aspx.

Second-line therapies for ED include prostaglandin E_1 (alprostadil) administered either via intracavernosal or intraurethral routes, with the former being more effective and better tolerated. Additional therapies include use of penile pumps and placement of penile prostheses. Testosterone therapy appears to be effective in men with ED and androgen deficiency (see below).

Premature Ejaculation

Premature ejaculation, ejaculation that occurs sooner than desired, is diagnosed by obtaining a thorough sexual history. Treatment should be individualized and include a discussion with the patient of risks and benefits of each option. Pharmacologic therapies can be either oral or topical. Oral therapies function by causing anorgasmia and include several selective serotonin reuptake inhibitors (fluoxetine, paroxetine, and sertraline) and clomipramine, a tricyclic antidepressant. Topical anesthetic agents, such as lidocaine or prilocaine cream, function by reducing stimulation and can be used with or without a condom.

Decreased Libido

Decreased libido, a decreased desire for sexual activity, is less common in men than in women but often is more disabling. When decreased libido is associated with marked distress and interferes with relationships, the term hypoactive sexual desire disorder is used. Causes include hypogonadism, hyperprolactinemia, medications, relationship difficulties, and psychiatric disorders (most commonly depression). Decreased libido also is more common as men age. Treatment is frequently directed toward the underlying cause, if one is identifiable. It is also important to explore the quality of the relationship with the patient's sexual partner, as relationship difficulties may be the underlying issue rather than decreased libido.

KEY POINTS

- First-line therapy for erectile dysfunction consists of lifestyle modifications, psychosexual counseling, and pharmacotherapy with a phosphodiesterase type 5 inhibitor.
- Men with erectile dysfunction (ED) and three or more cardiac risk factors require cardiac evaluation before initiating treatment for ED or resuming sexual activity.
- The use of phosphodiesterase type 5 inhibitors is contraindicated in patients taking nitrates owing to the potential for profound hypotension.

Androgen Deficiency

Androgen deficiency in the setting of male hypogonadism is suggested by the signs and symptoms listed in **Table 36**. Men with specific signs and symptoms of androgen deficiency should be evaluated by measuring morning total testosterone level as the initial diagnostic test. However, because the less specific symptoms of potential androgen deficiency overlap considerably with many other common symptoms, testing in men with these symptoms should be approached judiciously, particularly those without more definitive findings on history or examination that suggest the diagnosis. The assessment of men for androgen deficiency should include a general health evaluation to exclude systemic illness and a review of medications (including opioids and high-dose corticosteroid therapy) and recreational drugs (such as marijuana) that affect testosterone production or metabolism. Eating disorders and excessive exercise can transiently lower testosterone levels. Clinical guidelines published by the Endocrine Society recommend against screening of asymptomatic men in the general population for androgen deficiency, regardless of age.

Men with low-normal testosterone levels should have confirmatory testing before initiating testosterone therapy, and further evaluation of the cause of hypogonadism should be pursued before treatment is started, if indicated (see

TABLE 36. Symptoms and Signs Suggestive of Androgen Deficiency in Men

More specific symptoms and signs
Incomplete or delayed sexual development, eunuchoidism
Reduced sexual desire (libido) and activity
Decreased spontaneous erections
Breast discomfort, gynecomastia
Loss of body (axillary and pubic) hair, reduced shaving
Very small (especially <5 mL) or shrinking testes
Inability to father children, low or zero sperm count
Height loss, low-trauma fracture, low bone mineral density
Hot flushes, sweats

Less specific symptoms and signs
Decreased energy, motivation, initiative, and self-confidence
Feeling sad or blue, depressed mood, dysthymia
Poor concentration and memory
Sleep disturbance, increased sleepiness
Mild anemia (normochromic, normocytic, in the female range)
Reduced muscle bulk and strength
Increased body fat, BMI
Diminished physical or work performance

Adapted with permission from Bhasin S, Cunningham GR, Hayes FJ, et al; Task Force, Endocrine Society. Testosterone therapy in men with androgen deficiency syndromes: an Endocrine Society clinical practice guideline. J Clin Endocrinol Metab. 2010;95(6):2537. [PMID: 20525905] Copyright 2010, The Endocrine Society.

MKSAP 16 Endocrinology and Metabolism). Testosterone therapy for men is recommended with symptomatic androgen deficiency to induce and maintain secondary sex characteristics and to improve sexual function, sense of well-being, muscle mass and strength, and bone mineral density. Because of potential adverse effects of testosterone therapy, the Endocrine Society recommends against its use in patients with breast or prostate cancer, a palpable prostate nodule or induration, a prostate-specific antigen (PSA) level greater than 4 ng/mL (or >3 ng/mL in men at high risk for prostate cancer), a hematocrit greater than 50%, untreated severe obstructive sleep apnea, severe lower urinary tract symptoms, or uncontrolled or poorly controlled heart failure. Management of patients on testosterone replacement therapy is addressed in more detail in MKSAP 16 Endocrinology and Metabolism.

KEY POINTS

- Men with symptoms of androgen deficiency and low-normal testosterone levels should have confirmatory testing before initiating testosterone therapy.
- Guidelines recommend against screening of asymptomatic men in the general population for androgen deficiency, regardless of age.

Benign Prostatic Hyperplasia

Benign prostatic hyperplasia (BPH) is a common cause of lower urinary tract symptoms (LUTS) in men. LUTS can be classified as related to overactive bladder symptoms versus bladder outlet obstruction (BOO). Overactive bladder symptoms, caused by BPH and detrusor muscle hyperactivity, include nocturia and urinary frequency and urgency. BOO symptoms, caused by physical obstruction, include decreased urinary stream, urinary retention, incomplete bladder emptying, and incontinence. The differential diagnosis of BPH includes neurologic conditions (stroke, multiple sclerosis, spinal cord conditions) as well as effects of certain medications, such as diuretics. Guidelines from the American Urological Association (AUA) recommend performing a digital rectal examination and obtaining a baseline AUA symptom index score (questionnaire available at http://www2.niddk.nih.gov/NR/rdonlyres/8E99FCF4-8A92-43EE-8E47-5B70D634938A/0/AUABPH.pdf) to track progression and effectiveness of treatment. A urinalysis should be obtained when evaluating BPH symptoms to rule out underlying infection.

Treatment modalities include watchful waiting and conservative measures for mild symptoms, drug therapy (**Table 37**), and surgical interventions for severe or refractory symptoms. Conservative measures include reduced fluid intake, timed voiding, limiting caffeine and alcohol, discontinuing exacerbating medications, and improving mobility.

TABLE 37. Medical Therapies for Patients with Moderate to Severe Symptoms of Benign Prostatic Hyperplasia

α-Blockers
Alfuzosin
Doxazosin
Tamsulosin
Terazosin
Silodosin
5α-Reductase inhibitors
Dutasteride
Finasteride
Anticholinergic agents
Oxybutynin
Tolterodine
Combination therapy
α-Blocker and 5α-reductase inhibitor
α-Blocker and anticholinergic agents
Phosphodiesterase type 5 inhibitor
Tadalafil

Information adapted from AUA Guidelines: www.auanet.org/content/guidelines-and-quality-care/clinical-guidelines.cfm?sub=bph. Accessed August 3, 2012.

Peripheral α-blockers and 5α-reductase inhibitors (5-ARIs) are the two most common drugs used for BPH, either alone or in combination. α-Blockers, effective in 70% of patients, have more immediate clinical effect, whereas 5-ARIs may lead to clinical shrinkage of the enlarged prostate gland. Coexisting overactive bladder symptoms can be treated with combination α-blocker and anticholinergic therapy (tolterodine, oxybutynin). Anticholinergic drugs should be avoided in those with post-void residual volumes greater than 250 mL.

When BPH coexists with BOO symptoms, combination α-blocker and 5-ARI therapy has shown the highest efficacy compared with other treatments when the prostate is enlarged. Data from two trials indicate that combination therapy may be better in the short term than treatment with either drug individually, although 5-year outcomes remain similar. Although commonly used by patients, complementary or alternative medications, such as saw palmetto, have not been found to have benefit in recent clinical trials.

The PDE-5 inhibitor tadalafil has been FDA-approved for treatment of lower urinary tract symptoms in BPH. No long-term studies have compared outcomes with tadalafil to those with α-blockers or 5-ARIs.

Indications for surgical interventions in patients with BPH include refractory lower urinary tract symptoms, recurrent urinary retention with or without urinary tract infection, bladder stones, and kidney failure with hydronephrosis. Open prostatectomy is indicated for a severely enlarged prostate; however, those with less severe enlargement may benefit from less invasive techniques. Transurethral resection of the prostate (TURP) has been the usual surgery of choice, with studies showing symptom improvement in 70% of men and average time to recurrent treatment of 3 years. Although long-term results from trials of minimally invasive surgical interventions, such as transurethral needle ablation (TUNA) and transurethral microwave thermotherapy (TUMT) show good initial results, the time to recurrent intervention is shorter, and the choice of procedure should balance the risk of recurrence with the decreased invasiveness and fewer side effects associated with these procedures. Studies are not sufficient to recommend any particular intervention.

KEY POINT

- Overactive bladder symptoms related to benign prostatic hyperplasia include nocturia and urinary frequency and urgency; bladder outlet obstruction symptoms include decreased urinary stream, urinary retention, incomplete bladder emptying, and incontinence.

Acute Testicular and Scrotal Pain

Diagnosis of acute scrotal pain can often be made on the basis of history and physical examination. The main sources of such symptoms are testicular torsion and epididymitis. Orchitis is painful inflammation of the testicle itself and can be virally

CONT.

induced (mumps) or an extension of bacterial infections of the urinary tract or epididymis. Other causes of scrotal pain may include referred pain from abdominal aneurysm, inguinal hernia with strangulation of bowel or omentum, nephrolithiasis, lumbosacral nerve impingement, and retroperitoneal inflammation.

The patient should be asked about the onset (sudden or gradual), quality and severity of pain, history of trauma, and recent sexual activity, as well as lower urinary tract symptoms such as urinary frequency, urgency, and dysuria. Physical examination should include inspection and palpation and transillumination of the testes. The cremasteric reflex (obtained by stroking the upper inner thigh and observing a rise in the ipsilateral testicle) is absent in most patients with testicular torsion. Urinalysis is indicated in the evaluation of acute scrotal pain to assess for infection. Doppler ultrasonography to assess blood flow can be a useful adjunct aiding in diagnosis and in one study was 82% sensitive and 100% specific for torsion.

Testicular Torsion

Testicular torsion constitutes an emergency and occurs when the testes twist on the spermatic cord, leading to decreased blood flow and ischemia. It is more common in children and in men younger than 30 years. Pain is usually sudden in onset and often accompanied by nausea and vomiting. Physical examination often reveals an elevated, high-riding testis with longitudinal access abnormally oriented transversely. Considerable edema may be present. Elevation of the testis hurts more in torsion, whereas epididymal pain may be relieved by this maneuver. Treatment of torsion includes rapid surgical decompression to resume blood flow. In the absence of rapid access to surgery, manual decompression may be attempted.

Epididymitis

Infection or inflammation of the epididymis often causes pain localized to the superior and posterior aspect of the testicle. The onset may be acute, subacute, or chronic, and pain may occur more gradually compared with torsion. Pain may be accompanied by lower urinary tract symptoms of dysuria, urgency, or frequency. Epididymitis may be infectious or noninfectious, with infectious epididymitis more likely to be acute. Patients with acute infectious epididymitis may be quite sick, with high fevers and leukocytosis. There may be concomitant prostatitis. Subacute presentations are more common and may not be accompanied by lower urinary tract symptoms.

Risk factors for epididymitis include recent sexual activity, heavy exertion, and bicycle riding. Distribution is bimodal, with occurrences highest in those younger than 35 years and older than 55 years. In younger patients, sexually transmitted diseases such as chlamydial infection and gonorrhea are the most likely causes (see MKSAP 16 Infectious

Disease). Older men and men who practice anal intercourse are more susceptible to *Escherichia coli*, Enterobacteriaceae, and pseudomonal infection and should be treated with ceftriaxone and a fluoroquinolone. A 21-day course of a fluoroquinolone antibiotic is appropriate for most other causes of infectious epididymitis.

Noninfectious epididymitis is caused by reflux of urine into the epididymis, which causes inflammation. Treatment is conservative, with scrotal support, application of ice, and NSAIDs.

KEY POINTS

- Urinalysis is indicated in the evaluation of acute scrotal pain to assess for infection.
- Testicular torsion, characterized by sudden pain and an elevated, high-riding, abnormally oriented testis, is a surgical emergency.

Hydrocele and Varicocele

One percent of adult males have a hydrocele, which is a fluid collection between the layers of the tunica vaginalis. A communicating hydrocele occurs when a patent processus vaginalis allows fluid to pass from the peritoneal space into the scrotum, whereas a simple hydrocele has no such connection. Hydroceles vary in size and often develop gradually. Although most are asymptomatic, larger hydroceles can become painful. Physical examination usually reveals a tense, smooth, scrotal mass that is easily transilluminated. Transillumination can help distinguish a hydrocele from a hernia, varicocele, or solid mass. If a question remains, ultrasonography is the preferred modality for evaluation.

In adults, hydroceles that are small and do not bother the patient do not require intervention. Large or painful hydroceles can be treated either surgically or with aspiration and sclerotherapy. Communicating hydroceles usually require correction.

Epididymal Cyst

Epididymal cysts are often palpated at the head of the epididymis. Cysts larger than 2 cm are considered spermatoceles. Cysts can be palpated separately from the testis and usually are not painful. Ultrasonography is the study of choice for definitive diagnosis. Surgical repair is recommended only in rare cases of chronic pain related to the cyst.

Varicocele

A varicocele is a dilation of the testicular vein and pampiniform plexus within the scrotum; 90% occur on the left side. Varicoceles are one of the most commonly identified scrotal abnormalities, found in 15% of adult men and in 40% of men with infertility. The classic description is a scrotal mass on the left side with a "bag of worms" consistency that increases in size with standing and decreases while supine. Varicoceles are often painless and discovered during adolescence by self-examination. Ultrasonography is the test of choice if the diagnosis is in question.

Varicoceles are a leading cause of infertility. Repair may be warranted in men with abnormal sperm counts who desire children, although a Cochrane review did not confirm increased fertility with repair. Conservative care is adequate for men who do not desire children and are otherwise asymptomatic.

Surgical repair techniques include open inguinal varicocelectomy, laparoscopic varicocelectomy, and subinguinal microscopic varicocelectomy. All of these techniques are effective at reversing abnormal sperm parameters but not necessarily fertility. Sclerotherapy is a less invasive option that is associated with fewer complications but may be less effective in reducing symptoms.

KEY POINT

- In adult men, asymptomatic hydroceles and varicoceles can usually be diagnosed clinically and generally do not require advanced imaging or treatment.

Acute and Chronic Prostatitis and Pelvic Pain

Acute and chronic prostatitis and pelvic pain are common, with up to 2 million physician visits annually attributed to these syndromes. Symptoms fall into two categories: pain symptoms, which may include the perineum, testes, penis, or suprapubic area; and urinary symptoms, including dysuria, urinary frequency, and incomplete bladder emptying. The NIH's Chronic Prostatitis Symptom Index can aid in diagnosis and can be used to follow symptoms objectively over time (www.prostate.net/wp-content/uploads/pdf/chronic-prostatitis-symptom-test.pdf).

The diagnosis of chronic prostatitis and pelvic pain is one of clinical exclusion. Examination should rule out active urethritis, urethral stricture, testicular sources of pain, rectal masses, hemorrhoids, and neurologic diseases of the bladder. Urinalysis and urine culture should be performed, although the results are usually negative. Leukocytes may be found in post–prostatic massage urine, expressed prostatic secretions, or semen, but the presence of leukocytes is not correlated with treatment response.

A four-stage classification system was developed by the NIH to describe prostate syndromes (**Table 38**). Patients with acute bacterial prostatitis (class I) present with fever and urinary symptoms and often have an exquisitely tender prostate gland upon digital rectal examination. These infections generally respond well to standard antibiotic treatment (fluoroquinolones, trimethoprim-sulfamethoxazole). Chronic bacterial prostatitis (class II) presents with pain and urinary symptoms with recurrent bacterial infection; an extended course (1 month) of a fluoroquinolone is typically the first-line treatment.

Treatment of class III syndromes, which present with pain or LUTS, is difficult and often refractory to intervention. α-Blockers may help control urinary symptoms but have less of an effect on pain. Antibiotics are often used in the treatment of inflammatory chronic pelvic pain syndrome (CPPS) despite studies that fail to show long-term efficacy. For inflammatory CPPS, AUA guidelines recommend one course of antibiotics but not recurrent courses if the first is ineffective. NSAIDs have also been recommended based on a trial of rofecoxib, which provided some reduction in symptoms.

Other agents that have been studied for the treatment of CPPS include muscle relaxants and finasteride. Agents used in the treatment of neuropathic pain, such as gabapentin, have been recommended when primary therapies are ineffective. Complementary therapies that may be helpful in some patients include cernilton, a pollen extract; quercetin, a natural bioflavonoid; and saw palmetto extract, but the efficacy of these agents has not been determined. Surgical interventions for CPPS should be avoided unless there is a structural cause for symptoms, such as urethral stricture or BOO.

TABLE 38. Classification of Prostatitis	
Category	**Definition**
I. Acute bacterial prostatitis	Acute infection of the prostate
II. Chronic bacterial prostatitis	Recurrent infection of the prostate
III. Chronic abacterial prostatitis/chronic pelvic pain syndrome (CPPS)	No demonstrable infection
IIIA. Inflammatory CPPS	Leukocytes in semen, expressed prostatic secretions, or post-prostatic massage urine
IIIB. Noninflammatory CPPS	No leukocytes in semen, expressed prostatic secretions, or post-prostatic massage urine
IV. Asymptomatic inflammatory prostatitis	No symptoms; detected either by prostate biopsy, or the presence of leukocytes in semen samples during evaluation for other disorders

Adapted from Litwin MS, McNaughton-Collins M, Fowler FJ Jr., et al. The National Institutes of Health chronic prostatitis symptom index: development and validation of a new outcome measure. Chronic Prostatitis Collaborative Research Network. J Urol. 1999;162(2)369–375. [PMID: 10411041] with permission from American Urological Association. Copyright 1999, American Urological Association.

- Acute (class I) and chronic bacterial (class II) prostatitis are treated with antibiotic therapy.
- Chronic prostatitis/pelvic pain syndromes (class III) are often refractory to intervention; treatment options include α-blockers, a single course of antibiotics, and NSAIDs.

Hernia

A hernia occurs when an organ bulges through an area of weakness in muscle or connective tissue. They most commonly occur in the groin, and the incidence is higher in men than women. Hernias also may occur in the abdomen (ventral and umbilical) and at incision sites. Hernias may be caused by acquired or congenital weakness of connective or muscle tissue and by increased intra-abdominal pressure owing to straining, heavy lifting, or cough.

There are two types of inguinal hernia, direct and indirect. Direct inguinal hernias occur when intra-abdominal contents herniate through a weak spot in the fascia between the rectus abdominis and the inguinal ligament. Indirect inguinal hernias occur when intra-abdominal contents protrude through the internal inguinal ring. The less common femoral hernia occurs when intra-abdominal contents protrude through the femoral canal. The vast majority of inguinal hernias are indirect.

Clinical presentations of inguinal hernias can vary from an asymptomatic bulge, to a feeling of groin or abdominal pressure, to severe pain owing to movement of abdominal contents into the inguinal canal and occasionally into the scrotum. Hernias may be complicated by incarceration or strangulation, which can also lead to bowel obstruction. Direct hernias tend to present with a low abdominal bulge and cause less pain and less frequently develop incarceration, whereas femoral hernias more commonly develop these complications.

Diagnosis is made by physical observation and digital examination of the inguinal canal, with a bulge that is often visible or palpable and is usually more prominent upon standing.

Asymptomatic inguinal hernias may be monitored, whereas symptomatic hernias may require surgical repair. There is evidence that watchful waiting in asymptomatic patients may be acceptable, but patients should be warned of potential complications, such as incarceration and strangulation. The optimal type of surgery (laparoscopic versus open surgical repair) remains controversial, although reviews indicate lower recurrence rates when polypropylene mesh is used. Potential complications of repair include early recurrence, infection, seroma, hematoma, chronic neuropathic pain, and late recurrence.

- Asymptomatic inguinal hernias may be monitored; symptomatic hernias require surgical repair.

Women's Health

Female Sexual Dysfunction

Approach to the Patient

Female sexual dysfunction, defined as sexual difficulties that are persistent and personally distressing to the patient, affects up to 35% of sexually active women, peaking in middle-age. Because women are often uncomfortable initiating discussions about sexual problems, it is incumbent upon the practitioner to routinely ask about sexual function, even during brief office visits. Asking if a patient is sexually active and if there are any related problems, including pain with intercourse, is appropriate. For individuals with potential issues, a complete sexual history should be obtained, including a thorough review of medical problems, psychiatric disorders, and reproductive surgeries that can contribute to sexual dysfunction. Patients should be queried about the use of medications that may interfere with sexual function. **Table 39** lists additional questions that aid in identifying problems with desire, arousal, orgasm, or pain, which may help in determining cause and potential treatment strategies. A pelvic examination is important and may be helpful in identifying specific areas of pain, vaginal atrophy, inadequate lubrication, and vaginismus. Laboratory testing is recommended only if there is suspicion for a particular diagnosis, such as a prolactinoma, thyroid abnormalities, or adrenal disease.

Classification of Female Sexual Disorders

The DSM-IV identifies six disorders that correspond to abnormalities in the female sexual response cycle: hypoactive

TABLE 39. Essential Questions to Include in an Assessment for Female Sexual Dysfunction
How does the patient describe the problem?
How long has the problem been present?
Was the onset sudden or gradual?
Is the problem specific to a situation/partner or is it generalized?
Were there likely precipitating events (biologic or situational)?
Are there any problems in the woman's primary sexual relationship (or any relationship in which the sexual problem is occurring)?
Are there current life stressors that might be contributing to sexual problems?
Is there guilt, depression, or anger that is not being directly acknowledged?
Are there physical problems such as pain?
Are there problems in desire, arousal, or orgasm?
Is there a history of physical, emotional, or sexual abuse?
Does the partner have any sexual problems?

With kind permission from Springer Science+Business Media: Int Urogynecol J Pelvic Floor Dysfunct, Evaluation and treatment of female sexual disorders, 2009;20 Suppl 1:S33-S43, Kingsberg S, Althof SE. [PMID: 19440781] Copyright 2009, Springer Science+Business Media.

sexual desire disorder and sexual aversion disorder (sexual desire disorders), sexual arousal disorder, orgasmic disorder, and dyspareunia and vaginismus (sexual pain disorders).

The Female Sexual Function Index (www.fsfi-questionnaire.com) is a validated 19-item, patient-completed questionnaire that assesses each of these areas of sexual functioning and can be used as an adjunct in the clinical assessment. Women who score less than 26 are considered to be at risk for sexual dysfunction.

Sexual Desire Disorders

Hypoactive sexual desire disorder (HSDD) is diagnosed if a woman reports a persistent lack of sexual thoughts or desire for or receptiveness to sexual activity. HSDD is the most common female sexual disorder, affecting 12% to 19% of U.S. women. Desire encompasses three separate components—drive, cognition, and motivation. Drive, perceived as spontaneous sexual interest, is biological and is based on neuroendocrine functions. Cognition refers to the belief and value framework that a patient has regarding sex. Motivation is the willingness to engage in sexual activity and may be influenced by the quality of the relationship and several psychosocial factors.

Testosterone is essential for normal sex drive and may also play a role in sexual motivation. Levels of testosterone decline progressively with age in women; however, measured testosterone levels have not been shown to correlate meaningfully with sexual functioning. Despite this, treatment with testosterone has been shown to increase sexual function scores and the number of satisfying sexual episodes but is associated with adverse effects, including excess hair growth and acne, and altered lipoprotein levels with oral therapy. In 2006, the Endocrine Society acknowledged the short-term efficacy of testosterone therapy for the treatment of sexual dysfunction in women but recommended against generalized use because of the lack of long-term safety data. The low estradiol levels that characterize surgical and natural menopause may also be linked to lack of desire and sexual responsiveness. Although study results are inconsistent, systemic estrogen or estrogen-progesterone therapy (EPT) may increase sexual desire, enjoyment, and orgasmic frequency.

To date, the FDA has not approved any medication for the treatment of female HSDD. Individual and couples sex therapy or psychotherapy may be beneficial.

Sexual aversion disorder is defined as a persistent or recurrent aversion to any genital contact with a sexual partner. Women with sexual aversion usually experience feelings of abhorrence and revulsion; panic may accompany specific sexual situations. Avoidance of sexual behavior typically reinforces the aversion, so treatment often involves graduated reintroduction of sexual behavior and relaxation exercises, which may be augmented by therapy with a selective serotonin reuptake inhibitor.

Orgasmic Disorder

Female orgasmic disorder is the persistent or recurrent delay or absence of orgasm following a normal excitement phase. Cognitive-behavioral therapy is most effective for teaching a woman to be comfortable, minimizing negative attitudes, and decreasing anxiety.

Sexual Arousal Disorder

Female sexual arousal disorder is the inability to complete sexual activity with adequate lubrication and absent or impaired genital responsiveness to sexual stimulation. Cognitive-behavioral therapy with sensate focus and training to improve partner communication are effective strategies. Systemic or local estrogen therapy can increase lubrication in postmenopausal women; in premenopausal women, vaginal moisturizers can be helpful.

Sexual Pain Disorders

Dyspareunia is persistent urogenital pain that occurs around intercourse and is not related exclusively to inadequate lubrication or vaginismus. Therapy is aimed at identifying and treating the underlying cause, which may include vulvodynia, interstitial cystitis, pelvic adhesions, infections, endometriosis, and pelvic venous congestion. Coexisting vaginal atrophy and inadequate lubrication may worsen the pain syndrome and usually can be diagnosed on physical examination. Vaginal estrogen frequently improves atrophy, whereas systemic estrogen or estrogen-progesterone therapy can increase vaginal blood flow and lubrication. Successful treatment strategies must address the complex psychological and behavioral changes that accompany this syndrome, as well as the desire and arousal disorders that often develop as a result of the painful sexual experience.

Vaginismus is the involuntary, recurrent, and persistent spasm of the outer third of the vagina, preventing desired vaginal penetration. Episodes may be situation-specific, for example, pelvic examinations or intercourse. The anticipation of pain with vaginal entry underpins this diagnosis and may result in sexual avoidance. Treatment involves cognitive-behavioral therapy to help the patient feel safe, calm, and in control of the encounter, thereby reducing her anticipatory response. Systematic desensitization teaches deep muscle relaxation and uses objects of increasing diameter, such as dilators, to achieve gradual vaginal tolerance.

KEY POINT

- Laboratory testing is recommended in the evaluation of female sexual dysfunction only if there is suspicion for a particular diagnosis.

Evaluation of a Breast Mass

Breast symptoms in women are common. In a retrospective study of 2400 primary care patients followed for 10 years, 16% of women ages 40 to 79 years presented with a "breast lump" or "lumpiness." Whether discovered by the patient or detected by a physician, a palpable breast mass requires a systematic and logical evaluation. The performance of a careful history and physical examination may lead to a likely diagnosis. However, in most cases, further testing (imaging, tissue sampling) is necessary.

Clinical Presentation

A breast mass or lump is a discrete, firm, three-dimensional abnormality that is different from the surrounding breast tissue. The differential diagnosis of a palpable breast mass is outlined in **Table 40**. The critical challenge in evaluating a breast mass is distinguishing benign from malignant disease. Risk factors for breast cancer should be determined (see MKSAP 16 Hematology and Oncology). History and physical examination features that favor a benign lesion include younger age, absence of breast cancer risk factors, normal overlying skin, a milky (vs. bloody) nipple discharge, change in size during menstrual cycles, and a mass that is round, mobile, and soft. Whereas pain is more likely to be associated with a benign lesion, the presence of pain does not rule out malignancy.

Although most breast masses (up to 90%) are benign cysts or fibroadenomas, neither the history nor the physical examination can definitively rule in or rule out underlying malignancy with sufficient accuracy. In a study of 201 referral patients with palpable solid breast masses, the sensitivity of the physical examination for the detection of breast cancer was 88%. The positive and negative predictive values for breast cancer were 73% and 87%, respectively. Therefore, a palpable breast mass requires further evaluation, including imaging and/or tissue sampling, for definitive diagnosis. Physicians should pursue all breast findings until resolution.

Evaluation

Mammography and ultrasonography are the best imaging modalities for evaluating a palpable breast mass. The choice of ultrasonography versus diagnostic mammography in evaluating a breast mass depends in part on the patient's age. The increased density of breast tissue in women younger than 30 to 35 years may limit the utility of mammography, making ultrasound a better first choice. Ultrasonography may also be a better choice in the pregnant patient as ultrasonography avoids potentially harmful radiation exposure. The main utility of ultrasonography is its ability to differentiate cystic from solid lesions. A simple cyst with symmetric round borders and no internal echoes that, with aspiration, drains nonbloody fluid and disappears completely, is likely to be benign. If bloody fluid is obtained from cyst aspiration, it should be sent for cytology. A solid lesion with uniform borders and uniformly sized internal echoes is most likely a benign fibroadenoma. Fibroadenomas should be followed to assure that they spontaneously regress or decrease in size. Alternatively, depending on the preference of the patient, they can be surgically removed.

TABLE 40. Differential Diagnosis of Breast Mass
Cysts
Simple
Complex
Infection
Abscess
Mastitis
Tuberculosis
Trauma
Fat necrosis
Hematoma
Benign tumors
Fibroadenoma
Hamartoma
Papilloma
Phyllodes tumor (benign variant)
Lipoma
Adenoma (tubular or lactating)
Granular cell tumor
Neurofibroma
Hemangioma
Malignant tumors
Ductal carcinoma in situ
Invasive ductal or lobular carcinoma
Phyllodes tumor (malignant variant)
Squamous cell carcinoma
Sarcoma
Angiosarcoma
Leukemia
Lymphoma
Other
Diabetic mastopathy
Sarcoidosis
Granulomatosis with polyangiitis (also known as Wegener granulomatosis)
Idiopathic granulomatous mastitis
Gynecomastia (in men)

Reproduced with permission from Ganschow PS, et al. Breast Health and Common Breast Problems. American College of Physicians. Philadelphia, PA. 2004:159. Copyright 2004, American College of Physicians.

In women older than 30 to 35 years, the test of choice is diagnostic mammography. An irregular mass with microcalcifications and spiculations is suspicious for malignant disease, and biopsy is mandatory in these cases (see below).

Approximately 10% to 20% of palpable breast cancers are undetected by ultrasonography or mammography. Therefore, the evaluation of a palpable breast mass suspicious for malignancy should continue with biopsy even if the mammogram or ultrasound is unrevealing.

After palpation and imaging, definitive diagnosis is obtained through tissue sampling. Tissue sampling procedures include fine needle aspiration, core needle biopsy with or without stereotactic or ultrasound guidance, or excisional biopsy. Fine needle aspiration, generally reserved for cystic lesions, is operator-dependent and requires an experienced cytopathologist for interpretation. Core needle biopsy, although more costly and with a greater risk for postprocedure hematoma, provides better tissue sampling for pathologic examination and hormone receptor status (if positive for cancer) and can distinguish in situ versus invasive cancer. Core needle biopsy is the test of choice for most solid lesions. Excisional biopsy is used when core needle biopsy is nondiagnostic or when biopsy and imaging studies are not in agreement. Further management of abnormal pathology requires consultation with a breast surgeon and oncologist.

KEY POINT

- When imaging a palpable breast mass, ultrasonography is preferred for pregnant women or women younger than 30 to 35 years; mammography is preferred for women older than 30 to 35 years.

Breast Pain

Clinical Presentation

Breast pain may be characterized as cyclical, noncyclical, or extramammary. Although most women experience mild breast discomfort with the onset of menses, cyclical mastalgia typically lasts for several days and is moderate to severe in intensity. Noncyclical mastalgia has no relationship to the menstrual cycle and may be caused by pregnancy, medications (nicotine, hormone therapy), stretching of Cooper ligaments (secondary to large breasts), or cancer. Extramammary breast pain may be caused by musculoskeletal, cardiac, gastrointestinal, or spinal disorders. Chest wall inflammation, a common cause of extramammary pain, typically presents with unilateral, localized, burning discomfort.

Evaluation

Breast cancer may be associated with mastalgia; therefore, a thorough physical examination is essential in all women presenting with breast pain. Women with a palpable breast mass should be referred for diagnostic imaging. Chest wall pain is typically reproduced by palpation or by examination maneuvers that place stress on the inflamed musculoskeletal structures. All women who are evaluated for mastalgia should be up to date on routine mammographic screening, according to age and personal risk factors for breast cancer.

Treatment

Women with cyclical mastalgia benefit from education and reassurance, as most will experience spontaneous resolution of their symptoms. Medical treatment may be considered for women with severe and persistent pain that interferes with quality of life. Danazol (100 mg twice daily) is the only therapy that has been FDA-approved for the treatment of cyclical mastalgia, but side effects, including menorrhagia and weight gain, often limit its use. Patients with cyclical mastalgia experience benefit with tamoxifen (10 mg/d), and treatment-associated hot flushes and menstrual irregularities are relatively infrequent.

Contraception

Nearly half of pregnancies in the United States are unintended. Adherence to contraception may be improved by counseling patients at risk for unintended pregnancy regarding appropriate contraceptive options, especially patients with serious medical conditions in whom the risk of adverse events of unintended pregnancy is high. Contraceptive options are compared in **Table 41**.

Oral Contraceptive Pills

Oral contraceptive pills (OCPs) include combination estrogen-progesterone products and progesterone-only pills. Differences in combination preparations lie in the type and strength of estrogen and in the androgenicity of their progesterone component. Combinations with lower estrogen dose are as effective with fewer side effects. The mechanisms of action of combination pills include inhibition of ovulation, alteration of the cervical mucus to an environment less conducive to sperm migration, and inhibition of endometrial proliferation. Most hormonal methods are highly effective; annual failure rates are 0.3% with "perfect" use, 8% with typical use. Combined products are also available as a patch and a vaginal ring. Contraindications to combination products include history of thrombosis, liver disease, breast cancer, migraine with aura, and uncontrolled hypertension. Women older than 35 years who smoke more than 15 cigarettes a day should not be prescribed estrogen-containing preparations. Progesterone-only pills, also called the "mini-pill," may be used by women with contraindications to estrogen.

Medications that induce the CYP3A class of liver enzymes may reduce the effectiveness of hormonal contraceptives. Common drugs with this effect include barbiturates, carbamazepine, many antiseizure medications, rifampin, and certain antiretroviral agents. In addition, some antibiotics and some other neurologic medications may alter efficacy of combination preparations via other mechanisms. Additional contraception or barrier methods should be used concurrently and for 4 weeks after discontinuing such drugs.

TABLE 41.	Comparison of Contraceptive Options		
Agent	**Failure Rate[a] (perfect use/ typical use[b])**	**Advantages**	**Disadvantages**
Combination estrogen-progesterone preparations		Decreased incidence of endometrial, ovarian cancers	Increased risk of myocardial infarction, ischemic stroke, VTE, hypertension
		Decreased dysmenorrhea, menorrhagia, symptomatic ovarian cysts	Increased risk of cancers of the cervix, liver, breast
		Less iron-deficiency anemia	Breakthrough bleeding.
Oral	0.3/8		May worsen acne, exacerbate migraine
Patch	0.3/8	Easier compliance	Local skin reaction
			Increased estrogen dose, thus higher VTE risk
Vaginal ring	0.3/8	Easier compliance	Requires self-insertion
		Lowest level of systemic estrogen	
Progesterone-only preparations		Use when estrogen is contraindicated	May worsen acne
Mini-pill			Must maintain precise daily dosing schedule
Long-acting preparations			Irregular bleeding, amenorrhea, decreased bone mineral density (especially in adolescents)
Depot medroxyprogesterone acetate (IM or SQ)	0.3/8	Administered every 3 months	Delayed return to ovulation (10 months)
		Decreased risk of endometrial cancer, PID	
		Improves endometriosis	
Progesterone implants	0.8-1/—	Effective up to 3 years	Delayed return to ovulation (6 months)
Intrauterine devices		Least dependence on user	Bleeding, pain, expulsion (rare); no protection from STIs
Copper	0.6/0.8	Nonhormonal	
		Effective up to 10 years	
Levonorgestrel	0.1/0.1	Decreased blood loss, decreased anemia	
		Effective up to 5 years	
Barrier methods		Only use when needed	Most user-dependent
Cervical cap	9-26/16-32		Requires spermicide
Diaphragm	6/16		Requires spermicide
Male condom	2/15	Protection from STIs	
Female condom	5/21	Protection from STIs	
Vaginal sponge	6-9/16-32		
Sterilization			
Female (tubal ligation)	2% in 10 years	May reduce ovarian cancer risk	Surgical complications
			Regret
			Increased risk of ectopic if pregnancy occurs
Male (vasectomy)	<1% in 10 years	Lower costs, fewer complications, and more effective than tubal ligation	Surgical complications

PID = pelvic inflammatory disease; SQ = subcutaneous; STI = sexually transmitted infection; VTE = venous thromboembolism.

[a]Per 100 women/year.

[b]Perfect use implies correct and consistent use exactly as directed/intended. Typical use reflects rates in actual practice with patients.

Long-Acting Contraceptives

Long-acting progesterone compounds include depot medroxyprogesterone acetate (DMPA) injections, subcutaneous progesterone implants, and progesterone-containing intrauterine devices (IUDs). DMPA may be administered either intramuscularly or subcutaneously following a negative pregnancy test. Etonogestrel implants are small rods inserted subdermally in the upper inner arm and are effective for 3 years. These long-acting progesterone methods are less reliant on user compliance, and therefore may be particularly effective in patients who may have difficulty with daily treatment or barrier methods. They are not recommended for women desiring pregnancy in the subsequent 2 years after cessation of treatment because of potential contraceptive-associated delayed fertility.

Intrauterine Devices

IUDs are the most commonly used form of reversible contraception worldwide. The copper IUD and the levonorgestrel-containing IUD may be placed at any time (except during pregnancy) in an office setting without need for anesthesia. IUDs combine the highest efficacy (typical failure rate <1%) with the lowest cost. The copper IUD may be implanted within 7 days of unprotected intercourse for use as emergency contraception.

Barrier Methods

Barrier methods (see Table 41) allow for "as-needed" contraception but are much less reliable than hormonal methods. All barrier methods are more effective when used with spermicides; spermicides alone are not considered reliable. All barrier methods reduce risk of sexually transmitted infection (STI); evidence is strongest for prevention of HIV infection with male condoms. Limited evidence suggests barrier methods protect future fertility, perhaps by reducing STIs. Combining a barrier method with a hormonal method is recommended when pregnancy must be avoided (for example, during use of teratogenic agents) and in adolescents, in whom risk of both unintended pregnancy and STI is very high.

Emergency Contraception

Emergency contraception refers to contraception administered after intercourse but before implantation. Efficacy for all products increases the earlier they are used. Four methods are available in the United States: levonorgestrel tablets, combined contraceptive tablets, the copper IUD, and progesterone modulators.

The levonorgestrel-only, single-dose (1.5 mg) regimen is the most widely used and most effective option, and is available over-the-counter (by prescription for adolescents younger than 17 years). Other options include two-dose levonorgestrel (0.75 mg taken 12 hours apart), or two tablets of a high-dose combination OCP (100 micrograms ethinyl estradiol, taken twice, 12 hours apart). Levonorgestrel has greater efficacy and fewer side effects (nausea, vomiting, dizziness, headache). If vomiting occurs within 2 hours of taking emergency contraception, the dose should be repeated, given vaginally, or given after an antiemetic has been used. These methods work by delaying or preventing ovulation, and are not abortifacients. They may be taken up to 5 days (120 hours) post-intercourse. The copper IUD is inserted up to 5 days after intercourse. It functions primarily by stopping fertilization and interfering with implantation. It may remain in place as long-term contraception.

Mifepristone, a progesterone-receptor modulator, is approved by the FDA as an abortifacient, but has been used outside the United States as emergency contraception. Ulipristal, another progesterone-receptor modulator with agonist and antagonist effects, has been approved for use as emergency contraception in the United States.

Sterilization

Sterilization is highly effective, with an annual failure rate of 1 in 1000. Female sterilization (tubal ligation) incurs more risk and cost than vasectomy and is less effective. Incidence of regret and requests for reversal of tubal ligation are significantly higher in women younger than 30 years and in those who are postpartum or postabortion at the time of the procedure.

KEY POINTS

- Women older than 35 years who smoke more than 15 cigarettes a day should not be prescribed estrogen-containing contraceptives.
- Intrauterine devices are highly effective at preventing pregnancy and are low cost.

Preconception Counseling

Adequate preconception care can significantly reduce the risk for preterm birth and birth anomalies. Each health care visit with a reproductive-age woman represents an opportunity for preconception counseling; providers should routinely ask if a patient is either considering pregnancy or could possibly become pregnant. For patients considering pregnancy, preconception risk should be assessed (**Table 42**) and brief interventions undertaken to optimize reproductive health, including encouraging a healthy lifestyle; stressing the importance of tobacco, alcohol, and drug cessation; and referring underweight or overweight patients for formal nutritional evaluation. Prescription medications should be changed, if possible, to minimize exposure to potential teratogens (**Table 43**). Consultation with specialists for co-management of specific diseases in pregnancy, such as diabetes mellitus and epilepsy, may be indicated.

A physical examination and focused laboratory testing can provide additional information regarding a patient's reproductive health and preconception risk. Measurements of

TABLE 42. Preconception Risk Assessment

Risk Category	Specific Items to Assess
Reproductive awareness	Desire for pregnancy, number and timing of desired pregnancies, age-related changes in fertility, sexuality, contraception
Environmental hazards and toxins	Exposure to radiation, lead, mercury
Nutrition and folic acid consumption	Healthy diet, daily consumption of folic acid, restricting consumption of shark, swordfish, king mackerel, and tilefish to fewer than 2 servings weekly (owing to high mercury content)
Genetics	Family history of inherited genetic disorders
Substance abuse	Use of tobacco, alcohol, illicit drugs
Medical conditions	Seizure disorder, diabetes mellitus, hypertension, thyroid disease, asthma, HIV infection, systemic lupus erythematosus
Medications	Over-the-counter and prescription medications, potential teratogens
Infectious diseases and vaccinations	Immunity to varicella, rubella, pertussis, tetanus; risk for hepatitis B
Psychosocial concerns	Depression, interpersonal/family relationships, risk for abuse (physical, sexual, emotional)

Based on Johnson K, Posner SF, Biermann J, et al.; CDC/ATSDR Preconception Care Work Group; Select Panel on Preconception Care. Recommendations to improve preconception health and health care—United States. A report of the CDC/ATSDR Preconception Care Work Group and the Select Panel on Preconception Care. MMWR Recomm Rep. 2006;55(RR-6):1-23. [PMID: 16617292]

TABLE 43. Teratogenic Medications Commonly Prescribed by Internists

ACE inhibitors

Androgens, testosterone derivatives

Carbamazepine

Fluoxetine, paroxetine

Folic acid antagonists

Lithium

Phenytoin

Primidone

Statins

Tetracycline

Valproic acid

Vitamin A derivatives: isotretinoin, retinoids, etretinate

Warfarin

Adapted from Berghella V, Buchanan E, Pereira L, Baxter JK. Preconception Care. Obstet Gynecol Surv. 2010;65(2):119-131. [PMID: 20100361]

BMI and blood pressure are essential, and the pelvic examination may include collecting specimens for cervical cytology and chlamydial testing (if indicated per screening recommendations for these tests). All women who are considering pregnancy should be routinely assessed for immunity to varicella and rubella, and screening for HIV may be considered.

Certain interventions optimize pregnancy outcomes in all reproductive-age women, including appropriate vaccinations, daily folic acid, and proper diet and exercise. Vaccination for rubella and varicella to nonimmune women should be administered at least 4 weeks before conception to minimize risks to the fetus. Influenza vaccination is appropriate for those who will be pregnant during flu season, and pertussis vaccination,

in combination with tetanus and diphtheria, is recommended for all persons who have not been immunized as adults. Supplementation with folic acid (400 micrograms/d) reduces the risk of neural tube defects. Because these defects occur very early in gestation, when a woman might not even know she is pregnant, folic acid supplementation is generally recommended for all women who are of reproductive age. Higher doses of folic acid may be appropriate in women who have prior children with a neural tube defect, take antiseizure medications, or who are obese.

KEY POINT

- Preconception counseling should include risk assessment in the following areas: reproductive awareness, environmental hazards and toxins, nutrition and folic acid supplementation, genetics, substance abuse, medical conditions, medications, infectious diseases and vaccinations, and psychosocial concerns.

Menopause

Overview

Menopause is defined as the permanent cessation of menses and is diagnosed retrospectively, after a woman has experienced amenorrhea for 12 months. Menopause occurs through a series of stages characterized according to variations in the menstrual cycle and alterations in follicle-stimulating hormone (FSH) levels. Women typically begin to experience irregular menses in early perimenopause, with cycles of variable length, and then progress into late perimenopause, with intervals of amenorrhea lasting more than 60 days and two or more skipped cycles. FSH levels begin to rise in this perimenopausal transition but may fluctuate significantly depending on the frequency of anovulation. After 1 year of amenorrhea (menopause), a woman is considered to be early postmenopausal, and FSH levels become very elevated (FSH >40 units/L, estradiol <20 ng/mL). Late postmenopause starts 5 years after the last menstrual period. On average, women in the United States experience menopause at the age of 51 years.

The hallmark symptoms of the menopausal transition are hot flushes and night sweats (vasomotor symptoms) and vaginal dryness and dyspareunia (urogenital symptoms). A hot flush is characterized by the sudden onset of intense warmth that starts in the face or chest and then spreads throughout the body; it is usually associated with sweating and palpitations. Night sweats are hot flushes that occur during sleep and often result in nocturnal awakenings. Up to 50% of women experience hot flushes during the menopausal transition, but symptoms typically resolve spontaneously within a few years of onset. Conversely, vaginal dryness and dyspareunia, which result from progressive estrogen depletion and subsequent urogenital atrophy, become much more prevalent in late postmenopause. Mood changes, cognitive difficulties, and primary sleep disorders may be more common in menopausal women, but these symptoms have not been definitely linked to changes in hormone levels. The differential diagnosis of menopausal symptoms includes thyroid disease, elevated prolactin levels, and pregnancy, and testing for these conditions may be considered in selected patients.

Management of Vasomotor Symptoms

Women should be reassured that hot flushes and night sweats are common in the menopausal transition and that spontaneous resolution typically occurs within a few years. As smoking, obesity, and sedentary lifestyle are all risk factors associated with hot flushes, behavioral changes may result in symptom improvement.

Systemic Hormone Therapy

Systemic hormone therapy is the most effective treatment for moderate to severe vasomotor symptoms, and has FDA approval for this indication. It may be considered as a treatment option for women who have a thorough understanding of the risks and benefits associated with therapy. Several formulations of estrogen are currently available and include conjugated equine estrogen, micronized 17 β-estradiol, and transdermal 17 β-estradiol. Most experts recommend starting with the lowest dose of estrogen that effectively relieves symptoms and titrating up as necessary to achieve maximal relief. Although supporting data are limited, transdermal estrogen, as compared with oral estrogen, may be associated with less thromboembolic risk as it avoids the hepatic first-pass effect. Moreover, transdermal and oral estrogen seem to be equally effective for treating vasomotor symptoms. Common adverse effects of systemic estrogen therapy are breast tenderness and uterine bleeding.

All women with an intact uterus who are treated with hormone therapy must receive progesterone to avoid estrogen-induced endometrial hyperplasia and cancer. Several preparations are available and may be given continuously or cyclically. Women treated with cyclic progesterone may have occasional withdrawal bleeding and should be counseled regarding this effect. Absolute contraindications to hormone therapy include pregnancy; unexplained vaginal bleeding; a history of coronary artery disease, stroke, thromboembolic disease, or breast or endometrial cancer; hypertriglyceridemia; recent vascular thrombosis or cardiovascular event; and immobilization.

Table 44 lists a stepwise approach for initiating hormone therapy in women aged 50-59 years who have experienced menopause at the median age (51 years). In general, women should be treated with the lowest possible dose of estrogen for the shortest amount of time necessary; treatment for longer than 5 years is not advised. Systemic hormone therapy can be discontinued abruptly or tapered gradually; there is no difference in the rates of vasomotor symptom recurrence. The North American Menopause Society (NAMS) suggests that bone density be measured if hormone therapy is discontinued after several years of treatment.

Benefits and Risks of Systemic Hormone Therapy

The Women's Health Initiative (WHI) demonstrated that combination estrogen and progesterone therapy (EPT) decreased the risk of osteoporotic fractures and colorectal cancer but increased the risk of coronary heart disease (CHD), venous thromboembolism, invasive breast cancer, and stroke. In contrast, estrogen-only therapy increased the risk for stroke, but no other outcomes. Notably, the absolute benefits and risks associated with treatment were quite small; among 10,000 women treated with EPT, there were five fewer hip fractures and eight additional strokes.

Additional analyses of data from the WHI suggest that while the overall risk of CHD in postmenopausal women on hormone therapy is increased, the greatest risk is in older women (ages 70-79 years) and is minimal in younger women (ages 50-59 years) treated earlier in menopause. This has led NAMS to recommend that hormone therapy not be used as primary prophylaxis for CHD among women at any age. Hormone therapy may be used to treat menopausal symptoms in women ages 50 to 59 years or those within 10 years of menopause as there is minimal CHD risk; hormone therapy should not be initiated in women older than 60 years.

In contrast to CHD risk, the increased risk of stroke observed with hormone therapy does not vary according to length of time since menopause onset. Notably, the risk of stroke with hormone therapy use among women aged 50 to 59 years did not differ significantly from that among women older than 60 years.

In a follow-up study of more than 12,000 women who participated in the WHI, investigators found that EPT, as

TABLE 44. Initiating Systemic Hormone Therapy in Women Ages 50-59 Years[a]

Step 1: Confirm that hot flushes/night sweats are moderate-severe in intensity and/or vaginal symptoms are moderate-severe in intensity and have been refractory to local therapies.

Step 2: Assess for absolute contraindications to systemic hormone therapy.

Step 3: Assess the patient's baseline risk for stroke, cardiovascular disease, and breast cancer (consider using the Framingham stroke risk score, Framingham CHD risk score, and Gail risk score to quantify this risk). If the Framingham stroke or CHD risk score is >10% or Gail risk score is elevated, consider avoiding systemic hormone therapy.[b,c]

Step 4: Use the lowest dose of estrogen that relieves menopausal symptoms.

Step 5: Add systemic progesterone therapy to estrogen therapy in women who have an intact uterus.

Step 6: Assess symptoms and side effects within 4-6 weeks of initiating therapy. Increase the dose of estrogen if symptoms are persistent.

Step 7: Reassess symptoms and risk factors for cardiovascular disease, stroke, and breast cancer regularly. Ideally, treatment with systemic hormone therapy should continue for no more than 5 years.

Step 8: Discontinue systemic hormone therapy if the risks of treatment outweigh the benefits, if symptoms resolve spontaneously, or according to patient preference. Therapy does not need to be tapered.

CHD = coronary heart disease.

[a]According to North American Menopause Society, systemic hormone therapy should be avoided in women older than 60 years who have experienced menopause at the median age (51 years). If a woman has experienced menopause later than the median age, these guidelines apply within the first 10 years of menopause.

[b]Some authors indicate that systemic hormone therapy is safe in women who have experienced menopause within the last 5 years and have a Framingham CHD risk score of 10%-20%.

[c]The majority of participants in the Women's Health Initiative had a Gail risk score of less than 2%.

compared with placebo, increases the risk of node-positive invasive breast cancer and breast cancer mortality. The timing of hormone therapy initiation may be influential: exposure to EPT during the early postmenopause is associated with an increased incidence of breast cancer, whereas exposure during late postmenopause is not. The increased breast cancer risk associated with therapy (8 excess cases per 10,000 person years) becomes apparent after 3 to 5 years of exposure to hormone therapy. Moreover, EPT increases breast density and may impede the interpretation of mammograms. Post-hoc analysis of the WHI data suggests that EPT may promote lung cancer among older smokers, but these results need further validation.

The low absolute risk of adverse events supports the option to prescribe hormone therapy for women with moderate to severe vasomotor or urogenital symptoms who are at low risk for CHD, stroke, and invasive breast cancer.

Nonhormonal Therapy

Several nonhormonal therapies are available for women who have contraindications to hormone therapy or want to avoid its attendant risks. Certain antidepressants (selective serotonin reuptake inhibitors and serotonin-norepinephrine reuptake inhibitors), gabapentin, and clonidine may reduce hot flush frequency by one or two per day as compared with placebo. Red clover extract and black cohosh are ineffective for treating hot flushes, and study results suggest mixed benefits with soy isoflavone extracts.

Management of Urogenital Symptoms

Progressive estrogen depletion during the menopausal transition leads to thinning of the vaginal epithelium and vaginal atrophy. Clinically, women may report vaginal dryness, itching, dyspareunia, dysuria, and frequent urinary tract infections. Mild to moderate symptoms can be effectively treated with vaginal moisturizers, and lubrication may ease pain with intercourse. The FDA has approved the use of vaginal estrogen therapy for women who do not respond to these measures or who have moderate to severe urogenital symptoms. Several preparations are currently available and include conjugated estrogen vaginal cream, estradiol vaginal cream, vaginal estradiol tablets, and an estradiol vaginal ring. Although each of these treatments is equally effective in relieving symptoms, low-dose vaginal estradiol tablets (10-25 micrograms) and the estradiol vaginal ring (8-9 micrograms) are preferred over vaginal estrogen creams, as they result in minimal systemic estrogen absorption. According to the NAMS guidelines, progesterone therapy is typically not indicated when low-dose local estrogen therapy is used to treat vaginal atrophy.

KEY POINTS

- Women with vasomotor menopausal symptoms that warrant hormone therapy should be treated with the lowest possible dose of estrogen for the shortest amount of time necessary.

- To minimize cardiovascular risk, hormone therapy should not be initiated in women older than 60 years who have not previously received hormone therapy and who experienced menopause at the median age.

- Hormone therapy does not increase the risk for coronary heart disease among women aged 50-59 years who have experienced menopause at the median age.

Abnormal Uterine Bleeding

Clinical Presentation and Evaluation

Abnormal uterine bleeding refers to bleeding that is excessive in frequency, duration, or amount, and is often described by the pattern of occurrence and degree of flow. *Polymenorrhagia* is bleeding occurring more than once every 24 days, the lower limit of the average menstrual cycle. *Oligomenorrhea* is bleeding less frequently than every 35 days, although women are more likely to complain of too frequent than infrequent menses. *Metrorrhagia* is irregular or intermenstrual bleeding. *Menorrhagia* refers to regular cycles with excessive bleeding, defined as monthly menstrual loss of more than 80 mL or bleeding for more than 7 days. *Menometrorrhagia* is bleeding at irregular intervals with excessive flow.

Abnormal bleeding is usually characterized as ovulatory or anovulatory. Ovulatory bleeding is cyclical and may be caused by anatomic abnormalities (polyps, leiomyomas), bleeding disorders, medications that interfere with hemostasis, or uterine cancer. Anovulatory bleeding is usually unpredictable and of variable flow and duration owing to loss of cyclical hormonal influences on the endometrium; if no anatomic or medical cause is identified for bleeding, anovulatory bleeding may be referred to as dysfunctional uterine bleeding (DUB). Anovulatory cycles are characterized by estrogen-mediated endometrial proliferation without the stabilizing effects of progesterone, resulting in endometrial desquamation and erratic bleeding. Anovulation has many potential causes, but also commonly occurs in women without underlying medical or anatomic issues.

These terms apply only to women of reproductive age; in postmenopausal women (absence of menses for 1 year), any uterine bleeding is abnormal and warrants further evaluation, especially for endometrial cancer. Perimenarchal and perimenopausal stages are often characterized by abnormal bleeding patterns and are usually not cause for concern.

Initial evaluation includes history with attention to stressors, diet, exercise, weight changes, trauma, medications, and substance abuse. Important historical factors for estimating changes in blood loss include change in pattern with flow excessive for the patient, increase in number of pads or tampons used, leaking despite use of pads or tampons, and presence of clots. Additional history may give clues to an underlying endocrine or bleeding disorder, chronic liver or kidney disease, or STI. Physical examination should include a complete pelvic examination with attention to pelvic pathology; screening for cervical malignancy should be up-to-date. Pregnancy testing should be performed in all women with abnormal uterine bleeding as pregnancy is the most common cause of a divergence from a normal bleeding pattern. An assessment for chronic diseases, including liver, kidney, thyroid, autoimmune, and bleeding diathesis, should be performed as indicated. In adolescents and young adults, coagulation disorders are most common. Pelvic ultrasonography should be performed in women with structural abnormalities noted on examination, abnormal bleeding despite evidence of ovulatory cycles, or new-onset intermenstrual bleeding.

In women with prolonged anovulation, exposure to unopposed estrogen increases risk for endometrial carcinoma. Therefore, pelvic ultrasonography is indicated in women older than 35 years to assess endometrial stripe thickness; an endometrial stripe 5 mm or thicker warrants endometrial biopsy before initiation of medical therapy. Ultrasonography is also indicated in younger women in whom empiric medical therapy has failed to control bleeding.

Management

Management of abnormal uterine bleeding should be directed toward the underlying cause. Anatomic or structural abnormalities causing ovulatory bleeding generally require directed therapy.

Management of anovulatory bleeding is directed toward restoring the hormonal balance and stabilizing the endometrium. Treatment depends on the contraceptive plans of the patient. For women desiring fertility, a progestin such as medroxyprogesterone acetate may be used for the last 2 weeks of each cycle to promote withdrawal bleeding. For women not desiring pregnancy, OCPs may be used, as well as other contraceptive methods, including depot medroxyprogesterone, the vaginal contraceptive ring, and levonorgestrel IUD. For severe bleeding, short courses of gonadotropin-releasing hormone (GnRH) agonists or intravenous high-dose estrogens may be used. For patients who do not respond to medical treatment, evaluation for alternative causes or surgical treatment is appropriate.

For patients with chronic diseases not otherwise amenable to therapy (for example, chronic kidney disease), treatment is symptomatic. NSAIDs can decrease uterine bleeding by up to 40% owing to the high concentrations of prostaglandins in the endometrium. Danazol (200-400 mg/d) is approved for the treatment of heavy or irregular bleeding.

KEY POINT

- In postmenopausal women, any uterine bleeding is abnormal and warrants further evaluation, especially for endometrial cancer.

Dysmenorrhea

Dysmenorrhea is complicated or painful menstruation. It is usually seen in adolescents and young adults and is the most common gynecologic symptom in this age group. In 90% of cases, dysmenorrhea is associated with normal ovulatory cycles and no pelvic pathology (primary dysmenorrhea). In the remaining 10% of cases, a secondary cause, such as endometriosis, fibroids, or uterine pathology may be found. Symptoms of dysmenorrhea include abdominal cramps, headache, nausea, and vomiting. Symptoms coincide with onset of menses and last 1 to 2 days. Severity typically correlates with the amount and duration of menstrual blood flow.

Initial evaluation includes a thorough history, with particular attention to sexual activity and risks for abuse or infection. Unless pelvic pathology is suspected (previous radiation, trauma, infection, foreign body), treatment may begin without further evaluation. Effective treatments include NSAIDs and cyclooxygenase-2 inhibitors. These agents block prostaglandins in the endometrial lining, inhibiting the inflammation, vasoconstriction, and uterine ischemia thought to be the etiology. For patients with incomplete relief of symptoms, use of combined contraceptive therapy is effective; pills, patches, or the vaginal ring may be used. Extended-cycle combined OCPs may be particularly useful for this indication. Other treatment options include long-acting progesterones; these options should be used with caution in adolescents owing to the risk for osteoporosis from estrogen deficiency.

Women not responding to therapy should be suspected of having a secondary cause. The most common of these is endometriosis, which causes both cyclic and noncyclic pain. Treatment options are similar; additionally, GnRH agonists and aromatase inhibitors have been used but require calcium and vitamin D supplementation. If pelvic pathology is suspected or if symptoms are refractory, gynecologic referral may be appropriate.

Chronic Pelvic Pain

Chronic pelvic pain (CPP) in women is defined as noncyclic pain of at least 6 months' duration that localizes to the anatomic pelvis, anterior abdominal wall at or below the umbilicus, the lumbosacral back, or the buttocks, and is of sufficient severity to cause functional disability or necessitate medical care. Approximately 15% to 20% of reproductive-age women have experienced CPP for more than 1 year. The most common causes of CPP are endometriosis, pelvic adhesions, pelvic varices, interstitial cystitis, and irritable bowel syndrome (IBS); many women have more than one diagnosis. Fifty percent to 80% of women with CPP have symptoms consistent with IBS. Risk factors for CPP include physical and sexual abuse, pelvic inflammatory disease, a difficult obstetric delivery, a history of abdominopelvic surgery, and other chronic pain syndromes, such as fibromyalgia. Endometriosis, interstitial cystitis, and IBS all tend to worsen during the menstrual cycle; additional historical clues and tests that aid in diagnosis are listed in **Table 45**. Laboratory studies should include a complete blood count, serum chemistries, erythrocyte sedimentation rate, urinalysis and urine culture, and vaginal/endocervical swabs for culture. Transvaginal ultrasonography is helpful for identifying anatomic pelvic pathology, and a normal study aids in providing reassurance. Laparoscopy may be indicated for evaluation of severe symptoms of unclear etiology or identified pathology on examination or ultrasonography.

NSAIDs can be used as first-line short-term therapy for most women with moderate CPP. Although evidence to support the use of antidepressants is limited, psychotherapy and writing about the stress of pelvic pain may be helpful.

TABLE 45.	Diagnosis and Treatment Strategies for the Most Common Causes of Chronic Pelvic Pain[a]			
Etiology	Characteristic History	Diagnostic Strategies	Treatment Strategies	Prevalence
Endometriosis	Pain that may worsen with menstruation, dyspareunia, dysmenorrhea	Empiric treatment with GnRH agonist therapy; diagnostic laparoscopy	GnRH agonist therapy; combination OCPs for women with significant dysmenorrhea; laparoscopic surgical destruction of endometriosis lesions (stages I-III endometriosis)	Up to two-thirds of women with CPP have endometriosis
Pelvic adhesions	History of PID, endometriosis, abdominal or pelvic surgery	Diagnostic laparoscopy	Surgical adhesiolysis for severe adhesions	25%-50% of women with CPP have adhesions, although causality is usually not clear
Pelvic varices	Dull, chronic pain worsened with prolonged standing, improved by lying down and elevating legs	Combined transabdominal and transvaginal ultrasound	Medroxyprogesterone acetate	May cause pain in up to 42% of women with CPP
Interstitial cystitis	Dysuria, urgency, frequency, repeatedly negative urine cultures	Interstitial cystitis symptom index; cystoscopy	Pentosan polysulfate sodium; tricyclic antidepressants; GnRH agonist therapy may be helpful	38%-85% of women presenting to gynecologists with CPP may have this diagnosis

CPP = chronic pelvic pain; GnRH = gonadotropin-releasing hormone; OCP = oral contraceptive pill; PID = pelvic inflammatory disease.

[a]Irritable bowel syndrome, a common cause of CPP, is discussed in MKSAP 16 Gastroenterology and Hepatology.

Condition-specific treatment strategies are listed in Table 45. GnRH agonists are effective in treating women with CPP associated with endometriosis or IBS and may improve pain control in women with interstitial cystitis. The American College of Obstetricians and Gynecologists (ACOG) guidelines recommend empiric treatment with GnRH agonists in women with undiagnosed CPP; benefit may obviate the need for diagnostic laparoscopy. Add-back therapy with estrogen or progesterone can mitigate the detrimental effects that GnRH agonist therapy has on bone density without affecting treatment efficacy.

Surgical options for treatment include laparoscopic excision of endometriotic implants, adhesiolysis, sacral nerve stimulation, presacral neurectomy, and uterine nerve ablation. Hysterectomy is an effective treatment for CPP, although a substantial proportion of young women with normal pelvic anatomy at surgery will continue to experience pain. Except for pathology-directed interventions (such as for endometriosis), surgical treatment is generally pursued only after failure of medical therapy.

Vaginitis

Clinical Presentation and Evaluation

Vaginitis comprises a spectrum of infectious and noninfectious conditions that produce characteristic vulvovaginal symptoms, including vaginal discharge, vulvar itching, burning, and irritation. The most common causes of vaginitis are bacterial vaginosis, trichomoniasis, and vulvovaginal candidiasis. Less frequently, vaginal irritation can result from atrophy, allergic reactions, or certain dermatologic conditions.

All patients should be queried about the duration of symptoms; relationship to the menstrual cycle, douching, and sexual activity; discharge odor; and associated vulvar itching, irritation, burning, and swelling. The vulva and vagina should be inspected carefully for erythema, excoriations, and tenderness, and vaginal wall secretions should be collected for pH, amine testing, and saline and 10% potassium hydroxide microscopy. Additional point-of-care testing may aid in the diagnosis.

Bacterial Vaginosis

Bacterial vaginosis (BV) is a polymicrobial infection characterized by an overgrowth of multiple anaerobic bacteria (*Gardnerella vaginalis*, *Ureaplasma*, *Mycoplasma*, and *Bacteroides* species, among others), resulting in a reduction of the normal vaginal hydrogen peroxide–producing *Lactobacillus* species. Risk factors include douching, lack of condom use, and multiple or new sexual partners (although BV may also be diagnosed in women who have never been sexually active). BV infection increases the risk of complications in pregnancy and obstetric surgery, and affected women are more likely to acquire HIV, gonorrhea, chlamydial infection, and genital herpes. Symptomatic patients may report a thin, white or gray homogeneous discharge that has a "fishy" smell.

BV can be diagnosed if at least three of the four Amsel criteria are present: homogenous, thin, white discharge; vaginal pH greater than 4.5; fishy odor before or after the addition of 10% potassium hydroxide to vaginal secretions ("whiff" test); and the presence of clue cells on saline microscopy. Clue cells are squamous vaginal epithelial cells with a large number of coccobacillary organisms densely attached to their surface, giving them a granular appearance (**Figure 18**). The Amsel criteria have a sensitivity of 92% and a specificity of 77% for diagnosis of BV. Other diagnostic options include a point-of-care test card that detects proline aminopeptidase and has a sensitivity of 90% and a specificity of 97%. Culture for *G. vaginalis* is not recommended owing to low specificity.

Treatment is with either oral (7 days) or topical (5-7 days) metronidazole or clindamycin (oral or topical). Metronidazole is safe in pregnancy, but topical clindamycin should be avoided as it may increase the risk of adverse outcomes. Approximately 30% of women will experience a recurrence of BV within 3 months.

Trichomoniasis

Women who have multiple sexual partners, exchange sex for payment, or use injected drugs are at particularly high risk for trichomoniasis, an STI caused by infection with the protozoan *Trichomonas vaginalis*. Although some infected women are asymptomatic, many experience a profuse malodorous yellow-green discharge with vulvar itching, burning, and postcoital bleeding. Trichomoniasis is associated with a vaginal pH greater than 4.5 and the presence of motile trichomonads on saline microscopy, but the specificity of an abnormal vaginal pH and the sensitivity of saline microscopy for identifying motile trichomonads are both low. If point-of-care tests are unavailable, vaginal secretions may be sent for culture.

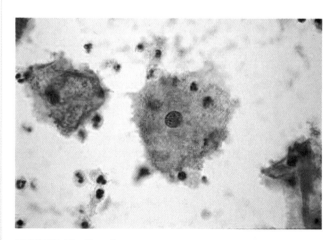

FIGURE 18. Clue cells.

Oral single-dose metronidazole therapy is associated with a high rate of cure and should be provided to all symptomatic women; in addition, treatment of the sexual partner is essential for preventing reinfection. Metronidazole may be safely given at any stage in pregnancy. Inadequate response to treatment may be caused by reinfection (up to 17% of treated women are reinfected within 3 months) or diminished responsiveness to metronidazole. If the latter is suspected, a 7-day course of metronidazole (500 mg twice daily) often results in clinical resolution. Subsequent diagnostic testing to confirm treatment success should be considered for women who are HIV-positive as they may be less responsive to single-dose metronidazole. Persistent coinfection with *T. vaginalis* can increase HIV shedding and viral transmission.

Vulvovaginal Candidiasis

Most women experience at least one episode of vulvovaginal candidiasis (VVC) in their lifetime, and more than one third will have two or more infections. Pregnancy, diabetes, and treatment with antibiotics or corticosteroids increase the risk for VVC. Although VVC produces classic symptoms, such as vulvar pruritus, external dysuria, and a thick, "cottage-cheese" discharge, studies have shown that the history alone is insufficient for reliably establishing the diagnosis. On examination, vulvar edema, erythema, and excoriations are suggestive of disease, but VVC is confirmed only if symptoms are accompanied by the presence of yeasts, hyphae, or pseudohyphae on microscopy or Gram stain, or if a vaginal culture is positive for yeast. Vaginal pH is normal in VVC. As the sensitivity of microscopy may be as low as 65%, empiric treatment for VVC can be considered if vaginal culture is unavailable and symptoms are accompanied by characteristic physical examination findings. Culture for *Candida* in the absence of symptoms is not recommended, as 10% to 20% of women are colonized.

Once the diagnosis of VVC is made, infection is characterized as uncomplicated or complicated and treatment is prescribed accordingly. Uncomplicated VVC responds well to therapy with over-the-counter topical imidazoles or a single dose of oral fluconazole. Complicated VVC, which is diagnosed in women who are severely symptomatic, pregnant, immunosuppressed, or diabetic, necessitates more aggressive treatment, including topical imidazole treatment for up to 14 days or two doses of oral fluconazole given 3 days apart. In pregnant women, VVC is treated with a 7-day course of topical imidazole. Recurrent VVC is defined as more than four symptomatic episodes per year. Recurrence is treated initially with a 7- to 14-day course of topical imidazole therapy or oral fluconazole every third day for a total of three doses, followed by oral fluconazole weekly for 6 months. Twenty percent of cases of recurrent VVC are caused by *Candida* species other than *C. albicans,* and these may be treated with a 2-week course of intravaginal boric acid.

Eye Disorders

Red Eye

Clinical Evaluation

Red eye is the most common eye condition seen in primary care. Most cases of red eye can be safely managed by the primary care physician, but it is important to know when to refer to an ophthalmologist. During the initial evaluation, the history should focus on the acuity of onset of symptoms, whether one or both eyes are involved, history of trauma or risk factors for foreign bodies or abrasion, other accompanying symptoms (nausea, vomiting, photophobia, headache), presence of systemic disease, and whether the vision is intact. The physical examination should begin with assessment of visual acuity, location and distribution of redness, presence or absence of discharge, and pupillary shape. Funduscopy has little diagnostic yield in evaluating the red eye.

Conjunctivitis

Conjunctivitis, inflammation of the thin, usually transparent outermost lining of the eye, is the most common cause of red eye. When inflamed, the conjunctiva appears pink or red and the conjunctival blood vessels may be seen. Conjunctivitis is caused by viruses, bacteria, allergies, or contact lens wear. The history is usually helpful in distinguishing these etiologies. Viral conjunctivitis (**Figure 19**) is usually caused by an adenovirus; a history of a preceding upper respiratory tract infection and recent exposure to a person with conjunctivitis are clues to this diagnosis. Onset is usually acute, with unilateral redness and watery discharge. Other symptoms include itching, mild photophobia, a diffuse foreign body sensation, and crusting of the eyelids after sleep. Persons with viral conjunctivitis are contagious for up to 2 weeks after the second eye becomes involved and, therefore, should perform frequent hand washing and avoid sharing personal items. Food handlers and health care providers should not return to work until eye discharge ceases. The treatment for viral conjunctivitis is largely supportive, including cold compresses and artificial tears. There is no role for antibiotic eye drops in the treatment of viral conjunctivitis.

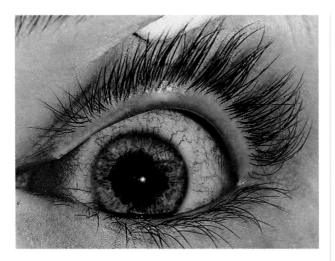

FIGURE 19. Viral conjunctivitis.

Eye with Viral Conjunctivitis. Digital image. Wikimedia Commons. 1 Feb. 2010. Web. 16 May 2012. <http://commons.wikimedia.org/wiki/File:An_eye_with_viral_conjunctivitis.jpg>.

Bacterial conjunctivitis (**Figure 20**) is also highly contagious and is categorized as hyperacute, acute, and chronic. Acute bacterial conjunctivitis, the most common form of bacterial conjunctivitis seen in the outpatient setting, is usually caused by *Staphylococcus aureus*; but *Streptococcus pneumoniae* and *Haemophilus influenzae* can also be culprit organisms. Bacterial conjunctivitis is usually distinguished from viral conjunctivitis by the presence of mucopurulent discharge that is worse when waking in the morning and when dried may form a significant crust, whereas viral conjunctivitis has clearer discharge and may be preceded by an upper respiratory tract infection. Hyperacute bacterial conjunctivitis is associated with a copious purulent discharge, pain, and diminished vision. In sexually active adults, hyperacute bacterial conjunctivitis may be caused by *Neisseria gonorrhoeae*. Gonococcal conjunctivitis is sudden in onset and can rapidly progress to corneal perforation. Patients with gonococcal conjunctivitis

should be treated systemically for *N. gonorrhoeae* as well as *Chlamydia trachomatis* infection, as one-third of patients with gonorrhea are coinfected with *C. trachomatis*.

Bacterial cultures and Gram staining are not generally performed in the evaluation of bacterial conjunctivitis. Exceptions include when gonococcal infection is suspected, the patient is immunocompromised, wears contact lenses, has hyperacute bacterial conjunctivitis, or has failed to improve after 1 week of therapy. Broad-spectrum antibiotic eyedrops should be prescribed for use for 5 to 7 days. Bacterial conjunctivitis that persists for at least 4 weeks is considered chronic; these patients should be evaluated by an ophthalmologist.

Allergic conjunctivitis is a clinical diagnosis. It may resemble viral conjunctivitis in terms of clear discharge; however, it tends to be associated with seasonal allergies, with itching in one or both eyes as the predominant symptom. Treatment includes oral antihistamines, topical antihistamines, and artificial tears; antibiotic treatment is not indicated.

Subconjunctival Hematoma

Subconjunctival hematoma (**Figure 21**) occurs when subconjunctival vessels bleed into the subconjunctival space. This can occur spontaneously or result from trauma, a Valsalva maneuver, cough, or antiplatelet or antithrombotic agents. Subconjunctival hematomas are painless and do not affect vision but are sometimes frightening for the patient. Patients should be reassured and informed that resolution occurs gradually over several weeks. Although most subconjunctival hemorrhages are benign, other causes of this finding include endocarditis, bleeding disorders, and medications (such as imatinib mesylate); these causes should be considered if appropriate.

Corneal Conditions

Corneal abrasions cause a foreign body sensation, photophobia, tearing, and pain. They often result from trauma caused by foreign bodies or fingernails. To examine the cornea, fluorescein dye should be instilled into the eye and the eye

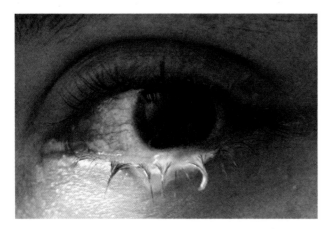

FIGURE 20. Bacterial conjunctivitis.

Swollen Eye with Conjunctivitis. Digital image. Wikimedia Commons. 8 Feb. 2008. Web. 16 May 2012. <http://commons.wikimedia.org/wiki/File:Swollen_eye_with_conjunctivitis.jpg>.

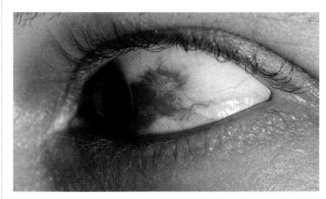

FIGURE 21. Subconjunctival hematoma. A well-localized superficial collection of extravasated blood is visible; the sclera and conjunctiva are not involved.

Subconjunctival Hemorrhage. Digital image. Wikimedia Commons. 28 Jun. 2011. Web. 16 May 2012. <http://commons.wikimedia.org/wiki/File:Subconjunctival_hemorrhage_eye.jpg>.

examined under a Wood lamp or with a slit lamp. The area underneath the upper lid should be examined to rule out a foreign body, which should be removed if present. Although there is little supporting evidence that topical antibiotics improve outcomes, many practitioners still prescribe a short course (48-72 hours). Eye patches have not been shown to speed healing or improve patient symptoms. Most abrasions improve markedly within 24 to 48 hours owing to rapid epithelial cell proliferation.

Corneal ulcers can result from bacterial infection, herpes simplex virus infection, contact lens wear, or trauma. The ulcer can be detected with fluorescein dye; herpes infection classically causes a dendritic-appearing ulcer. Corneal ulcers can erode and cause corneal perforation and permanent visual loss. Patients should be seen by an ophthalmologist early for antimicrobial therapy and consideration of corneal scraping.

Episcleritis and Scleritis

Episcleritis (**Figure 22**) is inflammation of the superficial vessels of the episclera, the vascular membrane that underlies the conjunctiva. The inflammation tends to be more localized than with conjunctivitis, which tends to be diffuse. Its etiology is unclear. It typically is not associated with pain, visual changes, or tearing, and it usually resolves without specific treatment.

Scleritis is inflammation of the fibrous layer of the eye underlying the conjunctiva and episclera. Anterior scleritis, involving the superficial sclera and the deep vessels within the episclera, is the most common form. Posterior scleritis involves the deeper structures of the eye. Patients presenting with this disorder usually have severe, dull pain that may have awoken them from sleep. There may be visual loss, particularly

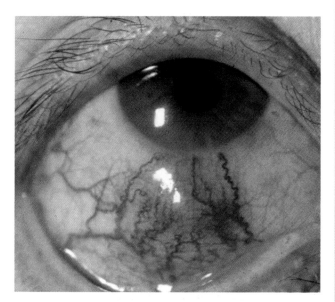

FIGURE 22. Episcleritis. Superficial dilated blood vessels are seen, with white sclera visible between the blood vessels.

Image courtesy of Linda Lippa, MD, University of California, Irvine.

with posterior scleritis. Patients with scleritis should be referred emergently to an ophthalmologist as this can be a sight-threatening condition.

The history is important for differentiating scleritis (pain, vision impairment) from episcleritis (less pain, vision unaffected); however, it is challenging to differentiate the two entities by physical examination. If there is uncertainty whether the patient has scleritis or episcleritis, an urgent referral should be made to an ophthalmologist for clarification.

Approximately 50% of patients with scleritis have an underlying systemic disease, such as rheumatoid arthritis, or an infectious disease, such as tuberculosis or syphilis. Treatment depends upon the underlying cause but may include NSAIDs for mild scleritis and systemic corticosteroids or tumor necrosis factor inhibitors for severe disease.

Uveitis

Uveitis, inflammation of the uvea, commonly presents as a red eye with pain, photophobia, and blurred vision. Anterior uveitis, or iridocyclitis, is inflammation of the iris and ciliary body and is more common than posterior uveitis. It is characterized by circumferential redness (ciliary flush) at the corneal limbus (junction of the cornea and sclera). Vision is usually normal in anterior uveitis. The classic finding upon slit lamp examination is the presence of inflammatory "flare cells" in the anterior chamber. The differential diagnosis for causes of uveitis includes infection (syphilis, tuberculosis), autoimmune disorders, sarcoidosis, and malignancy, although no cause is identified in more than 50% of patients. Anterior uveitis is usually idiopathic but can be associated with herpes simplex virus infection, trauma, or the presence of HLA-B27 antigen. Patients with uveitis should be urgently referred to an ophthalmologist for treatment.

Blepharitis

Blepharitis is inflammation of the eyelid margins. It is usually caused by *S. aureus* infection or seborrheic dermatitis, and occasionally by rosacea. It is treated with warm compresses and cleansing of the eyelid margins with diluted nontearing shampoo using a cotton tip applicator. Topical antibiotic ointment may also be used for staphylococcal blepharitis. Oral tetracyclines may be prescribed when blepharitis is associated with rosacea.

KEY POINTS

- Conjunctivitis, most often caused by a viral infection, is the most common cause of red eye; antibiotic therapy is not indicated for viral conjunctivitis.
- Both viral and bacterial conjunctivitis are highly contagious, and hand hygiene and other measures should be emphasized to minimize transmission.
- Corneal ulceration, scleritis, and uveitis should be evaluated by an ophthalmologist if diagnosed or if there is diagnostic uncertainty.

Macular Degeneration

Pathophysiology and Clinical Presentation

Age-related macular degeneration (AMD) is a leading cause of visual loss, particularly in the elderly. Progression of disease can lead to difficulty driving, reading, and performing activities of daily living, and may increase the risk of falling.

There are two types of AMD, dry (atrophic) and wet (neovascular) (**Figure 23**). In dry AMD (approximately 85% of cases), soft drusen (deposits of extracellular material) form in the area of the macula. Dry AMD may present in one or both eyes. It may be asymptomatic in the early stages and subsequently progress, with the gradual loss of central vision. Wet AMD is usually more aggressive and sight-threatening than dry AMD. It is caused by neovascularization of the macula with subsequent bleeding or scar formation. Visual loss may be more sudden (over a period of weeks) and is often more severe. It most frequently presents in one eye.

The strongest risk factors for AMD are age, smoking, family history, and cardiovascular disease. Quitting smoking reduces the risk of developing AMD. No antioxidant or other supplement has been proved conclusively to prevent AMD; however, some studies report that diets high in antioxidants may be protective.

The diagnosis of either wet or dry AMD is made with dilated funduscopic examination and fluorescein angiography performed by an ophthalmologist.

Treatment

There are no proven treatments for dry AMD. Patients with advanced dry AMD may benefit from antioxidant agents (vitamin C, vitamin E, β-carotene) and zinc; smokers should avoid β-carotene owing to risk of increased lung cancer. Laser phototherapy for dry AMD and drusen is not recommended as it may increase the incidence of neovascularization.

Several inhibitors of vascular endothelial growth factor (VEGF) have been used to slow the neovascularization of wet AMD. Laser photocoagulation therapy is no longer routinely recommended for wet AMD owing to potential complications outweighing possible benefits, except in patients with extrafoveal lesions.

KEY POINT
- Quitting smoking reduces the risk of developing age-related macular degeneration.

Glaucoma

Primary Open Angle Glaucoma

Primary open angle glaucoma (POAG) is a progressive optic neuropathy associated with increased intraocular pressure (IOP) without an identifiable blockage of the normal drainage pathways of the aqueous humor. It is the most common form of glaucoma and is the leading cause of irreversible blindness in the world. POAG is characterized by painless, gradual loss of peripheral vision in both eyes, which may be unnoticed by the patient. It is often asymmetric. In later stages, it may progress to involve central visual acuity. Clinical findings include an increased optic cup:disc ratio (>0.5), disc hemorrhages, and vertical extension of the central cup. Risk factors include age older than 40 years, race (incidence in blacks is four times higher than in whites), and positive family history.

Lowering IOP has been shown to delay or prevent the progression of POAG symptoms over time. Pharmacologic agents are the mainstay of glaucoma treatment, but adverse effects can be significant (**Table 46**). Laser therapy to increase

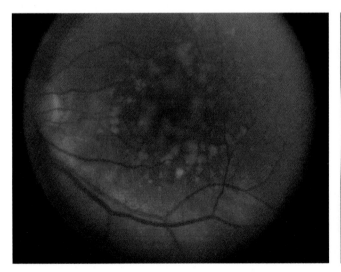
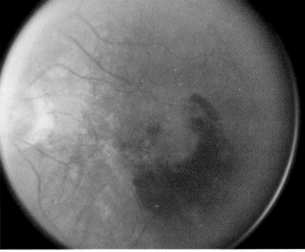

FIGURE 23. Age-related macular degeneration. The dry form (*left*), is characterized by distinct yellow-white lesions (drusen) surrounding the macular region and areas of pigment mottling. The wet form (*right*), is characterized by clumps of hyperpigmentation, hypopigmentation, and evidence of subretinal hemorrhage.

Images courtesy of Edward A. Jaeger, MD, Jefferson Medical College, Wills Eye Institute, Philadelphia, PA.

TABLE 46. Drug Treatment for Primary Open Angle Glaucoma

Agent	Mechanism of Action	Systemic Side Effects
β-Blockers (timolol)	Decreases inflow	Bradycardia, heart block, bronchospasm, decreased libido, central nervous system depression, mood swings
Nonselective adrenergic agonists (epinephrine)	Decreases inflow and increases outflow	Hypertension, headaches, extrasystole
Selective α₂-adrenergic agonists (brimonidine)	Decreases inflow and increases outflow	Hypotension, vasovagal attack, dry mouth, fatigue, insomnia, depression, syncope, dizziness, anxiety
Parasympathomimetic agents (pilocarpine, echothiophate iodide)	Increases outflow	Increased salivation, increased gastric secretion, abdominal cramps, urinary frequency, shock
Oral carbonic anhydrase inhibitors (acetazolamide)	Decreases inflow	Acidosis, depression, malaise, hirsutism, paresthesias, numbness, blood dyscrasias, diarrhea, weight loss, kidney stones, loss of libido, bone marrow suppression, hypokalemia, bad taste, increased serum urate level
Topical carbonic anhydrase inhibitors (dorzolamide)	Decreases inflow	Lower incidence of systemic effects compared with oral carbonic anhydrase inhibitors
Prostaglandin analogues (latanoprost)	Increases outflow	Flu-like symptoms, joint and muscle pain
Hyperosmotic agents (mannitol)	Reduces vitreous and aqueous volume	Headache, heart failure, expansion of blood volume, nausea, vomiting, diarrhea, electrolyte disturbance, kidney failure

Adapted from Smith OU, Seligsohn AL, Khan SJ, Spaeth GL. Primary open angle glaucoma. http://pier.acponline.org/physicians/diseases/d602/tables/d602-tables.html (login required). In PIER (online database). Philadelphia: American College of Physicians, 2009. Accessed July 7, 2009.

aqueous outflow, although able to lower the IOP, may lose efficacy over time. Surgical options, such as trabeculectomy or iridectomy, have attendant risks of complications, including blindness.

Acute Angle Closure Glaucoma
Acute angle closure glaucoma results from blocked drainage of the aqueous humor. Patients present with red eye with severe pain and headache and occasionally nausea and vomiting and visual halos. Visual acuity is usually reduced. It is caused by increased IOP owing to blocked drainage of the aqueous humor. Physical examination reveals a semidilated, nonreactive pupil with an IOP greater than 50 mm Hg. Acute angle closure glaucoma is an immediate threat to vision, and urgent referral to an ophthalmologist is important to avert optic nerve atrophy.

KEY POINT
- Pharmacologic agents are the mainstay of primary open angle glaucoma treatment, but adverse effects can be significant.

Cataract
A cataract is an opacity of the lens. Cataracts are the leading cause of blindness and low vision globally, and the prevalence in the United States approaches 20% in those older than 40 years. Risk factors include older age, ultraviolet B radiation exposure, smoking, diabetes mellitus, a family history of cataracts, and systemic corticosteroid use. Symptoms include

painless decreased visual acuity, decreased night vision, glare, and diplopia. On ophthalmoscopic examination, there is a decrease or absence of the red reflex, and opacification of the lens can be visualized.

Treatment is surgical removal of the cataract. Surgery is indicated if symptoms from the cataract interfere with the patient's ability to meet his or her needs of daily living; there are no criteria based upon the level of visual acuity. The posterior capsule is left intact, and a corrective replacement intraocular lens may be inserted to restore normal vision. Perioperative consultation is not required for those undergoing a procedure under local anesthesia and sedation as the surgery is considered low risk; aspirin and warfarin can be continued.

Complications from surgery are rare but include inflammation, corneal edema, and macular edema. Rarely, infective endophthalmitis develops (see Eye Emergencies). A common late-stage complication is opacification of the posterior capsule, leading to decreased visual acuity; this may be managed surgically.

Dry Eye
Dry eye (keratoconjunctivitis sicca) causes symptoms of gritty irritation, dryness, and burning of the eyes. Symptoms usually occur gradually and may worsen over the course of the day. Symptoms can be caused by any process that disrupts the tear film, either by decreasing tear production and secretion or by increasing tear evaporation. Symptoms may be aggravated by environmental irritants (smoke, allergens, low humidity) and relieved with eye closing and increased humidity.

Decreased tear secretion is usually caused by inflammation of the lacrimal gland, which may be a localized process or associated with a systemic disease, such as Sjögren syndrome or rheumatoid arthritis. Additionally, decreased corneal sensation, which may occur with diabetes, hard contact lens wearing, herpes zoster infection, or laser-assisted in situ keratomileusis (LASIK) eye surgery, causes reduced tear secretion. Increased tear evaporation may be caused by increased size of the palpebral fissure (as seen in Graves ophthalmopathy) or by meibomian gland dysfunction, which reduces the protective lipid layer of the tear film. Other risk factors for dry eyes include increasing age, female sex, decreased androgen levels, and certain medications, including anticholinergic agents, antihistamines, selective serotonin reuptake inhibitors, nicotinic acid, and isotretinoin. Patients with persistent or severe dry eye, as with Sjögren syndrome, Graves disease, or Bell palsy, may suffer corneal damage.

Treatment of dry eye is directed at decreasing inflammation and addressing any lid pathology disrupting the tear film. Artificial tears are helpful for lubrication. Warm compresses may also be helpful. Lid inflammation may be treated with oral tetracyclines. Meibomianitis may respond to gentle scrubs with mild nontearing shampoo. Punctal or canalicular plugs may lower tear film osmolality and thus decrease evaporation. Topical corticosteroid drops (short-term use only) and topical cyclosporine have also been used in patients with dry eye caused by systemic illness.

Excessive Tearing

Excessive tearing results from either overproduction of tears (lacrimation) or impaired drainage through the lacrimal duct system (epiphora). Lacrimation is often bilateral and painless, whereas epiphora may be unilateral and can be painful, particularly if infection of the ductal system is involved (dacryocystitis). The eyes should be examined for evidence of foreign body or acute conjunctivitis. The lids should be examined for ectropion and adequate lid closure and the punctum examined for blockage, inflammation, or purulence.

Treatment is focused on the underlying cause, with ophthalmologic referral for mechanical intervention for patients with lacrimal drainage problems.

Retinal Detachment

Retinal detachment occurs when the neurosensory layer of the retina separates from the retinal pigment epithelial layer and choroid. This can result from either fluid accumulation behind or vitreous traction on the retina. Separation can cause ischemia in the retina or a tear that may lead to visual loss. Retinal detachment occurs predominantly in myopic patients. Patients may report floaters, squiggly lines, flashes of light, and then a sudden visual defect that is peripheral,

appearing as a black curtain, which then progresses across the visual field. Funduscopic examination usually visualizes the detachment (**Figure 24**). The treatment is surgical. Prognosis depends upon the extent of the detachment or tear and time to surgery, so early recognition and emergent referral is crucial.

Posterior vitreous detachment (PVD), in which contraction of the vitreous places traction on the retina, is the most common type of retinal detachment and typically occurs in persons aged 50 to 75 years. Patients with PVD can be asymptomatic but most often present with floaters or flashes of light (photopsias). Most photopsias are benign and idiopathic, becoming more common as age progresses.

Symptoms of PVD usually progress over a period of 1 week to 3 months and can progress to visual loss. Patients with uncomplicated PVD have less than a 5% chance of developing a full retinal tear within 6 weeks, and symptomatic patients should simply be reassured and educated about potential symptoms of visual loss. Symptoms in patients without full tears usually resolve over 3 to 12 months. No specific limits on activity are necessary. For those patients with PVD who develop retinal tears, one half go on to full retinal detachment. A full retinal detachment may present with cobweb-like floaters with acute visual loss or with a monocular decreased visual field; these patients should be evaluated acutely. Those with full detachments will require ophthalmologic intervention.

KEY POINT

- Patients with cobweb-like floaters with acute visual loss or who are found to have a monocular decreased visual field may have a full retinal detachment and should be seen urgently by an ophthalmologist.

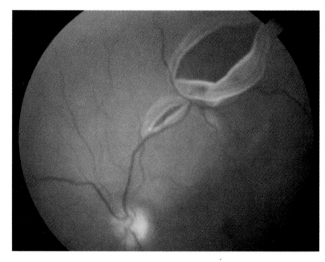

FIGURE 24. Retinal detachment, with characteristic folding and tearing of the retina.

Image courtesy of Edward A. Jaeger, MD, Jefferson Medical College, Wills Eye Institute, Philadelphia, PA.

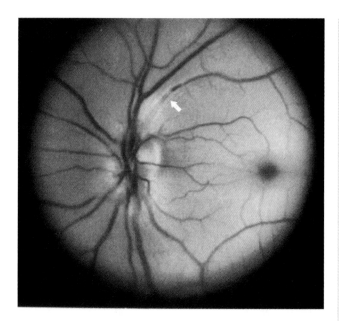

FIGURE 25. Occlusion of the central retinal artery (*arrow*) characterized by the appearance of an opalescent retina, retinal pallor, and "cherry-red spot" defining the fovea.

Image courtesy of Edward A. Jaeger, MD, Jefferson Medical College, Wills Eye Institute, Philadelphia, PA.

Retinal Vascular Occlusion
Central Retinal Vein Occlusion

Patients with central retinal vein occlusion (CRVO) typically report a sudden, unilateral loss of vision. This differs from occlusion of a branch retinal vein, which is often asymptomatic. The etiology of CRVO is usually a thrombus occluding the central retinal vein. Risk factors include age, hypertension, diabetes, hyperlipidemia, smoking, obesity, hypercoagulable states, glaucoma, and retinal arteriolar abnormalities. Diagnosis is based on the history of abrupt onset of monocular blindness coupled with classic funduscopic examination findings of congested, tortuous retinal veins; scattered intraretinal hemorrhages; and cotton wool spots in the area of the vein occlusion. An afferent pupillary defect may be seen.

Suspicion of CRVO warrants rapid ophthalmologic consultation. Clinical outcomes usually correlate well with visual acuity level at presentation, and those with severe visual loss are less likely to regain normal function.

Central Retinal Artery Occlusion

Arterial occlusions are usually seen in the elderly and may be caused by embolic or thrombotic events or vasospasm. Patients present with sudden, painless visual loss in one eye, an afferent pupillary defect, and a pale retina with a cherry red fovea that appears accentuated in color owing to the pale retinal background (**Figure 25**). Visual acuity at the time of presentation predicts final visual acuity, and irreversible vision loss tends to occur after 4 hours of ischemia. Attempts can be made to lower IOP while awaiting emergent ophthalmology consultation. **H**

- Abrupt onset of painless monocular blindness may indicate a retinal vascular occlusion and warrants emergent ophthalmologic consultation.

Eye Emergencies

Indications for urgent or emergent ophthalmology consultation are listed in **Table 47**. Any patient with acute vision loss should be seen emergently by an ophthalmologist. Important causes of acute visual loss include retinal artery occlusion, retinal vein occlusion, temporal arteritis, retinal detachment, and optic neuritis.

Nearly all patients with globe trauma should be seen emergently by an ophthalmologist. Orbital fractures do not need to be seen emergently unless there is globe penetration, visual loss, or impairment of extraocular muscles. Direct trauma or laceration to the eyelid, nasolacrimal system, lid margin, or tarsal plate should be seen by either an ophthalmologist or plastic surgeon.

Chemical injuries to the eye are an ocular emergency. The eye should be irrigated for at least 30 minutes using normal saline solution or lactated Ringer solution while an ophthalmology consultation is occurring.

Endophthalmitis is inflammation of the aqueous and vitreous humors and usually results from infection, most often as a postoperative complication of eye surgery. It may also be associated with endocarditis. Treatment may include intravitreal antibiotics. Orbital cellulitis involves the periocular tissues and eyelids and usually results from contiguous sinus or dental infection. Patients present with marked ocular and eyelid erythema, swelling, pain, and fever. To differentiate preseptal cellulitis from orbital cellulitis, extraocular muscles and pupillary reflexes should be carefully evaluated. A CT scan is usually performed to evaluate for deeper infection. Any patient presenting

TABLE 47. Indications for Urgent or Emergent Ophthalmology Consultation

Condition
Acute angle closure glaucoma
Acute vision loss
Central retinal vascular occlusion
Corneal ulceration
Endophthalmitis
Herpes zoster ophthalmicus
Optic neuritis
Orbital cellulitis
Retinal detachment
Scleritis
Trauma to globe or lid
Uveitis

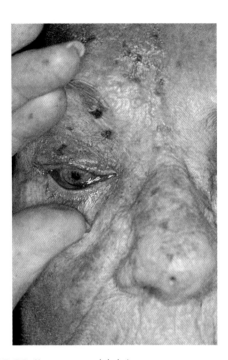

FIGURE 26. Herpes zoster ophthalmicus.

with herpes zoster involving the tip of the nose (Hutchinson sign) should be seen by an ophthalmologist to rule out herpes zoster ophthalmicus (**Figure 26**). The Hutchinson sign has a fairly high correlation with the presence of corneal involvement, which can cause permanent visual loss.

Optic neuritis occurs predominantly in middle-aged, white persons, and affects women more than men. Patients present with pain with eye movement, blurred vision, visual field deficits, and change in color perception. The optic disc usually appears normal. Optic neuritis is usually self-limited, but an ophthalmology consultation and a brain MRI should be obtained. Optic neuritis can be an early harbinger of multiple sclerosis. Intravenous corticosteroids may help speed recovery. H

KEY POINTS

- Any patient with acute vision loss should be seen emergently by an ophthalmologist.

- Globe trauma, chemical injury, orbital cellulitis, endophthalmitis, and optic neuritis are ocular emergencies, and urgent ophthalmologic evaluation should be obtained.

Ear, Nose, Mouth, and Throat Disorders

Evaluation of Hearing Loss

Causes of hearing loss are generally categorized as conductive or sensorineural (**Table 48**). Conductive hearing loss is caused by a mechanical problem preventing the transmission of acoustic vibrations from external sources to the cochlea and may originate in the ear canal, tympanic membrane, or the ossicles of the middle ear. Sensorineural hearing loss involves the perception and transmission of acoustic vibrations and may reflect a cochlear problem or an issue with the acoustic nerve.

If hearing loss is unilateral, the Weber and Rinne tests can help to differentiate between conductive and sensorineural hearing loss. A 256 Hz tuning fork is commonly used for the Weber test and a 512 Hz fork for the Rinne test, although a 512 Hz fork may be used for both. In the Weber test, the vibrating tuning fork is placed in contact with the forehead or scalp in the midline equidistant from both ears. In conductive hearing loss, the fork will be heard more loudly in the affected ear, and in sensorineural hearing loss, it will be louder in the unaffected ear. In the Rinne test, the vibrating tuning fork is held against the mastoid process of the affected ear until it can no longer be heard; it is then removed and held outside the ear. If the tuning fork can be heard after removal, the conductive system is likely intact, favoring a sensorineural cause of hearing loss. If the tuning fork is better heard in contact with the mastoid bone, conductive hearing loss is more likely.

In practice, patients who report hearing loss and lack an obvious cause on physical examination (such as cerumen impaction or middle ear effusion) should be referred for formal audiometry, which is better able to discriminate between conductive and sensorineural hearing loss, and help determine which patients will likely benefit from amplification.

Imaging of the central nervous system is not considered part of a routine evaluation for hearing loss. A clinical setting in which imaging should be considered is the progressive onset of unilateral sensorineural hearing loss; a small but significant number of these patients have retrocochlear pathology as a cause of their hearing loss, such as an acoustic neuroma. If imaging is pursued, MRI is the study of choice to evaluate the posterior fossa and internal auditory canal.

Sudden sensorineural hearing loss, defined as a 30 dB loss over a period of 3 days or less, is a discrete and poorly understood clinical syndrome. Viral infection, bacterial meningitis, Lyme disease, migraine, Meniere disease, acoustic neuroma, head injury, drug reactions, and neurosarcoidosis can all cause sudden hearing loss; however, a cause is identified in only approximately 10% of these patients. Most cases are idiopathic and unilateral and otoscopy is normal; acute otorhinolaryngologic evaluation is appropriate. Limited data suggest that corticosteroid therapy may improve the likelihood of hearing recovery. Fortunately, more than half of patients recover completely within 2 weeks.

KEY POINT

- Patients who report hearing loss and lack an obvious cause on physical examination should be referred for formal audiometry.

TABLE 48. Common Causes of Hearing Loss

Disease	Notes
Conductive	
Cerumen impaction	Cerumen may completely obstruct ear canal, causing conductive hearing loss. Impacted cerumen can be removed with gentle irrigation or an ear curette. No removal needed if asymptomatic.
Otosclerosis	Bony overgrowth of the stapes footplate with eventual fixation. Family history of otosclerosis is common. Treatment is stapedectomy or stapedotomy. Hearing aid may be helpful.
Tympanic membrane perforation	Often heals without intervention. Ear should be kept dry. Refer for possible repair if associated with significant hearing loss or possible middle ear pathology.
Cholesteatoma	An expanding mass composed of keratinizing squamous epithelial cells that may contain cholesterol crystals. Although histologically benign, it may erode extensively into local structures, including the cochlea, ossicles, tympanic membrane, and facial nerve. Treatment is surgical removal.
Sensorineural	
Presbycusis	Age-related hearing loss; typically symmetric high-frequency hearing loss. Hearing aids are mainstay of treatment.
Sudden sensorineural hearing loss	Unclear etiology; presents as a sudden loss of hearing that is sensorineural in nature. Rapid treatment with corticosteroids may improve outcome, although one study showed little difference whether treatment was initiated within 24 hours or 7 days.
Meniere disease	Classically presents as a triad of sensorineural hearing loss, tinnitus, and vertigo, although all three are not necessarily present in each patient. Symptoms may fluctuate, and attacks are often precipitated by high salt intake.
Vestibular schwannoma (acoustic neuroma)	Benign neoplasm, usually causing sensorineural hearing loss, tinnitus, and sometimes vertigo. A family or personal history of neurofibromatosis 2 puts patients at high risk for these tumors, often bilaterally.
Noise-induced	History of chronic noise exposure or sudden, short exposure to noise blast. Prevention is mainstay of treatment; hearing aids if condition is already advanced.
Drug-induced	History of ototoxic medication use (aminoglycosides, chemotherapeutic agents [irreversible], aspirin and NSAIDs [partially reversible], antimalarials [reversible], loop diuretics [sometimes irreversible]).
Both conductive and sensorineural	
Infection	Middle ear infection may impair movement of the tympanic membrane or ossicles, producing reversible conductive hearing loss. Viral cochleitis may cause reversible sensorineural hearing loss. Chronic ear infection may lead to conductive hearing loss.
Head trauma	May produce a conductive hearing loss from ossicular disruption and hemotympanum or a sensorineural hearing loss from cochlear fracture or auditory nerve injury.

Tinnitus

Tinnitus is the perception of sound that is not audible. Patients frequently characterize it as "ringing," "buzzing," or "whistling," although it may manifest as other sounds. It may be unilateral or bilateral, depending on the nature of the underlying disorder. Although tinnitus is part of the defining triad for Meniere disease, it is not specific to Meniere disease and can occur with virtually any cause of sensorineural hearing loss, such as presbycusis, noise exposure, or acoustic neuroma. It can also occur with conductive hearing loss, such as from eustachian tube dysfunction or cerumen impaction, although this is less common.

Pulsatile tinnitus (tinnitus synchronized with the patient's pulse) and objective tinnitus (tinnitus that can be heard by an external observer, for example with a stethoscope) may be indicators of an underlying vascular etiology such as arteriovenous malformation, atherosclerosis, carotid artery disease, or a paraganglioma (glomus tumor). Physical examination for pulsatile tinnitus includes auscultation for bruits over the ear and eye as well as the neck. Pulsatile tinnitus of indeterminate etiology should be evaluated by an otorhinolaryngologist.

Absent a treatment for the underlying cause, treatment for tinnitus is challenging. Medications are largely ineffective, and the mainstay of therapy is neurocognitive interventions to help patients cope with the problem and diminish dysfunctional cognitive processes associated with the experience of tinnitus. External noise generators are sometimes used to mask the sound of tinnitus, but evidence supporting their efficacy is sparse.

KEY POINTS

- Tinnitus can occur with virtually any cause of sensorineural hearing loss, including Meniere disease, presbycusis, noise exposure, or acoustic neuroma.
- Pulsatile tinnitus and objective tinnitus may be indicators of an underlying vascular etiology.

- Medications are largely ineffective in the treatment of tinnitus; the mainstay of therapy is neurocognitive interventions to help patients cope with the problem.

Otitis Media

Acute otitis media is inflammation of the middle ear. It occurs predominantly in children. Despite the fact that it is diagnosed more than 5 million times each year in the United States, there is a paucity of quality studies of the disorder in children and remarkably little substantive literature about acute otitis media in adults. In some countries, such as the Netherlands, management is frequently observation only, in contrast to the United States, where this diagnosis is the leading cause of antibiotic prescriptions for children.

Otitis media usually follows an upper respiratory tract infection and is frequently accompanied by ear pain for 24 to 48 hours. Fever, although less common than ear pain, increases the likelihood of otitis media. In the pediatric literature, tympanic membrane bulging has the highest likelihood ratio for acute otitis media, followed by tympanic membrane cloudiness and immobility. Other signs include erythema of the tympanic membrane, with the likelihood ratio increasing for greater degrees of redness. Complications of acute otitis media include hearing loss, tympanic membrane perforation, mastoiditis, and meningitis. However, suppurative complications may occur in as few as 0.12% of untreated children.

There are no adequate trials of treatment in adults, but in children, the American Academy of Pediatrics and the American Academy of Family Practice currently recommend observation along with analgesic therapy in cases in which there is diagnostic uncertainty or in milder cases of otitis media. In patients in whom a decision is made to treat, amoxicillin should be used in patients who are not allergic to penicillin-containing antibiotics, with escalation to amoxicillin-clavulanate in 48 to 72 hours if the patient fails to improve or worsens. A macrolide antibiotic should be used as initial therapy in penicillin-allergic patients. An anti-inflammatory agent should be recommended for pain relief.

KEY POINT

- Complications of otitis media include hearing loss, tympanic membrane perforation, mastoiditis, and meningitis.

Otitis Externa

Otitis externa, a diffuse inflammation of the outer ear canal, may be acute or chronic. The acute form, which accounts for approximately 90% of cases of otitis externa, is usually caused by bacteria. The chronic form, which lasts 3 or more months, is usually caused by fungal infection, allergy, or a systemic dermatitis. Manifestations of otitis externa include pain, itching, and erythema early in the course but may progress to include edema, otorrhea and conductive hearing loss. Risk factors for the development of otitis externa include increased moisture, use of cotton-tipped swabs or bobby pins to clean the ear canal, use of hearing aids, and decreased production of cerumen, which contains an antimicrobial lysozyme and has a pH of 6.9, helping to inhibit bacterial growth.

Acute otitis externa can range from mild inflammation of the external canal to a severe and life-threatening infection if the temporal bone becomes involved. Onset is usually over a few days to a week and is initially manifested by pruritus, erythema, and discomfort, which progresses to edema of the canal, serous or purulent secretions, and pain with tugging on the pinna or moving the tragus. Approximately 50% of bacterial cases are caused by *Pseudomonas aeruginosa* and the remainder by *Staphylococcus aureus* and other aerobic and anaerobic bacteria. Fungi cause 10% or fewer cases of acute otitis externa; other etiologies, such as herpes zoster, cause fewer than 5% of cases. Hospital admission is usually not required, but is indicated if disease progresses to necrosis of the ear canal and osteomyelitis of the underlying bone (malignant otitis externa) or to involve the temporal or mastoid bones. These patients usually have disproportionate pain along with fever higher than 39.0 °C (102.2 °F); skin necrosis, facial paralysis, vertigo, and meningeal signs also may be present.

Chronic otitis externa is frequently caused by allergic contact dermatitis from earrings, cosmetics, soaps, shampoos, or the plastic components in hearing aids. Ironically, some patients initially treated for acute otitis externa develop a type IV delayed hypersensitivity reaction to the otic solutions used to treat the acute infection. Fungal infections causing otitis externa usually can be identified by the presence of white, cotton-like strands (*Candida*) with or without white or black fungal balls (*Aspergillus*).

Management of acute otitis externa involves clearing the canal of as much debris as possible to optimize penetration of ototopical agents as well as to visualize the tympanic membrane to ensure it is intact before initiating an ototopical agent. Most forms of otitis externa may be effectively treated with topical therapy. Mild otitis externa can be treated with a dilute acetic acid solution, although many practitioners still choose to prescribe a 7- to 10-day course of an ototopical agent containing neomycin, polymyxin B, and hydrocortisone for both mild and more severe forms. However, ototoxicity can occur from topical aminoglycosides when use is prolonged or the tympanic membrane is not intact; in addition, these agents can cause contact dermatitis in 5% to 18% of patients. Topical fluoroquinolones are more expensive but are approved for use when the tympanic membrane is not intact. Oral antibiotics should be considered for extra-canal involvement, for older patients, for those who have not responded to topical treatment, and for immunocompromised or diabetic patients. Patients with malignant otitis externa or disease involving the temporal or mastoid bones should be hospitalized and given intravenous antibiotics.

Fungal infections are usually treated with 2% acetic acid or isopropyl alcohol. Severe fungal infections may require treatment with topical antifungal agents, such as 1% clotrimazole.

KEY POINTS

- Management of otitis externa involves clearing the canal of as much debris as possible before initiating an ototopical agent.
- Patients with malignant otitis externa or involvement of the temporal or mastoid bones usually have disproportionate pain and fever higher than 39.0 °C (102.2 °F); hospital admission and intravenous antibiotics are indicated.

Cerumen Impaction

Cerumen cleans, protects, and lubricates the external auditory canal. Cerumen is normally eliminated by a mechanism involving jaw motion, causing it to migrate out of the ear canal. Accumulation of cerumen occurs when this self-cleaning mechanism is inadequate. Excess cerumen is present in 1 in 20 adults and one third of geriatric patients and is a common cause of visits to physicians for ear symptoms. Cerumen impaction refers to a collection of cerumen sufficiently large that it is either symptomatic or blocks visualization of the ear canal or tympanic membrane. Cerumen-related symptoms include pain, itching, tinnitus, odor, drainage, vertigo, and hearing loss. Hearing loss can range from 5 to 40 dB, depending on the degree of impaction.

Treatment options for cerumen impaction include observation without specific treatment, use of ceruminolytic agents, manual removal of cerumen, and irrigation. Evidence-based guidelines indicate that it is not necessary to remove the cerumen unless the patient is symptomatic or the canal or tympanic membrane needs to be evaluated. Patients should be reassured that cerumen is naturally occurring and has beneficial effects, and that specific efforts to cleanse the ear canals are not needed. Complications of treatment, which occur in approximately 1 in 1000 treated patients, include tympanic membrane perforation, ear canal laceration, infection, and hearing loss.

KEY POINT

- It is not necessary to remove cerumen from the ear canal unless the patient is symptomatic or the canal or tympanic membrane needs to be evaluated.

Upper Respiratory Tract Infections

Sinusitis

Acute sinusitis is a challenging clinical domain because the correlation between symptoms, pathophysiology, and treatment is tenuous. Evidence about diagnosis of sinusitis is limited. A history of cigarette smoking, allergic rhinitis, or previous episodes of sinusitis may indicate patients at increased risk. Common symptoms associated with sinusitis such as headache, facial pain and pressure that increases when bending forward, fever, and toothache have not been well assessed in comparison with gold standard tests such as sinus aspiration or radiography. Physical examination findings that have been shown to add diagnostic value include purulent rhinorrhea with unilateral predominance, local pain with unilateral predominance, bilateral purulent rhinorrhea, and pus in the nasal cavity. The presence of three or more of these symptoms has a positive likelihood ratio of 6.75. Imaging is rarely necessary in an average-risk patient, but should be considered in immunocompromised patients at risk for unusual organisms, such as fungal or pseudomonal sinusitis.

Initial treatment of patients with symptoms suggestive of acute sinusitis is largely symptomatic. Systemic antihistamines, intranasal corticosteroids, and topical decongestants have all been shown to be helpful. Topical decongestants should be limited to a few days of use to avoid rebound rhinitis (rhinitis medicamentosa). Evidence in acute sinusitis suggests a small increase in the number of patients whose symptoms resolve if antibiotics are used in patients with symptoms that have been present for at least 7 days. However, the cure rate is high in placebo-treated patients (80%); therefore, the number needed to treat is also high: between 8 and 15 patients would need to be treated with antibiotics to produce one additional cure. Because of this, some guidelines and clinicians recommend initial symptomatic treatment with initiation of antibiotics only in patients with 3 to 4 days of severe symptoms (such as fever ≥39.0 °C [102.2 °F], purulent drainage, and facial pain), worsening of symptoms that were initially improving following a typical upper respiratory tract infection, or failure to improve after 10 days. If antibiotics are used, there is no evidence of superiority for any particular antibiotic in patients without risk for infection with resistant organisms. Amoxicillin-clavulanate and doxycycline are both appropriate first-line agents.

Allergic Rhinitis

Allergic rhinitis should be strongly considered in a patient with rhinitis symptoms (sneezing, congestion, rhinorrhea) associated with a particular season, environment (for example, home or work), or exposure (such as pets). A detailed history of when and where symptoms occur can often point to a probable allergen. Although not a part of routine evaluation, either in vitro specific IgE antibody testing or skin testing can confirm an allergy to specific antigens if needed. Such testing is most valuable when considering allergen immunotherapy but should also be considered if the patient is considering expensive or difficult lifestyle changes to reduce allergen exposure.

Initial therapy should include an assessment of the options to reduce exposure to allergens; for example, closing windows and doors and using an air filter at home to mitigate pollen exposure. These measures can be cumbersome, however, and patients, especially those with mild or transient symptoms, may prefer pharmacotherapy. Treatment options include intranasal corticosteroids, oral antihistamines, intranasal antihistamines, oral leukotriene inhibitors, and intranasal cromolyn. Intranasal corticosteroids are considered first line therapy because of superior effectiveness in controlled trials. Cost and frequency of dosing are also important to consider in developing a treatment plan. Combining intranasal corticosteroids and oral antihistamines may be helpful in patients who have persistent symptoms with a single agent. Patients with specific allergies confirmed by testing may be candidates for allergen immunotherapy. Immunotherapy reduces symptoms and medication use but is expensive, requires multiple injections or sublingual administrations over a long period of time, and carries a small risk of systemic reactions with each injection.

Nonallergic Rhinitis

Patients with chronic rhinitis symptoms without an associated exposure may have nonallergic or vasomotor rhinitis. Nonallergic rhinitis may also have specific triggers, such as odors, spicy foods, and changes in temperature. The diagnosis is often evident by clinical history but may be confirmed by allergy testing, which reveals either no specific allergies or allergies that correlate poorly with the patient's symptoms. Treatments for nonallergic rhinitis include intranasal corticosteroids, antihistamines, and anticholinergic agents; oral medications are less effective for nonallergic rhinitis. Nasal saline irrigation may also be helpful.

Rhinitis medicamentosa is the syndrome of chronic rhinitis resulting from long-term use of topical nasal decongestants. Withdrawal of the offending medication is the only effective therapy, but management of the resulting rebound rhinitis is notoriously difficult. Intranasal corticosteroids may be helpful.

Many anatomic conditions and systemic illnesses should be considered in the differential diagnosis of chronic rhinitis. Anatomic conditions include deviated septum, nasal polyps, hypertrophic turbinates, and cerebrospinal fluid leak; systemic illnesses include sarcoidosis, granulomatosis with polyangiitis (also known as Wegener granulomatosis), cystic fibrosis, and hypothyroidism. Pregnancy also may be associated with chronic rhinorrhea and congestion.

Pharyngitis

Most cases of acute pharyngitis are viral and require no specific intervention other than symptomatic therapy. Because of the association between group A streptococcal (GAS) pharyngitis and rheumatic fever, however, GAS pharyngitis should be identified and treated to prevent rheumatic heart disease. However, empiric antimicrobial treatment not based on a clinical decision tool incorporating specific clinical information is discouraged as this has been shown to lead to significant inappropriate antibiotic use. The four-point Centor criteria are widely used to identify patients at risk of GAS pharyngitis: (1) fever (subjective or measured >38.1 °C [100.5 °F]); (2) absence of cough; (3) tonsillar exudates; and (4) tender anterior cervical lymphadenopathy. Patients with zero or one Centor criterion are low-risk and do not need additional testing. Patients with two or three criteria should have a confirmatory test (either a rapid GAS antigen test or throat culture; both studies are not necessary) and be treated based on the result. Patients meeting all four criteria should also have a confirmatory test but may be treated empirically while awaiting results.

Penicillin is the treatment of choice for GAS pharyngitis: options include a 10-day course of oral penicillin or a single intramuscular injection of penicillin G. The latter is a particularly good option in high-risk situations (for example, secondary prevention of rheumatic fever) or if there is concern about the patient completing a full course of oral therapy. A 10-day course of erythromycin or a 5-day course of azithromycin are alternatives in patients who are allergic to penicillin.

Group C and group G streptococci can cause a clinical syndrome similar to GAS pharyngitis, although often less severe. Although they have been associated with glomerulonephritis and reactive arthritis, group C and G streptococci are not known to cause acute rheumatic fever. Treatment with antibiotics may shorten the duration of symptoms, but controlled trials are lacking.

Lemierre Syndrome

Acute pharyngitis is rarely complicated by septic thrombosis of the internal jugular vein (Lemierre syndrome). This is most often caused by *Fusobacterium necrophorum*, an anaerobic gram-negative rod that is part of the normal oropharyngeal flora. Infection is thought to occur by contiguous spread through the tissues of the pharynx. The diagnosis should be suspected in anyone with antecedent pharyngitis and persistent fever despite antimicrobial therapy. Anterior neck pain and tenderness are frequently but not universally present. Soft tissue CT of the neck with contrast typically shows a jugular vein thrombus with surrounding tissue enhancement. Empiric therapy should be directed at both streptococci and anaerobes and should be active against β-lactamase–producing organisms. Therapy typically lasts at least 4 weeks.

- Initial treatment of patients with symptoms suggestive of acute sinusitis is largely symptomatic, including systemic antihistamines, intranasal corticosteroids, and topical decongestants.
- First-line therapy for the treatment of allergic rhinitis is an intranasal corticosteroid.
- Patients with pharyngitis with zero or one of the Centor criteria (fever, absence of cough, tonsillar exudates, tender anterior cervical lymphadenopathy) have a low risk of group A streptococcal infection, and do not need additional testing or antibiotic therapy.

Epistaxis

Epistaxis is a common occurrence, affecting 60% of the population some time in their lifetime; approximately 6% seek medical treatment. More than 90% of nosebleeds occur along the anterior portion of the nasal septum (the Kiesselbach area). This area receives its blood supply from branches of both the internal and external carotid arteries. Most episodes of anterior epistaxis can be controlled with patient-exerted direct pressure. The other 10% of epistaxis episodes occur posteriorly, along the nasal septum and lateral wall. This area's blood supply is from the external carotid artery via the sphenopalatine branch of the maxillary artery. Posterior epistaxis is more common in older patients.

The most common cause of epistaxis in children is nose picking; other causes in adults include the administration of intranasal medications such as corticosteroids or decongestants, dry nasal mucosa during winter months, viral or bacterial rhinosinusitis, and neoplasms. Systemic diseases associated with epistaxis include hematologic malignancies, hemophilia, and acquired bleeding disorders from liver or kidney disease. Iatrogenic causes associated with epistaxis include anticoagulant and antiplatelet medications and possibly *Ginkgo biloba* and ginseng supplements. Patients with epistaxis frequently have hypertension upon presenting to a health care provider; however, it is unclear whether chronic hypertension is associated with epistaxis or whether the hypertension is simply the result of anxiety owing to the epistaxis. Nosebleeds are rarely life threatening.

Evaluation of epistaxis begins with a history focused on frequency, location, whether the nosebleed is unilateral or bilateral, and evaluation of risk factors that may be associated with the bleeding. Ideally, the site of the bleed should be visualized in order to localize the epistaxis as anterior or posterior. Anesthetic or vasoconstrictor topical sprays (lidocaine with oxymetazoline, for example) may be needed both to control bleeding and allow visual localization of the bleeding site.

Unless the patient has severe epistaxis or has an associated systemic disease such as a coagulopathy or hematologic malignancy or is on medications that affect clotting, laboratory studies are usually not necessary. If these studies are obtained, a complete blood count and coagulation panel should be ordered. These studies, however, are normal in nearly 80% of patients, including those with systemic conditions that predispose to a coagulopathy. Imaging is also not required in most patients with epistaxis; in patients with recurrent unilateral epistaxis, particularly in those who smoke, a malignant or benign sinonasal neoplasm should be considered as a diagnostic possibility and radiographic imaging should be obtained.

Most anterior nosebleeds do not require any medical treatment and respond to compression of the nasal ala against the septum by the patient for at least 15 minutes. The head position while applying pressure can be either forward or backward depending on which is more comfortable. Vasoconstrictor topical agents may also be useful. If bleeding fails to resolve, cautery can be carried out with chemicals such as silver nitrate or electrical cautery by an otorhinolaryngologist. Anterior nasal packing (which is extremely uncomfortable for patients) for 1 to 3 days can be performed with either nondegradable products or absorbable or biodegradable products. These maneuvers work in 60% to 80% of patients in whom pressure and vasoconstrictor agents do not control bleeding. Patients with posterior epistaxis should be seen by an otorhinolaryngologist who may need to insert posterior packing which will stop 70% of posterior epistaxis. Patients for whom these maneuvers are unsuccessful may require surgical ligation or embolization of persistently bleeding nasal arteries.

Many physicians prescribe topical or oral antibiotics while packing is in place in either the anterior or posterior locations to prevent toxic shock syndrome. The true risk of developing toxic shock syndrome from nasal packing, however, is unknown.

- Most anterior nosebleeds do not require any medical treatment and respond to compression of the nasal ala against the septum for at least 15 minutes.

Oral Health

Various oral conditions can impact the overall health of the patient. Dental disease can cause pain and discomfort and result in nutritional compromise if the ability to chew is impaired. Periodontal disease has been associated with increased prevalence of coronary heart disease. Mucosal lesions can cause pain and discomfort, and oral cancers pose a direct threat to health. Xerostomia, common in elderly patients, is frequently exacerbated by medication adverse effects. Gingival hyperplasia is also strongly associated with exposure to medications: anticonvulsant agents (especially phenytoin), cyclosporine, and nifedipine are most frequently implicated.

The U.S. Preventive Services Task Force concluded in 2004 that the evidence is insufficient to recommend for or against screening adults for oral cancer. Some patients have poor access to dental care, however, and for these patients, and for patients at high risk of oral disease (tobacco, alcohol, or methamphetamine use; bulimia; family history of oral cancer), some groups recommend that screening oral examinations be performed. This examination should include inspection of the teeth and oral mucosa, looking for evidence of caries, periodontal disease, and leukoplakia or ulcerative lesions of the mucosa. Palpation of the neck and submandibular area for masses or lymphadenopathy is also appropriate.

Oral Infections and Ulcers

Oral lesions can be caused by infection, neoplasm, and systemic conditions. Common infectious causes of mucosal lesions include *Candida*, herpes simplex virus, coxsackievirus, HIV (bacillary angiomatosis, Kaposi sarcoma, hairy leukoplakia), and syphilis. The most common malignancy in the oral cavity is squamous cell carcinoma (particularly in tobacco users); melanoma can also occur. Systemic diseases associated with oral findings include lichen planus, bullous pemphigoid and pemphigus vulgaris, erythema multiforme and Stevens-Johnson syndrome, and Behçet syndrome. More information about oral mucosal lesions is provided in MKSAP 16 Dermatology.

Dental Infection

Dental infections may involve either the tooth and underlying bony structures or the gingiva and periodontal tissues. Infections of the tooth structure are typically asymptomatic until they involve the pulp cavity, at which point the patient develops a toothache. Infection frequently extends into the underlying bone, forming a periapical abscess. Definitive treatment of these types of infection requires either endodontic removal of diseased pulp (root canal) or extraction of the infected tooth. In patients without cellulitis or symptoms of systemic infection, antibiotic therapy is not necessary if dental intervention can be performed within several days.

Periodontal disease involves the gum, connective tissue, and bone supporting the teeth. Most periodontal disease is a chronic, indolent condition that poses a long-term risk of tooth loss. Periodontal disease has also been associated with atherosclerotic cardiovascular disease. Oral hygiene (including toothbrushing and flossing) and removal of plaque are the mainstay of therapy. Oral antimicrobial rinses may also be helpful in preventing progression of disease, although evidence is limited.

Halitosis

Eighty percent to 90% of cases of halitosis (bad breath) originate in the mouth. The remainder are attributed to other conditions, including chronic sinusitis, nasal polyps, and tonsillar stones. Some systemic conditions, such as ketoacidosis, advanced kidney failure, and advanced liver disease, can produce characteristic breath odors. Esophageal diverticula and chronic pulmonary infections (abscess, bronchiectasis) may also cause halitosis. A clinician can sometimes differentiate oral, nasal, and other causes of halitosis by positioning his or her nose in front of the patient's face and asking the patient to exhale several breaths through the mouth, then several through the nose. Oral halitosis should have a stronger odor coming from the mouth, and nasal from the nose; if both are equal it raises concern of a systemic, esophageal, or pulmonary cause of halitosis. Treatment for bad breath should focus on oral hygiene, particularly flossing between the teeth and cleaning (and possible scraping) the posterior tongue, both common sites of origin of halitosis. Patients with primary dental disorders (caries, abscesses, periodontal disease) should be referred for appropriate dental care. Chlorhexidine mouthwashes may reduce odor.

Tongue Syndromes

Geographic tongue manifests as patchy areas of atrophy of the filiform papillae, leading to erythematous patches on the tongue with white borders. Lesions typically recur and regress in various areas over time. Patients are usually asymptomatic, although tongue discomfort is occasionally reported.

Atrophic glossitis, a bright red, smooth, sometimes tender tongue without visible taste buds, can be seen in patients with vitamin B_{12} deficiency and has been reported in those with iron deficiency and with celiac disease. Treatment should be directed at the underlying disorder.

Burning Mouth Syndrome

Burning mouth syndrome is characterized by a burning sensation in the mouth or tongue in the absence of an explanatory diagnosis. Patients frequently have other oral symptoms such as dryness or taste alterations. It appears to be most prevalent in postmenopausal women. It is typically managed by addressing xerostomia, if present, and excluding other possible causes, such as atrophic candidiasis, herpes virus infection, post-herpetic neuralgia, local reaction to dental products, and nutritional deficiencies. Medications directed at neuropathic pain, such as anticonvulsant agents and tricyclic antidepressants, may be helpful.

Temporomandibular Disorders

Temporomandibular disorders are a group of pain problems that involve the temporomandibular joint (TMJ) and associated structures. Typical features include jaw pain and headache and clicking, grinding, or grating at the TMJ. Although temporomandibular symptoms are common, most are self-limiting; fewer than 5% of adults with temporomandibular symptoms develop chronic symptoms. Temporomandibular disorders are classified into articular disorders, which include derangements of the intra-articular disk that normally sits between the mandibular condyle and its articulation in the glenoid fossa, and masticatory muscle disorders, which include myofascial pain syndrome.

Diagnostic evaluation of temporomandibular disorders should focus on eliminating alternative diagnoses, such as dental pain, otitis and mastoiditis, salivary gland disorders, temporal arteritis, trigeminal neuralgia, and herpes zoster. Palpation of the TMJ by applying mild anterior pressure with a finger placed posteriorly to each tragus may reveal tenderness, clicking, or crepitus. Side-to-side jaw movement with the fingers palpating the TMJ may also show similar abnormalities or asymmetry in findings. The jaw muscles should also be palpated for evidence of asymmetry or tenderness. Although not indicated in most patients, diagnostic imaging may be helpful in excluding dental disease if suspected and assessing TMJ anatomy to distinguish articular disorders from muscle disorders in complex cases. CT is particularly helpful in the diagnosis of osteoarthritis of the TMJ, whereas MRI provides additional information about the soft tissues, vascularization, and cartilaginous structures. In general, the therapeutic value of imaging is modest, and most patients are managed conservatively regardless of the underlying etiology.

Initial treatment of temporomandibular disorders focuses on noninterventional, nonpharmacologic strategies. Jaw relaxation, heat, and therapeutic exercises may be helpful. For patients with chronic temporomandibular disorders, cognitive-behavioral therapy has been shown to reduce pain, depression, and interference with activities. Biofeedback may also be of value. Jaw appliances and occlusal splints have been a prominent part of temporomandibular disorder therapy for years despite questionable evidence of benefit. Evidence is limited on the benefit of pharmacotherapy, but NSAIDs and tricyclic antidepressants are sometimes used.

Patients with anatomic abnormalities of the TMJ, such as osteoarthritis or disk derangements, may benefit from intra-articular injections of corticosteroids or hyaluronic acid, although neither is recommended for long-term use. Arthrocentesis, arthroscopy, and joint replacement may be helpful, but controlled trials are few and of poor quality.

KEY POINT

- Initial treatment of temporomandibular disorders focuses on noninterventional, nonpharmacologic strategies, such as jaw relaxation, heat, and therapeutic exercises.

Anorectal Disorders

Approach to the Patient with Anorectal Disorders

Patients with anorectal disorders should be questioned regarding bowel frequency and consistency, bleeding, pain,

and itching. Weight loss may suggest underlying inflammatory bowel disease or malignancy. Fever may be associated with abscess. Hard stools can contribute to the formation of hemorrhoids and anal fissures, and history of sharp pain following instrumentation or an unusually hard bowel movement should increase suspicion of anal fissure. Pain with defecation is typical of anal fissures and anorectal abscesses but can also occur with hemorrhoids. A palpable mass on defecation suggests a prolapsed internal hemorrhoid or overt anal prolapse.

Physical examination should include inspection for external masses, thrombosed external hemorrhoids, skin lesions, and excoriations. Having the patient bear down during the examination can sometimes reveal prolapsed internal hemorrhoids. Digital rectal examination is valuable to exclude perirectal abscess and anorectal neoplasia. Anoscopy allows for visualization of internal hemorrhoids, anal fissures, and cancers of the anal canal.

Hemorrhoids and Rectal Bleeding

Hemorrhoids are dilated veins in the hemorrhoidal plexus surrounding the anal canal. They are classified as internal or external depending on whether they are above or below the dentate line. Internal hemorrhoids are more frequently associated with painless bleeding, whereas external hemorrhoids more often cause pain; thrombosed external hemorrhoids are particularly painful. Internal hemorrhoids may prolapse and only be externally visible or palpable during a bowel movement or Valsalva maneuver.

Hemorrhoids are a common cause of bright red blood from the rectum, and further evaluation should be based on risk for colon cancer and other gastrointestinal diseases. Visualizing a hemorrhoid or other source of bleeding in a low-risk patient younger than 40 years without other symptoms to suggest inflammatory bowel disease or colon cancer may spare the patient further endoscopic evaluation as the risk of malignancy is low in this age group. Patients 40 to 50 years old with typical hemorrhoidal symptoms but at low risk for colon cancer should probably have at least sigmoidoscopy. In patients older than 50 years, rectal bleeding should not be considered hemorrhoidal without additional investigation. These patients should undergo colonoscopy to evaluate the source of bleeding provided that routine screening has not been recently performed.

Initial treatment of hemorrhoids should focus on interventions to soften bowel movements, sitz baths, and topical anesthetics or topical corticosteroids to relieve pain and itching. Recurrent hemorrhoids that fail to respond to conservative therapy can be treated with sclerotherapy, banding, photocoagulation, or surgical resection.

KEY POINT

- In patients older than 50 years, rectal bleeding should not be considered hemorrhoidal without additional investigation.

Anal Fissure

Anal fissures are tears in the anal skin distal to the dentate line, and may therefore be exquisitely painful, particularly with defecation. They are most often caused by local trauma such as hard stools or anal instrumentation. High-fiber diets and other measures that soften stools may help to reduce the risk of anal fissures, although the specific causes are poorly understood, particularly of fissures that are persistent or recurrent. Anoscopy typically reveals a small mucosal tear, most often in the posterior midline.

Acute anal fissures often heal spontaneously; treatment should start with warm sitz baths for symptom relief, increased dietary fiber to soften stools, and topical anesthetics to decrease pain with bowel movements. Chronic anal fissures are more challenging to treat. Topical nitroglycerin has the most evidence of benefit but must be compounded at a lower concentration for anorectal use (0.2% instead of 2%, the standard concentration). Topical calcium channel blockers (also compounded) and botulinum toxin injections may also be helpful, but evidence is limited. Internal anal sphincterotomy is occasionally used for refractory anal fissures but carries an increased risk of incontinence.

Anorectal Abscess

Anorectal abscesses typically originate in one of the anal crypt glands surrounding the anal canal at the dentate line. Pain and tenderness to palpation are typical, and fluctuance may be noted either on palpation of the external anus or internally on digital rectal examination.

Definitive management involves surgical drainage, which can often be accomplished in an outpatient setting with local anesthesia. Antibiotics are generally unnecessary unless there are specific risk factors, such as extensive cellulitis, diabetes mellitus, or the patient is immunocompromised.

Chronic Anorectal Pain

Chronic anorectal pain syndromes include chronic proctalgia (levator ani syndrome), characterized by chronic pain or aching, with episodes lasting more than 20 minutes, and proctalgia fugax, characterized by sudden severe pain that disappears completely within seconds or minutes. Neither condition is well understood. The approach to chronic proctalgia is similar to other chronic pain syndromes. Proctalgia fugax rarely requires specific treatment because of the brief nature of symptoms.

Pruritus Ani

Many conditions, including infection, primary skin diseases, local irritants, and malignancy, can cause anal itching. Dietary factors, including caffeine, alcohol, spices, citrus foods, milk products, tomatoes, and peanuts, have been implicated in pruritus ani; dietary modification is frequently recommended, although its effectiveness has not been established.

For some patients, anal itching becomes a primary and self-perpetuating problem. Patients should have a careful external and digital rectal examination; endoscopic evaluation should be considered in patients with a history of rectal bleeding or change in bowel movements. Patients without an apparent underlying cause should be counseled on proper anal hygiene (fecal soiling can cause irritation), including the avoidance of excessive cleaning or astringent cleansers. Protective ointments such as zinc oxide and limited short-term use of topical corticosteroids may be helpful.

Mental and Behavioral Health

Depression

The prevalence of depression in the United States is 15%, and depression is the second most common cause of primary care visits. Patients with chronic medical disorders, such as diabetes mellitus, heart disease, stroke, and cancer, have an increased risk of developing depression, and depression can negatively influence morbidity and mortality outcomes in these patients.

Despite its high prevalence and severe negative effects, depression often goes undiagnosed in the primary care setting. Brief screening tools have been validated, with the simplest being a two-question instrument (see Routine Care of the Healthy Patient). It is imperative to assess the presence of suicidal ideation and level of functional impairment, which may guide treatment decisions. Patients with active suicidal plans warrant urgent referral to a psychiatrist or emergency hospitalization in order to immediately treat their depression.

Diagnosis of Depressive Disorders

A major depressive episode is diagnosed according to the DSM-IV by the presence of five or more of the following symptoms during the same 2-week period, at least one of which is either (1) depressed mood or (2) loss of interest or pleasure:

1. Depressed mood most of the day, nearly every day

2. Loss of interest or pleasure in all or almost all activities most of the day, nearly every day

3. Significant weight loss when not dieting, or weight gain; or decrease or increase in appetite nearly every day

4. Insomnia or hypersomnia nearly every day

5. Psychomotor agitation or retardation nearly every day

6. Fatigue or loss of energy nearly every day

7. Feelings of worthlessness or inappropriate guilt nearly every day

8. Diminished ability to think or concentrate nearly every day

9. Recurrent thoughts of death, recurrent suicidal ideation with or without a specific plan; suicide attempt

The nine-item Patient Health Questionnaire (PHQ-9) is a validated instrument for identifying and assessing severity of depression, with a sensitivity of 80% and specificity of 92%. Each of the nine symptoms is scored from 0 (not bothered by the symptom at all) to 3 (bothered by the symptom nearly every day), for a maximum score of 27. A score of 10 or greater indicates the diagnosis of depression.

Minor (subsyndromal) depression is characterized by the presence in the preceding 2 weeks of two to four depressive symptoms associated with impaired social functioning, mental health, and health perceptions. Dysthymia has a similar level of symptoms as minor depression but symptoms must be present most of the time for a duration of 2 years or more. Depressive symptoms are common after the loss of a loved one; treatment should be considered if the bereaved person meets the criteria for major depression 2 months after the loss.

Seasonal affective disorder is a cyclical depression usually occurring in the fall and winter months with improvement in spring and summer. Lack of exposure to sunlight seems to be the triggering factor.

Premenstrual dysphoric disorder occurs in 3% to 5% of menstruating women. It is characterized by recurrent symptoms of depression, anxiety, or emotional lability within 1 week of menstruation and resolving within 1 week after menstruation. Postpartum depression occurs in up to 15% of women within 6 months of giving birth and can lead to significant negative outcomes in both mother and child, such as decreased effectiveness at home and work, increased risk of maternal suicide, and poorer infant-mother bonding.

Management of Depression

Most patients with mild to moderate depression can be diagnosed and treated by primary care physicians. Before initiating treatment the physician should rule out underlying medical illnesses causing depressive symptoms and evaluate any comorbid conditions. Treatment can be multimodal and may include medication, psychotherapy, or a combination of both. Psychiatric referral is recommended for any patient with (1) suicidal or homicidal ideation, (2) bipolar disorder, (3) psychotic symptoms, or (4) symptoms refractory to at least two medications.

Response rates with cognitive-behavioral therapy (CBT), interpersonal therapy, or psychodynamic therapy are similar to those with medication alone; the best outcomes occur with the combination of medication and formal psychotherapy, which is usually performed by a trained psychotherapist.

There are several classes of antidepressant agents with proven efficacy in relieving depressive symptoms (**Table 49**). The choice of agent is primarily based on side effect profile, cost, prominent symptoms, and patient preference. Treatment should be to full remission of symptoms, and symptoms should be monitored regularly. The American College of Physicians recommends that treatment for a first episode continue for 4 to 9 months after full remission of symptoms, and that patients with recurrent depression consider lifelong therapy.

Antidepressants have been associated with a risk of precipitating suicidal ideation in children, adolescents, and young adults; therefore, close monitoring is required. The risk of suicide in untreated depression, however, is likely much greater.

The most commonly prescribed antidepressants are currently the selective serotonin reuptake inhibitors (SSRIs), which have good efficacy and also treat anxiety syndromes. SSRIs have an excellent safety profile compared with tricyclic antidepressants, but sexual side effects are common. Serotonin-norepinephrine reuptake inhibitors (SNRIs) may be especially helpful in patients with concomitant pain syndromes. Bupropion may be a good alternative for those with sexual side effects on SSRI or SNRI therapy but may lower seizure threshold in higher doses and thus is contraindicated in patients with seizure disorders. Because of potential interactions with other medications, monoamine oxidase inhibitors (MAOIs) are not frequently used relative to other agents. However, a transdermal preparation of selegiline is available that is the only nonoral antidepressant available. All SSRIs, SNRIs, and MAOIs can cause serotonin syndrome, which is characterized by mental status changes, neuromuscular hyperactivity, and autonomic instability and is potentially lethal.

Patients refractory to a single SSRI may respond to a change in therapy, which may include replacement with another antidepressant, either from the same or a different class; addition of a second antidepressant; or a psychotherapeutic intervention. Patients with severe or refractory depressive symptoms (suicidality, poor cognitive functioning, interference with activities of daily living) should be referred to psychiatric providers, who may employ electroconvulsive and other multimodality interventions.

The treatment of seasonal affective disorder involves full-spectrum light therapy in addition to antidepressants and CBT.

Treatment of premenstrual and postpartum depression is similar to that of other forms of depression. There are no contraindications to breastfeeding while on antidepressants; however, SSRIs and SNRIs are FDA pregnancy category C, which warrants consideration of risks and benefits of treating maternal depression versus theoretical risks to the fetus.

TABLE 49. Characteristics of Selected Antidepressants

Drug	Advantages	Disadvantages
SSRIs		
Citalopram	Few drug interactions	Gastrointestinal, sexual side effects
Escitalopram	Few drug interactions	Gastrointestinal, sexual side effects
Fluoxetine	Long half-life reduces risk of withdrawal syndrome; effective for anxiety disorders, OCD, PMDD	Long half-life can lead to accumulation, drug interactions common (cytochrome P-450 inhibitor)
Paroxetine	Effective for anxiety disorders, panic disorder, PTSD, OCD	High risk in pregnancy (class D), drug interactions (cytochrome P-450 inhibitor), weight gain; high risk for withdrawal syndrome
Sertraline	Few drug interactions; effective for panic disorder, PTSD, OCD, PMDD	
SNRIs		
Venlafaxine	Effective in anxiety disorders	Nausea, can increase blood pressure
Desvenlafaxine	Effective in anxiety disorders	Nausea, can increase blood pressure
Duloxetine	Effective in pain conditions, generalized anxiety disorder	Nausea, urinary retention
Tricyclic antidepressants		
Nortriptyline	Drug level monitoring possible, analgesic effect	Cardiac toxicity with overdose, anticholinergic effects
Amitriptyline	Analgesic effect, sedating effect	Cardiac toxicity with overdose, anticholinergic effects, sedation, weight gain
Serotonin antagonist/norepinephrine agonist		
Mirtazapine	Sedating, increased appetite; available as orally disintegrating tablet	Weight gain, sedation
Norepinephrine and dopamine reuptake inhibitor		
Bupropion	Fewer sexual side effects than SSRIs, improved concentration, less weight gain	Seizure risk
MAOIs		Oral formulation can cause hypertensive crisis, serotonin syndrome
Tranylcypromine	Good for atypical symptoms	Dietary restrictions, hypertensive crisis, hypotension, serotonin syndrome
Selegiline transdermal system	Fewer dietary restrictions than other MAOIs, transdermal	Hypotension, serotonin syndrome

GAD = generalized anxiety disorder; MAOI = monoamine oxidase inhibitor; OCD = obsessive-compulsive disorder; PMDD = premenstrual dysphoric disorder; PTSD = posttraumatic stress disorder; SNRI = serotonin-norepinephrine reuptake inhibitor; SSRI = selective serotonin reuptake inhibitor.

KEY POINTS

- Psychiatric referral is recommended for any patient with depression associated with suicidal or homicidal ideation, bipolar disorder, psychotic symptoms, or refractory symptoms.
- In the treatment of depression, the best outcomes are achieved with a combination of medication and psychotherapy.

Anxiety Disorders

Anxiety disorders are among the most common psychiatric disorders in the general population; of these, generalized anxiety disorder (GAD) is the most common, with a prevalence of approximately 4% to 6%. GAD is characterized by excessive anxiety and worry about various events or activities on most days for at least 6 months, with difficulty controlling worrying. Associated symptoms include fatigue, irritability, restlessness, insomnia, and difficulty concentrating. Patients with GAD often have comorbid anxiety disorders, depression, or substance abuse. Patients with GAD often have somatoform symptoms, which can make them high utilizers of health care resources. Most patients with GAD or panic disorder present to their primary care physician or the emergency department rather than a mental health professional. The history should include inquiries into underlying medical conditions that can cause anxiety symptoms as well as any history of comorbid psychiatric disorders, substance abuse, recent stressors, coping skills, and family history of psychiatric disorders.

Panic disorder is a syndrome characterized by sudden panic attacks with the sudden onset of somatic symptoms, which may include chest pain, palpitations, sweating, nausea, dizziness, dyspnea, and numbness. These symptoms usually last from 5 to 60 minutes. The diagnosis of panic disorder requires that an attack be followed by at least 1 month of worry about a recurrence of an attack. The incidence of panic disorder is twice as high in women as in men. About one half of patients with panic disorder also have associated agoraphobia, with fears of being in crowds or in places from which escape would be difficult. Studies have shown higher suicide attempt rates in those with panic disorder compared with the general population. Although not common, medical disorders potentially presenting with anxiety-like symptoms need to be considered, including cardiac disease, thyroid disease, or pheochromocytoma.

Treatment options for GAD and panic disorder include medication and psychotherapy. CBT has been shown to be the most effective psychotherapeutic intervention in controlled trials, appears to be equal in efficacy to pharmacologic interventions, and has a lower relapse rate. SSRIs and SNRIs have been shown to be effective for both GAD and panic disorder. Buspirone is another pharmacologic option, although it may take several weeks to show clinical effect. Benzodiazepines are frequently used, either alone or in conjunction with other treatments, although they carry a risk of dependence and should not be used in those with a history of substance abuse. Panic disorder that is severe or refractory appears to be most amenable to the combination of CBT and pharmacotherapy compared with either treatment alone.

Posttraumatic Stress Disorder

Clinical Presentation

Posttraumatic stress disorder (PTSD) occurs in response to exposure to a traumatic event that involves serious threat to oneself or others. PTSD is characterized by at least 1 month of symptoms that include intrusive thoughts about the trauma, nightmares or flashbacks, avoidance of reminders of the event, and hypervigilance with sleep disturbance. To meet DSM-IV criteria, the symptoms must be in each of three areas: re-experiencing the event, avoiding reminders of the event, and heightened arousal. Risk factors for PTSD include lower socioeconomic status, parental neglect, a family or personal history of a psychiatric condition, poor social support, and initial severity of reaction to the traumatic event. Common events precipitating PTSD include military combat, sexual assault, mass displacement or disaster, and severe physical illness. PTSD most commonly presents within 1 month of the traumatic event, but symptoms can be delayed for more than 6 months. Comorbid psychiatric conditions may include depression, anxiety, and substance abuse. Traumatic brain injury (TBI) and postconcussion syndrome are often coexistent as

well (see MKSAP 16 Neurology). A study of returning U.S. veterans reported that patients with mild TBI had a 6-fold greater prevalence of PTSD versus those without such an injury. Patients with PTSD have a higher incidence of marital and occupational problems and a higher incidence of suicide than the general population.

Treatment

PTSD symptoms are complex and often require multimodal treatments. Early intervention may prevent chronicity of symptoms. No advantage has been identified for either psychotherapy or pharmacotherapy, although, for patients with refractory PTSD, combination therapy may be most useful. Trauma-focused CBT focuses on cognitively reframing distorted thinking patterns while gradually re-exposing the patient to the traumatic experience to allow desensitization of triggered symptoms. Simple stress management interventions can also be helpful in alleviating some symptoms. The most effective medications for PTSD are SSRIs, with positive symptoms (hyperarousal, flashbacks) responding best. Tricyclic antidepressants may also be used. Benzodiazepines have not been shown to be effective despite their anxiolytic effect. Finally, the α-blocker prazosin has been demonstrated to reduce the incidence and severity of nightmares but not other associated symptoms.

Social Anxiety Disorder

Social anxiety disorder is one of the most common anxiety disorders, with a lifetime prevalence estimated at 2.4%. It is characterized by a severe, persistent fear of social or performance situations, such as public speaking, test taking, or parties. In these situations, autonomic symptoms of anxiety occur, including blushing, dyspnea, palpitations, and emotional distress. Social anxiety disorder can be generalized or specific to a single activity. Patients generally realize their fear is excessive and often avoid trigger situations, which may lead to impairment in social function. Effective treatments include CBT as well as SSRI pharmacotherapy. Pharmacotherapy, particularly with an SSRI, has been demonstrated effective for both short- and long-term use. MAOIs have shown efficacy, although to a lesser extent.

Obsessive-Compulsive Disorder

Patients with obsessive-compulsive disorder (OCD) report recurrent obsessions or compulsions sufficiently severe to occupy 1 hour daily or result in marked distress or impaired social function. Obsessions are persistent ideas, thoughts, impulses, or images experienced as intrusive and are associated with significant anxiety or distress. Examples include fears of having left doors unlocked and fears of germ contamination. Compulsions are repetitive behaviors, such as handwashing, checking, ordering, or counting, that are repeated to decrease the anxiety related to the obsessions.

CBT, with exposure and response prevention interventions, is the preferred primary treatment for OCD. Pharmacotherapy is used in conjunction with CBT in patients with severe symptoms or in those with an incomplete response to CBT alone. SSRIs in higher doses are the primary pharmacotherapy, although clomipramine may be effective; some antipsychotic agents may also be useful as adjunctive therapy in severe cases.

KEY POINTS

- Cognitive-behavioral therapy is the most effective nonpharmacologic intervention for generalized anxiety disorder and panic disorder and may be equal in efficacy to pharmacologic interventions and have lower relapse rates.
- Cognitive-behavioral therapy, with exposure and response prevention interventions, is the preferred primary treatment for obsessive-compulsive disorder.

Intermittent Explosive Disorder

Intermittent explosive disorder (IED), an impulse control disorder, may affect 0.3% of the U.S. population. It is characterized by repeated episodes of aggressive violent behaviors grossly out of proportion to the situation. Examples include road rage, severe temper tantrums, and domestic abuse. Explosive episodes may be accompanied by feelings of irritability or rage and by physical symptoms of tingling, tremors, palpitations, or head pressure. Outbursts may result in injury. Persons with IED often later express remorse or embarrassment. Episodes may occur in clusters or be separated in time.

Treatment is achieved through both CBT and pharmacotherapy. Mood stabilizers and anticonvulsant agents (such as carbamazepine, phenytoin, and lithium) may be effective in decreasing aggressive behavior. SSRIs are helpful in treating comorbid depression in these patients.

Bipolar Disorder

Bipolar disorder is characterized by manic or hypomanic mood episodes and depressive episodes and affect up to 2% of the general population. A manic episode is marked by a persistent period of elevated mood, irritability, lack of need for sleep, racing thoughts, high energy levels, increased talkativeness, spending sprees, hypersexuality, and increased self-confidence, with possible delusions of grandeur or psychosis. Bipolar disorder is a leading cause of suicide, and is highly associated with substance abuse problems. Bipolar disorder is thought to be underdiagnosed; many patients presenting with symptoms of major depression are not asked about manic symptoms and are therefore not recognized as having bipolar disease.

Treatment of bipolar disorder is more complex than unipolar depression and is optimally managed in conjunction with a psychiatrist. Treatment is mainly with mood-stabilizing drugs (lithium, valproate, carbamazepine) or lamotrigine and is vital given the high recurrence of both depressive and manic symptoms in the absence of treatment. Although lithium has long been the mainstay of maintenance therapy, it has a narrow therapeutic window with long-term negative effects on the thyroid and kidneys; in addition, it is teratogenic. For acute manic episodes, the combination of either lithium or valproate with an atypical antipsychotic agent such as olanzapine, quetiapine or aripiprazole appears to be more effective than either mood stabilizer alone. Adjunctive psychotherapy may help patients adjust to having this chronic illness and may enhance compliance with maintenance pharmacotherapy. It is important that the history be assessed for manic symptoms in any patient being considered for initiation of pharmacologic treatment for depression, both to identify the presence of the disorder and to avoid triggering a manic episode, which may occur with treatment with SSRIs.

Somatoform Disorders

Clinical Presentation and Evaluation

Somatization refers to the presence of medically unexplained symptoms (MUSs). MUSs are seen in all populations, although they are more common in women, minorities, and those with less education or lower socioeconomic status. MUSs are relatively common in primary care offices, accounting for up to 50% of all symptom-related visits. Although 10% to 20% of patients in primary care practices have four or more unexplained symptoms, only a small number of these patients have a true somatoform disorder. True somatoform disorders are psychiatric diseases that involve persistent medically unexplained symptoms or symptoms that are out of proportion to medically expected findings and significantly affect a patient's ability to function. Somatoform disorders can cause great distress to patients, families, and physicians; in addition, patients suffering from these diseases are often high utilizers of the medical system, subjecting them to batteries of costly and potentially dangerous diagnostic tests.

Somatization disorder requires that multiple MUSs be present for years in multiple organ systems, although each symptom can wax and wane and all need not be present simultaneously. To fulfill the diagnostic criteria, symptoms need to have started before age 30 years and include gastrointestinal, pain, pseudoneurologic, and sexual symptoms. *Undifferentiated somatoform disorder* requires only a single somatic symptom that is present for at least 6 months (for example, nausea). Patients with *conversion disorder* have a single pseudoneurologic symptom that is not explained by a medical evaluation and often follows lay understanding of neurology (for example, hemiparesis that does not follow crossed corticospinal tracts). In *hypochondriasis*, patients misinterpret normal bodily sensations and are afraid these symptoms are manifestations of serious illness. Patients with *body dysmorphic disorder* are preoccupied with a real (usually minor) or imagined physical finding (for example, swelling of the face when examination reveals no edema).

The evaluation of possible somatoform disorders requires the consideration of both a medical and psychiatric differential diagnosis. Even when somatoform disorders are strongly suspected, clinicians should perform a thorough history and physical examination to construct a differential diagnosis that could explain a patient's symptoms medically. Laboratory and other testing should be ordered logically to evaluate plausible medical diagnoses; extensive and elaborate testing to explore unsupported or very unlikely diagnoses should be avoided despite a patient's concerns and requests. Testing should not be ordered to reassure a patient, as tests, even those with normal results, rarely help patients improve their level of function and increase the risk of iatrogenic complications. It is also important to screen for psychiatric comorbidities, including depression, panic disorder, and substance abuse. In addition, clinicians must carefully rule out malingering and factitious disorders. In these conditions, a patient purposely adopts a physical symptom. Patients with malingering do this for external gain (such as avoidance of work), whereas those with a factitious disorder do so in order to remain in the sick role.

Management

Patients with a somatoform disorder are psychologically dependent on potential illness, and unlike conversion or malingering, the symptoms expressed are not consciously fabricated. Treatment for somatoform disorders starts with an honest discussion of the diagnosis. Comorbid medical or psychiatric diseases should be treated. Regular office visits should be scheduled at frequent intervals. Some patients will need limits on visits or between-visit communications. Visits should focus on new or changed symptoms. These should be thoroughly evaluated to exclude new medical problems, although the disorder may require an increased reliance on physical signs rather than symptoms. Otherwise, primary care encounters should focus on functioning with symptoms rather than elimination of the symptoms.

No therapy has been shown to be consistently helpful in treating somatoform disorders. Reassurance can be helpful; however, it rarely leads to a resolution of symptoms. Although antidepressants have shown benefit in patients with medically unexplained symptoms, they have not been consistently shown to benefit patients with somatoform disorders. Several studies have shown a benefit from CBT, and psychiatric evaluation is often appropriate. Such referrals must be handled with care because patients with somatoform disorders can be sensitive to feelings of abandonment.

KEY POINT

- In patients with somatoform disorders, primary care visits should focus on the evaluation of new or changed symptoms and functioning with somatic symptoms rather than elimination of the symptoms.

Eating Disorders

Types of Eating Disorders

Anorexia nervosa is defined by four diagnostic criteria: an abnormally low body weight (<85% of expected) in association with an intense fear of gaining weight, an overemphasis of body weight on self-evaluation, and, in women and girls, amenorrhea for at least three consecutive menstrual cycles. It is classified as either restricting (with regular caloric restriction) or binge-eating/purging (binge eating that may or may not be associated with self-induced vomiting or the misuse of laxatives, diuretics, or enemas). The lifetime prevalence of anorexia nervosa is 1.0% to 3.7%, with adolescent girls and young women disproportionately affected. A family history of eating disorders or a diagnosis of childhood anxiety or OCD increases the risk for developing anorexia nervosa. The SCOFF questionnaire is a brief five-question instrument that can be used in the primary care setting to screen for anorexia nervosa (**Table 50**).

Physical signs of anorexia nervosa may be obvious on general inspection, as patients may present with parotid gland hyperplasia, dry and brittle hair, lanugo, yellowing skin, and

TABLE 50.	SCOFF Questionnaire for Screening for Eating Disorders
S	Do you make yourself Sick because you feel uncomfortably full?
C	Do you worry that you have lost Control over how much you eat?
O	Have you recently lost more than One stone (6.4 kg [14 lb]) in a 3-month period?
F	Do you believe yourself to be Fat when others say you are too thin?
F	Would you say Food dominates your life?

Score one point for each yes. A score of two or more points indicates a likely diagnosis of anorexia nervosa or bulimia.

Adapted with permission from Morgan JF, Reid F, Lacey JH. The SCOFF questionnaire: assessment of a new screening tool for eating disorders. BMJ. 1999;319(7223):1467-1468. [PMID: 10582927] Copyright 1999, BMJ Publishing Group Ltd.

xerosis. Other signs include a low BMI (usually <18.5), bradycardia, orthostatic hypotension, and hypothermia. Cognitive impairment and a depressed or anxious mood are common in patients with anorexia nervosa, and these patients are also at high risk for suicide.

In a study reviewing the prognosis of 5590 patients treated for anorexia nervosa, the mortality rate was 5%. Among survivors, approximately 47% experienced a full recovery, whereas 33% improved and 20% remained chronically ill. Younger age (<19 years) and treatment within 3 years of diagnosis may be associated with improved recovery rates.

Although bulimia nervosa is more common than anorexia nervosa, affecting approximately 1% to 1.5% of women, it may be more difficult to diagnose. This disorder is characterized by recurrent episodes of binge eating with compensatory behavior aimed at preventing weight gain, including self-induced vomiting and misuse of medications (purging type) or fasting and excessive exercise (nonpurging type). Additional diagnostic criteria include the presence of these behaviors at least twice a week for 3 months and the excessive influence of body weight and shape on the patient's self-perception. Patients with bulimia nervosa are usually ashamed of and secretive about their abnormal eating patterns and may not seek medical treatment; nor may bulimia be suspected in typically normal-weight patients. The SCOFF screening tool, as well as subtle physical findings, such as dental caries and enlarged salivary glands, may aid in the diagnosis of bulimia nervosa. Scarring on the dorsum of the hand (Russell sign) caused by repeated abrasions during self-induced vomiting, is highly suggestive. As with anorexia nervosa, additional psychiatric illnesses may accompany bulimia nervosa, including anxiety and depression.

Eating disorder not otherwise specified (EDNOS) is diagnosed in patients who have disordered eating but do not fulfill the diagnostic criteria for anorexia nervosa or bulimia nervosa. The most common subtype of EDNOS is binge-eating disorder, which has a prevalence of about 2% to 3% in the general population; approximately one third of diagnosed patients are male. Characteristic behavior includes consumption of large quantities of food in a 2-hour period with an associated sense of lack of control. Although the binge episodes often occur in secret and patients feels disgust afterward, there is no compensatory behavior after the binge. Characteristic physical findings include an increased BMI; some patients may be severely obese. The Eating Attitudes Test (www.eat-26.com) is a useful screen for binge-eating disorder in the primary care setting.

Medical Complications of Eating Disorders

Hypokalemia, hypomagnesemia, and metabolic alkalosis may be seen in patients with anorexia nervosa or bulimia nervosa. A patient with severe anorexia nervosa may experience significant cardiovascular complications, including bradycardia and orthostatic hypotension; hospitalization is necessary if these

abnormalities are noted. The hypoestrogenic state that is characteristic of anorexia nervosa results in amenorrhea and low bone mineral density, and current guidelines recommend obtaining a dual-energy x-ray absorptiometry scan if menses are absent for more than 6 months. The most worrisome complication of anorexia nervosa is refeeding syndrome, which occurs when a severely malnourished patient receives aggressive oral, enteral, or parenteral nutritional repletion. This syndrome is associated with large volume shifts and sudden changes in electrolyte levels, resulting in edema, hypomagnesemia, hypophosphatemia, hypokalemia, and in rare cases, death. Close monitoring and repletion of electrolytes are essential for avoiding this complication.

Treatment of Eating Disorders

There is limited evidence to indicate the optimal therapeutic approach in patients with anorexia nervosa. Individual psychotherapy may be most beneficial during acute refeeding, and there is weak evidence that CBT is efficacious in preventing relapse after weight has been restored. There is no role for monotherapy with psychotropic medications in anorexia nervosa, although they are indicated to treat comorbid psychiatric disorders and may have an adjunctive role in severely ill patients. As underweight patients are at increased risk for adverse effects, specific agents should be avoided, including bupropion, tricyclic antidepressants, and MAOIs.

In patients with bulimia nervosa and binge-eating disorder, in contrast to those with anorexia nervosa, there is strong evidence to support the use of CBT. Pharmacotherapy is a useful adjunct to CBT, and SSRI antidepressants have been shown to be effective and safe for treatment. Fluoxetine has been FDA-approved for the treatment of bulimia nervosa, and sertraline may also be effective. Topiramate has been shown to reduce binge eating and promote weight loss.

KEY POINTS

- Psychotherapy and nutritional support are the primary treatments for acutely ill patients with anorexia nervosa.
- Cognitive-behavioral therapy is an effective treatment for bulimia nervosa and binge-eating disorder.

Schizophrenia

Schizophrenia has a prevalence of 1% in the general population and affects women and men equally. It usually begins in the teenage years or in the early 20s; the strongest risk factor for its development is family history. First-degree relatives of persons with schizophrenia have a 6% to 17% lifetime incidence of the disease. It is manifested by positive and negative symptoms. Positive symptoms include paranoid delusions, hearing voices, and hallucinations; negative symptoms include flat affect, social withdrawal, and lack of interest or enjoyment in life. Thought tends to be disorganized, with confused speech and rapid shifts in topic. No symptom or sign is pathognomonic for schizophrenia. Diagnosis is based on the presence of signs and symptoms for at least 1 month in duration, with some manifestations of the disease present for at least 6 months. The onset of schizophrenia can be abrupt or insidious. Schizophrenia is thought to have several inciting factors, but genetics appears to play the biggest role in its development. It is important to consider other psychiatric diagnoses (depression with psychotic features, bipolar disorder) or medical diseases (substance abuse and withdrawal, delirium, central nervous system tumors) in the differential diagnosis, as 22% of those initially diagnosed with schizophrenia have their diagnosis changed during subsequent hospitalizations. Patients with schizophrenia should be co-managed with psychiatrists and other mental health professionals whenever possible.

Atypical antipsychotic agents, such as clozapine and olanzapine, have less risk of extrapyramidal side effects than traditional antipsychotic agents, such as haloperidol and chlorpromazine. However, adverse effects of these newer agents confer a higher risk of diabetes, lipid disorders, and weight gain. There is little consensus about the frequency of how often these metabolic parameters should be monitored, but most recommendations suggest monitoring periodically.

KEY POINT

- It is important to consider other psychiatric diagnoses and medical diseases in the differential diagnosis of schizophrenia, as 22% of those initially diagnosed with schizophrenia have their diagnosis changed during subsequent hospitalizations.

Attention-Deficit/Hyperactivity Disorder

Attention-deficit/hyperactivity disorder (ADHD) first manifests in childhood and is characterized by inattention, hyperactivity, and impulsivity accompanied by functional impairment in at least two settings (home, work, school). Although many children with ADHD show improvement as they age, symptoms of inattention may persist into adulthood. Prevalence in adults is estimated at 4%. ADHD is more likely in first-degree relatives of persons with ADHD. It may be associated with neurodevelopmental disorders (cerebral palsy, autism, learning disabilities) and with psychiatric disorders (substance abuse, mood disorders).

There are no diagnostic tests for ADHD. The DSM-IV-TR includes criteria for ADHD in children but may be applicable to adults if adapted. For example, functional impairment manifests differently in adult patients, who can have problems at both work and school. Adults with ADHD are more likely to have traffic infractions, vehicular accidents, and spousal separation and divorce than the general population.

Diagnosing ADHD in an adult patient can be challenging but should be considered in a patient with a history of inattention or impulsive behavior and significant functional impairment beginning in early childhood. About 10% to 20% of adults with substance abuse or mood disorders have ADHD; it is therefore important to review the patient's history for evidence of ADHD in childhood.

The first-line treatment for childhood ADHD is stimulants, such as amphetamine and methylphenidate. These agents may be effective in adults but must be used more cautiously, particularly in patients with hypertension or cardiovascular disease. The increased risk of substance use disorders is also of concern in adults with ADHD, as stimulants are controlled substances with high potential for abuse or diversion. Atomoxetine is a selective norepinephrine reuptake inhibitor specifically approved for treatment of ADHD in adults and has shown benefit. Bupropion and tricyclic antidepressants may also be beneficial. Because the natural history of ADHD usually shows gradual improvement with age, it is important to regularly verify the ongoing need for medication with periodic "drug holidays" in well controlled patients. CBT has been reported to be effective for ADHD but may be most helpful as an adjunct to medications.

KEY POINT

- Because attention-deficit/hyperactivity disorder usually shows gradual improvement with age, it is important to regularly verify the need for medication in adults.

Autism Spectrum Disorders

Autism spectrum disorders are characterized by difficulties in social interactions and repetitive behaviors or narrow interests. Severe autism accompanied by developmental delay is evident in early childhood, while those with milder symptoms and no cognitive deficits may not be diagnosed until later in life. Approximately 0.9% of children have an autism spectrum disorder, according to Centers for Disease Control and Prevention estimates, and autism spectrum disorders are thought to be equally prevalent in adults.

DSM-IV-TR diagnostic criteria for autistic disorder are based on childhood behavior and include impairment in social interaction; impairment in communication; and repetitive patterns of behavior, interests, or activities, with onset before age 3 years. Patients with these symptoms without significant delay in language or cognitive development may meet criteria for Asperger disorder. The current draft version of the DSM-V, however, has eliminated Asperger disorder in favor of a broader definition of autism spectrum disorder that no longer requires the presence of developmental delay but includes impairment of everyday functioning. The new definition also specifies that symptoms must be present in early childhood but may not become fully manifest until later in life, when social demands exceed capacities. Persons with Asperger disorder frequently come to medical attention later than autistic children because of their lesser developmental deficits. Making the formal diagnosis of an autism spectrum disorder in adults is difficult and frequently requires a specialized clinical evaluation using a number of diagnostic tools.

Managing adults with autism spectrum disorders is highly influenced by individual patient characteristics. For those with difficulty with physical contact, physical examination should be limited only to essential maneuvers, performed slowly, and explained in detail before proceeding. Efforts should be made to communicate with patients who are unable to speak as they frequently are able to comprehend and participate in decision making; alternative methods of communication (pen and paper, pictures, assistive devices) should be considered. Repetitive and stereotyped behaviors are calming for many patients with autism and should not be interrupted unless they are harmful or disruptive. The assistance of a caregiver or colleague who is familiar with the individual patient and how best to interact with him or her is invaluable.

KEY POINT

- Because patients with autism generally have difficulty with physical contact, physical examination should be limited only to essential maneuvers, performed slowly, and explained in detail before proceeding.

Difficult Patient Encounters

Several studies indicate that physicians experience about 15% of patient encounters as difficult. Difficult encounters often involve patients who have a depressive or anxiety disorder, poorer functional status, unmet expectations, reduced satisfaction, and greater use of health care services. Physicians often report the most difficulty with patients by whom they feel manipulated or frustrated, patients who are time consuming and have unrealistic demands, patients who do not follow recommendations, patients who express anger, and those who interrupt physician routine and make extra work. Patients who have somatization disorder, chronic pain, substance abuse, or an undiagnosable medical problem are often labeled as difficult. Patients with identifiable personality disorders, such as borderline, dependent, histrionic, obsessive, or antisocial personality disorders, also are frequently labeled as difficult.

Physician characteristics also play a role in generating a difficult patient encounter. Physicians who are fatigued or harried or develop a dislike for a patient are more likely to consider a patient difficult. Additional physician characteristics include having less experience, having a higher perceived workload, and having poor communication skills.

It is vital for a physician to identify the underlying emotion that is creating difficulty in order to best address it. Frequent negative emotions in providers include anger, fear of losing control, fear of displeasing, and fear of harming the patient, as well as those stemming from unique personal issues, such as fear of incompetence, fear of death, or reminders of illnesses in the provider's personal life.

One of the first steps in improving a difficult patient interaction is recognizing the underlying emotion at work in the situation. Often, being open with the patient about any patient behaviors that are eliciting the negative reaction can be helpful in alleviating the underlying tension. It is important that the physician take responsibility for managing his or her own negative emotion rather than expecting the patient to respond, however, as the physician may be better able to overcome the inherent conflicts in the situation.

Depending on the clinical situation, it may be important for the physician to specifically address certain behaviors, such as limit setting with borderline patients or setting expectations for frequency of visits with high utilizers. Being observant of and compassionate about the underlying emotions that drive patients to become "difficult" is one of the best ways to remedy unpleasant interactions. If a complete lack of trust develops or it becomes obvious that a therapeutic relationship is not possible, the physician should consider transferring care of the patient to another provider.

KEY POINT

- Both patient and physician factors contribute to difficult patient encounters.

Geriatric Medicine

Functional Assessment

In older patients, functional status is as important as medical illness in determining overall well-being. Function in geriatric patients is a predictor of independent living as well as the development of future medical illnesses. Therefore, functional assessment and treatment of disorders associated with functional decline must be incorporated into the evaluation and care of elderly patients in both office and hospital settings.

Aids to functional assessment, beyond history and physical examination, may include screening instruments and a multidisciplinary assessment involving occupational and physical therapists as well as physicians trained in geriatric medicine. Activities of daily living (ADLs) are basic self-care activities, including bathing, dressing, and feeding, that help determine a patient's required level of support (**Table 51**). Instrumental activities of daily living (IADLs) are activities that are associated with independent living, including shopping for food, administering one's own medications, and handling finances. To

TABLE 51. Indices to Assess Basic and Instrumental Activities of Daily Living

Index (time to complete)	Functional Activities Assessed
Katz Index of Independence in Activities of Daily Living[a] (5-10 min)	Bathing
	Dressing
	Toileting
	Transferring
	Continence
	Feeding
Barthel Index[b] (5-10 min)	Feeding
	Bathing
	Grooming
	Dressing
	Bowels
	Bladder
	Toilet use
	Transfers
	Mobility
	Stairs
Lawton and Brody Instrumental Activities of Daily Living Scale[c] (5-10 min)	Ability to use a telephone
	Shopping
	Food preparation
	Housekeeping
	Laundry
	Mode of transportation
	Responsibility for own medications
	Ability to handle finances
Direct Assessment of Functional Status[d] (30-35 min)	Time orientation
	Communication
	Transportation
	Finance
	Shopping
	Eating
	Dressing and grooming

[a]The Katz index is scored by assigning a score of 1 to each activity if it can be completed independently, which is defined as having no supervision, direction, or personal assistance; scores are then added for a range of 0 to 6.

[b]Each item on the Barthel index is assigned a 0 to 10 value, resulting in a score of 0 to 100, with higher scores reflecting independence.

[c]The Lawton and Brody scale results in a score of 0 to 8, with a score of 8 representing independence and 0 representing total dependence for activities of daily living.

[d]The Direct Assessment of Functional Status is a more complex 85-item instrument that evaluates individual tasks for each of the skills using direct observation.

ensure accuracy and objectivity, assessment of these activities should include direct observations of patients by health care personnel when possible. Assessing ADLs and IADLs in the hospital can facilitate discharge planning.

Fall Prevention and Home Safety

Falls are a serious problem for older adults and occur in approximately one third of community-dwelling adults who are 65 years or older and half of similarly aged hospitalized adults. Falling is most often related to patient and environmental factors. Those at greatest risk include persons with gait imbalance, stroke, or dementia, or who use an assistive device to walk. Chronic conditions associated with falls include arthritis, depression, orthostatic hypotension, and visual deficits. Leg muscle weakness, Parkinson disease, and peripheral neuropathy also can increase risk. Falls are associated with increased morbidity and mortality, a decline in functional abilities, and a loss of independence.

Because of the high prevalence of falls, as well as the associated burden of illness and cost and the potential to improve outcomes, the Institute of Medicine has identified prevention of falls as a priority area. Screening for fall risk and institution of fall prevention strategies has been proposed as a way to limit the impact of falls in the geriatric population. The American Geriatrics Society recommends that physicians ask adults aged 75 years and older if they have difficulty with walking and balance and if they have fallen in the past year. For patients who have fallen, the history should include a description of the circumstances of the fall as well as a review of current medications. Psychotropic medications increase the risk of falling, and their gradual withdrawal reduces the rate of falls. Educating physicians about modifying medications in the elderly has been shown to reduce the risk of falling.

Physical examination for patients with a history of falling in the past year should include assessment of gait and mobility; this can be facilitated by using the timed "Up & Go" (TUG) test. The patient is asked to rise from a chair, walk 10 feet, turn around, walk back, and sit down again in the same chair. The physician observes the patient for ease of performance, speed, and balance. Patients should perform the task using any routine assistive devices, such as a cane or walker. The average healthy adult can complete the task in less than 10 seconds; those completing the task in more than 14 seconds are considered to be at high risk for subsequent falls. A recent pooled analysis of nine cohort studies including nearly 35,000 community-dwelling adults with a mean age of 73.5 years found that increased gait speed was associated with increased survival. In these studies, patients were asked to walk at their usual pace. The walk distance varied from 2.4 m (8 ft) to 6 m (20 ft), and speed was calculated as meters per second. For men between 75 and 84 years old, mean 10-year survival was 15% for gait speeds slower than 0.4 m/s and 50% for gait speeds 1.4 m/s or faster. For women the same age, the corresponding 10-year survival rates were 35% and 92%, respectively. This model, using age, sex, and gait speed, performed as well in predicting survival as more complex models based on several factors, including chronic conditions, smoking, and blood pressure.

Physical examination should also include assessment for visual deficits and lower extremity joint examination to detect arthritis. Cardiovascular evaluation should include assessment for orthostatic hypotension, arrhythmia, and, when syncope or presyncope is suspected, for carotid sinus hypersensitivity. Neurologic examination should include evaluation of cognitive function, lower extremity weakness, and peripheral neuropathy.

Finally, the home environment should be evaluated for falling hazards. Environmental hazards are responsible for 25% to 66% of falls in the home, and hazards can be found in two thirds or more of homes. Common environmental hazards include throw rugs; low toilet seats; no grab bar for bathtub, shower, or toilet; no nightlight in the bedroom, kitchen, or living room; uneven lighting of stairway or poorly visible step edges; and difficult-to-reach kitchen storage. Other hazards include slippery bathing areas, general clutter, difficult-to-reach light switches, and unsafe handrails. Recommendations to improve home safety include installing nonslip stripping to noncarpeted steps, removing all unevenness in floors (thresholds) and changing chair seat height so that the patient's upper and lower legs are at 90-degree angles when sitting. If the physician or family member has a concern about the patient's living environment, a home nurse evaluation for home safety should be arranged. The USPSTF, however, was not able to find sufficient evidence for or against home hazard modification.

Persons with a history of falls should undergo the assessment detailed above followed by individually tailored interventions to reduce the risk for future falling. Evidence-based interventions include prescribing gait, exercise, and balance training. A Cochrane Database review of interventions to prevent falls in elderly persons living in the community also found evidence for use of anti-slip shoes in icy conditions, pacemaker installation in patients with carotid sinus hypersensitivity, and cataract surgery in the first eye affected.

A recent systematic review and meta-analysis recommends prescribing vitamin D at a dose of 800 IU daily for elderly patients who have vitamin D deficiency, for those residing in long-term care facilities, and potentially for all elderly adults at increased risk for falling. The Institute of Medicine recommends a vitamin D intake of 600 units/d for all men and women aged 51 to 70 years old and 800 units/d for men and women older than 70 years. In a meta-analysis of adults aged 60 years or older, vitamin D supplementation for at least 6 months resulted in a 14% relative risk reduction for falls (number needed to treat = 15). The proposed mechanism of action of vitamin D is its beneficial effect on muscle strength and function and on gait. The USPSTF recommends exercise or physical therapy and vitamin D supplementation to prevent falls in community-dwelling adults aged 65 years or older who are at increased risk for falls.

Mild Cognitive Impairment and Dementia

Mild cognitive impairment (MCI), or cognitive impairment without dementia, is associated with decreased quality of life and functional status, loss of independence, and increased health care costs. MCI is present in about one fifth of patients older than 70 years and may be present in nearly one third of hospitalized patients older than 75 years. The most common subtypes include prodromal Alzheimer disease, vascular cognitive impairment, and MCI due to medical conditions and stroke. (In vascular cognitive impairment, cardiovascular or cerebrovascular disease is present, but the cognitive impairment is not temporally linked to a single stroke). MCI may be more common in older patients with depression, neurologic conditions, alcohol abuse, and low baseline intellect. Patients who develop essential tremor after age 65 years may be more likely to have MCI than either those without essential tremor or those who develop tremor before age 65 years. Progression from MCI to dementia is about 12% annually but is higher (17%-20%) in those with stroke and prodromal Alzheimer disease. Researchers are evaluating cerebrospinal fluid markers and genetic markers as predictors for progression to Alzheimer disease. A recent study found that a genetic variation in the caspase-1 gene predicted accelerated progression from MCI to Alzheimer disease over a 2-year period, but the clinical utility of this genetic test is unknown at this time.

The Mini–Mental State Examination (MMSE) has been the standard screening instrument for cognitive function, with a sensitivity of 76% and specificity of 88% for detecting cognitive impairment. Scores of 24 to 25 out of 30 suggest mild impairment, scores of 19 to 24 suggest mild dementia, and scores of 10 to 19 suggest moderate dementia. The MMSE may under-diagnose those with high intellect and may over-diagnose those with low intellect or with delirium. A briefer screening tool, the Mini-Cog (sensitivity 76%, specificity 89%), performs comparably to the MMSE and employs a three-item recall test followed by the clock-drawing test if any one of the three items is missed. If all three items are recalled, no further testing is necessary. The Sweet 16 (sensitivity 80%, specificity 70%) is a newer instrument that is easier to administer than the MMSE and can be completed in 2 to 3 minutes. The 16 items include eight orientation items, three immediate-recall and three delayed-recall items, and two backward digit span items. When screening for dementia, it is also extremely important to ask a family member or caregiver about memory loss, personality change, word-finding difficulties, changes in activity level, getting lost, and difficulty in performing ADLs to place testing results into a clinical context.

Although there is no widely accepted treatment for MCI, cognitive rehabilitation has been shown to have some effectiveness in improving functioning in some patients. Cognitive rehabilitation is performed by neuropsychologists and occupational therapists and involves using external memory aids as well as teaching patients organizational and attention skills. A randomized trial of cognitive rehabilitation for patients with MCI with a mean age of 79 years demonstrated improved memory at 2 weeks and 4 months.

Depression

Depression is common in older adults, with major depressive disorder being present in 6% to 9% of patients older than 60 years presenting to physicians' offices and some form of depression in 25% of persons older than age 60 years. Depression in older adults may present with somatic and vegetative symptoms rather than dysphoria. Depression is more common in patients residing in institutions and in those with acute or chronic illnesses, including cardiovascular and cerebrovascular disease, cognitive decline and dementia, and bereavement. Medical conditions associated with depression include hypothyroidism, hyperthyroidism ("apathetic hyperthyroidism"), chronic pain, Parkinson disease, cancer, diabetes mellitus, vitamin B_{12} deficiency, alcohol abuse, and use of corticosteroids or interferon. Depressed patients presenting with cognitive decline (pseudodementia) may display delayed responses to cognitive test questions compared with patients with true dementia. Treatment of the depression improves cognitive function in these patients. Because depression in older adults is often perceived as an expected consequence of chronic illness, it is frequently undiagnosed and untreated.

The PHQ-9 (see Mental and Behavioral Health) can be used to identify and assess severity of depression in older adults. When tested in adults aged 65 years and older, its sensitivity and specificity for diagnosing major depressive disorder were 100% and 77%, respectively. The Geriatric Depression Scale consists of 15 questions, and a score of 5 or greater indicates depression. Its sensitivity is 80% to 90% and its specificity is 70% to 85%.

The USPSTF has found good evidence that treatment of depression in older adults who are identified through screening in primary care settings decreases clinical morbidity. Treatment may include antidepressants, psychotherapy, or both. Relapse may occur more frequently in older compared with younger adults. Patients older than 70 years receiving selective serotonin reuptake inhibitor (SSRI) therapy may have fewer recurrences of depression if treated for 2 years. Evidence is fair that SSRI use is associated with an increased risk for upper gastrointestinal bleeding in older patients, with risk increasing with age. SSRIs can also cause the syndrome of inappropriate antidiuretic hormone secretion (SIADH). The use of stimulants can be considered for some older patients with apathetic major depressive illness. For elderly patients with insomnia and weight loss, mirtazapine may be preferred because of its beneficial effect on these symptoms. For patients with refractory severe depression, electroconvulsive therapy (ECT) can be considered in medically stable patients.

Hearing

Hearing loss is present in one third of patients aged 65 years and older and in 80% of those 80 years or older. The most common cause of hearing loss is presbycusis, or age-related hearing loss. Presbycusis results in high-frequency hearing loss, which typically impairs sound localization and hearing the spoken voice (particularly in noisy environments). Hearing impairment can lead to depression, limited activity, and social isolation. Among the available screening tests, the whispered voice test, in which the examiner stands 2 feet behind a seated patient and assesses the ability of the patient to repeat a whispered combination of numbers and letters, or a single question about whether the patient has hearing difficulty seem to be nearly as accurate as hand-held audiometry or a detailed hearing loss questionnaire. The USPSTF concludes that evidence is insufficient to weigh the benefits and harms of screening for hearing loss in older adults. The Canadian Task Force on the Periodic Health Examination has recommended screening older adults for hearing impairment using single-question screening, the whispered voice test, or audiometry. The use of hearing aids does not result in normal hearing but can improve communication abilities. Only 20% of patients who could potentially benefit from using a hearing aid actually use one. Cochlear implants can be considered for patients who are not able to distinguish more than 50% of words in a test sentence using the worst ear with a hearing aid in place.

Vision

Visual impairment, defined as best corrected vision worse than 20/40, is present in 1% of persons aged 65 to 69 years and increases to 17% in those older than 80 years. The most common causes of visual impairment in older persons are refractive errors, cataracts, and age-related macular degeneration (AMD). Diabetic retinopathy and glaucoma are also important causes of visual impairment.

The USPSTF found insufficient evidence to recommend for or against screening adults for glaucoma and also concluded that the current evidence is insufficient to recommend for or against screening for visual acuity in older adults. Although evidence was adequate that early treatment of refractive error, cataracts, and AMD improves or prevents loss of visual acuity, evidence that these improvements would enhance functional outcomes was inadequate. The American Academy of Ophthalmology recommends comprehensive eye examinations every 1 to 2 years for persons 65 years or older who have no risk factors. When screening is performed by primary care physicians, use of a visual acuity test (such as the Snellen eye chart) is recommended.

Some evidence suggests that the use of multifocal lenses may increase risk for falls in older adults, probably because looking down through the reading segment of the lens causes the ground to be out of focus.

The Older Driver

The risk for automobile accidents is increased among older drivers, and both patients and physicians have a responsibility to reduce this risk. Although patients often self-restrict their driving as they become aware of driving difficulties, "low mileage" drivers may be at the greatest risk. Medical conditions most likely to cause problems include those affecting vision, motor function, and cognition. Specific medical conditions that increase risk include cataract, arthritis, dizziness, history of falls, arrhythmia, and seizure disorders, as well as substance abuse and use of sedating medications. Dementia is associated with a two-fold risk for driving accidents. Although some studies have shown impaired driving in older adults with MCI, there are not enough data to make clear recommendations regarding assessing or restricting drivers with MCI. The American Medical Association (AMA) recommends that physicians assess patients for physical or mental impairments that might adversely affect driving abilities. In addition, older drivers can be evaluated by driver rehabilitation specialists (associated with hospital occupational therapy departments) who can also make recommendations for safer driving. State-specific physician reporting requirements, along with tools for patients and physicians, can be found in the AMA's *Physician's Guide to Assessing and Counseling Older Drivers* (available at www.ama-assn.org/ama/pub/physician-resources/public-health/promoting-healthy-lifestyles/geriatric-health/older-driver-safety/assessing-counseling-older-drivers.page).

KEY POINTS

- Adults aged 75 years and older should be assessed for fall risk by asking if they have difficulty with walking and balance and if they have fallen in the past year.
- Evidence-based interventions to reduce falls in older adults include supplemental vitamin D; modification of risk factors in the home; reducing or eliminating psychoactive medications; and prescribing gait, exercise, and balance training to patients with abnormal gait or balance.
- Depression in older adults may present with somatic and vegetative symptoms rather than dysphoria.

Levels of Care

For patients who cannot live independently at home, either following a hospitalization or as a result of progressive decline, various care options may be available. Levels of care can be divided into postacute and long-term care. Postacute care options following hospitalization include inpatient rehabilitation (for patients with stable medical issues able to participate in ≥3 hours/d of therapy); skilled nursing facilities, for patients requiring care that must be administered by trained nursing personnel or needing rehabilitation services but are unable to participate in at least 3 hours/day of therapy

(sometimes called subacute rehabilitation); long-term acute care hospitals (LTACHs), which provide long-term complex care following hospital discharge, including ventilator care and weaning; advanced health care services provided in the home (home health care); and hospice or palliative care. Long-term care options include supportive home care, which includes assistance in performing ADLs; assisted living, which provides institution-based care in semi-independent units with variable levels of assistance available; nursing homes, which provide ongoing nursing-level care; and adult day care, in which care services are provided during the day. It is not uncommon, particularly in elderly patients being discharged from the hospital, for patients to receive postacute care but ultimately require a higher level of chronic care than before admission. It is, therefore, imperative that physicians have a basic understanding of various care options so that they can help patients or their representatives make the best possible decisions for both long-term and transitional care.

Pressures to discharge patients as soon as medical conditions requiring hospitalization are resolved may interfere with the process of determining the best long-term living situation for a patient. Primary care physicians are particularly important advocates for their patients and can provide valuable input to hospitalists to ensure optimal post-discharge planning. Care managers, funded either privately or through public agencies, can also be valuable assets in configuring the best living situation for a patient.

Polypharmacy

Polypharmacy refers to the use of many medications together, and it tends to be a term used almost exclusively in the context of elderly patients. Ninety percent of noninstitutionalized patients older than 65 years take at least one medication, and approximately 50% take five or more medications each week. Twelve percent of patients older than 65 years take ten or more medications each week. As more medications are prescribed, rates of adverse drug reactions and medication errors rise. More drugs being taken together increases the risk of drug-drug interactions.

Many drugs used in the elderly have been studied primarily in younger patients with significantly longer life expectancies, and their safety and efficacy in older patients are not well established. Drug metabolism may be altered in the elderly owing to decreased glomerular filtration or underlying illness as well as to altered pharmacokinetics related to aging. A recent study found that four medications were responsible for two thirds of emergency hospitalizations for adverse drug events. Hospitalizations involving three of them (warfarin, insulin, and oral hypoglycemic agents) were related to unintentional overdose. Warfarin was implicated most frequently, accounting for one third of emergency hospitalizations. The fourth class of drugs, oral antiplatelet agents, were implicated by acting alone or by interacting with warfarin.

CONT.

Frequent, routine review to verify need for medication and appropriate dosing is an important aspect of optimal geriatric care. Many strategies have been studied to monitor and reduce polypharmacy. Biannual review (or more frequently for higher numbers of medications taken) of medication lists helps to prevent duplication of medication classes. The "Good Palliative–Geriatric Practice" (GP-GP) algorithm for drug discontinuation (available at http://archinte.jamanet work.com/article.aspx?doi=10.1001/archinternmed .2010.355) has been shown to be effective in reducing polypharmacy and improving mortality and morbidity in nursing home inpatients and has been studied in smaller populations of community-dwelling outpatients and found to be effective. **H**

KEY POINTS

- Altered pharmacodynamics, multiple medications, and increased susceptibility to adverse effects make polypharmacy a major problem in geriatric patients.

- Frequent, routine review to verify need for medication and appropriate dosing is an important aspect of optimal geriatric care.

Urinary Incontinence

Epidemiology

Urinary incontinence, or involuntary urine leakage, affects one third of middle-aged and older women and 20% of older men. These numbers likely underestimate its true prevalence, however, as many patients do not report incontinence to their physician. In addition to female sex, risk factors include age, diabetes mellitus, obesity, history of vaginal childbirth, history of gynecologic surgery, pelvic floor muscle weakness, high caffeine intake, tobacco use, menopause, and impairment in cognition or mobility. Urinary incontinence in men may result from benign prostatic hyperplasia (overflow incontinence) or from surgery or radiation therapy for prostate cancer.

Urinary incontinence is associated with excess health care expenditures. It increases the risk of falls and may lead to social isolation, embarrassment, decreased quality of life, functional decline, and admission to a nursing home. Effective treatment is available and improves quality of life. Although much of the evidence regarding management of incontinence comes from studies enrolling only women, most principles can be generalized to men.

Evaluation

Urinary incontinence is categorized as (1) urge incontinence (loss of urine accompanied by sense of urgency; caused by detrusor overreactivity); (2) stress incontinence (loss of urine with effort, coughing, or sneezing; caused by sphincter incompetence); (3) mixed urge and stress incontinence; and (4) overflow incontinence (caused by outlet obstruction).

Functional incontinence, defined as simply not getting to the toilet quickly enough, may occur in patients with significant mobility and cognitive impairments. Determining the type (or types) of incontinence guides management.

Because patients may not report incontinence spontaneously, the Agency for Healthcare Research and Quality recommends routine screening for all frail older men and women; some groups also recommend screening women aged 65 years and older for incontinence. Standardized questionnaires can distinguish urge from stress incontinence, including the 3 Incontinence Questions (3IQ) (**Figure 27**). For urge incontinence, the 3IQ has a sensitivity of 75%, specificity of 77%, positive likelihood ratio of 3.29, and negative likelihood ratio of 0.32. The 3IQ's metrics for stress incontinence are similar (86%, 60%, 2.13, and 0.24, respectively).

The evaluation should include a targeted history, including surgeries, instrumentations, and other relevant interventions; medication review; and physical examination, including a pelvic examination in women and a digital rectal examination in men. Men should be asked about prostate symptoms. Reversible causes should be noted, including delirium, urinary tract infection, atrophic vaginitis, medications, depression, hyperglycemia, impaired mobility, and fecal impaction. Urinalysis should be performed. Unless there is high clinical suspicion for neurologic disease or bladder outlet obstruction, a post-void residual urine volume determination is not necessary.

Treatment

General recommendations for all patients with urinary incontinence include caffeine restriction and, if overweight or obese, weight reduction. Excess fluid intake should be avoided, especially at nighttime, but not at the expense of adequate hydration. Any underlying causes should be addressed. Further treatment depends on the type of urinary incontinence.

Behavioral Therapy

Pelvic floor muscle training (PFMT, or Kegel exercises) and bladder training/urge suppression techniques are the two most effective behavioral therapies. PFMT is considered first-line therapy for patients with stress incontinence and is of likely benefit in patients with mixed urge and stress incontinence. PFMT exercises, if performed correctly and diligently, strengthen the pubococcygeus muscles that form the pelvic floor and enhance urinary retention by increasing the tone of the supporting structures of the urethra. The patient is instructed to contract the pelvic muscles as if trying to interrupt urination. In women, correct technique may be assessed by inserting a finger into the vagina and feeling the circumvaginal muscles tighten and the pelvic floor move upward. Patients should work up to three or four sets of ten contractions daily, with contractions lasting 10 seconds. Bladder

1. During the last 3 months, have you leaked urine (even a small amount)?

❑ Yes   ❑ No

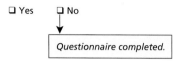

        Questionnaire completed.

2. During the last 3 months, did you leak urine:
(Check all that apply.)

  ❑ a. When you were performing some physical activity, such as coughing, sneezing, lifting, or exercise?
  ❑ b. When you had the urge or the feeling that you needed to empty your bladder, but you could not get to the toilet fast enough?
  ❑ c. Without physical activity and without a sense of urgency?

3. During the last 3 months, did you leak urine *most often*:
(Check only one.)

  ❑ a. When you were performing some physical activity, such as coughing, sneezing, lifting, or exercise?
  ❑ b. When you had the urge or the feeling that you needed to empty your bladder, but you could not get to the toilet fast enough?
  ❑ c. Without physical activity and without a sense of urgency?
  ❑ d. About equally as often with physical activity as with a sense of urgency?

Definitions of type of urinary incontinence are based on responses to question 3:

Response to Question 3	Type of Incontinence
a. Most often with physical activity	Stress only or stress predominant
b. Most often with the urge to empty the bladder	Urge only or urge predominant
c. Without physical activity or sense of urgency	Other cause only or other cause predominant
d. About equally with physical activity and sense of urgency	Mixed

FIGURE 27. The 3 Incontinence Questions (3IQ) for evaluation of urinary incontinence.

Reprinted with permission from Brown JS, Bradley CS, Subak LL, et al; Diagnostic Aspects of Incontinence Study (DAISy) Research Group. The sensitivity and specificity of a simple test to distinguish between urge and stress urinary incontinence. Ann Intern Med. 2006;144:715-723. [PMID: 16702587] Copyright 2006, American College of Physicians.

training and suppressive therapy are indicated for urge and mixed incontinence. Patients are instructed to void regularly throughout the day, regardless of urge, and progressively increase the interval between voids. Urge to void outside of the schedule is managed by suppression techniques. The patient is instructed to contract pelvic floor muscles quickly three or four times, use a distraction technique (counting backwards from 100), and, when the urge passes, walk to the bathroom to urinate.

A systematic review of 96 randomized controlled trials of nonsurgical treatments for urinary incontinence concluded that PFMT alone improved stress incontinence compared with usual care. The pooled relative risk ratio for continence was 7.1. Individual therapy, biofeedback, and use of skilled therapists improved outcomes. Bladder training alone improved symptoms but not continence rates. In studies of stress and urge incontinence, PFMT coupled with bladder training increased continence rates (pooled relative risk ratio, 13).

Prompted voiding (periodically asking the patient about incontinence, reminding and assisting the patient to go to the toilet, and providing positive reinforcement for continence) is effective in elderly nursing home residents with functional incontinence.

Pharmacologic Therapy

Effective pharmacologic therapy is available for treatment of incontinence. Data on long-term continence rates are lacking, however, and adverse effects may limit long-term tolerability.

In patients with stress incontinence for whom PFMT has not been successful, duloxetine, a serotonin and norepinephrine reuptake inhibitor, is an option. In a systematic review of randomized, controlled trials, duloxetine improved incontinence rates and quality of life but did not cure incontinence.

For urge incontinence, anticholinergic antimuscarinic medications are first-line therapy. Options include oxybutynin, tolterodine, fesoterodine, darifenacin, solifenacin, and trospium. High-quality head-to-head trials comparing individual antimuscarinics are limited. However, all of these drugs appear to provide similar small benefits in continence rates without clear superiority of newer agents relative to older medications, except for a slightly lower incidence of anticholinergic side effects. Anticholinergic agents are contraindicated in patients with angle-closure glaucoma.

Treatment of prostate-related lower urinary tract symptoms is addressed in further detail in Men's Health.

Medications that have been found to be ineffective for incontinence are pseudoephedrine (an α-agonist), oral estrogens (may worsen incontinence), and transdermal and vaginal estrogens. Conclusive long-term data for imipramine, a tricyclic antidepressant with α-agonist and anticholinergic properties, are lacking.

Combined use of behavioral therapy with pharmacologic therapy has not been shown to be more effective than medication alone in women with urge incontinence. Although behavioral therapy may reduce incontinence frequency during active treatment, it does not improve ability to stop the medication.

Devices, Injectable Bulking Agents, and Surgery
For stress incontinence, medical devices (pessaries, intravaginal devices, urethral plugs, vaginal cones) are available. Pessaries are most effective but require fitting by experienced practitioners. The most effective surgeries for stress incontinence are sling procedures for intrinsic sphincter deficiency (success rate, 80%-90%), retropubic suspension, needle bladder neck suspension, and anterior vaginal repair with plication of the bladder neck (success rates 79%, 74%, and 65%, respectively). Although increasingly used, results of studies of periurethral injection of bulking agents (collagen, porcine dermal implant, myoblasts, fibroblasts, and dextran) for treatment of stress incontinence have been variable.

For urge incontinence, studies of intradetrusor botulinum toxin injection report complete continence in 32% to 86% of patients, with mean duration of 6 months. Variable cure rates are seen with sacral nerve stimulation and augmentation cystoplasty.

Condom or indwelling (Foley) urinary catheters increase risk of urinary tract infections. Their use, except as palliative or temporizing measures, is not advised.

KEY POINTS
- Pelvic floor muscle training and bladder training/urge suppression techniques are effective behavioral therapies for stress urinary incontinence.
- Pharmacologic options for urinary incontinence treatment include oxybutynin or tolterodine for urge incontinence and duloxetine for stress incontinence.

Pressure Ulcers
Clinical Presentation
Pressure ulcers are a common condition, particularly in persons who are acutely hospitalized, admitted to nursing homes, or receiving home health care. More than 2.5 million pressure ulcers are reported nationally in acute care settings alone. Annual treatment costs are estimated at $11 billion. They result from continuous pressure, friction, and shearing forces to the skin. Risk factors include increased age, reduced mobility, reduced level of consciousness, malnutrition, peripheral vascular disease, incontinence, and poor skin condition.

Pressure ulcers most commonly occur on bony prominences, usually on the hips and lower extremities. One study reported that 36% of patients with hip fractures developed pressure ulcers. It is important to differentiate pressure ulcers from ulcers related to diabetic neuropathy or venous or arterial insufficiency, as treatments for these conditions vary.

Prevention and Management
Preventive interventions are much more cost effective than the prolonged and intensive efforts required to treat pressure ulcers. Patients should be assessed at each hospital or nursing home admission for risks of development of ulcers. Skin inspection of those at high risk should be conducted regularly. Preventive efforts should focus on avoiding friction, shear, and heavy moisture, which are often a result of wound drainage or incontinence. Various types of support surfaces, including beds, mattresses and overlays, have been studied to evaluate their ability to prevent pressure ulcers. Foam mattresses that distribute pressure over a larger area (relative risk [RR], 0.40; 95% CI, 0.21 to 0.74) and medical grade sheepskin (RR, 0.56; 95% CI, 0.32 to 0.97) are beneficial in preventing ulcers in hospitalized patients compared with standard mattresses. The effectiveness of alternating and constant low-pressure mattresses and overlays is not clear. Scientific evidence for nutritional supplements, seat cushions, and lotions is minimal.

Treatment of existing ulcers can be informed by staging (Table 52). Treatment should be provided by interdisciplinary teams, with a focus on addressing predisposing and exacerbating factors that initially led to the ulcer. In general, a wide variety of dressings, barriers, and gels may be used, with a focus on maintaining a clean and moist wound environment and managing exudates. Higher-stage ulcers with eschar may require surgical or nonsurgical debridement. Attention to superinfection, frank cellulitis, and potential underlying osteomyelitis is vital. The presence of infectious complications is an indication for systemic antibiotic therapy.

Stage I ulcers can generally be treated with transparent films and do not require debriding. Emphasis should be placed on prevention of further progression. Stage II ulcers can be treated using an occlusive dressing to keep the area moist. Wet-to-dry dressings should be avoided because debridement is usually unnecessary at this stage. Stage III and IV ulcers generally require surgical or nonsurgical debridement, treatment of wound infection, and appropriate dressings based on the wound environment. For nonhealing wounds that are stage III or higher, imaging to rule out underlying osteomyelitis is indicated. Surgical wound intervention may be necessary in severe or nonhealing ulcers if conservative measures fail.

Although often used, there is no evidence that supplementation with either vitamin C or zinc is helpful in the absence of deficiency. Adequate nutrition to maintain a positive anabolic balance should be provided. Negative-pressure

TABLE 52.	Classification of Pressure Ulcers
Stage	**Description**
Suspected deep tissue injury	Purple or maroon localized area of discolored, intact skin or blood-filled blister due to damage of underlying soft tissue from pressure and/or shear. May be difficult to detect in persons with dark skin tones.
Stage I	Intact skin with nonblanchable redness of a localized area, usually over a bony prominence. Darkly pigmented skin may not have visible blanching; its color may differ from the surrounding area.
Stage II	Partial-thickness loss of dermis presenting as a shallow open ulcer with a red-pink wound bed, without slough. May also present as an intact or open/ruptured serum-filled blister.
Stage III	Full-thickness tissue loss. Subcutaneous fat may be visible but bone, tendon, or muscle is not exposed. Slough may be present but does not obscure the depth of tissue loss. May include undermining and tunneling. Depth varies by anatomic location and may be extremely deep in areas of significant adiposity.
Stage IV	Full-thickness tissue loss with exposed bone, tendon, or muscle. Slough or eschar may be present on some parts of the wound bed. Often includes undermining and tunneling.
Unstageable	Full-thickness tissue loss in which the base of the ulcer is covered by slough (yellow, tan, gray, green, or brown) and/or eschar (tan, brown, or black) in the wound bed.

Adapted with permission from National Pressure Ulcer Advisory Panel. Pressure ulcer stages revised by NPUAP. http://npuap.org/pr2.htm. Published February 2007. Accessed October 6, 2011. Copyright 2007, National Pressure Ulcer Advisory Panel.

wound therapy using a vacuum-assisted closure device has been shown to enhance patient comfort and is less labor intensive than standard therapy, but in three controlled trials, it has not been shown to improve objective measures of wound healing. [H]

KEY POINTS

- Skin inspection should be conducted regularly in patients at high risk of pressure ulcer.

- Foam alternatives to standard mattresses and medical grade sheepskin support surfaces are effective in preventing pressure ulcers.

- Staging of existing pressure ulcers is helpful in guiding appropriate therapy.

Perioperative Medicine

General Recommendations

The preoperative risk assessment allows the internist to identify and mitigate, if possible, complications from surgery for which the patient is at higher-than-baseline risk. In addition, the preoperative risk assessment can serve an important patient safety role by aiding with medication reconciliation, noting baseline abnormalities in physical examination, and, if appropriate, outlining goals of care. Although there is no set time to perform a preoperative risk assessment, scheduling a visit 3 to 4 weeks before a proposed procedure allows time to complete a diagnostic evaluation and implement preoperative management without delaying surgery.

Internists are also consulted to assist in the postoperative care of patients; these internists may be hospitalists or other consultants who did not perform the preoperative evaluation.

However, preoperative and in-hospital management should ideally be linked through close communication, particularly in complex, high-risk patients, in whom coordination and consistency of care may lead to avoidance of unexpected problems and improved transition from inpatient to outpatient settings.

Perioperative Testing

Patients undergoing even minor surgeries are often asked to obtain a comprehensive battery of laboratory and other testing. However, results of up to 5% of tests can be abnormal given chance alone, and this prevalence is increased in older, medically ill patients who often undergo surgery. Thus, this approach uncovers a relatively high number of abnormal test results that are of no clinical significance or are falsely positive. Each abnormal test typically requires further testing, which delays surgery, adds expense, rarely influences perioperative care, and may lead to potentially dangerous and low-value care. For example, comprehensive preoperative testing has not been shown to be helpful in cataract surgery and is not endorsed by any major specialty society or payer.

Preoperative tests should be based on known or suspected comorbidities and should only be ordered when a result will alter management. For example, pregnancy testing should be conducted in women of reproductive age, cervical spine radiographs should be ordered to assess for odontoid-axial stability in patients with rheumatoid arthritis, serum creatinine and calculated glomerular filtration rate should be measured in patients with or at risk for chronic kidney disease, and serum potassium level should be obtained in patients taking diuretics. In each case, the test is performed to evaluate for evidence of a condition that can have a silent presentation or assess an important physiologic variable likely to be abnormal.

Perioperative Medication Management

The preoperative evaluation should explicitly address perioperative medication management. The internist should collect a comprehensive medication list that includes herbal and over-the-counter medications. This list is essential for both perioperative management and medication reconciliation.

Medication reconciliation, or ensuring continuity of medications from the preoperative period until full recovery, is an important component of perioperative management. Alterations in medication associated with surgery or other interventions are a source of potential medication errors but also represent an opportunity to review a patient's medication regimen for need and for appropriate dosing.

There is a relative paucity of either evidence or consensus regarding perioperative medication use. Specific recommendations exist for the management of aspirin, clopidogrel, anticoagulants, antihypertensive agents, oral hypoglycemic agents, and short-acting insulins (see individual sections and **Table 53**). For other medications, management is usually based on an individualized assessment of the need for the treatment and the potential consequences of either continuing, stopping, or adjusting the dose of the medication in the perioperative period.

Patients are routinely advised to fast on the morning of surgery. The true risk of perioperative aspiration in nonfasting patients, however, is unclear, and medications deemed necessary can be taken with a small amount of water on the day of surgery. **H**

KEY POINTS

- Preoperative imaging and laboratory tests should be ordered only when an abnormal result is suspected on the basis of known or suspected comorbidities and when such a result would alter management.

- As part of the preoperative evaluation, a list of all medications taken by the patient should be generated; those for which risk outweighs benefit during the perioperative period should be temporarily discontinued.

Cardiovascular Perioperative Management

Unexpected perioperative myocardial infarction in patients undergoing noncardiac surgery is a much feared complication, although it impacts less than 5% of patients. Searching for undiagnosed coronary artery disease (CAD) in unselected patients, therefore, is a costly and low-yield strategy that places patients at risk for delayed surgery and complications from diagnostic procedures. Prevention of perioperative myocardial infarction now emphasizes cardiac evaluation in patients at highest risk for these complications.

Although a number of risk stratification schemas have been developed, the Revised Cardiac Risk Index (RCRI) is the most widely used. This risk score was developed in 1999 based on a cohort of patients undergoing noncardiac surgery. Clinicians can quickly calculate a RCRI score based on history and easily available laboratory testing (**Table 54**, page 128). The RCRI is considered to be the best available prognostic scoring system to distinguish low- versus high-risk patients.

Recommendations from the American College of Cardiology/American Heart Association (ACC/AHA) regarding perioperative cardiovascular evaluation for noncardiac surgery are presented in **Figure 28** (page 127). Regardless of their cardiac risk, patients who need emergent surgery should not delay surgery for preoperative testing. Consultation for these patients will necessarily focus on managing postoperative complications. Conversely, patients with "active cardiac conditions" (see Figure 28) are at extremely high risk for perioperative cardiac complications. Elective surgery for these patients, including minor surgery, should be deferred until these conditions have been treated.

ACC/AHA recommendations highlight three groups of patients in whom the risk of perioperative cardiac complications is low enough that preoperative cardiac evaluation is rarely, if ever, warranted: patients undergoing low-risk surgery, those who have at least moderate exercise capacity (>4 metabolic equivalents [METs]), and those who have low exercise capacity but no RCRI risk factors. However, preoperative noninvasive cardiac testing should be considered in patients with poor or unknown exercise tolerance based on the presence and number of RCRI risk factors and the nature of the surgery, provided that the results will impact management. For patients in whom cardiac testing is pursued, exercise stress testing is preferred. In general, exercise stress tests provide additional information, specifically exercise tolerance, compared with pharmacologic stress tests. However, many patients requiring preoperative stress testing have limited exercise tolerance and thus require a pharmacologic stress test. Although both nuclear stress tests and dobutamine stress echocardiograms can predict perioperative cardiac events, data from meta-analyses suggest that dobutamine stress echocardiography is superior.

Coronary revascularization is not routinely recommended for patients with CAD before noncardiac surgery. Coronary artery bypass grafting has considerable risks (which may be more than the proposed surgery) and should be reserved for patients who already meet criteria for revascularization, including those with stable angina with high-risk lesions, such as left main or three-vessel disease. Similarly, percutaneous coronary intervention (PCI) generally is reserved for patients already meeting criteria for PCI, such as those with unstable angina, and mostly has not been shown to be helpful preoperatively in patients without such conditions. If PCI is performed preoperatively, the choice of intervention (balloon angioplasty, bare metal stent, drug-eluting stent) should take into account both the nature of the atherosclerotic lesion and urgency of the surgery, as

TABLE 53. Suggested Perioperative Medication Management

Medication Class	Recommendation	Comments
Anticoagulant	Continue for minor surgery. Discontinue before major surgery: 6 h for intravenous heparin; 12-24 h for LMWH; 3-5 d for warfarin; 1-2 d (normal kidney function), 3-5 d (creatinine clearance <50 mL/min) for dabigatran.	Bridging with heparin indicated for high-risk patients and possibly moderate-risk patients (see text, Table 57, and Table 58).
Antiplatelet	Clopidogrel: discontinue 5-7 d before surgery; patients with cardiac stent may require continuation.	Aspirin and clopidogrel use in patients with cardiac stent and/or at high risk is controversial.
	Aspirin: continue if minor surgery. Continue if indication is recent myocardial infarction (up to 6 months), cardiac stent, or high risk for coronary event; otherwise, discontinue 7-10 d before major surgery (other than CABG)	Aspirin should be started before CABG.
Cardiovascular	Continue β-blockers, calcium channel blockers, nitrates, antiarrhythmia agents. ACEIs and ARBs should be used with caution. Diuretics optional (usually withheld).	ACEIs and ARBs can promote intraoperative hypotension, especially in patients with hypovolemia; perioperative use, especially in persons with left ventricular dysfunction, is controversial.
Lipid lowering	Continue statins; hold cholestyramine.	
Pulmonary	Continue controller and rescue inhalers as well as systemic corticosteroids (if used). Probably continue leukotriene antagonists and lipoxygenase inhibitors.	
Gastrointestinal	Continue H_2 receptor blockers and proton pump inhibitors.	
Hypoglycemic agents	Oral hypoglycemic agents: discontinue 12-72 h before surgery depending upon half-life of the drug and risk of hypoglycemia.	Hypoglycemia is more dangerous than hyperglycemia; caution to always have some basal insulin in patients with type 1 diabetes.
	Short-acting insulin: hold morning of surgery; may need dose reduction preoperatively if modified diet (e.g., gastrointestinal surgery).	
	Long-acting insulin: reduce dose, typically to one-half to two-thirds of usual dose.	
Thyroid	Continue thyroid replacement, propylthiouracil, methimazole.	
Corticosteroids	Continue; increase to stress doses if indicated.	Stress-dose corticosteroids for patients taking >10 mg/d prednisone for >3 weeks.
Estrogen	Discontinue several weeks before surgery. May continue oral contraceptives and increase level of deep venous thrombosis prophylaxis.	
Psychiatric	Discontinue MAOIs 10-14 d before surgery; SSRIs and TCAs can either be continued or tapered 2-3 weeks before surgery. Continue antipsychotic medications. Can continue lithium, although some experts taper and discontinue several days before surgery.	Paucity of evidence, although most agents confer at least some theoretical risk. Risk of serotonin syndrome with some anesthetic agents. Must weigh risks of continuing vs. stopping. May wish to consult with psychiatrist.
Neurologic	Continue anticonvulsants. May continue antiparkinsonian agents, although some experts may discontinue the night before surgery. Discontinue Alzheimer drugs.	
Herbal	Discontinue up to 1 week before surgery.	
Analgesic	NSAIDs and COX-2 inhibitors are usually discontinued 7 d before surgery. Long-acting narcotics continued or dose reduced.	
Immunomodulators	Methotrexate should be continued; other agents have not been studied but are usually continued.	Paucity of data; risk of disease flare balanced against risk of adverse reaction from medication.

ACEI = angiotensin-converting enzyme inhibitor; ARB = angiotensin receptor blocker; CABG = coronary artery bypass grafting; COX-2 = cyclooxygenase-2; LMWH = low-molecular-weight heparin; MAOI = monoamine oxidase inhibitor; SSRI = selective serotonin reuptake inhibitor; TCA = tricyclic antidepressant.

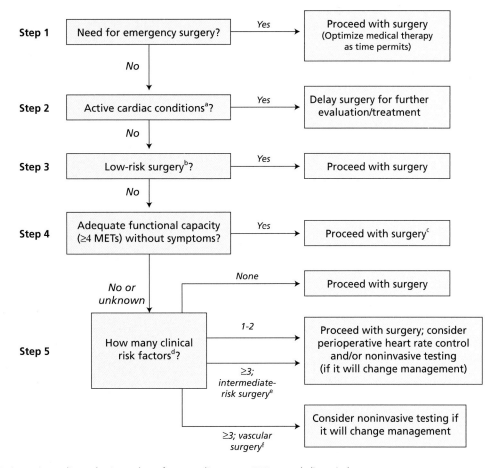

FIGURE 28. Perioperative cardiac evaluation and care for noncardiac surgery. MET = metabolic equivalent.

[a]Active cardiac conditions: unstable coronary syndromes (myocardial infarction <30 days ago, unstable or severe angina), decompensated heart failure, significant arrhythmia, severe valvular disease.

[b]Low-risk surgical procedure examples: endoscopic, superficial, breast, cataract, ambulatory.

[c]Consider noninvasive testing in patients undergoing vascular surgery with ≥1-2 risk factors if it will change management.

[d]Clinical risk factors: (1) history of heart disease, (2) history of compensated or prior heart failure, (3) history of cerebrovascular disease, (4) kidney insufficiency, (5) diabetes mellitus. Unlike the Revised Cardiac Risk Index (RCRI), the ACC/AHA guidelines do not limit diabetes to insulin-requiring to be considered a risk factor.

[e]Intermediate-risk surgery: intraperitoneal, intrathoracic, endovascular aortic aneurysm repair, carotid endarterectomy, head/neck, orthopedic, prostate.

[f]Vascular surgery: aortic or other major vascular surgery; peripheral vascular surgery.

Recommendations from Fleisher LA, Beckman JA, Brown KA, et al. 2009 ACCF/AHA focused update on perioperative beta blockade incorporated into the ACC/AHA 2007 guidelines on perioperative cardiovascular evaluation and care for noncardiac surgery: a report of the American College of Cardiology Foundation/American Heart Association Task Force on Practice Guidelines. Circulation. 2009;120(21):e180. [PMID: 19884473]

CONT.

stenting requires postprocedural antiplatelet therapy that will likely delay surgery (see Hematologic Perioperative Management, below).

β-Blockers have been studied extensively in the context of perioperative care, with sometimes conflicting results. According to recommendations from the ACC/AHA, patients who are already using a β-blocker should not stop this medication preoperatively. The ACC/AHA recommends β-blocker use for patients with CAD who are undergoing vascular surgery. It also recommends β-blockers in patients undergoing intermediate or higher risk surgeries, including vascular surgeries, who have more than one RCRI risk factor. If used, β-blockers should ideally be started a few weeks before surgery at a low dose, and then titrated to control heart rate and blood pressure without hypotension or bradycardia. Although there are no recommendations on the duration of β-blocker therapy started in the perioperative period, most of these patients have other reasons to be on β-blockers and should be continued on these medications indefinitely.

Preoperative heart failure is an independent risk factor for perioperative cardiac morbidity even in the absence of CAD. In general, patients with decompensated heart failure should have surgery deferred if possible. Beyond this there are no specific consensus recommendations for the perioperative management of patients with heart failure. **H**

TABLE 54. Revised Cardiac Risk Index (RCRI)

Assign 1 point each for:
History of ischemic heart disease
Compensated or prior chronic heart failure
Diabetes mellitus requiring insulin
Chronic kidney disease (creatinine >2.0 mg/dL [176.8 µmol/L])
History of cerebrovascular disease
Higher risk surgery (intrathoracic, intraperitoneal, supra-inguinal vascular)

Risk by RCRI Score[a]

Number of Points	Risk
0	0.4%
1	1.0%
2	2.4%
≥3	5.4%

[a]Risk of perioperative cardiac death, nonfatal myocardial infarction, or nonfatal cardiac arrest.

Adapted from Devereaux PJ, Goldman L, Cook DJ, Gilbert K, Leslie K, Guyatt GH. Perioperative cardiac events in patients undergoing noncardiac surgery: a review of the magnitude of the problem, the pathophysiology of the events and methods to estimate and communicate risk. CMAJ. 2005;173(6):627-634. [PMID: 16157727]

TABLE 55. Risk factors for Perioperative Pulmonary Complications

Patient-Related	Surgery-Related
Major	**Major**
Older age	Intrathoracic, intra-abdominal surgeries
COPD	Surgeries lasting >3 hours
Chronic heart failure	Emergency surgery
Poor general health status and/or functional dependence	
Smoking	
Low serum albumin level	
Kidney dysfunction	
Minor or Possible	**Minor or Possible**
Obesity	General anesthesia
Sleep apnea	

KEY POINTS

- Preoperative cardiac stress testing should be reserved for patients with reduced exercise tolerance and multiple cardiovascular risk factors.
- In patients not already on a β-blocker, perioperative β-blocker use is recommended only for those with coronary artery disease who are undergoing vascular surgery and for those undergoing other intermediate or higher risk surgery who have more than one cardiac risk factor.

Pulmonary Perioperative Management

Perioperative pulmonary complications, including prolonged and unexpected intubation, occur after 3% to 13% of surgical procedures. Many risk factors are associated with perioperative pulmonary complications (**Table 55**). Patients with COPD are two to five times more likely to experience such complications, and patients with more severe COPD are likely at higher risk.

The type of surgery is an extremely important predictor of perioperative pulmonary complications. The highest-risk surgeries are thoracic surgeries, abdominal aortic aneurysm repairs, and abdominal surgeries, especially open procedures near the diaphragm. General anesthesia may slightly increase the risk of pulmonary complications compared with spinal anesthesia. However, the added risk is

small and not apparent in every study, and the risk of pulmonary complications should not drive the selection of type of anesthesia. There is no correlation between FEV_1 or FVC and perioperative pulmonary complications. Therefore, preoperative spirometry should be reserved for patients with unexplained dyspnea.

Few interventions have been shown to reduce the risk of perioperative pulmonary complications. Pre- and postoperative lung volume expansion, either via deep breathing or incentive spirometry, reduces the risk for pulmonary complications. In patients with poorly controlled asthma, systemic corticosteroids can be used perioperatively. Patients with suboptimally controlled COPD should be treated aggressively with inhaled bronchodilators and probably systemic corticosteroids. Patients should have adequate pain control postoperatively to minimize atelectasis. Smoking is clearly associated with postoperative complications, including both pulmonary and nonpulmonary complications. However, there is mixed evidence regarding the benefit of smoking cessation less than 2 months before surgery, with some studies suggesting recent quitters may have higher rates of perioperative pulmonary complications. Smoking cessation at least 8 weeks before surgery, however, is clearly beneficial. In patients at highest risk for perioperative pulmonary complications, the internist, surgeon, and anesthesiologist should collaborate closely to assess the risk/benefit ratio for surgery and consider alternative surgical or nonsurgical interventions for the patient.

Obstructive sleep apnea (OSA) is associated with difficult intubation and an increased risk of postoperative apnea. The importance of OSA in the perioperative period may be underappreciated, in part because of the high prevalence of undiagnosed OSA in the community. The STOP-BANG questionnaire, a series of eight yes-or-no

CONT.

questions, is an easy-to-use screening tool for OSA (**Table 56**). Three or more positive responses have a sensitivity of 92% and specificity of 63% for predicting perioperative pulmonary complications. In patients with known or suspected OSA, this information should be made known to the anesthesiologist preoperatively and the patient monitored closely postoperatively, possibly with extended observation in an intensive care or step-down unit. These patients may also require continuous or bilevel positive airway pressure. [H]

KEY POINTS

- Preoperative spirometry should be reserved for patients with unexplained dyspnea.

- Pre- and postoperative lung volume expansion, either via deep breathing or incentive spirometry, reduces the risk for pulmonary complications.

- Obstructive sleep apnea (OSA) is associated with perioperative pulmonary complications, and preoperative screening for OSA is warranted because of the high prevalence of undiagnosed OSA in the community and its potential for causing perioperative pulmonary complications.

[H] Hematologic Perioperative Management

Venous Thromboembolism Prophylaxis

Perioperative venous thromboembolism (VTE) is a major preventable surgical complication. The risk of VTE is related to clinical risk factors and proposed surgery (**Table 57**). Preoperative evaluation should focus on assessing for clinical risk factors.

Early ambulation is often sufficient postoperative prophylaxis in patients with a low risk of VTE. In patients with a high risk of bleeding or for whom postoperative bleeding could be catastrophic (for example, neurosurgery patients), postoperative mechanical prophylaxis with pneumatic compression devices can be used alone; elastic graduated compression stockings are not recommended owing to lack of clear efficacy and risk for lower extremity skin damage. For the remainder of patients, drug prophylaxis for VTE with low-molecular-weight heparin (LMWH), fondaparinux, subcutaneous unfractionated heparin (UFH), or warfarin should be provided unless the assessed risk of bleeding outweighs the likely benefits (see MKSAP 16 Hematology and Oncology). Prophylactic anticoagulants should be withheld until the risk of postoperative bleeding is low, at least 12 hours after surgery. In general, prophylaxis should be continued until discharge. Patients with orthopedic surgeries, abdominal or gynecologic surgery for malignancy, or previous VTE should receive prophylaxis for up to 5 weeks after surgery.

Inferior vena cava (IVC) filters have been used for VTE prophylaxis in selected patients at high risk of VTE, especially those who have had a VTE within 1 to 3 months before surgery and for whom anticoagulants will be contraindicated postoperatively. Removable IVC filters are reasonable for these patients. There is no evidence supporting the use of prophylactic IVC filters in other populations, including patients undergoing bariatric surgery, and their routine use is discouraged.

Perioperative Management of Warfarin Therapy

Depending on the patient's thrombotic risk and the type of procedure, perioperative management options for patients using warfarin are to stop the warfarin during the perioperative period, stop the warfarin and bridge with a parenteral anticoagulant, or continue the warfarin throughout the perioperative period. Patients undergoing procedures considered low risk for bleeding, including cataract surgery, dental procedures, and biopsy of non-major organs, should continue warfarin during the perioperative period, with a target INR of 1.3 to 1.5 at the time of surgery. In patients using warfarin who are undergoing other surgeries, management of anticoagulant therapy is guided by the patient's risk of perioperative thrombosis (**Table 58**). Patients at low risk for thrombosis should usually discontinue warfarin 4 to 5 days preoperatively without bridging therapy. In patients at intermediate or high risk for perioperative thrombosis, warfarin also should be discontinued 4 to 5 days preoperatively; intermediate-risk patients should be considered for bridging,

TABLE 56.	STOP-BANG Screening Tool for Obstructive Sleep Apnea
Parameter	**Question**
Snoring	Do you snore loudly (louder than talking or loud enough to be heard through closed doors)?
Tired	Do you often feel tired, fatigued, or sleepy during daytime?
Observed	Has anyone observed you stop breathing during your sleep?
Blood pressure	Do you have or are you being treated for high blood pressure?
BMI	BMI more than 35?
Age	Age over 50 years?
Neck circumference	Neck circumference greater than 40 cm?
Gender	Gender male?

Scoring: High risk of obstructive sleep apnea: answering *yes* to three or more items; low risk of OSA: answering *yes* to less than three items.

Adapted with permission from Chung F, Yegneswaran B, Liao P, et al. STOP questionnaire: a tool to screen patients for obstructive sleep apnea. Anesthesiology. 2008;108(5):812-821. [PMID: 18431116] Copyright 2008, Lippincott Williams & Wilkins.

TABLE 57. Surgical Risk Stratification and Associated VTE Incidence

Patient Risk	Risk Factor Stratification	VTE Incidence Without Prophylaxis
Low	Minor surgery in patients younger than 40 years with no additional risk factors[a]	Calf vein DVT: 2% Proximal vein DVT: 0.4% Clinical PE: 0.2% Fatal PE: 0.002%
Moderate	Nonmajor surgery in patients aged 40-60 years with no clinical risk factors Minor surgery lasting <30 min in patients with clinical risk factors Major surgery in patients younger than 40 years with no clinical risk factors	Calf vein DVT: 10%-20% Proximal DVT: 2%-4% Clinical PE: 1%-2% Fatal PE: 0.1%-0.4%
High	Nonmajor surgery in patients older than 60 years or with clinical risk factors Major surgery in patients older than 40 years or with clinical risk factors	Calf vein DVT: 20%-40% Proximal DVT: 4%-8% Clinical PE: 2%-4% Fatal PE: 0.4%-1%
Very high	Major surgery in patients older than 40 years with history of VTE, cancer, or certain hypercoagulable states Hip or knee arthroplasty Hip fracture surgery Major trauma Spinal cord injury	Calf vein DVT: 40%-80% Proximal DVT: 10%-20% Clinical PE: 4%-10% Fatal PE: 0.2%-5%

DVT = deep venous thrombosis; PE = pulmonary embolism; VTE = venous thromboembolism.

[a]Potential risk factors include heart failure, nephrotic syndrome, pregnancy, estrogen use, use of general anesthesia, acute respiratory failure, active cancer, stroke with paresis, history of VTE, acute infectious illness, age >60 years, thrombophilia, acute rheumatic disease, inflammatory bowel disease, obesity, trauma, institutionalization, and immobility.

Adapted from PIER. Venous thromboembolism prophylaxis in the surgical patient. http://pier.acponline.org/physicians/diseases/periopr830/periopr830.html. Accessed 8 December 2011.

and high-risk patients should be bridged with either LMWH at therapeutic doses or UFH. Bridging should be started 1 to 2 days after the last dose of warfarin. For patients at intermediate thrombotic risk, LMWH at prophylactic doses is an option, especially for patients with intermediate risk of thrombosis. The decision of which agent to use and at what dosage should be based on patient-specific risks and benefits.

Bridging therapy with LMWH should be stopped 24 hours preoperatively and UFH 4 to 6 hours preoperatively. Patients with an intermediate thrombotic risk who are receiving LMWH for bridging can be given a half dose for the last injection before surgery to minimize the risk of intraoperative bleeding. LMWH or UFH can be resumed as early as 12 to 24 hours after surgery, although the exact timing should depend on the patient's indication for anticoagulation and bleeding risk. Patients at intermediate risk for thrombosis can restart LMWH at prophylactic doses; those at high risk should be treated at therapeutic doses. Warfarin should be restarted once the patient is at low risk for bleeding, and bridging therapy is stopped once the INR is therapeutic.

Perioperative Management of Antiplatelet Medications, Coagulopathies, and Thrombocytopenia

Patients undergoing surgeries with low risk for bleeding can continue aspirin and/or clopidogrel therapy. Patients receiving antiplatelet therapy for recent myocardial infarction or cardiac stent placement should not have this therapy interrupted for 6 weeks for a bare metal stent or myocardial infarction or for 1 year for a drug-eluting stent. Low-risk surgery can usually be performed while the patient is on antiplatelet therapy, whereas most other surgeries should be delayed if possible. Antiplatelet therapy is usually avoided in patients undergoing neurosurgery or other surgeries in which the sequelae of postoperative hemorrhage could be catastrophic. Conversely, aspirin therapy is recommended before coronary artery bypass grafting (CABG), although other antiplatelet agents should be discontinued before elective CABG. There is little evidence or consensus regarding antiplatelet therapy in other instances, and decisions regarding clinical care should be based on a patient's individualized risks and benefits. Aspirin therapy may be safe in patients undergoing other surgeries, although it is often stopped 7 to 10 days before

TABLE 58.	Perioperative Bridging Strategies for Patients Using Warfarin	
Risk	**Conditions**	**Bridging Strategy**
Low	VTE >12 months ago and no additional risk factors	Discontinue warfarin; no bridging
	Atrial fibrillation with CHADS$_2$ score ≤2 without prior CVA	
Intermediate	VTE within 3-12 months or history of recurrent VTE	Discontinue warfarin; consider bridging with LMWH (therapeutic or prophylactic dose) or UFH based on assessment of individual patient and surgery-related factors
	Active malignancy (treated within 6 months or palliatively)	
	Known hypercoagulable state	
	Atrial fibrillation with CHADS$_2$ score of 3 or 4 without prior CVA	
	Newer mechanical heart valve in nonmitral position	
High	VTE <3 months ago or VTE with thrombophilia	Discontinue warfarin; bridge with LMWH (therapeutic dose) or UFH
	CVA <6 months ago	
	Atrial fibrillation with CHADS$_2$ score >4 or prior CVA	
	Mechanical heart valve in mitral position or older aortic prosthesis	

CVA = cerebrovascular accident; LMWH = low-molecular-weight heparin; UFH = unfractionated heparin; VTE = venous thromboembolism.

elective surgery. Antiplatelet therapy is usually restarted 24 hours after surgery unless there is evidence of or elevated risk for postoperative bleeding.

All patients should be carefully screened preoperatively for signs or symptoms of underlying bleeding disorders and anemia. Laboratory testing should be reserved for patients in whom there is a reasonable probability of an abnormal test, and is not required as a routine component of preoperative evaluation. A complete blood count, and possibly coagulation studies, can be obtained in patients undergoing surgery with a high risk for significant bleeding as well as in patients with known or suspected hepatic dysfunction. A preoperative prothrombin time may also be reasonable in Ashkenazi Jews, approximately 3% of whom have low factor XI levels from a hereditary deficiency.

In patients with known quantitative platelet deficiencies, the platelet count should be increased to above 50,000/µL (50×10^9/L) before elective surgery, if possible. Patients with immune thrombocytopenic purpura should receive corticosteroids, intravenous immune globulin, or Rho(D) immune globulin preoperatively. Patients with thrombotic thrombocytopenic purpura (TTP) should receive plasmapheresis. Platelet transfusion is unlikely to be helpful in patients with TTP; however, other patients with persistent thrombocytopenia are typically transfused with platelets just before surgery. Patients with qualitative platelet dysfunction (for example, from kidney or liver disease) can be given desmopressin acetate 1 hour preoperatively for lower-risk procedures for bleeding. Patients undergoing higher-risk procedures should receive a platelet transfusion. Hematology consultation is often helpful in the perioperative management of these patients.

Perioperative Management of Anemia

Patients with a preoperative hemoglobin concentration below 6 g/dL (60 g/L) or a postoperative hemoglobin concentration below 7 g/dL (70 g/L) have worse outcomes than those with higher hemoglobin levels. Patients with either known anemia or anemia discovered as part of the preoperative evaluation should be evaluated for an underlying cause. Patients who require iron, vitamin B$_{12}$, or folic acid supplements should receive these therapies perioperatively. Patients with anemia of kidney disease or other anemias that are potentially responsive to exogenous erythropoietin should be treated preoperatively only if blood losses are expected to be large and transfusion is contraindicated.

Transfusion is reserved for patients with symptomatic anemia, a preoperative hemoglobin concentration below 6 g/dL (60 g/L), postoperative hemoglobin concentration below 7 g/dL (70 g/L), or patients with symptomatic cardiovascular disease and hemoglobin concentrations between 6 and 10 g/dL (60 and 100 g/L). Transfusing asymptomatic patients with known CAD to achieve a hemoglobin level of greater than 10 g/dL (100 g/L) is frequently done, although the data supporting this practice remain controversial. Patients with sickle cell disease are at high risk for perioperative sickle cell crisis, which can be reduced by reducing the percentage of sickle-cell variant erythrocytes in total blood volume. Consultation with an experienced hematologist is advisable to determine the extent of transfusion needed for these patients. **H**

- Patients on chronic warfarin undergoing low-risk procedures, including cataract surgery, dental procedures, and biopsy of nonmajor organs, can continue warfarin, with a target INR of 1.3 to 1.5 perioperatively.

- Patients on chronic warfarin undergoing intermediate- or high-risk procedures should discontinue warfarin 4 to 5 days before surgery; patients with a low thrombotic risk typically do not require bridging anticoagulant therapy, whereas those with an intermediate or high thrombotic risk should receive heparin bridging therapy perioperatively.

- Aspirin and/or clopidogrel should be continued in patients undergoing low-risk surgery and in patients with recent cardiac stent placement or myocardial infarction; in most other patients, antiplatelet therapy can be safely discontinued 7 to 10 days preoperatively.

Perioperative Management of Endocrine Diseases

Diabetes Mellitus

Patients with diabetes mellitus are at higher risk for perioperative complications, although many of these are related to end-organ damage from the diabetes rather than hypo- or hyperglycemia. Patients with type 1 diabetes mellitus will need to have some insulin continued at all times to prevent the development of diabetic ketoacidosis; this warning should be emphasized in preoperative consultations and in communications with the surgeon and anesthesiologist.

Hyperglycemia increases the risk of infectious and other postoperative complications. Hemoglobin A_{1c} and kidney function should be measured preoperatively in patients with diabetes if these have not been measured recently. Patients found to have poorly controlled diabetes should usually have elective surgeries delayed until their glycemic control is improved, ideally to a fasting plasma glucose level below 220 mg/dL (12.21 mmol/L).

Diabetes medications require adjustment on the morning of surgery. Metformin is usually discontinued at least the night before surgery; other oral hypoglycemic medications should be withheld on the morning of surgery. In general, short-acting insulins should be withheld the morning of surgery. Long-acting insulins are usually dose adjusted, although the exact amount depends on the patient's baseline control and regimen. Typically one-half to two-thirds of the usual dose of long-acting insulin is given in the 12 hours before surgery, with a lesser reduction in patients who are poorly controlled at baseline or who are taking corticosteroids or other agents expected

to raise glucose levels. Given the complexities of preoperative medication adjustment, a patient's plasma glucose level should be measured the morning of surgery, and insulin or dextrose may be needed to keep the patient euglycemic.

Oral agents are challenging to use perioperatively because of risk of hypoglycemia given their long half-lives and variable oral intake in the postoperative patient. In addition, metformin confers a risk of lactic acidosis while thiazolidinediones promote fluid retention. Thus, many patients with diabetes, even those who have previously been well controlled with diet or oral medications, may need insulin during the perioperative period. Intensive insulin therapy (IIT) using continuous insulin infusions has been extensively investigated in the postoperative setting with mixed results. Current evidence does not support IIT as part of routine postoperative care. Approaches to glycemic management in hospitalized patients are discussed in MKSAP 16 Endocrinology and Metabolism.

Thyroid Disease

Patients with thyroid disease who have not had recent thyroid function testing and those in whom thyroid disease is suspected should have thyroid function tested preoperatively. Hyperthyroidism can predispose patients to perioperative complications, including atrial fibrillation, cardiomyopathy, respiratory failure, and thrombocytopenia. These risks are highest in patients undergoing thyroid surgery. Patients with hyperthyroidism should be made euthyroid prior to surgery, typically with antithyroid drugs. In patients whose surgery cannot be delayed, β-blockers, iodine, and corticosteroids can be added, although the risks of these medications should be balanced by the degree of thyroid dysfunction and nature of the surgery. In contrast, for patients with hypothyroidism, surgery should be delayed only for severe hypothyroidism; mild or subclinical hypothyroidism does not significantly increase the risk of perioperative complications.

Adrenal Insufficiency

The incidence of acute adrenal insufficiency is relatively low in the perioperative period, even in patients treated with chronic corticosteroids. Patients using chronic low-dose corticosteroids (prednisone ≤10 mg/d), short-term corticosteroids, or inhaled corticosteroids have a low risk for adrenal crisis and do not need preoperative testing or treatment. Patients who chronically use higher doses of corticosteroids (>10 mg/d prednisone for at least 3 weeks) or who have known adrenal insufficiency should take their usual daily dose on the day of surgery. These patients should be well hydrated and can receive supplemental hydrocortisone on the day of surgery, with low doses (for example, 25 mg) for minor surgery and higher doses (up to 150 mg) for major surgery. These doses should be

CONT.

tapered rapidly back to baseline over the first 2 postoperative days unless signs or symptoms of adrenal crisis develop. Adrenocorticotropic hormone stimulation testing should be reserved for patients in whom primary adrenal insufficiency is suspected or in whom empiric supplemental corticosteroids could be harmful.

KEY POINTS

- Many patients with diabetes mellitus, even those who have previously been well controlled with diet or oral medications, need insulin during the perioperative period.

- For patients with hypothyroidism, surgery should be delayed only for severe hypothyroidism; mild or subclinical hypothyroidism does not significantly increase the risk of perioperative complications.

Perioperative Management of Kidney Disease

Patients with chronic kidney disease (CKD) have a higher incidence of perioperative complications than those without, although many of these complications are attributable to cardiovascular disease. Preoperative evaluation of patients with CKD should include laboratory testing to assess the stage of kidney disease. Patients with significant anemia may benefit from preoperative exogenous erythropoietin if more than minimal blood loss is expected as these patients are unable to physiologically respond to acute blood loss. ACE inhibitors and angiotensin receptor blockers, commonly used in patients with CKD, can cause intraoperative hypotension and may be withheld on the day of surgery.

No agents have been shown to be protective against intraoperative acute kidney injury. In general, patients with CKD should be adequately hydrated perioperatively with anesthetic and other agents selected specifically to avoid hypotension. Intraoperative urine output is not a good predictor of postoperative acute kidney injury, and fluid intake should not be titrated to urine output.

Postoperatively, patients with CKD are at risk for volume overload, electrolyte imbalance, and acute kidney injury. NSAIDs and other nephrotoxic agents should be avoided. Care should be taken that all medications are adjusted for the patient's glomerular filtration rate. Patients with uremia are at risk for platelet dysfunction and postoperative bleeding. In patients on dialysis, the timing of dialysis perioperatively should be coordinated between anesthesiologist, surgeon, and nephrologist.

KEY POINT

- In patients with chronic kidney disease, care should be taken that all medications are adjusted for the patient's glomerular filtration rate.

Perioperative Management of Liver Disease

Both acute hepatitis and chronic liver disease with cirrhosis are associated with an elevated risk of perioperative complications and death. Surgery can worsen liver disease because of hepatic ischemia and hepatic hypoxemia. The half-life of many medications, including sedatives, opioids, and anesthetic agents, may be prolonged in patients with hepatic dysfunction, causing further hypoxia and hypotension. Poor liver function predisposes to hepatic failure, bleeding, poor wound healing, and infections. The internist should be alert for signs and symptoms of hepatic dysfunction, especially in patients who have risk factors for liver disease. Patients whose history and physical examination suggest ongoing liver disease should receive preoperative liver chemistry tests.

Elective surgery should be deferred to evaluate newly diagnosed liver disease and postponed in patients with acute hepatitis from any cause. Patients with chronic liver disease without evidence of cirrhosis appear to be at no excess perioperative risk. Patients with hemochromatosis should be carefully evaluated for cardiomyopathy. In patients being treated for hepatitis B, the danger of temporary cessation of antiretroviral therapy causing a disease flare should be emphasized to the surgeon.

In patients with chronic liver disease with evidence of cirrhosis, surgical risk is based on both the extent of liver disease and the type of surgery. The Child-Turcotte-Pugh (CTP) score has been used to assess risk: patients with CTP class A liver disease have a 10% risk of death after general surgery; those with class B disease have a 30% risk; and those with class C disease have a 75% to 80% risk. The Model for End-stage Liver Disease (MELD) score, American Society of Anesthesia (ASA) risk score, and patient age are all independent predictors of mortality. These variables have been linked into a single calculator that can be used to estimate postoperative mortality risk (www.mayoclinic.org/meld/mayomodel9.html).

Intrabdominal surgeries, especially hepatic surgery and gallbladder surgery, are high risk in patients with cirrhotic liver disease associated with portal hypertension. The combination of coagulopathy and internal varices makes these surgeries technically challenging. Estimating operative risk in biliary surgery is especially difficult as the jaundice in these patients is multifactorial, confounding the risk prediction models. Coronary artery bypass grafting is also higher risk in patients with cirrhotic liver disease. Herniorrhaphy, in contrast, is average risk.

Preoperative management of cirrhotic liver disease involves optimizing liver function. Patients with coagulopathy are typically treated with oral vitamin K to reverse any nutritional deficiencies. Vitamin K, however, does not typically normalize these patients' coagulopathy, and they may need fresh frozen plasma, cryoprecipitate, or activated factor VIIa. Ascites predisposes to perioperative pulmonary

CONT.

complications, poor wound healing of abdominal surgeries, and excess death. Ascites should primarily be managed with diuretics, as large-volume paracentesis is effective only for a short period of time. Placement of a transjugular intrahepatic portosystemic shunt (TIPS) may be indicated preoperatively in patients with refractory ascites. TIPS may also be appropriate for patients with known esophageal varices undergoing major surgery.

Perioperative management should focus on preventing complications of chronic liver disease. Blood pressure and volume status should be carefully monitored to minimize a renal insult that could precipitate a hepatorenal syndrome. Sedatives and narcotics that are hepatically metabolized should be dosed carefully. Patients with ileus or other causes of slowed intestinal transit should be observed closely for signs of hepatic encephalopathy. If encephalopathy develops, the patient should receive lactulose orally or, if on NPO status (nothing by mouth), via retention enema. Patients with advanced liver disease are at risk for hypoglycemia postoperatively because of impaired gluconeogenesis.

KEY POINT

- Patients with examination findings suggesting ongoing liver disease should receive preoperative liver chemistry tests; elective surgery should be deferred to evaluate newly diagnosed liver disease.

Perioperative Management of Neurologic Disease

Patients with neurologic diseases present specific challenges in the perioperative period. Patients with neuromuscular diseases, including amyotrophic lateral sclerosis, muscular dystrophy, and myasthenia gravis, are at high risk for respiratory failure. Preoperative pulmonary function testing is sometimes done in these patients, although there are no specific risk prediction models for respiratory failure. Close consultation among surgeon, anesthesiologist, internist, and neurologist is essential in safely managing patients with neuromuscular diseases.

Patients with a seizure disorder should have their therapy optimized preoperatively, and anticonvulsant drug levels should be therapeutic. Patients should continue the anticonvulsant drugs through the morning of surgery. The presence of a seizure disorder will usually influence an anesthesiologist's choice of agents. Postoperatively, patients with a seizure disorder may require parenteral medication.

Patients with multiple sclerosis may experience an acute exacerbation after anesthesia. Interferon is typically continued for these patients perioperatively, while baclofen, which is only available orally, may need to be transitioned to a benzodiazepine to prevent postoperative withdrawal seizures.

Patients with Parkinson disease should continue antiparkinsonian agents through the morning of surgery.

Perioperative management of patients who use short-acting dopamine agonists is challenging, as abrupt withdrawal of these agents can produce severe muscle rigidity that can interfere with ventilation and mimic neuroleptic malignant syndrome. Patients with Parkinson disease are also at risk for aspiration secondary to hypersalivation and poor respiratory mechanics.

Perioperative stroke impacts 0.3% to 0.8% of postsurgical patients and is further discussed in MKSAP 16 Neurology. Risk factors for delirium in the postoperative setting are similar to those in medically hospitalized patients and include pain, immobilization, anemia, hypoxemia, and sedative and opioid use. Early consultation by an internist or geriatrician for patients at risk for postoperative delirium may be helpful. Delirium is further discussed in MKSAP 16 Pulmonary and Critical Care Medicine.

Bibliography

Interpretation of the Medical Literature

Guyatt G, Rennie D, Meade MO, Cook DJ, eds. Users' Guides to the Medical Literature: A Manual for Evidence-Based Clinical Practice. 2nd ed. New York, NY: McGraw-Hill; 2008.

Ho PM, Peterson PN, Masoudi FA. Evaluating the evidence: is there a rigid hierarchy? Circulation. 2008;118(16):1675-1684. [PMID: 18852378]

Lin KW, Slawson DC. Identifying and using good practice guidelines. Am Fam Physician. 2009;80(1):67-70. [PMID: 19621847]

Sox HC, Greenfield S. Comparative effectiveness research: a report from the Institute of Medicine. Ann Intern Med. 2009;151(3):203-205. [PMID: 19567618]

Routine Care of the Healthy Patient

2008 PHS Guideline Update Panel, Liasons, and Staff. Treating tobacco use and dependence: 2008 update U.S. Public Health Service Clinical Practice Guideline executive summary. Respir Care. 2008;53(9):1217-1222. [PMID: 18807274]

Berg AO, Baird MA, Botkin JR, et al. National Institutes of Health State-of-the-Science Conference Statement: Family History and Improving Health. Ann Intern Med. 2009;151(12):872-877. [PMID: 19884615]

Fiore MC, Baker TB. Clinical practice. Treating smokers in the health care setting. N Engl J Med. 2011;365(13):1222-1231. [PMID: 21991895]

Heshka JT, Palleschi C, Howley H, Wilson B, Wells PS. A systematic review of perceived risks, psychological and behavioral impacts of genetic testing. Genet Med. 2008;10(1):19-32. [PMID: 18197053]

Kahn JA. HPV vaccination for the prevention of cervical intraepithelial neoplasia. New Engl J Med. 2009;361(3):271-278. [PMID: 19605832]

Lambert LC, Fauci AS. Influenza vaccines for the future. New Engl J Med. 2010;363(21):2036-2044. [PMID: 21083388]

Lin JS, O'Connor E, Whitlock EP, Beil TL. Behavioral counseling to promote physical activity and a healthful diet to prevent cardiovascular disease in adults: a systematic review for the U.S. Preventive Services Task Force. Ann Intern Med. 2010;153(11):736-750. [PMID: 21135297]

Long EF, Brandeau ML, Owens DK. The cost-effectiveness and population outcomes of expanded HIV screening and antiretroviral treatment in the United States. Ann Intern Med. 2010;153(12):778-789. [PMID: 21173412]

Porter ME. What is value in health care? N Engl J Med. 2010;363(26):2477-2481. [PMID: 21142528]

Powers BJ, Olsen MK, Smith VA, Woolson RF, Bosworth HB, Oddone EZ. Measuring blood pressure for decision making and quality reporting: where and how many measures? Ann Intern Med. 2011;154(12):781-788. [PMID: 21690592]

Rollnick S, Butler CC, Kinnersley P, Gregory J, Mash B. Motivational interviewing. BMJ. 2010;340:c1900. [PMID: 20423957]

Saitz R, Alford DP, Bernstein J, Cheng DM, Samet J, Palfai T. Screening and brief intervention for unhealthy drug use in primary care settings: randomized clinical trials are needed. J Addict Med. 2010;4(3):123-130. [PMID: 20936079]

Schousboe J, Kerlikowski K, Loh A, Cummings SR. Personalizing mammography by breast density and other risk factors for breast cancer: analysis of health benefits and cost-effectiveness. Ann Intern Med. 2011;155(1):10-20. [PMID: 21727289]

Smith PC, Schmidt SM, Allensworth-Davies D, Saitz R. A single-question screening test for drug use in primary care. Arch Intern Med. 2010;170(13):1155-1159. [PMID: 20625025]

Thompson SG, Ashton HA, Gao L, Scott RA; Multicentre Aneurysm Screening Study Group. Screening men for abdominal aortic aneurysm: 10 year mortality and cost effectiveness results from the randomised Multicentre Aneurysm Screening Study. BMJ. 2009;338:b2307. [PMID: 19553269]

U.S. Preventive Services Task Force. Behavioral counseling to prevent sexually transmitted infections: U.S. Preventative Services Task Force recommendation statement. Ann Intern Med. 2008;149(7):491-496, W95. [PMID: 18838729]

Zolotor AJ, Denham AC, Weil A. Intimate partner violence. Prim Care. 2009;36(1):167-179, x. [PMID: 19231608]

Patient Safety

Chassin MR, Loeb JM, Schmaltz SP, Wachter RM. Accountability measures—using measurement to promote quality improvement. N Engl J Med. 2010;363(7):683-688. [PMID: 20573915]

Schiff GD, Bates DW. Can electronic clinical documentation help prevent diagnostic errors? N Engl J Med. 2010;362(12):1066-1069. [PMID: 20335582]

Swensen, SJ, Meyer GS, Nelson EC, et al. Cottage industry to postindustrial care—the revolution in health care delivery. N Engl J Med. 2010;362(5):e12. [PMID: 20089956]

Professionalism and Ethics

Braddock CH 3rd, Edwards KA, Hasenberg NM, Laidley TL, Levinson W. Informed decision making in outpatient practice: time to get back to basics. JAMA. 1999;282(24):2313-2320. [PMID: 10612318]

Castillo LS, Williams BA, Hooper SM, Sabatino CP, Weithorn LA, Sudore RL. Lost in translation: the unintended consequences of advance directive law on clinical care. Ann Intern Med. 2011;154(2):121-128. [PMID: 21242368]

DesRoches CM, Rao SR, Fromson JA, et al. Physicians' perceptions, preparedness for reporting, and experiences related to impaired and incompetent colleagues. JAMA. 2010;304(2):187-193. [PMID: 20628132]

Gallagher TH, Studdert D, Levinson W. Disclosing harmful medical errors to patients. N Engl J Med. 2007;356(26):2713-2719. [PMID: 17596606]

Localio AR. Patient compensation without litigation: a promising development. Ann Intern Med. 2010;153(4):266-267. [PMID: 20713794]

Owens DK, Qaseem A, Chou R, Shekelle P; Clinical Guidelines Committee of the American College of Physicians. High-value, cost-conscious health care: concepts for clinicians to evaluate the benefits, harms, and costs of medical interventions. Ann Intern Med. 2011;154(3):174-180. [PMID: 21282697]

Quill T, Arnold RM. Evaluating requests for hastened death #156. J Palliat Med. 2008;11(8):1151-1152. [PMID: 18980457]

Snyder L; American College of Physicians Ethics, Professionalism, and Human Rights Committee. American College of Physicians Ethics Manual: sixth edition. Ann Intern Med. 2012;156(1 Pt 2):73-104. [PMID: 22213573]

Palliative Care

Bakitas M, Lyons KD, Hegel MT, et al. Effects of a palliative care intervention on clinical outcomes in patients with advanced cancer: the Project ENABLE II randomized controlled trial. JAMA. 2009;302(7):741-749. [PMID: 19690306]

Lorenz KA, Lynn J, Dy SM, et al. Evidence for improving palliative care at the end of life: a systematic review. Ann Intern Med. 2008;148(2):147-159. [PMID: 18195339]

Morrison RS, Penrod JD, Cassel JB, et al. Cost savings associated with US hospital palliative care consultation programs. Arch Intern Med. 2008;168(16):1783-1790. [PMID: 18779466]

Reville B, Axelrod D, Maury R. Palliative care for the cancer patient. Prim Care. 2009;36(4):781-810. [PMID: 19913186]

Swetz KM, Kamal AH. Palliative care. Ann Intern Med. 2012;156(3):ITC21. [PMID: 22312158]

Temel JS, Greer JA, Muzikansky, et al. Early palliative care for patients with metastatic non-small-cell lung cancer. N Engl J Med. 2010;363(8):733-742. [PMID: 20818875]

Common Symptoms

American Geriatrics Society Panel on the Pharmacologic Management of Persistent Pain in Older persons. Pharmacologic management of persistent pain in older persons. J Am Geriatr Soc. 2009;57(8):1331-1346. [PMID: 19573219]

Anderson JL, Adams CD, Antman EM, et al; American College of Cardiology; American Heart Association Task Force on Practice Guidelines (Writing Committee to Revise the 2002 Guidelines for the Management of Patients With Unstable Angina/Non-ST-Elevation Myocardial Infarction); American College of Emergency Physicians; Society for Cardiovascular Angiography and Interventions; Society of Thoracic Surgeons; American Association of Cardiovascular and Pulmonary Rehabilitation; Society for Academic Emergency Medicine. ACC/AHA 2007 guidelines for the management of patients with unstable angina/non-ST-Elevation myocardial infarction: a report of the American College of Cardiology/American Heart Association Task Force on Practice Guidelines (Writing Committee to Revise the 2002 Guidelines for the Management of Patients With Unstable Angina/Non-ST-Elevation Myocardial Infarction) developed in collaboration with the American College of Emergency Physicians, the Society for Cardiovascular Angiography and Interventions, and the Society of Thoracic Surgeons endorsed by the American Association of Cardiovascular and Pulmonary Rehabilitation and the Society for Academic Emergency Medicine. J Am Coll Cardiol. 2007;50(7):e1-e157. [PMID: 17692738]

Bittner ML, Marcus DA, Tenzer P, Romito K. Using Opioids in the Management of Chronic Pain Patients: Challenges and Future Options. American Academy of Family Physicians. 2010.

Bohnert AS, Valenstein M, Bair MJ, et al. Association between opioid prescribing patterns and opioid overdose-related deaths. JAMA. 2011;305(13):1315-1321. [PMID: 21467284]

Cooper PN, Westby M, Pitcher DW, Bullock I. Synopsis of the National Institute for Health and Clinical Excellence Guideline for management of transient loss of consciousness. Ann Intern Med. 2011;155(8):543-549. [PMID: 21930835]

Dunn KM, Saunders KW, Rutter CM, et al. Opioid prescriptions for chronic pain and overdose: a cohort study. Ann Intern Med. 2010;152(2):85-92. [PMID: 20083827]

Eccleston C, Williams AC, Morley S. Psychological therapies for the management of chronic pain (excluding headache) in adults. Cochrane Database Syst Rev. 2009;(2):CD007407. [PMID: 19370688]

Fife TD, Iverson DJ, Lempert T, et al; Quality Standards Subcommittee, American Academy of Neurology. Practice parameter: therapies for benign paroxysmal positional vertigo (an evidence based review): report of the Quality Standards Subcommittee of the American

Academy of Neurology. Neurology. 2008;70(22):2067-2074. [PMID: 18505980]

Gilron I, Bailey JM, Tu D, Holden RR, Jackson AC, Houlden RL. Nortriptyline and gabapentin, alone and in combination for neuropathic pain: a double-blind, randomised controlled crossover trial. Lancet. 2009;374(9697):1252-1261. [PMID: 19796802]

Gonzales R, Bartlett JG, Besser RE, et al; American Academy of Family Physicians; American College of Physicians-American Society of Internal Medicine; Centers for Disease Control; Infectious Diseases Society of America. Principles of appropriate antibiotic use for treatment of uncomplicated acute bronchitis: background. Ann Intern Med. 2001;134(6):521-529. [PMID: 11255532]

Hess EP, Dipti A, Chandra S, et al. Diagnostic accuracy of the TIMI risk score in patients with chest pain the emergency department: a meta-analysis. CMAJ. 2010;182(10):1039-1044. [PMID: 20530163]

Hotson JR, Baloh RW. Acute vestibular syndrome. N Engl J Med. 1998;339(10):680-685. [PMID: 9725927]

Irwin RS, Baumann MH, Bolser DC, et al; American College of Chest Physicians (ACCP). Diagnosis and management of cough executive summary: ACCP evidence-based clinical practice guidelines. Chest. 2006;129(1 suppl):1S-23S. [PMID: 16428686]

Moore RA, Straube S, Wiffen PJ, Derry S, McQuay HJ. Pregabalin for acute and chronic pain in adults. Cochrane Database Syst Rev. 2009;(3):CD007076. [PMID: 19588419]

Moya A, Sutton R, Ammirati F, et al; Task Force for the Diagnosis and Management of Syncope; European Society of Cardiology (ESC); European Heart Rhythm Association (EHRA); Heart Failure Association (HFA); Heart Rhythm Society (HRS). Guidelines for the diagnosis and management of syncope (version 2009). Eur Heart J. 2009;30(21):2631-2671. [PMID: 19713422]

Nijrolder I, van der Horst H, van der Windt D. Prognosis of fatigue: a systematic review. J Psychosom Res. 2008;64(4):335-349. [PMID: 18374732]

Ouyang H, Quinn J. Diagnosis and evaluation of syncope in the emergency department. Emerg Med Clin North Am. 2010;28(3):471-485. [PMID: 20709239]

Parry SW, Tan MP. An approach to the evaluation and management of syncope in adults. BMJ. 2010;340:c880. [PMID: 20172928]

Schroeder K, Fahey T. Over-the-counter medications for acute cough in children and adults in ambulatory settings. Cochrane Database Syst Rev. 2004;(4):CD001831. [PMID: 15495019]

Schutte-Rodin S, Broch L, Buysse D, Dorsey C, Sateia M. Clinical guideline for the evaluation and management of chronic insomnia in adults. J Clin Sleep Med. 2008;4(5):487-504. [PMID: 18853708]

Sloane PD, Coeytaux RR, Beck RS, Dallara J. Dizziness: state of the science. Ann Intern Med. 2001;134(9 Pt 2):823-832. [PMID: 11346317]

Swap CJ, Nagurney JT. Value and limitations of chest pain history in the evaluation of patients with suspected acute coronary syndromes. JAMA. 2005;294(20):2623-2629. [PMID: 16304077]

Wilson JF. In the clinic. Insomnia. Ann Intern Med. 2008;148(1):ITC13-1-ITC13-16. [PMID: 18166757]

Musculoskeletal Pain

Chou R, Qaseem A, Snow V, et al; Clinical Efficacy Assessment Subcommittee of the American College of Physicians; American College of Physicians; American Pain Society Low Back Pain Guidelines Panel. Diagnosis and treatment of low back pain: a joint clinical practice guideline from the American College of Physicians and the American Pain Society. Ann Intern Med. 2007;147(7):478-491. [PMID: 17909209]

Chou R, Shekelle P. Will this patient develop persistent disabling low back pain? JAMA. 2010;303(13):1295-1302. [PMID: 20371789]

Coombes BK, Bisset L, Vicenzino B. Efficacy and safety of corticosteroid injections and other injections for management of tendinopathy: a

systematic review of randomised controlled trials. Lancet. 2010;376(9754):1751-1767. [PMID: 20970844]

Gaujoux-Viala C, Dougados M, Gossec L. Efficacy and safety of steroid injections for shoulder and elbow tendonitis: a meta-analysis of randomised controlled trials. Ann Rheum Dis. 2009;68(12):1843-1849. [PMID: 19054817]

Jarvik JG, Comstock BA, Kliot M, et al. Surgery versus non-surgical therapy for carpal tunnel syndrome: a randomised parallel-group trial. Lancet. 2009;374(9695):1074-1081. [PMID: 19782873]

Kuijper B, Tans JTJ, Beelen A, Nollet F, de Visser M. Cervical collar or physiotherapy versus wait and see policy for recent onset cervical radiculopathy: randomised trial. BMJ. 2009;339:b3883. [PMID: 19812130]

Nikolaidis I, Fouyas IP, Sandercock PA, Statham PF. Surgery for cervical radiculopathy or myelopathy. Cochrane Database Syst Rev. 2010;(1):CD001466. [PMID: 20091520]

Ottenheijm RP, Jansen MJ, Staal JB, et al. Accuracy of diagnostic ultrasound in patients with suspected subacromial disorders: a systematic review and meta-analysis. Arch Phys Med Rehabil. 2010;91(10):1616-1625. [PMID: 20875523]

Seida JC, LeBlanc C, Schouten JR, et al. Systematic review: nonoperative and operative treatments for rotator cuff tears. Ann Intern Med. 2010;153(4):246-255. [PMID: 20621893]

Young C. In the clinic. Plantar fasciitis. Ann Intern Med. 2012;156(1 Pt 1):ITC1-1-ITC1-16. [PMID: 22213510]

Dyslipidemia

Ginsberg HN, Elam MB, Lovato MC, et al; ACCORD Study Group. Effects of combination lipid therapy in type 2 diabetes mellitus. N Engl J Med. 2010;362(17):1563-1574. [PMID: 20228404]

Blaha MJ, Bansal S, Rouf R, Golden SH, Blumenthal RS, Defilippis AP. A practical "ABCDE" approach to the metabolic syndrome. Mayo Clin Proc. 2008;83(8):932-941. [PMID: 18674478]

Calderon RM, Cubeddu LX, Goldberg RB, Schiff ER. Statins in the treatment of dyslipidemia in the presence of elevated liver aminotransferase levels: a therapeutic dilemma. Mayo Clin Proc. 2010;85(4):349-356. [PMID: 20360293]

Egan A, Colman E. Weighing the benefits of high-dose simvastatin against the risk of myopathy. N Engl J Med. 2011;365(4):285-287. [PMID: 21675881]

Hayward RA, Krumholz HM, Zulman DM, Timbie JW, Vijan S. Optimizing statin treatment for primary prevention of coronary artery disease. Ann Intern Med. 2010;152(2):69-77. [PMID: 20083825]

Joy TR, Hegele RA. Narrative review: statin-related myopathy. Ann Intern Med. 2009;150(12):858-868. [PMID: 19528564]

Kromhout D, Giltay EJ, Geleijnse JM; Alpha Omega Trial Group. n-3 fatty acids and cardiovascular events after myocardial infarction. N Engl J Med. 2010;363(21):2015-2026. [PMID: 20929341]

Mottillo S, Filion KB, Genest J, et al. The metabolic syndrome and cardiovascular risk a systematic review and meta-analysis. J Am Coll Cardiol. 2010;56(14):1113-1132. [PMID: 20863953]

Ray KK, Seshasai SRK, Erqou S, et al. Statins and all-cause mortality in high-risk primary prevention: a meta-analysis of 11 randomized controlled trials involving 65,229 participants. Arch Intern Med. 2010;170(12):1024-1031. [PMID: 20585067]

Taylor AJ, Villines TC, Stanek EJ, et al. Extended-release niacin or ezetimibe and carotid intima-media thickness. N Engl J Med. 2009;361(22):2113-2122. [PMID: 19915217]

Tota-Maharaj R, Defilippis AP, Blumenthal RS, Blaha MJ. A practical approach to the metabolic syndrome: review of current concepts and management. Curr Opin Cardiol. 2010;25(5):502-512. [PMID: 20644468]

Obesity

Adams TD, Gress RE, Smith SC, et al. Long-term mortality after gastric bypass surgery. N Engl J Med. 2007;357(8):753-761. [PMID: 17715409]

Foster GD, Wyatt HR, Hill JO, et al. Weight and metabolic outcomes after 2 years on a low-carbohydrate versus low-fat diet: a randomized trial. Ann Intern Med. 2010;153(3):147-157. [PMID: 20679559]

Lang IA, Llewellyn DJ, Alexander K, Melzer D. Obesity, physical function, and mortality in older adults. J Am Geriatr Soc. 2008;56:1474-1478. [PMID: 18662211]

Leblanc ES, O'Connor E, Whitlock EP, Patnode CD, Kapka T. Effectiveness of primary care-relevant treatments for obesity in adults: a systematic evidence review for the U.S. Preventive Services Task Force. Ann Intern Med. 2011;155(7):434-477. [PMID: 21969342]

Li Z, Maglione M, Tu W, et al. Meta-analysis: pharmacologic treatment of obesity. Ann Intern Med. 2005;142(7):532-546. [PMID: 15809465]

Maciejewski ML, Livingston EH, Smith VA, et al. Survival among high-risk patients after bariatric surgery. JAMA. 2011;305(23):2419-2526. [PMID: 21666276]

Maggard MA, Shugarman LR, Suttorp M, et al. Meta-analysis: surgical treatment of obesity. Ann Intern Med. 2005;142(7):547-559. [PMID: 15809466]

Silk AW, McTigue KM. Reexamining the physical examination for obese patients. JAMA. 2011;305(2):193-194. [PMID: 21191004]

Men's Health

Greco KA, McVary KT. The role of combination medical therapy in benign prostatic hyperplasia. Int J Impot Res. 2008;20(suppl 3):S33-S43. [PMID: 19002123]

Gupta BP, Murad MH, Clifton MM, Prokop L, Nehra A, Kopecky SL. The effect of lifestyle modification and cardiovascular risk factor reduction on erectile dysfunction: a systematic review and meta-analysis. Arch Intern Med. 2011;171(20):1797-1803. [PMID: 21911624]

Qaseem A, Snow V, Denberg TD, et al; Clinical Efficacy Assessment Subcommittee of the American College of Physicians. Hormonal testing and pharmacologic treatment of erectile dysfunction: a clinical practice guideline from the American College of Physicians. Ann Intern Med. 2009;151(9):639-649. [PMID: 19884625]

Rosen RC, Cappelleri JC, Smith MD, et al. Development and evaluation of an abridged, 5-item version of the International Index of Erectile Function (IIEF-5) as a diagnostic tool for erectile dysfunction. Int J Impot Res. 1999;11(6):319-326. [PMID: 10637462]

Shah NR, Mikami DJ, Cook C, et al. A comparison of outcomes between open and laparoscopic surgical repair of recurrent inguinal hernias. Surg Endosc. 2011;25(7):2330-2337. [PMID: 21298523]

Touma NJ, Nickel JC. Prostatitis and chronic pelvic pain in men. Med Clin North Am. 2011;95(1):75-86. [PMID: 21095412]

Traish AM, Miner MM, Morgentaler A, Zitzmann M. Testosterone deficiency. Am J Med. 2011;124(7):578-587. [PMID: 21683825]

Tsertsvadze A, Fink HA, Yazdi F, et al. Oral phosphodiesterase-5 inhibitors and hormonal treatments for erectile dysfunction: a systematic review and meta-analysis. Ann Intern Med. 2009;151(9):650-661. [PMID: 19884626]

Wampler SM, Llanes M. Common scrotal and testicular problems. Prim Care. 2010;37(3):613-626. [PMID: 20705202]

Women's Health

Amy JJ, Tripathi V. Contraception for women: an evidence based overview. BMJ. 2009;339:b2895. [PMID: 19666684]

Berghella V, Buchanan E, Pereira L, Baxter JK. Preconception care. Obstet Gynecol Surv. 2010;65(2):119-131. [PMID: 20100361]

Casablanca Y. Management of dysfunctional uterine bleeding. Obstet Gynecol Clin North Am. 2008;35(2):219-234. [PMID: 18486838]

Chlebowski RT, Andersonn GL, Gass M, et al; WHI Investigators. Estrogen plus progestin and breast cancer incidence and mortality in postmenopausal women. JAMA. 2010;304(15):1684-1692. [PMID: 20959578]

Harel Z. Dysmenorrhea in adolescents and young adults: from pathophysiology to pharmacological treatments and management strategies. Expert Opin on Pharmacother. 2008;9(15):2661-2672. [PMID: 18803452]

Kingsberg S, Althof SE. Evaluation and treatment of female sexual disorders. Int Urogynecol J Pelvic Floor Dysfunct. 2009;(20)(suppl 1):S33-S43. [PMID: 19440781]

Lanston A. Emergency contraception: update and review. Semin Reprod Med. 2010;28(2):95-102. [PMID: 20352558]

Martin KA, Manson JE. Approach to the patient with menopausal symptoms. J Clin Endocrinol Metab. 2008;93(12):4567-4575. [PMID: 19056840]

Nappi RE, Martini E, Terreno E, et al. Management of hypoactive sexual desire disorder in women: current and emerging therapies. Int J Womens Health. 2010;2:167-175. [PMID: 21072309]

Rossouw JE, Prentice RL, Manson JE, et al. Postmenopausal hormone therapy and risk for cardiovascular disease by age and years since menopause. JAMA. 2007;297(13):1465-1477. [PMID: 17405972]

Rungruang B, Kelley JL 3rd. Benign breast diseases: epidemiology, evaluation, and management. Clin Obstet Gynecol. 2011;54(1):110-124. [PMID: 21278510]

Santen RJ, Mansel R. Benign breast disorders. N Engl J Med. 2005;353(3):275-285. [PMID: 16034013]

Vercellini P, Somigliana E, Viganò P, Abbiati A, Barbara G, Fedele L. Chronic pelvic pain in women: etiology, pathogenesis, and diagnostic approach. Gynecol Endocrinol. 2009;25(3):149-158. [PMID: 19347704]

Wilson, JF. In the clinic. Vaginitis and cervicitis. Ann Intern Med. 2009;151(5):ITC3-1-ITC3-15; Quiz ITC3-16. [PMID: 19721016]

Eye Disorders

Ahmed R, Foroozan R. Transient monocular visual loss. Neurol Clin. 2010;28(3):619-629. [PMID: 20637992]

Arroyo JG. A 76-year-old man with macular degeneration. JAMA. 2006;295(20):2394-2406. [PMID: 16720825]

Asbell PA, Dualan I, Mindel J, Brocks D, Ahmad M, Epstein S. Age-related cataract. Lancet. 2005;365(9459):599-609. [PMID: 15708105]

Cronau H, Kankanala RR, Mauger T. Diagnosis and management of red eye in primary care. Am Fam Physician. 2010;81(2):137-144. [PMID: 20082509]

Hollands H, Johnson D, Brox AC, Almeida D, Simel DL, Sharma S. Acute-onset floaters and flashes: is this patient at risk for retinal detachment? JAMA. 2009;302(20):2243-2249. [PMID: 19934426]

Magauran B. Conditions requiring emergency ophthalmologic consultation. Emerg Med Clin North Am. 2008;26(1):233-238, viii. [PMID: 18249265]

Weinreb RN, Khaw PT. Primary open-angle glaucoma. Lancet. 2004;363(9422):1711-1720. [PMID: 15158634]

Ear, Nose, Mouth, and Throat Disorders

Calderon MA, Alves B, Jacobson M, Hurwitz B, Sheikh A, Durham S. Allergen injection immunotherapy for seasonal allergic rhinitis. Cochrane Database Syst Rev. 2007;(1):CD001936. [PMID: 17253469]

Chow AW, Benninger MS, Brook I, et al. IDSA clinical practice guideline for acute bacterial rhinosinusitis in children and adults. Clin Infect Dis. 2012;54(8):e72-e112. [PMID: 22438350]

Coco A, Vernacchio L, Horst M, Anderson A. Management of acute otitis media after publication of the 2004 AAP and AAFP clinical practice guideline. Pediatrics. 2010;125(2):214-220. [PMID: 20100746]

Douglass AB, Gonsalves W, Maier R, et al. Smiles for Life: A National Oral Health Curriculum for Family Medicine. A model for curriculum development by STFM groups. Fam Med. 2007;39(2):88-90. [PMID: 17273948]

Friedewald VE, Kornman KS, Beck JD, et al; American Journal of Cardiology; Journal of Periodontology. The American Journal of Cardiology and Journal of Periodontology Editors' Consensus: periodontitis and atherosclerotic cardiovascular disease. Am J Cardiol. 2009;104(1):59-68. [PMID: 19576322]

Hobson J, Chisholm E, El Refaie A. Sound therapy (masking) in the management of tinnitus in adults. Cochrane Database Syst Rev. 2010;(12):CD006371. [PMID: 21154366]

Osguthorpe DJ, Nielsen DR. Otitis externa: Review and clinical update. Am Fam Physician. 2006;74(9):1510-1516. [PMID: 17111889]

Powers JH. Diagnosis and treatment of acute otitis media: evaluating the evidence. Infect Dis Clin North Am. 2007;21(2):409-426, vi. [PMID: 17561076]

Roland PS, Smith TL, Schwartz SR, et al. Clinical practice guideline: Cerumen impaction. Otolayngol Head Neck Surg. 2008;139(3)(suppl 2):S1-S21. [PMID: 18707628]

Schlosser RJ. Clinical practice. Epistaxis. N Engl J Med. 2009;360(8):784-789. [PMID: 19228621]

Schreiber BE, Agrup C, Haskard DO, Luxon LM. Sudden sensorineural hearing loss. Lancet. 2010;375(9721):1203-1211. [PMID: 20362815]

Scrivani SJ, Keith DA, Kaban LB. Temporomandibular disorders. N Engl J Med. 2008;359(25):2693-2705. [PMID: 19092154]

Stachler RJ, Chandrasekhar SS, Archer SM, et al; American Academy of Otolaryngology-Head and Neck Surgery. Clinical practice guideline: sudden hearing loss. Otolaryngol Head Neck Surg. 2012;146(3 suppl):S1-35. [PMID: 22383545]

Young J, De Sutter A, Merenstein D, et al. Antibiotics for adults with clinically diagnosed acute rhinosinusitis: a meta-analysis of individual patient data. Lancet. 2008;371(9616):908-914. [PMID: 18342685]

Anorectal Disorders

Schubert MC, Sridhar S, Schade RR, Wexner SD. What every gastroenterologist needs to know about common anorectal disorders. World J Gastroenterol. 2009;15(26):3201-3209. [PMID: 19598294]

Mental and Behavioral Health

American Psychiatric Association Work Group on Eating Disorders. Practice guideline for the treatment of patients with eating disorders (revision). Am J Psychiatry. 2000;157(1 suppl):1-39. [PMID: 10642782]

Belmaker RH. Treatment of bipolar depression. N Engl J Med. 2007;356(17):1771-1773. [PMID: 17392296]

Brugha TS, McManus S, Bankart J, et al. Epidemiology of autism spectrum disorders in adults in the community in England. Arch Gen Psychiatry. 2011;68(5):459-465. [PMID: 21536975]

Bulik CM, Berkman ND, Brownley KA, Sedway JA, Lohr KN. Anorexia nervosa treatment: a systematic review of randomized controlled trials. Int J Eat Disord. 2007;40(4):310-320. [PMID: 17370290]

Fancher TL, Kravitz RL. In the clinic. Depression. Ann Intern Med. 2010;152(9):ITC51-15; quiz ITC5-16. [PMID: 20439571]

Franklin ME, Foa EB. Treatment of obsessive compulsive disorder. Annu Rev Clin Psychol. 2011;7:229-243. [PMID: 21443448]

Gammicchia C, Johnson C. Autism Information for Paramedics and Emergency Room Staff. Autism Society. Available at www.autism-society.org/about-us/publications/resource-materials.html. Accessed July 9, 2012.

Gartlehner G, Hansen RA, Morgan LC, et al. Comparative benefits and harms of second-generation antidepressants for treating major depressive disorder: an updated meta-analysis. Ann Intern Med. 2011;155(11):772-785. [PMID: 22147715]

Gartlehner G, Hansen RA, Morgan LC, et al. Second-Generation Antidepressants in the Pharmacologic Treatment of Adult Depression: An Update of the 2007 Comparative Effectiveness Review [Internet]. Rockville (MD): Agency for Healthcare Research and Quality (US); 2011 Dec. (Comparative Effectiveness Reviews, No. 46.) Peer Reviewers. Available at www.effectivehealthcare.ahrq.gov/index.cfm/search-for-guides-reviews-and-reports/?pageaction=displayproduct&productid=862. Accessed July 9, 2012.

Jones RM, Arlidge J, Gillham R, Reagu S, van den Bree M, Taylor PJ. Efficacy of mood stabilisers in the treatment of impulsive or repetitive aggression: systematic review and meta-analysis. Br J Psychiatry. 2011;198(2):93-98. [PMID: 21282779]

Kroenke K, Spitzer RL, Williams JB, Monahan PO, Löwe B. Anxiety disorders in primary care: prevalence, impairment, comorbidity, and detection. Ann Intern Med. 2007;146(5):317-325. [PMID: 17339617]

Kroenke K. Unburdening the difficult clinical encounter. Arch Intern Med. 2009;169(4):333-334. [PMID: 19237715]

Schultz SH, North SW, Shields CG. Schizophrenia: a review. Am Fam Physician. 2007;75(12):1821-1829. [PMID: 17619525]

Sim LA, McAlpine DE, Grothe KB, Himes SM, Cockerill RG, Clark MM. Identification and treatment of eating disorders in the primary care setting. Mayo Clin Proc. 2010;85(8):746-751. [PMID: 20605951]

Stein MB, Goin MK, Pollack MH, et al. Practice guideline for the treatment of patients with panic disorder. Arlington, VA: American Psychiatric Association, 2009.

Wilens TE, Faraone SV, Biederman J. Attention-deficit/hyperactivity disorder in adults. JAMA. 2004;292(5):619-623. [PMID: 15292088]

Geriatric Medicine

Budnitz DS, Lovegrove MC, Shehab N, Richards CL. Emergency hospitalizations for adverse drug events in older Americans. N Engl J Med. 2011;365:2002-2012. [PMID: 22111719]

Burgio KL, Kraus SR, Menefee S, et al; Urinary Incontinence Treatment Network. Behavioral therapy to enable women with urge incontinence to discontinue drug treatment: a randomized trial. Ann Intern Med. 2008;149(3):161-169. [PMID: 18678843]

Carr DB, Ott BR. The older adult driver with cognitive impairment: "It's a very frustrating life". JAMA. 2010;303(16):1632-1641. [Erratum in: JAMA. 2010;303(23):2357]. [PMID: 20424254]

Fong TG, Jones RN, Rudolph JL, et al. Development and validation of a brief cognitive assessment tool: the sweet 16. Arch Intern Med. 2011;171(5):432-427. [PMID: 21059967]

Garfinkel D, Mangin D. Feasibility study of a systematic approach for discontinuation of multiple medications in older adults: addressing polypharmacy. Arch Intern Med. 2010;170(18):1648-1654. [PMID: 20937924]

Gillespie LD, Robertson MC, Gillespie WJ, et al. Interventions for preventing falls in older people living in the community. Cochrane Database Syst Rev. 2009;(2):CD007146. [PMID: 19370674]

Hayes BD, Klein-Schwartz W, Barrueto F. Polypharmacy and the geriatric patient. Clin Geriatr Med. 2007;23:371-390. [PMID: 17462523]

Kalyani RR, Stein B, Valiyil R, Manno R, Maynard JW, Crews DC. Vitamin D treatment for the prevention of falls in older adults: systematic review and meta-analysis. J Am Geriatr Soc. 2010;58(7):1299-1310. [PMID: 20579169]

Kane RL. Finding the right level of posthospital care: "We didn't realize there was any other option for him". JAMA. 2011;305(3):284-293. [PMID: 21245184]

Kinsella GJ, Mullaly E, Rand E, et al. Early intervention for mild cognitive impairment: a randomised controlled trial. J Neurol Neurosurg Psychiatry. 2009;80(7):730-736. [PMID: 19332424]

Li C, Friedman B, Conwell Y, Fiscella K. Validity of the Patient Health Questionnaire 2 (PHQ-2) in identifying major depression in older people. J Am Geriatr Soc. 2007;55(4):596-602. [PMID: 17397440]

McInnes E, Dumville JC, Jammali-Blasi A, Bell-Syer SE. Support surfaces for treating pressure ulcers. Cochrane Database Syst Rev. 2011;(12):CD009490. [PMID: 22161450]

McInnes E, Jammali-Blasi A, Bell-Syer SE, Dumville JC, Cullum N. Support surfaces for pressure ulcer prevention. Cochrane Database Syst Rev. 2011;(4):CD001735. [PMID: 21491384]

Panel on Prevention of Falls in Older Persons; American Geriatrics Society and British Geriatrics Society. Summary of the Updated American Geriatrics Society/British Geriatrics Society clinical practice guideline for prevention of falls in older persons. J Am Geriatr Soc. 2011;59(1):148-157. [PMID: 21226685]

Plassman BL, Langa KM, Fisher GG, et al. Prevalence of cognitive impairment without dementia in the United States. Ann Intern Med. 2008;148(6):427-434. [PMID: 18347351]

Reddy M, Gill SS, Kalkar SR, Wu W, Anderson PJ, Rochon PA. Treatment of pressure ulcers: a systematic review. JAMA. 2008;300(22):2647-2662. [PMID: 19066385]

Shamliyan T, Wyman JF, Ramakrishnan R, Sainfort F, Kane RL. Systematic Review: Benefits and Harms of Pharmacologic Treatment for Urinary Incontinence in Women. Ann Intern Med. 2012 Apr 9 [Epub ahead of print] [PMID: 22492633]

Studenski S, Perera S, Patel K, et al. Gait speed and survival in older adults. JAMA. 2011:305(1):50-58. [PMID: 21205966]

Wyman JF, Croghan CF, Nachreiner NM, et al. Effectiveness of education and individualized counseling in reducing environmental hazards in the homes of community-dwelling older women. J Am Geriatr Soc. 2007;55(10):1548-1556. [PMID: 17908058]

Perioperative Medicine

Carson JL, Grossman BJ, Kleinman S, et al; for the Clinical Transfusion Medicine Committee of the AABB. Red Blood Cell Transfusion: A Clinical Practice Guideline From the AABB*. Ann Intern Med. 2012;157(1):49-58. [PMID: 22751760]

Douketis JD, Berger PB, Dunn AS, et al; American College of Chest Physicians. The perioperative management of antithrombotic therapy: American College of Chest Physicians Evidence-Based Clinical Practice Guidelines (8th Edition). Chest. 2008;133(6 suppl):299S-339S. [PMID: 18574269]

Douketis JD, Spyropoulos AC, Spencer FA, et al; American College of Chest Physicians. Perioperative management of antithrombotic therapy: Antithrombotic Therapy and Prevention of Thrombosis, 9th ed: American College of Chest Physicians Evidence-Based Clinical Practice Guidelines. Chest. 2012;141(2 suppl):e326S-e350S. [PMID: 22315266]

Eilers H, Liu KD, Gruber A, Niemann CU. Chronic kidney disease: implications for the perioperative period. Minerva Anestesiol. 2010;76(9):725-736. [PMID: 20820151]

Ford MK, Beattie WS, Wijeysundera DN. Systematic review: prediction of perioperative cardiac complications and mortality by the revised cardiac risk index. Ann Intern Med. 2010;152(1):26-35. [PMID: 20048269]

Hepner DL. The role of testing in the preoperative evaluation. Cleve Clin J Med. 2009;76(suppl 4):S22-S27. [PMID: 19880831]

Lieb K, Selim M. Preoperative evaluation of patients with neurological disease. Semin Neurol. 2008;28(5):603-610. [PMID: 19115168]

Lipshutz AK, Gropper MA. Perioperative glycemic control: an evidence-based review. Anesthesiology. 2009;110(2):408-421. [PMID: 19194167]

Marik PE, Varon J. Requirement of perioperative stress doses of corticosteroids: a systematic review of the literature. Arch Surg. 2008;143(12):1222-1226. [PMID: 19075176]

O'Leary JG, Yachimski PS, Friedman LS. Surgery in the patient with liver disease. Clin Liver Dis. 2009;13(2):211-231. [PMID: 19442915]

Patel MS, Carson JL. Anemia in the preoperative patient. Med Clin North Am. 2009;93(5):1095-1104. [PMID: 19665622]

Qaseem A, Humphrey LL, Chou R, Snow V, Shekelle P; Clinical Guidelines Committee of the American College of Physicians. Use of intensive insulin therapy for the management of glycemic control in hospitalized patients: a clinical practice guideline from the American College of Physicians. Ann Intern Med. 2011;154(4):260-267. [PMID: 21320941]

Smetana GW, Lawrence VA, Cornell JE; American College of Physicians. Preoperative pulmonary risk stratification for noncardiothoracic surgery: systematic review for the American College of Physicians. Ann Intern Med. 2006;144(8):581-595. [PMID: 16618956]

Vasu TS, Doghramji K, Cavallazzi R, et al. Obstructive sleep apnea syndrome and postoperative complications: clinical use of the STOP-BANG questionnaire. Arch Otolaryngol Head Neck Surg. 2010;136(10):1020-1024. [PMID: 20956751]

General Internal Medicine Self-Assessment Test

This self-assessment test contains one-best-answer multiple-choice questions. Please read these directions carefully before answering the questions. Answers, critiques, and bibliographies immediately follow these multiple-choice questions. The American College of Physicians is accredited by the Accreditation Council for Continuing Medical Education (ACCME) to provide continuing medical education for physicians.

The American College of Physicians designates MKSAP 16 General Internal Medicine for a maximum of 24 *AMA PRA Category 1 Credits*™. Physicians should claim only the credit commensurate with the extent of their participation in the activity.

Earn "Same-Day" CME Credits Online

For the first time, print subscribers can enter their answers online to earn CME credits in 24 hours or less. You can submit your answers using online answer sheets that are provided at mksap.acponline.org, where a record of your MKSAP 16 credits will be available. To earn CME credits, you need to answer all of the questions in a test and earn a score of at least 50% correct (number of correct answers divided by the total number of questions). Take any of the following approaches:

> ➢ Use the printed answer sheet at the back of this book to record your answers. Go to mksap.acponline.org, access the appropriate online answer sheet, transcribe your answers, and submit your test for same-day CME credits. There is no additional fee for this service.

> ➢ Go to mksap.acponline.org, access the appropriate online answer sheet, directly enter your answers, and submit your test for same-day CME credits. There is no additional fee for this service.

> ➢ Pay a $10 processing fee per answer sheet and submit the printed answer sheet at the back of this book by mail or fax, as instructed on the answer sheet. Make sure you calculate your score and fax the answer sheet to 215-351-2799 or mail the answer sheet to Member and Customer Service, American College of Physicians, 190 N. Independence Mall West, Philadelphia, PA 19106-1572, using the courtesy envelope provided in your MKSAP 16 slipcase. You will need your 10-digit order number and 8-digit ACP ID number, which are printed on your packing slip. Please allow 4 to 6 weeks for your score report to be emailed back to you. Be sure to include your email address for a response.

If you do not have a 10-digit order number and 8-digit ACP ID number or if you need help creating a username and password to access the MKSAP 16 online answer sheets, go to mksap.acponline.org or email custserv@acponline.org.

CME credit is available from the publication date of December 31, 2012, until December 31, 2015. You may submit your answer sheets at any time during this period.

*Each of the numbered items is followed by lettered answers. Select the **ONE** lettered answer that is **BEST** in each case.*

Item 1

A 32-year-old man is evaluated during a routine examination. He is in good health, has no concerning symptoms, and takes no medications. He does not smoke, seldom drinks alcohol, and exercises 30 minutes daily 5 days per week. He ingests a heart-healthy diet. All of his immunizations are up to date. The patient has no symptoms or health problems.

Which of the following is the most reasonable next screening step for genetic disease in this patient?

(A) Obtain a family history of disease
(B) Obtain a three-generation pedigree
(C) Refer for genetic counseling
(D) Screen for common genetic mutations

Item 2

A 58-year-old woman is evaluated for a 7-week history of tingling pain involving the first, second, and third digits of the left hand. The pain is worse at night and radiates into the thenar eminence. The pain does not radiate into the proximal forearm. She has hypothyroidism and her only current medication is levothyroxine.

On physical examination, the patient reports pain with plantar flexion at the wrist with the elbow extended. She also reports pain with percussion over the median nerve at the level of the wrist. There is no thenar or hypothenar eminence atrophy. Strength is 5/5 with thumb opposition. A hand diagram is completed (shown) demonstrating the location of the patient's paresthesia.

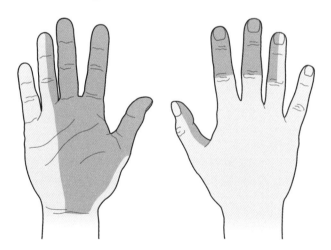

In addition to avoidance of repetitive wrist motions, which of the following is the most appropriate initial treatment?

(A) Local corticosteroid injection
(B) Oral ibuprofen
(C) Surgical intervention
(D) Wrist splinting

Item 3

A 40-year-old woman is evaluated for having difficulty at work. She is a nurse, and over the past 6 months she has become very zealous about avoiding infection. She washes her hands six or seven times before entering patients' rooms and then again afterwards. She is having difficulty completing tasks on time. She showers multiple times daily and has scrubbed her skin raw in several areas. She recognizes that these actions are unreasonable but she no control over them. She has no history of psychiatric disease, bipolar disorder, or schizophrenia.

On physical examination, vital signs are normal. Both hands are raw and there are several areas of denuded skin on her arms and legs.

In addition to cognitive-behavioral therapy, which of the following is the most appropriate pharmacologic treatment?

(A) Fluoxetine
(B) Haloperidol
(C) Lorazepam
(D) Quetiapine

Item 4

A 24-year-old man is evaluated for a 2-hour history of epistaxis, which began after blowing his nose. The bleeding is controlled by placing pressure on the anterior portion of the nose for 3 minutes but then recurs. The bleeding is from the left nostril only. He has severe seasonal rhinitis that has been active recently. He has no history of bleeding, bruising, or clotting, and there is no family history of bleeding disorders. Current medications are loratadine and an intranasal corticosteroid.

On physical examination, he is afebrile, blood pressure is 138/88 mm Hg, and pulse rate is 82/min. Blood pressure and pulse are without significant change from supine to standing positions. He is holding a tissue against his nose. Examination of the left naris with a nasal speculum after the removal of dried blood reveals a small oozing vessel in the septum in the Kiesselbach area. The right naris is clear of blood, and a skin examination demonstrates no petechiae or bruises.

Which of the following is the most appropriate management of this patient?

(A) Arterial embolization
(B) Cauterization and nasal packing
(C) Complete blood count and coagulation studies
(D) Uninterrupted nasal pressure for 15 to 30 minutes
(E) Urgent otorhinolaryngology evaluation

Item 5

A 54-year-old woman is evaluated during a routine examination. She is very concerned by her lack of interest in sexual intercourse. The patient feels like she "just doesn't want to be touched." She used to enjoy intercourse and does not know why she feels this way now, but she acknowledges that it is causing tremendous stress in her marriage. She has been menopausal for the past 2 years. She uses lubrication for intercourse, which is successful in reducing discomfort. She has no previous history of menstrual irregularities, pelvic surgeries, sexual trauma, or sexually transmitted infections. She currently takes calcium and vitamin D supplements daily.

On physical examination, external genitalia are normal, with no pain with vulvar palpation or with speculum insertion. The vaginal walls are pale with decreased rugae and petechial hemorrhages. Decreased vaginal lubrication is noted. The remainder of the physical examination is normal.

Which of the following is the most likely diagnosis?

(A) Dyspareunia
(B) Hypoactive sexual desire disorder
(C) Sexual aversion disorder
(D) Vaginismus

 Item 6

An 88-year-old man in hospice care is evaluated for dyspnea. He has advanced dementia, severe COPD, and coronary artery disease. Based on prior discussions with his family regarding the goals of care, it was decided that his treatment should consist of comfort care measures only. All of his medications except as-needed albuterol and ipratropium have been discontinued.

On physical examination, he is afebrile, blood pressure is 108/76 mm Hg, pulse rate is 110/min, and respiration rate is 26/min. Oxygen saturation is satisfactory. He is cachectic and tachypneic and is disoriented and in moderate respiratory distress. Heart sounds are distant and tachycardic but an S_3 is not present. Chest examination reveals decreased breath sounds as well as diffuse, fine inspiratory crackles consistent with prior examinations. Extremities are warm and dry.

In addition to continuing his bronchodilator therapy, which of the following is the most appropriate next step in the treatment of this patient?

(A) Ceftriaxone and azithromycin
(B) Lorazepam
(C) Methylprednisolone
(D) Morphine

Item 7

A 55-year-old woman is evaluated for fatigue for the past 9 months. She used to be an avid runner, but now can only walk 1 mile before experiencing severe muscle aches, joint pain and fatigue for the next several days. She reports no insomnia but describes her 8 hours of nightly sleep as unrefreshing. She does not smoke, drink, or use illicit drugs. She describes tender lymph nodes in her neck and axillae. She reports having "the flu" last winter and believes her fatigue

began after that. She has undergone several comprehensive medical evaluations with no explanation for her symptoms. Recent records from previous physicians reveal normal complete blood count, comprehensive metabolic panel, and thyroid function studies.

On physical examination, vital signs are normal. BMI is 24. There is no lymphadenopathy, but the patient notes tenderness when lymph node areas are palpated. There is tenderness to joint movement but no evidence of synovitis or restricted movement. There is generalized tenderness to muscle palpation; strength is normal. The remainder of the physical examination is unremarkable. Mini–Mental State Examination score is 29/30; a two-question depression screen is negative.

Which of the following should be done next to help diagnose this patient's symptoms?

(A) Epstein-Barr virus titer
(B) Erythrocyte sedimentation rate
(C) Parvovirus B19 titer
(D) No additional testing

Item 8

A 29-year-old woman is evaluated preoperatively before elective breast reduction and liposuction. She feels well and has no symptoms or pertinent medical history. She exercises regularly. Her last menstrual period was 3 weeks ago. She drinks alcohol socially and does not smoke cigarettes. She has no family history of premature heart disease or abnormal bleeding. The procedure will be done under general anesthesia. She takes no medications or supplements. Results of the physical examination are normal.

Which of the following is the most appropriate preoperative test to perform next?

(A) Chest radiography
(B) Coagulation studies
(C) Electrocardiography
(D) Pregnancy testing
(E) No further testing

Item 9

A 66-year-old woman is evaluated for several months of a "whistling" or "swishing" sound in her right ear. She notes that it gets faster and louder when she exercises and thinks it is timed to her heartbeat. She does not notice any hearing loss, dizziness, or vertigo.

On physical examination, temperature is 37.4 °C (99.3 °F), blood pressure is 138/84 mm Hg, and pulse rate is 84/min. Auditory acuity to normal conversation appears normal, and otoscopic examination is unremarkable bilaterally. Neurologic examination is normal.

Which of the following is the most appropriate next step in the management of this patient?

(A) Audiometry
(B) Auscultation over the right ear, eye, and neck

(C) Trial of a sound-masking device

(D) Trial of a nasal corticosteroid spray

Item 10

A 46-year-old woman is evaluated during a routine examination. Her 72-year-old mother was just diagnosed with lung cancer, so the patient asks you for help with quitting smoking. She has a 27-pack-year smoking history. She made one previous quit attempt several years ago using over-the-counter nicotine gum, but she was unable to quit for more than a few days. Medical history is significant for seizure disorder. Review of systems discloses mild shortness of breath with exertion and occasional wheezing. Medications are a multivitamin and phenytoin.

On physical examination, vital signs are normal. Lung examination reveals occasional wheezing and a prolonged expiratory phase. The rest of the examination is normal.

In addition to counseling regarding tobacco use, which of the following is an appropriate adjunct to increase her likelihood of successful smoking cessation?

(A) A benzodiazepine

(B) Bupropion

(C) Electronic smokeless cigarette use

(D) Nicotine replacement therapy

Item 11

A 23-year-old man is evaluated for a 3-day history of redness and itchiness of the right eye. He had an upper respiratory tract infection 3 days before the eye symptoms began. Each morning he has awoken with crusting over the lids. He is otherwise healthy, with no ocular trauma or recent medical problems.

On physical examination, he is afebrile, blood pressure is 122/72 mm Hg, pulse rate is 66/min, and respiration rate is 16/min. Right eye conjunctival injection is present, with some crusting at the lids. Bilateral vision is 20/20. Pupils are equally round and reactive to light.

Which of the following is the most appropriate management of this patient?

(A) Cool compresses to the affected eye

(B) Oral antihistamine

(C) Topical antibiotics

(D) Topical corticosteroids

Item 12

A 67-year-old man is evaluated for right groin pain. The pain began spontaneously 2 days ago. Yesterday, he was evaluated in the emergency department and was diagnosed with groin strain and discharged home. He is reevaluated today because the groin pain has continued without improvement. He has well-controlled hypertension and a 30-pack-year smoking history. Medications are hydrochlorothiazide and aspirin.

On physical examination, he is afebrile. Blood pressure is 100/62 mm Hg and pulse rate is 104/min. Respiration rate is 16/min. The abdomen is slightly distended but nontender. There is no focal tenderness over the hip or pelvis. Active and passive range of motion testing of his right hip does not exacerbate his groin pain. The patient is reassured that a groin muscle strain is the likely cause of his discomfort. He is advised to take more fluids and rest.

12 hours later he is brought to the emergency department because of diffuse severe abdominal pain. A CT scan of the abdomen shows a rupturing 8.2-cm abdominal aortic aneurysm.

Which of the following categories of diagnostic error is responsible for missing the correct diagnosis at the follow-up examination?

(A) Anchoring heuristic

(B) Availability heuristic

(C) No-fault error

(D) Representativeness heuristic

Item 13

A 32-year-old man is evaluated for a 3-day history of productive cough, sore throat, coryza, rhinorrhea, nasal congestion, generalized myalgia, and fatigue. His sputum is slightly yellow. His two children (ages 3 years and 1 year) had similar symptoms 1 week ago. He is a nonsmoker and has no history of asthma.

On physical examination, temperature is 37.5 °C (99.4 °F), blood pressure is 128/76 mm Hg, pulse rate is 92/min, and respiration rate is 14/min. There is bilateral conjunctival injection. The nasal mucosa is boggy, with clear drainage. The oropharynx is erythematous without tonsillar enlargement or exudates. The tympanic membranes and external auditory canals are normal. Lungs are clear to auscultation. There is no rash or lymphadenopathy.

Which of the following is the most appropriate treatment?

(A) Albuterol

(B) Amoxicillin

(C) Chlorpheniramine

(D) Codeine

Item 14

A 48-year-old man is evaluated for a 2-day history of episodic dizziness with nausea. He noted the onset abruptly and compares the feeling to "being on a roller coaster." His most severe episodes occurred while arising from bed and when parallel parking his car. The symptoms lasted 30 to 40 seconds and were followed by two episodes of emesis. He has no recent fever, headache, tinnitus, hearing loss, double vision, dysarthria, weakness, or difficulty walking. He had a similar episode 5 years ago. Medical history is significant for depression. His only medication is citalopram.

On physical examination, vital signs are normal. Results of cardiac and neurologic examinations are normal. The

Dix-Hallpike maneuver precipitates severe horizontal nystagmus after about 20 seconds. With repeated maneuvers, the nystagmus is less severe.

Which of the following is the most likely diagnosis?

(A) Benign paroxysmal positional vertigo
(B) Cerebellar infarction
(C) Meniere disease
(D) Vestibular neuronitis

Item 15

A 47-year-old woman is evaluated for an abnormal complete blood count obtained as part of a life insurance physical examination. She has no active medical problems. She underwent Roux-en-Y gastric bypass surgery 10 years ago and has successfully kept off the weight she lost after the surgery. She has not seen a physician for more than 7 years. She has no family history of hematologic disorders or colon cancer.

On physical examination, temperature is normal, blood pressure is 124/80 mm Hg, and pulse rate is 78/min. BMI is 24. Cardiovascular, pulmonary, and neurologic examinations are all normal. There is no thyromegaly. Abdominal examination shows a well-healed surgical scar. The remainder of the examination is unremarkable. A stool sample is guaiac-negative. The laboratory results obtained by the patient are shown.

Laboratory studies:

Leukocyte count	4200/µL (4.2×10^9/L)
Hemoglobin	10.9 g/dL (109 g/L)
Mean corpuscular volume	107 fL
Platelet count	122,000/µL (122×10^9/L)
Reticulocyte count	1.5%

Which of the following is the most appropriate test to establish the diagnosis?

(A) Bone marrow biopsy
(B) Colonoscopy
(C) Serum thyroid-stimulating hormone level
(D) Serum vitamin B_{12} level

Item 16

A 28-year-old woman is evaluated during a routine examination. Her 52-year-old mother was recently diagnosed with Huntington disease. The patient has no symptoms. She is planning on starting a family. Physical examination, including complete neurologic examination, is normal.

Which of the following should be done next?

(A) Obtain genetic testing for Huntington disease
(B) Order brain MRI
(C) Reassure the patient that she is unlikely to develop Huntington disease
(D) Refer for genetic counseling

Item 17

An 85-year-old man is admitted to a nursing home. He has diabetes mellitus, coronary artery disease, chronic heart failure, and dementia. On physical examination, vital signs are normal. He has a full thickness 5×8 cm pressure ulcer on his left buttock covered with a thick eschar. There is visible subcutaneous fat beneath the eschar; no bone or tendon is exposed. His skin is dry and there is evidence of mild dehydration and malnutrition. He has urinary but not fecal incontinence. His current medications are lisinopril, metformin, hydrochlorothiazide, glipizide, and carvedilol.

Which of the following is the most appropriate management of this patient's ulcer?

(A) Debridement
(B) Hyperbaric oxygen therapy
(C) Negative-pressure wound vacuum therapy
(D) Oral vitamin C and zinc supplementation
(E) Surgical flap therapy

Item 18

An 80-year-old man is evaluated for a 1-year history of progressive urinary symptoms including weak stream, hesitancy, and nocturia four times nightly. He has coronary artery disease and chronic heart failure. His current medications are lisinopril, isosorbide dinitrate, aspirin, and metoprolol.

On physical examination, vital signs are normal. He has mild suprapubic tenderness and a symmetrically enlarged prostate without nodules or tenderness. The remainder of the physical examination is normal.

Which of the following is the most appropriate diagnostic test to perform next?

(A) Postvoid residual urinary volume measurement
(B) Plasma glucose level
(C) Prostate-specific antigen testing
(D) Transrectal ultrasound
(E) Urinalysis

Item 19

A 58-year-old man recently diagnosed with multiple myeloma with bony metastases is evaluated before hospital discharge. He is being discharged today on hospice care after receiving melphalan and prednisone and having a poor response to therapy. He is currently on intravenous morphine as needed for pain and has requested 10 mg every 4 hours over the last 24 hours. On physical examination, vital signs are normal.

Which of the following is the most appropriate treatment of this patient's pain?

(A) Fentanyl transdermal patch
(B) Methadone
(C) Short-acting hydromorphone
(D) Sustained-release morphine

Item 20

A 29-year-old man is evaluated for the gradual onset of right-sided hearing loss. He reports a continuous high-pitched ringing in his right ear that has been present for 3 to 4 months.

On physical examination, vital signs are normal. When a vibrating 512 Hz tuning fork is placed on the top of his head, it is louder in the left ear. When placed adjacent to his right ear, it is heard better when outside the ear canal than when touching the mastoid bone. Otoscopic examination is normal bilaterally. Neurologic examination is normal other than right-sided hearing loss.

Which of the following is the most appropriate management of this patient?

(A) Biofeedback therapy
(B) Immediate treatment with oral corticosteroids
(C) MRI of the posterior fossa and internal auditory canal
(D) Otolith repositioning maneuver

Item 21

A 72-year-old woman is evaluated in the emergency department after an episode of syncope. While watching a movie, the patient felt palpitations; the next thing she remembers is being on the floor. She experienced a similar episode about 1 month ago. History is significant for hypertension, hypothyroidism, osteoporosis, and chronic kidney disease. Medications are amlodipine, lisinopril, levothyroxine, and calcium supplements. She currently feels well.

On physical examination, temperature is normal, blood pressure is 148/78 mm Hg, pulse rate is 84/min and regular, and respiration rate is 12/min. Oxygen saturation on ambient air is normal. There is no thyromegaly, carotid upstrokes are +2 without bruits, and there is no jugular venous distention. Cardiac auscultation reveals a grade 2/6, early peaking, crescendo-decrescendo systolic murmur at the right upper sternal border with occasional extra beats. The remainder of the physical examination is normal.

A resting electrocardiogram and rhythm strip show a sinus rate of 85/min with occasional premature ventricular contractions but no sustained arrhythmia, normal axis and intervals, and no ischemic changes.

Which of the following is the most likely cause of this patient's syncope?

(A) Aortic stenosis
(B) Cardiac arrhythmia
(C) Myocardial ischemia
(D) Transient ischemic attack

Item 22

A 56-year-old woman is evaluated for a 6-month history of symmetric bilateral lower extremity edema. She notices no leg swelling upon arising in the morning; her symptoms appear by midday and worsen thereafter. She does not have pain but notes her legs feel heavy and her shoes leave indentations in her skin with prolonged standing. She has no periorbital or upper extremity edema, chest pain, shortness of breath, paroxysmal nocturnal dyspnea, orthopnea, change in urinary habits, or abdominal fullness. She has no history of malignancy, immobility, or hormone replacement therapy.

On physical examination, vital signs are normal. BMI is 34. Results of the cardiovascular examination and abdominal examination are normal. The lungs are clear. There is no inguinal lymphadenopathy, lower extremity rash, or erythema. There is 1+ pitting ankle edema bilaterally.

Laboratory studies:

Creatinine	0.8 mg/dL (70.7 µmol/L)
Albumin	4.1 g/dL (41 g/L)
Alanine aminotransferase	28 units/L
Aspartate aminotransferase	24 units/L
Bilirubin	1.1 mg/dL (18.8 µmol/L)
Sodium	140 meq/L (140 mmol/L)
Potassium	3.9 meq/L (3.9 mmol/L)

Results of thyroid function testing are normal. Urinalysis shows no protein or blood.

Which of the following is the most appropriate next step in management?

(A) Compression stockings
(B) CT scan of abdomen and pelvis
(C) Furosemide
(D) Lower extremity venous duplex ultrasonography

Item 23

A 29-year-old man is evaluated for a 1-day history of left shoulder pain. He was throwing a football approximately 30 yards when the pain began. The pain is located over the left lateral deltoid muscle. He notes weakness with abduction. He has no previous history of shoulder problems, no history of trauma, and no paresthesia. He has been taking ibuprofen as needed for pain.

On physical examination, he is afebrile, blood pressure is 126/80 mm Hg, and pulse rate is 96/min. There is pain in the left shoulder with active abduction beginning at approximately 60 degrees, and he has difficulty actively abducting the left arm beyond 60 degrees. The patient is unable to slowly lower his left arm to his waist (positive drop-arm test). He has no pain with his left arm in full flexion (negative Neer test). When the patient is asked to hold the arm extended anteriorly at 90 degrees with the forearm bent to 90 degrees (at 12 o'clock), he does not have pain with the arm internally rotated to cross in front of the body (negative Hawkins test). There is no pain with forward elevation of the left arm to 90 degrees with active adduction of the arm (negative cross-arm test). Strength (other than during abduction) is intact.

Which of the following is the most appropriate next step in management?

(A) MRI of the left shoulder
(B) NSAID therapy
(C) Physical therapy
(D) Subacromial corticosteroid injection

Item 24

A 70-year-old man is admitted to the hospital for peritonitis. He has Alzheimer disease, hypertension, type 2 diabetes mellitus, cirrhosis, and ascites. He has been falling frequently at home. His current medications are metformin, donepezil, lisinopril, and propranolol.

On physical examination, temperature is 38.5 °C (101.3 °F), blood pressure is 130/70 mm Hg, pulse rate is 80/min, and respiration rate is 12/min. He is oriented to person and is in no acute distress. There is shifting dullness on abdominal examination and diffuse abdominal tenderness with palpation. There are areas of blanching erythema on the lower back and buttocks. There is no ulceration or skin breakdown. Laboratory studies show serum albumin level of 2.8 g/dL (28 g/L).

Which of the following interventions is most appropriate for preventing pressure ulcers in this patient?

(A) Doughnut-type device
(B) Free ambulation
(C) Indwelling urinary catheter
(D) Pressure-distributing mattress

Item 25

A 56-year-old woman is evaluated for severe vaginal itching and discomfort. Her symptoms have progressively worsened for the past 4 months. There is no associated vaginal discharge or vaginal odor. She is experiencing significant vaginal dryness and intercourse has become painful despite the use of lubricants. She has been menopausal since age 53 years. Her only medications are calcium and vitamin D.

On physical examination, vital signs are normal. BMI is 29. She has pale, dry vaginal walls with decreased rugae and petechial hemorrhages. There is scant vaginal discharge. Vaginal pH is 6.0. Wet mount shows occasional leukocytes. "Whiff" test is negative. There are no clue cells and no hyphae on potassium hydroxide preparation.

Which of the following is the most appropriate management of this patient?

(A) Oral conjugated estrogen with medroxyprogesterone acetate
(B) Oral metronidazole
(C) Vaginal clotrimazole
(D) Vaginal estradiol

Item 26

A 58-year-old man is evaluated for an 8-month history of slowly progressive right shoulder pain. The pain is located over the anterior shoulder and is worse with moving his arm across his chest and also when he fully abducts his arm. His only medication is acetaminophen.

On physical examination, vital signs are normal. He has pain when he forward elevates his right arm to 90 degrees and actively adducts his arm across his chest wall (positive cross-arm test). There is pain with shoulder abduction beyond 120 degrees. He exhibits normal shoulder internal

and external range of motion. There is pain with palpation of the acromioclavicular joint. He has no pain with his left arm in full flexion (negative Neer test). He is able to slowly lower his right arm to his waist (negative drop-arm test).

Which of the following is the most likely diagnosis?

(A) Acromioclavicular joint degeneration
(B) Adhesive capsulitis
(C) Rotator cuff tear
(D) Rotator cuff tendinitis

Item 27

A 59-year-old man is evaluated during a follow-up examination. He has COPD and hypertension. He has an 80-pack-year history of cigarette use, but has recently decreased his smoking to a half pack of cigarettes daily. Medications are ipratropium and amlodipine.

On physical examination, temperature is 37.3 °C (99.2 °F), blood pressure is 138/92 mm Hg, pulse rate is 96/min, and respiration rate is 22/min. BMI is 29. He is barrel-chested with diffuse wheezing on lung examination. The remainder of the physical examination is normal.

Which of the following is the most appropriate management regarding this patient's tobacco use?

(A) Assess his interest in smoking cessation
(B) Prescribe bupropion
(C) Prescribe nicotine replacement therapy
(D) Refer for smoking cessation counseling

Item 28

A 45-year-old woman is evaluated in the hospital after radical hysterectomy for cervical carcinoma. Aside from postoperative pain, she has no symptoms. She has no history of venous thromboembolism or excessive bleeding. Her only current medication is morphine as needed.

On physical examination, temperature is normal, blood pressure is 110/72 mm Hg, and pulse rate is 84/min. There is trace edema in the legs. Prothrombin time, activated partial thromboplastin time, and INR are normal.

In addition to early ambulation, which of the following interventions is the most appropriate in this patient for thromboembolism prophylaxis?

(A) Enoxaparin for 5 weeks
(B) Inferior vena cava filter placement
(C) Unfractionated heparin until discharge
(D) Warfarin for 3 months

Item 29

A 55-year-old man is evaluated for a 1-day history of seeing flashing lights, "squiggly" lines, and floating objects in his left eye followed by loss of vision at the outer periphery of the eye shortly after having breakfast this morning. He now describes seeing what looks like a curtain coming down in that location. He has myopia requiring prescription glasses.

On physical examination, vital signs are normal. Vision in the right eye is 20/100 uncorrected and 20/40 with glasses. Vision in the left eye is 20/100 uncorrected and 20/40 with glasses. Pupils are equally reactive to light and accommodation. There is no conjunctival injection. Findings on funduscopic examination are shown.

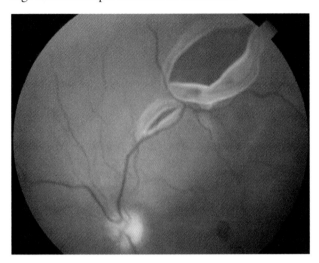

Which of the following is the most likely diagnosis?

(A) Central retinal artery occlusion
(B) Central retinal vein occlusion
(C) Ocular migraine
(D) Retinal detachment
(E) Temporal arteritis

Item 30

A 73-year-old woman is admitted to the hospital for drug-related hypersensitivity syndrome. She was hospitalized 2 weeks ago for a right ankle fracture and subsequently underwent open reduction and internal fixation. On the day of discharge she was noted to have a urinary tract infection and was prescribed trimethoprim-sulfamethoxazole despite a previously documented allergy to this agent in her internist's office chart, which was paper based and not linked to the hospital's electronic order entry system and drug allergy alert system.

After admitting the patient to the hospital and stopping her antibiotic, which of the following is the most appropriate immediate next step to reduce the likelihood of future similar errors?

(A) Discuss with the patient's internist the need to emphasize to patients the importance of communicating medication allergies with other caregivers
(B) Emphasize to the patient the importance of knowing and communicating her known allergies with caregivers
(C) Encourage hospital administration to consider implementation of an electronic health record
(D) Plan an intervention to improve communication of medication allergies from outpatient to inpatient records

Item 31

A 30-year-old woman is evaluated during a follow-up examination. She has had recurrent episodes of presyncope and syncope over the past few months. She continues to have an episode every 3 to 4 weeks, with no discernible pattern or trigger. She reports becoming light-headed and feeling faint, without other associated symptoms, followed by transient loss of consciousness for several seconds followed by spontaneous recovery without residual symptoms. On previous evaluation, an electrocardiogram (ECG) and echocardiogram were normal. Results of 24-hour continuous ambulatory ECG monitoring were unremarkable, and a cardiac event recorder showed no arrhythmia associated with presyncopal symptoms. History is significant for anxiety and intermittent insomnia; the patient takes no medications for these conditions. There is no history of prior head trauma. She does not use drugs or alcohol.

On physical examination, temperature is normal. Blood pressure is 122/68 mm Hg and pulse rate is 72/min while supine. After three minutes of standing, blood pressure is 112/84 mm Hg and pulse rate is 88/min, without reproduction of syncope or symptoms. The remainder of the examination is normal. Serum electrolytes, kidney function, and thyroid function studies are normal.

Which of the following is the most appropriate next step in the evaluation of this patient?

(A) Electroencephalography
(B) Exercise cardiac stress test
(C) Signal-averaged electrocardiogram
(D) Tilt-table testing

Item 32

A 32-year-old woman is evaluated as a new patient. She is planning to attempt conception with her partner. She has a history of systemic lupus erythematosus complicated by chronic kidney disease that has been inactive for several years off of treatment. She has had borderline blood pressure elevations since the diagnosis of kidney disease. She was also diagnosed with impaired fasting glucose and mild hyperlipidemia 2 years ago, both of which have been treated with dietary changes. Her current medications are calcium and vitamin D supplements.

On physical examination, blood pressure is 156/92 mm Hg and her vital signs are otherwise normal. BMI is 26. The remainder of the physical examination, including a gynecologic examination, is normal.

Laboratory studies:

Electrolytes	Normal
Blood urea nitrogen	12 mg/dL (4.2 mmol/L)
Creatinine	1.2 mg/dL (106.0 µmol/L)
Total cholesterol	250 mg/dL (6.4 mmol/L)
LDL cholesterol	160 mg/dL (4.1 mmol/L)
HDL cholesterol	34 mg/dL (0.8 mmol/L)
Triglycerides	200 mg/dL (2.26 mmol/L)
Spot urine albumin/ creatinine ratio	300 mg/g
Hemoglobin A$_{1c}$	7.5%

In addition to a daily prenatal vitamin, which of the following is the most appropriate treatment?

(A) Aspirin
(B) Lisinopril
(C) Metformin
(D) Simvastatin

Item 33

A 78-year-old woman living in a nursing home is evaluated for incontinence. Over the past year, she has had progressive decline in her cognitive status and now spends most of the day in bed. She requires coaxing to join the other residents in their communal meals and requires assistance for eating and bathing. When accompanied by an aide or family member, she is able to walk slowly to the bathroom without leakage and to urinate. Medical history is significant for dementia and depression treated with citalopram.

She is a frail, elderly woman in no acute distress. On physical examination, temperature is normal, blood pressure is 132/88 mm Hg, and pulse rate is 68/min. BMI is 23. Her score on the Mini–Mental State Examination is 14/30. Her gait is slow and she requires assistance. Abdominal examination is without suprapubic fullness. Rectal examination reveals normal sphincter tone. Results of urinalysis are normal.

Which of the following is the most appropriate management of this patient?

(A) Cystoscopy
(B) Indwelling Foley catheter
(C) Pelvic floor muscle training
(D) Prompted voiding
(E) Tolterodine

Item 34

A 31-year-old woman is evaluated during a routine office visit. She is married and in a monogamous relationship with her husband of 10 years. She has been getting annual Pap smears since the age of 20 years, all of which have been within normal limits, including the most recent, 1 year ago. She has no family history of cervical cancer. On physical examination, vital signs are normal.

Which of the following is the most appropriate management of this patient?

(A) Obtain human papillomavirus DNA testing
(B) Obtain Pap smear in 2 years
(C) Obtain Pap smear now
(D) Discontinue Pap smears

Item 35

A 78-year-old man is evaluated for a 1-year history of forgetfulness and not being able to remember names. He is a retired attorney. He reports no problems with performing activities of daily living, planning his day, or managing his finances. He is frustrated but not depressed and is still able to enjoy life. He has hypertension and hyperlipidemia, controlled with hydrochlorothiazide and simvastatin.

On physical examination, he is afebrile, blood pressure is 140/82 mm Hg, and pulse rate is 78/min. Mini–Mental State Examination score is 25. The lungs are clear. The heart is without murmur. Neurologic, motor, and sensory examinations are normal.

Which of the following is the most likely diagnosis?

(A) Alzheimer disease
(B) Mild cognitive impairment
(C) Pseudodementia
(D) Vascular dementia

Item 36

A 76-year-old woman was evaluated 10 days ago for weight loss and occasional hemoptysis. Non–small cell lung cancer was subsequently diagnosed. In addition to a 4×5 cm single lesion in the left upper lobe of her lung, there are metastatic lesions in the left humerus, as well as a single lesion in the left lobe of the liver. She does all of her own activities of daily living and is able to walk 1 mile before stopping because of fatigue. Her only medications are a daily multivitamin and a calcium supplement.

On physical examination, vital signs are normal. She appears comfortable and in no distress and is interested in life-prolonging therapy.

Which of the following is the most appropriate time to begin palliative care discussions with this patient?

(A) After she develops symptoms
(B) At the current visit
(C) When admitted to hospice care
(D) When she no longer desires active treatment

Item 37

A 58-year-old woman is evaluated for a 2-day history of burning, stinging pain in her posterior neck that radiates down her left arm and began after she spent several hours painting the ceiling of her home. She reports no trauma or other symptoms. She feels mild numbness and paresthesias on the back of her left hand.

On physical examination, vital signs are normal. Neck range of motion is limited by pain, especially in extension. Axial loading of the neck increases pain. There is slightly diminished sensation on the back of the left hand. There are no motor deficits. Reflexes are symmetric.

Which of the following is the most appropriate management of this patient?

(A) Analgesics and avoidance of provocative activities
(B) Cervical traction
(C) Electromyography/nerve conduction study
(D) MRI of cervical spine

Item 38

A 55-year-old man is evaluated during a follow-up appointment for a 6-month history of nonproductive cough. The cough predictably comes after meals, at bedtime, or any time he lies down, but it can occur at other times as well. He experiences heartburn throughout the day. He has no shortness of breath, dyspnea on exertion, fever, chills, postnasal drip, recent upper respiratory tract infection, or wheezing. Omeprazole was prescribed 2 weeks ago but he reports no change in his cough or heartburn symptoms. He is a nonsmoker, does not drink alcohol, and takes no other medications.

Vital signs are normal, as is the remainder of the physical examination. Chest radiograph is normal.

Which of the following is the most appropriate treatment?

(A) Amoxicillin-clavulanate
(B) Continue omeprazole
(C) Inhaled albuterol
(D) Loratadine with pseudoephedrine

Item 39

A 42-year-old woman is evaluated for chest pain that started a few days ago. It is midsternal, sharp, constant, and worsens with deep inspiration and recumbency. It does not radiate to the back and does not worsen with physical activity. The pain has increased slightly over the past day. She has no recent fevers or chills, cough, joint pain, or rash. Two weeks ago, she had symptoms consistent with acute tracheobronchitis.

On physical examination, temperature is 37.5 °C (99.5 °F), blood pressure is 122/80 mm Hg, pulse rate is 88/min, and respiration rate is 17/min. BMI is 32. She is uncomfortable lying down and prefers to sit forward for the examination. Cardiac auscultation demonstrates normal heart sounds with no murmur or rub. The remainder of the examination is normal.

Electrocardiogram is shown. Chest radiograph is normal.

Which of the following is the most likely diagnosis?

(A) Acute coronary syndrome
(B) Acute pericarditis
(C) Acute pleuritis
(D) Acute pulmonary embolism

Item 40

A 60-year-old man is evaluated for a 1-year history of generalized fatigue and lack of energy. He has had erectile dysfunction for the past 9 months. He has chronic low back pain and hypertension. Current medications are metoprolol, hydrochlorothiazide, hydrocodone, and naproxen.

On physical examination, vital signs are normal. Cardiac, lung, and thyroid examinations are all normal. Laboratory studies show a morning total serum testosterone level of 180 ng/dL (6.2 nmol/L). Complete blood count, metabolic panel, and thyroid-stimulating hormone level are all normal.

Which of the following is the most appropriate next step in the management of this patient?

(A) Discontinue hydrocodone
(B) Discontinue metoprolol
(C) Recheck testosterone level
(D) Start testosterone replacement therapy

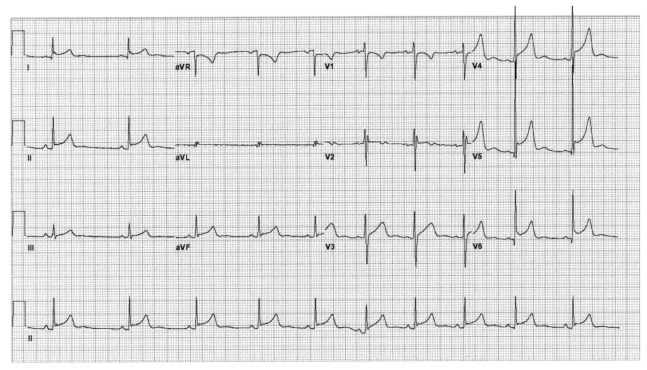

ITEM 39

Item 41

A 67-year-old man is evaluated during a routine examination. He has hypertension and obesity. He also has a history of gout, but has not had an attack in more than 1 year. His current medications are lisinopril and a daily aspirin.

On physical examination, blood pressure is 140/82 mm Hg; vital signs are otherwise normal. BMI is 32. His waist circumference is 107 cm (42 in). There is no hepatomegaly.

Laboratory studies:

Total cholesterol	192 mg/dL (4.97 mmol/L)
HDL cholesterol	27 mg/dL (0.70 mmol/L)
LDL cholesterol (directly measured)	68 mg/dL (1.76 mmol/L)
Triglycerides	554 mg/dL (6.26 mmol/L)
Glucose	100 mg/dL (5.5 mmol/L)
Creatinine	1.1 mg/dL (97.2 µmol/L)

In addition to recommending weight loss and exercise, which of the following is the most appropriate treatment for his lipid abnormalities?

(A) Colesevelam
(B) Extended-release nicotinic acid
(C) Fenofibrate
(D) Omega-3 fatty acids

Item 42

A 65-year-old man is evaluated for a 3-day history of scrotal pain. He notes some pain with urination and tenderness in the left testicular region. He has felt febrile at home with some nausea and generalized weakness. He has not had similar symptoms before and has not had any trauma. He has no nocturia, urinary frequency, or weak urinary stream. He takes no medications.

On physical examination, temperature is 38.7 °C (101.6 °F), blood pressure is 140/80 mm Hg, pulse rate is 90/min, and respiration rate is 14/min. He is in moderate distress. The left scrotum shows erythema with mild fullness. The testicle itself is nontender, but there is fullness superior to it that is extremely tender to palpation, with some discomfort to palpation over the posterior aspect of the testicle. The left testicle is lower in the scrotum than the right testicle. The prostate is normal in size and nontender. Leukocyte count is 14,000/µL (14 × 10⁹/L) with 18% band forms.

Which of the following is the most likely diagnosis?

(A) Acute prostatitis
(B) Epididymitis
(C) Indirect hernia
(D) Orchitis
(E) Testicular torsion

Item 43

An 82-year-old man was admitted to the hospital 2 days ago with pneumonia, sepsis, and acute kidney injury. Medical history is significant for recurrent lung cancer, for which he previously underwent lobectomy, now with adrenal metastases. He has remained anuric since admission. This morning his serum potassium level was 7.2 meq/L (7.2 mmol/L) with electrocardiographic changes. It is clear that dialysis is indicated. The patient is unable to give consent, and his wife is his surrogate decision maker. She says that he was aware of the poor prognosis from his lung cancer and expressed a desire not to be kept alive on machines for a long period of time. However, he was looking forward to his great-grandson's graduation from college in 3 weeks and hoped that he could be able to attend. The wife is willing to consent to dialysis.

On physical examination, temperature is 38.1 °C (100.5 °F), blood pressure is 110/64 mm Hg, pulse rate is 112/min, and respiration rate is 28/min.

Which of the following is the most appropriate management of this patient?

(A) Start long-term hemodialysis
(B) Start temporary hemodialysis
(C) Withdraw all life-sustaining treatment
(D) Withhold dialysis and continue medical treatment

Item 44

A 38-year-old woman is evaluated for gritty, burning eyes that worsen over the course of the day. She reports her eyes are often dry and are worse on windy days. She also reports dry mouth with difficulty salivating at times. She has no other symptoms.

On physical examination, vital signs are normal. The conjunctiva is irritated. She has normal vision by Snellen chart. Fundi are normal. Decreased tear production is documented with the Schirmer test. The remainder of the physical examination is normal.

The antinuclear antibody test, rheumatoid factor, and anti-Ro/SSA and anti-La/SSB tests are positive.

Which of the following is the most likely diagnosis?

(A) Meibomianitis
(B) Primary Sjögren syndrome
(C) Rheumatoid arthritis
(D) Systemic lupus erythematosus

Item 45

A 28-year-old woman is evaluated for a painful lump in her left breast of 6 weeks' duration. There is neither discharge from the nipple nor skin changes over the area. Her last normal menstrual period was 3 weeks ago and she thinks that the lump became slightly larger right before and during her menses. She is on low-dose oral contraceptives. She has no history of breast disease or breast biopsy. Menarche was at age 12 years. She has never been pregnant. A maternal aunt had breast cancer.

On physical examination, vital signs are normal. BMI is 24. There is a 1.5-cm mobile, soft, slightly tender mass in the lower mid quadrant of the left breast. There is no nipple discharge and no abnormalities of the overlying skin. The right breast has no masses. There is no axillary lymphadenopathy. The remainder of the examination is unremarkable.

Which of the following is the most appropriate management of this patient?

(A) Core needle biopsy
(B) Mammography
(C) Repeat clinical breast examination in 6 months
(D) Ultrasonography

Item 46

A 94-year-old woman is brought to the emergency department by her daughter for a 5-day history of progressive weakness, anorexia, dizziness, and mild confusion. She was hospitalized 2 weeks ago for an acute exacerbation of chronic heart failure that was treated with intravenous diuretics and an increase in her daily oral diuretic dose. She initially did well following discharge, and a follow-up appointment with her primary care physician is scheduled for next week. She has a history of chronic atrial fibrillation, upper gastrointestinal bleeding owing to a duodenal ulcer 18 months ago, COPD, hypertension, post-herpetic neuralgia, chronic kidney disease, depression, anxiety, and seasonal rhinitis. Medications are furosemide, potassium chloride, aspirin, omeprazole, ipratropium and albuterol inhalers, metoprolol, gabapentin, loratadine, and as-needed lorazepam.

On physical examination, she is a pleasant but frail-appearing woman who is arousable but mildly confused. Temperature is 37.3 °C (99.1 °F), blood pressure is 108/56 mm Hg, pulse rate is 95/min, and respiration rate is 16/min. Oxygen saturation is 94% on ambient air. The mucous membranes are dry. The pupils are symmetric and reactive. Heart examination is significant for an irregularly irregular rate and a grade 3/6 crescendo-decrescendo murmur at the right upper sternal border. The lungs are clear to auscultation. The abdomen is scaphoid without hepatosplenomegaly. There is no peripheral edema. Her neurologic examination is nonfocal except for her cognitive deficits.

Laboratory studies show normal serum electrolytes and a plasma glucose level of 110 mg/dL (6.1 mmol/L). Her serum creatinine level is 1.4 mg/dL (123.8 μmol/L), increased from 1.2 mg/dL (106.1 μmol/L) at the time of hospital discharge. Her complete blood count reveals a leukocyte count of 7500/μL (7.5×10^9/L) with a normal differential, a hematocrit of 35%, and normal platelet count. A urinalysis shows trace ketones but no cells. A chest radiograph is significant for severe kyphoscoliosis and changes consistent with emphysema, but not pneumonia or heart failure.

Which of the following is the most likely cause of the patient's clinical presentation?

(A) Acute kidney injury
(B) Medication effect
(C) Occult infection
(D) Recent stroke

Item 47

A 60-year-old man is admitted to the hospital with a traumatic hip fracture. A total hip arthroplasty under general anesthesia is planned. He has COPD and reports that he is significantly limited in his exercise tolerance because of dyspnea, although his functional capacity has remained stable over the past 4 to 6 months. He has a cough with occasional white sputum, unchanged for the past 6 months. He has no other acute respiratory symptoms. He smokes 1 pack per day of cigarettes. Current medications are tiotropium, albuterol, and fluticasone/salmeterol.

On physical examination, temperature is normal, blood pressure is 108/72 mm Hg, pulse rate is 78/min, and respiration rate is 18/min. Oxygen saturation is 96% on ambient air. Pulmonary examination demonstrates scattered crackles and wheezing, unchanged from his baseline findings. Cardiac examination shows regular rate and rhythm and a normal S_1 and S_2.

Which of the following should be recommended before surgery?

(A) Nocturnal continuous positive airway pressure
(B) Chest radiograph
(C) Incentive spirometry
(D) Pulmonary function testing

Item 48

A 46-year-old man is evaluated for a 3-week history of occasional painless bright red rectal bleeding. He has no fatigue, lightheadedness, weight loss, or abdominal pain. His stools are frequently firm, occasionally hard, and there is no change in the frequency or consistency of his bowel movements. He has never been screened for colorectal cancer.

On physical examination, temperature is 37.2 °C (98.9 °F), blood pressure is 132/78 mm Hg, and pulse rate is 84/min. Digital rectal examination yields a stool sample that is positive for occult blood; the examination is otherwise normal. Anoscopy reveals a few internal hemorrhoids without active bleeding. Laboratory studies show a blood hemoglobin level of 14 g/dL (140 g/L).

Which of the following is the most appropriate management of this patient?

(A) Banding of hemorrhoids
(B) Colonoscopy
(C) Fiber supplementation without further evaluation
(D) Home fecal occult blood testing

Item 49

A 52-year-old man is evaluated during a periodic health examination. He has benign prostatic hyperplasia, and his father died of prostate cancer at the age of 74 years. His only current medication is tamsulosin. He has no urinary symptoms. Vital signs are normal, as is the remainder of the physical examination.

Which of the following is the most appropriate management?

(A) Discuss the risks and benefits of prostate cancer screening

(B) Obtain a prostate-specific antigen level

(C) Perform a digital rectal examination

(D) Perform a digital rectal examination and obtain a prostate-specific antigen level

Item 50

A 72-year-old man is evaluated in the emergency department for a 12-hour episode of dizziness, described as a "spinning sensation" when he opens his eyes. He has nausea without vomiting, has had no loss of consciousness, no palpitations, and no other neurologic symptoms. He requires assistance to walk. He prefers to keep his eyes closed but has no diplopia. He has hypertension, hyperlipidemia, and type 2 diabetes mellitus. He had an upper respiratory tract infection 2 weeks ago. Medications are hydrochlorothiazide, lisinopril, simvastatin, and metformin.

On physical examination, vital signs are normal. There are no orthostatic changes. Results of a cardiovascular examination are normal. He has no focal weakness. He cannot stand without assistance. Vertical nystagmus occurs immediately with the Dix-Hallpike maneuver. It persists for 90 seconds and does not fatigue. Electrocardiogram is consistent with left ventricular hypertrophy and shows no acute changes.

Which of the following is the most appropriate next step in management?

(A) CT scan of the head without contrast

(B) MRI with angiography of the brain

(C) Otolith repositioning

(D) Trial of vestibular suppressant medication

Item 51

A 48-year-old woman is evaluated during a routine examination. She is concerned about her gradual weight gain over the years and requests counseling on how she can most effectively lose weight.

Over 8 years, she has gained approximately 18 kg (40 lb). With several commercial diets, she has lost weight but always gains it back. She has a sedentary job, and often skips breakfast or eats dinner on the run. She states she cannot fit exercise into her busy day. She takes no medications and has no allergies.

On physical examination, temperature is normal, blood pressure is 132/70 mm Hg, pulse rate is 80/min, and respiration rate is 12/min. BMI is 32. There is no thyromegaly. The abdomen is obese, soft, nontender, and without striae. Fasting plasma glucose level is 106 mg/dL (5.9 mmol/L) and thyroid function test results are normal.

Which of the following is the most appropriate next step to help this patient achieve long-term weight reduction?

(A) Exercise 15-30 minutes 5 days/week

(B) Laparoscopic adjustable band surgery

(C) Orlistat

(D) Reduce current caloric intake by 500-1000 kcal/d

Item 52

A 75-year-old woman is evaluated during a follow-up examination for recently diagnosed symptomatic peripheral arterial disease. The patient has hypothyroidism, hypertension, atrial fibrillation, and smokes cigarettes (30-pack-year history). Her current medications are diltiazem, warfarin, hydrochlorothiazide, levothyroxine, calcium, and vitamin D.

On physical examination, she is afebrile, blood pressure is 140/82 mm Hg, pulse rate is 66/min, and respiration rate is 12/min. BMI is 21. Posterior tibialis and dorsalis pedis pulses are diminished bilaterally (1+); the skin on the anterior aspect of the lower legs is shiny and hairless. Heart rhythm is irregularly irregular and without murmurs. Neurologic and musculoskeletal examinations are normal.

Laboratory studies:

Total cholesterol	238 mg/dL (6.16 mmol/L)
HDL cholesterol	36 mg/dL (0.93 mmol/L)
LDL cholesterol	165 mg/dL (4.27 mmol/L)
Triglycerides	205 mg/dL (2.32 mmol/L)
Serum creatinine	0.9 mg/dL (79.6 µmol/L)

In addition to strongly recommending smoking cessation, which of the following is the safest treatment for this patient?

(A) Atorvastatin

(B) Pravastatin

(C) Rosuvastatin

(D) Simvastatin

Item 53

A 42-year-old woman is evaluated for a 6-month history of heavy menstrual bleeding. She has been menstruating for the last 8 days and is still going through 10 pads or more daily with frequent clots. She has fatigue but no dizziness. Previous evaluation for this problem has included normal thyroid function and prolactin testing. She has no other medical problems and takes no medications. Pelvic ultrasonography has demonstrated a large posterior submucosal fibroid. A surgical treatment is planned in 2 weeks.

On physical examination, vital signs are normal. Abdominal examination is benign, and the pelvic examination reveals a moderate amount of blood in the vaginal vault.

Hemoglobin level is 10.5 g/dL (105 g/L). Pregnancy test is negative.

Which of the following is the most appropriate next management step?

(A) Estrogen/progesterone multiphasic oral contraceptive

(B) Intravenous estrogen

(C) Oral medroxyprogesterone acetate

(D) Reevaluation in 1 week

Item 54

A 31-year-old woman is evaluated for a 4-week history of anterior knee pain. It developed insidiously and has progressively worsened. The pain worsens with prolonged sitting and with walking up and down stairs. There is no morning stiffness. She has no history of trauma. She is taking acetaminophen as needed for the pain.

On physical examination, vital signs are normal. The pain is reproduced by applying pressure to the surface of the patella with the knee in extension and moving the patella both laterally and medially. There is no effusion, swelling, or warmth. Range of knee motion is normal, without crepitus or pain.

Which of the following is the most likely diagnosis?

(A) Knee osteoarthritis
(B) Patellofemoral pain syndrome
(C) Pes anserine bursitis
(D) Prepatellar bursitis

Item 55

An 87-year-old woman is evaluated for dizziness of 1 year's duration. She describes feeling lightheaded and unsteady when she walks but has not fallen. She denies vertigo, tinnitus, headache, loss of consciousness, chest pain, palpitations, or focal weakness. Medical history is significant for hypertension, glaucoma, and left eye cataract. Current medications are lisinopril and latanoprost ophthalmic drops.

On physical examination, blood pressure is 142/72 mm Hg supine and 136/66 mm Hg standing, pulse rate is 72/min supine and 76/min standing. BMI is 22. On neurologic examination, she has 20/50 vision, decreased auditory acuity, and 4+/5 motor strength throughout. Vibration and position sensation are normal. There is no tremor, cogwheeling, or bradykinesia, and her gait is not ataxic, although she feels safer holding on to the wall. There is no nystagmus. The lungs are clear. Cardiovascular examination is normal.

Laboratory studies, including a metabolic profile and complete blood count, are normal.

Which of the following is the most appropriate management of this patient?

(A) Physical therapy with gait evaluation
(B) Replace latanoprost with timolol
(C) Replace lisinopril with losartan
(D) Vestibular rehabilitation therapy

Item 56

A 50-year-old woman is evaluated during a follow-up appointment for moderate depression. Eight weeks ago, she was started on bupropion; 4 weeks ago, the dose was increased to the maximal dose. At this time, her PHQ-9 score has not improved over baseline, and she confirms that her symptoms have not improved. She has no suicidal ideation and does not have hallucinations or other psychotic features. She has no previous episodes of high energy,

spending sprees, lack of need of sleep, or previous psychiatric problems. She is not interested in psychotherapy at this time.

Which of the following is the most appropriate next step in treatment?

(A) Add buspirone
(B) Continue bupropion at current dose for an additional 8 weeks
(C) Discontinue bupropion, begin sertraline
(D) Refer for electroconvulsive therapy

Item 57

A 44-year-old man is evaluated during a routine examination. He is concerned about his general health and risk of diabetes mellitus. He has no medical problems. Both parents and his sister have type 2 diabetes mellitus.

On physical examination, temperature is normal, blood pressure is 130/79 mm Hg, pulse rate is 66/min, and respiration rate is 14/min. BMI is 28. The remainder of the physical examination is normal.

Laboratory studies:

Glucose (fasting)	104 mg/dL (5.8 mmol/L)
Total cholesterol	247 mg/dL (6.40 mmol/L)
HDL cholesterol	50 mg/dL (1.30 mmol/L)
LDL cholesterol	177 mg/dL (4.58 mmol/L)
Triglycerides	100 mg/dL (1.13 mmol/L)

Which of the following interventions is the most appropriate initial strategy to decrease this patient's chance of developing type 2 diabetes mellitus?

(A) Acarbose
(B) Metformin
(C) Pioglitazone
(D) Weight loss and exercise

Item 58

A physician is asked to advise the Pharmacy and Therapeutics Committee of the hospital regarding a new drug to prevent deep venous thrombosis (DVT), drug "Z." The physician reviews a recent randomized controlled trial of 5000 patients that compared drug Z with drug C, which is commonly used and is on the hospital's formulary. The following data are abstracted from the trial:

Study results:

Drug	DVT Cases
Drug Z (n = 2500)	25
Drug C (n = 2500)	50

Based on these data, how many patients need to be treated (number needed to treat, NNT) with drug Z, compared with drug C, to prevent one extra case of DVT?

(A) 1
(B) 2
(C) 25
(D) 100
(E) 167

Item 59

A 21-year-old man is evaluated in the emergency department for left ankle pain that began 6 hours ago when he inverted his left ankle while playing soccer. He was unable to bear weight immediately after the injury, but is now able to bear weight with some difficulty.

There is ecchymosis and swelling around the entire ankle joint, with tenderness to palpation of the anterior talofibular ligament. He is able to bear weight but finds it painful to do so. There is no tenderness to palpation of bony structures (lateral and medial malleolus, base of fifth metatarsal) or the Achilles tendon. There is no ankle instability. Compression of the distal tibia and fibula does not cause any discomfort (negative squeeze test).

Which of the following is the most appropriate management for this patient?

(A) Ankle joint corticosteroid injection
(B) Ankle MRI
(C) Ankle radiograph
(D) Ankle splinting
(E) Urgent surgical evaluation

Item 60

A 61-year-old woman is evaluated for hot flushes, which have been persistent for the last 10 years. They occur at least 7 times per day, last for approximately 60 seconds, and are associated with severe sweating, palpitations, and occasional nausea. She is awakened several times per night. She has tried herbal medications, including soy and black cohosh, but has not experienced any benefit. She has hypertension, type 2 diabetes mellitus, and hyperlipidemia. Five years ago, she developed deep venous thrombosis after hip replacement surgery. Her current medications are ramipril, metformin, atorvastatin, calcium, and vitamin D.

On physical examination, vital signs are normal. BMI is 29. The remainder of the examination is normal.

Which of the following is the most appropriate treatment?

(A) Citalopram
(B) Oral estrogen therapy
(C) Oral estrogen/progesterone therapy
(D) Topical (vaginal) estrogen
(E) Venlafaxine

Item 61

A 60-year-old man is evaluated for new-onset monocular cloudy vision of the left eye that began 4 hours ago. He has type 2 diabetes mellitus and coronary artery disease. His current medications are aspirin, simvastatin, lisinopril, metoprolol, and metformin.

On physical examination, vital signs are normal. When a light is shined into his left eye it is not reactive, but shining a light in his right eye causes his left pupil to contract (left afferent pupillary defect). The visual acuity of the right eye is 20/30, that of the left eye is 20/120. Retinal findings are shown. The remainder of the examination is normal.

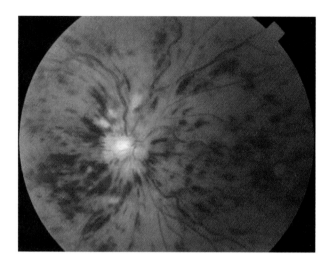

Which of the following is the most likely diagnosis?

(A) Acute angle closure glaucoma
(B) Central retinal artery occlusion
(C) Central retinal vein occlusion
(D) Retinal detachment

Item 62

A 62-year-old man is evaluated before elective total hip arthroplasty. He reports no prior medical problems aside from hip osteoarthritis. His only medications are ibuprofen and oxycodone. He drinks 1 pint of liquor daily.

On physical examination, temperature is normal, blood pressure is 100/62 mm Hg, and pulse rate is 92/min. He is alert and oriented. He has gynecomastia and multiple spider angiomata. He is jaundiced. There is ascites but no hepatomegaly or splenomegaly.

Laboratory studies:

Platelet count	52,000/µL (52×10^9/L)
Bilirubin (total)	2.3 mg/dL (39.3 µmol/L)
Alanine aminotransferase	68 units/L
Aspartate aminotransferase	90 units/L
INR	1.8

Abdominal ultrasound shows a cirrhotic liver and ascites. The patient's Child-Turcotte-Pugh (CTP) score is class C.

Which of the following is the best management of this patient?

(A) Administer prednisolone for 1 week prior to surgery
(B) Administer vitamin K for 3 days prior to surgery
(C) Nonoperative management
(D) Proceed with surgery

Item 63

A 52-year-old man is evaluated during a routine examination. He is asymptomatic but is concerned about his weight. Medical history is significant for prediabetes and elevated cholesterol levels. He smokes one or two cigars a week. He drinks one or two alcoholic beverages a few nights each week. He does not get any regular exercise.

On physical examination, vital signs are normal. BMI is 33. The examination is otherwise unremarkable. The patient indicates he is ready to make important lifestyle changes to improve his health.

Which of the following is the best initial management?

(A) Assess the patient's confidence in making lifestyle changes

(B) Determine which lifestyle change the patient believes is most important

(C) Inform the patient he needs to lose weight

(D) Provide advice on smoking cessation

Item 64

A 56-year-old woman is evaluated during a follow-up visit after presenting as a new patient 2 weeks ago. At that time, her blood pressure was found to be elevated (156/88 mm Hg) and follow-up laboratory tests were ordered. She has had no major illnesses. Her father had type 2 diabetes mellitus and died at age 52 years of a myocardial infarction. She is currently taking no medications.

On physical examination, blood pressure is 156/92 mm Hg in the left arm and 160/90 mm Hg in the right arm. Pulse rate is 86/min and respiration rate is 16/min. BMI is 34. Waist circumference is 39 in (99 cm). Results of a funduscopic examination are normal.

Laboratory studies:

Blood urea nitrogen	16 mg/dL (5.7 mmol/L)
Creatinine	0.9 mg/dL (79.6 µmol/L)
LDL cholesterol (fasting)	162 mg/dL (4.19 mmol/L)
HDL cholesterol (fasting)	32 mg/dL (0.83 mmol/L)
Triglycerides (fasting)	148 mg/dL (1.67 mmol/L)
Glucose (fasting)	98 mg/dL (5.4 mmol/L)
Urinalysis	Trace protein, no glucose

In addition to hypertension and obesity, which of the following is the most likely diagnosis?

(A) Hypertriglyceridemia

(B) Impaired fasting glucose

(C) Metabolic syndrome

(D) No additional diagnoses

Item 65

An 85-year-old man is evaluated following a recent diagnosis of non–small cell lung cancer with metastatic disease to the liver, spine, multiple ribs, and sternum. He has declined treatment. The patient describes pain in his ribs that is present throughout the day and wakes him from sleep. He rates his pain as a 2 or 3 on a 10-point pain scale. His only medication is acetaminophen, 1000 mg every 6 hours, but this is not entirely effective in relieving his pain. Palpation of the right anterior chest and sternum reproduces his pain.

Which of the following is the most appropriate treatment?

(A) Gabapentin

(B) Ibuprofen

(C) Meperidine, orally

(D) Morphine, intramuscularly

Item 66

A 52-year-old man presents for routine care. Several years ago he was told that his cholesterol level was borderline. He is a vegetarian and a marathon runner, does not smoke, and drinks alcohol only socially. He takes a daily multivitamin. His father had a myocardial infarction at the age of 42 years.

On physical examination, vital signs are normal. BMI is 22. The remainder of the examination is normal.

Laboratory studies:

Total cholesterol	325 mg/dL (8.42 mmol/L)
HDL cholesterol	50 mg/dL (1.30 mmol/L)
LDL cholesterol	196 mg/dL (5.08 mmol/L)
Triglycerides	185 mg/dL (2.09 mmol/L)
Glucose	72 mg/dL (3.9 mmol/L)
Thyroid-stimulating hormone	0.52 µU/mL (0.52 mU/L)

Which of the following is the most appropriate management?

(A) Calculate the non-HDL cholesterol level

(B) Measure high-sensitivity C-reactive protein

(C) Initiate fibrate therapy

(D) Initiate statin therapy

Item 67

A 72-year-old woman is evaluated for a fall three nights ago. She lives in a single-floor apartment. At about 2 AM, she got up to go to the bathroom and fell after bumping into a wall. She had no lightheadedness or loss of consciousness and has not fallen before. Her home has no rugs and no thresholds between rooms. She normally has no problems walking and does not use an assistive device.

On physical examination, vital signs are normal. BMI is 23. She is alert and oriented. There are no orthostatic blood pressure changes or pulse changes. Visual testing using a Snellen chart reveals 20/20 distance vision in both eyes. The remainder of the physical examination, including a motor examination, is normal. In the Timed "Up & Go" test, she walks 10 feet in 10 seconds (normal, ≤14 sec).

Which of the following is the most appropriate next step in this patient's management?

(A) Ask about use of night lights

(B) Begin an individualized exercise program

(C) Ophthalmology evaluation

(D) Provide patient with a walker

Item 68

A 28-year-old woman is evaluated after being brought to the office by her boyfriend. He reports that she has been hearing voices and exhibiting increasingly paranoid behavior, believing that the mailman is trying to poison her. She has not gone to work in 4 weeks and spends most of her day alone in her bedroom wearing head phones and listening to heavy metal rock music. Her boyfriend reports that she has had several other episodes of paranoid behavior over the past 8 months but none as bad as the current one. The patient is minimally interactive. She previously drank two beers daily (none recently) and smoked marijuana at parties. Her father was diagnosed with schizophrenia at age 18 years. Her mother died of breast cancer 2 years ago after a long illness.

On physical examination, vital signs are normal. She appears disheveled and withdrawn. She is a thin woman, staring straight ahead and not making eye contact. She declines to talk to the physician or undress to be examined. A urine toxicology screen is positive for cannabinoids. A complete blood count and basic chemistry panel are normal.

Which of the following is the most likely diagnosis?

(A) Bipolar disorder
(B) *Cannabis* abuse with psychosis
(C) Major depressive disorder with psychotic features
(D) Schizophrenia

Item 69

A 20-year-old woman presents for a gynecologic examination and discussion of contraception. She has been sexually active for the past 3 years and has been using condoms. However, she finds condom use inconvenient, although she admits she is bad about remembering to take pills. She has had four partners in the past, currently has a new partner, has no history of sexually transmitted infection, and has never been pregnant. Medical history and family history are noncontributory. She drinks 2 to 4 beers on the weekends and does not smoke cigarettes.

Physical examination, including pelvic examination, is normal.

Which of the following is the most appropriate contraceptive recommendation for this patient?

(A) Condom use with combination estrogen-progesterone pills
(B) Condom use with subcutaneous progesterone implants
(C) Depot medroxyprogesterone acetate
(D) Estrogen-progesterone vaginal ring

Item 70

A 68-year-old man is evaluated for continuing urinary frequency and nocturia. His symptoms have been slowly progressive over the past 1 to 2 years with a weak urinary stream and hesitancy. He was started on doxazosin 6 months ago, which he tolerates well and initially provided some improvement. However, his symptoms have continued and are beginning to interfere with his quality of life, particularly the urinary frequency and nocturia. His only other medical problem is hypertension, for which he takes lisinopril and metoprolol.

On physical examination, he is afebrile, blood pressure is 140/85 mm Hg, pulse rate is 70/min, and respiration rate is 14/min. BMI is 25. He has a symmetric moderately enlarged prostate gland with no prostate nodules or areas of tenderness. A urinalysis is normal.

Which of the following is most appropriate next step in treatment of this patient's benign prostatic hyperplasia?

(A) Add finasteride
(B) Change doxazosin to finasteride
(C) Change doxazosin to tamsulosin
(D) Prescribe a fluoroquinolone antibiotic for 4 weeks

Item 71

A 30-year-old woman is evaluated during a routine examination in November. She received a routine tetanus, diphtheria, and acellular pertussis (Tdap) booster 5 years ago. She is sexually active with a single lifetime sexual partner. She has had no history of sexually transmitted infection. She was born in the United States and reports getting "routine shots" in childhood. She has had regular Pap smears without any abnormal results; her most recent was 3 years ago. She does not smoke cigarettes. She works as an attorney in a large corporate law firm. Findings on physical examination are unremarkable.

Which of the following vaccinations should be administered?

(A) Hepatitis B vaccine series
(B) Human papillomavirus vaccine series
(C) Influenza vaccine
(D) Tetanus and diphtheria (Td) vaccine

Item 72

A 32-year-old woman is evaluated following a diagnosis of chronic fatigue syndrome. She has a several-year history of chronic disabling fatigue, unrefreshing sleep, muscle and joint pain, and headache. A comprehensive evaluation has not identified any other medical condition, and a screen for depression is normal. Her only medications are multiple vitamins and dietary supplements. Physical examination is normal.

Which of the following is the most appropriate management for this patient's symptoms?

(A) Acyclovir
(B) Evening primrose oil
(C) Graded exercise program
(D) Growth hormone
(E) Sertraline

Item 73

A 36-year-old woman comes for her fifth visit in the past 3 months. She has a history of chronic abdominal pain and reports continued excruciating, diffuse, chronic abdominal pain and bloating. She has intermittent diarrhea and constipation, but reports no weight loss or other localizing symptoms. She is able to carry out routine activities of daily living. She has tried multiple over-the-counter medications as well as previous prescriptions for omeprazole, psyllium fiber supplements, dicyclomine, loperamide, and NSAIDs, all of which she states "do not touch" her pain. She states that she tried her friend's acetaminophen-oxycodone and had good relief. A previous workup (including complete blood count, comprehensive metabolic panel, amylase, lipase, anti-transglutaminase antibodies, and abdominal CT scan) was negative. She reports several episodes of abuse as a child and has been in a number of difficult and disruptive relationships as an adult. Although she smokes cigarettes, she denies any past or present alcohol or drug use. She is currently on no medications.

Results of the physical examination are normal. When her request for acetaminophen-oxycodone is denied, she becomes angry and upset, stating that all she needs is a medicine that works.

Which of the following is the most appropriate approach to this patient?

(A) Initiate an ongoing discussion of the causes and significance of her pain
(B) Prescribe a limited number of acetaminophen-oxycodone tablets
(C) Refer to a gastroenterologist
(D) Request that her care be transferred to another physician

Item 74

A 58-year-old man is evaluated as a new patient. A review of his previous records shows he received a pneumococcal vaccination 6 years ago when he was admitted to the hospital with community-acquired pneumonia. He feels well with no acute symptoms. He has type 2 diabetes mellitus, hypertension, and hyperlipidemia. Medications are insulin glargine, metformin, lisinopril, and simvastatin. Results of the physical examination are unremarkable.

When should this patient receive an additional pneumococcal vaccination?

(A) Today
(B) Today and repeat every 5 years
(C) Today and at age 65 years
(D) At age 65 years
(E) No further pneumococcal vaccinations are required

Item 75

A 30-year-old woman is evaluated for hyperlipidemia. Medical history is significant for type 1 diabetes mellitus, hypothyroidism, and hypertension. She is planning pregnancy. Her father was diagnosed with coronary artery disease at the age of 47 years. Her current medications are levothyroxine, hydrochlorothiazide, insulin glargine, and insulin aspart.

On physical examination, vital signs and the remainder of the physical examination are normal.

Laboratory studies:

Hemoglobin A_{1c}	8.1%
Total cholesterol	223 mg/dL (5.78 mmol/L)
HDL cholesterol	67 mg/dL (1.74 mmol/L)
LDL cholesterol	140 mg/dL (3.63 mmol/L)
Triglycerides	90 mg/dL (1.02 mmol/L)

In addition to recommending therapeutic lifestyle changes, which of the following is the most appropriate management of this patient's lipid levels?

(A) Colesevelam
(B) Ezetimibe
(C) Gemfibrozil
(D) Simvastatin

Item 76

A 67-year-old woman is admitted to the hospital with shortness of breath and is found to have a pulmonary embolus. She is begun on low-molecular-weight heparin. Upon further evaluation, a large left breast mass is found along with a malignant left-sided pleural effusion. Biopsy of the breast mass reveals poorly differentiated adenocarcinoma. Although she has a limited social support system and minimal understanding of her disease, she is interested in evaluating possible treatment options for her condition. She continues to have mild shortness of breath and marked anxiety related to her newly diagnosed condition, but otherwise feels well.

In addition to oncology and surgery consultations, which of the following is the most appropriate next step in this patient's care?

(A) Antidepressant therapy
(B) Hospice care referral
(C) Long-acting morphine
(D) Palliative care consultation

Item 77

A 32-year-old woman is evaluated for a 6-month history of nonproductive cough. She has no history of recurrent upper respiratory tract infections and has never smoked cigarettes. She has no fever, dyspnea on exertion, hemoptysis, heartburn, or wheezing. She has worked in the same office for 7 years and has lived in the same house for the past 20 years. She has not traveled out of the area for more than 2 years. She has no pets at home, no occupational or other exposure to toxic chemicals, and no family history of pulmonary disease. She takes no medications.

The vital signs and results of the physical examination are normal.

A complete blood count with differential is normal. Chest radiograph is normal. Pulmonary function tests are normal and a methacholine challenge test is negative.

Which of the following is the most appropriate diagnostic test to perform next?

(A) Bronchoscopy
(B) 24-hour esophageal pH manometry
(C) Sinus imaging
(D) Sputum testing for eosinophils

Item 78

A 78-year-old woman is evaluated after she tripped while carrying a garbage bag to the trash bin in her kitchen. She remembers falling but did not injure herself. She has had no previous falls. She reports no loss of consciousness, light-headedness, or dizziness. She has no history of seizures. She lives in a one-floor apartment with no steps, no loose rugs, and good lighting. She has a history of hypertension. Her daughter heard the fall and immediately came into the kitchen; when she entered, her mother was already getting back up and was not confused. Her only current medication is lisinopril.

On physical examination, blood pressure is 138/85 mm Hg, without orthostatic changes. There are no ecchymoses or tenderness over the hips and no pain on ambulation. The physical examination is otherwise normal.

Which of the following is the most appropriate management of this patient?

(A) Assess gait and mobility
(B) Discontinue lisinopril
(C) Prescribe an exercise program
(D) Provide a standard walker

Item 79

A 38-year-old woman is evaluated for left knee pain. The pain has been present for the past 3 weeks. Before onset, she had been preparing for a 5-kilometer race by running approximately 2 miles per day, 6 days per week, for the past 6 months. Walking up steps makes the pain worse; she also notes pain at night. She has never had this pain before.

On physical examination, vital signs are normal. There is tenderness to palpation located near the anteromedial aspect of the proximal tibia. A small amount of swelling is present at the insertion of the medial hamstring muscle. There is no medial or lateral joint line tenderness.

Which of the following is the most likely diagnosis?

(A) Iliotibial band syndrome
(B) Patellofemoral pain syndrome
(C) Pes anserine bursitis
(D) Prepatellar bursitis

Item 80

A 32-year-old woman at 30 weeks' gestation is evaluated for a 1-week history of thick, white vaginal discharge as well as severe vaginal itching and discomfort. She was diagnosed with vulvovaginal candidiasis 8 weeks ago, treated, and had symptom resolution at that time. Her only medication is a prenatal vitamin.

On physical examination, vital signs are normal. There is vulvar edema, erythema, and excoriations with a thick, white, "cottage cheese" discharge present in the vaginal vault. There is no cervical motion or adnexal tenderness. Vaginal pH is 4.5; potassium hydroxide preparation shows yeast and hyphae. There are no clue cells or motile trichomonads on saline microscopy.

Which of the following is the most appropriate treatment?

(A) Boric acid, topically
(B) Clotrimazole, topically
(C) Fluconazole, orally
(D) Voriconazole, orally

Item 81

A 56-year-old woman is evaluated for an 8-week history of persistent nonproductive cough. The cough is paroxysmal and is preceded by a tickle in the back of her throat. She has no shortness of breath, hemoptysis, fever, chills, sore throat, myalgia, otalgia, wheezing, or rhinorrhea. Approximately 3 months ago, she was diagnosed with type 2 diabetes mellitus and hypertension and was started on metformin, hydrochlorothiazide, lisinopril, and atorvastatin. She has a 10-pack-year history of tobacco use, but stopped smoking 5 years ago.

On physical examination, vital signs are normal. There is no conjunctival injection, oropharyngeal erythema, or cobblestoning. The lungs are clear and cardiovascular examination is unremarkable. Chest radiograph is normal.

Which of the following is the most appropriate treatment?

(A) Albuterol inhaler
(B) Discontinue lisinopril
(C) Loratadine
(D) Omeprazole

Item 82

A 70-year-old man is evaluated before elective cataract surgery. Aside from decreased vision he has no symptoms. He has coronary artery disease and a seizure disorder. He does not have chest pain, dyspnea, or recent seizures. He had a myocardial infarction 6 months ago and was treated with a drug-eluting stent placed in the left anterior descending coronary artery. Current medications are aspirin, clopidogrel, simvastatin, metoprolol, and phenytoin.

On physical examination, temperature is normal, blood pressure is 142/88 mm Hg, and pulse rate is 64/min. The remainder of the examination is normal.

Which of the following is the best perioperative management of this patient's medications?

(A) Continue all medications
(B) Discontinue clopidogrel 1 week before surgery
(C) Hold metoprolol the morning of surgery
(D) Hold phenytoin on the morning of surgery

Item 83

A 54-year-old man is evaluated for a long-standing history of COPD. Although he had previously done well, his lung function has progressively declined over the past year. He is oxygen dependent and is unable to perform even minor physical activity without severe dyspnea. He is not a transplant candidate and is unhappy with his quality of life and prognosis. He requests a prescription that he can take that will cause him to die at the time of his choosing.

Which of the following is the most appropriate next step in management of this patient's request?

(A) Assess the adequacy of his current treatment
(B) Consult legal counsel about state law in such cases
(C) Decline the request
(D) Prescribe sedating medication that could ensure a comfortable death

Item 84

A 37-year-old woman is evaluated for right forefoot pain on the plantar surface. She describes the pain as burning in character and worsening with standing. She feels as if she is "walking on a marble." The pain began 2 to 3 months ago. She has never had this problem before. She frequently wears high heels.

On physical examination, there is tenderness to palpation on the plantar surface of the foot in the space between the third and fourth toes. There is no tenderness to palpation of the plantar surface of the metatarsal head, no tenderness to palpation of the metatarsophalangeal joint, and no dorsal metatarsal tenderness to palpation.

Which of the following is the most likely diagnosis?

(A) Hammer toe
(B) Metatarsal stress fracture
(C) Morton neuroma
(D) Tarsal tunnel syndrome

Item 85

A 25-year-old woman presents as a new patient for re-evaluation of an abdominal mass. She reports finding a right lower quadrant mass 9 months ago. She reports that the mass has been stable in size, does not vary with meals or a Valsalva maneuver, and is not tender. She has had no change in bowel habits. A review of her chart reveals that she has been seen by two internists, a gastroenterologist, and a general surgeon since her initial presentation. All reported normal physical examination findings. She has no history of colorectal cancer. She has been unable to work because of the mass.

On physical examination, her affect is normal, with no evidence of delusional thinking or hallucinations. Vital signs are normal. Abdominal examination shows no masses or hernia. Results of a metabolic panel are normal. An abdominal ultrasound 5 months ago and a CT scan of the abdomen and pelvis 3 months ago both were normal.

Which of the following is the most appropriate management?

(A) Cognitive-behavioral therapy
(B) Diazepam
(C) MRI of the abdomen
(D) Olanzapine

Item 86

A 42-year-old woman is evaluated in the emergency department after fainting earlier in the evening. She was at a dinner party and reports having two glasses of wine. After standing for approximately 35 minutes, she felt warm, diaphoretic, and anxious; as she moved toward a chair, she lost consciousness. She recovered spontaneously within 2 minutes and has been completely lucid ever since. Medical history is significant only for hypothyroidism and perennial allergies; medications are levothyroxine and fexofenadine.

On physical examination, she is alert and oriented. Vital signs are normal without orthostatic changes. Thyroid is normal. The remainder of the physical examination is normal. A 12-lead electrocardiogram is normal.

Which of the following is the most appropriate next step in the management of this patient?

(A) Admit to hospital for observation and telemetry
(B) Head CT scan
(C) Obtain echocardiography
(D) Perform tilt-table testing
(E) No further testing

Item 87

A 78-year-old-woman is evaluated in the emergency department after she fell at home last night. She has long-standing sleeping difficulties and last night got out of bed and fell in her hallway. She had no loss of consciousness and notes left hip pain. She has hypertension, hyperlipidemia, and gastroesophageal reflux disease. Her current medications are lisinopril, simvastatin, and omeprazole.

On physical examination, she is afebrile. Blood pressure is 142/82 mm Hg supine and 138/76 mm Hg standing, and pulse rate is 76/min supine and 78/min standing. She appears frail with generalized weakness. There is mild tenderness in the left lateral hip and weakness of the quadriceps muscles bilaterally. There are no ecchymoses in the left hip area. She is slow getting up from a chair and has a slow walking speed but no ataxia. Distance vision using glasses without bifocal lenses evaluated with a Snellen chart is normal. There is mild difficulty with near vision evaluated using a near-vision testing card. Lungs are clear. The heart rhythm is regular with no murmur. There is no focal neurologic deficit. Radiograph of the left hip and femur reveals no fracture.

Acetaminophen is prescribed for pain. Arrangements are made for home physical therapy and for a visiting nurse to perform a home safety evaluation.

Which of the following is the most appropriate additional management of this patient?

(A) Discontinue lisinopril
(B) Prescribe vitamin D
(C) Prescribe zolpidem at bedtime
(D) Refer for prescription glasses with bifocal lenses

Item 88

A 69-year-old woman is evaluated for involuntary leakage of urine with coughing, sneezing, laughing, or when lifting heavy boxes at work. She has no dysuria, frequency, or urgency and she has no mobility problems. She is gravida 4, para 4, and underwent a total abdominal hysterectomy 20 years ago for uterine fibroids. She has type 2 diabetes mellitus. Medications are metformin and lisinopril. She has no known drug allergies.

On physical examination, vital signs are normal. BMI is 31. There is bulging of the anterior vaginal wall when the patient is asked to cough, accompanied by leakage of urine. Bimanual examination is unremarkable. The remainder of her examination is normal.

Laboratory studies show fasting plasma glucose level of 89 mg/dL (5.0 mmol/L) with hemoglobin A_{1c} of 6.5%. Urinalysis is normal.

Which of the following is the most appropriate treatment?

(A) Pelvic floor muscle training
(B) Prompted voiding
(C) Pubovaginal sling
(D) Tolterodine

Item 89

A 97-year-old woman was hospitalized with jaundice, abdominal pain, weight loss, nausea, and intermittent vomiting 1 week ago. She was found to have poorly differentiated metastatic pancreatic adenocarcinoma. She lives with her daughter. Current medications are morphine, a stool softener, and a laxative. On physical examination, vital signs are normal. She is a depressed-appearing woman in no distress who appears cachectic but comfortable.

During bedside discussions, the patient has deferred all medical decision-making to her family. They have asked that "everything be done" and have declined to place the patient on do-not-resuscitate status. They have requested that a surgeon be consulted to remove the cancer and that an oncologist be consulted for initiation of chemotherapy. The health care team has arranged a family meeting to address end-of-life care.

Which of the following is the best initial communication strategy for the family meeting?

(A) Ask the patient's opinion about an advanced directive
(B) Explain that curative therapy is futile
(C) Explain the diagnosis and the prognosis
(D) Explore the family's understanding about the patient's condition

Item 90

A 62-year-old woman is evaluated for a 3-month history of a palpable nonpainful breast mass. She has no nipple discharge. She underwent menarche at age 14 years and menopause at age 55 years. She has no history of previous breast biopsies and no family history of breast, ovarian, or colorectal cancer. Her current medications are calcium and vitamin D. She took hormone replacement therapy for 1 year after menopause because of vasomotor symptoms.

On physical examination, temperature is 37.4 °C (99.3 °F), blood pressure is 135/80 mm Hg, pulse rate is 80/min, and respiration rate is 14/min. There is a firm, nontender mass in the upper outer quadrant of the right breast, approximately 2 cm at its largest dimension. There is no nipple discharge or change in or fixation to the overlying skin. There is no axillary lymphadenopathy. A diagnostic mammogram obtained 2 days before the visit revealed no masses or calcifications.

Which of the following is the most appropriate management of this patient?

(A) Breast MRI
(B) Breast ultrasonography
(C) Core needle biopsy
(D) Reassurance

Item 91

A 44-year-old man is evaluated for low back pain. Five days ago he was playing racquetball when he felt a popping sensation in his back and felt a shooting pain down his leg. The pain worsened over the next 2 to 3 days, causing some difficulty with sleeping. He started taking ibuprofen on day 2, and has improved slightly since then. He currently rates his pain as 5 or 6 out of 10. He has no numbness, weakness, or bladder/bowel incontinence.

On physical examination, vital signs are normal. BMI is 31. Straight leg raise test on both the left and right sides reproduces pain in the left leg. The ankle reflex is diminished on the left side compared with the right side. He is able to walk with some discomfort. No motor or sensory deficits are observed. Saddle anesthesia is not present. Rectal tone is normal.

Which of the following is the most appropriate management of this patient?

(A) Analgesics and mobilization as tolerated
(B) Complete blood count and erythrocyte sedimentation rate
(C) Epidural corticosteroid injection
(D) Lumbar spine MRI
(E) Lumbar spine radiograph

Item 92

A 75-year-old man is hospitalized with sepsis leading to multi-organ failure. A meeting with family members is convened to discuss goals of care for the patient. The treatment team, including infectious disease and critical care consultants, has indicated that the patient is deteriorating despite optimized therapy, and the prognosis is poor. The daughter brings an Internet printout of a trial of a new medication for sepsis. The abstract states "We gave drug 'X' to 100 consecutive patients with refractory sepsis in our five intensive care units located in the same geographic region. Eight percent were alive at 30 days." Although drug "X" is marketed in the United States, it is not FDA-approved for treatment of sepsis. A quick literature search reveals no other studies of drug "X" in the treatment of sepsis.

Which of the following is the main reason that it is difficult to determine the effectiveness of drug "X" based on the published study?

(A) No comparison group
(B) Outcome assessment not blinded
(C) Patients not randomly assigned to treatment
(D) Small study size

Item 93

A 37-year-old man is seen as a new patient. He requests a refill of dexamphetamine, which he takes for attention-deficit/hyperactivity disorder (ADHD). He was diagnosed in childhood when he had difficulty in school and has been on the medication ever since. His symptoms are generally well controlled with occasional impulsive behavior (traffic ticket 3 years ago, confrontation with his boss 5 years ago). He has had no problems over the past 2 years. He is otherwise healthy and drinks three or four beers per week. He smokes socially, less than one pack per week. He does not use illicit drugs. His only medication is dexamphetamine.

On physical examination, temperature is 36.6 °C (97.8 °F), blood pressure is 149/92 mm Hg, pulse rate is 96/min, and respiration rate is 14/min. BMI is 23. The remainder of the physical examination is normal.

Which of the following is the most appropriate management?

(A) Continue dexamphetamine
(B) Switch to atomoxetine
(C) Switch to fluoxetine
(D) Switch to methylphenidate
(E) Stop medications and reassess

Item 94

An 85-year-old woman is evaluated before hospital discharge after a 2-week hospitalization for a traumatic right hip fracture treated with open reduction and internal fixation complicated by a pulmonary embolism, catheter-associated urosepsis, and acute delirium. She has improved steadily but continues to require low-level supplemental oxygen, remains significantly debilitated, and is able to participate in only 30 minutes of physical therapy daily. Medical history is significant for type 2 diabetes mellitus, hypertension, depression, and obesity. Her daughter meets with the treating internist to discuss discharge planning. She feels her mother has been failing for several years and

is no longer able to live independently as she had before hospitalization. She asks that the patient be transferred back to the hospital or emergency department if she develops more acute medical issues following discharge, and requests that the patient receive everything short of aggressive resuscitation with cardiopulmonary resuscitation and intubation if this situation were to arise. The treating internist meets separately with the patient and she agrees that these are her preferences.

Based on the patient's medical status and the wishes of the patient and her family, which of the following postdischarge care options is most appropriate?

(A) Inpatient rehabilitation facility
(B) Long term acute care hospital
(C) Residential hospice facility
(D) Skilled nursing facility

Item 95

A 76-year-old woman is evaluated for a 1-day history of headache, left eye pain, nausea and vomiting, seeing halos around lights, and decreased visual acuity of the left eye. She has type 2 diabetes mellitus, hypertension, and atrial fibrillation. Medications are metformin, digoxin, metoprolol, hydrochlorothiazide, and warfarin.

On physical examination, temperature is 36.8 °C (98.2 °F), blood pressure is 148/88 mm Hg, pulse rate is 104/min, and respiration rate is 16/min. Visual acuity wearing glasses is 20/40 (right eye) and 20/100 (left eye). The left eye has conjunctival erythema. The right pupil is reactive to light, the left pupil is sluggish and constricts in response to light from 6 mm to 4 mm. On palpation of the ocular globe, the left globe feels firm as compared with the right.

Which of the following is the most likely diagnosis?

(A) Acute angle-closure glaucoma
(B) Central retinal artery occlusion
(C) Ocular migraine
(D) Temporal arteritis

Item 96

A 28-year-old man is evaluated for pain on the radial aspect of the right wrist that occurs with use of the thumb. The pain has been present for 2 weeks. He has never had this pain before and has not had any trauma. He works as a computer programmer and plays video games for 3 to 4 hours each night when he gets home from work.

On physical examination, vital signs are normal. Localized tenderness to palpation is present over the distal radial styloid; pain is present with resisted thumb abduction and extension, and the patient has pain on the radial side of the thumb when he is asked to make a fist over the fully flexed thumb and then to ulnar deviate the hand (positive Finkelstein test). There are no palpable masses; there is no joint pain, bogginess, or swelling; sensation is intact throughout the wrist and hand, strength is 5/5 throughout.

Which of the following is the most likely diagnosis?

(A) Carpometacarpal arthritis

(B) de Quervain tenosynovitis

(C) Flexor carpi radialis ganglion cyst

(D) Scaphoid fracture

Item 97

A 32-year-old woman is evaluated for a 3-month history of left-sided jaw pain and clicking below her left ear when she chews. She reports no joint problems elsewhere, no visual changes, and no headache other than the jaw pain. She has some trouble sleeping at night, but the pain is more likely to affect her at work. Once or twice a month she goes home early because of jaw pain.

On physical examination, temperature is 37.3 °C (99.1 °F), blood pressure is 118/72 mm Hg, and pulse rate is 60/min. There is mild tenderness and palpable crepitus over the left temporomandibular joint. Otoscopy is normal bilaterally. She has no lymphadenopathy, rash, or salivary gland masses. Oropharynx is normal. Thyroid is normal. She has no tooth pain when teeth are tapped with a tongue blade.

Which of the following is the most appropriate next step in management?

(A) Fluoxetine

(B) Ibuprofen

(C) Jaw MRI

(D) Jaw relaxation, heat, and therapeutic exercises

(E) Radiography of the teeth

Item 98

A 49-year-old woman is evaluated for vertigo of 1 week's duration. She was seen 1 week ago in the emergency department. During that visit, she described severe vertigo that predictably occurred while abruptly turning her head to the right and lasted less than 1 minute. She had no antecedent viral illness, headache, hearing loss, tinnitus, diplopia, dysarthria, dysphagia, or weakness. She was diagnosed with benign paroxysmal positional vertigo and given instructions for head tilting exercises (Epley maneuver). Her symptoms improved but have not abated. She is afraid to drive because of the symptoms. She has no history of hypertension, diabetes mellitus, hyperlipidemia, or tobacco use.

On physical examination, vital signs are normal. With the Dix-Hallpike maneuver, she develops horizontal nystagmus and nausea after 15 seconds. The nystagmus lasts approximately 1 minute. The Epley maneuver is unsuccessful in relieving symptoms. The remainder of the examination is normal, including the neurologic examination.

Which of the following is the most appropriate management?

(A) Brain MRI

(B) Hydrochlorothiazide

(C) Meclizine

(D) Vestibular rehabilitation

Item 99

An 84-year-old man who resides in a skilled nursing facility is brought to the office by his daughter, who reports that he has become less active in the past few months. The patient does not have a change in mood. He has multiple somatic symptoms including headache, scalp pain, and constipation, all of which are long-standing, intermittent, of brief duration, and not associated with any positive physical examination or laboratory test findings. There has been no weight loss. He has osteoarthritis but has no difficulty with ambulation and has had no falls. His wife died 4 months ago. His only medication is acetaminophen.

On physical examination, he is afebrile, blood pressure is 148/92 mm Hg, and pulse rate is 68/min. He is slow to respond but answers questions appropriately. He is alert and oriented. His gait is slow but otherwise unremarkable. The remainder of the physical examination is normal.

Complete blood count, comprehensive metabolic profile, and serum thyroid-stimulating hormone level are normal.

Which of the following is the most appropriate diagnostic test to perform next?

(A) Dix-Hallpike maneuver

(B) Mini–Mental State Examination

(C) PHQ-9 depression assessment

(D) Timed "Up & Go" test

Item 100

A 60-year-old woman is evaluated for increased irritability and anxiety. She was in an automobile accident 3 months ago in which she was rear-ended by a car at a stop light. Since that time she has nightmares about the incident and states she has not returned to driving for fear of being in another accident. Her sleep is poor and her husband states she is becoming more socially isolated since she has stopped driving. She has continued to perform her usual hobbies at home. She has no suicidal thoughts. On physical examination, all vital signs are normal.

Which of the following is the most likely diagnosis?

(A) Generalized anxiety disorder

(B) Major depressive disorder

(C) Obsessive-compulsive disorder

(D) Posttraumatic stress disorder

Item 101

A 59-year-old woman is evaluated in the emergency department for midsternal chest pain. The pain began several hours ago as a vague ache in her left upper sternal region that progressed in intensity and severity. The pain abated spontaneously after approximately 45 minutes. She had no further chest pain until several hours later, when it recurred unprovoked by exertion. She has no shortness of breath, nausea or vomiting, syncope, previous history of chest pain, or known cardiac disease or risk factors for venous thromboembolism. Medical history is significant for hyperlipidemia and hypertension. She does not smoke cigarettes. Medications are simvastatin, aspirin, lisinopril, and hydrochlorothiazide.

On physical examination, she is afebrile, blood pressure is 110/70 mm Hg, pulse rate is 68/min, and respiration rate is 22/min. BMI is 28. Oxygen saturation on ambient air is 97%. Estimated central venous pressure is 8 cm H_2O and carotid pulses are without bruits. Lungs are clear. Heart sounds are normal. There is a grade 2/6 holosystolic murmur at the left sternal border with radiation to the apex. There is no lower extremity edema. The remainder of the examination is normal.

Electrocardiogram is shown. Chest radiograph is normal.

Which of the following is the most appropriate initial management of this patient?

(A) Adenosine stress test
(B) Admit to the coronary care unit
(C) CT pulmonary angiography
(D) Ibuprofen administration

Item 102

A 36-year-old man is evaluated during a routine health examination. He has no family history of hypertension, hyperlipidemia, or cardiovascular disease. He has never used tobacco, drinks approximately two beers each week, and does not use illicit drugs. He is fairly sedentary but feels well and is without cardiovascular or other symptoms.

On physical examination, he is afebrile, blood pressure is 112/70 mm Hg, and pulse rate is 76/min. BMI is 25.

Laboratory studies:

Total cholesterol	148 mg/dL (3.83 mmol/L)
LDL cholesterol	96 mg/dL (2.48 mmol/L)
HDL cholesterol	44 mg/dL (1.14 mmol/L)
Triglycerides	88 mg/dL (0.99 mmol/L)

Which of the following is the recommended interval for follow-up screening for hypertension in this patient?

(A) 1 year
(B) 2 years
(C) 3 years
(D) 4 years
(E) 5 years

Item 103

A 72-year-old woman is evaluated for short-term memory loss. She has trouble remembering names, where she placed certain items such as her keys, and occasionally, what she did earlier in the day. She avoids some social situations and feels lower self esteem because of memory problems and decreased social contact, but notes no depression, low energy, or sleep disturbance, and she still enjoys playing cards with her husband. She does not need help with eating, dressing, or bathing. She has hypertension, well controlled with hydrochlorothiazide. She has no history of stroke. She is concerned about her condition and wants to know if anything can be done about it.

On physical examination, temperature is 37.2 °C (98.9 °F), blood pressure is 135/84 mm Hg, and pulse rate is 72/min. She is conversant, with a normal range of affect. Neurologic examination is without focal deficit. The remainder of the physical examination is normal. Mini–Mental State Examination score is 26.

Which of the following is the most appropriate management of this patient?

(A) Anticholinesterase inhibitor
(B) Cognitive rehabilitation

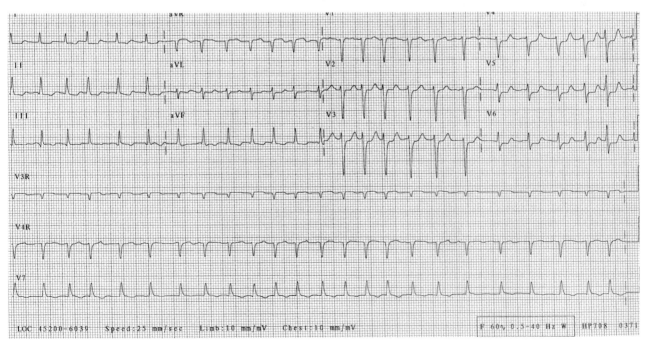

ITEM 101

(C) PET scan

(D) Reassurance that progression to dementia is unlikely

Item 104

A 70-year-old man is evaluated for sharp left-sided pleuritic chest pain and shortness of breath that began suddenly 24 hours ago. The pain has been persistent over the past 24 hours and does not worsen or improve with exertion or position. History is significant for severe COPD, hypertension, and hyperlipidemia. He is a current smoker with a 52-pack-year history of smoking. Medications are ipratropium, albuterol, lisinopril, simvastatin, and aspirin.

On physical examination, temperature is normal, blood pressure is 128/80 mm Hg, pulse rate is 88/min, and respiration rate is 18/min. BMI is 24. Oxygen saturation on ambient air is 89%. Cardiac examination reveals distant heart sounds but no S_3. Lung examination reveals hyper-resonance, decreased chest wall expansion, and decreased breath sounds on the left. The trachea is midline.

Which of the following is the most appropriate diagnostic test to perform next?

(A) Chest CT

(B) Chest radiography

(C) Echocardiography

(D) Electrocardiography

Item 105

A 28-year-old man is evaluated for a 6-week history of intractable nausea. He states he is nauseated all day although he is able to eat if he forces himself. He has had no vomiting, weight loss, or change in stool pattern. He went to an emergency department last week because of his symptoms, and the results of laboratory testing at that time were normal.

He reports a 1-year history of intermittent episodes of severe right upper quadrant abdominal pain and bloating, as well as separate episodes of intermittent numbness of the right side of his face and body. He says that he has had neck and back pain, dysuria, intermittent odynophagia, and loss of libido for the past 3 years. He does not have sleep disturbance, anhedonia, or crying spells. Prior laboratory testing, upper endoscopy, colonoscopy, CT scan of the abdomen and pelvis, and MRI of the cervical and lumbar spine were normal. Current medications are acetaminophen, odansetron, and tramadol. He is currently unemployed.

On physical examination, vital signs are normal. The abdomen shows diffuse tenderness to palpation but is otherwise normal. Neurologic examination is normal. A two-question depression screen is normal.

Which of the following is the most likely diagnosis?

(A) Celiac disease

(B) Malingering

(C) Multiple sclerosis

(D) Somatization disorder

Item 106

A 28-year-old man is evaluated for a 6-month history of pelvic pain, urinary frequency, and painful ejaculation. He has been treated with antibiotics for urinary tract infections three times in the past 6 months, each time with temporary relief of symptoms but recurrence shortly after completion of antibiotics.

On physical examination, vital signs are normal. There is minimal suprapubic tenderness with palpation. The prostate is of normal size with minimal tenderness and no nodules. Urinalysis shows multiple leukocytes, bacteria, and no erythrocytes.

Which of the following is the most appropriate treatment of this patient?

(A) 1-week course of trimethoprim-sulfamethoxazole

(B) 1-month course of ciprofloxacin

(C) Cognitive-behavioral therapy

(D) Finasteride

Item 107

A 28-year-old woman is evaluated for headache, purulent nasal discharge, and left unilateral facial and maxillary tooth pain present for 4 days.

On physical examination, temperature is 37.3 °C (99.1 °F); vital signs are otherwise normal. There is mild tenderness to palpation over the maxillary sinus on the left. Nasal examination shows inflamed turbinates bilaterally with a small amount of purulent discharge. Maxillary trans-illumination is darker on the left than on the right. Oto-scopic examination is normal bilaterally. There is no lymphadenopathy in the head or neck.

Which of the following is the most appropriate next step in management?

(A) Amoxicillin

(B) Chlorpheniramine

(C) Nasal culture

(D) Sinus CT

(E) Systemic corticosteroids

Item 108

A 72-year-old woman is evaluated for sudden hearing loss in the left ear with moderate ringing that started yesterday. She has no vertigo or dizziness.

On physical examination, vital signs are normal. Otoscopic examination is initially obscured by cerumen bilaterally. Once cerumen is removed, the tympanic membranes appear normal and there is some redness in the canals bilaterally. When a 512 Hz tuning fork is placed on top of the head, it is louder in the right ear. When placed adjacent to the left ear, it is heard better when outside the ear canal than when touching the mastoid bone. Neurologic examination is normal other than left-sided hearing loss.

Which of the following is the most appropriate management of this patient?

(A) Acyclovir

(B) Neomycin, polymyxin B, and hydrocortisone ear drops

(C) Triethanolamine ear drops

(D) Urgent audiometry and referral

Item 109

A 78-year-old man is brought to the emergency department with a 1-hour history of vomiting bright red blood. Despite profuse hematemesis, he clearly states that he does not want a blood transfusion for religious reasons. Four minutes after he arrives, he starts to have new severe substernal chest pain and 2 minutes later loses consciousness. His wife, who he appointed his agent with durable power of attorney for health care, confirms his long-standing religious beliefs against transfusion. Medical history is significant for coronary artery disease, hypertension, and hyperlipidemia. There is no history of cognitive decline or impaired judgment. His current medications are aspirin, simvastatin, and amlodipine.

On physical examination, temperature is 36.8 °C (98.2 °F), blood pressure is 80/40 mm Hg, pulse rate is 156/min, and respiration rate is 24/min. His skin is pale, clammy, and cool to touch. The chest is clear to auscultation. Cardiac examination reveals tachycardia but is otherwise normal. The abdomen is soft and nondistended.

Complete blood count shows a hemoglobin level of 6 g/dL (60 g/L) and hematocrit of 18%. Electrocardiogram shows 2- to 3-mm ST-segment depression in leads V_3 through V_6.

Which of the following is the most appropriate management?

(A) Immediate blood transfusion

(B) Obtain an emergency court-appointed guardian

(C) Seek permission from the patient's wife to transfuse

(D) Treat without transfusion

Item 110

A 24-year-old man is evaluated in the emergency department for a 6-hour history of acute scrotal pain. The pain occurred suddenly while mowing the lawn. The patient is not sexually active and has no recent trauma, history of penile discharge, urinary urgency, frequency, or dysuria.

On physical examination, he is afebrile, blood pressure is 160/100 mm Hg, pulse rate is 100/min, and respiration rate is 12/min. The right testicle rides high in the scrotum and is exquisitely tender. The cremasteric reflex is absent on the right side. There is no abnormal mass in the scrotum or inguinal area. There is no penile discharge. A urinalysis is normal.

Which of the following is the most likely diagnosis?

(A) Epididymitis

(B) Strangulated inguinal hernia

(C) Orchitis

(D) Testicular torsion

Item 111

A 25-year-old woman is evaluated for a 1-week history of malodorous vaginal discharge associated with vulvar itching and burning. She is sexually active and has had three partners in the past 6 months. She has no history of sexually transmitted infection.

On physical examination, vital signs are normal. BMI is 22. There is a thin, gray, homogeneous discharge coating the vaginal walls. There are no external genital lesions and no vulvar erythema or excoriations. The cervix appears normal. There is no cervical motion tenderness or adnexal tenderness. Vaginal pH is 6.0, "whiff" test is positive. Results of saline microscopy are shown. Microscopy after the addition of potassium hydroxide does not show hyphae or pseudohyphae. A urine pregnancy test is negative.

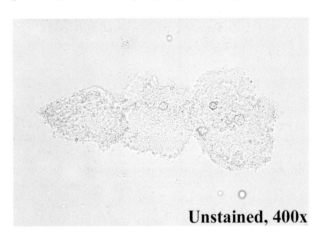

Unstained, 400x

Which of the following is the most appropriate treatment?

(A) Clotrimazole cream, 7-day topical regimen

(B) Fluconazole, single-dose oral regimen

(C) Metronidazole, 7-day oral regimen

(D) Metronidazole, single-dose oral regimen

Item 112

A 56-year-old man is evaluated for a 7-month history of difficulty maintaining erections. He has difficulty with sexual intercourse and achieving orgasm. He reports that sexual desire is good. He does not have penile curvature, genital pain, depressed mood, or anxiety. He has not tried anything for this problem. He is active, jogging for 30 minutes 4 to 5 times per week. He has type 2 diabetes mellitus, which is diet controlled, and hyperlipidemia. He does not use alcohol, tobacco, or illicit drugs. Current medications are aspirin and simvastatin.

On physical examination, he is afebrile, blood pressure is 124/70 mm Hg, and pulse rate is 76/min. BMI is 24. The testes are bilaterally descended and normal in size and consistency, the penis is normal in appearance, and there is normal distribution of male secondary hair. Rectal examination reveals a normal-sized prostate. Posterior tibialis and dorsalis pedis pulses are palpable bilaterally and the neurologic examination is normal.

Serum thyroid-stimulating hormone level is 2.95 µU/mL (2.95 mU/L) and early morning serum total testosterone level is 320 ng/dL (11 nmol/L).

Which of the following is the most appropriate treatment?

(A) Intracavernosal alprostadil
(B) Penile pump
(C) Sildenafil
(D) Testosterone therapy

Item 113

A 78-year-old woman was recently admitted to the hospital for an acute exacerbation of chronic heart failure. She has coronary artery disease and hypertension. During that admission she was treated with intravenous diuretics, with reduction of her weight to slightly below her established optimal weight goal and resolution of her heart failure symptoms. Upon discharge her dosages of lisinopril and oral furosemide were increased from their preadmission level, and spironolactone was started. She was scheduled for a follow-up appointment with her internist in 1 week.

Four days after discharge she presents to the emergency department because of worsening shortness of breath since hospital discharge and is readmitted for further treatment. She has no chest pain but has noticed increased swelling in her lower extremities. She states that she has been taking her medications as directed.

On physical examination, temperature is 37.4 °C (99.3 °F), blood pressure is 115/78 mm Hg, and respiration rate is 18/min. Oxygen saturation on ambient air is 89%. The chest examination reveals mild bilateral crackles at the lung bases. Heart examination shows a regular rate without murmur. There is trace lower extremity edema. The remainder of the examination is unremarkable.

Laboratory studies are significant for normal serum electrolyte levels and a serum creatinine level of 1.2 mg/dL (106 µmol/L) (unchanged from discharge). A chest radiograph shows bilateral hilar infiltrates consistent with pulmonary edema.

Which of the following is the most likely cause of her readmission?

(A) Diuretic resistance
(B) Inadequate hospital follow-up
(C) Medication nonadherence
(D) Spironolactone intolerance

Item 114

An 84-year-old man is evaluated for a 5-day history of rhinitis, nasal congestion, sneezing, and nonproductive cough. The symptoms began with a sore throat, which resolved after 24 hours. He has mild ear pain when blowing his nose or coughing. He has a history of coronary artery disease and hypertension. Medications are aspirin, metoprolol, and hydrochlorothiazide.

On physical examination, temperature is 36.5 °C (97.7 °F), blood pressure is 130/72 mm Hg, pulse rate is 82/min, and respiration rate is 16/min. He has nasal congestion and has an occasional cough. There is mild clear nasal discharge with no sinus tenderness. The oropharynx is without injection or exudate. There is no lymphadenopathy. External auditory canals are normal. The tympanic membranes are dull bilaterally but without injection. A small left middle ear effusion is noted.

Which of the following is the most appropriate management?

(A) Amoxicillin
(B) Erythromycin
(C) Referral to an otorhinolaryngologist
(D) Reassurance and observation

Item 115

A 32-year-old man is evaluated for daytime fatigue of 9 months' duration. He has never fallen asleep at the wheel, but falls asleep at other times during the day. He does not think he snores, but his wife is unavailable to confirm this. He reports no leg symptoms. He has no significant medical history and takes no medications. He does not smoke. He drinks two or three beers on Friday and Saturday nights. He does not exercise regularly, and has gained 9.1 kg (20 lb) since getting married 18 months ago.

On physical examination, temperature is normal, blood pressure is 128/76 mm Hg, and pulse rate is 82/min. BMI is 32. Neck circumference is 43 cm (17 in). Pharynx is normal. The thyroid is difficult to palpate owing to the patient's large neck size. The lungs are clear, and the cardiovascular and neurologic examinations are normal.

In addition to counseling regarding sleep hygiene and weight loss, which of the following is the most appropriate management for this patient?

(A) Advise alcohol abstinence
(B) Initiate therapy with zolpidem
(C) Order iron studies
(D) Refer for polysomnography

Item 116

A 46-year-old man is evaluated for dull, aching, right groin pain. He says it has been present for the past 3 months. The pain was initially severe, improved for a few weeks, but slowly has been worsening since that time. He is now walking with a limp. He has no history of trauma. He drinks six beers a day and has done so for the past 25 years. He is a current smoker, with a 30-pack-year history.

On physical examination, vital signs are normal. He has limited internal and external rotation of the right hip. Internal rotation is limited to a greater degree than external rotation and pain is present with rotating the thigh medially and laterally (log-rolling). Radiographs of the right hip are normal.

Which of the following is the most likely diagnosis?

(A) Hip osteoarthritis
(B) L1 radiculopathy

(C) Osteonecrosis of the hip

(D) Septic arthritis of the hip

Item 117

A 33-year-old woman is evaluated for chronic pain. She has a history of fibromyalgia and reports widespread musculoskeletal pain involving her hips, knees, back, and neck with significant worsening in recent weeks. The pain in her neck and back is 7/10 in intensity and is constant. She participated in a 3-month course of physical therapy with little improvement in her symptoms. The patient reports that she is sleeping about 3 to 4 hours per night because her pain is keeping her awake. Previously she had been able to work, but now she has difficulty getting out of bed every day. Her current medications are gabapentin and duloxetine.

On physical examination, vital signs are normal. BMI is 28. She has several tender trigger points. Her neck has limited range of motion secondary to pain. There is tenderness to palpation over the paravertebral muscles of the lower lumbar spine. Strength is 5/5 in all extremities, reflexes are 2+ and symmetric, sensation to light touch and pinprick is normal throughout, and a straight leg raise test is negative. Her affect is flat.

Which of the following is the most appropriate management?

(A) Electromyogram/nerve conduction velocity study

(B) Evaluate for intimate partner violence

(C) High-dose ibuprofen

(D) Oxycodone/acetaminophen

Item 118

A 78-year-old man is evaluated for routine follow up of hypertension. He reports that he is able to perform all activities of daily living and that he only drives in the neighborhood and to nearby stores. He has used a cane while walking since he fell 3 months ago. His only medication is chlorthalidone.

On physical examination, vital signs are normal. His corrected vision with glasses is 20/20 in both eyes. His gait is somewhat slow and he needs some assistance getting on to the examination table. The remainder of the physical examination is normal. He scores 25/30 on the Mini–Mental State Examination.

Which of the following is the most appropriate management of this patient?

(A) Advise the patient that he should no longer drive

(B) Advise the patient to continue to drive only locally

(C) Ask about any driving difficulties

(D) Report the patient to the state department of transportation

Item 119

A 24-year-old man is evaluated for a 6-month history of episodic substernal chest pain. Episodes occur four to seven times per week and are accompanied by palpitations and sweating, as well as a "sense of doom." They resolve spontaneously after approximately 30 minutes. His symptoms are unrelieved with antacids, can occur at rest or with exertion, and are nonpositional. There are no specific precipitating factors. He is a nonsmoker. His lipid levels, which were checked recently at a school wellness fair, are normal. He has no personal or family history of coronary artery disease, diabetes mellitus, hyperlipidemia, or hypertension. He is not taking any medications.

On physical examination, vital signs are normal. He has no cardiac murmurs and no abdominal pain. Complete blood count, serum thyroid-stimulating hormone level, and electrocardiogram are all normal.

Which of the following is the most appropriate management of this patient?

(A) Cardiac event monitor

(B) Cardiac stress test

(C) Empiric trial of proton pump inhibitor

(D) Selective serotonin reuptake inhibitor

Item 120

A 47-year-old woman is evaluated during a follow-up appointment. She had been hospitalized for acute pancreatitis secondary to alcohol abuse. She has had no previous primary medical care. She takes no medications and is currently unemployed. She has been arrested one time for driving while intoxicated, but no longer drives. She smokes one pack of cigarettes daily and does not currently use illicit drugs; she did use marijuana when she was younger. She tells you she only drinks when she can afford it, which may be once a week or less, and usually has 6 or 7 drinks when she does. She has never had withdrawal symptoms.

Physical examination reveals a thin woman in no apparent distress; vital signs are normal. Sclera and skin are anicteric. The liver edge is felt 4 cm below the right costal margin. There is mild epigastric tenderness but no ascites or other stigmata of chronic liver disease.

Which of the following is the most appropriate management for this patient?

(A) Connect her drinking habits with the negative consequences

(B) Identify that she is an alcoholic and needs to abstain from drinking

(C) Initiate therapy with disulfiram

(D) Initiate therapy with naltrexone

Item 121

A 54-year-old man is evaluated after urgent transfer to the intensive care unit following an elective hemicolectomy. His surgery was performed under general anesthesia and he was extubated before leaving the operating room. After several hours of observation in the postanesthesia care unit, he was reported by nursing staff to be drowsy but awake and responsive with stable vital signs, and was transferred to a general surgical ward.

CONT.

A few hours later he was noted to be in respiratory distress, was intubated, and placed on mechanical ventilation. He is currently awake and alert while being ventilated. His wife reports that he is a nonsmoker, has hypertension but no known lung or heart problems, and had been doing well prior to surgery except for chronic tiredness.

On physical examination, temperature is normal, blood pressure is 150/90 mm Hg, pulse rate is 98/min, and respiration rate is 12/min. BMI is 39. Oxygen saturation by pulse oximetry is 99% on 40% F_{IO_2}. Heart and lung examinations are normal. There is no lower extremity edema.

Laboratory studies performed just before intubation included an arterial blood gas measurement with a pH of 7.24 and a P_{CO_2} of 75 mm Hg (10 kPa). Serum bicarbonate level was 28 meq/L (28 mmol/L). CT angiogram shows no pulmonary embolism and normal lungs. Electrocardiogram shows sinus tachycardia with no ST- or T-wave changes.

Which of the following is the most likely cause of his respiratory failure?

(A) Myocardial ischemia
(B) Obstructive sleep apnea
(C) Premature extubation
(D) Sepsis

Item 122

A 42-year-old woman is evaluated for a 10-day history of right shoulder pain, located posteriorly and superiorly, that becomes worse with overhead activities. She has no history of trauma. She recently painted her basement ceiling. She has no weakness or paresthesia of her right arm and has never had this problem before. She has been taking ibuprofen as needed for the pain.

On physical examination, vital signs are normal. There is no shoulder asymmetry and no tenderness to palpation of bony structures or soft tissue structures. There is full range of motion (other than with internal rotation, which is limited by pain) and strength is 5/5 throughout the right arm, with sensation intact. She is able to slowly lower her extended arm from over her head to her side (negative drop-arm test). There is pain with abduction of the right arm between 60 and 120 degrees. The patient is asked to hold the arm extended anteriorly at 90 degrees with the forearm bent to 90 degrees (at 12 o'clock), as if holding a shield. When the arm is internally rotated to cross in front of the body, the patient feels pain in the shoulder (positive Hawkins test).

Which of the following is the most likely diagnosis?

(A) Acromioclavicular joint degeneration
(B) Adhesive capsulitis
(C) Rotator cuff impingement
(D) Rotator cuff tear

Item 123

A 30-year-old man is evaluated during a routine examination. He is asymptomatic. He is a nonsmoker and has no history of illicit drug use. He has had two lifetime female sexual partners and is sexually active in a monogamous relationship with a woman for the past 5 years. His father is 58 years old and has hypertension; his mother is 57 years old and has hyperlipidemia. Results of the physical examination, including vital signs, are normal. Results of a fasting lipid panel 4 years ago were normal.

Which of the following is the most appropriate screening test to obtain?

(A) Fasting lipid panel
(B) Fasting plasma glucose
(C) HIV enzyme immunoassay antibody testing
(D) Thyroid-stimulating hormone level

Item 124

A physician unexpectedly encounters a colleague at a pub on a Friday night. They enjoy four or five drinks together while watching the first hour of a baseball game. Suddenly, the colleague's pager goes off. Annoyed, she looks at it, and says, slurring her words, "It's the hospital. I have to go admit a patient." When he tries to stop her, she gets angry and shakes him off.

Which of the following is the most appropriate course of action for this physician to take regarding his colleague?

(A) Contact the hospital chief of staff and report his concerns immediately
(B) Report his concerns to state authorities on Monday
(C) Take his colleague aside later and discuss his concerns with her
(D) No obligation to intervene

Item 125

A 55-year-old man is evaluated before scheduled endoscopic sinus surgery. In addition to symptoms of chronic sinusitis, he has chronic knee pain that limits his activity to below 4 metabolic equivalents (METs). He has no chest pain, dyspnea, or lower extremity edema. He has type 2 diabetes mellitus, coronary artery disease, chronic kidney disease, hypertension, hyperlipidemia, osteoarthritis, and chronic sinusitis. He had a myocardial infarction 5 years ago and was treated with a single bare metal stent. Medications are insulin glargine, metoprolol, aspirin, simvastatin, lisinopril, and acetaminophen.

On physical examination, temperature is normal, blood pressure is 142/84 mm Hg, and pulse rate is 56/min. The electrocardiogram is consistent with a previous lateral myocardial infarction and is unchanged from 1 year ago. Serum creatinine level is 2.1 mg/dL (186 µmol/L).

Which of the following is the most appropriate preoperative management of this patient?

(A) Discontinue metoprolol
(B) Obtain dobutamine stress echocardiogram
(C) Refer for cardiac catheterization
(D) Proceed to surgery without further testing

Item 126

A 32-year-old woman presents for emergency department follow-up. She was seen 1 week ago for a facial laceration. She tells you she cannot remember the incident. She had a humeral fracture 1 year ago, and has had bruising on her arms and legs on several visits. History is significant for depression and recurrent urinary tract infection. Her only current medication is citalopram. Upon questioning about intimate partner violence, the patient admits that her husband often beats her.

Physical examination is significant for normal vital signs; a healing, sutured, 4-cm laceration across the left zygomatic arch; and several 5- to 6-cm ecchymoses on her upper extremities.

Which of the following is the most appropriate next step in management?

(A) Advise the patient to leave her current living situation immediately

(B) Ask her to bring her husband to her next appointment

(C) Assess her immediate safety and develop a safety plan

(D) Report the husband to the police

(E) Request psychiatry consultation

Item 127

A 50-year-old woman is evaluated for nonischemic cardiomyopathy. Her exercise tolerance is not limited. She takes an ACE inhibitor daily. She took a β-blocker briefly but discontinued because of fatigue. Results of the physical examination are normal.

The patient inquires whether she should receive drug "H". Drug H was studied in 2000 patients ages 40 to 80 years (mean age 63 years) with New York Heart Association functional class III or IV heart failure. Patients were randomized to receive drug H or a placebo in addition to usual medications. Eighty percent of patients in the trial also took a β-blocker and 70% an ACE inhibitor. At the end of 3 years, patients taking drug H had a significantly reduced rate of a composite outcome of death or heart failure exacerbations. Approximately 5% of the patients taking drug H had serious adverse events, compared with 2% in the placebo group.

Which of the following is the main reason why this patient should not be treated with drug H?

(A) Her heart failure is too mild

(B) She is too young

(C) She should be treated with a β-blocker first

(D) The drug's adverse event rate is too high

Item 128

A 16-year-old patient is brought to the office by his mother for an evaluation. His mother notes that he has been "strange" since a very young age. He did not start speaking until age 3 years. Since that time, he has been home-schooled but has avoided other children and adults in social contexts. He is prone to emotional outbursts, and frequently repeats back what is said to him many times over. Currently he spends most of his time in his room, and is unwilling to help with routine chores at home. However, he is fascinated by trains, and when he is engaged will recite numerous details about trains.

Which of the following is the most likely diagnosis?

(A) Autism spectrum disorder

(B) Obsessive-compulsive disorder

(C) Schizophrenia

(D) Social anxiety disorder

Item 129

A 25-year-old woman is evaluated in October before starting a certified nursing assistant degree program. She was diagnosed with HIV infection 3 months ago. She reports having received "all my shots as a child," and specifically recalls having chickenpox as a child. Before starting school she needs to provide proof of her immunization status. Her only medication is an oral contraceptive. Findings on physical examination are unremarkable.

Which of the following is the most appropriate next step in this patient's immunization management?

(A) Administer a single measles, mumps, and rubella booster now

(B) Administer live, attenuated, intranasal influenza vaccine now

(C) Begin hepatitis B immunization series

(D) Certify her as immune to varicella given her clinical history

(E) Obtain a CD4 cell count

Item 130

A 38-year-old man is evaluated in the emergency department for a 2-week history of nonpleuritic, sharp, anterior chest pain. Each episode of pain lasts 3 to 10 hours. He states that the pain is to the left of the sternum but at times it radiates across the entire chest. It does not radiate to the shoulders, arms, or back. The pain can be present at rest. It is worsened with lateral movement of the trunk. He does not notice any change in intensity with walking or other activity. He has no other symptoms and no other medical problems. He does not use drugs and takes no medications.

On physical examination, temperature is 37.0 °C (98.6 °F), blood pressure is 132/70 mm Hg, pulse rate is 90/min, and respiration rate is 14/min. BMI is 26. There is reproducible point tenderness along the sternum. The remainder of the examination, including the cardiovascular examination, is normal.

Which of the following is the most likely diagnosis?

(A) Acute pericarditis

(B) Aortic dissection

(C) Costochondritis

(D) Unstable angina

Item 131

A 19-year-old woman is evaluated for painful menses. She usually misses one or two days of school each month owing to these symptoms, which include cramps and nausea. Menarche occurred at age 12 years. Menses have been regular for the past 2 years, occurring every 29 days. The patient is not sexually active, and her medical history is noncontributory. She takes no medications.

Physical examination, including external pelvic examination, is normal.

Which of the following is the most appropriate management option for this patient?

(A) Combined estrogen-progesterone contraceptive

(B) Depot medroxyprogesterone acetate

(C) Ibuprofen

(D) Measurement of follicle-stimulating hormone and luteinizing hormone levels

(E) Pelvic ultrasound

Item 132

A 42-year-old man is evaluated for a 4-month history of left elbow pain. The pain radiates to his hand and is worse at night, with flexion of the arm at the elbow, and with wrist flexion. The pain is accompanied by an intermittent tingling sensation in the fourth and fifth fingers. He has no weakness and has never had this problem before.

On physical examination, vital signs are normal. Pain is elicited in the left elbow with flexion of the arm at the elbow. There is decreased light touch sensation involving both palmar and dorsal surfaces of the fourth and fifth fingers to the level of the wrist. No tenderness to palpation of any of the structures of the elbow is elicited.

Which of the following is the most likely diagnosis?

(A) Lateral epicondylitis

(B) Medial epicondylitis

(C) Olecranon bursitis

(D) Ulnar nerve entrapment

Item 133

A 48-year-old man is evaluated for watery bowel movements. The patient is having 8 to 12 watery bowel movements daily. Several days before the diarrhea began, the patient went to an urgent care clinic with a sinus headache. He was diagnosed with bacterial sinusitis and given a 7-day course of antibiotics. He was asked to return to the urgent care center if he experienced any problems or did not improve. He says there was no discussion of adverse effects or alternatives to antibiotic therapy. Stool assay is positive for *Clostridium difficile* toxin.

Which of the following can be concluded about informed consent in this case?

(A) Acceptance of the antibiotics fulfilled requirements for informed consent

(B) Informed consent is only needed for invasive procedures

(C) Informed consent only applies when signing a consent form

(D) Informed consent was not properly obtained

Item 134

A 47-year-old man is evaluated for follow-up of left-sided cervical radiculopathy. He presented 2 weeks ago with severe arm and hand pain that developed shortly after doing yard work; no trauma was noted. He was treated with NSAIDs and rest. Although his pain symptoms have improved, he has developed progressive difficulty opening jars because he has trouble holding onto the lid. On two occasions over the past several days, he has dropped a coffee cup without intending to.

On physical examination, vital signs are normal. There is normal bulk and tone of the trapezius muscle on the left. Triceps strength is normal on the left, although the biceps muscle group shows 4/5 strength relative to the right. There are also diminished biceps and brachioradialis reflexes on the left. The remainder of the examination is unremarkable.

An MRI of the cervical spine shows herniation of the C5-C6 disk with compression of the left C6 nerve root and increased signal in the area of compression.

Which of the following is the most appropriate next step in management?

(A) Continued analgesics and rest

(B) Epidural corticosteroid injection

(C) Physical therapy for strengthening

(D) Surgical evaluation

Item 135

A 33-year-old woman is evaluated for chronic lower pelvic pain. It has been persistent for the past year but has worsened in recent months. She describes it as a constant, aching discomfort centered over her lower pelvis that persists during her menstrual cycle and has prevented her from being sexually active with her partner. She also reports a 4-month history of urinary urgency and frequency. She has been empirically treated twice for urinary tract infections, but her urinary symptoms improve for only a few days and then recur. She has no history of pelvic surgeries or pelvic infections and has never been pregnant. She has no associated constipation, diarrhea, abdominal distention, or flank pain. She currently takes ibuprofen as needed for pain.

On physical examination, vital signs are normal. BMI is 24. There is mild tenderness to palpation over the pelvic floor muscles with significant tenderness over the anterior vaginal wall. External genitalia are normal in appearance; there is no tenderness to palpation over the vulva. There is no cervical motion tenderness, adnexal tenderness, or discomfort with palpation of the uterus.

Laboratory studies show normal electrolytes, kidney function, and a complete blood count. Erythrocyte sedimentation rate is 4 mm/h. Urinalysis is without erythrocytes or leukocytes and is negative for nitrite and leukocyte esterase. Urine culture is negative. Tests for chlamydial infection and gonorrhea are negative.

Transvaginal/transabdominal ultrasonography is negative for endometrial or ovarian masses and no abnormalities are noted.

Which of the following is the most likely diagnosis?

(A) Endometriosis

(B) Interstitial cystitis

(C) Irritable bowel syndrome

(D) Pelvic adhesions

Item 136

A 66-year-old man with diabetic neuropathy is evaluated for increasing pain in his lower extremities. The pain is 7/10 in intensity, constant, and keeps him awake at night. He has been treated with trials of NSAIDs, amitriptyline, pregabalin, gabapentin, and duloxetine, both individually and in various combinations, without significant control of his symptoms. He presented to an outside emergency department 3 weeks ago and was prescribed oxycodone-acetaminophen 5 mg/325 mg. He has been taking 2 tablets every 6 hours as recommended and has experienced good relief of his pain, although his symptoms worsen with late or missed doses. Medical history is also significant for hypertension, hyperlipidemia, and ischemic cardiomyopathy. He has no personal or family history of drug or alcohol abuse. Current medications are gabapentin, amitriptyline, insulin glargine, insulin aspart, lisinopril, aspirin, simvastatin, carvedilol, and oxycodone-acetaminophen.

On physical examination, temperature is 36.7 °C (98.2 °F), blood pressure is 122/76 mm Hg, pulse rate is 64/min, and respiration rate is 12/min. BMI is 28. He has decreased sensation to light touch and pinprick in a stocking-glove distribution, and reflexes are 1+ and symmetric. Romberg test is positive. There is no hepatomegaly, scleral icterus, or jaundice.

Laboratory studies are significant for normal electrolytes, liver chemistry studies, vitamin B_{12} level, and complete blood count. The serum creatinine level is 1.3 mg/dL (115 μmol/L).

A previous resting electrocardiogram showed first-degree atrioventricular block and small Q waves in an anterolateral distribution without active ischemia.

Which of the following is the most appropriate treatment for this patient's neuropathic pain?

(A) Continue oxycodone-acetaminophen at the current dose

(B) Discontinue oxycodone-acetaminophen and start tramadol

(C) Transition to methadone

(D) Transition to sustained-release morphine

Item 137

An 81-year-old man is evaluated for a 3-week history of shortness of breath, chest pain, palpitations, difficulty sleeping, early morning awakening, and lack of interest in getting

out of bed in the morning. The patient's wife died of cancer 9 months ago. He says that he has been seeing her face at night when he closes his eyes and frequently awakes at night thinking that she is next to him in bed. Medical history is significant for hypertension and hyperlipidemia. Medications are hydrochlorothiazide, atorvastatin, and diphenhydramine at bedtime as needed for sleep. Results of the physical examination are normal.

Chemistry panel and complete blood count are normal. Electrocardiogram reveals normal sinus rhythm with left ventricular hypertrophy without ischemic changes. Chest radiograph is normal. Exercise treadmill test is negative for cardiac ischemia.

Which of the following is the most likely diagnosis?

(A) Anticholinergic drug side effect

(B) Complicated grief

(C) Generalized anxiety disorder

(D) Major depression with psychotic features

Item 138

A 34-year-old woman is evaluated for a 6-month history of allergies that have not responded to treatment. She normally has hay fever in the spring, but it typically subsides after 1 to 2 months and the symptoms can be controlled with antihistamines and decongestants. Now she reports intractable nasal congestion and rhinorrhea present for months. She does not have sinus pain or dental pain. She lives in a 10-year old house with no known mold problems and has no pets. She does not think her symptoms are worse or better when she leaves the house or travels. She notes no sneezing or itchy eyes. Current medications are oxymetazoline nasal spray, pseudoephedrine, cetirizine, and diphenhydramine at bedtime. She has no other medical problems.

On physical examination, temperature is 36.8 °C (98.2 °F), blood pressure is 124/72 mm Hg, pulse rate is 96/min, and respiration rate is 16/min. BMI is 23. Nasal mucosa is hyperemic and slightly edematous with clear nasal drainage. The pharynx is normal without tonsillar enlargement or cobblestoning.

Which of the following is the most likely diagnosis?

(A) Chronic rhinosinusitis

(B) Chronic vasomotor rhinitis

(C) Granulomatosis with polyangiitis (Wegener granulomatosis)

(D) Rhinitis medicamentosa

Item 139

A 34-year-old woman is evaluated for significant breast pain. She says her breasts are generally very "sensitive" but she develops more pronounced discomfort shortly before she has her menstrual period, when both breasts seem to ache and throb. She has not noticed any associated skin discoloration, nipple discharge, or breast masses. She is obese and has gastroesophageal reflux disease. She does not use tobacco or alcohol. She otherwise feels well and has increased her exercise level to help her lose weight. She has no shortness of breath, nausea, vomiting, difficulty swallowing, or recent rashes. Her menses are regular and occur every 28 days. Her mother was diagnosed with breast cancer at age 53 years and her sister had a benign breast biopsy. Her current medications are omeprazole and a daily multivitamin.

On physical examination, vital signs are normal. BMI is 32. Her breasts are symmetric in shape and appearance. There are no palpable masses in either breast, and there is no supraclavicular or axillary lymphadenopathy. There is no nipple discharge or skin discoloration or dimpling. There is diffuse tenderness to palpation over both breasts, most prominent in the upper outer quadrants. Cardiovascular, pulmonary, and abdominal examinations are normal. There is no tenderness to palpation over the chest wall.

Which of the following is the most appropriate management?

(A) Danazol
(B) Diagnostic mammography
(C) Support bra
(D) Tamoxifen

Item 140

A 26-year-old man is evaluated for a 2-month history of depressed mood, lack of energy, and increased sleep. He has had less interest in his usual hobby of woodworking and has found it more difficult to perform well at his job at a law firm. In the past, he has had periods of high energy requiring little sleep without getting tired. During these periods he recalls going on spending sprees and having many sexual partners. He does not have any suicidal ideation. His mother has a history of alcohol abuse. The physical examination, including the mental status examination, is normal.

Which of the following is the most appropriate treatment?

(A) Duloxetine
(B) Lamotrigine
(C) Lorazepam
(D) Sertraline

Item 141

A 55-year-old woman is evaluated during a follow-up appointment. She has hypertension and hyperlipidemia. She does not use alcohol. Review of systems is notable for fatigue and occasional constipation. She is menopausal. Her family history is noncontributory. Her medications are simvastatin (40 mg/d), aspirin, and lisinopril.

On physical examination, she is afebrile, blood pressure is 140/82 mm Hg, pulse rate is 66/min, and respiration rate is 12/min. BMI is 25. She has mildly dry skin. There is no evidence of xanthomas and no hepatomegaly.

Laboratory studies:

Total cholesterol	284 mg/dL (7.36 mmol/L)
LDL cholesterol	231 mg/dL (5.98 mmol/L)
HDL cholesterol	55 mg/dL (1.42 mmol/L)
Triglycerides	113 mg/dL (1.28 mmol/L)
Glucose (fasting)	100 mg/dL (5.5 mmol/L)

Additional laboratory results reveal normal kidney and liver function.

In addition to recommending diet and exercise therapy, which of the following is the most appropriate management?

(A) Add gemfibrozil
(B) Increase simvastatin to 80 mg/d
(C) Measure hemoglobin A_{1c} level
(D) Measure thyroid-stimulating hormone level

Item 142

A 54-year-old woman is evaluated before an elective cholecystectomy. Medical history is significant for atrial fibrillation, type 2 diabetes mellitus, chronic heart failure, hypertension, and a transient ischemic attack 2 months ago. Medications are warfarin, insulin glargine, insulin lispro, metoprolol, lisinopril, furosemide, and simvastatin.

On physical examination, temperature is normal, blood pressure is 142/88 mm Hg, and pulse rate is 88/min and irregularly irregular. The remainder of the physical examination is normal. INR is 2.5.

Which of the following is the most appropriate treatment?

(A) Administer half the usual dose of warfarin for 5 days before surgery
(B) Continue warfarin
(C) Discontinue warfarin 5 days before surgery
(D) Discontinue warfarin 5 days before surgery and administer enoxaparin until the morning of surgery

Item 143

A 22-year-old woman is evaluated during a routine examination. She has a history of anorexia nervosa but has been in remission for the past 2 years. She has recently been under significant stress related to her parents' divorce, and has started restricting her caloric intake because she is worried about gaining weight. She has not had a menstrual period for 4 months (previously she had regular menses) and she has lost 13.6 kg (30 lb) in the last 12 weeks. Medical history is significant for depression and osteopenia. Current medications are calcium and vitamin D.

On physical examination, temperature is 36.4 °C (97.6 °F), blood pressure is 100/60 mm Hg, pulse rate is 60/min, and respiration rate is 12/min. There is no orthostasis. BMI is 16. There is fine, soft hair covering the arms, chest, and abdomen. The heart rate is slow with a regular rhythm. The abdomen is scaphoid. The skin is pale and there is no edema. Pulmonary, abdominal, and musculoskeletal examinations are normal. Blood chemistry studies are normal except for a sodium level of 132 meq/L (132 mmol/L) and a phosphorus level of 2.5 mg/dL (0.81 mmol/L). A pregnancy test is negative.

In addition to referring the patient for nutritional rehabilitation, which of the following is the most appropriate treatment?

(A) Amitriptyline
(B) Bupropion
(C) Cognitive-behavioral therapy
(D) Megestrol acetate
(E) Oral contraceptive pills

Item 144

A 75-year-old man is evaluated for low back pain. The pain began several months ago and is getting worse. Its intensity is now 6 or 7 (on a scale of 1-10) most days. It worsens with activity and improves with sitting. He has been unable to walk or exercise because of the pain and has gained 9.0 kg (20 lb) in the past year. He has not experienced any bowel or bladder incontinence or lower extremity numbness or tingling, and has not had fevers or chills. Medical history is significant for hypertension, hyperlipidemia, and peptic ulcer disease. He does not use tobacco or alcohol. His current medications are hydrochlorothiazide, lisinopril, simvastatin, omeprazole, and aspirin. He has been taking additional aspirin, which has been providing modest pain relief.

On physical examination, vital signs are normal. BMI is 34. There is mild tenderness to palpation over the lower lumbar paravertebral muscles. Patellar and ankle jerk reflexes are 1+ and symmetric. Sensation to light touch and pinprick is symmetric, and strength is 5/5 in the lower extremities. Complete blood count and metabolic panel are normal.

A radiograph of the lumbar spine shows degeneration of the L4 and L5 vertebrae, osteophyte formation, and facet arthropathy with narrowing of the spinal canal.

Which of the following is the most appropriate treatment for this patient's symptoms?

(A) Acetaminophen
(B) Amitriptyline
(C) Cyclobenzaprine
(D) Ibuprofen

Item 145

A 60-year-old woman is evaluated during a routine examination. She has hyperlipidemia. She has a 5-pack-year smoking history but is not actively using tobacco and has no history of illicit drug use. She is married and in a monogamous relationship with her husband of 25 years. She has no family history of breast, colon, or cervical cancer. Her only medication is simvastatin.

On physical examination, she is afebrile, blood pressure is 118/76 mm Hg, and pulse rate is 74/min. BMI is 25. Pap smear and mammography, both performed 11 months ago, were within normal limits.

Which of the following conditions should also be screened for in this patient?

(A) Abdominal aortic aneurysm
(B) Depression

(C) Hepatitis B virus infection
(D) Osteoporosis

Item 146

A 38-year-old woman is evaluated for a 2-year history of irritability and frequent headaches, accompanied by nausea and sweating. She is a housecleaner and has had increasing difficulty concentrating at work over the past year, and it takes her much longer to clean houses lately. She has a difficult time getting to sleep and frequently arises after 2 to 3 hours of fitful sleep in bed. Her mood is good. She worries frequently about her ability to pay her bills and what she will do for retirement. She has cut back on activities with friends and does not like to go out in social situations anymore. She has asthma, and her only current medication is albuterol as needed.

On physical examination, she is afebrile, blood pressure is 130/72 mm Hg, pulse rate is 98/min, and respiration rate is 14/min. BMI is 22. Serum thyroid-stimulating hormone level, complete blood count, and urinalysis are normal.

Which of the following is the most likely diagnosis?

(A) Attention-deficit/hyperactivity disorder
(B) Bipolar disorder
(C) Generalized anxiety disorder
(D) Major depressive disorder

Item 147

A 56-year-old woman is evaluated during a routine examination. On review of systems, she reports a 2-year history of decreased interest in sexual intercourse. Her lack of interest is gradually worsening and starting to cause problems in her marriage. She has no history of sexual trauma, sexually transmitted infection, or pelvic surgery. Her last menstrual period was 2 years ago.

On physical examination, vital signs are normal. Gynecologic examination shows pink, well-lubricated vaginal walls; there is no cervical motion or adnexal tenderness and no discomfort with speculum insertion.

Which of the following is the most appropriate treatment of this patient?

(A) Sex therapy
(B) Sildenafil
(C) Systemic estrogen and progesterone therapy
(D) Systemic testosterone therapy

Item 148

A 70-year-old woman is evaluated for a 3-month history of vision problems. She reports that objects may appear blurry or distorted, particularly in the central field. She has difficulty reading and recognizing faces. She has no eye pain or recent eye trauma. She is a smoker. Her only medication is tiotropium.

On physical examination, vital signs are normal. Funduscopic findings are shown (see next page). The remainder of the eye examination is normal.

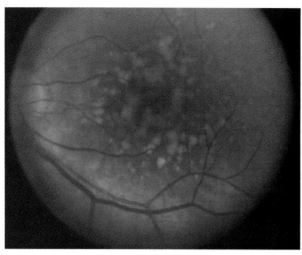

ITEM 148

Which of the following is the most likely diagnosis?

(A) Age-related macular degeneration

(B) Cataracts

(C) Primary open angle glaucoma

(D) Retinal detachment

Item 149

A 70-year-old man is evaluated preoperatively before elective total hip arthroplasty. He is able to ambulate on a level surface slowly but is unable to carry laundry or groceries up stairs because of his hip pain. He has had no recent chest pain or pressure. He has no orthopnea. Other than his hip pain, he feels well. He has hypertension and hyperlipidemia. Current medications are metoprolol, losartan, and simvastatin.

On physical examination, temperature is 36.8 °C (98.3 °F), blood pressure is 132/78 mm Hg, pulse rate is 64/min, and respiration rate is 14/min. Results of the remainder of the examination are normal. Serum creatinine level is 1.3 mg/dL (115 µmol/L). An electrocardiogram shows sinus rhythm with no ST- or T-wave abnormalities.

Which of the following is the most appropriate diagnostic test to perform next?

(A) Cardiac catheterization

(B) CT coronary angiography

(C) Dobutamine stress echocardiography

(D) No further testing needed before surgery

Item 150

A 42-year-old-man is evaluated for obesity. His weight has gradually increased over the past two decades and is currently 168.2 kg (370 lb). Five years ago, he was diagnosed with type 2 diabetes mellitus, hypertension, and hyperlipidemia. Over the past 6 months, he has unsuccessfully tried diet and exercise therapy for his obesity. He tried over-the-counter orlistat but could not tolerate the gastrointestinal side effects. Medications are metformin, lisinopril, and simvastatin. His total weight loss goal is 45.4 kg (100 lb).

On physical examination, temperature is normal, blood pressure is 130/80 mm Hg, pulse rate is 80/min, and respiration rate is 14/min. BMI is 48. Waist circumference is 121.9 cm (48 in). There is no thyromegaly. Heart sounds are normal with no murmur. There is no lower extremity edema.

Results of complete blood count, thyroid studies, and urinalysis are unremarkable.

Which of the following is the most appropriate management of this patient?

(A) Bariatric surgery evaluation

(B) Prescribe phentermine

(C) Reduce caloric intake to below 800 kcal/d

(D) Refer to an exercise program

Item 151

A 66-year-old man is evaluated during a routine examination. He is asymptomatic and walks for 2 miles on the treadmill three times a week. He has hypertension. He drinks three or four beers three times per week and has done so for the past 30 years. He is a former smoker, smoking one pack per day for 2 years between the ages of 20 and 25 years. Current medications are hydrochlorothiazide and aspirin.

On physical examination, he is afebrile, blood pressure is 124/76 mm Hg, and pulse rate is 72/min. BMI is 23. The examination is otherwise unremarkable. A fasting lipid profile last year was within normal limits. His most recent colonoscopy was performed 5 years ago and was negative for any polyps.

Which of the following is the most appropriate screening test?

(A) Abdominal ultrasonography

(B) Chest radiography

(C) Coronary artery calcium score determination

(D) Fasting lipid profile

(E) No additional testing

Item 152

A 44-year-old man is evaluated for chronic back pain. Six months ago he underwent decompressive spinal laminectomy for treatment of refractory pain secondary to spinal stenosis. He was discharged on oxycodone-acetaminophen, 5 mg/325 mg, and despite taking 2 tablets every 6 hours, he continues to report severe discomfort. He has been taking ibuprofen and cyclobenzaprine to help with the pain and has been using hot compresses intermittently. His surgeon has been satisfied with his operative treatment and has recommended that he start a physical therapy program, but the patient reports that he is in too much pain to exercise. Medical history is significant for mild depression and tobacco use. His father abused alcohol and his mother has COPD secondary to smoking.

On physical examination, vital signs are normal. BMI is 32. There is mild tenderness to palpation over the lumbar paravertebral muscles. A complete neurologic examination of the lower extremities and a straight leg raise test cannot be performed because of patient discomfort, although there are no abnormalities noted on limited testing.

In addition to starting the patient on a good bowel regimen, which of the following is the most appropriate management?

(A) Amitriptyline
(B) Change analgesic to extended-release morphine
(C) Evaluate for opioid dependency
(D) MRI of the lumbar spine

Item 153

A 42-year-old man is evaluated for difficulty sleeping the past several months. He reports trouble both falling asleep and staying asleep. He has not tried any over-the-counter medications. He drinks two or three beers on the weekends only and this has not changed; he also drinks two cups of coffee in the mornings. His wife, who is present, has not heard any snoring, gasping, or other breathing problems at night. He reports no leg symptoms. They have recently moved to a new apartment; he reports that the bedroom may be hotter than the previous one, although his wife reports feeling comfortable.

Results of the physical examination are unremarkable. Vital signs are normal, BMI is 26, and mood and mental status are normal.

Which of the following is the best initial management for this patient?

(A) Advise alcohol abstinence
(B) Benzodiazepine
(C) Counseling regarding sleep hygiene
(D) Over-the-counter antihistamine

Item 154

A 28-year-old woman is evaluated for a 3-month history of fatigue and muscle cramps. She states that she is eating well, drinking plenty of fluids, and exercising regularly, but the fatigue is starting to interfere with her ability to complete her daily 3-mile run. She has a previous history of anorexia nervosa diagnosed at age 16 years requiring two inpatient hospitalizations. She has had a normal weight and menstrual cycle for the last 4 years. She currently takes daily calcium and vitamin D supplements.

On physical examination, temperature is 36.6 °C (98.0 °F), blood pressure is 106/64 mm Hg, pulse rate is 66/min, and respiration rate is 12/min. BMI is 22. She has poor dentition with multiple dental caries. The remainder of the examination is normal. Pregnancy test is negative.

Laboratory studies:

Complete blood count	Normal
Electrolytes	
Sodium	132 meq/L (132 mmol/L)
Potassium	3.2 meq/L (3.2 mmol/L)
Chloride	95 meq/L (95 mmol/L)
Bicarbonate	31 meq/L (31 mmol/L)
Blood urea nitrogen	6 mg/dL (2.1 mmol/L)
Creatinine	0.8 mg/dL (70.7 µmol/L)
Thyroid-stimulating hormone	2.5 µU/mL (2.5 mU/L)

Which of the following is the most likely diagnosis?

(A) Anorexia nervosa, binge-eating/purging subtype
(B) Binge-eating disorder
(C) Bulimia nervosa, purging subtype
(D) Night-eating syndrome

Item 155

A 48-year-old man is evaluated for pain located on his lateral thigh. He describes the pain as a burning sensation that has been present for 3 weeks. He has never had this pain before and has no associated leg weakness or back pain.

On physical examination, vital signs are normal. BMI is 34. Dysesthesia is present in the anterolateral thigh. There is no tenderness to palpation of the lateral femoral epicondyle. Knee and hip examinations are normal. A straight leg raising test is negative bilaterally and strength is 5/5 in both extremities.

Which of the following is the most likely diagnosis?

(A) Greater trochanteric bursitis
(B) Iliotibial band syndrome
(C) L5 radiculopathy
(D) Meralgia paresthetica

Item 156

A 78-year-old man is evaluated in the emergency department after a witnessed episode of syncope. The patient reports that, while eating dinner, he experienced a pounding in his chest and then fell to the floor. His wife estimates he was unconscious for approximately 30 seconds, had no head trauma, and was oriented and alert upon regaining consciousness. He has not experienced any similar episodes in the past, although he has felt the pounding previously. Medical history is significant for hypertension, COPD, osteoarthritis, and benign prostatic hyperplasia. Medications are chlorthalidone, lisinopril, celecoxib, ipratropium-albuterol inhaler, and tamsulosin. He currently feels well except for pain in his right thigh where he fell.

On physical examination, temperature is normal. Blood pressure is 138/88 mm Hg and pulse rate is 82/min, without orthostatic changes. Respiration rate is 16/min. Oxygen saturation on ambient air is normal. Carotid upstrokes are +2 without bruits, and there is no jugular venous distention. Cardiac examination is normal, with the exception of occasional extra beats. The remainder of the examination, including neurologic examination, is normal. 12-Lead electrocardiogram shows a few premature ventricular contractions without evidence of ischemia.

Which of the following is the most appropriate next step in this patient's management?

(A) Carotid Doppler ultrasonography
(B) Echocardiography
(C) Inpatient cardiac monitoring
(D) Noncontrast CT of head

Item 157

A 26-year-old woman is evaluated in the emergency department for an 8-day history of sore throat, fever, and neck pain. She has severe pain on the left side of her neck with swallowing. She has had fevers for the past week with rigors starting today. Over the past 3 to 4 days she has had increasing cough. She was previously healthy and takes no medications.

On physical examination, temperature is 39.1 °C (102.3 °F), blood pressure is 108/68 mm Hg, pulse rate is 116/min, and respiration rate is 20/min. BMI is 19. She is toxic-appearing. The neck is tender to palpation along the left side without lymphadenopathy. The pharynx is erythematous with tonsillar enlargement and no exudates. The chest is clear to auscultation. Other than tachycardia, the cardiac examination is normal.

Chest radiograph is shown. Leukocyte count is 18,400/µL (18.4 × 10⁹/L) with 17% band forms. Serum creatinine level is 0.8 mg/dL (70.7 µmol/L).

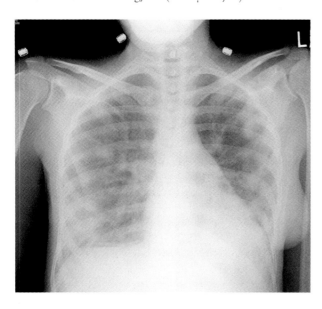

Which of the following tests is most likely to establish the diagnosis?

(A) CT of the chest with contrast
(B) CT of the neck with contrast
(C) Radiography of the pharyngeal soft tissues
(D) Transthoracic echocardiography

Item 158

A 56-year-old man presents for evaluation of elevated liver chemistry test results that were obtained during an application for life insurance. At an office visit 12 weeks ago, he was started on simvastatin for dyslipidemia. He has not experienced any side effects with this medication and specifically does not have nausea, vomiting, or abdominal pain.

On physical examination today, blood pressure is 140/80 mm Hg; vital signs are otherwise normal. BMI is 29. There is no scleral icterus, hepatomegaly, or abdominal tenderness.

Laboratory studies:

	12 Weeks Ago	Current
Alanine aminotransferase	28 units/L	76 units/L
Aspartate aminotransferase	21 units/L	63 units/L
Total bilirubin	0.8 mg/dL (13.6 µmol/L)	1 mg/dL (17.1 µmol/L)

Which of the following is the most appropriate management?

(A) Discontinue simvastatin
(B) Measure serum antibodies to hepatitis B and C
(C) Order liver ultrasonography
(D) No change in management

Item 159

A 30-year-old man was admitted to the hospital 2 days ago with an acute exacerbation of asthma. He was placed on a regimen of corticosteroids and inhaled β-agonists. He has responded well and is ready for discharge today with plans for a short course of oral corticosteroids as well as inhaled corticosteroids and β-agonists. He reports receiving "all his shots" while growing up. He does not smoke cigarettes. He is in a monogamous relationship with his wife and reports no illicit drug use.

Which of the following vaccines should this patient receive?

(A) Hepatitis B
(B) Human papillomavirus
(C) Meningococcal
(D) Pneumococcal

Item 160

A 66-year-old woman is evaluated in the hospital 12 hours after a total knee arthroplasty. She is experiencing anorexia and some nausea and is not eating. She has a history of type 2 diabetes mellitus treated with glimepiride.

On physical examination, vital signs are normal. BMI is 35. Her preoperative hemoglobin A₁c concentration was 6.9%, and plasma glucose level 6 hours postoperatively is 250 mg/dL (13.9 mmol/L).

Which of the following is the most appropriate treatment of her diabetes?

(A) Glimepiride
(B) Long- and short-acting insulin
(C) Sliding scale insulin
(D) No treatment at this time

Item 161

A 19-year-old man is evaluated for a 2-day history of sore throat, cough, fever, and chills. On physical examination, temperature is 38.9 °C (102.0 °F), blood pressure is 122/82 mm Hg, pulse rate is 88/min, and respiration rate is 14/min. The pharynx is erythematous with tonsillar enlargement and exudates bilaterally. There is no cervical lymphadenopathy.

Which of the following is the most appropriate management?

(A) Obtain throat culture and start penicillin therapy
(B) Perform rapid antigen detection testing
(C) Start penicillin therapy
(D) No further testing or treatment indicated

Item 162

A 42-year-old man is seen for follow-up of hepatitis C. Three years ago, serologic tests were positive for hepatitis A virus and negative for hepatitis B virus. He received a single dose of hepatitis B vaccine but was lost to follow-up. He feels well today without specific symptoms. Findings on physical examination are unremarkable.

Which of the following is the most appropriate management of this patient's hepatitis B vaccination?

(A) Complete the hepatitis B vaccine series
(B) Measure hepatitis B surface antibody
(C) Restart the hepatitis B vaccine series
(D) No further vaccination or serologic testing for hepatitis B is needed

Item 163

A 19-year-old woman is evaluated for a 1-week history of left ear canal pruritus, redness, and pain. She swims 1 mile each day and has recently started wearing plastic ear plugs to keep water out of her ears while swimming.

On physical examination, she is afebrile, blood pressure is 98/66 mm Hg, pulse rate is 62/min, and respiration rate is 16/min. She appears healthy and in no distress. There is pain with tugging on the pinna and compression or movement of the tragus. The left ear canal is shown. With irrigation,

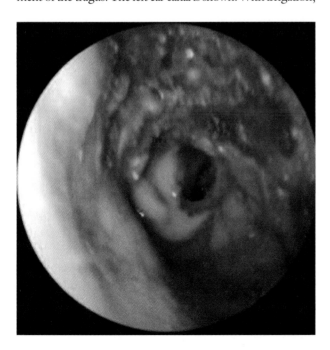

the left tympanic membrane appears normal. There is no preauricular or cervical lymphadenopathy.

Which of the following is the most likely diagnosis?

(A) Acute otitis externa
(B) Delayed-type hypersensitivity reaction to ear plugs
(C) Malignant otitis externa
(D) Otitis media

Item 164

A 38-year-old woman is evaluated during a routine examination. She has recently divorced and is interested in some form of hormonal contraception, as her ex-husband had a vasectomy after their last child, and she does not want to use condoms. She has no history of deep venous thrombosis, hypertension, or heart disease. She drinks one glass of wine 4 or 5 nights per week, and smokes a pack of cigarettes daily. Family history is significant for stroke in her mother at age 72 years. All previous Pap smears have been negative.

Physical examination, including pelvic examination, is normal. A Pap smear is obtained.

Which of the following is the most appropriate hormonal contraceptive option for this patient?

(A) Estrogen patch
(B) Estrogen-progesterone combination
(C) Progesterone contraceptive
(D) No hormonal-based method

Item 165

A 70-year-old man is evaluated for a 6-month history of low energy and decreased libido. He is not in a depressed mood and is still interested in daily activities. He has glaucoma and hypertension. Over the past year his vision has decreased and his ophthalmologist has adjusted his medications repeatedly. His current medications are timolol drops, latanoprost drops (a prostaglandin analogue), dorzolamide drops (a topical carbonic anhydrase inhibitor), lisinopril, and amlodipine.

On physical examination, temperature is 37.6 °C (99.7 °F), blood pressure is 138/84 mm Hg, pulse rate is 48/min and regular, and respiration rate is 12/min. BMI is 28. Other than bradycardia, the results of the physical examination are normal. An electrocardiogram shows only sinus bradycardia.

Which of this patient's medications should be discontinued?

(A) Amlodipine
(B) Dorzolamide
(C) Latanoprost
(D) Lisinopril
(E) Timolol

Item 166

A 65-year-old man is evaluated for a 6-month history of inability to achieve a successful erection. He is otherwise asymptomatic. He has coronary artery disease and hyperlipidemia. A bare metal stent was placed 5 years ago to his mid–left anterior descending coronary artery after he experienced exertional chest pain. Currently, he exercises in the form of brisk walking 3 to 4 times per week. He does not smoke. His current medications are aspirin, metoprolol, and simvastatin. He has no family history of early coronary artery disease.

On physical examination, he is afebrile, blood pressure is 114/80 mm Hg, pulse rate is 84/min, and respiration rate is 16/min. BMI is 29. Results of the cardiac examination are normal. He has no gynecomastia, the testes are normal in size, and sensation is intact in both lower extremities. The dorsalis pedis and posterior tibialis pulses are palpable bilaterally.

An electrocardiogram is normal. Laboratory investigation reveals a serum thyroid-stimulating hormone level of 2.75 µU/mL (2.75 mU/L) and an 8 AM total testosterone level of 425 ng/dL (15 nmol/L).

Which of the following is the most appropriate management for this patient?

(A) Begin sildenafil
(B) Begin testosterone replacement therapy
(C) Perform exercise stress testing
(D) Stop metoprolol

Item 167

A 22-year-old woman is evaluated during a follow-up appointment for plantar fasciitis. She has been doing appropriate stretching exercises for the past 8 weeks and has been using acetaminophen, 1000 mg every 8 hours, with some improvement in pain. The pain is still present, however, and interferes with her job. She has never had pain like this before.

On physical examination, there is tenderness to palpation of the plantar medial calcaneal tuberosity and 1 to 2 cm distally along the plantar fascia. Passive dorsiflexion of the toes increases the patient's pain. Pes planus is present. There is no ecchymosis, tenderness, or swelling over the plantar fascia and no tenderness of the calcaneus with medial or lateral pressure. The calcaneal tuberosity is neither prominent nor tender. Sensation is intact on the plantar surface of the foot.

Which of the following is the most appropriate treatment?

(A) Arch supports
(B) Corticosteroid injection
(C) Extracorporeal shock wave therapy
(D) Plantar fascia release surgery

Item 168

A 60-year-old woman is admitted to the hospital for abdominal pain. A subsequent evaluation has revealed a large cecal mass, and hemicolectomy is planned. She is able to walk her dog at a brisk pace, actively garden, and shovel light snow. She has had no chest pain or dyspnea on exertion. She has type 2 diabetes mellitus, hypertension, hyperlipidemia, and chronic kidney disease. Current medications are insulin, lisinopril, and simvastatin.

On physical examination, temperature is normal, blood pressure is 132/88 mm Hg, and pulse rate is 78/min. Heart rate and rhythm are regular with no murmurs or gallops. Laboratory studies show a serum creatinine level of 2.4 mg/dL (212 µmol/L). Electrocardiogram shows normal sinus rhythm without ST- or T-wave abnormalities.

Which of the following is the most appropriate diagnostic test to perform prior to surgery?

(A) Adenosine thallium stress test
(B) Cardiac catheterization
(C) Exercise stress test
(D) Proceed to surgery without further testing

Answers and Critiques

Item 1 Answer: A

Educational Objective: Identify appropriate genetic counseling strategies.

The most appropriate screening step for genetic diseases in this patient is to inquire about any diseases that "run in the family" and, specifically, to inquire about family history of the more common and important inherited diseases, including breast, ovarian, prostate, and colon cancer, as well as early cardiovascular disease. A detailed family history should follow for those conditions identified through this preliminary questioning. Patient-reported family histories for first-degree relatives have been shown to be accurate and valuable for breast and colon cancer, but a negative family history for ovarian and endometrial cancer is less accurate. Although few diseases follow strict Mendelian genetics that allow for a relatively certain prediction of disease, knowledge regarding the frequency of disease occurrence in a given family cohort is helpful in assessing individual risk for developing specific disorders with a genetic predisposition.

Genetic counseling with the option for testing should be offered when: (1) the patient has a personal or family history suggestive of a genetic susceptibility condition; (2) the genetic test can be adequately interpreted; and (3) the test results will aid in diagnosis or influence the medical or surgical management of the patient or family at hereditary risk. It is premature to refer for genetic counseling without first determining if there is concern for a genetic disorder.

The process of taking a family history typically employed by medical genetics professionals is both labor- and time-intensive. It typically involves a three-generation pedigree and may require hours to complete. Given the multiple demands on the internist during the clinical encounter, this degree of detail is not feasible.

Although it is standard of care to perform genetic testing for certain mutations in unselected preconception, prenatal, and newborn populations, and direct-to-consumer genomic kits are commercially available, at least three important issues make it unwise to perform genetic testing in unselected populations seen by internists: (1) the clinical validity of such a test may be lacking, (2) there may be a high likelihood of false-positive tests, and (3) the harms of performing a genetic test may outweigh any benefits.

KEY POINT

- The most appropriate first screening step for genetic diseases is to inquire about any diseases that "run in the family" and to inquire specifically about family history of the more common and important inherited diseases, including breast, ovarian, prostate, and colon cancer, as well as early cardiovascular disease.

Bibliography

Berg AO, Baird MA, Botkin JR, et al. National Institute of Health State-of-the-Science Conference Statement: Family History and Improving Health. Ann Intern Med. 2009; 151(12):872-877. [PMID: 19884615]

Item 2 Answer: D

Educational Objective: Treat carpal tunnel syndrome.

This patient has carpal tunnel syndrome, and the most appropriate initial treatment, in addition to the avoidance of repetitive wrist motions, is wrist splinting. Wrist splinting appears to be most effective when done in the neutral position compared with 20 degrees of extension. In one prospective study, full-time splinting was superior to nocturnal splinting at 6 weeks in terms of nerve latencies, although there was significant cross-over of patients between groups in this study. Nocturnal splinting has the advantage of being more convenient to patients in comparison with full-time splinting.

Local corticosteroid injection has been shown to provide short-term (up to 3 months) pain relief, although the effect does not appear to be durable. Contraindications to local corticosteroid injections include thenar weakness and atrophy, profound sensory loss, and acute carpal tunnel syndrome.

Owing to possible adverse effects, drug therapy should be reserved for patients in whom wrist splinting has failed. Although NSAIDs are frequently used as first-line therapy, evidence is lacking as to their effectiveness.

Surgical intervention should be reserved for patients in whom both nonpharmacologic and pharmacologic conservative therapies have failed. Other indications include progressive sensory or motor deficits and moderate to severe findings on electrodiagnostic studies. In one randomized controlled trial of 116 patients, those with carpal tunnel syndrome who underwent surgical intervention had better outcomes (function and symptoms) than those who underwent nonsurgical management, although clinically, the benefit was modest.

KEY POINT

- Initial therapy for carpal tunnel syndrome is wrist splinting and avoidance of repetitive wrist motions.

Bibliography

Jarvik JG, Comstock BA, Kliot M, et al. Surgery versus non-surgical therapy for carpal tunnel syndrome: a randomised parallel-group trial. Lancet. 2009;374(9695):1074-1081. [PMID: 19782873]

Item 3   Answer: A

Educational Objective: Treat obsessive-compulsive disorder.

In addition to cognitive-behavioral therapy (CBT), the pharmacologic treatment of choice for this patient is a selective serotonin reuptake inhibitor (SSRI) such as fluoxetine. She has the hallmark features of obsessive-compulsive disorder (OCD), including recurrent obsessions or compulsions sufficiently severe to occupy 1 hour daily or result in marked distress or impaired social function. Obsessions are persistent ideas, thoughts, impulses, or images experienced as intrusive and are associated with significant anxiety or distress. Examples include fears of having left doors unlocked and fears of germ contamination. Compulsions are repetitive behaviors, such as handwashing, checking, ordering, or counting, that are repeated to decrease the anxiety related to the obsessions. Cognitive-behavioral therapy (CBT) with an exposure therapy element is the treatment of choice for OCD. SSRIs are the most effective pharmacotherapy and should be used in patients who are resistant or only partially responsive to CBT and in those with more severe OCD or in whom a rapid response is critical. Higher SSRI doses are often needed to treat OCD as compared with depression, and the dose may be escalated at 2- to 4-week intervals. Adjunctive use of antipsychotics has some evidence of benefit.

Haloperidol, a typical antipsychotic agent, has been shown to be effective in combination with an SSRI for OCD in patients who are refractory to initial treatment. Haloperidol has many serious adverse effects, including QT-interval prolongation and extrapyramidal symptoms that further limit its use as a first-line agent.

Benzodiazepines, such as lorazepam, are not effective for treating OCD and should be avoided given their lack of efficacy and high risk for dependence.

Quetiapine is an atypical antipsychotic agent that has not been shown to improve OCD symptoms in patients who are refractory to serotonin reuptake inhibitor monotherapy.

KEY POINT

- **Cognitive-behavioral therapy (CBT) with an exposure element is the treatment of choice for obsessive-compulsive disorder (OCD); high-dose selective serotonin reuptake inhibitors should be used in patients who are resistant or only partially responsive to CBT and in those with more severe OCD or in whom a rapid response is critical.**

Bibliography

Soomro GM, Altman D, Rajagopal S, Oakley-Browne M. Selective serotonin re-uptake inhibitors (SSRIs) versus placebo for obsessive compulsive disorder (OCD). Cochrane Database Syst Rev. 2008;(1):CD001765. [PMID: 18253995]

Item 4   Answer: D

Educational Objective: Manage epistaxis.

This patient should be told to apply uninterrupted nasal pressure for 15 to 30 minutes, to not remove the clot or blow his nose, and to temporarily discontinue nasal corticosteroids. More than 90% of epistaxis cases occur at the anterior nasal septum in the Kiesselbach area, the anteroinferior aspect of the nasal septum where multiple arteries anastomose to form a plexus. These episodes of bleeding almost always stop with consistent pressure for at least 15 minutes. Direct causes of epistaxis include nose picking, dry air during winter months, intranasal corticosteroids and decongestants, bacterial or viral rhinosinusitis, and less commonly tumors.

Nasal arterial embolization is reserved for severe refractory epistaxis, which this patient does not have.

The patient would not require cauterization and anterior nasal packing unless the bleeding fails to resolve with at least 15 to 30 minutes of pressure. Nasal packing with or without nasal constrictive agents is effective (60%-80%) but uncomfortable for the patient given that the packing is left in for 1 to 3 days.

Based upon the patient's history, it is unlikely that he has a bleeding disorder as a systemic cause of his epistaxis and is unlikely to have developed a significant anemia from 2 hours of epistaxis. Laboratory studies are rarely helpful in healthy patients with epistaxis. Even in patients with known bleeding disorders, laboratory studies and coagulation studies are normal in 80% of patients.

It is not necessary to consult an otorhinolaryngologist because the patient reports that the bleeding stops with pressure and the examiner has identified an oozing vessel in the anterior nasal septum. Posterior bleeds warrant referral because they can be difficult to control by application of direct external pressure.

KEY POINT

- **Anterior nosebleeds almost always stop with consistent pressure for at least 15 minutes.**

Bibliography

Schlosser R. Epistaxis. N Engl J Med. 2009;360(8):784-789. [PMID: 19228621]

Item 5   Answer: B

Educational Objective: Diagnose hypoactive sexual desire disorder.

The most likely diagnosis is hypoactive sexual desire disorder (HSDD). Female sexual dysfunction, defined as sexual difficulties that are persistent and personally distressing to the patient, affects up to 35% of sexually active women and is common among middle-aged women. HSDD is defined as a persistent lack of desire for or receptiveness to sexual activity or a persistent lack of sexual thoughts. HSDD is one of the most common causes of female sexual dysfunction, and prevalence ranges from 12% to 19%. Natural and surgical menopause may contribute to the development of HSDD, as the associated decline in testosterone levels may decrease sexual motivation and desire. There is no FDA-approved medication for the treatment of female HSDD; individual and couples sex therapy or psychotherapy may be beneficial.

Dyspareunia is persistent urogenital pain that occurs around intercourse and is not related exclusively to inadequate lubrication or vaginismus. Several conditions may cause dyspareunia, including interstitial cystitis, pelvic adhesions, infections, endometriosis, pelvic venous congestion, and vulvodynia. Treatment is aimed at correcting the underlying abnormality. This patient's absence of sexual pain, history of previously normal sexual intercourse, and lack of symptoms and signs associated with any of the aforementioned conditions (no urinary symptoms, no history of pelvic surgeries or sexually transmitted infections) make dyspareunia an unlikely etiology for her current sexual problems.

Sexual aversion disorder is a persistent or recurrent aversive response to any genital contact with a sexual partner. Physiologic responses often accompany these feelings, with associated nausea and shortness of breath. Frequently there is a history of a painful or traumatic sexual event. Although this patient is avoiding intercourse, this is related to low sexual desire and motivation. Patients with sexual aversion disorder avoid intercourse because of feelings of revulsion and disgust.

Vaginismus is involuntary and recurrent spasm of the outer third of the vaginal musculature that interferes with vaginal penetration. Pain may accompany this involuntary spasm, and there is often associated avoidance and anticipatory fear of penetration. Prevalence ranges between 1% and 6%. On examination, this patient easily tolerated insertion of the vaginal speculum without any evidence of muscular spasm, although it should be noted that some women experience vaginismus only during sexual activity (situation-specific).

KEY POINT

- **Hypoactive sexual desire disorder, a common cause of female sexual dysfunction, is defined as a persistent lack of desire for or receptiveness to sexual activity or a persistent lack of sexual thoughts.**

Bibliography
Kingsberg S, Althof SE. Evaluation and treatment of female sexual disorders. Int Urogynecol J Pelvic Floor Dysfunct. 2009;20(suppl 1):S33-S43. [PMID: 19440781]

Item 6   Answer: D
Educational Objective: Treat dyspnea at the end of life.

This patient on comfort care should be given morphine. Dyspnea is one of the most common symptoms encountered in palliative care. It is most often the result of direct cardiothoracic pathology, such as pleural effusion, heart failure, COPD, pulmonary embolism, pneumonia, or lung metastases. Dyspnea can also be caused by systemic conditions, such as anemia, muscle weakness, or conditions causing abdominal distention. Patients with underlying lung disease on bronchodilator therapy should have this therapy continued to maintain comfort. Opioids are effective in reducing dyspnea in patients with underlying cardiopulmonary disease and malignancy. In patients already receiving opioids, using the breakthrough pain dose for dyspnea and increasing this dose by 25% if not fully effective may be helpful. A 5-mg dose of oral morphine given four times daily has been shown to help relieve dyspnea in patients with end-stage heart failure. Low-dose (20 mg) extended-release morphine given daily has been used to relieve dyspnea in patients with advanced COPD.

Antibiotics and corticosteroids are appropriately used in patients with exacerbations of severe COPD. However, neither would be expected to provide immediate relief of the patient's respiratory distress and would also be inconsistent with care focusing primarily on comfort measures at the end of life.

In contrast to opioids, benzodiazepines have not demonstrated consistent benefit in treating dyspnea. However, they may be useful in specific patients who have significant anxiety associated with their dyspnea.

KEY POINT

- **Opioids are effective in reducing dyspnea in patients with underlying cardiopulmonary disease and malignancy.**

Bibliography
Swetz KM, Kamal AH. Palliative care. Ann Intern Med. 2012;156(3):ITC21. [PMID: 22312158]

Item 7   Answer: D
Educational Objective: Diagnose chronic fatigue syndrome.

This patient requires no additional testing. Chronic fatigue syndrome (CFS) is defined as medically unexplained fatigue that persists for 6 months or more, accompanied by at least four of the following symptoms: subjective memory impairment, sore throat, tender lymph nodes, muscle or joint pain, headache, unrefreshing sleep, and postexertional malaise lasting longer than 24 hours.

There is no diagnostic test for CFS. An appropriate history and physical examination should include an assessment for common causes of fatigue, including a sleep history; those with a history of loud snoring, apneic spells, or frequent limb movements during sleep should undergo a sleep study to evaluate for sleep apnea or restless legs syndrome. All patients with fatigue should be assessed for depression and anxiety disorders. Patients with hypothyroidism may present with fatigue in the absence of other findings; it is reasonable to order a thyroid-stimulating hormone level. If significant weight loss, lymphadenopathy, or fever is found, assessment for malignancy and chronic infections should ensue. A complete blood count should be obtained to rule out anemia and to look for evidence of lymphoma or leukemia. A metabolic panel is reasonable to rule out diabetes mellitus, kidney disease, and liver disease. An erythrocyte sedimentation rate can help assess for an active inflammatory process. Additional studies may be warranted in selected patients based on the history and physical examination findings. This patient, however, has no findings on physical examination that warrant additional testing and her previous laboratory evaluation was appropriate and normal; repeating previously normal laboratory tests is not indicated.

Although CFS has been associated with certain viruses, such as Epstein-Barr virus and parvovirus B19, these associations have not been reproduced consistently in studies. Thus, obtaining titers for these viruses would neither definitely identify etiology nor result in a treatable diagnosis.

KEY POINT

- There is no test that is diagnostic for chronic fatigue syndrome; in addition to a complete history and physical examination, reasonable tests to consider are a complete blood count, comprehensive metabolic panel, and thyroid-stimulating hormone level.

Bibliography
Holgate ST, Komaroff AL, Mangan D, Wessely S. Chronic fatigue syndrome: understanding a complex illness. Nat Rev Neurosci. 2011;12(9):539-544. [PMID: 21792218]

Item 8   Answer: D

Educational Objective: Manage preoperative testing in a patient without comorbidities.

The only diagnostic test appropriate to perform preoperatively in this young woman is a pregnancy test. A preoperative pregnancy test is recommended in all women for whom pregnancy is still possible. Any additional preoperative testing should be selective, based on the likelihood of finding an abnormality and, more importantly, that the result will change management. The results of most screening tests will be normal, and any abnormalities found usually do not affect management. Additionally, patients with previously normal laboratory studies in the 4 months prior to surgery and no change in their clinical condition rarely warrant repeat testing. However, most hospital policies continue to require preoperative screening tests despite the evidence to the contrary. This approach is not endorsed by any major physician groups and, owing to chance alone, will yield 1 abnormal result for every 20 tests ordered, which are typically either false-positive results or of no clinical significance.

This patient has no symptoms or signs of pulmonary disease. In the absence of this, chest radiography has a low pretest probability of abnormality and should not be ordered.

In the absence of a personal or family history of abnormal bleeding, liver disease, significant alcohol use, malabsorption, or anticoagulation therapy, the likelihood of a bleeding disorder is low, and no further preoperative testing is required.

This patient is young, has no signs or symptoms of cardiac disease, and no risk factors for early or silent myocardial infarction. Preoperative electrocardiography should be limited to patients in whom a silent or previously unrecognized myocardial infarction is possible.

KEY POINT

- **Perioperative testing should be limited to tests that have a reasonable pretest probability of being abnormal, and whose abnormal result would directly impact perioperative care.**

Bibliography
Hepner DL. The role of testing in the preoperative evaluation. Cleve Clin J Med. 2009;76 (suppl 4):S22-7. [PMID: 19880831]

Item 9   Answer: B

Educational Objective: Evaluate pulsatile tinnitus.

Tinnitus that is timed with the patient's pulse (pulsatile tinnitus) is concerning for an intracranial vascular anomaly, such as stenosis, arteriovenous malformation, or glomus tumor, although patients with middle ear congestion may report a pulsatile sensation as part of their symptom complex. It is valuable to listen over the patient's ears, eyes, and neck, because if a vascular abnormality is present, the bruit causing tinnitus may sometimes be detected externally (objective tinnitus). If a bruit is present, or there is other significant concern for a vascular cause of tinnitus, imaging of the cranial vasculature (Doppler ultrasonography or magnetic resonance angiography) is the definitive study to rule out these diagnoses.

Audiometry would be appropriate if the patient had decreased auditory acuity, but this patient's physical examination findings do not suggest hearing loss.

External noise generators to mask the sound of tinnitus are helpful for some patients and may be reasonable to consider in this patient if no reversible cause is found. Evidence supporting their efficacy is sparse, however. The mainstay of therapy for tinnitus is neurocognitive interventions to help patients cope with the problem and diminish dysfunctional cognitive processes associated with the experience of tinnitus.

Nasal corticosteroid sprays can be helpful in patients with eustachian tube dysfunction, although this is an uncommon cause of tinnitus associated with conductive hearing loss. This patient does not demonstrate conductive hearing loss and has no evidence of middle ear congestion on examination. Thus, nasal corticosteroids are not indicated as the next step in management.

KEY POINT

• Patients with pulsatile tinnitus should be evaluated for the possible presence of an intracranial vascular anomaly, such as stenosis, arteriovenous malformation, or glomus tumor as a cause of their symptoms.

Bibliography

Liyanage SH, Singh A, Savundra P, Kalan A. Pulsatile tinnitus. J Laryngol Otol. 2006;120(2):93-97. [PMID: 16359136]

Item 10   Answer: D

Educational Objective: Counsel a patient regarding methods for smoking cessation.

Although both counseling and pharmacotherapy are effective strategies for smoking cessation, the combination of counseling with medication use is more effective than either intervention alone. Nicotine replacement is effective for smoking cessation; its availability in multiple formulations (gum, lozenge, patch, aerosol) allows for alternative options in patients who have not benefited from one type of therapy, as in this patient. Although centrally acting agents (bupropion, varenicline) are also effective treatment options, bupropion would be contraindicated in this patient with an underlying seizure disorder. The choice of cessation method is less important than that an effective method is used correctly by the patient; the array of treatment options allows for individualization based on patient preference, previous experience, cost, and potential side effects. Counseling may be brief or intensive; the two most effective counseling components include practical problem-solving skills and social support.

Many smokers indicate that stress reduction is a primary reason for their tobacco use. Although selected individuals with true anxiety disorders may benefit from anxiolytic therapy, the use of benzodiazepines as a smoking cessation medication has not been documented.

Electronic smokeless cigarettes deliver a warmed aerosol through a cigarette-like device that bears the appearance, physical sensation, and possibly the taste of tobacco smoke, with the intention of helping smokers maintain the activities associated with smoking but without the harmful effects. However, their use in smoking cessation has not been established.

KEY POINT

• Smoking cessation is achieved more effectively with a combination of counseling and anti-smoking medication use than with either intervention alone.

Bibliography

2008 PHS Guideline Update Panel, Liasons, and Staff. Treating tobacco use and dependence: 2008 update U.S. Public Health Service

Clinical Practice Guideline executive summary. Respir Care. 2008;53(9):1217-1222. [PMID: 18807274]

Item 11   Answer: A

Educational Objective: Manage viral conjunctivitis.

The most appropriate management is the application of cool compresses to the affected eye. This patient has symptoms and signs most consistent with viral conjunctivitis. Onset is usually acute, with unilateral redness, watery discharge, itching, crusting, a diffuse foreign body sensation, and mild photophobia. This patient's preceding upper respiratory tract infection, normal vision, and unilateral eye involvement are supportive of this diagnosis. Viral conjunctivitis is managed conservatively with cool compresses. The patient should be told not to share towels or other personal items with family members and should wash his hands frequently throughout the day. He should also be warned that the infection may spread to the other eye before resolving.

Allergic conjunctivitis may be recurrent and seasonal and presents with itching, conjunctival edema, and cobblestoning under the upper lid. It usually responds to topical antihistamines, short-course topical NSAIDs (3 days maximum), and compresses. Oral antihistamines have no role in the treatment of viral conjunctivitis.

Bacterial conjunctivitis usually has a mucopurulent discharge, in contrast to the clear, watery discharge seen in viral conjunctivitis. Topical antibiotics are not efficacious for viral conjunctivitis and can be associated with adverse effects, including the development of contact dermatitis and antibiotic resistance. If a lubricant is required, nonantibacterial lubricating agents may be used.

Topical corticosteroids are not indicated despite the patient's discomfort and should rarely, if ever, be used by physicians other than ophthalmologists. If used inappropriately for herpes simplex, fungal, or bacterial conjunctivitis, topical corticosteroids can lead to corneal scarring, melting, and perforation.

KEY POINT

• Viral conjunctivitis, characterized by acute onset and unilateral redness, watery discharge, itching, crusting, a diffuse foreign body sensation, and mild photophobia, is managed conservatively with cool compresses.

Bibliography

Galor A, Jeng BH. Red eye for the internist: when to treat, when to refer. Clev Clin J Med. 2008;75(2):137-144. [PMID: 18290357]

Item 12   Answer: A

Educational Objective: Identify anchoring as a source of diagnostic error.

This case illustrates an error resulting from an anchoring heuristic. Heuristics are cognitive shortcuts that clinicians employ in an attempt to efficiently reach a diagnosis. Anchoring occurs when a diagnostician latches onto a diagnosis and fails to consider other possibilities for the presenting symptoms. The physician in this case settled on a diagnosis because another physician previously diagnosed the patient. Despite the fact that there are other pieces of data that do not fit the diagnosis—tachycardia, relative hypotension, abdominal distention, and lack of reproducibility of pain with musculoskeletal examination contrary to the diagnosis of "groin strain"—the clinician remains anchored to the diagnosis established in the emergency department. This type of error can be avoided by explicitly looking for findings that do not fit the diagnosis as well as by using a "worst case scenario" approach to patient care—considering the diagnoses that would be most life-threatening to the patient, such as an abdominal aortic aneurysm in a patient with risk factors for this condition.

The availability heuristic is used when a clinician attempts to make a diagnosis based upon what is available in the physician's mind rather than what is most probable. For example, if the physician had seen a similar patient with a groin strain from physical activity the previous week and decided that this was the most likely diagnosis, the clinician would be missing the diagnosis because of the availability heuristic.

A no-fault error is one in which the presentation is misleading and the clinician has little opportunity to pick up clues based on any data that there is an underlying problem.

The representativeness heuristic is used when the clinician applies pattern recognition in making a diagnosis. This source of diagnostic error occurs when the patient's clinical presentation appears to fit a typical case with similar features but the clinician fails to consider other disease processes that may also present in this manner.

KEY POINT

- **Anchoring heuristic errors occur when a clinician holds to an initial impression, such as might occur when a referring physician has provided a diagnosis that is then accepted at face value.**

Bibliography
Trowbridge RL. Twelve tips for teaching avoidance of diagnostic errors. Med Teach. 2008;30(5):496-500. [PMID: 18576188]

Item 13   Answer: C
Educational Objective: Treat acute rhinosinusitis.

Treatment with chlorpheniramine may be considered for this patient. The common cold, or rhinosinusitis, presents with acute cough, nasal congestion, rhinorrhea, and occasionally, low-grade fever. Targeted treatment is aimed at symptom relief. Antihistamines, such as chlorpheniramine, and antihistamine-decongestant combinations have been shown to decrease congestion and rhinorrhea with variable

effects on cough suppression. Second-generation nonsedating antihistamines are generally ineffective for rhinosinusitis symptoms.

Albuterol does not relieve symptoms of rhinosinusitis unless wheezing is present. The patient did not report wheezing or shortness of breath, and wheezes were not heard on examination.

Because rhinosinusitis is caused by viruses, routine antibiotic treatment in immunocompetent hosts is not recommended. Antibiotics do not improve symptoms, illness duration, or patient satisfaction with medical care. Contrary to common belief, purulent sputum does not reliably predict bacterial infection or superinfection. Therefore, sputum purulence should not be used as a criterion for antibiotic administration. Evidence-based guidelines from the Infectious Diseases Society of America suggest that if bacterial rhinosinusitis is highly suspected, based on the presence of persistent symptoms or signs lasting more than 10 days without evidence of clinical improvement, onset with severe symptoms (fever >39.0 °C [102.2 °F]), or onset with worsening symptoms or signs (new fever, headache, or upper respiratory tract infection symptoms that were initially improving), the antibiotic of choice is amoxicillin-clavulanate.

Multiple studies have found little if any improvement in acute cough associated with acute upper respiratory tract infections by using codeine, dextromethorphan, or moguisteine antitussive therapy. The American College of Chest Physicians does not recommend treatment with these medications. Codeine may be effective in patients with chronic cough; however, it is not indicated in this patient with acute rhinosinusitis.

Other treatments that may relieve symptoms of rhinosinusitis include intranasal ipratropium (rhinorrhea and sneezing), intranasal cromolyn (rhinorrhea, cough, throat pain), and short-term topical nasal decongestants (nasal obstruction). Consistent high-quality data on the use of zinc, echinacea, and vitamin C do not support the use of these over-the-counter products for the treatment or prevention of rhinosinusitis.

KEY POINT

- **Antibiotics are not recommended for the treatment of acute rhinosinusitis.**

Bibliography
Siamasek M, Blandino DA. Treatment of the common cold. Am Fam Physician. 2007;75(4):515-520. [PMID: 17323712]

Item 14   Answer: A
Educational Objective: Diagnose benign paroxysmal positional vertigo.

This patient has benign paroxysmal positional vertigo (BPPV). The first step in the evaluation of the patient with dizziness is to distinguish among its major causes: vertigo, presyncope, dysequilibrium, and other nonspecific causes.

This patient describes classic vertigo, a sensation that his stationary environment is spinning around him (or that one is spinning around in one's environment).

There are two major categories of vertigo, peripheral and central. Peripheral causes of vertigo include BPPV, vestibular neuronitis, Meniere disease, aminoglycoside toxicity, and herpes zoster. Patients with all causes of peripheral vertigo have similar findings on the Dix-Hallpike maneuver, in which the examiner supports the patient's head in 20 degrees of extension while sitting, then assists the patient rapidly to the supine position with the head turned to one side and hanging over the edge of the examining table; the test is repeated with the head turned to the other side. A positive test results in horizontal nystagmus with latency of 2 to 40 seconds and duration less than 1 minute, with reproduction of symptoms that will fatigue and habituate. Patients with BPPV describe episodes of vertigo lasting less than 1 minute that occur with a rapid change in head position, as in this patient. Nervous system imaging or other testing is not required for diagnosis in patients with classic findings and an otherwise normal neurologic examination.

Central vertigo may result from ischemia, infarction, or hemorrhage of the brainstem or cerebellum. It is accompanied by diplopia, dysarthria, dysphagia, focal weakness, numbness, or gait abnormalities, depending on the involved area of the brain. On the Dix-Hallpike maneuver, the induced nystagmus has no latency, lasts more than 1 minute, and can have a vertical direction. The Dix-Hallpike maneuver findings in this patient are consistent with peripheral, not central, vertigo. As he has neither cardiovascular risk factors nor focal neurologic abnormalities, cerebellar infarction is unlikely.

The classic triad of Meniere disease is vertigo, unilateral hearing loss, and tinnitus. The vertigo in Meniere disease is usually not positional, as in this patient, and he does not have hearing loss or tinnitus.

Vestibular neuronitis is frequently associated with a viral infection. Symptoms generally last much longer than they do in BPPV (days) but can be more severe. Although symptoms typically resolve within 1 week, residual dizziness can last for months. The recurrent, intense, and brief nature of this patient's episodes of vertigo makes BPPV a more likely diagnosis.

KEY POINT

- Benign paroxysmal positional vertigo is characterized by brief episodes of severe vertigo brought on by a rapid change in head position and Dix-Hallpike maneuver findings of delayed horizontal nystagmus with a rotatory component concurrent with symptoms of vertigo.

Bibliography
Bhattacharyya N, Baugh RF, Orvidas L, et al. Clinical practice guideline: benign paroxysmal positional vertigo. Otolaryngol Head Neck Surg. 2008;139(5)(suppl 4):S47-81. [PMID: 18973840]

Item 15   Answer: D

Educational Objective: Diagnose vitamin B_{12} deficiency in a patient who has undergone gastric bypass surgery.

This patient's serum vitamin B_{12} level should be measured. Macrocytic anemia, thrombocytopenia, mild neutropenia, and an inappropriately low reticulocyte count are the hallmark hematologic findings in vitamin B_{12} deficiency. Vitamin B_{12} deficiency is one the most common nonoperative complications of Roux-en-Y gastric bypass surgery. It results from decreased absorption of vitamin B_{12}, mainly through lack of intrinsic factor production from the bypassed gastric mucosa. It is essential for patients who undergo a roux-en-Y gastric bypass procedure to participate in postoperative monitoring of vitamin B_{12} levels and to maintain lifelong adequate vitamin B_{12} supplementation (500-1000 micrograms/d orally or 1000 micrograms intramuscularly monthly). Recent guidelines recommend that serum vitamin B_{12} levels, along with ferritin, folate, vitamin D, and calcium, be monitored twice yearly for the first 2 years after Roux-en-Y gastric bypass surgery and yearly thereafter.

A bone marrow biopsy, a relatively invasive and costly test, is premature at this point. Bone marrow biopsy is indicated for unexplained anemia, leukopenia, thrombocytopenia, or pancytopenia. The patient has a high likelihood of vitamin B_{12} deficiency that can explain the patient's hematologic findings, and a performing a bone marrow biopsy prior to measuring the serum vitamin B_{12} level would be inappropriate.

With no gastrointestinal symptoms, no family history of colorectal cancer, a benign abdominal examination, guaiac-negative stool, and a macrocytic (not microcytic) anemia with neutropenia and thrombocytopenia, the suspicion for gastrointestinal malignancy or other lower gastrointestinal tract disease is very low. Therefore, a colonoscopy is not indicated at this point.

Based on history and physical examination, there is no strong clinical suspicion for thyroid disease. Although hypothyroidism can be associated with mild macrocytosis, the presence of neutropenia and thrombocytopenia is inconsistent with this diagnosis. Therefore, measuring the serum thyroid-stimulating hormone level is not indicated.

KEY POINT

- Vitamin B_{12} deficiency is common after Roux-en-Y gastric bypass surgery.

Bibliography
Buchwald H, Ikramuddin S, Dorman RB, Schone JL, Dixon JB. Management of the metabolic/bariatric surgery patient. Am J Med. 2011;124(12):1099-1105. [PMID: 22014789]

Item 16   Answer: D

Educational Objective: Manage a patient's request for genetic testing.

This patient should be referred for genetic counseling. Huntington disease is an autosomal dominant disorder caused by a CAG repeat within the gene on chromosome 4. Because of the potential harms from genetic test information and the need for patients and their families to receive appropriate information for decision-making, patients with possible inherited diseases should undergo genetic testing only in the context of genetic counseling. Genetic counseling should include discussion of possible risks and benefits of early detection and prevention modalities. Genetic counseling with the option for testing should be offered when: (1) the patient has a personal or family history suggestive of a genetic susceptibility condition; (2) the genetic test can be adequately interpreted; and (3) the test results will aid in diagnosis or influence the medical or surgical management of the patient or family at hereditary risk.

Brain MRI in patients with well-defined findings of Huntington disease demonstrates caudate atrophy. Such imaging is unlikely to be helpful in an asymptomatic patient and is not preferred to genetic counseling in estimating the likelihood of disease.

Symptoms of Huntington disease typically begin in the fourth and fifth decades, but 10% of patients have symptoms in the second decade. It is premature to reassure the patient, considering her young age and absence of genetic test data.

KEY POINT

- Patients with possible inherited diseases should be referred for genetic testing only in the context of genetic counseling.

Bibliography

Berg AO, Baird MA, Botkin JR, et al. National Institute of Health State-of-the-Science Conference Statement: Family History and Improving Health. Ann Intern Med. 2009; 151(12):872-877. [PMID: 19884615]

Item 17   Answer: A
Educational Objective: Manage a pressure ulcer.

This patient has a stage III or IV pressure ulcer, and debridement is the most appropriate management. Both stage III and stage IV pressure ulcers include full-thickness tissue loss. In stage III ulcers, subcutaneous fat may be visible but bone, tendon, and muscle are not exposed, whereas in stage IV ulcers, bone, tendon, or muscle is exposed and undermining and tunneling are often present. The eschar covering this patient's wound precludes the definitive differentiation of a stage III from a stage IV ulcer.

Treatment of pressure ulcers is best managed with an interdisciplinary team approach, with a care plan directed toward addressing the factors that predisposed to the development of the ulcer. Dressings should be chosen to maintain a moist wound environment and manage exudates. When present, infection should be controlled with topical therapies and the addition of systemic antibiotics

when cellulitis is present. The possibility of underlying osteomyelitis should be considered. Surgical or nonsurgical debridement of eschar and nonviable tissue may be needed. Wet-to-dry dressings may aid in debridement but caution must be used to avoid removing excessive viable tissue with dressing changes.

Cochrane reviews do not support a role for electromagnetic therapy, ultrasound therapy, or hyperbaric oxygen therapy in pressure ulcer treatment.

Negative-pressure wound vacuum healing has been used for stage IV ulcers. However, three clinical trials have not shown superiority to standard therapy. Wound vacuum therapy may be more convenient due to less frequent dressing changes but is also very costly. It is not the recommended first line therapy.

Although frequently utilized, vitamin C and zinc oral supplements have not been shown to aid in ulcer healing.

Referral for surgical flap and repair may be necessary for refractory pressure ulcers but is usually reserved for patients in whom conservative treatment has failed.

KEY POINT

- Stage III pressure ulcers, defined by full-thickness tissue loss but without exposure of bone, tendon, or muscle, generally require debridement, proper dressing selection, and treatment of infection, if present.

Bibliography

Reddy M, Gill SS, Kalkar SR, et al. Treatment of pressure ulcers: a systematic review. JAMA. 2008;300(22):2647-2662. [PMID: 19066385]

Item 18   Answer: E
Educational Objective: Diagnose benign prostatic hyperplasia.

The most important diagnostic test to perform next in this patient is urinalysis. Benign prostatic hyperplasia (BPH) is an extremely common cause of lower urinary tract symptoms in men, such as nocturia, urinary frequency and urgency, decreased urinary stream, urinary retention, incomplete bladder emptying, and incontinence. Symptoms may worsen with increasing size of the prostate. The American Urological Association (AUA) recommends screening and following the AUA symptom score to assess need for and effectiveness of treatment. Diagnostic work-up for BPH includes the necessity to rule out underlying infection. Although this patient does not have specific symptoms or clinical findings suggestive of a urinary tract infection, abnormal bladder emptying increases the risk for infection, and even subclinical infection may exacerbate BPH symptoms. Therefore, urinalysis (and if positive, a subsequent urine culture) is indicated in this patient.

Postvoid residual urinary volumes are measured via in-and-out catheterization or by ultrasonography after a patient spontaneously voids. This test is not indicated for routine management of BPH but is useful in evaluation of overflow incontinence or neurogenic bladder. As neither of these conditions is present in this patient, postvoid residual urinary volume measurement is not indicated.

Elevated plasma glucose levels may cause urinary frequency and nocturia due to osmotic diuresis but are unlikely to cause weak stream or urinary hesitancy. Additionally, urinary incontinence due to neurogenic bladder can be seen in late-stage diabetes mellitus with neuropathic complications; however, this patient has no history of diabetes mellitus and is not incontinent.

The U.S. Preventive Services Task Force has concluded that the harms of screening for prostate cancer outweigh the benefits in men of any age regardless of risk factors. Other guidelines, including those of the AUA, recommend offering periodic screening to men older than 50 years who have a life expectancy of at least 10 years. The presence of BPH symptoms does not affect indications for prostate cancer screening.

Transrectal ultrasound of the prostate is most commonly used for evaluation of prostate cancer. Prostate cancer itself rarely causes lower urinary tract symptoms as seen in this patient.

KEY POINT

- Diagnostic work-up for benign prostatic hyperplasia (BPH) includes urinalysis to rule out underlying infection; neither post-void residual urinary volume measurement nor prostate-specific antigen testing is indicated in the routine evaluation of BPH.

Bibliography
McVary KT, Roehrborn CG, Avins AL, et al. Update on AUA guideline on the management of benign prostatic hyperplasia. J Urol. 2011;185(5):1793-1803. [PMID: 21420124]

Item 19   Answer: D
Educational Objective: Treat cancer-related pain.

Sustained-release morphine should be started to better control this patient's cancer-related pain. Long-acting morphine is indicated in cancer patients who develop persistent pain throughout the day or beyond 24 hours of treatment with shorter-acting opioids. The initial dose is usually 30% to 50% of a patient's current 24-hour usage of short-acting opioid. He should also be prescribed short-acting oral morphine for breakthrough pain, and his long-acting morphine should be gradually titrated upward until his pain is well controlled.

A fentanyl patch is convenient and reduces frequency of dosing but will take 24 hours to begin working. Therefore, used alone it would not be the correct choice for this patient who is being discharged today.

Methadone, a long-acting opioid, has an unpredictable half-life that varies from patient to patient making it

challenging to dose-adjust. It has also been linked to QT-interval prolongation and other arrhythmias. It should be used with caution, with monitoring of the QT interval. For these reasons, methadone is generally a less ideal choice for long-term pain control in cancer patients.

Short-acting hydromorphone has a rapid onset of action and is dosed every 4 to 6 hours. This would not be optimal in this patient as he requires sustained relief from his pain and would require repeated doses for adequate control, including during hours of sleep. Extended-release hydromorphone preparations are now available, and in conjunction with short-acting hydromorphone for breakthrough pain, these formulations would also be a reasonable treatment option.

KEY POINT

- Long-acting morphine is indicated in cancer patients who develop persistent pain throughout the day or beyond 24 hours of treatment with shorter-acting opioids; the initial dose is usually 30% to 50% of a patient's current 24-hour usage of short-acting opioid.

Bibliography
Swetz KM, Kamal AH. Palliative care. Ann Intern Med. 2012;156(3):ITC2-1-TC2-16. [PMID: 22312158]

Item 20   Answer: C
Educational Objective: Manage unilateral sensorineural hearing loss.

This patient should undergo MRI of the posterior fossa and internal auditory canal. His sensorineural hearing loss is confirmed on physical examination, which demonstrates lateralization of the Weber test to the left ear and demonstration of better hearing with air conduction than bone conduction with the Rinne test. The Rinne test is about 80% sensitive in diagnosing sensorineural hearing loss. In patients with asymmetric sensorineural hearing loss that is not clearly due to Meniere disease, contrast-enhanced MRI of the posterior fossa and internal auditory canal should be considered to exclude acoustic neuroma and meningioma.

Continuous tinnitus most often originates within the auditory system and is usually a consequence of sensorineural hearing loss. A high-pitched continuous tone is most common. Low-pitched tinnitus may be seen in patients with Meniere disease. Other causes are noise exposure, ototoxic medications, presbycusis, otosclerosis, acoustic neuroma, and barotrauma. Treatment of tinnitus should first be directed at the underlying disorder. Behavioral therapies include biofeedback, stress reduction, and cognitive-behavioral therapy directed at improving the patient's ability to cope with tinnitus. Behavioral therapy is not appropriate until other remediable causes of tinnitus are excluded.

Sudden sensorineural hearing loss is defined as hearing loss occurring in 3 days or less. Ninety percent of patients have unilateral hearing loss, and some have tinnitus, ear fullness, and vertigo. It is considered an otologic emergency, and oral corticosteroids are usually given, although randomized trials differ in their conclusions regarding efficacy. This patient's hearing loss has occurred over a period of months, and oral corticosteroids are not indicated.

Benign paroxysmal positional vertigo (BPPV) is the most common cause of vestibular dizziness. BPPV is thought to be caused by otolith debris within the semicircular canal. Otolith repositioning has been shown helpful in resolving symptoms of BPPV, however this patient does not have symptoms compatible with BPPV and therefore this intervention is not warranted.

KEY POINT

- **In patients with asymmetric sensorineural hearing loss that is not clearly due to Meniere disease, contrast-enhanced MRI of the posterior fossa and internal auditory canal should be considered to exclude acoustic neuroma and meningioma.**

Bibliography

McDonald R. Acoustic neuroma: what the evidence says about evaluation and treatment. J Fam Pract. 2011;60(6):E1-4. [PMID: 21647465]

Item 21   Answer: B
Educational Objective: Diagnose the cause of a syncopal episode.

In this elderly woman, given the short prodrome, palpitations, and history of a previous event, a cardiac arrhythmia is the most likely cause of syncope. Arrhythmias are the most common causes of syncope in the elderly population. Patients with an arrhythmogenic cause of syncope usually have had only one or two episodes. A prodrome is usually brief or absent. The patient often experiences palpitations immediately preceding the episode.

Aortic stenosis may cause syncope; however, despite a low-grade systolic murmur, this patient's carotid upstrokes are normal and her episode occurred at rest and not with exertion, making aortic stenosis unlikely.

Myocardial ischemia is a rare cause of syncope, especially in the absence of typical ischemic symptoms. Myocardial ischemia is a consideration in patients with an arrhythmia leading to presyncope or syncope as ischemic myocardium may be arrhythmogenic. However, myocardial ischemia as a cause of hypoperfusion in a patient without symptoms at rest would likely not account for her clinical presentation.

This patient has several risk factors for a possible transient ischemic attack (TIA). However, TIAs typically present with focal neurologic symptoms and findings, and are rarely a cause of syncope.

KEY POINT

- **Arrhythmia is a common cause of syncope in the elderly; arrhythmogenic syncope is characterized by a brief or absent prodrome and palpitations immediately preceding the event.**

Bibliography

Moya A, Sutton R, Ammirati F, et al; Task Force for the Diagnosis and Management of Syncope; European Society of Cardiology (ESC); European Heart Rhythm Association (EHRA); Heart Failure Association (HFA); Heart Rhythm Society (HRS). Guidelines for the diagnosis and management of syncope (version 2009). Eur Heart J. 2009;30(21):2631-2671. [PMID: 19713422]

Item 22   Answer: A
Educational Objective: Treat bilateral symmetric lower extremity edema due to venous stasis.

The most appropriate treatment for this patient is use of compression stockings. This obese woman has dependent symmetric bilateral lower extremity edema caused by venous insufficiency. Her normal cardiovascular and abdominal examinations, along with normal creatinine and albumin levels, urinalysis, and liver chemistry tests, rules out significant heart, lung, kidney, or liver disease as causative. The most effective treatments for edema due to chronic venous stasis are weight reduction, sodium restriction, leg elevation, and compression stockings. External compression decreases accumulation of tissue fluid in the lower extremities that is unable to be removed through the venous system. Compression stockings are particularly effective when used for extended periods when in the upright position to prevent dependent pooling of fluid.

Lower abdominal and pelvic imaging may be useful in assessing for lesions obstructing venous and lymphatic return as a cause of bilateral lower extremity edema. However, this is an uncommon cause of swelling in an otherwise healthy individual with a typical clinical picture of venous insufficiency.

According to expert opinion, diuretics should be avoided in patients with chronic venous insufficiency because they do not predictably lead to mobilization of fluid from the interstitial to the vascular space. Instead, diuretics may lead to decreased intravascular volume followed by orthostatic hypotension and prerenal azotemia.

Lower extremity venous duplex ultrasonography is useful in evaluating for the presence of venous thrombosis. In this patient there is no suspicion of deep vein thrombosis, and imaging is not necessary for a diagnosis of venous insufficiency without additional concerning signs or symptoms.

KEY POINT

- **The most effective treatments for edema due to chronic venous stasis are sodium restriction, leg elevation, weight reduction, and compression stockings; diuretics should be avoided.**

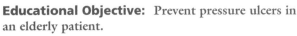

Bibliography

O'Brien JG, Chennubhotla SA, Chennubhotla RV. Treatment of edema. Am Fam Physician. 2005;71(11):2111-2117. [PMID: 15952439]

Item 23   Answer: A

Educational Objective: Manage a suspected rotator cuff tear.

This patient should undergo MRI of the left shoulder. He most likely has a complete left supraspinatus rotator cuff tear. The diagnosis is suggested by his difficulty with abducting the left arm and the positive drop-arm test. The drop-arm test can be performed by the examiner passively abducting the patient's arm and then having the patient slowly lower the arm to the waist. When a complete supraspinatus tear is present, the patient's arm often drops to the waist. Although imaging is not necessary in most patients with uncomplicated shoulder pain, because of the high likelihood of a complete supraspinatus tear by history and examination, it is appropriate to obtain an MRI to confirm the diagnosis. MRI has a high sensitivity (>90%) and specificity in the diagnosis of rotator cuff tears. Not all rotator cuff tears require surgical intervention and many respond to conservative therapy; however, establishing the diagnosis and obtaining more detailed anatomic information are necessary in making the decision about whether surgery would be indicated.

Medication with an NSAID may form a component of the initial treatment plan but a confirmed diagnosis is necessary to make definitive treatment decisions.

Although referral to physical therapy is appropriate for suspected or confirmed incomplete tears, it would not be the appropriate first step in this patient with a suspected complete tear who is young and has no medical comorbidities.

Performing a subacromial corticosteroid injection would not be the most appropriate option in this patient who is suspected of having a complete supraspinatus tear. Subacromial corticosteroid injections have been shown to provide pain relief that lasts up to 9 months in patients with rotator cuff tendinitis or an impingement syndrome, but a significant tear may require surgical intervention, and this should be determined as an initial step in management.

KEY POINT

- **MRI has a high sensitivity and specificity for diagnosing a rotator cuff tear.**

Bibliography

Seida JC, LeBlanc C, Schouten JR, et al. Systematic review: nonoperative and operative treatments for rotator cuff tears. Ann Intern Med. 2010;153(4):246-255. [PMID: 20621893]

Item 24   Answer: D

Educational Objective: Prevent pressure ulcers in an elderly patient.

The most appropriate intervention for preventing pressure ulcers in this patient is use of a pressure-distributing mattress. He was admitted to the hospital with peritonitis and has a very high risk for pressure ulcer given his limited mobility, ascites, and low serum albumin level. The blanching erythematous patches on his lower back and buttocks must be watched carefully because they are at-risk areas for ulceration. A nonblanching erythematous patch is a stage I pressure ulcer. There is evidence that pressure reduction, accomplished through frequent patient repositioning and use of pressure-distributing support surfaces, is effective in reducing the risk of ulcers. The strongest evidence of benefit exists for higher-specification foam mattresses compared with standard hospital mattresses; beds or mattresses that actively alternate pressure by shifting air or water are of unclear benefit, but may be useful in clinical situations in which prolonged bedrest is required. Medical-grade sheepskin overlays also have some evidence of benefit compared with standard hospital mattresses. Bed overlays made of foam, gel, or water or air-filled pockets are commonly used, although their efficacy in preventing ulcer development has not been established and there is some evidence that they may contribute to additional skin irritation.

Air-filled vinyl boots, water-filled gloves, regular sheepskin, and doughnut-type devices are likely to be harmful and should not be used for prevention of pressure ulcers.

Indwelling urinary catheters increase the risk of urinary tract infection if left in place. Although they are frequently placed specifically to avoid urine contact with skin areas at high risk of ulceration, other mechanisms to avoid moisture contact with the area at risk for breakdown are preferred.

KEY POINT

- **Pressure-distributing mattresses and medical-grade sheepskin overlays reduce the incidence of pressure ulcers in high-risk patients.**

Bibliography

McInnes E, Jammali-Blasi A, Bell-Syer SE, Dumville JC, Cullum N. Support surfaces for pressure ulcer prevention. Cochrane Database Syst Rev. 2011;(4):CD001735. [PMID: 21491384]

Item 25   Answer: D

Educational Objective: Treat menopausal vaginal symptoms.

The most appropriate management of this patient is vaginal estradiol. The clinical history and physical examination are most helpful for making the diagnosis of vaginal atrophy; pale vaginal walls, decreased rugae, and petechiae are characteristic findings. Approximately 10% to 40% of menopausal women experience symptoms related to vaginal atrophy, which include vulvar itching, vaginal dryness, and dyspareunia. In contrast to menopausal vasomotor symptoms, which may last for a few years and resolve spontaneously, vaginal atrophy is frequently progressive and often requires treatment. Mild to moderate symptoms can be treated with vaginal moisturizers and lubricants, but more severe symptoms, as experienced by this patient, are best treated with vaginal estrogen. Low-dose vaginal estradiol tablets (10-25 micrograms) and the estradiol vaginal ring (8-9 micrograms) are preferred over vaginal estrogen creams, as they result in minimal systemic estrogen absorption.

Although oral estrogen therapy is effective for relieving vaginal atrophy symptoms, it has been associated with several adverse outcomes, including increased rates of coronary heart disease, stroke, venous thromboembolism, and invasive breast cancer. For that reason, current guidelines recommend the use of low-dose local, rather than systemic, estrogen therapy for the treatment of patients who only have vaginal symptoms.

Bacterial vaginosis is characterized by a vaginal discharge, an increased vaginal pH, and clue cells on normal saline preparation and a positive "whiff" test; the absence of these findings in this patient argues against this diagnosis. Treatment for bacterial vaginosis with metronidazole would therefore not be indicated.

Yeast infections are often accompanied by a thick white discharge that is potassium hydroxide–positive. This patient does not have discharge and no hyphae are seen on potassium hydroxide preparation; therefore, she is unlikely to respond to vaginal clotrimazole therapy.

KEY POINT

- **Vaginal estrogen is the recommended therapy for severe symptoms of vaginal atrophy that have not responded to vaginal moisturizers and lubricants.**

Bibliography

North American Menopause Society. The role of local vaginal estrogen for treatment of vaginal atrophy in postmenopausal women: 2007 position statement of The North American Menopause Society. Menopause. 2007;14(3 Pt 1):355-369. [PMID: 17438512]

Item 26   Answer: A

Educational Objective: Diagnosis acromioclavicular joint degeneration.

This patient's pain is originating from his acromioclavicular joint. Given his age, his pain is most likely due to osteoarthritis. Acromioclavicular joint degeneration typically results from trauma (in younger patients) or osteoarthritis (in older patients). Bilateral involvement should raise concern for rheumatoid arthritis. On examination, there is typically pain to palpation of the acromioclavicular joint. Pain on palpation is a very sensitive but not specific sign of acromioclavicular joint disease; absent pain on palpation makes acromioclavicular joint disease unlikely. Palpable osteophytes may be present. Pain

characteristically occurs with shoulder adduction and abduction above 120 degrees.

Adhesive capsulitis is caused by thickening of the capsule surrounding the glenohumeral joint. Pain is characteristically slow in onset and is located near the insertion of the deltoid muscle, and patients often avoid lying on the affected side. On examination, there is loss of both active and passive range of motion. Although this patient's symptoms have been insidious in onset, which could be consistent with adhesive capsulitis, he does not have limited range of motion in all or most planes of motion, which argues against adhesive capsulitis.

Examination findings of a rotator cuff tear include supraspinatus weakness, weakness with external rotation, evidence of impingement, and a positive drop-arm test (inability to slowly and steadily lower the arm completely; the arm drops to the side). The patient has a negative drop-arm sign, which argues against rotator cuff tear.

The patient does not have pain between 60 to 120 degrees of abduction, has normal internal/external rotation, and has a negative Neer and Hawkins sign, all of which argue against the diagnosis of rotator cuff tendinitis.

KEY POINT

- **Acromioclavicular joint degeneration is characterized by pain to palpation of the acromioclavicular joint and pain that occurs with shoulder adduction and abduction above 120 degrees.**

Bibliography

House J, Mooradian A. Evaluation and management of shoulder pain in primary care clinics. South Med J. 2010;103(11):1129-1135. [PMID: 20890250]

Item 27   Answer: A

Educational Objective: Counsel a patient regarding smoking cessation.

Current recommendations are that all clinicians assess tobacco use at every visit, encourage every patient to make a quit attempt, and counsel patients appropriately. Patients who exhibit medical illnesses related to smoking present an opportunity for clinicians to increase the patient's awareness of the connection between the unhealthy behavior and its negative consequences. Even if time does not allow for an in-depth counseling session, all patients should be asked about their smoking at every visit, and a brief, clear message about quitting should be provided to all patients. A recommended strategy for counseling is to follow the "five A's": Ask every patient at every visit about their smoking; Advise all smokers to quit; Assess their current interest in quitting; Assist by offering resources and/or medications, and Arrange for follow-up.

It is not clear yet whether this patient is truly interested in quitting. Thus it would be inappropriate to prescribe either smoking cessation aids or counseling until the physician has determined that the patient is indeed ready to quit.

- Tobacco use should be assessed at every visit, and patients who smoke should be encouraged to make a quit attempt and counseled appropriately.

Bibliography

2008 PHS Guideline Update Panel, Liasons, and Staff. Treating tobacco use and dependence: 2008 update U.S. Public Health Service Clinical Practice Guideline executive summary. Respir Care. 2008;53(9):1217-1222. [PMID: 18807274]

Item 28   Answer: A

Educational Objective: Manage postoperative venous thromboembolism prophylaxis in a high-risk patient.

The most appropriate treatment for this patient is venous thromboembolism (VTE) prophylactic therapy for up to 5 weeks with a low-molecular-weight heparin (LMWH), such as enoxaparin. VTE is a major preventable postoperative complication, and nearly all surgical patients should receive some VTE prophylaxis postoperatively. Patients at high risk for VTE, including patients with previous VTE, patients who have undergone orthopedic surgery, and patients with some cancers (especially gynecologic malignancy) should receive extended (up to 5 weeks) prophylaxis with LMWH.

Nonpharmacologic prophylaxis against VTE, such as early ambulation, should be encouraged in all postsurgical patients. Other nonpharmacologic treatments include elastic compression stockings and pneumatic compression devices. However, these treatments are only suitable as the sole modality when either the risk of VTE is very low (outpatient surgery) or the morbidity from excess bleeding is unacceptably high (such as in patients undergoing neurosurgery). This patient's surgery for a gynecologic malignancy places her in a high-risk category, and pharmacologic prophylaxis is indicated.

Inferior vena cava (IVC) filters are sometimes used perioperatively, especially in patients with known VTE or patients with a high risk for VTE who cannot receive prophylaxis because of bleeding risk. This patient does not have an excessive bleeding risk, and IVC placement is not indicated. Although newer IVC filters are thought to be extractable following a procedure, the retrieval rate is not typically 100%, and a filter that cannot be removed postoperatively may complicate ongoing care.

Unfractionated subcutaneous heparin is an accepted medication to prevent VTE. However, in this high-risk patient, extended prophylaxis is indicated; therefore, providing prophylaxis only until the patient is discharged is incorrect.

Warfarin, in both fixed doses and adjusted doses, has been studied for VTE prophylaxis, primarily in the orthopedic setting, and been found to be effective in preventing venous thromboembolism in the perioperative period. However, 3 months of prophylaxis would not be indicated

and would substantially increase the risk of bleeding once the perioperative thromboembolism risk has resolved.

- Surgical patients at high risk for venous thromboembolism, including those with previous venous thromboembolism, patients who have undergone orthopedic surgery, and patients with some cancers (especially gynecologic malignancy), should receive extended (up to 5 weeks) prophylaxis.

Bibliography

Gould MK, Garcia DA, Wren SM, et al; American College of Chest Physicians; Prevention of VTE in nonorthopedic surgical patients: Antithrombotic Therapy and Prevention of Thrombosis, 9th ed: American College of Chest Physicians Evidence-Based Clinical Practice Guidelines. Chest. 2012;141(2 suppl):e227S-e77S.

Item 29   Answer: D

Educational Objective: Diagnose acute retinal detachment.

This patient presents with symptoms consistent with a retinal detachment. Retinal detachment occurs predominantly in myopic patients and is a separation of the retina from underlying retinal epithelium and choroid as fluid from the vitreous cavity enters a tear in the retina and dissects underneath the retina. As with this patient, patients may experience floaters, squiggly lines, flashes of light, and then a sudden peripheral visual defect, appearing as a black curtain that progresses across the visual field. Funduscopic examination usually visualizes the tear and folding of the retina. Treatment is surgical. Prognosis depends upon the extent of the tear and time to surgery, so early recognition and emergent referral are crucial.

Central retinal artery occlusion is marked by painless loss of vision and occurs most frequently in the elderly. It is usually caused by emboli or thrombosis. Examination demonstrates a pale fundus with a cherry-red fovea (accentuated by the pale background).

Central retinal vein occlusion is characterized by abrupt monocular visual loss, and may present with transient episodes of monocular blindness, which can last 2 to 4 hours, longer than is typical for transient arterial retinal ischemia. Patients may report cloudiness of vision rather than frank visual loss. Examination of the retina will show congested, tortuous veins; retinal hemorrhages; and cotton wool spots in the area of the vein occlusion.

Ocular migraine, with or without headache, can cause floaters and squiggly lines but would not cause a visual field defect or a retinal tear and folding seen on funduscopic examination.

The most common presenting symptom in patients with temporal arteritis is a new headache, which this patient does not have. Although visual loss can be sudden and irreversible in the setting of temporal arteritis, it is not preceded by floaters, squiggly lines, or peripheral field defects.

- Patients with a retinal detachment may experience floaters, squiggly lines, flashes of light, and then a sudden peripheral visual defect, appearing as a black curtain that progresses across the visual field.

Bibliography

Magauran B. Conditions requiring emergency ophthalmologic consultation. Emerg Med Clin North Am. 2008;26(1):233-238. [PMID: 18249265]

Item 30   Answer: D

Educational Objective: Implement the Plan-Do-Study-Act (PDSA) cycle in quality improvement.

A specific plan to improve communication of medication allergies from outpatient to inpatient medical records should be developed to attempt to avoid subsequent occurrences. The Plan-Do-Study-Act (PDSA) cycle is a quality improvement approach in which a specific change is planned and implemented on a limited scale, the results are observed, and action is taken based on what is learned. The first step in a PDSA cycle in this case would be to plan an intervention that would remedy the communication deficit between the internist's office records and the hospital's electronic order system and drug allergy alert system. The next steps are to institute the planned intervention in a limited fashion and then to study the outcome of the intervention. The "act" step involves refining the intervention to achieve the ideal outcome based upon what is learned by evaluating the limited intervention. This approach to quality improvement works well in a small-scale health care environment, such as a small office, as well as in a large-scale environment, such as a hospital or health care system.

Most physicians are aware of the importance of patient engagement in their care, but greater involvement by patients may not be adequate in overcoming issues regarding consistent and reliable communication of key medical information across different caregivers in different settings.

Although it is important for patients to know, understand, and communicate their important medical information to other caregivers, not all patients are able to do so in a reliable manner, and this intervention will not address larger systemic issues related to improving quality of care and patient safety.

Electronic health records may be of immeasurable help in improving communication of medical information. However, implementing such systems in institutions and communities is costly, complex, and not easily accomplished, and is not the next step in this case. Clear interventions to avoid known patient safety issues should occur as possible within existing systems, with overall system change to optimize quality of care being the long-term goal.

- The Plan-Do-Study-Act (PDSA) cycle is a quality improvement approach in which a specific change is planned and implemented on a limited scale, the results are observed, and action is taken based on what is learned.

Bibliography

Institute of Medicine of the National Academies. Crossing the Quality Chasm: A New Health System for the 21st Century. www.iom.edu/Reports/2001/Crossing-the-Quality-Chasm-A-New-Health-System-for-the-21st-Century.aspx. Published March 1, 2001. Accessed July 12, 2012.

Item 31   Answer: D

Educational Objective: Evaluate a patient with recurrent syncope.

The most appropriate next step in the evaluation of this patient is tilt-table testing. Tilt-table testing is useful in evaluating recurrent syncope in the absence of heart disease, to discriminate neurocardiogenic from orthostatic syncope, and to evaluate frequent syncope in patients with psychiatric disease. This patient continues to have recurrent syncopal episodes despite normal cardiac and metabolic evaluations without definitive evidence of orthostasis or other explanation for her symptoms.

Electroencephalography may be useful in patients in whom a seizure is suspected as a cause of syncope. However, this patient has no risk factors for seizure and her episodes are without a prodromal aura, evidence of seizure activity, or postictal symptoms suggestive of seizure activity.

Exercise cardiac stress testing has a low yield for syncope in patients at low risk for ischemic heart disease. In this patient with a normal electrocardiogram and echocardiogram, cardiac stress testing would not be expected to contribute significant diagnostic information.

Signal-averaged electrocardiography is a technique designed to detect altered depolarization through the myocardium that could lead to reentrant arrhythmias that may not be evident on surface electrocardiography. It has been studied primarily in patients following myocardial infarction to assess for risk of developing sustained tachyarrhythmias. Its use in evaluating syncope has not been established, however, and its routine use is not recommended.

- Tilt-table testing is useful in evaluating recurrent syncope in the absence of heart disease, to discriminate neurocardiogenic from orthostatic syncope, and to evaluate frequent syncope in patients with psychiatric disease.

Bibliography

Moya A, Sutton R, Ammirati F, et al; Task Force for the Diagnosis and Management of Syncope; European Society of Cardiology (ESC);

European Heart Rhythm Association (EHRA); Heart Failure Association (HFA); Heart Rhythm Society (HRS). Guidelines for the diagnosis and management of syncope (version 2009). Eur Heart J. 2009;30(21):2631-2671. [PMID: 19713422]

Item 32   Answer: C

Educational Objective: Manage medications in a woman who may become pregnant.

The most appropriate treatment for this woman is metformin to treat her type 2 diabetes mellitus. Each visit with a reproductive-age woman represents an opportunity for preconception counseling, as adequate preconception care can reduce the risks for preterm birth and birth anomalies, particularly in a woman actively contemplating pregnancy. If this patient were to become pregnant, her poorly controlled diabetes and hypertension increase her risk for adverse maternal and fetal outcomes. This patient should be counseled about her risk factors for potential medical complications of pregnancy, and she should be referred to a high-risk obstetrician for co-management of her medical and gynecologic issues should she become pregnant. It is essential to avoid prescribing teratogenic medications to reproductive-age women who may become pregnant. Metformin is an FDA pregnancy class B medication and is a reasonable option for controlling this patient's hyperglycemia before pregnancy. If she were to become pregnant, consideration may be given to discontinuing the metformin and starting insulin therapy, which is the preferred treatment of diabetes in pregnancy.

The risk of premature fetal loss is increased in women with systemic lupus erythematosus, particularly in those with the antiphospholipid antibody syndrome. Low-dose aspirin has been used in these patients to attempt to lower this risk, although the effectiveness of this intervention is not clear. As aspirin may interfere with implantation when used near the time of conception and this patient has no clear indication for aspirin therapy at present, it should not be prescribed.

Lisinopril and simvastatin, and all ACE inhibitors and statins, are teratogenic medications and can cause serious fetal anomalies. They are FDA pregnancy class X medications and should not be prescribed to this patient who is anticipating pregnancy. Additionally, although this patient might benefit from treatment with an angiotensin receptor blocker because of her diabetes and proteinuria, this class of medication is also contraindicated in pregnancy owing to its potential teratogenic effects. Labetalol or methyldopa is safely used for the treatment of hypertension in pregnant women, and may be considered for this patient. Bile acid resins, such as colestipol, are not orally absorbed and are FDA pregnancy class B medications. They may be a useful adjunct to diet and lifestyle therapy for managing this patient's dyslipidemia.

> **KEY POINT**
> - Avoidance of potentially teratogenic medications is important when treating medical conditions in reproductive-age women contemplating pregnancy.

Bibliography

Berghella V, Buchanan E, Pereira L, Baxter JK. Preconception care. Obstet Gynecol Surv. 2010;65(2):119-131. [PMID: 20100361]

Item 33   Answer: D

Educational Objective: Treat functional urinary incontinence.

This patient would be best managed by establishing a prompted voiding protocol. Urinary incontinence affects more than 50% of nursing home patients and is associated with significant morbidity and cost. Most of these patients have limited mobility or significant cognitive impairment, leading to a high prevalence of functional incontinence, defined as simply not getting to the toilet quickly enough. In a systematic review of 14 randomized controlled studies involving 1161 nursing home patients, the use of prompted voiding (periodically asking the patient about incontinence, reminding the patient to go to the toilet, and providing praise for maintaining continence and using the toilet) was associated with modest short-term improvement in urinary incontinence.

History, focused examination, and urinalysis are often adequate to classify urinary incontinence. Postvoid residual urine volume determination is most useful if overflow incontinence due to outlet obstruction or a flaccid neurogenic bladder is suspected. Detailed urologic evaluations, such as cystoscopy and urodynamic testing, are unnecessary in uncomplicated urinary incontinence.

An indwelling Foley catheter is not advised as a first-line measure to manage urinary incontinence owing to an increased risk of urinary tract infection, resultant antibiotic treatment, and the development of antibiotic complications and resistance.

Pelvic floor muscle training is effective for stress incontinence, which may be coexistent in this patient, but successful implementation requires a cooperative and cognitively intact patient who can understand and participate in the exercise program.

Tolterodine, a selective anticholinergic antimuscarinic medication, is primarily indicated for urge incontinence and is of no benefit in functional incontinence. In addition, adverse side effects, such as dry mouth and worsening cognitive function, render its use in this patient ill advised.

> **KEY POINT**
> - Prompted voiding is an effective management strategy for patients with functional urinary incontinence.

Bibliography

Fink HA, Taylor BC, Tacklind JW, Rutks IR, Wilt TJ. Treatment interventions in nursing home residents with urinary incontinence: a systematic review of randomized trials. Mayo Clin Proc. 2008;83(12):1332-1343. [PMID: 19046552]

Item 34   Answer: B

Educational Objective: Screen for cervical cancer.

The patient should have a Pap smear in 2 years. Because she has had multiple normal consecutive satisfactory Pap smears, the most appropriate interval for cervical cancer screening is every 3 years (this patient had a Pap smear 1 year ago and should undergo repeat screening in 2 years). Although the U.S. Preventive Services Task Force (USPSTF), the American College of Obstetrics and Gynecology (ACOG), and the American Cancer Society (ACS) each differ slightly in their specific recommendations, each agrees that the screening interval can be extended beyond 1 year for this patient. The USPSTF recommends screening at least once every 3 years following the initiation of screening. In contrast, the ACOG recommends that screening occur every 2 years between the ages of 21 and 29 years and every 3 years beginning at the age of 30 years if the patient has had three normal consecutive satisfactory Pap smears and has no history of in utero diethylstilbestrol exposure, is not immunocompromised, is not HIV-positive, and does not have a history of cervical intraepithelial neoplasia grade 2 or 3. The ACS recommends that screening should be performed every 3 years between the ages of 21 and 29 years. Between the ages of 30 and 65 years, the preferred method of screening is the combination of a Pap smear and human papillomavirus (HPV) DNA testing every 5 years. Alternatively, a Pap smear alone can be performed every 3 years.

Although medical providers can consider using HPV DNA testing along with cervical cytology in women aged 30 years and older to help guide the appropriate screening interval, it should not be used alone owing to poor specificity.

Discontinuation of screening for cervical cancer at the age of 31 years would not be appropriate despite the patient's having multiple previous normal satisfactory Pap smears. It is generally agreed that screening should be continued into the seventh decade, although controversy exists regarding the exact age to stop screening.

KEY POINT

- **In women older than 30 years with no risk factors for cervical cancer or history of abnormal Pap smears, the cervical cancer screening interval can be extended to 3 years with cytology or 5 years with cytology and human papillomavirus DNA testing.**

Bibliography

Moyer VA. Screening for cervical cancer: U.S. Preventive Services Task Force recommendation statement. Ann Intern Med. 2012;156(12):880-891. [PMID: 22711081]

Item 35   Answer: B

Educational Objective: Diagnose mild cognitive impairment.

This patient most likely has mild cognitive impairment (MCI). Memory is the only cognitive domain that is impaired. Impairment of other domains that might suggest dementia would include impairment of language, apraxia (for example, problems with dressing not related to motor dysfunction), and impaired executive functioning, none of which are abnormal in this patient. Patients with MCI have a single or few areas of cognitive impairment, and this patient's deficit is limited to forgetfulness and recalling names. His age is typical for MCI and about one-fifth of patients older than age 70 years have this condition. His Mini–Mental State Examination (MMSE) score is within the expected range of 24-25 for MCI and may even be falsely elevated because of his high intellectual level.

Alzheimer disease is less likely in this patient because there are no impairments in other domains, such as activities of daily living and instrumental activities of daily living; other language difficulties; or personality changes. MMSE scores of 19 to 24 suggest mild dementia, and scores of 10 to 19 suggest moderate dementia. His MMSE score of 25 suggests MCI rather than dementia.

Pseudodementia is a condition in which the cognitive impairment is secondary to depression. Treatment of the depression leads to improvement in cognition. Whereas this patient is frustrated with his condition, he is not depressed.

Although he has risk factors for cerebrovascular disease, vascular dementia would be less likely with his MMSE score of 25 and normal neurologic examination. In addition, vascular dementia would not affect memory in isolation and would likely affect additional cognitive domains and neurologic functioning.

KEY POINT

- **Patients with mild cognitive impairment have a single or few areas of cognitive impairment, and the Mini–Mental State Examination score is typically 24 or 25.**

Bibliography

Plassman BL, Langa KM, Fisher GG, et al. Prevalence of cognitive impairment without dementia in the United States. Ann Intern Med. 2008;148(6):427-434. [PMID: 18347351]

Item 36   Answer: B

Educational Objective: Manage palliative care discussion.

Palliative care discussions with this patient should begin now. It is important to stress to patients that a palliative care discussion is not a discussion of withholding or withdrawal of treatment or patient abandonment. The primary focus of palliative care is to relieve patient suffering and to improve the quality of patients' lives and those of their caregivers.

Palliative care is often thought of as end-of-life care only, but palliative care addresses pain, suffering, and quality of life across all stages of treatment and does not exclude life-prolonging treatment and rehabilitation. Palliative care may be offered along with curative or life-prolonging therapies for patients with complex, life-threatening disorders. Recent literature suggests that early referral for palliative care improves quality of life and decreases depressive symptoms as compared with patients who only receive standard oncologic care. In a study of 151 patients with metastatic non–small cell lung cancer, patients referred for early palliative care had longer median survival than those referred for oncologic care only.

Waiting until the patient develops symptoms, refuses active treatment, or is admitted to hospice care does not take full advantage of the benefits of early and appropriately administered palliative care.

KEY POINT

• Early referral for palliative care in addition to oncologic care improves quality of life and decreases depressive symptoms as compared with standard oncologic care only.

Bibliography

Temel JS, Greer JA, Muzikansky A, et al. Early palliative care for patients with metastatic non-small-cell lung cancer. N Engl J Med. 2010;363(8):733-742. [PMID: 20818875]

Item 37   Answer: A
Educational Objective: Manage acute cervical radiculopathy.

This patient should be treated with analgesics and avoidance of provocative activities. The initial approach to patients with cervical spine radiculopathy, typically due to nerve root compression, is assessment for weakness and possible involvement of the spinal cord (myelopathy). Weakness due to nerve root compression will be seen in the muscles in the area of distribution of the affected nerve(s); myelopathy is seen as additional neurologic symptoms at and below the affected level of the spinal cord. In patients with acute cervical radiculopathy without appreciable motor deficits, imaging and nerve conduction studies are not initially necessary, even if there are mild focal sensory findings. Management should focus on relief of symptoms, as many patients experience complete resolution without intervention.

A variety of nonsurgical treatments are used for management of cervical radiculopathy in addition to nonnarcotic analgesics, including a short course of systemic corticosteroids, hard and soft cervical collars, and cervical pillows, although evidence that these interventions are effective relative to analgesics and rest alone is of poor quality. Cervical traction has also not been documented to be effective and is not recommended as initial treatment for acute cervical radiculopathy.

Imaging studies should be directed based on suspicions raised during history and physical examination. Except in cases of acute trauma, mechanical neck pain rarely requires imaging. Patients with weakness, hyporeflexia, or symptoms or signs of spinal cord involvement should be evaluated with MRI or CT myelography. An electromyelogram and nerve conduction studies are most helpful in patients with radiculopathy that is poorly defined or in those for whom surgery is being considered to localize the specific area of nerve compression. These studies are not indicated in the initial management of cervical spine radiculopathy.

KEY POINT

• Conservative treatment of acute cervical radiculopathy without imaging or further testing is appropriate in patients without trauma or evidence of weakness or myelopathy.

Bibliography

Carette S, Fehlings MG. Clinical practice. Cervical radiculopathy. N Engl J Med. 2005;353:392-399. [PMID: 16049211]

Item 38   Answer: B
Educational Objective: Treat chronic cough due to gastroesophageal reflux disease.

Omeprazole should be continued in this patient. He presents with chronic cough (>8 weeks) most likely due to gastroesophageal reflux disease (GERD). Although typical heartburn symptoms are absent in more than one-third of patients with GERD-related cough, this patient's clinical profile and symptoms of heartburn and cough exacerbated by the recumbent position are classic for GERD. The treatment of chronic cough due to GERD is challenging. If lifestyle modification (weight loss, elevation of the head of the bed, avoidance of tobacco and alcohol) is unsuccessful, targeted and prolonged treatment with histamine blockers or proton pump inhibitors (PPIs) is recommended. In a recent Cochrane review, patients who were treated with PPIs experienced a significant improvement in cough scores. There was no significant difference in total resolution of cough, however (odds ratio [OR] 0.46, 95% CI 0.19-1.15, intention to treat analysis). The duration of therapy was 2 to 3 months. As this patient has been on therapy for only 2 weeks and his clinical picture is without any interim change, continuation for 8 to 12 weeks would be recommended.

The American College of Chest Physicians recommends a symptom-guided, systematic, algorithmic approach to chronic cough. There is no evidence of infection, and therefore, antibiotics are not indicated. The patient does not present with symptoms or signs of upper airway cough syndrome (postnasal drainage, frequent throat clearing, nasal discharge, cobblestone appearance of the oropharyngeal mucosa, or mucus dripping down the oropharynx). The use of antihistamines and decongestants, such as loratadine with pseudoephedrine, should be reserved until the empiric trial of treatment for GERD is completed and found to be ineffective.

Cough-variant asthma (cough is the predominant symptom) occurs in up to 57% of patients with asthma. Cough-variant asthma is suggested by the presence of airway hyperresponsiveness and confirmed when cough resolves with asthma medications. The treatment of cough-variant asthma is the same as asthma in general, but the maximum symptomatic benefit may not occur for 6 to 8 weeks in cough-variant asthma. This patient does not have asthma and has a reasonable alternative explanation for his chronic cough; therefore treatment with an inhaled bronchodilator such as albuterol is not indicated at this time.

KEY POINT

- **The duration of empiric proton pump inhibitor therapy for a patient with gastroesophageal reflux disease–related cough is 8 to 12 weeks.**

Bibliography

Chang AB, Lasserson TJ, Gaffney J, Connor FL, Garske LA. Gastro-oesophageal reflux treatment for prolonged non-specific cough in children and adults. Cochrane Database Syst Rev. 2011;(1): CD004823. [PMID: 21249664]

Item 39   Answer: B
Educational Objective: Diagnose acute pericarditis.

This patient most likely has acute pericarditis. Characteristic findings in acute pericarditis include sharp, pleuritic retrosternal chest pain that is more prominent in the recumbent position, a pericardial friction rub, widespread ST-segment elevation or PR-segment depression on electrocardiogram (ECG), and new or worsening pericardial effusion. This patient has pleuritic chest pain that worsens with recumbency and improves with sitting forward and widespread concave-upward ST-segment elevation, making acute pericarditis the likely diagnosis. The presence of a friction rub is helpful if present but its absence does not exclude the diagnosis. Etiologies of acute pericarditis include infection (especially viral infection, as is likely in this patient), autoimmune disease, neoplasia, uremia, and trauma.

The patient has no risk factors for ischemic heart disease and her description of her chest pain is atypical for that of coronary artery disease. The widespread concave-upward ST-segment ECG changes are more consistent with acute pericarditis rather than ischemia, in which changes localized to leads associated with the specific regions of the involved myocardium would be expected.

Like pericarditis, the pain of acute pleuritis worsens with inspiration, may be positional, and can be accompanied by dyspnea. However, pleuritic chest pain is not confined to the retrosternal area, as it is in pericarditis, and ECG changes would not be expected with pleuritis.

Although the chest pain that accompanies a pulmonary embolism is typically pleuritic, pulmonary embolism is not associated with widespread ST-segment elevation or PR-segment depression on ECG.

KEY POINT

- **The chest pain of acute pericarditis is typically sharp, pleuritic, retrosternal, worsened by recumbency, and improved by sitting forward.**

Bibliography

Khandaker MH, Espinosa RE, Nishimura RA, et al. Pericardial disease: diagnosis and management. Mayo Clin Proc. 2010;85(6):572-593. [PMID: 20511488]

Item 40   Answer: A
Educational Objective: Manage androgen deficiency.

This patient's hydrocodone should be discontinued. Low testosterone levels can lead to decreased energy and libido, fatigue, and erectile dysfunction. Once discovered, low testosterone levels should be investigated further. Many drugs, including opioids, high-dose corticosteroids, and hormonal therapies, can lower testosterone levels, and a review of medications is an important initial step in the evaluation of men with low testosterone levels. It is also important to test morning levels of testosterone as opposed to random levels, as secretion is cyclical. In this patient, hydrocodone may be decreasing testosterone levels and should be discontinued, and the testosterone level should subsequently be retested before any testosterone replacement therapy is given.

Whereas metoprolol and other β-blockers may cause erectile dysfunction and fatigue, they do not generally lower testosterone levels.

While repeat morning testing of testosterone levels is recommended to confirm low values, it would be more appropriate to first discontinue the potential offending agent before retesting the testosterone level.

As testosterone replacement therapy is usually a long-term treatment intervention, it should only be initiated after definitive confirmation of testosterone deficiency in the absence of testosterone-lowering therapies and after weighing the risks and benefits and discussing the multiple potential delivery options for the hormone with the patient.

KEY POINT

- **In men with low testosterone levels, a review of medications should be undertaken; many drugs, including opioids, high-dose corticosteroids, and hormonal therapies, can lower testosterone levels.**

Bibliography

Bhasin S, Cunningham GR, Hayes FJ, et al; Task Force, Endocrine Society. Testosterone therapy in men with androgen deficiency syndromes: an Endocrine Society clinical practice guideline. J Clin Endocrinol Metab. 2010;95(6):2536-2559. [PMID: 20525905]

Item 41   Answer: C
Educational Objective: Treat isolated hypertriglyceridemia.

Among the options listed, fenofibrate is the best treatment option for this patient. His serum triglyceride level is classified as "very high" (≥500 mg/dL [5.65 mmol/L]) according to the National Cholesterol Education Program Adult Treatment Panel III (ATP III) guidelines. He also has a significantly low HDL cholesterol level. The non-HDL cholesterol level (calculated as total cholesterol – HDL cholesterol) correlates closely with elevated LDL and VLDL concentrations, and is considered a secondary target of therapy when triglycerides are elevated. In patients with an LDL cholesterol goal of 130 mg/dL (3.37 mmol/L) or less, as with this patient, the non-HDL cholesterol goal is 160 mg/dL (4.14 mmol/L [30 points higher than the LDL cholesterol goal]). This patient's calculated non-HDL cholesterol level is 165 mg/dL (4.27 mmol/L), and so medical therapy should be initiated. Fenofibrate is very effective for reducing serum triglyceride levels, with observed decreases of 20% to 50%. Additionally, several trials have demonstrated the benefit of fibrate therapy in the primary and secondary prevention of cardiovascular outcomes.

Colesevelam, a bile acid resin, would not be indicated for treatment in this patient with hypertriglyceridemia. Bile acid resins are effective alone or in combination with statins for lowering LDL cholesterol level but may raise serum triglycerides, especially in patients with serum triglyceride levels greater than 400 mg/dL (4.52 mmol/L). These agents should be avoided as monotherapy in patients with triglyceride levels above 200 mg/dL (2.26 mmol/L).

Nicotinic acid will reduce serum triglyceride level by 20% to 50%, decrease LDL cholesterol level by 5% to 25%, and increase the HDL cholesterol level by 15% to 35%. Treatment with nicotinic acid has been shown to reduce cardiovascular outcomes in both primary and secondary prevention trials. However, treatment with nicotinic acid can precipitate gouty attacks, and so should be avoided in patients, such as this one, with a known history of gout.

Omega-3 fatty acids reduce hepatic secretion of triglyceride-rich lipoproteins and thereby lower serum triglyceride levels. However, their effectiveness in reducing cardiovascular risk in high-risk patients has not been established, and these agents thus should be considered alternative therapies for treatment of patients with hypertriglyceridemia who cannot tolerate fibric acids or nicotinic acid.

KEY POINT
- For patients with hypertriglyceridemia, fibric acid derivatives, such as fenofibrate, reduce triglyceride levels and provide benefit in primary and secondary cardiovascular prevention.

Bibliography
McCullough PA, Ahmed AB, Zughaib MT, Glanz ED, Di Loreto MJ. Treatment of hypertriglyceridemia with fibric acid derivatives: impact on lipid subfractions and translation into a reduction in cardiovascular events. Rev Cardiovasc Med. 2011;12(4):173-185. [PMID: 22249508]

Item 42   Answer: B
Educational Objective: Diagnose epididymitis.

This patient most likely has epididymitis. Infection or inflammation of the epididymis often causes pain localized to the superior and posterior aspect of the testicle. The onset may be acute, subacute, or chronic, and pain may occur more gradually compared with torsion. Pain may be accompanied by lower urinary tract symptoms of dysuria, urgency, or frequency. Patients with acute epididymitis may be quite sick, with high fevers and leukocytosis. Risk factors for epididymitis include recent sexual activity, heavy exertion, and bicycle riding. Distribution is bimodal, with occurrences highest in those younger than 35 years and older than 55 years. In younger patients, sexually transmitted infections such as chlamydial infection and gonorrhea are the most likely causes. Older men and men who engage in receptive anal intercourse are more susceptible to *Escherichia coli*, Enterobacteriaceae, and pseudomonal infection.

Acute prostatitis usually presents with pelvic pain and lower urinary tract symptoms, such as dysuria, urgency, and frequency. It may cause fever and leukocytosis, but on examination, the prostate gland is usually exquisitely tender, which is not the case with this patient.

An indirect hernia may lead to discomfort and fullness in the scrotum unilaterally, and also cause palpable changes along the course of the inguinal canal on the affected side. An indirect hernia is unlikely in this patient given lack of a scrotal mass or other physical findings consistent with a hernia; in addition, hernias do not cause fever or leukocytosis.

Orchitis, or inflammation of the testicle, can present as a febrile illness with testicular pain but pain would be expected with direct palpation of the testicle and potentially testicular enlargement.

Testicular torsion, which occurs when the testicle twists on the spermatic cord, usually occurs quite acutely. It leads to decreased blood flow and ischemia and is a surgical emergency. Physical findings usually include severe pain, often accompanied by nausea and vomiting, and a high-riding testicle. This patient's presentation is not consistent with testicular torsion.

KEY POINT
- Epididymitis is characterized by pain localized to the superior and posterior aspect of the testicle; patients may be quite sick, with high fevers and leukocytosis.

Bibliography
Wampler SM, Llanes M. Common scrotal and testicular problems. Prim Care. 2010;37(3):613-626, x. [PMID: 20705202]

Item 43   Answer: B

Educational Objective: Manage life-sustaining care in a critically ill patient.

It is unclear from the clinical scenario whether or not the patient will need dialysis for an extended period of time. However, with the information given, the best course of action is to dialyze temporarily with the hope that the patient will either regain kidney function or improve sufficiently to participate in decision making about long-term dialysis. Although it may be more difficult and resource intensive to initiate dialysis now and stop later if the patient fails to improve, it is the course of action that is most likely to meet both his short-term goal of seeing his great-grandson graduate and his long-term goal of not being dependent on machines. It is important to recognize that from an ethical and legal perspective, stopping a life-sustaining therapy is no different from not starting it, although evidentiary standards among states and cultural and religious beliefs regarding withdrawing or withholding treatment may vary. Interventions should not be withheld for fear they cannot be withdrawn if necessary.

Placing a long-term dialysis catheter may reflect a reasonable assessment of this patient's likelihood of regaining normal kidney function, but implies disregard for his wish not to be dependent on a machine for a long period of time.

Withdrawing all treatment would be in conflict with the wishes of both the patient and his wife so this is not an appropriate choice at this time. However, it would be important to meet with the wife and family to set realistic expectations given the patient's wishes, age, comorbidities, and the severity of illness. They need to be informed that his survival to discharge even with maximal medical support and dialysis is highly unlikely.

Withholding dialysis now would honor his wish not to be dependent on machines, but he would be unlikely to survive. Because it is unclear how long he will need dialysis, it is difficult to tell if it will conflict with his desire not to be on machines for "a long period of time." Although dialysis will not help his poor prognosis from his cancer, it may help him meet his short-term goal of surviving until his great-grandson's graduation, so it is not futile.

KEY POINT

- **From an ethical and legal perspective, stopping a life-sustaining therapy is no different from not starting it; interventions should not be withheld for fear they cannot be withdrawn if necessary.**

Bibliography

Snyder L; American College of Physicians Ethics, Professionalism, and Human Rights Committee. American College of Physicians Ethics Manual: sixth edition. Ann Intern Med. 2012;156(1 Pt 2):73-104. [PMID: 22213573]

Item 44   Answer: B

Educational Objective: Diagnose primary Sjögren syndrome.

This patient has primary Sjögren syndrome. Sjögren syndrome is characterized by keratoconjunctivitis sicca, which causes xerophthalmia (dry eyes), and xerostomia (dry mouth). The absence of oral mucosal moisture often causes difficulty with mastication and swallowing and increases the risk for dental caries and periodontal disease. Vaginal dryness and parotid gland enlargement are frequently present, and fatigue and arthralgia are common. Some patients with Sjögren syndrome also may develop an inflammatory polyarthritis. Additional systemic features of Sjögren syndrome include cutaneous vasculitis, peripheral neuropathy, vasculitis that may be associated with mononeuritis multiplex, and interstitial nephritis with associated distal renal tubular acidosis. Pulmonary involvement may develop in patients with Sjögren syndrome and most commonly manifests with interstitial lung disease; however, bronchial and bronchiolar disease also may occur. Abnormal findings on the Schirmer test, which measures moisture under the lower eyelids, are consistent with Sjögren syndrome. Approximately 50% of patients with this syndrome are antinuclear antibody positive and 60% to 75% of patients with primary Sjögren syndrome are anti-Ro/SSA antibody positive, and approximately 40% of these patients are anti-La/SSB antibody positive. A total of 60% to 80% of patients with this condition are rheumatoid factor positive. The presence of xerophthalmia and xerostomia accompanied by anti-Ro/SSA and anti-La/SSB antibody positivity and abnormal findings on the Schirmer test have a 94% sensitivity and specificity for primary Sjögren syndrome.

Meibomianitis is caused by dysfunction of the meibomian glands responsible for production of the lipid portion of the tear film. Given that this patient also has dry mouth and positive anti-Ro/SSA and anti-La/SSB serology, meibomianitis is unlikely.

Both rheumatoid arthritis and systemic lupus erythematosus can be associated with Sjögren syndrome, in which case, multiple systemic symptoms and findings such as joint involvement, pleuritis, cerebritis, lung dysfunction, and skin changes may all occur. Despite this patient's positive antinuclear antibody and rheumatoid factor test results, her lack of systemic symptoms and a normal physical examination (except for xerophthalmia and xerostomia) argue against rheumatoid arthritis or systemic lupus erythematosus as a cause of secondary Sjögren syndrome.

KEY POINT

- **The presence of xerophthalmia and xerostomia accompanied by anti-Ro/SSA and anti-La/SSB antibody positivity and abnormal findings on the Schirmer test have a 94% sensitivity and specificity for primary Sjögren syndrome.**

Bibliography

Latkany R. Dry eyes: etiology and management. Curr Opin Ophthalmol. 2008;19(4):287-291. [PMID: 185450008]

Item 45   Answer: D

Educational Objective: Evaluate a breast mass in a young woman.

This patient should undergo ultrasonography. A slightly tender, discrete, round, soft, and mobile breast mass, with no nipple discharge and no overlying skin changes, is consistent with a fibroadenoma or benign cyst and not breast cancer. However, no single clinical factor by history or physical examination has sufficient accuracy to rule in or rule out underlying malignancy, and diagnostic imaging should be performed. Ultrasonography serves to distinguish cystic from solid masses. A cystic mass should be aspirated and the fluid sent for cytologic evaluation if bloody or recurrent. A solid mass requires biopsy by fine-needle aspiration, core needle, or excision. A benign biopsy in a woman with a normal mammogram still requires close follow-up, as documented by a study in which breast cancer developed in 707 of 9087 women with previous benign breast biopsies followed for a median of 15 years.

In general, imaging should precede core needle biopsy. A core needle biopsy will not be necessary if the mass is definitively cystic by ultrasonography.

The increased density of breast tissue in women 30 to 35 years of age and younger may limit the utility of mammography, making ultrasonography a better first choice. Ultrasonography can readily distinguish cystic from solid lesions and guide further evaluation, such as aspiration, if needed.

Clinical observation and follow-up in 6 months is not appropriate for a palpable breast mass, which should be evaluated until diagnosis or resolution.

KEY POINT

- **A palpable breast mass should be evaluated until diagnosis or resolution.**

Bibliography

Rungruang B, Kelley JL 3rd. Benign breast diseases: epidemiology, evaluation, and management. Clin Obstet Gynecol. 2011;54(1):110-124. [PMID: 21278510]

Item 46   Answer: B

Educational Objective: Recognize a medication-related adverse effect in an elderly patient.

The patient's clinical presentation is likely the result of overmedication in an elderly patient who has significant medical comorbidities and is taking numerous medications. She was recently hospitalized and had medication adjustments made in the setting of chronic kidney disease, including an increase in her diuretic dose, that have led to volume depletion, which, in turn, may have led to changes in her kidneys' ability to metabolize drugs that are renally cleared.

Polypharmacy is becoming more common as the population ages. Twelve percent of patients in the United States older than 65 years take 10 or more medications each week, and adverse drug reactions in the elderly account for 10% of emergency department visits and up to 17% of acute hospitalizations. Numerous medications on this patient's list could cause adverse reactions. For example, gabapentin can cause dizziness and weakness and needs to be dose-adjusted in the setting of kidney disease. A review of every patient's medications, particularly in the elderly, should be a part of routine care to avoid polypharmacy and potential medication-related adverse events.

Although this patient has an apparent decline in her kidney function as estimated by her serum creatinine level, there is no clear evidence of acute kidney injury being the primary cause of her altered mental status.

Infection should always be a primary consideration in elderly patients presenting with mental status changes and failure to thrive. However, in this patient there is no evidence of infection as a cause of her symptoms.

The patient has atrial fibrillation and is not receiving anticoagulation therapy. She does, therefore, have an increased risk for thromboembolic disease. However, her neurologic examination is nonfocal, which would be less consistent with stroke as the underlying cause of her presentation.

KEY POINT

- **Polypharmacy, particularly in elderly patients with multiple comorbid medical conditions, is a frequent cause of adverse events; ongoing review of the need and appropriate dosing of medications should be a part of routine care.**

Bibliography

Hayes BD, Klein-Schwartz W, Barrueto F Jr. Polypharmacy and the geriatric patient. Clin Geriatr Med. 2007;23(2):371-390. [PMID: 17462523]

Item 47   Answer: C

Educational Objective: Manage preoperative care of a patient with COPD scheduled for an intermediate-risk procedure.

This patient with COPD undergoing hip surgery should begin performing incentive spirometry preoperatively to reduce his risk of perioperative pulmonary complications (PPCs). Risk factors for PPCs including chronic lung disease, older age, use of spinal or general anesthesia, and surgery around the diaphragm. Patients with COPD are two to five times more likely to experience PPCs. The only therapy proved effective for reducing the risk of PPCs in the immediate postoperative period is pre- and postoperative lung volume expansion, either via deep breathing or incentive spirometry.

CONT.

Positive airway pressure can be used postoperatively to minimize atelectasis in patients unable to adequately perform incentive spirometry (such as those with musculoskeletal or neuromuscular limitations to full lung expansion). However, there is no clear role for perioperative positive airway pressure in those who are able to perform incentive spirometry. Additionally, continuous positive airway pressure (CPAP) is not indicated during the day, nocturnally, or both, in the preoperative management of patients with COPD unless they already have an indication for treatment or are unable to use an incentive spirometer.

Chest radiographs are often ordered preoperatively. Only 1% to 3% show a clinically significant abnormality, however, of which only approximately 0.1% affect clinical care. Furthermore, most clinically significant chest radiograph abnormalities can be predicted by history and physical examination. Given this patient's unchanged clinical symptoms and stable pulmonary examination, imaging would not be expected to lead to an improved clinical outcome associated with surgery.

Results of pulmonary function testing do not predict the risk of PPCs, and these tests have no role in routine preoperative evaluation. Pulmonary function testing should be reserved for the evaluation of dyspnea when the cause is not known.

KEY POINT

- **The only therapy proved effective for reducing the risk of postoperative pulmonary complications in the immediate perioperative period is pre- and postoperative lung volume expansion, either via deep breathing or incentive spirometry.**

Bibliography

Qaseem A, Snow V, Fitterman N, et al; Clinical Efficacy Assessment Subcommittee of the American College of Physicians. Risk assessment for and strategies to reduce perioperative pulmonary complications for patients undergoing noncardiothoracic surgery: a guideline from the American College of Physicians. Ann Intern Med. 2006;144(8):575-580. [PMID: 16618955]

Item 48 Answer: B
Educational Objective: Manage rectal bleeding.

In this average-risk patient, the most appropriate next step would be to proceed to endoscopic evaluation, such as colonoscopy, to rule out colonic neoplasia as a source of bleeding. Typically, patients with hemorrhoidal bleeding report streaks of bright red blood on the toilet paper or on the outside of a firm stool. There is usually pain associated with defecation. However, the hemorrhoids themselves are not painful because there is no innervation to the colonic mucosa proximal to the dentate line. Hemorrhoids are unlikely to cause serious bleeding. Although hemorrhoids are a common cause of bright red blood from the rectum, rectal bleeding should not be considered hemorrhoidal without additional investigation in older patients. Most authorities

agree that the nature of the evaluation is governed by the patient's risk for colon cancer. In young patients (age <40 years) with typical symptoms of hemorrhoid bleeding and low risk for colon cancer, additional evaluation of the colon is unnecessary. Because of the increasing incidence of colon cancer with age, patients 40 to 50 years old with typical hemorrhoidal symptoms but at low risk for colon cancer should probably have at least sigmoidoscopy. Patients aged 50 years and older should undergo colonoscopy to evaluate the source of bleeding provided that routine screening has not been recently performed.

If colon cancer is excluded by colonoscopy, his hemorrhoids can be treated conservatively. Banding and other invasive procedures are reserved for patients whose hemorrhoids do not respond to conservative therapy.

Fiber supplementation is an appropriate treatment for this patient with hard stools but as the only management for his hematochezia is inappropriate, as this option potentially puts him at risk for a missed diagnosis of colon cancer.

Home fecal occult blood testing would likely be positive, but whether positive or negative, the recommendation for this 46-year-old patient remains the same; colonoscopy or sigmoidoscopy based upon the report of bright red rectal bleeding.

KEY POINT

- **Patients older than 40 years with hematochezia should undergo colon cancer evaluation with colonoscopy or sigmoidoscopy.**

Bibliography

Schubert MC, Sridhar S, Schade RR, Wexner SD. What every gastroenterologist needs to know about common anorectal disorders. World J Gastroenterol. 2009;15(26):3201-3209. [PMID: 19598294]

Item 49 Answer: A
Educational Objective: Manage prostate cancer screening.

The most appropriate management is to have an informed discussion with the patient regarding the risks and benefits of prostate cancer screening. The European Randomized Study of Screening for Prostate Cancer included 162,243 men aged 55 to 69 years. During a median of 9 years, the rate of diagnosis of prostate cancer was higher in the prostate-specific antigen (PSA)–screened group (8.2%) compared with the control (non-screened) group (4.8%) and there was an absolute, albeit small, mortality benefit (1410 men would need to be screened and an additional 48 men would need to be treated for prostate cancer to prevent one death from prostate cancer). In contrast, the Prostate, Lung, Colorectal, and Prostate Cancer Screening Trial found no benefit for annual concurrent PSA and digital rectal examination (DRE) after 7 to 10 years of follow up. Given the conflicting evidence regarding the benefit of prostate cancer screening, the decision of whether or not to screen an individual patient should begin with the clinician having an informed discussion with the patient regarding the risks and benefits of screening and the limitations of the methods used to screen. Based on the conflicting results of these trials, it is not surprising that there is little consensus in terms of screening recommendations. The American Cancer Society supports the need for men to be involved in the decision of whether or not to be screened. In 2012, the U.S. Preventive Services Task Force (USPSTF) published a formal recommendation statement based on a review of existing evidence advising against PSA testing for prostate cancer screening in all men.

Performing a DRE alone is not recommended for screening owing to the poor test characteristics (positive likelihood ratio, 0.53-1.33; negative likelihood ratio, 0.65-14.9).

Although obtaining a PSA level alone and performing a DRE in combination with obtaining a PSA level are frequently employed in screening for prostate cancer, neither approach should be performed without first having an informed discussion with the patient.

KEY POINT

- **The decision of whether or not to screen for prostate cancer in an individual man should begin with an informed discussion regarding the risks and benefits of screening and the limitations of the methods used to screen.**

Bibliography

Chou R, Croswell JM, Dana T, et al. Screening for prostate cancer: a review of the evidence for the U.S. Preventive Services Task Force. Ann Intern Med. 2011;155(11):762-771. Epub 2011 Oct 7. [PMID: 21984740]

Item 50   Answer: B

Educational Objective: Diagnose central vertigo.

This patient demonstrates vertigo of central origin, a medical emergency. He should undergo MRI with angiography of the brain. Acute vertigo accompanied by vertical nystagmus and nystagmus that is immediate, prolonged (>1 min), and nonfatigable on the Dix-Hallpike maneuver is characteristic of a central origin. Central vertigo may be caused by ischemia or infarct in the brainstem or cerebellum. The patient's inability to stand without support and the absence of diplopia or dysarthria likely puts his lesion in the cerebellum. Up to one quarter of patients with traditional risk factors for stroke who present with severe vertigo and nystagmus and who are unable to stand without support have ischemia or infarction of the cerebellum.

Diffusion-weighted MRI is recommended over CT scanning as the first-line evaluation for stroke within 12 hours of symptom onset owing to its superior sensitivity. Although CT scanning without contrast has excellent sensitivity for intracranial hemorrhage, is widely available, and,

in most cases, can be performed more quickly and with less cost, it is less sensitive than MRI for acute ischemic stroke and does not provide adequate imaging of the vasculature of the posterior circulation.

Otolith repositioning, commonly known as the Epley maneuver, has been shown helpful in resolving symptoms of benign paroxysmal positional vertigo (BPPV). BPPV is the most common cause of vestibular (peripheral) dizziness. Patients with BPPV describe vertigo lasting minutes in duration, with multiple episodes occurring over weeks to months. Tinnitus, ear pain, and hearing loss are absent, and nausea that is sufficiently severe or prolonged to cause vomiting is rare. The patient's findings are not consistent with BPPV.

Symptomatic treatment with vestibular suppressants is generally reserved for peripheral causes. The patient's recent upper respiratory tract infection is a risk factor for vestibular neuritis. However, his history and bedside examination are inconsistent with peripheral vertigo. On the Dix-Hallpike maneuver, vertigo of peripheral origin is usually severe, lasts less than 1 minute, has a latency of 2 to 40 seconds, and fatigues with time. The direction of peripheral nystagmus is not vertical but is horizontal with a rotational component.

KEY POINT

- **Acute vertigo accompanied by vertical nystagmus and nystagmus that is immediate, prolonged, and nonfatigable on the Dix-Hallpike maneuver is characteristic of central vertigo.**

Bibliography

Post RE, Dickerson LM. Dizziness: a diagnostic approach. Am Fam Physician. 2010;82(4):361-368, 369. [PMID: 20704166]

Item 51   Answer: D

Educational Objective: Counsel an obese patient regarding weight reduction.

This patient should reduce her current caloric intake by 500 to 1000 kcal/d. Consistent reduction in daily dietary caloric intake is the most successful long-term and safest weight loss strategy in obese and overweight patients. Patients who follow a diet that reduces their caloric intake by 500 to 1000 kcal/d as compared with their intake that is currently maintaining weight will lose an average of 0.45 to 0.91 kg (1-2 lb) per week. The initial goal should be a loss of 10% of total body weight. If this patient adheres to this recommendation, she should lose 9.1 kg (20 lb) in 4 to 5 months. This degree of weight loss has been shown to decrease the health-related consequences of obesity, including diabetes mellitus. Because she already has prediabetes, weight loss is important to her long-term health.

Exercise is an important part of a comprehensive weight loss program that focuses on lifestyle modification.

However, without attention to eating habits and caloric restriction, exercise alone is not adequate for weight loss.

Current National Institutes of Health and Veterans Affairs guidelines recommend consideration of bariatric interventions, such as laparoscopic band surgery, in patients with a BMI greater than 40 or patients with a BMI of 35 to 40 with obesity-related comorbidities, such as diabetes mellitus, obstructive sleep apnea, or severe joint disease. This patient does not meet these recommendations.

Orlistat is a lipase inhibitor that leads to fat malabsorption. It is FDA approved when used in conjunction with a reduced calorie diet. It is moderately effective in weight loss (2.9 kg [6.4 lb] at 12 months) but gastrointestinal side effects are common. More serious adverse effects, such as severe liver injury and malabsorption of fat-soluble vitamins, have been reported. Lifestyle management with diet and exercise should be the first step in any weight loss program. Medications can be used in conjunction with, but not as a substitute for, diet and exercise.

KEY POINT

- Consistent reduction in daily dietary caloric intake is the most successful long-term and safest weight loss strategy in obese and overweight patients.

Bibliography

Management of Overweight and Obesity Working Group. VA/DoD clinical practice guideline for screening and management of overweight and obesity. Washington (DC): Department of Veterans Affairs, Department of Defense; 2006.

Item 52   Answer: B

Educational Objective: Treat elevated LDL cholesterol level.

Pravastatin is the safest choice for lowering LDL cholesterol level in this patient. She has recently diagnosed peripheral arterial disease, which is associated with atherosclerosis; her goal LDL cholesterol level is, therefore, less than 100 mg/dL (2.59 mmol/L). Pravastatin is one of the preferred statins in patients who are being treated with multiple medications.

Statins should be considered first-line therapy for lowering LDL cholesterol levels in this patient, as studies have shown that older patients (ages 65-80 years) derive similar benefit as younger patients for secondary prevention of cardiovascular disease. However, advanced age is also a risk factor for statin-related myopathy, and therapy should be chosen carefully to minimize this risk. Female sex, small body frame, hypothyroidism, statin dosage, and treatment with multiple medications also influence the likelihood of developing statin-related myopathy. Pravastatin is metabolized by the kidneys; therefore, its concentration will be unaffected by cytochrome isoenzymes that affect the metabolism of other statins or warfarin.

In contrast, atorvastatin, lovastatin, and simvastatin are primarily metabolized through the cytochrome P-450 3A4 isoenzyme, and treatment with these medications in combination with diltiazem can increase serum statin levels, placing the patient at higher risk for statin myopathy. These statins should not be combined with diltiazem in a patient who is at already high risk for statin-induced myopathy based on her age, small body frame, hypothyroidism, and multiple medications.

Rosuvastatin and fluvastatin are metabolized through the cytochrome P-450 CYP2C9 isoenzyme, and would effectively lower this patient's LDL cholesterol level. However, rosuvastatin may affect the metabolism of warfarin, leading to an increased INR. Caution is therefore necessary when combining these medications, and this is not the safest choice for this patient.

KEY POINT

- In patients who require lipid-lowering therapy and who are taking multiple medications, a statin that is renally metabolized, such as pravastatin, has a lower risk of drug-drug interactions.

Bibliography

Joy TR, Hegele RA. Narrative review: statin-related myopathy. Ann Intern Med. 2009;150(12):858-868. [PMID: 19528564]

Item 53   Answer: C

Educational Objective: Treat heavy menstrual bleeding.

The most appropriate next management step is oral medroxyprogesterone acetate. In patients who present with menorrhagia (heavy menstrual bleeding) with a known etiology, several therapeutic agents can decrease bleeding. For moderate bleeding that can be managed on an outpatient basis, a progestational agent such as medroxyprogesterone acetate can be given for 10 to 21 days. The progesterone will typically act to stabilize the endometrium and stop uterine blood flow.

Estrogen/progesterone-containing oral contraceptives may be useful in decreasing menstrual blood loss, although the doses of both agents in most typical formulations would likely be inadequate to control the degree of bleeding in this patient, particularly with a multiphasic preparation. If a specific progestational agent is not available, a monophasic oral contraceptive may be dosed four times daily for 5 to 7 days, and subsequently reduced to daily dosing until definitive treatment is undertaken.

If the patient were orthostatic or dizzy from blood loss, intravenous estrogen would be appropriate. Parenteral conjugated estrogens are approximately 70% effective in stopping the bleeding entirely. Pulmonary embolism and venous thrombosis are complications of intravenous estrogen therapy.

Monitoring the patient for an additional week of observation is not appropriate given her significant, ongoing blood loss.

KEY POINT

- Medroxyprogesterone acetate for 10 to 21 days is effective treatment for moderate menstrual bleeding.

Bibliography
Fazio SB, Ship AN. Abnormal uterine bleeding. South Med J. 2007;100(4):376-382; quiz 383, 402. [PMID: 17458397]

Item 54   Answer: B
Educational Objective: Diagnose patellofemoral pain syndrome.

This patient most likely has patellofemoral pain syndrome, the most common cause of knee pain in patients younger than 45 years. Patellofemoral pain syndrome is a clinical diagnosis and further diagnostic testing such as radiographs is not necessary. Patellofemoral pain syndrome is more common in women than in men and is characterized by anterior knee pain that is made worse with prolonged sitting and with going up and down stairs. The pain is reproduced by applying pressure to the patella with the knee in extension and moving the patella both medially and laterally (patellofemoral compression test).

According to the American College of Rheumatology's clinical criteria, osteoarthritis of the knee can be diagnosed if knee pain is accompanied by at least three of the following features: age greater than 50 years, stiffness lasting less than 30 minutes, crepitus, bony tenderness, bony enlargement, and no palpable warmth. These criteria are 95% sensitive and 69% specific but have not been validated for clinical practice. Crepitus of the knee is common in patients with osteoarthritis between the patella and the femur. Passive range of motion of the knee often elicits pain at the extremes of flexion and extension. Palpation of the knee discloses only mild tenderness. This patient has no clinical evidence of knee osteoarthritis.

Pes anserine bursitis characteristically produces pain that is located near the anteromedial aspect of the proximal tibia. On examination, tenderness is elicited at the level of the tibial tuberosity (approximately 3.8 cm [1.5 in] below the level of the medial joint line). Swelling may be present at the insertion of the medial hamstring muscles. This patient's presentation is not consistent with pes anserine bursitis.

Prepatellar bursitis is often caused by recurrent trauma, such as repeated kneeling ("housemaid's knee") but can also be caused by infection or gout. Although the pain is located anteriorly, examination reveals swelling, tenderness to palpation (usually localized near the lower pole of the patella), and erythema, all of which are lacking in this patient.

KEY POINT

- Patellofemoral pain syndrome is more common in women than in men and is characterized by anterior knee pain that is made worse with prolonged sitting and with going up and down stairs.

Bibliography
Collado H, Fredericson M. Patellofemoral pain syndrome. Clin Sports Med. 2010;29(3):379-398. [PMID: 20610028]

Item 55   Answer: A
Educational Objective: Manage chronic dizziness in an elderly patient.

This elderly woman with chronic dizziness should receive physical therapy with gait evaluation. Chronic dizziness is a common problem in the elderly. Although not associated with excess mortality, chronic dizziness is associated with falls, syncope, and self-rated health decline. It is often multifactorial and exhaustive work-ups are costly and often unrewarding, particularly in the absence of suggestive or supporting findings on history or physical examination. Common contributing factors, including medications, sensory impairments, neuropathy, muscle weakness, deconditioning, anxiety, depression, and postural hypotension, should be identified and addressed. This patient specifically presents with dysequilibrium, a nonvertiginous feeling of imbalance or unsteadiness while standing or walking. She has impairments in vision and hearing. She is at high risk for falls. In addition to evaluation for visual and hearing aids, referral to physical therapy for balance and gait training is an appropriate first step. In a recent systematic review and meta-analysis of community- and residential care–dwelling older adults, programs that included exercise and that focused on exercises that challenge balance had the greatest relative effects on fall rates (RR = 0.58, 95% CI = 0.48-0.69).

Administration of topical ophthalmic medication carries some risk of systemic absorption. This patient is being treated with latanoprost, a prostaglandin analogue that typically has minimal systemic effects. β-Blocker ophthalmic drops, such as timolol, are associated with systemic absorption, which may worsen her symptoms.

Although medication side effects and polypharmacy can contribute to dizziness, this patient is not orthostatic, and changing from an ACE inhibitor to an angiotensin receptor blocker would not likely relieve her symptoms.

Vestibular rehabilitation therapy is most useful for patients with benign paroxysmal positional vertigo. This patient presents with nonspecific dizziness and not true vertigo.

KEY POINT

- Physical therapy is an effective intervention to decrease fall risk in elderly patients with dysequilibrium.

Bibliography

Sherrington C, Whitney JC, Lord SR, Herbert RD, Cumming RG, Close JC. Effective exercise for the prevention of falls: a systematic review and meta-analysis. J Am Geriatr Soc. 2008;56(12):2234-2243. [PMID: 19093923]

Item 56   Answer: C
Educational Objective: Treat depression.

The most appropriate next treatment step for this patient is to discontinue bupropion and begin a different antidepressant, such as sertraline. She has moderate depression that is refractory to initial single-agent treatment. The goal of treatment is to achieve complete remission within 6 to 12 weeks and continue treatment for 4 to 9 months thereafter. Patients should be assessed 2 and 4 weeks after starting therapy for adherence, adverse drug reactions, and suicide risk, and again at 6 to 8 weeks for response to therapy. Using a formal tool for severity assessment (such as the PHQ-9) helps quantify the nature of the response; patients are considered to have at least a partial response if a 50% or greater decrease in symptom score has occurred. Using the PHQ-9, patients can be classified as complete responders, partial responders, or nonresponders. Complete responders should continue the same therapy modality for an additional 4 to 9 months. Treatment options for partial responders and nonresponders include using a higher dose of the same agent (ineffective in this patient), adding a second agent, switching to a new drug, or adding psychotherapy (patient not interested). Any change in therapy requires periodic follow-up as outlined above.

Buspirone is an anxiolytic. Given the patient's lack of anxiety symptoms and her total lack of response to bupropion, adding this medication is not appropriate.

This patient remains unresponsive to treatment with bupropion following a dose escalated to the maximal dose. Waiting an additional 8 weeks is unlikely to change management and will slow this patient's recovery. Switching to a new drug, either of the same class (unavailable in this case) or different class, is indicated. Selective serotonin reuptake inhibitors (SSRIs), such as sertraline, are the most commonly prescribed class of antidepressants. In general, SSRIs are well tolerated with low toxicity; however, sexual side effects are common.

Electroconvulsive therapy is indicated in severely depressed patients, such as those with profound suicidal ideation or psychotic features in whom a rapid response to therapy is particularly desirable. This patient has no indication for electroconvulsive therapy.

KEY POINT

- **Patients refractory to a single antidepressant may respond to a change in therapy, which may include replacement with another antidepressant, either from the same or a different class; addition of a second antidepressant; or a psychotherapeutic intervention.**

Bibliography

Fancher TL, Kravitz RL. In the clinic. Depression. Ann Intern Med. 2010;152(9):ITC51-15; quiz ITC5-16. [PMID: 20439571]

Item 57   Answer: D
Educational Objective: Prevent type 2 diabetes mellitus in an overweight patient.

The most appropriate therapies to prevent type 2 diabetes mellitus in this patient are weight loss and exercise. This patient has a strong family history of type 2 diabetes mellitus and impaired fasting glucose, defined as a fasting plasma glucose level of 100 to 125 mg/dL (5.6 to 7.0 mmol/L). Based on multiple clinical trials, lifestyle modification has been shown to be the most effective intervention to prevent type 2 diabetes and its associated cardiovascular consequences. The Finnish Diabetes Prevention Study and the U.S. Diabetes Prevention Program (USDPP) both demonstrated a 58% relative risk reduction in the progression to diabetes with these methods in generally obese, middle-aged persons with impaired glucose tolerance. The American Diabetes Association recommends that lifestyle modifications continue to be the standard approach in diabetes prevention, with the goal being to increase regular physical activity by approximately 30 minutes on most days of the week and to reduce calories (to reduce weight) by 7%.

The USDPP reported a 31% risk reduction in the development of diabetes in patients treated with metformin. Acarbose reduced the risk of diabetes by 25% in the Study to Prevent Non–Insulin-Dependent Diabetes Mellitus (STOP-NIDDM) trial but had a high drop-out rate owing to gastrointestinal adverse effects. Other studies have shown a 62% reduction in progression to diabetes with rosiglitazone in patients with impaired glucose tolerance or impaired fasting glucose and an 82% reduction in the progression to diabetes with pioglitazone. However, the thiazolidinediones are associated with significant potential adverse effects, and the harm of these drugs may outweigh the benefit of their use in this patient population. Despite these findings, currently no drugs are FDA-approved for the prevention of diabetes. In patients with impaired fasting glucose and other risk factors (BMI ≥35, a strong family history, elevated triglyceride level, reduced HDL cholesterol level, hypertension, hemoglobin A_{1c} >6.0%), some clinicians will use metformin if lifestyle modifications have not been successful.

KEY POINT

- **The most appropriate therapies to prevent type 2 diabetes mellitus are weight loss and exercise.**

Bibliography

Knowler WC, Fowler SE, Hamman RF, et al; Diabetes Prevention Program Research Group. 10-year follow-up of diabetes incidence and weight loss in the Diabetes Prevention Program Outcomes Study. Lancet. 2009;374(9702):1677-1686. [PMID: 19878986]

Item 58   Answer: D

Educational Objective: Evaluate relative versus absolute risk.

The number needed to treat (NNT) with drug Z compared with drug C to prevent one additional case of deep venous thrombosis (DVT) is 100.

Absolute risk (AR) is the risk of a specific disease based on its actual occurrence, or its event rate (ER), in a group of patients being studied, and is expressed as:

$$AR = \frac{\text{patients with event in group}}{\text{total patients in group}}$$

As seen in the table, in this study, the AR for DVT in the group treated with drug Z is 25/2500, or 1%, and the AR for the group treated with drug C is 50/2500, or 2%.

Often, the event rate of a disease in an experimental group (EER) is compared with the event rate in a control group (CER). When the risk between groups is reduced, this difference is termed the absolute risk reduction (ARR), or if the outcome is of benefit, the difference is called the absolute benefit index (ABI). In this case, patients treated with drug Z (EER) appear to benefit from treatment with a lower risk of DVT than patients in the group treated with drug C (CER). This is expressed as:

$$ABI = |\, EER - CER \,|$$
$$ABI = |1\% - 2\%| = 1\% \text{ or } 0.01$$

This means that treatment with drug Z benefits patients compared with drug C by lowering the risk of DVT from 2% to 1%, or an absolute difference of 1%.

Assessing treatment studies using absolute measures also allows determination of "numbers needed," which are estimates of the clinical magnitude of the differences between treatments. In this case, the NNT indicates the number of patients needed to be treated with drug Z, compared with drug C, to obtain one additional beneficial outcome. The NNT is calculated as:

$$NNT = 1/ABI$$
$$NNT = 1 \div 0.01 = 100$$

This means that 100 patients would need to be treated with drug Z compared with drug C in order to prevent one additional case of DVT.

Treatment study results may also be reported as relative measures; these measures compare the ratio of two outcomes without regard to the actual frequency of the outcome in a given study population. In this case, treatment with drug Z leads to a 50% reduction in risk of DVT compared with treatment with drug C (25 compared with 50 events), even though the actual frequency of DVT in the study populations does not exceed 2%. Therefore, outcomes expressed in relative terms usually appear of greater magnitude than when expressed in absolute terms; they also do not allow calculations of number needed to estimate clinical impact.

KEY POINT

- Treatment study outcomes reported in absolute terms reflect the frequency of a disease in the study population and allow estimation of "numbers needed"; outcomes reported in relative terms tend to appear to be of greater magnitude.

Bibliography

Guyatt GH, Sackett DL, Cook DJ. Users' guides to the medical literature. II. How to use an article about therapy or prevention. B. What were the results and will they help me in caring for my patients? Evidence-Based Medicine Working Group. JAMA. 1994;271(1):59-63. [PMID: 8258890]

Item 59   Answer: D

Educational Objective: Manage ankle sprain.

The most appropriate management of this patient's ankle sprain is splinting. This patient most likely has a grade II ankle sprain. Correct grading of ankle sprains is important both in terms of predicting prognosis and for helping to ensure appropriate treatment. Grade II ankle sprains involve partial tears of one or more ankle ligaments and manifest clinically with moderate pain and some difficulty with bearing weight, which is occurring in this patient. Mild ankle instability and limited range of motion may also be present. In addition to conservative therapy (rest, ice, compression, elevation) and NSAIDs, joint stabilization is indicated and may be achieved with an elastic bandage and ankle splint. Adequate splinting will also support early ambulation and help protect against repeat injury. The optimal duration of splinting is unclear, although several weeks is reasonable with improvement of symptoms. Formal rehabilitation, including proprioceptive training, may be helpful in preventing chronic instability in grade II sprains.

Corticosteroid injections do not have a role in acute ankle injuries and should not be performed.

Although MRI may provide more detailed information than plain radiographs, they offer no advantage if acute imaging is indicated. MRIs are reserved primarily for evaluation of ankle sprains that fail to respond to a course of standard therapy or complex ankle injuries.

An inability to bear weight, although common with severe sprains, should raise concern for the possibility of a fracture. Fractures of the base of the fifth metatarsal are associated with tenderness to palpation of this area on examination. Lateral malleolar fractures are associated with tenderness to palpation of the lateral malleolus. According to the Ottawa ankle rules, ankle radiographs should be obtained only in patients with ankle pain who are unable to bear weight or who have bony tenderness to palpation at the posterior edge of either the lateral or medial malleoli. One systematic review found this set of criteria to be almost 100% sensitive in diagnosing fractures. Thus, it would not be appropriate to obtain ankle radiographs in this patient.

Answers and Critiques

Urgent surgical referral would be appropriate for a patient with a grade III ankle sprain, which is characterized by complete rupture of one or more ligaments and presents with severe swelling, ecchymosis, instability, and the inability to bear weight. Urgent surgical referral is not needed in a patient with a grade II ankle sprain.

KEY POINT

- Ankle radiographs should only be obtained in patients with acute ankle pain who are unable to bear weight or who have bony tenderness to palpation at the posterior edge of either the lateral or medial malleoli.

Bibliography

Seah R, Mani-Babu S. Managing ankle sprains in primary care: what is best practice? A systematic review of the last 10 years of evidence. Br Med Bull. 2011;97:105-135. [PMID: 20710025]

Item 60   Answer: E

Educational Objective: Treat menopausal vasomotor symptoms.

This 61-year-old woman with cardiovascular risk factors and a history of deep venous thrombosis should be started on a nonhormonal therapy for her hot flushes. Certain antidepressants, including serotonin-norepinephrine reuptake inhibitors such as venlafaxine, are effective nonhormonal medications for reducing menopausal vasomotor symptoms.

Approximately 10% of menopausal women experience hot flushes for 7 to 10 years after the cessation of menses. This patient is continuing to experience frequent and severe hot flushes which have been refractory to conservative therapy and are decreasing her quality of life; thus, pharmacologic therapy is warranted. Systemic estrogen therapy is the most effective treatment for the relief of menopausal hot flushes and must be coadministered with progesterone in women with an intact uterus. However, combined estrogen and progesterone therapy has been shown to increase the risk of several adverse outcomes, including coronary heart disease, stroke, invasive breast cancer, and venous thromboembolism. The North American Menopause Society guideline notes that women older than 60 years who experienced natural menopause at the median age and have never used hormone therapy will have elevated baseline risks of cardiovascular disease, venous thromboembolism, and breast cancer; hormone therapy, therefore, should not be initiated in this population without a compelling indication and only after appropriate counseling and attention to cardiovascular risk factors. Moreover, this patient has a history of deep venous thrombosis, which is an absolute contraindication to initiating hormone therapy.

Several nonhormonal medications have been found to be effective for the treatment of menopausal hot flushes. Notably, there is a significant placebo effect: in most studies, approximately one-third of women will experience relief of hot flushes, even if they do not receive active treatment. In numerous studies, venlafaxine, administered at doses of 37.5 mg/d to 150 mg/d, decreases hot flush severity and frequency in approximately 60% of patients (as compared with 30% who experienced benefit with placebo treatment). Paroxetine is similarly beneficial; in contrast, few studies have shown efficacy with fluoxetine or citalopram. Gabapentin and clonidine are two additional nonhormonal treatments that reduce hot flushes, but attendant side effects may limit their use in some patients.

Vaginal estrogen therapy is typically used for the isolated treatment of vaginal dryness, pruritus, and dyspareunia. Treatment with vaginal estrogen tablets will improve local vaginal symptoms, but will not improve menopausal vasomotor symptoms.

KEY POINT

- Owing to cardiovascular and thromboembolic risks, systemic hormone therapy is not recommended for treatment of menopausal vasomotor symptoms in women older than 60 years who experienced menopause at the median age.

Bibliography

Nelson HD, Vesco KK, Haney E, et al. Nonhormonal therapies for menopausal hot flashes: systematic review and meta-analysis. JAMA. 2006;295(17):2057-2071. [PMID: 16670414]

Item 61   Answer: C

Educational Objective: Diagnose central retinal vein occlusion.

This patient most likely has central retinal vein occlusion (CRVO). Patients with CRVO experience acute onset of painless blurry vision due to reduced venous outflow and vascular edema in the eye. CRVO is characterized by optic disc swelling, dilated and tortuous veins, flame-shaped retinal hemorrhages, and cotton-wool spots ("blood and thunder"). Because the nerve supply to the eye remains intact but vision is decreased, an afferent pupillary defect in the affected eye may be present. CRVO is most commonly encountered in older patients with hypertension and atherosclerotic vascular disease. Cases have also been associated with acute carotid artery dissection and conditions associated with increased blood viscosity, such as polycythemia vera, sickle cell disease, and leukemia. Prognosis depends on the degree of visual impairment at the onset of symptoms. There is no generally accepted acute management, but a thorough investigation into possible etiologies should be undertaken.

Acute angle closure glaucoma is characterized by narrowing or closure of the anterior chamber angle, which impedes the trabecular drainage system in the anterior chamber, resulting in elevated intraocular pressure and damage to the optic nerve. Typical signs and symptoms include significant pain, diminished visual acuity, seeing halos around lights, a red eye, headache, and a dilated pupil.

The globe may feel firm owing to increased intraocular pressure (often to 30 mm Hg or higher). Retinal examination may be normal or demonstrate optic cupping if chronic narrow-angle glaucoma is present.

Central retinal artery occlusion (CRAO) classically presents in a 50- to 70-year-old patient as a painless, abrupt blurring or loss of vision that occurs in the early morning hours—usually between midnight and 6 AM. It results from an embolic or thrombotic event in the ophthalmic artery. It is typically unilateral. On examination, visual acuity is markedly diminished in the affected eye to either finger counting or light perception. There is an afferent pupillary defect. On funduscopic examination, the retina appears pale, either segmentally or completely. The fovea may appear as a cherry red spot. Interruption of the venous blood columns may be recognized with the appearance of "box-carring"—rows of slowly moving corpuscles separated by clear intervals. These findings are not present in this patient.

Symptoms of retinal detachment include diminished vision, photopsia (flashes of light), abrupt onset of multiple floaters in the vision, and metamorphopsia (wavy vision). Retinal detachment may result from trauma or occur spontaneously, particularly in persons with myopia. It is typically unilateral. On funduscopic examination, retinal detachment is characterized by distortion, folding, and tearing of the retina, which were not seen in this patient.

KEY POINT

- **Central retinal vein occlusion is characterized by acute onset of painless blurry vision and optic disc swelling, dilated and tortuous veins, flame-shaped retinal hemorrhages, and cotton-wool spots ("blood and thunder").**

Bibliography
Ahmed R, Foroozan R. Transient monocular visual loss. Neurol Clin. 2010;28(3):619-629. [PMID: 20637992]

Item 62   Answer: C

Educational Objective: Manage a perioperative patient with cirrhosis.

This patient has cirrhotic liver disease, placing him at a high risk of perioperative complications, and nonoperative management of his hip osteoarthritis should be recommended. Patients with cirrhosis have an increased risk of perioperative morbidity and mortality. Surgery and anesthesia in these patients are risk factors for fulminant hepatic failure, and cirrhosis itself can predispose to bleeding, infection, adverse reactions to drugs, and poor wound healing. The risk of perioperative complications can be quantified using a number of scales, including Child-Turcotte-Pugh (CTP) classification. The CTP score is based on the presence of ascites and encephalopathy, as well as serum bilirubin, albumin, and INR values. Patients with CTP class A (0-6 points), class B (7-9 points), and class C (≥10 points) scores have postoperative mortality rates of approximately 10%, 30%, and 80%, respectively. Patients with a CTP class C score are usually advised to avoid elective surgery.

Patients with acute alcoholic hepatitis may present with leukocytosis, jaundice, hepatomegaly, and right upper quadrant pain. In addition to abstinence from alcohol and nutritional therapy, pharmacologic therapy with corticosteroids may be beneficial in patients with severe alcoholic hepatitis. However, this patient's cirrhosis is a result of long-term chronic alcohol use, and there is no indication for corticosteroid therapy.

Patients with cirrhosis are predisposed to bleeding because of quantitative and qualitative platelet dysfunction as well as a deficiency of hepatically produced clotting factors. The INR elevation in these patients is usually not caused by vitamin K deficiency. Although patients with coagulopathy are sometimes treated with oral vitamin K to reverse any nutritional deficiencies, administration of vitamin K would only minimally change the inherent risks of surgery in this patient.

KEY POINT

- **Patients with a Child-Turcotte-Pugh class C score are usually advised to avoid elective surgery.**

Bibliography
O'Leary JG, Yachimski PS, Friedman LS. Surgery in the patient with liver disease. Clin Liver Dis. 2009;13(2):211-231. [PMID: 19442915]

Item 63   Answer: B

Educational Objective: Counsel a patient using motivational interviewing.

It would be appropriate to determine which lifestyle change this patient believes is most important to implement. Key features of motivational interviewing are that the patient chooses the agenda, the provider is not in "control" and does not tell the patient what he or she should do, and the provider assesses the patient's sense of the importance of issues for them and their level of confidence in making these changes, which should be small and incremental. Physicians can support the patient's choice and provide advice on how to overcome barriers to implementation.

The patient has indicated a willingness to make important lifestyle changes; he now needs to be empowered to identify those changes he wishes to make and identify barriers and facilitators to those changes. He does not need to be told to lose weight; the patient has already acknowledged the need to make lifestyle changes. After the patient identifies the changes that are important to him, it would be appropriate to ascertain his confidence in making those changes, but to do so prior to this step would be premature. Having the patient control the agenda and select the changes he believes are most important and identify the

Answers and Critiques

associated barriers and facilitators is more likely to be effective than the physician providing advice on smoking or other lifestyle changes that the patient may deem as less important.

KEY POINT

- Key features of motivational interviewing are that the patient chooses the agenda, the provider is not in "control" and does not tell the patient what he or she should do, and the provider assesses the patient's sense of the importance of issues and level of confidence in making changes.

Bibliography
Rollnick S, Butler CC, Kinnersley P, Gregory J, Mash B. Motivational interviewing. BMJ. 2010;340:1242-1245. [PMID: 20423957]

Item 64   Answer: C
Educational Objective: Diagnose metabolic syndrome.

Given this patient's hypertension, lipid profile, and abdominal obesity, she meets the criteria for metabolic syndrome. The diagnosis of metabolic syndrome (Adult Treatment Panel III criteria) is made by the presence of three or more of the following five criteria: (1) waist circumference >40 in (102 cm) in men and >35 in (88 cm) in women; (2) systolic blood pressure ≥130 mm Hg or diastolic blood pressure ≥85 mm Hg; (3) HDL cholesterol level <40 mg/dL (1.04 mmol/L) in men and <50 mg/dL (1.30 mmol/L) in women; (4) triglyceride level ≥150 mg/dL (1.70 mmol/L); and (5) fasting plasma glucose level ≥110 mg/dL (6.1 mmol/L).

The clinical importance of identifying the metabolic syndrome is the increased risk for cardiovascular disease and type 2 diabetes mellitus in those with this diagnosis. Persons with the metabolic syndrome should receive aggressive intervention focused on lifestyle modification to decrease weight, increase physical activity, and implement a nonatherogenic diet, in addition to treating the significant metabolic abnormalities that define the syndrome. The metabolic syndrome is frequently identified in patients with polycystic ovary syndrome, and has also been associated with the development of other disorders, including fatty liver disease, obstructive sleep apnea, hyperuricemia, and gout.

The patient does not meet the criteria for hypertriglyceridemia, although American Heart Association guidelines recommend an optimal triglyceride level of below 100 mg/dL (1.13 mmol/L), and this would be an appropriate goal for this patient for lifestyle modifications.

Impaired fasting glucose (prediabetes) is defined as a fasting blood glucose level of 100 to 125 mg/dL (5.6-6.9 mmol/L). She does not have this diagnosis, and the diagnosis of the metabolic syndrome does not strictly require abnormalities in glucose metabolism.

KEY POINT

- Metabolic syndrome is diagnosed by the presence of three or more of five abnormalities: increased waist circumference, elevated systolic or diastolic blood pressure, decreased HDL cholesterol level, elevated triglyceride level, and elevated fasting plasma glucose level.

Bibliography
Tota-Maharaj R, Defilippis AP, Blumenthal RS, Blaha MJ. A practical approach to the metabolic syndrome: review of current concepts and management. Curr Opin Cardiol. 2010;25(5):502-512. [PMID: 20644468]

Item 65   Answer: B
Educational Objective: Manage advanced cancer pain.

The next step in the treatment protocol for this patient would be a NSAID, such as ibuprofen. The World Health Organization analgesic ladder represents a useful framework for pharmacologic treatment of pain. Nonnarcotic treatments, such as aspirin, acetaminophen, or NSAIDs, are used for mild pain (score of 1-3 on the 0-10 pain intensity scale). Moderate pain (pain score 4-6) is treated with a combination of opioids and nonnarcotic pain relievers. If these agents are combined in a single pill (such as oxycodone and acetaminophen) to reduce polypharmacy, care must be taken to avoid inadvertent overdosing of the nonnarcotic component when the need for the opioid ingredient increases. The daily cumulative acetaminophen dose (<4 g) limits the dosing of the opioid in combination medications. Severe pain (pain score 7-10) is mainly treated with opioids. Adjunctive therapies (antidepressants, anticonvulsants, corticosteroids, muscle relaxants) can be used at all levels of the analgesic ladder. NSAIDs can be especially effective in patients with bone pain, particularly if there is an inflammatory component.

The use of gabapentin, an anticonvulsant, is a useful adjuvant pain medication and may be particularly helpful in patients with neuropathic pain but would be a poor choice for this patient with bone pain.

Meperidine is rarely appropriate for oral use owing to variable oral bioavailability and the accumulation of active metabolites with prolonged use at high doses or in kidney failure. Such accumulation lowers the seizure threshold and causes central nervous system symptoms, such as tremors, twitching, and nervousness.

Oral administration is the preferred route for opioid analgesics because of its convenience, low cost, and ability to produce stable opioid blood levels. Intramuscular injections are not recommended because of the associated pain, unreliable absorption, and relatively long interval to peak drug concentrations. This patient should be tried on a NSAID prior to an opioid medication.

KEY POINT

- Nonopioid agents are the first step in the management of mild cancer pain and should be initiated before progressing to an opioid agent.

Bibliography

Swetz KM, Kamal AH. Palliative care. Ann Intern Med. 2012;156(3):ITC21. [PMID: 22312158]

Item 66   Answer: D
Educational Objective: Treat dyslipidemia.

This patient should be started on statin therapy. He has a very high LDL cholesterol level despite a healthy diet and regular vigorous exercise. According to the National Cholesterol Education Program (NCEP) Adult Treatment Panel III guidelines, persons with two or more cardiovascular risk factors, such as this patient, should have an LDL cholesterol goal of below 130 mg/dL (3.37 mmol/L), and drug therapy should be considered in those with LDL cholesterol levels of 160 mg/dL (4.14 mmol/L) or above.

The non-HDL cholesterol level is calculated by subtracting the measured HDL cholesterol from the total cholesterol level. In patients with elevated triglycerides, the non-HDL level correlates with high concentrations of atherogenic lipoproteins, including VLDL remnants. The NCEP guidelines designate the non-HDL cholesterol level as a secondary target for therapy, after goal LDL cholesterol levels have been achieved. Calculation of the non-HDL cholesterol level will not alter this patient's current management strategy.

The U.S. Preventive Services Task Force (USPSTF) has recently reviewed the utility of adding several novel cardiac risk markers to traditional methods of cardiac risk stratification. According to their guidelines, there is insufficient evidence to recommend for or against the use of high-sensitivity C-reactive protein levels for assessing cardiovascular risk. Measurement of the high-sensitivity C-reactive protein level in this patient is not likely to affect management.

Fibric acid derivatives are effective at lowering triglyceride levels, but have a lesser effect on LDL cholesterol level. Although this patient has borderline-high triglyceride levels, lowering his LDL cholesterol level would significantly reduce his cardiovascular risk, and some reduction in his triglyceride levels would be expected with statin therapy.

KEY POINT

- In moderate-risk patients with LDL cholesterol levels of 160 mg/dL (4.14 mmol/L) or above, therapeutic lifestyle changes and pharmacologic lipid-lowering therapy are warranted.

Bibliography

U.S. Preventive Services Task Force. Using nontraditional risk factors in coronary heart disease risk assessment: U.S. Preventive Services Task Force recommendation statement. Ann Intern Med. 2009;151(7):474-482. [PMID: 19805770]

Item 67   Answer: A
Educational Objective: Manage fall risk in an elderly patient.

This patient appears to have had a fall without any indication of gait abnormality, visual deficit, or weakness. Her bumping into a wall at night may have caused the fall. It would be important to know if she has night lights in each room, because lack of proper lighting would contribute to her risk for falls. Installing night lights in each room is a simple and inexpensive fall prevention strategy. Additionally, an evaluation for home safety is always an appropriate consideration for patients who have fallen, because hazards can be found in two-thirds of homes. Other causes for falls, such as the presence of rugs and thresholds between rooms, have been ruled out. If the patient was already using night lights, then a home safety evaluation for other hazards, including general clutter, uneven lighting, and unsafe or absent hand rails, would be important.

In the Timed "Up & Go" (TUG) test, the patient is asked to arise from a chair, walk 10 feet, turn around, and sit in the same chair. Those completing the task in more than 14 seconds are considered high risk for subsequent falling. This patient's gait and TUG test are normal. An individualized exercise program is probably unnecessary in this patient with normal gait and motor examination. Additionally, meta-analyses have shown some harm with exercise programs in the elderly, especially in frail patients.

This patient's normal gross visual acuity on office testing suggests against an ophthalmologic contribution to her fall. Her normal gait and timed Up & Go test indicate that she does not require a walker.

KEY POINT

- An evaluation for home safety is important for patients who have fallen and may include the presence of rugs and thresholds between rooms, use of night lights, general clutter, uneven lighting, and unsafe or absent hand rails.

Bibliography

Wyman JF, Croghan CF, Nachreiner NM, et al. Effectiveness of education and individualized counseling in reducing environmental hazards in the homes of community-dwelling older women. J Am Geriatr Soc. 2007;55(10):1548-1556. [PMID: 17908058]

Item 68   Answer: D
Educational Objective: Diagnose schizophrenia.

This patient's negative symptoms of social withdrawal and flat affect and positive symptoms of paranoia and hearing voices are consistent with schizophrenia. Signs and symptoms should be present for at least 1 month and some for at least 6 months, as in this patient. Her family history of schizophrenia in a first-degree relative puts this patient's lifetime risk for developing this disorder between 6% and

Answers and Critiques

17%. Positive symptoms of schizophrenia include paranoid delusions, hearing voices, and hallucinations; negative symptoms include flat affect, social withdrawal, and lack of interest or enjoyment in life. Thought tends to be disorganized, with confused speech and rapid shifts in topic. No symptom or sign is pathognomonic for schizophrenia. Women tend to present later in life than males, who tend to present in their teenage years or early twenties.

Both bipolar disorder and major depressive disorder should be included in the differential diagnosis at this time. Up to 22% of patients diagnosed with schizophrenia will have their diagnosis changed during subsequent hospitalizations, so it is important to keep other medical and psychiatric causes of paranoia, auditory hallucinations, and social withdrawal in the differential diagnosis. This patient requires urgent psychiatric evaluation and possibly admission to the hospital for further evaluation.

Although this patient has been using marijuana, there is little evidence that *Cannabis* dependence or abuse leads to psychosis to the degree she is experiencing.

KEY POINT

- To make a diagnosis of schizophrenia, signs and symptoms should be present for at least 1 month and some for at least 6 months.

Bibliography

Schultz SH, North SW, Shields CG. Schizophrenia: a review. Am Fam Physician. 2007;75(12):1821-1829. [PMID: 17619525]

Item 69   Answer: B

Educational Objective: Recommend contraception options for a young woman.

Given this patient's demographic profile and behavior pattern, her risks of unintended pregnancy and sexually transmitted infection (STI) are very high, and a combination of barrier and hormonal methods is recommended. Condom use with a repository form of progesterone would both help prevent STIs and minimize the risk of contraceptive failure due to medication noncompliance.

Although condom use with combination estrogen-progesterone pills would be an effective regimen for both prevention of STIs and contraception, it would require daily medication adherence.

Although long-acting progesterone compounds such as depot medroxyprogesterone acetate are recommended in adolescents and young adults in whom user compliance may be unreliable, they do not offer protection from STIs.

A contraceptive vaginal ring containing estrogen and progesterone is a method of non–coitally based contraception that many users find more convenient than daily pills. It is an effective means of contraception, although it does require that the user be able to properly place the ring. It does not, however, confer protection against STIs, and therefore would not be a method of choice in this patient.

KEY POINT

- Contraception with a combination of a barrier method and a hormonal method is recommended in patients in whom the risks of unintended pregnancy and STIs are high.

Bibliography

Workowski KA, Berman S; Centers for Disease Control and Prevention (CDC). Sexually transmitted diseases treatment guidelines, 2010. MMWR Recomm Rep. 2010;59(RR-12):1-110. [PMID: 21160459]

Item 70   Answer: A

Educational Objective: Treat benign prostatic hyperplasia.

This patient has classic findings of symptomatic benign prostatic hyperplasia (BPH), and combination therapy with both an α-blocker and a 5α-reductase inhibitor is indicated. The American Urological Association (AUA) guideline on treatment of BPH recommends that patients with an AUA symptom score greater than 7 (questionnaire available at www2.niddk.nih.gov/NR/rdonlyres/8E99FCF4-8A92-43EE-8E47-5B70D634938A/0/AUABPH.pdf) or who are bothered by their symptoms receive treatment for BPH. 5α-Reductase inhibitors (5-ARIs), such as finasteride and dutasteride, may be suitable in patients who have failed to respond to or do not tolerate α-antagonists and those with severe symptoms. The Medical Therapy of Prostate Symptoms Study demonstrated that in the long term, among men with larger prostates, combination therapy is superior to either α-blocker or 5-ARI therapy in preventing progression and improving symptoms. Similarly, the ComBAT trial demonstrated that combination therapy resulted in significantly greater improvements than single-agent therapy. Combination therapy was associated with a higher incidence of adverse effects than monotherapy.

5-ARIs decrease the production of dihydrotestosterone, thereby arresting prostatic hyperplasia. Because shrinkage is slow, symptoms often do not improve until after 6 months of therapy. Therefore, these agents are not typically used as initial monotherapy for BPH, and switching this patient from an α-antagonist to a 5-ARI would not be indicated. Side effects include erectile and ejaculatory dysfunction, reduced libido, gynecomastia, and breast tenderness.

α-Antagonists (terazosin, doxazosin, alfuzosin, tamsulosin, silodosin) relax the prostatic smooth muscle in the bladder outflow tract, act rapidly (usually within 48 hours), and are considered first-line treatment, producing a clinical response in 70% of men. All drugs in this class have similar efficacy and tend to improve symptoms by 30% to 40%. Although some agents are more selective for prostate-specific α-receptors and therefore have less effect on systemic blood pressure, there is not a significant difference in effectiveness in treating BPH. Therefore, there is no benefit in switching between α-antagonists in this patient, as he has tolerated his current treatment well. Abnormal ejaculation is a side effect and appears similar for all α-antagonists. Elderly patients are less likely to discontinue treatment because of ejaculatory dysfunction than because of cardiovascular side effects, such as postural hypotension, dizziness, and headaches.

A 4-week course of a fluoroquinolone antibiotic would be appropriate therapy for chronic bacterial prostatitis. However, this patient has no symptoms or signs of prostatitis on examination and a normal urinalysis, making this diagnosis unlikely.

> **KEY POINT**
> • In patients with symptomatic benign prostatic hyperplasia, the combination of an α-blocker and a 5α-reductase inhibitor is associated with greater improvement in symptoms and more side effects than treatment with either agent alone.

Bibliography

Juliao AA, Plata M, Kazzazi A, Bostanci Y, Djavan B. American Urological Association and European Association of Urology guidelines in the management of benign prostatic hypertrophy: revisited. Curr Opin Urol. 2012;22(1):34-39. [PMID: 22123290]

Item 71   Answer: C
Educational Objective: Manage influenza vaccination in a healthy woman.

This healthy 30-year-old woman should receive a seasonal influenza vaccination. The Centers for Disease Control and Prevention currently recommends that all adults be vaccinated annually against influenza, regardless of risk factors. Vaccination usually takes place between September and March in the Northern hemisphere. Healthy adults can be vaccinated with either an inactivated vaccine injected intramuscularly or a live attenuated intranasal vaccine.

The hepatitis B vaccine is indicated for all children and adolescents through age 18 years, persons with HIV or other recent sexually transmitted infections, persons who are sexually active but not monogamous, workers with occupational exposure to blood, clients and staff of institutions for the developmentally disabled, correctional facility inmates, illicit drug users, persons with diabetes mellitus who are younger than 60 years, and persons with advanced chronic kidney disease who are approaching hemodialysis. Hepatitis B vaccination is also indicated for those planning travel to an endemic area and those with an increased risk for morbidity related to the disease, as well as for persons who request vaccination. This patient has no indication for hepatitis B vaccination.

The human papillomavirus vaccine is licensed for males and females aged 9 through 26 years and is recommended for females between the ages of 11 and 26 years and males

between the ages of 11 and 21 years. The vaccine is not indicated for this 30-year-old woman.

Current recommendations are that a tetanus and diphtheria (Td) vaccine be routinely administered every 10 years. Owing to an increased incidence of pertussis, thought in part to be related to waning immunity from childhood vaccination, all adults are recommended to receive a single tetanus, diphtheria, and acellular pertussis (Tdap) vaccination regardless of the interval since their last Td booster (although it may be given in place of a decennial Td booster if scheduled); this is a particularly important recommendation for persons aged 65 years or older because of the high burden of associated disease in this patient population. In addition, all postpartum women, health care workers, and adults who have close contact with infants younger than 12 months should receive a one-time Tdap booster if not already given. This patient is not due for a routine repeat Td booster for another 5 years and has no indications to receive either a Td or Tdap vaccination at this time.

> **KEY POINT**
> • Annual seasonal influenza vaccination is recommended for all adults, regardless of risk factors.

Bibliography

National Center for Immunization and Respiratory Diseases. General recommendations on immunization — recommendations of the Advisory Committee on Immunization Practices (ACIP). MMWR Recomm Rep. 2011;60(2):1-64. [PMID: 21293327]

Item 72   Answer: C
Educational Objective: Manage chronic fatigue syndrome.

The most appropriate management for this patient is to begin a graded exercise program. Chronic fatigue syndrome (CFS) is defined as medically unexplained fatigue that persists for 6 months or more and is accompanied by at least four of the following symptoms: subjective memory impairment, sore throat, tender lymph nodes, muscle or joint pain, headache, unrefreshing sleep, and postexertional malaise lasting longer than 24 hours. Management of CFS is challenging and is geared toward managing symptoms and maintaining function, rather than seeking cure. A comprehensive, individually tailored approach is required, typically based on nonpharmacologic therapy, such as lifestyle modification and sleep hygiene. Specific treatment options that have been demonstrated to improve symptoms include graded exercise programs and cognitive-behavioral therapy (CBT). CBT in this setting is targeted in part at breaking the cycle of effort avoidance, decline in physical conditioning, and increase in fatigue, and can work well in combination with graded exercise in this regard. CBT reduces fatigue and improves functional status.

Although Epstein-Barr virus and a host of other infectious agents have been considered in the pathogenesis of

CFS, none have been borne out by careful study; therefore, antiviral therapy, including acyclovir, has no role in the treatment of CFS. A variety of other medications have been tried, including corticosteroids, mineralocorticoids, growth hormone, and melatonin, but with no clear evidence of benefit, and are not indicated for this patient.

Current evidence is not sufficiently robust to recommend dietary supplements, herbal preparations (evening primrose oil), homeopathy, or even pharmacotherapy. Patients with concomitant depression should be treated with antidepressants. Although no specific class of antidepressant is recommended in this setting, tricyclic antidepressants are often utilized in patients with CFS and depression owing to their adjunct effectiveness in treating muscle pain.

KEY POINT

- Effective treatment options for chronic fatigue syndrome include graded exercise programs and cognitive-behavioral therapy.

Bibliography

Reid S, Chalder T, Cleare A, Hotopf M, Wessely S. Chronic fatigue syndrome. Clin Evid (Online). 2011;05:(1101)1-52. [PMID: 21615974]

Item 73   Answer: A

Educational Objective: Manage a difficult clinical encounter.

In this case of a patient with persistent symptoms not attributable to a specific cause and who is angry and demanding, an appropriate response is to provide empathetic supportive care at relatively frequent intervals. This would be best accomplished by initiating an ongoing discussion with the patient to better understand the potential causes and significance of her pain symptoms.

Multiple studies indicate that physicians classify about 15% of clinical encounters as difficult. Difficult encounters often involve patients who have a depressive or anxiety disorder, poorer functional status, unmet expectations, reduced satisfaction, and greater use of health care services. Physicians often report the most difficulty with patients by whom they feel manipulated or frustrated, patients who are time consuming and have unrealistic demands, patients who express anger, patients who do not follow the physician's recommendations, and those who interrupt physician routine and make extra work. Patients who have somatization disorder, chronic pain, substance abuse, or have an undiagnosable medical problem are often labeled as difficult. Patients with identifiable personality disorders such as borderline, dependent, histrionic, obsessive, or antisocial personality disorders also are frequently labeled as difficult.

It would be inappropriate to treat this patient's nonspecific pain with opioid medications based only on a patient's request without a better understanding of its etiology. Although this is an expedient way of dealing with a

difficult situation, it would not address the potentially complex causes of her symptoms or allow identification of more appropriate therapeutic interventions.

Patients with physical complaints that are inconsistent or without evidence of underlying pathology are particularly difficult to manage, especially in the context of a busy medical practice. These persons are often evaluated by multiple subspecialist physicians and undergo extensive testing, both as an attempt to achieve a diagnosis and because of time considerations. In this patient, while not inappropriate, gastroenterology evaluation would likely not be of high yield given her nonspecific clinical symptoms and examination findings, and would likely not address the issues underlying her complaints.

Transferring the care of the patient to another physician would not be desirable. One of the most important aspects of dealing with patients seen as difficult is to recognize the potential psychosocial and emotional factors that may be contributing to a patient's symptoms, even if they are not recognized as such by the individual. Equally important is for physicians to understand their own, potentially negative, emotions about the patient. Having some insight into these factors will hopefully allow the patient and physician to work together collaboratively to develop an appropriate diagnostic and treatment plan.

KEY POINT

- When involved in a difficult clinical encounter, an understanding of the patient's psychosocial and emotional factors potentially contributing to his or her symptoms as well as the physician's own feelings about the patient is essential in establishing and maintaining an effective therapeutic relationship.

Bibliography

Kroenke K. Unburdening the difficult clinical encounter. Arch Intern Med. 2009;169(4):333-334. [PMID: 19237715]

Item 74   Answer: D

Educational Objective: Appropriately administer the pneumococcal vaccine in a patient who has been previously vaccinated.

This man should receive a single pneumococcal polysaccharide vaccination at age 65 years. Adults 65 years and older should be immunized against pneumococcal pneumonia. The vaccine contains 23 antigen types of *Streptococcus pneumoniae* and protects against 60% of bacteremic disease. The vaccine is also recommended in some populations of younger patients, including Alaskan natives and certain American Indian populations; residents of long-term care facilities; patients who are undergoing radiation therapy or are on immunosuppressive medication; patients who smoke; and patients with chronic pulmonary disorders (including asthma), diabetes mellitus, cardiovascular disease, chronic liver or kidney disease, cochlear implants, asplenia, immune disorders, or malignancies. There is no information on vaccine safety during pregnancy. The vaccine is reasonably effective, with high levels of antibody typically found for at least 5 years. Currently, immunocompetent persons vaccinated after age 65 years are not recommended to receive a booster. Immunocompetent persons vaccinated before age 65 years, such as this patient, should receive a single booster vaccination at age 65 years, or 5 years after their first vaccination if they were vaccinated between the ages of 60 and 64 years.

Immunocompromised patients (including those with HIV infection and kidney disease) as well as patients with asplenia should receive a single pneumococcal vaccine booster 5 years after their first vaccine. This strategy would be inappropriate for this patient.

Current recommendations do not support more than a single booster after initial pneumococcal vaccination for any persons. Hence, a strategy of vaccination every 5 years would be inappropriate.

All patients vaccinated before age 65 years need a booster at some point. Hence, withholding further pneumococcal vaccination is inappropriate.

KEY POINT

- Immunocompetent persons who received the pneumococcal polysaccharide vaccine before age 65 years should receive a single booster vaccination at age 65 years, or 5 years after their first vaccination if they were vaccinated between the ages of 60 and 64 years.

Bibliography
Targonski PV, Poland GA. Pneumococcal vaccination in adults: recommendations, trends, and prospects. Cleve Clin J Med. 2007;74(6):401-406, 408-410, 413-414. [PMID: 17569198]

Item 75   Answer: A

Educational Objective: Treat hyperlipidemia in a woman who desires pregnancy.

This patient should be started on colesevelam. She has several risk factors for cardiovascular disease, including poorly controlled diabetes mellitus, hypertension, dyslipidemia, and a family history of premature myocardial infarction. Her goal LDL cholesterol level is below 100 mg/dL (2.59 mmol/L). Therapeutic lifestyle changes, which include a low-saturated fat diet and at least 120 minutes of aerobic exercise weekly, will reduce LDL cholesterol levels by 7% to 15%. Thus, this patient needs additional therapy to achieve her LDL cholesterol goal.

Ezetimibe is a cholesterol absorption inhibitor that can reduce LDL cholesterol levels by up to 19%. Treatment with ezetimibe has not been shown to have beneficial effects on cardiovascular morbidity or mortality. Moreover, ezetimibe is FDA pregnancy class X, and should be avoided in women who may become pregnant.

Gemfibrozil is a fibric acid that is typically used for the treatment of hypertriglyceridemia. It reduces LDL cholesterol levels by 10% or less; in addition, gemfibrozil monotherapy in patients with hypertriglyceridemia can actually raise LDL cholesterol levels. Gemfibrozil is not contraindicated in pregnancy (FDA pregnancy class C) but would not be effective for achieving this patient's LDL cholesterol goal.

Although statins (such as simvastatin) are typically the first-line treatment for lowering LDL cholesterol levels, statins are teratogenic (FDA pregnancy class X) and should be avoided in women who may be or wish to become pregnant. Colesevelam, which is a bile acid sequestrant that lowers LDL cholesterol levels by up to 18%, is the best initial treatment option for this patient. Colesevelam is FDA pregnancy class B and so is safe to use in premenopausal women who are sexually active. Bile acid sequestrants have been shown to reduce the risk of coronary heart disease in primary prevention trials. The most common side effects associated with bile acid sequestrants include constipation, abdominal pain and bloating, and flatulence. Bile acid sequestrants can bind to and reduce the absorption of other drugs; this effect can be minimized by administering the other drugs 1 hour before or 4 hours after taking a bile acid sequestrant.

KEY POINT

- Bile acid sequestrants are an option for reducing LDL cholesterol levels in women with hyperlipidemia who wish to become pregnant.

Bibliography
Pande RL. Approach to lipid therapy in the patient with atherosclerotic vascular disease. Curr Treat Options Cardiovasc Med. 2012;14(2)177-183. [PMID: 22270374]

Item 76   Answer: D

Educational Objective: Initiate nonhospice palliative care in a patient with newly diagnosed cancer.

In this patient with a newly diagnosed advanced malignancy, palliative care consultation is an important component of her care. Palliative care focuses on improving and maintaining the quality of life in individuals with any severe illness. Palliative care is a multidisciplinary, boarded specialty that focuses on preventing and relieving suffering and establishing goals of treatment that are consistent with the patient's wishes. This often involves efforts at pain and symptom control and encouraging and enabling patients to be actively involved in the decisions regarding their care. Nonhospice palliative care does not exclude testing, treatment, or hospitalization, but seeks to ensure that these interventions are consistent with what the patient wants and the expected goals and outcomes of care. Whereas care in a hospice setting may be palliative in nature, not all palliative care takes place in patients with terminal illness. Palliative care input may be particularly valuable in assisting this patient, who has a new diagnosis of severe

CONT.

disease, with understanding her illness and making key decisions regarding her care. Although studies are limited, palliative care has been shown to improve overall quality of life in the setting of various diseases relative to usual care for severely ill individuals.

Although depression may be seen in some patients with severe illness, starting therapy for depression without clear evidence the patient is having significant depressive symptoms or that pharmacologic treatment is indicated would be inappropriate.

It is not clear that this patient is either medically or emotionally ready for hospice care. Although her newly diagnosed malignancy may carry a poor prognosis, her currently stable condition and expressed desire to explore possible treatment options would make a decision to pursue hospice care premature without further characterization of her disease and discussion of her long-term treatment goals.

Opioid therapy is commonly used in cancers and particularly malignancies involving the respiratory tract to reduce both pain and dyspnea. However, this patient does not have significant pain and has only mild shortness of breath, which should improve as her pulmonary embolism resolves. Therefore, initiation of ongoing opioid therapy is not indicated.

KEY POINT

- Palliative care focuses on improving and maintaining the quality of life in any patient with severe illness; it is not limited to those with terminal illness or inpatient settings.

Bibliography
Bakitas M, Lyons KD, Hegel MT, et al. Effects of a palliative care intervention on clinical outcomes in patients with advanced cancer: the Project ENABLE II randomized control trial. JAMA. 2009;302(7):741-749. [PMID: 19690306]

Item 77 Answer: D
Educational Objective: Diagnose nonasthmatic eosinophilic bronchitis.

This patient's presentation is consistent with nonasthmatic eosinophilic bronchitis (NAEB), and the next diagnostic step would be sputum testing for eosinophils. NAEB is an increasingly recognized cause of chronic cough, particularly in patients such as this one who lack risk factors or findings for the more common causes of chronic cough (smoking, cough-variant asthma, gastroesophageal reflux disease, upper airways disease). Patients with NAEB do not exhibit symptoms of or pulmonary function testing evidence of airflow obstruction or hyperresponsiveness, with or without provocation with methacholine, which differentiates this entity from asthma. The diagnosis is supported by airway eosinophilia in an induced sputum sample (greater than 3%), bronchial washings, or biopsy. Although bronchial mucosal biopsies are required to definitively diagnose eosinophilic bronchitis, most experts recommend a therapeutic trial of

inhaled corticosteroid therapy as initial therapy, as most patients with NAEB will respond to this intervention.

Targeted and optimized empiric treatment of common causes of chronic cough is generally recommended prior to more invasive or costly testing. Treatment with antihistamines or decongestants should begin first, without need for sinus radiographs to evaluate for sinus disease in patients with suspected upper airway cough syndrome. Similarly, diet and lifestyle modification plus proton pump inhibitors for 1 to 3 months should be prescribed prior to considering 24-hour esophageal pH manometry to evaluate for acid reflux disease.

KEY POINT

- A diagnosis of nonasthmatic eosinophilic bronchitis should be considered in patients with chronic, nonproductive cough without an apparent cause, including asthma; sputum examination for eosinophils is useful in establishing the diagnosis.

Bibliography
Desai D, Brightling C. Cough due to asthma, cough-variant asthma and non-asthmatic eosinophilic bronchitis. Otolaryngol Clin North Am. 2010;43(1):123-130, x. [PMID: 20172262]

Item 78 Answer: A
Educational Objective: Evaluate an elderly patient with a recent fall.

This patient who has recently fallen should be assessed for gait and mobility. The Timed "Up & Go" (TUG) is a validated test for mobility that can be easily performed in the clinic and may be useful in predicting the likelihood of future falls. The test is performed by asking the patient to arise from a chair, walk 10 feet, turn around, and sit back down in the same chair. A time of more than 14 seconds indicates an increased risk for future falls. The sensitivity and specificity for one or more falls during the 6 months after the TUG test are 96% and 32%, respectively. In patients who have fallen, it is important to get a detailed history of the circumstances of the fall and whether the patient has fallen before or has problems with balance. A complete list of medications, particularly psychotropic medications, should be obtained. This patient had what sounds like a mechanical fall, without any evidence of syncope, lightheadedness, or dizziness. She remembers the entire event and was not confused after the fall, making a seizure unlikely.

Discontinuing lisinopril is not likely to reduce this patient's risk for falls because her blood pressure is not low, she has no orthostatic blood pressure changes, and she has no symptoms of lightheadedness or dizziness. Discontinuing antihypertensive medication would be indicated if it were deemed likely that hypotension or orthostatic hypotension were present and a possible cause for her fall.

Prescribing an exercise program would be indicated if physical examination revealed weakness or poor balance.

Some studies have shown that there may be harms associated with exercise programs in the frail older adult, so all such programs should be supervised.

Whereas providing an assistive device such as a walker would be indicated for patients with weakness, poor balance, or gait disturbance, assessment of gait and mobility should be performed first. If the TUG were abnormal, further assessment by a physical therapist could be performed to determine if an assistive device is indicated and which assistive device might be most helpful.

KEY POINT

- The Timed "Up & Go" (TUG) test for evaluating gait and mobility is performed by asking the patient to arise from a chair, walk 10 feet, turn around and sit back down in the same chair; a time of more than 14 seconds indicates an increased risk for future falls.

Bibliography

Nordin E, Lindelöf N, Rosendahl E, Jensen J, Lundin-Olsson L. Prognostic validity of the Timed Up-and-Go test, a modified Get-Up-and-Go test, staff's global judgement and fall history in evaluating fall risk in residential care facilities. Age Ageing. 2008;37(4):442-448. [PMID: 18515291]

Item 79   Answer: C
Educational Objective: Diagnose pes anserine bursitis.

This patient most likely has pes anserine bursitis. Although pes anserine bursitis most commonly occurs in patients with medial compartment osteoarthritis, it also occurs in the setting of overuse, as is the case with this patient. The pain is typically located along the anteromedial aspect of proximal tibia distal to the joint line of the knee. Pain is worse with climbing steps and frequently worsens at night.

Iliotibial band syndrome is a common cause of knife-like lateral knee pain that occurs with vigorous flexion-extension activities of the knee, such as running. It is treated conservatively with rest and stretching exercises. This patient's presentation is not consistent with iliotibial band syndrome as the patient's pain is located medially. Also, the pain with iliotibial band syndrome is characteristically worsened with walking both up and down steps, which this patient does not report.

The most common cause of knee pain in persons younger than 45 years, especially in women, is the patellofemoral syndrome. The pain is peripatellar and exacerbated by overuse (such as running), descending stairs, or prolonged sitting. On examination, pain and apprehension can often be elicited by applying pressure on the patella (the patellofemoral compression test).

Prepatellar bursitis presents with pain in the anterior aspect of the knee. On examination, swelling and tenderness to palpation are frequently present near the lower pole of the patella.

KEY POINT

- The pain of pes anserine bursitis is typically located along the anteromedial aspect of the proximal tibia distal to the joint line of the knee and characteristically worsens with step climbing and at night.

Bibliography

Schraeder TL, Terek RM, Smith CC. Clinical evaluation of the knee. New Engl J Med. 2010;363(4):e5. [PMID: 20660399]

Item 80   Answer: B
Educational Objective: Treat vulvovaginal candidiasis in a pregnant patient.

The most appropriate treatment for this pregnant woman is a topical imidazole, such as clotrimazole. She has classic symptoms and signs of vulvovaginal candidiasis (VVC), including itching, discomfort, and a thick, white vaginal discharge with evidence of vulvar edema and erythema on examination. The vaginal pH is normal, and potassium hydroxide preparation shows evidence of hyphae and yeast, supporting this diagnosis. Uncomplicated VVC is diagnosed when an otherwise healthy, nonpregnant patient has mild to moderate symptoms and suspected *Candida albicans* infection. Complicated VVC is diagnosed in women with severe symptoms (extensive vulvar erythema, edema, excoriation, and fissure formation), immunosuppression, multiple recurrences, or diabetes mellitus; and in women who are pregnant. As compared with treatment of uncomplicated VVC, patients with complicated VVC, such as this pregnant woman, typically require longer and more aggressive therapy. Regimens for treatment of complicated *C. albicans* vulvovaginitis include topical imidazole therapy for up to 14 days or two 150-mg doses of oral fluconazole given in two sequential doses 72 hours apart (compared with single-dose therapy). Topical imidazole therapy should be used preferentially in pregnant women, and a variety of regimens are available for treatment. Seven days of topical clotrimazole cream is an appropriate option in this patient.

Oral fluconazole is an appropriate treatment for uncomplicated VVC, and is associated with high treatment success rates. However, it should not be given in pregnancy as the effect on the fetus is unknown (FDA pregnancy category C medication), and topical therapy is equally efficacious.

Although 30% of women will experience two or more episodes of VVC, recurrent VVC is diagnosed if a patient experiences more than four symptomatic episodes per year. Frequently, recurrent VVC is associated with non-*albicans Candida* infection. Initial treatment of culture-proven non-*albicans* VVC includes 7 to 14 days of an oral or topical non-imidazole therapy, such as voriconazole, a second-generation triazole antifungal agent; recurrent VVC may be treated with intravaginal boric acid for 2 weeks. Because this patient has had only one previous episode of symptomatic VVC, which responded well to treatment, she can be empirically treated for *Candida albicans* infection again.

KEY POINT

• Treatment of *Candida albicans* vulvovaginal candidiasis in pregnant women typically requires longer and more aggressive therapy; topical imidazole therapy for 7 days is the preferred treatment.

Bibliography

ACOG Committee on Practice Bulletins—Gynecology. ACOG Practice Bulletin. Clinical management guidelines for obstetrician-gynecologists, Number 72, May 2006: Vaginitis. Obstet Gynecol. 2006;107(5):1195-1206. [PMID: 16648432]

Item 81   Answer: B

Educational Objective: Treat cough in a patient taking an ACE inhibitor.

In this patient with a nonproductive cough, the best option is to discontinue lisinopril. Clinical evaluation of chronic cough (>8 weeks in duration) includes a careful history and physical examination focusing on the common causes of chronic cough. All patients should undergo chest radiography. Smoking cessation and discontinuation of ACE inhibitors should be recommended for 4 weeks before additional workup. Cough is a common side effect of ACE inhibitors. Approximately 15% of patients who are prescribed these medications will develop a nonproductive cough. Reported causative factors include bradykinin and substance P, which are metabolized by angiotensin-converting enzyme and prostaglandins. The onset may be delayed, as in this patient, and may take up to 4 weeks to resolve upon discontinuation of the drug (rarely, up to 3 months). Although the cough is frequently mild, in some patients it is significant enough to interfere with quality of life, and alternate therapy needs to be considered. Substitution of an angiotensin receptor blocker, such as losartan, is a good alternative in this patient; these medications generally do not cause cough (incidence is similar to that of placebo) and evidence supports their renal protective benefits in patients with diabetes mellitus.

Because this patient's cough has been present for 8 weeks, other causes of chronic cough should be considered. As the clinical picture is most consistent with ACE inhibitor–induced cough and there is no symptom predominance to support bronchospasm (history of asthma, wheezing and cough with exertion, exposure to allergens or cold air), upper airway cough syndrome (postnasal drip with frequent nasal discharge, a sensation of liquid dripping into the back of the throat, and frequent throat clearing), or gastroesophageal reflux disease (heartburn or regurgitation), initial empiric treatment with albuterol, an antihistamine, intranasal corticosteroids, or omeprazole is not indicated at this time. ACE inhibitor–induced cough generally abates within 4 weeks

after the drug is discontinued. If this patient's cough persists beyond this time, a systemic approach to treatment of chronic cough should ensue.

KEY POINT

• In patients with chronic cough and a normal chest radiograph, smoking cessation and discontinuation of ACE inhibitors should be recommended for 4 weeks before additional evaluation for the cough.

Bibliography

Dicpinigaitis PV. Angiotensin-converting enzyme inhibitor-induced cough: ACCP evidence-based clinical practice guidelines. Chest. 2006;129(1 suppl):169S-173S. [PMID: 16428706]

Item 82   Answer: A

Educational Objective: Manage medications perioperatively.

This patient should continue all of his current medications. Antiplatelet therapy (including aspirin and clopidogrel), antihypertensive medications, and anticonvulsant drugs can be continued during low-risk surgeries, such as cataract surgery, if the benefit outweighs the risk. In a preoperative evaluation each medication should be assessed for its individual risk and benefit. Those for which risk outweighs benefit should be temporarily discontinued perioperatively.

Dual antiplatelet therapy with clopidogrel and aspirin should be continued for at least 1 year in patients who have received a drug-eluting stent. This patient's drug-eluting stent was inserted only 6 months ago; therefore, the patient remains at increased risk for in-stent thrombosis if clopidogrel is discontinued and at no increased risk of bleeding related to the cataract surgery if clopidogrel is continued.

The use of β-blockers in the perioperative period is controversial, with well-designed randomized controlled trials showing both benefit and harm. Current recommendations are that patients currently on a β-blocker should continue taking it. Thus, metoprolol should not be discontinued.

Any medication that can produce withdrawal symptoms, such as benzodiazepines, long-acting narcotics, and antiseizure drugs, are typically continued the morning of surgery.

KEY POINT

• In a preoperative evaluation, each medication should be assessed for its individual risk and benefit, and those for which risk outweighs benefit should be temporarily discontinued perioperatively.

Bibliography

Whinney C. Perioperative medication management: general principles and practical applications. Cleve Clin J Med. 2009;76(suppl 4):S126-32. [PMID: 19880829]

Answers and Critiques

Item 83   Answer: A

Educational Objective: Manage a request for physician-assisted suicide.

When approached with a request for assistance in dying, it is best to respond to the request with empathy and compassion, and assess whether or not the patient is receiving adequate palliative interventions. Optimizing care interventions focused on maintaining or improving the quality of life may not always occur in the context of treating the underlying disease process; thus, reviewing the patient's overall care to address comfort and functional issues in severe illness is essential to appropriate management. Involving physicians trained specifically in palliative care medicine may also be helpful in such situations.

Physician-assisted suicide is a controversial area of ethics. Most ethicists agree that it is acceptable to consider interventions that may hasten the death of a terminally ill patient if the primary intent is therapeutic (the principle of "double effect"). However, physician-assisted suicide using prescriptions or interventions with the specific intent to kill the patient is illegal in most states. The American Medical Association and the American College of Physicians have both taken positions against the practice.

Seeking legal counsel may be advisable if one intends to provide the patient assistance in dying, as states in which it is legal have specific protocols that must be followed. However, this step would not be appropriate until alternatives such as improved palliative care were assessed.

Categorically refusing to discuss a request for physician-assisted suicide can close the door to a discussion of why the patient is making the request and may jeopardize the therapeutic relationship with the patient.

Writing a prescription for medication to assist a patient in dying without a detailed assessment of the patient's situation and motives would be irresponsible.

KEY POINT

- When approached with a request for assistance in dying, it is best to respond to the request with empathy and compassion, and assess whether or not the patient is receiving adequate palliative care.

Bibliography

Snyder L, Sulmasy DP; Ethics and Human Rights Committee, American College of Physicians-American Society of Internal Medicine. Physician-assisted suicide. Ann Intern Med. 2001;135(3):209-216. [PMID: 11487490]

Item 84   Answer: C

Educational Objective: Diagnose Morton neuroma.

This patient most likely has Morton neuroma, which is thought to be caused by inflammation, edema, and scarring of the small interdigital nerves. It commonly occurs in overuse syndromes (such as running) and with wearing tight shoes. It classically presents with burning pain on the plantar surface in the space between the third and fourth toes but may also occur between the second and third toes. Women are more commonly affected than men, and the wearing of high heels is a recognized risk factor. Treatment is typically conservative, with the goal of reducing pressure across the metatarsal heads through the use of padding, orthotics, and the removal of likely inciting footwear or activities. If conservative measures fail, a local corticosteroid injection is usually successful.

A hammer toe is characterized by a flexion deformity of the proximal interphalangeal joints with normal distal interphalangeal joints and metatarsophalangeal joints. Presenting symptoms include pain and difficulty wearing shoes because of the resulting toe structure. A corn may also develop on the dorsal surface of the proximal interphalangeal joint.

In metatarsal stress fractures, the examination is notable for tenderness to palpation of the fracture site. It would not be expected to cause pain between toes, as is the case in this patient.

Tarsal tunnel syndrome is entrapment of the posterior tibial nerve or one of its branches as it travels behind the medial malleolus. Although this may cause pain and a burning sensation, symptoms tend to occur on the medial plantar aspect of the foot, occasionally mimicking plantar fasciitis.

KEY POINT

- Morton neuroma is characterized by burning pain on the plantar surface in the space between the third and fourth toes.

Bibliography

Wu KK. Morton neuroma and metatarsalgia. Curr Opin Rheumatol. 2000;12:131-142. [PMID: 10751016]

Item 85   Answer: A

Educational Objective: Manage body dysmorphic disorder.

Cognitive-behavioral therapy (CBT) would be appropriate in the management of this patient. This patient's presentation is consistent with body dysmorphic disorder, a somatoform disorder in which a patient is focused on a single real or imagined symptom. In order to qualify as a psychiatric disorder, somatoform symptoms need to be medically unexplained or out of proportion to medically expected findings, should persist over time, and cause impairment in a patient's ability to function. Although no therapy has been shown to be consistently helpful in treating somatoform disorders, multiple trials have found benefit in patients who undergo CBT.

Benzodiazepines such as diazepam have not been shown to be of benefit for somatoform disorders, and would likely be a poor choice because of their ability to induce tolerance and long-term dependence.

It is unlikely that this patient would have any additional abnormal findings on further abdominal imaging. As patients with somatoform disorders have a true psychiatric disease, additional normal diagnostic tests are ineffective in alleviating symptoms.

Psychosis encompasses delusions, hallucinations, disorganized speech, and disorganized or catatonic behavior. Psychotic features may occur in depression as well as other psychiatric or organic disorders, but schizophrenia is a disorder in which psychosis is a defining feature. The diagnosis requires at least 6 months of symptoms, including 1 month or more of at least two active-phase symptoms, such as hallucinations, delusions, disorganized speech, grossly disorganized or catatonic behavior; and negative symptoms, such as flattened affect. This patient is not psychotic and treatment with an antipsychotic medication such as olanzapine is not indicted.

KEY POINT

- Although no therapy has been shown to be consistently helpful in treating somatoform disorders, multiple trials have found benefit in patients who undergo cognitive-behavioral therapy.

Bibliography

Kroenke K. Efficacy of treatment for somatoform disorders: a review of randomized controlled trials. Psychosom Med. 2007;69(9):881-888. [PMID: 18040099]

Item 86   Answer: E

Educational Objective: Evaluate vasovagal syncope.

No further testing is required for this patient. Her symptoms are consistent with the most common form of syncope, vasovagal neurocardiogenic syncope, the common "faint." Suggestive features of vasovagal syncope include any of the "3 P's": Posture (occurrence during prolonged standing, or similar previous episodes that have been aborted by lying down); Provoking factors (e.g., pain, a medical procedure); and Prodromal symptoms (sweating, feeling warm before loss of consciousness). Persons with an uncomplicated faint, situational syncope, or orthostatic hypotension should undergo electrocardiography but do not otherwise require immediate further investigation or specialist referral.

Admission to the hospital for telemetry should be considered in patients with undiagnosed syncope but with known structural heart disease and at high risk for arrhythmia. Even in this selected group, however, the diagnostic yield is low (approximately 16%), and there is no benefit for patients with symptoms compatible with vasovagal syncope in the absence of known heart disease.

Neuroimaging, such as CT scanning, is of limited use in evaluating syncope. It has the highest yield in patients who are older than 65 years and have neurologic symptoms, such as headache, neurologic examination abnormalities, head trauma, or are on anticoagulants. This patient has no features to suggest a neurologic cause of syncope and a head CT scan is not indicated.

If structural heart disease is suspected, further assessment should include cardiac imaging, usually by echocardiography, as the first diagnostic test. There is nothing in the patient's history or physical examination that suggests structural heart disease, and echocardiography is not indicated.

Tilt-table testing is reserved for patients with suspected neurocardiogenic syncope not confirmed by history and physical examination, those with recurrent episodes, and those with a suspected cardiac cause. As this patient's history and physical examination are consistent with vasovagal syncope and there is no history of recurrent episodes, tilt-table testing is not indicated.

KEY POINT

- Persons with uncomplicated faint, situational syncope, or orthostatic hypotension do not require further investigation if the initial physical examination and electrocardiogram are normal.

Bibliography

Cooper PN, Westby M, Pitcher DW, Bullock I. Synopsis of the National Institute for Health and Clinical Excellence Guideline for management of transient loss of consciousness. Ann Intern Med. 2011;155(8):543-549. [PMID: 21930835]

Item 87   Answer: B

Educational Objective: Manage a fall in an elderly patient.

In this patient with generalized weakness as well as leg muscle weakness, slow gait, and a recent fall, it is appropriate to prescribe vitamin D. Vitamin D deficiency increases the risk for falls in the elderly and vitamin D supplementation reduces this risk. According to U.S. Preventive Services Task Force recommendations, vitamin D supplementation can be prescribed without first obtaining a serum vitamin D level for patients with an increased risk of falling. The proposed mechanism of action of vitamin D is its beneficial effect on muscle strength and function and on gait. Although calcium supplementation may have a beneficial effect on bone loss, there is no clear benefit to adding calcium in reducing falls.

Discontinuing lisinopril is not appropriate because she does not demonstrate orthostatic blood pressure changes that would account for her fall, and discontinuing antihypertensive medication would likely result in elevated blood pressure.

Zolpidem is a nonbenzodiazepine sedative hypnotic with a short half-life that can be prescribed for a limited time period for insomnia. Caution must be exercised, however, because of adverse effects, including an increased risk for falls, especially among older adults. Reviewing sleep hygiene would be a better first step in managing her insomnia.

Although this patient demonstrates a mild near-vision deficit, it is not likely that this deficit contributed significantly to her fall. Furthermore, bifocal lenses are associated with an increased risk for falling. If needed, reading glasses could be obtained.

KEY POINT

- Vitamin D supplementation reduces the risk for falls in elderly patients, and can be prescribed without obtaining a serum vitamin D level in patients with an increased risk of falling.

Bibliography
Kalyani RR, Stein B, Valiyil R, et al. Vitamin D treatment for the prevention of falls in older adults: systematic review and meta-analysis. J Am Geriatr Soc. 2010;58(7):1299-1310. [PMID: 20579169]

Item 88   Answer: A
Educational Objective: Treat stress urinary incontinence.

This patient has stress urinary incontinence and should receive pelvic floor muscle training (PFMT). Stress urinary incontinence, defined as loss of urine with physical activity, cough, or sneeze, is caused by sphincter incompetence. Findings on physical examination include weakened anterior or posterior vaginal wall support (cystocele or rectocele, respectively). PFMT is considered first-line therapy for urinary stress incontinence. In PFMT, women learn repetitive exercises (Kegel exercises) to strengthen the voluntary urethral sphincter and levator ani muscles. For PFMT to be effective, it is important that the patient learn to correctly contract her muscles without straining, which increases abdominal pressure. Each contraction is held for approximately 10 seconds, followed by an equal relaxation period. The number of repetitions should be increased weekly until the patient is performing 8 to 12 repetitions three times daily, every day or at least 3 to 4 days per week. In a systematic review of nonsurgical therapy, PFMT improved stress urinary incontinence episodes. Outcomes were even better when PFMT was combined with biofeedback and when skilled therapists directed the treatment.

Prompted voiding is indicated in and is effective in patients with significant mobility or cognitive impairments that may hinder the patient's ability to reach the toilet in time, neither of which this patient has.

Sling procedures are effective for moderate to severe stress incontinence, but surgery is usually reserved for patients who do not benefit from more conservative approaches, including behavioral or appropriate pharmacologic therapy.

Tolterodine, a selective antimuscarinic anticholinergic medication, is most effective for patients with urge, rather than stress, incontinence. This patient does not experience the classic sense of urinary urgency with her incontinence episodes, and, therefore, tolterodine would not be an appropriate first choice.

KEY POINT

- Pelvic floor muscle training is first-line treatment for stress urinary incontinence.

Bibliography
Shamliyna TA, Kane RL, Wyman J, Wilt TJ. Systematic review: randomized, controlled trials of nonsurgical treatments for urinary incontinence in women. Ann Intern Med. 2008;148(6):459-473. [PMID: 18268288]

Item 89   Answer: D

Educational Objective: Initiate a discussion about palliative care with the family of a cancer patient.

The cornerstone of establishing goals of care in the end-of-life setting is to communicate in a patient-centered, open-ended format. This is true regardless of whether a patient or patient's family is angry or is requesting inappropriately aggressive care. The first step in this process in this case is to ask the family to tell you what they understand about the patient's condition. Active, empathic listening allows the caregiver to establish what the patient and family understand about the diagnosis and prognosis. It also shows respect for the myriad ways in which loved ones process information about medical conditions and helps to establish trust. The family should be allowed to vent their frustration and to articulate what they believe the patient's condition and chance of meaningful recovery to be. Given the feelings of distress about the patient's condition, it is entirely possible that one meeting may not be enough to establish clearly defined goals of care. Asking open-ended questions and being comfortable with silences are important in building a trusting relationship with the patient and family.

The upcoming dialogue with the family is likely to be emotionally charged, and a series of visits may be needed to cover all appropriate areas. It would not be appropriate to initiate the discussion with the patient and family about advanced directives until it is learned what the family knows about the diagnosis and prognosis.

It would not be helpful to begin a meeting with a distraught family or patient by stating curative therapy would be futile. This approach is likely to further alienate a family struggling with a distressing diagnosis.

Although explaining the diagnosis and prognosis may be an important goal for a family meeting, it is usually more effective to begin the meeting with an open-ended question that allows the physician to better understand the family's

CONT.

perspective. Explanations can then be better tailored to what the family knows and understands about the patient's condition.

> **KEY POINT**
> • The cornerstone of establishing goals of care in the end-of-life setting is to communicate in a patient-centered, open-ended format.

Bibliography

Swetz KM, Kamal AH. Palliative care. Ann Intern Med. 2012;156(3):ITC21. [PMID: 22312158]

Item 90   Answer: C

Educational Objective: Evaluate a breast mass in a postmenopausal woman.

This patient should undergo core needle biopsy of the mass. She presents with a normal mammogram but with suspicious findings on physical examination for breast cancer. The palpable mass is nonpainful, persistent, and firm. Although her normal mammogram could be interpreted as reassuring, approximately 10% to 20% of palpable breast cancers can be missed by either ultrasonography or screening mammography. She requires further evaluation to definitively rule in or rule out malignancy. Core needle biopsy, with or without ultrasonographic or stereotactic guidance, provides excellent tissue sampling for pathology and receptor status. It is the test of choice for most solid lesions.

Breast MRI would likely better define the breast lesion radiographically that was not visualized on mammography, but would not replace the need for a tissue diagnosis in this patient.

Breast ultrasonography is particularly useful in defining possible cystic lesions identified on examination or mammography. However, given the highly suspicious nature of this patient's breast mass, ultrasonography would not be indicated.

Reassurance is inappropriate as definitive diagnosis of the mass via tissue sampling is imperative in this postmenopausal woman.

> **KEY POINT**
> • Core needle biopsy is the test of choice for most solid breast masses.

Bibliography

Barlow WE, Lehman CD, Zheng Y, et al. Performance of diagnostic mammography for women with signs or symptoms of breast cancer. J Natl Cancer Inst. 2002;94(15):1151-1159. [PMID: 12165640]

Item 91   Answer: A

Educational Objective: Manage acute low back pain.

In this patient presenting with uncomplicated low back pain and examination findings suggesting radiculopathy,

initial treatment with nonopioid analgesics and mobilization as tolerated is most appropriate. The overall prognosis for acute musculoskeletal low back pain is excellent; most patients without sciatica show substantial improvement within 2 weeks, and three quarters of those with sciatica are substantially better after 3 months; therefore, therapeutic interventions should focus on mitigating symptoms and maintaining function while the patient recovers.

Complete blood count and erythrocyte sedimentation rate are helpful in assessing for infection, inflammatory spondylitis, and malignancy. This patient has no signs or symptoms suggestive of systemic illness, and specific laboratory testing is therefore not indicated at this time.

Epidural corticosteroid injection is sometimes considered in patients with chronic radiculopathy, although the literature is mixed regarding its value. This patient has an excellent prognosis without intervention, so invasive treatments would be inappropriate as initial therapy.

Lumbar spine imaging is not indicated for most patients with acute lumbosacral back pain with radiculopathy as it does not add clinically significant information. Situations in which imaging is necessary include patients with rapidly progressing neurologic symptoms, evidence of cord compression, cauda equina syndrome, or if infection or malignancy is a possible cause of the patient's symptoms and examination findings.

Lumbar spine radiography is helpful to assess for possible malignancy or compression fracture. In this younger patient without evidence of systemic illness, radiography is not indicated. An MRI would likely demonstrate the disk herniation and nerve root compression that are already evident on physical examination, but the management plan would still be analgesics and gentle mobilization.

> **KEY POINT**
> • Therapeutic interventions for most patients with acute low back pain should focus on mitigating symptoms and maintaining function while the patient recovers.

Bibliography

Chou R, Qaseem A, Snow V, et al; Clinical Efficacy Assessment Subcommittee of the American College of Physicians; American College of Physicians; American Pain Society Low Back Pain Guidelines Panel. Diagnosis and treatment of low back pain: a joint clinical practice guideline from the American College of Physicians and the American Pain Society. Ann Intern Med. 2007;147(7):478-491. [PMID: 17909209]

Item 92   Answer: A

Educational Objective: Recognize threats to validity in a medical study.

The main reason that it is difficult to determine the effectiveness of this drug based on the published study is that there is no comparison, or control, group. When evaluating the medical literature, it is important to consider the quality of the study design. Studies assessing treatment effectiveness should always have a control group, which can receive either an alternative treatment or a placebo. A control group is critical because it tells the investigators what would have happened if the intervention had not been done. Depending on the study type, patients can be assigned to a control group (in an experimental study), or be part of a "natural" control (observational study). The primary threat to validity of this study is the absence of a control group; that is, there is no group with which the patients taking "drug X" can be compared.

In general, it is always best for outcomes in any study to be assessed by an independent evaluator who is unaware of treatment assignment ("blinded"). In the case of unambiguous outcomes such as death, however, an unblinded outcomes assessment is permissible.

In experimental study designs, investigators often randomly assign patients to a therapy in order to equalize the group for measured and unmeasured confounding variables. This trial has no comparison group, so randomization would not be possible.

Increased numbers of patients in studies generally yield greater precision in measurement. In this trial, however, the key threat to validity is not trial size but absence of a control group.

KEY POINT

- The primary threat to validity in a case series is the absence of a control group.

Bibliography
Ho PM, Peterson PN, Masoudi FA. Evaluating the evidence: is there a rigid hierarchy? Circulation. 2008;118(16):1675-1684. [PMID: 18852378]

Item 93   Answer: E

Educational Objective: Manage attention-deficit/hyperactivity disorder in an adult.

The most appropriate management for this patient with attention-deficit/hyperactivity disorder (ADHD) is to stop his ADHD medication and reassess his need for treatment. ADHD is characterized by difficulty paying attention, impulsivity, and motor restlessness or hyperactivity, with onset before the age of 7 years. There must also be some impairment in social, occupational, or academic functioning, and the symptoms must be manifest in at least two different environments, such as school and home. There are three subtypes: predominantly inattentive, predominantly hyperactive, and a combined type. The presence of symptoms in childhood is crucial to the diagnosis of ADHD, and this patient gives a history that is compatible with ADHD. However, he also has new-onset hypertension and a heart rate at the higher end of normal, which could be related to sympathomimetic drug use. He has had relatively few symptoms related to ADHD for the past 2 years. Periodic "drug holidays" for adult patients with ADHD may be useful to assess

need for ongoing medications; this would be an opportune moment for a drug holiday in this patient.

Atomoxetine is a selective norepinephrine reuptake inhibitor that is specifically approved for treatment of ADHD in adults. It is not associated with hypertension and would be a reasonable option after his drug holiday if there is a need for ongoing medications; however, first it should be ascertained whether he still needs pharmacologic treatment for his ADHD. Atomoxetine carries a black box warning of increased suicidal ideation in the pediatric population and has been associated with rare but serious hepatotoxicity.

Fluoxetine and other selective serotonin reuptake inhibitors have not been shown to be useful for the treatment of ADHD. Bupropion and tricyclic antidepressants may be helpful for ADHD, although this is an off-label use of these drugs.

Methylphenidate has sympathomimetic properties, and could contribute to his hypertension. Therefore, switching to this agent would not be beneficial.

KEY POINT

- In adult patients with attention-deficit/hyperactivity disorder (ADHD), it is important to reassess the need for ADHD medications periodically.

Bibliography
Okie S. ADHD in Adults. N Engl J Med. 2006;354:2637-2641. [PMID: 16790695]

Item 94   Answer: D

Educational Objective: Manage a transition of care in an elderly patient undergoing hospital discharge.

The patient should be evaluated for placement in a skilled nursing facility. Although discharge home is preferable if a patient is safe and medically stable for care in that setting, this patient is not able to return home to a setting in which she was not doing well prior to admission. Her complicated hospitalization has left her significantly debilitated. Skilled nursing facilities provide nursing level services, such as intravenous medications and medication management, wound care, and other medical services in addition to low-level rehabilitation services. With further recovery, her long-term care options may be reassessed and the most appropriate type pursued.

Inpatient rehabilitation is focused on intensive physical and occupational therapy and other forms of rehabilitative treatment as needed. Although patients with active medical issues may be candidates for inpatient rehabilitation, these issues need to be stable, and patients are generally required to participate in therapy for a minimum of 3 hours daily.

Long-term acute care hospitals (LTACHs) provide care similar to that in an acute hospital setting but for patients who are considered stable with the need for hospital-based

CONT.

testing or interventions and with few anticipated changes in the care plan. This setting is overseen by physicians and is appropriate for patients who require significant medical monitoring but are expected to have a more prolonged (more than 25 days) time to recovery. This patient's medical needs are minimal and could be appropriately provided in a skilled nursing setting.

Although this patient may have been declining for several years, she does not have a diagnosis or condition indicative of a prognosis of less than 6 months. To qualify for hospice care, her physician must feel that her expected prognosis is less than 6 months of life remaining.

Establishing appropriate discharge care plans involves close coordination with the physician, patient and family, and the care coordination staff. Understanding the patient's medical needs is critical in determining the appropriate options available, and this process should be started as early as possible in the course of hospitalization.

KEY POINT

- Understanding a patient's medical needs in conjunction with the wishes and resources available to the patient and family is critical in determining appropriate posthospital care, and this process should be started as early as possible in the course of hospitalization.

Bibliography
Kane RL. Finding the right level of posthospital care: "We didn't realize there was any other option for him". JAMA. 2011;305(3):284-293. [PMID: 21245184]

Item 95   Answer: A
Educational Objective: Diagnose acute angle-closure glaucoma.

This patient most likely has acute angle-closure glaucoma. Angle-closure glaucoma is characterized by narrowing or closure of the anterior chamber angle, which impedes the trabecular drainage system in the anterior chamber, resulting in elevated intraocular pressure and damage to the optic nerve. Acute angle-closure glaucoma is an ophthalmologic emergency. Symptoms depend upon the rapidity of the elevation of intraocular pressure. Typical history of acute angle-closure glaucoma may include seeing halos around lights, severe unilateral eye pain, headache, and nausea and vomiting. Occasionally, patients may present with only nausea and vomiting and be mistaken as having cardiac or abdominal pathology. Physical examination may show conjunctival erythema; a sluggish or nonreactive, mid-range dilated pupil; corneal cloudiness; and, on funduscopic examination, cupping of the optic nerve. Treatment in this case would be immediate referral to an ophthalmologist or emergency department for initiation of topical β-adrenergic antagonists and pilocarpine and carbonic anhydrase inhibitors.

Central retinal artery occlusion (CRAO) classically presents in a 50- to 70-year-old patient as a painless, abrupt loss of vision that occurs in the early morning hours—usually between midnight and 6 AM and, second most commonly, between 6 AM and noon. It results from an embolic or thrombotic event in the ophthalmic artery. Although this patient is at risk for CRAO owing to her atrial fibrillation, CRAO would not cause red eye, a firm globe, ocular pain, nausea, or vomiting.

Ocular migraine, also known as retinal migraine, typically occurs in persons with a family history or personal history of migraine, which this patient does not have. Symptoms include flashing lights, scintillating scotomas, visual blurring, and even total unilateral vision loss. Patients with ocular migraine tend to be younger than 40 years, making this diagnosis highly unlikely in this 76-year-old patient.

Temporal arteritis should be considered in patients older than 50 years presenting with a severe new headache. Visual loss in temporal arteritis is painless, however, and would not cause a red eye, nausea, or vomiting.

KEY POINT

- Acute angle-closure glaucoma is characterized by severe unilateral eye pain, headache, nausea and vomiting, and seeing halos around lights; physical examination findings include conjunctival erythema; a sluggish or nonreactive, mid-range dilated pupil; corneal cloudiness; and cupping of the optic nerve.

Bibliography
Magauran B. Conditions requiring emergency ophthalmologic consultation. Emerg Med Clin North Am. 2008;26(1):233-238. [PMID: 18249265]

Item 96   Answer: B
Educational Objective: Diagnose de Quervain tenosynovitis.

This patient's presentation is most consistent with de Quervain tenosynovitis, which refers to swelling or stenosis of the abductor pollicis longus and extensor pollicis brevis tendon sheaths at the level of the wrist. It is most commonly caused by repetitive motion of the thumb but can also be associated with underlying conditions including pregnancy and rheumatoid arthritis. This condition commonly presents with pain and swelling located over the radial styloid. The pain occurs with use of the thumb. On examination, there is localized tenderness of the distal radial styloid. Pain is elicited with both resisted thumb abduction and extension. The Finkelstein test is frequently positive (as with this patient).

Carpometacarpal arthritis presents with pain at the base of the thumb that occurs with thumb gripping and pinching. This pain may radiate into the distal forearm. On examination, there is tenderness to palpation on both the dorsal and palmar surfaces of the joint. Compressing the joint by applying a longitudinal load frequently produces pain. In advanced cases, joint stiffness and loss of range of motion may be present. The absence of these findings, as well as the patient's young age, argues against carpometacarpal arthritis as the cause of his pain.

A ganglion is a cyst that forms on the tendon sheath and results from inflammation, often following trauma. The anatomic location of the patient's pain and the absence of a palpable cystic structure do not support this diagnosis.

Patients with a scaphoid fracture usually have a history of an injury that involves wrist dorsiflexion. Pain is located in the anatomic snuffbox (the radial side of the wrist between the abductor and long thumb extensor tendons just distal to the radial styloid). On examination, there is significant tenderness to palpation of the anatomic snuffbox.

KEY POINT

- de Quervain tenosynovitis is pain that occurs with thumb use, characterized by pain and swelling over the radial styloid that is is elicited with both resisted thumb abduction and extension.

Bibliography

Moore JS. De Quervain's tenosynovitis. Stenosing tenosynovitis of the first dorsal compartment. J Occup Environ Med. 1997;39(10):990-1002. [PMID: 9343764]

Item 97   Answer: D

Educational Objective: Manage temporomandibular joint disorder.

This patient likely has a temporomandibular disorder. Initial treatment of temporomandibular disorders focuses on non-interventional, nonpharmacologic strategies. Jaw relaxation, heat, and therapeutic exercises may be helpful. Temporomandibular disorders are more common in women and typically present in the third or fourth decade of life. Patients typically report unilateral jaw discomfort in the masticatory muscles, often with radiation to the ear or posterior neck; chewing almost always makes the pain worse. Some patients report a history of clicking with jaw movement.

There is insufficient evidence for or against the effectiveness of simple analgesics such as ibuprofen or the use of tricyclic drugs to treat temporomandibular disorders. Evidence for the effectiveness for selective serotonin reuptake inhibitors such as fluoxetine is lacking. Furthermore, fluoxetine and paroxetine should be avoided as they can sometimes cause bruxism and exacerbate the problem.

The diagnosis of temporomandibular disorders is primarily clinical. Radiography is usually not helpful but may be considered when dental disease is suspected based on visual inspection or tooth percussion or if the patient does not respond to conservative therapy. If structural (nondental) changes of the jaw are suspected and the patient has not responded to conservative therapy or jaw locking is present,

jaw MRI is the imaging procedure of choice but is not indicated in most patients.

For patients with chronic temporomandibular disorders, cognitive-behavioral therapy has been shown to reduce pain, depression, and interference with activities. Biofeedback may also be of value. Jaw appliances and occlusal splints have been a prominent part of temporomandibular disorder therapy for years despite questionable evidence of benefit.

KEY POINT

- Initial treatment of temporomandibular disorders focuses on noninterventional, nonpharmacologic strategies.

Bibliography

Mujakperuo HR, Watson M, Morrison R, Macfarlane TV. Pharmacological interventions for pain in patients with temporomandibular disorders. Cochrane Database Syst Rev. 2010;(10):CD004715. [PMID: 20927737]

Item 98   Answer: D

Educational Objective: Manage peripheral vertigo.

This patient should be referred for vestibular rehabilitation, which involves balance exercises and physical therapy. She presents with persistent symptoms of benign paroxysmal positional vertigo (BPPV), the most common cause of vertigo. Patients with BPPV classically report recurrent episodes of vertigo with rapid change in head position. The Dix-Hallpike maneuver is performed by having the examiner support the patient's head in 20 degrees of extension while sitting, then assisting the patient rapidly to the supine position with the head turned to one side and hanging over the edge of the examining table; the test is repeated with the head turned to the other side. A positive test results in horizontal nystagmus with latency 2 to 40 seconds and duration less than 1 minute with reproduction of symptoms that will fatigue and habituate.

BPPV is thought to be caused by movement of debris in the semicircular canals and resultant perturbation of sensory receptors. The Epley maneuver is a particle repositioning procedure intended to move the debris within the semicircular canal; it can successfully relieve symptoms in more than 60% of patients. In this patient, however, the maneuver was unsuccessful, and, based on her symptoms, further treatment is warranted. Vestibular rehabilitation, especially if initiated early, is effective in treating peripheral vertigo. Studies have shown improvement in symptoms, balance, and activities of daily living. Referral to a therapist trained in vestibular rehabilitation is recommended.

With a classic presentation for BPPV and no focal neurologic findings, brain imaging is not indicated in this patient. The severity of vertiginous symptoms is highly concerning for many patients, who seek reassurance that their condition is benign by undergoing imaging. However, such testing is typically of very low yield and does not alter the course of clinical management.

Meniere disease is characterized by the symptomatic triad of vertigo, tinnitus, and hearing loss, although it can present with vertigo alone. The vertigo is usually episodic and may not be positional. It can be accompanied by a sensation of aural fullness. Diuretic therapy (hydrochlorothiazide) is advocated for patients with this disease by some experts, but robust efficacy data are lacking. This patient's presentation is most consistent with BPPV, and therapeutic interventions should be targeted toward this diagnosis.

In general, medications are ineffective for the treatment of BPPV. Benzodiazepines and centrally acting anticholinergic antihistamines (meclizine) may modify the intensity of symptoms for some patients, particularly those with vestibular neuritis. When medications are used, they should be prescribed for less than 24 to 48 hours, since longer use may prolong symptoms by suppressing vestibular feedback and central compensation mechanisms.

KEY POINT

• Vestibular rehabilitation is effective in treating peripheral vertigo.

Bibliography

Bhattacharyya N, Baugh RF, Orvidas L, et al. Clinical practice guideline: benign paroxysmal positional vertigo. Otolaryngol Head Neck Surg. 2008;139(5)(suppl 4):S47-S81. [PMID: 18973840]

Item 99   Answer: C
Educational Objective: Diagnose depression in an older adult.

This patient should be assessed for depression. Elderly patients with depression may present with somatic and vegetative symptoms rather than dysphoria. The PHQ-9 is a validated depression assessment tool with a sensitivity of 80% and specificity of 92% for major depression using a score 10 or above as a cut off value. Administering the PHQ-9 in this patient is appropriate because depression in older adults is often underdiagnosed as changes in mood or behavior are often perceived as a consequence of underlying chronic illnesses. This patient's risk factors for depression include living in an institutional facility, chronic illness, and the recent death of his wife. The PHQ-9 assesses anhedonia, depressed mood, sleeping difficulties, decreased energy, changes in appetite, feelings of guilt or worthlessness, concentration impairment, psychomotor changes, and suicidal ideation. Alternatively, the Geriatric Depression Scale, consisting of 15 questions, could be administered. Its sensitivity of 80% to 90% and specificity of 70% to 85% are similar to the sensitivity and specificity of the PHQ-9.

The Dix-Hallpike maneuver is often performed in patients with dizziness to assess for benign paroxysmal positional vertigo. To perform the maneuver, the patient is directed to assume the supine position with the head

allowed to lie below the horizontal and turned to one side. The maneuver is repeated with the head turned to the other side. The examiner observes for nystagmus and vertigo. Dizziness is not a symptom in this patient.

The Mini–Mental State Examination (MMSE) is a validated instrument to test cognition. Although the MMSE is an appropriate screening test in older adults, this patient's normal orientation and lack of symptoms regarding cognition would make this test less of a priority at this time. Furthermore, false-positive MMSE results can be seen in patients with untreated depression.

In the Timed "Up & Go" (TUG) test, the patient is asked to arise from a chair, walk 10 feet, turn around, and return to sit in the same chair. Those completing the task in more than 14 seconds are considered to be at high risk for subsequent falling. Although the TUG test is appropriate for assessing fall risk, it would not address the causes of his diminished activity or his somatic symptoms.

KEY POINT

• Elderly patients with depression may present with somatic and vegetative symptoms rather than dysphoria.

Bibliography

Kroenke K, Spitzer RL, Williams JB. The PHQ-9: validity of a brief depression severity measure. J Gen Intern Med. 2001;16(9):606-613. [PMID: 11556941]

Item 100   Answer: D
Educational Objective: Diagnose posttraumatic stress disorder.

This patient most likely has posttraumatic stress disorder (PTSD). PTSD occurs in response to exposure to a traumatic event that involves serious threat to oneself or others. PTSD is characterized by at least 1 month of symptoms that include intrusive thoughts about the trauma, nightmares or flashbacks, avoidance of reminders of the event, and hypervigilance with sleep disturbance. To meet DSM-IV criteria, the symptoms must be in each of three areas: re-experiencing the event, avoiding reminders of the event, and heightened arousal. Comorbid psychiatric conditions are common, so screening for depression, anxiety, and substance abuse is essential. PTSD symptoms often require multimodal treatments, and early intervention may prevent chronicity of symptoms. Trauma-focused cognitive-behavioral therapy focuses on cognitively reframing distorted thinking patterns while gradually re-exposing the patient to the traumatic experience. Simple stress management interventions can also be helpful in alleviating some symptoms. The most effective pharmacotherapy is selective serotonin reuptake inhibitors. However, no advantage has been identified for either psychotherapy or pharmacotherapy.

Generalized anxiety disorder is characterized by excessive anxiety and worry about a variety of events or activities on most days for at least 6 months, with difficulty controlling worrying. Physical symptoms of headache, nausea, and tremulousness may occur. In generalized anxiety disorder there is usually not a link to a particular inciting incident, and interfering nightmares are not a hallmark.

A major depressive episode is diagnosed according to the DSM-IV by the presence of five or more of the nine cardinal symptoms of depression during the same 2-week period, at least one of which is either depressed mood or loss of interest or pleasure. Symptoms should represent a change from previous functioning and cause clinically significant distress or impairment in functioning. This patient does not have significant mood disturbance or anhedonia.

Patients with obsessive-compulsive disorder report recurrent obsessions or compulsions sufficiently severe to occupy 1 hour daily or result in marked distress or impaired social function. Obsessions are persistent ideas, thoughts, impulses, or images experienced as intrusive and are associated with significant anxiety or distress. Examples include fears of having left doors unlocked and fears of germ contamination. Compulsions are repetitive behaviors, such as handwashing, checking, ordering, or counting, that are repeated to decrease the anxiety related to the obsessions. This patient's presentation is not consistent with obsessive-compulsive disorder.

KEY POINT

- **Posttraumatic stress disorder is characterized by at least 1 month of symptoms that include intrusive thoughts about the trauma, nightmares or flashbacks, avoidance of reminders of the event, and hypervigilance with sleep disturbance; symptoms must be in each of three areas: re-experiencing the event, avoiding reminders of the event, and heightened arousal.**

Bibliography

Ravindran LN, Stein MB. Pharmacotherapy of PTSD: premises, principles, and priorities. Brain Res. 2009;1293:24-39. [PMID: 19332035]

Item 101   Answer: B

Educational Objective: Manage chest pain due to an acute coronary syndrome.

This patient should be admitted to the coronary care unit for further treatment. Because chest pain is a common clinical symptom and may have noncardiac causes, assessment of the probability that chest pain has a cardiac etiology is critical to pursuing appropriate diagnosis and treatment. This is done through an understanding of existing cardiac risk factors, the nature of the presenting symptoms, findings on physical examination, and the results of specific initial diagnostic studies, such as chest radiography and electrocardiography. Her cardiac risk factors include her age, hypertension, and hyperlipidemia, and the substernal nature of her chest pain places her in an intermediate risk

category for cardiac-related pain. Coupled with her electrocardiogram (ECG) showing anterolateral ST-segment depression, her clinical picture is consistent with coronary ischemia as the cause of her chest pain. She therefore requires emergent treatment for coronary ischemia and admission to a coronary care unit.

Low-risk patients without evidence of myocardial infarction can be evaluated with an exercise or pharmacologic stress test. However, a stress test in a patient with probable acute coronary syndrome could provoke an extension of her myocardial infarction or a life-threatening arrhythmia.

CT pulmonary angiography would be helpful if there were a high probability of acute pulmonary embolism. Because this patient has symptoms and ECG findings of acute coronary syndrome and the probability of pulmonary embolism is low (she has no risk factors or physical examination findings to support the diagnosis of venous thromboembolism and her symptoms can be explained by an alternative diagnosis), a CT pulmonary angiogram is not indicated.

NSAIDs are indicated for the treatment of acute pericarditis or musculoskeletal chest wall pain. The pain of pericarditis is characteristically pleuritic in nature. In addition, the characteristic ECG finding in pericarditis is ST-segment elevation throughout the precordial and limb leads rather than regional ST-segment depression, as in this patient. ECG changes are not present in musculoskeletal chest pain.

KEY POINT

- **Assessment of chest pain is based on preexisting risks for cardiac or other diseases, elements of the history and physical examination, and appropriate, directed testing based on the likely cause of chest symptoms.**

Bibliography

Panju AA, Hemmelgarn BR, Guyatt GH, Simel DL. The rational clinical examination. Is this patient having a myocardial infarction? JAMA. 1998;280(14):1256-1263. [PMID: 9786377]

Item 102   Answer: B

Educational Objective: Screen for essential hypertension.

It is recommended that this patient be screened again for hypertension in 2 years. Although there are not strong data on outcomes with different screening intervals, the Seventh Report of the Joint National Committee on Prevention, Detection, Evaluation, and Treatment of High Blood Pressure (JNC 7) recommends that persons with blood pressure below 120/80 mm Hg should be screened every 2 years. The mean of two or more seated clinic measurements should be used to evaluate for possible hypertension.

The JNC 7 recommends that yearly screening should be reserved for patients with systolic blood pressures of 120 mm Hg to 139 mm Hg and diastolic blood pressures of 80 mm Hg to 89 mm Hg.

Benefits of screening for hypertension at intervals longer than 2 years have not been established.

KEY POINT

- All adults aged 18 years and older should be screened for hypertension; screening every 2 years is appropriate for those with blood pressure below 120/80 mm Hg.

Bibliography

Chobanian AV, Bakris GL, Black HR, et al; Joint National Committee on Prevention, Detection, Evaluation, and Treatment of High Blood Pressure; National Heart, Lung, and Blood Institute; National High Blood Pressure Education Program Coordinating Committee. Seventh report of the Joint National Committee on Prevention, Detection, Evaluation, and Treatment of High Blood Pressure. Hypertension. 2003;42(6):1206-1252. [PMID: 14656957]

Item 103   Answer: B

Educational Objective: Manage mild cognitive impairment.

This patient has mild cognitive impairment (MCI) as evidenced by reported memory loss, some impaired functioning, and no involvement of other cognitive domains. Her Mini–Mental State Examination (MMSE) score of 26 is typical for MCI. She does not demonstrate involvement of other domains of mental impairment that might suggest dementia, including problems with executive functioning, language difficulties, or activities of daily living. Patient concern about memory loss is more likely with MCI than it is with dementia, in which concerns are usually raised by family members. Although there is no widely accepted treatment for MCI, cognitive rehabilitation has been shown to have some effectiveness in improving functioning in some patients. Cognitive rehabilitation is performed by neuropsychologists and occupational therapists and involves using external memory aids as well as teaching patients organizational and attention skills.

In patients with Alzheimer disease, anticholinesterase inhibitors, such as donepezil, galantamine, and rivastigmine, may be tried because their use may result in modest improvement of cognition, performance of activities of daily living, and functioning, as determined by global assessment. However, the use of anticholinesterase inhibitors has not been shown to delay the progression from MCI to dementia.

Although PET scanning can detect pathologic levels of amyloid in patients with MCI and dementia, and possibly differentiate between the two, its use at this time is still investigational.

Reassurance that the patient will not progress to dementia is not appropriate because persons with MCI appear to be at increased risk for further declines in

cognition relative to those with normal cognitive function. The annual incidence rate of dementia in the general elderly population is 1% to 3%, whereas the annual incidence rate of dementia in patients with a diagnosis of MCI is approximately 12%, suggesting a significant increased risk of progression to dementia from their baseline level of cognitive impairment.

KEY POINT

- Although there is no widely accepted treatment for mild cognitive impairment, cognitive rehabilitation has been shown to have some effectiveness in improving functioning in some patients.

Bibliography

Kinsella GJ, Mullaly E, Rand E, et al. Early intervention for mild cognitive impairment: a randomised controlled trial. J Neurol Neurosurg Psychiatry. 2009;80(7):730-736. [PMID: 19332424]

Item 104   Answer: B

Educational Objective: Evaluate a patient with pleuritic chest pain.

This patient should undergo radiography of the chest. He has severe COPD and findings consistent with spontaneous secondary pneumothorax. These findings include sudden, sharp, nonradiating pleuritic chest pain and shortness of breath with hyperresonance, decreased breath sounds, and decreased chest wall expansion on the side of the pneumothorax in a patient with underlying lung disease. Pneumothorax should be considered in any patient with sudden onset of pleuritic chest pain and dyspnea. The diagnostic test of choice if pneumothorax is suspected is an upright chest radiograph. Findings on chest radiograph include separation of the parietal and visceral pleura by a collection of gas and the absence of vessels in this space. The diagnosis of pneumothorax may be difficult in patients with COPD because the pleural line may be difficult to visualize in hyperlucent lung tissue, and a pneumothorax may be difficult to distinguish from a large bulla.

Chest CT also can be used to diagnose a pneumothorax. Chest CTs may be more sensitive in delineating smaller collections of gas in the pleural space and in providing more information about the pulmonary parenchyma and pleura. Plain film radiography remains the initial test of choice for most patients, however, and CT of the chest should be reserved for patients in whom the chest radiograph does not provide information to guide further treatment or evaluation.

The patient's history and physical examination are classic for pneumothorax and his pain descriptors do not strongly suggest ischemia or other primary cardiovascular disease. An electrocardiogram or echocardiogram, tests of choice to evaluate ischemic heart disease, valvular heart disease or cardiomyopathy, would not be the first diagnostic test of choice for suspected pneumothorax.

KEY POINT

- Pneumothorax should be considered in any patient with sudden onset of pleuritic chest pain and dyspnea, and the diagnostic test of choice if pneumothorax is suspected is an upright chest radiograph.

Bibliography

Noppen M. Spontaneous pneumothorax: epidemiology, pathophysiology and cause. Eur Respir Rev. 2010;19(117):217-219. [PMID: 20956196]

Item 105   Answer: D

Educational Objective: Diagnose somatization disorder.

This patient most likely has somatization disorder. Although medically unexplained symptoms are common, as are patient concerns and anxiety regarding the possible presence of disease for which they seek evaluation, somatization disorder is a relatively rare psychiatric disease related to an extreme focus on medical symptoms and their evaluation. DSM-IV criteria for somatization disorder include a constellation of symptoms, including two gastrointestinal symptoms, four pain symptoms, one pseudoneurologic symptom, and one sexual symptom. The symptoms must start before age 30 years, persist (although they often wax and wane), and cause significant impairment for the patient. In addition, each symptom must be medically unexplained after evaluation. Somatization disorder should always be distinguished from depression with somatic features; the latter will meet diagnostic criteria for depression. This patient meets DSM-IV criteria for somatization disorder.

Celiac disease may be difficult to diagnose and may cause diffuse symptoms, including nausea, but would most likely cause weight loss and other gastrointestinal symptoms. In addition, celiac disease would not fully explain the focal neurologic and other symptoms experienced by the patient.

Patients who are malingering consciously fabricate symptoms for some secondary gain, whereas patients with somatoform disorders are unaware that their symptoms are a manifestation of psychiatric disease. This patient's history gives no suggestion of secondary gain.

Patients with multiple sclerosis can have nausea. However, this patient's neurologic symptoms affect the right face and body and thus do not follow neuroanatomy. Furthermore, multiple sclerosis is an unlikely cause of the patient's multiple somatic symptoms, and the patient's recent neuroimaging study did not show evidence of demyelination.

KEY POINT

- Criteria for somatization disorder include a constellation of medically unexplained, persistent symptoms, including gastrointestinal, pain, pseudoneurologic, and sexual, that begin before age 30 years and cause significant impairment for the patient.

Bibliography

Oyama O, Paltoo C, Greengold J. Somatoform disorders. Am Fam Physician. 2007;76(9):1333-1338. [PMID: 18019877]

Item 106   Answer: B

Educational Objective: Treat chronic bacterial prostatitis.

The most appropriate treatment for this patient is a 1-month course of a fluoroquinolone antibiotic. This patient has chronic bacterial prostatitis (National Institutes of Health category II), which presents with pain and urinary symptoms with recurrent bacterial infection. The prostate in patients with chronic bacterial prostatitis may be less inflamed than with acute prostatitis. The recommendation for treatment of category II prostatitis is a prolonged (1 month) course of a fluoroquinolone antibiotic such as ciprofloxacin, which covers common bacterial infections of the prostate with good penetration of the prostate.

A 1-week course of trimethoprim-sulfamethoxazole would be appropriate for acute bacterial prostatitis (category I prostatitis) or urinary tract infection; however, this patient has had short-course antibiotics for three prior infections, placing him in category II and warranting a longer course of antibiotics.

Category III prostatitis (chronic abacterial prostatitis/chronic pelvic pain syndrome) is noninfectious and therefore does not respond to antibiotics. This patient's urinary findings of bacteria and leukocytes support an infectious cause of his symptoms, and not this form of prostatitis. There is some evidence that cognitive-behavioral therapy may provide some benefit to patients with chronic pelvic pain syndrome, although there is not a role for this intervention in bacterial prostatitis. Symptoms of category III chronic pelvic pain syndrome are often refractory, and empathetic supportive care is often required.

Finasteride is a 5-α-reductase inhibitor that decreases prostate volume and is used primarily in the treatment of benign prostatic hyperplasia. It does not have an established use in either acute or chronic bacterial prostatitis.

KEY POINT

- The recommended treatment for chronic bacterial prostatitis is a prolonged course of a fluoroquinolone antibiotic.

Bibliography

Touma NJ, Nickel JC. Prostatitis and chronic pelvic pain syndrome in men. Med Clin North Am. 2011;95:75-86. [PMID: 21095412]

Item 107   Answer: B

Educational Objective: Manage acute sinusitis.

This patient with clinical findings typical of acute sinusitis should be observed and given symptomatic treatment, such as chlorpheniramine. Most cases of acute sinusitis are caused by viruses and typically resolve in 7 to 10 days without directed therapy. The clinical presentation is not helpful in determining whether the cause of symptoms is viral or bacterial. However, because most cases of viral or bacterial sinusitis resolve spontaneously within 10 days, observation and treatment of the associated symptoms with analgesics and decongestants is appropriate.

Antibiotics are generally reserved for sinusitis accompanied by high or continued fever or worsening symptoms, and even in this setting, their efficacy is not well documented. When used, an antibiotic focused on common respiratory organisms is reasonable.

Nasal cultures have not been shown to be helpful in diagnosing a bacterial etiology for sinusitis or in guiding antibiotic therapy.

Sinus imaging is not part of the initial management of acute sinusitis because imaging results are frequently abnormal in symptomatic patients with either a viral or bacterial sinusitis, and also in a high percentage of asymptomatic patients. Imaging is generally indicated in patients with a complicated presentation, such as those with visual changes or severe headache.

Inhaled nasal corticosteroids are frequently prescribed for acute symptom relief for sinusitis and have some efficacy in this setting; however, the role of systemic corticosteroids in acute sinusitis is not clear, and they are not recommended.

KEY POINT

- Most cases of viral or bacterial sinusitis resolve spontaneously within 10 days, and observation and treatment of the associated symptoms with analgesics and decongestants is appropriate.

Bibliography

Chow AW, Benninger MS, Brook I, et al. IDSA clinical practice guideline for acute bacterial rhinosinusitis in children and adults. Clin Infect Dis. 2012;54(8):e72-e112. [PMID: 22438350]

Item 108   Answer: D

Educational Objective: Manage sudden sensorineural hearing loss.

This woman with sudden-onset unilateral sensorineural hearing loss requires urgent audiometry and otorhinolaryngology referral because early diagnosis and treatment may be associated with improved outcomes. Based on the initial examination, this patient does not have conductive hearing loss because she hears better when sound is transmitted via air (through the external ear canal and middle ear) than when it is transmitted via bone vibration. Sudden sensorineural hearing loss (SSNHL) is an alarming problem that is defined as sensorineural hearing loss occurring in 3 days or less. Patients often report immediate or rapid hearing loss or loss of hearing upon awakening. Ninety percent have unilateral hearing loss, and some have tinnitus, ear fullness, and vertigo. SSNHL constitutes a considerable diagnostic challenge because it may be caused by many conditions, including infection, neoplasm, trauma, autoimmune disease, vascular events, and ototoxic drugs. Immediate otorhinolaryngologic referral is required. Improvement occurs in about two thirds of patients. Oral or intratympanic corticosteroids are usually given, although randomized trials differ in their conclusions regarding efficacy.

Otic herpes zoster (Ramsay Hunt syndrome) is characterized by herpetic lesions in the external canal and ipsilateral facial palsy neither of which is seen in this patient. Acyclovir may be considered in a clear case of Ramsay Hunt syndrome but has been shown to be unhelpful in idiopathic SSNHL.

Neomycin, polymyxin B, and hydrocortisone ear drops are a possible treatment for acute otitis externa. This patient is unlikely to have otitis externa because she does not have otalgia, otorrhea, itching, or pain intensified by jaw motion. She does not have internal tenderness when the tragus or pinna is pushed or pulled. Her ear canal erythema is most likely secondary to the trauma of recent cerumen removal than otitis externa.

Triethanolamine ear drops may help to treat or prevent cerumen impaction, but cerumen impaction causes conductive hearing loss, not sudden sensorineural hearing loss. After her cerumen was successfully removed, the patient's conductive hearing was intact, making this an unlikely cause of her sudden hearing loss in her left ear. Cerumen impaction is also unlikely to cause tinnitus.

KEY POINT

- Patients with sudden sensorineural hearing loss should be urgently evaluated by audiometry and considered for oral or intratympanic corticosteroid treatment by an otorhinolaryngologist.

Bibliography

Stachler RJ, Chandrasekhar SS, Archer SM, et al; American Academy of Otolaryngology-Head and Neck Surgery. Clinical practice guideline: sudden hearing loss. Otolaryngol Head Neck Surg. 2012;146(3 suppl):S1-S35. [PMID: 22383545]

Item 109   Answer: D

Educational Objective: Employ the principle of substituted judgment in managing care of a patient without decisional capacity.

Although the patient is unconscious and unable to make his own decisions, the ethical obligation of both the practitioner and the surrogate decision maker (his wife) is to continue to make decisions that are consistent with his previously expressed wishes and values. The principle, called "substituted judgment," essentially asks, "What would the patient want if he or she could decide?"

In patients who present to the emergency department unable to make decisions, lifesaving therapy is both ethical and necessary under the principle of implied consent. However, once a patient's wishes are known, it is unethical to specifically defy those wishes simply because the patient has lost decisional capacity; therefore, it would be unethical to transfuse the patient knowing that he specifically did not want transfusion.

Obtaining a court-appointed guardian is not indicated in this case because the patient clearly stated his views, and subsequent care decisions will be made by his duly appointed surrogate based on his wishes.

Seeking the permission of the patient's wife to allow transfusion or attempting to convince her that transfusion would be in her husband's best interest is ethically unacceptable; all available evidence suggests that he was consistent in his wishes to avoid transfusion, and it would be inappropriate to place her in a difficult ethical position, especially in this stressful situation.

KEY POINT

• When a patient is unable to make his or her own decisions, the ethical principle of substituted judgment obliges surrogate decision makers to make decisions that are consistent with the patient's previously expressed wishes and values.

Bibliography
Snyder L; American College of Physicians Ethics, Professionalism, and Human Rights Committee. American College of Physicians Ethics Manual: sixth edition. Ann Intern Med. 2012;156(1 Pt 2):73-104. [PMID: 22213573]

Item 110   Answer: D
Educational Objective: Diagnose testicular torsion.

This patient has testicular torsion, which occurs when the testicle twists on the spermatic cord, leading to decreased blood flow and ischemia. It is more common in children and in men younger than 30 years. Pain is usually sudden in onset and examination often reveals a high-riding testicle with the longitudinal axis abnormally oriented transversely. Absence of the cremasteric reflex on the affected side is nearly 99% sensitive for torsion. Treatment of torsion includes rapid surgical decompression to resume blood flow. In the absence of rapid access to surgery, manual decompression may be attempted.

Men with epididymitis typically present with subacute onset of scrotal pain, dysuria, urinary frequency, and fever. Inflammation and infection of the epididymis cause pain localizing to the posterior and superior aspect of the testicle. The scrotum may be edematous and erythematous. It

does not result in malpositioning of the testicle or an absent cremasteric reflex.

Clinical presentations of inguinal hernias can vary from an asymptomatic bulge to a feeling of groin or abdominal pressure to severe pain when incarceration or strangulation occurs. A strangulated hernia may present as a painful mass in the scrotum or as a tender bulge in the inguinal area; signs of bowel obstruction may also be present. This patient does not have findings consistent with a strangulated inguinal hernia.

Orchitis, an inflammation of the testicle, is usually caused by viral infection (mumps) or extension of a bacterial infection from epididymitis or urinary tract infection; in mumps, parotiditis begins about 5 days prior to orchitis. The testicle is diffusely tender and may be swollen; the position of the testicle in the scrotum is normal and the cremasteric reflex is present.

KEY POINT

• Testicular torsion is characterized by severe pain and an elevated high-riding testicle with the longitudinal axis abnormally oriented transversely and an absent cremasteric reflex.

Bibliography
Wampler SM, Llanes M. Common scrotal and testicular problems. Prim Care. 2010;37(3):613-626, x. [PMID: 20705202]

Item 111   Answer: C
Educational Objective: Treat bacterial vaginosis.

The most appropriate treatment for this patient is a 7-day oral regimen of metronidazole (500 mg twice daily). She has bacterial vaginosis (BV), a polymicrobial infection characterized by an overgrowth of multiple anaerobic bacteria. Although BV is not a sexually transmitted infection, risk factors include lack of condom use and multiple or new sexual partners. BV can be diagnosed clinically using Amsel criteria, which include the following symptoms or signs: (1) homogeneous thin discharge that coats the vaginal walls; (2) clue cells (epithelial cells with borders obscured by small bacteria) on saline microscopy; (3) pH of vaginal fluid >4.5; and (4) fishy odor of vaginal discharge before or after the addition of 10% potassium hydroxide to the secretions (the "whiff" test). The presence of at least three of these clinical findings has a high sensitivity and specificity for diagnosing BV when compared with Gram stain of collected secretions, which is the gold standard. Because this woman is symptomatic, treatment should be offered with either oral metronidazole, vaginal metronidazole gel, or vaginal clindamycin cream; patient preference should dictate treatment choice. Topical clindamycin should be avoided during pregnancy as it may increase the risk of adverse outcomes. Women treated with oral metronidazole should be cautioned to avoid alcohol, which can cause a disulfiram-like reaction.

This patient's abnormal vaginal pH and lack of yeast and hyphae on potassium hydroxide preparation make vulvovaginal candidiasis an unlikely explanation for her symptoms. Treatment with oral fluconazole or topical clotrimazole cream, effective therapies for vulvovaginal candidiasis, is not warranted.

This patient has multiple sexual partners, increasing her risk for trichomoniasis. Characteristic symptoms and signs include a malodorous discharge with vulvar itching, burning, and postcoital bleeding. Although the vaginal pH will be elevated and the whiff test may be positive (as noted with this patient), clue cells are not a characteristic finding on saline microscopy, making trichomoniasis an unlikely diagnosis in this patient.

Oral metronidazole is also used for the treatment of trichomoniasis, but it is typically given as a single 2-g dose, which would not be appropriate for treatment of BV.

KEY POINT

- Bacterial vaginosis is the likely diagnosis in women with at least three of the following features: (1) homogeneous thin discharge that coats the vaginal walls; (2) clue cells on saline microscopy; (3) pH of vaginal fluid >4.5; and (4) fishy odor of vaginal discharge (positive "whiff" test).

Bibliography

Wilson, JF. In the clinic. Vaginitis and cervicitis. Ann Intern Med. 2009;151(5):ITC3-1-ITC3-15. [PMID: 19721016]

Item 112   Answer: C
Educational Objective: Treat erectile dysfunction.

Since this patient has not yet taken anything for his erectile dysfunction (ED), it would be most appropriate to treat him with sildenafil, a phosphodiesterase type 5 (PDE-5) inhibitor. PDE-5 inhibitors are generally considered first-line pharmacologic therapy for ED and include sildenafil, vardenafil, and tadalafil. These agents increase penile cyclic guanosine monophosphate (cGMP), facilitating smooth muscle relaxation and allowing inflow of blood. All of these drugs have been shown to improve erectile function, as measured by successful sexual intercourse attempts and improved scores on various survey instruments. There are no direct comparisons to support superiority of any one agent, as the populations studied differ in various characteristics.

The PDE-5 inhibitors vary in their duration of action, interaction with food and other medications, and adverse effects. Treatment failure may result from lack of patient education or improper use (timing, taking with food, inadequate sexual stimulation, inadequate dose, inadequate trial), performance anxiety or unrealistic expectations, hypogonadism, or an incorrect diagnosis

(premature ejaculation or hypoactive sexual desire disorder). An adequate trial is generally deemed to constitute patient reeducation and gradual escalation of the dose to maximum dose and at least six attempts on maximum-dose therapy. PDE-5 inhibitors should be avoided in patients receiving any form of nitrate therapy.

Second-line therapies for ED should be reserved for men who fail to improve with lifestyle modifications or with use of PDE-5 inhibitors. These include alprostadil (either intraurethral or intracavernosal), penile pumps, and penile prostheses. Intraurethral alprostadil is more effective than that administered intracavernosally and is associated with fewer side effects.

Testosterone replacement therapy should be limited to patients with clinical symptoms and signs consistent with androgen deficiency and a subnormal serum testosterone level (generally an 8 AM total testosterone level <200 ng/dL [7 nmol/L]).

KEY POINT

- First-line pharmacologic therapy for erectile dysfunction consists of phosphodiesterase type 5 inhibitors.

Bibliography

Tsertsvadze A, Fink HA, Yazdi F, et al. Oral phosphodiesterase-5 inhibitors and hormonal treatments for erectile dysfunction: a systematic review and meta-analysis. Ann Intern Med. 2009;151(9):650-661. [PMID: 19884626]

Item 113   Answer: C
Educational Objective: Prevent medication errors from occurring during a transition in care.

The most likely cause for this patient's readmission is a medication error stemming from her medication changes at discharge. It is likely that she either did not receive or did not take the medications at the increased dosages. One in five patients discharged from the hospital will suffer an adverse event related to medical management within 3 weeks of hospital discharge, with 66% of these being adverse events related to medications. Most medication errors result from inadequate communication by hospital caregivers with patients and their primary care clinicians. Medication reconciliation is the process by which medications are reviewed at every step of the care process, with a focus on ensuring that the patient is taking only those medications intended, and that this is clear to the patient and all others involved in that patient's care. Patients should receive a list of medications at the time of discharge, be informed of previous medications that have been discontinued or changed, any new medications that have been added, and the reasons for these changes.

True diuretic resistance is uncommon, although the bioavailability of oral diuretics may be highly variable, particularly in the edematous state. She responded to intravenous diuretics as an inpatient with a return of her weight to a nonedematous level, and her oral diuretic dose was appropriately increased at the time of discharge. Her rapid decompensation from her normal baseline weight on an increased dose of diuretic with the addition of a second agent at the time of discharge makes clinically significant resistance to diuretics unlikely.

Inadequate post-hospital follow-up is a potential cause for readmission, particularly with complex patients who have had extended hospitalizations and multiple changes to their treatment regimen. In general, for most patients admitted for heart failure exacerbation, a follow-up appointment in 1 week should be scheduled at the time of discharge, preferably with direct contact with the primary care physician. This patient was scheduled for a 1-week follow-up, but worsening of her symptoms shortly after discharge suggests an issue with treatment of her initial problem, or development of an additional medical complication.

Spironolactone has been shown to decrease mortality in selected patients with systolic heart failure. Its primary complications are hyperkalemia and other effects of aldosterone blockade. However, it is unlikely to be an independent cause of her acute heart failure decompensation.

KEY POINT

- Hospitalized patients should receive a list of medications at the time of discharge and be informed of previous medications that have been discontinued or changed.

Bibliography

Kripalani S, Jackson AT, Schnipper JL, Coleman EA. Promoting effective transitions of care at hospital discharge: a review of key issues for hospitalists. J Hosp Med. 2007;2(5):314-323. [PMID: 17935242]

Item 114   Answer: D

Educational Objective: Manage upper respiratory tract infection with ear pain.

This patient presents with signs and symptoms of a viral upper respiratory tract infection (URI). The recent development of ear pain and the findings of a dull tympanic membrane with a small middle ear effusion are compatible with either otitis media or a viral URI without otitis media. Treatment of otitis media in adults has not been well studied. There are no guidelines for antibiotic use in adults separate from those for children. In children older than 2 years without severe illness, outcomes appear to be similar for observation without antibiotics compared with antibiotic treatment. This strategy to reduce use of antimicrobials has not been evaluated in adults, and it is not known if antibiotics are associated with improved short- or long-term outcomes. However, antibiotic use is associated with adverse effects and higher levels of antibiotic resistance that should be considered in conjunction with the lack of evidence regarding benefit. Considering the patient's equivocal

diagnosis of otitis media and mild symptoms, it would be reasonable to withhold antibiotic therapy.

If an antibiotic was prescribed, amoxicillin is recommended as first-line therapy in adults. Erythromycin could be used in a penicillin-allergic patient, but there is no evidence that it is more efficacious.

An otorhinolaryngology consultation is not indicated at this time because the patient only has a URI.

KEY POINT

- Do not routinely prescribe antibiotic therapy for adults with otitis media.

Bibliography

Coco A, Vernacchio L, Horst M, Anderson A. Management of acute otitis media after publication of the 2004 AAP and AAFP clinical practice guideline. Pediatrics. 2010;125(2):214-220. [PMID: 20100746]

Item 115   Answer: D

Educational Objective: Manage secondary insomnia.

This patient's history of daytime fatigue and obesity and large neck size put him at risk for obstructive sleep apnea, which can be diagnosed with an overnight polysomnography study. It would be helpful to obtain corroborating information from his wife regarding symptoms of snoring, gasping, other breathing problems, or abnormal leg movements. Referral for polysomnography is indicated when a primary sleep disorder is suspected (obstructive sleep apnea, restless legs syndrome, periodic limb movement disorder). A sleep study may also include multiple sleep latency testing, in which a patient takes four or five 20-minute naps, and sleep latency (the time from deciding to sleep to actually falling asleep) is measured. Sleep latency of less than 8 minutes is associated with hypersomnia, which occurs with sleep disorders such as narcolepsy, insufficient sleep syndrome, medication adverse effects, sleep apnea syndromes, and periodic limb movements of sleep.

Although alcohol can contribute to insomnia, this patient's pattern of alcohol use does not support its having a role in his symptoms, since he is having daily fatigue symptoms despite only using alcohol on weekends.

Pharmacotherapy would not be appropriate in this patient until a secondary cause of insomnia is ruled out. Prescription drug therapy for insomnia is reserved for patients with primary insomnia who have not benefited from nonpharmacologic and behavioral therapies.

Restless legs syndrome is a clinical diagnosis. Besides an urge to move the legs, other symptoms that patients may exhibit in support of this diagnosis include an uncomfortable or unpleasant sensation in the legs that may begin or worsen during periods of rest or inactivity, is partially or totally relieved by movement as long as activity continues, and is worse in the evening or night or is present only at night. Restless legs syndrome can be divided into primary and secondary forms. The primary form refers to patients without another condition known to be associated with restless legs syndrome. Conditions associated with secondary restless legs syndrome include pregnancy, end-stage kidney disease, and iron deficiency. Since this patient does not have restless legs syndrome, iron studies are not indicated.

> **KEY POINT**
> - Referral for polysomnography is indicated when a primary sleep disorder is suspected (obstructive sleep apnea, restless legs syndrome, periodic limb movement disorder).

Bibliography
Wilson JF: In the clinic: Insomnia. Ann Intern Med. 2008;148(1): ITC13-1-ITC13-16. [PMID: 18166757]

Item 116   Answer: C
Educational Objective: Diagnose osteonecrosis of the hip.

This patient's presentation is most consistent with osteonecrosis of the hip. Osteonecrosis of the hip commonly presents with dull, aching groin pain (most commonly) or thigh or buttock pain that is indolent in onset. Occasionally, as is the case in this patient, severe pain may be reported in the early stages as bone death is occurring. Corticosteroid use and excessive use of alcohol account for more than 90% of hip osteonecrosis cases. On examination, patients have limited range of motion of the hip. During the early stages of this disease, radiographic imaging may be normal. Eventually, patchy areas of sclerosis and lucency may be seen. Hip MRI is the most sensitive imaging test for osteonecrosis and is typically positive early in the course of the disease.

Osteoarthritis of the hip can be established in patients with a history of chronic pain in the groin and medial thigh that worsens with activity and is relieved by rest. Although osteoarthritis of the hip can present with slowly progressive hip pain, severe pain at the onset of symptoms does not usually occur. Radiographs in patients with osteoarthritis may show joint-space narrowing, subchondral sclerosis, and osteophyte formation. Although there is a poor correlation between radiographic evidence of osteoarthritis and symptoms, it would be unusual for a patient with osteoarthritis of the hip to have a normal radiographic series.

L1 radiculopathy is rare. Symptoms include pain, paresthesia, and sensory loss in the groin. On examination, this patient has limited internal and external range of motion and pain with log-rolling of the hip. Each of these findings supports a joint etiology of this patient's hip pain and argues against lumbar disk disease at the L1 level.

Septic arthritis would be expected to present acutely with fever and limited range of motion. This patient's slow

onset of symptoms and prolonged course are not consistent with septic arthritis.

> **KEY POINT**
> - Osteonecrosis of the hip commonly presents with dull, aching groin pain that is indolent in onset; risk factors include corticosteroid use and excessive alcohol use.

Bibliography
Amanatullah DF, Strauss EJ, Di Cesare PE. Current management options for osteonecrosis of the femoral head: part 1, diagnosis and nonoperative management. Am J Orthop (Belle Mead NJ). 2011;40(9):E186-92. [PMID: 22022684]

Item 117   Answer: B
Educational Objective: Manage a patient with a chronic pain syndrome.

This patient should be evaluated for possible intimate partner violence. It is essential to perform a comprehensive assessment in the evaluation of patients with chronic pain syndromes. This patient has a chronic pain syndrome, fibromyalgia that had previously been well controlled but has worsened recently, significantly affecting her functional status. In patients with chronic pain conditions, overlying psychosocial stressors, including domestic violence, may exacerbate or destabilize symptoms. Therefore, in addition to questioning the patient more thoroughly about pain onset and relieving and exacerbating factors, the provider should also inquire about threats to the patient's safety as well as other potential psychosocial events or situations that may be contributing to her worsened clinical status.

There is no specific role for diagnostic testing or imaging in the evaluation of patients with most chronic pain syndromes in the absence of objective physical examination findings or laboratory abnormalities suggesting a specific underlying disorder. Although various studies are frequently obtained in patients with chronic pain, they are typically not revealing, and abnormalities that are identified on diagnostic testing may not be the source of the patient's pain. This patient is experiencing worsening of her typical fibromyalgia pain, and obtaining muscle and nerve conduction studies without focal symptoms or clinical findings is unlikely to change management.

NSAIDs are most effective for treating the pain associated with rheumatoid arthritis, inflammatory arthropathies, and musculoskeletal pain. They are generally ineffective in the management of neuropathic and muscular pain syndromes, such as fibromyalgia, and can be associated with significant gastrointestinal and cardiovascular toxicities. Adding high-dose ibuprofen to this patient's pain regimen is unlikely to significantly improve her symptoms.

Opioid therapy should generally be avoided in patients with chronic pain syndromes given the expected chronicity of use, lack of demonstrated efficacy, and the potential for significant side effects and dependency.

KEY POINT

- Patients with chronic pain syndromes should be evaluated for concurrent psychosocial stressors, particularly in those in whom symptoms have worsened without explanation.

Bibliography

Bradley LA. Pathophysiology of fibromyalgia. Am J Med. 2009;122(12 suppl):S22-30. [PMID: 19962493]

Item 118   Answer: C

Educational Objective: Manage risk for motor vehicle accidents in an older adult driver.

This patient has a number of factors that increase his risk of being involved in a motor vehicle accident and his physician has a responsibility to reduce this risk. This patient's risk factors for a motor vehicle accident include his age, likely visual deficits, decreased motor function (including a history of falling), and decreased cognitive function. The first step in assessing driving ability in older adults is to ask the patient and family members about driving difficulties. This assessment should include questions about whether friends and family members are worried about their driving, getting lost while driving, near misses, and recent accidents. A more complete set of questions to assess driving risk can be found in the "Am I a Safe Driver" self-assessment tool (www.ama-assn.org/ama1/pub/upload/mm/433/am_i _a_safe_driver.pdf). A positive response to any of the questions suggests unsafe driving.

It would be premature to advise this patient to stop driving before assessing driving-related skills, providing the patient with information on safe driving, and suggesting that the patient enroll in a driving course designed to improve skills. Referral to a driver rehabilitation specialist can also assist in assessment and skill improvement.

Advising the patient to drive only locally is not advised because so-called "low-mileage" drivers may be at the greatest risk. Older drivers who are having driving difficulties often self-restrict their driving, but local roads often have more hazards, including more signs and signals and confusing and congested intersections.

Guidelines for reporting patients to the department of transportation vary by state and include immediate threats to driving safety such as new seizures. Even in states that require reporting of immediate threats to driving safety, there is no indication to report this patient before a more complete evaluation is performed.

KEY POINT

- The first step in assessing driving ability in older adults is to ask the patient and family members about driving difficulties, including whether friends and family members are worried about their driving, getting lost while driving, near misses, and recent accidents.

Bibliography

Carr DB, Schwartzberg JG, Manning L, Sempek J. Physician's Guide to Assessing and Counseling Older Drivers. 2nd edition. Washington, DC. NHTSA. 2010. Available at www.ama-assn .org/ama/pub/physician-resources/public-health/promoting -healthy-lifestyles/geriatric-health/older-driver-safety/assessing -counseling-older-drivers.page.

Item 119   Answer: D

Educational Objective: Manage panic disorder.

The most appropriate management of this patient is to prescribe a selective serotonin reuptake inhibitor. Panic disorder is a syndrome characterized by sudden panic attacks with the acute onset of somatic symptoms, which may include chest pain, palpitations, sweating, nausea, dizziness, dyspnea, and numbness. These symptoms usually last from 5 to 60 minutes. About 50% of patients with panic disorder also have associated agoraphobia, with fears of being in crowds or in places from which escape would be difficult. Diagnosis is based on clinical descriptors and setting, but care should be made to consider underlying medical disorders, such as cardiac disease, thyroid disease, or pheochromocytoma, particularly in patients at increased risk for one of these disorders. However, extensive testing is not necessary in most patients with a characteristic presentation and normal physical examination and basic laboratory studies. Treatment options for panic disorder include medication and psychotherapy. Cognitive-behavioral therapy (CBT) has been shown to be the most effective psychotherapeutic intervention in controlled trials. Selective serotonin reuptake inhibitors and serotonin-norepinephrine reuptake inhibitors have been shown to be effective. Panic disorder that is severe or refractory appears to be most amenable to the combination of CBT and pharmacotherapy compared with either treatment alone.

This patient has classic symptoms of panic disorder and no cardiac risk factors. It would be inappropriate to order further cardiac testing in the setting of a normal electrocardiogram and classic symptoms. This patient's symptoms are also atypical for gastroesophageal reflux disease, rendering empiric proton pump inhibitor therapy an incorrect choice.

KEY POINT

- Panic disorder is characterized by sudden panic attacks with the acute onset of somatic symptoms, which may include chest pain, palpitations, sweating, nausea, dizziness, dyspnea, and numbness.

Bibliography

Work Group on Panic Disorder; American Psychiatric Association; Practice guideline for the treatment of patients with panic disorder. Am J Psychiatry. 1998;155(5 suppl):1-34. [PMID: 9585731]

Answers and Critiques

Item 120   Answer: A

Educational Objective: Manage a patient with harmful alcohol use.

This patient is exhibiting harmful use of alcohol and should be counseled appropriately, including connecting her drinking habits with the negative consequences that she has recently experienced. Harmful drinking is drinking that causes physical or psychological harm. This patient's drinking has resulted in serious illness as well as an arrest for driving while intoxicated. Optimal management would include a discussion of appropriate amounts of alcohol, negative consequences, and agreement of goals for reducing alcohol intake. This should be performed in the setting of frequent follow-up and reassessment and should incorporate the patient's ideas about her drinking behaviors and ways to change them, barriers she may face in reducing her alcohol consumption, and previous experiences with attempting to stop or reduce her drinking.

Labeling a patient an alcoholic is neither productive nor a medically useful term. Goals of managing this patient may not require complete abstinence, and abstinence may be difficult for the patient to accomplish immediately.

Adjunct management strategies may include medications or referral to Alcoholics Anonymous or psychiatry, but these measures are more effective when done in combination with primary counseling.

The National Institute on Alcohol Abuse and Alcoholism defines at-risk drinking as more than 14 drinks per week or 4 drinks per occasion in men and more than 7 drinks per week or 3 drinks per occasion in women. However, harmful drinking is defined by consequences and not by the quantity consumed.

KEY POINT

- **Management of harmful drinking patterns includes counseling to help patients connect the negative consequences to their drinking, discussion of appropriate amounts of alcohol, and agreement of goals for reducing alcohol intake, performed in a patient-centered manner in a setting of frequent follow-up and reassessment.**

Bibliography

U.S. Preventive Services Task Force. Screening and behavioral counseling interventions in primary care to reduce alcohol misuse: recommendation statement. Ann Intern Med. 2004;140(7):554-556. [PMID: 15068984]

Item 121   Answer: B

Educational Objective: Manage a patient with suspected obstructive sleep apnea in the postoperative period.

This patient most likely has undiagnosed obstructive sleep apnea (OSA). OSA is a major risk factor for perioperative pulmonary complications, although a large number of patients in the community have unrecognized OSA. Patients with more than a negligible risk for OSA should be screened preoperatively. One instrument that may be used is the STOP-BANG questionnaire, a screen based on eight parameters: Snoring, Tired, Observed stopping breathing during sleep, high blood Pressure, BMI (>35), Age (>50 years), Neck circumference (>40 cm), and Gender (male). Patients with three or more positive responses have a high risk of OSA. Had he been screened, this patient would have scored at least 5 points (tiredness, hypertension, high BMI, age >50 years, male), and would have qualified for evaluation for possible OSA.

Although myocardial ischemia may lead to transient respiratory failure, this patient has a negative cardiac history, no chest pain, and a normal electrocardiogram, making this less likely than OSA.

Extubation following surgery is typically performed after careful assessment of stability following removal of sedating and paralyzing medications, with subsequent monitoring in a postanesthesia care unit. It is likely that he met criteria for extubation following his procedure, but patients with unrecognized OSA can develop acute respiratory failure induced by the sleep apnea combined with the respiratory depression caused by narcotics for postoperative analgesia and the lingering effects of anesthesia.

Sepsis can cause perioperative respiratory failure; however, patients with sepsis are typically febrile, hypotensive, and show evidence of a metabolic acidosis. The absence of any of these findings makes sepsis a less likely cause of his respiratory failure.

KEY POINT

- **Patients with more than a negligible risk for obstructive sleep apnea (OSA) should be screened preoperatively; those with three or more of the following parameters have a high risk of OSA: snoring, tired, observed stopping breathing during sleep, hypertension, BMI >35, age >50 years, neck circumference >40 cm, and male sex.**

Bibliography

Vasu TS, Doghramji K, Cavallazzi R, et al. Obstructive sleep apnea syndrome and postoperative complications: clinical use of the STOP-BANG questionnaire. Arch Otolaryngol Head Neck Surg. 2010;136(10):1020-1024. [PMID: 20956751]

Item 122   Answer: C

Educational Objective: Diagnose rotator cuff tendinitis.

This patient most likely has rotator cuff impingement syndrome from underlying tendinitis. She presented with pain in her shoulder that began after performing the repetitive overhead motion of painting, and her pain is most pronounced with abduction of her arm. On examination, her pain occurs between 60 and 120 degrees of abduction, which supports the diagnosis of rotator cuff tendinitis. She also has a positive Hawkins test, which has a high sensitivity (92%) but poor specificity (25%) for rotator cuff impingement.

Acromioclavicular joint degeneration is typically associated with trauma (in younger patients) or osteoarthritis (in older patients). Palpable osteophytes may be present, and radiographs, if obtained, may demonstrate degenerative changes. It characteristically presents with pain that occurs with shoulder adduction and abduction above 120 degrees. This diagnosis is unlikely in this patient given that she has no history of trauma and that there is no acromioclavicular joint tenderness on examination.

Adhesive capsulitis is caused by thickening of the capsule surrounding the glenohumeral joint. Adhesive capsulitis presents with loss of both passive and active range of motion in multiple planes and patient reports of stiffness, which are not present in this patient. Also, pain is typically slow in onset and is located near the insertion of the deltoid muscle.

Rotator cuff tears are usually accompanied by weakness and loss of function. Examination findings include supraspinatus weakness, weakness with external rotation, and a positive drop-arm test. The absence of weakness along with the negative drop-arm test argues against the presence of a rotator cuff tear in this patient.

KEY POINT

- **Rotator cuff impingement syndrome due to underlying tendinitis is a common cause of nontraumatic shoulder pain; characteristic findings are pain with arm abduction and a positive Hawkins test.**

Bibliography

House J, Mooradian A. Evaluation and management of shoulder pain in primary care clinics. South Med J. 2010;103(11):1129-1135. [PMID: 20890250]

Item 123   Answer: C
Educational Objective: Screen for HIV infection.

According to guidelines published by the Centers for Disease Control and Prevention (CDC), this man should be screened for HIV infection using enzyme immunoassay antibody (EIA) testing. The guidelines recommend that all persons between the ages of 13 and 64 years be screened for HIV infection. This recommendation is based on evidence from several studies that have demonstrated that screening for HIV is effective even in low-prevalence settings. This is particularly true when screening is coupled to the availability of antiretroviral therapy. All positive results using EIA testing should be confirmed by Western blot testing. Western blot testing should not be used as the initial screening test owing to its high rate of false-positive and false-negative results. In contrast to the CDC guidelines, the U.S. Preventive Services Task Force (USPSTF) assigns

a C grade to HIV screening, making no recommendation for or against routine HIV screening.

The National Cholesterol Education Program (NCEP) recommends that screening be initiated at the age of 20 years and then continued at least every 5 years thereafter if normal. This patient's lipid levels were normal 4 years ago; therefore, it would not be appropriate to screen him according to the NCEP guideline. The USPSTF recommends lipid screening for all men 35 years or older and for men 20 to 35 years of age with increased cardiovascular risk. Because this patient is not at increased risk for atherosclerotic heart disease, according to the USPSTF guidelines, screening for hyperlipidemia should begin at the age of 35 years.

The USPSTF recommends diabetes screening for all adults with a sustained blood pressure of 135/80 mm Hg or greater. In contrast, the American Diabetes Association recommends screening all adults who are 45 years and older and all adults who have a BMI of 25 or greater who have one or more additional risk factors (gestational diabetes, hypertension, hyperlipidemia, family history of type 2 diabetes mellitus in a first-degree relative). Screening for diabetes would be inappropriate in this patient owing to his age, absence of hypertension or obesity, and lack of other risk factors.

There is no agreement among major groups related to screening for hypothyroidism. The American Academy of Family Physicians and the American Association of Clinical Endocrinologists recommend screening for hypothyroidism in older women. The American Thyroid Association recommends screening adults by measuring thyroid-stimulating hormone (TSH) beginning at age 35 years, but the USPSTF does not recommend routine screening. This patient is not in a high-risk group defined by either age or sex, and screening for thyroid disease with a TSH level is not appropriate.

KEY POINT

- **The Centers for Disease Control and Prevention recommend that all persons between the ages of 13 and 64 years be screened for HIV infection.**

Bibliography

Qaseem A, Snow V, Shekelle P, Hopkins R Jr, Owens DK; Clinical Efficacy Assessment Subcommittee, American College of Physicians. Screening for HIV in health care settings: a guidance statement from the American College of Physicians and HIV Medicine Association. Ann Intern Med. 2009;150(2):125-131. [PMID: 19047022]

Item 124   Answer: A

Educational Objective: Manage an encounter with an impaired colleague.

In this situation, there is considerable evidence that the colleague's judgment is impaired by both the amount and rate

CONT.

of alcohol consumption and her response to an expression of concern. The ethical obligation is to prevent her from potentially harming a patient, which means contacting the hospital tonight.

Reporting to state authorities on Monday may help this physician and her future patients but would not protect the patient she is admitting tonight.

Taking her aside later is unlikely to be helpful, and puts the unimpaired physician in the position of monitoring whatever action she may take to address the issue.

Members of the medical profession have an obligation to protect the welfare of patients, which includes taking action when a colleague puts patients at risk. Many states have mandatory reporting statutes. Nevertheless, almost 75% of respondents in a 2009 survey did not believe they had a duty to report a known impaired colleague to the relevant authority, raising significant concerns about physicians' understanding of their personal and professional ethical obligations.

KEY POINT

- **Members of the medical profession have an obligation to protect the welfare of patients, which includes taking action when a colleague puts patients at risk.**

Bibliography

DesRoches CM, Rao SR, Fromson JA, et al. Physicians' perceptions, preparedness for reporting, and experiences related to impaired and incompetent colleagues. JAMA. 2010;304(2):187-193. [PMID: 20628132]

Item 125   Answer: D

Educational Objective: Manage a patient undergoing low-risk surgery.

This patient undergoing endoscopic sinus surgery should proceed to surgery without further testing. Patients undergoing low-risk surgery, which includes endoscopic surgery, cataract surgery, superficial surgery, breast surgery, and ambulatory surgery, do not need perioperative cardiac testing unless they have high-risk ("active") conditions such as an unstable coronary syndrome (myocardial infarction <30 days ago, unstable or severe angina), decompensated heart failure, significant arrhythmia, or severe valvular disease. Although this patient has three clinical risk factors (coronary artery disease, chronic kidney disease, diabetes mellitus requiring insulin) for a major perioperative cardiac complication, he does not require further cardiac testing because the anticipated surgery is low risk.

The use of β-blockers in the perioperative period is controversial, with well-designed randomized controlled trials showing both benefit and harm. Current recommendations are that patients currently on a β-blocker should continue taking it. Thus, metoprolol should not be discontinued.

Cardiac testing is reserved for patients undergoing surgery at the highest risk of a perioperative cardiac event

as predicted by their Revised Cardiac Risk Index (clinical risk factors), exercise tolerance, and the nature of the proposed surgery. Patients with a low or unknown exercise tolerance who have three or more clinical risk factors undergoing intermediate- or higher-risk surgery should be considered for preoperative cardiac testing if it will change management; however, in this patient who is undergoing low-risk surgery, no testing is needed.

Percutaneous cardiac interventions have no demonstrated value in the perioperative setting. Thus, perioperative cardiac risk assessment, if needed, should be done through noninvasive stress testing. In general, the overriding theme of perioperative cardiac risk assessment is that testing should only be done if the results will affect management, and prophylactic revascularization is rarely necessary just to get a patient through surgery. This patient has no indications for cardiac catheterization.

KEY POINT

- **In patients without active cardiac conditions undergoing low-risk surgery, preoperative cardiovascular testing is not routinely needed.**

Bibliography

Fleisher LA, Beckman JA, Brown KA, et al. 2009 ACCF/AHA focused update on perioperative beta blockade incorporated into the ACC/AHA 2007 guidelines on perioperative cardiovascular evaluation and care for noncardiac surgery: a report of the American College of Cardiology Foundation/American Heart Association Task Force on Practice Guidelines. Circulation. 2009;120(21):e169-276. [PMID: 19884473]

Item 126   Answer: C

Educational Objective: Manage a patient who is a victim of intimate partner violence.

The primary responsibility of the provider for a patient who is a victim of intimate partner violence is to assist with health; assess for safety; and provide validation, support, and empathy.

Leaving the abuser is neither necessary nor recommended without a well thought-out plan unless the patient is in imminent danger, in which case immediate intervention is indicated. Advising victims of intimate partner violence to simply leave the situation, to utilize a shelter, contact an intimate partner violence counseling service, or press criminal charges is generally not helpful as the circumstances surrounding intimate partner abuse relationships are complex, and the abused individual may have significant reasons for not pursuing these actions that need to be understood. An appreciation of the individual circumstances in the context of a supportive relationship will help in developing a plan that may ultimately involve the use of these valuable resources.

It is not recommended that the potential abuser be confronted directly or legal action be undertaken as an initial step in most cases as this may potentially put the victim in greater danger.

Psychiatry intervention may be necessary for refractory depression, or when the patient is deemed a risk to harm herself or others. However, this would not be an appropriate next step in management of this patient.

A substantial number of patients remain in adverse relationships yet demonstrate improved health and health outcomes after disclosure of their situation with appropriate support and management.

KEY POINT

- The primary responsibility of the provider for a patient who is a victim of intimate partner violence is to assist with health; assess for safety; and provide validation, support, and empathy.

Bibliography

Zolotor AJ, Denham AC, Weil A. Intimate partner violence. Prim Care. 2009;36(1):167-179. [PMID: 19231608]

Item 127   Answer: A

Educational Objective: Evaluate a randomized controlled trial for generalizability.

This patient with cardiomyopathy is asymptomatic, placing her in the category of New York Heart Association (NYHA) functional class I heart failure. Therefore, her heart failure is too mild for her to take drug H, which was tested on patients with NYHA class III and IV heart failure.

Randomized controlled trials (RCTs) are often considered the "gold standard" for evaluating new therapies because their experimental design allows confounding variables that might obscure the benefit of a therapy to be balanced between groups. Thus, any finding in a well-designed RCT is typically considered valid. In order to maximize the ability of a given study to find a meaningful result, RCTs are typically restricted to relatively homogeneous individuals who meet rigidly defined inclusion and exclusion criteria. The proscribed nature of patient selection and intervention in RCTs therefore make their conclusions narrow. Clinicians must use caution when generalizing these results to other populations. Drug H was shown to be effective for patients with NYHA class III or IV heart failure, and it may not be effective for a patient with more mild heart failure, such as this patient.

Although the mean age of participants in the trial was 63 years, the drug was tested on patients between the ages of 40 and 80 years. Thus, based on her age, the patient would have been eligible for the trial, and age alone is not a reason to withhold the drug from her.

Despite rigid criteria for inclusion and exclusion in a RCT, there will still likely be some variability between individual patients included in a particular study, such as concurrent medications being used. Even with these differences, however, a net benefit of treatment was found in the study population. Although most patients in the study were already on a β-blocker, it cannot be inferred from the study whether this treatment is required to see the benefit of drug H.

There is no arbitrary level of risk of harm that would impact a decision to use a medication; rather, each medication should be evaluated according to its risk and benefit profile. Furthermore, in this trial, drug H had net benefit despite its rate of serious adverse events.

KEY POINT

- Caution should be used when generalizing the results of randomized controlled trials to populations other than those who would meet the inclusion and exclusion criteria of the study.

Bibliography

Ho PM, Peterson PN, Masoudi FA. Evaluating the evidence: is there a rigid hierarchy? Circulation. 2008;118(16):1675-1684. [PMID: 18852378]

Item 128   Answer: A

Educational Objective: Diagnose an autism spectrum disorder.

The diagnosis is autism spectrum disorder. Autism is characterized by a triad of impaired communication; impaired social interactions; and restrictive, repetitive, and stereotyped behaviors and interests. In addition, classic autism is often associated with some degree of learning disability or mental retardation and is typically diagnosed in early childhood. Less severe variants include high-functioning autism (HFA) and Asperger syndrome, which may not be diagnosed until adolescence or even adulthood. HFA is a category of autistic disorder with less severe clinical features and without cognitive impairment. Asperger syndrome differs from HFA in that early language development is not delayed. Many experts believe that autism, HFA, and Asperger syndrome are variants along a single spectrum.

The hallmark of obsessive-compulsive disorder is the presence of recurrent obsessions or compulsions that are of sufficient severity to occupy at least 1 hour per day or to result in marked distress or functional impairment. The person should recognize that the obsessions or compulsions are excessive or unreasonable. Obsessions are defined as persistent ideas, thoughts, impulses, or images that are experienced as intrusive, inappropriate, and associated with significant anxiety or distress. This patient has compulsions but has additional symptoms not characteristic of obsessive-compulsive disorder.

Schizophrenia is defined by the presence of psychosis. Psychosis encompasses delusions, hallucinations, disorganized speech, and disorganized or catatonic behavior. The diagnosis requires at least 6 months of symptoms, including 1 month or more of at least two active-phase symptoms, such as hallucinations, delusions, disorganized speech, grossly disorganized or catatonic behavior; and negative symptoms, such as flattened affect. There must also be significant impairment in social or occupational function. This patient's symptoms are not consistent with schizophrenia.

The primary feature of social anxiety disorder is a severe and persistent fear of social or performance situations, such as public speaking or taking an examination. Persons with more generalized social anxiety disorder avoid many occupational and social situations because of fears of interacting with other people. This patient's symptoms of emotional outbursts, echolalia, and stereotyped interest in trains do not suggest social anxiety disorder.

KEY POINT

- **Autism is characterized by a triad of impaired communication; impaired social interactions; and restrictive, repetitive, and stereotyped behaviors and interests.**

Bibliography

Rao S, Salmon G. Autism spectrum disorders. Br J Hosp Med (Lond). 2010;71(12):699-703. [PMID: 21135768]

Item 129   Answer: E

Educational Objective: Select an appropriate vaccination strategy for an HIV-positive patient.

A CD4 cell count should be obtained in this patient before any vaccines are administered. This woman is entering school to become a certified nursing assistant; all health care workers should be vaccinated against or have serologic evidence of immunity to hepatitis B, varicella, measles, mumps, and rubella. In addition, health care workers should receive a one-time tetanus, diphtheria, and acellular pertussis (Tdap) vaccine as well as annual influenza vaccination. In general, vaccines can either be inactivated viral proteins or live attenuated viruses. Inactivated viral proteins are safe to administer in all patients, including those with HIV infection, except those with a documented allergy to the vaccine or its growth media (such as eggs). Live attenuated vaccines, on the other hand, should be withheld in patients with immune deficiency, including HIV-positive patients with a CD4 cell count below 200/microliter. Therefore, before administering any vaccines, however, it is important to determine whether or not she is functionally immunodeficient.

The measles, mumps, and rubella vaccine contains live, attenuated virus, and for this patient, it would be inappropriate to administer it before verifying that she is immunocompetent and also that she needs revaccination (based on negative serologic studies).

Live, attenuated influenza vaccine should be avoided in patients with immunodeficiency. Regardless of her CD4 cell count, the inactivated influenza vaccine would likely be preferred for this patient.

Hepatitis B vaccination is indicated in health care workers and in HIV-positive patients, as well as in patients with unknown hepatitis B status for whom hepatitis B vaccination is needed. As for other vaccines, it would be best to determine this patient's immune status before providing the vaccine.

Persons born after 1980, health care workers, and those born before 1980 who have a high risk for disseminated varicella should receive a two-dose varicella vaccination series unless they have serologic evidence of varicella immunity or physician-documented evidence of either varicella or varicella vaccination. Patient or parent self-report is not considered reliable.

KEY POINT

- **In patients who are HIV-positive, CD4 cell counts should be obtained before administering live attenuated vaccines.**

Bibliography

Advisory Committee on Immunization Practices; Centers for Disease Control and Prevention (CDC). Immunization of health-care personnel: recommendations of the Advisory Committee on Immunization Practices (ACIP). MMWR Recomm Rep. 2011;60(RR-7):1-45. [PMID: 22108587]

Item 130   Answer: C

Educational Objective: Diagnose costochondritis.

This patient most likely has costochondritis. The etiology of chest pain can be determined in most cases after a careful history and physical examination. Musculoskeletal chest pain has an insidious onset and may last for hours to weeks. It is most recognizable when sharp and localized to a specific area of the chest; however, it can also be poorly localized. The pain may be worsened by turning, deep breathing, or arm movement. Chest pain may or may not be reproducible by chest palpation (pain reproduced by palpation does not exclude ischemic heart disease), and the cardiovascular examination is often normal. Importantly, his findings are not consistent with an alternative cause of chest pain.

The chest pain associated with acute pericarditis is typically pleuritic in nature and is worsened when the patient lies down. A two- or three-component friction rub is often present. This patient does not have any risk factors for pericarditis; specifically, there is no history of recent viral infection, myocardial infarction, trauma, malignancy, medications, connective tissue disease, or uremia. Pericarditis, therefore, is highly unlikely.

Aortic dissection is generally described as a tearing or ripping pain with radiation to the back. It is more commonly seen in patients with a history of hypertension. Although physical examination findings may be missed, asymmetric intensity of peripheral pulses has a positive likelihood ratio of 5.7. This patient's chest pain description, physical examination, and absence of risk factors are inconsistent with aortic dissection.

This patient has no risk factors for cardiac disease. His history is inconsistent with descriptors that increase the probability of ischemic chest pain, including unstable angina. Specifically, there is no radiation to the arms, exertional component, relief with rest, diaphoresis, nausea, vomiting, or pressure description. Considering the patient's age and description of his chest pain, the probability of unstable angina or an acute coronary syndrome is low.

KEY POINT

- Musculoskeletal chest pain has an insidious onset and may last for hours to weeks; it is most recognizable when sharp and localized to a specific area of the chest; and the pain may be worsened by turning, deep breathing, or arm movement.

Bibliography
Stochkendahl MJ, Christensen HW. Chest pain in focal musculoskeletal disorders. Med Clin North Am. 2010;94(2):259-273. [PMID: 20380955]

Item 131   Answer: C
Educational Objective: Manage primary dysmenorrhea.

The most appropriate management option for this patient is a trial of NSAID therapy, such as ibuprofen. This patient has dysmenorrhea associated with normal menstrual cycles and no pelvic pathology. Initial treatment options for primary dysmenorrhea include NSAIDs and cyclooxygenase-2 inhibitors, which inhibit the inflammation, vasoconstriction, and uterine ischemia that are thought to cause the symptoms.

If symptoms are not relieved with NSAID therapy or the patient requests contraception or is sexually active, a combination estrogen-progesterone contraceptive would be appropriate. Extended-cycle formulations are particularly useful for this indication.

Depot medroxyprogesterone acetate (DMPA) is a long-acting progesterone compound, administered intramuscularly or subcutaneously every 12 to 14 weeks. Long-acting progesterone therapy is a treatment option for dysmenorrhea, and also provides contraception. For adolescents and young adults, however, long-term use of progesterone therapy decreases bone mineral density owing to prolonged estrogen deficiency. Therefore, such treatment should be used with caution for dysmenorrhea or for contraception in younger women based on the risks and benefits of treatment in a given patient. In general, NSAIDs should be tried before hormonal therapy.

In the absence of worrisome symptoms such as severe pelvic pain or significant bleeding abnormalities, treatment for dysmenorrhea may be initiated without further evaluation, such as pelvic imaging, hormonal testing, or gynecologic referral.

KEY POINT

- The first-line treatment for primary dysmenorrhea is NSAID therapy.

Bibliography
Harel Z. Dysmenorrhea in adolescents and young adults: from pathophysiology to pharmacological treatment and management strategies. Expert Opin Pharmacother. 2008;9(15):2661-2672. [PMID: 18803452]

Item 132   Answer: D
Educational Objective: Diagnose ulnar nerve entrapment at the level of the elbow.

This patient's presentation is consistent with ulnar nerve entrapment at the elbow (cubital tunnel syndrome). The cubital tunnel is the path followed by the ulnar nerve as it passes around the elbow toward the hand. In this region, the nerve is near the surface of the skin and therefore susceptible to injury. Injury may occur from mild and often unrecognized trauma, sustained pressure on the nerve as may occur during sleep, or activities that involve sustained flexion of the elbow and stretching of the nerve. Diagnostically, maneuvers that compress or stretch the injured nerve, such as flexing the arm (as seen in this patient), result in elbow pain. Paresthesias are also commonly present in the ulnar nerve distribution in the hand. These paresthesias are characteristically located on both the palmar and dorsal surfaces of the hand, which contrasts with entrapment of the ulnar nerve at the wrist, which only involves the palmar surface.

Patients with lateral epicondylitis (tennis elbow) typically present with pain in the lateral elbow that radiates down the forearm to the dorsal hand. On examination, there is tenderness to palpation at the location of the insertion of extensor muscles on the lateral epicondyle. Pain is reproduced by forced extension of the wrist.

Patients with medial epicondylitis (golfer's elbow) typically present with pain in the medial elbow and proximal forearm. On examination, there is tenderness to palpation from the medial epicondyle to the pronator teres and flexor carpi radialis muscles. Pain can be reproduced with wrist flexion and resisted forearm supination.

Olecranon bursitis is characterized by pain in the posterior elbow and swelling of the bursal sac that overlies the olecranon process. Range of motion of the elbow is not limited.

KEY POINT

- Ulnar nerve entrapment at the elbow is characterized by pain that occurs with flexion of the arm and paresthesias on both the palmar and dorsal surfaces of the hand, in the distribution of the ulnar nerve.

Bibliography
Caliendro P, La Torre G, Padua R, Giannini F, Padua L. Treatment for ulnar neuropathy at the elbow. Cochrane Database Syst Rev. 2011;(2):CD006839. [PMID: 21328287]

Item 133   Answer: D
Educational Objective: Understand the principles of informed consent.

The principles of informed consent were not followed in this case. The three key elements of informed consent are: understanding of the proposed treatment, understanding of alternatives to the proposed treatment, and understanding the risks and benefits of both the treatment and the alternatives. In this case, the patient says he was not given either information about risks of antibiotics or alternative options. This calls into question whether he received adequate information to give informed consent.

Informed consent applies to all health care decisions, not only to invasive procedures. It requires an active dialogue around the three key elements.

Many practitioners obtain written informed consent for invasive procedures because this entails documentation of consent, but it does not exempt physicians from having a discussion of risks, benefits, and alternatives for all treatments that have the potential to cause harm.

KEY POINT

- **The three key elements of informed consent are: understanding of the proposed treatment, understanding of alternatives to the proposed treatment, and understanding the risks and benefits of both the treatment and the alternatives.**

Bibliography

Snyder L; American College of Physicians Ethics, Professionalism, and Human Rights Committee. American College of Physicians Ethics Manual: sixth edition. Ann Intern Med. 2012;156(1 Pt 2):73-104. [PMID: 22213573]

Item 134   Answer: D

Educational Objective: Treat chronic cervical radiculopathy with neurologic deficits.

This patient should be referred for surgical evaluation. He has clinical and imaging evidence of cervical radiculopathy, and progressive weakness in the affected arm that correlates with his disk herniation. Surgical intervention is generally indicated in patients with progressive neurologic symptoms resulting from a defined anatomic abnormality to preserve and avoid permanent loss of function.

In the absence of progressive motor deficits, a conservative approach is indicated as most patients experience improvement in symptoms without more aggressive imaging or intervention. Local corticosteroid injections may provide faster pain relief, although long-term outcomes are similar to conservative therapy. Physical therapy is also a useful intervention in patients with uncomplicated cervical radiculopathy to decrease discomfort and possibly strengthen the neck muscles to prevent recurrent episodes. However, these interventions, including continued analgesics and rest, would not be appropriate in this patient with worsening neurologic function.

KEY POINT

- **Surgical referral is indicated for patients with cervical radiculopathy with progressive motor deficits.**

Bibliography

Nikolaidis I, Fouyas IP, Sandercock PA, Statham PF. Surgery for cervical radiculopathy or myelopathy. Cochrane Database Syst Rev. 2010;(1):CD001466. [PMID: 20091520]

Item 135   Answer: B

Educational Objective: Diagnose interstitial cystitis as a cause of chronic pelvic pain.

This most likely diagnosis in this patient with chronic pelvic pain is interstitial cystitis. Chronic pelvic pain is defined as noncyclic pain of at least 6 months' duration that localizes to the anatomic pelvis, the anterior abdominal wall at or below the umbilicus, the lumbosacral back, or the buttocks, and is of sufficient severity to impair quality of life. Potential causes of chronic pelvic pain include interstitial cystitis, endometriosis, pelvic adhesions, and irritable bowel syndrome. In this patient, the combination of chronic pelvic pain in association with unexplained urinary symptoms is most consistent with a diagnosis of interstitial cystitis. Interstitial cystitis is a chronic inflammatory condition of the bladder that causes symptoms of urinary urgency, frequency, and pelvic discomfort. The pelvic discomfort may be worsened by sexual intercourse, and patients may urinate numerous times per day. Although urinalysis and urine cultures are almost always negative, most women with interstitial cystitis have been treated empirically several times for urinary tract infections.

Endometriosis is a common cause of chronic pelvic pain, and patients typically report severe dysmenorrhea, cyclic pain, and dyspareunia. The absence of severe dysmenorrhea and the noncyclic nature of this patient's pelvic pain make endometriosis a less likely diagnosis. Similarly, irritable bowel syndrome is unlikely to explain her symptoms in the absence of any associated gastrointestinal symptoms.

Adhesions are diagnosed in 25% to 50% of women with chronic pelvic pain. Pelvic adhesions typically form in the setting of acute or chronic inflammatory processes, such as infection, or surgery. This patient has no history of pelvic infection and has never had pelvic surgery, making this an unlikely cause of her symptoms.

KEY POINT

- **Interstitial cystitis is a likely diagnosis in women with chronic pelvic pain associated with unexplained urinary symptoms; most women with interstitial cystitis have been treated empirically several times for urinary tract infections.**

Bibliography

Vercellini P, Somigliana E, Viganò P, Abbiati A, Barbara G, Fedele L. Chronic pelvic pain in women: etiology, pathogenesis, and diagnostic approach. Gynecol Endocrinol. 2009;25(3):149-158. [PMID: 19347704]

Item 136   Answer: D
Educational Objective: Treat chronic neuropathic pain with opioid therapy.

Long-acting opioid therapy, such as sustained-release morphine, would be the best treatment option in this patient. Although opioid medications are generally not recommended for use in patients with chronic noncancer pain, they are appropriately considered in patients with moderate to severe neuropathic pain that has not responded to adequate trials of multiple nonopioid therapies. As with all patients being considered for long-term opioid treatment, he should have a thorough understanding of its risks and benefits and should work together with the physician to develop an opioid management plan, or pain contract, that outlines agreed-upon goals and rules of treatment.

Long-acting opioids provide more consistent serum drug levels and are generally preferred to intermittent dosing of shorter-acting agents that may lead to significant fluctuations in pain level. Although this patient's pain is reasonably well controlled on his current regimen of oxycodone-acetaminophen, it is also a short-acting preparation and is less desirable for long-term use. When used chronically, the overall daily dose of acetaminophen needs to be taken into account; daily doses should be below 4 g and less in patients with liver disease, significant alcohol use, or those being treated with other potentially hepatotoxic medications.

Tramadol is a weak opioid agonist and may be effective for mild, episodic neuropathic pain, although it may require a relatively high daily dose with an increased risk of associated side effects, such as gastrointestinal symptoms. It also has a short period of action and requires multiple daily dosing, which would not be preferable in this patient.

Methadone is a long-acting opioid that can be very effective for pain control but can be associated with significant adverse cardiovascular outcomes, such as QT-interval prolongation, hypotension, and cardiac arrhythmias. It should be avoided in this patient with a history of ischemic cardiomyopathy and conduction defects noted on the electrocardiogram.

KEY POINT
- Long-acting opioid therapy should be considered in a patient with moderate to severe neuropathic pain that has not responded to nonopioid therapies.

Bibliography
Bril V, England J, Franklin GM, et al; American Academy of Neurology; American Association of Neuromuscular and Electrodiagnostic Medicine; American Academy of Physical Medicine and Rehabilitation. Evidence-based guideline: Treatment of painful diabetic neuropathy: report of the American Academy of Neurology, the American Association of Neuromuscular and Electrodiagnostic Medicine, and the American Academy of Physical Medicine and Rehabilitation. Neurology. 2011;76:1758-1765. [PMID: 21482920]

Item 137   Answer: B
Educational Objective: Diagnose complicated grief.

This patient is likely suffering from complicated grief stemming from his wife's death 9 months ago. Complicated grief, also referred to as complicated bereavement, is an abnormal response to bereavement persisting more than 6 months, at least 6 months after a death. Its chief symptom is yearning for a loved one so intensely that all other desires are incapacitated. Although interventions have been attempted to prevent this severe grief reaction, none have proved beneficial. It is important for health care providers to be watchful for this disorder in bereaved survivors.

Drugs with the potential for anticholinergic adverse effects, such as diphenhydramine, are generally not a good choice in the elderly. Although the anticholinergic properties of diphenhydramine could be responsible for acute confusion and hallucinations, this patient's persistent symptoms, such as anhedonia and early morning wakening, would not be explained by such a short-acting agent.

Generalized anxiety disorder is characterized by excessive anxiety and worry about a variety of events or activities over at least a 6-month period; difficulty exercising control over worrying; several symptoms associated with the anxiety, such as fatigue, irritability, restlessness, sleep disturbance, and difficulty concentrating; and functional impairment. Although an anxiety disorder should also be considered in the differential diagnosis of this patient given his sleep disturbance, his lack of excessive anxiety and worry make it less likely.

Although this patient could also have major depression, his intense feelings that his wife is beside him are more indicative of complicated grief marked by an unwillingness to accept her death. His sense that his wife is beside him when he wakes up in the middle of the night and his visions of his wife's face when he closes his eyes are not consistent with hallucinations because the patient is aware that they are not real. Patients with true psychosis are convinced their hallucinations and delusions are real.

KEY POINT
- Complicated grief is grief persisting more than 6 months, at least 6 months after a death; its chief symptom is yearning for a loved one so intensely that all other desires are incapacitated.

Bibliography
Wittouck C, Van Autreve S, De Jaegere E, Portzky G, van Heeringen K. The prevention and treatment of complicated grief: a meta-analysis. Clin Psychol Rev. 2011;31(1):69-78. [PMID: 21130937]

Item 138   Answer: D
Educational Objective: Diagnose rhinitis medicamentosa.

This patient most likely has rhinitis medicamentosa. The key clue in this patient's presentation is ongoing use of a topical nasal vasoconstrictor (oxymetazoline). In some patients, this produces a syndrome of tolerance (rhinitis medicamentosa) in which continued use of the vasoconstrictor produces diminishing returns, but withdrawal of it causes severe nasal congestion. Withdrawal of the offending agent is the only reliable way to treat this condition. Sometimes, use of nasal corticosteroids or nasal saline rinses can mitigate symptoms of decongestant withdrawal.

A 2011 trial randomized 60 patients with perennial allergic rhinitis to fluticasone, oxymetazoline, a combination of both agents, and placebo. After 4 weeks of treatment, no evidence of rhinitis medicamentosa was seen in either of the oxymetazoline-treated groups, raising the possibility that rhinitis medicamentosa is much less common than previously thought.

Chronic rhinosinusitis is characterized by mucopurulent drainage or facial pain or pressure typical of sinusitis. In the absence of these findings and the presence of ongoing oxymetazoline use, rhinitis medicamentosa is the more likely diagnosis.

Chronic nonallergic (vasomotor) rhinitis is a syndrome characterized by the presence of at least one typical symptom of rhinitis (sneezing, rhinorrhea, nasal congestion, postnasal drainage) in the absence of a specific etiology. Chronic nonallergic rhinitis is a possibility in this patient, but the diagnosis cannot be made until the oxymetazoline is stopped.

Granulomatosis with polyangiitis (Wegener granulomatosis) is a necrotizing vasculitis that typically affects the respiratory tract and the kidneys. More than 70% of patients present with upper airway symptoms, particularly sinusitis. Up to 90% of patients have pulmonary manifestations that can include cough, hemoptysis, or pleurisy. The patient's findings are not consistent with granulomatosis with polyangiitis.

KEY POINT

- **Ongoing use of a topical nasal vasoconstrictor may cause rhinitis medicamentosa, in which continued use of the vasoconstrictor produces diminishing returns, but withdrawal of it causes severe nasal congestion.**

Bibliography

Doshi J. Rhinitis medicamentosa: what an otolaryngologist needs to know. Eur Arch Otorhinolaryngol. 2009;266(5):623-625. [PMID: 19096862]

Item 139   Answer: C

Educational Objective: Manage cyclical mastalgia.

This patient has cyclical mastalgia, which affects up to 40% of premenopausal women. It is most prominent during the luteal phase of the menstrual cycle and is typically described as a bilateral, throbbing discomfort. Education, reassurance, and the use of a well-fitting bra are recommended for all women with cyclical mastalgia, and 20% of patients will experience resolution of their pain without any intervention. This patient has recently increased her level of physical activity, and lack of a supportive sports bra may have exacerbated her discomfort.

Medical treatment is typically reserved for women who have severe and persistent pain that interferes with their quality of life. Danazol is the only treatment that has been approved by the FDA for cyclical mastalgia, although it would not be appropriate in this patient without a trial of nonmedical therapy.

A thorough history and physical examination are typically sufficient to rule out more serious causes of breast discomfort. A patient can be diagnosed with benign mastalgia if there is no evidence of extramammary causes of breast discomfort, such as pneumonia, pleuritis, myocardial ischemia, infection, or costochondritis. In the absence of a palpable breast mass or skin changes suggestive of malignancy, there is no role for diagnostic mammography in the management of cyclical mastalgia.

Tamoxifen has been used off-label for treatment of benign mastalgia, and rarely can be associated with hot flushes and menstrual irregularities. It could be considered for this patient, but only if she does not benefit from conservative measures, including use of a well-fitting bra.

KEY POINT

- **Conservative measures, including education, reassurance, and the use of a well-fitting support bra, are recommended for all women with cyclical mastalgia and should be tried before initiating medical treatment.**

Bibliography

Miltenburg DM, Speights VO Jr. Benign breast disease. Obstet Gynecol Clin North Am. 2008;35(2):285-300, ix. [PMID: 18486842]

Item 140   Answer: B

Educational Objective: Treat a depressive episode of bipolar disorder.

The most appropriate treatment for this patient is lamotrigine. He most likely is having a depressive episode of bipolar disorder. Careful questioning of patients who present with depressive symptoms to elucidate a history of hypomanic or manic episodes is important in order to identify bipolar disorder. The Mood Disorders Questionnaire (MDQ) is a relatively brief, validated questionnaire to screen for bipolar disorder. A cut-off of seven or more positive responses out of the thirteen items on question 1 yields a sensitivity of 73% and specificity of 90%. Pharmacotherapy for bipolar disorder is more complicated than for unipolar depression, and a psychiatrist should be involved in the care of most patients with the disorder. Lithium has long been a mainstay of bipolar disorder therapy; however, it has a narrow therapeutic window and is teratogenic, nephrotoxic, and can cause hypothyroidism. Alternative first-line therapies include mood stabilizing agents, such as lamotrigine, valproic acid, or carbamazepine. In addition, atypical antipsychotic agents, such as aripiprazole or quetiapine, can be used for frank mania. Simply prescribing antidepressants alone places the patient at risk for experiencing a frank manic episode.

Duloxetine, a serotonin-norepinephrine reuptake inhibitor, is an appropriate therapy for the treatment of depressive disorders. Most classes of antidepressants have equal efficacy (about 70% in most studies) and should be chosen on the basis of previous patient response, side-effect profile, and cost. This patient has bipolar disorder, and an antidepressant alone would not be the appropriate treatment.

Benzodiazepines, such as lorazepam, are ineffective single agents for depression or bipolar disorder, but may be used as an adjunct therapy in patients with mania or hypomania. This patient is having a depressive episode, and there is no role for lorazepam in treating his condition.

Selective serotonin reuptake inhibitors (SSRIs), such as sertraline, may trigger a manic episode in patients with bipolar disease and should not be used in this population. For this reason, in any patient being considered for initiation of SSRIs for depression, it is important that the history be assessed for manic symptoms.

KEY POINT

- **In patients with depressive symptoms, it is important to elucidate a history of hypomanic or manic episodes in order to identify bipolar disorder, which is treated with mood stabilizers rather than antidepressants.**

Bibliography

Belmaker RH. Treatment of bipolar depression. N Engl J Med. 2007;356(17):1771-1773. [PMID: 17392296]

Item 141   Answer: D

Educational Objective: Diagnose secondary causes of dyslipidemia.

This patient's serum thyroid-stimulating hormone level should be measured. Her total cholesterol and LDL cholesterol levels are markedly elevated despite adherence to treatment with simvastatin. Secondary causes of dyslipidemia should be considered, as statin therapy may be ineffective in the setting of untreated hypothyroidism, diabetes mellitus, obstructive liver disease, or nephrotic syndrome. There are several clinical clues that suggest the diagnosis of hypothyroidism in this patient, including symptoms of fatigue and constipation and dry skin noted on physical examination. Undiagnosed thyroid disease is likely contributing to this patient's apparent treatment-refractory dyslipidemia.

Gemfibrozil is a fibric acid derivative that is typically used for the treatment of hypertriglyceridemia. Adding

gemfibrozil to this patient's regimen will likely reduce her triglyceride levels by up to 50%, but will not substantially decrease her LDL cholesterol (typical reductions of 5%-20%). Moreover, gemfibrozil raises the serum concentration of statins by two-fold, thereby increasing the risk for statin-induced myopathy. The risks adding gemfibrozil to her statin therapy, therefore, outweigh the benefits for this patient.

A review of data from several large clinical trials found that the risk of myopathy with the 80-mg dose of simvastatin was significantly higher than the risk observed with other statin therapies. In patients who have not achieved goal LDL cholesterol levels with a 40-mg dose of simvastatin, the FDA has now recommended that therapy be switched to atorvastatin or rosuvastatin. These statins are more potent and can achieve LDL cholesterol goals at lower doses, thereby decreasing the risk for statin-induced myopathy. Increasing the simvastatin dose to 80 mg/d, therefore, is inappropriate for this patient's management.

Undiagnosed diabetes mellitus should be considered in patients with unresponsive hyperlipidemia and may be diagnosed by a hemoglobin A_{1c} level of 6.5% or greater. In this patient, her fasting glucose and triglyceride levels are normal, making a diagnosis of diabetes less likely; therefore, obtaining a hemoglobin A_{1c} level would not be an appropriate next step in management.

KEY POINT

- **In patients with hyperlipidemia that is refractory to medical therapy, secondary causes, including hypothyroidism, diabetes mellitus, nephrotic syndrome, and obstructive liver disease, should be considered.**

Bibliography

Alwaili K, Alrasadi K, Awan Z, Genest J. Approach to the diagnosis and management of lipoprotein disorders. Curr Opin Endocrinol Diabetes Obes. 2009;16(2):132-140. [PMID: 19306526]

Item 142   Answer: D

Educational Objective: Manage warfarin perioperatively in a high-risk patient.

For this patient with a high risk for a perioperative thromboembolic event, the most appropriate treatment is to discontinue warfarin 5 days before surgery and provide bridging anticoagulation with a low-molecular-weight heparin (LMWH), such as enoxaparin, until the morning of surgery. In general, patients using warfarin have three possible preoperative treatment options: stop warfarin, receive bridging therapy with a parenteral anticoagulant, or continue the warfarin. This patient has atrial fibrillation with a high $CHADS_2$ score (1 point each for diabetes mellitus, heart failure, and hypertension, and 2 points for previous stroke or transient ischemic attack [TIA] = 5) and her TIA is recent, placing her at a high risk for thrombosis; such patients should not have anticoagulation withheld for a prolonged period of time. Thus, warfarin should be changed to an agent with a shorter and more predictable half-life, usually LMWH. This agent is then withheld just before surgery and restarted after surgery, thus minimizing the amount of time the patient is not therapeutically anticoagulated.

The effect of dose adjustment of warfarin on INR is hard to predict. Thus, it would be inappropriate to recommend a fixed half dose of warfarin. This may result in an inappropriately high INR level for surgery (as would continuing the current dose of warfarin up to surgery) or a prolonged period of time with an inadequate INR, putting the patient at risk for thromboembolism.

In patients taking warfarin who have a low risk of thromboembolism, including those with a history of venous thromboembolism more than 12 months ago and those with atrial fibrillation with a $CHADS_2$ score of 2 or less, stopping warfarin without providing bridging anticoagulation is acceptable. However, this patient's $CHADS_2$ score is 5, and withholding anticoagulation for 5 days preoperatively is not recommended.

KEY POINT

- Patients taking warfarin who are at high risk of postoperative venous thromboembolism and are undergoing intermediate- or high-risk surgery should have warfarin discontinued 5 days before surgery and receive bridging anticoagulation, usually with low-molecular-weight heparin.

Bibliography

Douketis JD, Spyropoulos AC, Spencer FA, et al; American College of Chest Physicians. Perioperative management of antithrombotic therapy: Antithrombotic Therapy and Prevention of Thrombosis, 9th ed: American College of Chest Physicians Evidence-Based Clinical Practice Guidelines. Chest. 2012;141(2 suppl):e326S-e50S. [PMID: 22315266]

Item 143   Answer: C
Educational Objective: Treat anorexia nervosa.

The most appropriate treatment for this patient with anorexia nervosa is cognitive-behavioral therapy (CBT). Anorexia nervosa is characterized by an abnormally low body weight (<85% of expected) in association with a fear of gaining weight, an excessive emphasis of body weight on self-perception, and amenorrhea for at least three menstrual cycles. Overall recovery rates range from 35% to 85%, and many patients relapse. The goals of treatment are to restore healthy weight, treat physical and metabolic complications, address abnormal attitudes and feelings related to eating, and treat associated psychiatric conditions. Behavioral interventions include CBT, cognitive analytic therapy, and family therapy; among these, CBT appears to be the most effective for reducing relapse after weight restoration has been initiated.

Antidepressants, when used as monotherapy for anorexia nervosa, have not been shown to increase weight gain or improve the underlying attitudes or behaviors associated with anorexia nervosa. In particular, amitriptyline and bupropion should be avoided in patients with anorexia nervosa because of the high risk of adverse effects of these agents when given in the setting of metabolic derangements, which are common in this patient population.

Megestrol acetate is an appetite stimulant that is approved for palliative treatment of patients with cancer and AIDS complicated by anorexia and significant weight loss. It is not approved for patients with anorexia nervosa and has not been studied in this population.

Amenorrhea is a diagnostic criterion for anorexia nervosa, and oral contraceptive pills will restore menses. However, there are no convincing data to support this practice, and restoration of menses through hormonal manipulation may decrease a patient's motivation for weight gain.

KEY POINT

- In patients with anorexia nervosa, cognitive-behavioral therapy can be effective for reducing relapse after weight restoration has been initiated.

Bibliography

Bulik CM, Berkman ND, Brownley KA, Sedway JA, Lohr KN. Anorexia nervosa treatment: a systematic review of randomized controlled trials. Int J Eat Disord. 2007;40(4):310-320. [PMID: 17370290]

Item 144   Answer: A
Educational Objective: Treat chronic pain in an elderly patient.

Acetaminophen is the best medication for the initial treatment of this patient's chronic pain secondary to spinal stenosis, and is recommended as first-line therapy for chronic noncancer pain by the American Geriatrics Society. It is effective for the relief of mechanical/compressive pain and has an excellent safety profile. This patient has no underlying liver disease and does not drink alcohol, so he has no contraindications to this medication. He should not exceed a dose of 4 g in 24 hours; the FDA has recently limited the dose of prescription acetaminophen to 325 mg to decrease the risk of toxicity.

Several medications are effective for treating mechanical/compressive pain, including tricyclic antidepressants, NSAIDs, acetaminophen, and duloxetine. However, older patients are more likely to experience medication-related side effects, and comorbid conditions may predispose to impaired drug metabolism. Careful selection of pain medications is therefore essential. Tricyclic antidepressants, such as amitriptyline, should be avoided in the elderly owing to their potential for adverse effects, including cardiac conduction abnormalities, orthostasis, and anticholinergic effects.

Muscle relaxants, such as cyclobenzaprine, have demonstrated limited effectiveness in the treatment of mechanical/compressive pain.

Although NSAIDs can be very effective for the relief of pain, their associated risks for gastrointestinal, cardiovascular, and renal toxicities limit their use in older patients with comorbidities. This patient has a history of peptic ulcer disease, and the addition of ibuprofen to his medication regimen may increase his risk for gastrointestinal bleeding.

KEY POINT

- First-line therapy for chronic pain in the elderly is acetaminophen.

Bibliography

American Geriatrics Society Panel on the Pharmacologic Management of Persistent Pain in Older Persons. Pharmacologic management of persistent pain in older persons. J Am Geriatr Soc. 2009;57(8):1331-1346. [PMID: 19573219]

Item 145   Answer: B

Educational Objective: Screen for depression.

This woman should be screened for depression. The U.S. Preventive Services Task Force (USPSTF) recommends screening all adults for depression provided that adequate resources are available to ensure adequate treatment and follow up. Little evidence supports using one screening method over another. However, asking two questions, "During the past 2 weeks, have you felt down, depressed, or hopeless?" and "During the past 2 weeks, have you felt little interest or pleasure in doing things?" appears to have similar effectiveness compared with longer instruments.

One-time abdominal ultrasonography to screen for abdominal aortic aneurysm (AAA) is recommended only for men between the ages of 65 to 75 years who have previously smoked. The USPSTF recommends against screening women for AAA regardless of age or whether or not they have ever smoked.

The USPSTF strongly recommends screening for hepatitis B virus infection in all pregnant women at their first prenatal visit. Owing to the low prevalence of hepatitis B in the general population in the United States, however, routine screening is not cost effective and is not recommended.

The USPSTF recommends screening for osteoporosis in all women age 65 years or older and also in younger women with an elevated fracture risk. Screening this patient for osteoporosis would not be appropriate as she is younger than 65 years and does not have a fracture risk that is equal to or greater than that of a 65-year-old woman without additional risk factors, such as alcoholism, corticosteroid use for more than 3 months, low body mass, current tobacco use, dementia, or use of anticonvulsants.

KEY POINT

- Screening for depression is recommended for all adults as long as appropriate supports are in place to ensure adequate treatment and follow up.

Bibliography

O'Connor EA, Whitlock EP, Beil TL, Gaynes BN. Screening for depression in adult patients in primary care settings: a systematic evidence review. Ann Intern Med. 2009;151(11):793-803. [PMID: 19949145]

Item 146   Answer: C

Educational Objective: Diagnose generalized anxiety disorder.

This patient most likely has generalized anxiety disorder (GAD). Anxiety disorders are among the most common psychiatric disorders in the general population; of these, GAD is the most common, occurring in approximately 4% of the population. GAD is characterized by excessive anxiety and worry about a variety of events or activities on most days for at least 6 months, with difficulty controlling worrying. Associated symptoms include fatigue, irritability, restlessness, insomnia, and difficulty concentrating. Patients with GAD often have comorbid anxiety disorders, depression, or substance abuse. Patients with GAD often have somatoform symptoms, which can make them high utilizers of health care resources.

Attention-deficit/hyperactivity disorder first manifests in childhood and is characterized by inattention, hyperactivity, and impulsivity accompanied by functional impairment in at least two settings (home, work, school). This patient's presentation is not consistent with attention-deficit/hyperactivity disorder.

Bipolar disorder is characterized by manic or hypomanic mood episodes and depressive episodes. A manic episode is marked by a persistent period of elevated mood, irritability, lack of need for sleep, racing thoughts, high energy levels, increased talkativeness, spending sprees, hypersexuality, and increased self confidence, with possible delusions of grandeur or psychosis.

A major depressive episode is diagnosed by the presence of five or more of the following symptoms occurring nearly every day during the same 2-week period, at least one of which is either depressed mood or loss of interest or pleasure: depressed mood most of the day, loss of interest or pleasure in most activities, significant unintentional weight or appetite gain or loss, insomnia or hypersomnia, psychomotor agitation or retardation, fatigue or loss of energy, feelings of worthlessness or guilt, diminished concentration, or recurrent thoughts of death or suicide without a specific plan or prior attempt. This patient's symptom complex does not fit with a diagnosis of depression.

KEY POINT

- Generalized anxiety disorder is characterized by excessive anxiety and worry about a variety of events or activities on most days for at least 6 months, with difficulty controlling worrying.

Bibliography

Kroenke K, Spitzer RL, Williams JB, Monahan PO, Löwe B. Anxiety disorders in primary care: prevalence, impairment, comorbidity, and detection. Ann Intern Med. 2007;146(5):317-325. [PMID: 17339617]

Item 147   Answer: A

Educational Objective: Manage hypoactive sexual desire disorder.

This woman has hypoactive sexual desire disorder (HSDD), which is diagnosed if a patient reports personal distress associated with a persistent lack of sexual thoughts, desire for, or receptiveness to sexual activity. HSDD is the most common female sexual disorder, with prevalence ranging from 12% to 19%. In studies of menopausal women, predictors of sexual function included feelings for partner, change in partner status, and previous level of sexual function. As this patient's current feelings about the relationship with her partner may be causing distress, individual or couples sex therapy, which provides information about the normal female sexual response and facilitates communication about sexual issues, may be beneficial. There is no FDA-approved medication for the treatment of female HSDD.

Sildenafil is an effective treatment for male erectile dysfunction but generally is not indicated for the treatment of sexual disorders in women. It was found to be no better than placebo for increasing the frequency of enjoyable sexual encounters or improving any aspect of sexual function in women. It may be used to improve sexual arousal and orgasm in women experiencing sexual dysfunction related to selective serotonin reuptake inhibitor therapy but does not impact sexual desire.

Systemic estrogen and progesterone therapy improves many symptoms associated with menopause, including hot flushes and vaginal atrophy (unresponsive to topical therapy). This patient has no signs or symptoms of vaginal atrophy and does not report vasomotor symptoms, so this treatment is not indicated.

Several studies have shown that systemic testosterone therapy, either as monotherapy or in combination with estrogen therapy, increases sexual function scores and number of satisfying sexual episodes in menopausal women but has significant adverse effects. Treated women experienced unwanted hair growth, vaginal bleeding, and had a trend toward an increased incidence of breast cancer. The FDA has not approved any testosterone therapy for the treatment of sexual dysfunction.

KEY POINT

- For women with hypoactive sexual desire disorder, individual or couples sex therapy may be beneficial.

Bibliography

Nappi RE, Martini E, Terreno E, et al. Management of hypoactive sexual desire disorder in women: current and emerging therapies. Int J Womens Health. 2010;2:167-175. [PMID: 21072309]

Item 148   Answer: A

Educational Objective: Diagnose macular degeneration.

This patient has age-related macular degeneration (AMD). In the early stages, AMD is often asymptomatic. Common symptoms, when present, include distortion of vision or a notable loss of central vision. Those with advanced AMD and profound visual loss may experience visual hallucinations (Charles Bonnet syndrome). In both dry and wet AMD, drusen are common findings. Drusen are amorphous deposits behind the retina that lead to visual loss through direct (space occupying) and indirect (inflammatory response) means. A few small, hard drusen are common as people age, but numerous large, soft drusen are a harbinger of severe AMD. Wet AMD, which is less common than dry AMD and typically more aggressive, is characterized by neovascularization with subsequent vessel leakage and hemorrhage. Smoking is a risk factor for AMD.

Cataract, or any opacification of the otherwise optically clear lens behind the pupil and iris, is the most common cause of blindness and low vision worldwide. Vision loss is slowly progressive and is usually worse in bright light or at night, with glaring headlights while driving. This patient's clear lens is not consistent with cataract.

Primary open angle glaucoma (POAG) is a progressive optic neuropathy associated with increased intraocular pressure. POAG is characterized by painless, gradual loss of peripheral vision in both eyes that may go unnoticed by the patient. In later stages, the central vision may also be affected. This patient's vision distortion and central vision loss and the funduscopic findings are not consistent with POAG.

Retinal detachment is a separation of the neurosensory layer of the retina from the choroid beneath. It may result from trauma or occur spontaneously, particularly in persons with myopia. Symptoms include diminished vision, photopsia (flashes of light), abrupt onset of multiple floaters in the vision, or metamorphopsia (wavy vision). Funduscopic examination reveals the folds of the retinal tear and detachment, which are not present in this patient.

KEY POINT

- Age-related macular degeneration causes painless progressive vision loss, characterized by distortion of vision and loss of central vision.

Bibliography
Jager RD, Mieler WF, Miller JW. Age-related macular degeneration. N Engl J Med. 2008;358(24):2606-2617. [PMID: 18550876]

Item 149   Answer: D

Educational Objective: Assess cardiac risk in a patient scheduled for intermediate-risk surgery.

This patient needs no further testing before surgery. Current recommendations are to reserve preoperative cardiac evaluation for patients at highest risk for perioperative cardiac events undergoing intermediate- or high-risk surgeries when testing would influence patient management. These are typically patients with both a low exercise tolerance and multiple risk factors. (Adequate exercise tolerance is defined as the ability to perform physical exertion of ≥4 metabolic equivalents [METs] without symptoms.) The Revised Cardiac Risk Index (RCRI) is a validated risk assessment tool that assigns one point each for a history of ischemic heart disease, compensated or prior chronic heart failure, diabetes mellitus requiring insulin, chronic kidney disease, or history of cerebrovascular disease. Although this patient has poor exercise tolerance and is undergoing an intermediate-risk procedure (orthopedic surgery), he has no RCRI risk factors. The American Heart Association/American College of Cardiology guidelines on perioperative cardiac evaluation recommend that patients with no RCRI risk factors undergoing an intermediate-risk procedure proceed to surgery without further cardiac evaluation. Cardiac complications occur in less than 1% of patients with zero or one RCRI risk factors. Thus, despite this patient's age and comorbidities, the current recommendations are for no preoperative cardiac testing.

Cardiac catheterization is not recommended as an initial preoperative cardiac evaluation, because of the good test performance characteristics of stress tests and the invasive nature a cardiac catheterization.

CT coronary angiography is a noninvasive means of defining cardiac anatomy. It has not been studied for perioperative cardiac risk assessment.

Noninvasive pharmacologic stress testing, either dobutamine stress echocardiography or nuclear perfusion stress tests, are recommended for patients in whom preoperative cardiac testing is indicated. However, this patient's cardiovascular risk is estimated to be low enough to not warrant stress testing.

KEY POINT

- Low-risk patients who are not undergoing higher-risk surgery can proceed to surgery without preoperative cardiac testing.

Bibliography
Fleisher LA, Beckman JA, Brown KA, et al. 2009 ACCF/AHA focused update on perioperative beta blockade incorporated into the ACC/AHA 2007 guidelines on perioperative cardiovascular evaluation and care for noncardiac surgery: a report of the American College of Cardiology Foundation/American Heart Association Task Force on Practice Guidelines. Circulation. 2009;120(21):e169-276. [PMID: 19884473]

Item 150   Answer: A

Educational Objective: Manage obesity with bariatric surgery.

This patient should be referred for bariatric surgery. For patients with class III obesity (BMI ≥40) or class II obesity (BMI 35.0-39.9) with obesity-related complications, the National Institutes of Health Consensus Development Conference recommends consideration of bariatric surgery if diet, exercise, and/or medication are ineffective. Patients should be motivated and well informed about this option and undergo multidisciplinary evaluation by a medical, surgical, psychiatric, and nutritionist team. The most common procedure is gastric bypass surgery, but laparoscopic banding is becoming common, as well. Bariatric surgery results in more dramatic and sustained weight loss than nonsurgical interventions and leads to improvement in obesity-related complications (diabetes mellitus, obstructive sleep apnea, hypertension, and hyperlipidemia). This patient has not attained his goal weight loss after a 6-month trial of diet and medication and has obesity-related complications that likely will improve with weight loss.

Phentermine is a sympathomimetic drug that is FDA-approved for short-term use (up to 12 weeks) as an adjunctive treatment of obesity. This patient's weight loss goal is 45.4 kg (100 lb), which will take much longer than 12 weeks. In addition, most persons regain any weight that is lost with this medication upon its discontinuation.

Restricting caloric intake to below 800 kcal/d (a very-low-calorie diet) is no more effective for long-term weight loss than a moderate strategy of restricting intake to 500-1000 kcal/d below what is estimated to maintain current body weight. In addition, long-term compliance with a very-low-calorie diet is nearly impossible.

Exercise is an important part of a comprehensive weight loss program that focuses on lifestyle modification. However, the patient has already not benefited from an exercise program. It is unlikely that exercise alone will meet his weight loss goals.

KEY POINT

- Bariatric surgery should be considered for patients with BMI of 40 or greater or BMI of 35.0 to 39.9 with obesity-related complications in whom diet, exercise, and/or medication are ineffective.

Bibliography
Colquitt JL, Picot J, Loveman E, Clegg AJ. Surgery for obesity. Cochrane Database Syst Rev. 2009;(2):CD003641. [PMID: 19370590]

Item 151   Answer: A

Educational Objective: Screen for abdominal aortic aneurysm.

This patient should undergo one-time abdominal ultrasonography to screen for an abdominal aortic aneurysm

(AAA) because he is a man between the ages of 65 to 75 years who has ever smoked (defined as 100 lifetime cigarettes). In the Multicentre Aneurysm Screening Study, a population-based sample of 67,770 men between the ages of 65 and 74 years were offered either screening for AAAs with an abdominal ultrasound or no screening. After 10 years of follow up, it was determined that screening offered a 14% absolute risk reduction in mortality from AAAs and a reduction in all-cause mortality that was of borderline significance.

Coronary artery calcium (CAC) determination by electron beam CT has high sensitivity for detecting stenoses of greater than 50% but low specificity. Because of this low specificity, a 2007 American College of Cardiology Foundation/American Heart Association consensus document states that determination of CAC by electron beam CT is not recommended in asymptomatic persons. Therefore, it would not be appropriate to order this screening test in this patient.

Although this patient is a former smoker, the U.S. Preventive Services Task Force (USPSTF) concludes that there is insufficient evidence to recommend for or against screening for lung cancer with either chest radiography, low-dose CT, sputum cytology, or a combination of these tests.

The USPSTF recommends screening for lipid disorders in men aged 35 years and older and in men or women aged 20 years and older who are at increased risk for cardiovascular disease. The Adult Treatment Panel of the National Cholesterol Education Program (ATP III) guidelines recommend that patients with 0 to 1 risk factor and a normal fasting lipid profile or normal nonfasting total cholesterol and HDL cholesterol levels do not have to be screened again for 5 years; the USPSTF acknowledges that the optimal screening interval is uncertain but that every 5 years is reasonable for low-risk persons. The patient's only risk factor is hypertension and his lipid levels were normal 1 year ago; therefore, there is no reason to repeat the test annually.

KEY POINT

- One-time abdominal ultrasonography to screen for an abdominal aortic aneurysm is recommended in men between the ages of 65 to 75 years who have ever smoked (defined as 100 lifetime cigarettes).

Bibliography
Thompson SG, Ashthon HA, Gao L, Scott RA; Multicentre Aneurysm Screening Study Group. Screening men for abdominal aortic aneurysm: 10 year mortality and cost effectiveness results from the randomised Multicentre Aneurysm Screening Study. BMJ. 2009;338:b2307. [PMID: 19553269]

Item 152   Answer: C
Educational Objective: Avoid adverse outcomes associated with opioid treatment for chronic pain.

This patient should be evaluated for opioid dependency. He has received definitive surgical treatment for chronic lower back pain secondary to spinal stenosis, and has continued to experience pain out of proportion to usual postoperative pain without evidence of ongoing spinal or nerve compression. Additionally, his not participating in further treatment, including physical therapy and home exercise, is concerning. He is currently on opioid therapy, which he has not tapered downward, and has risk factors that have been associated with aberrant drug-taking behaviors, including age younger than 45 years, cigarette smoking, a history of depression, and a family history of alcohol abuse. The possibility of opioid dependency should be discussed directly with the patient and a plan for managing his opioid use developed and mutually agreed upon, possibly including development of a pain management contract.

Amitriptyline can be a useful adjunctive therapy in the management of chronic pain, and might be a useful adjunctive treatment in this patient, although it would be inappropriate to start this therapy before addressing his opioid use.

It is generally preferable to avoid long-term opioid use for chronic pain. In situations in which they must be used, long-acting opioids, such as sustained-release morphine sulfate, are preferable to short-acting agents as they avoid the serum peaks and troughs that occur with short-acting opioids and provide more stable pain control.

Although this patient is post–spinal surgery, his surgical course has been uneventful and he has no focal findings suggestive of an operative complication or intervening issue, such as infection. Therefore, further imaging is not indicated.

KEY POINT

- Opioid dependency should be suspected in patients with risk factors for aberrant drug use and an inability to stop opioid medications after being treated with these agents for legitimate indications.

Bibliography
Dunn KM, Saunders KW, Rutter CM, et al. Opioid prescriptions for chronic pain and overdose, a cohort study. Ann Intern Med. 2010;152(2):85-92. [PMID: 20083827]

Item 153   Answer: C
Educational Objective: Manage chronic primary insomnia.

This patient should be counseled regarding sleep hygiene, which refers to behavioral and environmental factors that affect sleep. This patient is experiencing a primary sleep disturbance likely related to environmental factors in his new apartment. Although sleep hygiene alone is often ineffective in completely relieving insomnia, it provides a foundation of good sleep habits to which other therapies may be added. In the case described, resolution may be as simple as adjusting the temperature in the bedroom; other environmental factors that may be contributing include noise level, bed comfort, and the patient's psychosocial adjustment in the new apartment.

Although alcohol can contribute to insomnia or be used inappropriately to treat insomnia, this patient's pattern of alcohol use does not suggest either of these. He is not using alcohol to help him fall asleep, and he is having nightly insomnia despite only using alcohol on weekends.

When nonpharmacologic approaches such as improving sleep hygiene are unsuccessful in treating insomnia, pharmacotherapy may be indicated. Although many patients take over-the-counter antihistamines as sleep aids, they are not recommended owing to their potential anticholinergic side effects and next-day drowsiness. If this patient requires medication, the nonbenzodiazepine hypnotics zolpidem or zaleplon are considered first line because they do not alter sleep architecture and have a favorable side-effect profile. Benzodiazepines, such as diazepam, may be used as second-line agents, preferably for short-term use only.

KEY POINT

- The first-line treatment of insomnia is counseling regarding sleep hygiene.

Bibliography
Wilson JF. In the clinic: Insomnia. Ann Intern Med. 2008;148(1):ITC13-1-ITC13-16. [PMID: 18166757]

Item 154   Answer: C
Educational Objective: Diagnose bulimia nervosa.

This patient most likely has bulimia nervosa, which is an eating disorder characterized by recurrent episodes of binge eating with subsequent compensatory behavior aimed at preventing weight gain. The compensatory behaviors may include self-induced vomiting and misuse of medications, such as laxatives (purging subtype), or fasting and excessive exercise. The purging subtype of bulimia nervosa may be suspected by metabolic abnormalities, including hypokalemia, hypomagnesemia, and metabolic alkalosis, as seen in this patient. Diagnostic behavior includes engaging in bingeing and compensatory behaviors at least twice a week for 3 months, and having one's self-perception be excessively influenced by body weight and shape. Most patients with bulimia nervosa have a normal weight; the presence of dental caries, enlarged salivary glands, and scarring on the dorsum of the hand are highly suggestive of purging behaviors.

Anorexia nervosa is characterized by an abnormally low body weight (<85% of expected) in association with an intense fear of gaining weight, an overemphasis of body weight on self-evaluation, and amenorrhea for three consecutive menstrual cycles. The restricting subtype of anorexia nervosa is associated with regular caloric restriction; the binge-eating/purging subtype is characterized by

binge-eating, which may or may not be associated with self-induced vomiting or the misuse of medications. This patient's normal body weight and regular menses are more suggestive of bulimia nervosa rather than anorexia nervosa. Notably, 30% of patients with the restricting subtype of anorexia nervosa go on to develop bulimia nervosa, as seen with this patient.

Binge-eating disorder is more common than either anorexia nervosa or bulimia nervosa, affecting 2% to 3% of the general population. It is differentiated from bulimia nervosa in that there is no associated compensatory behavior after the binge.

Night-eating syndrome is characterized by excessive eating at night, difficulty sleeping, and morning anorexia. It is a prevalent disorder in obese patients and those seeking bariatric surgery.

KEY POINT

- **Bulimia nervosa is an eating disorder characterized by recurrent episodes of binge eating with subsequent compensatory behavior aimed at preventing weight gain.**

Bibliography
Sim LA, McAlpine DE, Grothe KB, Himes SM, Cockerill RG, Clark MM. Identification and treatment of eating disorders in the primary care setting. Mayo Clin Proc. 2010;85(8):746-751. [PMID: 20605951]

Item 155   Answer: D
Educational Objective: Diagnose meralgia paresthetica.

This patient most likely has meralgia paresthetica, or entrapment of the lateral femoral cutaneous nerve beneath the inguinal ligament. Meralgia paresthetica is characterized by paresthesia (burning/numbness) located over the anterolateral thigh. There are no motor symptoms because the lateral femoral cutaneous nerve is a purely sensory nerve. Risk factors for developing meralgia paresthetica include diabetes mellitus, obesity, and the wearing of tight-fitting pants or belts. On examination, dysesthesia or hypoesthesia is present in the distribution of the lateral femoral cutaneous nerve. The remainder of the examination is typically normal.

Patients with greater trochanteric bursitis report pain in the region of the greater trochanter that is made worse with lying on the affected side. On examination, there is tenderness to palpation approximately 2.5 cm (1 in) posterior and superior to the greater trochanter.

Iliotibial band syndrome typically presents with pain in the anterolateral knee that is worse with running downhill or cycling. The pain is typically absent during rest. On examination, patients frequently have pain to palpation of the lateral femoral epicondyle.

Lumbar disk herniation at L5 typically presents with back pain that radiates down the lateral thigh to the foot. There is weakness in foot dorsiflexion, toe extension, foot inversion, and foot eversion. The straight leg raising test is more than 90% sensitive for lumbar radiculopathy and its absence is strong evidence against lumbar disk disease. Deep tendon reflexes are typically normal in L5 radiculopathy. This patient's findings are not compatible with L5 radiculopathy.

KEY POINT

- **Meralgia paresthetica is a nerve entrapment syndrome of the lateral femoral cutaneous nerve of the anterior thigh typified by pain and burning.**

Bibliography
Plante M, Wallace R, Busconi BD. Clinical diagnosis of hip pain. Clin Sports Med. 2011;30(2):225-238. [PMID: 21419954]

Item 156   Answer: C

Educational Objective: Manage syncope in an elderly patient.

Cardiac arrhythmia is the most likely cause of syncope in this patient, given his prodrome, time course, and complete recovery immediately following the event. Cardiac causes of syncope carry a high mortality, and patients with suspected cardiac causes warrant further evaluation in the hospital regardless of age. High-risk patients requiring immediate in-hospital telemetry are those with exertional or supine syncope, palpitations prior to the event, a family history of sudden death, nonsustained ventricular tachycardia, and abnormal electrocardiographic findings. Thus, monitoring by telemetry in the hospital is appropriate for this high-risk patient.

Neurologic abnormalities are uncommon causes of syncope. Therefore, studies to assess for an intracranial or carotid process are very low yield in patients without new neurologic findings; thus, neither carotid Doppler ultrasonography nor head CT scan is indicated. Brain imaging may be appropriate to assess head trauma associated with his syncopal event, but not as a routine component of syncope evaluation.

Echocardiography for evaluation of syncope is also low yield except in patients suspected of having structural heart disease or with significant findings on cardiovascular examination, neither of which is the case in this patient.

KEY POINT

- **Cardiac causes of syncope carry a high mortality, and patients with suspected cardiac causes warrant further evaluation in the hospital.**

Bibliography
Mendu ML, McAvay G, Lampert R, Stoehr J, Tinetti ME. Yield of diagnostic tests in evaluating syncopal episodes in older patients. Arch Intern Med. 2009;169(14):1299-1305. [PMID: 19636031]

Item 157   Answer: B

Educational Objective: Diagnose Lemierre syndrome.

This patient should undergo CT of the neck with contrast. She has fever, leukocytosis, sore throat, unilateral neck tenderness, and multiple densities on her chest radiograph, suggestive of septic emboli. The combination of these factors points strongly toward Lemierre syndrome, which is septic thrombosis of the internal jugular vein. The diagnosis should be suspected in anyone with pharyngitis, persistent fever, neck pain, and septic pulmonary emboli. CT of the affected vessel with contrast would confirm the diagnosis. Treatment should include intravenous antibiotics that cover streptococci, anaerobes, and β-lactamase–producing organisms. Penicillins with β-lactamase inhibitors and carbapenems are both reasonable choices (such as ampicillin-sulbactam, piperacillin-tazobactam, and ticarcillin-clavulanate).

Chest CT would better characterize the pulmonary infiltrates, but such information would not provide specific diagnostic information that would guide therapy.

Soft tissue radiography of the neck is incapable of detecting jugular vein filling defects or thromboses, which are diagnostic of septic thrombophlebitis.

Echocardiography would be helpful to rule out right-sided endocarditis as a cause of septic emboli; however, there is nothing in the history or on the cardiac examination to suggest a cardiac source of septic emboli.

KEY POINT

- **The diagnosis of septic thrombosis of the jugular vein (Lemierre syndrome) should be suspected in anyone with pharyngitis, persistent fever, neck pain and septic pulmonary emboli.**

Bibliography
Centor RM, Samlowski R. Avoiding sore throat morbidity and mortality: when is it not "just a sore throat?". Am Fam Physician. 2011;83(1):26, 28. [PMID: 21888123]

Item 158   Answer: D

Educational Objective: Manage elevated liver chemistry test results in a patient on statin therapy.

No change in management of this patient's lipid levels is indicated, including repeat liver chemistry testing or change in statin medication. Statins work by inhibiting the hepatic HMG-CoA reductase enzyme, and can be associated with an elevation of aminotransferase levels, and rarely hepatotoxicity and acute liver failure. Aminotransferase elevations less than three times the upper limit of normal may occur in up to 3% of statin-treated patients. Conversely, statin-related hepatotoxicity (defined as alanine aminotransferase level more than three times the upper limit of normal and total bilirubin level more than twice the upper limit of normal) and acute liver failure are very rare. Acknowledging this, the FDA has recently recommended that baseline liver chemistry tests be measured prior to initiating statin therapy and then only as clinically indicated thereafter.

This patient has minor elevations of aminotransferase levels that were discovered incidentally. Statin-related minor elevation of aminotransferase levels is usually asymptomatic, occurs within the first 12 weeks of therapy, and resolves spontaneously without discontinuation of therapy. It is thought to represent a "leak" of liver enzymes related to increased hepatocyte permeability; there are no associated histopathologic changes. This phenomenon has been observed with all of the statins but is more common with higher doses.

Simvastatin should only be discontinued if there is clinical evidence of drug-related hepatotoxicity. This occurs most commonly in the setting of underlying liver conditions or as a result of drug interactions (such as acetaminophen).

In the setting of possible hepatotoxicity on treatment, persistent elevations of liver chemistry test results after discontinuation of the statin warrant further evaluation. Common causes of liver disease should be sought, including hepatitis C virus infection, nonalcoholic fatty liver disease, and autoimmune hepatitis. Serum antibody studies and liver ultrasonography may be helpful in this situation, and statin therapy should be withheld until investigations are complete.

KEY POINT

- **Baseline liver chemistry tests should be obtained in patients prior to starting statin therapy; however, routine follow-up of liver chemistry testing is not needed and is indicated only if there is clinical evidence of liver dysfunction.**

Bibliography
FDA Drug Safety Communication: Important safety label changes to cholesterol-lowering statin drugs. Additional Information for Healthcare Professionals. Available at: www.fda.gov/Drugs/DrugSafety/ucm293101.htm#hcp. Accessed June 7, 2012.

Item 159   Answer: D
Educational Objective: Appropriately administer the pneumococcal vaccine in a young adult.

This young man with asthma should receive the pneumococcal polysaccharide vaccine. Pneumococcal vaccination is currently indicated for adults aged 65 years and older and for adults younger than 65 years who have risk factors for acquisition of pneumococcal disease or morbidity from it. This includes persons with chronic cardiovascular disease (including hypertension), chronic pulmonary disease (including asthma), chronic liver disease, diabetes mellitus, alcoholism, and persons who smoke. Vaccination is generally considered safe in patients with mild to moderate illness and should not be routinely withheld in hospitalized patients. In fact, pneumococcal vaccination is routinely administered to inpatients and is part of the Joint Commission's Core Measures for patients with pneumonia.

Hepatitis B vaccination is reserved for persons at highest risk for either hepatitis B acquisition or its sequelae, as well as persons who request the vaccine. This includes travelers to endemic regions as well as persons with an increased risk of sexual, percutaneous, and mucosal transmission, such as those with multiple sex partners or men who have sex with men, injection drug users, and health care workers. This patient has none of these risk factors and should not be routinely vaccinated.

Human papillomavirus (HPV) vaccination is recommended for males between the ages of 11 and 21 years, and is permitted in men ages 22 to 26 years. The rationale for vaccinating men is the prevention of genital warts, anal carcinoma (in men who have sex with men), and transmission of HPV to women. This patient is 30 years old and the vaccination is not indicated.

Meningococcal vaccination is reserved for adolescents and for adults living in college dormitories or military barracks or who are asplenic. It is not indicated in this patient.

KEY POINT

- **The pneumococcal polysaccharide vaccine is indicated for adults with asthma; it is considered safe in patients with mild to moderate illness and should not be routinely withheld in hospitalized patients.**

Bibliography
Advisory Committee on Immunization Practices. Recommended adult immunization schedule: United States, 2012. Ann Intern Med. 2012;156(3):211-217. [PMID: 22298576]

Item 160   Answer: B

Educational Objective: Manage a patient with type 2 diabetes mellitus postoperatively.

This patient with type 2 diabetes mellitus should be given long- and short-acting insulin postoperatively to control her glucose level. Both the stress of surgery and anesthesia independently contribute to intra- and postoperative hyperglycemia. Therefore, many patients, even those who have previously been well controlled with diet or oral medications, may need insulin during the perioperative period.

Oral agents are challenging to use perioperatively owing to variability in the patient's ability to eat as well as the long-acting nature of these agents; in general, these medications should be avoided during the perioperative period.

Sliding scale insulin, the administration of short-acting insulin in a dose based on periodic blood glucose measurements (usually every 4-6 hours), has been a traditional method of treating patients with diabetes in acute care and perioperative settings. However, because basal hypoglycemic treatment is not provided and the dosing of insulin is "retrospective" based on current glucose levels, control with this approach is typically poor,

CONT.

with the potential for significant fluctuations in glucose levels. Providing a basal level of long-acting insulin with as-needed short-acting insulin is the preferred method of glucose control in acute care settings.

The optimal plasma glucose level postoperatively is controversial. Overt hyperglycemia likely contributes to postoperative dehydration as well as poor wound healing, although there is no reduction in mortality when intensive insulin therapies are used to lower plasma glucose level to a target of 80 to 180 mg/dL (4.4 to 10.0 mmol/L) among patients in the postoperative period. Therefore, most experts advocate using insulin to keep random glucose level below 180 mg/dL. As this patient's plasma glucose level is 250 mg/dL (13.9 mmol/L), she should be treated to reduce her glucose level.

KEY POINT

- Owing to the stresses of surgery and the potential adverse effects of oral diabetic agents, many patients with type 2 diabetes mellitus require insulin during the perioperative period even if their diabetes was well controlled with diet or oral medications previously.

Bibliography
Lipshutz AK, Gropper MA. Perioperative glycemic control: an evidence-based review. Anesthesiology. 2009;110(2):408-421. [PMID: 19194167]

Item 161   Answer: B
Educational Objective: Manage acute pharyngitis.

This patient should be given a rapid streptococcal antigen test before beginning antibiotic therapy. The patient's primary symptoms (fever, cough, and sore throat) are compatible with either a viral upper respiratory tract infection or streptococcal pharyngitis. The Centor criteria (presence of fever >38.1 °C [100.5 °F], tonsillar exudates, tender cervical lymphadenopathy; absence of cough) predict the likelihood of streptococcal pharyngitis and is a reasonable way to triage patients with pharyngitis to empiric treatment with antibiotics, symptomatic treatment only, or testing with treatment if the test is positive. Patients with all four criteria have a 40% or greater chance of having group A β-hemolytic streptococcal (GABHS) pharyngitis; patients with zero or one criterion have a low (<3%) probability of GABHS pharyngitis. Patients with two criteria, such as this patient, or three criteria have an intermediate probability of GABHS pharyngitis; for these patients, some guidelines recommend throat culture and others recommend the rapid antigen detection test (RADT) with confirmation of negative results. The advantage of RADT is the immediate availability of the results. RADT has comparable sensitivity and specificity to throat culture. The throat swab for either culture or RADT should be obtained from both tonsils or tonsillar fossae and the posterior

pharyngeal wall. In high-risk patients, a negative antigen test should be confirmed by throat culture.

No guidelines recommend antibiotic treatment without further testing. Some recommend treating patients with three or four Centor criteria while test results are pending, although guidelines differ on this point.

KEY POINT

- Use of the four-point Centor criteria is a reasonable way to triage patients with pharyngitis to empiric treatment with antibiotics, symptomatic treatment only, or testing with treatment if the test is positive.

Bibliography
Wessels MR. Clinical practice. Streptococcal pharyngitis. N Engl J Med. 2011;364(7):648-655. [PMID: 21323542]

Item 162   Answer: A
Educational Objective: Manage vaccination in a patient in whom a multidose vaccination series has been interrupted.

This patient who received only the first of a three-dose series of hepatitis B vaccine 3 years ago should finish the series. Many vaccines require multiple doses to achieve an optimal immune response. However, the interval between doses is a minimum interval, not a maximum, and a longer than desired interval is not thought to reduce the overall antibody concentration following completion of the series. Thus, in patients with a prolonged interval since the previous dose of vaccine, the series does not need to be restarted but should be resumed with the next injection as soon as possible after the missed prescribed interval and completed as recommended.

An adequate response to immunization against hepatitis B virus is suggested by the presence of greater than 10 milliunits/mL of anti-HBs antibody in the blood. However, because the seroconversion rate in a general patient population is approximately 95%, antibody titer testing to confirm an adequate response following completion of a vaccination series is not routinely indicated except in certain high-risk patient populations (such as health care workers at high risk for exposure to bodily fluids, hemodialysis patients, and those who may be repeatedly exposed to hepatitis B virus). As this patient has not yet completed the vaccination series, antibody titer testing is not currently indicated and would not affect the recommendation to complete his remaining injections. He would require post-vaccination antibody testing only if he is in a known high-risk group or if there are concerns regarding his ability to generate an immune response owing to his existing liver disease.

Hepatitis B vaccine is currently indicated for adults at increased risk of seroconversion or increased risk of complications for hepatitis, such as patients with chronic liver disease. The patient has chronic liver disease and thus should complete a vaccination series against hepatitis B.

- In patients with a prolonged interval since the previous dose of a multiple-dose vaccine, the series should be resumed rather than restarted.

Bibliography

Poland GA, Jacobson RM. Clinical practice: prevention of hepatitis B with the hepatitis B vaccine. N Engl J Med. 2004;351(27):2832-2838. [Erratum in: N Engl J Med. 2005;352(22):2362 and N Engl J Med. 2005;352(7):740]. [PMID: 15625334]

Item 163 Answer: A
Educational Objective: Diagnose acute otitis externa.

This patient most likely has uncomplicated acute otitis externa. Her swimming puts her at risk for otitis externa owing to moist conditions created by daily water immersion. Symptoms include otalgia, itching or fullness with or without hearing loss, and pain intensified by jaw motion. Signs include internal tenderness when the tragus or pinna is pushed or pulled and diffuse ear canal edema, purulent debris, and erythema, with or without otorrhea. Otitis externa can cause erythema of the tympanic membrane and mimic otitis media. In otitis externa, however, pneumatic otoscopy shows good tympanic membrane mobility. Management consists of clearing the canal of as much debris as possible to optimize penetration of ototopical agents as well as to visualize the tympanic membrane to ensure it is intact before initiating treatment. Topical agents have been the mainstay of therapy for uncomplicated otitis, although there is a paucity of data regarding the effectiveness of one topical treatment compared with another. An ototopical agent containing neomycin, polymyxin B, and hydrocortisone is frequently used and is effective when given for 7 to 10 days. Mild otitis externa can be treated with a dilute acetic acid solution.

Whereas an allergic reaction to plastic ear plugs should be considered, the purulent discharge and the much higher likelihood of this being bacterial acute otitis externa make a delayed type (type IV) hypersensitivity reaction unlikely. Delayed hypersensitivity reactions (contact dermatitis) are typically characterized by erythema and edema with vesicles or bullae that often rupture, leaving a crust. Allergic reactions to the plastic in hearing aids, metal in earrings, or even to otic suspension drops used to treat otitis externa should always be considered in the differential diagnosis of an inflamed external auditory canal.

Malignant otitis externa is a much more serious entity in which the infection in the ear canal spreads to the cartilage and bones nearby. It is frequently accompanied by fever, significant pain, and otorrhea, and patients usually appear much more ill than this healthy-appearing woman with localized ear discomfort. On physical examination, granulation tissue is often visible along the inferior margin of the external canal.

Pain with tugging on the pinna and movement of the tragus and an inflamed external auditory canal make otitis media highly unlikely as a diagnostic possibility. In addition, acute otitis media is associated with signs of middle ear effusion and middle ear inflammation (erythema of the tympanic membrane), which are not present in this patient.

- Symptoms of otitis externa include otalgia, itching or fullness, and pain intensified by jaw motion; signs include internal tenderness when the tragus or pinna is pushed or pulled and diffuse ear canal edema, purulent debris, and erythema.

Bibliography

Osguthorpe JD, Nielsen DR. Otitis externa: Review and clinical update. Am Fam Physician. 2006;74(9):1510-1516. [PMID: 17111889]

Item 164 Answer: C
Educational Objective: Recommend contraception options for a woman who smokes.

The best hormonal contraception option for this 38-year-old woman who smokes is a progesterone-only preparation. Women older than 35 years who smoke more than 15 cigarettes daily should not be prescribed estrogen-containing preparations because of the increased risk of thromboembolic disease. A family history of stroke itself is not a contraindication to the use of estrogen-containing preparations, although a personal history of stroke or thromboembolic disease is; progesterone-only contraceptives are considered safe in these women. Progesterone-only options for women with contraindications to estrogen include the "mini-pill," long-acting progesterone compounds (such as depot medroxyprogesterone acetate), subcutaneous progesterone implants, and progesterone-containing intrauterine devices.

Estrogen-only patches are never appropriate for contraception; they may be used as hormone replacement therapy in postmenopausal women without an intact uterus.

Combined estrogen-progesterone preparations are available in the form of patches and vaginal rings, which avoid first-pass hepatic metabolism and may limit estrogen's effects on the liver and on lipids. These products do not negate the thrombogenic effects of estrogen, however, and so they are still contraindicated in women who smoke.

- Estrogen-containing contraceptives are contraindicated in women older than 35 years who smoke more than 15 cigarettes daily because of the increased risk of thromboembolic disease.

Bibliography

ACOG Committee on Practice Bulletins-Gynecology. ACOG practice bulletin. No. 73: Use of hormonal contraception in women with coexisting medical conditions. Obstet Gynecol. 2006;107(6):1453-1472. [PMID: 16738183]

Item 165   Answer: E

Educational Objective: Recognize the adverse effects of glaucoma treatment options.

This patient's timolol drops should be discontinued. Glaucoma is a frequent cause of blindness in the elderly and is characterized by increased intraocular pressure causing damage to the optic nerve. Many classes of drugs, local and systemic, have been used to reduce intraocular pressure, by either decreasing inflow or increasing outflow of the aqueous humor. Timolol decreases the inflow of aqueous humor and is generally well tolerated, but even locally applied drugs can have systemic side effects. Most adverse reactions of timolol are manifestations of its therapeutic effect and may include heart block, sinus bradycardia, and hypotension; most reactions are not serious and can be alleviated by eliminating the drug or decreasing the dosage. Other associated adverse effects of topical β-blocker therapy include bronchospasm, decreased libido, central nervous system depression, and mood swings.

Amlodipine, a systemic antihypertensive agent, has the main side effects of hypotension, peripheral edema, dizziness, and headache. Fewer than 1% of patients taking amlodipine experience bradycardia, but a cause and effect relationship has not been established.

Carbonic anhydrase inhibitors, which may be administered orally or topically, reduce intraocular pressure by decreasing aqueous humor inflow. Dorzolamide, a topical carbonic anhydrase inhibitor, has fewer side effects than systemic carbonic anhydrase inhibitors, such as acetazolamide, which can cause acidosis, malaise, hirsutism, diarrhea, and blood dyscrasias.

Latanoprost, a topical prostaglandin analogue, increases outflow of the aqueous humor. It can cause flu-like symptoms and muscle aches.

ACE inhibitors, such as lisinopril, have adverse effects of cough, hyperkalemia, and kidney failure but not bradycardia.

KEY POINT

- Timolol, a topically applied β-blocker for treatment of glaucoma, may have systemic adverse effects, including bradycardia and heart block.

Bibliography
Foganolo P, Rossetti L. Medical treatment of glaucoma: present and future. Expert Opin Investig Drugs. 2011;20(7):947-959. Epub 2011 May 3. [PMID: 21534887]

Item 166   Answer: A

Educational Objective: Manage erectile dysfunction in a patient with coronary artery disease.

The most appropriate treatment for this man with erectile dysfunction is initiation of a phosphodiesterase type 5 (PDE-5) inhibitor, such as sildenafil. Cardiovascular disease is common in men with erectile dysfunction (ED), and ED is a warning sign of future cardiovascular events similar in magnitude to smoking or a family history of myocardial infarction. It is essential to accurately assess cardiovascular risk prior to treating ED. According to the Second Princeton Consensus Conference risk classification for sexual activity, this patient would be classified as having low cardiovascular risk as he is asymptomatic and has fewer than three of the following major cardiovascular risk factors: age, hypertension, diabetes mellitus, smoking, dyslipidemia, sedentary lifestyle, and family history of premature coronary artery disease. Although he underwent prior coronary revascularization, this intervention was successful, it was performed more than 8 weeks ago, and he is currently asymptomatic. As a result of his low cardiovascular risk classification, it is appropriate to initiate therapy for his ED without performing further cardiac evaluation. Because he is not on a nitrate drug, first-line therapy with a PDE-5 inhibitor would be most appropriate.

Testosterone replacement therapy should only be initiated in patients with ED who have symptoms and signs of hypogonadism and whose testosterone level is measured and found to be low.

Although stopping his metoprolol may improve his ED, the cardiovascular mortality benefit of this medication makes it unwise to stop.

KEY POINT

- Patients with coronary artery disease who have successfully undergone previous coronary revascularization, are without cardiovascular symptoms, and have fewer than three major cardiovascular risk factors are considered to be at low risk and can safely engage in sexual activity without cardiac evaluation.

Bibliography
Schwartz BG, Kloner RA. Clinical cardiology: physician update: erectile dysfunction and cardiovascular disease. Circulation. 2011;123(1):98-101. [PMID: 21200016]

Item 167   Answer: A

Educational Objective: Treat plantar fasciitis.

The most appropriate next step in the management of this patient is arch supports. Plantar fasciitis is the most common cause of heel pain in adults. Initial therapy for plantar fasciitis should focus on nonpharmacologic measures with acetaminophen or NSAIDs for pain control. Although this patient has been doing heel stretches and has been using acetaminophen, her pes planus has not yet been addressed. Pes planus, the loss of the arch of the foot, leads to decreased cushioning with standing and walking and allows the redistribution of forces across the foot and ankle, commonly resulting in pain and exacerbation of other foot issues. Arch supports to correct her pes planus should therefore be tried. The patient should also be educated that the expected period of time until recovery is long and is often measured in months.

Although corticosteroid injections (15 to 30 mg of methylprednisolone injected into the origin of the plantar fascia) appear to provide short-term improvement in symptoms, one meta-analysis found that there was no improvement in long-term outcomes. Given the lack of proven benefit in long-term outcomes, corticosteroid injection is best reserved for patients who do not respond to a conservative management plan that has included addressing pes planus, if present.

Multiple studies have investigated the role of extracorporeal shock wave therapy in the treatment of plantar fasciitis with conflicting results. In a meta-analysis that only included studies considered to be of high quality, there was no statistically significant benefit observed. Consequently, although extracorporeal shock wave therapy is well tolerated (the only significant side effect is a temporary increase in pain), it should not be routinely recommended owing to a lack of evidence supporting its use.

Plantar fascia release surgery should be reserved for patients with refractory plantar fasciitis.

KEY POINT

- Initial therapy for plantar fasciitis should focus on nonpharmacologic measures with acetaminophen or NSAIDs for pain control.

Bibliography

Young C. In the clinic. Plantar fasciitis. Ann Intern Med. 2012;156(1 pt 1):ITC1-1-16. [PMID: 22213510]

Item 168   Answer: D

Educational Objective: Manage perioperative risk in a patient undergoing intermediate-risk surgery.

This patient can proceed to surgery without further testing. The American College of Cardiology/American Heart Association recommendations for perioperative cardiac risk assessment suggest that preoperative stress testing be reserved for patients at greatest likelihood of a perioperative cardiac event. Risk is based on the nature of the planned surgery as well as the patient's clinical risk for a perioperative cardiac event, usually derived from the number of Revised Cardiac Risk Index (RCRI) risk factors present and exercise tolerance. Stress testing is reserved for patients undergoing non–low risk surgeries who have three or more RCRI risk factors and are unable to achieve four metabolic equivalents (METs) of exercise without symptoms suggestive of angina, and in whom testing will result in changes in management. Although this patient will be undergoing an intermediate-risk procedure, she has two RCRI risk factors (diabetes mellitus, chronic kidney disease with serum creatinine level >2.0 mg/dL [177 μmol/L]) and a good self-reported level of exercise. Therefore, no further testing is required.

Electrocardiographic stress testing, and pharmacologic stress testing for those unable to physically exercise, can be used for perioperative risk stratification. However, based on this patient's good functional capacity, as seen by her ability to exercise to a reasonable rate without significant difficulty, no further cardiovascular testing is needed.

Preoperative percutaneous coronary interventions have not been shown to improve postoperative outcomes and are not routinely indicated preoperatively even in high-risk patients. In patients for whom testing is required, stress testing is preferred. In addition, coronary angiography would put this patient at risk for worsening kidney injury and should be avoided unless absolutely necessary.

KEY POINT

- In patients undergoing non–low risk surgeries, preoperative stress testing is reserved for those who have three or more clinical cardiac risk factors and are unable to achieve four metabolic equivalents (METs) of exercise without symptoms suggestive of angina.

Bibliography

Fleisher LA, Beckman JA, Brown KA, et al. 2009 ACCF/AHA focused update on perioperative beta blockade incorporated into the ACC/AHA 2007 guidelines on perioperative cardiovascular evaluation and care for noncardiac surgery: a report of the American College of Cardiology Foundation/American Heart Association Task Force on Practice Guidelines. Circulation. 2009;120(21):e169-276. [PMID: 19884473]

Index

Note: Page numbers followed by f and t denote figures and tables, respectively. Test questions are indicated by Q.

A   NAME AND ADDRESS (Please complete.)

_____
Last Name   First Name   Middle Initial

_____
Address

_____
Address cont.

_____
City   State   ZIP Code

_____
Country

_____
Email address

B   Order Number
(Use the Order Number on your MKSAP materials packing slip.)

C   ACP ID Number
(Refer to packing slip in your MKSAP materials
for your ACP ID Number.)

ACP
AMERICAN COLLEGE OF PHYSICIANS
INTERNAL MEDICINE | Doctors for Adults

Medical Knowledge Self-Assessment Program® 16

TO EARN *AMA PRA CATEGORY 1 CREDITS*™ YOU MUST:

1. Answer all questions.
2. Score a minimum of 50% correct.

===

TO EARN *FREE* SAME-DAY *AMA PRA CATEGORY 1 CREDITS*™ ONLINE:

1. Answer all of your questions.
2. Go to **mksap.acponline.org** and access the appropriate answer sheet.
3. Transcribe your answers and submit for CME credits.
4. You can also enter your answers directly at **mksap.acponline.org** without first using this answer sheet.

To Submit Your Answer Sheet by Mail or FAX for a $10 Administrative Fee per Answer Sheet:

1. Answer all of your questions and calculate your score.
2. Complete boxes A–F.
3. Complete payment information.
4. Send the answer sheet and payment information to ACP, using the FAX number/address listed below.

COMPLETE FORM BELOW ONLY IF YOU SUBMIT BY MAIL OR FAX

Last Name															First Name																	MI

Payment Information. Must remit in US funds, drawn on a US bank.

The processing fee for each paper answer sheet is $10.

☐ Check, made payable to ACP, enclosed

Charge to   ☐ **VISA**   ☐ **MasterCard**   ☐ **AMERICAN EXPRESS**   ☐ **DISCOVER**

Card Number _____

Expiration Date _____ / _____   Security code (3 or 4 digit #s) _____
                    MM   YY

Signature _____

Fax to: 215-351-2799

Questions?
Go to **mskap.acponline.org** or email **custserv@acponline.org**

Mail to:
Member and Customer Service
American College of Physicians
190 N. Independence Mall West
Philadelphia, PA 19106-1572

1 Ⓐ Ⓑ Ⓒ Ⓓ Ⓔ
2 Ⓐ Ⓑ Ⓒ Ⓓ Ⓔ
3 Ⓐ Ⓑ Ⓒ Ⓓ Ⓔ
4 Ⓐ Ⓑ Ⓒ Ⓓ Ⓔ
5 Ⓐ Ⓑ Ⓒ Ⓓ Ⓔ

6 Ⓐ Ⓑ Ⓒ Ⓓ Ⓔ
7 Ⓐ Ⓑ Ⓒ Ⓓ Ⓔ
8 Ⓐ Ⓑ Ⓒ Ⓓ Ⓔ
9 Ⓐ Ⓑ Ⓒ Ⓓ Ⓔ
10 Ⓐ Ⓑ Ⓒ Ⓓ Ⓔ

11 Ⓐ Ⓑ Ⓒ Ⓓ Ⓔ
12 Ⓐ Ⓑ Ⓒ Ⓓ Ⓔ
13 Ⓐ Ⓑ Ⓒ Ⓓ Ⓔ
14 Ⓐ Ⓑ Ⓒ Ⓓ Ⓔ
15 Ⓐ Ⓑ Ⓒ Ⓓ Ⓔ

16 Ⓐ Ⓑ Ⓒ Ⓓ Ⓔ
17 Ⓐ Ⓑ Ⓒ Ⓓ Ⓔ
18 Ⓐ Ⓑ Ⓒ Ⓓ Ⓔ
19 Ⓐ Ⓑ Ⓒ Ⓓ Ⓔ
20 Ⓐ Ⓑ Ⓒ Ⓓ Ⓔ

21 Ⓐ Ⓑ Ⓒ Ⓓ Ⓔ
22 Ⓐ Ⓑ Ⓒ Ⓓ Ⓔ
23 Ⓐ Ⓑ Ⓒ Ⓓ Ⓔ
24 Ⓐ Ⓑ Ⓒ Ⓓ Ⓔ
25 Ⓐ Ⓑ Ⓒ Ⓓ Ⓔ

26 Ⓐ Ⓑ Ⓒ Ⓓ Ⓔ
27 Ⓐ Ⓑ Ⓒ Ⓓ Ⓔ
28 Ⓐ Ⓑ Ⓒ Ⓓ Ⓔ
29 Ⓐ Ⓑ Ⓒ Ⓓ Ⓔ
30 Ⓐ Ⓑ Ⓒ Ⓓ Ⓔ

31 Ⓐ Ⓑ Ⓒ Ⓓ Ⓔ
32 Ⓐ Ⓑ Ⓒ Ⓓ Ⓔ
33 Ⓐ Ⓑ Ⓒ Ⓓ Ⓔ
34 Ⓐ Ⓑ Ⓒ Ⓓ Ⓔ
35 Ⓐ Ⓑ Ⓒ Ⓓ Ⓔ

36 Ⓐ Ⓑ Ⓒ Ⓓ Ⓔ
37 Ⓐ Ⓑ Ⓒ Ⓓ Ⓔ
38 Ⓐ Ⓑ Ⓒ Ⓓ Ⓔ
39 Ⓐ Ⓑ Ⓒ Ⓓ Ⓔ
40 Ⓐ Ⓑ Ⓒ Ⓓ Ⓔ

41 Ⓐ Ⓑ Ⓒ Ⓓ Ⓔ
42 Ⓐ Ⓑ Ⓒ Ⓓ Ⓔ
43 Ⓐ Ⓑ Ⓒ Ⓓ Ⓔ
44 Ⓐ Ⓑ Ⓒ Ⓓ Ⓔ
45 Ⓐ Ⓑ Ⓒ Ⓓ Ⓔ

46 Ⓐ Ⓑ Ⓒ Ⓓ Ⓔ
47 Ⓐ Ⓑ Ⓒ Ⓓ Ⓔ
48 Ⓐ Ⓑ Ⓒ Ⓓ Ⓔ
49 Ⓐ Ⓑ Ⓒ Ⓓ Ⓔ
50 Ⓐ Ⓑ Ⓒ Ⓓ Ⓔ

51 Ⓐ Ⓑ Ⓒ Ⓓ Ⓔ
52 Ⓐ Ⓑ Ⓒ Ⓓ Ⓔ
53 Ⓐ Ⓑ Ⓒ Ⓓ Ⓔ
54 Ⓐ Ⓑ Ⓒ Ⓓ Ⓔ
55 Ⓐ Ⓑ Ⓒ Ⓓ Ⓔ

56 Ⓐ Ⓑ Ⓒ Ⓓ Ⓔ
57 Ⓐ Ⓑ Ⓒ Ⓓ Ⓔ
58 Ⓐ Ⓑ Ⓒ Ⓓ Ⓔ
59 Ⓐ Ⓑ Ⓒ Ⓓ Ⓔ
60 Ⓐ Ⓑ Ⓒ Ⓓ Ⓔ

61 Ⓐ Ⓑ Ⓒ Ⓓ Ⓔ
62 Ⓐ Ⓑ Ⓒ Ⓓ Ⓔ
63 Ⓐ Ⓑ Ⓒ Ⓓ Ⓔ
64 Ⓐ Ⓑ Ⓒ Ⓓ Ⓔ
65 Ⓐ Ⓑ Ⓒ Ⓓ Ⓔ

66 Ⓐ Ⓑ Ⓒ Ⓓ Ⓔ
67 Ⓐ Ⓑ Ⓒ Ⓓ Ⓔ
68 Ⓐ Ⓑ Ⓒ Ⓓ Ⓔ
69 Ⓐ Ⓑ Ⓒ Ⓓ Ⓔ
70 Ⓐ Ⓑ Ⓒ Ⓓ Ⓔ

71 Ⓐ Ⓑ Ⓒ Ⓓ Ⓔ
72 Ⓐ Ⓑ Ⓒ Ⓓ Ⓔ
73 Ⓐ Ⓑ Ⓒ Ⓓ Ⓔ
74 Ⓐ Ⓑ Ⓒ Ⓓ Ⓔ
75 Ⓐ Ⓑ Ⓒ Ⓓ Ⓔ

76 Ⓐ Ⓑ Ⓒ Ⓓ Ⓔ
77 Ⓐ Ⓑ Ⓒ Ⓓ Ⓔ
78 Ⓐ Ⓑ Ⓒ Ⓓ Ⓔ
79 Ⓐ Ⓑ Ⓒ Ⓓ Ⓔ
80 Ⓐ Ⓑ Ⓒ Ⓓ Ⓔ

81 Ⓐ Ⓑ Ⓒ Ⓓ Ⓔ
82 Ⓐ Ⓑ Ⓒ Ⓓ Ⓔ
83 Ⓐ Ⓑ Ⓒ Ⓓ Ⓔ
84 Ⓐ Ⓑ Ⓒ Ⓓ Ⓔ
85 Ⓐ Ⓑ Ⓒ Ⓓ Ⓔ

86 Ⓐ Ⓑ Ⓒ Ⓓ Ⓔ
87 Ⓐ Ⓑ Ⓒ Ⓓ Ⓔ
88 Ⓐ Ⓑ Ⓒ Ⓓ Ⓔ
89 Ⓐ Ⓑ Ⓒ Ⓓ Ⓔ
90 Ⓐ Ⓑ Ⓒ Ⓓ Ⓔ

91 Ⓐ Ⓑ Ⓒ Ⓓ Ⓔ
92 Ⓐ Ⓑ Ⓒ Ⓓ Ⓔ
93 Ⓐ Ⓑ Ⓒ Ⓓ Ⓔ
94 Ⓐ Ⓑ Ⓒ Ⓓ Ⓔ
95 Ⓐ Ⓑ Ⓒ Ⓓ Ⓔ

96 Ⓐ Ⓑ Ⓒ Ⓓ Ⓔ
97 Ⓐ Ⓑ Ⓒ Ⓓ Ⓔ
98 Ⓐ Ⓑ Ⓒ Ⓓ Ⓔ
99 Ⓐ Ⓑ Ⓒ Ⓓ Ⓔ
100 Ⓐ Ⓑ Ⓒ Ⓓ Ⓔ

101 Ⓐ Ⓑ Ⓒ Ⓓ Ⓔ
102 Ⓐ Ⓑ Ⓒ Ⓓ Ⓔ
103 Ⓐ Ⓑ Ⓒ Ⓓ Ⓔ
104 Ⓐ Ⓑ Ⓒ Ⓓ Ⓔ
105 Ⓐ Ⓑ Ⓒ Ⓓ Ⓔ

106 Ⓐ Ⓑ Ⓒ Ⓓ Ⓔ
107 Ⓐ Ⓑ Ⓒ Ⓓ Ⓔ
108 Ⓐ Ⓑ Ⓒ Ⓓ Ⓔ
109 Ⓐ Ⓑ Ⓒ Ⓓ Ⓔ
110 Ⓐ Ⓑ Ⓒ Ⓓ Ⓔ

111 Ⓐ Ⓑ Ⓒ Ⓓ Ⓔ
112 Ⓐ Ⓑ Ⓒ Ⓓ Ⓔ
113 Ⓐ Ⓑ Ⓒ Ⓓ Ⓔ
114 Ⓐ Ⓑ Ⓒ Ⓓ Ⓔ
115 Ⓐ Ⓑ Ⓒ Ⓓ Ⓔ

116 Ⓐ Ⓑ Ⓒ Ⓓ Ⓔ
117 Ⓐ Ⓑ Ⓒ Ⓓ Ⓔ
118 Ⓐ Ⓑ Ⓒ Ⓓ Ⓔ
119 Ⓐ Ⓑ Ⓒ Ⓓ Ⓔ
120 Ⓐ Ⓑ Ⓒ Ⓓ Ⓔ

121 Ⓐ Ⓑ Ⓒ Ⓓ Ⓔ
122 Ⓐ Ⓑ Ⓒ Ⓓ Ⓔ
123 Ⓐ Ⓑ Ⓒ Ⓓ Ⓔ
124 Ⓐ Ⓑ Ⓒ Ⓓ Ⓔ
125 Ⓐ Ⓑ Ⓒ Ⓓ Ⓔ

126 Ⓐ Ⓑ Ⓒ Ⓓ Ⓔ
127 Ⓐ Ⓑ Ⓒ Ⓓ Ⓔ
128 Ⓐ Ⓑ Ⓒ Ⓓ Ⓔ
129 Ⓐ Ⓑ Ⓒ Ⓓ Ⓔ
130 Ⓐ Ⓑ Ⓒ Ⓓ Ⓔ

131 Ⓐ Ⓑ Ⓒ Ⓓ Ⓔ
132 Ⓐ Ⓑ Ⓒ Ⓓ Ⓔ
133 Ⓐ Ⓑ Ⓒ Ⓓ Ⓔ
134 Ⓐ Ⓑ Ⓒ Ⓓ Ⓔ
135 Ⓐ Ⓑ Ⓒ Ⓓ Ⓔ

136 Ⓐ Ⓑ Ⓒ Ⓓ Ⓔ
137 Ⓐ Ⓑ Ⓒ Ⓓ Ⓔ
138 Ⓐ Ⓑ Ⓒ Ⓓ Ⓔ
139 Ⓐ Ⓑ Ⓒ Ⓓ Ⓔ
140 Ⓐ Ⓑ Ⓒ Ⓓ Ⓔ

141 Ⓐ Ⓑ Ⓒ Ⓓ Ⓔ
142 Ⓐ Ⓑ Ⓒ Ⓓ Ⓔ
143 Ⓐ Ⓑ Ⓒ Ⓓ Ⓔ
144 Ⓐ Ⓑ Ⓒ Ⓓ Ⓔ
145 Ⓐ Ⓑ Ⓒ Ⓓ Ⓔ

146 Ⓐ Ⓑ Ⓒ Ⓓ Ⓔ
147 Ⓐ Ⓑ Ⓒ Ⓓ Ⓔ
148 Ⓐ Ⓑ Ⓒ Ⓓ Ⓔ
149 Ⓐ Ⓑ Ⓒ Ⓓ Ⓔ
150 Ⓐ Ⓑ Ⓒ Ⓓ Ⓔ

151 Ⓐ Ⓑ Ⓒ Ⓓ Ⓔ
152 Ⓐ Ⓑ Ⓒ Ⓓ Ⓔ
153 Ⓐ Ⓑ Ⓒ Ⓓ Ⓔ
154 Ⓐ Ⓑ Ⓒ Ⓓ Ⓔ
155 Ⓐ Ⓑ Ⓒ Ⓓ Ⓔ

156 Ⓐ Ⓑ Ⓒ Ⓓ Ⓔ
157 Ⓐ Ⓑ Ⓒ Ⓓ Ⓔ
158 Ⓐ Ⓑ Ⓒ Ⓓ Ⓔ
159 Ⓐ Ⓑ Ⓒ Ⓓ Ⓔ
160 Ⓐ Ⓑ Ⓒ Ⓓ Ⓔ

161 Ⓐ Ⓑ Ⓒ Ⓓ Ⓔ
162 Ⓐ Ⓑ Ⓒ Ⓓ Ⓔ
163 Ⓐ Ⓑ Ⓒ Ⓓ Ⓔ
164 Ⓐ Ⓑ Ⓒ Ⓓ Ⓔ
165 Ⓐ Ⓑ Ⓒ Ⓓ Ⓔ

166 Ⓐ Ⓑ Ⓒ Ⓓ Ⓔ
167 Ⓐ Ⓑ Ⓒ Ⓓ Ⓔ
168 Ⓐ Ⓑ Ⓒ Ⓓ Ⓔ
169 Ⓐ Ⓑ Ⓒ Ⓓ Ⓔ
170 Ⓐ Ⓑ Ⓒ Ⓓ Ⓔ

171 Ⓐ Ⓑ Ⓒ Ⓓ Ⓔ
172 Ⓐ Ⓑ Ⓒ Ⓓ Ⓔ
173 Ⓐ Ⓑ Ⓒ Ⓓ Ⓔ
174 Ⓐ Ⓑ Ⓒ Ⓓ Ⓔ
175 Ⓐ Ⓑ Ⓒ Ⓓ Ⓔ

176 Ⓐ Ⓑ Ⓒ Ⓓ Ⓔ
177 Ⓐ Ⓑ Ⓒ Ⓓ Ⓔ
178 Ⓐ Ⓑ Ⓒ Ⓓ Ⓔ
179 Ⓐ Ⓑ Ⓒ Ⓓ Ⓔ
180 Ⓐ Ⓑ Ⓒ Ⓓ Ⓔ

MKSAP® 16

Medical Knowledge Self-Assessment Program®

Pulmonary and Critical Care Medicine

Welcome to the Pulmonary and Critical Care Medicine Section of MKSAP 16!

Here, you will find updated information on pulmonary diagnostic tests, asthma, COPD, diffuse parenchymal lung disease, pleural disease, pulmonary thromboembolism, pulmonary hypertension, lung cancer, sleep medicine, high-altitude illness, respiratory failure, shock, mechanical ventilation, sepsis, and anaphylaxis. All of these topics are uniquely focused on the needs of generalists and subspecialists *outside* of pulmonary and critical care medicine.

The publication of the 16th edition of Medical Knowledge Self-Assessment Program heralds a significant event, culminating 2 years of effort by dozens of leading subspecialists across the United States. Our authoring committees have strived to help internists succeed in Maintenance of Certification, right up to preparing for the MOC examination, and to get residents ready for the certifying examination. MKSAP 16 also helps you update your medical knowledge and elevates standards of self-learning by allowing you to assess your knowledge with 1,200 all-new multiple-choice questions, including 108 in Pulmonary and Critical Care Medicine.

MKSAP began more than 40 years ago. The American Board of Internal Medicine's examination blueprint and gaps between actual and preferred practices inform creation of the content. The questions, refined through rigorous face-to-face meetings, are among the best in medicine. A psychometric analysis of the items sharpens our educational focus on weaknesses in practice. To meet diverse learning styles, we offer MKSAP 16 online and in downloadable apps for PCs, tablets, laptops, and smartphones. We are also introducing the following:

High-Value Care Recommendations: The Pulmonary and Critical Care Medicine section starts with several recommendations based on the important concept of health care value (balancing clinical benefit with costs and harms) to address the needs of trainees, practicing physicians, and patients. These recommendations are part of a major initiative that has been undertaken by the American College of Physicians, in collaboration with other organizations.

Content for Hospitalists: This material, highlighted in blue and labeled with the familiar hospital icon (🏥), directly addresses the learning needs of the increasing number of physicians who work in the hospital setting. MKSAP 16 Digital will allow you to customize quizzes based on hospitalist-only questions to help you prepare for the Hospital Medicine Maintenance of Certification Examination.

We hope you enjoy and benefit from MKSAP 16. Please feel free to send us any comments to mksap_editors@acponline.org or visit us at the MKSAP Resource Site (mksap.acponline.org) to find out how we can help you study, earn CME, accumulate MOC points, and stay up to date. I know I speak on behalf of ACP staff members and our authoring committees when I say we are honored to have attracted your interest and participation.

Sincerely,

Patrick Alguire, MD, FACP
Editor-in-Chief
Senior Vice President
Medical Education Division
American College of Physicians

Pulmonary and Critical Care Medicine

Committee

Craig E. Daniels, MD, Editor[2]
Assistant Professor of Medicine
Program Director, Pulmonary and Critical Care
  Fellowship
Section Head, Critical Care
Division of Pulmonary and Critical Care Medicine
College of Medicine, Mayo Clinic
Rochester, Minnesota

Richard S. Eisenstaedt, MD, FACP, Associate Editor[1]
Clinical Professor of Medicine
Temple University School of Medicine
Chair, Department of Medicine
Abington Memorial Hospital
Abington, Pennsylvania

Rendell W. Ashton, MD, FACP[1]
Associate Director, Medical ICU
Program Director, Pulmonary and Critical Care Fellowship
Respiratory Institute, Cleveland Clinic
Cleveland, Ohio

Sean M. Caples, DO[2]
Assistant Professor of Medicine
Division of Pulmonary and Critical Care Medicine
College of Medicine, Mayo Clinic
Rochester, Minnesota

Stanley B. Fiel, MD, FACP[2]
Professor of Medicine
Mount Sinai School of Medicine
New York, New York
Chairman, Department of Medicine
Morristown Medical Center/Atlantic Health System
Morristown, New Jersey

Jeffrey Glassroth, MD, MACP[2]
Professor of Medicine
Division of Pulmonary and Critical Care Medicine
Northwestern University Feinberg School of Medicine
Chicago, Illinois

Nizar N. Jarjour, MD, FACP[2]
Professor and Head
Allergy, Pulmonary and Critical Care Division
Department of Medicine
School of Medicine and Public Health
Clinical Science Center
Madison, Wisconsin

Robert Kempainen, MD[1]
Associate Professor
Department of Medicine
Pulmonary and Critical Care Medicine
University of Minnesota School of Medicine
Hennepin County Medical Center
Minneapolis, Minnesota

David E. Midthun, MD, FACP[1]
Professor of Medicine
Section Head, Bronchoscopy and Interventional Pulmonary
Consultant, Division of Pulmonary and Critical Care
  Medicine
College of Medicine, Mayo Clinic
Rochester, Minnesota

Otis B. Rickman, DO[1]
Director of Bronchoscopy
Assistant Professor of Medicine and Thoracic Surgery
Vanderbilt University Medical Center
Nashville, Tennessee

Timothy Whelan, MD[2]
Associate Professor of Medicine
Medical Director of Lung Transplantation
Medical University of South Carolina
Charleston, South Carolina

Consulting Contributor

John Mullon, MD, FACP[1]
Assistant Professor of Medicine
Division of Pulmonary and Critical Care Medicine
College of Medicine, Mayo Clinic
Rochester, Minnesota

Editor-in-Chief

Patrick C. Alguire, MD, FACP[1]
Senior Vice President, Medical Education
American College of Physicians
Philadelphia, Pennsylvania

Deputy Editor-in-Chief

Philip A. Masters, MD, FACP[1]
Senior Medical Associate for Content Development
American College of Physicians
Philadelphia, Pennsylvania

Senior Medical Associate for Content Development

Cynthia D. Smith, MD, FACP[2]
American College of Physicians
Philadelphia, Pennsylvania

Pulmonary and Critical Care Medicine Clinical Editor

Richard S. Eisenstaedt, MD, FACP[1]

Pulmonary and Critical Care Medicine Reviewers

Rabeh Elzuway, MD[1]
Lois J. Geist, MD, FACP[1]
Nora F. Goldschlager, MD, MACP[1]
Dan L. Longo, MD, MACP[1]
Joseph J. Padinjarayveetil, MD[1]
Michael W. Peterson, MD, FACP[1]

Pulmonary and Critical Care Medicine Reviewers Representing the American Society for Clinical Pharmacology & Therapeutics

Ahmed D. Abdalrhim, MD, FACP[1]

Pulmonary and Critical Care Medicine ACP Editorial Staff

Katie Idell[1], Senior Staff Editor
Sean McKinney[1], Director, Self-Assessment Programs
Margaret Wells[1], Managing Editor
John Haefele[1], Assistant Editor

ACP Principal Staff

Patrick C. Alguire, MD, FACP[1]
Senior Vice President, Medical Education

D. Theresa Kanya, MBA[1]
Vice President, Medical Education

Sean McKinney[1]
Director, Self-Assessment Programs

Margaret Wells[1]
Managing Editor

Valerie Dangovetsky[1]
Program Administrator

Becky Krumm[1]
Senior Staff Editor

Ellen McDonald, PhD[1]
Senior Staff Editor

Katie Idell[1]
Senior Staff Editor

Randy Hendrickson[1]
Production Administrator/Editor

Megan Zborowski[1]
Staff Editor

Linnea Donnarumma[1]
Assistant Editor

John Haefele[1]
Assistant Editor

Developed by the American College of Physicians

---

1. Has no relationships with any entity producing, marketing, re-selling, or distributing health care goods or services consumed by, or used on, patients.

2. Has disclosed relationships with entities producing, marketing, re-selling, or distributing health care goods or services consumed by, or used on, patients. See below.

Conflicts of Interest

The following committee members, reviewers, and ACP staff members have disclosed relationships with commercial companies:

Sean M. Caples, DO
Research Grants/Contracts
ResMed Foundation, Ventus Medical

Craig E. Daniels, MD
Research Grants/Contracts
Boehringer Ingelheim

Stanley Fiel, MD, FACP
Other
PTC Therapeutics, Gilead, Pfizer, Novartis Research Grant, Vertex, DSMB
Advisory Board
Novartis, Boehringer Ingelheim, Pfizer, Gilead, Bayer
Speakers Bureau
Novartis, Boehringer Ingelheim, Pfizer, Gilead, Milan
Research Grants/Contracts
Cystic Fibrosis Foundation, Gilead, Vertex, CFF, Novartis, Bayer, MPEX, Transave, Boehringer Ingelheim

Jeffrey Glassroth, MD, MACP
Other/Advisory Board
Merck Pharmaceuticals

Nizar N. Jarjour, MD, FACP
Consultantship
Asthmatx
Research Grants/Contracts
GlaxoSmithKline, Merck, Genentech

Cynthia D. Smith, MD, FACP
Stock Options/Holdings
Merck and Company

Timothy Whelan, MD
Consultantship
InterMune
Research Grants/Contracts
InterMune, Celgene, Actelion, Centocor, Genzyme,
   SanofiAventis, Boehringer Ingelheim

Acknowledgments

The American College of Physicians (ACP) gratefully
acknowledges the special contributions to the development
and production of the 16th edition of the Medical
Knowledge Self-Assessment Program® (MKSAP® 16) made
by the following people:

Graphic Services: Michael Ripca (Technical
Administrator/Graphic Designer) and Willie-Fetchko
Graphic Design (Graphic Designer).

Production/Systems: Dan Hoffmann (Director, Web
Services & Systems Development), Neil Kohl (Senior
Architect), and Scott Hurd (Senior Systems
Analyst/Developer).

MKSAP 16 Digital: Under the direction of Steven Spadt,
Vice President, ACP Digital Products & Services, the digital
version of MKSAP 16 was developed within the ACP's
Digital Product Development Department, led by Brian
Sweigard (Director). Other members of the team included
Sean O'Donnell (Senior Architect), Dan Barron (Senior
Systems Analyst/Developer), Chris Forrest (Senior Software
Developer/Design Lead), Jon Laing (Senior Web
Application Developer), Brad Lord (Senior Web
Developer), John McKnight (Senior Web Developer),
and Nate Pershall (Senior Web Developer).

The College also wishes to acknowledge that many other
persons, too numerous to mention, have contributed to the
production of this program. Without their dedicated efforts,
this program would not have been possible.

Introducing the MKSAP Resource Site (mksap.acponline.org)

The MKSAP Resource Site (mksap.acponline.org) is a con-
tinually updated site that provides links to MKSAP 16
online answer sheets for print subscribers; access to
MKSAP 16 Digital, Board Basics® 3, and MKSAP 16
Updates; the latest details on Continuing Medical
Education (CME) and Maintenance of Certification
(MOC) in the United States, Canada, and Australia;
errata; and other new information.

ABIM Maintenance of Certification

Check the MKSAP Resource Site (mksap.acponline.org) for
the latest information on how MKSAP tests can be used to
apply to the American Board of Internal Medicine for
Maintenance of Certification (MOC) points.

RCPSC Maintenance of Certification

In Canada, MKSAP 16 is an Accredited Self-Assessment
Program (Section 3) as defined by the Maintenance of
Certification Program of The Royal College of Physicians
and Surgeons of Canada (RCPSC) and approved by the
Canadian Society of Internal Medicine on December 9,
2011. Approval of Part A sections of MKSAP 16 extends
from July 31, 2012, until July 31, 2015. Approval of Part B
sections of MKSAP 16 extends from December 31, 2012,
to December 31, 2015. Fellows of the Royal College may
earn three credits per hour for participating in MKSAP 16
under Section 3. MKSAP 16 will enable Fellows to earn up
to 75% of their required 400 credits during the 5-year
MOC cycle. A Fellow can achieve this 75% level by earning
100 of the maximum of 174 *AMA PRA Category 1
Credits*™ available in MKSAP 16. MKSAP 16 also meets
multiple CanMEDS Roles for RCPSC MOC, including that
of Medical Expert, Communicator, Collaborator, Manager,
Health Advocate, Scholar, and Professional. For information on how to apply MKSAP 16 CME credits to RCPSC
MOC, visit the MKSAP Resource Site at
mksap.acponline.org.

The Royal Australasian College of Physicians CPD Program

In Australia, MKSAP 16 is a Category 3 program that
may be used by Fellows of The Royal Australasian College
of Physicians (RACP) to meet mandatory CPD points.
Two CPD credits are awarded for each of the 174 *AMA
PRA Category 1 Credits*™ available in MKSAP 16. More
information about using MKSAP 16 for this purpose is
available at the MKSAP Resource Site at mksap.acponline
.org and at www.racp.edu.au. CPD credits earned
through MKSAP 16 should be reported at the MyCPD
site at www.racp.edu.au/mycpd.

Continuing Medical Education

The American College of Physicians is accredited by the
Accreditation Council for Continuing Medical Education
(ACCME) to provide continuing medical education for
physicians.

The American College of Physicians designates this enduring material, MKSAP 16, for a maximum of 174 *AMA
PRA Category 1 Credits*™. Physicians should claim only the

credit commensurate with the extent of their participation in the activity.

Up to 16 *AMA PRA Category 1 Credits*™ are available from December 31, 2012, to December 31, 2015, for the MKSAP 16 Pulmonary and Critical Care Medicine section.

Learning Objectives

The learning objectives of MKSAP 16 are to:
- Close gaps between actual care in your practice and preferred standards of care, based on best evidence
- Diagnose disease states that are less common and sometimes overlooked and confusing
- Improve management of comorbid conditions that can complicate patient care
- Determine when to refer patients for surgery or care by subspecialists
- Pass the ABIM Certification Examination
- Pass the ABIM Maintenance of Certification Examination

Target Audience

- General internists and primary care physicians
- Subspecialists who need to remain up-to-date in internal medicine
- Residents preparing for the certifying examination in internal medicine
- Physicians preparing for maintenance of certification in internal medicine (recertification)

Earn "Same-Day" CME Credits Online

For the first time, print subscribers can enter their answers online to earn CME credits in 24 hours or less. You can submit your answers using online answer sheets that are provided at mksap.acponline.org, where a record of your MKSAP 16 credits will be available. To earn CME credits, you need to answer all of the questions in a test and earn a score of at least 50% correct (number of correct answers divided by the total number of questions). Take any of the following approaches:

1. Use the printed answer sheet at the back of this book to record your answers. Go to mksap.acponline.org, access the appropriate online answer sheet, transcribe your answers, and submit your test for same-day CME credits. There is no additional fee for this service.

2. Go to mksap.acponline.org, access the appropriate online answer sheet, directly enter your answers, and submit your test for same-day CME credits. There is no additional fee for this service.

3. Pay a $10 processing fee per answer sheet and submit the printed answer sheet at the back of this book by mail or fax, as instructed on the answer sheet. Make sure you

calculate your score and fax the answer sheet to 215-351-2799 or mail the answer sheet to Member and Customer Service, American College of Physicians, 190 N. Independence Mall West, Philadelphia, PA 19106-1572, using the courtesy envelope provided in your MKSAP 16 slipcase. You will need your 10-digit order number and 8-digit ACP ID number, which are printed on your packing slip. Please allow 4 to 6 weeks for your score report to be emailed back to you. Be sure to include your email address for a response.

If you do not have a 10-digit order number and 8-digit ACP ID number or if you need help creating a username and password to access the MKSAP 16 online answer sheets, go to mksap.acponline.org or email custserv@acponline.org.

Permission/Consent for Use of Figures Shown in MKSAP 16 Pulmonary and Critical Care Medicine Multiple-Choice Questions

Figure shown in Self-Assessment Test Item 60 appears courtesy of Dr. James Ravenel.

Disclosure Policy

It is the policy of the American College of Physicians (ACP) to ensure balance, independence, objectivity, and scientific rigor in all of its educational activities. To this end, and consistent with the policies of the ACP and the Accreditation Council for Continuing Medical Education (ACCME), contributors to all ACP continuing medical education activities are required to disclose all relevant financial relationships with any entity producing, marketing, re-selling, or distributing health care goods or services consumed by, or used on, patients. Contributors are required to use generic names in the discussion of therapeutic options and are required to identify any unapproved, off-label, or investigative use of commercial products or devices. Where a trade name is used, all available trade names for the same product type are also included. If trade-name products manufactured by companies with whom contributors have relationships are discussed, contributors are asked to provide evidence-based citations in support of the discussion. The information is reviewed by the committee responsible for producing this text. If necessary, adjustments to topics or contributors' roles in content development are made to balance the discussion. Further, all readers of this text are asked to evaluate the content for evidence of commercial bias and send any relevant comments to mksap_editors@acponline .org so that future decisions about content and contributors can be made in light of this information.

Resolution of Conflicts

To resolve all conflicts of interest and influences of vested interests, the ACP precluded members of the content-creation committee from deciding on any content issues that involved generic or trade-name products associated with proprietary entities with which these committee members had relationships. In addition, content was based on best evidence and updated clinical care guidelines, when such evidence and guidelines were available. Contributors' disclosure information can be found with the list of contributors' names and those of ACP principal staff listed in the beginning of this book.

Hospital-Based Medicine

For the convenience of subscribers who provide care in hospital settings, content that is specific to the hospital setting has been highlighted in blue. Hospital icons (🏥) highlight where the hospital-only content begins, continues over more than one page, and ends.

Educational Disclaimer

The editors and publisher of MKSAP 16 recognize that the development of new material offers many opportunities for error. Despite our best efforts, some errors may persist in print. Drug dosage schedules are, we believe, accurate and in accordance with current standards. Readers are advised, however, to ensure that the recommended dosages in MKSAP 16 concur with the information provided in the product information material. This is especially important in cases of new, infrequently used, or highly toxic drugs. Application of the information in MKSAP 16 remains the professional responsibility of the practitioner.

The primary purpose of MKSAP 16 is educational. Information presented, as well as publications, technologies, products, and/or services discussed, is intended to inform subscribers about the knowledge, techniques, and experiences of the contributors. A diversity of professional opinion exists, and the views of the contributors are their own and not those of the ACP. Inclusion of any material in the program does not constitute endorsement or recommendation by the ACP. The ACP does not warrant the safety, reliability, accuracy, completeness, or usefulness of and disclaims any and all liability for damages and claims that may result from the use of information, publications, technologies, products, and/or services discussed in this program.

Publisher's Information

Unauthorized Use of This Book Is Against the Law

MKSAP 16 ISBN: 978-1-938245-00-8
(Pulmonary and Critical Care Medicine) ISBN: 978-1-938245-11-4

Printed in the United States of America.

For order information in the U.S. or Canada call 800-523-1546, extension 2600. All other countries call 215-351-2600. Fax inquiries to 215-351-2799 or email to custserv@acponline.org.

Errata and Norm Tables

Errata for MKSAP 16 will be available through the MKSAP Resource Site at mksap.acponline.org as new information becomes known to the editors.

MKSAP 16 Performance Interpretation Guidelines with Norm Tables, available July 31, 2013, will reflect the knowledge of physicians who have completed the self-assessment tests before the program was published. These physicians took the tests without being able to refer to the syllabus, answers, and critiques. For your convenience, the tables are available in a printable PDF file through the MKSAP Resource Site at mksap.acponline.org.

Table of Contents

Pulmonary and Critical Care Medicine High-Value Care Recommendations

The American College of Physicians, in collaboration with multiple other organizations, is embarking on a national initiative to promote awareness about the importance of stewardship of health care resources. The goals are to improve health care outcomes by providing care of proven benefit and reducing costs by avoiding unnecessary and even harmful interventions. The initiative comprises several programs that integrate the important concept of health care value (balancing clinical benefit with costs and harms) for a given intervention into various educational materials to address the needs of trainees, practicing physicians, and patients.

To integrate discussion of high-value, cost-conscious care into MKSAP 16, we have created recommendations based on the medical knowledge content that we feel meet the below definition of high-value care and bring us closer to our goal of improving patient outcomes while conserving finite resources.

High-Value Care Recommendation: A recommendation to choose diagnostic and management strategies for patients in specific clinical situations that balances clinical benefit with cost and harms with the goal of improving patient outcomes.

Below are the High-Value Care Recommendations for the Pulmonary and Critical Care Medicine section of MKSAP 16.

- Omalizumab is recommended only for patients with severe asthma who have allergies, an elevated IgE level, and persistent symptoms despite optimizing therapy with combination therapy of high-dose inhaled corticosteroids and a long-acting β_2-agonist (see Item 73).
- Smoking cessation is the single most clinically effective and cost-effective way to prevent COPD, slow progression of established disease, and improve survival.
- Spirometry is essential for the diagnosis of COPD, although testing for airflow limitation should not be performed in asymptomatic individuals as a screening intervention (see Item 81).
- Roflumilast is a very expensive medication with significant side effects (diarrhea, weight loss, nausea, headache, anxiety, insomnia, and depression), and it should be reserved for patients with severe disease not adequately controlled on other COPD medications (see Item 85).
- In multiple randomized trials, noninvasive positive pressure ventilation reduced the need for intubation,

shortened hospital stays, and decreased mortality in patients with moderate to severe COPD exacerbations (see Item 61).
- In the intensive care unit, daily interruption of sedation and spontaneous breathing trials lead to sooner extubation and lower rate of mechanical ventilation.
- Ventilator-associated pneumonia can be prevented by the routine use of protocols that require elevating the head of the bed by 30 degrees and hastening time to extubation.
- In patients with septic shock, the efficacy of crystalloid or colloid is likely equivalent; however, colloid is far more expensive (see Item 26).
- High-dose corticosteroids are of no benefit in sepsis and have been shown to harm patients in earlier studies; intravenous hydrocortisone is appropriate in septic shock only if blood pressure is poorly responsive to fluid resuscitation and vasopressor therapy (see Item 26).
- The combination of history, physical examination, serology, and characteristic radiographic studies can often lead to a firm diagnosis and obviate the need for an open lung biopsy in up to 60% or more of patients with diffuse parenchymal lung disease.
- Examination of previous chest imaging is critical in pulmonary nodule evaluation and may show that a nodule is stable, growing, or shrinking over time.
- Solid pulmonary nodules that remain stable in size for 2 years on chest radiograph or CT scan are considered benign, and no further follow-up is indicated; this is known as the 2-year stability rule.
- Calcification in a benign pattern (central, diffuse, lamellar) indicates that a pulmonary nodule is a granuloma and requires no further investigation (see Item 6).
- In order to limit unnecessary invasive testing, the diagnosis and staging of lung cancer is best done simultaneously.
- PET scanning and integrated PET-CT are valuable tools in the evaluation of non–small cell lung cancer; they have been shown to be cost effective owing to avoidance of unnecessary surgery in one out of five patients whose disease was previously considered resectable.
- Thoracentesis is not necessary in patients who develop small pleural effusions associated with heart failure, pneumonia, or heart surgery.
- Chest CT exposes patients to doses of radiation that are forty times higher than chest radiography; therefore, the

benefit of CT in clinical evaluation should be weighed against the radiation exposure, especially in younger patients who are more vulnerable to radiation-induced malignancy (see Item 34).

- The use of well-validated scoring systems to generate pretest clinical probability of pulmonary embolism is essential to guide diagnostic test selection (see Item 79, Item 89, and Item 94).
- In clinically stable patients with a low pretest probability of pulmonary embolism, a normal D-dimer assay effectively excludes pulmonary embolism and eliminates the need for further testing (see Item 79).

Pulmonary Diagnostic Tests

Pulmonary Function Testing

Pulmonary function tests are used to evaluate patients with pulmonary symptoms (most frequently dyspnea). They provide information on the degree of impairment and potential causes. These tests are typically obtained in patients with known lung disease or unexplained pulmonary symptoms; they are also used to establish a baseline in patients who are starting a job or a treatment that may cause lung dysfunction. They should be performed during preoperative evaluation, especially in patients undergoing thoracic surgery (particularly lung resection). Pulmonary function tests are essential in these patients to assess the feasibility of lung resection and calculate predicted lung function after resection.

Spirometry

Spirometry is the most widely used pulmonary function test. It can be performed in the outpatient setting with relative simplicity using small, hand-held devices that can be connected to a personal computer for immediate display and storage of test results. Spirometry is obtained by measurement of forced expiratory volume over time after the patient has taken a deep inspiration (**Table 1**). Coaching the patient throughout the

---

TABLE 1. Guidelines for Performance of Office Spirometry

Spirometry should be performed by a trained medical technician using an approved spirometer that is calibrated regularly

The patient is seated comfortably and is asked to:

  inhale completely

  position the mouthpiece in the mouth and close lips around it

  exhale with maximal force

Coach the patient to perform the expiratory volumes tracing for 6-12 seconds

Three technically adequate curves should be obtained

The FVC and FEV_1 values in at least two of these curves should not vary by more than 5% (reproducible curve)

The highest FEV_1 and FVC from any of the reproducible curves can be used

Compare the results to predicted values based on age, height, gender, and race

Data from: Standardization of Spirometry, 1994 Update. American Thoracic Society. Am J Respir Crit Care Med. 1995;152(3):1107-1136. [PMID: 7663792]

---

maneuver is critical to obtaining an optimal result. The patient may have to repeat the maneuver up to eight times to generate a reproducible and maximum effort. The maximum volume exhaled in this maneuver is referred to as the forced vital capacity (FVC); the maneuver should last 6 to 12 seconds to obtain an accurate measurement. The forced expiratory volume exhaled in the first second is called the FEV_1. An FEV_1/FVC ratio of less than 70% indicates airway obstruction. Spirometry can be repeated after giving an inhaled bronchodilator to assess reversibility, which is defined as an improvement in FEV_1 of 12% or greater compared with baseline (provided the increase in FEV_1 is actually greater than 200 mL). An important aspect of examining spirometry is reviewing the flow-volume curve for evidence of hesitation, cough, or a slow start, all of which could influence the accuracy of the results.

A flow-volume loop can help determine the cause of airway obstruction (**Figure 1**).

Bronchial Challenge Testing

Bronchial challenge testing is performed to assess airway hyperresponsiveness. This test is very sensitive for asthma, but it is not very specific. Many conditions, including viral infections, allergy, smoking, bronchitis, and cystic fibrosis, can increase airway responsiveness. Bronchial challenge testing requires the support of a skilled technician to obtain serial spirometry measurements while administering increasing concentrations of an inhaled medication that promotes bronchoconstriction. Because the test may trigger significant bronchospasm, it should be performed in a controlled setting with personnel trained to manage provoked airway obstruction. A test is diagnostically positive if the FEV_1 falls 20% from baseline. It is important to understand that this degree of bronchospasm seen on a challenge test is not diagnostic of asthma, given the many potential causes of a positive test. Patients with asthma may have a false-negative test if they have recently used their bronchodilator, if the test is not performed appropriately, or if the patient has seasonal or occupational asthma without recent exposures. The most appropriate use of this test is to exclude asthma in patients with normal spirometry and symptoms consistent with, but not typical of, asthma.

The direct airway stimulants methacholine and histamine are the most commonly used agents for bronchial challenge testing. The FDA recently approved the use of inhaled mannitol to evaluate airway responsiveness. Mannitol is regarded as an indirect challenge that leads to release of endogenous mediators when inhaled, which in turn causes airway smooth

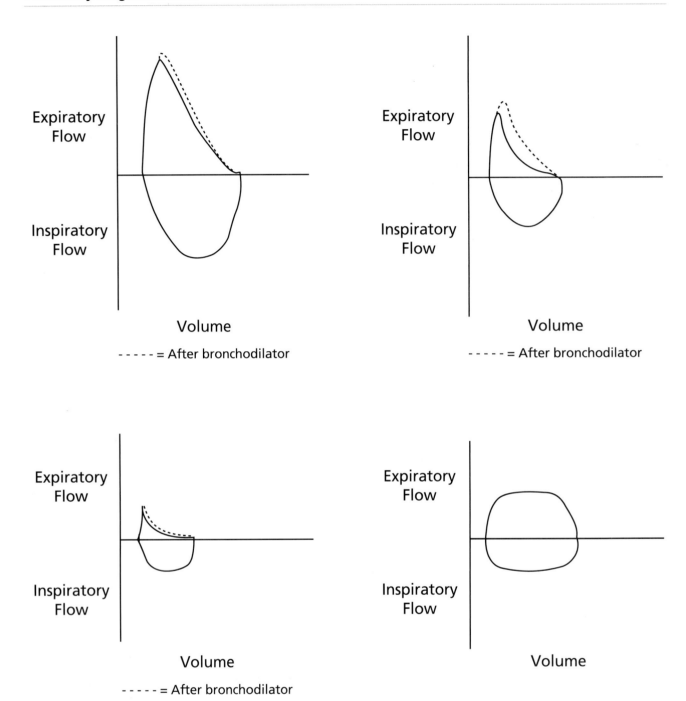

FIGURE 1. *Top left panel:* Flow-volume loop demonstrating normal spirometry, with similar maximum inspiratory and expiratory flows; no significant change is seen after bronchodilator administration. *Top right panel:* Flow-volume loop demonstrating asthma, with a reduction in peak expiratory flow and concave curvature for the expiratory limb while the inspiratory limb remains normal; improvement is seen in expiratory flows (particularly the increase in peak flow) after bronchodilator administration. *Bottom left panel:* Flow-volume loop demonstrating COPD, with a significant reduction in peak expiratory flow and concave appearance of the expiratory limb; no significant change is seen after bronchodilator administration. *Bottom right panel:* Flow-volume loop demonstrating fixed obstruction/tracheal stenosis, with flattening of the peak inspiratory and expiratory flows.

muscle constriction. Use of mannitol challenge testing is likely to increase as an alternative to methacholine and histamine owing to its technical simplicity and accuracy in reflection of underlying airway inflammation.

Lung Volumes

Lung volumes are obtained in specialized pulmonary function diagnostic laboratories and include total lung capacity (TLC), inspiratory capacity (IC), expiratory reserve volume (ERV), and residual volume (RV). Reduced TLC (<80% of predicted) indicates chest restriction. Restriction can be secondary to a parenchymal lung disease such as pulmonary fibrosis, in which a parallel reduction in all lung volumes, including RV, is seen. In such patients, DLCO is also reduced. Chest restriction may also result from respiratory muscle weakness due to neuromuscular disease, where TLC is reduced and RV is increased (owing to the patient's inability to fully exhale). Chest restriction can be suspected based on spirometry when FVC and FEV_1 are reduced with a normal or higher-than-normal FEV_1/FVC ratio. However, chest restriction is ideally confirmed with measurement of TLC.

Diffusing Capacity for Carbon Monoxide

Diffusing capacity for carbon monoxide (DLCO) measures the lungs' ability to transfer gas across the alveolar-capillary membrane. DLCO testing involves asking the patient to inhale a very low known concentration of carbon monoxide (CO) and measuring the amount of CO in exhaled breath to calculate its uptake.

There are several causes of reduced DLCO, including loss of surface for gas exchange (emphysema), fibrosis (idiopathic pulmonary fibrosis), or parenchymal infiltration (diffuse pneumonia). Because CO uptake is dependent on the concentration and volume of available hemoglobin, anemia and pulmonary vascular diseases (pulmonary hypertension) can result in a low DLCO measurement in the absence of lung disease. Patients with asthma may have an increased DLCO related to increased blood volume and inflammation. Patients with pulmonary hemorrhage syndrome may also have an increased DLCO owing to faster uptake of CO by erythrocytes present in the airspace. Reduced DLCO below 50% of predicted is associated with significant dyspnea on exertion and potential need for supplemental oxygen.

6-Minute Walk Test

The 6-minute walk test is a very useful indicator of a patient's functional capacity. This is particularly helpful in patients with advanced lung or heart disease. Measurements of pulse oximetry during the test can help determine the need for supplemental oxygen. The patient should be monitored for symptoms that may warrant discontinuation of exercise, such as significant dyspnea, severe leg cramps, or chest pain. The distance walked is the most important result of the 6-minute walk test, and its change over time can be used to assess response to therapy or disease progression.

Pulse Oximetry

Pulse oximetry provides a simple, noninvasive measurement of oxygen saturation in the peripheral capillaries. Pulse oximeters are accurate within 2% to 3% of arterial oxygen saturation determined directly; however, factors such as excessive ambient light, significant peripheral vasoconstriction, and cardiac arrhythmias can lead to a falsely low reading. In contrast, carboxyhemoglobinemia can cause a falsely elevated oxygen saturation reading because oxyhemoglobin and carboxyhemoglobin waves are not distinguishable by most pulse oximeters. Therefore, pulse oximetry should not be used in patients who are victims of fire or smoke inhalation.

Pulse oximetry has several limitations when evaluating patient oxygenation status: (1) partial pressure of oxygen (Po_2) may decrease well below "normal" before oxygen saturation is significantly impacted; and (2) oxygen saturation may also remain normal or near normal in patients who are hypoventilating with evolving hypercapnic respiratory failure. In these cases and in other situations where there is uncertainty about adequacy of patient oxygenation, arterial blood gas measurements should be obtained. **H**

KEY POINTS

- An FEV_1/FVC ratio of less than 70% on spirometry indicates airway obstruction.
- Bronchial challenge testing is sensitive for asthma but is not very specific.
- DLCO measures the lungs' ability to transfer gas across the alveolar-capillary membrane.
- Pulse oximetry provides a simple, noninvasive measurement of oxygen saturation in the peripheral capillaries.

Imaging and Bronchoscopy

Chest Radiography

The chest radiograph provides a rapid, global assessment of the chest anatomy. A single chest radiograph summarizes the depth of the thorax and is greatly limited in resolution compared with CT. For this reason, chest radiographs are often more helpful in ruling in some conditions than excluding them (**Table 2**). In diffuse parenchymal lung disease, the chest radiograph can provide diagnostic clues by identifying the distribution of the abnormality. Upper-lobe distribution of opacities is typically seen in conditions such as sarcoidosis, silicosis, cystic fibrosis, Langerhans cell histiocytosis, and reactivation tuberculosis (**Figure 2**). Lower lung zone predominance is typical in pulmonary fibrosis, cryptogenic organizing pneumonia, asbestosis, and heart failure.

TABLE 2. Common Clinical Indications for Imaging Tests	
Imaging Modality	**Disorder**
Chest radiograph	Rib fracture
	Pneumothorax
	Pleural effusion
	Heart failure
	Pneumonia
	Line, device, and tube placement
	Follow-up of recognized disorder
CT	Diffuse parenchymal lung disease
	Bronchiolitis
	Bronchiectasis
	Lung mass
	Lymphadenopathy
	Nodule
	Pulmonary embolism
	Guide for aspiration or biopsy
PET-CT	Lung cancer staging
	Nodule/mass evaluation

Short-term response to treatment, as in the setting of pneumonia, pneumothorax, and heart failure, may be confirmed by chest radiography. The chest radiograph often provides little helpful information in conditions such as pulmonary embolism, COPD, and asthma.

Computed Tomography

The superior resolution of anatomic structures provided by CT compared with chest radiography makes it a valuable diagnostic tool to evaluate chest disease. Subtle abnormalities on chest radiography are often seemingly dramatic on subsequent CT. Classic features on CT may eliminate the need for biopsy in the diagnosis of idiopathic pulmonary fibrosis (**Figure 3**). Imaging pulmonary nodules with CT frequently identifies calcification, other nodules, or lymphadenopathy and directs the diagnostic approach. Intravenous contrast enhancement is used with CT to distinguish between lymph nodes and vessels (particularly in the hilar areas), to evaluate the liver and adrenals for metastases, and to identify vascular abnormalities such as dissections and thrombosis. The development of CT angiography has largely replaced ventilation-perfusion scanning and direct pulmonary arteriography in evaluating suspected pulmonary embolism. However, contrast-induced nephrotoxicity is a concern with the use of CT angiography.

CT exposes the patient to significantly higher doses of radiation than chest radiography. The effective dose for CT is approximately 40 times that of a chest radiograph. The benefit of CT in clinical evaluation should be weighed against the radiation exposure, especially in younger patients who are more vulnerable to radiation-induced malignancy. However, the risk is usually acceptable when a CT study is the most appropriate test.

Positron Emission Tomography

PET scanning is based on the principle that cancer cells have a high rate of glycolysis compared with non-neoplastic cells.

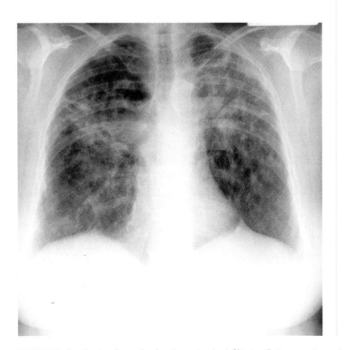
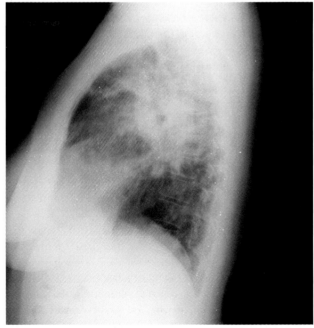

FIGURE 2. Chest radiographs showing extensive infiltrates that are most prominent in the upper lung zones and are associated with hilar enlargement. Bronchoscopic biopsy confirmed sarcoidosis.

PET-CT integrates simultaneously acquired CT and PET images and has been shown to have higher sensitivity and specificity for assessing lung cancer stage than CT and PET done separately. Although expensive and associated with radiation exposure, PET-CT may be an important and cost effective study in specific clinical circumstances; for example, it has been shown to detect distant metastases in 10% to 20% of patients with known or suspected lung cancer who were otherwise thought to be candidates for surgery (**Figure 4**). Because of the possibility of false-positive PET scans, a positive PET scan is not the same as a tissue diagnosis, and a biopsy of distant metastasis should be obtained before determining that a patient has unresectable disease.

KEY POINTS

- Chest radiography remains a valuable initial investigation in the evaluation of a variety of chest disorders and can suggest a differential based on the distribution of disease.
- CT allows for far superior resolution than chest radiography but at a cost of greater radiation and the potential to induce cancer.
- PET is most often integrated with CT and is cost effective in the staging evaluation of known or suspected lung cancer.

Bronchoscopy

Bronchoscopy is an effective method for sampling central airway lesions, mediastinal lymph nodes, and parenchymal masses. Diagnostic yields with bronchoscopy using fluoroscopy for peripheral pulmonary nodules less than 2 cm in diameter are in the range of 10% to 50%, and CT-guided percutaneous biopsy may be preferred. Recently developed techniques of radial ultrasound and electromagnetic navigation have increased the yield to 50% to 75% for peripheral nodules. Yields for masses (larger than 3 cm) are 60% to 80%, and they approach 100% for endobronchial abnormalities. The addition of endobronchial ultrasound has made endoscopic lung cancer staging similar in yield to mediastinoscopy, and it is often preferred owing to the avoidance of a skin incision and general anesthesia (**Figure 5**).

Bronchoscopy is often used to further evaluate diffuse parenchymal lung diseases detected on chest radiography and CT. Transbronchoscopic biopsies are often diagnostic in sarcoidosis, silicosis, hypersensitivity pneumonia, organizing pneumonia, lymphangitic metastases, and lymphangioleiomyomatosis. The normal cell differential of a bronchoscopic lavage is about 95% alveolar macrophages; the finding of lymphocytosis, neutrophilia, or eosinophilia can be a clue to the diagnosis. Diagnosis of infection in immunocompromised patients by bronchoalveolar lavage is a frequent indication for bronchoscopy. A therapeutic role for bronchoscopy is established for mucus clearance,

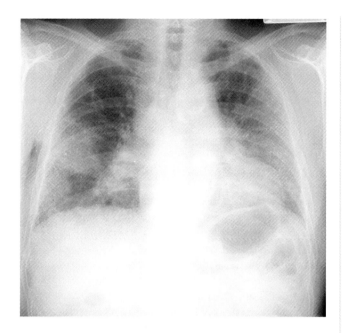

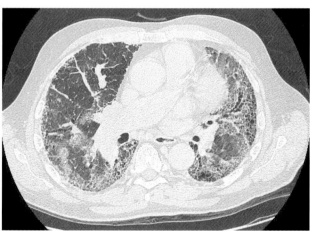

FIGURE 3. Chest radiograph (*top panel*) showing nonspecific lower lung zone infiltrates. High-resolution CT image (*bottom panel*) showing peripheral subpleural interstitial infiltrates, honeycombing, and traction bronchiectasis consistent with a clinical diagnosis of idiopathic pulmonary fibrosis.

The PET tracer 18-fluoro-deoxyglucose is taken up into cells, is metabolically trapped, and accumulates. For evaluation of mediastinal lymph node metastasis, PET has a sensitivity and specificity of approximately 90% and 85%, respectively; it compares favorably with standard CT, which has approximately a 30% to 40% rate of both false-positive and false-negative results. False-positive PET scans have been reported with tuberculosis, fungal diseases, other infections, sarcoidosis, and other inflammatory conditions. False-negative PET scans may occur with low-grade tumors such as adenocarcinoma in situ (formerly known as bronchioloalveolar cell carcinoma), carcinoid tumor, and malignancies less than 1 cm in diameter.

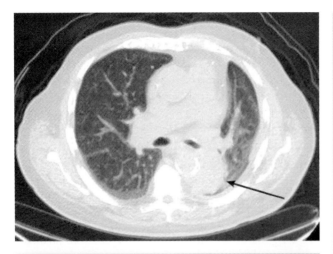

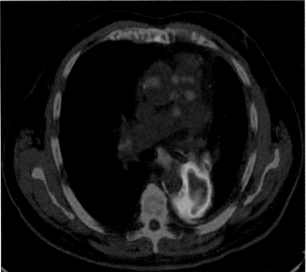

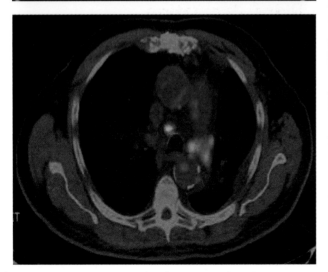

FIGURE 4. CT of the chest (*top panel*) shows a left lower lobe mass consistent with malignancy, and PET-CT, done for preoperative staging, showed enhanced uptake of the 18-fluoro-deoxyglucose marker in the left lower lobe mass (*middle panel*) and mediastinal lymph nodes (*bottom panel*). Endobronchial ultrasound sampling confirmed nodal metastases in both the contralateral (N3) and ipsilateral (N2) nodes, establishing stage IIIB disease.

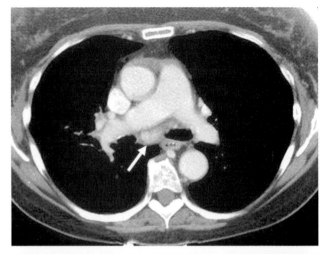

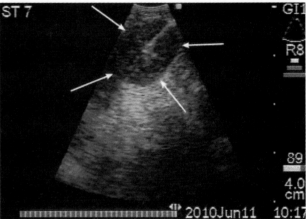

FIGURE 5. CT of the chest (*top panel*) showing a 4-cm right upper lobe mass and evidence of subcarinal mediastinal node enlargement (*arrow*). At endobronchial ultrasound *(bottom panel)*, the 16-mm node is shown with the needle in the node at sampling. A diagnosis of adenocarcinoma of the lung with metastatic (N2) node involvement (stage IIIA) is established with a single procedure.

foreign body removal, debulking central tumors, and airway dilation and stent placement for a variety of mechanisms of stenosis.

Bronchoscopy has historically been considered a very safe procedure. Retrospective series have reported that major complications such as bleeding, respiratory depression, cardiorespiratory arrest, arrhythmia, and pneumothorax occur in less than 1% of cases. Mortality is rare, with a reported death rate of 0.01% to 0.03%. **H**

KEY POINTS

- Bronchoscopy allows for evaluation of the larger airways and endobronchial, mediastinal node, and parenchymal sampling.

- Therapeutic indications for bronchoscopy include mucus clearance, foreign body removal, and dilation and stenting of stenosis.

Asthma

Overview

Asthma manifests with episodic cough, chest tightness, shortness of breath, and wheezing. Patients with asthma have increased nonspecific airway responsiveness that results in increased sensitivity to inhaled bronchoconstrictive agents (such as methacholine) and airway obstruction that is typically reversible. An underlying problem in asthma is airway inflammation, which is often related to allergies. When patients with asthma are exposed to relevant allergens, they develop an early-phase response that manifests 15 to 30 minutes after the exposure and resolves in 1 to 2 hours. Roughly half of patients develop a late-phase response 3 to 8 hours following the exposure. Uncontrolled inflammation or repeat exacerbations can potentially be associated with development of structural airway changes known as remodeling. Although asthma can be managed very effectively in most cases, a minority of patients have severe disease that can result in frequent exacerbations and may lead to death. Up to 4000 deaths from asthma are reported annually in the United States, many of which are believed to be preventable.

Epidemiology and Natural History

Asthma is one of the most common diseases. It affects 5% of the adult population in the United States, with greater prevalence in some other industrialized countries. There is a disparity in asthma prevalence between developed and developing countries. Decreased prevalence in developing countries has been ascribed to early childhood infections that alter the immune response of inflammatory T lymphocytes toward increasing host defenses against infectious diseases (termed the Th1 response) and away from one that triggers allergic inflammation (the Th2 response). Air pollution and Western lifestyle are also believed to be contributing factors to increased asthma incidence. In most cases, asthma starts in childhood; however, adult onset is well recognized even in the elderly. Between 70% and 90% of patients with asthma have allergies demonstrated with skin testing and confirmed by relevant history. There is a genetic predisposition, but no single gene explains asthma. Gene and environment interaction is likely; this confirms the importance of environmental factors such as pollution, viral infections, and tobacco smoke. Although airway obstruction in asthma is reversible, there is a greater decline in lung function over time among patients with asthma compared with healthy controls. This decline is more prominent in patients who smoke.

KEY POINTS

- Asthma is one of the most common diseases, affecting 5% of the adult population in the United States.
- Between 70% and 90% of patients with asthma have allergies demonstrated with skin testing and confirmed by relevant history.

Pathogenesis

Airway inflammation in asthma is marked by infiltration with eosinophils, mast cells, lymphocytes, and neutrophils; subepithelial fibrosis; mucus gland hyperplasia; and increased airway smooth muscle mass (**Figure 6**). The numbers and activation status of various inflammatory cells are increased in the airways, particularly when asthma is symptomatic. A large number of cytokines and mediators (histamines, tryptase, and leukotrienes) are released from inflammatory cells, such as mast cells, upon activation by inhaled allergens. The mediators play a role in the early-phase response, while the cytokines promote airway inflammation, which is an important feature of the late-phase response.

Ongoing airway inflammation or repeated asthma exacerbations may contribute to persistent airway injury with development of structural changes, known collectively as airway remodeling. These features include increased subepithelial fibrosis, increased smooth muscle mass, and mucus gland hyperplasia. The role of airway remodeling in asthma is not fully defined, because some of the features (such as fibrosis) may have a protective effect by stiffening the airway and preventing excessive constriction, while others (such as smooth muscle hyperplasia) can lead to excessive constriction and airway lumen narrowing.

An important feature that has received limited attention is mucus gland and goblet cell hyperplasia, which leads to the production of large amounts of tenacious sputum. This contributes significantly to asthma symptoms during exacerbation, particularly severe exacerbations that lead to hospitalization or intensive care admissions.

Clinical Evaluation

Patients with asthma typically present with episodic cough, dyspnea, wheezing, and chest tightness. The cough can be dry but is often productive of thick, clear sputum. The majority of patients with asthma have a personal and family history

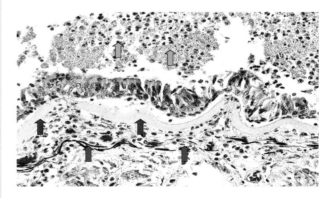

FIGURE 6. Airway tissue in a patient with severe asthma demonstrating sub-basement membrane thickening (*red arrows*), disruption of elastic fibers (*blue arrows*), and infiltration with inflammatory cells and filling of the airway lumen with mucus and inflammatory cells (*green arrows*)

of allergies, and their exposure to relevant allergens often provokes asthma symptoms. Other triggers include viral upper respiratory tract infections, cold air, stress, and exercise. Asthma is generally worse at night. Most patients report increased asthma symptoms at night or in the early morning at least once a month. The differential diagnosis of asthma is described in **Table 3**. Several comorbid conditions (sinusitis, rhinitis, gastroesophageal reflux disease [GERD], obstructive sleep apnea, obesity, and vocal cord dysfunction) can worsen asthma and its symptoms. Between attacks, patients with asthma can have a normal examination. Symptomatic patients typically have tachypnea, polyphonic wheezing, and signs of nasal allergies. Certain signs suggest an alternative diagnosis; for example, bilateral crackles and leg edema suggest heart failure, and clubbing suggests cystic fibrosis.

On initial evaluation of patients who are suspected of having asthma, spirometry should be performed to confirm the diagnosis with demonstrated airway obstruction (low FEV_1/FVC ratio) and reversibility (12% or greater improvement in FEV_1 after administration of bronchodilators) (**Figure 7**). Patients who have normal spirometry should undergo a bronchial challenge test to assess for airway hyperresponsiveness. The vast majority of patients with asthma have a positive test; therefore, a negative bronchial challenge test makes an alternative diagnosis more likely. See Pulmonary Diagnostic Tests for further discussion of spirometry and bronchial challenge testing.

Allergy skin testing can determine patient sensitization. The results of skin testing should be interpreted in light of the clinical history to determine the important allergens contributing to symptoms. Many patients with asthma would benefit from confirming their sensitization by allergy skin testing to better understand triggers, focus their avoidance measures, and guide immune therapy in those whose disease is difficult to manage. If skin testing is not feasible owing to dermatologic conditions, concomitant medications, or lack of

clinical expertise, a radioallergosorbent test can be used to determine allergen-specific serum IgE levels.

Exhaled nitric oxide measurements are now available in many pulmonary laboratories and asthma clinics. This noninvasive measurement reflects active airway inflammation and generally correlates with airway eosinophilia. Exhaled nitric oxide levels are decreased in response to corticosteroid therapy and can be used to determine adherence to therapy.

KEY POINTS

- Spirometry should be performed in patients with suspected asthma to confirm airway obstruction and reversibility.
- Patients with suspected asthma who have normal spirometry should undergo a bronchial challenge test to assess for airway hyperresponsiveness; a negative test generally excludes asthma.

Asthma Syndromes

Occupational Asthma

Exposure to irritants, allergens, and sensitizing chemicals can be an important contributor to the development or worsening of asthma. Therefore, any patient with asthma should be asked about work-related exposures, keeping in mind that some exposures may be in the home environment. Allergic sensitization typically develops over a period of exposure. Once sensitized, patients typically experience asthma symptoms shortly after exposure to the offending agent. This early-phase response can resolve in about an hour; however, a late response, which is marked by return of the asthma symptoms 3 to 8 hours after exposure, is known to occur in about half of patients. Patients with occupational asthma report feeling better when away from the offending environment, such as on weekends or vacations; however, symptoms may still

TABLE 3. Differential Diagnosis of Asthma	
Condition	**Characteristics**
COPD	Airway obstruction is less reversible; typically seen in older patients with smoking history
Vocal cord dysfunction	Abrupt onset and end of symptoms; monophonic wheeze; more common in younger patients; confirm with laryngoscopy or flow-volume loop
Heart failure	Dyspnea and often wheezing; crackles on auscultation; limited response to asthma therapy; cardiomegaly; edema; elevated BNP; other features of heart failure
Bronchiectasis	Cough productive of large amount of purulent sputum; rhonchi and crackles are common; may have wheezing and clubbing; confirmed by CT imaging
Allergic bronchopulmonary aspergillosis	Recurrent infiltrates on chest radiograph; eosinophilia; high IgE levels; frequent need for corticosteroid treatment
Cystic fibrosis	Cough productive of large amount of purulent sputum; rhonchi and crackles are common; prominent clubbing; may have wheezing
Mechanical obstruction	More localized wheezing; if central in location, flow-volume loop may provide a clue

BNP = B-type natriuretic peptide.

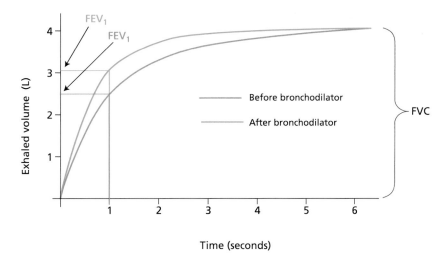

FIGURE 7. Spirometry before and after an inhaled bronchodilator showing reversible airway obstruction

occur even when away from the work environment because of underlying airway hyperresponsiveness.

In addition to the history, measurement of spirometry or peak flow rate before and after work exposure over a period of a few weeks (which ideally would include at least 1 week away from work) may help establish a relationship between changes in lung function and workplace exposure. It should be noted that lung function in patients with asthma has a diurnal pattern, with highest lung function in the midafternoon and lowest lung function in the early morning hours. Confirmation of nonspecific airway hyperresponsiveness with a bronchial challenge test can help support the diagnosis. A negative test can occur when patients are away from occupational exposure. When a specific agent is highly suspected to cause an allergic response, a skin test can be obtained to establish sensitization.

Avoidance of exposure to the offending agent (by changing jobs, changing the work environment, or using protective equipment) is recommended. Patients with occupational asthma can show improvement in lung function, symptoms, and airway hyperresponsiveness over time and can return to normal if they have no further exposure to the offending agent.

Reactive Airways Dysfunction Syndrome

Reactive airways dysfunction syndrome (RADS) is a distinct type of occupational asthma that results from a single accidental exposure to high levels of irritant vapors, gases, or fumes such as chlorine gas, bleach, or ammonia. This exposure leads to significant airway injury with persistent airway inflammation, dysfunction, and hyperresponsiveness. Patients with RADS typically do not have a history of asthma and do not have "allergic sensitization" to the offending irritant prior to the accidental exposure. Their symptoms start within minutes to hours after the exposure and include cough, dyspnea,

and chest tightness. Symptoms can persist for years afterward. Patients with RADS have a positive bronchial challenge test and may or may not have airway obstruction on spirometry. Similar to occupational asthma, patients with RADS can show improvement over time.

Virus-Induced Asthma

Infections with respiratory viruses such as rhinovirus, respiratory syncytial virus, and influenza virus are associated with asthma exacerbations. Respiratory syncytial virus and influenza virus routinely infect the lower airway, whereas rhinovirus mostly infects the upper airway. Patients with asthma often develop increased asthma symptoms with loss of asthma control 2 to 4 days after the onset of the upper respiratory tract infection. These exacerbations can range from mild to very severe and have been blamed for increased asthma hospitalizations and school and work absenteeism during the fall and spring seasons. In mild exacerbations, patients can achieve control by increasing the frequency of inhaled bronchodilator medication, starting inhaled corticosteroids, increasing the dose of inhaled corticosteroids, or adding a long-acting β_2-agonist bronchodilator. However, for more severe exacerbations, systemic corticosteroids, given for 5 to 7 days, are the recommended therapy. Patients with viral respiratory tract infections typically have increased airway responsiveness that lasts 4 to 6 weeks following the infection, leading to increased asthma symptoms.

Cough-Variant Asthma

Cough-variant asthma is present in patients who have cough as their main symptom. The cough is typically dry and is sometimes the only symptom of asthma. The diagnosis is confirmed with spirometry that demonstrates airway obstruction with improvement following inhaled bronchodilator administration or with bronchial challenge testing that demonstrates airway hyperresponsiveness. The syndrome should be distinguished from other causes of chronic cough, such as rhinitis, sinusitis, or GERD. Patients with chronic cough can have more then one cause for their cough; therefore, a comprehensive evaluation and management approach is essential (see MKSAP 16 General Internal Medicine).

Gastroesophageal Reflux Disease and Asthma

Patients with asthma often have associated GERD that can contribute to symptoms (typically cough) or increased frequency of exacerbations. It is important to recognize that many patients with GERD can be asymptomatic; therefore, GERD should be considered in patients who have asthma that is difficult to control (see MKSAP 16 Gastroenterology and Hepatology for a discussion of evaluation for GERD). In patients with asymptomatic GERD, interventions targeting GERD have not resulted in consistent improvement in lung function, asthma symptoms, or need for medications. However, a subset of patients with clear GERD symptoms, a positive 24-hour esophageal pH study, and a temporal relationship between heartburn and asthma symptoms are candidates for trials of GERD-targeting approaches; asthma symptoms may improve in some of these patients.

Allergic Bronchopulmonary Aspergillosis

Radiologic chest evaluation should be performed in patients who have difficulty achieving asthma control with the usual therapy or who have frequent exacerbations requiring systemic corticosteroids. Patients who have recurrent pulmonary infiltrates or bronchiectasis may have allergic bronchopulmonary aspergillosis (ABPA), which is a result of sensitization to *Aspergillus fumigatus*. This ubiquitous fungus colonizes abnormal airways in patients with asthma or cystic fibrosis, with subsequent development of specific immune responses that can lead to pulmonary inflammation, bronchiectasis, and fibrosis. The diagnosis of ABPA is confirmed by demonstrating elevated serum levels of IgE (total and specific *Aspergillus* IgE), a positive skin test to *A. fumigatus*, and eosinophilia. High-resolution chest CT scan demonstrates proximal bronchiectasis, often with mucus occluding airways or leading to atelectasis. Achieving disease control in these patients requires systemic corticosteroids in addition to inhaled corticosteroids and bronchodilator rescue therapy. Once disease is under control, systemic corticosteroids can be tapered off, as guided by evaluation of symptoms, pulmonary function testing, levels of circulating eosinophils, chest radiograph, and IgE levels. However, continued monitoring is essential to achieving optimal long-term outcome. Left untreated, ABPA can result in progressive pulmonary fibrosis and loss of lung function.

Exercise-Induced Bronchospasm

The majority of patients with asthma have exercise-induced bronchoconstriction (EIB) that manifests a few minutes after intense exercise. EIB is enhanced when breathing cold, dry air. The mechanism for EIB is dryness and cooling of the airways that is directly related to the magnitude of increased ventilation associated with exercise. Bronchial obstruction in EIB peaks 5 to 10 minutes after cessation of exercise and resolves within 30 minutes; symptoms are at their worst not during exercise but immediately following cessation of exercise. Symptoms should be distinguished from vocal cord dysfunction and exercise-induced GERD. Patients with typical EIB usually demonstrate a 15% or greater reduction in FEV_1 within 5 to 10 minutes following exercise challenge. Treatment with short-acting β_2-agonists given 15 minutes before exercise prevents EIB in most patients. The protection lasts up to 3 hours, allowing most patients to engage fully in desired physical activity. Leukotriene-modifying drugs can also be used to prevent EIB; however, they are not as effective as inhaled β_2-agonists. Nonpharmacologic approaches to prevent EIB include gradual warmup before intense exercise, using a mask over the nose and mouth during cold weather, and avoidance of high-intensity intermittent exercise.

Vocal Cord Dysfunction

When patients with asthma present with prominent wheezing that is more notable during inspiration (stridor), vocal cord dysfunction (VCD) should be suspected. Typically, patients with VCD have abrupt onset of symptoms that are felt in the neck, but these symptoms are often difficult to distinguish from symptoms of typical asthma. Patients with VCD may or may not have other associated asthma symptoms. Because a significant proportion of patients with VCD have concomitant asthma, distinguishing between the two is often difficult. Patients with VCD who do not have asthma are often on similar therapies as patients with severe asthma. Clinical evaluation of VCD demonstrates monophonic wheezing that is loudest over the neck, as opposed to polyphonic wheezing over the chest as is seen in patients with asthma. Abrupt onset and termination of the episode is characteristic of VCD and is atypical for asthma. Further confirmation can be obtained with laryngoscopy, which shows marked adduction of the vocal cords with severe airway narrowing. Flow-volume loops show inspiratory flow cutoff and preserved expiratory flow, in contrast to what is seen in asthma (**Figure 8**). Treatment of VCD includes patient education, behavior modification, and speech therapy. GERD, which is often present in patients with VCD, may also need to be treated. During acute attacks, inhaled helium-oxygen mixture and/or continuous positive airway pressure can relieve acute symptoms of VCD.

Aspirin-Sensitive Asthma

A small percentage of adults with asthma are aspirin sensitive. A subset of these patients has severe asthma, aspirin sensitivity, and nasal polyps (Samter triad). Aspirin sensitivity should be considered in patients with difficult-to-control disease and should be confirmed based on history and aspirin challenge.

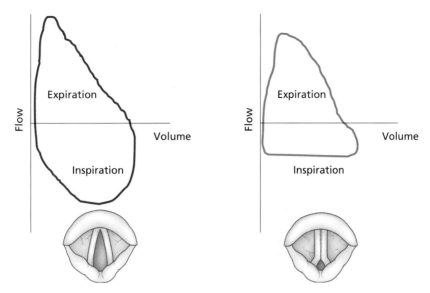

FIGURE 8. Flow-volume loops showing maximum inspiratory and expiratory flow-volume relationships in a patient with vocal cord dysfunction during asymptomatic (*left*) and symptomatic (*right*) periods. Note also the marked adduction of the vocal cords with severe reduction of the glottic aperture during a symptomatic period of airway obstruction (*right*).

Patients who must use aspirin should be referred for desensitization. Once patients are desensitized and taking aspirin regularly, aspirin sensitivity remains quiescent; however, it could become symptomatic again if there is a hiatus in aspirin use. Aspirin-induced asthma is probably related to increased leukotriene levels. Therefore, the use of leukotriene-modifying drugs should be considered in these patients. Other NSAID medications may also provoke asthma symptoms in these patients and should be avoided.

> **KEY POINTS**
>
> - Infections with respiratory viruses such as rhinovirus, respiratory syncytial virus, and influenza virus are associated with asthma exacerbations.
> - Bronchial obstruction in exercise-induced bronchoconstriction peaks 5 to 10 minutes after cessation of exercise and resolves within 30 minutes; symptoms are at their worst not during exercise but immediately following cessation of exercise.

Management

Despite asthma's prevalence and the availability of widely disseminated guidelines, management of many patients remains less than optimal. Effective management of asthma requires a multifaceted approach that includes patient education, agreement on goals of therapy in partnership with patients, and providing asthma action plans that guide patients in self-management of this chronic illness. Additional components of asthma management include assessment and monitoring, control of environmental factors and comorbid conditions, and pharmacologic therapy. The goals of asthma management are to (1) maintain a normal functional status; (2) preserve normal lung function; (3) reduce the need for rescue albuterol to less than twice weekly; (4) reduce symptom flares that require more intensive therapy; and (5) decrease the side effects of treatment. Asthma is classified as intermittent or persistent; persistent asthma is further classified as mild, moderate, or severe (**Table 4**). These different categories are associated with a stepwise approach to asthma management aimed at reducing impairment and risk (**Figure 9**). Asthma control can be evaluated by inquiring about the frequency of day and night symptoms, exacerbations, and the need for rescue therapy. The Asthma Control Test is a validated questionnaire that can be easily adapted to clinical practice and helps determine the level of asthma control over the preceding 4 weeks (www.asthma.com/resources/asthma-control-test.html).

> **KEY POINT**
>
> - Despite the availability of widely disseminated guidelines, management of many patients with asthma remains less than optimal.

Pharmacotherapy

Medications for asthma can be divided into relievers (used to treat acute symptoms) and controllers (used to maintain long-term control and prevent exacerbations). Relievers include short-acting β_2-agonists and short-acting anticholinergics and are used intermittently as needed. Controllers are used on a regular basis and work via anti-inflammatory (inhaled corticosteroids, leukotriene-modifying drugs, and anti-IgE therapy) or bronchodilator (inhaled long-acting β_2-agonists and sustained-release theophylline) effects. If possible, the inhaled

TABLE 4. Classification of Asthma Severity

Components of Severity	Intermittent	Persistent		
		Mild	**Moderate**	**Severe**
Impairment[a]				
Symptoms	≤2 days/week	>2 days/week but not daily	Daily	Throughout the day
Nighttime awakenings	≤2 ×/month	3-4 ×/month	>1 ×/week but not nightly	Often 7 ×/week
SABA use for symptom control (not prevention of EIB)	≤2 days/week	>2 days/week but not more than 1 ×/d	Daily	Several times a day
Interference with normal activity	None	Minor limitation	Some limitation	Extremely limited
Lung function	Normal FEV_1 between exacerbations	FEV_1 >80% of predicted	FEV_1 >60% but <80% of predicted	FEV_1 <60% of predicted
	FEV_1 >80% of predicted	FEV_1/FVC normal	FEV_1/FVC reduced 5%	FEV_1/FVC reduced >5%
	FEV_1/FVC normal			
Risk				
Exacerbations (consider frequency and severity)[b,c]	0-1/year	>2/year	>2/year	>2/year
Recommended step for initiating treatment (see Figure 9 for treatment steps)[d]	Step 1	Step 2	Step 3; consider short courses of systemic corticosteroids	Step 4 or 5; consider short courses of systemic corticosteroids

EIB = exercise-induced bronchospasm; SABA = short-acting β_2-agonist.

[a]Normal FEV_1/FVC ratio: 8-19 years old, 85%; 20-39 years old, 80%; 40-59 years old, 75%; 60-80 years old, 70%.

[b]Frequency and severity may fluctuate over time for patients in any severity category.

[c]Relative annual risk for exacerbations may be related to FEV_1.

[d]In 2 to 6 weeks, evaluate the level of asthma control that is achieved and adjust therapy accordingly.

Source: National Heart, Lung, and Blood Institute; National Institutes of Health; U.S. Department of Health and Human Services. National Asthma Education and Prevention Program. Expert Panel Report 3 (EPR-3): Guidelines for the Diagnosis and Management of Asthma-Summary Report 2007. J Allergy Clin Immunol. 2007;120(5 suppl):S94-138. [PMID: 17983880]

route for asthma medications is preferred to achieve the highest airway concentration while minimizing systemic side effects. Pressurized metered-dose inhalers (MDIs) are the most commonly used devices. They deliver the medication mixed with a propellant from a pressurized canister. The use of a spacer provides more leeway in coordinating inspiration and activation of the MDI. This can enhance lower airway deposition and reduce oral and systemic absorption of the medication, particularly in patients who do not fully master the inhaler technique. Dry powder inhalers (DPI) are another type of inhalation device and are increasingly replacing propellant inhalers to decrease the release of chlorofluorocarbons into the atmosphere; these are breath activated and contain no propellant. They tend to be lighter and more compact than MDIs; however, DPIs require fast inhalation of high enough flow for optimal drug delivery. Patients should be instructed on the proper technique for inhalation devices at the initial clinic visit, and their technique should be reviewed

at subsequent visits. Poor inhaler technique is a common cause of lack of response to asthma therapy, particularly in patients with neurologic or musculoskeletal disorders, and should be evaluated when starting or before adjusting inhaled medications.

β_2-Agonists

Short-acting β_2-agonists should be provided to all patients with asthma. These are the most effective bronchodilator medications available and have a rapid onset of action. They prevent exercise- and cold-air–induced asthma and relieve bronchoconstriction from other causes such as exposure to allergens. With appropriate, as-needed use of these medications, benefits are maintained and side effects are minimized.

Long-acting β_2-agonists, such as salmeterol and formoterol, are frequently added to an inhaled corticosteroid controller medication if symptoms are not adequately controlled.

| Intermittent asthma | Persistent asthma: Daily medication
Consult with asthma specialist if step 4 care or higher is required
Consider consultation at step 3 | | | | |

Step 1

Preferred:
SABA PRN

Step 2

Preferred:
Low-dose ICS

Alternative:
Cromolyn, LTRA, nedocromil, or theophylline

Step 3

Preferred:
Low-dose ICS + LABA

OR

Medium-dose ICS

Alternative:
Low-dose ICS + LTRA, theophylline, or zileuton

Step 4

Preferred:
Medium-dose ICS + LABA

Alternative:
Medium-dose ICS + LTRA, theophylline, or zileuton

Step 5

Preferred:
High-dose ICS + LABA

AND

Consider omalizumab for patients who have allergies

Step 6

Preferred:
High-dose ICS + LABA + oral corticosteroid

AND

Consider omalizumab for patients who have allergies

Step up if needed

(first check adherence, environmental control, and comorbid conditions)

Assess control

Step down if possible

(and asthma is well controlled at least 3 months)

| **Each step: Patient education, environmental control, and management of comorbidities**
Steps 2-4: Consider subcutaneous allergen immunotherapy for patients who have allergic asthma |

Quick relief medication for all patients:

- SABA as needed for symptoms. Intensity of treatment depends on severity of symptoms: up to 3 treatments at 20-minute intervals as needed. Short course of oral systemic corticosteroids may be needed.

- Use of SABA >2 days a week for symptom relief (not prevention of EIB) generally indicates inadequate control and the need to step up treatment.

FIGURE 9. Stepwise approach to asthma therapy. EIB = exercise-induced bronchospasm; ICS = inhaled corticosteroids; LABA = long-acting β_2-agonist; LTRA = leukotriene receptor antagonist; PRN = as needed; SABA = short-acting β_2-agonist.

Source: National Heart, Lung, and Blood Institute; National Institutes of Health; U.S. Department of Health and Human Services. National Asthma Education and Prevention Program. Expert Panel Report 3 (EPR-3): Guidelines for the Diagnosis and Management of Asthma-Summary Report 2007. J Allergy Clin Immunol. 2007;120(5 suppl):S94-138. [PMID: 17983880]

Formoterol has a rapid onset and 12-hour duration of action, whereas salmeterol has a slower onset and equal duration of effect. The addition of a long-acting β_2-agonist generally results in better asthma control compared with increasing the dose of inhaled controller corticosteroids. Because long-acting β_2-agonists control asthma symptoms but provide no anti-inflammatory effects, treatment with long-acting β_2-agonists as single-agent therapy in asthma is not appropriate; it can mask worsening of airway inflammation and lead to increased risk of asthma-related complications.

Several studies have revealed an increased risk of asthma-related complications, including death, in patients who are on long-acting β_2-agonist therapy; this has raised questions about the safety of long-acting β_2-agonists and has led to an FDA-required black box warning. The majority of the reported complications occurred in patients treated with long-acting β_2-agonists without concomitant use of inhaled corticosteroids. Studies to address these safety concerns are ongoing; in the meantime, long-acting β_2-agonists should be added only after inhaled corticosteroid therapy has been optimized, and a short-acting β_2-agonist should be provided to treat acute bronchospasm that might occur during the delayed onset of the long-acting medication.

Anticholinergic Agents

Anticholinergic agents have been used mainly in COPD. Short-acting anticholinergics (such as ipratropium) have been used to enhance the bronchodilator effect of short-acting β_2-agonists in acute asthma exacerbations or as a rescue inhaler in patients with excessive sensitivity to β_2-agonists. A recent study showed that a long-acting anticholinergic drug (tiotropium) added to corticosteroids can improve lung function and asthma symptoms in patients whose symptoms are less than adequately controlled on inhaled corticosteroids; the study also showed that this effect is equivalent to that of salmeterol. Given the concerns about the use of long-acting β_2-agonists in asthma, tiotropium may be an appropriate alternative in some patients.

Inhaled Corticosteroids

Inhaled corticosteroids are the mainstay controller therapy for asthma. They have a potent anti-inflammatory function, reducing the numbers and activity of inflammatory cells (eosinophils, mast cells, and lymphocytes). Neutrophils increase in patients who are taking long-term inhaled corticosteroids; however, their presence is not believed to be associated with airway injury. Inhaled corticosteroids blunt the late-phase response to allergens that is linked to inflammation, but they also enhance the effectiveness of β_2-agonists by upregulating their receptor function. Regular use of inhaled corticosteroids reduces asthma exacerbations, hospitalizations, and asthma-related mortality.

Although inhaled corticosteroids are very well tolerated, there are side effects associated with regular use, particularly at high doses. Local side effects include hoarseness, cough, and oral thrush. These side effects can be reduced or eliminated by including an inhalation aid, carefully rinsing the mouth after each use, and lowering the corticosteroid dose. However, patients may sometimes be unable to tolerate inhaled corticosteroids or may require topical antifungal therapy for thrush. Regular use of high-dose inhaled corticosteroids, particularly in elderly patients, can result in systemic side effects including weight gain, adrenal gland suppression, osteopenia, skin thinning, glaucoma, and cataracts. Although the incidence and severity of these side effects are considerably less than those noted with systemic corticosteroids, patients should be evaluated at regular intervals for appropriateness of stepping down therapy to use the lowest inhaled corticosteroid dose consistent with adequate disease control.

Leukotriene-Modifying Drugs

Leukotrienes contribute to asthma by promoting mucus secretion, vasodilation, and inflammation. Leukotriene-modifying agents have been developed to block their receptors (montelukast and zafirlukast) or production by inhibiting 5-lipoxygenase (zileuton). Leukotriene receptor antagonists and zileuton have a modest anti-inflammatory and bronchodilator effect and have been shown to reduce asthma symptoms, improve quality of life, prevent exercise-induced asthma, and reduce the need for albuterol. They are used primarily as add-on or alternative therapy to corticosteroid or β_2-agonist therapy and are most appropriate in patients with mild persistent asthma who are intolerant of inhaled corticosteroids

or in those with aspirin sensitivity. There may also be a subset of patients with preferential response to leukotriene receptor antagonists as opposed to inhaled corticosteroids as a long-term controller therapy.

Leukotriene receptor antagonists have been reported to cause neuropsychologic events (agitation, anxiety, hallucination, depression, and suicidal ideation). Although these events are rare and may not be directly related to these drugs, there is an FDA-mandated warning associated with their use. Owing to concern about liver toxicity, zileuton use has been limited.

Theophylline

Theophylline is one of the oldest drugs for asthma. Its advantages include ease of use and low cost. However, its disadvantages are weak bronchodilator effect and narrow therapeutic margin. Targeting a lower serum concentration (5-12 micrograms/mL [28-67 micromoles/L]) may enhance the benefit-to-risk ratio. It is important to educate patients about potential drug interactions; circulating levels may increase severalfold when other drugs such as fluoroquinolones are used. Therefore, dose adjustment and drug level monitoring should be done when patients are started on such medications or if they exhibit symptoms of potential toxicity (tremor, headache, nausea, palpitations). More serious, life-threatening side effects include cardiac arrhythmias and seizure, which are seen at concentrations greater than 20 micrograms/mL (111 micromoles/L). Theophylline is not recommended for use in acute asthma exacerbations and is considered a second-line alternative to inhaled corticosteroids for chronic asthma management.

Anti-IgE Antibody

The cross-linking of IgE antibody on the surface of mast cells and basophils with antigen results in release of active mediators including histamine and leukotrienes, initiating the allergic inflammatory response. Omalizumab blocks IgE with a recombinant antibody against its F_C (fragment crystallizable) portion and is effective in improving asthma control. Treatment with omalizumab reduces exacerbations and allows tapering of the inhaled and systemic corticosteroid dose. Omalizumab is recommended for selected patients with severe asthma who have evidence of allergies, have an IgE level between 30 and 700 international units/mL (30 and 700 kilounits/L) (normal range, 0-90 international units/mL), and remain symptomatic despite optimizing treatment with combination therapy (high-dose inhaled corticosteroids and a long-acting β_2-agonist). Omalizumab is very expensive and should generally be administered by an asthma specialist. Because of the risk of serious anaphylactoid reactions (roughly 1 in 1000 patients), patients should be observed for at least 2 hours after the initial three doses and 1 hour after subsequent treatments.

- Patients with asthma should be instructed on the use of inhalation devices at the initial clinic visit, and their technique should be reviewed at subsequent visits.
- Short-acting β_2-agonists are the most effective bronchodilator medications available and have a rapid onset of action.
- Long-acting β_2-agonists should be added to other asthma medications only after inhaled corticosteroid therapy has been optimized.
- Inhaled corticosteroids are the mainstay controller therapy for asthma.
- Regular use of inhaled corticosteroids can result in systemic side effects; patients should be evaluated at regular intervals for appropriateness of stepping down therapy to the lowest inhaled corticosteroid dose consistent with adequate asthma control.

Allergen Immunotherapy and Allergen Avoidance

Allergen avoidance is recommended in patients who have sensitivity to known offending agents. However, approaches to control house dust mite exposure (such as encasing mattresses with impermeable fabric) have resulted in limited benefits. Immunotherapy is most effective in patients with allergic rhinitis and can be used in those with asthma when other approaches have failed. The development of sublingual administration of allergen extract may allow for wider use of these approaches; however, efficacy needs to be confirmed in controlled clinical trials.

Alternative and Complementary Therapies

Several drugs have been tried in patients with corticosteroid-dependent asthma in attempts to reduce the corticosteroid dose and associated side effects and improve asthma control; however, there is no evidence to support the use of methotrexate, azathioprine, and cyclosporine in asthma. Their effects are modest and side effects are significant. Complementary approaches, including acupuncture, homeotherapy, herbal interventions, breathing techniques, relaxation, and yoga, have been tried. However, most of the studies are small, have variable quality, and lack appropriate controls, making it difficult to recommend these approaches for asthma therapy.

Management of Asthma Exacerbations

Increasing short-acting β_2-agonists and consideration of a short course of systemic corticosteroids is recommended to initiate treatment of exacerbation at home. If symptoms do not respond to these measures, the patient should be evaluated in a clinical setting. Spirometry and/or peak expiratory flow rate (PEFR) measurement is recommended. Patients

with moderate (PEFR 40%-69% of predicted or personal best) or severe (PEFR <40%) exacerbations should be treated with frequent short-acting β_2-agonists and systemic corticosteroids. In patients with severe exacerbations, bronchodilator medications (short-acting β_2-agonists and ipratropium) should be given by nebulization, whereas in mild attacks an MDI with a holding chamber can be used. The intravenous route is preferred for corticosteroids in severe attacks, whereas the oral route is used in milder cases. Most patients should receive 5 to 7 days of oral corticosteroids (40 mg/d of prednisone) to ensure resolution and reduce chances for recurrence. Pulse oximetry should be monitored, and supplemental oxygen should be given to maintain saturation above 92%. Follow-up pulmonary function tests should be obtained in 1 hour; patients without significant improvement should be considered for hospitalization (see Critical Care), and patients with a good response (PEFR >70%) that is sustained for 1 hour can be discharged.

Difficult-to-Manage Asthma

A subset of patients with asthma (generally <10%) require chronic use of systemic corticosteroids to achieve adequate control of their disease. Factors associated with corticosteroid dependency include nonadherence to inhaled medications, continued exposure to tobacco smoke and other respiratory irritants, psychosocial problems, and comorbidities (such as severe allergies or chronic sinusitis). Addressing these barriers through patient education, close follow-up, and possible involvement of an asthma specialist can help reduce or eliminate the need for chronic corticosteroid therapy. All patients with asthma, particularly those with more severe disease, should have a written, personalized asthma action plan that they can follow if they have increased symptoms or decreased PEFR.

Bronchial thermoplasty, which was approved by the FDA in 2010 for patients with severe asthma, consists of applying heat to the airway with a catheter that is inserted via a bronchoscope connected to a radiofrequency generator. Bronchial thermoplasty is proposed to reduce smooth-muscle hypertrophy, which has been reported in patients with asthma. The treatment requires three bronchoscopies and modestly improves several asthma-related outcomes. Its long-term efficacy and safety remain to be established.

Asthma and Pregnancy

Asthma (particularly poorly controlled asthma) is one of the most common medical problems that complicates pregnancy. Dyspnea of pregnancy should be distinguished from that related to asthma. When asthma is suspected, it should be confirmed with spirometry to demonstrate obstruction and reversibility with inhaled bronchodilators. Other diagnostic techniques are not recommended (such as skin testing) or are contraindicated (such as bronchial challenge testing) during pregnancy. Asthma can lead to low birth weight, preeclampsia, premature labor, and increased infant mortality. Therefore, better asthma control is likely to reduce the risk to both mother and fetus. During pregnancy, one third of patients have improvement in asthma control, another third have worsening asthma, and another third have no change.

Pregnant patients with asthma should have regular monitoring to evaluate disease control and attempt stepping down of asthma therapy. There are limited studies of efficacy of asthma medications during pregnancy; therefore, the majority of the recommendations are based on extrapolated data from nonpregnant patients. Short-acting β$_2$-agonists (albuterol) are recommended for quick relief of asthma symptoms during pregnancy, while inhaled corticosteroids are the mainstay controller medications. Among corticosteroids, budesonide has the most safety data available during gestation and is recommended for use in pregnant patients; however, patients who are already doing well on other inhaled corticosteroids can continue them after they become pregnant because there has been no evidence of harm from the use of these medications. The preferred second-line therapy is long-acting β$_2$-agonists.

Alternative drugs that can be used during pregnancy include leukotriene receptor antagonists and theophylline. Although systemic corticosteroids have been linked to a small risk of congenital abnormalities, their use is recommended in patients with acute severe asthma. Left untreated, acute asthma exacerbations can have serious morbidity for the mother and outcome of pregnancy.

KEY POINT

- Asthma is one of the most common medical problems that complicates pregnancy; better asthma control is likely to reduce the risk to both mother and fetus.

Chronic Obstructive Pulmonary Disease

Epidemiology

COPD is the third most common cause of death for both men and women worldwide. Evidence suggests that up to 50% of the population with COPD has not yet been diagnosed and that patients who smoke or have other risk factors for COPD may currently be asymptomatic. COPD mortality rates increased 22% over the last decade. Worldwide COPD deaths in women, which have risen steadily since 1970, reached parity with COPD deaths in men by 2000. By 2007, prevalence of COPD in women surpassed that of men in all

racial groups in patients under 65 years of age. The substantial increase in COPD morbidity and mortality is, in part, due to increased tobacco use and changing global demographics that have enabled a greater number of smokers to survive long enough to develop COPD, especially in developing countries.

Pathophysiology

COPD is a slowly progressive inflammatory disease of the airways and lung parenchyma. It is characterized by gradual loss of lung function with increasing obstruction to expiratory airflow. Obstruction is caused by inflammatory narrowing of the small airways (bronchiolitis) and proteolytic digestion of lung tissue adjacent to these airways (emphysema). Inflammation intensifies as the disease progresses and increases the risk of exacerbations, which affect health status, exercise tolerance, and quality of life.

Inflammation from COPD damages and thickens small airways and disrupts normal repair mechanisms, causing small-airway fibrosis. Proteases are released and dissolve some of the adjacent supporting lung tissue that tethers the small airways, resulting in a decrease in the elastic recoil of the lungs that normally keeps airways open during exhalation. The decreased elasticity of the lung parenchyma, associated with emphysema, causes static hyperinflation, which has only a modest impact on overall hyperinflation in most patients. In contrast, dynamic hyperinflation occurs when patients begin to inhale before full exhalation has been completed, such that inspiratory air volume exceeds expiratory volume and air is trapped within the lungs with each successive breath. The ability to fully exhale is dependent on the degree of airflow obstruction (for example, increases in cholinergic tone, inflammation, and mucus plugging) and rate of breathing. Both can vary and cause greater hyperinflation during periods of exacerbation and exertion. When the demand for greater minute ventilation increases tidal volume and respiration rate, the available time for exhalation can become insufficient. A vicious cycle of air trapping and progressive dynamic hyperinflation occurs (**Figure 10**). Hyperinflation flattens and reduces the effectiveness of the diaphragm, making use of accessory muscles of breathing more crucial while also markedly increasing the work of breathing as chest wall compliance decreases. Impaired gas diffusion (as reflected by decreased D$_{LCO}$ on pulmonary function testing) correlates with the degree of emphysema as the capillary bed is reduced by loss of lung parenchyma.

The ability to increase minute ventilation is severely compromised in patients with COPD. As the disease progresses, dynamic hyperinflation occurs even during quiet breathing, causing worsening dyspnea. Various pulmonary complications can result from the chronic inflammation and tissue destruction in COPD (**Table 5**).

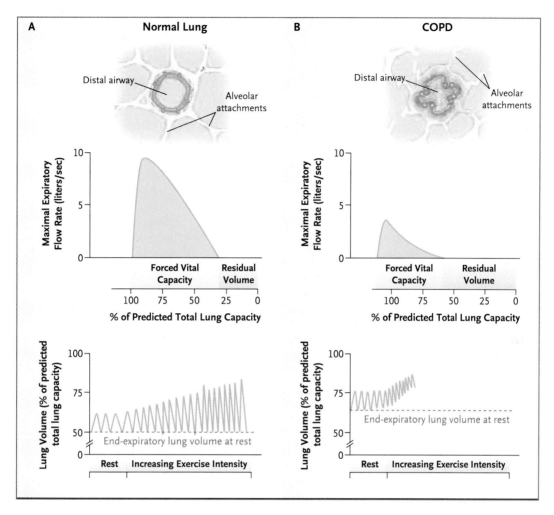

FIGURE 10. Pathophysiological features of airflow obstruction in COPD. Airflow obstruction in COPD is largely due to disruption of the alveolar walls, along with inflammation of lung tissue, fibrosis, and mucus plugging in the distal airways (*A*, normal distal airway surrounded by intact alveolar walls; *B*, abnormal distal airway surrounded by disrupted alveolar walls). Alveolar attachments provide a radial tethering effect that is essential for keeping small airways patent in the normal lung. Decreased lung elasticity and weaker tethering cause the airways to narrow as lung volumes decrease, reducing airflow with expiration with lengthening of the expiratory phase (*A*, normal flow; *B*, reduced flow). Residual volume may account for as much as 60% to 70% of predicted total lung capacity. Patients with COPD must breathe at larger lung volumes to optimize expiratory airflow, but this requires greater respiratory work because the lungs and chest wall become stiffer at larger volumes. In situations when the respiration rate is increased, because of insufficient expiratory time, breaths become increasingly shallow and end-expiratory lung volume progressively enlarges. This results in an increase in the residual volume, which results in increased air trapping, termed dynamic hyperinflation (*A*, normal response to exercise; *B*, response with COPD).

Reproduced with permission from Niewoehner DE. Clinical practice. Outpatient management of severe COPD. N Engl J Med. 2010;362(15):1407-1416. [PMID: 20393177]. Copyright 2010, Massachusetts Medical Society.

TABLE 5. Pulmonary Complications of COPD
Pulmonary hypertension
Cor pulmonale
Pneumonia
Pneumothorax
Bronchiectasis
Atelectasis
Lung cancer

Risk Factors

Essentially all risk for COPD results from an interaction between patient factors and environmental factors. Risk factors for COPD include exposure to tobacco smoke (including second-hand smoke), dust and chemicals (vapors, irritants, fumes), outdoor air pollution, and environmental (biomass) smoke, as well as genetic factors such as α_1-antitrypsin deficiency (**Table 6**).

Inhalation of cigarette smoke and other noxious particles causes lung inflammation. Patients who smoke have a higher

TABLE 6.	Risk Factors Associated with COPD

Tobacco smoking

History of pulmonary tuberculosis

History of chronic asthma

Low educational attainment

Poor socioeconomic status

Poor nutrition

Indoor air pollution (smoke from the combustion of wood, charcoal, coal, and other materials)

Outdoor air pollution
   Respirable particulate matter
   Nitrogen dioxide
   Carbon monoxide

Occupational exposures
   Crop farming (grain dust and other types of dust)
   Animal farming (organic dust, ammonia, hydrogen sulfide)
   Dust exposure (coal mining, hard-rock mining, tunneling, concrete manufacturing, construction, brick manufacturing, gold mining, iron and steel founding)
   Chemical exposure (plastic, textile, and rubber industries; leather manufacturing; manufacturing of food products)
   Pollutant exposure (transportation, trucking, automotive repair)

prevalence of respiratory symptoms and lung function abnormalities, a greater annual rate of decline in FEV_1, and a greater COPD mortality rate than nonsmokers. Risk for COPD is dose related. The age when the patient started to smoke, total pack-years smoked, and current smoking status are predictive of COPD mortality. Smoking cessation is the single most clinically effective and cost-effective way to prevent COPD, slow progression of established disease, and improve survival.

It is estimated that up to 20% or more of all COPD cases in the United States occur in never-smokers; the cause may relate to one or a combination of factors identified in Table 6. Conversely, it is not well understood why only a subset (up to 20%) of chronic heavy smokers develop COPD. Genetic predisposition other than α_1-antitrypsin deficiency may account for some of the predisposition, but cofactors unrelated to genetics, such as childhood viral respiratory infections, childhood asthma, and environmental and occupational pollution undoubtedly contribute to the increased susceptibility of this subset. Chronic, poorly controlled asthma can cause a degree of fixed airflow obstruction similar to COPD. Tuberculosis can result in airflow obstruction secondary to destruction of lung tissue.

Worldwide, about 50% of all households and 90% of rural households use biomass fuels (wood, charcoal, vegetable matter, and animal dung) as the main source of domestic energy. Exposure to smoke from combustion of biomass fuels may potentially represent a greater global risk factor for the development of COPD than tobacco smoking.

COPD development is also related to hereditary factors, but these remain poorly defined. Although there is no clear mendelian pattern of inheritance, data show that relatives of patients with COPD have a higher prevalence of the disease that cannot be attributed to environmental risk factors. There also is a higher prevalence of reduced lung function among children of patients with COPD than those of the spouses of patients with COPD.

COPD is affected by multiple genes. The best documented genetic influence is hereditary deficiency of α_1-antitrypsin (a circulating inhibitor of serine protease); deficiency should be considered in patients diagnosed with COPD at a young age (≤ 45 years), in nonsmokers, in patients with predominantly basilar lung disease, and in patients with concurrent liver disease. Other genes, including those for α_1-antichymotrypsin, α_2-macroglobulin, vitamin D–binding protein, and blood group antigens, also have been associated with the development of COPD.

The current classification structure of COPD fails to account for the substantial heterogeneity among patients with COPD. For example, among a select, matched group of patients who have similarly staged COPD, there will be a subgroup of patients who, for no apparent reason, experience more frequent and severe pulmonary exacerbations than others (worsening bronchitis, bronchospasm, and possibly respiratory failure). There also may be patients within that same group who, over time, will experience a more rapid rate of decline in pulmonary function than others, and some will become cachectic. In fact, among any similarly staged, matched group of patients with COPD, there will be a great deal of heterogeneity in individual expression of COPD. This heterogeneity in COPD implies that there are inadequately understood underlying genetic, biologic, or behavioral mechanisms that determine individual susceptibility to the previously mentioned conditions, independent of disease severity.

KEY POINTS

- Smoking cessation is the most clinically effective and cost-effective way to prevent COPD, slow progression of established disease, and improve survival.

- In developing countries, exposure to smoke from the indoor burning of biomass fuels (such as wood, charcoal, and vegetable matter) may be an important risk factor for COPD.

Extrapulmonary Effects and Comorbid Conditions

The extrapulmonary or systemic consequences of COPD can be particularly debilitating for patients with severe disease. Weight loss, muscle wasting, and weakness are common in severe COPD as a result of deconditioning and malnutrition. Extrapulmonary effects of COPD have a negative cumulative impact on respiratory morbidity, which results in diminished functional status and decreased survival.

In the presence of chronic inflammation and smoking-related toxins, comorbid conditions further complicate disease management and significantly affect COPD morbidity and mortality. Frequently observed comorbid conditions seen with COPD are shown in **Table 7**. As patients age, the comorbid conditions associated with COPD increase and require concurrent management along with COPD in internal medicine settings.

Awareness, prompt diagnosis, and effective management of the comorbid conditions of COPD can have a profound impact on patients' quality of life and their continuing ability to participate in activities of daily living. Early interventions in COPD should be directed at preventing and aggressively treating comorbid conditions and complications of COPD and should be an integral component of the comprehensive treatment plan.

KEY POINTS

- Weight loss, muscle wasting, and weakness are common in severe COPD as a result of deconditioning and malnutrition.

- As patients age, the comorbid conditions associated with COPD increase and require concurrent management along with COPD in internal medicine settings.

Assessment and Monitoring of Disease Progression

Assessment and Classification

A clinical diagnosis of COPD should be considered in any patient who has dyspnea, chronic cough, intermittent wheezing, sputum production, decreased exercise tolerance, a history of significant exposure to tobacco smoke, and/or a history of other risk factors for the disease. Physical examination may be normal; however, in more advanced disease there may be evidence of dynamic hyperinflation characterized by hyperresonance and distant breath sounds.

Spirometry is essential for the diagnosis of COPD, although testing for airflow limitation should not be performed in asymptomatic individuals as a screening intervention. When indicated, diagnostic spirometry should be performed after administration of an inhaled bronchodilator because this will improve the accuracy of the study results.

Guidelines from both the American College of Physicians (ACP) and the Global Initiative for Chronic Obstructive Lung Disease (GOLD) define airflow obstruction as a postbronchodilator FEV_1/FVC ratio less than 70%. The GOLD guidelines further classify COPD based on the level of airflow obstruction assessed by spirometry (**Table 8**) and also based on several additional functional criteria, including clinical symptoms as documented by the Modified Medical Research Council (MMRC) Dyspnea Scale (**Table 9**) and the frequency of exacerbations. This method of classifying the severity of disease may be more clinically useful than spirometry alone (**Table 10**).

Another means of assessing disease severity is the BODE (BMI, Obstruction, Dyspnea, Exercise) Index (**Table 11**), which is a composite disease marker that takes into account the systemic nature of COPD. The index incorporates spirometry, MMRC scores, and other parameters and is useful in evaluating the risk for hospitalization and estimating the long-term prognosis for patients with COPD. A higher score is associated with worse outcomes. Pulmonologists also may use BODE scores in the assessment of patients for lung transplantation. Patients with a BODE index score of 7 or higher will have a 4-year survival rate of 20% or lower.

There are several other tests that may be useful in characterizing the severity of COPD, including measurement of lung volume, D_{LCO}, arterial blood gases, and pulse oximetry; however, these tests are not routinely recommended for diagnostic confirmation. Chest radiographs may be useful to

---

TABLE 7. Comorbid Conditions Commonly Observed in Patients with COPD

Cardiovascular disease (including angina, acute myocardial infarction, fibrillation, heart failure, blood clots)
High cholesterol
Gastroesophageal reflux disease
Depression
Osteoporosis
Diabetes mellitus
Glaucoma
Erectile dysfunction
High blood pressure
Arthritic symptoms
Sinus symptoms
Cataracts
Sleep apnea
Stroke
Cancer

TABLE 8. Classification of Severity of Airflow Limitation in COPD (Based on Postbronchodilator FEV_1)

In patients with FEV_1/FVC <70%:

GOLD 1	Mild	$FEV_1 \geq 80\%$ of predicted
GOLD 2	Moderate	$50\% \leq FEV_1 < 80\%$ of predicted
GOLD 3	Severe	$30\% \leq FEV_1 < 50\%$ of predicted
GOLD 4	Very severe	$FEV_1 <30\%$ of predicted

GOLD = Global Initiative for Chronic Obstructive Lung Disease.

From the Global Strategy for Diagnosis, Management, and Prevention of COPD, 2011, Global Initiative for Chronic Obstructive Lung Disease (GOLD). Copyright 2011, Global Initiative for Chronic Obstructive Lung Disease. Available at: www.goldcopd.org. Accessed June 20, 2012.

TABLE 9. Modified Medical Research Council Questionnaire for Assessing Severity of Dyspnea

Severity	Score	Level of Breathlessness
None	0	Not troubled with breathlessness except with strenuous exercise
Mild	1	Troubled by shortness of breath when hurrying or walking up a slight hill
Moderate	2	Walks slower than people of the same age owing to breathlessness or has to stop for breath when walking at own pace on level ground
Severe	3	Stops for breath after walking approximately 100 meters (328 feet) or after a few minutes on level ground
Very severe	4	Too breathless to leave the house or breathless when dressing or undressing

Data from Bestall JC, Paul EA, Garrod R, Garnham R, Jones PW, Wedzicha JA. Usefulness of the Medical Research Council (MRC) dyspnoea scale as a measure of disability in patients with chronic obstructive pulmonary disease. Thorax. 1999;54(7):581-586. [PMID: 10377201]

TABLE 11. BODE Index for COPD[a]

Variable	Points			
	0	1	2	3
FEV_1 (% of predicted)[b]	≥65	50-64	36-49	≤35
6-Minute walking distance (meters)	≥350	250-349	150-249	≤149
MMRC[c]	0-1	2	3	4
BMI[d]	>21	≤21		

BODE = BMI, Obstruction, Dyspnea, Exercise.

[a]The cutoff values for the assignment of points are shown for each variable. The total possible values range from 0 to 10.

[b]The FEV_1 categories are based on stages identified by the American Thoracic Society.

[c]Scores on the Modified Medical Research Council (MMRC) dyspnea scale can range from 0 to 4, with a score of 4 indicating that the patient is too breathless to leave the house or becomes breathless when dressing or undressing.

[d]The values for BMI were 0 or 1 because of the inflection point in the inverse relation between survival and BMI at a value of 21.

Reprinted from Celli BR, Cote CG, Marin JM, et al. The body-mass index, airflow obstruction, dyspnea, and exercise capacity index in chronic obstructive pulmonary disease. N Engl J Med. 2004;350(10):1005-1012. [PMID: 14999112]. Copyright 2004, Massachusetts Medical Society.

assess flattening of the diaphragm, and CT may be useful to show destruction of pulmonary parenchyma in patients who have emphysema. Echocardiography may be appropriate in evaluating patients with pulmonary hypertension. Exercise testing may be useful in patients with dyspnea to differentiate whether symptoms are from pulmonary or cardiac causes.

Ongoing Monitoring

COPD monitoring consists of assessment of symptoms and measures of airflow limitation. These measures help determine if therapy should be adjusted and if complications are present. As at the initial assessment, follow-up visits should include a physical examination and discussion of symptoms, particularly any new or worsening ones. Periodic spirometry should be performed to track a patient's lung function.

Dosages of medications, adherence to the therapeutic regimen, inhaler technique, effectiveness of symptom control, and side effects of treatment should all be monitored, and therapy should be adjusted as appropriate and as the disease progresses. Inhaled medications are a mainstay of COPD management; if inhaler technique is poor, the response to such therapy is not optimal. Therefore, in a patient with suboptimal response to therapy, inhaler technique should be evaluated before therapy is adjusted.

Exacerbation frequency and severity should be assessed with patient history and evaluation of symptoms. Likely triggers for exacerbations should be assessed, and the patient's psychological well being should be evaluated. Increased sputum volume, acutely worsening dyspnea, and the presence of purulent sputum should be noted. These

TABLE 10. GOLD Classification System for COPD Severity

Patient Group	Severity	Definition
A	Low risk/fewer symptoms	Mild or moderate airflow limitation (previously GOLD stage 1 or 2) and/or ≤1 exacerbation per year *and* MMRC[a] score <2
B	Low risk/more symptoms	Mild or moderate airflow limitation (previously GOLD stage 1 or 2) and/or ≤1 exacerbation per year *and* MMRC[a] score ≥2
C	High risk/fewer symptoms	Severe or very severe airflow limitation (previously GOLD stage 3 or 4) and/or ≥2 exacerbations per year *and* MMRC[a] score <2
D	High risk/more symptoms	Severe or very severe airflow limitation (previously GOLD stage 3 or 4) and/or ≥2 exacerbations per year *and* MMRC[a] score ≥2

GOLD = Global Initiative for Chronic Obstructive Lung Disease.

[a]See Table 9.

Data from: Global Strategy for Diagnosis, Management, and Prevention of COPD, 2011, Global Initiative for Chronic Obstructive Lung Disease (GOLD). Available at: www.goldcopd.org. Accessed June 20, 2012.

actions may aid in prescribing antibiotics for early symptoms of exacerbation in outpatients and may reduce the need for subsequent hospitalizations.

Interactive questioning and listening to patients can be highly effective in determining the impact of COPD on an individual's quality of life; however, when patients are reticent or not fully informative, there are additional tools available to internists that can provide incremental information. These include the Clinical COPD Questionnaire that measures COPD-related symptoms, functional status, and mental health (www.ccq.nl), and the COPD Assessment Test (CAT), which correlates very closely with health status and can provide a reliable score to identify patients with frequent exacerbations (www.catestonline.org).

Referral

Internists may consider referral to a pulmonary specialist in the presence of disease onset before 40 years of age, a rapidly progressive course of disease, severe COPD despite optimal treatment, need for oxygen therapy, onset of a comorbid condition, diagnostic uncertainty, symptoms disproportionate to the severity of airway obstruction, confirmed or suspected α_1-antitrypsin deficiency, a request for a second opinion, possibility for lung transplantation or lung volume reduction surgery, very severe disease requiring elective surgery that may impair respiratory function, or frequent exacerbations and persistent symptoms despite adequate treatment.

KEY POINTS

- A clinical diagnosis of COPD should be considered in any patient who has dyspnea, chronic cough or sputum production, decreased exercise tolerance, a history of significant exposure to tobacco smoke, and/or a history of risk factors for the disease.

- Spirometry is essential for the diagnosis of COPD; a postbronchodilator FEV_1/FVC ratio less than 70% is generally considered the diagnostic threshold.

- Monitoring to adjust COPD therapy should focus on doses of medications, adherence to the regimen, inhaler technique, effectiveness of symptom control, and the side effects of treatment.

Management

A comprehensive treatment plan facilitates achieving the basic goals of management of stable COPD, which are to reduce symptoms, prevent exacerbations, enhance quality of life, and reduce disease morbidity and mortality. The components of a COPD management plan are (1) identification and reduction of risk factors, (2) assessment and monitoring of disease progression, (3) managing stable COPD, and (4) managing exacerbations.

The frequency of exacerbations increases as the severity of COPD increases. Patients who experience frequent exacerbations are also likely to have more symptoms, worsened health status, faster disease progression, and an increased risk of death. To maximize outcomes, treatment regimens must be sustained for the long term and reassessed periodically to monitor for efficacy and side effects.

Pharmacologic Therapy

Although no medication has been shown to reduce the progressive decline in lung function in COPD, pharmacologic interventions may reduce symptoms, diminish the frequency and severity of exacerbations, reduce the frequency of hospitalization, and improve exercise tolerance and health status. Medications used to treat COPD are listed in **Table 12**.

Inhaled medications are the mainstay of therapy in COPD. Short-acting, as-needed bronchodilators (β_2-agonists or anticholinergic agents), either alone or in combination, are usually the first treatment intervention implemented for mild disease ($FEV_1 \geq 60\%$ of predicted) for alleviation of intermittent symptoms. However, their use is appropriate for all levels of COPD for treatment of "breakthrough" symptoms that may occur on daily maintenance therapy and for treatment of acute exacerbations.

The ACP guidelines recommend instituting daily bronchodilator treatment in symptomatic patients when the FEV_1 is below 60% of predicted (**Table 13**). A long-acting β_2-agonist or long-acting anticholinergic agent as monotherapy is recommended as first-line maintenance therapy, with the choice of agent based on patient and physician preference, potential side effects, and cost.

If patients do not achieve adequate symptom control with inhaled monotherapy, switching between these classes of medication is appropriate. If a patient remains symptomatic with monotherapy with either class of medication, combination therapy is typically pursued. Various combinations are possible, including the use of a β_2-agonist and anticholinergic medication together, or using an inhaled corticosteroid with either a β_2-agonist or anticholinergic medication. In advanced, poorly controlled disease, the triple combination of a β_2-agonist, an anticholinergic agent, and an inhaled corticosteroid is common. Treatment with different inhaled agents as monotherapy and in combination with other medications is discussed later in this section.

For patients who do not respond optimally to inhaled therapy, adherence should be verified and inhaler technique should be assessed before therapeutic changes are made. Metered-dose inhalers, dry powder inhalers, and nebulizers are equally effective devices; however, patients will require instruction regarding proper technique to ensure adequate drug delivery. Although nebulizers also require additional equipment maintenance, they may be appropriate and useful in elderly patients or those who have cognitive impairment, difficulty with hand coordination, or difficulty controlling actions of breathing.

TABLE 12. Drug Treatment for Chronic Obstructive Pulmonary Disease		
Agent	**Side Effects**	**Notes**
Bronchodilators		
Inhaled short-acting β_2-agonists (albuterol, fenoterol, levalbuterol, metaproterenol, pirbuterol, terbutaline)	Sympathomimetic symptoms such as tremor and tachycardia	Generally used as needed for mild disease with few symptoms
Inhaled short-acting anticholinergic agents (ipratropium)	Dry mouth, mydriasis on contact with eye, tachycardia, tremors, rarely acute narrow angle glaucoma	Not to be used with tiotropium; generally used as needed for mild disease with few symptoms; avoid using both short- and long-acting anticholinergics
Inhaled long-acting anticholinergic agents (tiotropium, aclidinium)	Dry mouth, mydriasis on contact with eye, tachycardia, tremors, rarely acute narrow angle glaucoma	Not to be used with ipratropium; use when short-acting bronchodilators provide insufficient control of symptoms for patients with an FEV_1 <60% of predicted
Inhaled long-acting β_2-agonists (salmeterol, formoterol, arformoterol, indacaterol)	Sympathomimetic symptoms such as tremor and tachycardia; overdose can be fatal	Use as maintenance therapy when short-acting bronchodilators provide insufficient control of symptoms for patients with an FEV_1 <60% of predicted; not intended to be used for treatment of exacerbations of COPD or acute bronchospasm
Methylxanthines (theophylline, aminophylline; sustained and short-acting)	Tachycardia, nausea, vomiting, disturbed pulmonary function, and disturbed sleep; narrow therapeutic index; overdose can be fatal with seizures and arrhythmias	Used as maintenance therapy; generally use only after long-acting bronchodilator treatment to provide additional symptomatic relief of exacerbations; may also improve respiratory muscle function
Oral β_2-agonists (albuterol, metaproterenol, terbutaline)	Sympathomimetic symptoms such as tremor and tachycardia	Used as maintenance therapy; rarely used because of side effects but may be beneficial to patients who cannot use inhalers
Oral Phosophodiesterase-4 Inhibitor		
Roflumilast	Diarrhea, nausea, backache, decreased appetite, dizziness	Used to reduce risk for exacerbations in patients with severe COPD (blood levels not required) with chronic bronchitis and history of exacerbations; roflumilast should not be used with methylxanthines owing to potential toxicity; very expensive and should be used only in selected patients
Anti-inflammatory Agents		
Inhaled corticosteroids (fluticasone, budesonide, mometasone, ciclesonide, beclomethasone)	Dysphonia, skin bruising, oral candidiasis, rarely side effects of oral corticosteroids (see below)	Most effective in patients with a history of frequent exacerbations and when used in conjunction with long-acting bronchodilators; not approved by the FDA for treatment for COPD
Oral corticosteroids (prednisone, prednisolone)	Skin bruising, adrenal suppression, glaucoma, osteoporosis, diabetes mellitus, systemic hypertension, pneumonia, cataracts, opportunistic infection, insomnia, mood disturbance	Use for significant exacerbations of COPD with taper; avoid, if possible, in stable COPD to limit corticosteroid toxicity; consider inhaled corticosteroids to facilitate weaning of systemic corticosteroids
Combination Agents		
Combined inhaled long-acting β_2-agonist and inhaled corticosteroid in a single inhaler (fluticasone/salmeterol, budesonide/formoterol)	Same/combined effects of both drug classes	Fluticasone/salmeterol is approved by the FDA as maintenance therapy and for prevention of exacerbations; budesonide/formoterol metered-dose inhaler is approved by the FDA as maintenance therapy; combinations are not to be used for treatment of acute bronchospasm

(continued on next page)

TABLE 12. Drug Treatment for Chronic Obstructive Pulmonary Disease *(continued)*

Agent	Side Effects	Notes
Combination Agents (*continued*)		
Combination short-acting β_2-agonists plus anticholinergic in a single inhaler (fenoterol/ipratropium, salbutamol/ipratropium)	Same/combined effects of both drug classes	Not to be used with tiotropium; generally used as needed for mild disease with few symptoms; avoid using both short- and long-acting anticholinergics; this combination therapy may be used for maintenance therapy only if patients have well-controlled disease on this combination treatment and do not require rescue therapy if/when expense is a determining factor

In patients who have more advanced disease or inadequate control with inhaled treatments, additional medications are frequently added. Methylxanthines have traditionally been used in addition to inhaled therapy, although their use has been declining owing to their limited effectiveness, narrow therapeutic window, and potential side effects. Other medications for add-on therapy, including several new agents, are available for use in selected patients, as discussed later in this section.

Bronchodilators

Bronchodilators relax the smooth muscles of the airways, resulting in widening of the airways. This improves emptying of the lungs during exhalation and tends to reduce dynamic hyperinflation. There are no available data to support the superiority of any bronchodilator over another, but inhaled β_2-agonists or anticholinergic agents, administered alone or in combination, are preferred to methylxanthines. The general approach to therapy is described in **Figure 11**.

Short-Acting Bronchodilators

Short-acting bronchodilators are prescribed initially as monotherapy for patients with mild COPD, intermittent and/or exertional symptoms of COPD, or for rescue therapy in acute exacerbations of COPD or breakthrough symptoms in patients who are already taking long-acting bronchodilator medications. Inhaled short-acting β_2-agonists (albuterol, levalbuterol, metaproterenol, pirbuterol) provide 3 to 6 hours of action. The inhaled short-acting anticholinergic agent ipratropium has a duration of action of 4 to 5 hours in most patients. Although the onset of action is slower than a short-acting β_2-agonist, ipratropium can be used for rescue as monotherapy or in combination with albuterol. Combination therapy with a short-acting β_2-agonist plus ipratropium provides a greater and more sustained improvement in FEV_1 than either drug alone and can be used when symptoms are not relieved with monotherapy.

Long-Acting Bronchodilators

Two classes of long-acting bronchodilators may be administered as monotherapy. Long-acting β_2-agonists (salmeterol, formoterol; duration of action approximately 12 hours) and long-acting anticholinergic agents (tiotropium; duration of action approximately 24 hours) significantly reduce frequency of exacerbations and improve respiratory health status but do not have a significant impact on the reduction of hospitalizations or

TABLE 13. Therapy for Stable, Symptomatic COPD Based on Level of Airflow Obstruction[a]

Level of Airflow Obstruction	Recommended Therapy[b]
FEV_1 60%-80% of predicted	Consider inhaled bronchodilator therapy (anticholinergic or β_2-agonist) (weak recommendation, low-quality evidence)
FEV_1 <60% of predicted	Daily monotherapy with an inhaled bronchodilator (long-acting anticholinergic or long-acting β_2-agonist), with the choice of therapy based on patient preference, cost, and side-effect profile (strong recommendation, moderate-quality evidence)
	Consider combination inhaled therapy (long-acting anticholinergic, long-acting β_2-agonist, or corticosteroid) (weak recommendation, moderate-quality evidence)
FEV_1 <50% of predicted	Consider adding pulmonary rehabilitation (weak recommendation, moderate-quality evidence)

[a]In patients with an FEV_1/FVC ratio <70%.

[b]Occasional use of short-term bronchodilators for breakthrough symptoms or exacerbation is appropriate at any level of pulmonary function in COPD.

Data from Qaseem A, Wilt TJ, Weinberger SE, et al; American College of Physicians; American College of Chest Physicians; American Thoracic Society; European Respiratory Society. Diagnosis and management of stable chronic obstructive pulmonary disease: a clinical practice guideline update from the American College of Physicians, American College of Chest Physicians, American Thoracic Society, and European Respiratory Society. Ann Intern Med. 2011;155(3):179-191. [PMID: 21810710]. Copyright 2011, American College of Physicians.

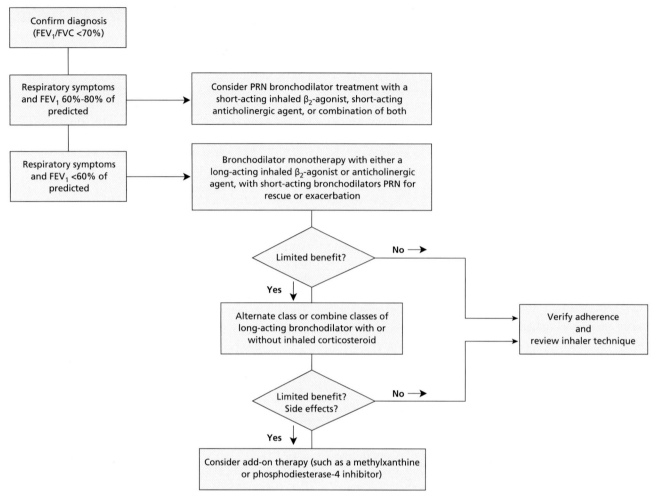

FIGURE 11. Step therapy for patients with COPD. PRN = as needed.

Adapted from Littner MR. In the clinic. Chronic obstructive pulmonary disease. Ann Intern Med. 2011;154(7):ITC4-1-ITC4-15; quiz ITC4-16. [PMID: 21464346]. Copyright 2010, American College of Physicians.

mortality. The FDA recently approved indacaterol, an inhaled long-acting β_2-agonist, for once-daily maintenance treatment of airflow obstruction in patients with COPD.

When monotherapy with either agent is insufficient for symptomatic relief or symptoms worsen and/or become more persistent, combination therapy using a long-acting β_2-agonist and a long-acting anticholinergic agent is sometimes prescribed. The benefits and risks of dual therapy with these agents have not yet been definitively established. A short-acting bronchodilator should always be prescribed to patients treated with long-acting agents for use as rescue therapy, because the slow onset of bronchodilation with long-acting drugs, if used alone, may lead to respiratory decompensation in patients with acute symptoms.

Inhaled Corticosteroids

Inhaled corticosteroids are widely prescribed for COPD and are frequently added to long-acting bronchodilators when patients remain symptomatic or have repeated exacerbations.

Inhaled corticosteroids should not be used alone as the primary therapy for patients with COPD.

As with combination therapy with long-acting β_2-agonists and long-acting anticholinergic agents, the effectiveness of adding an inhaled corticosteroid to either of these medications alone has not been established. In some patients with severe COPD and inadequately controlled symptoms, the combination of a long-acting β_2-agonist, long-acting anticholinergic agent, and an inhaled corticosteroid is used. There is some evidence that triple therapy may be beneficial, but similar to other combinations, the efficacy and safety of this intervention remain to be definitively proved.

Older patients and those with more advanced disease may have an increased risk of pneumonia following therapy with inhaled corticosteroids. Regular treatment with inhaled corticosteroids does not alter the long-term decline of FEV_1 in patients with COPD, and the safety of long-term use is not known. All patients using inhaled corticosteroids should be monitored for adverse effects associated with long-term corticosteroid use, including osteopenia, hyperglycemia, and cataracts.

Oral and Intravenous Corticosteroids
Oral corticosteroids should be reserved for limited periodic use to treat acute exacerbations in patients with COPD. Long-term oral corticosteroid therapy has been shown to have limited, if any, benefits in COPD. In addition, oral corticosteroid therapy has a high risk for significant side effects, including muscle weakness and decrease in functional status in addition to the side effects observed with inhaled corticosteroids.

Intravenous corticosteroids are recommended for management of acute exacerbations of COPD severe enough to warrant hospitalization. The effective dose is not known. Patients who respond to therapy should be switched to oral corticosteroids and the dose should be tapered following discharge. Prolonged treatment does not result in greater efficacy and increases the risk of side effects.

Methylxanthines
Although methylxanthines (aminophylline, theophylline) are effective in COPD, the potential toxicity of this drug class has led to increasingly limited use. Use of these drugs is most often relegated to selected patients with late-stage, advanced COPD. Inhaled bronchodilators with or without inhaled corticosteroid therapy are preferred for routine treatment, and methylxanthines are usually administered only after these other therapeutic approaches have been tried. The mechanism of action in methylxanthines is not fully known, but they may act as nonselective inhibitors of phosphodiesterase. The therapeutic effect lasts up to 24 hours. They are available in both oral and intravenous formulations. They have a narrow therapeutic window, effects are relatively modest, there can be multiple interactions with other medications, and higher plasma levels of theophylline are poorly tolerated in the geriatric population.

Phosphodiesterase-4 Inhibitors
The most recent addition to pharmacotherapy for COPD, roflumilast, has shown efficacy and tolerability in patients with severe COPD. Roflumilast is an oral selective phosophodiesterase-4 inhibitor (a new drug class). It is indicated to reduce the risk and frequency of exacerbations or to improve symptoms in patients with severe COPD associated with chronic bronchitis and a history of exacerbations. Roflumilast is not a bronchodilator, but it provides a measurable but modest improvement in FEV_1 independent of the patient's smoking status or use of concomitant medications.

Roflumilast is not indicated for the relief of acute bronchospasm or rescue therapy, and it is not intended for the treatment of primary emphysema. It is an expensive medication and is used primarily as add-on therapy in patients with severe disease not adequately controlled on other COPD medications. Common adverse events include diarrhea, weight loss, nausea, and headache. Psychiatric adverse events such as anxiety,

insomnia, and depression were reported more frequently with roflumilast compared with placebo. This agent is contraindicated in patients with liver impairment, and its use with strong cytochrome P-450 enzyme inducers (rifampin, phenobarbital, carbamazepine, phenytoin) is not recommended.

Other Agents
α_1-Antitrypsin replacement therapy may be used in the rare patient whose COPD is related to α_1-antitrypsin deficiency. Mucolytic agents (mucokinetic, mucoregulatory) may provide minor benefit to few patients with viscous sputum; however, their use cannot currently be recommended. Early data created speculation that antioxidant agents (particularly *N*-acetylcysteine) might have a role in treatment of COPD in patients with recurrent exacerbations, but further studies have not shown efficacy for this treatment approach. Routine use of antitussives is not recommended in patients with stable COPD because cough has a significant protective role. Based on available evidence, the use of pulmonary vasodilators (such as phosphodiesterase-5 inhibitors, calcium channel blockers, and nitric oxide) has not shown benefit and may worsen oxygenation; these agents are therefore contraindicated in COPD. Narcotics (morphine), when given either orally or parenterally, are effective for treating dyspnea in advanced COPD, although in high doses they may have a hypoventilatory effect. Nedocromil and leukotriene modifiers have not been adequately tested in COPD.

Antibiotic Agents
Antibiotic therapy is most beneficial in treating infectious exacerbations of COPD that are characterized by increases in dyspnea, sputum volume, and sputum purulence. Antibiotic therapy also is indicated in patients with severe exacerbations of COPD who require mechanical ventilation, whether invasive or noninvasive. Although the inciting factor of an exacerbation may be unknown, a fluoroquinolone such as levofloxacin or the combination of a third-generation cephalosporin plus a macrolide antibiotic will usually cover the most common bacterial pathogens (*Haemophilus influenzae*, *Streptococcus pneumoniae*, and *Moraxella catarrhalis* as well as causes of "atypical" pneumonia). Even when the cause of the exacerbation is viral, patients with COPD are often colonized with bacteria. Antibiotics in this setting have been demonstrated to improve air flow, reduce mortality, and reduce treatment failure, especially in patients experiencing more severe exacerbations. A number of meta-analyses and systematic reviews support the use of antibiotic treatment for acute exacerbations of COPD. Although there is some evidence of their effectiveness, more definitive data are awaited regarding the use of prophylactic antibiotics to prevent repeat exacerbations.

Vaccines
Influenza and pneumococcal vaccinations are recommended for patients with COPD. The newer 7-valent diphtheria-conjugated pneumococcal polysaccharide vaccine appears to

induce a superior immune response than the 23-valent pneumococcal polysaccharide vaccine.

Nonpharmacologic Therapy

Smoking Cessation

Smoking cessation and oxygen therapy are the only interventions demonstrated to reduce COPD risk and positively affect decline in pulmonary function. Smoking cessation is the most important goal in the management of COPD in patients who smoke, and it should be addressed at every visit. Active smokers lose pulmonary function at a higher rate than sustained quitters. Passive exposure to cigarette smoke also may contribute to respiratory symptoms. Although cigarette smoking has declined in recent years, there has been a substantial increase in pipe and cigar smoking. Cessation of smoking reduces the rate of death from any cause, and the benefits of quitting smoking are more pronounced when quitting sooner or earlier. Supportive counseling and pharmacotherapy can be effective tools to increase success rates in cessation of smoking (see MKSAP 16 General Internal Medicine).

Pulmonary Rehabilitation

Pulmonary rehabilitation can be considered for all symptomatic patients with an FEV_1 less than 50% of predicted. It involves a combination of education, nutritional counseling, exercise training, assessment, and follow-up to reinforce behaviors and techniques. When added to other forms of therapy, the exercise training component (30 minutes or more three times weekly for at least 6 to 8 weeks) helps to improve endurance, flexibility, and strength in the upper and lower extremities. Pulmonary rehabilitation has been shown to reduce the perceived intensity of breathlessness, decrease dyspnea and fatigue, increase participation in daily activities, improve quality of life (including a reduction of anxiety and depression associated with COPD), and reduce the number of hospitalizations and lengths of stay. Pulmonary rehabilitation is less likely to achieve those goals in patients who are not able to walk at baseline, who have the most severe breathlessness, or who have additional psychological or medical comorbidities that limit their motivation. In general, patients should have quit smoking or be in smoking cessation programs to participate in pulmonary rehabilitation. Sustained benefit requires continued participation in the program, and this may be a limiting factor for some patients from a resource perspective.

Oxygen Therapy

Oxygen therapy is a major component of treatment for patients with very severe COPD and is indicated for patients who have resting hypoxemia, defined as an arterial Po_2 of 55 mm Hg (7.3 kPa) or lower or arterial oxygen saturation of 88% or lower. Although resting oxygen saturation may not meet those criteria, patients may still benefit from supplemental oxygen if they desaturate at night while sleeping or during exercise. Oxygen criteria may be more liberal in patients with overt cor pulmonale or polycythemia.

In patients who qualify for continuous therapy because of resting hypoxemia, duration of oxygen treatment should be greater than 15 hours per day and preferably longer. The use of long-term oxygen therapy in patients with chronic respiratory failure improves survival and has a beneficial effect on hemodynamics, hematologic characteristics, exercise capacity, mental status, general alertness, motor speed, and hand grip. Studies have shown that delivering oxygen during exercise can increase the duration of endurance and/or reduce the intensity of breathlessness at the end of exercise.

Oxygen therapy is the cornerstone of hospital treatment of COPD exacerbations. Achieving adequate levels of oxygenation (arterial Po_2 greater than 60 mm Hg [8.0 kPa] or oxygen saturation greater than 90%) in an uncomplicated exacerbation may be relatively straightforward; however, carbon dioxide retention can occur insidiously with little change in symptoms. Arterial blood gas levels should be measured 30 to 60 minutes after oxygen therapy is started to ensure that oxygenation is adequate without carbon dioxide retention or acidosis. ◨

Noninvasive Mechanical Ventilation

Noninvasive positive pressure ventilation (NPPV) is appropriate and useful in spontaneously breathing patients with severe COPD during acute exacerbation and/or acute respiratory infection, such as pneumonia or chronic bronchitis (**Table 14**). In these patients, NPPV improves the breathing pattern, reduces dyspnea, improves oxygenation, and may be

TABLE 14. Noninvasive Positive Pressure Ventilation in Patients with COPD Exacerbations

Purpose

Improves respiratory acidosis

Increases pH

Decreases need for endotracheal intubation

Reduces arterial P_{CO_2}, respiratory rate, severity of breathlessness, length of hospital stay, and mortality

Indications

Moderate-to-severe dyspnea with use of accessory muscles of breathing and paradoxical abdominal motion

Moderate to severe acidosis (pH <7.35) and/or hypercapnia (arterial P_{CO_2} >45 mm Hg [6.0 kPa])

Respiration rate >25/min

Contraindications

Respiratory arrest

Cardiovascular instability (hypotension, arrhythmias, myocardial infarction)

Change in mental status or uncooperative patient

High aspiration risk

Viscous or copious secretions

Recent facial or gastroesophageal surgery

Craniofacial trauma or burns

Fixed nasopharyngeal abnormalities

TABLE 15. Indications for Endotracheal Intubation with Mechanical Ventilation in Patients with COPD

Inability to tolerate or failure of noninvasive ventilation

Severe dyspnea with a respiration rate greater than 35/min despite aggressive medical treatment

Life-threatening hypoxia (persistent despite increased F_{IO_2})

Severe acidosis (pH <7.25) and/or hypercapnia (arterial P_{CO_2} >60 mm Hg [8.0 kPa])

Respiratory arrest

Somnolence or impaired mental status

Cardiovascular complications (hypotension, shock)

Other complications such as metabolic abnormalities, sepsis, pneumonia, pulmonary embolism, barotrauma, and massive pleural effusion

---

of benefit in these very sick patients to avoid intubation (see Critical Care). In selected stable patients with advanced COPD, NPPV may be a helpful adjunctive treatment, particularly at night. Similar to obstructive sleep apnea, in some patients it can improve sleep continuity, daytime symptoms of sleepiness and exertional dyspnea, and awake arterial P_{CO_2}.

Endotracheal Intubation with Mechanical Ventilation
Endotracheal intubation with mechanical ventilation, generally administered in hospital and critical care settings, is indicated for patients presenting with very severe disease and/or life-threatening hypoxia, progressive hypercapnia, somnolence, or significantly altered mental status (**Table 15**) (see Critical Care). The decision to initiate intubation is influenced by the likelihood of reversing the precipitating event and the patient's advance directives and current wishes. Patients who have advance care directives but who remain alert and interactive should continue to actively participate in such decisions.

Preoperative Patient Management
Effective preoperative preparation of patients with COPD can decrease the incidence of serious postoperative complications. Patients who smoke should be advised to quit smoking before surgery. Although there are no definitive data

regarding an optimal period of preoperative smoking cessation, it is clear that smoking has a negative effect on surgical outcomes, and longer periods of smoking cessation appear to be more effective in reducing the incidence and risk of postoperative complications.

Pulmonary function should be optimized before any surgical intervention; elective procedures should be delayed in the presence of a COPD exacerbation. Additionally, close communication with the surgical team and associated care providers is essential to maintaining consistent care and ensuring stable treatment of the patient's lung disease.

Lung Volume Reduction Surgery
Lung volume reduction surgery (LVRS) involves resecting up to 30% of diseased or nonfunctioning parenchyma to reduce hyperinflation and allow the remaining lung to function more efficiently. This type of surgery makes respiratory muscles more effective by improving their mechanical efficiency and improves expiratory flow rates by increasing the elastic recoil pressure of the lung. LVRS is a high-risk, expensive, palliative surgical procedure and is recommended only in a clearly defined group of patients. LVRS is indicated in patients with advanced COPD (maximum FEV_1 ≤45% and >20% of predicted and D_{LCO} >20% of predicted with bilateral predominant upper-lobe emphysema) who remain symptomatic despite maximal pharmacologic therapy. In eligible patients (**Table 16**), LVRS increases chances for improvements in exercise capacity, lung function, dyspnea, and quality of life, but overall survival is not improved when compared with medical therapy alone. Patients who have an FEV_1 less than or equal to 20% of predicted and either homogeneous emphysema on CT scan or D_{LCO} less than or equal to 20% of predicted should not be considered for LVRS. It is unlikely they will benefit and their risk for perioperative mortality is high.

Current research is focused on endobronchial approaches to reduce lung volume by creating atelectasis of

TABLE 16. Lung Volume Reduction Surgery Eligibility Criteria
Severe COPD
Received maximal medical treatment
Completed pulmonary rehabilitation
Evidence of bilateral predominant upper-lobe emphysema on CT scan
Postbronchodilator total lung capacity of >150% AND residual lung volume >100% of predicted
Maximum FEV$_1$ >20% and ≤45% of predicted
Ambient air arterial Pco$_2$ ≤60 mm Hg (8.0 kPa) AND arterial Po$_2$ ≥45 mm Hg (6.0 kPa)

CONT.

the emphysematous portion of the lung. Techniques for this may include one-way valves, introduction of biologic materials, or creation of a nonanatomic pathway to decompress the hyperinflated portions of the lung; however, none of these techniques has been approved to date. ▣

Lung Transplantation

In appropriately selected patients (**Table 17**) with very advanced COPD, lung transplantation has been shown to improve quality of life and functional capacity, although it does not appear to confer a survival benefit in patients with end-stage emphysema after 2 years. Survival data for single-lung transplantation is approximately 83%, 60%, and 43% for patients with COPD at 1, 3, and 5 years, respectively. Data for double-lung transplant survival have been found to be similar or slightly higher. The leading cause of long-term morbidity at 5 years posttransplant is chronic allograft rejection (obliterative bronchiolitis), which occurs in as many as 50% to 70% of survivors. Patients should be referred for lung

TABLE 17. Lung Transplantation Eligibility Criteria
Patients must have a BODE Index of 7 to 10 AND at least one of the following:
History of hospitalization for an exacerbation associated with acute hypercapnia (Pco$_2$ >50 mm Hg [6.7 kPa])
Pulmonary hypertension, cor pulmonale, or both despite oxygen therapy
FEV$_1$ <20% of predicted and one of the following:
Dlco <20% of predicted
Homogeneous distribution of emphysema
Arterial Po$_2$ <55 mm Hg (7.3 kPa)
Exclusion Criteria
Advanced age and comorbid conditions
Demand for suitable organs outstrips availability
Expense
BODE = BMI, Obstruction, Dyspnea, Exercise.

transplantation when they have an FEV$_1$ less than 20% of predicted, arterial Po$_2$ less than 55 to 60 mm Hg (7.3 to 8.0 kPa), arterial Pco$_2$ of 50 mm Hg (6.7 kPa) or greater, and secondary pulmonary hypertension. Referral is advisable when patients have less than 50% 2- to 3-year predicted survival or have New York Heart Association class III or IV level of function.

Absolute contraindications to lung transplantation include continued smoking, substance addiction (alcohol, tobacco, or narcotics) that is current or active within the last 6 months, malignancy in the last 2 years, untreated advanced dysfunction of another major organ system, noncurable chronic extrapulmonary infection, significant chest wall or spinal deformity, untreated psychiatric issues, inability to comply with medical therapy, and absence of a reliable social support system.

KEY POINTS

- Smoking cessation and oxygen therapy are the only interventions demonstrated to reduce COPD risk and positively affect decline in pulmonary function; smoking cessation is the most important goal in the management of COPD in patients who smoke, and it should be addressed at every visit.

- Pulmonary rehabilitation (consisting of education, nutritional counseling, exercise training, assessment, and follow-up) can be considered for all symptomatic patients with COPD who have an FEV$_1$ less than 50% of predicted.

- Oxygen therapy is a major component of treatment for patients with very severe COPD and is indicated for patients who have hypoxemia (arterial Po$_2$ ≤55 mm Hg [7.3 kPa] or arterial oxygen saturation ≤88%).

Managing Exacerbations of COPD

Although there is no single definition of an acute exacerbation of COPD, there is a set of major and additional criteria that are useful in making the diagnosis (**Table 18**). Exacerbations of COPD may be caused by many factors but frequently result from an upper respiratory infection, and prompt recognition and treatment are important to prevent worsening. Exacerbations cause bronchoconstriction, airway inflammation, increased secretions, and hyperinflation with decreased chest wall compliance, all of which increase the work of breathing. Treatment may involve additions or adjustments to bronchodilator therapy, inhaled or systemic corticosteroid therapy, initiation of antibiotic treatment, and possibly mechanical ventilation. When exacerbations are severe, patients must be evaluated for the need for hospitalization.

There are several factors that determine a patient's risk for exacerbation, and these should be assessed to best tailor a COPD treatment regimen. Two or more exacerbations in the past year are the greatest predictor of future exacerbations.

TABLE 18. Criteria and Classification of Acute COPD Exacerbation

Major Criteria

Increase in sputum volume

Increase in sputum purulence (generally yellow or green)

Worsening of baseline dyspnea

Additional Criteria

Upper respiratory infection in the past 5 days

Fever of no apparent cause

Increase in wheezing and cough

Increase in respiration rate or heart rate 20% above baseline

Various nonspecific signs and symptoms may accompany these findings, such as fatigue, insomnia, depression, and confusion

Degree of Exacerbation

Mild exacerbation = 1 major criterion + 1 or more additional criteria

Moderate exacerbation = 2 major criteria

Severe exacerbation = all 3 major criteria

Other indicators include a baseline FEV_1 less than 50% of predicted and a history of gastroesophageal reflux disease or heartburn. Preliminary data suggest that treatment with a proton pump inhibitor in older patients who have COPD may be helpful in preventing exacerbations. Other adjunctive therapies, including relaxation techniques, nutrition support, pulmonary rehabilitation, and chest physiotherapy, also are commonly used, although data supporting their effectiveness are limited. Patients with COPD who have concomitant heart disease also may have heart failure contributing to and/or causing an exacerbation. Differentiation may be required using chest radiography, physical examination, and echocardiography.

Home Management

Home care is increasingly common for the treatment of mild-to-moderate exacerbations of COPD as well as for patients with end-stage disease. This may require changes and additions to usual care, home care support, and in some cases, noninvasive mechanical ventilation (see Table 14). In addition to usual care (which most commonly will already include treatment with a long-acting bronchodilator), management of an acute exacerbation can include the addition of or increase in dose and/or frequency of a short-acting bronchodilator, specifically a short-acting β_2-agonist, with or without a short-acting anticholinergic agent. Inhaled corticosteroids plus long-acting β_2-agonist or long-acting anticholinergic therapy can shorten recovery time and improve lung function and hypoxemia and may reduce the risk of early relapse, treatment failure, and potential hospitalization. There

is a slight increase in risk for pneumonia in patients using inhaled corticosteroids. Oral corticosteroids should be added if the patient's baseline FEV_1 is less than 50% of predicted. When a patient experiences a COPD flare that does not require hospitalization, treatment with lower-dose oral corticosteroids, tapered more quickly than would be done in a more critically ill patient, is appropriate. Antibiotics are used for patients with some combination of purulent secretions, increased volume of secretions, and/or fever.

Hospital Management

Risk of death from an exacerbation of COPD closely correlates with development of respiratory acidosis, the presence of significant comorbidities, and requirement for ventilatory support. Patients with COPD exacerbations should be hospitalized in the presence of underlying severe COPD, advanced patient age, significant comorbidities, marked increase in intensity of symptoms, newly occurring arrhythmias, diagnostic uncertainty, insufficient home support, onset of new physical signs, or failure to respond adequately to initial medical management. Admission of patients with severe exacerbations to intermediate or special respiratory care units may be appropriate if personnel, skills, and equipment exist to successfully identify and manage acute respiratory failure. Some patients may require direct admission to the intensive care unit (**Table 19**).

Hospital Discharge and Follow-up

After hospitalization for an acute exacerbation of COPD, patients should be discharged when they no longer require short-acting inhaled β_2-agonist therapy more frequently than every 4 hours, are clinically stable and have demonstrated stable arterial blood gas levels for 12 to 24 hours, and can understand the correct use of medications (either personally or through a caretaker). In addition, home nurse visits will often be valuable, especially for elderly patients and those with advanced disease or significant comorbidity. A follow-up visit should occur 2 to 4 weeks after hospital discharge or sooner if clinically necessary. Subsequent treatment is the same as for

TABLE 19. Indications for Immediate Admission to the Intensive Care Unit for COPD Exacerbations

Severe dyspnea that responds inadequately to initial emergency therapy

Changes in mental status (confusion, lethargy, coma)

Despite supplemental oxygen and noninvasive ventilation, the patient has:

Persistent or worsening hypoxemia (arterial Po_2 <40 mm Hg [5.3 kPa]), and/or

Severe/worsening hypercapnia (arterial Pco_2 >60 mm Hg [8.0 kPa]), and/or

Severe/worsening respiratory acidosis (pH <7.25) and requires endotracheal intubation with mechanical ventilation

Hemodynamic instability (need for vasopressors)

CONT.

stable COPD. If the patient required oxygen in the hospital and still needs it at discharge, follow-up at approximately 2 weeks with evaluation of the oxygen level on ambient air should be done to determine continuing need. Pharmacotherapy that includes long-acting inhaled bronchodilators, inhaled corticosteroids, and combination inhalers, in addition to physiotherapy, pulmonary rehabilitation, and patient education, may help to prevent and/or delay future exacerbations and hospitalizations. H

KEY POINTS

- Treatment of COPD exacerbations may involve additions or adjustments to bronchodilator therapy, inhaled or systemic corticosteroid therapy, initiation of antibiotic treatment, possibly mechanical ventilation, or hospitalization in severe exacerbations.
- Home care is increasingly common for the treatment of mild-to-moderate exacerbations of COPD as well as for patients with end-stage disease.
- After hospitalization for a COPD exacerbation, early follow-up is important to reduce hospital readmission rates.

Diffuse Parenchymal Lung Disease

Overview

Diffuse parenchymal lung disease (DPLD) and interstitial lung disease are processes that are grouped together based on similar clinical, radiographic, physiologic, or pathologic findings. The term interstitial lung disease is confusing because these processes often affect airways, vasculature, and pleura in addition to affecting the lung parenchyma. The general rule for these disorders is that they are noninfectious and affect the distal lung parenchyma in varying degrees. These diseases typically present with dyspnea, and imaging studies show abnormalities that are more diffuse than focal. The term DPLD excludes pulmonary hypertension and COPD.

Classification and Epidemiology

Greater than one hundred DPLDs exist, and each of these disorders is rare, particularly when compared with the prevalence of dyspnea associated with heart disease or COPD. The large number of these disorders is often daunting to the general internist and pulmonologist. In clinical practice, it is useful to classify DPLDs into those with known cause or association and those with unknown cause (**Table 20**).

The most common classification of idiopathic DPLD, using the consensus statement of the American Thoracic Society and the European Respiratory Society published in 2001, has led to confusion among clinicians because its histologic basis for diagnosis relies on open lung biopsy and is coupled to an unfamiliar, nonclinical nomenclature (**Table 21**). Clinical diagnosis of DPLD can be complex and should be based on combined information gathered from the history, physiologic testing, imaging, and pathology (when appropriate). A basic understanding of diagnosis and prognosis for the common DPLDs is relevant to the practicing internist.

Previous estimates of DPLD prevalence probably grossly underestimated the true prevalence of these diseases, likely owing to the difficulty of obtaining accurate and complete data from death certificates. Although adult disease estimates vary, overall prevalence rates for DPLD are approximately 70 per 100,000 persons. Approximately 30% to 40% of cases do not have a clear cause.

Diagnostic Approach and Evaluation

History and Examination Features

Evaluation of DPLDs should include a careful history, physical examination, pulmonary function testing, and imaging, which allows the clinician to narrow the differential and identify the potential cause.

The typical time course of DPLD is progressive, with gradually worsening pulmonary symptoms (typically cough and shortness of breath) for greater than 3 months. Because DPLD is rare, a patient with diffuse radiographic changes and symptoms over a 2- to 4-week period should first undergo evaluation for more common causes such as infectious or cardiogenic pulmonary edema. If these causes are ruled out or if the patient does not have an appropriate therapeutic response to medical interventions (such as failure to respond to antibiotic or diuretic therapy), the DPLDs should be considered. The differential diagnosis for DPLDs with acute onset is relatively short (**Table 22**). For patients with the typical gradual time course, progression of disease can be gauged by comparing current exercise tolerance with that from 6 months to 1 year ago.

The cause of disease may be inferred if the patient can relate the onset of symptoms to a specific event; for example, the start of a new medication may cause drug-induced lung disease, or a viral illness may cause bronchiolitis obliterans organizing pneumonia.

Patients should be questioned about exposures, including work- and hobby-related exposures (see Occupational Lung Disease); current and past medications or therapies (radiation exposure, chemotherapy, methotrexate, amiodarone); and exposure to tobacco smoke, dust, birds, mold (water damage in the home may signal underlying mold), or indoor hot tubs.

Family history may provide clues to a potential cause, such as familial pulmonary fibrosis or autoimmune disease.

The pulmonary physical examination should evaluate for basal inspiratory crackles (common in idiopathic pulmonary fibrosis [IPF]), wheezing suggestive of airflow obstruction, and cardiac features of pulmonary hypertension and right-sided

TABLE 20. Classification of the Diffuse Parenchymal Lung Diseases

Known Causes

Connective tissue disease–associated (for example, rheumatoid arthritis, polymyositis, systemic sclerosis)

Hypersensitivity pneumonitis (for example, farmer's lung, hot tub lung, bird fancier's lung)

Pneumoconioses (for example, asbestosis, silicosis, coal worker's pneumoconiosis)

Drug-induced (for example, chemotherapeutic agents, amiodarone, nitrofurantoin)

Smoking-related
   Pulmonary Langerhans cell histiocytosis
   Respiratory bronchiolitis interstitial lung disease
   Desquamative interstitial pneumonia

Acute eosinophilic pneumonia

Radiation-induced

Toxic inhalation–induced (for example, cocaine, zinc chloride [smoke bomb], ammonia)

Unknown Causes: Classified Based on Pathologic Findings	Comments
Idiopathic pulmonary fibrosis	Usual interstitial pneumonia without a cause
Sarcoidosis	
Other idiopathic diffuse parenchymal lung diseases	
Cryptogenic organizing pneumonia	Bronchiolitis obliterans organizing pneumonia without a cause
Nonspecific interstitial pneumonia	
Lymphocytic interstitial pneumonia	
Acute interstitial pneumonia	Diffuse alveolar damage without a risk factor
Chronic eosinophilic pneumonia	
Pulmonary vasculitides	
Pulmonary lymphangioleiomyomatosis	Almost exclusively affects women; lung findings similar to those seen in tuberous sclerosis complex but without skin or central nervous system involvement
Pulmonary alveolar proteinosis	Idiopathic form associated with antibodies to granulocyte-macrophage colony-stimulating factor; also occurs in the setting of occupational exposures (for example, silica dust)
Many other rare disorders	

Adapted from Ryu JH, Daniels CE, Hartman TE, Yi ES. Diagnosis of interstitial lung diseases. Mayo Clin Proc. 2007;82(8):976-986. [PMID: 17673067]. Copyright 2007, Elsevier.

heart failure. Extrapulmonary physical findings include clubbing (common in IPF), arthritis, tenosynovitis, sclerodactyly, and other features of autoimmune disease (especially rheumatoid arthritis and systemic sclerosis).

KEY POINTS

- Evaluation of diffuse parenchymal lung disease should include a careful history, physical examination, pulmonary function testing, and imaging.

- The typical time course of diffuse parenchymal lung disease is progressive, with gradually worsening pulmonary symptoms (typically cough and shortness of breath) for greater than 3 months; acute onset of symptoms should raise suspicion for infectious or cardiogenic pulmonary edema.

High-Resolution CT

High-resolution CT (HRCT) is the gold standard for evaluating parenchymal opacities seen on a plain radiograph. In addition, approximately 20% of patients with DPLD have subtle interstitial abnormalities not detectable on a chest radiograph. For this reason, HRCT should even be considered in symptomatic patients with a normal chest radiograph. The patterns seen on CT correlate with pathologic findings on an open lung biopsy. In certain instances, a thoracic radiologist can confidently identify characteristic radiographic features associated with specific underlying pathology, which will help limit the differential diagnosis. The combination of history, physical examination, serology, and characteristic radiographic studies can often lead to a firm diagnosis and obviate the need for an open lung biopsy in up

TABLE 21. Classification of Idiopathic Diffuse Parenchymal Lung Disease by Histopathologic Features[a]

Histologic Pattern	Clinical-Radiologic-Pathologic Diagnosis
Usual interstitial pneumonia	Idiopathic pulmonary fibrosis/cryptogenic fibrosing alveolitis
Nonspecific interstitial pneumonia	Nonspecific interstitial pneumonia (provisional)[b]
Organizing pneumonia	Cryptogenic organizing pneumonia[c]
Diffuse alveolar damage	Acute interstitial pneumonia
Respiratory bronchiolitis	Respiratory bronchiolitis interstitial lung disease
Lymphoid interstitial pneumonia	Lymphoid interstitial pneumonia

[a]Some cases are unclassifiable for various reasons.

[b]This group represents a heterogeneous group with poorly characterized clinical and radiologic features that needs further study.

[c]Cryptogenic organizing pneumonia is the preferred term, but it is synonymous with bronchiolitis obliterans organizing pneumonia.

Reprinted with permission of the American Thoracic Society. Copyright © 2012 American Thoracic Society. International Multidisciplinary Consensus Classification of the Idiopathic Interstitial Pneumonias. This joint statement of the American Thoracic Society (ATS), and the European Respiratory Society (ERS) was adopted by the ATS board of directors, June 2001 and by the ERS Executive Committee, June 2001 [erratum in Am J Respir Crit Care Med. 2002;166(3):426]. Am J Respir Crit Care Med. 2002;165(2):277-304. [PMID: 11790668]. Official journal of the American Thoracic Society.

TABLE 22. Diffuse Parenchymal Lung Diseases with Acute Onset

Acute interstitial pneumonia
Acute eosinophilic pneumonia
Acute hypersensitivity pneumonitis
Drug-induced pneumonitis
Bronchiolitis obliterans organizing pneumonia
Diffuse alveolar hemorrhage syndromes
Vasculitis

to 60% or more of patients. For those in whom the diagnosis remains unclear, consideration of an open lung biopsy is appropriate.

Pattern and Distribution

The HRCT should be examined for both the pattern and distribution of disease. DPLDs cause the following radiologic patterns, which are readily visualized on HRCT: septal, reticular, nodular, reticulonodular, and ground-glass (**Table 23**). Once the predominant pattern has been determined, the next important consideration is distribution of disease, which may be a clue to the diagnosis (**Table 24**).

Associated Findings

Beyond the lung parenchyma seen on the CT scan, the soft tissue windows help identify associated findings within the mediastinum and pleura that can narrow the differential. Associated findings of pleural plaques may suggest asbestosis. Mediastinal and hilar lymphadenopathy are commonly seen in patients with sarcoidosis, whereas these are rare findings in patients with IPF. Pleural effusions are also rare in patients with IPF. Bony abnormalities may give further clues to other underlying causes such as ankylosing spondylitis.

KEY POINT

- High-resolution CT is the gold standard for evaluating diffuse parenchymal lung disease.

Surgical Lung Biopsy

For patients who have disparate findings on history, physical examination, laboratory studies, or imaging, surgical lung biopsy should be considered. Open lung biopsy via video-assisted thoracoscopic surgery is well tolerated by most patients. Although there are case reports of patients worsening after biopsy, there remains no clear evidence that surgical lung biopsy results in progression of disease. Nonetheless, patients should be screened carefully for perioperative risk, including assessment of lung function, cardiovascular risk, and pulmonary hypertension.

Biopsies should preferably be obtained from areas of the lung that appear grossly normal to the surgeon as well as from grossly abnormal areas. Upper and lower lobes should be biopsied if possible.

An experienced pulmonary pathologist is key to interpretation of the results. It has been shown that communication between the pulmonologist, radiologist, and pathologist often leads to a change in diagnosis that can affect treatment and prognosis discussions with the patient. **H**

KEY POINT

- For patients with diffuse parenchymal lung disease who have disparate findings on history, physical examination, laboratory studies, or imaging, surgical lung biopsy should be considered.

Idiopathic Interstitial Pneumonias

Idiopathic Pulmonary Fibrosis

IPF is the most common idiopathic interstitial pneumonia and has an increased prevalence with increasing age. The

TABLE 23. Pattern of High-Resolution CT Findings in Diffuse Parenchymal Lung Disease

Pattern	Characteristics	Comments
Septal	Short lines that extend to the pleura in the periphery of the lung or as polygonal arcades that outline the pulmonary lobules more centrally	Seen with lymphatic enlargement, most often from pulmonary edema or lymphangitic spread of cancer
Reticular	Interlacing lines that suggest a mesh or lattice	
Nodular	Spherical lesions (<1 cm) that accumulate within the interstitium	Commonly seen in sarcoidosis
Reticulonodular	Intersection of reticular lines or nodules on top of a reticular pattern or vice versa	Seen in sarcoidosis, pulmonary Langerhans cell histiocytosis, and lymphangitic carcinomatosis
Ground-glass	Hazy increased opacity that does not obscure the underlying vascular markings	Seen in desquamative interstitial pneumonia
Consolidation	Denser opacity that obscures vascular markings, unlike ground-glass opacity	
Honeycomb change	Septal lines are coarse and adjacent to cystic areas that stack in the peripheral portion of the lung	Septal lines and honeycomb change are characteristic of but not specific for IPF

IPF = idiopathic pulmonary fibrosis.

hallmark of IPF is peripheral- and basal-predominant disease on CT imaging in a patient with progressive pulmonary symptoms. Physical examination is notable for inspiratory crackles at the bases. Pathologic specimens from open lung biopsy reveal patchy involvement of the lung parenchyma with subpleural predominance, collagen deposition with temporal heterogeneity, and fibroblastic foci as well as areas of normal lung. Inflammation is not a predominant feature of the findings on open lung biopsy. As the disease progresses, cystic areas with epithelial transformation or honeycomb change develop. The parenchymal destruction also leads to a decreased vascular bed, and pulmonary hypertension is common late in the disease course.

Diagnosis is dependent on exclusion of other known causes of DPLD. Characteristic clinical features and CT findings seen in IPF (reticular opacities and honeycombing with a peripheral or basilar predominance and minimal ground-glass opacification) may be adequate to establish the diagnosis without the need for lung biopsy.

The prognosis for patients with IPF remains poor, with a median survival of 3 to 5 years. Multiple studies have failed to demonstrate any benefit of corticosteroid therapy for IPF. Chronic corticosteroids should be avoided because of their extensive side effects.

Patients with IPF are at significant risk for comorbid conditions such as gastroesophageal reflux disease, pulmonary hypertension, obstructive sleep apnea, obesity, and emphysema. Therapies directed toward those comorbidities are appropriate. Because many patients have extensive dyspnea and resultant deconditioning, pulmonary rehabilitation is a reasonable treatment option, with multiple small studies showing improvements in the 6-minute walk test as well as quality of life. In addition, supplemental oxygen for patients with oxygen saturations less than 89% breathing ambient air is appropriate to help improve exercise tolerance.

Patients with IPF have progressive decline in lung function leading to respiratory failure. Disease course is variable; most patients experience slow, steady decline, while a smaller percentage of previously stable patients can experience an acute decline over less than 30 days. The only intervention shown to improve survival in selected patients with IPF is lung transplantation. Given the average age of onset of disease

TABLE 24. Distribution of High-Resolution CT Findings in Diffuse Parenchymal Lung Disease

Distribution	Lung Disease	Comments
Basal predominant	IPF, asbestosis, NSIP	
Upper-lobe predominant	Hypersensitivity pneumonitis, sarcoidosis	
Peripheral	IPF, chronic eosinophilic pneumonia, cryptogenic organizing pneumonia	
Central	Sarcoidosis, pulmonary alveolar proteinosis	
Mosaic attenuation	Pulmonary vascular disease, small airways disease (hypersensitivity pneumonitis, respiratory bronchiolitis–associated interstitial lung disease)	Neighboring lobules have varying density and with small airways disease this is accentuated on expiratory images

IPF = idiopathic pulmonary fibrosis; NSIP = nonspecific interstitial pneumonia.

and the increased comorbidities associated with increasing age, this intervention is only available to a small portion of patients with IPF.

Acute exacerbations in patients with IPF may occur, and the appearance of new ground-glass opacities on chest CT is characteristic. In these patients, evaluation for infection or another treatable cause of the exacerbation (such as pulmonary embolism) is indicated. In patients with advanced disease with a poor prognosis and remote likelihood of recovery from an exacerbation, evidence-based guidelines recommend reducing unnecessary suffering by avoidance of mechanical ventilation and initiating palliation with opioids to decrease dyspnea.

KEY POINTS

- Idiopathic pulmonary fibrosis is the most common idiopathic interstitial pneumonia.

- The hallmark of idiopathic pulmonary fibrosis is peripheral- and basal-predominant disease on CT imaging in a patient with progressive pulmonary symptoms.

- The prognosis for patients with idiopathic pulmonary fibrosis remains poor, with a median survival of 3 to 5 years.

- The only intervention shown to improve survival in selected patients with idiopathic pulmonary fibrosis is lung transplantation.

Nonspecific Interstitial Pneumonia

Nonspecific interstitial pneumonia is most often associated with an underlying connective tissue disease. For example, lung disease related to systemic sclerosis is most often a form of nonspecific interstitial pneumonia. Similar to IPF, the disease is basal predominant but has radiographic ground-glass predominance without evidence of honeycombing.

Open lung biopsy is necessary to make the diagnosis. Findings include a lymphoplasmacytic interstitial infiltration that is uniform and disrupts the normal lung architecture. Pathology may be predominantly cellular with an extensive inflammatory infiltrate or may have areas of collagen deposition with a less predominant cellularity. Varying degrees of both patterns also exist.

When nonspecific interstitial pneumonia is identified on open lung biopsy, a careful history, physical examination, and laboratory evaluation should be performed to rule out an underlying connective tissue disease.

Nonspecific interstitial pneumonia is often responsive to corticosteroids with or without cytotoxic therapy, although recurrence of disease is common with the tapering of immunosuppressive treatment. The cellular form has a significantly better prognosis and response to immunosuppressive regimens. For patients with idiopathic nonspecific interstitial pneumonia, follow-up should include repeat evaluation for

the development of systemic symptoms, because systemic connective tissue disease can present after the development of lung involvement.

KEY POINT

- Nonspecific interstitial pneumonia is most often associated with an underlying connective tissue disease.

Cryptogenic Organizing Pneumonia

Cryptogenic organizing pneumonia (COP) is the idiopathic form of bronchiolitis obliterans organizing pneumonia (BOOP). Many underlying conditions, including infectious diseases, collagen vascular diseases, and drug-induced reactions, are associated with BOOP histopathology and best respond to specific treatment of the primary disease process.

Patients with COP initially present with cough and other symptoms suggestive of community-acquired pneumonia. The diagnosis of COP is more likely to be considered 6 to 8 weeks later, as symptoms and clinical findings persist despite one or more courses of antibiotics. The vast majority of patients have symptoms for less than 3 months, and very few have symptoms for more than 6 months. Radiographic appearance classically consists of bilateral, diffuse alveolar opacities in the presence of normal lung volume. COP can also present with focal consolidation or multiple large nodules or masses, and half of these are peripheral predominant. Although these findings are suggestive of BOOP, they are not specific. Lung biopsy confirms the diagnosis.

Prognosis is typically favorable with a good response to systemic corticosteroids. Recurrences are fairly common with tapering of corticosteroids, but they typically respond to an increase in therapy and slow subsequent taper.

KEY POINT

- Patients with cryptogenic organizing pneumonia initially present with cough and other symptoms suggestive of community-acquired pneumonia; the diagnosis of cryptogenic organizing pneumonia is more likely to be considered 6 to 8 weeks later, as symptoms and clinical findings persist despite one or more courses of antibiotics.

Acute Interstitial Pneumonia

Acute interstitial pneumonia (also known as Hamman-Rich syndrome or idiopathic diffuse alveolar damage) is characterized by rapid onset of disease over days to weeks that results in progressive hypoxemic respiratory failure. Pathology specimens demonstrate diffuse alveolar damage. The clinical presentation is consistent with that of patients with a risk factor for the development of acute respiratory distress syndrome (ARDS). Acute interstitial pneumonia is a diagnosis of exclusion that requires ruling out other potential causes for ARDS (sepsis, pneumonia, inhalational injury) and the other DPLDs that may present acutely. Treatment with corticosteroids is

CONT.

advocated, although data to support this are anecdotal. In addition to corticosteroids, supportive care in the intensive care unit with low tidal volume ventilation is appropriate. Prognosis is poor, with an estimated 50% short-term mortality rate. Patients who recover may relapse or develop chronic interstitial lung disease. **H**

> **KEY POINT**
>
> - Acute interstitial pneumonia is characterized by rapid onset of disease over days to weeks that results in progressive respiratory failure.

Diffuse Parenchymal Lung Disease of Known Cause

Smoking-Related Parenchymal Lung Disease

In a recent review of CT scans from current and past smokers with at least a 10-pack-year history, 8% of scans had evidence of interstitial abnormalities. Of these, 40% had findings of centrilobular micronodules, and current smokers were at the greatest risk for these findings. HRCT imaging findings in smoking-related parenchymal lung disease can range from indistinct centrilobular micronodular disease that is mildly symptomatic (respiratory bronchiolitis–associated interstitial lung disease) to more prevalent micronodular disease to diffuse ground-glass opacities that are present extensively throughout all lung fields (desquamative interstitial pneumonia). Pulmonary Langerhans cell histiocytosis demonstrates thin-walled cysts that are upper-lung predominant with accompanying nodules. All of these diseases typically present in active smokers with subacute, progressive cough and dyspnea. Pulmonary function tests reveal an obstructive pattern with decreased D$_{LCO}$ in patients with severe disease. For those with milder disease, pulmonary function tests can be restrictive, normal, or obstructive. The primary treatment is smoking cessation. Corticosteroids are used in more severe disease but are of uncertain efficacy.

> **KEY POINTS**
>
> - Smoking is associated with several forms of parenchymal lung disease in addition to usual smoking-related findings, and these diseases typically present in active smokers with subacute, progressive cough and dyspnea.
> - The primary treatment for smoking-related parenchymal lung disease is smoking cessation.

Connective Tissue Disease

Pulmonary complications associated with connective tissue diseases are common and can affect the lung parenchyma, pleura, airways, pulmonary vasculature, and musculoskeletal structures of the chest. DPLD typically affects patients with known underlying connective tissue disease, but it can

occasionally be the presenting manifestation. Although controversial, a recent consensus statement placed value in screening patients diagnosed with DPLD but without associated symptoms for underlying connective tissue disease, as identifying an underlying process may affect prognosis and determine treatment strategies for pharmacologic interventions.

For patients who present with pulmonary symptoms, have a history of connective tissue disease, and are being treated with immunomodulating or cytotoxic therapy (such as methotrexate), drug-induced lung disease is part of the differential, as are atypical pulmonary infections. In patients whose pulmonary findings are believed to be associated with their underlying connective tissue disease, treatment is typically with agents that are known to have disease-modifying effects for other features of the patient's connective tissue disease. For patients with stable pulmonary function, treatment strategies are focused on addressing their other systemic symptoms.

For patients with systemic sclerosis, progressive DPLD is the leading cause of mortality. Histopathologic findings are most often consistent with nonspecific interstitial pneumonia; however, oral corticosteroids have not consistently proved to be beneficial. Cyclophosphamide may have some short-term benefit; however, routine treatment with cyclophosphamide or other cytotoxic or immunosuppressive agents has not been established.

Pulmonary disease in rheumatoid arthritis is common, with potential for pleural disease, nodules, bronchitis, bronchiectasis, and acute lung injury. Rheumatoid-associated interstitial lung disease is more common in men than women and may precede musculoskeletal disease. It is typically gradually progressive; patients with rheumatoid arthritis and a definite usual interstitial pneumonia pattern on CT scan have as poor a prognosis as those with IPF. Treatment consists of corticosteroids and disease-modifying agents, but efficacy of these agents remains unclear.

> **KEY POINTS**
>
> - For patients with systemic sclerosis, progressive diffuse parenchymal lung disease is the leading cause of mortality.
> - Pulmonary disease in rheumatoid arthritis is common, with potential for pleural disease, nodules, bronchitis, bronchiectasis, and acute lung injury.

Hypersensitivity Pneumonitis

Hypersensitivity pneumonitis (HP) is caused by repeated inhalation of finely dispersed antigens. The pathogenesis of the disease process remains poorly understood. Antigens can be fungal, bacterial, or protozoal; they may also be animal or insect proteins or small molecular chemical compounds. HP is most frequently caused by thermophilic actinomycetes, fungi, and bird droppings (**Table 25**).

TABLE 25. Hypersensitivity Pneumonitis: Antigen Sources and Associated Diseases

Antigen Source	Associated Disease
Organic Antigens: Bacteria, Fungi, Mycobacteria	
Moldy hay, silage, or grain	Farmer's lung
Potatoes packed in moldy hay	Potato worker's lung
Moldy typesetting water	Bible printer's lung
Moldy cheese	Cheese washer's lung
Aerosolized hot tub water	Hot tub lung
Stagnant humidifier water	Humidifier lung
Moldy cork	Suberosis
Moldy wood dust	Wood dust or wood trimmer's lung
Organic Antigens: Animal Protein	
Bird feathers and droppings	Bird fancier's lung
Processed turkey or chicken serum	Turkey or chicken handler's lung
Animal pelts	Furrier's lung
Laboratory animal dander, serum, excrement	Laboratory worker's lung
Inorganic Antigens	
Diisocyanate(s)	Chemical lung
Aerosolized machine lubricants	Machine operator's lung
Pyrethrum	Pesticide lung

Patients with the acute form of hypersensitivity pneumonitis present with flulike symptoms 4 to 8 hours after intense exposure to the offending antigen. Symptoms include fever, chills, malaise, frontal headache, arthralgia, and myalgia. Pulmonary symptoms include dyspnea, chest tightness, and dry cough. Chest imaging demonstrates bilateral hazy opacities, and HRCT imaging reveals ground-glass opacities with centrilobular nodules in a predominantly upper- and mid-lung distribution. Symptoms resolve after 24 to 48 hours but recur with reexposure to the antigen.

Subacute and chronic forms of hypersensitivity pneumonitis typically occur with chronic low-level exposure to an inhaled antigen. The classic example is exposure to domestic caged birds. The disease process is often insidious with few acute symptoms. Patients ultimately present with dyspnea, cough, fatigue, anorexia, malaise, and weight loss. HRCT demonstrates a similar distribution and pattern as in acute hypersensitivity pneumonitis but also includes evidence of fibrosis with reticular lines, traction bronchiectasis, architectural distortion, and honeycomb change with severe disease.

Pulmonary function testing may show obstructive and restrictive defects. Diagnosis is based on careful history and documentation of an offending antigen. In chronic hypersensitivity pneumonitis, the antigen is often not clearly determined, and the disease process can mimic IPF. In this case, the distribution of findings on the CT scan and histopathologic examination of lung tissue can help differentiate the disease.

Treatment consists of removal of the offending antigen. For patients with modest symptoms, this alone may lead to complete resolution. For those with more severe symptoms, oral corticosteroids should be used in addition to antigen avoidance. In patients with fibrosis and chronic hypersensitivity pneumonitis, treatment initially includes corticosteroids. If there is no response, consideration of cytotoxic therapy is reasonable along with referral of select patients for possible lung transplantation.

KEY POINTS

- Hypersensitivity pneumonitis is caused by repeated inhalation of finely dispersed antigens.
- Treatment of hypersensitivity pneumonitis consists of removal of the offending antigen; oral corticosteroids may be used for patients with severe symptoms.

Drug-Induced and Radiation-Induced Parenchymal Lung Disease

Drug-induced DPLDs are becoming more common owing to the development of new pharmacologic therapies. It may be difficult to determine the culprit drug, and decisions about empirically stopping a medication may be complicated if that drug has an important therapeutic benefit.

Typically, there is a temporal association between the initiation of a drug or offending agent and the development of pulmonary symptoms.

Amiodarone

Amiodarone, a widely used antiarrhythmic agent, has a high incidence of pulmonary toxicity, which is one of the leading causes for discontinuation of the drug. It occurs more commonly in elderly patients, those on higher doses, and those who have accumulated higher doses over time. The pneumonitis may occur within a few days to more than 10 years after continued therapy. However, it typically presents within the first year of treatment. There are several radiographic presentations of amiodarone toxicity (**Table 26**).

Clearance of the drug from the pulmonary parenchyma is very slow; autopsy studies demonstrate the presence of the drug and the metabolite 1 year after discontinuation of amiodarone. As a result, parenchymal abnormalities rarely improve with discontinuation of the drug alone and can recur with tapering of corticosteroids 2 to 3 months after an initial response in some patients.

Methotrexate

Pneumonitis occurs in less than 5% of patients treated with methotrexate. Patients present with insidious onset of fever, cough, and dyspnea with diffuse pulmonary infiltrates. Time to presentation is unpredictable, and there is no correlation between the dose and clinical severity. Radiographs demonstrate diffuse reticular and/or ground-glass attenuation; with more severe cases there can be dense consolidation. Mild to moderate peripheral eosinophils are seen in the peripheral blood in up to two thirds of patients but are not necessarily seen in the pulmonary tissue of those who have undergone biopsy. The pathologic findings most typically show interstitial pneumonitis with granuloma formation resembling hypersensitivity pneumonitis. Other pathologic patterns have been described (although less commonly), including bronchiolitis obliterans organizing pneumonia, diffuse alveolar damage, and bland fibrosis.

Prognosis is generally favorable with discontinuation of the drug and treatment with corticosteroids. As with other drug-induced lung diseases, the dosage and duration of treatment with corticosteroids are based on response and toxicity assessment.

Nitrofurantoin

Nitrofurantoin toxicity presents with acute and chronic forms; the acute form is much more common. It can occur within several days of starting nitrofurantoin and can occur even after previously uneventful treatment courses. It presents with fever, chills, dyspnea, cough, wheezing, myalgia, and chest pain, and a cutaneous rash can occur in 10% to 20% of cases. Peripheral eosinophils are common but are not prominent in lung tissue. Imaging studies demonstrate faint, discrete, bibasilar markings or Kerley B lines; moderate pleural effusions are occasionally present.

The chronic form does not develop after the acute form of the disease but is rather a separate entity that develops months to years after chronic exposure. Patients develop a chronic cough and progressive dyspnea. Imaging studies reveal reticular infiltrates, coarse central lines converging to the hila, subpleural lines, or thickened peribronchovascular areas, and sometimes reduced lung volumes.

Treatment requires discontinuation of the drug; the abnormalities will return if nitrofurantoin is restarted. The benefits of corticosteroid use are not clear for the acute presentation, as it will often resolve on its own with discontinuation of nitrofurantoin. For the chronic form, there is anecdotal evidence that corticosteroids are of benefit.

Radiation Pneumonitis

Patients with radiation pneumonitis present with cough and/or dyspnea approximately 6 weeks after the exposure. CT imaging typically shows hazy opacities with ground-glass attenuation. Affected areas are most commonly found in the field of radiation but can occasionally occur outside the field. For example, patients who have undergone radiation

TABLE 26. Amiodarone Pulmonary Toxicity	
Condition	**Characteristics**
Subacute pneumonitis	Patchy ground-glass diffuse opacities on CT imaging
Single or multiple subpleural masses	Typically abut the pleura and may be associated with chest pain/pleural rub
Pulmonary fibrosis	Dense bibasilar reticular opacities in a patient with dyspnea, hypoxemia, and weight loss; response to corticosteroids is poor
Organizing pneumonia	Migratory fixed alveolar opacities/nodules
Diffuse alveolar damage	Rapidly progressive respiratory failure with diffuse bilateral opacities consistent with pulmonary edema
Alveolar hemorrhage	Unusual presentation; diffuse bilateral opacities on chest radiograph/CT imaging
Subclinical pneumonitis	Normal chest radiograph; patient taking chronic amiodarone; HRCT shows ground glass, septal lines; patients are asymptomatic

HRCT = high-resolution CT.

Adapted from Schwarz MI, King TE. Interstitial lung disease. 4th ed. Hamilton, Ont.; Lewiston, N.Y.: B.C. Decker; 2003. Copyright 2003, Talmadge E. King, Jr., MD.

treatment for breast cancer are known to develop areas of organizing pneumonia in the contralateral lung. The abnormalities in classic radiation pneumonitis typically resolve within 6 months but can progress to a well-demarcated area of fibrosis with volume loss and bronchiectasis. Infections, including opportunistic disease in immunosuppressed patients, should be considered. Treatment of radiation pneumonitis often involves corticosteroids when it is identified early. Corticosteroids, however, are not necessary for all patients and treatment should be determined based on the severity of disease.

KEY POINTS

- Amiodarone, a widely used antiarrhythmic agent, has a high incidence of pulmonary toxicity, which is one of the leading causes for discontinuation of the drug.

- Patients with radiation pneumonitis present with cough and/or dyspnea approximately 6 weeks after the exposure.

Miscellaneous Diffuse Parenchymal Lung Diseases

Sarcoidosis

Sarcoidosis is a multiorgan inflammatory disease characterized by tissue infiltration by mononuclear phagocytes, lymphocytes, and noncaseating granulomas. The cause remains unknown, but there is increasing evidence to suggest it is the end result of interactions among a persistent antigen, HLA class II molecules, and T-cell receptors.

Sarcoidosis presents with varying time courses, ranging from acute disease with erythema nodosum, fever, arthralgia, and hilar lymphadenopathy (Löfgren syndrome) to a more indolent course. Ninety percent of patients will have pulmonary involvement; however, diagnosis is often difficult because symptoms can be nonspecific and may be attributed to other common diseases such as asthma or bronchitis. Pulmonary function tests often show restriction, but obstruction can be seen as well; these findings are not specific to sarcoidosis. Sarcoidosis is a diagnosis of exclusion based on multisystem involvement and histologic evidence of noncaseating granulomas when all other causes are ruled out. Most patients require a tissue diagnosis, but there are some exceptions that do not warrant histologic confirmation. These include classic clinical presentations of known sarcoid syndromes such as Löfgren syndrome and Heerfordt syndrome (uveitis, parotid gland enlargement, and fever).

For patients who require a tissue biopsy, lymphadenopathy is a common presenting manifestation. Multiple studies have shown that endobronchial ultrasound is useful for making a diagnosis and has a sensitivity of greater than 85%. In addition, bronchoscopy with transbronchial biopsies combined with endobronchial biopsies has been shown to have sensitivities as high as 90%.

Sarcoidosis often spontaneously resolves. Staging based on the chest radiography findings can be useful (**Table 27**). Patients with stage II disease have spontaneous remission rates of 90%, while patients with stage III disease have spontaneous remission rates of less than one third. This system's utility is limited by the lack of agreement among radiologists' interpretations. The decision to treat or not should ultimately be based on symptoms. Enthusiasm for treatment is tempered by the potential side effects of therapy and the lack of clear data on the natural history of disease. Corticosteroids are the treatment of choice. A recent report suggested that much lower dosages of corticosteroids may be equally effective for patients with acute respiratory exacerbations of sarcoidosis. This approach may have the benefit of decreased acute side effects and may allow for more rapid tapering.

For a discussion of the musculoskeletal manifestations of sarcoidosis, see MKSAP 16 Rheumatology.

KEY POINTS

- Ninety percent of patients with sarcoidosis will have pulmonary involvement; however, diagnosis is often difficult because symptoms can be nonspecific and may be attributed to other common diseases such as asthma or bronchitis.

- Sarcoidosis is a diagnosis of exclusion based on multisystem involvement and histologic evidence of noncaseating granulomas when all other causes are ruled out.

Lymphangioleiomyomatosis

Lymphangioleiomyomatosis (LAM) is a rare cystic lung disease that occurs sporadically in women of childbearing age or in association with tuberous sclerosis. Advancements in the understanding of the pathophysiology of LAM have identified pulmonary parenchymal infiltration of smooth muscle cells that have inactivating mutations of the tuberous sclerosis complex (TSC) gene. These mutations lead to activation of the mammalian target of the rapamycin (mTOR) pathway. These findings, coupled with

TABLE 27.	Staging of Sarcoidosis
Stage	**Radiographic Pattern**
0	Normal
I	Hilar lymphadenopathy with normal lung parenchyma
II	Hilar lymphadenopathy with abnormal lung parenchyma
III	No lymphadenopathy with abnormal lung parenchyma
IV	Parenchymal changes with fibrosis and architectural distortion

disease recurrence after transplantation, suggest that LAM is a low-grade, metastatic neoplasm that selectively targets the lung.

The diagnosis is based on imaging studies in conjunction with the appropriate clinical context. Although the disease is rare and often initially diagnosed as emphysema, spontaneous pneumothorax and/or chylothorax in a young woman with dyspnea and chest radiography demonstrating hyperinflation should prompt consideration of LAM. Suspicion of LAM should lead to HRCT, which can be diagnostic, with findings of diffuse, thin-walled, small cysts. In addition, elevated vascular endothelin growth factor-D (VEGF-D) can be a specific marker for the diagnosis of LAM compared with other cystic lung diseases.

Originally LAM was thought to be associated with limited survival, but more recent studies demonstrate significant variability in disease progression and survival. The disease is progressive, and lung transplantation remains a therapeutic option for selected patients. Hormonal manipulation and progestin therapy have not been effective. There is some evidence of benefit with biologic immunosuppressant agents, although the safety and efficacy for their routine use are not yet established.

KEY POINT

- Lymphangioleiomyomatosis (LAM) is a rare cystic lung disease that occurs sporadically in women of childbearing age or in association with tuberous sclerosis.

Occupational Lung Disease

Overview

Occupational lung diseases affect all aspects of the pulmonary tree, including the upper airways (rhinitis, laryngitis), lower airways (tracheitis, bronchitis, bronchiolitis, asthma, and COPD), interstitium, parenchyma, and pulmonary vasculature. They are caused by repeated or single, often severe, exposures to irritating or toxic substances. Occupational lung disease includes de novo respiratory ailments as well as exposure-related exacerbations of chronic lung disease. The four broad categories of occupational lung disease are occupational asthma (see Asthma), pneumoconiosis (restrictive lung diseases due to mineral dust inhalation), hypersensitivity pneumonitis (see Diffuse Parenchymal Lung Disease), and acute toxic inhalation syndromes (see Critical Care).

Although many exposure-related respiratory diseases are incurable, all are preventable. Although some patients may have the classic presentation of disease (for example, asbestosis in a retired ship builder with bilateral pleural plaques,

restrictive disease, and interstitial opacities that are basal predominant), it is far more common for occupational exposures to be more difficult to identify. The biologic significance of some exposures may not be known, and new products that may have unknown implications are consistently introduced to the workplace. Clear improvements have been made in occupational safety and health surveillance, but occupational lung disease remains a concern.

When to Suspect an Occupational Lung Disease

Suspicion for exposure-related respiratory disease should increase and the clinical history should be expanded in the following situations:

1. The patient raises concerns that symptoms or signs may be related to an occupational exposure.
2. The patient reports a temporal pattern that follows the work routine (symptoms are aggravated during work and resolve or significantly improve when away from work).
3. The patient's history includes several coworkers with similar symptoms.
4. The patient reports a known hazard at work.
5. There is a lack of therapeutic response to appropriate medical therapy or recurrence of symptoms after an appropriate response.
6. A disorder is diagnosed in a patient without associated risk factors for the disease or who is outside of typical epidemiologic parameters for the disease.
7. Multiple cases of a rare disease are identified in one practice or one geographic area (clustering).

Key Elements of the Exposure History

Obtaining a comprehensive and clinically relevant exposure history is a challenge. It is often difficult to identify all exposures and estimate the concentration of the exposure. In addition, the time until the onset of symptoms or clinical findings following exposure may be prolonged, and the manifestations of occupational lung disease may be highly variable. For example, patients with distant exposure to coal dust are at significant risk for accelerated obstructive lung disease, even without symptoms or evidence of typical coal-associated lung disease and without a smoking history. Therefore, for patients with suspected pneumoconiosis, the history should focus on dust exposures that date back many years; pulmonary function tests should be performed to evaluate for obstructive lung disease if it is suspected. For patients with suspected occupational asthma, the history can focus on the initial onset of symptoms. Questions that constitute a thorough patient history are shown in **Table 28**.

TABLE 28. Elements of a Thorough Patient History for Suspected Occupational Lung Disease

Understand the Occupation

What tasks do you perform at your current job?

How long have you been working at your current job?

What other jobs have you had in the past and for how long?

Understand the Type and Extent of Exposure

Are you exposed to vapors, gases, dust, or fumes in your work?

Do you know the amount and type of chemicals used?

Do you have Material Safety Data Sheets (MSDS) from your workplace?

Is your work environment well ventilated?

Does your employer require you to wear protective equipment? Do you wear it for the full duration of your exposure?

Is there visible dust in the air or on surrounding equipment?

Understand the Temporal Relationship of Symptoms to the Work Environment

Were there any changes to your work process prior to the onset of symptoms?

Do symptoms improve when you are away from the work environment? With vacation?

Understand Other Relevant Exposures

What are your hobbies?

Do you have pets in the home?

What is your travel history?

For patients who work with potentially harmful substances, the U.S. Occupational Safety and Health Administration (OSHA) requires that employers maintain and make available to employees Material Safety Data Sheets (MSDS) that outline potential health risks of specific substances. They may be helpful in assessing the risk of lung disease related to exposure in the workplace.

If the history is unrevealing but there are still concerns that a patient's symptoms may be related to occupational or environmental exposures, referral to an occupational/environmental lung disease specialist should be considered.

KEY POINT

- A thorough history for suspected occupational lung disease includes information on the work process, type and extent of exposure, temporal relationship of symptoms to work, and non–work-related exposures.

Management

Management of these illnesses depends on correct identification of the offending agent and its removal from the environment. Supportive and pharmacologic therapies are often used as well. Workplace or public health response may be appropriate if other individuals are at risk. For the affected employee, worker's compensation needs arise, and assessment of the symptoms attributed to occupational exposure is often challenging. Referral to a specialist may be appropriate for assistance in these areas.

KEY POINT

- Management of occupational lung disease depends on correct identification of the offending agent and its removal from the environment.

Surveillance

Primary prevention through control or removal of adverse exposures in the workplace remains the priority. Surveillance to ensure prevention is of paramount importance. Spirometry can be used in several ways to monitor safety. Longitudinal spirometry measurements can monitor patients who are at high risk owing to their exposures. It can also be used to ensure that primary prevention strategies are effective. Finally, longitudinal spirometry can follow individuals exposed to unclear risk. This allows for early intervention and identification of future safety concerns.

Asbestos-Related Lung Diseases

Epidemiology

Asbestos is a hydrated silicate fiber that occurs naturally and is resistant to acid, alkaline solutions, and heat; it was used extensively in the past as insulation. Respiratory diseases associated with asbestos exposure are shown in **Table 29**. Between 1940 and 1979, approximately 20 million workers in the United States were exposed to asbestos. Owing to the latency of asbestos-related disease (15 to 35 years), it will remain a concern in the United States well into the current century. The incidence of mesothelioma was expected to peak in the United States in 2010; however, asbestos is still used in developing countries.

TABLE 29. Respiratory Diseases Associated with Asbestos Exposure

Pleural Disease

Pleural plaques (localized, often partially calcified)

Diffuse pleural thickening

Rounded atelectasis

Benign pleural effusion

Mesothelioma

Parenchymal Lung Disease

Asbestosis

Lung cancer

Risk Factors

The single most important risk factor for the development of asbestos-related lung disease is the extent of exposure, which, in turn, is closely related to the nature of the industrial exposure. The construction, automotive servicing, and shipbuilding industries are most commonly affected.

KEY POINTS

- The single most important risk factor for the development of asbestos-related lung disease is the extent of exposure.
- The construction, automotive servicing, and shipbuilding industries are most commonly affected by asbestos exposure.

Pathophysiology

Asbestos fiber deposition occurs at airway bifurcations and in the alveolus. Alveolar epithelial cells will transport some fibers to the interstitium, while others will migrate to the pleura through lymphatic channels. The mechanism behind pleural disease is poorly understood. It is likely that well-circumscribed pleural plaques and diffuse pleural fibrosis are distinct entities. Fiber deposition in the lung parenchyma elicits a chronic inflammatory response. This chronic inflammation ultimately leads to proliferation of mesenchymal cells, intra-alveolar fibrosis, and loss of alveolar capillary units; this is known as asbestosis, a form of diffuse parenchymal lung disease.

Pleural Diseases

Pleural plaques are the most common radiographic finding in patients exposed to asbestos (**Figure 12**). Ninety percent of asbestos-induced pleural abnormalities are due to pleural plaques (well-circumscribed lesions) and diffuse pleural thickening. Pleural plaques alone are rarely associated with symptomatic disease and are most often seen as an incidental finding on chest radiograph. Diffuse pleural thickening, on the other hand, is much more likely to be associated with restrictive pulmonary physiology. Very extensive disease can lead to respiratory failure. Surgical decortication is not of clear benefit in these patients and is generally not recommended.

Pleural fibrosis may also lead to the development of rounded atelectasis, which occurs when the lung becomes atelectatic in the region beneath pleural thickening. As the pleural fibrosis continues, the atelectatic lung forms a rounded, mass-like lesion that includes the bronchi and blood vessels; this may be asymptomatic or, if extensive, may lead to pulmonary impairment. These mass-like lesions must be distinguished from malignancy, which can often be done based on radiographic features. Similar to diffuse pleural thickening, surgical intervention is of little benefit.

Benign asbestosis pleural effusion is a diagnosis of exclusion, and it can occur both early and late after exposure. It is often asymptomatic but can be associated with pleuritic chest pain. It is an exudative, often hemorrhagic pleural effusion, and eosinophils are present in 30% of cases. The differential diagnosis includes infection, malignancy (especially mesothelioma), and pulmonary embolism. Most benign effusions resolve spontaneously without further clinical complications.

Asbestos exposure significantly increases the risk of lung cancer (small cell and non–small cell carcinoma) and mesothelioma. Asbestos exposure acts synergistically with

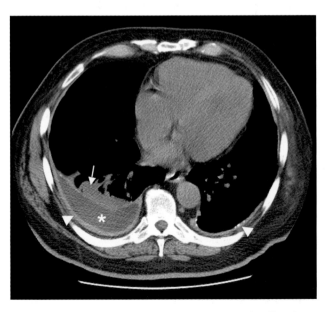
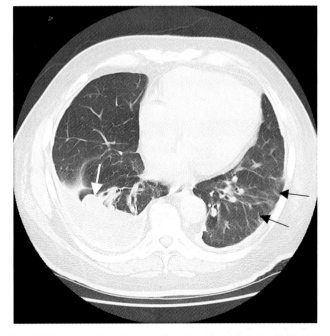

FIGURE 12. Chest CT scan showing complex asbestos-related lung disease. Mediastinal (*left panel*) and lung (*right panel*) windows show bilateral partially calcified pleural thickening (*arrowheads*), asbestosis (*black arrows*), rounded atelectasis on the right with a classic "comet tail" (*white arrows*), and a loculated right-sided benign pleural effusion (*star*).

exposure to tobacco to increase the risk of lung cancer 60-fold compared with patients who do not smoke and who have not had asbestos exposure. For mesothelioma, the latency period is approximately 30 to 40 years (see Lung Tumors).

KEY POINTS

- Asbestos exposure significantly increases the risk of lung cancer (small cell and non–small cell carcinoma) and mesothelioma.

- Asbestos exposure acts synergistically with exposure to tobacco to increase the risk of lung cancer 60-fold compared with patients who do not smoke and who have not had asbestos exposure.

Silicosis

Silicosis is a spectrum of pulmonary diseases related to inhalation of crystalline silicon dioxide (silica). Silica is the most abundant mineral on earth, and the most common form is quartz. Any occupation that disturbs the earth's crust or uses or processes silica-containing rock or sand has potential risks. Several clinical presentations of silicosis are outlined in **Table 30**. Radiographic abnormalities range from simple silicosis to progressive massive fibrosis (**Table 31**).

Silicosis is associated with an increased risk for tuberculosis. Silicosis may also lead to alterations in immune function that have been associated with an increased risk of autoimmune disease, including systemic sclerosis, rheumatoid arthritis, and systemic lupus erythematosus. Silica dust exposure and silicosis may also increase the risk for lung cancer, although this association and magnitude of potential risk are controversial.

There are no specific proven therapies for silicosis. Treatment is symptomatic with inhaled bronchodilators, antibiotics for infections, and supplemental oxygen in patients with hypoxemia. Patients should be screened for tuberculosis. Given the increased risk for infection, corticosteroids are

TABLE 31. Radiologic Findings Associated with Silicosis

Radiographic Abnormality	Characteristics
Simple silicosis	Profusion of small (<10 mm in diameter), rounded nodules that are upper-lung predominant
Progressive massive fibrosis	Enlarging nodules that coalesce to form larger, upper- or mid-lung opacities of >10 mm in diameter; hilar retraction with upper-lobe volume loss and lower-lung hyperinflation

of unclear benefit. For patients who progress to chronic respiratory failure, lung transplantation should be considered.

KEY POINT

- Treatment of silicosis is symptomatic with inhaled bronchodilators, antibiotics for infections, and supplemental oxygen in patients with hypoxemia.

Pleural Disease

Pleural disease is the abnormal accumulation of fluid, air, or tissue within the pleural space.

Pleural Effusion

Approximately 1.5 million pleural effusions are diagnosed in the United States annually. Two thirds of these are caused by heart failure, pneumonia, or malignancy (**Table 32**).

History and Physical Examination

The most common symptoms associated with pleural effusions are dyspnea, pleuritic chest pain, and nonproductive

TABLE 30. Types of Silicosis

Type	Onset and Radiographic Findings	Symptoms, Signs, and Prognosis
Acute silicosis	Develops several weeks to 4-5 years after exposure to high concentrations of respirable crystalline silica; radiographs show alveolar filling process	Cough, weight loss, fatigue, and pleuritic pain; PFTs show mixed obstruction and restriction; PE typically shows crackles; mycobacterial and fungal infections typically complicate course; survival is often less than 4 years from first symptoms
Chronic silicosis	Develops after decades of repeated exposure and is the most common clinical presentation of silicosis; upper-lobe predominant; small nodular is the most common radiographic pattern; minority develop PMF	Occasionally asymptomatic; often with cough and dyspnea; PFTs show mixed obstruction and restriction; PE shows clear breath sounds to increased adventitial sounds, crackles are rare; patients with PMF have increased progression to chronic respiratory failure and cor pulmonale
Accelerated silicosis	Develops less than 10 years after initial exposure; same radiographic appearance as chronic silicosis; higher risk for the development of PMF	Same as chronic silicosis

PE = physical examination; PFT = pulmonary function test; PMF = progressive massive fibrosis.

TABLE 32. Approximate Annual Incidence of Causes of Pleural Effusions in the United States[a]

Cause	Incidence	Percentage
Heart failure	500,000	36.1%
Parapneumonic	300,000	21.7%
Malignant pleural effusion	200,000	14.5%
Pulmonary embolism	150,000	10.9%
Viral illness	100,000	7.3%
Cirrhosis with ascites	50,000	3.6%
Post–coronary artery bypass surgery	50,000	3.6%
Gastrointestinal disease (for example, hepatic hydrothorax, pancreatitis, esophageal rupture)	25,000	1.8%
Tuberculosis	2500	0.19%
Mesothelioma	2300	0.16%
Benign asbestos disease	2000	0.15%

[a]Approximately 1.5 million pleural effusions are diagnosed in the United States annually. The sum of less common causes makes up the remaining roughly 120,000 cases of pleural effusion diagnosed annually.

CONT.

cough. Additional features such as weight change, fever, arthralgia, and orthopnea help further narrow the differential diagnosis. History of malignancy, cardiac or abdominal surgery, myocardial infarction, tuberculosis, asbestos exposure, medications, and travel should be elicited.

Examination clues include digital clubbing, joint deformities, synovitis, and stigmata of end-stage liver or heart failure. Most pleural effusions are initially identified on plain radiography. Chest radiographs and chest CT are useful in identifying air within the pleural space and defining pulmonary infiltrates and masses that may be pertinent to the evaluation of the effusion. Thoracic ultrasound is also useful in the evaluation of a pleural effusion. Ultrasound localization of the effusion enhances the safety and success of thoracentesis, and ultrasound characterization can also offer clues to the underlying cause of the effusion. Septations and fluid echo density approaching that of the liver suggest an exudative process, and pleural-based nodules suggest a malignant process. Ultrasound is also effective in differentiating fluid from lung consolidation and assessing diaphragmatic dysfunction and pleural thickening.

Pleural fluid testing is rarely diagnostic but, rather, supports or refutes the prethoracentesis differential diagnosis and points to additional studies that may be needed.

KEY POINTS

- Heart failure, pneumonia, and malignancy are the most common causes of pleural effusions.

- Pleural fluid testing is rarely diagnostic but, rather, supports or refutes the prethoracentesis differential diagnosis and points to additional studies that may be needed.

Pleural Fluid Analysis

Thoracentesis is not necessary in patients who develop small pleural effusions associated with heart failure, pneumonia, or heart surgery. Unexplained effusions measuring greater than 1 cm (1 cm between the lung and chest wall on chest radiograph) should be aspirated.

The initial pleural fluid analysis is used to define the fluid as either transudative or exudative; this is usually done by testing for concurrent serum and pleural fluid protein and lactate dehydrogenase levels. Additional initial studies are used to further characterize the fluid and usually include the pH, glucose, cell count with differential, Gram stain, and cultures. Further studies are used to assess for specific diagnoses and should not routinely be obtained initially unless there is a high degree of clinical suspicion. These tests include cytology, triglycerides, amylase, N-terminal pro–B-type natriuretic peptide, adenosine deaminase, and specific tumor markers.

Transudate or Exudate Characterization

The criteria most frequently used to determine whether pleural fluid is transudative or exudative are (1) pleural fluid total protein to serum total protein ratio greater than 0.5; and (2) pleural fluid lactate dehydrogenase level greater than two thirds the upper limit of normal. If either of these criteria is met, the fluid is almost always an exudate; if neither criterion is met, the fluid is almost always a transudate (**Table 33**). The specificity of these measures decreases in the setting of a transudative process with ongoing diuresis, which may make the fluid appear more exudative. In this instance it is reasonable to determine the serum to pleural fluid protein or albumin gradient (the difference between the serum and pleural values). If the total protein gradient is greater than 3.1 g/dL (31 g/L)

TABLE 33. Causes of Transudative Pleural Effusions	
Diagnosis	**Comment**
Common Causes	
Heart failure	Most common cause of transudative effusion; diuresis can cause borderline exudative chemical characteristics
Atelectasis	Small effusion caused by negative transpleural pressure
Hepatic hydrothorax	Most are right-sided; occurs in 6%-12% of patients with end-stage liver disease and clinical ascites; can occur in the absence of ascites
Hypoalbuminemia	Small bilateral effusions with evidence of generalized anasarca, from decreased intravascular oncotic pressure
Constrictive pericarditis	Usually bilateral with normal heart size; 95% have jugular venous distention
Trapped lung	Unilateral as a result of remote pleural inflammation and resultant unexpandable lung; caused by negative transpleural pressure
Uncommon Causes	
Cerebrospinal fluid leak into pleural space (duropleural fistula)	Caused by trauma or thoracic spinal surgery
Urinothorax	Unilateral effusion caused by ipsilateral obstructive uropathy; the only low-pH transudate
Iatrogenic	Caused by a central venous catheter misdirected into the pleural space
Superior vena cava obstruction	From acute systemic venous hypertension or lymphatic congestion
Peritoneal dialysis	Massive effusion; develops within 48 hours of initiating dialysis due to dialysate crossing into the chest because of congenital or acquired defects

or the albumin gradient is greater than 1.2 g/dL (12 g/L), then the underlying process is likely transudative.

Cell Counts and Differential

Although pleural fluid cell counts are neither sensitive nor specific, they are helpful in narrowing the differential diagnosis. Pleural fluid appears red if 5000 to 10,000 erythrocytes per microliter (5.0 to 10×10^9/L) are present. Frank hemothorax is diagnosed if the pleural fluid hematocrit is greater than 50% of the peripheral hematocrit. Transudates can be tinged with blood, although grossly bloody effusions are associated with trauma, cancer, or tuberculosis.

A leukocyte count greater than 10,000 per microliter (10×10^9/L) implies infection, but such levels can also be seen in noninfectious processes. Transudative processes typically have a leukocyte count less than 1000 per microliter (1.0×10^9/L).

The presence of neutrophils implies acute inflammation or infection. Pneumonia may be associated with a pleural effusion, which is termed a parapneumonic effusion. These are classified as either uncomplicated or complicated. An uncomplicated parapneumonic effusion represents the influx of interstitial lung fluid and neutrophils into the pleural space; although exudative, uncomplicated parapneumonic effusions do not require drainage and tend to resolve with improvement of the pneumonia. A complicated parapneumonic effusion additionally involves bacterial invasion of the pleural space; these effusions may respond to antibiotics alone but often require drainage to speed recovery and decrease the risk

of long-term pleuropulmonary complications. An empyema is pus in the pleural space and invariably requires drainage and antibiotic therapy. Other causes of inflammation on pleural fluid analysis include pancreatitis, pulmonary embolus, subphrenic abscess, or early tuberculosis.

Lymphocyte predominance is most often seen in cancer or tuberculosis but may be noted in a broad differential diagnosis. If no diagnosis is established in an exudative, lymphocyte-predominant effusion by pleural fluid analysis, pleural biopsy is indicated to exclude tuberculosis or malignancy. Approximately one third of transudative effusions are lymphocyte predominant, which is of no significance.

The presence of greater than 10% eosinophils is usually due to air or blood in the pleural space. If pleural fluid eosinophilia is not due to air or blood, other causes (including medications, fungal infections, parasitic disease, eosinophilic pneumonia, Churg-Strauss syndrome, and benign asbestos pleural effusions) should be considered. As many as 35% of patients with pleural fluid eosinophilia will not have an identifiable cause.

Chemistries

A pleural fluid glucose level less than 60 mg/dL (3.33 mmol/L) is most commonly due to tuberculosis, parapneumonic effusion, malignant effusion, or rheumatoid disease. In parapneumonic effusions, a low glucose level implies the need for chest tube drainage. In malignant effusions, a low glucose level predicts a high yield on cytology, poor result of pleurodesis, and a poorer prognosis. A low glucose level has the

CONT.

same implications as a low pH in parapneumonic and malignant disease, but unlike pH, accuracy is less dependent on sampling technique and handling.

A pleural fluid pH less than 7.2 is seen in complicated parapneumonic effusions, esophageal rupture, rheumatoid and tuberculous pleuritis, malignant pleural disease, systemic acidosis, paragonimiasis, lupus pleuritis, or urinothorax. The pH correlates with the glucose level but tends to fall before the glucose. Collection and processing of samples for pH must be done carefully. Analysis must be run on a blood gas analyzer within 1 hour. Even miniscule amounts of air raise the pH, and very small amounts of lidocaine (as small as 0.2 mL) lower it.

A pleural fluid triglyceride level greater than 110 mg/dL (1.2 mmol/L) suggests the diagnosis of a chylothorax, which is further confirmed by finding chylomicrons on lipoprotein analysis. Chylothorax is further suggested by a milky white pleural fluid appearance, which is seen in about half of patients with chylothorax. A triglyceride level less than 50 mg/dL (0.6 mmol/L) makes chylothorax unlikely.

Tests for Tuberculous Effusions

Worldwide, tuberculosis is the leading cause of exudative pleural effusion. In the United States, 1000 cases of tuberculous effusion are diagnosed annually, and they occur in 3% to 5% of patients with tuberculosis. Only 20% have active parenchymal disease at the time effusion is diagnosed. The effusions spontaneously resolve within 2 to 4 months, but most of these patients progress to active tuberculosis within 5 years. Any lymphocyte-predominant exudate in the presence of a positive purified protein derivative test is considered tuberculous until proved otherwise, and this may be an indication for antituberculous therapy while diagnostic studies are pending. Those studies include pleural biopsy (with either granulomas or positive culture results in 80%-90%), pleural fluid smear (positive in <5%), and culture (positive in approximately 25%). Adenosine deaminase is elevated in many inflammatory conditions, but it is highest (>70 units/L) in tuberculosis and has a negative predictive value approaching 100% when less than 40 units/L. Other pleural fluid clues to tuberculosis are absence of mesothelial cells and eosinophils and a protein level greater than 5 g/dL (50 g/L).

Tests for Pleural Malignancy

A massive, unilateral effusion increases the likelihood of malignancy. Diagnostic yield increases with sequential samplings in patients with a malignant effusion. Approximately 65% of malignant effusions are positive after a single thoracentesis with cytology. Repeating thoracentesis for cytology in those with a negative result will diagnose malignancy in an additional 27% with the second sampling, and 5% with the third. Diagnostic yield does not increase appreciably following the third thoracentesis or with closed pleural biopsy.

Thoracoscopic pleural biopsy is indicated for all undiagnosed exudative pleural effusions following three pleural fluid samplings. Thoracoscopic biopsy is more than 90% sensitive for pleural malignancy. Closed pleural biopsy is less sensitive than cytology for pleural malignancy and should not be performed.

Flow cytometry is useful with lymphocyte-predominant effusions when lymphoma is a diagnostic consideration.

KEY POINTS

- Thoracentesis is not necessary in patients who develop small (<1 cm) pleural effusions associated with heart failure, pneumonia, or heart surgery.
- The initial pleural fluid analysis should focus on characterizing the fluid as either transudative or exudative.

Management
Parapneumonic Effusions and Empyema

Pleural space infections are on the rise worldwide and carry a 15% to 20% mortality rate. Causative bacteria vary regionally, although they mimic the bacteria that cause pneumonia. Common causative bacteria include *Streptococcus pneumoniae*, *Streptococcus milleri*, *Staphylococcus aureus*, and Enterobacteriaceae. Anaerobic bacteria are isolated in up to 36% to 76% of empyemas. Small (<1 cm), free-flowing parapneumonic effusions can be safely managed with antibiotics and can be followed serially. Most of these will resolve without consequences. Factors associated with a more complicated course include large effusions (greater than one half of a hemithorax), septations and areas of loculation, pleural fluid pH less than 7.2, glucose level less than 60 mg/dL (3.33 mmol/L), and positive pleural fluid Gram stain or culture. Effusions with any of these complicating factors should be treated with antibiotics and pleural drainage. Smaller thoracostomy tubes are effective and are less uncomfortable for the patient. Intrapleural tissue plasminogen activator combined with deoxyribonuclease has been shown to increase pleural drainage, decrease hospital length of stay, and decrease need for surgery in empyema. Effusions refractory to antibiotics and drainage with or without tissue plasminogen activator and deoxyribonuclease require surgical debridement.

Malignant Pleural Effusion

The primary objective in managing malignant pleural effusions is to palliate symptoms. For slowly reaccumulating effusions, serial therapeutic thoracentesis is reasonable. For symptomatic effusions that reaccumulate rapidly, more definitive management is required. Worldwide, chemical pleurodesis with talc, applied via chest tube or thoracoscopically, is most common. The success rate is greater than 90% when the lung is shown to fully re-expand. More recently, placement of a tunneled indwelling pleural catheter has gained popularity owing to its ability to provide symptom palliation while avoiding

CONT.

hospitalization. Other options, such as placement of a pleuroperitoneal shunt or surgical pleurectomy, are rarely used. H

KEY POINTS

- Small (<1 cm), free-flowing parapneumonic effusions can be safely managed with antibiotics and can be followed serially.
- Complicated parapneumonic effusions are large, have septations and areas of loculation, positive Gram stain or culture, and low pH and glucose; they should be treated with antibiotics and pleural drainage.

H Pneumothorax

Pneumothorax can occur spontaneously or iatrogenically. Spontaneous pneumothorax is classified as primary if lung disease is absent and as secondary if lung disease is present.

The most important risk factor for primary spontaneous pneumothorax is smoking. Other risk factors include family history, Marfan syndrome, and thoracic endometriosis. Lifetime recurrence rate ranges between 25% and 50%, with most recurrences coming in the first year.

Chronic obstructive lung disease is the most common risk factor for secondary spontaneous pneumothorax. Other causes include cystic fibrosis, tuberculosis, and *Pneumocystis jirovecii* infection. Secondary pneumothorax is more likely to be symptomatic, life threatening, and recurrent owing to underlying lung disease.

Initial management for a large, hemodynamically significant pneumothorax is the same regardless of whether it is primary or secondary. Patients require high-flow supplemental oxygen, emergent needle thoracostomy, and chest tube placement. All of these patients require hospitalization.

Smaller pneumothoraces are managed differently depending on whether they are primary or secondary spontaneous pneumothoraces. For primary spontaneous pneumothoraces, small pneumothoraces (defined as <2 cm between the lung and chest wall on chest radiograph) with minimal symptoms may be managed with observation and serial chest radiography. If the pneumothorax is greater than 2 cm or has more than minimal symptoms, a simple aspiration may be attempted, and a chest tube should be placed if reaccumulation is seen on repeat chest radiograph. If the chest tube sufficiently vacates the pneumothorax, then outpatient follow-up with a chest physician is reasonable. Referral to a thoracic surgeon should be made for persistent air leaks. No additional therapy is needed until a second episode occurs.

For secondary spontaneous pneumothoraces, inpatient management is indicated. Even small (<2 cm) secondary pneumothoraces are more safely observed in the inpatient setting. Pneumothoraces larger than 2 cm should be managed with simple aspiration or chest tube placement as for primary spontaneous pneumothoraces; however, given the higher risk for recurrence and a poor outcome, definitive management to

prevent recurrence is recommended after a single event. Definitive management to prevent recurrence typically consists of chemical pleurodesis via thoracostomy, which is shown to reduce lifetime recurrence to 25%, or thoracoscopic repair with pleurodesis, which reduces recurrence to approximately 5%. The same therapy would be used for recurrent episodes of primary pneumothorax.

Tension pneumothorax can occur with any form of pneumothorax, whether it be iatrogenic, traumatic, or primary or secondary spontaneous. Patients with tension pneumothorax will often present with dyspnea and chest pain in the setting of hemodynamic instability. Tracheal deviation, jugular venous distention, and subcutaneous crepitus may or may not be evident. Management of tension pneumothorax consists of high-flow supplemental oxygen, immediate thoracic decompression (by insertion of a cannula into the pleural space at the second intercostal space along the midclavicular line and aspiration until clinical stability is achieved), and immediate placement of a thoracostomy tube. H

KEY POINTS

- Initial management for a large, hemodynamically significant pneumothorax is the same regardless of whether it is primary or secondary and consists of high-flow supplemental oxygen, emergent needle thoracostomy, and chest tube placement.
- For primary spontaneous pneumothoraces, small pneumothoraces with minimal symptoms may be managed with observation alone.
- For secondary spontaneous pneumothoraces, inpatient management is indicated; even small (<2 cm) pneumothoraces are more safely observed in the inpatient setting.

Pulmonary Vascular Disease

Acute Pulmonary Thromboembolism

Pathophysiology and Epidemiology

The vast majority of acute pulmonary emboli (PE) arise from deep venous thrombosis (DVT) involving the veins at or above the popliteal fossae. The thrombus dislodges and migrates to the pulmonary arterial circulation as PE. Approximately 10% to 30% of untreated DVT leads to PE. The physiologic impact of acute PE depends on the patient's underlying cardiopulmonary condition, the total volume of the pulmonary vascular bed obstructed by thromboses, and the rapidity of the occlusion. The most important clinical effects are acute increases in pulmonary arterial and right ventricular pressures, decrease in cardiac output, and ventilation/perfusion mismatching that produces gas exchange perturbations.

Acute PE incidence is estimated at 1 to 2 per thousand person-years, but it may be as high as 1% in persons 75 years or older and is significantly higher in hospitalized patients. Its incidence may be increasing. As many as 300,000 persons die annually in the United States from acute PE. An increasing proportion of fatal PE may arise from hospital-acquired DVT, raising the possibility of improved outcomes with more aggressive prevention strategies (see MKSAP 16 Hematology and Oncology).

Risk Factors

Risk factors for thromboembolism (**Figure 13**) are summarized in the Thrombotic Disorders chapter of MKSAP 16 Hematology and Oncology. Beyond those specific examples, the risk for thromboembolism approximately doubles for each decade beyond age 60 years. Lengthy air travel has also been established as a risk factor for thromboembolism; the magnitude is generally low but increases by approximately 18% for each 2-hour increment in a trip.

Diagnosis

Clinical Assessment

Diagnosis of PE is complicated by its variable clinical presentation and the lack of sensitivity and specificity of PE symptoms and signs. Many patients with confirmed PE have few symptoms, and symptoms may be nonspecific. The most common symptoms and signs are tachypnea (92%), chest or pleuritic pain (85%), dyspnea (84%), anxiety (59%), crackles (58%), cough (53%), and increased intensity of the pulmonic component of S_2 (53%). The presence and severity of these clinical manifestations are not good indicators of the size or extent of the PE; however, the absence of dyspnea or tachycardia reduces the likelihood of PE. Despite these diagnostic challenges, well-validated clinical risk prediction scores such as the Wells (**Table 34**) or Revised Geneva (**Table 35**) scores can generate a pretest probability of PE. Assessment of PE pretest probability (low, intermediate, or high) and hemodynamic status is essential to guide additional cost-effective evaluation and may aid in the interpretation of subsequent tests.

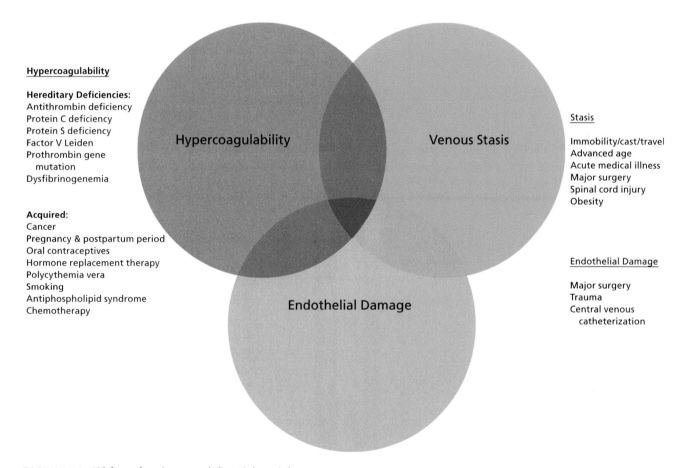

Hypercoagulability

Hereditary Deficiencies:
Antithrombin deficiency
Protein C deficiency
Protein S deficiency
Factor V Leiden
Prothrombin gene
  mutation
Dysfibrinogenemia

Acquired:
Cancer
Pregnancy & postpartum period
Oral contraceptives
Hormone replacement therapy
Polycythemia vera
Smoking
Antiphospholipid syndrome
Chemotherapy

Stasis

Immobility/cast/travel
Advanced age
Acute medical illness
Major surgery
Spinal cord injury
Obesity

Endothelial Damage

Major surgery
Trauma
Central venous
  catheterization

FIGURE 13. Risk factors for pulmonary embolism: Virchow triad

Data from Tapson VF. Acute pulmonary embolism. N Engl J Med. 2008;358(10):1037-1052. [PMID: 18322285]

TABLE 34. Wells Prediction Score for Pretest Probability of Pulmonary Embolism

Variable	Points
DVT symptoms and signs	3.0
PE as likely as or more likely than alternative diagnosis	3.0
Heart rate >100/min	1.5
Immobilization or surgery within the past 4 weeks	1.5
Previous DVT or PE	1.5
Hemoptysis	1.0
Cancer	1.0

Clinical (Pretest) Probability Estimate of PE[a]	Total Score
Low	<2.0
Moderate	2.0-6.0
High	>6.0

DVT = deep venous thrombosis; PE = pulmonary embolism.

[a]A Modified Wells Scoring System provides a dichotomous approach as follows:

Score >4 indicates that PE is "likely" (consider imaging for confirmation).

Score ≤4 indicates that PE is "unlikely" (consider D-dimer for further evaluation).

Adapted from Wells PS, Anderson DR, Rodger M, et al. Derivation of a simple clinical model to categorize patients probability of pulmonary embolism: increasing the models utility with the SimpliRED D-dimer. Thromb Haemost. 2000;83(3):416-420. [PMID: 10744147]. Copyright 2000, International Society on Thrombosis and Haemostasis.

TABLE 35. Revised Geneva Scoring System for Pretest Probability of Pulmonary Embolism

Variable	Points
Risk Factors	
Age >65 years	1
Previous DVT or PE	3
Surgery under general anesthesia or fracture of lower limbs within 1 month	2
Active cancer (solid or hematologic, currently active or considered cured <1 year)	2
Symptoms	
Unilateral lower limb pain	3
Hemoptysis	2
Clinical Signs	
Heart rate 75-94/min	3
Heart rate ≥95/min	5
Pain on lower-limb deep venous palpation and unilateral edema	4

Clinical (Pretest) Probability Estimate of PE	Total Score
Low	0-3
Intermediate	4-10
High	≥11

DVT = deep venous thrombosis; PE = pulmonary embolism.

Reprinted from Le Gal G, Righini M, Roy PM, et al. Prediction of pulmonary embolism in the emergency department: the revised Geneva score. Ann Intern Med. 2006;144(3):165-171. [PMID: 16461960]. Copyright 2006, American College of Physicians.

KEY POINTS

- Diagnosis of pulmonary embolism is complicated by its variable clinical presentation and the lack of sensitivity and specificity of symptoms and signs.

- The use of well-validated scoring systems to generate pretest clinical probability of pulmonary embolism is essential to guide diagnostic test selection.

Biomarker Assays

Measurement of blood D-dimer using a highly sensitive quantitative enzyme-linked immunosorbent assay (ELISA) is helpful in assessing clinically stable patients with a low pretest likelihood of PE using one of the validated scoring approaches. In this setting, a negative test indicates a low enough likelihood of PE and DVT that no further testing is indicated. Using this method, up to 30% of patients with suspected PE will require no further study. In patients with intermediate or high pretest probability of PE, however, a negative D-dimer test is not sufficient to rule out the disease. Conversely, a positive D-dimer test is not specific for PE and is seen in other conditions that are prevalent in hospitalized patients. For these reasons, D-dimer tests should generally not be done for patients with a moderate or high risk of PE or in hospitalized patients.

Although not useful in establishing or excluding the diagnosis and not routinely obtained in the evaluation for PE, an elevated B-type natriuretic peptide (BNP) level, elevated serum troponin level, hyponatremia, and cardiac ultrasound showing acute right-sided heart strain all suggest a worse prognosis; however, the use of such risk markers in choosing more aggressive (and more toxic) primary treatment with thrombolytic agents rather than heparin remains controversial.

KEY POINTS

- In clinically stable patients with a low pretest probability of pulmonary embolism, a normal D-dimer assay effectively excludes pulmonary embolism and eliminates the need for further testing.

- In patients with intermediate or high pretest probability of pulmonary embolism, a D-dimer assay adds little information, and further evaluation is usually required.

Chest Radiography and Electrocardiography

Findings on chest radiography and electrocardiography are nonspecific and are most useful for excluding other conditions such as pneumonia, pneumothorax, and acute myocardial infarction. Plain radiography abnormalities (including atelectasis, elevated hemidiaphragm, small pleural effusion, and findings of underlying chronic lung disease), when they occur, are usually too nonspecific to be clinically useful. Pleural effusions tend to be unilateral, small to moderate (one third of the hemithorax or smaller), and typically do not recur if drained. The Westermark sign of focal oligemia distal to a PE and Hampton hump (a peripheral conical density with the base apposed to the chest wall) are more specific but are not commonly seen.

The electrocardiogram is most likely to be normal or show nonspecific changes like tachycardia. Signs of right-sided heart strain (P-pulmonale, right axis deviation, right bundle branch block, S1Q3T3 pattern) are uncommon but may suggest the presence of a large clot burden.

Other Imaging Studies

CT angiography (CTA), using a multidetector spiral scanning system, is increasingly being used as the primary diagnostic method for suspected PE. Although somewhat dependent on radiologic interpretation and the size and location of the embolus, the sensitivity and specificity for detection of PE are typically greater than 90%. CTA may also provide clues to possible alternative diagnoses in patients with symptoms consistent with PE. CTA is particularly helpful when the chest radiograph is abnormal, which would make interpretation of a ventilation/perfusion (V/Q) scan more difficult. Potential drawbacks of CTA include availability, significant radiation dose, and exposure to contrast dye. Morbidly obese patients may require an open scanner and results may be suboptimal. CTA has the potential to be extended to allow imaging of the venous phase and the lower extremities (CT venography), but the exact role of such extended study is uncertain at this time. Alternatively, magnetic resonance angiography and thigh magnetic resonance venography may be considered for patients with contraindication (such as dye allergy) to these other studies and at centers with experience in these techniques.

V/Q lung scanning remains an option and can be used when CTA is not available or is contraindicated. V/Q scanning has the advantages of relatively low radiation dose and no requirement for contrast dye. V/Q scanning is most useful in patients with normal cardiopulmonary status prior to the acute illness; V/Q test results may be unreliable in patients with COPD and other conditions in which there is structural lung disease or if holding the breath is difficult. Interpretation of V/Q scanning is highly dependent on the pretest likelihood of the presence of PE. Because of this, the sensitivity may range from 50% to 98% and specificity from 20% to 60%. The highest specificity is attained with multiple large (lobar or segmental) perfusion defects without anatomically matching ventilation abnormalities. Normal results effectively exclude PE; multiple, large, mismatched results in

the setting of high pretest probability confirm PE. Other results are usually considered nondiagnostic.

Because of the close relationship between lower-extremity DVT and PE, compression ultrasonography of the legs to detect evidence of clots has an important role in evaluating patients with high pretest probability of acute PE. Ultrasonography may be especially useful in situations in which dye or radiation exposure is undesirable (for example, dye allergy or pregnancy, respectively). If DVT is identified on ultrasonography, therapy should be initiated for DVT and the presumed PE because treatment for both conditions is similar. If no DVT is identified or when direct confirmation of PE is required (such as when a patient is a candidate for thrombolysis of PE or when there is uncertainty in some aspect of the clinical picture), chest imaging will be needed. Conversely, if the diagnosis of PE is initially made with chest imaging (CT or V/Q scanning), lower extremity ultrasonography is not necessary to evaluate for DVT.

Conventional pulmonary angiography, usually with digital subtraction, is invasive; therefore, it is reserved for patients in whom uncertainty remains after CTA or when direct measurement of hemodynamic parameters is needed to guide management.

Echocardiography can be a useful adjunct in assessing selected patients with suspected or confirmed PE. In patients who are too unstable for CTA or V/Q scanning, echocardiographic findings such as elevated pulmonary artery systolic pressure, right ventricular dilatation/hypokinesis, paradoxical septal motion, and/or diminished left ventricular size support a diagnosis of acute PE, particularly when pretest probability is intermediate or high.

KEY POINTS

- Pulmonary CT angiography is becoming the primary method for diagnosis of pulmonary embolism because of high sensitivity and specificity.
- Alternative diagnostic methods for pulmonary embolism, including ventilation/perfusion scanning, are options when CT angiography is not available or is contraindicated owing to kidney disease or sensitivity to contrast media.

Acute Treatment

The initial focus of PE treatment is stabilization with assessment of hemodynamic stability and hypotension.

Hemodynamically Stable Patients

For patients who are hemodynamically stable, the next step is generally prevention of additional clot formation through treatment with anticoagulants while natural lysis of the existing clots occurs over a period of weeks.

When treating acute PE, it is essential to initiate anticoagulation immediately and achieve therapeutic levels of anticoagulation within 24 hours; failure to do so correlates with an increased risk of clinical progression and recurrence. Anticoagulation can be achieved with unfractionated heparin (either intravenous or subcutaneous), subcutaneous low-molecular-weight heparin (LMWH), or the pentasaccharide fondaparinux (**Table 36**). Contraindications to anticoagulation (such as active internal bleeding, recent hemorrhagic stroke) pertain to all anticoagulant agents, whereas drug allergies are class specific. Other conditions such as bleeding diathesis, history of gastrointestinal bleeding, brain metastasis, or recent surgery are best considered in terms of the risk/benefit ratio of anticoagulation and on an individual basis.

Unfractionated heparin should be administered in a fixed-dose, weight-adjusted manner, typically via continuous intravenous infusion in the hospital. Activated partial thromboplastin time (aPTT) should be monitored and the dose should be adjusted appropriately.

Comparable anticoagulation may be achieved using a fixed dose of LMWH, which does not require aPTT monitoring and is administered subcutaneously. Avoiding the need for monitoring and intravenous access for a continuous intravenous infusion may make LMWH preferable to unfractionated heparin for initial therapy in some patients with acute PE. LMWH also is preferred when patients with PE no longer require hospitalization but continue to require heparin treatment because they have not yet achieved a therapeutic warfarin effect. LMWH is cleared by the kidneys and should not be used when there is significant reduction in kidney function, unless plasma Xa levels can be monitored and dose adjustments can be made according to those levels. A similar approach should be taken in patients with morbid obesity. LMWH has a long half-life and should be avoided if heparin will likely need to be withheld for procedures or if the patient is unstable or has a high risk of bleeding.

Fondaparinux also requires no coagulation monitoring. Fondaparinux is also cleared by the kidneys and should not be used in patients with kidney disease.

Unfractionated heparin and LMWH should not be used in the setting of suspected or proven heparin-induced thrombocytopenia (HIT). Treatment with fondaparinux in patients with HIT is uncertain because there is currently insufficient clinical evidence to recommend its routine use.

Warfarin is generally begun at the time one of the previously mentioned agents is started and is usually continued for 4 to 5 days, including several days after achieving a therapeutic INR. Overlapping therapy with warfarin and one of the previously mentioned agents should be continued until a therapeutic INR is documented for 2 or more consecutive days; this ensures that all vitamin K–dependent factors have declined and physiologic anticoagulation has been reliably achieved.

With appropriate early risk stratification, it is possible to identify patients who might be candidates to have most or all of their treatment as outpatients. This includes hemodynamically stable patients with normal biomarkers/cardiac ultrasound, no significant comorbidities (such as cancer, heart failure, COPD) or need for supplemental oxygen, younger age (<75-80 years), low risk of anticoagulation complications, and ability to adhere to prescribed treatment.

TABLE 36. Anticoagulation Agents	
Agent	**Comments**
Unfractionated heparin	Much experience in use; requires monitoring and usually IV access for continuous infusion; inexpensive
Low-molecular-weight heparin, dalteparin, enoxaparin	Generally no coagulation monitoring required; renal clearance; less reliable dosing in very obese patients; less experience treating PE with hemodynamic instability; expensive
Fondaparinux	Synthetic pentasaccharide; no coagulation monitoring required; renal clearance; less experience treating PE with hemodynamic instability; expensive, but generic version available
Rivaroxaban, apixaban	Direct factor Xa inhibitor; extended anticoagulation effect; no coagulation monitoring required; partial hepatic metabolism; renal clearance (both drugs should be dose modified in the setting of kidney disease and avoided in advanced kidney or hepatic impairment); rivaroxaban is FDA approved for prevention of CVA in patients with nonvalvular atrial fibrillation and for DVT prophylaxis in patients undergoing knee and hip replacement surgery; expensive
Hirudin, bivalirudin, argatroban	Not used for primary treatment; may be used for acute anticoagulation in patients with HIT; expensive
Dabigatran	Oral; no coagulation monitoring required; prompt therapeutic effect; long half-life; no clear antidote for toxicity and bleeding; FDA approved only for prevention of CVA in nonvalvular atrial fibrillation; raises INR; expensive
Warfarin	Oral; much experience in use; requires 4-5 days of heparin therapy before continuing warfarin alone; less predictable dosing requires close INR monitoring; many drug-drug and diet-drug interactions may reduce efficacy and/or increase toxicity; inexpensive

CVA = cerebrovascular accident; DVT = deep venous thrombosis; HIT = heparin-induced thrombocytopenia; IV = intravenous; PE = pulmonary embolism.

CONT.

Although not yet approved for treatment of DVT or PE, new direct thrombin inhibitors such as dabigatran and factor Xa inhibitors such as rivaroxaban may facilitate ambulatory treatment of some patients with PE. Ease of use via the oral route, no requirement for overlap with heparin, and no requirement for anticoagulation monitoring are factors that favor such use. Important drawbacks may include long half-life, lack of antidote, and inability to determine when the anticoagulant effect has worn off if invasive procedures are planned. These agents are currently reserved for special situations such as management of patients with HIT. ⊞

KEY POINTS

- It is essential to achieve therapeutic levels of anticoagulation within 24 hours of starting treatment to prevent pulmonary embolism progression and recurrence.

- In patients with pulmonary embolism, warfarin may be started at the time of initial anticoagulation.

- Heparin therapy (unfractionated or low-molecular-weight) should be continued for at least 4 to 5 days in patients with pulmonary embolism who are started on warfarin therapy, and should include an overlap of several days with a stable, therapeutic INR to ensure reliable anticoagulation.

Hemodynamically Unstable Patients

Hemodynamic instability reflects substantial elevation in pulmonary vascular resistance and pulmonary artery pressure, which compromises right ventricular function and cardiac output via decreased left ventricular filling, with consequent decrease in systemic blood pressure. Hemodynamically unstable patients usually require supplemental oxygen and may require mechanical ventilation. Fluid resuscitation may improve right ventricular function; however, rapid fluid infusion may exacerbate pulmonary hypertension and compromise right ventricular function. In the setting of otherwise refractory hypotension, vasoconstrictors should be administered to raise systemic arterial pressure, a key determinant of coronary blood flow. There is no clearly preferable vasopressor agent.

Because of their higher risk for complications and mortality, patients with refractory hypotension should be treated with thrombolytic therapy (unless contraindicated), followed by anticoagulation. If thrombolytic therapy is contraindicated (**Table 37**), surgical or catheter embolectomy should be considered if available. Rapid clot lysis must be considered against the risk of bleeding complications; use of thrombolytics for PE has been associated with a 2.1% risk for intracranial hemorrhage and a 1.6% risk for fatal nonintracranial hemorrhage. Current risk-benefit and cost-effectiveness studies do not generally support the initial use of thrombolytics except when there is clear evidence of hemodynamic instability. There is controversy whether thrombolytics should be used

TABLE 37.	Contraindications to Thrombolytic Therapy
Absolute
History of intracranial bleeding
CVA within the past 3 months (ischemic CVA within the past 3 hours)
Closed head or facial trauma within the past 3 months
Suspected aortic dissection
Active internal bleeding
Uncontrolled hypertension (systolic >180 mm Hg or diastolic >100 mm Hg)
Relative
Current anticoagulation or bleeding diathesis
Surgery or invasive procedures within the past 2 weeks
Prolonged CPR ≥10 minutes
Controlled severe hypertension
Diabetic or hemorrhagic retinopathy
Pregnancy

CPR = cardiopulmonary resuscitation; CVA = cerebrovascular accident.

to treat patients with normal blood pressure and CT or echocardiographic findings of right ventricular strain, such as dilatation or hypokinesis. Biomarker abnormalities may be useful to enhance accuracy of risk stratification. In selected patients at high risk for hemodynamic instability (as suggested by cardiac ultrasound findings and/or elevated biomarkers such as troponin and BNP) and with low risk of bleeding, thrombolytic therapy may be a reasonable consideration. ⊞

KEY POINT

- Because of their higher risk for complications and mortality, patients with refractory hypotension due to pulmonary embolism should be treated with thrombolytic therapy, followed by anticoagulation.

Ongoing Management and Prevention of Recurrent Pulmonary Embolism

Anticoagulation

Patients with acute PE are at substantial risk for recurrent episodes of DVT and PE. Anticoagulation has traditionally been continued (unless contraindicated) for 3 months following an episode of acute PE, after which the likely cause and the risks and benefits of treatment are reassessed. The standard of therapy has been warfarin in doses sufficient to maintain an INR of 2.0 to 3.0. PE risk factors that are short term and reversible such as surgery or trauma might call for shorter duration of anticoagulation, whereas a longer or indefinite duration would be desirable when greater or continuing risks such as cancer, history of proximal DVT, or idiopathic PE are present.

In selected patients who have completed a course of anticoagulation for acute PE, a D-dimer assay performed 3 to 4 weeks after stopping anticoagulation may be helpful in assessing the need for longer-term treatment. An elevated high-sensitivity D-dimer assay result suggests up to a four-fold higher risk of recurrent PE compared with a normal D-dimer result.

In patients requiring long-term anticoagulation for PE, the role of new oral anticoagulants in postacute PE care is uncertain.

Inferior Vena Cava Interruption

Inferior vena cava filters have been used to prevent embolization of clots from the iliofemoral veins in patients who are not candidates for acute and/or chronic anticoagulation, have had unsuccessful anticoagulant therapy, are at high risk for recurrent emboli, or are at high risk for mortality from recurrent PE because of reduced cardiopulmonary reserve and/or pulmonary hypertension.

Long-term use of filters may facilitate clot formation on or around the filter, venous collateralization with embolization, and DVT formation below the filter. For these reasons, the use of removable filters (extracted when the indication for use has passed) and concomitant anticoagulation (if not contraindicated) while the filter is in place have been advocated. ⬚

KEY POINT

- Patients with ongoing risk for pulmonary embolism may require extended or indefinite periods of anticoagulation.

Pulmonary Hypertension

Pathophysiology and Epidemiology

Pulmonary hypertension (PH) is defined by an elevation of mean pulmonary artery pressure of 25 mm Hg or greater during rest. The pulmonary vascular tree is normally a low-pressure, low-resistance system, and when PH develops it may lead to secondary effects on right-sided heart function and patient symptoms.

PH encompasses five distinct disease groups that differ in pathology, cause, and treatment (**Table 38**). In group 1 (pulmonary arterial hypertension [PAH]), the underlying

---

TABLE 38. Classification of Pulmonary Hypertension

1. PAH (resting mPAP ≥25 mm Hg and PCWP ≤15 mm Hg)
   Idiopathic PAH
   Heritable (including *BMPR2*, *ALK1*, endoglin with or without hereditary hemorrhagic telangiectasia)
   Drug- and toxin-induced (e.g., anorexigens, methamphetamine, rapeseed oil)
   Associated with connective tissue diseases (e.g., scleroderma), HIV infection, portal hypertension, congenital heart diseases, schistosomiasis, chronic hemolytic anemia

1'. Pulmonary veno-occlusive disease and/or pulmonary capillary hemangiomatosis

2. Pulmonary hypertension owing to left-sided heart disease (mPAP >25 mm Hg with elevated PCWP and left-sided heart dysfunction)
   Systolic dysfunction
   Diastolic dysfunction
   Valvular disease

3. Pulmonary hypertension owing to lung diseases and/or hypoxia (mPAP >25 mm Hg with underlying lung disease)
   COPD
   Interstitial lung disease
   Other pulmonary diseases with mixed restrictive and obstructive pattern
   Sleep-disordered breathing
   Alveolar hypoventilation disorders
   Chronic exposure to high altitude

4. Chronic thromboembolic pulmonary hypertension

5. Pulmonary hypertension with unclear or multifactorial causes
   Hematologic disorders: myeloproliferative disorders, sickle cell disease
   Systemic disorders: sarcoidosis, pulmonary Langerhans cell histiocytosis, vasculitis
   Metabolic disorders: glycogen storage disease, Gaucher disease, thyroid disorders
   Others: tumoral obstruction, fibrosing mediastinitis, chronic kidney failure on dialysis

ALK1 = activin receptor-like kinase type 1; *BMPR2* = bone morphogenic protein receptor type 2; mPAP = mean pulmonary artery pressure; PAH = pulmonary arterial hypertension; PCWP = pulmonary capillary wedge pressure.

Modified from Simonneau G, Robbins IM, Beghetti M, et al. Updated clinical classification of pulmonary hypertension. J Am Coll Cardiol. 2009;54(1 Suppl):S43-54. [PMID: 19555858]. With permission from Elsevier. Copyright 2009, Elsevier.

pathophysiology relates to restricted flow through the pulmonary vasculature with elevation in vascular resistance. An uncommon but important subgroup is idiopathic PAH, which has an approximately 2-to-1 female-to-male predominance and an estimated prevalence of only about 6 cases per million adult population. Management of PAH differs from that of most other causes of PH because treatment is focused on vasodilator therapy.

Over 80% of cases of PH are due to conditions causing elevation of left-sided heart filling pressures or pulmonary disease (groups 2 and 3, respectively). Treatment in these cases typically consists of addressing the underlying cause.

PH is associated with substantial morbidity and mortality. PH usually portends a worse prognosis when it complicates the diseases in each of groups 2 through 5. The prognosis among the types of PAH (group 1) varies. Right-sided heart function/pressures and functional status (as determined by tests such as the 6-minute walk test) are better predictors of prognosis than the actual value of pulmonary artery pressure. With mild PH, right ventricular function may be preserved and patients may be asymptomatic. As disease worsens, however, right-sided heart function deteriorates and symptoms progress.

KEY POINTS

- Pulmonary hypertension is defined by an elevation of mean pulmonary artery pressure of 25 mm Hg or greater during rest.

- Most cases of pulmonary hypertension arise secondary to left-sided heart dysfunction or underlying chronic lung disease.

Diagnosis

Fatigue and dyspnea with exertion are the most common symptoms. Patients may have palpitations or chest pain that may be ill defined or angina-like. With advanced PH, symptoms and signs of right ventricular decompensation, including syncope, edema, ascites, and hepatomegaly, may be noted. Depending on the severity of the PH, the cardiac examination may show a left parasternal lift; augmentation of the jugular a wave and the pulmonic component of S_2 or a single S_2; murmurs of tricuspid regurgitation or pulmonic insufficiency; and right ventricular S_3 or S_4 gallops. Signs and symptoms of underlying conditions may be present and may suggest the underlying cause of PH.

The evaluation is similar for most patients with PH, but certain considerations may require special studies. Chest imaging studies suggest the diagnosis when pulmonary artery enlargement is noted. A diagnosis of PH can be confirmed only by right heart catheterization and direct measurement of mean pulmonary artery pressure. Cardiac ultrasonography, with systolic mean pulmonary artery pressure of 40 mm Hg or greater, is highly suggestive and provides information regarding left and right ventricular function and

valvular abnormalities. However, cardiac ultrasound findings may underestimate pulmonary artery pressures; this is a particular problem in the setting of advanced diffuse parenchymal lung disease. Right heart catheterization is required to confirm the diagnosis and to assess its cause if therapy for PH is to be considered.

Once PH is confirmed, evaluation is generally directed at determining the specific cause (if not already apparent) and the anatomic location and extent of vascular involvement. An array of studies (such as imaging of the chest to assess parenchymal lung disease; V/Q scanning to assess potential chronic thromboembolic disease; pulmonary function testing with D$_{LCO}$; serologic studies for connective tissue disease, liver disease, and HIV; and sleep studies) may be helpful in selected patients. Biomarkers such as BNP or troponins may provide prognostic information. Some patients with PH and all patients suspected of having PAH should be considered for right heart/pulmonary artery catheterization to confirm the diagnosis and guide therapy.

Six-minute walk studies provide a simple and important functional assessment. Repeat 6-minute walk, cardiac ultrasound, and/or catheterization studies are useful in assessing progression of disease and response to therapy.

KEY POINTS

- Pulmonary hypertension may be definitively diagnosed via right heart catheterization; this study should be performed in all patients with suspected pulmonary arterial hypertension, in those with an uncertain cause of pulmonary hypertension, or in those in whom specific therapy for pulmonary hypertension is being considered.

- Functional assessment with cardiac ultrasound and 6-minute walk test is useful for evaluating progression of pulmonary hypertension and response to therapy.

Treatment

Treatment of most forms of PH without isolated PAH (groups 2, 3, 4, and 5 in Table 38) is directed at the underlying condition. This may include optimal treatment of systolic and diastolic heart failure; oxygen therapy for patients with resting, exercise, or sleep-related desaturation; appropriate treatment of COPD; and evaluation and management of obstructive sleep apnea.

In rare instances, despite aggressive treatment of underlying heart and lung disease, PH may persist and contribute to patient morbidity. The benefits of vasodilator therapy in this population remain unproved, and potential adverse effects of vasodilator therapy (including fluid retention, hypotension, and worsening hypoxemia from V/Q mismatch) underscore the need for careful patient selection and referral to a specialist with expertise in this area.

- Treatment of most forms of pulmonary hypertension without isolated pulmonary arterial hypertension is directed at the underlying condition.

Chronic Thromboembolic Pulmonary Hypertension

Most patients who survive acute PE have complete or near-complete resolution of clots with normalization of any pulmonary artery pressure abnormalities within 1 month of the acute event; however, some will develop chronic thromboembolic pulmonary hypertension (CTEPH). Estimates of CTEPH incidence range from 0.1% to almost 4% of patients surviving acute PE. The pathologic lesions of CTEPH are white-yellow, organized, and endothelialized, in marked contrast to the red free thrombi of acute PE. CTEPH is associated with vascular remodeling similar to that seen in other forms of PH.

Diagnosis

Symptoms associated with CTEPH, like those of acute PE, are nonspecific, are often misdiagnosed, and appear to correlate with the degree of PH and related right ventricular decompensation. As many as 50% of patients with CTEPH may not report a prior episode of diagnosed acute DVT/PE. In patients in whom a prior PE was identified, factors associated with increased risk for CTEPH include larger perfusion defects, younger age at prior diagnosis, and elevated D-dimer 3 months after initial diagnosis.

Patients with CTEPH may have findings of PH and cor pulmonale and invariably have defects on V/Q lung scan, which remains the recommended initial test for evaluating potential CTEPH. CTA is useful for localizing the site and surgical accessibility of the obstructing lesions. If these studies are inconclusive and CTEPH remains a concern, right heart catheterization and angiography should be considered. Pulmonary angiography permits direct measurement of pulmonary artery and right ventricular hemodynamics and will reveal vascular obstruction and changes of remodeling, indicating the chronic nature of the process.

Management

Management includes general supportive care, anticoagulation to prevent further PE or in situ clot formation, and inferior vena cava interruption in patients at risk for hemodynamic instability or new emboli (those with lower extremity ultrasound studies showing DVT). Pulmonary vasodilator therapy may improve right ventricular function and symptoms, but the impact on survival is not clear. Definitive treatment is surgical and involves thromboendarterectomy to remove the organized clots. Results are best when patients have fair functional capacity (New York Heart Association functional class III or better), the target lesions are central, and when surgery is performed at

an experienced center. In the absence of clear contraindication, anticoagulation should be continued indefinitely and a vena cava filter should be considered. **H**

KEY POINTS

- Chronic thromboembolic pulmonary hypertension is estimated to occur in up to 4% of patients who have survived acute pulmonary embolism, but half of these patients will not report a prior episode of diagnosed acute deep venous thrombosis or pulmonary embolism.
- Chronic thromboembolic pulmonary hypertension is characterized by organization of acute thromboemboli and pulmonary vascular remodeling; it is best treated by thromboendarterectomy when surgically amenable clots are present.
- Patients with chronic thromboembolic pulmonary hypertension should receive anticoagulation if not contraindicated.

Pulmonary Arterial Hypertension

Epidemiology and Categorization

PAH is a subset of PH (see group 1 in Table 38) with elevated mean pulmonary artery pressure, normal pulmonary capillary wedge pressure (≤15 mm Hg), and elevated pulmonary vascular resistance. The mechanisms underlying PAH are unclear but may involve underexpression of vasodilators such as prostacyclin and nitric oxide, overexpression of vasoconstrictors such as endothelin, and overexpression of angiogenic mediators such as vascular endothelial-derived growth factor and platelet-derived growth factor. Heritable forms, with low penetrance, appear to be linked to mutations in at least two members of the transforming growth factor-β family (*BMPR2* and *ALK1*). The common histologic features among the conditions in group 1 are intimal fibrosis, increased medial thickness, vascular occlusion, and plexiform lesions within small pulmonary arteries and arterioles; lung biopsy is generally avoided and is not used for diagnosis. Within group 1 are three entities: idiopathic PAH (formerly primary pulmonary hypertension), heritable PAH, and PAH associated with other conditions such as connective tissue diseases. PAH associated with other conditions is, in aggregate, most common. Although prognosis varies, most cases of PAH are likely to be progressive if left untreated (in the absence of effective therapy, median survival of idiopathic PAH is 2.8 years). Even with current therapy, mortality for all PAH is 15% within 1 year of diagnosis.

Diagnosis

Although evaluation of these patients will be similar in many respects to other patients with PH, it is important to emphasize that all patients considered for vasodilator therapy should undergo right heart catheterization for confirmation of the diagnosis, to establish baseline physiologic measurements, and to assess vasodilator responsiveness. Although genetic testing and counseling may be useful in patients with apparent heritable PAH (cluster of cases, early-onset PAH), it has no clear role at this time for most patients.

Treatment
Treatment of PAH involves supportive and PAH-specific therapy. Given the high mortality and complexity of management, most patients with PAH are treated by experienced specialists. Supportive therapy consists of diuretics, anticoagulants to prevent in situ clot formation common in many forms of PAH, cardiac glycosides to augment right-sided heart function, and supplemental oxygen when hypoxemia is present (may also produce pulmonary vasodilation). PAH-specific therapy may be given with single agents or combinations of agents from different classes. Single agents are used with patients in better functional classes, and combination therapy is generally reserved for more advanced disease or when single-agent therapy is ineffective. There are currently four classes of drugs available for PAH-specific therapy (**Table 39**). Patients with vasodilator responsiveness demonstrated at the time of cardiac catheterization have a better prognosis and are the only appropriate candidates for a trial of treatment with calcium channel blockers. Although these therapies are associated with improved symptoms, quality of life, and survival, many patients continue to require lung transplantation.

Lung (or heart-lung) transplantation is indicated for some patients with end-stage pulmonary or pulmonary vascular disease in whom available therapy has been unsuccessful or for whom no therapies are available.

KEY POINTS
- Pulmonary arterial hypertension is a subset of pulmonary hypertension characterized by elevated mean pulmonary artery pressure, normal pulmonary capillary wedge pressure (<15 mm Hg), and elevated pulmonary vascular resistance.

- Right heart catheterization should be performed to confirm the pulmonary arterial hypertension and assess acute vasodilator responsiveness before long-term vasodilator therapy is attempted.
- Pulmonary arterial hypertension–specific therapy has been shown to improve symptoms and performance, and it may improve survival.

Lung Tumors
Pulmonary Nodule Evaluation
Evaluation of a pulmonary nodule should balance the goal of early detection and treatment of malignancy against the goal of avoiding invasive procedures for benign processes. A pulmonary nodule is defined as a focal, nodular opacity that is up to 3 cm in diameter, is surrounded by normal lung, and is not associated with lymphadenopathy. Lesions larger than 3 cm are considered lung masses; the high likelihood of a malignancy in masses reduces the consideration of differential processes. Pulmonary nodules may be single or multiple.

The increased use of CT to evaluate symptoms both inside and outside the chest has led to frequent identification of small nodules below the resolution of a chest radiograph. CT screening studies for lung cancer suggest that 25% to 50% or more of patients who have a CT of the chest will have one or more lung nodules detected.

Assessment of Risk for Malignancy
The likelihood of malignancy is based on the size and surface characteristics of the nodule, patient age, smoking history, and history of prior malignancy. Nodule size is often the most important feature in predicting malignancy. Screening studies have shown that more than 98% of nodules smaller than 8 mm are benign, whereas the majority of nodules larger than 2 cm are malignant. A smooth border is

TABLE 39. Pharmacologic Therapy for Pulmonary Arterial Hypertension	
Class	**Comments**
Calcium channel blockers	Only for patients with acute vasodilator response at catheterization; acute response does not assure chronic response
Prostanoids (epoprostenol, treprostinil, iloprost)	Supplements endogenous levels of prostacyclin (PGI$_2$); a vasodilator with anti–smooth muscle proliferative properties
Endothelin-1 receptor antagonists (bosentan, ambrisentan)	Blocks action of endogenous vasoconstrictor and smooth muscle mitogen endothelin; class-wide risk of liver injury and teratogenicity, liver chemistry testing and pregnancy testing for reproductive-aged women are required[a]
Phosphodiesterase-5 inhibitors (sildenafil, tadalafil)	Prolongs effect of intrinsic vasodilator cyclic GMP by inhibiting hydrolysis by phosphodiesterase 5

GMP = guanosine monophosphate.

[a]Although not required for ambrisentan, some experts suggest that it is prudent to perform liver chemistry tests at the outset of treatment for pulmonary arterial hypertension and at periodic intervals thereafter at the discretion of the managing physician.

an indication a nodule is more likely benign; a spiculated border indicates a high likelihood of malignancy (**Figure 14**). Risk from smoking increases with earlier age at onset of smoking, duration of smoking, and number of cigarettes smoked per day. Risk for lung cancer increases with age, and the age-specific lung cancer incidence rates for both women and men are highest after age 70 years. Lung cancers are less frequent in persons younger than 45 years; only about 10% of all lung cancers occur in this age group and only about 1% occur in persons younger than 35 years. A history of another malignancy increases the likelihood that a pulmonary nodule is malignant. Metastasis to the lung is common; surgical series identify that approximately one third of resected nodules are metastases.

Management

The Fleischner Society for Thoracic Imaging and Diagnosis recommendations for follow-up of various nodule sizes are described in **Table 40**. No follow-up is necessary for nodules

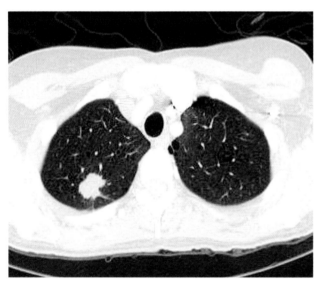

FIGURE 14. The CT scan shown discloses a 2-cm spiculated nodule. A nodule of this size with a spiculated border is highly likely to be malignant. Resection showed it was a grade 4, stage IA adenocarcinoma.

that are smaller than 4 mm in never-smokers with no other known risk factors for malignancy (history of a first-degree relative with lung cancer or significant radon or asbestos exposure). Nodules 4 mm or larger should be further evaluated according to the recommendations in the guideline. A new, noncalcified nodule larger than 8 mm for which there are no old images should prompt a calculation of the probability of malignancy and consideration of additional imaging or biopsy.

Examination of previous chest imaging studies is critical in nodule evaluation and may show that a nodule is stable, growing, or shrinking over time. In addition to reviewing previous chest radiographs and chest CT scans, other sources of lung images such as abdominal CT, shoulder films, and CT of the coronary arteries may also be helpful. Solid nodules that remain stable in size for 2 years on chest radiograph or CT scan are considered benign, and no further follow-up is indicated; this is known as the 2-year stability rule. Growth is a strong indicator that the nodule may be malignant, although some benign nodules will also show growth. Lung cancers tend to grow rapidly. Volume doubling times range from 1 month to 1 year, with most cancers doubling in 50 to 100 days. Benign nodules such as granulomas or focal pneumonias may grow; however, they typically grow faster (for focal pneumonia) or slower (for benign, noninfectious neoplasms) than a malignant nodule.

CT is more sensitive than chest radiography at identifying calcification, which is another factor that can help determine that the nodule is likely benign. Calcification in a benign pattern (central, diffuse, lamellar) indicates that the nodule is a granuloma and requires no further investigation. A nodule that has eccentric or off-center calcification may be either benign or malignant, and further evaluation or follow-up is advised. The presence of fat (and often the combination of fat and calcification) indicates that a nodule is a hamartoma and is benign; hamartomas should be removed only if they cause symptoms. CT may show other small nodules called satellite nodules in the region of a dominant nodule; this suggests a benign process due to a fungus or mycobacterium.

TABLE 40. Recommendations for Pulmonary Nodule Evaluation Based on Risk		
Nodule Size (mm)	**Low-Risk[a] Follow-up**	**High-Risk[b] Follow-up**
<4	None	12 months; if unchanged, stop
4-6	12 months; if unchanged, stop	6-12 months; if unchanged, 18-24 months
6-8	6-12 months; if unchanged, 18-24 months	3-6 months; if unchanged, 9-12 and 24 months
>8	Consider contrast CT study, PET scan, or biopsy; if followed, 3, 9, and 24 months	Same as low risk

[a]Low risk: Never-smoker and no other risk factors.

[b]High risk: Current or former smoker or other risk factors.

Modified from MacMahon H, Austin JH, Gamsu G, et al; Fleischner Society. Guidelines for management of small pulmonary nodules detected on CT scans: a statement from the Fleischner Society. Radiology. 2005;237(2):395-400. [PMID: 16244247] Copyright 2005, Radiological Society of North America.

Further radiographic evaluation of a nodule may include PET-CT imaging. PET-CT combines a radiotracer (usually 18-fluoro-deoxyglucose) with CT scanning to provide anatomically localized information on the metabolic activity of a lesion based on uptake of the radiotracer. It has a sensitivity of about 95% and a specificity of 85% for identifying a nodule as malignant (**Figure 15**). It is a technically complex and expensive procedure and is not indicated for the routine evaluation of all lung nodules. PET scanning has a low sensitivity for small nodules and is not useful for nodules smaller than 1 cm. It may be useful in a patient with a nodule that remains indeterminate after CT imaging and that is 1 cm or greater in size. A nodule that exhibits intense activity on PET-CT usually prompts resection as long as there is no evidence of regional or distant spread. Nodules with no or low activity on PET-CT are followed with CT to confirm lack of change over 2 years.

Ground-glass opacities (GGO) are nodules of low density (attenuation) that are generally only visible by CT scan (**Figure 16**). They deserve special mention because they may represent low-grade adenocarcinomas that behave differently than most malignancies presenting as solid nodules. The differential diagnosis for GGOs includes focal inflammation or fibrosis, atypical adenomatous hyperplasia (thought to be a precursor of malignancy), adenocarcinoma in situ (previously called bronchioloalveolar carcinoma), and invasive adenocarcinoma. Malignant GGOs typically exhibit slow growth with average doubling times over 400 days; for this reason, the 2-year stability rule for solid nodules does not apply and a longer period of follow-up is recommended. PET scanning is not helpful to distinguish malignancy owing to the low density of the lesions, and needle biopsy is often nondiagnostic. GGOs may grow or stay the same size; they may become solid or partly solid as they progress. Limited resection (wedge resection or segmentectomy) rather than lobectomy is usually performed for resection of GGOs found to be adenocarcinoma in situ or minimally invasive adenocarcinoma owing to the low likelihood of recurrence.

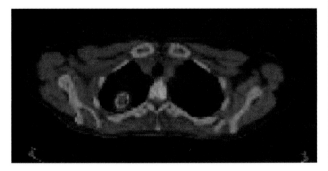

FIGURE 15. Preoperative staging PET-CT scan showing a markedly enhancing nodule, indicating a high likelihood of malignancy. No abnormal 18-fluoro-deoxyglucose uptake was seen elsewhere in the body. Resection showed an adenocarcinoma with no evidence of spread to hilar or mediastinal nodes.

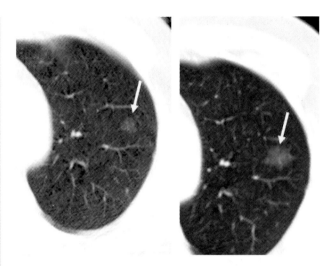

FIGURE 16. A CT scan of the chest shows a 13-mm ground-glass opacity (*arrow*) (*left panel*). Serial CT follow-up showed it to grow slowly over 5 years to 20 mm (*right panel*). Limited resection via segmentectomy showed adenocarcinoma in situ (formerly called bronchioloalveolar carcinoma) with negative nodes.

KEY POINTS

- The likelihood of malignancy of a pulmonary nodule is based on the size, surface characteristics, patient age, smoking history, and history of prior malignancy.

- No follow-up is necessary for pulmonary nodules that are smaller than 4 mm in never-smokers with no other known risk factors for malignancy (history of a first-degree relative with lung cancer or significant radon or asbestos exposure).

- Examination of previous chest imaging studies is critical in pulmonary nodule evaluation and may show that a nodule is stable, growing, or shrinking over time.

Lung Cancer

Epidemiology

Lung cancer (also referred to as bronchogenic carcinoma) is the most common cause of cancer mortality worldwide for both men and women; there are approximately 1.6 million new cases and 1.4 million deaths per year. More people die annually of lung cancer than of colon, breast, and prostate cancer combined.

Lung cancer is classified primarily into two types: non–small cell lung cancer (NSCLC) and small cell lung cancer (SCLC). Approximately 95% of all cancers originating in the lung fall into these two subtypes. Determining the cell type is essential for staging, treatment, and prognosis of lung cancer. NSCLC, which comprises more than 80% of all cases of lung cancer, consists of three primary histologic subtypes: adenocarcinoma, squamous cell carcinoma, and large cell carcinoma. Bronchioloalveolar carcinoma was considered a subtype of adenocarcinoma; however, this term is no longer favored. Lepidic-predominant pattern replaces the descriptor of bronchioloalveolar carcinoma. Adenocarcinoma is now described as preinvasive, minimally invasive, or invasive.

Risk Factors

Although smoking rates have declined to approximately 20% of men and 15% of women, approximately 90% of all cases of lung cancer are caused by smoking. Reflecting the decline in smoking popularity, more lung cancers are currently diagnosed in former smokers than in current smokers. Lung cancer risk for a current smoker with a 40-pack-year history is approximately 20 times that of someone who has never smoked. Quitting smoking is the most effective method to reduce risk. Following smoking cessation, risk for lung cancer remains elevated based on duration and quantity of smoking, but it does not continue to rise as in a continuing smoker. After controlling for smoking, evidence of airway obstruction on pulmonary function testing reflects a four- to sixfold increase in risk for lung cancer. Patients with a history of both smoking and asbestos exposure have an increased risk for lung cancer that is 50 to 90 times that of a never-smoker. Other exposures that increase risk include second-hand smoke, asbestos, radon, metals (arsenic, chromium, and nickel), ionizing radiation, and polycyclic aromatic hydrocarbons. Pulmonary fibrosis appears to be associated with an increased risk for lung cancer.

KEY POINTS

- More people die annually of lung cancer than of colon, breast, and prostate cancer combined.
- Determining the cell type (non–small cell lung cancer or small cell lung cancer) is essential for staging, treatment, and prognosis of lung cancer.
- Quitting smoking is the most effective method to reduce risk for lung cancer.

Screening and Primary Prevention

Primary prevention for lung cancer consists of smoking cessation, never starting smoking, and avoidance of second-hand smoke.

Randomized trials have not shown mortality benefit of screening for lung cancer with plain chest radiography. However, CT has been shown to be more sensitive for detecting lung cancer than chest radiography. Recently, the National Lung Screening Trial (NLST) showed fewer lung cancer deaths from screening with low-dose spiral CT; this is the first indication that any test can reduce deaths from lung cancer. Based on this study, the American Lung Association and the American College of Chest Physicians/American Society of Clinical Oncology have released guidelines recommending that low-dose spiral CT screening for lung cancer be recommended to patients meeting the admission criteria for the NLST. However, despite the encouraging results of the NLST, significant questions remain concerning which patients will benefit from CT screening, the number of patients needed to screen to detect each new case of lung cancer, the necessary duration of screening to be effective, the risks of overdiagnosis and other harms, the personal and societal cost-effectiveness of screening, and reimbursement for testing. Therefore, widespread adoption of low-dose spiral CT screening for lung cancer should await additional information; for patients at high risk who seek screening, these outstanding issues should be carefully discussed before deciding to proceed.

KEY POINTS

- Primary prevention for lung cancer consists of smoking cessation, never starting smoking, and avoidance of second-hand smoke.
- Plain chest radiography has been shown to be ineffective in screening for lung cancer.
- Preliminary evidence suggests that screening for lung cancer with low-dose spiral CT may have potential to reduce mortality in high-risk patients, although more information is needed before this intervention is widely adopted.

Diagnosis and Evaluation

Lung cancer is usually discovered during the evaluation of symptoms. By the time cancer causes symptoms, approximately three out of four lung cancers are at an advanced stage when they are no longer resectable. Because the lung does not have pain sensation, presence of symptoms often reflects invasion into local or distant structures. Symptoms stemming from local effects on the airway include cough, hemoptysis, and dyspnea. Chest pain can result from mediastinal, pleural, or rib invasion. Metastasis can occur to almost any body tissue, but the most frequent sites of metastasis are the hilar and mediastinal lymph nodes, pleura, liver, adrenal glands, bones, and brain. Spread may occur by direct extension, hematogenously, or through the lymphatic system.

Paraneoplastic syndromes occur in approximately 10% of patients with lung cancer and are generally associated with specific cell types (**Table 41**). See MKSAP 16 Neurology for a discussion of the neurologic paraneoplastic syndromes.

Evaluating a patient with known or suspected lung cancer begins with a careful history and physical examination. Patients should be asked about new bone pain or neurologic symptoms such as headaches or unsteadiness, as these may be an indication of metastases. Laboratory investigation includes a complete blood count, serum liver chemistry studies, and measurement of serum calcium. There are currently no tumor markers that are routinely measured for lung cancer. The chest CT scan should include the liver and adrenals to assess these common sites of metastasis. New headaches, visual changes, or unsteadiness should prompt a CT or MRI of the

TABLE 41. Common Paraneoplastic Syndromes Associated with Lung Cancer

System	Paraneoplastic Syndrome	Most Common Cell Type
Neurologic	Lambert-Eaton syndrome	Small cell
	Peripheral neuropathy	Small cell
	Encephalomyelitis	Small cell
Hematologic	Thrombophlebitis	Various
	Nonbacterial thrombotic endocarditis	
	Thrombocytosis	
	Leukemoid reaction	
Musculoskeletal	Hypertrophic osteoarthropathy	Various
	Digital clubbing	
	Polymyositis, dermatomyositis	
Endocrinologic	Cushing syndrome	Small cell
	Syndrome of inappropriate secretion of antidiuretic hormone (SIADH)	Small cell
	Hypercalcemia	Squamous cell
Miscellaneous	Anorexia, cachexia	Various

brain. New sites of bone pain should be imaged. Pulmonary function testing should be done in all patients who are considered for surgical or radiation treatment.

In order to limit unnecessary invasive testing, the diagnosis and staging of lung cancer are best done simultaneously. When advanced disease is suggested by CT or PET-CT, the diagnosis and staging are best accomplished with a single invasive test, usually of the location that would confirm the most advanced stage (**Table 42**). For example, in a patient with a 4-cm lung mass and mediastinal lymphadenopathy on CT, biopsy should start with the mediastinal nodes to establish a diagnosis and a more advanced stage than would be established with a needle biopsy of the mass.

In early-stage disease, clinical circumstances should dictate whether a diagnosis is needed before surgery. For example, a 2-cm, growing peripheral nodule in a former smoker with a PET-CT showing uptake only in the lesion may not require biopsy before resection, because the likelihood of identifying a specific benign diagnosis in this setting is low, and a nonspecific result would still lead to resection because of the high likelihood of malignancy. In contrast, a new 2-cm nodule in a never-smoker might prompt CT-guided biopsy or bronchoscopy of the nodule as a next step to establish a diagnosis before resection, because the likelihood of a benign diagnosis is higher.

KEY POINTS

- By the time cancer causes symptoms, approximately three out of four lung cancers are at an advanced stage.
- In order to limit unnecessary invasive testing, the diagnosis and staging of lung cancer are best done simultaneously.
- Pulmonary nodules with features highly suggestive of malignancy may not require biopsy before resection.

Staging

Staging for NSCLC should be done to identify appropriate treatment for patients with resectable disease and avoid unnecessary surgery in patients with advanced disease.

TABLE 42. Clinical Findings and Actions in Evaluating Patients with Confirmed Non–Small Cell Lung Cancer

Finding	Action	Referral
Lung nodule or mass with otherwise negative PET-CT (stage I or II)	Assess functional status and pulmonary function	Thoracic surgery for resection candidates; radiation oncology if disease is localized and patient is not a surgical candidate owing to poor function
Evidence of mediastinal lymphadenopathy on PET-CT	Mediastinal node staging by EBUS or EUS guided-needle biopsy or mediastinoscopy	Medical oncology if mediastinal involvement confirmed; thoracic surgery if no mediastinal involvement confirmed
Distant organ involvement by CT or PET-CT	Biopsy to confirm diagnosis and advanced stage	Medical oncology
Painful bone involvement by imaging	Biopsy to confirm diagnosis and advanced stage	Radiation oncology and medical oncology for palliative treatment
Localized disease with pleural effusion	Thoracentesis	Medical oncology if positive for malignancy; thoracic surgery if negative for malignancy
Evidence of a single brain metastasis	Assess operability of disease in the chest	Neurosurgery

EBUS = endobronchial ultrasound; EUS = esophageal ultrasound.

Staging of NSCLC is done with the T (tumor) N (node) M (metastasis) system (**Table 43**).

Staging of SCLC may be done using the TNM classification but is traditionally still done using the Veterans Administration Lung Study Group designations of limited and extensive disease. Limited disease consists of disease confined to one hemithorax and therefore one radiation port. Extensive disease extends beyond one hemithorax.

PET scanning and integrated PET-CT are valuable tools in the evaluation of NSCLC. Randomized controlled trials have shown the cost effectiveness of adding PET-CT to preoperative staging. Approximately one in five patients thought to have resectable disease prior to PET-CT will have evidence of mediastinal or distant spread and unnecessary surgery can be avoided. PET-CT is most often pursued in the preoperative staging of NSCLC; however, it is frequently also used by oncologists for treatment planning in nonresectable disease, and it may be helpful in determining limited versus extensive disease in SCLC.

Use of ultrasound guidance has greatly improved yields of bronchoscopic sampling of paratracheal, subcarinal, and hilar lymph nodes identified by CT or PET-CT. Endobronchial ultrasonography provides real-time imaging of the mediastinal nodes and enables the operator to see the needle in the node at the time of sampling. Yields of greater than 90% for the paratracheal and subcarinal nodes and negative predictive values of greater than 90% have been reported. Randomized trials have shown that the combination of ultrasound-guided endobronchial and esophageal needle aspiration is comparable if not superior to mediastinoscopy for preoperative staging of N2 (ipsilateral mediastinal) and N3 (contralateral mediastinal) nodes.

KEY POINTS

- PET scanning (or integrated PET-CT) is cost effective for preoperative staging of patients with known or suspected non–small cell lung cancer.
- Where available, endoscopic ultrasound-guided needle aspiration through the trachea or esophagus is an accurate and less invasive alternative to staging with mediastinoscopy.

Treatment

Curative-intent surgery is the best treatment for NSCLC in stages I or II for those patients who can withstand surgery. Patients with good performance status, no major cardiovascular risk (recent myocardial infarction, unstable angina, uncompensated heart failure, or severe valvular disease), and an FEV_1 and D_{LCO} at or above 80% of predicted are candidates for resection.

For patients with an FEV_1 of less than 80% of predicted, calculating the predicted postoperative pulmonary function helps identify which patients are otherwise acceptable surgical candidates. The postoperative predicted pulmonary function is calculated by subtracting the approximate percentage of lung function to be lost with surgical removal (segment, lobe, or pneumonectomy) from the preoperative function. If the postoperative predicted FEV_1 and D_{LCO} are greater than 40%, surgery is generally well tolerated. A quantitative perfusion scan or an exercise assessment, specifically measuring

Stage Subset	TNM	Descriptors
IA	T1a,bN0M0	T1a: ≤2 cm T1b: >2 cm but ≤3 cm
IB	T2aN0M0	T2a: >3 cm but ≤5 cm
IIA	T1a,bN1M0	N1: metastasis to an ipsilateral hilar or intrapulmonary node
	T2aN1M0	T2b: >5 cm but ≤7cm
	T2bN0M0	
IIB	T2bN1M0	T3: >7 cm, or invasion of chest wall or diaphragm, or <2 cm from carina, or a metastatic nodule in the same lobe
	T3N0M0	
IIIA	T1,2N2M0	N2: metastasis to an ipsilateral mediastinal node and/or subcarinal node
	T3N1,2M0	T4: metastatic nodule on the ipsilateral side in a different lobe
	T4N0,1M0	
IIIB	T4N2M0	N3: metastasis to a contralateral mediastinal or hilar node or a supraclavicular node
	AnyTN3M0	
IV	Any T, Any N, M1a,b	M1a: metastatic nodule contralateral lobe, pleural effusion, or pleural nodules
		M1b: distant metastasis

TABLE 43. Stage Grouping for Non–Small Cell Lung Cancer

Data from Rami-Porta R, Crowley JJ, Goldstraw P. The revised TNM staging system for lung cancer. Ann Thorac Cardiovasc Surg. 2009;15:4-9. [PMID: 19262443]

CONT.

aerobic capacity, may help determine whether surgery is appropriate in patients who have a predicted postoperative FEV$_1$ or D$_{LCO}$ of less than 40%.

Lobectomy is still considered the best standard surgical approach to resection of stage I or II NSCLC. For patients who have marginal pulmonary reserve, limited resection such as a segmentectomy or wedge may be a more appropriate surgical option. Lobectomy and lesser resections are increasingly being performed by video-assisted thoracic surgery (VATS), with the advantages of less pain and shorter hospitalization compared with standard thoracotomy. Surgical node dissection should be performed in all patients for proper staging regardless of type of resection. Operative mortality is lower in centers with the highest volumes and focused expertise. Surgical mortality rates are approximately 1% for lobectomy and 6% for pneumonectomy. Patients with stage I disease who are not surgical candidates or who refuse surgery may be candidates for standard radiotherapy, stereotactic body radiotherapy, radiofrequency ablation, or cryoablation. Stereotactic body radiotherapy uses higher doses of radiation delivered more precisely and allows for fewer fractions (usually 3 to 5 treatments) than traditional radiotherapy. Patients with resected stage II cancers are offered postoperative (adjuvant) chemotherapy, as this has been shown to improve chances for long-term survival.

Patients recognized to have stage IIIA NSCLC on preoperative staging are usually offered chemotherapy rather than resection as a first step in treatment. Select patients with single station N2 node involvement, having a good response to chemotherapy, may be offered resection after chemotherapy (neoadjuvant). Patients with stage IIIB and stage IV NSCLC are treated with chemotherapy, and radiation may be used for local control of disease in situations of bone or brain involvement. Increasingly, lung cancer specimens are being tested for genetic mutations such as epidermal growth factor receptor (*EGFR*) and anaplastic lymphoma kinase (*ALK*) to allow selective tailoring of therapy for the individual.

Limited-stage SCLC is treated primarily with combination chemotherapy and radiotherapy, and extensive-stage disease is treated with chemotherapy alone.

Palliation of symptoms of airway involvement may be achieved by bronchoscopic techniques. Rigid bronchoscopy under general anesthesia and use of laser therapy, cautery, or cryotherapy can be used to clear the airway in patients with bulky, centrally obstructing tumors (**Figure 17**). Candidates for airway treatment include those who have not responded to other treatment modalities, have an identifiable bronchial lumen, and show evidence of functioning lung beyond the level of the endobronchial obstruction. Improvement of dyspnea is often immediate, and median survival after laser resection is about 6 months.

Placement of an airway stent helps maintain airway patency after obstructing tumor removal and for patients with extrinsic airway compression. Stent complications include migration, mucus obstruction, and granulation tissue formation.

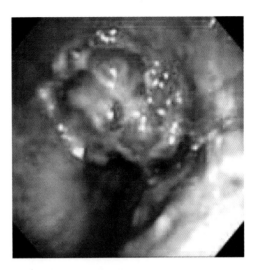

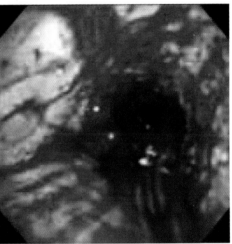

FIGURE 17. A polypoid squamous cell carcinoma nearly completely occluding the tracheal lumen (*top panel*). Rigid bronchoscopy (along with cautery for hemostasis and forceps for removal) was used to debulk the tumor and reestablish the tracheal lumen (*bottom panel*). The patient later received external-beam radiation therapy and had no recurrent tracheal obstruction.

For patients who have had maximal external-beam radiation therapy and have recurrent airway compromise, brachytherapy (the application of intraluminal radiation) may provide relief. ◧

KEY POINTS

- Surgical resection is the appropriate treatment for stages I or II non–small cell lung cancer when the patient is a surgical candidate.
- Stage III and IV lung cancer is treated with chemotherapy alone or in combination with radiotherapy.

Prognosis and Follow-up

Stage at presentation is the greatest indicator of prognosis for lung cancer. Survival decreases progressively with more advanced disease from a median of 59 months for patients with surgically resected stage IA disease to only 4 months for those with stage IV disease. Poor performance status and weight loss have also been associated with shortened survival. Patients with stage I cancers detected with screening have a 5-year survival rate over 80%. Patients who have had curative-intent surgical resection are generally followed every 6 months for the first year or two and then annually with a clinic visit and CT scan.

KEY POINT

- The most important factors in the prognosis of a patient with lung cancer are stage at presentation and performance status.

Other Pulmonary Neoplasia

Carcinoid Tumors

Carcinoid tumor in the lung is a low-grade malignancy consisting of cells of neuroendocrine origin. They account for only about 2% of all tumors in the lung and have no association with smoking. Owing to the tendency for carcinoid tumors to have an endobronchial location, patients frequently present with hemoptysis or evidence of bronchial obstruction resulting in atelectasis or focal bronchiectasis (**Figure 18**). Carcinoid tumors are classified as typical or atypical. In the absence of nodal metastasis, the 10-year survival rate for patients with typical carcinoid tumors is greater than 90%. Atypical carcinoid tumors are associated with a higher rate of mitosis and metastasis, poorer survival, and larger size at diagnosis than typical carcinoid tumors. The 5-year survival rate for patients with atypical carcinoid tumors is approximately 60% to 70%. Surgical resection is the treatment of choice for both typical and atypical carcinoid tumors and is often curative. Patients with typical carcinoid tumors have excellent prognosis with surgery. Carcinoid syndrome (flushing and diarrhea) rarely occurs with carcinoid tumor in the lung.

Mesothelioma

Mesothelioma is a neoplasm that arises from the mesothelial surfaces of the pleural and peritoneal cavities (about 80% are pleural in origin). Inhalation of asbestos is the predominant cause and about 75% of patients with mesothelioma will have a history of significant asbestos exposure. The annual incidence of mesothelioma in the United States and worldwide continues to rise and reflects the long latency period between exposure and disease manifestation. The prognosis of mesothelioma is poor, with a median survival of about 6 to 18 months.

The pattern of growth of mesothelioma is to ensheathe the lung. Pain is the most common symptom owing to parietal pleural involvement; characteristically this is a dull pain that is unrelenting. As the process progresses and more of the pleural space is involved, shortness of breath develops. Chest imaging often shows a large pleural effusion and diffuse

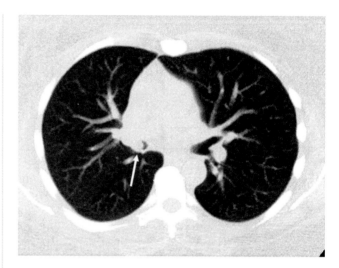

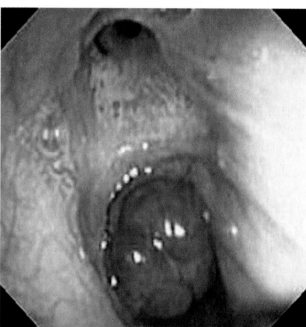

FIGURE 18. A 36-year-old woman who never smoked presented with a 3-year history of cough that had not responded to treatments for asthma, gastroesophageal reflux, and cough suppression. Chest radiograph showed volume loss, and CT showed an obstructing lesion in the bronchus intermedius (*arrow, top panel*). At bronchoscopy a polypoid lesion was seen (*bottom panel*), and biopsies confirmed a typical carcinoid tumor. Sleeve bronchoplasty was performed and she remained disease free 8 years later.

pleural thickening. Mesothelioma may be difficult to diagnose; although thoracentesis and/or closed pleural biopsy may be diagnostic, a larger biopsy (usually obtained with video-assisted thoracic surgery) is often required. Histologically, mesotheliomas are categorized as predominantly epithelial or sarcomatous (spindle cell morphology), but mixed variants are common.

Chemotherapy is the usual treatment, but it is not often effective. For localized disease of the epithelioid type, extrapleural pneumonectomy (removal of the entire pleural surface along with the lung) may be an option in highly select patients and usually follows chemotherapy. Pleural catheter placement or pleurodesis is often needed to palliate symptoms for large recurrent effusions due to mesothelioma. For a discussion of other types of asbestos-related lung disease, see Occupational Lung Disease.

Neoplasms Metastatic to the Lung

The lung is a common site of metastases from cancers originating in other organs. Frequent sources for pulmonary metastases include cancers of the head and neck, colon, kidney, breast, thyroid, and skin (melanoma). Metastases are often suspected based on the history of malignancy and the pattern of involvement in the lung. Presence of innumerable nodules, multiple nodules of 1 cm or larger, or multiple masses in a patient with a history of malignancy suggests metastases (**Figure 19**). Lymphangitic metastasis, or tumor spread through the lymphatic system, presents with a pattern of nodular thickening of the septa of pulmonary lobules. Malignant pleural effusions may be caused by metastatic disease from primary lung cancer as well as malignancies outside the chest. Surgical resection may be appropriate for solitary pulmonary metastasis when there is no evidence of spread elsewhere. Improvement in survival has been demonstrated for patients who have resection of solitary pulmonary metastasis from sarcomas, renal cell carcinoma, breast cancer, and colon cancer.

Mediastinal Masses

The mediastinum lies between the two pleural surfaces in the center of the chest and is divided into anterior, middle, and posterior compartments. These categories are helpful clinically in determining a differential diagnosis. Patients with mediastinal tumors may present with cough, venous distention, hoarseness, back pain, or chest pain, or they may be

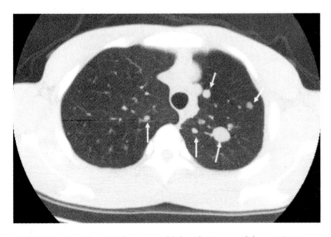

FIGURE 19. Chest CT showing multiple pulmonary nodules consistent with metastases (*arrows*)

asymptomatic. Imaging with CT, MRI, and sometimes additional studies such as a thyroid scan or endoscopic ultrasound are used for further characterization.

If images strongly indicate that a lesion is a cyst, follow-up is indicated. A mediastinal mass that remains indeterminate after imaging studies is usually an indication for biopsy or removal.

Anterior Mediastinal Masses

Masses in the anterior mediastinum are most commonly lymphoma, thyroid (or parathyroid) tumors, thymoma (or thymic carcinoma), or teratoma (or germ cell tumor). Substernal thyroid glands should be managed with observation unless symptomatic. Teratomas have all three germ cell lines present and may be distinguishable on plain chest radiograph or CT scan if contents such as teeth are radiographically visible. Thymomas may be malignant or benign. Benign thymomas are generally well encapsulated. Malignant thymomas typically invade the adjacent tissues, but the distinction of malignancy is made histologically. If thymoma is suggested by imaging studies, resection is often performed. There are several paraneoplastic syndromes that can be associated with thymoma; the most common is myasthenia gravis. Approximately 35% to 50% of patients with a thymoma will develop myasthenia gravis and exhibit the typical changes on electromyography and have elevated serum acetylcholine receptor antibodies. Other paraneoplastic syndromes associated with thymoma include pure red cell aplasia and hypogammaglobulinemia.

Middle Mediastinal Masses

Causes of middle mediastinal masses include enlarged lymph nodes from metastasis, lymphoma, granulomatous disease (sarcoidosis, fungal infections, tuberculosis), or giant lymph node hyperplasia (Castleman disease). Other causes of a mass in the middle compartment include diaphragmatic hernia, pericardial or bronchogenic cysts, and vascular masses and enlargements.

Posterior Mediastinal Masses

Masses in the posterior mediastinum originate most often from neural tissue or the esophagus. Common neural tumors include neurofibroma and neurilemmoma (schwannoma). Esophageal lesions include leiomyomas, fibromas, lipomas, and carcinoma.

KEY POINTS

- Carcinoid tumors are histologically described as typical and atypical; typical carcinoid has an excellent prognosis with surgery.

- The lung is a common site of metastases from cancers originating in other organs (common sources are the head and neck, colon, kidney, breast, thyroid, and skin).

- Determining the location of a mass in the mediastinum (anterior, middle, or posterior compartment) is a diagnostic clue to its cause.

Sleep Medicine

Excessive Daytime Sleepiness

Excessive daytime sleepiness (EDS) refers to difficulty staying awake and alert during daytime hours. EDS is typically most prominent during permissive situations, such as reading, watching television, driving, or meetings. Sleepiness should be distinguished from fatigue, which is a sense of exhaustion that prevents mental or physical activity at the intensity and/or pace desired. Fatigue is rarely the result of a primary sleep disorder. More commonly, fatigue is due to medical conditions (chronic infections, malignancies, autoimmune disorders, endocrinopathies), neurologic diseases (myasthenia gravis, multiple sclerosis, Parkinson disease), psychiatric conditions (mood disorders), and chronic fatigue syndrome.

Causes of excessive sleepiness can be categorized as extrinsic (circumstantial) or intrinsic (disease-related) processes (**Table 44**).

Insufficient sleep duration (or sleep deprivation) is the most common cause of EDS and plays an important role in motor vehicle and occupational accidents. It has also been implicated as a cause of medical errors by residents in training. Because insufficient sleep duration is pervasive in our society, the evaluation of EDS should include a thorough history of the sleep-wake schedule to ensure that opportunities for adequate sleep time (7 to 8 hours for most people) exist before pursuing additional testing. This may be accomplished simply by having a patient keep a 1- or 2-week sleep diary that identifies the number of hours spent awake and asleep. A more objective assessment of sleep and wakefulness can be obtained with an actigraph, a wristwatch-shaped device that measures movement and ambient light over a 1- or 2-week period.

Subjective questionnaires (for example, the Epworth Sleepiness Scale) may be helpful in quantifying EDS. Polysomnography, a sleep laboratory–based study, is useful if a primary sleep disorder such as sleep-disordered breathing is suggested by the history and physical examination. Mean sleep latency testing (MSLT), another sleep laboratory–based study, measures the time to sleep in a series of brief naps. MSLT provides an objective measure of sleepiness and is key to establishing the diagnoses of narcolepsy and idiopathic hypersomnia. MSLT may also aid in the evaluation of patients with persistent EDS despite standard therapy (for example, a patient with obstructive sleep apnea who is compliant with continuous positive airway pressure therapy). On MSLT, a mean sleep latency of more than 15 minutes is considered normal and less than 5 minutes is indicative of pathologic sleepiness.

Therapy for EDS, regardless of the cause, should include counseling to maintain a firm sleep-wake schedule that allows for 8 hours of sleep. Specific treatment depends on the underlying condition (for example, continuous positive airway pressure for obstructive sleep apnea or stimulants for narcolepsy). Short-term management may include naps or caffeinated beverages. Patients with EDS should be instructed to avoid driving or engaging in potentially hazardous activities when drowsy.

Common Conditions that Disrupt Circadian Rhythm

Jet Lag

Jet lag results when the internal circadian clock is out of phase with the local time following air travel across multiple (more than five) time zones. Symptoms are proportional to the distance traveled and may include insomnia, daytime sleepiness, and neuropsychiatric impairment. Jet lag is usually self limited, but the several days required to realign the internal and external clocks may be unacceptably long for the frequent business traveler or the infrequent vacationer. Management includes general measures (avoidance of sleep deprivation and dehydration before travel; hypnotic medications if needed during flight; and naps, caffeinated beverages, and/or stimulant drugs after flight) and specific interventions (bright light exposure and/or melatonin) given at specific times depending upon the direction traveled.

Shift Work Sleep Disorder

It is estimated that as much as one fifth of the American work force maintains a job schedule outside the usual day shift hours. Notwithstanding recent changes in medical trainee work hours, shift work is intrinsic to the health care industry, and it has been associated with an increased risk of motor vehicle accidents. Shift work sleep disorder (SWSD), associated mainly with the night shift, is mechanistically similar to jet lag in that the internal circadian clock is desynchronized

---

TABLE 44. Extrinsic and Intrinsic Causes of Excessive Sleepiness

Extrinsic Causes
Insufficient sleep duration (or inadequate opportunity for sleep)
Circadian rhythm disturbance (shift work sleep disorder, jet lag)
Drug-, substance-, or medical condition–related hypersomnia
Environmental sleep disorder (ambient noise, pets)

Intrinsic Causes
Sleep-disordered breathing syndromes, such as obstructive sleep apnea and central sleep apnea
Narcolepsy
Idiopathic hypersomnia
Restless legs syndrome and periodic limb movement disorder
Circadian rhythm sleep disorders

with the 24-hour clock; however, the persistence of this misalignment distinguishes SWSD from jet lag. SWSD is characterized by insomnia during the daytime sleep period and resultant sleepiness during the nighttime work period. Management may include bright light treatment in the evening before the night shift, caffeinated beverages or stimulants during work hours, planned napping during work breaks, and bright light avoidance with or without hypnotic medications in the morning in anticipation of the daytime sleep period.

KEY POINTS

- Insufficient sleep duration (or sleep deprivation) is the most common cause of excessive daytime sleepiness and plays an important role in motor vehicle and occupational accidents.
- Therapy for excessive daytime sleepiness, regardless of the cause, should include counseling to maintain a firm sleep-wake schedule that allows for a minimum of 7 to 8 hours of sleep.

Obstructive Sleep Apnea

Obstructive sleep apnea (OSA) is defined by repetitive narrowing and/or occlusion of the upper airway during sleep. During polysomnography monitoring, upper airway events are classified as apneas (characterized by complete cessation of airflow) or hypopneas (reductions in airflow), known as disordered breathing events. The apnea-hypopnea index (AHI) is the number of disordered breathing events per hour of sleep, and it is the standard by which severity of OSA is measured. An AHI of 5 to 15 indicates mild OSA; an AHI of more than 30 indicates severe OSA.

Pathophysiology

OSA is characterized by upper airway instability, where neuromuscular mechanisms that maintain airway patency during sleep are overcome by forces that promote collapse. Snoring is usually present and occurs as inspired air collides with redundant soft tissue. Disordered breathing events are particularly prominent during sleep in the supine position, when airway narrowing is promoted by gravitational forces, and during rapid eye movement (REM), a stage of sleep characterized by muscle atonia. Lack of airflow may persist for several seconds, but efforts to breathe against the occlusion continue, resulting in episodes of markedly negative intrathoracic pressure. Disordered breathing events are usually terminated with a brief awakening from sleep (called a microarousal), where upper airway patency is restored, ventilation resumes, and reoxygenation occurs.

Classically, obstructive breathing events result in an acute surge in peripheral vascular resistance along with slowing of heart rate; this response to hypoxemia is called the diving reflex, as a similar cascade of events are observed in diving

mammals such as sea lions. Adrenergic tone and inflammatory markers are often elevated in patients with OSA. As airway narrowing or collapse may persist for several seconds, oxyhemoglobin desaturations can be marked, particularly in those who have coexistent cardiopulmonary disease. These nightly repetitive physiologic stressors are believed to be important in the development of other disorders. Observational studies have shown OSA to be an established independent risk factor for hypertension. OSA is also associated with heart failure, cardiac arrhythmias, and diabetes mellitus, but shared underlying risk factors such as obesity, aging, and male gender make cause and effect difficult to establish.

Risk Factors

The most important risk factor for OSA is obesity, particularly in patients with prominent distribution of adipose tissue in the trunk and neck. Men are at higher risk than women; however, rates are similar between genders following menopause. Alcohol and sedative drugs can exacerbate OSA. Tonsillar hypertrophy, macroglossia, retrognathia/micrognathia, and upper airway mass lesions can contribute to upper airway narrowing.

Clinical Features and Diagnosis

Loud snoring, gasping, and breathing pauses are commonly observed by a bed partner in patients with OSA. Subjective symptoms include frequent awakenings, snorting, and nonrestorative sleep. Morning headaches are uncommon and are a nonspecific symptom.

EDS is the classic consequence of OSA. EDS is not present in all patients with OSA, but the absence of self-reporting should not take the place of a careful history (including collateral history from a family member), which often reveals some degree of impaired daytime alertness. Other neuropsychiatric symptoms are common, including mood alterations, difficulty in concentrating, and problems completing tasks at school or the workplace.

Occasionally, OSA first comes to medical attention immediately following a surgical procedure involving general anesthesia and/or narcotic analgesia, when repeated apneas, acute respiratory failure, and even death unexpectedly occur.

Objective testing is required for a diagnosis of OSA. The current gold standard is polysomnography; however, its cost and limited availability in some regions have spurred interest in multichannel portable home monitoring, which will likely continue to gain interest in the future. Overnight oximetry alone is not sufficiently sensitive or specific in patients with moderate to high pretest probability of OSA; however, normal oximetry may be helpful in ruling out OSA and avoiding polysomnography in patients with a low pretest probability.

Treatment

Strong indications for treatment of OSA include EDS or other daytime neurocognitive symptoms, particularly in patients who perform mission critical work (truck drivers, pilots). The role of treatment in otherwise healthy individuals or patients with comorbid cardiovascular disease without such symptoms is not clear.

Weight Loss and Conservative Measures

Because even small reductions in body weight are associated with clinically significant improvements in the AHI, weight loss should be recommended to overweight patients with OSA. Other lifestyle or conservative measures may include curbing alcohol intake before bedtime and avoiding a supine posture if OSA is position dependent.

Positive Airway Pressure

Positive airway pressure (PAP) remains the most proven and effective therapy for OSA. By delivering ambient air at a constant pressure, continuous positive airway pressure (CPAP) acts as a pneumatic splint, holding the airway open and thereby eliminating upper airway flow limitation in the vast majority of patients. It is associated with improvements in daytime symptoms, objective sleepiness, and quality of life. Occasionally, bilevel PAP (BPAP), which delivers separate inspiratory and expiratory pressures (the gradient is referred to as pressure support) to augment alveolar ventilation, is used in patients with an underlying hypoventilation syndrome (see Sleep-Related Hypoventilation Syndromes) or for patients in whom the constant pressure of CPAP is uncomfortable. However, the efficacy of BPAP for routine management of OSA compared with CPAP has not been established.

Traditionally, PAP devices have been manually titrated by a trained technician in the polysomnography laboratory to eliminate apneas and hypopneas. An alternative to this resource-intensive approach is the autotitrating PAP machine, which uses a computer algorithm to detect upper airway narrowing and responds with pressures sufficient to overcome it; this approach might be used as part of a portable testing program in lieu of a clinical sleep laboratory.

The effectiveness of PAP therapy depends upon user compliance, which may be negatively affected by side effects such as rhinitis and nasal congestion. In-line heated humidification, nasal saline sprays, or corticosteroid sprays may alleviate nasal symptoms, although the benefits of these interventions in increasing compliance have not been documented. Claustrophobia can be managed by proper mask fitting and a desensitization program, where the patient gradually increases mask time application during longer intervals while awake. A trial of alternative delivery systems, such as different mask types, may also help in increasing compliance.

Surgery

Upper airway surgeries have been performed for decades as a treatment for OSA with varying reports of success. Soft-palatal procedures such as uvulopalatopharyngoplasty (UPPP) result in only very modest reductions in the AHI. Maxillomandibular advancement (MMA), which may be performed in conjunction with a soft-palatal procedure, may be more effective at reducing the AHI. Tonsillectomy is the treatment of choice in children with tonsillar hypertrophy and significant airway obstruction, although this is rarely curative in adults. Because the surgical literature consists mostly of case reports and series, objective data regarding surgical outcomes and risks in OSA are limited. Therefore, surgical procedures are not recommended as primary therapy for OSA. Although surgery can be considered in those who fail to respond to or refuse CPAP and/or weight loss, recent analyses of the surgical literature have failed to conclusively identify which preoperative variables predict surgical success. If surgery is performed, reassessment of the AHI by polysomnography should be performed within 3 to 6 months of surgical intervention to assess evidence of benefit.

Tracheostomy, which bypasses the entire upper airway, is an effective treatment for OSA, but it is limited by patient acceptance, aesthetics, an increased risk of infection, and the need for maintenance.

Oral Appliances

Mandibular advancement devices (oral appliances that pull the mandible forward to increase upper airway caliber and reduce posterior displacement of the tongue) are modestly effective for patients with mild to moderate OSA. Some form of objective confirmation of efficacy should be performed with the oral appliance in place, which could include polysomnography or oximetry.

Other Therapies

Novel nasal end-expiratory PAP technology has recently been developed that is applied to the nasal openings by way of an adhesive. The device generates pressure upon exhalation and has been shown to reduce the AHI. However, there is insufficient evidence that it is more effective than CPAP or that compliance is greater than with standard therapy. No drug therapy is currently available for OSA. Supplemental oxygen is not recommended as primary therapy for OSA.

KEY POINTS

- Obstructive sleep apnea is defined by repetitive narrowing and/or occlusion of the upper airway during sleep.
- The most important risk factor for obstructive sleep apnea is obesity.
- Polysomnography is the gold standard for diagnosis of obstructive sleep apnea.
- Weight loss should be recommended to overweight patients with obstructive sleep apnea.
- Positive airway pressure remains the most proven and effective therapy for obstructive sleep apnea.

Central Sleep Apnea Syndromes

Classification and Pathophysiology

Central sleep apnea (CSA) syndromes were previously classified into two general categories based upon the presence or absence of hypercapnia during wakefulness. However, in the modern classification the term CSA denotes nonhypercapnic disorders, which are discussed here. For conditions associated with hypercapnia, see Sleep-Related Hypoventilation Syndromes.

CSA is characterized by loss of ventilatory output from the central respiratory generator in the brainstem to the respiratory pump, which manifests on polysomnography with the absence of respiratory effort associated with loss of airflow for at least 10 seconds.

Compared with wakefulness, ventilation decreases during sleep and is primarily determined by blood carbon dioxide tension (arterial P_{CO_2}); increases in arterial P_{CO_2} cause a near-linear increase in ventilation (as opposed to a weaker influence from decreasing blood oxygen levels). A key mechanistic feature of CSA is the tendency to hyperventilate and drive down the arterial P_{CO_2} to a level near the apneic threshold (the point at which respiratory effort ceases).

Not all central apneas are pathologic. Sleep-onset central apneas are physiologic and occur during transitions from wakefulness to sleep. Sleep-onset central apnea by definition is transient, persisting until arterial P_{CO_2} rises to a steady state as sleep deepens and ventilation stabilizes. In contrast, pathologic CSA occurs throughout the sleep cycle, particularly during non-REM sleep.

Risk Factors

Risk factors for CSA include comorbid illnesses (particularly heart failure, atrial fibrillation, stroke, brainstem lesions, and kidney failure), and the use of opiate analgesics. Men may be at higher risk than women. A small percentage of patients with OSA who are treated with CPAP develop CSA (known as CPAP-emergent CSA or complex apnea). CSA often occurs with ascension to higher altitude (see High-Altitude–Related Illnesses). In a small proportion of patients with CSA, no risk factors are identified; this is known as primary or idiopathic CSA.

The most common type of CSA is Cheyne-Stokes breathing (also referred to as periodic breathing), characterized by a crescendo-decrescendo pattern of ventilation (periods of gradually waxing and waning tidal volume). It is strongly associated with heart failure, in which there is an exaggerated ventilatory response to carbon dioxide. It may indicate worse survival in patients with heart failure, although it is not clear whether CSA is a marker of more severe heart failure or an independent risk factor for death.

Symptoms and Diagnosis

Symptoms of CSA may include frequent awakenings from sleep, insomnia, nonrestorative sleep, EDS, and paroxysmal nocturnal dyspnea. These symptoms can mimic those of OSA, and it is often the clinical context of comorbid disease (central nervous system disease or heart failure) that heightens the suspicion for CSA. However, many patients with CSA do not report sleep-related symptoms, particularly those with heart failure. Polysomnography is required to accurately diagnose CSA. Oximetry alone, if abnormal, does not reliably discriminate between OSA and CSA.

Treatment

Treatment is indicated for patients with sleep-related symptoms and should first target management of the comorbid condition. Medical optimization of heart failure has been shown to attenuate Cheyne-Stokes breathing. Reduction or withdrawal of opioids improves CSA.

Although there is interest in treating CSA as a means of adjunctively managing comorbid conditions such as heart failure or atrial fibrillation, interventional trials are currently lacking to show benefit of such a practice. There is further uncertainty in patients who have no sleep-related symptoms, and little evidence exists to guide whether such patients should be screened or targeted for therapy directed at CSA.

In patients with an indication for treatment of CSA, various forms of PAP therapy are used. CPAP may be useful, particularly if there is overlapping OSA; however, in many cases, CSA may be exacerbated by CPAP. Under these circumstances and in patients with CPAP-emergent CSA, adaptive servoventilation (ASV) is often effective at stabilizing ventilation. The computer algorithm governing ASV promotes ventilatory stability with timed delivery of pressure support that is synchronized to the patient's breathing effort. Despite the immediate apparent efficacy of ASV in the laboratory setting, there is currently little data on clinical outcomes related to ASV use in CSA.

Small studies have shown supplemental oxygen to attenuate CSA. Emerging evidence supports the efficacy of treatment with low levels of inhaled carbon dioxide. The carbonic anhydrase inhibitor acetazolamide has been shown to reduce CSA in patients with and without heart failure and in those at high altitude. The respiratory stimulant theophylline may stabilize ventilatory rhythm in CSA, but potential proarrhythmic effects in patients with heart failure may limit its usefulness.

KEY POINTS

- Risk factors for central sleep apnea include heart failure, atrial fibrillation, stroke, brainstem lesions, kidney failure, opiate use, and travel to high altitudes.

- Treatment of central sleep apnea is indicated for patients with symptoms and should first target management of the comorbid condition.

Sleep-Related Hypoventilation Syndromes

The most common sleep-related hypoventilation syndromes are those associated with other medical conditions. Most notable are COPD, obesity hypoventilation syndrome, and restrictive lung diseases related to kyphoscoliosis or neuromuscular disorders (**Table 45**). Documented hypercapnia during sleep is generally required to confirm hypoventilation, but such measurements are rarely practical. Instead, sustained reductions in oxyhemoglobin saturations (<90% for at least 5 minutes or more than 30% of total sleep time by oximetry or polysomnography) in the setting of a compatible medical condition signify a hypoventilation syndrome. Obstructive or central disordered breathing events may or may not be an associated feature, and it is the sustained reductions in oxyhemoglobin saturations that distinguish hypoventilation syndromes from the brief, repetitive deoxygenation-reoxygenation cycles typical of OSA or CSA.

Chronic Obstructive Pulmonary Disease

Patients with chronic airflow obstruction have exaggerations of the normally mild reductions in blood oxygen and increases in carbon dioxide levels associated with the sleep state. These are particularly evident during REM sleep, where muscle atonia can result in severe oxyhemoglobin desaturations. The overlap syndrome is characterized by OSA superimposed upon gas exchange abnormalities related to the underlying pulmonary disease. In addition to optimization of COPD therapy, the pressure support of BPAP is often required to bolster ventilation, sometimes with supplemental oxygen if gas exchange derangements are severe.

Obesity Hypoventilation Syndrome

Previously referred to as the pickwickian syndrome, the obesity hypoventilation syndrome (OHS) is an increasingly recognized disorder. The epidemiology of OHS is not well described, and the disorder likely remains underappreciated or misdiagnosed as asthma or COPD. It is estimated that nearly one third of persons with a BMI of 35 or higher and one half with a BMI of 50 or higher exhibit sleep-related hypoventilation.

Daytime hypercapnia (arterial P_{CO_2} >45 mm Hg [6.0 kPa]) is a cardinal sign of OHS, reflecting reduced ventilation during wakefulness as well as sleep, which is believed to result from a combination of mechanical load imposed by obesity and attenuation of both hypoxic and hypercapnic ventilatory drive. Cardiopulmonary morbidity in OHS is very high, and there are high rates of biventricular failure and pulmonary hypertension.

Because OSA often coexists with OHS, first-line therapy is usually CPAP; however, in patients with resistant hypoventilation and hypoxemia, the addition of supplemental oxygen or BPAP may be required. Clinical trials comparing different treatment options are currently lacking, but weight loss (possibly including bariatric surgical intervention) should be universally recommended.

Neuromuscular Diseases

Because many neuromuscular disorders (see Table 45) have no known treatment, assisted breathing devices are often prescribed to alleviate sleep-related symptoms and to support blood oxygen levels. CPAP may be effective in isolated cases of OSA without respiratory pump impairment; however, in more advanced cases in which there is hypercapnic respiratory impairment due to neuromuscular disease, BPAP with or without supplemental oxygen should be considered, particularly in patients with associated pulmonary hypertension, right-sided heart failure, or polycythemia. Tracheostomy and home mechanical ventilation may be appropriate in some patients. Importantly, supplemental oxygen may further depress ventilation in patients with respiratory muscle weakness and should generally not be prescribed without adjunctive ventilatory support, either by noninvasive means or by tracheostomy.

TABLE 45. Sleep-Related Hypoventilation Syndromes
COPD
Obesity hypoventilation syndrome
Myxedema
Neuromuscular disease
Muscular dystrophy
Amyotrophic lateral sclerosis
Myasthenia gravis
Guillain-Barré syndrome
Phrenic nerve injury
Poliomyelitis, post-polio syndrome
Cervical spine injury
Kyphoscoliosis

KEY POINTS

- The most common sleep-related hypoventilation syndromes are those associated with COPD, obesity hypoventilation syndrome, and restrictive lung diseases related to kyphoscoliosis or neuromuscular disorders.

- It is estimated that nearly one third of persons with a BMI of 35 or higher and one half with a BMI of 50 or higher exhibit obesity hypoventilation syndrome.

- Because many neuromuscular disorders have no known treatment, assisted breathing devices are often prescribed to alleviate sleep-related symptoms and to support blood oxygen levels.

High-Altitude–Related Illnesses

Sleep Disturbances and Periodic Breathing

Nearly everyone who ascends to elevations greater than 7500 meters (approximately 25,000 feet) will experience high-altitude periodic breathing (HAPB), characterized by cyclic central apneas and hyperpneas associated with repetitive arousals from sleep, often with paroxysms of dyspnea. The onset of HAPB coincides with ascension and usually occurs the first night at elevation. Significant symptoms can occur at lesser elevations but usually do not occur below 2500 meters (approximately 8200 feet). The pathophysiologic mechanism appears to be an exaggerated ventilatory response to the reduced ambient partial pressure of inspired oxygen (known as hypobaric hypoxia), leading to hypocapnia and ventilatory instability. The best method of management is prevention. A gradual rather than rapid ascent allows acclimatization. Acetazolamide, which accelerates the acclimatization process, is sometimes used prophylactically, particularly in patients with a history of altitude illness. Supplemental oxygen, if available, often relieves symptoms of disrupted sleep and paroxysmal nocturnal dyspnea.

Acute Mountain Sickness and High-Altitude Cerebral Edema

Acute mountain sickness is diagnosed clinically based on nonspecific symptoms of varying intensity (headache, fatigue, nausea, vomiting, and disturbed sleep) in a person who lives at low altitude and has recently ascended to a high altitude. There are wide individual differences in susceptibility to the effects of altitude, but mountain sickness tends to occur at elevations greater than 2000 meters (approximately 6500 feet). Symptoms, which may be mistaken or dismissed as an expected result of physical activity, are typically delayed for 6 to 12 hours after ascent and usually resolve within 24 hours, provided no further ascent occurs. Prevention and treatment are similar to HAPB.

An extreme and more serious manifestation of acute mountain sickness is high-altitude cerebral edema, where encephalopathy (characterized by altered mental status) and ataxia occur in response to vasogenic brain swelling. Because the risk of coma and death is high, suspicion of cerebral edema should prompt immediate intervention. Definitive treatment is descent from altitude; dexamethasone, supplemental oxygen, and hyperbaric therapy may be used as temporizing measures.

High-Altitude Pulmonary Edema

A leaky pulmonary vasculature, thought to arise from elevations in pulmonary artery pressures in response to hypoxia, appears to play a role in high-altitude pulmonary edema. Symptoms of cough, dyspnea, chest tightness, fatigue, and decreased exercise capacity occur insidiously, usually over 2 to 4 days at high altitude. Other features of acute mountain sickness may or may not be present. The onset may occasionally be acute, particularly during sleep. On examination, affected patients have tachypnea and tachycardia. Crackles or wheezing are present, occasionally as a unilateral finding. As disease progresses, pink frothy sputum or frank hemoptysis may be evident, followed by worsening gas exchange and respiratory failure. The treatment of choice is supplemental oxygen. If oxygen is not available, descent should ensue. Salvage therapies in the absence of supplemental oxygen and transport include vasodilators such as nifedipine or phosphodiesterase-5 inhibitors (sildenafil).

Air Travel in Pulmonary Disease

Commercial airline cabins are pressurized to the equivalent of 1500 to 2500 meters (approximately 5000 to 8200 feet) in altitude, which results in an inspired oxygen tension between 110 and 120 mm Hg (normal levels are 150 to 160 mm Hg at sea level). In persons with underlying pulmonary disease (COPD or pulmonary hypertension), such levels may cause substantial reductions in arterial oxygenation during flight. Screening for prospective travelers with lung disease should consist of pulse oximetry at sea level; an oxyhemoglobin saturation of less than 92% indicates a probable need for in-flight supplemental oxygen. Simulators that mimic altitude hypoxia, available at some centers, can be used to better define oxygenation in at-risk patients. Established indications for hypoxia altitude simulation testing include patients with equivocal oximetry (92% to 95%) or an arterial Po_2 of less than 70 mm Hg (9.3 kPa) and patients with COPD who have hypercapnia on chronic oxygen therapy, previous in-flight symptoms, or a recent exacerbation. Patients who are already on supplemental oxygen will likely need an increase in flow rates for air travel.

Because the cabins of commercial airlines are partially pressurized, the risk of a pneumothorax or pneumomediastinum developing during flight is generally believed to be low. In theory, those with bullae, blebs, or cystic lung disease may have a higher risk, and such patients should be questioned about any history of pneumothorax. Furthermore, an exacerbation of COPD, where air trapping is more pronounced, should prompt a delay in any planned air travel. An existing pneumothorax, even if small enough that it may not require hospitalization or active therapy, is a contraindication to flight, because the reduction in barometric pressure during flight (even in pressurized cabins) causes the air inside a pneumothorax cavity to expand, which could result in tension physiology.

- High-altitude periodic breathing is characterized by cyclic central apneas and hyperpneas associated with repetitive arousals from sleep, often with paroxysms of dyspnea.

- Acute mountain sickness is a clinical diagnosis based upon nonspecific symptoms of varying intensity (headache, fatigue, nausea, vomiting, and disturbed sleep) in a person who lives at low altitude and has recently ascended to a high altitude.

- An extreme and more serious manifestation of acute mountain sickness is high-altitude cerebral edema, where encephalopathy and ataxia occur in response to vasogenic brain swelling.

- Screening of prospective air travelers with lung disease should consist of pulse oximetry at sea level; an oxyhemoglobin saturation of less than 92% indicates a probable need for in-flight supplemental oxygen.

Critical Care

Recognizing the Critically Ill Patient

Survival of the critically ill patient depends on initiating life-saving measures in a timely fashion. However, recognizing serious illness before the onset of overt instability can be challenging. For example, younger patients with sepsis or calcium channel blocker overdose can appear deceptively well but may develop multiorgan failure within hours. A systematic approach to patient assessment minimizes the likelihood of delayed recognition of critical illness.

The initial evaluation should consist of a brief bedside history and focused examination to discern whether immediate action is needed to stabilize the patient's airway, breathing, or circulation. Review of vital signs over the preceding hours often provides valuable information on the patient's overall trajectory and current stability. Common early interventions include intravenous fluid boluses for hypotension, oxygen and noninvasive ventilatory support for respiratory distress, and naloxone or dextrose (D50) for encephalopathy due to narcosis and hypoglycemia, respectively. Studies that may be useful for diagnosing the cause and determining severity of illness include arterial or venous blood gases; plasma glucose, hemoglobin, and serum lactate levels; electrocardiography; and portable chest radiography. The use of limited bedside echocardiography by intensivists to assess the hemodynamic status of unstable patients has increased in recent years. After imminently life-threatening issues are addressed, a more comprehensive secondary assessment should be performed with an emphasis on identifying less obvious evidence of organ hypoperfusion. This includes changes in mental status (confusion, agitation), decreased urine output, skin changes (pallor, diaphoresis, cyanosis, cool extremities), and increased work of breathing.

Respiratory Failure

Admission to the intensive care unit (ICU) for respiratory insufficiency is prompted by three basic conditions: (1) hypoxemic respiratory failure; (2) ventilatory, or hypercapnic, respiratory failure; and (3) impaired upper airway.

Hypoxemic Respiratory Failure

Acute hypoxemic respiratory failure is characterized by an abrupt, severe decline in oxyhemoglobin saturation that does not readily correct with supplemental oxygen. Generally, the ambient air arterial P_{O_2} is 60 mm Hg (8.0 kPa) or less and the arterial P_{O_2}/F_{IO_2} is 200 mm Hg (26.6 kPa) or less; the arterial P_{CO_2} is typically normal or reduced. Hypoxemia is caused by ongoing perfusion of lung units that are no longer receiving ventilation owing to alveolar collapse or flooding with edema, pus, or blood. This creates intrapulmonary shunt physiology that does not correct with increased alveolar ventilation or supplemental oxygen. Rather, hypoxemia is reversed by application of positive end-expiratory pressure (PEEP) to the lung, which opens up, or "recruits," flooded or collapsed alveoli.

Acute Respiratory Distress Syndrome

Pathophysiology, Epidemiology, and Diagnosis
The acute respiratory distress syndrome (ARDS) is a noncardiogenic form of pulmonary edema characterized by acute, persistent, diffuse lung inflammation that is injurious to alveolar epithelial cells and pulmonary capillary endothelial cells. The consequent increased vascular permeability and cytokine release result in leakage of protein, fluid, and neutrophils into the interstitium and alveoli. This, in turn, shifts the oncotic gradient in favor of further movement of fluid out of the vasculature. Atelectasis due to decreased surfactant function further impairs gas exchange. Alveolar flooding and atelectasis reduce lung compliance and thereby markedly increase the work of breathing. The pathologic correlate of ARDS is diffuse alveolar damage, although the diagnosis usually is made clinically rather than histologically.

Previously, patients with this type of lung injury and an arterial P_{O_2}/F_{IO_2} of ≤300 mm Hg (39.9 kPa) were defined as having acute lung injury (ALI); the subset of patients with more severe hypoxia (an arterial P_{O_2}/F_{IO_2} ≤200 mm Hg [26.6 kPa]) were classified as having ARDS. However, the 2012 Berlin definition of ARDS, a validated consensus by the European Society of Intensive Care Medicine, the American Thoracic Society, and Society of Critical Care Medicine, recommended defining and classifying ARDS into mild, moderate, and severe by the level of oxygenation and eliminating the term ALI. The Berlin criteria for the diagnosis of ARDS

CONT.

include: (1) acute onset within 1 week of an apparent clinical insult or development and progression of respiratory symptoms; (2) bilateral opacities on chest imaging not explained by other pulmonary pathology (such as pleural effusions, lung collapse, or nodules); (3) respiratory failure not explained by heart failure or volume overload. Mild ARDS is defined by an arterial P_{O_2}/F_{IO_2} ratio between 201 and 300 mm Hg (26.7 and 39.9 kPa). In moderate ARDS, the ratio is between 101 and 200 mm Hg (13.4 and 26.6 kPa), and severe ARDS is defined by a ratio of 100 mm Hg (13.3 kPa) or less. All three categories require that measurement of the arterial P_{O_2}/F_{IO_2} ratio be performed with a PEEP level of at least 5 cm H_2O, which may be delivered noninvasively with CPAP in the mild ARDS group. The new definition also explicitly defines the acuity criterion, recognizes that both chest radiograph and chest CT scans can fulfill the radiographic requirement, and eliminates pulmonary artery wedge pressure measurement from the definition. The use of pulmonary artery catheters has declined significantly owing to substantial evidence that their routine use does not improve outcomes in patients with lung injury. Furthermore, cardiac failure and volume overload can coexist with ARDS. According to the new definition, the exclusion of cardiogenic edema does not require objective assessment (with echocardiography or possibly measurement of pulmonary artery wedge pressure) unless the patient presents without a risk factor for developing ARDS.

More than 60 disorders can precipitate ARDS by direct or indirect injury to the lung, but severe sepsis from pneumonia or nonpulmonary sources constitutes the majority of cases (**Table 46**). Lung injury typically manifests 48 to 72 hours after risk-factor exposure. The approximate mortality rate of ARDS is 40%; trauma-associated lung injury has the best prognosis, and severe sepsis from a pulmonary source has the worst prognosis. Deaths are primarily caused by the underlying precipitant of lung injury or subsequent nosocomial infections rather than directly by lung injury.

Non–Ventilator-Related Management
Mechanical ventilation is the primary supportive treatment in ARDS. For details on ventilator management of ARDS, see the Invasive Mechanical Ventilation section later in this chapter.

The key pathologic event of ARDS is flooding of alveoli by disruption of alveolar capillary membranes. Because the increased capillary permeability allows greater intravascular leak at any given hydrostatic pressure, limiting intravascular volume to the level necessary to maintain tissue perfusion is optimal. A multicenter study of lung-injury patients with hemodynamic stability and normal kidney function found a relatively complex conservative fluid strategy improved lung function and shortened the duration of mechanical ventilation and ICU stay, but it did not change mortality. The conservative strategy utilized lower target central venous filling pressures. As a result, patients in the conservative group received fewer intravenous fluid boluses and more furosemide than patients in the liberal group.

Many other therapies have been tried in ARDS, and most have shown an improvement in oxygenation but not survival (**Table 47**). These include the use of pulmonary vasodilators and corticosteroids. Inhaled pulmonary vasodilators such as nitric oxide and prostaglandins have been shown to provide dramatic short-term increases in oxygenation and pulmonary artery pressures but no differences in mortality. Currently there is no clear evidence that corticosteroids benefit patients with ARDS, and they are not recommended routinely. Many

TABLE 46. Common Causes of Acute Respiratory Distress Syndrome	
Direct Pulmonary Injury	
Pneumonia	
Aspiration	
Near drowning	
Inhalational injury	
Trauma or lung contusion	
Indirect Pulmonary Injury	
Sepsis	
Severe trauma	
Multiple blood transfusions	
Pancreatitis	

TABLE 47. Nonventilator Management of Acute Respiratory Distress Syndrome	
Intervention	**Comments**
Inhaled vasodilators	↑ O_2 saturation; no proven survival benefit
Systemic corticosteroids	↑ O_2 saturation; may reduce duration of invasive ventilation; no survival benefit; optimal patient selection, timing, dose, and duration uncertain
Neuromuscular blockade	Used in early severe ARDS; may improve mortality but limited published experience and not widely used in North America
Conservative fluid strategy	↑ O_2 saturation and reduced duration of invasive mechanical ventilation in single large National Institutes of Health study
Prone positioning	↑ O_2 saturation; no survival benefit in individual trials
Extracorporeal membrane oxygenation	May improve mortality in severe ARDS but limited published experience, limited availability

ARDS = acute respiratory distress syndrome.

CONT.

therapies (inhaled vasodilators, prone positioning, occasionally corticosteroids) are still used in the minority of patients with life-threatening hypoxemia despite aggressive ventilator support even though there is no proven survival benefit.

A recent study found that pharmacologic paralysis of patients with severe ARDS for 48 hours early in the course of lung injury improved 90-day survival when adjusted for differences in baseline characteristics and did not increase the risk of residual neuromuscular weakness. However, these results will likely require replication before this approach would gain widespread acceptance. Experience managing patients with ARDS during the H1N1 influenza epidemic has renewed interest in the use of extracorporeal membrane oxygenation (ECMO) for severe refractory hypoxemia, but few centers offer this therapy and identifying patients most likely to benefit remains a challenge.

Heart Failure

Patients with left ventricular systolic dysfunction are prone to acute cardiogenic pulmonary edema, but the ejection fraction is normal in approximately half of patients admitted for heart failure. Diastolic dysfunction, myocardial ischemia, hypertension, valve disease, and a variety of tachyarrhythmias are important considerations in the absence of systolic failure. Regardless of the underlying cause, left-sided heart failure can produce bilateral pulmonary infiltrates that are radiographically indistinguishable from ARDS. Unlike ARDS, cardiogenic edema can rapidly improve with aggressive medical management, and therefore early differentiation of the two disorders is important. Echocardiography is the primary means of diagnosing systolic and diastolic failure and valve disease. Evaluation for myocardial ischemia includes measuring troponin levels and review of electrocardiograms for ischemic changes. Electrocardiograms are also used to evaluate arrhythmias. B-type natriuretic peptide levels can be useful in distinguishing cardiogenic from noncardiogenic edema in ambiguous cases, but they do not reliably diagnose or exclude heart failure when evaluated in isolation.

Atelectasis

Atelectasis is very common following general anesthesia. It accounts for approximately half of severe postoperative hypoxemia and can persist for days. Morbidly obese patients are particularly vulnerable to atelectasis, and respiratory failure is an important cause of perioperative mortality in patients undergoing bariatric surgery. Chest physiotherapy, incentive spirometry, early mobilization, and continuous positive airway pressure (CPAP) are commonly used in the perioperative period to prevent respiratory complications. Atelectasis is also common in patients receiving invasive mechanical ventilation. Supine position, absence of intermittent larger sigh breaths, and low tidal volumes predispose patients to bibasilar atelectasis. Mucus plugging and right-mainstem intubation can precipitate lobar collapse.

Pneumonia

Lung consolidation due to pneumonia creates a physiologic shunt similar to cardiogenic and ARDS-related edema. Pneumonia is the most common trigger for ARDS among nonhospitalized patients, and differentiating bilateral pneumonia from pneumonia that has evolved into ARDS can be difficult. Unilateral pneumonia occasionally causes profound hypoxemia. This is especially difficult to manage because focal areas of flooded and atelectatic lung are less amenable to recruitment with PEEP. In fact, PEEP can exacerbate hypoxemia in this setting by overdistending normal lung. Positioning the patient in the lateral decubitus position with the "good" lung dependent is a temporizing measure that may reduce intrapulmonary shunt. **H**

KEY POINTS

- Positive end-expiratory pressure is the first-line approach to correcting shunt-associated hypoxemia in patients with acute respiratory distress syndrome, but it is less applicable in the setting of focal disease.

- The diagnosis of acute respiratory distress syndrome (ARDS) is predominantly made on clinical grounds, and pulmonary artery catheters infrequently play a role in the diagnosis or management of ARDS.

- Atelectasis is an important cause of hypoxemia in surgical and mechanically ventilated patients.

Ventilatory (Hypercapnic) Respiratory Failure **H**

Ventilatory respiratory failure stems from inadequate alveolar ventilation relative to CO_2 production. Although the primary gas exchange abnormality in ventilatory failure is hypercapnia, patients typically have concomitant hypoxemia. Elevation of arterial P_{CO_2} arises from increased carbon dioxide production (V_{CO_2}) and/or decreased alveolar ventilation. Increased V_{CO_2} in critically ill patients usually stems from increased metabolic demands from fever or increased muscle activity related to the patient's respiratory efforts and/or agitation. Causes of decreased alveolar ventilation fall into one of three basic categories: (1) decreased respiratory drive, as seen with sedating drugs; (2) respiratory muscle weakness or excessive mechanical work of breathing, as seen in neuromuscular disease and severe kyphoscoliosis; and (3) lung diseases in which much of the inhaled gas does not participate in gas exchange. For instance, patients with COPD and severe ARDS have increased dead space, or "wasted" ventilation, resulting from ongoing ventilation of lung units that have injured capillary beds.

Reduced oxygen saturation accompanies CO_2 elevation in patients with ventilatory failure, but in contrast to patients with physiologic shunt, the hypoxemia corrects with supplemental oxygen. However, hypoxemic respiratory failure and ventilatory respiratory failure often occur concomitantly. For example, patients with severe ARDS have hypoxemic failure from shunt but may also be hypercapnic despite twice-normal

CONT.

minute ventilation as a result of increased work of breathing (elevated V_{CO_2}) and elevated dead-space ventilation. Dead-space ventilation, which normally constitutes 30% of each breath, can more than double in ARDS and is an independent predictor of mortality in ARDS.

Decreased Respiratory Drive

Illicit and iatrogenic drug overdoses are the most common causes of respiratory failure due to insufficient drive. Sedating drugs can be particularly problematic in patients with obesity hypoventilation syndrome and other conditions associated with baseline reduced ventilatory drive and CO_2 retention. Opioids are especially potent respiratory depressants, but any sedating medication taken in sufficient quantity can precipitate respiratory failure. Hypoglycemia must be excluded in patients with suspected drug overdose. In general, obtunded patients with ventilatory failure require intubation and mechanical ventilation to prevent aspiration and normalize gas exchange. Suspected opioid intoxication is an important exception, as excess sedation can be rapidly reversed with the opioid antagonist naloxone. Signs of opioid intoxication include miosis, encephalopathy, hypotension, hypothermia, and hyporeflexia. Alternative diagnoses should be sought in patients who do not respond to a total naloxone dose of 10 mg. The mean half-life of naloxone is only 1 hour, and continuous infusion may be necessary in patients who require frequent repeat dosing for recurrent respiratory depression. Chronic opioid users receiving naloxone should be closely monitored for signs of withdrawal, including delirium, agitation, diaphoresis, tremulousness, hypertension, fever, and seizures. The benzodiazepine antagonist flumazenil can rapidly reverse respiratory depression in patients with benzodiazepine overdose, but it is not routinely administered in this setting owing to the risk of precipitating seizures in chronic benzodiazepine users. Furthermore, benzodiazepine overdose generally does not cause life-threatening respiratory depression in the absence of coingestion of other drugs such as narcotics that suppress ventilatory drive. Strokes infrequently cause respiratory depression unless there is secondary intracranial hypertension. Decreased respiratory drive as well as muscle weakness can cause ventilatory failure in patients with severe hypothyroidism, but this is rare.

Neuromuscular Disease

Decreased ventilatory drive, impaired respiratory muscle strength, and chest wall disorders may cause ventilatory failure even in the absence of intrinsic lung disease, an effect referred to as bellows failure. Typical physical examination findings in patients with neuromuscular weakness include use of accessory respiratory muscles, weak cough, orthopnea, and a rapid, shallow breathing pattern. Diaphragmatic weakness causes paradoxical inward motion of the abdomen with inspiration.

Evaluation and Management of Respiratory Muscle Weakness

Respiratory failure due to neuromuscular weakness typically includes an acute component of decompensation, even in patients with previously diagnosed neuromuscular diseases. Patients with advanced baseline weakness may poorly tolerate even relatively modest respiratory challenges such as fever, focal atelectasis, or small pulmonary emboli. Ventilatory failure is an obvious concern in this population, but weakness causes a variety of other respiratory complications including atelectasis, aspiration, and pneumonia (**Table 48**). Often the most urgent concern in the ICU setting is determining the need for, as well as the best approach to, mechanical ventilatory support. Patients who are persistently obtunded, are in marked respiratory distress, or have profound gas exchange abnormalities require immediate ventilatory support. In patients with less overt failure, bedside measurement of vital capacity, maximal inspiratory pressure, and maximal expiratory pressure can help to correctly identify patients who need mechanical ventilatory support. Reduced vital capacity predisposes patients to atelectasis and CO_2 elevation, and values less than 15 to 20 mL/kg indicate a high risk of respiratory failure. Maximal inspiratory pressure tests diaphragmatic and accessory inspiratory muscle strength; more negative values indicate greater strength. Failure to generate more than 30 cm H_2O of negative inspiratory force indicates an elevated risk of

TABLE 48. Respiratory Complications of Neuromuscular Weakness		
Complication	**Risk Factors**	**Treatment**
Chronic ventilatory failure		
Pulmonary hypertension	Chronic ↓arterial P_{O_2}, ↑arterial P_{CO_2}	Ventilatory support
Sleep-disordered breathing	↓↓Arterial P_{O_2}, ↑↑arterial P_{CO_2} with sleep	Ventilatory support
	Upper airway obstruction due to bulbar dysfunction	Ventilatory support
Atelectasis	Reduced lung volumes	Ventilatory support
	Mucus plugging	Chest physiotherapy
Pneumonia	Dysphagia with aspiration	Dietary modification
	Impaired cough, atelectasis	Chest physiotherapy

ventilatory failure. Maximal expiratory pressure tests the strength of the expiratory muscles, including the abdominal and internal intercostal muscles. Values less than +40 cm H_2O are associated with impaired cough and secretion retention.

Notably, none of these tests have optimal predictive value, and the decision to initiate ventilatory support should be guided by serial values used in combination rather than isolated values. Furthermore, neuromuscular diseases such as amyotrophic lateral sclerosis can cause bulbar dysfunction that precludes accurate testing of respiratory muscle strength. Monitoring such patients is especially challenging because their bulbar dysfunction places them at greater risk of rapid deterioration due to aspiration events. Arterial blood gas analysis can be useful in the initial assessment, but serial pulmonary function tests are better suited for detecting declining strength over time.

Many additional factors merit consideration when formulating a care plan, including the underlying cause and reversibility of the weakness, the precipitant of acute deterioration, the tempo of decline, and the specific muscle groups involved. Airway clearance regimens and interventions to minimize aspiration risk are other integral aspects of management. Chest physiotherapy (including incentive spirometry, postural drainage, and manually and mechanically assisted cough) reduces the risk of mucus plugging, atelectasis, and pneumonia. However, an endotracheal tube is often required in the acute setting to ensure airway patency. Tracheostomy is a consideration in patients requiring long-term ventilator support.

Causes of Ventilatory Failure from Respiratory Muscle Weakness

Spinal Cord Injury. The phrenic nerve arises from cervical spinal roots 3, 4, and 5 (C3-C5) and innervates the diaphragm. Complete spinal cord injury above the C3 level results in nearly complete loss of ventilatory muscle function. Such patients require lifelong ventilatory support or diaphragmatic pacing and remain at high risk of atelectasis and pneumonia. Patients with incomplete injury above C3 or with complete injury at levels C3-C5 most often require mechanical ventilation initially. However, reduced spinal cord inflammation, recruitment of accessory muscles, conversion from flaccid to rigid paralysis, and recovery of muscle strength allow most of these patients to eventually recover independent ventilation. Patients with lower cervical and upper thoracic spinal cord injuries have preserved diaphragm function, but paralysis of the intercostal and abdominal muscles prevents forceful exhalation and to a lesser degree impairs inspiration. The resulting reduced lung volumes and weak cough predispose this population to atelectasis, mucus plugging, and pneumonia.

Generalized Neuromuscular Weakness. Guillain-Barré syndrome (GBS) encompasses a spectrum of acute immune-mediated polyneuropathies that can cause ventilatory failure

and bulbar dysfunction. Acute inflammatory demyelinating polyneuropathy, which accounts for approximately 90% of GBS cases in the United States, presents with progressive, symmetric weakness and hyporeflexia, typically with the lower extremities affected first. Bulbar dysfunction can further compromise patients' respiratory status, and approximately 25% of patients with GBS require invasive mechanical ventilation. Myasthenic crisis refers to weakness due to myasthenia gravis, which causes respiratory insufficiency or failure. As with GBS, oropharyngeal weakness often accompanies respiratory muscle weakness and contributes to the need for invasive mechanical ventilation. Myasthenic crisis is most often triggered by infection but can also be precipitated by medications, surgery, or pregnancy. It may also occur as part of the natural history of myasthenia gravis. Acute treatment of GBS and respiratory failure in myasthenic crisis is comprised of plasmapheresis or intravenous immune globulin. Immune-modulating medications such as systemic corticosteroids are used to establish sustained control of myasthenia but do not have a role in the treatment of GBS. Motor neuron diseases such as amyotrophic lateral sclerosis may also present with acute ventilatory failure, most often in the context of well-established disease.

Restrictive Lung Disease

Extrapulmonary

A number of conditions substantially increase the mechanical work of breathing such that ventilatory failure can occur in the absence of intrinsic lung disease or weakness. Pulmonary function tests in this population have a restrictive pattern. Patients with kyphoscoliosis may develop slowly progressive ventilatory failure and hypercapnia with secondary pulmonary hypertension, but admission to the ICU is usually precipitated by an acute event such as infection, thromboembolism, or volume overload. Adults are not suitable candidates for surgical correction, but noninvasive positive pressure ventilation is an effective means of compensating for the increased mechanical load caused by kyphoscoliosis, particularly during sleep when accessory muscle activity is decreased. Although pleural effusions are common in the ICU, only occasionally are they sufficiently large for drainage to result in significant improvement in gas exchange or work of breathing. Conditions that increase intra-abdominal pressure, including ascites, bowel edema, and gas insufflation, also place the respiratory musculature at a significant mechanical disadvantage.

Pulmonary

The predominant gas exchange abnormality in most patients with underlying fibrotic lung disease and acute respiratory failure is hypoxemia rather than hypercapnia. Systemic corticosteroids and other immunosuppressive medications generally are ineffective, and the overall prognosis is poor. However, patients should be evaluated for reversible causes of their deterioration, including infection, venous thromboembolism, and chronic heart failure. Acute exacerbation of

CONT. idiopathic pulmonary fibrosis, which is characterized by diffuse alveolar damage superimposed on baseline fibrosis, is increasingly recognized as a cause of death in patients with even mild baseline decrements in pulmonary function tests. **H**

KEY POINTS

- Ventilatory respiratory failure is characterized by hypoventilation and hypercapnia caused by excess mechanical load, decreased respiratory drive, respiratory muscle weakness, increased dead-space ventilation, and neuromuscular weakness.

- Management of critically ill patients with neuromuscular weakness should consist of early identification and treatment of ventilatory failure, minimizing aspiration risk, and assisting with airway clearance.

Obstructive Lung Disease

Pathophysiology

Acute ventilatory failure in patients with exacerbations of asthma and COPD is primarily caused by increased mechanical work of breathing rather than refractory hypoxemia. These patients commonly have a combination of worsening airflow obstruction and elevated minute ventilation that leads to incomplete expiration between breaths, a phenomenon referred to as air trapping or dynamic hyperinflation, which produces acute increases in end-expiratory lung volumes and higher positive end-expiratory pressure (auto-PEEP or intrinsic PEEP). Elevated intrathoracic pressure from severe air trapping places the patient at risk of pneumothorax from alveolar rupture as well as hypotension from markedly reduced venous return to the right heart. Chronic ventilatory failure is common in advanced COPD owing to high airway resistance, reduced chest-wall compliance from hyperinflation, and elevated dead-space ventilation at baseline. Such patients are especially vulnerable to developing acute-on-chronic ventilatory failure during exacerbations, as their respiratory muscles fatigue in the presence of worsening lung mechanics and the demand for increased minute ventilation.

Upper airway disease is a less common cause of obstructive ventilatory failure. Infectious causes include epiglottitis and deep space infections of the neck such as Ludwig angina, retropharyngeal abscess, and peritonsillar abscess. Trauma, thermal injury, anaphylactic reactions, and angioedema associated with ACE inhibitor therapy or C1 inhibitor deficiency can also critically narrow the airway. Inspiratory stridor, retractions, and cyanosis indicate the need for immediate endotracheal intubation; drooling, dysphagia, and hoarseness are less overt signs of upper airway obstruction. It is imperative to maintain close monitoring and a low threshold for intubation given the difficulty of endotracheal tube placement in this population. Paradoxical vocal cord motion is a cause of upper airway obstruction that mimics asthma exacerbation but does not cause the sustained blockage of the upper airway that makes endotracheal intubation so technically challenging.

Management

COPD and asthma exacerbations produce hypoxemia that is readily correctable with supplementary oxygen. Therefore, patients requiring a large amount of supplemental oxygen to maintain saturations greater than 90% should be evaluated for concomitant and alternative diagnoses. Heart failure, pneumonia, pneumothorax, and pulmonary embolism may accompany or mimic exacerbations. Nearly 25% of COPD exacerbations result in hospitalization, and the mortality rate among patients requiring ICU admission is approximately 25%. For management of COPD exacerbations, see Chronic Obstructive Pulmonary Disease. For noninvasive and invasive mechanical ventilatory management of exacerbations, see the Noninvasive Mechanical Ventilation and Invasive Mechanical Ventilation sections later in this chapter.

Patients with severe asthma exacerbations usually present with accessory muscle use, decreased breath sounds, limited ability to speak, severely reduced pulmonary function test results, and paradoxical pulse greater than 25 mm Hg. However, some patients with life-threatening exacerbations may not appear overtly ill. Serial spirometry or measurement of peak expiratory flow can identify deceptively severe, as well as rapidly improving, cases. Patients with persistent FEV_1 or peak expiratory flow less than 40% of predicted after 1 hour of aggressive bronchodilator therapy are suitable candidates for ICU admission. If severe respiratory distress precludes reliable measurement of pulmonary function, mechanical ventilation should be started without delay unless there is rapid improvement with maximal medical therapy. Typically, patients with an exacerbation initially present with respiratory alkalosis. Slightly elevated or even normal arterial PCO_2 levels often indicate imminent respiratory arrest rather than recovery, and clinical correlation is critical for interpreting arterial blood gas results in this setting. Indications for invasive mechanical ventilation include decreased level of consciousness, agonal respirations, and escalating work of breathing and fatigue despite aggressive bronchodilator therapy.

Patients presenting with a severe asthma exacerbation require prompt institution of aggressive bronchodilator therapy as well as supplemental oxygen if hypoxemic (**Table 49**). High-dose inhaled short-acting β_2-agonists are the first-line treatment for bronchoconstriction. Inhaled anticholinergics modestly augment the bronchodilation achieved with β_2-agonists alone when used early in the course of illness. Systemic corticosteroids do not provide immediate relief to the patient but are necessary for reversing the underlying inflammatory process and are recommended for all patients requiring hospital admission. There is little evidence to support routine use of magnesium sulfate or helium-oxygen mixtures (heliox), but both are safe and are more likely to offer a clinically meaningful benefit in the most severely affected patients. Antibiotics, methylxanthines, aggressive hydration, chest physiotherapy, mucolytics, and sedatives

TABLE 49. Initial Management of Life-Threatening Asthma Exacerbations

Established Interventions	Comment
Supplemental O_2	Titrate to keep saturation >90%
Inhaled bronchodilators[a]	
High-dose selective SABA	For example, albuterol, 2.5-5 mg by nebulizer every 20 min × 3, then 2.5-10 mg every 1-4 hours as needed
Anticholinergic agent[b]	For example, ipratropium, 0.5 mg every 20 min × 3
Systemic corticosteroids[a]	For example, methylprednisolone, 60 mg/d intravenously
Adjunct Interventions[c]	
Magnesium	For example, 2 g magnesium sulfate intravenously × 1
Helium-oxygen mixtures (heliox)	For example, 60% helium, 40% oxygen
Noninvasive ventilation	Limited reported clinical experience

SABA = short-acting β_2-agonist.

[a]Supported by randomized trials and uniformly included in treatment guidelines

[b]Effective early in course of treatment; not recommended after hospital admission

[c]Less evidence to support use; inconsistently included in treatment guidelines

CONT.

are not recommended in the routine management of asthma exacerbations.

KEY POINTS

- Increased work of breathing due to high airway resistance and air trapping, combined with increased ventilatory demands, may lead to ventilatory failure in patients with obstructive lung disease.

- The need for large amounts of supplemental oxygen in patients with exacerbations of COPD or asthma should prompt consideration of alternative diagnoses.

- Patients with acute upper airway obstruction should be closely monitored and there should be a low threshold for intubation given the difficulty of endotracheal tube placement in this population.

- Patients with a severe asthma exacerbation that does not respond to 1 hour of aggressive bronchodilator therapy are candidates for admission to the intensive care unit.

- A slightly elevated, or even normal, arterial P_{CO_2} in a patient with an asthma exacerbation may indicate impending respiratory arrest.

Shock

Shock is a state of decreased tissue perfusion, which can result in inadequate oxygen delivery for cellular needs (tissue ischemia). Ischemia in tissues often results in organ or system dysfunction if severe or prolonged. Patients develop shock when there is a problem with one or more of the key hemodynamic parameters that contribute to perfusion, outlined in **Figure 20**. Clinical signs and symptoms of shock, listed in **Table 50**, can be seen in any form of shock and can range in severity from barely perceptible to lethal. The three main types of shock are cardiogenic, distributive, and hypovolemic (**Table 51**). Understanding the cause of shock alerts the clinician to which parameter needs to be supported or corrected, as well as the underlying problems that require therapy.

In all types of shock, the therapeutic goals are to support tissues and organs that are dysfunctional or at risk of damage due to hypoperfusion and to restore perfusion if possible. Perfusion can often be improved by administering some combination of intravenous fluids, vasopressors, and inotropic agents. Understanding the cause of shock and reversing the cause of the abnormal physiologic parameter is the key to successful outcomes. Such directed treatments could include lysis of a massive pulmonary embolism causing cardiogenic shock or treatment of an infection causing septic shock. The pulmonary artery catheter, with its ability to measure cardiac output and the pulmonary artery occlusion pressure (the "wedge pressure") as a surrogate for left ventricular filling pressure, has been used to differentiate different shock states; however, owing to the lack of supporting outcomes data, pulmonary artery catheters are not recommended in the diagnosis or routine care of patients in shock.

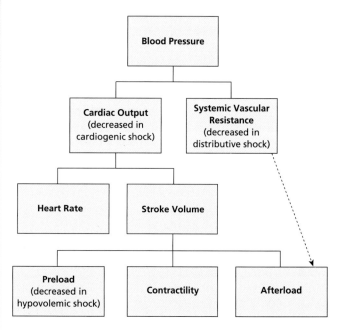

FIGURE 20. Key hemodynamic parameters of shock

TABLE 50. Common Clinical Features of Shock

Hypotension

SBP <90 mm Hg

MAP <60 mm Hg

Acute decrease in SBP of >40 mm Hg

Lack of MAP response to initial fluid challenge

End-Organ Dysfunction Due to Hypoperfusion

Decreased urine output

Change in mental status

Increased serum lactic acid level

MAP = mean arterial blood pressure; SBP = systolic blood pressure.

TABLE 51. Types of Shock

Type of Shock	Decreased Parameter	Examples
Cardiogenic	Cardiac output	Acute heart failure, massive pulmonary embolism
Distributive	Systemic vascular resistance	Sepsis, anaphylaxis
Hypovolemic	Preload	Acute hemorrhage, severe dehydration

CONT.

If increased fluid volume is likely to improve perfusion, intravenous fluids should be given liberally as boluses with immediate clinical reassessment. The adoption of guidelines using physiologic parameters, such as central venous pressure, as targets for resuscitation has improved outcomes by encouraging more timely administration of needed fluids. No conclusive evidence exists to favor colloid over crystalloid fluids for resuscitation in shock; therefore, it is reasonable to recommend crystalloids owing to their favorable cost compared with colloids. Aggressive volume expansion is most important in patients with hypovolemic shock and has also been associated with improved outcomes in patients with septic shock. Concern about precipitating heart failure and pulmonary edema should not modify the need for large bolus volume administration.

Vasopressors are medications that increase blood pressure by increasing smooth muscle tone in vascular walls. Some vasopressors also affect cardiac output by augmenting myocardial contractility and heart rate. Vasopressor therapy must be given systemically, and nearly all systemic vasopressors have some effect on more than one cellular receptor, which frequently leads to adverse effects such as cardiac arrhythmias and ischemia of extremities or mesentery. Clinical response to vasopressor agents and optimum doses may vary between patients. **Table 52** compares common vasopressors. Vasopressor agents should be administered through a central venous catheter, owing to serious complications of local tissue ischemia if these agents extravasate into tissue around a peripheral intravenous catheter site.

In addition to definitive treatment of the cause of shock and physiologic goal-directed use of fluids and vasopressors, there is some evidence for the use of other therapies in certain shock situations. Corticosteroids are advocated by some for septic shock, but their use is controversial and the most recent evidence does not support their routine use. Current guidelines recommend use of low-dose corticosteroids in septic shock refractory to vasopressor therapy. Transfusion of erythrocytes can improve perfusion and, along with aggressive crystalloid or colloid volume expansion, is a mainstay in the therapy of hemorrhagic shock. Transfusion triggers for patients with cardiogenic or septic shock are not universally agreed upon. Critically ill patients who are not bleeding and who do not have acute coronary syndrome appear to do better with a more conservative threshold (hemoglobin level of ≤7 g/dL [70 g/L]) for blood transfusion.

TABLE 52. Vasopressor Agents and Their Physiologic Effects

Agent (Dose)	Receptors	Clinical Use	Common Side Effects or Contraindications
Norepinephrine	$\alpha_1 > \beta_1$	First-line in septic shock, other refractory shock	Some arrhythmias, digital ischemia
Dopamine (low)	$DA > \beta_1$	Historically used for kidney failure, but no evidence of effectiveness for this indication	Highest arrhythmia risk, ischemia
Dopamine (medium)	$\beta_1 > \beta_2$	Septic or cardiogenic shock	Highest arrhythmia risk, ischemia
Dopamine (high)	$\alpha_1 > \beta_1$	First-line for septic shock, other refractory shock	Highest arrhythmia risk, ischemia
Epinephrine (low)	$\beta_1 > \beta_2$	Second-line for septic or cardiogenic shock	Arrhythmias, ischemia
Epinephrine (high)	$\alpha_1 = \beta_1$	Second-line for septic shock, other refractory shock	Arrhythmias, ischemia
Phenylephrine	α_1	Milder shock states, least risky through peripheral IV line	Lowest arrhythmia risk, not as powerful as other vasopressors
Vasopressin	Vasopressin receptors	Second vasopressor for septic shock only, add to catecholamine vasopressor	Splanchnic ischemia, no indication for nonseptic shock

$\alpha_1 = \alpha_1$ adrenergic receptor; $\beta_1 = \beta_1$ adrenergic receptor; $\beta_2 = \beta_2$ adrenergic receptor; DA = dopaminergic receptor; IV = intravenous.

CONT.

Shock can develop in a variety of settings, both inside and outside the hospital. As in many acute conditions, the timing of therapy is critical, and the sooner perfusion can be restored, even partially, the better a patient's chance for survival. Studies involving early and aggressive resuscitation of patients in shock, by prehospital emergency medical personnel, physicians in the emergency department, and rapid response teams in non-ICU areas of the hospital have shown promise for improved outcomes due to earlier restoration of perfusion in the early stages of shock. Even in cases in which shock can be quickly reversed, patients should be cared for in an ICU, at least initially, where their hemodynamic status can be closely monitored and where timely intervention is available as needed. H

KEY POINTS

- Shock is a state of decreased tissue perfusion that can result in inadequate oxygen delivery for cellular needs (tissue ischemia).

- In all types of shock, the therapeutic goals are to support tissues and organs that are dysfunctional or at risk of damage due to hypoperfusion and to restore perfusion if possible.

- Perfusion can often be improved in patients with shock by administering some combination of intravenous fluids, vasopressors, and inotropic agents.

- Understanding the cause of shock and reversing the cause of the abnormal physiologic parameter is the key to successful outcomes.

Noninvasive Mechanical Ventilation

Noninvasive positive pressure ventilation (NPPV) consists of delivery of positive airway pressure breaths without the use of an endotracheal tube or tracheostomy. In general, the interface between the critically ill patient and NPPV device is a tight-fitting mask, most often fitting over the mouth and nose. NPPV settings include an inspiratory positive airway pressure (IPAP) and an end-expiratory positive airway pressure (EPAP). The driving pressure, which is the EPAP subtracted from the IPAP, offloads the work of breathing and results in less energy expenditure to support a patient's required minute ventilation. NPPV is analogous to the pressure support mode used in invasive mechanical ventilation. EPAP helps maintain upper airway patency and increases end-expiratory volume. EPAP is equivalent to CPAP used for sleep apnea and to PEEP used in a closed mechanical ventilator system in intubated patients. Unlike CPAP and PEEP, NPPV provides pressure during inspiration (IPAP), thereby reducing inspiratory effort. The EPAP component of NPPV recruits atelectatic or flooded alveoli and counters the increased workload imposed by high airway resistance. Patients generally

trigger NPPV inspiratory support by spontaneously initiating a breath, but a back-up rate can be used to ensure NPPV cycling between EPAP and IPAP a set number of times per minute in patients whose spontaneous rate is below target.

Indications

Noninvasive ventilation is widely used in patients with a variety of causes of acute respiratory failure in order to avoid intubation as well as to expedite weaning from invasive ventilation. The role of NPPV is particularly well established in patients with COPD exacerbations.

Obstructive Lung Disease

NPPV is the standard of care for managing moderate to severe COPD exacerbations (see Chronic Obstructive Pulmonary Disease). In several randomized trials, NPPV reduced the need for intubation, shortened hospital stays, and decreased mortality. These findings provide a strong rationale for using NPPV in patients with asthma exacerbations, and small trials suggest benefit in this population. However, the lack of compelling evidence is reflected in inconsistent recommendations on the use of NPPV in various asthma treatment guidelines.

Cardiogenic Pulmonary Edema

Several randomized trials indicate that NPPV and CPAP improve dyspnea and gas exchange in patients with respiratory failure due to acute cardiogenic pulmonary edema. Many studies and multiple meta-analyses also found that noninvasive support reduces mortality and the need for intubation, particularly in patients with hypercapnia. However, a recent large trial found that NPPV and CPAP did not reduce the need for intubation, shorten hospital stay, or improve mortality. The discordant outcome has been attributed to differences in the study population and study design.

Immunocompromised Patients

There is a strong rationale for avoiding intubation in immunocompromised patients given their increased risk of nosocomial infections, including ventilator-associated pneumonia. Several smaller trials among patients with a variety of immunocompromised states presenting with hypoxemic respiratory failure found that NPPV reduces the need for intubation as well as mortality. The greatest benefit appears to be achieved with early initiation of treatment and in patients with single-organ failure.

Following Extubation

NPPV can be used in various ways to facilitate weaning from invasive mechanical ventilation. One randomized study of patients with COPD in whom a ventilator weaning trial was unsuccessful found that extubation directly to NPPV shortened ICU stay and improved survival. However, these results were not replicated in a subsequent study, and this

CONT.

approach is appropriate only for highly selected patients. A more recent study found immediate application of prophylactic NPPV following extubation after a successful weaning trial reduced the need for reintubation among patients with chronic lung disease and hypercapnia. It appears that this population also benefits from NPPV following extubation even when it is not applied until after the patient has developed respiratory failure. In contrast, other studies indicate no benefit or worse outcomes with use of NPPV in unselected patients with postextubation respiratory failure. Taken together, the evidence suggests that the use of NPPV in patients in whom a trial of extubation has failed should be limited primarily to those with chronic lung disease and hypercapnia.

Other Populations with Hypoxemic Respiratory Failure

CPAP reduces the need for intubation in patients with hypoxemic respiratory failure complicating abdominal surgery as well as following lung resection, presumably by reducing atelectasis. Studies of NPPV in other groups with acute hypoxemic respiratory failure have not consistently shown benefit. Although many of the studies enrolled patients with heterogeneous causes of respiratory failure, it appears that NPPV does not improve survival or need for intubation in the setting of ARDS. NPPV may be beneficial in selected patients with pneumonia.

Patient Selection

Patients with acute respiratory failure who do not require immediate intubation are potential candidates for NPPV, but some potential contraindications should be considered before initiating a trial of noninvasive support (**Table 53**). Patients with an underlying condition such as COPD that is known to respond to noninvasive ventilation and in whom a prolonged period of ventilatory support is not anticipated are most likely to benefit. Use in other situations in which NPPV is not supported by robust evidence may be warranted based on individual patient characteristics, including severity of respiratory distress, cause of respiratory failure, and rate of clinical deterioration. However, NPPV has the potential to worsen outcomes by excessively delaying, rather than preventing, intubation in high-risk populations. Institutional expertise is important in determining whether higher-risk patients should undergo a trial of noninvasive support. To reduce the risk of respiratory arrest, elective intubation should be considered in patients who do not respond to a 1- to 2-hour trial of noninvasive support.

Application

A major challenge to the successful implementation of NPPV in critically ill patients is reaching physiologically beneficial pressures in a timely fashion while maintaining good patient tolerance. This process is time intensive and requires

TABLE 53. Potential Contraindications to Noninvasive Positive Pressure Ventilation
Medical Instability
Respiratory or cardiac arrest
Severe acidosis (pH <7.10)
Hemodynamic instability
Cardiogenic or septic shock
Cardiac arrhythmia
Upper gastrointestinal bleeding
Inability to Protect Airway
Excessive secretions
Severe bulbar dysfunction
Excessive somnolence/encephalopathy
Uncooperative patient requiring sedation
Mechanical Issues
Unable to fit mask/large air leak
Recent facial trauma or surgery
Facial deformity
Upper airway obstruction

trained personnel. Nasal masks allow speech and oral intake and are generally more comfortable; however, oronasal (full face) masks have fewer problems with air leaks and typically are used initially in unstable patients. Claustrophobia can also be problematic, but a variety of mask interfaces are available, which allows tailoring of mask selection to the patient's facial characteristics and preferences. Treatment is initiated with relatively low pressures and is gradually titrated upward with close monitoring of patient synchrony with breath delivery, comfort of fit, relief of dyspnea, vital signs, tidal volumes, and gas exchange. Complications include local skin breakdown, drying, sinus congestion, eye irritation, and gastric distention.

KEY POINTS

- Noninvasive positive pressure ventilation is the standard of care for managing moderate to severe COPD exacerbations.
- Noninvasive positive pressure ventilation has the potential to worsen outcomes by excessively delaying, rather than preventing, intubation in high-risk populations.
- Elective intubation is appropriate for patients with acute respiratory failure who do not respond to a 1- to 2-hour trial of noninvasive support.
- Successful implementation of noninvasive positive pressure ventilation is time intensive and requires trained personnel.

H Invasive Mechanical Ventilation

Invasive mechanical ventilation requires a device in the trachea (endotracheal tube) to secure the airway and deliver ventilation by either volume or pressure. The three most common modes of ventilation are assist/control, pressure support, and synchronized intermittent mandatory ventilation. Other parameters that allow clinicians to achieve goals of ventilation, oxygenation, and patient-ventilator synchrony include respiration rate, tidal volume, PEEP, oxygen fraction (FIO_2), inspiratory:expiratory ratio, inspiratory flow rates, and alarms.

Assist/control mode can deliver a preset volume or preset pressure. Volume preset mode delivers a preset tidal volume breath to the patient for each detected inspiratory effort by the patient. If there are no efforts by the patient, the same preset volume breath is delivered at a preset respiration rate. This is the most common mode of ventilation used for patients with ARDS. Advantages of this mode include maximal diaphragm rest and maximal control of minute ventilation through a preset volume and respiration rate. Disadvantages of assist/control volume preset mode include patient discomfort, overventilation in patients with a high respiration rate, and air trapping if there is insufficient expiratory time before the next delivered volume breath.

Pressure support mode is used to assist spontaneously breathing patients. In this mode, for each inspiratory effort by the patient the machine delivers a high rate of flow to achieve a preset pressure. This pressure-supported breath occurs when the ventilator senses patient-initiated inspiratory flow at the onset of inhalation. If the patient fails to initiate a breath or if the preset pressure is insufficient to support inspiratory flow, delivered minute ventilation may be inadequate.

Synchronized intermittent mandatory ventilation (SIMV) is a mixture of assist/control and pressure-supported ventilation. Machine breaths are delivered at a scheduled rate with preset tidal volume. Patient-triggered breaths are pressure supported, in contrast to the assist/control mode in which patient-triggered breaths are volume supported. This mode was developed for weaning, so that the number of mechanical breaths could be gradually reduced, allowing for increasing spontaneous ventilation. However, clinical trials have shown SIMV to be an inferior/ineffective weaning mode. Despite the lack of evidence to support its use, SIMV remains a popular mode in clinical practice because it allows clinicians to deliver a certain minute volume (unlike pressure support ventilation) with less air trapping and overventilation (associated with assist/control volume preset ventilation).

Acute Respiratory Distress Syndrome

For non–ventilator-related management of ARDS, see the Hypoxemic Respiratory Failure section.

The physiologic hallmark of ARDS is hypoxemia, which is typically corrected with mechanical ventilation combined with supplemental oxygen and PEEP. Limiting atelectrauma (lung injury that is presumed to arise from repetitive opening and closing of alveoli) and barotrauma may limit the potential for disruption of the alveolar capillary membrane by the ventilator, often referred to as ventilator-associated lung injury. This can be achieved by delivering tidal volumes of limited size, minimizing plateau pressure, optimizing PEEP, and reducing FIO_2 to less than 0.6 as described later in this section.

A landmark randomized study (ARMA) found that decreasing tidal volume from 12 mL/kg of ideal body weight to 6 mL/kg of ideal body weight while keeping plateau pressure less than 30 cm H_2O reduced mortality from 40% to 30%. Ideal body weight rather than actual body weight should be used to calculate tidal volume, because among patients who are overweight or edematous, using actual body weight will typically result in inappropriately large tidal volumes.

Reducing tidal volumes can result in alveolar hypoventilation and hypercapnia. This is called permissive hypercapnia and does not appear to be harmful; some evidence suggests that mild hypercapnia may decrease the degree of ventilator-induced lung injury.

PEEP increases functional residual capacity and is intended to recruit partially collapsed alveoli and act as a pneumatic splint to prevent atelectrauma. PEEP improves lung compliance, ventilation/perfusion (V/Q) matching, and oxygenation. Excessive PEEP due to increased intrathoracic pressure can cause hypotension by decreasing venous return and increasing pulmonary vascular resistance, resulting in decreased cardiac output. Barotrauma and pneumothorax are of particular concern when PEEP exceeds 15 cm H_2O. Several randomized trials have found no difference in survival using higher PEEP (approximately 15 cm H_2O) versus lower PEEP (approximately 8 cm H_2O); however, the patients with the most severe ARDS did show improvement in secondary endpoints, such as improved oxygenation and decreased need for rescue therapies, when treated with higher PEEP. Importantly, these studies found no evidence of significant harm or increased risk of barotrauma despite the use of higher PEEP. Current recommendations are to use a PEEP level that achieves adequate oxygenation with a FIO_2 of less than 0.6 and does not cause hypotension.

Randomized trials evaluating ventilation in the prone position have shown improvements in oxygenation, but there was no mortality difference and there was an increase in complications such as endotracheal tube obstruction, accidental extubation, and pressure ulcers. Ventilation in the prone position is recommended only in experienced centers and in patients with the most severe ARDS, in whom oxygenation by traditional methods is unsuccessful.

Obstructive Lung Disease

The primary and preferred method for managing respiratory failure secondary to obstructive lung disease is with NPPV (see Noninvasive Mechanical Ventilation). When NPPV fails or is contraindicated, invasive mechanical ventilation is used. The ventilator strategies discussed here are appropriate for both COPD exacerbation and asthma.

Markedly elevated airway pressures, severe dynamic hyperinflation, and ventilator-patient dyssynchrony make the management of intubated patients with obstructive lung disease particularly challenging. The primary ventilator strategy is to allow adequate time for exhalation before the next delivered breath and to minimize airway resistance through optimal PEEP. The result of this ventilator strategy is a relatively low minute ventilation with permissive hypercapnia.

PEEP is used to decrease dynamic expiratory airway collapse and minimize resistance to flow. Severe airway obstruction may result in breath stacking (delivery of a preset volume before full expiration) and auto-PEEP if sufficient time is not allowed for the preceding breath to be completely emptied. Checking end-expiratory pressure during an end-expiratory pause (no airflow) will allow pressure to equilibrate between the alveoli and airway and will confirm the presence or absence of auto-PEEP. Breath stacking can result in dangerous increases in intrathoracic pressure, with resultant barotrauma and hypotension. The ventilator should be set at high inspiratory flow rates to deliver a breath in a very short time and should allow the majority of the respiratory cycle for exhalation. If a patient has anxiety and triggers breaths more frequently than the set rate, sedation may be required to slow the respiration rate and avoid potential auto-PEEP. This is especially true with hypercapnia, as it is a potent stimulus to increase respiration rate. Using a large endotracheal tube facilitates exhalation and minimizes resistance.

Patients with obstructive lung disease often present with acute-on-chronic respiratory acidosis. When choosing the initial minute ventilation, it is important to ventilate to achieve the patient's baseline and not a normal P_{CO_2} level. Immediate respiratory correction can result in life-threatening metabolic alkalosis.

Weaning

Weaning is the process by which a patient is liberated from mechanical ventilation. Patients are candidates for weaning when they are hemodynamically stable and have recovered from respiratory failure. They should have a cough that is strong enough to clear secretions, a low secretion burden, and a patent upper airway.

The rapid shallow breathing index is a method to test the readiness of a patient for weaning and should be measured daily. It is defined as the ratio of the respiration rate to tidal volume (f/V_T). If the f/V_T is greater than 105, there is a 95% chance that a spontaneous breathing trial will be unsuccessful; if it is less than 105, there is an 80% chance of success.

Spontaneous breathing trials are done by placing the patient on a T-piece where no positive pressure is delivered (only supplemental oxygen) or by adjusting the ventilator so that it applies only enough pressure to overcome the resistance of the endotracheal tube.

Daily interruption of sedation and spontaneous breathing trials should be used as a standard of care for appropriate patients in critical care units. Their use will shorten the need for mechanical ventilation by an average of 1.5 days, dramatically decrease the number of patients who require mechanical ventilation for more than 3 weeks, decrease ICU length of stay, and lower 1-year mortality.

Direct extubation to NPPV is effective at weaning patients with obstructive lung disease from mechanical ventilation. However, it is not effective for patients with primarily hypoxemic respiratory failure.

Numerous trials have studied early versus late tracheostomy to facilitate weaning with mixed results, and optimal timing remains unclear. Current consensus is that tracheostomy should be performed within 14 to 21 days of intubation.

Ventilator-Associated Pneumonia

Ventilator-associated pneumonia (VAP) is a serious, preventable complication of mechanical ventilation. It is defined as pneumonia with onset at least 48 hours after endotracheal intubation. It affects 10% to 25% of ventilated patients and has an associated 25% to 50% mortality rate. In patients undergoing mechanical ventilation, pneumonia is difficult to diagnose because pulmonary infiltrates are frequently present, tracheal secretions may be colonized by bacteria, and signs such as fever and leukocytosis may be blunted. This makes clinical scores such as the clinical pulmonary infection score unreliable. The optimal approach to diagnosis is controversial, but general opinion is that all patients suspected of having VAP should undergo lower respiratory tract sampling, followed by microscopic analysis and culture of the specimen. There are various methods for sampling the lower respiratory tract, which are categorized based on the requirement for bronchoscopy. Nonbronchoscopic methods are simple suctioning of the endotracheal tube and mini–bronchoalveolar lavage (BAL). Bronchoscopic methods are formal BAL and protected specimen brush. There does not appear to be a difference in mortality between bronchoscopic and nonbronchoscopic methods. However, bronchoscopic methods may allow for narrower antibiotic choices and more rapid de-escalation of antibiotics. Quantitative cultures (with thresholds of 1,000,000 colony-forming units [cfu]/mL for samples obtained by simple aspiration, 10,000 cfu/mL for samples obtained by BAL, or 1000 cfu/mL for samples obtained by protected specimen brush) are more reliable than semiquantitative culture. Mortality may be reduced by employing a VAP bundle (see Approaches to Providing Best Practice). There is evidence that shortened antibiotic courses of 8 days are sufficient to treat VAP. If quantitative cultures are negative, antibiotics should be discontinued at 3 days. **H**

KEY POINTS

- The physiologic hallmark of acute respiratory distress syndrome is hypoxemia, which is typically corrected with mechanical ventilation combined with supplemental oxygen and positive end-expiratory pressure.

- In patients with acute respiratory distress syndrome, limiting tidal volumes, minimizing plateau pressure, optimizing positive end-expiratory pressure, and reducing F_{IO_2} to less than 0.6 may help prevent ventilator-associated lung injury.

- The primary ventilator strategy in patients with obstructive lung disease is to allow adequate time for exhalation before the next delivered breath and to minimize airway resistance through optimal positive end-expiratory pressure.

- The rapid shallow breathing index may be used to test the readiness of a patient for weaning.

- Daily interruption of sedation and spontaneous breathing trial lead to sooner extubation and lower rate of mechanical ventilation.

Sepsis

Epidemiology

Sepsis is an exaggerated inflammatory response to an infectious stimulus and is characterized by a severe catabolic reaction, widespread endothelial dysfunction, and release of inflammatory agents. The incidence of sepsis rises exponentially after age 65 years. Age-specific mortality rates are much higher in patients with comorbidities such as diabetes mellitus, chronic kidney disease, and chronic heart disease, as well as in those with continued systemic signs of sepsis (persistent hypotension despite multiple liters of fluids) and persistent deficits in oxygen delivery. The mortality rate of patients with sepsis complicated by multiorgan failure may be greater than 70% to 90%; mortality rate can be estimated by adding 15% to 20% predicted mortality for each sepsis-induced dysfunctional organ.

Pathophysiology

Sepsis is a complex dysregulation of both inflammation and coagulation. Primary cellular injury may result from infection or the host's immune response to the infection. Numerous cytokines such as tumor necrosis factor α and interleukin-1 activate leukocytes and promote leukocyte adhesion, diapedesis, and degranulation, with resultant endothelial cell damage. Endothelial damage leads to tissue factor expression and activation of the clotting cascade. The inflammatory cascade induced by sepsis results in vasodilation and capillary leak, with attendant decreases in effective circulating volume,

which initially leads to an increase in heart rate as a means to maintain blood pressure. Later in sepsis, there is myocardial dysfunction with decreased contractility, which exacerbates sepsis-induced hypotension. Hypotension, microthrombi, and cellular dysoxia (abnormal tissue oxygen utilization) result in further cellular ischemia, cell death, and release of additional inflammatory mediators.

Classification

In an attempt to achieve common terminology for clinical trials, the term systemic inflammatory response syndrome (SIRS) was introduced to describe findings of altered temperature, tachycardia, hyperventilation, and abnormal leukocyte count regardless of cause (inflammatory or infectious). Sepsis is defined as SIRS plus suspected infection. Severe sepsis is associated with systemic effects including hypotension, decreased urine output, or metabolic acidosis. Septic shock, signs of which are summarized in Table 50, is sepsis with persistent organ hypoperfusion despite adequate fluid resuscitation (that is, requires vasopressor agents to maintain blood pressure).

Management

The goals of sepsis management are to treat infection and optimize tissue perfusion. This is accomplished by controlling sources of infection, instituting early and appropriate antibiotic therapy, optimizing oxygen delivery by correcting hypoxia, using crystalloids to maintain adequate preload, starting vasoactive agents to maintain perfusion pressure for persistent hypotension despite fluids, and transfusion of erythrocytes if oxygen delivery is inadequate despite the previous measures.

Source Control and Antibiotic Therapy

The source of a patient's infection should be identified and controlled. Removal of infected devices and drainage of abscesses may be life-saving interventions. Blood and source cultures should be collected before administration of antibiotics when possible. Broad-spectrum empiric antibiotics, chosen based on the site of infection (lung, gastrointestinal, or unknown) should be implemented within 1 hour after recognition of sepsis. Even with early implementation, use of inappropriate antibiotics (that is, antibiotics to which bacteria are resistant) is associated with a mortality rate of 42%, whereas the mortality rate is 17% if appropriate antibiotics are used (**Table 54**). A delay in initiation or choice of inappropriate antibiotic agent is associated with an increased mortality rate. The broad-spectrum coverage that was initiated may be modified to address the culture results and should be continued for 7 to 10 days.

Management of Septic Shock

In addition to infection control, optimizing tissue perfusion is critical. Initial resuscitation should begin early and be

TABLE 54. Antibiotic Choice in Sepsis

Begin intravenous antibiotics as early as possible and always within the first hour of recognizing severe sepsis and septic shock

Broad-spectrum: one or more agents active against likely bacterial/fungal pathogens and with good penetration into presumed source

Reassess antimicrobial regimen daily to optimize efficacy, prevent resistance, avoid toxicity, and minimize costs

Consider combination therapy in *Pseudomonas* infections

Consider combination empiric therapy in patients with neutropenia

Combination therapy <3-5 days and de-escalation following culture and susceptibility results

Duration of therapy typically limited to 7-10 days; longer if response is slow or there are undrainable foci of infection or immunologic deficiencies

Stop antimicrobial therapy if cause is found to be noninfectious

Adapted from Dellinger RP, Levy MM, Carlet JM, et al. Surviving Sepsis Campaign: International Guidelines for management of severe sepsis and septic shock: 2008. Crit Care Med. 2008;36(1):296-327. [PMID: 18158437]. Copyright 2008, Lippincott Williams & Wilkins.

CONT.

aggressive. A landmark study of early goal-directed therapy started in an emergency department with transition into the ICU showed a significant mortality reduction.

Supplemental oxygen and endotracheal intubation with mechanical ventilation should be initiated as needed to maintain adequate oxygenation. The preload should be assessed by measuring central venous pressure or with bedside echocardiography. Crystalloids (for example, normal saline or lactated Ringer solution) should be given to achieve a central venous pressure of 8 to 12 mm Hg. If the mean arterial pressure is less than 65 mm Hg despite fluid challenge and adequate preload, vasoactive agents should be started and titrated as needed. The 2008 Surviving Sepsis guidelines recommend using measurement of the vena cava oxygen saturation ($Scvo_2$) to assess adequacy of resuscitation. The $Scvo_2$ can be measured continuously with a specialized central venous catheter or intermittently by direct measurement of a blood sample aspirated from a central venous catheter. If the $Scvo_2$ is less than 70%, packed red blood cell transfusion should be performed to achieve a hematocrit of greater than 30%. If the $Scvo_2$ is less than 70% despite transfusion, inotropic agents should be started to enhance cardiac contractility.

Repetitive fluid challenges are performed by giving a 500 to 1000 mL bolus of crystalloid over short intervals while assessing response to target central venous pressure. Most patients need 4 to 6 L of fluid in the first 6 hours, and a frequent error is underestimating the intravascular volume deficit and the amount of fluid required. The fluid input is typically greater than output owing to vasodilation and capillary leak. Use of crystalloid or colloid is likely equivalent; however,

colloid is far more expensive. Therefore, most practitioners use crystalloid such as lactated Ringer solution or normal saline. Albumin or other colloid infusions may have an advantage over crystalloid in situations of low oncotic pressure and extensive "third spacing" such as occurs in liver disease and burns.

Vasopressor therapy should be started immediately if the initial fluid challenge fails to restore adequate blood pressure and organ perfusion. Prolonged hypoperfusion results in worsening ischemia and organ failure. Vasopressor therapy with norepinephrine, vasopressin, or dopamine is frequently needed to restore perfusion during life-threatening hypotension. No trials have established a single superior vasopressor; norepinephrine and dopamine are first-line agents for correcting hypotension in septic shock. Vasopressor agents can be used concurrently with fluid resuscitation in life-threatening hypotension.

Activated Protein C

As noted previously, patients with septic shock have acquired thrombophilic and inflammatory derangements. Endogenous activation of protein C is impaired in sepsis. Recombinant activated protein C (drotrecogin alfa) has anti-inflammatory and profibrinolytic properties and was previously recommended for adult patients with sepsis-induced organ dysfunction associated with a clinical assessment of high risk of death. However, subsequent clinical trials failed to demonstrate benefit, and drotrecogin alfa is no longer available for use.

Corticosteroids

High-dose corticosteroids are of no benefit in sepsis and have been shown to harm patients in earlier studies. The Surviving Sepsis Campaign suggests that replacement-dose intravenous hydrocortisone be given only to adult patients with septic shock after blood pressure is found to be poorly responsive to fluid resuscitation and vasopressor therapy. This is a change from previous guidelines. Although corticosteroids appear to promote shock reversal, the lack of a clear improvement in mortality, coupled with known side effects of corticosteroids such as increased risk of infection and myopathy, have tempered enthusiasm for their broad use.

Hyperglycemia

Effective glucose control in the ICU has been shown to decrease morbidity and mortality across a large range of conditions. The traditional threshold for treatment of hyperglycemia has been a plasma glucose level greater than 215 mg/dL (11.9 mmol/L), as this level is associated with higher rates of infection. Intensive insulin therapy with a goal of maintaining plasma glucose level between 80 and 110 mg/dL (4.4 and 6.1 mmol/L) showed a reduction in mortality in a large single-center study of postoperative surgical patients. This was not reproducible using the same protocol and targets in the medical ICU. A large international randomized trial (NICE-SUGAR) found that intensive glucose control actually increased mortality; a more modest target of less than

CONT. 180 mg/dL (10 mmol/L) resulted in a lower mortality rate than did a target of 81 to 108 mg/dL (4.5 to 6.0 mmol/L). Following initial stabilization, patients with severe sepsis and hyperglycemia who are admitted to the ICU should receive intravenous insulin therapy to reduce plasma glucose levels to less than 180 mg/dL (10 mmol/L).

Mechanical Ventilation

The goal of mechanical ventilation in sepsis is to relieve hypoxemia. Sepsis is the most common cause for development of ARDS, and most patients with septic shock require mechanical ventilation. It is important to note that NPPV is not effective at avoiding invasive mechanical ventilation in patients with sepsis. It only delays the need for mechanical ventilation and may in fact be deleterious. A lung-protective strategy (low tidal volume) should be used (see Invasive Mechanical Ventilation).

Miscellaneous Issues

Other important aspects of sepsis management that are covered in more detail in other sections include avoiding malnutrition, employing therapist-driven weaning protocols, using sedation protocols with a daily interruption in ventilated patients, using intermittent or bolus sedation rather than continuous infusions, avoiding neuromuscular blockade, using sequential compression devices and either low-molecular-weight heparin or low-dose unfractionated heparin subcutaneously for venous thromboembolism prophylaxis, providing stress ulcer prophylaxis, and discussing advance care planning with patients and families. Intermittent dialysis and continuous renal replacement therapy are considered equivalent to one another for sepsis-associated kidney failure; however, continuous renal replacement therapy may offer easier management in unstable patients. Bicarbonate should not be used for the purpose of improving hemodynamics or reducing vasopressor requirement when treating lactic acidosis with a pH higher than 7.15.

KEY POINTS

- The goals of sepsis management are to treat infection and optimize tissue perfusion.

- Appropriate broad-spectrum empiric antibiotics should be implemented within 1 hour after recognition of sepsis.

- Initial resuscitation in septic shock should begin early and be aggressive.

- High-dose corticosteroids are of no benefit in sepsis and have been shown to harm patients in earlier studies; intravenous hydrocortisone is appropriate in septic shock only if blood pressure is poorly responsive to fluid resuscitation and vasopressor therapy.

- Following initial stabilization, patients in the intensive care unit with severe sepsis and hyperglycemia should receive intravenous insulin therapy to reduce plasma glucose levels to less than 180 mg/dL (10 mmol/L).

Emergent Disorders in Critical Care

Acute Inhalational Injuries

Inhalational injuries are common, especially in burn victims. Damage to the airways and lung parenchyma is responsible for the high morbidity and mortality rates in these patients. Approximately half of deaths associated with burns are due to complications of inhalational injury. Respiratory tract damage results from thermal and chemical toxicity. Chemical injury may also occur from exposures other than smoke.

When inhalational exposure is brief and the inhaled toxins are water soluble, tissue damage is greatest in the proximal airways, including the nose, mouth, and pharynx. Symptoms usually occur immediately following the exposure, and complications can include airway obstruction from edema and necrotic debris. These patients may need repeated bronchoscopy to maintain airway patency and usually must be intubated for airway protection.

When inhalational injury involves less-soluble toxins or prolonged heat exposure, the damage can extend into distal airways and lung parenchyma. Pulmonary edema is often seen acutely but may not be clinically or radiographically evident for 12 to 24 hours following the exposure. Other delayed effects may include airway stenosis, reactive airways dysfunction syndrome, bronchiolitis obliterans, bronchiectasis, and parenchymal fibrosis.

Airways may become bronchospastic after inhalational exposure, even in patients without a history of reactive airways disease. Other common dangers of inhalational injury include asphyxiation (due to other gases displacing oxygen in the lungs) and systemic effects of toxins absorbed through the lungs after inhalation. Carbon monoxide toxicity is common in patients with smoke inhalation and leads to carboxyhemoglobin formation and reduced oxygen delivery to tissues. Another inhaled and absorbed toxin is cyanide, which is produced in the combustion of some plastics and acrylics (see the Toxicology section for more information on carbon monoxide and cyanide toxicity). Significant cyanide levels are seen in 30% of patients treated for smoke inhalation from fires. Burn victims are at high risk of secondary infections; staphylococcal and pseudomonal infections are particularly common.

Supportive care of patients with acute inhalational injury may include intravenous fluids, intubation for mechanical ventilation, chest physiotherapy, bronchoscopic debridement and suctioning, inhaled racemic epinephrine (and other bronchodilators for bronchospasm and upper airway edema), and antibiotics.

Chemical effects from inhaled toxins may be subtle at first but should be identified early and treated specifically. Mental status changes or blood lactic acid level out of proportion to hypoxia can alert to these conditions. Pulse oximetry may be falsely reassuring in the setting of carboxyhemoglobinemia; blood gas analysis should be performed to confirm oxyhemoglobin saturation. Sodium thiosulfate should be used rather than nitrites for cyanide toxicity associated with smoke inhalation, although both are accepted antidotes for cyanide toxicity. There is a risk of methemoglobin formation with nitrites, which may compound coexisting carboxyhemoglobinemia.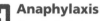

- Approximately half of deaths associated with burns are due to complications of inhalational injury.
- Supportive care of patients with acute inhalational injury may include intravenous fluids, intubation for mechanical ventilation, chest physiotherapy, bronchoscopic debridement and suctioning, inhaled racemic epinephrine (and other bronchodilators for bronchospasm and upper airway edema), and antibiotics.

Anaphylaxis

Anaphylaxis is a severe allergic reaction that occurs in response to food or environmental proteins, insect venom, drugs, latex, blood transfusions, or other allergens. It results from IgE activation on the surface of basophils and mast cells, causing release of histamine and other inflammatory mediators. Elevated histamine levels can be detected in serum and urine, but anaphylaxis is generally diagnosed clinically. Anaphylaxis requires previous sensitization to the allergen, but it often occurs in patients without a known or documented exposure history. Radiocontrast reaction is a special case in which the contrast agent directly activates mast cells without an IgE intermediary.

Clinical features may include urticaria, tachycardia (sometimes bradycardia), stridor, hoarseness, wheezing, and hypotension. Hypotension may be profound, as histamine increases vascular permeability and can lead to large losses of circulating plasma volume into the extravascular space. Gastrointestinal symptoms include cramping abdominal pain, vomiting, and diarrhea. Angioedema (localized tissue edema) may be associated with anaphylaxis and often affects the lips, tongue, upper airway, gastrointestinal tract, and extremities. Clinical manifestations of anaphylaxis usually occur immediately or soon after exposure to the allergen, especially when the offending agent has been introduced intravenously. However, the reaction may be delayed for hours or days. Rapid onset of symptoms usually indicates a more severe reaction.

Although angioedema may be a component of anaphylaxis, it may also occur alone without urticaria or other features of anaphylaxis; it is sometimes triggered by certain exposures (particularly ACE inhibitors), and it sometimes occurs without an identifiable cause. Familial angioedema is associated with C1 inhibitor deficiency and is characterized by episodes of angioedema that occur following trauma or illness and begin early in life. Patients who develop angioedema later in life may have an acquired C1 inhibitor deficiency associated with a lymphoproliferative disorder. These forms of angioedema are not mediated by IgE release and do not respond to usual anaphylaxis therapies, although airway management is essential owing to potential laryngeal edema.

With timely supportive care, anaphylaxis is rarely fatal. When fatalities do occur, the cause of death is usually airway closure due to laryngeal edema. Patients with a likely exposure and signs of anaphylaxis or a history of previous reactions should be monitored closely and should be given oxygen and intravenous fluids. They may receive epinephrine, usually by subcutaneous or intramuscular injection. High-dose or continuous epinephrine may be needed for severe reactions or patients taking β-blockers. If hypotension is refractory to treatment, intravenous vasopressors may be required. Although strong evidence is lacking, antihistamines and corticosteroids are sometimes used to prevent delayed worsening or recurrence. Inhaled bronchodilators and racemic epinephrine can reduce bronchospasm and airway edema. Noninvasive ventilatory support may be used, but intubation to prevent airway closure is needed if there is no immediate response to initial therapy. In such cases, airway management may be difficult, requiring advanced techniques and equipment, such as flexible or rigid fiberoptic scopes, videolaryngoscopes, or intubating laryngeal mask airway devices.

- Clinical features of anaphylaxis may include urticaria, angioedema, tachycardia (sometimes bradycardia), stridor, hoarseness, wheezing, and hypotension.
- Angioedema can occur as a component of anaphylaxis, but it may also occur alone, possibly triggered by certain exposures (particularly ACE inhibitors) or as an inherited or acquired disorder; these forms of angioedema do not respond to usual anaphylaxis therapies, although airway management is essential owing to potential laryngeal edema.
- With timely supportive care, anaphylaxis is rarely fatal.

Hypertensive Emergencies

Hypertensive emergencies are episodes of elevated blood pressure associated with acute end-organ damage or dysfunction. There is no absolute blood pressure that defines an emergency. For example, severely elevated pressure with diastolic values above 120 mm Hg but no end-organ effects is labeled hypertensive urgency. Hypertensive emergencies and urgencies occur most often in patients with poorly controlled essential hypertension, especially men, black patients, and elderly patients. Organ systems affected by severely elevated blood pressure include central nervous (presenting with stroke in 25% of cases), renal (acute kidney injury), and cardiovascular (ischemic chest pain or acute heart failure).

The initial evaluation of severely elevated blood pressure focuses on identifying end-organ damage or dysfunction. Blood pressure should be measured in both arms and in both supine and standing positions if possible. A careful neurologic

CONT.

examination that includes mental status and visual fields and acuity should be performed. Physical findings suggesting pulmonary and peripheral fluid overload, such as lung field crackles and edema, should be sought. Laboratory studies should include measurement of electrolytes, blood cell counts, blood urea nitrogen, creatinine, cardiac biomarkers, urinalysis, and drug levels (including cocaine and amphetamines). Electrocardiography and chest radiography should be performed. Brain imaging is appropriate if mental status is decreased or the neurologic examination suggests a stroke. Aortic dissection is always a possibility, and pulses should be assessed for asymmetry, a finding that should trigger further investigation with CT angiography, transesophageal echocardiography, and/or conventional aortic angiography.

In patients with hypertensive emergency, blood pressure must be lowered quickly with short-acting intravenous antihypertensive infusions to limit end-organ damage (**Table 55**). However, blood pressure should not be lowered to normal or any further than is required to stop end-organ damage acutely (generally, not more than 25% initially); more rapid blood pressure lowering may be indicated only if there is evidence of ongoing organ damage. Systolic and diastolic targets over the next 2 to 6 hours should be 160 mm Hg and 110 mm Hg, respectively, with gradual correction after that. Treatment of hypertensive urgencies is often done with oral medications, but patients must be evaluated and monitored

for end-organ damage. Long-term control of blood pressure is the goal to prevent future hypertensive crises. H

KEY POINTS

- Hypertensive emergencies are episodes of elevated blood pressure associated with end-organ damage or dysfunction.
- In hypertensive emergency, blood pressure must be lowered quickly with short-acting intravenous antihypertensive infusions to limit end-organ damage, but blood pressure should not be lowered to normal or any further than is required to stop end-organ damage acutely (generally, not more than 25% initially).

Hyperthermic Emergencies

Hyperthermia, a rise in core body temperature above 40.0 °C (104.0 °F), can be life threatening. Clinical features include altered mental status (including seizures), muscle rigidity, and rhabdomyolysis (with kidney failure). In severe cases, disseminated intravascular coagulation and ARDS also occur. Hyperthermia occurs most commonly owing to heat stroke, malignant hyperthermia, and neuroleptic malignant syndrome.

Heat stroke results from failure of the body's thermoregulatory system; the system may be impaired or overwhelmed. Thermoregulation may be impaired in the elderly and in patients who have or are being treated for conditions

Agent (Class)	Dose (Delivery)	Onset	Duration	Notes	Adverse Effects (All Cause Hypotension)
Nitroprusside (vasodilator)	0.25-10 μg/kg/min (IV)	Immediate	1-10 min	Easy to titrate; often first choice for acute situations	Risk of cyanide toxicity
Nitroglycerin (vasodilator)	0.25-5 μg/kg/min (IV)	Immediate	3-5 min	Used for myocardial ischemia; tolerance may develop	Headache, bradycardia
Hydralazine (vasodilator)	5-20 mg every 4-6 hours (IV)	1-5 min	1-4 hours	Safe in pregnancy	Nausea, headache, tachycardia
Labetalol (α- and β-blocker)	20 mg every 10 min (IV)	2-5 min	3-6 hours	Can be switched to oral	Bradycardia, heart block, nausea, bronchospasm
Enalaprilat (ACE inhibitor)	1.25 mg every 6 hours (IV)	15 min	6-12 hours	Can be switched to oral; good for left ventricular failure	Prolonged hypotension
Nicardipine (calcium channel blocker)	5 mg/hour titrated up to 15 mg/hour (IV)	1-5 min	3-6 hours	Often used for patients with stroke	Myocardial ischemia, tachycardia, headache
Fenoldopam (dopamine agonist)	0.03-0.1 μg/kg/min (IV)	10 min	1 hour	Can be titrated up slowly to 1.6 μg/kg/min; may be protective of kidneys	Flushing, headache, nausea, tachycardia, possibly increased myocardial ischemia
Phentolamine (α-blocker)	5-20 mg (IV)	15-20 min	30-45 min	Used for diagnosis of and surgery for pheochromocytoma	Nausea, arrhythmia

TABLE 55. Antihypertensive Agents for Hypertensive Crises

IV = intravenous.

that can lead to dehydration or anhidrosis. Diuretics and anticholinergic medications are commonly implicated. Overwhelmed thermoregulation is seen in athletes and military recruits who are required to exercise strenuously in hot and humid weather.

Patients with heat stroke have a high mortality rate (up to 60%), depending on the degree and duration of hyperthermia, the number of organ systems showing dysfunction, and other comorbidities. Patients with heat stroke should be cooled to lower their core temperature. They do not respond to centrally acting antipyretic medications. Evaporative cooling methods and ice packs are usually most effective. In severe cases, cold gastric or peritoneal lavage may be attempted. Benzodiazepines decrease discomfort and shivering during these treatments.

Malignant hyperthermia is a reaction to certain classes of drugs, including inhaled anesthetics (halothane and others) and depolarizing neuromuscular blockers (succinylcholine and decamethonium), resulting in markedly increased intracellular calcium, increased cellular metabolism, and sustained muscle tetany. Susceptibility to malignant hyperthermia is inherited. Severe muscle rigidity, masseter spasm, hyperthermia with core temperatures up to 45.0 °C (113.0 °F), cardiac tachyarrhythmias, and rhabdomyolysis usually manifest quickly when susceptible patients are exposed to one of the triggering agents, although symptoms may be delayed. Previous exposure without a reaction does not eliminate risk with subsequent exposure.

The mortality rate in malignant hyperthermia is approximately 10%. Treatment should begin immediately upon signs of the developing syndrome. The triggering agent should be stopped, and fluids and cooling measures should be initiated. Dantrolene is given as a muscle relaxant every 5 to 10 minutes until hyperthermia and rigidity resolve. Dantrolene can also prevent recurrence in patients with a history of malignant hyperthermia if given before administration of an agent that could trigger the syndrome.

Neuroleptic malignant syndrome is an idiosyncratic reaction to neuroleptic antipsychotic agents. It is characterized by muscle rigidity, hyperthermia, and autonomic dysregulation. Temperature may be only modestly elevated in some patients, and delirium is common. Potent "typical" neuroleptics such as haloperidol are most commonly implicated, but all neuroleptic agents have been associated with the syndrome. It often occurs at the time that medication is started or following rapid dose escalation; however, it occasionally occurs after years of apparently problem-free use. It is more common in men and with parenteral administration. Dehydration is commonly associated, but this may be an effect rather than a cause. Concomitant lithium use may be a risk factor, but this is controversial. It has occurred in patients with Parkinson disease when high-dose medications are discontinued abruptly.

The mortality rate in neuroleptic malignant syndrome is 10% to 20%. Treatment includes stopping the neuroleptic agent, maintaining blood pressure stability, replacing fluid volume, lowering the elevated temperature as in malignant hyperthermia, and administering benzodiazepines for agitation. Dantrolene and bromocriptine are also used, but the evidence for these agents is weak. Recurrence of neuroleptic malignant syndrome is variable and unpredictable. Patients who recover may be restarted on the neuroleptic medication after a waiting period of at least 2 weeks, generally at a lower dose of a low-potency agent. Concomitant lithium therapy and dehydration should be avoided, and patients should be monitored for recurrence of neuroleptic malignant syndrome. **H**

KEY POINTS

- Hyperthermia, a rise in core body temperature above 40.0 °C (104.0 °F), is characterized by altered mental status (including seizures), muscle rigidity, and rhabdomyolysis (with kidney failure).

- Hyperthermia occurs most commonly owing to heat stroke, malignant hyperthermia, and neuroleptic malignant syndrome.

Hypothermic Emergencies

Hypothermia is usually defined as core temperatures below 35.0 °C (95.0 °F); it occurs commonly with exposure to cold weather and with submersion in cold water. Patients with impaired thermoregulation or altered perception of cold are at greatest risk, including elderly and intoxicated persons. Hypothermia can develop in patients undergoing lengthy surgical procedures when exposure is prolonged and the patient cannot thermoregulate adequately owing to age, comorbid conditions, or the effects of anesthesia.

Hypothermia causes cellular dysfunction and electrolyte abnormalities, especially hyperkalemia. Mild hypothermia (32.0-35.0 °C [89.6-95.0 °F]) causes shivering, mental status changes, ataxia, and polyuria. Moderate hypothermia (28.0-32.0 °C [82.4-89.6 °F]) causes decreased heart rate and cardiac output, more severe mental status and other nervous system dysfunction, and cardiac arrhythmias. Patients may no longer shiver. Severe hypothermia (<28.0 °C [82.4 °F]) can cause pulmonary edema, coma, hypotension, areflexia, and ventricular arrhythmias, including cardiac arrest. Electrocardiogram may show a characteristic J wave (Osborne wave) (**Figure 21**), which should not be mistaken for acute myocardial infarction or intraventricular conduction delay.

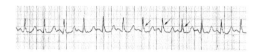

FIGURE 21. Electrocardiogram showing Osborne waves. Hypothermia is associated with bradycardia, either sinus or with atrial fibrillation, and the appearance of the classic Osborne waves at the QT interval. They are best seen in the inferior and lateral chest leads. Osborne waves are defined by the shoulder or "hump" between QRS and ST segments.

CONT.

The electrocardiogram may also show the shiver artifact, which should not be mistaken for atrial fibrillation/flutter and erroneously treated.

Hypothermic patients who are shivering generally can rewarm themselves passively if they are removed from the cold environment and kept dry and covered. Any patient who no longer shivers must be actively rewarmed using external warming techniques or invasive methods such as gastric, peritoneal, or pleural space lavage. Invasive rewarming techniques are indicated for patients with severely decreased core temperatures who exhibit signs of central nervous system depression or cardiac dysfunction. Rewarming therapy may be complicated by burns and organ system dysfunction, including rhabdomyolysis, disseminated intravascular coagulation, and pulmonary edema.

Therapeutic hypothermia is the intentional lowering of a patient's core temperature after cardiac arrest. This has been shown to improve neurologic outcomes in patients who recover circulation. See MKSAP 16 Cardiovascular Medicine for a discussion of therapeutic hypothermia. ◨

KEY POINTS

- Patients with impaired thermoregulation or perception of cold (including elderly and intoxicated persons) are at greatest risk for hypothermia.
- Patients with hypothermia who are shivering generally can rewarm themselves passively if they are removed from the cold environment and kept dry and covered.

Toxicology

In patients with toxic ingestion, the first challenge is discovering what substance has been ingested or taken. Symptoms and signs of one or more of the common toxic syndromes (**Table 56**) along with clinical laboratory results can usually determine the proper treatment approach. Coingestions are common in both accidental and intentional overdoses; therefore, other toxins must be ruled out in addition to the primary toxin identified.

TABLE 56.	Toxic Syndromes and Their Manifestations	
Syndrome	**Manifestations**	**Representative Drugs**
Sympathomimetic	Tachycardia	Cocaine
	Hypertension	Amphetamines
	Diaphoresis	Ephedrine
	Agitation	Caffeine
	Seizures	
	Mydriasis	
Cholinergic	"SLUDGE" (Salivation, Lacrimation, increased Urination and Defecation, Gastrointestinal upset, and Emesis)	Organophosphates (insecticides, sarin)
	Confusion	Carbamates
	Bronchorrhea	Physostigmine
	Bradycardia	Edrophonium
	Miosis	Nicotine
Anticholinergic	Hyperthermia	Antihistamines
	Dry skin and mucous membranes	Tricyclic antidepressants
	Agitation, delirium	Antiparkinson agents
	Tachycardia, tachypnea	Atropine
	Hypertension	Scopolamine
	Mydriasis	
Opioids	Miosis	Morphine and related drugs
	Respiratory depression	Heroin
	Lethargy, confusion	
	Hypothermia	
	Bradycardia	
	Hypotension	

Alcohols

The most common alcohol toxicity comes from excessive chronic or binge drinking of ethanol. Alcohol activates the same receptor as γ-aminobutyric acid, which is the major inhibitory neurotransmitter in the brain, causing central nervous system depression. If ethanol has been present frequently enough in a heavy drinker to develop tolerance and dependence, sudden withdrawal creates a state of central nervous system hyperactivity, which can be life threatening. Early symptoms include diaphoresis, insomnia, anxiety, tremor, palpitations, and headache. As withdrawal becomes more severe, patients may have seizures and/or hallucinations, known as delirium tremens. Onset is usually 48 to 96 hours after the last drink and sometimes persists for many days. Hypokalemia, hypomagnesemia, and hypophosphatemia are common and contribute to cardiac dysfunction and arrhythmias. Mortality rate is approximately 5%, usually owing to arrhythmias or other complications such as aspiration pneumonia. Patients at risk should be monitored closely for signs of withdrawal and treated as needed with benzodiazepines, fluid rehydration, and electrolyte correction. Benzodiazepines should be given as needed, rather than by scheduled dosing or continuous infusion. The benzodiazepine dose that is adequate to manage withdrawal without causing excessive sedation may be difficult to predict. Thiamine, glucose, and folate are supplemented routinely, and nutrition should be instituted early. A multidisciplinary team should address issues of alcohol dependence when the patient has recovered.

Other commonly ingested alcohols include ethylene glycol (antifreeze), methanol (wood alcohol), and isopropyl (rubbing) alcohol, which also have central nervous system depressant effects (**Table 57**). Ethylene glycol is converted by alcohol dehydrogenase to oxalic acid, which crystalizes in renal tubules and causes kidney injury. Methanol is converted to formic acid, which is toxic to the retina. Isopropyl alcohol is converted to acetone but has no toxic metabolite. Ketone levels are elevated with isopropyl alcohol, but there is no anion gap metabolic acidosis as there is with ethylene glycol and methanol toxicity. Conversion to toxic metabolites and clearance of these three alcohols is greatly diminished by ethanol or intravenous fomepizole. All can be removed rapidly with dialysis.

Carbon Monoxide

Carbon monoxide (CO) is colorless and odorless, so patients are often unaware of exposure. Because it cannot be detected by pulse oximetry, it may be undetected unless clinicians suspect it and test for it specifically with co-oximetry, as in routine blood gas analysis. CO binds hemoglobin avidly to produce carboxyhemoglobin. Nonsmokers typically have up to 3% of their hemoglobin bound by CO (carboxyhemoglobin), whereas heavy smokers may have up to 10% to 15%. With higher exposure, carboxyhemoglobin can reach toxic levels above 20%, shifting the oxyhemoglobin dissociation curve to the left, reducing oxygen transfer to the tissues, and resulting in dysfunction of high oxygen–requiring organs like the brain and heart. Headache, disorientation, and nausea occur with mild exposure; with more concentrated exposure, symptoms may progress to chest pain, more severe mental status changes, dyspnea, arrhythmias, muscle weakness, coma, and death. Days to months after recovery from the acute effects of CO toxicity, up to 40% of patients develop a delayed cognitive impairment syndrome. Hyperbaric oxygen treatment appears to reduce the risk of this delayed neuropsychiatric syndrome.

In cases of suspected CO toxicity, patients should be monitored closely for hypoxic organ effects, and co-oximetry and electrocardiogram should be obtained. Patients should be given 100% oxygen. If the carboxyhemoglobin level is high (>20%) and the patient is symptomatic, hyperbaric oxygen treatment should be initiated, if available. The half-life of carboxyhemoglobin is 300 minutes in a patient breathing ambient air, 90 minutes breathing 100% oxygen, and 30 minutes breathing hyperbaric oxygen. If the CO exposure is from smoke inhalation, concomitant cyanide toxicity must be considered because both toxins are common and together they have synergistic toxicity.

Cyanide

Cyanide toxicity occurs following inhalation or ingestion. For cyanide inhalation, see the Acute Inhalational Injuries section.

TABLE 57. Clinical Manifestations of Ethylene Glycol, Methanol, and Isopropyl Alcohol Ingestion

Alcohol	Common Name	Toxic Metabolite	Nontoxic Metabolite	Anion Gap	Osmolar Gap	Toxicity	Antidote
Methanol	Wood alcohol	Formic acid	-	Yes	Yes	Retina	Fomepizole, ethanol, dialysis
Ethylene glycol	Antifreeze	Glycolic, glyoxylic, and oxalic acids	-	Yes	Yes	Renal tubules	Fomepizole, ethanol, dialysis
Isopropyl alcohol	Rubbing alcohol	-	Acetone	No	Yes	CNS depression	Fomepizole, ethanol, dialysis

CNS = central nervous system.

Ingestion of potassium cyanide or sodium cyanide is usually associated with attempted suicide or homicide. Cyanide blocks oxidative phosphorylation by disabling cytochrome oxidase in the mitochondria. This leads to effective hypoxia, even in the presence of oxygen, resulting in lactic acidosis and depleted cellular energy stores. Chronic exposure causes headache, nausea, chest and abdominal pain, and anxiety. Acute exposure, depending on dose and duration, can cause severe organ dysfunction, particularly in the central nervous system and cardiovascular system. Treatment of cyanide toxicity uses agents that speed metabolism and elimination of cyanide, including nitrites, sodium thiosulfate, hydroxocobalamin, and others. Note that nitrites are not recommended for inhalational cyanide toxicity owing to the risk of methemoglobin formation.

Nitroprusside, a potent intravenous vasodilator used for hypertensive crises, contains cyanide, which can accumulate to toxic levels if the infusion is given at a high rate or for a prolonged time. High-dose infusions lasting 3 to 10 hours can result in fatal doses of cyanide. Toxicity can usually be avoided by shielding the drug from light (which breaks down the nitroprusside molecules in solution), limiting the rate and duration of the infusion, and by adding sodium thiosulfate to the infusion.

Toxicity of Drugs of Abuse

Amphetamines increase central catecholamine activity, resulting in anorexia, tachycardia, hypertension, hyperthermia, and psychomotor agitation. Organ system effects can include myocardial ischemia and infarction, strokes, seizures, acute kidney failure, fulminant hepatic failure, and psychosis. Recreational use of "ecstasy" or 3,4-methylenedioxymethamphetamine also commonly causes bruxism (sometimes leading to severe dental damage with chronic use) and hyponatremia, resulting in cerebral edema and other central nervous system effects. Management of amphetamine toxicity consists of benzodiazepines and supportive measures. Fluid repletion and nutrition are important in both binge and chronic users.

Cocaine is a potent stimulant that can be inhaled or administered through oral, intravenous, and transmucosal routes. It produces a classic sympathomimetic toxic syndrome with tachycardia, hypertension, mydriasis, hyperthermia, and agitation. Additional cardiac effects include atrial and ventricular arrhythmias, myocardial ischemia, aortic dissection, and even aortic rupture secondary to acute hypertension. It can cause seizures, strokes, bronchospasm, pulmonary edema, alveolar hemorrhage, and rhabdomyolysis. Management of cocaine toxicity is usually with benzodiazepines for sympathomimetic symptoms; calcium channel blockers are considered safe and effective for lowering the blood pressure and heart rate. Despite a lack of clinical data, some experts believe that patients with hypertensive crises suspected of cocaine toxicity should not receive β-blockers, as this could result in unopposed α-mediated vasoconstriction and more severe hypertension.

An alternative hypertensive treatment is a combined α- and β-receptor antagonist such as labetalol. Cocaine-related myocardial ischemia is treated with nitroglycerin and aspirin. Coronary spasm is common in acute cocaine toxicity, but plaque rupture and acute thrombosis are possible and must be ruled out in selected patients by coronary angiography.

Therapeutic Drug Overdoses

In therapeutic drug overdoses, it is important to ascertain whether the overdose was intentional (suicide attempt) or accidental and whether there were multiple agents ingested. **Table 58** outlines some of the therapeutic agents commonly taken in overdose.

Overdoses of over-the-counter analgesics are among the most common toxic ingestions. A search for the presence of acetaminophen and/or salicylate is prudent any time an overdose is discovered or suspected. Acetaminophen toxicity can occur even when ingestion has not exceeded the recommended limits when there is concomitant alcohol use or pre-existing liver disease. Aspirin overdose produces both an anion gap metabolic acidosis as well as respiratory alkalosis through central stimulation of the respiratory centers. Nomograms can be useful for estimating the dose ingested if the time of ingestion is known, but they are not valuable in many situations where toxicity has developed as a result of repeated or chronic ingestion. Another caveat affecting the pharmacokinetics of these agents after ingestion is that they are sometimes formulated for sustained release, which can delay the achievement of peak plasma levels for many hours and lead to underestimation of the dose ingested. Acetaminophen overdose is treated with *N*-acetylcysteine, which regenerates depleted glutathione and reduces the accumulation of toxic metabolites leading to liver damage. Aspirin overdose is managed with activated charcoal, intravenous glucose, and bicarbonate infusion. ▪

KEY POINTS

- Coingestions are common in both accidental and intentional overdoses; therefore, other toxins must be ruled out in addition to the primary toxin identified.

- Headache, disorientation, and nausea occur with mild carbon monoxide exposure; with more concentrated exposure, symptoms may progress to chest pain, more severe mental status changes, dyspnea, arrhythmias, muscle weakness, coma, and death.

- Days to months after recovery from the acute effects of carbon monoxide toxicity, up to 40% of patients develop a delayed cognitive impairment syndrome; hyperbaric oxygen treatment appears to reduce the risk.

Acute Abdominal Surgical Emergencies

Acute abdomen is characterized by abdominal pain and tenderness of less than 24 hours' duration. Conditions resulting in such pain require emergent medical evaluation and

TABLE 58. Therapeutic Drug Toxicities, Antidotes, and Management

Agent	Toxic Dose (or Serum Level)	Toxic Effect or Syndrome	Pharmaceutical Antidote	Other Interventions
Acetaminophen	7.5 g in 8 hours (nomogram for serum levels at 4 hours)	Acute hepatitis, fulminant hepatic failure	N-acetylcysteine PO or IV within 8 hours (may give later as well)	Charcoal within 4 hours
Benzodiazepines	Variable	CNS and respiratory suppression	Flumazenil (caution if risk of seizures)	Ventilatory and hemodynamic support
β-Blockers	Variable	Bradycardia, heart block, hypotension	Glucagon, calcium chloride	Transcutaneous or transvenous pacing
Calcium channel blockers	Variable	Bradycardia, heart block, hypotension	Calcium chloride, glucagon	Transcutaneous or transvenous pacing
Digoxin	>2 ng/mL [2.6 nmol/L] but serum levels have poor correlation with toxicity	Bradyarrhythmia and tachyarrhythmia; chronic toxicity; CNS and GI symptoms	Digoxin-specific antibody	Hemodialysis is not effective
Sulfonylureas	One tablet in a child or nondiabetic patient may cause hypoglycemia	Hypoglycemia and related symptoms	Dextrose, octreotide; glucagon for short term while dextrose is delayed	Beware recurrent hypoglycemia even after initial response
Lithium	Most overdoses are chronic (serum level upper limit is 1.2 mEq/L for acute mania, 0.8 mEq/L for maintenance; 3.0 mEq/L indicates severe toxicity); note that CNS penetration is slow	Tremor, nausea, polyuria, diabetes insipidus, arrhythmias, photosensitivity, cardiogenic shock due to CNS effects; neurologic sequelae may be permanent	No antidote for lithium; medical treatments for secondary arrhythmias, seizures, hypotension	Hemodialysis for altered mental status, anuria or seizures; IV fluid hydration with careful monitoring of electrolytes, especially in diabetes insipidus
Salicylates	Levels >30-40 mg/dL usually mean clinical toxicity; chronic toxicity is more common and more dangerous	Metabolic acidosis, hyperventilation, dehydration; severe intoxication can cause seizures, hypoglycemia, and electrolyte abnormalities	Sodium bicarbonate infusion to achieve urine output of >2 mL/kg/h and pH of >8.0 (pH is more important than diuresis)	Hemodialysis for severe toxicity or poorly tolerated medical therapy
Theophylline	Therapeutic range 10-20 µg/mL (56-111 µmol/L), but toxicity can occur in this range	Nausea, nervousness, tachycardia, CNS stimulation, hypertension, tachypnea, seizures, atrial arrhythmias, hypokalemia, hyperglycemia, ventricular arrhythmias, status epilepticus	Activated charcoal can be given	Charcoal hemoperfusion is treatment of choice, but hemodialysis can also be used if hemoperfusion is not available; cardioversion, seizure control, airway management, electrolyte correction
Tricyclic antidepressants	Levels do not correlate well with toxicity; better to follow clinical signs and symptoms	Sudden or delayed onset of seizures, severe arrhythmias, hypotension, rhabdomyolysis, and kidney failure	Bicarbonate infusion titrated to QT interval improvement on ECG (note that sodium loading is more important than alkalinization); benzodiazepines for seizures	Hemodialysis is not effective; monitor and correct electrolytes closely; defibrillation; pacing for bradycardia (avoid atropine or catecholamines)

CNS = central nervous system; ECG = electrocardiogram; GI = gastrointestinal; IV = intravenously; PO = by mouth.

CONT.

possibly surgery to avoid deterioration and death. The differential diagnosis of the acute abdomen is broad and heterogeneous (**Table 59**). Risk factors and clinical signs and symptoms direct the diagnostic evaluation to specific management, which can be life saving. In most cases, the most important clues to the cause of an acute abdomen come from the history and physical examination, although imaging and other testing play a crucial role.

Nonsurgical causes are suggested by features of the presentation or underlying illness, such as elevated glucose

TABLE 59. The Differential Diagnosis of the Acute Abdomen

Nonsurgical Causes

Metabolic
  Uremia
  Diabetic ketoacidosis
  Addisonian crisis
  Acute intermittent porphyria
  Hereditary Mediterranean fever

Hematologic
  Sickle cell or other hemoglobinopathy

Toxins and withdrawal
  Opioid withdrawal
  Lead and other heavy metal poisoning
  Black widow spider bite

Surgical Causes

Hemorrhage
  Solid organ laceration or fracture
  Ruptured arterial aneurysm
  Ectopic pregnancy
  Vascular enteric fistula

Obstruction
  Postsurgical adhesions
  Volvulus of sigmoid colon or cecum
  Incarcerated hernia
  Inflammatory bowel disease
  Obstructing tumor
  Intussusception

Ischemia
  Mesenteric thrombosis or embolism
  Ovarian or testicular torsion
  Ischemic colitis
  Incarcerated hernia
  Buerger disease

Infection/inflammation
  Appendicitis
  Cholecystitis/cholangitis
  Diverticulitis
  Abscess of solid organs or muscles
  Pancreatitis

Perforated viscus
  Peptic ulcer perforation
  Malignant perforation
  Diverticular perforation
  Boerhaave syndrome (esophageal rupture)

CONT. level, ketosis, abnormal hormone levels, blast cells on peripheral smear, or history of spider bite. The character and distribution of abdominal pain can be revealing. For example, pain that radiates to the back suggests aortic aneurysm or pancreatitis.

Vascular causes for acute abdominal pain become more common with advancing age and vascular disease risk factors. Abdominal pain from thrombosis or ischemia is often diffuse and out of proportion to history and physical examination findings. If ischemia is suspected, emergent surgery is usually needed, and antibiotics should be given (see MKSAP 16 Gastroenterology and Hepatology). Free air under the diaphragm on abdominal imaging is strongly suggestive of perforation unless there has been a recent abdominal procedure to introduce the air. Organs that commonly perforate include the appendix, stomach, colon, and duodenum. A perforated viscus requires surgical repair.

Intestinal obstruction is common and may be complete or partial. Partial small-bowel obstruction usually resolves without surgery, but surgery is nearly always needed for complete obstruction. In cases of partial obstruction, the patient may have diarrhea. High-pitched, hyperactive bowel sounds are typical of obstruction, and the associated pain is crampy. Symptoms begin more quickly after small-bowel obstruction than after colonic obstruction.

For a discussion of abdominal compartment syndrome, see MKSAP 16 Nephrology. **H**

KEY POINTS

- Acute abdomen is characterized by abdominal pain and tenderness of less than 24 hours' duration.
- In most cases, the most important clues to the cause of an acute abdomen come from the history and physical examination, although imaging and other testing play a crucial role.

Supportive Care in Critical Illness **H**
Pain, Anxiety, and Delirium

Pain, anxiety, and delirium are common in critical care and contribute significantly to patient suffering, regardless of whether the primary condition can be cured. Increased attention has been focused on evidence-based management, especially as research shows that pain, anxiety, and delirium contribute to mortality and morbidity in critically ill patients. Up to 80% of patients in the ICU experience delirium, which can be hyperactive (agitated), hypoactive (lethargic), or mixed (alternating agitation and lethargy).

Evidence supports routine and protocol-based assessment and management of pain, anxiety, and delirium. There is demonstrable improvement in hospital and posthospital morbidity and mortality when these conditions are controlled. Assessment should be regular, frequent, and objective and should use a validated instrument such as a visual analog scale for pain, the Richmond Agitation Sedation Scale (RASS) for anxiety, and the Confusion Assessment Method for the ICU (CAM-ICU) for delirium. These validated scales allow goal-directed titration of medication to treat each condition, with better control of the condition and less chance of oversedation. Often there are nonpharmacologic ways to provide orienting cues to patients in order to avoid delirium, such as verbal reorientation or conversation with a family member or other familiar person.

When sedative medications are used in the ICU, intermittent as-needed dosing or daily interruptions of continuous infusions are recommended and have been shown to shorten the overall length of sedation, decrease ventilator time, and shorten length of ICU stay. There are no FDA-approved medications for delirium, but haloperidol is recommended in guidelines for both agitated and lethargic delirium.

Intensive Care Unit–Acquired Weakness

More than 50% of patients with prolonged critical illness develop weakness out of proportion to deconditioning expected from immobility. These patients may have critical illness myopathy, critical illness polyneuropathy, or both. These two entities are associated with different risk factors, but distinguishing them clinically is difficult and usually not helpful; therefore, observed weakness is usually collectively described as ICU-acquired weakness. It complicates weaning from mechanical ventilation and prolongs length of ICU stay. Treatment options are disappointing, and prevention by limiting avoidable risk factors is best. Weakness may persist for many years or indefinitely.

Persistent Neuropsychiatric Disorders After Critical Illness

Neuropsychiatric impairment may persist for months, years, or indefinitely after critical illness. Up to 75% of patients with these illnesses experience cognitive impairment beyond the time of hospital discharge, and nearly half still have significant clinical impairment at 1 and 2 years after discharge. These deficits resemble acquired dementia and contribute to measurable decreases in quality of life. These syndromes are not well understood, but awareness and interest are growing and research has identified some associated risk factors in cohorts of patients with ARDS or severe sepsis. These studies have so far identified associations with age, duration of mechanical ventilation, and degree of hyperglycemia.

Depression, anxiety, and posttraumatic stress disorder are more than four times more common in survivors of critical illness than in the general population, with clinical effects documented in cohort studies up to 8 years after hospital discharge.

Nutrition

Historically, critically ill patients were not routinely given nutrition, sometimes for many days after admission to the ICU. Many critical illnesses create high energy requirements, and some are the result of nutritional deficiency in the first place. Feeding in the ICU may be difficult or risky. Poor nutrition contributes to immunosuppression and poor wound healing as well as complicating fluid and electrolyte balance. Some nutrition, when reasonably safe and tolerated, is recommended, but evidence suggests that critically ill patients may not need full nutritional support, especially early in their illness. Overfeeding, especially with high-fat formulations, may lead to increased CO_2 production and increased difficulty with ventilation.

In general, enteral feeding is preferred over parenteral routes if possible. Most patients with burns and those with airway injury can tolerate placement of an enteral feeding tube. Postpyloric feeding tube placement has not been shown to improve any clinically significant outcomes compared with gastric feeding. Specifically, there is no decrease in the risk of reflux, aspiration, pneumonia, length of ICU stay, or mortality. Delayed gastric emptying is common in critical illness and may respond to prokinetic agents like metoclopramide or erythromycin.

The Harris-Benedict equation can be used to estimate nutritional requirements in critically ill patients, as in other clinical situations. However, critically ill patients may have a number of conditions that limit the usefulness of the equation, including mechanical ventilation, morbid obesity, organ transplantation, fluid overload, ascites, limb amputation or plegia, and severe malnutrition. A more accurate assessment of nutritional needs is indirect calorimetry from exhaled breath analysis, but the equipment needed may not be widely available. Some common critical illnesses may require changes to routine nutritional formulations, outlined in **Table 60**.

TABLE 60.	Special Nutrition Situations in Critical Care	
Condition	**Protein Adjustment**	**Other Nutritional Adjustments**
Chronic kidney failure, not on dialysis	Decrease to 0.6-1.0 g/kg/d	
Chronic kidney failure, on dialysis	Increase to 1.2-1.3 g/kg/d	
Acute kidney failure	No protein restriction	
Hypercarbic respiratory failure		Decrease carbohydrate calories and increase fat calories
Burns	Increase to >2.5 g/kg/d	Increase total calories to 30 kcal/kg/d; supplement glutamine and arginine to decrease risk of infection
Pancreatitis		Elemental enteral formulation; alternatively total parenteral nutrition with limited lipids, keep serum triglyceride level <400 mg/dL (4.5 mmol/L)

CONT.

Serum prealbumin level less than 5 mg/dL (50 mg/L) is an indicator of severe protein and caloric malnutrition. **H**

KEY POINTS

- Up to 80% of patients in the intensive care unit experience delirium, which can be hyperactive (agitated), hypoactive (lethargic), or mixed (alternating agitation and lethargy).
- There is demonstrable improvement in hospital and posthospital morbidity and mortality when pain, anxiety, and delirium are controlled.
- More than 50% of patients with prolonged critical illness develop weakness out of proportion to deconditioning expected from immobility.
- Neuropsychiatric impairment may persist for months, years, or indefinitely after critical illness.

Approaches to Providing Best Practice

The goal of evidence-based practice and quality improvement is to create an environment in which mistakes are less likely to occur despite the complexity of care being provided in the ICU. The Institute for Healthcare Improvement recommends establishing an organized system of ICU care that includes daily rounds, daily goals, and improving clinical outcomes through the use of care "bundles" for patients requiring ventilators and central lines (see the Process Measures section). Specific care algorithms are also recommended for bladder catheter management, glucose control, transfusion management, and deep venous thrombosis prophylaxis. Strategies to reduce the risk of delirium and pressure ulcers should be implemented. Goals of care should be established and assessed daily, and multidisciplinary rounds should be coordinated by a clinician with both the expertise and dedicated time to spend in the critical care unit.

Structural Measures

The effectiveness of open versus closed ICU models remains controversial; however, consensus is that a closed model, led and managed by an intensivist, is associated with reduction in overall ICU mortality and has the greatest effect on patients admitted longer than 48 hours. It is believed that a closed-model ICU is associated with improved outcomes and less resource utilization. However, most ICUs use an open model owing to lack of specialized physicians.

Collaboration between physicians and nurses is an important component of effective care in the ICU. Multidisciplinary teams that include critical care nurses, pharmacists, respiratory therapists, social workers, and intensivists can improve care with collaborative decision-making. A daily goals assessment by the multidisciplinary team helps to keep track and verify completion of care plans.

Process Measures

Care bundles and checklists are examples of process measures. Care bundles are groups of best practices that improve patient care. Common care bundles used in the ICU are the ventilator bundle, central line bundle, sedation and analgesia bundle, delirium bundle, and urinary bundle (**Table 61**).

Rapid Response Team

The rapid response team (also known as the medical emergency team) is a team of clinicians who bring critical care expertise to the bedside outside the ICU. Failures in planning, recognition, and communication often lead to "failure to rescue." The goal of rapid response teams is to identify, treat, and transfer unstable patients prior to development of respiratory or cardiac arrest. Although reduction in overall hospital mortality following implementation of rapid response teams has not been definitively established, reductions in cardiac and respiratory arrests outside of the ICU setting are reduced following implementation.

Intensive Care Unit Prognosis

The use of severity-of-illness scoring systems is common in the ICU. These systems attempt to define overall risks for populations of patients. An accurate, quantifiable description of the pretreatment status of critically ill patients may allow for risk prognostication and evaluation of effectiveness of quality improvement processes. The Glasgow Coma Scale was developed in the 1970s as a triage tool for patients with head injury. The Glasgow Coma Scale has been shown to correlate with mortality and level of eventual brain function in patients with traumatic brain injury. Several multi-scoring systems

TABLE 61.	Care Bundles in the Intensive Care Unit
Bundle	**Key Components**
Ventilator	Elevation of the head of the bed, daily "sedation vacations" and assessment of readiness to extubate, peptic ulcer disease prophylaxis, deep venous thrombosis prophylaxis, daily oral care with chlorhexidine
Central line	Hand hygiene, maximal barrier precautions upon insertion, chlorhexidine skin antisepsis, optimal catheter site selection with avoidance of the femoral vein for central venous access in adult patients, daily review of line necessity with prompt removal of unnecessary lines
Sedation	Protocol-directed sedation, use of validated sedation scale, bolus doses of benzodiazepines instead of continuous infusion, use of sedatives with a short duration of action, daily interruption of sedation
Delirium	Daily assessment for delirium, minimize risk factors for delirium, use sedation protocols
Urinary	Daily assessment for catheter removal, utilize securement device, use reminder system

CONT.

have been developed for use in critically ill patients. They include the Acute Physiologic and Chronic Health Evaluation (APACHE) score, Simplified Acute Physiologic Score (SAPS), and Therapeutic Intervention Scoring System (TISS). The role for scoring systems in the care of individual patients is undefined. ▣

Bibliography

Pulmonary Diagnostic Tests

Barnes PJ, Dweik RA, Gelb AF, et al. Exhaled nitric oxide in pulmonary diseases: a comprehensive review. Chest. 2010;138(3):682-692. [PMID: 20822990]

Dooms C, Seijo L, Gasparini S, Trisolini R, Ninane V, Tournoy KG. Diagnostic bronchoscopy: state of the art. Eur Respir Rev. 2010;19(117):229-236. [PMID: 20956198]

Joos GF, O'Connor B, Anderson SD, et al; ERS Task Force. Indirect airway challenges [erratum in Eur Respir J. 2003;22(4):718]. Eur Respir J. 2003;21(6):1050-1068. [PMID: 12797503]

Kligerman S, Digumarthy S. Staging of non-small cell lung cancer using integrated PET/CT. AJR Am J Roentgenol. 2009;193(5):1203-1211. [PMID: 19843732]

Lange NE, Mulholland M, Kreider ME. Spirometry: don't blow it! Chest. 2009;136(2):608-614. [PMID: 19666760]

Mehta AC, Chua AP, Gleeson F, Meziane M. The debate on CXR utilization and interpretation is only just beginning: a Pro/Con debate. Respirology. 2010;15(8):1152-1156. [PMID: 20920120]

Rasekaba T, Lee AL, Naughton MT, Williams TJ, Holland AE. The six-minute walk test: a useful metric for the cardiopulmonary patient. Intern Med J. 2009;39(8):495-501. [PMID: 19732197]

Smith-Bindman R, Lipson J, Marcus R, et al. Radiation dose associated with common computed tomography examinations and the associated lifetime attributable risk of cancer. Arch Intern Med. 2009;169(22):2078-2086. [PMID: 20008690]

American Thoracic Society. Standardization of Spirometry, 1994 Update. Am J Respir Crit Care Med. 1995;152(3):1107-1136. [PMID: 7663792]

Verschakelen JA. The role of high-resolution computed tomography in the work-up of interstitial lung disease. Curr Opin Pulm Med. 2010;16(5):503-510. [PMID: 20644479]

Asthma

Lazarus SC. Clinical practice. Emergency treatment of asthma. N Engl J Med. 2010;363(8):755-764. [PMID: 20818877]

Lemanske RF Jr, Busse WW. Asthma: clinical expression and molecular mechanisms. J Allergy Clin Immunol. 2010;125(2)(suppl 2):S95-102. [PMID: 20176271]

Moore WC, Pascual RM. Update in asthma 2009. Am J Respir Crit Care Med. 2010;181(11):1181-1187. [PMID: 20516492]

Murphy DM, O'Byrne PM. Recent advances in the pathophysiology of asthma. Chest. 2010;137(6):1417-1426. [PMID: 20525652]

National Asthma Education and Prevention Program. Expert Panel Report 3 (EPR-3): Guidelines for the Diagnosis and Management of Asthma-Summary Report 2007 [erratum in J Allergy Clin Immunol. 2008;121(6):1330]. J Allergy Clin Immunol. 2007;120(5 suppl):S94-138. [PMID: 17983880]

Schatz M, Dombrowski MP. Clinical practice. Asthma in pregnancy. N Engl J Med. 2009;360(18):1862-1869. [PMID: 19403904]

Chronic Obstructive Pulmonary Disease

Calverley PM, Rabe KF, Goehring UM, Kristiansen S, Fabbri LM, Martinez FJ; M2-124 and M2-125 study groups. Roflumilast in symptomatic chronic obstructive pulmonary disease: two randomised clinical trials [erratum in Lancet. 2010;376(9747):1146]. Lancet. 2009;374(9691):685-694. [PMID: 19716960]

Casaburi R, ZuWallack R. Pulmonary rehabilitation for management of chronic obstructive pulmonary disease. N Engl J Med. 2009;360(13):1329-1335. [PMID: 19321869]

Fromer L, Goodwin E, Walsh J. Customizing inhaled therapy to meet the needs of COPD patients. Postgrad Med. 2010;122(2):83-93. [PMID: 20203459]

Global Strategy for Diagnosis, Management, and Prevention of COPD. December 2011. Available at: www.goldcopd.org/. Accessed June 27, 2012.

Littner MR. In the clinic. Chronic obstructive pulmonary disease. Ann Intern Med. 2011;154(7):ITC4-1-ITC4-15; quiz ITC4-16. [PMID: 21464346]

Mahler DA, Selecky PA, Harrod CG, et al. American College of Chest Physicians consensus statement on the management of dyspnea in patients with advanced lung or heart disease. Chest. 2010;137(3):674-691. [PMID: 2020294]

Orens JB, Estenne M, Arcasoy S, et al; Pulmonary Scientific Council of the International Society for Heart and Lung Transplantation. International guidelines for the selection of lung transplant candidates: 2006 update—a consensus report from the Pulmonary Scientific Council of the International Society for Heart and Lung Transplantation. J Heart Lung Transplant. 2006;25(7):745-755. [PMID: 16818116]

Qaseem A, Wilt TJ, Weinberger SE, et al; American College of Physicians; American College of Chest Physicians; American Thoracic Society; European Respiratory Society. Diagnosis and management of stable chronic obstructive pulmonary disease: a clinical practice guideline update from the American College of Physicians, American College of Chest Physicians, American Thoracic Society, and European Respiratory Society. Ann Intern Med. 2011;155(3):179-191. [PMID: 21810710]

Stoller JK, Panos RJ, Krachman S, Doherty DE, Make B; Long-term Oxygen Treatment Trial Research Group. Oxygen therapy for patients with COPD: current evidence and the long-term oxygen treatment trial. Chest. 2010;138(1):179-187. [PMID: 20605816]

Diffuse Parenchymal Lung Disease

American Thoracic Society; European Respiratory Society. American Thoracic Society/European Respiratory Society International Multidisciplinary Consensus Classification of the Idiopathic Interstitial Pneumonias. This joint statement of the American Thoracic Society (ATS), and the European Respiratory Society (ERS) was adopted by the ATS board of directors, June 2001 and by the ERS Executive Committee, June 2001 [erratum in: Am J Respir Crit Care Med. 2002;166(3):426]. Am J Respir Crit Care Med. 2002;165(2):277-304. [PMID: 11790668]

Baughman RP, Culver DA, Judson MA. A concise review of pulmonary sarcoidosis. Am J Respir Crit Care Med. 2011;183(5):573-581. [PMID: 21037016]

Collard HR, Moore BB, Flaherty KR, et al; Idiopathic Pulmonary Fibrosis Clinical Research Network Investigators. Acute exacerbations of idiopathic pulmonary fibrosis. Am J Respir Crit Care Med. 2007;176(7):636-643. [PMID: 17585107]

Flaherty KR, Andrei AC, King TE Jr, et al. Idiopathic interstitial pneumonia: do community and academic physicians agree on diagnosis? Am J Respir Crit Care Med. 2007;175(10):1054-1060. [PMID: 17255566]

Kim EJ, Elicker BM, Maldonado F, et al. Usual interstitial pneumonia in rheumatoid arthritis-associated interstitial lung disease. Eur Respir J. 2010;35(6):1322-1328. [PMID: 19996193]

McCormack FX, Inoue Y, Moss J, et al; National Institutes of Health Rare Lung Diseases Consortium; MILES Trial Group. Efficacy and safety of sirolimus in lymphangioleiomyomatosis. N Engl J Med. 2011;364(17):1595-1606. [PMID: 21410393]

McKinzie BP, Bullington WM, Mazur JE, Judson MA. Efficacy of short-course, low-dose corticosteroid therapy for acute pulmonary sarcoidosis exacerbations. Am J Med Sci. 2010;339(1):1-4. [PMID: 19996733]

Bibliography

Raghu G, Collard HR, Egan JJ, et al; ATS/ERS/JRS/ALAT Committee on Idiopathic Pulmonary Fibrosis. An official ATS/ERS/JRS/ALAT statement: idiopathic pulmonary fibrosis: evidence-based guidelines for diagnosis and management. Am J Respir Crit Care Med. 2011;183(6):788-824. [PMID: 21471066]

Washko GR, Hunninghake GM, Fernandez IE, et al; COPDGene Investigators. Lung volumes and emphysema in smokers with interstitial lung abnormalities. N Engl J Med. 2011;364(10):897-906. [PMID: 21388308]

Occupational Lung Disease

Aldrich TK, Gustave J, Hall CB, et al. Lung function in rescue workers at the world trade center after 7 years. N Engl J Med. 2010;362(14):1263-1272. [PMID: 20375403]

Banerjee D, Kuschner WG. Diagnosing occupational lung disease: a practical guide to the occupational pulmonary history for the primary care practitioner. Compr Ther. 2005;31(1):2-11. [PMID: 15793319]

Beckett WS. Occupational respiratory diseases. N Engl J Med. 2000;342(6):406-413. [PMID: 10666432]

Beeckman LA, Wang ML, Petsonk EL, Wagner GR. Rapid declines in FEV1 and subsequent respiratory symptoms, illnesses, and mortality in coal miners in the United States. Am J Respir Crit Care Med. 2001;163(3 Pt 1):633-639. [PMID: 11254516]

State of Lung Diseases in Diverse Communities 2010: Occupational Lung Diseases. Available at www.lungusa.org/finding-cures/our-research/solddc-index.html. Accessed June 27, 2011.

U.S. Department of Health and Human Services. Progress Review: Occupational Safety and Health. Healthy People 2010. February 21, 2008. Available at http://healthypeople.gov/2020/topics objectives2020/overview.aspx?topicid=30. Accessed June 27, 2012.

Pleural Disease

American Thoracic Society; Centers for Disease Control and Prevention; Infectious Diseases Society of America. American Thoracic Society/Centers for Disease Control and Prevention/Infectious Diseases Society of America: controlling tuberculosis in the United States. Am J Respir Crit Care Med. 2005;172(9):1169-1227. [PMID: 16249321]

Baumann MH, Strange C, Heffner JE, et al; AACP Pneumothorax Consensus Group. Management of spontaneous pneumothorax: an American College of Chest Physicians Delphi consensus statement. Chest. 2001;119(2):590-602. [PMID: 11171742]

Davies HE, Davies RJ, Davies CW; BTS Pleural Disease Guideline Group. Management of pleural infection in adults: British Thoracic Society Pleural Disease Guideline 2010. Thorax. 2010;65(suppl 2):ii41-53. [PMID: 20696693]

Janssen JP, Collier G, Astoul P, et al. Safety of pleurodesis with talc poudrage in malignant pleural effusion: a prospective cohort study. Lancet. 2007;369(9572):1535-1539. [PMID: 17482984]

Light RW. Clinical practice. Pleural effusion. N Engl J Med. 2002;346(25):1971-1977. [PMID: 12075059]

Maldonado F, Hawkins FJ, Daniels CE, Doerr CH, Decker PA, Ryu JH. Pleural fluid characteristics of chylothorax. Mayo Clin Proc. 2009;84(2):129-133. [PMID: 19181646]

Rahman NM, Mishra EK, Davies HE, Davies RJ, Lee YC. Clinically important factors influencing the diagnostic measurement of pleural fluid pH and glucose. Am J Respir Crit Care Med. 2008;178(5):483-490. [PMID: 18556632]

Roberts ME, Neville E, Berrisford RG, Antunes G, Ali NJ; BTS Pleural Disease Guideline Group. Management of a malignant pleural effusion: British Thoracic Society Pleural Disease Guideline 2010. Thorax. 2010;65(suppl 2):ii32-40. [PMID: 20696691]

Romero-Candeira S, Fernández C, Martín C, Sánchez-Paya J, Hernández L. Influence of diuretics on the concentration of proteins and other components of pleural transudates in patients with heart failure. Am J Med. 2001;110(9):681-686. [PMID: 11403751]

Tremblay A, Michaud G. Single-center experience with 250 tunneled pleural catheter insertions for malignant pleural effusion. Chest. 2006;129(2):362-368. [PMID: 16478853]

Pulmonary Vascular Disease

Agnelli G, Becattini C. Acute pulmonary embolism. N Engl J Med. 2010;363(3):266-274. [PMID: 20592294]

Farber HW, Loscalzo J. Pulmonary arterial hypertension. N Engl J Med. 2004;351(16):1655-1665. [PMID: 15483284]

Fedullo P, Kerr KM, Kim NH, Auger WR. Chronic thromboembolic pulmonary hypertension. Am J Respir Crit Care Med. 2011;183(12):1605-1613. [PMID: 21330453]

Guyatt GH, Akl EA, Crowther M, Gutterman DD, Schuünemann HJ; American College of Chest Physicians Antithrombotic Therapy and Prevention of Thrombosis Panel. Executive summary: Antithrombotic Therapy and Prevention of Thrombosis, 9th ed: American College of Chest Physicians Evidence-Based Clinical Practice Guidelines. Chest. 2012;141(2 suppl):7S-47S. [PMID: 22315257]

Hajduk B, Tomkowski WZ, Malek G, Davidson BL. Vena cava filter occlusion and venous thromboembolism risk in persistently anticoagulated patients: a prospective, observational cohort study. Chest. 2010;137(4):877-882. [PMID: 19880907]

Jaff MR, McMurtry MS, Archer SL, et al; American Heart Association Council on Cardiopulmonary, Critical Care, Perioperative and Resuscitation; American Heart Association Council on Peripheral Vascular Disease; American Heart Association Council on Arteriosclerosis, Thrombosis and Vascular Biology. Management of massive and submassive pulmonary embolism, iliofemoral deep vein thrombosis, and chronic thromboembolic pulmonary hypertension: a scientific statement from the American Heart Association. Circulation. 2011;123(16):1788-1830. [PMID: 21422387]

Jiménez D, Aujesky D, Moores L, et al; RIETE Investigators. Simplification of the pulmonary embolism severity index for prognostication in patients with acute symptomatic pulmonary embolism. Arch Intern Med. 2010;170(15):1383-1389. [PMID: 20696966]

Lucassen W, Geersing GJ, Erkens PM, et al. Clinical decision rules for excluding pulmonary embolism: a meta-analysis. Ann Intern Med. 2011;155(7):448-460. [PMID: 21969343]

McLaughlin VV, Archer SL, Badesch DB, et al; American College of Cardiology Foundation Task Force on Expert Consensus Documents; American Heart Association; American College of Chest Physicians; American Thoracic Society, Inc; Pulmonary Hypertension Association. ACCF/AHA 2009 expert consensus document on pulmonary hypertension a report of the American College of Cardiology Foundation Task Force on Expert Consensus Documents and the American Heart Association developed in collaboration with the American College of Chest Physicians; American Thoracic Society, Inc.; and the Pulmonary Hypertension Association. J Am Coll Cardiol. 2009;53(17):1573-1619. [PMID: 19389575]

Tapson VF. Acute pulmonary embolism. N Engl J Med. 2008;358(10):1037-1052. [PMID: 18322285]

Lung Tumors

Annema JT, van Meerbeeck JP, Rintoul RC, et al. Mediastinoscopy vs endosonography for mediastinal nodal staging of lung cancer: a randomized trial. JAMA. 2010;304(20):2245-2252. [PMID: 21098770]

Cao C, Yan TD, Kennedy C, Hendel N, Bannon PG, McCaughan BC. Bronchopulmonary carcinoid tumors: long-term outcomes after resection. Ann Thorac Surg. 2011;91(2):339-343. [PMID: 21256263]

Godoy MC, Naidich DP. Subsolid pulmonary nodules and the spectrum of peripheral adenocarcinomas of the lung: recommended interim guidelines for assessment and management. Radiology. 2009;253(3):606-622. [PMID: 19952025]

Gould MK, Fletcher J, Iannettoni MD, et al; American College of Chest Physicians. Evaluation of patients with pulmonary nodules:

when is it lung cancer? ACCP evidence-based clinical practice guidelines (2nd edition). Chest. 2007;132(3 suppl):108S-130S. [PMID: 17873164]

Jemal A, Bray F, Center MM, Ferlay J, Ward E, Forman D. Global cancer statistics. CA Cancer J Clin. 2011;61(2):69-90. [PMID: 21296855]

National Lung Screening Trial Research Team; Aberle DR, Berg CD, Black WC, et al. The National Lung Screening Trial: overview and study design. Radiology. 2011;258(1):243-253. [PMID: 21045183]

Pelosof LC, Gerber DE. Paraneoplastic syndromes: an approach to diagnosis and treatment. Mayo Clin Proc. 2010;85(9):838-854. [PMID: 20810794]

Ramalingam SS, Owonikoko TK, Khuri FR. Lung cancer: New biological insights and recent therapeutic advances. CA Cancer J Clin. 2011;61(2):91-112. [PMID: 21303969]

Rami-Porta R, Crowley JJ, Goldstraw P. The revised TNM staging system for lung cancer. Ann Thorac Cardiovasc Surg. 2009;15(1):4-9. [PMID: 19262443]

Scott WJ, Allen MS, Darling G, et al. Video-assisted thoracic surgery versus open lobectomy for lung cancer: a secondary analysis of data from the American College of Surgeons Oncology Group Z0030 randomized clinical trial. J Thorac Cardiovasc Surg. 2010;139(4):976-981. [PMID: 20172539]

Sleep Medicine

Caples SM, Rowley JA, Prinsell JR, et al. Surgical modifications of the upper airway for obstructive sleep apnea in adults: a systematic review and meta-analysis. Sleep. 2010;33(10):1396-1407. [PMID: 21061863]

Epstein LJ, Kristo D, Strollo PJ Jr, et al; Adult Obstructive Sleep Apnea Task Force of the American Academy of Sleep Medicine. Clinical guideline for the evaluation, management and long-term care of obstructive sleep apnea in adults. J Clin Sleep Med. 2009;5(3):263-276. [PMID: 19960649]

Mokhlesi B, Tulaimat A. Recent advances in obesity hypoventilation syndrome. Chest. 2007;132(4):1322-1336. [PMID: 17934118]

Morgenthaler TI, Aurora RN, Brown T, et al; Standards of Practice Committee of the AASM; American Academy of Sleep Medicine. Practice parameters for the use of autotitrating continuous positive airway pressure devices for titrating pressures and treating adult patients with obstructive sleep apnea syndrome: an update for 2007. An American Academy of Sleep Medicine report. Sleep. 2008;31(1):141-147. [PMID: 18220088]

Sack RL. Clinical practice. Jet lag. N Engl J Med. 2010;362(5):440-447. [PMID: 20130253]

Yumino D, Bradley TD. Central sleep apnea and Cheyne-Stokes respiration. Proc Am Thorac Soc. 2008;5(2):226-236. [PMID: 18250216]

High-Altitude–Related Illnesses

Schoene RB. Illnesses at high altitude. Chest. 2008;134(2):402-416. [PMID: 18682459]

Silverman D, Gendreau M. Medical issues associated with commercial flights. Lancet. 2009;373(9680):2067-2077. [PMID: 19232708]

West JB; American College of Physicians; American Physiological Society. The physiologic basis of high-altitude diseases. Ann Intern Med. 2004;141(10):789-800. [PMID: 15545679]

Critical Care

ARDS Definition Task Force, Ranieri V, Rubenfeld G, Thompson B, et al. Acute Respiratory Distress Syndrome: The Berlin Definition. JAMA. 2012;307(23):2526-2533. [PMID: 22797452]

Briel M, Meade M, Mercat A, et al. Higher vs lower positive end-expiratory pressure in patients with acute lung injury and acute respiratory distress syndrome: systematic review and meta-analysis. JAMA. 2010;303(9):865-873. [PMID: 20197533]

Brooks DE, Levine M, O'Connor AD, French RN, Curry SC. Toxicology in the ICU: Part 2: specific toxins. Chest. 2011;140(4):1072-1085. [PMID: 21972388]

Dellinger RP, Levy MM, Carlet JM, et al; International Surviving Sepsis Campaign Guidelines Committee; American Association of Critical-Care Nurses; American College of Chest Physicians; American College of Emergency Physicians; Canadian Critical Care Society; European Society of Clinical Microbiology and Infectious Diseases; European Society of Intensive Care Medicine; European Respiratory Society; International Sepsis Forum; Japanese Association for Acute Medicine; Japanese Society of Intensive Care Medicine; Society of Critical Care Medicine; Society of Hospital Medicine; Surgical Infection Society; World Federation of Societies of Intensive and Critical Care Medicine. Surviving Sepsis Campaign: international guidelines for management of severe sepsis and septic shock: 2008 [erratum in: Crit Care Med. 2008;36(4):1394-1396]. Crit Care Med. 2008;36(1):296-327. [PMID: 18158437]

Fan E, Needham DM, Stewart TE. Ventilatory management of acute lung injury and acute respiratory distress syndrome. JAMA. 2005;294(22):2889-2896. [PMID: 16352797]

Hill NS, Brennan J, Garpestad E, Nava S. Noninvasive ventilation in acute respiratory failure. Crit Care Med. 2007;35(10):2402-2407. [PMID: 17717495]

Institute for Healthcare Improvement. Changes for Improvement. www.ihi.org/knowledge/Pages/Changes/default.aspx. Accessed June 27, 2012.

Leaver SK, Evans TW. Acute respiratory distress syndrome. BMJ. 2007;335(7616):389-394. [PMID: 17717368]

Levine M, Brooks DE, Truitt CA, Wolk BJ, Boyer EW, Ruha AM. Toxicology in the ICU: Part 1: general overview and approach to treatment. Chest. 2011;140(3):795-806. [PMID: 21896525]

Levine M, Ruha AM, Graeme K, Brooks DE, Canning J, Curry SC. Toxicology in the ICU: part 3: natural toxins. Chest. 2011;140(5):1357-1370. [PMID: 22045882]

National Heart, Lung, and Blood Institute. National Asthma Education and Prevention Program. Expert Panel Report 3: Guidelines for the Diagnosis and Management of Asthma. August 28, 2007: www.nhlbi.nih.gov/guidelines/asthma/asthgdln.pdf. Accessed June 27, 2012.

Oddo M, Feihl F, Schaller MD, Perret C. Management of mechanical ventilation in acute severe asthma: practical aspects. Intensive Care Med. 2006;32(4):501-510. [PMID: 16552615]

Perrin C, Unterborn JN, Ambrosio CD, Hill NS. Pulmonary complications of chronic neuromuscular diseases and their management. Muscle Nerve. 2004;29(1):5-27. [PMID: 14694494]

Pronovost PJ, Thompson DA, Holzmueller CG, Lubomski LH, Morlock LL. Defining and measuring patient safety. Crit Care Clin. 2005;21(1):1-19, vii. [PMID: 15579349]

Putensen C, Theuerkauf N, Zinserling J, Wrigge H, Pelosi P. Meta-analysis: ventilation strategies and outcomes of the acute respiratory distress syndrome and acute lung injury [Erratum in: Ann Intern Med. 2009;151(12):897]. Ann Intern Med. 2009;151(8):566-576. [PMID: 19841457]

Rodrigo GJ, Rodrigo C, Hall JB. Acute asthma in adults: a review. Chest. 2004;125(3):1081-1102. [PMID: 15006973]

Schweickert WD, Hall J. ICU-acquired weakness. Chest. 2007;131(5):1541-1549. [PMID: 17494803]

Ventilation with lower tidal volumes as compared with traditional tidal volumes for acute lung injury and the acute respiratory distress syndrome. The Acute Respiratory Distress Syndrome Network. N Engl J Med. 2000;342(18):1301-1308. [PMID: 10793162]

Pulmonary and Critical Care Medicine Self-Assessment Test

This self-assessment test contains one-best-answer multiple-choice questions. Please read these directions carefully before answering the questions. Answers, critiques, and bibliographies immediately follow these multiple-choice questions. The American College of Physicians is accredited by the Accreditation Council for Continuing Medical Education (ACCME) to provide continuing medical education for physicians.

The American College of Physicians designates MKSAP 16 Pulmonary and Critical Care Medicine for a maximum of 16 *AMA PRA Category 1 Credits*™. Physicians should claim only the credit commensurate with the extent of their participation in the activity.

Earn "Same-Day" CME Credits Online

For the first time, print subscribers can enter their answers online to earn CME credits in 24 hours or less. You can submit your answers using online answer sheets that are provided at mksap.acponline.org, where a record of your MKSAP 16 credits will be available. To earn CME credits, you need to answer all of the questions in a test and earn a score of at least 50% correct (number of correct answers divided by the total number of questions). Take any of the following approaches:

➢ Use the printed answer sheet at the back of this book to record your answers. Go to mksap.acponline.org, access the appropriate online answer sheet, transcribe your answers, and submit your test for same-day CME credits. There is no additional fee for this service.

➢ Go to mksap.acponline.org, access the appropriate online answer sheet, directly enter your answers, and submit your test for same-day CME credits. There is no additional fee for this service.

➢ Pay a $10 processing fee per answer sheet and submit the printed answer sheet at the back of this book by mail or fax, as instructed on the answer sheet. Make sure you calculate your score and fax the answer sheet to 215-351-2799 or mail the answer sheet to Member and Customer Service, American College of Physicians, 190 N. Independence Mall West, Philadelphia, PA 19106-1572, using the courtesy envelope provided in your MKSAP 16 slipcase. You will need your 10-digit order number and 8-digit ACP ID number, which are printed on your packing slip. Please allow 4 to 6 weeks for your score report to be emailed back to you. Be sure to include your email address for a response.

If you do not have a 10-digit order number and 8-digit ACP ID number or if you need help creating a username and password to access the MKSAP 16 online answer sheets, go to mksap.acponline.org or email custserv@acponline.org.

CME credit is available from the publication date of December 31, 2012, until December 31, 2015. You may submit your answer sheets at any time during this period.

Directions

*Each of the numbered items is followed by lettered answers. Select the **ONE** lettered answer that is **BEST** in each case.*

Self-Assessment Test

Item 1

A 48-year-old man is evaluated for a 1-year history of cough. He has not had dyspnea, abdominal pain, heartburn, or change in appetite or weight. He has a 30-pack-year history of smoking. He does not have seasonal allergies. His medical history is significant for hypertension that is treated with losartan.

On physical examination, vital signs are normal. Pulmonary examination discloses normal breath sounds that are equal bilaterally with no wheezing. No nasal polyps are noted. Abdominal examination is unremarkable. There is no cyanosis, clubbing, or edema. Pulmonary function tests disclose an FEV_1 of 75% of predicted and an FEV_1/FVC ratio of 63%. Following administration of a bronchodilator, there is no significant change in the FEV_1/FVC ratio, and the FEV_1 is 83% of predicted. Chest radiograph shows no masses and normal lung markings.

Which of the following is the most likely cause of this patient's cough?

(A) Asthma
(B) COPD
(C) Gastroesophageal reflux disease
(D) Losartan

Item 2

A 66-year-old man is evaluated in the intensive care unit for possible extubation. He was admitted for a severe COPD exacerbation 3 days ago. His carbon dioxide remained markedly elevated despite a trial of noninvasive ventilation, and he was therefore intubated and placed on invasive mechanical ventilation. He has improved with treatment of his COPD. His medications are methylprednisolone, albuterol, ipratropium, propofol, and levofloxacin.

On physical examination, he is awake and responsive. Temperature is 37.0 °C (98.6 °F), blood pressure is 138/82 mm Hg, pulse rate is 96/min, and respiration rate is 20/min. Pulmonary examination reveals decreased breath sounds bilaterally with no wheezing. Accessory muscle use is noted. A small amount of thin secretions is noted with endotracheal suctioning.

Arterial blood gas levels have returned to baseline, with a pH of 7.36, a PCO_2 of 55 mm Hg (7.3 kPa), and a PO_2 of 70 mm Hg (9.3 kPa) on an FIO_2 of 0.35. He tolerates a weaning trial well and the decision is made to extubate.

Which of the following interventions will decrease this patient's risk for reintubation?

(A) Incentive spirometry every 2 hours
(B) Inhaled helium-oxygen mixture
(C) Nebulized *N*-acetylcysteine
(D) Noninvasive positive pressure ventilation

Item 3

A 78-year-old man is evaluated during a routine physical examination. One year ago, he was treated in the intensive care unit (ICU) for severe sepsis and respiratory failure due to community-acquired pneumonia. He was intubated for 9 days during the ICU stay and required treatment with corticosteroids, ceftriaxone, levofloxacin, lorazepam, vecuronium, and norepinephrine. A family member reports concern that the patient has not regained his ability to function independently since the illness. He is forgetful, has occasional difficulty finding words, gets lost easily in familiar places, and cannot seem to make decisions. The patient has successfully completed a physical therapy rehabilitation program and has regained his former muscle strength. There is no history of chronic illness such as coronary artery disease, diabetes mellitus, or hypertension, and he takes no medications.

On physical examination, vital signs are normal. He is alert but slow to answer questions. The cardiopulmonary examination is normal. The Mini–Mental State Examination score is 25/30. There are no focal neurologic deficits.

Which of the following factors associated with this patient's critical illness is the most likely cause of his clinical findings?

(A) Chronic disseminated intravascular coagulation
(B) Critical illness polyneuropathy
(C) Post-ICU neuropsychiatric impairment
(D) Prolonged neuromuscular blockade

Item 4

A 67-year-old man is evaluated for a 3-month history of pauses in breathing during sleep that have been witnessed by his wife. He has minimal snoring but occasional paroxysmal nocturnal dyspnea. His normal sleep schedule is 10:30 PM to 6:00 AM. He does not have insomnia or daytime sleepiness. He was recently diagnosed with heart failure. His current medications are aspirin, lisinopril, atorvastatin, and metoprolol.

On physical examination, temperature is 36.6 °C (97.9 °F), blood pressure is 128/78 mm Hg, pulse rate is 88/min, and respiration rate is 16/min; BMI is 24. Cardiac examination discloses an S_3 but no murmurs. Pulmonary examination shows a widely patent oropharyngeal airway and a few bibasilar crackles. There is trace bilateral lower extremity edema. Polysomnography discloses classic Cheyne-Stokes breathing. Oxygen saturation throughout the study is greater than 88%.

Which of the following is the most appropriate next step in treatment?

(A) Adaptive servoventilation
(B) Continuous positive airway pressure
(C) Diuresis
(D) Nocturnal oxygen
(E) Oral appliance

Item 5

A 70-year-old woman is evaluated during a routine examination. She has severe COPD with recurrent exacerbations and decreasing exercise capacity. She does not have cough or fever, but she has dyspnea with activities of daily living. She stopped smoking 1 year ago and is adherent to her medication regimen. Her inhaler technique is good. Her medications are fluticasone/salmeterol, tiotropium, and an albuterol inhaler as needed.

On physical examination, pulse rate is 80/min and respiration rate is 22/min; BMI is 22. Pulmonary examination reveals diminished breath sounds that are equal bilaterally. No wheezing or crackles are noted. FEV_1 is 45% of predicted. Oxygen saturation is 92% at rest and 90% after exertion breathing ambient air. Chest radiograph shows no infiltrate or mass.

Which of the following is the most appropriate management?

(A) Morphine
(B) Oxygen therapy
(C) Prednisone
(D) Pulmonary rehabilitation

Item 6

A 52-year-old woman is evaluated for a 1-month history of cough associated with yellow phlegm production. She has a 35-pack-year history of cigarette smoking but stopped smoking at the time of cough onset. She received albuterol, but the cough did not improve. A follow-up chest radiograph showed hyperinflation and a 2-cm nodular opacity in the left lower lobe. There are no old images available for comparison. A mammogram and Pap smear earlier this year were normal. She has not had colorectal cancer screening.

On physical examination, temperature is 37.0 °C (98.6 °F), blood pressure is 132/77 mm Hg, pulse rate is 76/min, and respiration rate is 18/min; BMI is 23. Pulmonary examination reveals diminished breath sounds bilaterally. No lymphadenopathy is noted.

Laboratory studies, including a complete blood count and metabolic profile, are normal. CT images (lung and mediastinal windows) of the 2.3-cm nodule in the left lower lobe are shown (see right column).

Which of the following is the most likely diagnosis?

(A) Carcinoid tumor
(B) Granuloma
(C) Metastatic cancer
(D) Non–small cell lung cancer

Item 7

A 55-year-old man is evaluated in the emergency department after being found unconscious on the ground outside of his home by family members. He was difficult to arouse and was confused. He was breathing spontaneously, but his breaths were rapid and shallow.

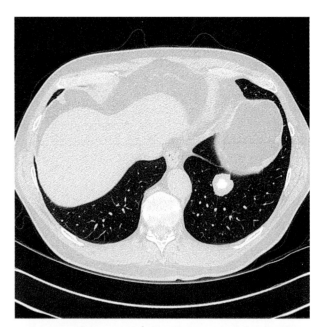

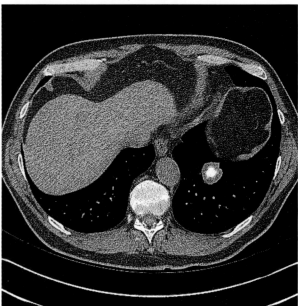

ITEM 6

On physical examination, temperature is 36.5 °C (97.7 °F), blood pressure is 135/91 mm Hg, pulse rate is 110/min, and respiration rate is 24/min. He is arousable only with noxious stimuli. Other than tachycardia, the cardiopulmonary examination is normal. The abdomen is soft, and there are no focal findings on neurologic examination.

Laboratory studies:

Blood urea nitrogen	14 mg/dL (5 mmol/L)
Creatinine	1.9 mg/dL (168 µmol/L)
Electrolytes:	
Sodium	138 meq/L (138 mmol/L)
Potassium	4.1 meq/L (4.1 mmol/L)
Chloride	90 meq/L (90 mmol/L)
Bicarbonate	12 meq/L (12 mmol/L)

Glucose	90 mg/dL (5.0 mmol/L)
Lactic acid	2.8 mg/dL (0.3 mmol/L)
Serum osmolality	390 mosm/kg (390 mmol/kg)
Blood gases:	
pH	7.24
Arterial P_{CO_2}	28 mm Hg (3.7 kPa)
Arterial P_{O_2}	102 mm Hg (13.6 kPa)

Toxicology screen is negative for ethanol, opioids, benzodiazepines, and common recreational drugs. Chest radiograph shows no lung infiltrates or masses. There is very little urine in the bladder, but urine obtained by catheterization contains many erythrocytes and envelope-shaped crystals.

Which of the following is the most appropriate treatment?

(A) Hemodialysis
(B) Intravenous ethanol
(C) Intravenous fomepizole
(D) Intravenous fomepizole and hemodialysis
(E) Supportive care

Item 8

A 67-year-old woman is evaluated for the abrupt onset of right-sided pleuritic chest pain and moderate dyspnea. She recently had symptoms typical of an upper respiratory infection (rhinorrhea, headache, sore throat, and nonproductive cough), and her chest pain and dyspnea seemed to be triggered by an episode of vigorous coughing. She has not had fever, chills, purulent sputum, or risk factors for thromboembolic disease. She smokes, and her medical history is significant for COPD without additional complications. Her medications are daily salmeterol and as-needed albuterol.

On physical examination, she appears uncomfortable but is not in respiratory distress. She is speaking in full sentences. Temperature is 37.0 °C (98.6 °F), blood pressure is 129/58 mm Hg, pulse rate is 78/min and regular, and respiration rate is 22/min. Oxygen saturation is 98% on 2 L of oxygen via nasal cannula. Pulmonary examination is significant for a prolonged expiratory phase but no wheeze; breath sounds are symmetric bilaterally. The trachea is midline. There is no accessory muscle use. Cardiac examination is normal with no murmurs. No edema is noted.

Electrocardiogram shows normal sinus rhythm without ischemic changes. Chest radiograph is shown (see top of right column).

In addition to hospital admission, which of the following is the most appropriate next step in management?

(A) Evaluation for pleurodesis
(B) Needle aspiration
(C) Serial chest radiography
(D) Tube thoracostomy

Item 9

A 28-year-old woman is evaluated for hoarseness. She was diagnosed with asthma 2 years ago. She has had two episodes of oral thrush over the past year. Control of her

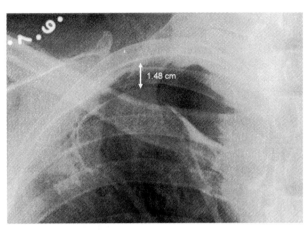

ITEM 8

asthma symptoms has been good, with no exacerbations for more than 1 year. She uses albuterol only as prophylaxis for exercise-induced asthma. She also takes a low-dose inhaled corticosteroid.

On physical examination, vital signs are normal. The lungs are clear. Spirometry results are normal.

Which of the following is the most appropriate next step in management?

(A) Add a long-acting β_2-agonist
(B) Discontinue inhaled corticosteroids
(C) Perform vocal cord examination
(D) Provide a spacer for use with inhaled corticosteroids

Item 10

A 74-year-old woman was evaluated in the emergency department for a urinary tract infection and hypotension. Antibiotics were administered in the emergency department, and she was admitted to the hospital. Six hours after admission, she is confused and lethargic.

On physical examination, temperature is 37.8 °C (100.0 °F), blood pressure is 88/50 mm Hg, pulse rate is 112/min, and respiration rate is 28/min. Other than tachycardia, the cardiopulmonary examination is normal. Her extremities are cool and mottled appearing. She has had no urine output since admission to the hospital.

Laboratory studies (from the emergency department):

Hemoglobin	10.5 g/dL (105 g/L)
Leukocyte count	16,700/µL (16.7 × 10⁹/L)
Platelet count	110,000/µL (110 × 10⁹/L)
Creatinine	Normal
Electrolytes	Normal

Electrocardiogram shows normal sinus rhythm with normal T-wave and ST-segment morphology.

Which of the following is the most appropriate next step in management?

(A) Corticosteroids
(B) Intravenous fluid bolus
(C) Norepinephrine
(D) Two units of packed red blood cells

Item 11

A 63-year-old man is evaluated for progressive dyspnea on exertion for the past several months. He is able to walk two to three blocks on a flat surface but becomes short of breath when going upstairs or uphill. He also notes shortness of breath when he lies down. He does not have cough or sputum production. He has a 7.5-pack-year history of smoking but quit 20 years ago. He takes no medications.

On physical examination, he is alert, oriented, and in no acute distress. Temperature is 37.0 °C (98.6 °F), blood pressure is 115/75 mm Hg, pulse rate is 78/min, and respiration rate is 22/min; BMI is 26. No jugular venous distention is noted. Pulmonary examination discloses minimal crackles and reduced breath sounds at the lung bases. Cardiac examination is normal. There is no leg edema.

Pulmonary function tests reveal an FEV_1 of 75% of predicted, an FVC of 68% of predicted with no change after administration of a bronchodilator, a total lung capacity of 68% of predicted, and a residual volume of 125% of predicted. FEV_1/FVC ratio is 82%. Chest radiograph shows low lung volumes with suggested bibasilar atelectasis.

Which of the following is the most likely diagnosis?

(A) COPD
(B) Heart failure
(C) Interstitial lung disease
(D) Respiratory muscle weakness

Item 12

A 24-year-old man is evaluated for daytime sleepiness. He is a graduate student who reports falling asleep during lectures or when reading online textbooks. He nearly had a car accident while driving home recently after working the evening at the campus bookstore. He notes that he goes to bed later than 1:00 AM on some school nights and wakes up for 8:00 AM classes, and on some weekends he will sleep until nearly noon. He reports no symptoms of cataplexy or restless legs syndrome. He sleeps alone, so he is unsure if he snores. He occasionally drinks alcohol on weekends but does not use illicit drugs. He has a history of seasonal allergies, and his father has obstructive sleep apnea. He takes loratadine as needed.

On physical examination, vital signs are normal, and BMI is 23. Examination of the upper airway is unremarkable, disclosing patent nares and no visible tonsils.

Which of the following is the most appropriate next step in management?

(A) Electroencephalography
(B) Multiple sleep latency testing
(C) Polysomnography
(D) Sleep diary

Item 13

A 56-year-old man is evaluated in follow-up for COPD, which was diagnosed last week with spirometry; his FEV_1 is 58% of predicted. He has a morning cough productive of sputum and dyspnea with moderate exertion. He quit

smoking at the time of diagnosis. His only medication is a nicotine patch. He is started on a short-acting bronchodilator and is given appropriate vaccinations.

On physical examination, vital signs are normal. The lungs are clear to auscultation, but prolonged expiration is noted. The remainder of the physical examination is normal.

Which of the following is the most appropriate management?

(A) Budesonide inhaler
(B) Oral montelukast
(C) Oral prednisone
(D) Tiotropium inhaler

Item 14

A 46-year-old man is evaluated for a new pleural effusion. He recently returned from a long trip to Cambodia. Shortly after arriving home, he noted the onset of left-sided pleuritic chest pain. A few days later he developed a nonproductive cough and low-grade fever. His medical history is unremarkable.

On physical examination, he is currently afebrile. Lung auscultation reveals a pleural rub at the left mid-lateral lung field. Dullness and decreased breath sounds are noted at the left base. The remainder of the examination is unremarkable.

A chest radiograph reveals a moderate-sized left pleural effusion. Thoracentesis is performed.

Laboratory studies:

Serum lactate dehydrogenase	78 units/L
Serum total protein	7.2 g/dL (72 g/L)
Pleural fluid lactate dehydrogenase	100 units/L
Pleural fluid total protein	5.2 g/dL (52 g/L)
Pleural fluid total nucleated cells	7200/µL (7.2×10^9/L) (14% neutrophils, 72% lymphocytes, 12% monocytes, 2% eosinophils)

Which of the following pleural fluid tests is most likely to establish the diagnosis?

(A) Adenosine deaminase measurement
(B) Culture for acid-fast bacilli
(C) Gram stain
(D) Stain for acid-fast bacilli

Item 15

A 34-year-old man is evaluated in the hospital for a 3-day history of bilateral lower extremity weakness with subsequent onset of exertional dyspnea and upper extremity weakness. He also notes difficulty swallowing in the past 24 hours. He had a self-limited upper respiratory infection 10 days before admission, but his medical history is otherwise unremarkable.

On physical examination, he is awake, alert, and speaking in full sentences. Temperature is 37.0 °C (98.6 °F), blood pressure is 168/96 mm Hg, pulse rate is 88/min, and respiration rate is 18/min. The lungs are clear to auscultation with use of accessory muscles and decreased breath sounds at both lung bases. Diffuse symmetric weakness and hyporeflexia are noted in the extremities. He develops a weak cough after being given ice chips. A diagnosis of acute inflammatory demyelinating polyneuropathy is made, and he is transferred to the intensive care unit for closer monitoring of his respiratory status.

Oxygen saturation is 96% breathing ambient air. Chest radiograph shows low lung volumes but is otherwise normal. Bedside vital capacity is 2.1 L (50% of predicted).

Which of the following is the best management strategy to prevent respiratory failure in this patient?

(A) Bilateral transcutaneous phrenic nerve pacing
(B) Continuous positive airway pressure
(C) Methylprednisolone
(D) Plasma exchange

Item 16

A 78-year-old man is evaluated for a 3-month history of increasing dry cough and dyspnea. His medical history is significant for atrial fibrillation with episodes of rapid ventricular response and hemodynamic instability; the last episode occurred 4 months ago. He is a former smoker with a 25-pack-year history, and he quit smoking at age 55 years. His medications are metoprolol and warfarin, initiated 5 years ago, and amiodarone, initiated 4 months ago.

On physical examination, vital signs are normal; BMI is 28. Oxygen saturation is 94% breathing ambient air. There is no evidence of jugular venous distention, and cardiac examination is normal. Pulmonary examination reveals occasional scattered crackles.

FVC is 72% of predicted, FEV_1 is 75% of predicted, FEV_1/FVC ratio is 78%, total lung capacity is 65%, and D_{LCO} is 50% of predicted. A chest radiograph is normal.

Which of the following is the most appropriate next step in management?

(A) Enroll in pulmonary rehabilitation
(B) Perform bronchoscopy
(C) Perform high-resolution CT imaging
(D) Prescribe inhaled albuterol and ipratropium

Item 17

A 39-year-old man is admitted to the hospital for new-onset agitation, fluctuating level of consciousness, and tremors. He is diagnosed with acute alcoholic hepatitis.

On physical examination, temperature is 38.8 °C (101.8 °F), blood pressure is 95/55 mm Hg, pulse rate is 130/min, and respiration rate is 30/min. Jaundice is noted. The abdomen is protuberant with ascites but is soft, with no abdominal rigidity or guarding. There is no blood in the stool. The patient is agitated and disoriented, is unable to maintain attention, and appears to be having visual hallucinations. He believes that the nurse has stolen his wallet (which is in his bedside drawer) in order to obtain his identity. He is diaphoretic and tremulous. Asterixis is absent, and the remainder of the neurologic examination is normal.

Which of the following is the most appropriate management?

(A) Ceftriaxone
(B) CT of the head
(C) Haloperidol
(D) Lactulose enema
(E) Lorazepam

Item 18

A 62-year-old woman is admitted to the hospital for a 2-week history of progressive dyspnea. Her medical history is significant for heart failure with an ejection fraction of 25%. Her current medications are carvedilol, lisinopril, spironolactone, and furosemide.

On physical examination, temperature is 37.1 °C (98.8 °F), blood pressure is 80/48 mm Hg, pulse rate is 106/min, and respiration rate is 30/min. Oxygen saturation is 89% on 70% oxygen delivered by a nonrebreather mask. She is confused and periodically removes the oxygen mask. Pulmonary examination reveals bilateral inspiratory crackles. Heart sounds are regular with a grade 2/6 holosystolic murmur and an S_3 gallop at the apex.

Laboratory studies:

Hemoglobin	12 g/dL (120 g/L)
Leukocyte count	8200/µL (8.2×10^9/L)
Platelet count	250,000/µL (250×10^9/L)
Blood urea nitrogen	52 mg/dL (18.6 mmol/L)
Creatinine	2.8 mg/dL (248 µmol/L)
Lactic acid	38 mg/dL (4.2 mmol/L)
Arterial blood gas studies (on F_{IO_2} of 0.7):	
pH	7.48
P_{CO_2}	30 mm Hg (4.0 kPa)
P_{O_2}	58 mm Hg (7.7 kPa)

Chest radiograph shows bilateral perihilar infiltrates, cardiomegaly, and bilateral effusions.

Which of the following is the most appropriate next step in treatment?

(A) Endotracheal intubation and mechanical ventilation
(B) Nitroglycerin infusion
(C) Noninvasive positive pressure ventilation
(D) Placement of a pulmonary artery catheter

Item 19

A 21-year-old man is evaluated in the emergency department for shortness of breath after a bee sting. He feels lightheaded and describes a sense of puffiness in his face.

On physical examination, temperature is 38.0 °C (100.4 °F), blood pressure is 98/60 mm Hg, pulse rate is 100/min, and respiration rate is 24/min. He is agitated. Bilateral wheezing is noted. There is no stridor and no evidence of facial, tongue, or oropharyngeal swelling. There is no rash. Chest radiograph shows hyperinflation.

Which of the following is the most appropriate treatment?

(A) Endotracheal intubation and mechanical ventilation
(B) Intramuscular epinephrine and inhaled albuterol
(C) Intravenous diphenhydramine and methylprednisolone
(D) Intravenous epinephrine, methylprednisolone, and diphenhydramine

Item 20

A 45-year-old woman is evaluated for worsening asthma symptoms. She has a lifelong history of asthma, which had been under good control. However, her symptoms have become severe over the past few years, with persistent productive cough, dyspnea, and wheezing. The symptoms have not been well controlled despite the use of an inhaled short-acting β_2-agonist, a long-acting β_2-agonist in combination with inhaled corticosteroid therapy, and low-dose oral corticosteroids. She has extensive allergies but is otherwise healthy.

On physical examination, temperature is 37.0 °C (98.6 °F), blood pressure is 110/70 mm Hg, pulse rate is 74/min, and respiration rate is 18/min; BMI is 33. Pulmonary examination discloses scattered wheezing and rhonchi, particularly over the upper lung fields. Examination is otherwise unremarkable.

Laboratory studies reveal a leukocyte count of 9200/μL (9.2×10^9/L) with 50% neutrophils, 30% lymphocytes, 13% eosinophils, and 7% monocytes. Chest radiograph shows a patchy upper-lobe infiltrate with increased bronchial markings. Chest CT reveals proximal bronchiectasis with suggestion of mucus plugging.

Which of the following is the most appropriate diagnostic test to perform next?

(A) Allergy skin testing for *Aspergillus*
(B) Bronchoscopy with bronchoalveolar lavage and biopsy
(C) Sputum Gram stain and culture
(D) Sweat chloride testing

Item 21

A 58-year-old man is evaluated for a 3-month history of loud snoring and "gasping" during sleep. He also frequently falls asleep in a chair while reading in the evening. His medical history is otherwise unremarkable.

On physical examination, temperature is 37.4 °C (99.3 °F), blood pressure is 130/82 mm Hg, pulse rate is 80/min, and respiration rate is 14/min; BMI is 34. Neck circumference is 45.7 cm (18 in), and a low-lying soft palate is noted. Polysomnography discloses severe obstructive sleep apnea, with an apnea-hypopnea index of 42 per hour.

Which of the following is the most appropriate next step in treatment?

(A) Continuous positive airway pressure
(B) Nocturnal oxygen therapy
(C) Oral appliance
(D) Upper airway surgery

Item 22

A 30-year-old woman is evaluated for a 2-week history of progressive dyspnea on exertion. Three months ago, she was involved in a motor vehicle accident with severe musculoskeletal injuries requiring a 1-week stay in the surgical intensive care unit with intubation and mechanical ventilation. She had an uneventful recovery and was discharged home 2 weeks later. She has a 7.5-pack-year smoking history. Her medical history is otherwise significant only for mild intermittent asthma for which she is treated with a daily low-dose inhaled corticosteroid and an as-needed albuterol metered-dose inhaler.

On physical examination, temperature is 37.4 °C (99.3 °F), blood pressure is 115/75 mm Hg, pulse rate is 84/min, and respiration rate is 20/min; BMI is 30. Pulmonary examination reveals wheezing during inspiration and expiration.

Oxygen saturation breathing ambient air is 97%. Spirometry shows an FEV_1 of 40% of predicted and an FEV_1/FVC ratio of 65%. There is no significant improvement following inhaled albuterol.

Which of the following is the most appropriate next step in management?

(A) Initiate a 2-week taper of oral corticosteroids
(B) Obtain flow-volume loops
(C) Obtain lung volume measurements
(D) Refer for voice and speech therapy

Item 23

A 47-year-old man is evaluated for worsening of asthma symptoms characterized by frequent daytime wheezing and cough, as well as nocturnal awakening related to asthma two to three times per week. He has been using his inhalers regularly without adequate relief. He has not had recent upper respiratory tract infection, sinusitis, postnasal drip, or new exposures. He is taking an inhaled corticosteroid and inhaled albuterol.

On physical examination, temperature is 37.0 °C (98.6 °F), blood pressure is 135/80 mm Hg, pulse rate is 80/min, and respiration rate is 18/min. Pulmonary examination reveals scattered bilateral wheezing. Spirometry shows an FEV_1 of 70% of predicted. Following an inhaled bronchodilator, FEV_1 improves to 90% of predicted.

Which of the following is the most appropriate next step in management?

(A) Add a leukotriene receptor antagonist
(B) Add prednisone
(C) Observe the patient using his inhalers
(D) Obtain a 2-week symptom and peak flow diary

Item 24

A 28-year-old woman is evaluated for a 12-week history of worsening cough, shortness of breath, and low-grade fevers. She was evaluated for these symptoms 6 weeks ago and was treated with an oral fluoroquinolone antibiotic for a presumed respiratory tract infection, but her symptoms did not improve. She has not had any recent travel or animal exposures. She is employed as a sheet metal worker at an automobile manufacturing plant. Her medical history is otherwise unremarkable, she does not smoke cigarettes, and she takes no medications.

On physical examination, temperature is 37.0 °C (98.6 °F), blood pressure is 120/82 mm Hg, pulse rate is 65/min, and respiration rate is 14/min; BMI is 24. The lungs are clear to auscultation with no wheezing, and the cardiac examination is normal.

Chest radiograph shows diffuse bilateral hazy opacity without nodules, no evidence of pleural effusions, and no cardiomegaly. CT scan shows diffuse centrilobular ground-glass opacity but is otherwise normal.

Which of the following is the most appropriate next step in management?

(A) Obtain detailed history of current work exposures
(B) Perform allergy testing
(C) Perform bronchial challenge testing
(D) Repeat chest CT with intravenous contrast

Item 25

A 45-year-old woman is evaluated in the emergency department for the acute onset of dyspnea, wheezing, and progressive respiratory distress. She has a history of severe persistent asthma with two previous admissions to the intensive care unit, one of which required intubation. Her medications are a high-dose inhaled corticosteroid, salmeterol, and as-needed albuterol. She has not responded to aggressive bronchodilation therapy and intravenous corticosteroids.

On physical examination, she is in marked distress and is anxious. Temperature is 37.0 °C (98.6 °F), blood pressure is 145/100 mm Hg, pulse rate is 120/min, and respiration rate is 25/min; BMI is 35. Cardiac examination reveals a rapid and regular rhythm with no murmurs. Pulmonary examination reveals very faint wheezing.

Arterial blood gas studies breathing ambient air show a P_{CO_2} of 80 mm Hg (10.6 kPa), a P_{O_2} of 50 mm Hg (6.7 kPa), and a pH of 7.08. Chest radiograph shows hyperinflation but no infiltrates.

She undergoes rapid sequence induction and intubation and is started on mechanical ventilation.

Which of the following strategies in establishing ventilator settings is most appropriate for this patient?

(A) Decreased inspiratory flow
(B) Increased minute ventilation
(C) Prolonged expiratory time
(D) Prolonged inspiratory time

Item 26

A 64-year-old woman is evaluated in the emergency department for a 3-day history of weakness, fever, chills, dyspnea, and cough. She has no other medical problems and takes no medications.

On physical examination, she appears ill, and the skin of the extremities is warm. Temperature is 38.9 °C (102.0 °F), blood pressure is 105/50 mm Hg, pulse rate is 125/min, and respiration rate is 28/min. Oxygen saturation is 92% while breathing 100% oxygen via a nonrebreather mask. Pulmonary examination reveals right lower posterior chest egophony and dullness to percussion. Cardiac examination reveals a bounding pulse.

Laboratory studies reveal a hematocrit of 32%, a leukocyte count of 18,000/μL (18×10^9/L) with 80% segmented neutrophils, and a serum creatinine level of 1.8 mg/dL (159 μmol/L); electrolyte levels are normal. Chest radiograph shows right lower lobe consolidation.

Intravenous ceftriaxone and levofloxacin are initiated.

Which of the following is the most appropriate additional initial treatment?

(A) Hydrocortisone
(B) Norepinephrine
(C) Normal saline
(D) Packed red blood cell transfusion

Item 27

A 62-year-old man is evaluated in follow-up after a recent CT scan of the abdomen for kidney stones revealed a 3-mm left lower lobe lung nodule. He is a former smoker with a 35-pack-year history, but he quit smoking 10 years ago.

On physical examination, vital signs are normal. The physical examination is unremarkable.

Follow-up CT of the chest shows only the 3-mm left lower lobe nodule and is otherwise normal. There are no other chest images available for comparison.

Which of the following is the most appropriate next step in management?

(A) CT of the chest in 3 months
(B) CT of the chest in 6 months
(C) CT of the chest in 12 months
(D) No follow-up imaging

Item 28

A 19-year-old woman is evaluated in the emergency department after taking an overdose of medication in an apparent suicide attempt.

On physical examination, she is intubated and on mechanical ventilation. She is obtunded. Temperature is 37.9 °C (100.2 °F), blood pressure is 96/60 mm Hg, pulse rate is 92/min, and respiration rate on assisted mode of ventilation is 18/min.

The remainder of the physical examination is normal.

Laboratory studies reveal a plasma glucose level of 100 mg/dL (5.6 mmol/L). Qualitative urine toxicology screen reveals the presence of benzodiazepines and tricyclic antidepressants. No other toxins are identified in her serum or urine. Initial electrocardiogram in the emergency department shows sinus tachycardia with a QRS duration of 90 ms.

Electrocardiogram in the intensive care unit several hours later shows a QRS duration of 130 ms.

CONT.

In addition to isotonic saline and vasopressors, which of the following is the most appropriate next step in management?

(A) Naloxone
(B) Procainamide
(C) Saline diuresis
(D) Sodium bicarbonate infusion

Item 29

A 28-year-old woman is evaluated for asthma symptoms that have worsened since she became pregnant 2 months ago. She now has frequent daytime symptoms with increased nighttime awakening owing to asthma. She has used her albuterol inhaler several times per week to achieve symptomatic relief. She has a history of mild persistent asthma that was well controlled before her pregnancy on an as-needed short-acting β_2-agonist and medium-dose inhaled corticosteroids.

On physical examination, vital signs are normal. The lungs are clear. Cardiac examination discloses a normal S_1 and S_2 with no gallops or murmurs. No leg edema is noted.

Spirometry shows an FEV_1 of 85% of predicted and an FEV_1/FVC ratio of 78%. Laboratory studies reveal a hemoglobin level of 11.5 g/dL (115 g/L).

Which of the following is the most appropriate next step in management?

(A) Add a long-acting β_2-agonist
(B) Add theophylline
(C) Double the inhaled corticosteroid dose
(D) Obtain a bronchial challenge test

Item 30

A 52-year-old man is evaluated in follow-up after starting nasal continuous positive airway pressure (CPAP) 6 weeks ago for obstructive sleep apnea. He reports inability to wear the mask for more than 3 or 4 hours per night because of nasal congestion. He continues to have residual sleepiness during the day. His wife notes that he does not snore or have apnea when the mask is on.

On physical examination, temperature is 37.4 °C (99.3 °F), blood pressure is 122/74 mm Hg, pulse rate is 76/min, and respiration rate is 14/min; BMI is 26. The nasal mucosa is boggy and erythematous with a clear mucoid discharge.

Which of the following management steps is most likely to improve this patient's compliance with CPAP therapy?

(A) Add heated humidification to the CPAP circuit
(B) Initiate oral modafinil
(C) Initiate oxymetazoline nasal spray
(D) Refer for nasal septal surgery

Item 31

A 70-year-old man is evaluated for a 3-month history of night sweats, weight loss, and increasing cough. He is a retired miner, and his medical history is significant for a diagnosis of pulmonary silicosis made 15 years ago based on exposure history and characteristic chest radiographic findings. He is a lifelong nonsmoker.

On physical examination, temperature is 37.9 °C (100.2 °F), blood pressure is 120/65 mm Hg, pulse rate is 84/min, and respiration rate is 22/min. Pulmonary examination reveals diffuse inspiratory crackles throughout all lung zones, unchanged from previous examinations.

Pulmonary function tests demonstrate mild obstruction with no change from 1 year ago. Chest radiograph shows multiple small nodules that appear throughout all lung zones but are upper-lobe predominant. There is no significant change in comparison with previous imaging studies.

Which of the following is the most appropriate next step in management?

(A) High-resolution CT of the chest
(B) Lung biopsy
(C) Prednisone
(D) Tuberculosis testing

Item 32

A 72-year-old woman is evaluated in follow-up for a 4-day history of a COPD exacerbation. She has severe COPD without resting hypoxemia and presented 1 week ago with fever, productive cough with green sputum, and mild dyspnea over her baseline. In addition to her current medications, her albuterol inhaler was increased to six times daily, and a β-lactam/β-lactamase inhibitor and a corticosteroid taper were started with scheduled follow-up today. She is still fatigued and dyspneic relative to baseline. Her medical history is notable for coronary artery disease and type 2 diabetes mellitus. Her baseline medications are tiotropium, fluticasone/salmeterol, albuterol, metformin, lisinopril, atorvastatin, and aspirin.

On physical examination, temperature is 37.8 °C (100.0 °F), blood pressure is 130/85 mm Hg, pulse rate is 95/min and regular, and respiration rate is 36/min. She is dyspneic at rest. Pulmonary examination discloses bilateral expiratory wheezing but no crackles. Oxygen saturation is 86% breathing ambient air and 92% on 2 L oxygen via nasal cannula.

Chest radiograph shows no infiltrate and no cardiomegaly.

Which of the following is the most appropriate next step in management?

(A) Add home oxygen
(B) Admit to the hospital
(C) Expand antibiotic spectrum
(D) Prolong corticosteroid taper

Item 33

A 19-year-old man is evaluated during a routine examination. He has a history of episodes of bronchitis since early childhood; symptoms include productive cough, wheezing, and shortness of breath. He is being treated for asthma, but his symptoms have not been well controlled. His current medications are a medium-dose inhaled corticosteroid and a long-acting β_2-agonist, with documented satisfactory inhaler technique.

On physical examination, temperature is 37.2 °C (99.0 °F), blood pressure is 110/65 mm Hg, pulse rate is 82/min, and respiration rate is 18/min; BMI is 20. Small nasal polyps are noted. Pulmonary examination reveals diffuse rhonchi and scattered wheezing. The neck veins are flat. Cardiac examination reveals a normal S_1 and S_2 with a soft grade 1/6 systolic murmur. Clubbing is noted. There is no pedal edema, and pulses are intact and symmetric. Oxygen saturation breathing ambient air is 93%.

Laboratory studies reveal a hemoglobin level of 11 g/dL (110 g/L) and a leukocyte count of 9800/µL (9.8 × 10^9/L). Chest radiograph shows increased bronchial markings consistent with bronchiectasis in the upper lung zones.

Which of the following is the most appropriate next step in management?

(A) Measure sweat chloride
(B) Perform bronchoscopy
(C) Perform echocardiography
(D) Record symptoms and medication use over 2 weeks

Item 34

A 66-year-old woman is evaluated for a 4-month history of nonproductive cough and exertional shortness of breath. Her medical history is notable for hypertension and gastroesophageal reflux disease. She is a former smoker with a 24-pack-year history, but she quit 22 years ago. There is no family history of lung problems. Her medications are atenolol and omeprazole.

On physical examination, temperature is 37.0 °C (98.6 °F), blood pressure is 136/86 mm Hg, pulse rate is 90/min, and respiration rate is 18/min; BMI is 28. Cardiac examination reveals normal heart sounds. Bilateral basilar crackles are noted on lung auscultation. Skin and joint examination findings are normal.

Laboratory studies, including a complete blood count, creatinine level, and urinalysis, are normal. Electrocardiogram is normal. Pulmonary function testing shows a mild reduction in lung volumes (mild restriction) and DLCO. Chest radiograph shows bibasilar interstitial opacities that were not present on an image obtained 5 years ago.

Additional radiographic study is recommended to further characterize the lung opacities, although the patient expresses concern regarding potential radiation exposure associated with imaging.

Given this patient's clinical status and concerns, which of the following is the most appropriate diagnostic study to recommend?

(A) Chest MRI
(B) High-resolution chest CT

(C) PET
(D) Ventilation/perfusion scan

Item 35

A 35-year-old woman is evaluated in an urgent care center for an acute exacerbation of asthma. She has a history of frequent asthma exacerbations requiring unscheduled visits; however, between these exacerbations, her examination and pulmonary function studies have been unremarkable. Her current medications are inhaled budesonide and inhaled albuterol.

On physical examination, she is in moderate distress with audible inspiratory and expiratory wheezing. Temperature is 37.0 °C (98.6 °F), pulse rate is 110/min, and respiration rate is 26/min. Monophonic inspiratory and expiratory wheezing is heard predominantly in the central lung fields. Other than tachycardia, the cardiac examination and remainder of the physical examination are normal.

She receives intravenous methylprednisolone and three nebulized albuterol-ipratropium bromide treatments. On follow-up evaluation 1 hour later, she still has wheezing, tachycardia, and tachypnea and is in moderate respiratory distress. Oxygen saturation is 96% breathing ambient air.

Which of the following is the most appropriate next step in management?

(A) Chest radiograph
(B) Intravenous magnesium sulfate
(C) Laryngoscopy
(D) Levofloxacin

Item 36

A 32-year-old woman is evaluated in the hospital for a 24-hour history of gradually worsening somnolence and hypoxemia. She underwent cholecystectomy 3 days ago. She has no other medical problems and takes no medications as an outpatient. She is receiving scheduled intravenous hydromorphone for pain management in the hospital.

On physical examination, she is able to open her eyes and move all extremities with painful stimuli, but she is not following commands. Temperature is 35.6 °C (96.1 °F), blood pressure is 94/50 mm Hg, pulse rate is 62/min, and respiration rate is 8/min. The pupils are pinpoint and minimally reactive. The chest is clear to auscultation, with decreased breath sounds at the lung bases bilaterally and no accessory muscle use. Deep tendon reflexes are normal and symmetric with plantar flexor response. There is no change in the examination after receiving naloxone.

Glucose level by fingerstick is 90 mg/dL (5.0 mmol/L). Oxygen saturation is 91% on 3 L/min of oxygen by nasal cannula. Arterial blood gas studies and a chest radiograph are pending.

Which of the following is the most appropriate next step in managing this patient's encephalopathy?

(A) Administration of naloxone at a higher dose
(B) Endotracheal intubation and mechanical ventilation
(C) Intravenous glucose
(D) Noncontrast CT of the head

Item 37

A 45-year-old man is evaluated in follow-up 16 weeks after an acute pulmonary embolism that was documented by CT angiography. Venous Doppler ultrasonography of the legs at that time showed no evidence of deep venous thrombosis. His anticoagulation initially consisted of low-molecular-weight heparin plus warfarin and then was continued with warfarin alone. His INR values were consistently between 2.5 and 3.0 until warfarin was discontinued 1 month ago. He feels well and is back working as a long-haul truck driver. He now takes no medications.

On physical examination, temperature is 36.8 °C (98.2 °F), blood pressure is 132/82 mm Hg, pulse rate is 82/min, and respiration rate is 16/min; BMI is 31. Cardiopulmonary examination is normal. No tenderness or swelling is seen in the legs.

Laboratory studies:

D-dimer	700 µg/mL (700 mg/L)
Hemoglobin	14 g/dL (140 g/L)
INR	1.1
Platelet count	160,000/µL (160 × 10⁹/L)

Which of the following is the most appropriate next step in management?

(A) Measure B-type natriuretic peptide
(B) Perform venous Doppler ultrasonography of the legs
(C) Repeat D-dimer study in 1 month
(D) Restart anticoagulation

Item 38

A 55-year-old woman is evaluated for a recent increase in asthma symptoms characterized by daily cough and dyspnea. She reports waking up two to three nights per week with asthma symptoms. She has no postnasal drip, nasal discharge, fever, or heartburn. Her current medications are medium-dose inhaled corticosteroids and albuterol as needed. She is able to demonstrate proper use of her metered-dose inhalers.

On physical examination, she appears comfortable and is in no respiratory distress. Pulse rate is 76/min, and respiration rate is 18/min. Pulmonary examination reveals bilateral wheezing. The remainder of the examination is normal.

Which of the following is the most appropriate treatment?

(A) Add a long-acting β_2-agonist inhaler
(B) Add an ipratropium metered-dose inhaler
(C) Double the dose of inhaled corticosteroids
(D) Start a 10-day course of a macrolide antibiotic

Item 39

A 78-year-old man was hospitalized 1 week ago for acute worsening of shortness of breath related to idiopathic pulmonary fibrosis (IPF), which was diagnosed 4 years ago. He has had a steady decline in pulmonary function since his diagnosis. He began to have significant worsening 6 weeks ago. Upon hospitalization he underwent extensive evaluation including CT scan, echocardiography, and bronchoscopy. There was no evidence of pulmonary embolism, heart failure, or infection. He was diagnosed with an acute exacerbation of IPF and was treated with high-dose intravenous methylprednisolone. His symptoms have steadily worsened on this therapy since his hospitalization, with more tachypnea and severe shortness of breath.

On physical examination, he appears acutely ill. Temperature is 37.2 °C (99.0 °F), blood pressure is 160/90 mm Hg, pulse rate is 135/min, and respiration rate is 34/min. No jugular venous distention is noted. Pulmonary examination reveals diffuse inspiratory crackles without wheezing or rhonchi. There is evidence of accessory muscle use. Cardiac examination reveals tachycardia with a normal S_1 and S_2 and no murmurs, rubs, or gallops. There is no lower extremity edema.

A sputum culture is negative.

Which of the following is the most appropriate treatment?

(A) Add antifungal therapy
(B) Initiate additional pulse-dose methylprednisolone
(C) Initiate continuous nebulized albuterol
(D) Initiate palliation with narcotics

Item 40

A 50-year-old man is evaluated in the hospital for low oxygen saturation 3 hours after undergoing bariatric surgery for morbid obesity. Oxygen saturation is 82% on 2 L/min of continuous oxygen by nasal cannula. His oxygen saturation improves to 89% on 10 L/min of oxygen delivered by a nonrebreather mask. He does not have dyspnea or chest pain. His operative course was uneventful.

On physical examination, he is alert. Temperature is 37.1 °C (98.8 °F), blood pressure is 168/98 mm Hg, pulse rate is 86/min, and respiration rate is 30/min; BMI is 42. Pulmonary examination reveals decreased breath sounds at the bases but is otherwise normal. The cardiac examination is normal. There is an intact, fresh abdominal surgical incision.

Arterial blood gas studies on 10 L/min of oxygen by nonrebreather mask reveal a pH of 7.44, a P_{CO_2} of 35 mm Hg (4.7 kPa), and a P_{O_2} of 60 mm Hg (8.0 kPa). Chest radiograph shows low lung volumes and linear bibasilar opacities.

Which of the following is the most appropriate next step in managing this patient's hypoxemia?

(A) Bronchoscopy
(B) Continuous nebulized albuterol
(C) Continuous positive airway pressure
(D) Naloxone

Item 41

A 62-year-old man is evaluated during a routine examination in October. He was recently diagnosed with COPD. His COPD is controlled with tiotropium and albuterol as needed. He receives an influenza vaccination every year. He has never received the pneumococcal vaccination, but all other immunizations are up-to-date.

On physical examination, vital signs are normal. The lungs are clear to auscultation.

Which of the following is the best influenza and pneumococcal immunization regimen for this patient?

(A) Influenza vaccine now
(B) Influenza and pneumococcal vaccines now
(C) Influenza vaccine now and pneumococcal vaccine at the next routine visit
(D) Influenza vaccine now and pneumococcal vaccine at age 65 years

Item 42

A 58-year-old woman is evaluated in the emergency department for an 8-hour history of worsening dyspnea and chest tightness. Her medical history is notable for hypertension, heart failure with an ejection fraction of 35% on echocardiography, and COPD with a baseline FEV_1 of 45% of predicted. Her current medications are lisinopril, metoprolol, furosemide, a budesonide/formoterol inhaler, and as-needed albuterol.

On physical examination, she appears anxious and is in moderate respiratory distress. Temperature is 38.0 °C (100.4 °F), blood pressure is 106/52 mm Hg, pulse rate is 110/min, and respiration rate is 22/min. Oxygen saturation is 90% breathing 6 L of oxygen by nasal cannula. There are bilateral end-expiratory wheezes, and there are no inspiratory crackles. Heart sounds are distant. There is trace bilateral lower extremity edema.

Electrolytes, kidney function tests, and complete blood count are normal. An electrocardiogram shows sinus tachycardia but no ischemic changes. A chest radiograph demonstrates hyperinflation and cardiomegaly but no effusions or infiltrate.

Her dyspnea and oxygen saturation do not improve after receiving two doses of nebulized ipratropium and albuterol.

Which of the following is the most appropriate next step in management?

(A) Administer aminophylline
(B) Obtain CT angiogram of the chest
(C) Obtain echocardiogram
(D) Start levofloxacin

Item 43

A 62-year-old man is evaluated in the emergency department for headache and confusion. He does not have chest pain or discomfort. His medical history is significant for essential hypertension, transient ischemic attack, type 2 diabetes mellitus (controlled by diet), and high cholesterol. His current medications are hydrochlorothiazide, amlodipine, aspirin, and atorvastatin.

On physical examination, temperature is normal, blood pressure is 220/135 mm Hg (same in both arms), pulse

rate is 88/min, and respiration rate is 20/min; BMI is 31. He is intermittently lethargic and agitated, and he is oriented to self and place but not date and time. Funduscopic examination cannot be performed owing to agitation. There is no focal weakness or loss of sensation, the cranial nerves are intact, and the gait is slow but otherwise normal. The lungs are clear. Pedal edema is noted.

Electrolytes, complete blood count, cardiac troponin level, and urinalysis are normal. Chest radiograph is normal. CT of the head shows evidence of an old lacunar infarction but no signs of acute stroke or bleeding.

Which of the following is the most appropriate initial target blood pressure for this patient?

(A) 130/80 mm Hg
(B) 140/90 mm Hg
(C) 185/110 mm Hg
(D) 200/120 mm Hg

Item 44

An 18-year-old man is evaluated for cough, chest tightness, and wheezing that occur after sprints that he runs for his school track team, particularly on cold days. Symptoms resolve after a few minutes of rest. He has no other daytime or nighttime symptoms. He has a history of hay fever with worsening of rhinitis symptoms during the fall and spring, but he is otherwise healthy. Several family members have allergies and/or asthma.

On physical examination, pulse rate is 70/min, respiration rate is 14/min, and BMI is 25. Lung examination findings are normal.

Spirometry shows an FEV_1 of 95% of predicted, and the FEV_1/FVC ratio is 85%. FEV_1 measured after intense exercise is 76% of predicted.

Which of the following is the most appropriate treatment?

(A) Avoidance of physical activity known to cause symptoms
(B) Inhaled short-acting β_2-agonist 15 minutes before exercise
(C) Low-dose inhaled corticosteroids
(D) Physical conditioning program

Item 45

A 35-year-old woman is evaluated for a 4-year history of increasing dyspnea on exertion with dry cough but no fever. Her medical history is significant for a spontaneous pneumothorax 3 years ago. She does not smoke.

On physical examination, temperature and blood pressure are normal, pulse rate is 105/min, and respiration rate is 22/min. Pulmonary examination reveals occasional scattered crackles bilaterally in all lung fields. Other than tachycardia, the cardiac examination is normal.

Laboratory studies reveal a normal complete blood count, normal comprehensive metabolic panel, and normal thyroid function studies. High-resolution CT of the chest is shown.

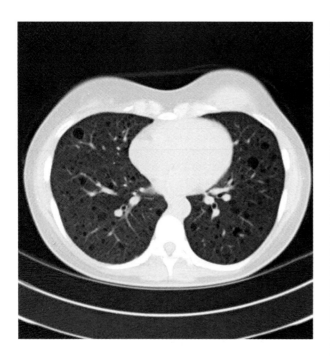

Which of the following is the most likely diagnosis?

(A) Lymphangioleiomyomatosis
(B) Organizing pneumonia
(C) Respiratory bronchiolitis–associated interstitial lung disease
(D) Sarcoidosis

 Item 46

A 62-year-old woman is admitted to the hospital for a 4-hour history of moderate dyspnea and right-sided pleuritic chest pain following an extended automobile trip. Her medical history is significant for long-standing type 2 diabetes mellitus for which she takes glipizide. She had transient hypotension on initial presentation that was corrected with a 500-mL bolus of normal saline.

On physical examination, she appears alert but anxious. Temperature is 37.8 °C (100.0 °F), blood pressure is 118/70 mm Hg, pulse rate is 108/min and regular, and respiration rate is 22/min. Oxygen saturation is 82% on ambient air and improves to 94% on 5 L/min of oxygen by nasal prongs. Pulmonary examination reveals no focal findings. Cardiac examination discloses sinus tachycardia with a prominent S_2; there are no murmurs or rubs.

Laboratory studies reveal a serum creatinine level of 2.5 mg/dL (221 μmol/L) and a B-type natriuretic peptide level of 500 pg/mL. CT angiography shows multiple bilateral segmental filling defects. An echocardiogram shows normal left and right ventricular systolic function with right ventricular dilatation; mean pulmonary artery pressure is estimated to be 20 mm Hg.

Which of the following is the most appropriate next step in management?

(A) Alteplase
(B) Low-molecular-weight heparin

(C) Thrombus extraction
(D) Unfractionated heparin

Item 47

A 64-year-old woman is evaluated in the intensive care unit after receiving invasive mechanical ventilation for the past 6 days. She has acute respiratory distress syndrome, which was precipitated by multiple fractures sustained in a motor vehicle collision. Ventilator weaning trials are limited by tachypnea and hypoxemia. Her medications are fentanyl infusion, propofol infusion, subcutaneous heparin, and ranitidine.

On physical examination during full ventilator support, she is lightly sedated and in no respiratory distress. Temperature is 37.0 °C (98.6 °F), blood pressure is 148/77 mm Hg, pulse rate is 78/min, and respiration rate is 18/min. Weight is 92.0 kg (202.8 lb), up 6.0 kg (13.2 lb) since admission. Pulmonary examination is notable for decreased breath sounds at the bases. Cardiac examination reveals a regular rhythm with no gallop. There is trace edema of the extremities.

Laboratory studies reveal a normal creatinine level. Central venous pressure is 12 cm H_2O. Oxygen saturation is 96% on an FIO_2 of 0.45 and positive end-expiratory pressure of 5 cm H_2O. Chest radiograph shows small bilateral pleural effusions but is otherwise unremarkable.

Which of the following interventions will most likely reduce the duration of this patient's mechanical ventilation?

(A) Administer cisatracurium for 48 hours
(B) Initiate scheduled doses of furosemide
(C) Place the patient in the prone position
(D) Treat with continuous inhaled nitric oxide

Item 48

A 45-year-old woman is admitted to the intensive care unit after a motor vehicle accident in which she sustained significant burns to 70% of her body. She is intubated and sedated.

On physical examination, temperature is 37.9 °C (100.2 °F), blood pressure is 145/85 mm Hg, and her ventilated respiration rate is 15/min. She has extensive burns involving nearly all of the face, neck, and trunk, with notable extravasation of tissue fluid through her dressings.

Which of the following is the most desirable approach to nutritional support in this patient?

(A) Enteral nutrition via nasogastric feeding tube
(B) Enteral nutrition via percutaneous jejunal feeding tube
(C) Parenteral nutrition via central access
(D) Parenteral nutrition via peripheral access

Item 49

A 75-year-old man is evaluated for a 12-month history of cough and dyspnea. He reports no other symptoms or medical problems and takes no medications. He is a former smoker with a 40-pack-year history, and he is a retired carpenter. He has no pets and no known environmental exposures other than wood dust.

On physical examination, blood pressure is 135/75 mm Hg, pulse rate is 88/min, and respiration rate is 24/min. Oxygen saturation is 88% breathing ambient air. There is no jugular venous distention. Cardiac examination is normal. Pulmonary examination discloses inspiratory crackles at the lung bases bilaterally. Digital clubbing is present.

Pulmonary function testing discloses a decreased FEV_1, decreased FVC, normal FEV_1/FVC ratio, and decreased DLCO. Chest CT scan is shown.

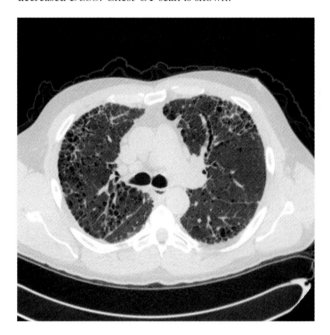

Which of the following is the most likely diagnosis?

(A) COPD
(B) Heart failure
(C) Hypersensitivity pneumonitis
(D) Idiopathic pulmonary fibrosis

Item 50

A 45-year-old man is evaluated for a 6-month history of increasing daily cough, sputum production, and dyspnea on exertion. He has been employed as a coal miner for 10 years. He has never smoked and does not have a history of diabetes mellitus, hypertension, or hyperlipidemia. His family history is negative for cardiopulmonary disease.

On physical examination, vital signs are normal. Pulmonary examination reveals mildly decreased breath sounds bilaterally with no wheezes, crackles, or rhonchi. Cardiac examination is normal.

A chest radiograph is normal.

Which of the following is the most appropriate next step in management?

(A) Annual chest radiography
(B) High-resolution CT of the chest

(C) PET chest imaging
(D) Pulmonary function studies

Item 51

A 25-year-old woman is evaluated in the emergency department for a 3-day history of sinus congestion, yellow nasal discharge, and progressively worsening cough, wheezing, and dyspnea despite using 16 puffs of her albuterol inhaler in the past 24 hours. She has a history of asthma and has not been taking her fluticasone/salmeterol inhaler since losing her insurance coverage 2 months ago. She received two doses of albuterol, 2.5 mg by nebulizer, in the ambulance on the way to the emergency department.

On physical examination, she is alert, appears anxious, and can speak only one word at a time. Temperature is 38.0 °C (100.4 °F), blood pressure is 98/62 mm Hg, pulse rate is 132/min, and respiration rate is 32/min. Pulmonary examination reveals markedly reduced breath sounds with minimal expiratory wheezes bilaterally. She is using neck and abdominal accessory muscles to breathe.

Arterial blood gas studies on 2 L of oxygen by nasal cannula reveal a pH of 7.34, a PCO_2 of 47 mm Hg (6.3 kPa), and a PO_2 of 62 mm Hg (8.2 kPa). Oxygen saturation is 92%.

Which of the following is the most appropriate next step in management?

(A) Continuous nebulized β_2-agonist
(B) Endotracheal intubation
(C) Intravenous methylprednisolone
(D) Lorazepam

Item 52

A 32-year-old woman is evaluated during a routine examination. She asks about preventing "altitude sickness" for an upcoming business and ski trip at an elevation of 3100 meters (10,171 feet). When she attended the same conference last year, she experienced 2 days and nights of exertional dyspnea, headache, fatigue, and repeated awakenings from sleep. The symptoms were severe enough that she did not feel up to skiing the first 2 days. Symptoms improved by day 4 of the trip. Her medical history is unremarkable.

On physical examination, temperature is 37.6 °C (99.7 °F), blood pressure is 126/74 mm Hg, pulse rate is 82/min, and respiration rate is 16/min; BMI is 27. Cardiac and pulmonary examinations are unremarkable. Pulse oximetry on ambient air reveals an oxygen saturation of 97%.

Which of the following is the most appropriate treatment to prevent recurrence of symptoms when this patient returns to altitude?

(A) Acetazolamide
(B) Dexamethasone
(C) Furosemide
(D) Zolpidem

Item 53

A 66-year-old woman is admitted to the hospital after falling at home and dislocating her artificial hip. The next day she becomes acutely short of breath and is transferred to the intensive care unit. She is diagnosed with acute pulmonary embolism and a heparin infusion is started. Her pain is managed with a patient-controlled intravenous analgesia pump. She undergoes closed reduction of her dislocated hip the following day, with temporary interruption of her anticoagulation. The day after her hip reduction, she is more comfortable and her pain medication requirements are lower. On day five, however, she becomes agitated and fearful, alternating with periods of inattention and somnolence.

On physical examination, vital signs are normal. She is awake but lethargic. It is difficult to obtain a history because of her inattentiveness. The cardiopulmonary examination is normal. There are no focal deficits on the neurologic examination. Results of arterial blood gas analysis are normal.

Which of the following is the most likely diagnosis?

(A) Acute hemorrhagic stroke
(B) Acute respiratory failure
(C) Delirium
(D) Opioid withdrawal
(E) Recurrent thromboembolism

Item 54

A 24-year-old woman is evaluated for increasing asthma symptoms. Her symptoms now require her to use her as-needed albuterol inhaler two to three times per week, and she has been waking up at night at least once a week with asthma symptoms that require her inhaler. She is still able to perform most of her daily activities, including regular exercise, if she uses albuterol for prevention. She is allergic to house dust mites, ragweed, grass, trees, and cats.

On physical examination, vital signs are normal. Pulmonary examination is normal with no wheezing. Spirometry shows an FEV_1 of 85% of predicted and an FEV_1/FVC ratio of 80% of predicted.

Which of the following is the most appropriate treatment?

(A) Add a long-acting β_2-agonist
(B) Add a long-acting β_2-agonist and a low-dose inhaled corticosteroid
(C) Add a low-dose inhaled corticosteroid
(D) Advise scheduled use of albuterol
(E) Refer for allergen immunotherapy

Item 55

A 33-year-old woman is evaluated for a 2-year history of progressive dyspnea on exertion accompanied by weakness and fatigue. There is no seasonal variation to her symptoms. She reports difficulty falling asleep but has no history of nocturnal awakening, snoring, or daytime somnolence. She does not have dizziness or syncope. Her medical history is otherwise normal, and she takes no medications.

On physical examination, temperature is 37.0 °C (98.6 °F), blood pressure 115/75 mm Hg, pulse rate is 108/min and regular, and respiration rate is 18/min at rest; BMI is 23. The neck veins are distended. Cardiac examination shows regular tachycardia and a prominent pulmonic component of S_2. The lungs are clear. There is edema of the legs bilaterally. There are no rashes, the joints appear normal, and there is no clubbing of the digits.

Laboratory studies, including a complete blood count, serum chemistries, and thyroid and coagulation studies, are normal. HIV testing is seronegative. Antinuclear antibody, rheumatoid factor, and ANCA studies are negative. Chest radiograph reveals prominent central pulmonary arteries, clear lungs, and normal heart size. Pulmonary function tests reveal a mildly decreased D_{LCO} without evidence of airway obstruction or decreased lung volumes. Electrocardiogram shows right axis deviation. Transthoracic echocardiogram shows normal left ventricular size and function, a dilated right ventricle, and an estimated right ventricular systolic pressure of 40 mm Hg. Ventilation/perfusion scan is normal.

Which of the following is the most appropriate diagnostic test to perform next?

(A) High-resolution chest CT scan
(B) Pulmonary angiography
(C) Right heart catheterization
(D) Sleep study
(E) Transesophageal echocardiography

Item 56

A 38-year-old woman is evaluated in follow-up for an abnormal chest radiograph, which was obtained during an emergency department visit for suspected pneumonia. She recovered from her acute respiratory symptoms and now feels well. She has been in excellent health and reports no current problems. She does note mild exertional dyspnea, but she does not think this is out of proportion for her level of conditioning.

On physical examination, vital signs are normal. No cervical, axillary, or inguinal lymphadenopathy is noted. Neurologic examination is normal.

The chest radiograph shows an abnormality at the right base. CT of the chest shows a 4-cm posterior mediastinal mass lateral to the midline that accounts for the abnormal findings on the chest radiograph.

Which of the following is the most likely tissue of origin of this tumor?

(A) Lymph
(B) Neural
(C) Thymus
(D) Thyroid

Item 57

A 62-year-old woman is evaluated in the emergency department for a 2-day history of increased dyspnea. She has advanced COPD, with an FEV_1 of 45% of predicted. She has a long-standing history of heavy smoking and continues to smoke one to two packs of cigarettes per day. Her current medications are tiotropium and as-needed albuterol.

On physical examination, she is difficult to arouse. Temperature is 37.0 °C (98.6 °F), blood pressure is 145/90 mm Hg, pulse rate is 95/min, and respiration rate is 25/min; BMI is 30. Pulmonary examination discloses prolonged expiration and wheezing. Bilateral pitting leg edema is noted. Oxygen saturation by pulse oximetry is 93%.

Which of the following is the most appropriate diagnostic test to perform next?

(A) Arterial blood gas studies
(B) Chest CT scan
(C) Complete blood count
(D) Echocardiography

Item 58

A 72-year-old man is evaluated for dyspnea at rest. He has end-stage COPD and is on a home hospice program. He has weight loss, reduced functional capacity, and muscle atrophy. His medications are ipratropium, salmeterol, fluticasone, albuterol as needed, and prednisone. He is uncomfortable, with chronic air hunger that has gradually increased over the past 2 weeks. Otherwise, his symptoms have been stable without change in cough, sputum production, or fever.

On physical examination, temperature is 37.0 °C (98.6 °F), blood pressure is 110/84 mm Hg, pulse rate is 102/min, and respiration rate is 30/min; BMI is 17. Breath sounds are decreased. Oxygen saturation on 2 L of oxygen via nasal cannula is 92%. Hematocrit is 36%.

Which of the following is the most appropriate management?

(A) Administer a blood transfusion
(B) Administer diazepam
(C) Administer morphine sulfate
(D) Increase oxygen flow

Item 59

A 52-year-old woman is evaluated in the emergency department for a 48-hour history of progressive dyspnea and weakness. Her oxygen saturation is 93% breathing ambient air and improves to 97% on 3 L/min of oxygen delivered by nasal cannula. Her medical history is significant for myasthenia gravis and alcohol dependence. Her baseline medication is pyridostigmine bromide, which she last took 2 weeks ago.

On physical examination, temperature is 37.0 °C (98.6 °F), blood pressure is 138/76 mm Hg, pulse rate is 102/min, and respiration rate is 25/min. Her weight is 68.0 kg (149.9 lb) and BMI is 22. She has clear speech and mild dysphagia but no pooling of oral secretions. Pulmonary examination reveals decreased breath sounds at the bases, accessory use of neck muscles, and paradoxical abdominal wall motion with inspiration.

She is admitted to the intensive care unit, and treatment of her myasthenia is restarted along with supplemental oxygen and supportive measures.

Which of the following serial tests is the most appropriate for assessing this patient's risk for respiratory failure?

(A) Arterial blood gas studies
(B) Bedside vital capacity
(C) Chest radiograph
(D) Rapid shallow breathing index

Item 60

A 73-year-old man is evaluated for a 14-month history of cough and increasing dyspnea on exertion. Although he is able to perform most daily activities, he becomes breathless with moderate exertion, and this has become gradually more apparent over the past several years. He reports no chest pain or other symptoms. His medical history is unremarkable and he takes no medications. He has been retired for 15 years after working as a ship builder in the Navy for 20 years. He has never smoked cigarettes.

On physical examination, temperature and blood pressure are normal, pulse rate is 95/min, and respiration rate is 22/min. Oxygen saturation is 93% breathing ambient air. There is no jugular venous distention. Pulmonary examination reveals mild inspiratory crackles at the bases. Cardiac examination is normal, and there is no peripheral edema.

A plain radiograph of the chest shows increased interstitial markings primarily at the bases, with thickened pleura and calcified pleural plaques.

Which of the following is the most likely cause of this patient's symptoms?

(A) Asbestosis
(B) Heart failure
(C) Hypersensitivity pneumonitis
(D) Idiopathic pulmonary fibrosis

Item 61

A 56-year-old man is evaluated in the emergency department for a 3-day history of increasing dyspnea, fever, and cough with purulent sputum. He has severe COPD with a history of exacerbations requiring hospitalization. He quit smoking 3 years ago. His medications are ipratropium, salmeterol, inhaled beclomethasone, and albuterol as needed.

On physical examination, temperature is 38.0 °C (100.4 °F), blood pressure is 134/84 mm Hg, pulse rate is 88/min, and respiration rate is 30/min; BMI is 23. He is awake and alert. He is dyspneic at rest and is using accessory muscles to breathe. Pulmonary examination reveals bilateral expiratory wheezes but no crackles. There is no edema.

Arterial blood gas studies breathing 2 L of oxygen via nasal cannula reveal a pH of 7.31, a P_{CO_2} of 53 mm Hg (7.0 kPa), and a P_{O_2} of 55 mm Hg (7.3 kPa). Oxygen saturation is 89%. Chest radiograph shows hyperinflation but no infiltrates.

In addition to antibiotics, corticosteroids, and bronchodilators, which of the following is the most appropriate management?

(A) Continuous positive airway pressure
(B) Increase in nasal oxygen

CONT.

(C) Intubation and mechanical ventilation

(D) Noninvasive positive pressure ventilation

Item 62

A 50-year-old man is evaluated for cough and hemoptysis. He has lost 6.8 kg (15.0 lb) over the past 6 months. He is a current smoker with a 25-pack-year history. His medical history is unremarkable.

On physical examination, temperature is 37.2 °C (99.0 °F), blood pressure is 128/80 mm Hg, pulse rate is 72/min, and respiration rate is 16/min; BMI is 24. Pulmonary examination reveals reduced breath sounds in the right lower lung field. Abdominal examination is normal. Clubbing is noted. There is no cervical, axillary, or inguinal lymphadenopathy.

Laboratory studies are normal except for a serum calcium level of 10.9 mg/dL (2.7 mmol/L). Sputum cytology is positive for squamous cell carcinoma. Chest radiograph shows a right hilar mass and collapse of the right lower lobe. CT shows a mass obstructing the right lower lobe bronchus. PET-CT images are shown.

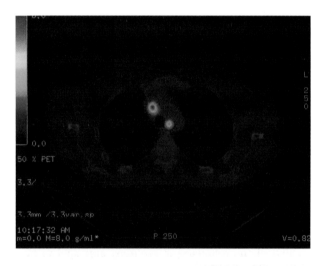

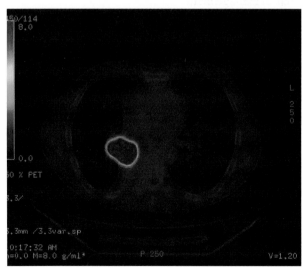

Which of the following is the most appropriate next step in management?

(A) Chemotherapy

(B) CT-guided needle biopsy of the mass

(C) Mediastinal lymph node sampling

(D) Surgical resection of the primary lesion

Item 63

A 72-year-old man is evaluated in follow-up after his first COPD exacerbation. He has moderate COPD. Prednisone was tapered and stopped 1 week ago. He is afebrile and his cough has decreased. He still has dyspnea despite adherence to his treatment regimen. He stopped smoking 6 months ago. His medications are enalapril, tiotropium, a salmeterol dry powder inhaler, and an albuterol metered-dose inhaler as needed. He is using albuterol up to six times daily.

On physical examination, vital signs are normal. Pulmonary examination discloses occasional expiratory wheezes. Oxygen saturation is 94% breathing ambient air.

Which of the following is the most appropriate next step in management?

(A) Add fluticasone inhaler

(B) Add oxygen therapy

(C) Check inhaler technique

(D) Restart prednisone

Item 64

A 62-year-old man is evaluated for a 3-week history of increasingly severe dyspnea and dry cough. He has idiopathic pulmonary fibrosis (IPF) that was diagnosed 3 years ago, and he normally uses 2 L/min of supplemental oxygen. He has no other medical problems and takes no medications.

On physical examination, temperature is 37.6 °C (99.7 °F), blood pressure is 140/84 mm Hg, pulse rate is 118/min, and respiration rate is 28/min; BMI is 27. Oxygen saturation is 88% on 3 L/min of oxygen by nasal cannula. Other than tachycardia, the cardiac examination is normal. Pulmonary examination reveals diffuse inspiratory crackles in all lung zones. Examination of the extremities reveals clubbing.

Laboratory studies:

Hemoglobin	15 g/dL (150 g/L)
Leukocyte count	12,000/µL (12 × 10⁹/L)
Platelet count	200,000/µL (200 × 10⁹/L)
B-type natriuretic peptide	10 pg/mL
Troponin I	0 ng/mL (0 µg/L)

Electrocardiogram shows sinus tachycardia and no evidence of ischemic changes. CT angiography shows new bilateral ground-glass opacities throughout all lung fields when compared with a previous chest CT performed 3 months ago. There is no evidence of pulmonary embolus. Bronchoalveolar lavage reveals clear fluid that has negative viral polymerase chain reaction studies, negative bacterial cultures, negative cytopathology review, and no evidence of hemorrhage.

Which of the following is the most likely diagnosis?

(A) Acute exacerbation of IPF
(B) Diffuse alveolar hemorrhage
(C) *Pneumocystis jirovecii* pneumonia
(D) Pulmonary edema due to tachycardia

Item 65

A 71-year-old woman is evaluated for a 2-month history of nonproductive cough that has not responded to a course of antibiotics. She has COPD. She is a former smoker with a 15-pack-year history, but she quit smoking 35 years ago. Her medications are tiotropium, albuterol as needed, aspirin, and a multivitamin.

On physical examination, vital signs are normal. Pulmonary examination reveals mildly reduced breath sounds bilaterally but is otherwise normal. Cardiac examination reveals a grade 2/6 crescendo-decrescendo systolic murmur. No lymphadenopathy is noted.

Laboratory studies, including a complete blood count and calcium, alkaline phosphatase, aspartate aminotransferase, and creatinine levels, are normal. Spirometry shows an FEV_1 of 60% of predicted and an FEV_1/FVC ratio of 65% with no change following administration of a bronchodilator. D_{LCO} is 58% of predicted. Chest radiograph shows a left upper lobe mass. Review of a chest radiograph from 2 years ago reveals a smaller nodular opacity in the same location. CT of the chest shows a 7-cm left upper lobe mass with no enlarged lymph nodes. PET-CT shows that the mass is moderately PET avid; there is no lymph node uptake, and there is only physiologic uptake elsewhere.

Which of the following is the most appropriate next step in management?

(A) Chemotherapy
(B) Radiation therapy
(C) Surgical resection
(D) Transthoracic needle biopsy

Item 66

A 71-year-old man is evaluated in the emergency department for septic shock secondary to a urinary tract infection.

On physical examination, he is lethargic and confused. Temperature is 38.5 °C (101.3 °F), blood pressure is 80/35 mm Hg, pulse rate is 122/min, and respiration rate is 23/min. Right costovertebral angle tenderness to percussion is noted.

Laboratory studies reveal a hematocrit of 33% and a leukocyte count of 15,600/µL (15.6 × 10⁹/L). Urinalysis shows innumerable leukocytes and gram-negative bacteria. Blood and urine culture results are pending.

Which of the following should be accomplished in the next hour?

(A) Attain hematocrit greater than 35%
(B) Begin low-dose dopamine
(C) Initiate antibiotic therapy
(D) Insert a pulmonary artery catheter

Item 67

A 50-year-old man is admitted to the hospital for pneumonia. He was started on antibiotics in the emergency department. He has a history of bipolar disorder that is controlled with lithium and risperidone.

On the evening of admission, he becomes agitated and confused. He is given intravenous haloperidol, and he develops fever and muscle rigidity.

On physical examination, temperature is 39.9 °C (103.8 °F), blood pressure is 187/108 mm Hg, pulse rate is 110/min, and respiration rate is 32/min. Diaphoresis, rigidity, and agitation are present. No stridor or signs of respiratory failure are noted.

In addition to intravenous fluid therapy, which of the following is the most appropriate initial treatment?

(A) Acetaminophen
(B) Atracurium
(C) Intubation and mechanical ventilation
(D) Lorazepam
(E) Nitroprusside

Item 68

A 72-year-old woman is evaluated during a routine examination. She has very severe COPD with multiple exacerbations. She has dyspnea at all times with decreased exercise capacity. She does not have cough or any change in baseline sputum production. She is adherent to her medication regimen, and she completed pulmonary rehabilitation 1 year ago. She quit smoking 1 year ago. Her medications are a budesonide/formoterol inhaler, tiotropium, and an albuterol inhaler as needed.

On physical examination, pulse rate is 94/min, and respiration rate is 26/min. Pulmonary examination reveals distant breath sounds and no wheezing. Oxygen saturation is 86% breathing ambient air. Pulmonary function testing reveals an FEV_1 of 26% of predicted and an FEV_1/FVC ratio of 41%.

Which of the following is the most appropriate next step in management?

(A) Oral antibiotics
(B) Oxygen therapy
(C) Prednisone taper
(D) Repeat pulmonary rehabilitation

Item 69

A 51-year-old man is evaluated for a 3-month history of worsening lower extremity edema and stable chronic dyspnea on exertion. His medical history is significant for dyslipidemia, hypertension, and type 2 diabetes mellitus. He does not drink alcohol. He has a 15-pack-year smoking history but has not used tobacco for the past 20 years. His current medications are simvastatin, lisinopril, aspirin, and insulin.

On physical examination, temperature is 37.6 °C (99.7 °F), blood pressure is 144/86 mm Hg, pulse rate is

94/min, and respiration rate is 18/min; BMI is 42. Neck circumference is 47 cm (18.5 in). Bilateral breath sounds are normal with no wheezing. Pigmented skin changes of chronic venous stasis are seen, and there is tense edema of both legs.

Laboratory studies reveal a hemoglobin level of 16.8 g/dL (168 g/L). Blood gas studies breathing ambient air reveal a pH of 7.36, an arterial P_{O_2} of 52 mm Hg (6.9 kPa), and an arterial P_{CO_2} of 53 mm Hg (7.0 kPa). Echocardiogram shows left ventricular hypertrophy and a normal ejection fraction of 65%. The right ventricle is dilated, and pulmonary artery systolic pressure is estimated at 78 mm Hg. There is moderate tricuspid regurgitation, but the valves are otherwise normal. Chest radiograph shows shallow inspiration but clear lung fields.

Which of the following is the most likely diagnosis?

(A) Cheyne-Stokes breathing
(B) COPD
(C) Interstitial lung disease
(D) Obesity hypoventilation syndrome

Item 70

A 32-year-old man is evaluated for persistent hypoxemia on mechanical ventilation in the intensive care unit. His medical history is significant for paraplegia and a chronic indwelling urinary catheter for neurogenic bladder. He presented to the emergency department 2 days ago with sepsis. At that time, he received piperacillin/tazobactam, normal saline, and vasopressors. He was endotracheally intubated for decreased level of consciousness. His initial chest radiograph was normal.

On physical examination on the second day of hospitalization, temperature is 37.1 °C (98.8 °F), blood pressure is 90/50 mm Hg, pulse rate is 96/min, and respiration rate is 26/min. His need for supplemental oxygen has steadily increased; his oxygen saturation on an F_{IO_2} of 0.8 is 89%. Pulmonary examination reveals bilateral inspiratory crackles. Cardiac examination reveals distant, regular heart sounds.

Laboratory studies:
Hemoglobin   13.2 g/dL (132 g/L)
Leukocyte count   10,000/µL (10×10^9/L)
Arterial blood gas studies
  (on an F_{IO_2} of 0.8):
  pH   7.48
  P_{CO_2} 30 mm Hg (4.0 kPa)
  P_{O_2} 60 mm Hg (8.0 kPa)

Urine and blood cultures are positive for *Escherichia coli*. A follow-up chest radiograph shows diffuse bilateral infiltrates without cardiomegaly. Central venous pressure is 8 mm Hg.

Which of the following is the most likely cause of this patient's hypoxemia?

(A) Acute respiratory distress syndrome
(B) *E. coli* pneumonia
(C) Heart failure
(D) Idiopathic acute eosinophilic pneumonia

Item 71

A 58-year-old man is evaluated for a nonproductive cough and weight loss of 8.2 kg (18.0 lb) over the last 2 months. He has had hoarseness for the last 3 weeks. He is a former heavy smoker; he quit 8 years ago. He takes no medications.

On physical examination, vital signs are normal. BMI is 21. Chest auscultation reveals decreased breath sounds and dullness to percussion on the right with prolonged expiration but no wheeze on the left. The remainder of the examination is unremarkable.

Chest radiograph shows a pleural effusion on the right and a right upper lobe mass. A chest CT scan is shown.

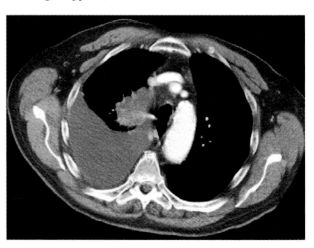

Diagnostic thoracentesis is performed, and 250 mL of fluid is removed.

Laboratory studies:

Serum lactate dehydrogenase	218 units/L
Serum total protein	6.2 g/dL (62 g/L)
Pleural fluid lactate dehydrogenase	286 units/L
Pleural fluid total protein	3.4 g/dL (34 g/L)
Pleural fluid cell counts:	
Erythrocyte count	3480/µL (3.5×10^9/L)
Total nucleated cells	1420/µL (1.4×10^9/L) (16% neutrophils, 66% lymphocytes, 6% monocytes, 12% atypical cells)
Pleural fluid cytology	Negative for malignancy

Which of the following is the most appropriate next step in the evaluation of this patient?

(A) Bronchoscopy
(B) Closed pleural biopsy
(C) Pleural fluid flow-cytometry
(D) Repeat thoracentesis and pleural fluid cytology

Item 72

A 48-year-old woman is evaluated in routine follow-up for idiopathic nonspecific interstitial pneumonia (NSIP), which was diagnosed 1 year ago after the onset of cough and dyspnea on exertion. The diagnosis was established with a high-resolution CT scan showing increased interstitial markings, traction bronchiectasis, and diffuse ground-glass opacities and with lung biopsy showing consistent pathologic findings. She does not have a history of drug or inhalational exposures, and testing for HIV and connective tissue diseases was negative. Her symptoms have been mild, and she has been on no directed treatment for NSIP. She continues to have mild dyspnea and cough that are unchanged since her last visit. She notes stiffness and mild pain in her joints, for which she takes NSAIDs as needed.

On physical examination, temperature is normal, blood pressure is 120/80 mm Hg, pulse rate is 85/min, and respiration rate is 18/min. Oxygen saturation on ambient air is 98%. Lung examination reveals decreased breath sounds bilaterally and mild bibasilar crackles, unchanged from previous examinations. The cardiac examination is normal. There is no digital clubbing. The joints of the proximal hands and wrists are mildly tender, but there is no effusion. The skin examination is normal.

A chest radiograph reveals increased bibasilar markings, unchanged from previous studies.

Which of the following is the most appropriate next step in the management of this patient's lung disease?

(A) Bronchoalveolar lavage
(B) Repeat connective tissue disease testing
(C) Repeat lung biopsy
(D) Clinical observation

Item 73

A 42-year-old man is evaluated during a routine examination. He has had lifelong asthma with significant environmental allergies and frequent exacerbations. Over the past year he has had daily symptoms with frequent nighttime awakenings requiring the use of rescue therapy. Six months ago, he was seen by an asthma educator who provided a written asthma action plan and reinforced the technique for proper use of his inhalers. His current medications are high-dose inhaled corticosteroids with a long-acting β_2-agonist and an as-needed short-acting β_2-agonist by metered-dose inhaler. He has required three extended courses of prednisone therapy for exacerbations over the past year. He is allergic to house dust mites, cats, molds, and trees. Allergen avoidance and desensitization have been attempted but have not been effective.

On physical examination, temperature is 37.0 °C (98.6 °F), blood pressure is 145/80 mm Hg, pulse rate is 82/min, and respiration rate is 18/min; BMI is 30. Pulmonary examination discloses scattered wheezing.

Laboratory studies reveal a leukocyte count of 8200/μL (8.2×10^9/L) with 8% eosinophils and an IgE level of 320 international units/mL (320 kilounits/L) (normal range, 0-90 international units/mL). Spirometry shows an FEV_1 of 65% of predicted. Chest radiograph is normal. A flow-volume loop shows a normal inspiratory limb.

Which of the following is the most appropriate treatment?

(A) Azathioprine
(B) Methotrexate

(C) Omalizumab
(D) Tumor necrosis factor α inhibitor

Item 74

A 78-year-old man was admitted to the hospital 5 days ago for worsening heart failure.

On physical examination at admission, temperature was normal, blood pressure was 150/88 mm Hg, pulse rate was 108/min, and respiration rate was 22/min. There were bibasilar crackles and dullness to percussion at both posterior lung bases. Jugular venous distention, an S_3, and lower extremity edema were present. Chest radiograph revealed cardiomegaly, vascular congestion, and moderate-sized bilateral pleural effusions. He was managed with furosemide and lisinopril. On the fourth hospital day, thoracentesis on the right was performed for further relief of dyspnea.

Pleural fluid analysis demonstrates a pleural fluid to serum lactate dehydrogenase (LDH) ratio of 61%, a pleural fluid LDH that is 46% of the upper limit of serum LDH, and a pleural fluid to serum total protein ratio of 0.51. Pleural fluid cultures and cytology are negative. The serum to pleural fluid total protein gradient is 3.3 g/dL (33 g/L).

Which of the following is the most likely cause of this patient's pleural effusion?

(A) Heart failure
(B) Malignancy
(C) Pneumonia
(D) Pulmonary embolism

Item 75

A 62-year-old man is evaluated during a routine examination. He has very severe COPD and has had multiple recent exacerbations and several hospitalizations over the past 2 years. During his last two hospitalizations he had acute hypercapnia requiring intubation. He has completed pulmonary rehabilitation twice, most recently 3 months ago, and his exercise capacity remains poor. He is adherent to his medication regimen. He used to smoke two packs per day but now only smokes two or three cigarettes per day. He is on 2 L of oxygen. His current medications are a fluticasone inhaler, salmeterol, tiotropium, roflumilast, and albuterol as needed.

On physical examination, temperature is 37.1 °C (98.8 °F), blood pressure is 130/85 mm Hg, pulse rate is 88/min and regular, and respiration rate is 22/min. Pulmonary examination discloses distant breath sounds without wheezing.

Oxygen saturation is 92% on 2 L of oxygen. Pulmonary function testing discloses an FEV_1 of 18% of predicted, an FEV_1/FVC ratio of 38%, and a D_{LCO} of 15% of predicted. Chest radiograph shows a flattened diaphragm and decreased lung markings.

Which of the following is the most appropriate next step in management?

(A) Increase oxygen
(B) Lung transplantation evaluation
(C) Lung volume reduction surgery evaluation

(D) Repeat pulmonary rehabilitation

(E) Smoking cessation

Item 76

A 25-year-old woman is admitted to the intensive care unit (ICU) for a 6-hour history of respiratory distress. She has acute lymphoblastic leukemia and received cytotoxic chemotherapy 2 weeks before ICU admission. She has had fever and leukopenia for 7 days.

On physical examination, she is in marked respiratory distress. Temperature is 39.0 °C (102.2 °F), blood pressure is 110/70 mm Hg, pulse rate is 130/min, and respiration rate is 42/min. Weight is 50.0 kg (110.2 lb). Ideal body weight is calculated as 50.0 kg (110.2 lb).

Acute respiratory distress syndrome is diagnosed. She is intubated and started on mechanical ventilation in the assist/control mode at a rate of 12/min, tidal volume of 300 mL, positive end-expiratory pressure (PEEP) of 5 cm H_2O, and FIO_2 of 1.0. An arterial blood gas study on these settings shows a pH of 7.47, PCO_2 of 30 mm Hg (4.0 kPa), and PO_2 of 45 mm Hg (6.0 kPa). Peak airway pressure is 26 cm H_2O, and the plateau pressure is 24 cm H_2O.

Which of the following is the most appropriate treatment to improve this patient's oxygenation?

(A) Increase PEEP to 10 cm H_2O

(B) Increase respiration rate to 18/min

(C) Increase tidal volume to 500 mL

(D) Start inhaled nitric oxide

Item 77

A 44-year-old woman is evaluated for a 1-week history of diffuse arthralgia with fever. She notes a new rash on the bilateral lower extremities associated with her other symptoms. She has no respiratory symptoms, and her medical history is unremarkable. She takes no medications.

On physical examination, temperature is 38.3° C (100.9 °F), blood pressure is 125/78 mm Hg, pulse rate is 88/min, and respiration rate is 12/min; BMI is 23. Physical examination reveals tenderness of the wrists bilaterally, normal range of motion of all joints, and no effusions. Examination of the bilateral lower extremities reveals erythematous nodules on the anterior shins that are best noted with palpation. The remainder of the physical examination, including eye, heart, lung, and lymph node examination, is normal.

Laboratory studies, including metabolic profile and complete blood count with differential, are normal. A chest radiograph obtained to evaluate her fever shows normal lung parenchyma but evidence of bilateral hilar lymphadenopathy.

Which of the following is the most appropriate next step in the management of this patient's chest radiograph findings?

(A) Bronchoscopy with transbronchial biopsy

(B) High-resolution CT scan of the chest

(C) Video-assisted thoracoscopic biopsy

(D) Observation

Item 78

A 54-year-old man is evaluated in the emergency department for a 24-hour history of progressive swelling of the lips. He does not have pruritus, but he has had hoarseness and difficulty swallowing. He has not had any recent insect stings, ingestion of new foods, or changes to his medications. His medical history is significant for hypertension and heart failure. Medications are carvedilol, hydrochlorothiazide, and lisinopril.

On physical examination, he is awake, alert, and able to speak in short sentences. Temperature is 37.0 °C (98.6 °F), blood pressure is 158/88 mm Hg, pulse rate is 98/min, and respiration rate is 18/min. Oxygen saturation is 96% breathing ambient air. The lips are edematous, and the posterior pharynx is difficult to visualize owing to an enlarged tongue. Inspiration is prolonged with audible stridor over the neck. The chest is clear to auscultation, but there is use of accessory respiratory muscles. No rash is noted.

Which of the following is the most appropriate next step in management?

(A) Endotracheal intubation

(B) Intravenous methylprednisolone

(C) Nebulized epinephrine

(D) Noninvasive positive pressure ventilation

Item 79

A 56-year-old woman is evaluated in the emergency department for a 4-hour history of nonproductive cough and shortness of breath. She does not have chest pain, hemoptysis, or other localizing signs. She underwent laparoscopic cholecystectomy under general anesthesia 6 weeks ago. Her medical history is notable for a childhood history of asthma, but she has not had asthma symptoms as an adult. Her sister and daughter both have asthma. She currently takes no medications.

On physical examination, temperature is 37.0 °C (98.6 °F), blood pressure is 140/86 mm Hg in both arms, pulse rate is 72/min and regular, and respiration rate is 18/min; BMI is 33. Mild injection of the pharynx is noted. Cardiac examination is normal. Pulmonary examination reveals rare scattered wheezes bilaterally over the chest with no tenderness to palpation. Surgical incisions are healing well. The abdomen is minimally tender, and bowel sounds are normal. There is no swelling or tenderness of the legs.

Laboratory studies reveal a D-dimer level of less than 0.5 µg/mL (0.5 mg/L) and a leukocyte count of 4,900/µL (4.9×10^9/L). Pulse oximetry is 93% breathing ambient air. Electrocardiogram and chest radiograph are normal.

Which of the following is the most appropriate next step in management?

(A) Abdominal CT

(B) CT angiography

(C) Duplex ultrasonography of the legs

(D) Peak flow measurement

Item 80

A 41-year-old woman is admitted to the intensive care unit for a 1-day history of progressively worsening altered mental status and jaundice. Her medical history is significant for autoimmune hepatitis, which was diagnosed 10 years ago.

On physical examination, temperature is 33.0 °C (91.4 °F), blood pressure is 105/55 mm Hg, pulse rate is 110/min, and respiration rate is 27/min; BMI is 18. She is unresponsive to sternal rub and is jaundiced. The lungs are clear, and cardiac examination is normal. Abdominal examination reveals a distended abdomen with a detectable fluid wave. The extremities are warm and well perfused.

Laboratory studies reveal a leukocyte count of 9800/µL (9.8×10^9/L), a serum creatinine level of 1.6 mg/dL (141 µmol/L), and a lactic acid level of 6 mg/dL (0.7 mmol/L).

A chest radiograph is normal, and examination of the urine is unremarkable. Blood and urine culture results are pending. Intravenous fluids and empiric broad-spectrum antibiotics are begun.

Which of the following is the most appropriate next step in management?

(A) Abdominal CT
(B) Diagnostic paracentesis
(C) Dopamine
(D) Hydrocortisone

Item 81

A 43-year-old man is evaluated for a 1-year history of cough with mucoid sputum and a 6-month history of progressive dyspnea. He has a 25-pack-year history of smoking. He has no history of asthma, allergies, or heart disease.

On physical examination, vital signs are normal. Pulmonary examination discloses decreased breath sounds bilaterally with no wheezing. Laboratory studies, including a complete blood count and complete metabolic panel, are normal. Oxygen saturation is 97% on ambient air. The electrocardiogram is normal.

Which of the following is the most appropriate management?

(A) Bronchial challenge testing
(B) CT of the chest without contrast
(C) Measurement of D$_{LCO}$
(D) Spirometry

Item 82

A 50-year-old man is evaluated in the intensive care unit for acute respiratory distress syndrome secondary to severe community-acquired pneumonia. He is intubated and placed on mechanical ventilation. He was previously healthy and took no medications before his hospitalization.

On physical examination, temperature is 38.3 °C (100.9 °F), blood pressure is 120/60 mm Hg, and pulse rate is 110/min. The patient weighs 60.0 kg (132.3 lb); ideal body weight is 60.0 kg (132.3 lb). He is sedated and is not using accessory muscles to breathe. Central venous pressure is 8 cm H_2O. Other than tachycardia, cardiac examination is normal. There are bilateral inspiratory crackles.

Initial ventilator settings are volume control with a rate of 18/min, a tidal volume of 360 mL, positive end-expiratory pressure (PEEP) of 10 cm H_2O, an FIO_2 of 0.8, a peak pressure of 34 cm H_2O, and a plateau pressure of 32 cm H_2O. Oxygen saturation by pulse oximetry is 96%.

Which of the following is the most appropriate next step in management?

(A) Decrease respiration rate
(B) Decrease tidal volume
(C) Increase FIO_2
(D) Increase PEEP

Item 83

A 30-year-old man is evaluated for chronic cough that has lasted nearly 1 year. He recalls noticing the cough initially after a "bad cold." At that time he received two courses of antibiotics (including a macrolide and a fluoroquinolone) with improvement in the acute symptoms. However, he subsequently noted persistent cough, particularly at nighttime and on cold days. Episodes of cough often occur after exercise or laughing. He is currently asymptomatic, with no postnasal drip, nasal congestion, or heartburn. He does not smoke. He has no history of occupational or other exposures. He has a remote history of hay fever. Multiple family members have seasonal allergies. His only medication is a proton pump inhibitor, which he has taken for the past 6 months without benefit.

On physical examination, vital signs are normal. The oropharynx appears normal, with no cobblestone appearance. There is no mucus in the nostrils or oropharynx. Pulmonary examination is normal. Spirometry shows an FEV$_1$ of 90% of predicted and an FEV$_1$/FVC ratio of 80%. Chest radiograph is normal.

Which of the following is the most appropriate diagnostic test to perform next?

(A) *Bordetella*-specific antibodies
(B) Bronchial challenge test
(C) Bronchoscopy
(D) Chest CT scan

Item 84

A 50-year-old man is evaluated during a routine examination. He feels well and has no current symptoms. He has no history of asthma and is a never-smoker. He was diagnosed with a rectal carcinoma 3 years ago. No metastatic disease was detected at that time, and he underwent surgical treatment for stage IIA (T3N0) disease. He has had no evidence of recurrent or metastatic disease since his initial treatment.

On physical examination, he appears well. Temperature is 37.4 °C (99.3 °F), blood pressure is 118/66 mm Hg, pulse rate is 66/min, and respiration rate is 12/min; BMI is 24. The lung fields are clear, and heart sounds are normal. Skin examination is normal.

The carcinoembryonic antigen level was normal at the time of his surgery 3 years ago and is now just above normal. A chest radiograph obtained for ongoing surveillance shows a right upper lobe nodule, a new finding since his last imaging study 1 year ago. CT of the chest shows a 1.5-cm right upper lobe nodule. PET-CT shows uptake within the nodule but is otherwise negative. The nodule is smoothly bordered and contains no calcium. CT-guided transthoracic needle biopsy of the lesion shows adenocarcinoma, and immunohistochemical staining is consistent with a gastrointestinal source. Colonoscopy shows postoperative changes but no evidence of local recurrence.

Which of the following is the most appropriate primary treatment of this patient's lung lesion?

(A) Chemotherapy
(B) External beam radiation
(C) Hospice care
(D) Surgical resection

Item 85

A 64-year-old man is evaluated following discharge from the hospital 1 week ago after an acute exacerbation of COPD. He completed a course of antibiotics in the hospital. He has severe COPD with chronic bronchitis, with multiple exacerbations over the past few years. He completed pulmonary rehabilitation 2 months ago and quit smoking 2 years ago. His medications are tiotropium, a budesonide/formoterol metered-dose inhaler, albuterol as needed, and a tapering dose of prednisone.

On physical examination, vital signs are normal. Pulmonary examination discloses scattered wheezes. Oxygen saturation is 93% breathing ambient air. Pulmonary function tests reveal an FEV_1 of 35% of predicted and an FEV_1/FVC ratio of 56%.

In addition to his current COPD therapies, which of the following is the most appropriate next step in treatment?

(A) Long-term oral corticosteroids
(B) Long-term oxygen therapy
(C) Oral N-acetylcysteine
(D) Roflumilast

Item 86

An 18-year-old woman is evaluated in the emergency department after being rescued from a burning house. She was unconscious for a few minutes at the scene and on the way to the hospital, but she regained consciousness in the emergency department.

On physical examination, she is agitated but follows commands and is oriented. Temperature is 37.4 °C (99.3 °F), blood pressure is 145/80 mm Hg, pulse rate is 90/min, and respiration rate is 20/min. Oxygen saturation on pulse oximetry is 98% breathing ambient air. She coughs frequently. There are no skin burns. No cyanosis, respiratory stridor, sputum production, or soot around airway orifices is noted.

Laboratory studies reveal a blood lactic acid level of 41 mg/dL (4.6 mmol/L).

Blood gas results in the emergency department:

	Initial Assessment	25 Minutes Later
pH	7.46	7.45
Arterial P_{CO_2}	27 mm Hg (3.6 kPa)	30 mm Hg (4.0 kPa)
Arterial P_{O_2}	86 mm Hg (11.4 kPa)	89 mm Hg (11.8 kPa)
Carboxyhemoglobin	29%	27%

Chest radiograph shows no lung infiltrates.

In addition to placing the patient on 100% oxygen, which of the following is the most appropriate next step in management?

(A) Blood cyanide level measurement
(B) Hyperbaric oxygen therapy
(C) Intubation and initiation of mechanical ventilation
(D) Pulse oximetry

Item 87

A 60-year-old man is evaluated during a routine examination, during which he expresses concern about smoking cessation and his risk for lung cancer. He has a 40-pack-year smoking history, and he has tried quitting smoking several times with nicotine gum and varenicline. Although he has not been able to completely stop smoking, he has recently decreased his use to about one-half pack per day. His brother died of lung cancer. He takes no medications.

On physical examination, vital signs are normal. Pulmonary examination reveals reduced lung sounds but is otherwise normal. Cardiac examination is normal. He had a normal chest radiograph 2 years ago for a persistent cough that has since resolved.

Which of the following is the most effective management to reduce this patient's lifetime risk of dying of lung cancer?

(A) Annual chest radiography
(B) β-Carotene supplementation
(C) Isotretinoin supplementation
(D) Smoking cessation

Item 88

A 29-year-old man is evaluated in the emergency department for chest pain.

On physical examination, temperature is 38.4 °C (101.1 °F), blood pressure is 155/95 mm Hg (identical in both arms), pulse rate is 112/min, and respiration rate is 20/min. He is alert, agitated, and uncomfortable owing to ongoing chest pain. The pupils are dilated but reactive. Electrocardiogram shows regular, narrow complex tachycardia. T-wave inversion and ST-segment depression are suggested in the lateral leads. Urine toxicology screen is positive for cocaine.

In addition to starting aspirin and nitroglycerin, which of the following is the most appropriate treatment?

(A) Alteplase followed by heparin infusion
(B) Intravenous diltiazem and lorazepam
(C) Intravenous metoprolol
(D) Intravenous nitroprusside

Item 89

A 63-year-old man is evaluated in the emergency department for a 4-hour history of acute worsening of dyspnea. He reports no fever, chest pain, hemoptysis, or other localizing symptoms. He has a cough associated with a history of bullous emphysema, but this is unchanged from baseline. He underwent resection of the right upper lobe for stage 1 adenocarcinoma of the lung 18 months ago. His medications are daily inhaled tiotropium/salmeterol and fluticasone.

On physical examination, temperature is 37.6 °C (99.7 °F), blood pressure is 110/72 mm Hg, pulse rate is 115/min and regular, and respiration rate is 20/min. Oxygen saturation is 89% on ambient air and improves to 96% on 2 L/min of oxygen by nasal prongs. He appears anxious and mildly dyspneic. There are healed scars on the right side of the chest from thoracoscopic lobectomy. The lung examination shows diminished breath sounds in the right upper lung field and occasional mild, diffuse expiratory wheezes but no other focal findings. Cardiac examination reveals sinus tachycardia but no murmur, gallops, or rubs. No digital clubbing or lymph node enlargement is seen. There is no tenderness in the legs.

Laboratory studies reveal normal serum chemistries, kidney function, and complete blood count. Serum cardiac troponin T level is less than 0.02 ng/mL (0.02 µg/L). Electrocardiogram shows no ischemic changes. Chest radiograph shows postoperative changes on the right and scattered bullous changes bilaterally with hyperinflation.

Which of the following is the most appropriate next step in management?

(A) CT angiography
(B) D-dimer measurement
(C) Duplex ultrasonography of the legs
(D) Ventilation/perfusion scan

Item 90

A 51-year-old man was admitted to the intensive care unit 3 days ago for septic shock with multisystem organ failure. Septic shock resulted from peritonitis following colon resection for a ruptured colonic diverticulum. He is on mechanical ventilation and had been treated with vasopressor agents, but these are no longer required. He is able to tolerate enteral nutrition with a standard commercial preparation (1 kcal/mL) at 10 mL/h via a soft nasogastric feeding tube.

On physical examination, temperature is 36.4 °C (97.5 °F), blood pressure is 120/70 mm Hg, pulse rate is 88/min, and respiration rate is 16/min. Weight is 80.0 kg (176.4 lb) and height is 177 cm (69.7 in).

Which of the following is the most appropriate next step in the management of this patient's nutrition?

(A) Begin supplemental total parenteral nutrition
(B) Change to an enhanced preparation of glutamine, arginine, antioxidants, and omega-3 fatty acids
(C) Increase the rate of the current nutritional preparation
(D) Supplement tube feeds with intravenous lipid formulation

Item 91

A 22-year-old woman is evaluated in the emergency department for a 3-day history of progressive dyspnea that is now severe. She has asthma and has a history of poor adherence to her medication regimen. Bedside spirometry reveals severe airflow obstruction with an FEV_1 of 25% of predicted. Her asthma medications are an inhaled corticosteroid and an albuterol inhaler as needed.

On physical examination, she is alert, appears anxious, and is speaking in partial sentences. Temperature is 37.0 °C (98.6 °F), blood pressure is 118/58 mm Hg, pulse rate is 116/min, and respiration rate is 30/min; BMI is 34. Oxygen saturation is 89% breathing ambient air and 93% breathing 2 L/min of oxygen by nasal cannula. Pulmonary examination reveals prolonged expiration and diffuse expiratory wheezes bilaterally. The abdominal muscles contract with expiration.

She is started on continuous nebulized albuterol, nebulized ipratropium, and methylprednisolone. After 2 hours of treatment, her bedside FEV_1 is 30% of predicted. Arterial blood gas studies reveal a pH of 7.48, a PCO_2 of 30 mm Hg (4.0 kPa), and a PO_2 of 70 mm Hg (9.3 kPa) on 2 L/min of oxygen. Chest radiograph shows hyperinflation without infiltrates.

Which of the following is the most appropriate next step in management?

(A) Administer antibiotics
(B) Admit to the intensive care unit
(C) Electively intubate
(D) Perform laryngoscopy

Item 92

A 67-year-old man is evaluated in the emergency department for a 2-day history of cough and shortness of breath. His medical history is significant for COPD, and he is a former smoker with a 120-pack-year history. His medications are fluticasone, tiotropium, and albuterol as needed.

On physical examination, temperature is 37.5 °C (99.5 °F), blood pressure is 145/90 mm Hg, pulse rate is 100/min, and respiration rate is 22/min. Lung auscultation reveals bibasilar crackles. Cardiac examination is normal. There is evidence of proximal muscle weakness and absent deep tendon reflexes in the extremities. Deep tendon reflexes returned after isometric exercise.

A CT of the chest is shown.

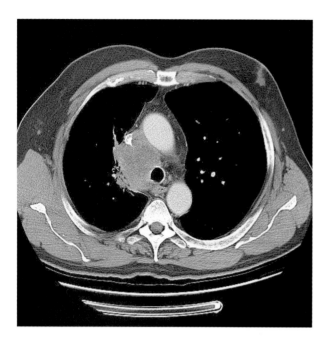

Which of the following is the most likely diagnosis?

(A) Carcinoid tumor
(B) Fibrosing mediastinitis
(C) Small cell lung cancer
(D) Thymoma

Item 93

A 38-year-old man is evaluated for a 1-year history of cough with mucoid sputum and a 6-month history of mildly progressive dyspnea. He has a 12-pack-year history of smoking. He has no history of asthma, allergies, skin disease, or liver disease.

On physical examination, vital signs are normal. Pulmonary examination discloses decreased breath sounds bilaterally with no wheezing.

Laboratory studies, including a complete blood count and complete metabolic panel, are normal. Oxygen saturation is 97% breathing ambient air. The electrocardiogram is normal. CT scan of the chest shows basilar lucency without bronchiectasis. Spirometry reveals an FEV_1 of 53% of predicted and an FEV_1/FVC ratio of 64%. The D_{LCO} is 67% of predicted. There is no significant improvement in airflow after bronchodilator administration.

Which of the following is the most appropriate next step in management?

(A) α_1-Antitrypsin level measurement
(B) Initiation of an inhaled corticosteroid
(C) Sweat chloride testing
(D) Z and S genotyping for α_1-antitrypsin alleles

Item 94

A 66-year-old man is evaluated in the emergency department for shortness of breath, which he first noted upon awakening this morning. He has not had chest pain, cough, or other localizing symptoms. He fractured his left leg in an automobile accident 7 weeks ago, and his short-leg cast was removed 2 weeks ago.

On physical examination, temperature is 37.8 °C (100.0 °F), pulse rate is 102/min, and respiration rate is 20/min. The chest is clear with good air movement in all lung fields. The legs are not swollen or tender, the toes of both feet are warm, and pedal pulses are normal. The remainder of the examination is unremarkable.

Laboratory studies show normal serum troponin levels and a normal leukocyte count. Oxygen saturation is 94% breathing oxygen at 2 L/min via nasal prongs. Electrocardiogram shows sinus tachycardia but is otherwise normal. Chest radiograph is normal.

Which of the following is the most appropriate and cost-effective next step in evaluation?

(A) CT angiography
(B) Duplex ultrasonography of the legs
(C) Echocardiography
(D) Serum D-dimer measurement

Item 95

A 67-year-old man is evaluated during a routine examination. He has severe COPD that was diagnosed 5 years ago. His exercise capacity is very low, and he has dyspnea that is not relieved by his medication regimen. He has had multiple exacerbations. He is adherent to his medication regimen, and his inhaler technique is good. He quit smoking 1 year ago. He has undergone pulmonary rehabilitation twice and completed the last one 3 months ago. His medications are tiotropium, salmeterol/fluticasone, roflumilast, albuterol as needed, and 2 L of oxygen via nasal cannula.

On physical examination, temperature is 37.8 °C (100.0 °F), blood pressure is 130/85 mm Hg, pulse rate is 95/min and regular, and respiration rate is 21/min. Pulmonary examination reveals reduced breath sounds but no wheezing.

Oxygen saturation is 90% on 2 L of oxygen via nasal cannula. Pulmonary function tests show an FEV_1 of 35% of predicted, an FEV_1/FVC ratio of 42%, a residual volume/total lung capacity ratio of 135%, and a D_{LCO} of 30%. Arterial blood gases on 2 L of oxygen reveal a P_{CO_2} of 46 mm Hg (6.1 kPa) and a P_{O_2} of 65 mm Hg (8.6 kPa). CT of the chest shows bilateral upper lobe emphysema.

Which of the following is the most appropriate next step in management?

(A) Increase oxygen to 3 L
(B) Long-term oral corticosteroids
(C) Lung volume reduction surgery evaluation
(D) Repeat pulmonary rehabilitation

Item 96

A 32-year-old man is evaluated for severe dyspnea and dry cough. He has had an 8-week history of increasing shortness of breath without fever or chills. He was treated with azithromycin when symptoms began, but there has been no improvement with treatment and his symptoms have continued to worsen. He has a 10-pack-year smoking history and was smoking until the onset of his current symptoms. His medical history is otherwise unremarkable and he takes no medications.

On physical examination, temperature is normal, blood pressure is 135/85 mm Hg, pulse rate is 105/min, and respiration rate is 28/min. Oxygen saturation is 88% breathing ambient air. There is no jugular venous distention. Pulmonary examination reveals bilateral crackles throughout the lungs. Cardiac examination is normal. There is no peripheral edema. No evidence of rash or arthritis is noted.

Chest radiograph shows peripheral-predominant consolidation and scattered hazy opacity and normal lung volumes. High-resolution CT demonstrates bilateral patchy ground-glass opacities and bilateral, lower lobe–predominant, subpleural consolidations.

Which of the following is the most likely diagnosis?

(A) Chronic pulmonary embolism
(B) COPD
(C) Cryptogenic organizing pneumonia
(D) Lymphangioleiomyomatosis

Item 97

A 58-year-old woman is admitted to the hospital for an 8-hour history of acute, moderately severe dyspnea and left lateral pleuritic chest pain. She has a history of hypertension and stage 4 chronic kidney disease. Her medications are atenolol and atorvastatin.

On physical examination, she is in moderate respiratory distress. Temperature is 37.6 °C (99.7 °F), blood pressure is 148/90 mm Hg, pulse rate is 88/min, and respiration rate is 22/min. Pulmonary examination reveals a left lateral pleural friction rub and inspiratory crackles at the left base. Cardiac examination is normal except for an S_4 gallop at the cardiac apex. There is no leg edema. Her rectal examination is heme negative.

Laboratory studies reveal a blood urea nitrogen level of 30 mg/dL (10.7 mmol/L) and a serum creatinine level of 2.8 mg/dL (248 µmol/L). Compete blood count, coagulation studies, and cardiac markers are normal. Oxygen saturation is 94% on 3 L/min of oxygen via nasal cannula. Electrocardiogram shows evidence of left ventricular hypertrophy. Echocardiogram shows left ventricular hypertrophy with normal function. The right ventricle is normal in size and function. CT angiography shows bilateral lobar and segmental pulmonary emboli.

Which of the following is the most appropriate treatment?

(A) Alteplase
(B) Argatroban plus warfarin
(C) Enoxaparin plus warfarin
(D) Fondaparinux plus warfarin
(E) Unfractionated heparin plus warfarin

Item 98

A 72-year-old man is evaluated during a routine examination. He has stage 3 COPD with limited exercise capacity, and he also has heart failure. He lives in New Jersey and asks about airline travel to visit his family in Phoenix, Arizona. His medications are lisinopril, hydralazine, isosorbide dinitrate, tiotropium, salmeterol, and albuterol as needed.

On physical examination, pulse rate is 88/min, and other vital signs are normal. Pulmonary examination reveals decreased breath sounds. Cardiac examination reveals a soft S_3. Oxygen saturation is 91% and arterial P_{O_2} is 68 mm Hg (9.0 kPa) breathing ambient air.

Which of the following is the most appropriate management related to airline travel for this patient?

(A) Advise the patient not to travel by airline
(B) Perform a hypoxia altitude simulation test
(C) Perform pulmonary exercise testing
(D) Perform pulmonary function testing with 6-minute walk test

Item 99

A 70-year-old woman is evaluated in follow-up for a pulmonary nodule that was discovered 2 years ago when she underwent a CT coronary study for evaluation of chest pain. This disclosed a 9-mm ground-glass nodule in the right upper lobe. The nodule has been followed by CT annually for the past 2 years, remains purely ground glass in character, and has not increased in size. She is asymptomatic and has no exertional dyspnea. She is a never-smoker. There is no family history of lung cancer.

On physical examination, vital signs are normal. Lung auscultation is normal, and the remainder of the examination is unremarkable.

Which of the following is the most appropriate management?

(A) Follow-up CT scan in 1 year
(B) PET-CT scan now
(C) Surgical removal now
(D) Transthoracic needle biopsy now
(E) No further evaluation

Item 100

A 46-year-old woman is evaluated for a 4-day history of fever, fatigue, and cough productive of purulent sputum and a 1-day history of left-sided pleuritic chest pain. She has a history of alcohol abuse and reports a 3-day binge that ended 2 days before the onset of symptoms.

On physical examination, she appears ill but is in no acute distress. Temperature is 38.6 °C (101.5 °F), blood pressure is 112/68 mm Hg, and pulse rate is 104/min. Oxygen saturation is 92% at rest breathing ambient air. Pulmonary examination demonstrates absent breath sounds and dullness to percussion over the left base. The remainder of the examination is unremarkable.

CONT.

Laboratory studies demonstrate a leukocyte count of 14,800/µL (14.8 × 10⁹/L) with neutrophil predominance. Chest radiograph demonstrates a dense infiltrate with consolidation at the left base and an adjacent left pleural effusion that is moderately sized and free flowing. Thoracic ultrasound shows a moderate effusion with increased echogenicity but no septations or loculations. Diagnostic thoracentesis is performed, and 450 mL of serosanguineous fluid is removed.

Laboratory studies:

Serum lactate dehydrogenase	85 units/L
Serum total protein	6.5 g/dL (65 g/L)
Pleural fluid lactate dehydrogenase	325 units/L
Pleural fluid total protein	3.3 g/dL (33 g/L)
Pleural fluid glucose	20 mg/dL (1.1 mmol/L)
Pleural fluid pH	7.1
Pleural fluid cell counts:	
Erythrocyte count	5880/µL (5.88 × 10⁹/L)
Total nucleated cells	11,489/µL (11.4 × 10⁹/L) (64% neutrophils, 22% lymphocytes, 4% monocytes, 10% mesothelial cells)
Pleural fluid cultures	Pending
Pleural fluid Gram stain	Negative

In addition to starting antibiotics, which of the following is the most appropriate next step in the management of this patient's pleural effusion?

(A) Repeat chest radiography in 1 week
(B) Surgical decortication
(C) Therapeutic thoracentesis
(D) Tube thoracostomy

Item 101

A 49-year-old woman is evaluated for a 6-month history of exertional dyspnea and nonproductive cough that had an insidious onset. She has not noticed any particular triggers for her cough. She has no history of asthma, airway disease, reflux, or aspiration. She has never smoked. She has had no chemical or industrial exposures, has not been in contact with birds, has not been in a hot tub recently, and has not had recent travel. She works as a computer programmer. She has no family history of atopy or asthma, and she takes no medications.

On physical examination, temperature is 37.6 °C (99.7 °F), blood pressure is 122/76 mm Hg, pulse rate is 84/min, and respiration rate is 16/min; BMI is 24. Auscultation of the heart and lungs is normal. There are no palpable lymph nodes and no notable skin findings.

Lung volumes and spirometry are normal; DLCO is mildly reduced at 75% of predicted. Chest radiographs are shown (see right column). The patient has not had any previous radiographs.

Which of the following is the most likely diagnosis?

(A) Asbestosis
(B) Cryptogenic organizing pneumonia
(C) Heart failure
(D) Idiopathic pulmonary fibrosis
(E) Sarcoidosis

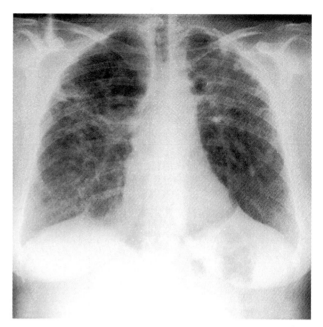

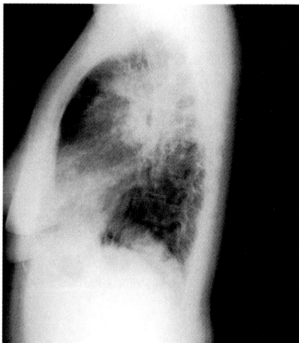

ITEM 101

Item 102

A 68-year-old man is evaluated for excessive daytime sleepiness. His wife has noted breathing pauses during sleep. He has amyotrophic lateral sclerosis.

On physical examination, temperature is 37.4 °C (99.3 °F), blood pressure is 116/74 mm Hg, pulse rate is 82/min, and respiration rate is 16/min; BMI is 23. The nares and oropharyngeal airway are widely patent. There is muscle atrophy of the extremities, particularly the arms. Prominent fasciculations of the tongue and the muscles of the arms and thighs are noted. Hyperreflexia and weakness are seen most prominently in the upper extremities. There is no sensory deficit.

Arterial blood gas studies with the patient awake and breathing ambient air reveal a pH of 7.39, a Po_2 of 61 mm Hg (8.1 kPa), and a Pco_2 of 53 mm Hg (7.0 kPa).

Which of the following is the most appropriate treatment?

(A) Bilevel positive airway pressure
(B) Continuous positive airway pressure
(C) Supplemental oxygen
(D) Tracheostomy

Item 103

A 63-year-old man with acute respiratory distress syndrome (ARDS) is evaluated in the intensive care unit. He has just been intubated and placed on mechanical ventilation for ARDS secondary to aspiration pneumonia. Before intubation, his oxygen saturation was 78% breathing 100% oxygen with a nonrebreather mask.

On physical examination, temperature is 37.0 °C (98.6 °F), blood pressure is 150/90 mm Hg, and pulse rate is 108/min. His height is 150 cm (59 in) and his weight is 70.0 kg (154.3 lb). Ideal body weight is calculated to be 52.0 kg (114.6 lb). Central venous pressure is 8 cm H_2O. Cardiac examination reveals normal heart sounds and no murmurs. Crackles are auscultated in the lower left lung field. The patient is sedated. Neurologic examination is nonfocal.

Mechanical ventilation is on the assist/control mode at a rate of 18/min. Positive end-expiratory pressure is 8 cm H_2O, and Fio_2 is 1.0.

Which of the following is the most appropriate tidal volume?

(A) 300 mL
(B) 450 mL
(C) 700 mL
(D) 840 mL

Item 104

A 32-year-old woman is evaluated in an urgent care center in Colorado for difficulty breathing during a weekend of hiking at an elevation of 3100 meters (10,171 feet). She reports shortness of breath during repeated awakenings from sleep. However, she is able to tolerate hiking on flat ground or modest inclines. She notes dryness of the eyes and mouth. She does not have any history of breathing problems. She has not had cough, sputum, headache, dizziness, visual changes, nausea, or vomiting. Her medical history is unremarkable.

On physical examination, she has a nontoxic general appearance. Temperature is 37.6 °C (99.7 °F), blood pressure is 126/74 mm Hg, pulse rate is 72/min, and respiration rate is 16/min; BMI is 24. The mucous membranes are dry. Mentation is normal, and neurologic and cardiopulmonary examinations are unremarkable. Pulse oximetry breathing ambient air reveals an oxygen saturation of 95%.

Which of the following is the most likely cause of this patient's symptoms?

(A) Asthma
(B) High-altitude cerebral edema

(C) High-altitude periodic breathing
(D) High-altitude pulmonary edema

Item 105

A 54-year-old woman is evaluated for a 1-year history of progressive dyspnea. Her symptoms have been progressively worsening, and she is now unable to walk more than a block without becoming significantly short of breath. Oxygen desaturation with ambulation was recently diagnosed, and she was prescribed supplemental oxygen during exertion. She recently developed ankle swelling but does not have chest pain, cough, lightheadedness, or other localizing symptoms. Medical history is significant only for a hysterectomy 3 years ago that was followed by a postoperative respiratory illness that was treated as pneumonia. Current medications are oxygen with exertion, 2 L/min by nasal prongs, and as-needed furosemide.

On physical examination, temperature is 37.0 °C (98.6 °F), blood pressure is 118/72 mm Hg, pulse rate is 100/min and regular, and respiration rate is 18/min. BMI is 27. The lungs are clear. Cardiac examination reveals sinus tachycardia, an increased pulmonic component of S_2, and no murmurs. The liver is not enlarged. There is no clubbing of the digits. Ankle edema is noted bilaterally, and there are no venous cords or tenderness in the legs.

Laboratory studies are normal except for a B-type natriuretic peptide level of 700 pg/mL. Arterial blood gas measurement breathing ambient air shows a pH of 7.41, a Pco_2 of 38 mm Hg (5.1 kPa), and a Po_2 of 62 mm Hg (8.2 kPa). Pulmonary function tests are normal except for a mild reduction in $Dlco$ to 70% of normal. Electrocardiogram discloses sinus tachycardia and right ventricular hypertrophy. A chest radiograph shows mildly increased interstitial markings, normal inflation, and no evidence of infiltrate or effusion. Echocardiogram shows a normal left ventricular ejection fraction and an estimated pulmonary artery systolic pressure of 35 to 45 mm Hg.

Which of the following is the most appropriate diagnostic study?

(A) Chest CT angiography
(B) D-dimer study
(C) Lower-extremity duplex ultrasonography
(D) Ventilation/perfusion scan

Item 106

A 78-year-old woman is treated in the intensive care unit (ICU) for a 24-hour history of altered mental status that has been progressively worsening. She is a resident of a nursing home, and her medical history is significant for Alzheimer disease.

On arrival to the emergency department, she was disoriented, febrile, tachycardic with a heart rate of 115/min, and hypotensive with a blood pressure of 82/40 mm Hg.

Laboratory studies showed a leukocyte count of 33,000/µL (33×10^9/L) and a hemoglobin level of 11 g/dL (110 g/L). A urine dipstick was positive for nitrites and leukocyte esterase. A chest radiograph was normal.

CONT.

Blood and urine culture results are pending. Central access was obtained and she was started on broad-spectrum antibiotics. A 1000-mL normal saline fluid challenge was administered over 30 minutes.

Current examination in the ICU shows the patient to have an unchanged mental status. Blood pressure is now 85/45 mm Hg and heart rate is 100/min. Her physical examination is unchanged.

Which of the following is the most appropriate immediate next step in management?

(A) Erythrocyte transfusion
(B) Hydrocortisone
(C) Norepinephrine
(D) Normal saline at 200 mL/h

Item 107

A 60-year-old man is evaluated prior to an elective hernia repair that is scheduled for next week. He has moderate COPD and has had a mild increase in cough, green sputum production, and dyspnea for the past 3 days. His last exacerbation was 6 months ago, at which time he quit smoking. His current medications are daily tiotropium and two puffs of albuterol four times daily.

On physical examination, temperature is 37.2 °C (99.0 °F), blood pressure is 128/78 mm Hg, pulse rate is 96/min and regular, and respiration rate is 20/min. Pulmonary examination discloses bilateral expiratory wheezing. Oxygen saturation is 92% breathing ambient air. Pulmonary function testing done 4 months ago revealed an FEV_1 of 55% of predicted and an FEV_1/FVC ratio of 60%.

In addition to treating the exacerbation of his COPD, which of the following is the most appropriate next step in management?

(A) Delay surgery
(B) Repeat pulmonary function testing
(C) Start roflumilast
(D) No further intervention

Item 108

A 37-year-old man is evaluated for a 3-year history of persistent cough. He has had four episodes of pneumonia in the last 3 years; each appeared to be in the right lower lobe. He experiences improvement temporarily with administration of antibiotics, but his symptoms return within weeks. He has fever at the time of worsening symptoms, but he has not had persistent fever. There has been no significant weight loss. He has no smoking history. He recently finished a 10-day course of a fluoroquinolone but takes no other medications.

On physical examination, temperature is 37.0 °C (98.6 °F), blood pressure is 127/68 mm Hg, pulse rate is 100/min, and respiration rate is 22/min; BMI is 25. Pulmonary examination reveals reduced breath sounds at the right base but no bronchial breath sounds or egophony.

Laboratory studies, including a complete blood count and calcium, creatinine, and alkaline phosphatase levels, are normal. Chest radiograph shows collapse of the right lower lobe. CT images are shown.

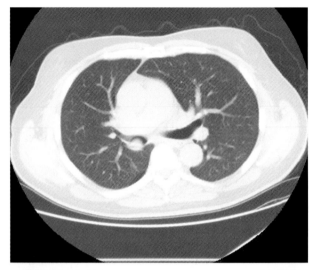

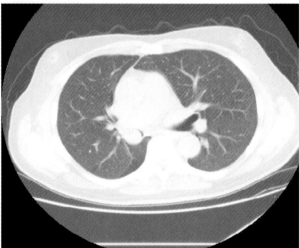

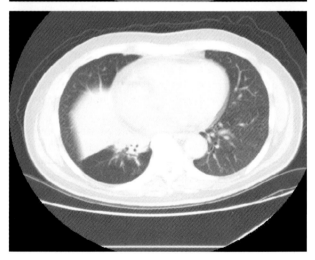

Which of the following is the most likely diagnosis?

(A) Adenocarcinoma
(B) Carcinoid tumor
(C) Small cell carcinoma
(D) Squamous cell carcinoma

Answers and Critiques

Item 1   Answer: B

Educational Objective: Diagnose COPD.

The most likely cause of this patient's cough is COPD. His postbronchodilator FEV_1/FVC ratio less than 70% confirms airflow limitation and a diagnosis of obstructive lung disease; his relatively preserved FEV_1 suggests that his COPD is mild. COPD should be considered in any patient older than 40 years who has dyspnea, chronic cough or sputum production, and/or a history of risk factors (such as exposure to tobacco smoke, dust, chemicals, outdoor air pollution, or biomass smoke). Spirometry is the gold standard for diagnosing COPD and monitoring its progress; it should be done to confirm the diagnosis and to exclude other diseases. The American College of Physicians and Global Initiative for Chronic Obstructive Lung Disease (GOLD) guidelines require an FEV_1/FVC ratio of less than 70% of predicted to establish the diagnosis of COPD. The GOLD guidelines use the degree of airflow obstruction as measured by the FEV_1 to further describe the level of disease. Level 1 (mild) COPD is characterized by an FEV_1 of 80% of predicted or greater; level 2 (moderate) COPD is characterized by an FEV_1 of 50% to 79% of predicted; level 3 (severe) COPD is characterized by an FEV_1 of 30% to 49% of predicted; and level 4 (very severe) COPD is characterized by an FEV_1 less than 30% of predicted.

Although asthma may present with cough, it is unlikely in this patient owing to the lack of atopy and history of respiratory symptoms as a child or any other clinical findings consistent with bronchospasm.

Gastroesophageal reflux disease may cause cough; however, COPD is the more likely cause of cough in this patient who does not have heartburn symptoms, has a history of smoking, and demonstrates airflow obstruction on pulmonary function testing.

ACE inhibitors may be associated with cough, but angiotensin receptor blockers (such as losartan) have a significantly lower rate of cough as a side effect and would not be a likely cause of this patient's cough given his other clinical parameters.

KEY POINT

- Spirometry is essential for the diagnosis of COPD and assessing its degree of severity; a postbronchodilator FEV_1/FVC ratio less than 70% confirms airflow limitation.

Bibliography

Global Strategy for Diagnosis, Management, and Prevention of COPD. December 2011. Available at: www.goldcopd.org. Accessed July 27, 2012.

Item 2   Answer: D

Educational Objective: Manage weaning from invasive ventilation with noninvasive positive pressure ventilation.

The most appropriate intervention at the time of extubation is noninvasive positive pressure ventilation (NPPV). Application of NPPV shortly after extubation for a 24-hour period reduced the need for reintubation in previous trials of intubated patients with chronic lung disease and hypercapnia after a successful weaning trial. This population also appears to benefit from NPPV even if it is not applied until after the patient has developed respiratory failure following extubation. However, studies enrolling unselected patients with postextubation respiratory failure indicate that the use of NPPV may actually increase mortality.

The use of incentive spirometry reduces the risk of postoperative pulmonary complications but does not have a role in the routine management of nonsurgical patients following extubation.

The reduced gas density of helium-oxygen mixtures (heliox) reduces resistance to airflow, and thereby the work of breathing, in patients with obstructive lung disease. However, there is insufficient evidence to support the routine use of heliox in the management of COPD exacerbations.

N-acetylcysteine is a mucolytic agent that has been used to thin secretions in patients with excess mucus production. However, *N*-acetylcysteine is less likely to benefit this patient because he had minimal secretions prior to extubation. Furthermore, nebulized *N*-acetylcysteine may trigger bronchospasm.

KEY POINT

- Application of noninvasive positive pressure ventilation shortly after extubation for a 24-hour period reduced the need for reintubation in trials of intubated patients with chronic lung disease and hypercapnia after a successful weaning trial.

Bibliography

Ferrer M, Sellarés J, Valencia M, et al. Non-invasive ventilation after extubation in hypercapnic patients with chronic respiratory disorders: randomised controlled trial. Lancet. 2009;374(9695):1082-1088. [PMID: 19682735]

Item 3   Answer: C

Educational Objective: Diagnose neuropsychiatric impairment as a common complication after critical illness.

The most likely long-term complication of critical illness is persistent neuropsychiatric impairment, which can affect up to 75% of critically ill patients, especially those with the diagnosis of either severe sepsis or acute respiratory distress syndrome. The syndrome appears clinically as acquired dementia. The factors in the intensive care unit (ICU) that are associated with the development of the syndrome include age, duration of mechanical ventilation, and glycemic control (hyperglycemia or hypoglycemia). There is some evidence that the degree of impairment correlates with hypoxemia in these patients.

A patient with chronic disseminated intravascular coagulation would most likely have problems related to low platelets and possibly thrombosis. Acquired dementia can be a result of microvascular thrombosis, but this is an unlikely explanation in the absence of other findings. Failure to provide appropriate prophylaxis in the ICU usually results in more acute complications, such as infection, peptic ulcer disease, or deep venous thrombosis.

Critical illness polyneuropathy is one type of ICU-acquired weakness, along with critical illness myopathy. ICU-acquired weakness is common with recognized risk factors, including corticosteroid use and neuromuscular blocking agents, but it does not affect cognition. By the time this patient's family member raised concerns, the patient had regained his former muscle strength. Therefore, ICU-acquired weakness is not the explanation for this patient's psychiatric disability.

Prolonged neuromuscular blockade is an uncommon condition associated with prolonged use of paralytic agents typically in patients with concomitant liver disease, but it does not cause cognitive impairment.

KEY POINT

- Persistent neuropsychiatric impairment can affect up to 75% of critically ill patients, and it is associated with the patient's age, duration of mechanical ventilation, and glycemic control (hyperglycemia or hypoglycemia).

Bibliography

Jackson JC, Mitchell N, Hopkins RO. Cognitive functioning, mental health, and quality of life in ICU survivors: an overview. Anesthesiol Clin. 2011;29(4):751-764. [PMID: 22078921]

Item 4   Answer: C

Educational Objective: Treat central sleep apnea in a patient with heart failure.

The most appropriate treatment is diuresis. This patient has Cheyne-Stokes breathing/central sleep apnea (CSA) related to underlying heart failure. Breathing pauses may be observed by a bed partner; however, in contrast with obstructive sleep apnea, snoring is not as common, and patients are not as likely to be sleepy or overweight or have a crowded oropharynx on examination. Cheyne-Stokes breathing/CSA is believed to occur as a consequence of heart failure, a condition that predisposes to hyperventilation. CSA severity tends to correlate with the degree of

cardiac dysfunction, such that improvements in cardiac function will have a concordant effect on CSA. Therefore, the usual first step in the management of CSA in the setting of heart failure is medical optimization of cardiac function. This patient has evidence of inadequately treated heart failure, with crackles, an S_3, and lower extremity edema on examination. Diuresis to improve fluid balance and manage heart failure would be the most appropriate next step before initiating additional therapies for his sleep-disordered breathing.

In cases where CSA persists after medical optimization, a form of positive airway pressure therapy called adaptive servoventilation (ASV) often effectively controls CSA, although clinical outcomes data are scant. The computer algorithm governing ASV promotes ventilatory stability with timed delivery of pressure support that is synchronized to the patient's breathing effort.

Continuous positive airway pressure (CPAP) may be effective, particularly if there is a mixed element of obstructive sleep apnea, but CPAP can also exacerbate or worsen CSA.

This patient had normal oxygen levels during polysomnography, so supplemental oxygen is not needed at this time. However, the use of supplemental oxygen could be considered in the setting of low oxyhemoglobin saturations due to impaired gas exchange from cardiac disease.

Oral appliances may be a useful adjunct in the treatment of obstructive sleep apnea. However, the use of a device in this patient without evidence of obstruction and a diagnosis of CSA would not be appropriate.

KEY POINT

- The most appropriate first-line treatment for central sleep apnea in a patient with heart failure is medical therapy to improve cardiac function.

Bibliography

Yumino D, Bradley TD. Central sleep apnea and Cheyne-Stokes respiration. Proc Am Thorac Soc. 2008;5(2):226-236. [PMID: 18250216]

Item 5   Answer: D

Educational Objective: Manage severe COPD with pulmonary rehabilitation.

Pulmonary rehabilitation is the most appropriate management for this patient. Current guidelines recommend pulmonary rehabilitation for symptomatic patients with an FEV_1 less than 50% of predicted. Pulmonary rehabilitation may be considered for symptomatic or exercise-limited patients with an FEV_1 greater than or equal to 50% of predicted, but this is a weaker recommendation based upon moderate-quality evidence. Exercise training improves skeletal muscle function and reduces dynamic hyperinflation. Benefits of pulmonary rehabilitation include improvement in exercise capacity, reduction in the perceived intensity of breathlessness, improvement in health-related quality of life, and reduction in anxiety and depression associated with COPD. It is not recommended for patients who cannot walk or who have unstable angina or recent myocardial infarction.

Morphine can be used in palliation for patients with severe dyspnea, especially at rest. However, this patient's dyspnea is not severe, so morphine is not appropriate at this time.

This patient's oxygenation is adequate, and supplemental oxygen is not required. Oxygen therapy is indicated for patients who have hypoxemia, arterial P_{O_2} of 55 mm Hg (7.3 kPa) or lower, or oxygen saturation of 88% or lower.

This patient has no indication for a short-term course of a systemic corticosteroid because she does not have evidence of an acute exacerbation. An exacerbation of COPD is defined as an acute event characterized by a change in baseline dyspnea, cough, and/or sputum production beyond normal daily variation. The main symptoms include increased dyspnea often accompanied by wheezing and chest tightness, increased cough and sputum production, change in the color and/or tenacity of sputum, and fever. Various nonspecific signs and symptoms such as fatigue, insomnia, depression, and confusion may accompany these findings.

KEY POINT

- Current guidelines recommend pulmonary rehabilitation for patients with symptomatic COPD who have an FEV_1 less than 50% of predicted.

Bibliography

Qaseem A, Wilt TJ, Weinberger SE, et al; American College of Physicians; American College of Chest Physicians; American Thoracic Society; European Respiratory Society. Diagnosis and management of stable chronic obstructive pulmonary disease: a clinical practice guideline update from the American College of Physicians, American College of Chest Physicians, American Thoracic Society, and European Respiratory Society. Ann Intern Med. 2011;155(3):179-191. [PMID: 21810710]

Item 6   Answer: B

Educational Objective: Evaluate a 2-cm calcified lung nodule in a former smoker.

The nodule in the CT images is densely, centrally calcified and smoothly bordered, consistent with a granuloma. The likelihood that a nodule is malignant depends on such factors as its size and surface characteristics and the patient's age, smoking history, and history of previous malignancy. Nodules with smooth borders are usually benign; nodules with spiculated borders have a high likelihood of being malignant. "Popcorn" (amorphous calcification in rings and arcs), lamellar (concentric rings), central, and diffuse patterns of calcification are associated with benign disease. Although this patient is at risk for lung cancer owing to her smoking history, this benign nodule needs no further evaluation. Not all patterns of calcification are associated with benign disease. A nodule that has eccentric or off-center calcification may be either benign or malignant, and further evaluation or follow-up is advised.

Bronchial carcinoid tumors are low-grade malignant neoplasms that consist of neuroendocrine cells and account for 1% to 2% of all tumors of the lung. Patients may present with hemoptysis, have evidence of bronchial obstruction, or be asymptomatic. Carcinoid tumors are often located within a central airway, have a smooth border, and are not calcified.

A history of malignancy is another indicator of possible cancer. The lung is a common site of metastasis from various tumors; the most common are tumors of the breast, head and neck, colon, thyroid gland, and kidney. This patient does not have a history of cancer, and metastases are usually multiple and smoothly bordered but not calcified.

Calcium within a non–small cell carcinoma is unusual and, when present, is eccentric (off-center).

KEY POINT

- Calcification in certain patterns (popcorn, central, diffuse, lamellar) indicates that a pulmonary nodule is probably benign and requires no further investigation.

Bibliography

Gould MK, Fletcher J, Iannettoni MD, et al; American College of Chest Physicians. Evaluation of patients with pulmonary nodules: when is it lung cancer?: ACCP evidence-based clinical practice guidelines (2nd edition). Chest. 2007;132(3 suppl):108S-130S. [PMID: 17873164]

Item 7   Answer: D

Educational Objective: Manage toxic alcohol (ethylene glycol) ingestion.

The most appropriate treatment is intravenous fomepizole and hemodialysis. This patient has acute toxicity from ingestion of ethylene glycol. Ethylene glycol is a component of antifreeze and solvents. Metabolism of ethylene glycol by alcohol dehydrogenase generates various acids, including glycolic, oxalic, and formic acids. Ethylene glycol poisoning initially causes neurologic manifestations similar to ethanol intoxication, and seizures and coma can rapidly develop. If this condition is not treated, noncardiogenic pulmonary edema and cardiovascular collapse may occur. Approximately 24 to 48 hours after ethylene glycol ingestion, patients may develop flank pain and kidney failure that are often accompanied by calcium oxalate crystals in the urine. Fomepizole is an inhibitor of alcohol dehydrogenase and should be given to decrease metabolism of ethylene glycol, which is itself not toxic. Hemodialysis should be started in this patient because there is evidence of end-organ damage to the kidney (elevated serum creatinine, oliguria, and hematuria), an osmolal gap (104 mosm/kg [104 mmol/kg]), and significant anion gap metabolic acidosis (anion gap, 36

CONT.

meq/L [36 mmol/L]), even though the acidosis may be masked by concomitant respiratory alkalosis and metabolic alkalosis from vomiting.

Hemodialysis plays a crucial role in ethylene glycol poisoning, particularly in patients with impending acute kidney failure. Hemodialysis alone would remove toxic metabolites, but without any competitive inhibition, ethylene glycol would continue to be converted into additional toxin.

Intravenous fomepizole or intravenous ethanol alone, without hemodialysis, would be insufficient to rapidly remove the toxic acid metabolites.

Supportive care alone will not be sufficient to prevent acute kidney failure, prevent cardiovascular complications, or correct the acid-base disorder.

KEY POINT
- **The most appropriate treatment for ethylene glycol toxicity is intravenous fomepizole and hemodialysis.**

Bibliography

Jammalamadaka D, Raissi S. Ethylene glycol, methanol and isopropyl alcohol intoxication. Am J Med Sci. 2010;339(3):276-281. [PMID: 20090509]

Item 8   Answer: C
Educational Objective: Manage secondary spontaneous pneumothorax.

The most appropriate next step in management is serial chest radiography. This patient presents with a small, spontaneous pneumothorax in the setting of known COPD. The pneumothorax is therefore classified as a secondary spontaneous pneumothorax. In this case, there is less than 2 cm between the chest wall and lung, and it is reasonable to observe the pneumothorax with serial chest radiography rather than intervene at this time. Given the decreased respiratory reserve and higher likelihood of progression and mortality in this patient group when compared with patients without known underlying structural lung disease (primary spontaneous pneumothorax), observation should be performed in the inpatient setting.

If a persistent air leak is noted after 3 to 5 days, it is reasonable to consider definitive treatment of the pneumothorax. Definitive management to prevent recurrence typically consists of chemical pleurodesis via thoracostomy (which is shown to reduce recurrence to 25%) or thoracoscopic repair with pleurodesis (which reduces recurrence to approximately 5%).

Needle aspiration is an option for treating secondary pneumothoraces, but it has been shown to be significantly less effective than tube thoracostomy in patients requiring therapeutic intervention.

If at any time the pneumothorax increases to greater than 2 cm, a small-bore chest tube should be placed, because the patient is experiencing dyspnea.

KEY POINT
- **For secondary spontaneous pneumothoraces, outpatient management is discouraged; even small (<2 cm) pneumothoraces are more safely observed in the inpatient setting.**

Bibliography

Baumann MH, Strange C, Heffner JE, et al; AACP Pneumothorax Consensus Group. Management of spontaneous pneumothorax: an American College of Chest Physicians Delphi consensus statement. Chest. 2001;119(2):590-602. [PMID: 11171742]

Item 9   Answer: B
Educational Objective: Manage asthma with step-down therapy.

The most appropriate next step in management is to discontinue inhaled corticosteroids and monitor this patient's asthma control over subsequent months. Although inhaled corticosteroids are generally safe, they can be associated with side effects, most commonly local ones such as oral thrush and hoarseness. Their long-term use, particularly in high doses, can lead to systemic side effects such as osteoporosis, cataracts, and glaucoma. When patients with persistent asthma are stable with an infrequent need for rescue medications, they should be evaluated for step-down therapy. This is particularly important when they are experiencing medication-related side effects. Treatment for oral thrush can also be provided.

Adding a long-acting β_2-agonist is not indicated in this patient, because her asthma is very well controlled.

Because hoarseness is most likely related to use of an inhaled corticosteroid, vocal cord examination is not necessary at this point. However, it could be considered if hoarseness persists following the discontinuation of the inhaled corticosteroid.

The addition of a spacer device would reduce the chance of oral deposition and decrease the chance of corticosteroid-related thrush. However, stopping the medication altogether is a better option for this patient.

KEY POINT
- **Regular use of inhaled corticosteroids can result in local and systemic side effects; patients should be evaluated at regular intervals for appropriateness of stepping down therapy to the lowest inhaled corticosteroid dose consistent with adequate disease control.**

Bibliography

National Asthma Education and Prevention Program. Expert Panel Report 3. Guidelines for the Diagnosis and Management of Asthma. Available at: www.nhlbi.nih.gov/guidelines/asthma/asthsumm.pdf. Accessed July 27, 2012.

Answers and Critiques

Item 10   Answer: B

Educational Objective: Manage shock in a hospitalized patient.

This patient should receive an intravenous fluid bolus. Initial resuscitation of a patient with severe sepsis and septic shock should begin early, with a goal of maintaining adequate tissue perfusion with intravenous fluid bolus administration. The defining features of inadequate tissue perfusion may include any of the following: low arterial or central venous pressure, tachycardia, tachypnea, central venous oxygen saturation less than 70%, oliguria, acidosis, delirium, cold extremities, and livedo reticularis.

Replacement-dose hydrocortisone is no longer recommended routinely for patients with septic shock who achieve a systolic blood pressure of at least 90 mm Hg with fluids and vasopressors, although corticosteroids may be useful for patients with more profound, refractory shock. Although an early study reported improved mortality rates in patients with relative adrenal insufficiency who were treated with hydrocortisone and fludrocortisone, the landmark CORTICUS study failed to demonstrate any survival advantage for patients in septic shock with a systolic blood pressure of at least 90 mm Hg. This patient needs a fluid bolus before considering the use of corticosteroids.

Vasopressor therapy with norepinephrine, vasopressin, or dopamine may be necessary when appropriate fluid challenge fails to restore adequate tissue perfusion or during life-threatening hypotension. Vasopressor therapy should not be administered before adequate volume replacement.

Patients with sepsis often are given packed red blood cell transfusion if they have tissue hypoperfusion marked by hypotension or lactic acidosis, active bleeding, profound anemia, or coronary artery disease. In the absence of these indications, erythrocyte transfusion strategies should be approached conservatively. A large, randomized trial showed that a target hemoglobin concentration of 7 to 9 g/dL (70 to 90 g/L) resulted in no additional mortality compared with the traditional target of 10 g/dL (100 g/L).

KEY POINT

- **Patients with shock should receive immediate volume resuscitation and monitoring in the intensive care unit.**

Bibliography

Dellinger RP, Levy MM, Carlet JM, et al; International Surviving Sepsis Campaign Guidelines Committee; American Association of Critical-Care Nurses; American College of Chest Physicians; American College of Emergency Physicians; Canadian Critical Care Society; European Society of Clinical Microbiology and Infectious Diseases; European Society of Intensive Care Medicine; European Respiratory Society; International Sepsis Forum; Japanese Association for Acute Medicine; Japanese Society of Intensive Care Medicine; Society of Critical Care Medicine; Society of Hospital Medicine; Surgical Infection Society; World Federation of Societies of Intensive and Critical Care Medicine. Surviving Sepsis Campaign: international guidelines for management of severe sepsis and septic shock: 2008 [erratum in: Crit Care Med. 2008;36(4):1394-1396]. Crit Care Med. 2008;36(1):296-327. [PMID: 18158437]

Item 11   Answer: D

Educational Objective: Diagnose respiratory muscle weakness.

The most likely diagnosis is respiratory muscle weakness. This patient has progressive dyspnea without other associated respiratory symptoms. He has a modest smoking history and is mildly overweight. His pulmonary function tests show a restrictive pattern without evidence of obstruction and with increased residual volume, which is typical for a patient with respiratory muscle weakness. Residual volume is increased owing to the patient's inability to fully exhale. This patient should be further evaluated with measurement of respiratory muscle forces and a detailed neurologic evaluation. It is important to recognize that dyspnea (related to respiratory muscle weakness) can be the presenting symptom for patients with neuromuscular disease.

Patients with COPD would have increased residual volume, but their total lung capacity would be increased at the same time. The chest radiograph shows low lung volumes, which is more consistent with respiratory muscle weakness.

Heart failure should be considered in patients such as this; however, there are no findings to suggest heart failure, because this patient has no jugular venous distention or edema and his cardiac examination is normal.

Interstitial lung diseases are associated with a reduction in both total lung capacity and residual volume.

KEY POINT

- **Respiratory muscle weakness due to neuromuscular disease is characterized by reduced total lung capacity and increased residual volume (owing to the patient's inability to fully exhale).**

Bibliography

Ambrosino N, Carpenè N, Gherardi M. Chronic respiratory care for neuromuscular diseases in adults. Eur Respir J. 2009;34(2):444-451. [PMID: 19648521]

Item 12   Answer: D

Educational Objective: Manage excessive daytime sleepiness.

The most appropriate next step is for the patient to keep a sleep diary. The most important initial step in the evaluation of the patient with excessive daytime sleepiness (EDS) is to ensure adequate quantities (near 8 hours) of sleep on a regular basis. The clinical history of a graduate student also carrying a part-time job suggests insufficient sleep syndrome. The simplest diagnostic step is a 1- or 2-week sleep diary that identifies the number of hours spent awake and asleep, alerting both patient and provider to the possibility of chronic sleep restriction. If desired, a more objective assessment of sleep schedule can be obtained by a wrist actigraph, a device worn around the wrist that can detect movement and ambient light and generates a report inferring wake and sleep cycles.

Electroencephalography might be useful if the clinical history was suggestive of seizures; however, this is not evident in this patient.

Multiple sleep latency testing can be useful in the evaluation of EDS and may help establish a diagnosis of narcolepsy, but it is resource intensive and expensive. It is usually performed after a sleep diary or actigraphy has excluded insufficient sleep and polysomnography (PSG) has ruled out common sleep disorders such as sleep apnea.

PSG would be indicated if the clinical history strongly suggested a primary sleep disorder such as obstructive sleep apnea (OSA). In this young, relatively thin man without obvious upper airway abnormalities, OSA is unlikely. PSG would be a reasonable next test if the diary or actigraphy suggested adequate sleep quantities.

KEY POINT

- **The most important initial step in the evaluation of the patient with excessive daytime sleepiness is to ensure adequate quantities (near 8 hours) of sleep on a regular basis.**

Bibliography

Kushida CA, Chang A, Gadkary C, Guilleminault C, Carrillo O, Dement WC. Comparison of actigraphic, polysomnographic, and subjective assessment of sleep parameters in sleep-disordered patients. Sleep Med. 2001;2(5):389-396. [PMID: 14592388]

Item 13   Answer: D

Educational Objective: Manage moderate COPD.

The most appropriate management is to begin a long-acting bronchodilator such as tiotropium. The 2011 American College of Physicians, American Thoracic Society, and European Respiratory Society guideline on the diagnosis and management of stable COPD recommends that for stable patients with symptomatic COPD and an FEV_1 of less than 60% of predicted, the treatment is an inhaled bronchodilator (strong recommendation, moderate-quality evidence). Further, the guideline recommends that clinicians prescribe monotherapy using either long-acting inhaled anticholinergics or long-acting inhaled β_2-agonists for symptomatic patients with COPD and FEV_1 less than 60% of predicted (strong recommendation, moderate-quality evidence). There is no evidence that one is superior to the other. Clinicians should base the choice of specific monotherapy on physician or patient preference, cost, and adverse effect profile. For patients with stable COPD with respiratory symptoms and FEV_1 between 60% and 80% of predicted, the guideline suggests that treatment with inhaled bronchodilators may be used (weak recommendation, low-quality evidence).

The guideline suggests that clinicians may administer combination inhaled therapies (long-acting inhaled anticholinergics,

long-acting inhaled β_2-agonists, or inhaled corticosteroids) for symptomatic patients with stable COPD and FEV_1 of less than 60% of predicted (weak recommendation, moderate-quality evidence). An inhaled corticosteroid such as budesonide as monotherapy is not recommended owing to its lack of clinical benefit compared with an inhaled bronchodilator.

Leukotriene modifiers such as montelukast have not been adequately tested in patients with COPD and are not recommended.

A short course of systemic corticosteroids is used in patients with an acute COPD exacerbation, but long-term use of systemic corticosteroids is not recommended owing to adverse effects.

KEY POINT

- **Symptomatic patients with COPD and an FEV_1 less than 60% of predicted should receive long-acting bronchodilator therapy.**

Bibliography

Qaseem A, Wilt TJ, Weinberger SE, et al; American College of Physicians; American College of Chest Physicians; American Thoracic Society; European Respiratory Society. Diagnosis and management of stable chronic obstructive pulmonary disease: a clinical practice guideline update from the American College of Physicians, American College of Chest Physicians, American Thoracic Society, and European Respiratory Society. Ann Intern Med. 2011;155(3):179-191. [PMID: 21810710]

Item 14   Answer: A

Educational Objective: Diagnose a tuberculous pleural effusion.

The most appropriate test to evaluate a possible tuberculous pleural effusion is pleural fluid adenosine deaminase measurement. This patient presents with subacute onset of fever, pleuritic chest pain, and nonproductive cough after traveling to a tuberculosis-endemic region. Pleural fluid analysis is consistent with a lymphocyte-predominant exudate with a low (<10%) eosinophil count and absence of mesothelial cells. All of these features are consistent with, although not specific for, a tuberculous pleural effusion. An adenosine deaminase level greater than 70 units/L is highly specific for tuberculous effusion, whereas a level less than 40 units/L all but excludes it. If pleural adenosine deaminase is elevated, empiric therapy for tuberculosis should be started and pleural biopsy should be performed. If left untreated, the tuberculous effusion will tend to resolve spontaneously over 2 to 4 months; however, up to 65% of these patients will develop active tuberculosis within 5 years.

A negative pleural fluid stain for acid-fast bacilli does not exclude tuberculous pleural involvement, because it is positive in less than 5% of cases in the non–HIV-positive population or in the absence of a tuberculous empyema. Likewise, pleural fluid cultures for tuberculosis are positive in as few as 24% of cases.

This patient's subacute presentation is not consistent with bacterial pneumonia with a parapneumonic effusion. Furthermore, cell counts greater than 10,000 per microliter $(10 \times 10^9/L)$ with a predominance of neutrophils occur most commonly in bacterial parapneumonic effusions. Gram staining the pleural fluid is unlikely to establish the diagnosis for this patient's pleural effusion.

Bibliography

Light RW. Pleural effusions. Med Clin North Am. 2011;95(6):1055-1070. [PMID: 22032427]

Item 15   Answer: D
Educational Objective: Manage ventilatory failure in a patient with Guillain-Barré syndrome.

The most appropriate next step in management is plasma exchange. Plasma exchange and intravenous immune globulin are both recommended treatment options for patients with Guillain-Barré syndrome (GBS), including its most common variant, acute inflammatory demyelinating polyneuropathy. Previous trials indicate plasma exchange reduces the need for and duration of mechanical ventilation in patients with GBS compared with supportive care alone.

Phrenic nerve pacing is not appropriate in the setting of impaired phrenic nerve function, including in patients with GBS and lower motor neuron diseases such as amyotrophic lateral sclerosis. Its use is generally limited to patients with complete high-cervical injuries (C1 and C2 levels) and select patients with brainstem dysfunction with respiratory failure of greater than 3 months' duration.

This patient is at high risk of further respiratory compromise requiring the institution of invasive mechanical ventilation, but he is not a suitable candidate for continuous positive airway pressure (CPAP). His examination, vital capacity, and ability to maintain adequate oxygenation indicate that he is not currently in need of mechanical ventilatory support, and his bulbar dysfunction places him at increased risk of aspiration with use of noninvasive ventilation. Furthermore, bilevel noninvasive ventilation rather than CPAP would be needed to improve his ventilation because the primary issue is respiratory muscle weakness.

Systemic corticosteroids are no longer recommended for the treatment of GBS because previous trials from the 1990s demonstrated no benefit. A more recent study found that the addition of methylprednisolone, 500 mg/d for 5 days, to intravenous immune globulin offers no advantage compared with immune globulin alone.

Bibliography

Raphaël JC, Chevret S, Hughes RA, Annane D. Plasma exchange for Guillain-Barré syndrome. Cochrane Database Syst Rev. 2002;(2):CD001798. [PMID: 12076424]

Item 16   Answer: C
Educational Objective: Diagnose amiodarone pulmonary toxicity.

The most appropriate next step in management is to perform high-resolution CT imaging. This patient presents with chronic dyspnea, dry cough, evidence of restriction on pulmonary function testing, and symptoms that are temporally related to the initiation of amiodarone, an agent that has a known association with pulmonary toxicity. Amiodarone is responsible for several forms of pulmonary toxicity, including chronic interstitial pneumonitis (the most common form), organizing pneumonia, acute respiratory distress syndrome, and a solitary pulmonary mass. Possible risk factors for pulmonary toxicity after initiation of amiodarone are increased age, dose and duration of therapy, and preexisting lung disease. Crude estimates of incidence of pulmonary toxicity secondary to amiodarone exposure versus nonusers are 3.8% and 1.3%, respectively. Owing to this patient's age and presenting symptoms, a high index of suspicion should remain for possible pulmonary toxicity. Up to 20% of patients with interstitial lung disease can present with a normal chest radiograph, so this finding does not preclude a diagnosis of amiodarone pulmonary toxicity. Further testing should be done to determine the extent of parenchymal disease; this is best done using the gold standard of high-resolution CT imaging.

Pulmonary rehabilitation may be helpful for patients with interstitial lung disease, but it will not identify the cause of this patient's symptoms or assist with the ultimate treatment.

Performance of bronchoscopy with bronchoalveolar lavage would be premature at this time. Although this diagnostic test is particularly useful to rule out infection, further imaging studies are required to clarify the extent of parenchymal lung disease.

Inhaled albuterol and ipratropium therapy is not appropriate because this patient's pulmonary function tests demonstrate restriction without evidence of obstructive lung disease.

KEY POINT

- Amiodarone has a high incidence of pulmonary toxicity, including chronic interstitial pneumonitis, organizing pneumonia, acute respiratory distress syndrome, and a solitary pulmonary mass.

Bibliography

Jackevicius CA, Tom A, Essebag V, et al. Population-level incidence and risk factors for pulmonary toxicity associated with amiodarone. Am J Cardiol. 2011;108(5):705-10. [PMID: 21704281]

Item 17   Answer: E

Educational Objective: Manage alcohol withdrawal in the hospital setting.

The most appropriate treatment is lorazepam for delirium tremens syndrome. The term delirium tremens is nearly universally used to refer to delirium due to alcohol withdrawal syndrome. The syndrome usually presents 48 to 96 hours after cessation of drinking, can last up to 2 weeks, and is usually exacerbated at night. The syndrome is characterized by impaired level of consciousness and disorientation (which may fluctuate significantly), reduced attention and global amnesia, impaired cognition and speech, and often hallucinations (usually tactile and/or visual) and delusions (persecutory). The condition can be rapidly fatal if not treated appropriately and aggressively. Seizure activity can occur. Benzodiazepines are the treatment of choice, with doses given as needed based on exhibited signs and symptoms consistent with alcohol withdrawal.

Empiric antibiotics would be appropriate if this patient developed sepsis, but sepsis is an unlikely cause of this patient's delirium, tremulousness, hallucinations, and paranoid ideation. His symptoms are much more suggestive of alcohol withdrawal than sepsis.

CT of the head would be the appropriate management for a suspected intracranial hemorrhage as the cause of this patient's deterioration in mental status. However, this patient does not have evidence of neurologic deficits, making alcohol withdrawal more likely than intracranial hemorrhage.

Haloperidol is used for general delirium, but it is a poor choice for delirium tremens in the setting of alcohol withdrawal because it can lower the seizure threshold and mask symptoms alerting the clinician to the severity of withdrawal.

Lactulose enema would be used in a patient with hepatic encephalopathy. Although hepatic encephalopathy is possible and can account for mental status changes, it cannot explain this patient's agitation, diaphoresis, hallucinations, and tremulousness. In addition, the patient does not manifest evidence of asterixis, typically associated with hepatic encephalopathy.

KEY POINT

- Delirium tremens is characterized by fluctuating level of consciousness, disorientation, reduced attention, global amnesia, impaired cognition and speech, and often hallucinations and delusions.

Bibliography

Amato L, Minozzi S, Davoli M. Efficacy and safety of pharmacological interventions for the treatment of the Alcohol Withdrawal Syndrome. Cochrane Database Syst Rev. 2011;(6):CD008537. [PMID: 21678378]

Item 18   Answer: A

Educational Objective: Treat a patient who has acute respiratory failure with mechanical ventilation.

The most appropriate next step in treatment is intubation and mechanical ventilation. This patient has cardiogenic shock and acute pulmonary edema due to acute decompensated heart failure. Her severe hypoxemia and respiratory distress are the first priority in stabilizing this patient, and therefore the next step in management should be endotracheal intubation and invasive mechanical ventilation. This patient is not a candidate for noninvasive mechanical ventilation. Contraindications to noninvasive ventilation include respiratory arrest, cardiovascular instability (hypotension, arrhythmias, myocardial infarction), change in mental status (lack of cooperation), high aspiration risk, viscous or copious secretions, recent facial or gastroesophageal surgery, craniofacial trauma, fixed nasopharyngeal abnormalities, burns, and extreme obesity. Early trials indicated that noninvasive positive pressure ventilation (NPPV) reduced the need for intubation in the setting of acute cardiogenic pulmonary edema. However, a recently published study found similar outcomes among patients with acute heart failure managed with continuous positive airway pressure, NPPV, and standard oxygen therapy alone, although the discordance with previous studies may be related to study population and design.

Nitroglycerin infusion is commonly used in managing acute decompensated heart failure, but in this instance its use could worsen the patient's hypotension and multiorgan failure. Regardless, stabilizing this patient's respiratory status is a higher priority.

Placement of a pulmonary artery catheter in selected patients can assist in addressing hemodynamic derangements; however, use of a pulmonary artery catheter does not ultimately appear to affect survival in critically ill patients or those with decompensated heart failure and should never take precedence over managing respiratory failure.

KEY POINT

- Contraindications for noninvasive ventilation include respiratory arrest, cardiovascular instability, change in mental status, high aspiration risk, viscous or copious secretions, recent facial or gastroesophageal surgery, craniofacial trauma, fixed nasopharyngeal abnormalities, burns, and extreme obesity.

Bibliography

Weng CL, Zhao YT, Liu QH, et al. Meta-analysis: noninvasive ventilation in acute cardiogenic pulmonary edema. Ann Intern Med. 2010;152(9):590-600. [PMID: 20439577]

Item 19   Answer: B
Educational Objective: Treat anaphylaxis.

The most appropriate treatment is intramuscular or subcutaneous epinephrine and an inhaled β_2-agonist such as albuterol. Initial treatment of anaphylaxis includes basic life support measures with high-flow oxygen, cardiac monitoring, and establishment of intravenous access. These measures are appropriate for asymptomatic patients with a history of a serious reaction and recent reexposure or for patients with local reactions only. This patient is experiencing anaphylaxis from a hypersensitivity reaction to insect venom. Concerns include airway obstruction, bronchospasm, and distributive shock. Of these, the patient has evidence of only bronchospasm at this time, but he should be monitored for the other manifestations of anaphylaxis. The initial treatment is intramuscular or subcutaneous epinephrine. Patients with wheezing should also receive treatment with an inhaled β_2-agonist such as albuterol. Patients with a history of anaphylactic reactions should carry an epinephrine autoinjector and wear an alert bracelet to let responders know of their hypersensitivity.

Mechanical ventilation is incorrect because the patient is showing no sign of respiratory failure or airway closure. If airway closure appears to be a threat and is not avoided by initial treatment with epinephrine, immediate intubation of the trachea is advisable. Signs of a threatened airway could include respiratory stridor, facial or tongue swelling, drooling, or inability to talk in a conscious patient. In some cases of anaphylaxis with airway compromise, intubation using conventional methods may be extremely challenging, and sometimes emergency cricothyrotomy is required to maintain an airway.

Neither antihistamines nor corticosteroids have been shown to improve outcomes in anaphylaxis, and neither agent would reverse this patient's bronchospasm quickly enough. When these agents are used, it is usually in an attempt to prevent a delayed recurrence of symptoms, but even this is not supported by strong evidence of efficacy.

Slow intravenous infusion of epinephrine may be indicated for patients with refractory hypotension. This patient has only mild hypotension; therefore, an intravenous infusion of epinephrine, with its associated risks of arrhythmia, rapid and uncontrolled rise in blood pressure, myocardial infarction, and stroke, is not warranted.

KEY POINT

- The initial treatment of anaphylaxis is with intramuscular or subcutaneous epinephrine.

Bibliography

Sheikh A, Shehata YA, Brown SG, Simons FE. Adrenaline for the treatment of anaphylaxis: cochrane systematic review. Allergy. 2009;64(2):204-212. [PMID: 19178399]

Item 20   Answer: A
Educational Objective: Diagnose allergic bronchopulmonary aspergillosis.

The most appropriate diagnostic test is allergy skin testing for *Aspergillus*. In patients with difficult-to-control asthma and a history of recurrent pulmonary infiltrates, allergic bronchopulmonary aspergillosis (ABPA) should be considered. ABPA is related to a hypersensitivity response to *Aspergillus fumigatus* in patients with asthma. It is characterized by persistent asthma symptoms and pulmonary infiltrate with bronchiectasis. Patients typically have elevated serum IgE levels and eosinophilia along with evidence of sensitization to *A. fumigatus* (high total IgE level, precipitating antibody to *A. fumigatus*). The classic syndrome also includes central bronchiectasis, which is best demonstrated on chest CT scan. All patients with ABPA have evidence of sensitization to *A. fumigatus* that is best demonstrated by allergy skin testing. A positive allergy skin test indicates sensitization, but sensitized patients do not necessarily have ABPA. Therefore, this test has a high sensitivity and negative predictive value. A positive test suggests ABPA and should prompt further evaluation. The next step is typically evaluation of IgE levels; a level greater than 1000 international units/mL (1000 kilounits/L) (normal range, 0-90 international units/mL) suggests ABPA, whereas a level less than 500 international units/mL (500 kilounits/L) argues against the diagnosis.

Bronchoscopy is invasive and carries unnecessary risk in this patient with asthma; therefore, it is not indicated unless there is evidence for an alternative diagnosis or superimposed opportunistic infection.

Sputum Gram stain and culture may confirm the presence of *A. fumigatus*, but it would not be adequate for making a diagnosis.

Sweat chloride testing is indicated to evaluate for cystic fibrosis in patients with a high likelihood of the disease. Cystic fibrosis is a remote possibility in this patient given her age (45 years), the course of her disease, lack of extrapulmonary manifestations (no clubbing or gastrointestinal symptoms), and lack of findings other than bronchiectasis on the chest CT. If the evaluation for ABPA is negative, cystic fibrosis would be reasonable to consider in the differential diagnosis.

KEY POINT

- The initial evaluation of allergic bronchopulmonary aspergillosis includes allergy skin testing for *Aspergillus*; a positive response should be followed by determination of IgE levels.

Bibliography

Agarwal R. Allergic bronchopulmonary aspergillosis. Chest. 2009;135(3):805-826. [PMID: 19265090]

Item 21   Answer: A

Educational Objective: Treat obstructive sleep apnea with continuous positive airway pressure.

The most appropriate next step in treatment is continuous positive airway pressure (CPAP). Obstructive sleep apnea (OSA) is defined by upper airway narrowing or collapse resulting in cessation (apnea) or reduction (hypopnea) in airflow despite ongoing efforts to breathe. The severity of OSA is commonly measured using the apnea-hypopnea index (AHI), the sum of apneas and hypopneas per hour of sleep. An AHI of 5 to 15 indicates mild OSA, an AHI of 16 to 30 indicates moderate sleep apnea, and an AHI of more than 30 indicates severe OSA. It is estimated that 24% of men aged 30 to 60 years and 9% of similarly aged women have OSA (AHI of at least 5/hour). CPAP should be considered first-line therapy in any patient who has OSA and associated symptoms, particularly excessive daytime sleepiness. Optimal positive airway pressure therapy may have salutary effects on cardiovascular diseases that are associated with OSA. Suboptimal adherence to CPAP and bilevel positive airway pressure devices is common in clinical practice, and rates of discontinuation are high. Therefore, objective monitoring of use and periodic follow-up are important to ensure adherence.

Nocturnal oxygen therapy alone is inadequate to prevent complications associated with OSA because it does not correct upper airway obstruction, which is the primary problem related to oxygen desaturation.

Oral devices may be considered for patients who cannot tolerate or are unwilling to use positive airway pressure therapy but should be reserved for patients with mild to moderate OSA.

Surgery may be indicated for patients with specific underlying surgically correctable craniofacial or upper airway abnormalities that contribute to OSA, including nasal polyps, nasal septal deviation, tonsillar enlargement, or retrognathia, although positive airway pressure therapy may still be preferred for such patients. Upper airway surgery may also be considered in selected patients with OSA who desire surgery, reject other therapeutic modalities, and can undergo the procedure.

KEY POINT

- Continuous positive airway pressure is first-line therapy in patients with obstructive sleep apnea and associated symptoms, particularly excessive daytime sleepiness.

Bibliography

Epstein LJ, Kristo D, Strollo PJ Jr, et al; Adult Obstructive Sleep Apnea Task Force of the American Academy of Sleep Medicine. Clinical guideline for the evaluation, management and long-term care of obstructive sleep apnea in adults. J Clin Sleep Med. 2009;5(3):263-276. [PMID: 19960649]

Item 22   Answer: B

Educational Objective: Diagnose fixed airway obstruction using flow-volume loops.

The most appropriate next step in management is to obtain flow-volume loops. This patient presents with significant dyspnea with stridor and evidence of reduced inspiratory as well as expiratory flows without improvement with an inhaled bronchodilator. The diagnosis will be further supported by a flow-volume loop that shows flattening of both inspiratory and expiratory limbs, which is typical of fixed airway obstruction. This is most likely secondary to tracheal stenosis related to recent endotracheal intubation. The diagnosis should be further confirmed with a CT scan (ideally one that includes reconstructed images of the trachea and large airway, also known as virtual bronchoscopy) or direct inspection with flexible fiberoptic bronchoscopy.

This patient's spirometry results and response to bronchodilators are not consistent with an asthma exacerbation. Poorly controlled asthma is associated with a low FEV_1, but there is typically no reduction in inspiratory flows. Therefore, treatment with systemic corticosteroids is not appropriate.

Measurement of lung volumes would likely show reduced total lung capacity because the patient is unable to take a full breath owing to tracheal stenosis. However, this would not provide evidence of a fixed airway obstruction as suspected.

Voice and speech therapy would be appropriate for a patient with confirmed vocal cord dysfunction (VCD). However, this patient's findings are not typical of VCD, which tends to cause more inspiratory wheezing that is generally best heard over the neck without a significant reduction in FEV_1. Flow-volume loops in patients with VCD show a preserved expiratory limb and an inspiratory limb with significant flattening.

KEY POINT

- A flow-volume loop can help determine the cause of airway obstruction; in patients with fixed airway obstruction (such as those with tracheal stenosis), the flow-volume loop shows flattening of both inspiratory and expiratory limbs.

Bibliography

Morshed K, Trojanowska A, Szymanski M, et al. Evaluation of tracheal stenosis: comparison between computed tomography virtual tracheobronchoscopy with multiplanar reformatting, flexible tracheofiberoscopy and intra-operative findings. Eur Arch Otorhinolaryngol. 2011;268(4):591-597. [PMID: 20848120]

Item 23   Answer: C

Educational Objective: Manage inadequately controlled asthma secondary to improper inhaler technique.

The most appropriate next step in management is to check the patient's inhaler technique. This patient's asthma appears to be refractory to his current therapy. Before adding more medications, it is important to ensure that the patient is using his current medications correctly. Poor inhaler technique is a common cause of lack of response to therapy. There are a number of devices on the market for delivery of asthma medications, including metered-dose inhalers and dry powder inhalers. Proper technique is essential for optimal drug delivery to the lungs and reducing side effects related to inhaled corticosteroids, such as oral thrush and dysphonia. A significant proportion of patients with asthma do not use their inhalers appropriately even after receiving instructions when the medications are first prescribed. Therefore, patient education on the proper technique for use of the inhaler should be a component of management of patients with persistent asthma.

Adding a leukotriene receptor antagonist might be appropriate if asthma control is not improved following the proper use of inhaled corticosteroids and β$_2$-agonists.

Prednisone therapy can be appropriate for refractory asthma but should only be used if symptoms and lung functions are not improved following proper inhaler usage. Although systemic corticosteroids are highly effective in management of asthma, they are associated with significant side effects when used on a long-term basis and, therefore, should not be used when topical therapy is adequate for disease control.

Peak flow meters can be used at home for serial measurement of lung function and to assess the relationship of lung function to symptoms. In patients with poor perception of airway obstruction, monitoring peak expiratory flow rate may help detect the loss of asthma control prior to the onset of symptoms. However, a symptom and peak flow diary will not be helpful in improving asthma management in a patient with poor inhaler technique.

KEY POINT

- Poor inhaler technique is a common cause of lack of response to asthma therapy; inhaler technique should be evaluated before therapy is adjusted.

Bibliography

Haughney J, Price D, Kaplan A, et al. Achieving asthma control in practice: understanding the reasons for poor control. Respir Med. 2008;102(12):1681-1693. [PMID: 18815019]

Item 24   Answer: A

Educational Objective: Diagnose occupational lung disease.

A detailed history of this patient's current work exposures should be obtained to evaluate for the possibility of a work-related occupational illness. The symptoms are occurring in an otherwise healthy 28-year-old woman without a clear cause; her exposure to industrial materials at her workplace should be considered as a potential source of occupational lung disease. Metal workers are at particular risk of exposure to metalworking fluids that are used to remove metal turnings and provide cooling and lubrication. These fluids have been associated with respiratory disorders such as lipoid pneumonia, hypersensitivity pneumonitis, and occupational asthma. The metalworking fluid itself, fluid additives, and contaminating bacteria have all been implicated as offending agents. There have been several epidemic presentations of workers with respiratory symptoms associated with metalworking fluid exposure. In addition to inquiring about specific exposures, the patient should be asked about similar symptoms in her co-workers and the temporal relationship of her symptoms to exposure to her work environment (including whether her symptoms improve when away from work for an extended period of time). Material Safety Data Sheets (MSDS) are an important resource for identifying exposures in the workplace and should be available to all employees working around industrial materials. They may be helpful in understanding the nature of materials to which a patient is exposed in the workplace.

Allergy and bronchial challenge testing may have a role in suspected occupational asthma, but linking or excluding the patient's symptoms with her work environment should be pursued before additional testing.

A CT scan of the chest with intravenous contrast is specifically done to evaluate the mediastinal and hilar structures, whereas a CT angiogram protocol is used to evaluate for evidence of pulmonary embolus. Because the findings in the initial high-resolution CT imaging were consistent with hypersensitivity pneumonitis, further imaging with contrast is not indicated.

KEY POINT

- Occupational lung disease should be suspected when symptoms are temporally related to presence in or absence from the workplace, symptoms fail to respond to usual medical therapy, or multiple co-workers have similar symptoms.

Bibliography

Zacharisen MC, Kadambi AR, Schlueter DP, et al. The spectrum of respiratory disease associated with exposure to metal working fluids. J Occup Environ Med. 1998;40(7):640-647. [PMID: 9675723]

Item 25   Answer: C

Educational Objective: Manage mechanical ventilation in a patient with a severe asthma exacerbation.

This patient has severe airflow obstruction caused by status asthmaticus and should be managed with ventilation with a prolonged expiratory time. Ventilation in patients with severe airway obstruction may result in breath stacking and auto–positive end-expiratory pressure (auto-PEEP) if sufficient time is not allowed for the preceding breath to be completely emptied. The goal of managing ventilation in patients with severe airway obstruction is to maximize ventilation by allowing adequate time for exhalation and avoid auto-PEEP with resultant increases in end-expiratory pressures, decreased venous return, hypotension, and barotrauma. Ventilation strategies that increase expiratory time include decreasing the tidal volume and respiration rate, increasing inspiratory flow rates, and judicious use of sedation and analgesia. Clinical suspicion of hemodynamic compromise caused by auto-PEEP should be immediately treated by disconnecting the ventilatory circuit at the endotracheal tube to allow trapped intrathoracic air and pressure to escape and venous return to improve. When ventilating patients with severe airflow obstruction, allowing hypercapnia is a permissible strategy.

Prolonging the inspiratory time will shorten the time spent in the expiratory cycle and worsen auto-PEEP and ventilation. Similarly, decreasing the rate of inspiratory flow will prolong inspiratory time. Increasing the minute ventilation (hyperventilation) may seem like an appropriate strategy in this patient with respiratory acidosis; however, the physiologic limitation of expiratory flow is the primary determinant of minute ventilation in patients with severe obstruction. Attempts to increase minute ventilation (through increases in respiration rate and/or tidal volume) increase the risk for development of auto-PEEP and hemodynamic compromise.

KEY POINT

- The primary ventilator strategy for patients with severe obstructive lung disease is to allow adequate time for exhalation before the next delivered breath and to minimize auto–positive end-expiratory pressure.

Bibliography
Oddo M, Feihl F, Schaller MD, Perret C. Management of mechanical ventilation in acute severe asthma: practical aspects. Intensive Care Med. 2006;32(4):501-510. [PMID: 16552615]

Item 26   Answer: C

Educational Objective: Treat sepsis.

The most appropriate initial treatment is administration of normal saline. The diagnostic criteria for sepsis are the presence of a known or suspected infection (documented positive cultures are not required) and the presence of at least two of the following criteria for the systemic inflammatory response syndrome: temperature greater than 38.0 °C (100.4 °F) or less than 36.0 °C (96.8 °F), leukocyte count greater than 12,000 per microliter (12×10^9/L) or less than 4000 per microliter (4.0×10^9/L), respiration rate greater than 20/min, and pulse rate greater than 90/min. Initial resuscitation of a patient with severe sepsis and septic shock should begin early, with a goal of maintaining adequate tissue perfusion. Most patients need at least 4 to 6 L of intravascular volume replacement within the first 6 hours, and one of the biggest pitfalls of management is underestimating the intravascular volume deficit. Early aggressive fluid resuscitation with intravenous crystalloid has been shown to improve mortality in these patients.

The 2008 Surviving Sepsis guidelines recommend that corticosteroids be avoided in sepsis in the absence of shock unless the patient's endocrine or corticosteroid history warrants it. Intravenous hydrocortisone may also be considered for adult septic shock when hypotension responds poorly to adequate fluid resuscitation and vasopressors.

The patient's blood pressure is stable and she has no signs of hypoperfusion, so there is no indication for vasopressor therapy at this time. In patients with known or suspected infection, persistent hypotension despite adequate fluid resuscitation mandates the use of vasopressors.

Although this patient is anemic, there is no evidence of active bleeding at this time. Transfusion is recommended for patients with sepsis if the central venous oxygen saturation is less than 70% after adequate fluid challenge or if the hematocrit is below 30%, but it would not be appropriate at this time. This patient has not yet received an adequate fluid challenge, and her hematocrit is 32%.

KEY POINT

- Initial resuscitation of a patient with severe sepsis and septic shock should begin early, with a goal of maintaining adequate tissue perfusion with intravascular volume replacement.

Bibliography
Dellinger RP, Levy MM, Carlet JM, et al; International Surviving Sepsis Campaign Guidelines Committee; American Association of Critical-Care Nurses; American College of Chest Physicians; American College of Emergency Physicians; Canadian Critical Care Society; European Society of Clinical Microbiology and Infectious Diseases; European Society of Intensive Care Medicine; European Respiratory Society; International Sepsis Forum; Japanese Association for Acute Medicine; Japanese Society of Intensive Care Medicine; Society of Critical Care Medicine; Society of Hospital Medicine; Surgical Infection Society; World Federation of Societies of Intensive and Critical Care Medicine. Surviving Sepsis Campaign: international guidelines for management of severe sepsis and septic shock: 2008 [erratum in Crit Care Med. 2008;36(4):1394-1396]. Crit Care Med. 2008;36(1):296-327. [PMID: 18158437]

Item 27　Answer:　C

Educational Objective: Manage a small pulmonary nodule in a patient at risk for lung cancer.

The most appropriate next step in management is a CT scan of the chest in 12 months. The Fleischner Society and the American College of Chest Physicians guidelines recommend a follow-up CT at 12 months for current or former smokers with pulmonary nodules less than 4 mm; if the nodule is unchanged at that point, no further follow-up is required. Studies evaluating the risk for lung cancer in patients at risk show that nodules of this size have a risk of malignancy of less than 1%. No follow-up is necessary for nodules that are smaller than 4 mm in never-smokers with no other known risk factors for malignancy (history of a first-degree relative with lung cancer or significant radon or asbestos exposure). Nodules 4 mm or larger should be further evaluated according to the recommendations in the guidelines. A new nodule larger than 8 mm for which there are no old images should prompt a calculation of the probability of malignancy and consideration of additional imaging or biopsy. Review of previous chest imaging studies is important in the evaluation of nodules to determine whether a nodule is stable, becoming larger, or shrinking. In addition to previous chest radiographs and chest CT scans, abdominal imaging (which shows the lower aspect of the chest) and CT scans done to assess the coronary arteries (which show the lungs) should be reviewed. A solid nodule that is stable on chest radiograph or CT scan for 2 years is considered benign. Growth of a nodule is a strong indicator that it may be malignant.

Follow-up at a shorter interval is not recommended for nodules of this size owing to the low risk of malignancy and to reduce unnecessary scanning and radiation exposure.

KEY POINT

- In former or current smokers, a pulmonary nodule that is less than 4 mm should be evaluated at 12 months with follow-up CT; if the nodule is unchanged, no further follow-up is required.

Bibliography

Gould MK, Fletcher J, Iannettoni MD, et al; American College of Chest Physicians. Evaluation of patients with pulmonary nodules: when is it lung cancer?: ACCP evidence-based clinical practice guidelines (2nd edition). Chest. 2007;132(3 suppl):108S-130S. [PMID: 17873164]

Item 28　Answer:　D

Educational Objective: Manage tricyclic antidepressant overdose.

The most appropriate management is sodium bicarbonate infusion. This patient has taken an overdose of a tricyclic antidepressant (TCA), which can have a wide variety of physiologic effects, including inhibition of presynaptic reuptake of norepinephrine and serotonin, blockade of cardiac muscle fast sodium channels, anticholinergic effects, peripheral α-receptor blockade, antihistamine activity, and γ-aminobutyric acid (GABA)–receptor blockade in the central nervous system. Most deaths due to TCA overdose are caused by cardiovascular collapse with refractory hypotension or lethal arrhythmias such as ventricular tachycardia or ventricular fibrillation. The best agent to use in this setting is sodium bicarbonate, given as boluses or as an infusion, which appears to narrow the QRS complex and decrease the risk of tachyarrhythmias. Although the mechanisms of bicarbonate therapy in TCA overdose are not well described, it is believed that the increased serum pH minimizes binding of the drug to sodium channels and that the increased serum sodium concentration alters the gradient across sodium channels, decreasing the risk of arrhythmic potentials in the myocardium. The electrocardiogram should be monitored for evidence of normalization of the typically widened QRS complex.

Naloxone is not appropriate because there is no evidence of opioid overdose. Naloxone is often given empirically in the early care of a patient with undiagnosed coma, but it would not have any effect on the electrocardiogram changes, which signal the possibility of an impending arrhythmia.

Procainamide, as well as most other antiarrhythmic medications, is contraindicated in TCA overdose. Class IA antiarrhythmics such as procainamide inhibit cardiac sodium channels just as TCAs do, and they would likely worsen the problems with arrhythmias. Class III agents such as amiodarone may prolong the QT interval and thereby exacerbate arrhythmias as well; however, torsades de pointes is an uncommon arrhythmia in this setting.

Saline diuresis, the administration of normal saline in conjunction with a diuretic to significantly increase urine output, is not appropriate because it does not increase the rate of clearance of lipophilic, highly bound molecules of TCA.

KEY POINT

- Sodium bicarbonate is the best therapeutic agent in the setting of tricyclic antidepressant overdose.

Bibliography

Body R, Bartram T, Azam F, Mackway-Jones K. Guidelines in Emergency Medicine Network (GEMNet): guideline for the management of tricyclic antidepressant overdose. Emerg Med J. 2011;28(4):347-368. [PMID: 21436332]

Item 29　Answer:　A

Educational Objective: Manage asthma during pregnancy.

The most appropriate next step in management is to add a long-acting β$_2$-agonist and continue inhaled corticosteroids. Approximately one third of patients with asthma experience worsening of disease control during pregnancy. Although this patient has had good control on medium-dose inhaled corticosteroids previously, the same regimen is not providing adequate control at this point. The recommendation for step-up therapy in pregnant patients is similar to that for nonpregnant patients, with the understanding that it is safer for pregnant women to be exposed to asthma medications with limited human safety data than it is to experience ongoing symptoms and exacerbations of asthma. Long-acting β_2-agonists are classified as pregnancy category C, meaning the evidence of some safety is lacking but the potential benefit of the drug may justify the potential risk. Despite this, the addition of a long-acting β_2-agonist is recommended when symptoms are not controlled with medium-dose inhaled corticosteroids because the addition of this medication results in better asthma control compared with doubling the dose of inhaled corticosteroids. This is based on studies performed in non-pregnant patients; large-scale studies have not been performed in pregnant patients.

Theophylline is also classified as a pregnancy category C drug. Theophylline is an alternative to adding a long-acting β_2-agonist as step-up therapy; however, because the drug's metabolism is altered during pregnancy and therefore requires more frequent monitoring of levels, a long-acting β_2-agonist is preferred over theophylline.

A bronchial challenge test (methacholine or mannitol) can be performed to evaluate patients whose symptoms are not clearly consistent with asthma, but methacholine challenge is contraindicated during pregnancy. Mannitol is listed as pregnancy category C; adequate information is not available on its safety during pregnancy. Furthermore, bronchial challenge is not likely to provide clinically useful information in this patient.

KEY POINT

- In pregnant patients with asthma, the addition of a long-acting β_2-agonist is recommended when symptoms are not controlled with medium-dose inhaled corticosteroids.

Bibliography

Schatz M, Dombrowski MP. Clinical practice. Asthma in pregnancy. N Engl J Med. 2009;360(18):1862-1869. [PMID: 19403904]

Item 30   Answer: A

Educational Objective: Treat continuous positive airway pressure–related rhinitis.

The most appropriate next step in management is to add heated humidification to the continuous positive airway pressure (CPAP) circuit. Nasal congestion is a common side effect of CPAP therapy, owing in part to desiccation of the nasal mucosa. The addition of in-line heated humidity, preferably with distilled water, is a simple, effective method to combat CPAP-associated nasal congestion.

Excessive daytime sleepiness may persist despite adherence to positive airway pressure therapy in some patients with obstructive sleep apnea (OSA). Modafinil, a wake-promoting agent, is an adjunctive therapy to improve residual daytime sleepiness in patients receiving optimal positive airway pressure therapy. Because full-night compliance has been limited by nasal congestion, this patient has not yet realized the full symptomatic benefits of CPAP, which can take as long as 3 months to fully appear. Therefore, it is premature to prescribe modafinil.

Oxymetazoline nasal spray should not be used to treat CPAP-associated congestion because of the risk of rhinitis medicamentosa. Rhinitis medicamentosa refers to the syndrome of rebound nasal congestion after discontinuing topical α-adrenergic decongestant sprays such as oxymetazoline. Symptoms may occur after using these sprays for 5 or more days and resolve with prolonged discontinuation of these agents.

Nasal surgery might be a treatment option for mild sleep apnea in patients with a substantial degree of nasal obstruction, but it would not be a primary therapy for CPAP-related nasal congestion. Surgery is indicated for patients with specific underlying surgically correctable craniofacial or upper airway abnormalities that contribute to OSA, including nasal polyps, nasal septal deviation, or tonsillar enlargement. Upper airway surgery may also be considered in selected patients with OSA who desire surgery, reject other therapeutic modalities, and can undergo the procedure.

KEY POINT

- **The addition of in-line heated humidity to continuous positive airway pressure (CPAP) therapy is a simple, effective method to combat CPAP-associated nasal congestion.**

Bibliography

Neill AM, Wai HS, Bannan SP, Beasley CR, Weatherall M, Campbell AJ. Humidified nasal continuous positive airway pressure in obstructive sleep apnea. Eur Respir J. 2003;22(2):258-262. [PMID: 12952257]

Item 31   Answer: D

Educational Objective: Evaluate for tuberculosis in a patient with pulmonary silicosis.

The most appropriate next step in management is evaluation for tuberculosis with purified protein derivative testing and sputum testing for acid-fast bacilli. Silicosis is a spectrum of pulmonary disease related to inhalation of crystalline silicon dioxide (silica). Silica is the most abundant mineral on earth, and the most common form is quartz. Any occupation that disturbs the earth's crust or uses or processes silica-containing rock or sand has potential risks. A number of other medical conditions are associated with silicosis and are believed to be due to immune dysfunction induced by silicon exposure. This includes an increased susceptibility to tuberculosis and autoimmune diseases such as systemic sclerosis, rheumatoid arthritis, and systemic lupus erythematosus. A recent investigation by the Centers for Disease Control and Prevention examined silicosis mortality rates associated with respiratory tuberculosis between the years of 1968 and 2006. Of the reported deaths, tuberculosis was on 14% of the death certificates. Seventy-three percent of these patients were older than 65 years, and greater than 99% were male. There has been a steady decline in the total number of deaths related to silicosis and concomitant tuberculosis infection. This is likely attributable to prevention and control measures to prevent silica dust exposure as well as to appropriately treat and contain tuberculosis.

A high-resolution chest CT would provide more detailed structural information concerning this patient's lung disease and might be abnormal if he has tuberculosis, but it would not be the appropriate next study to evaluate for that potential diagnosis.

In patients with a known exposure and characteristic radiographic findings, lung biopsy is generally not needed to establish the diagnosis of silicosis. Additionally, in this patient with a long-standing diagnosis, stable clinical course, and no radiographic changes from his stable baseline, a lung biopsy is not currently indicated.

Corticosteroids have been used in some trials to attempt to modulate the immune reaction to silica and may be of some benefit, particularly in patients with acute or severe disease; however, it is not considered an established therapy for chronic silicosis. In addition, it would be inappropriate therapy until tuberculosis is excluded as a cause of this patient's systemic symptoms.

KEY POINT

- Silicosis is a spectrum of pulmonary disease related to inhalation of crystalline silicon dioxide (silica), and it is associated with an increased risk for tuberculosis.

Bibliography

Nasrullah M, Mazurek JM, Wood JM, Bang KM, Kreiss K. Silicosis mortality with respiratory tuberculosis in the United States, 1968-2006. Am J Epidemiol. 2011;174(7):839-848. [PMID: 21828370]

Item 32   Answer: B
Educational Objective: Manage an acute exacerbation of COPD.

The most appropriate next step in management is hospital admission. Although many COPD exacerbations may be managed with in-home therapy, hospital admission should be considered in patients with severe disease, advanced age, significant comorbidities, a marked increase in intensity of symptoms, newly occurring arrhythmias, diagnostic uncertainty, insufficient home support, or onset of new physical signs, as well as failure to respond adequately to initial

medical management, as in this patient. This patient has multiple comorbidities, has not responded to appropriate outpatient treatment, and now has a mild oxygen requirement. She should be admitted to the hospital for more aggressive treatment with inhaled bronchodilators, continuous oxygen therapy, pulmonary toilet, antibiotics, corticosteroids, and monitoring for potential complications.

Home oxygen is frequently used in patients with COPD; however, this patient's new resting hypoxia suggests a lack of improvement or worsening of her current exacerbation. Therefore, providing home oxygen alone as a next therapeutic step would not be appropriate.

This patient has purulent sputum, an increase in sputum volume, and worsening dyspnea; therefore, antibiotic treatment is appropriate. The initial antibiotic choice was appropriate, but empiric expansion of antibiotic coverage is not indicated in the absence of additional risk factors.

Corticosteroids have been shown to be effective in treating acute COPD exacerbations. Although the ideal dose and duration of therapy are not well defined, prolonging this patient's treatment course alone in the context of her failure to improve would not be appropriate.

KEY POINT

- Patients with COPD exacerbations should be admitted to the hospital if they have underlying severe COPD and advanced age, significant comorbidities, marked increase in intensity of symptoms, failure to respond to initial medical management, newly occurring arrhythmias, diagnostic uncertainty, insufficient home support, or onset of new physical signs.

Bibliography

Global Strategy for Diagnosis, Management, and Prevention of COPD. December 2011. Available at: www.goldcopd.org. Accessed July 27, 2012.

Item 33   Answer: A
Educational Objective: Evaluate for cystic fibrosis in a patient whose disease mimics asthma.

The most appropriate management is measurement of sweat chloride. This young man has been diagnosed with asthma, but he is more likely to have cystic fibrosis based on his symptoms and the presence of clubbing and upper-lobe bronchiectasis. The diagnosis should be confirmed with measurement of sweat chloride, which is elevated (greater than 60 meq/L [60 mmol/L]) in patients with cystic fibrosis. Genetic testing for cystic fibrosis is recommended for patients who have positive sweat chloride tests and helps support the diagnosis. Most cases of cystic fibrosis are diagnosed during childhood; however, delayed diagnosis can occur in patients with a mild form of cystic fibrosis, who are often misdiagnosed as having asthma when the symptoms are limited to the respiratory tract.

Answers and Critiques

Diagnostic bronchoscopy can be helpful in patients with regional bronchiectasis to exclude proximal airway obstruction. However, in this patient bronchoscopy is unlikely to lead to additional information, and it is a more invasive test than the measurement of sweat chloride.

Echocardiography is helpful in evaluating patients with clubbing suspected of having congenital heart disease; however, this patient has no other stigmata to suggest congenital heart disease, such as a loud pathologic murmur, asymmetric pulses, evidence of heart failure, or cyanosis.

Keeping a home diary of asthma symptoms and/or peak expiratory flow rate can be helpful to assess asthma control; however, in this patient with good inhaler technique, the persistence of symptoms is not likely to be related to asthma. In addition, uncontrolled asthma cannot explain the presence of bronchiectasis and clubbing in this patient.

KEY POINT

- Delayed diagnosis can occur in patients with a mild form of cystic fibrosis; these patients are often misdiagnosed as having asthma when symptoms are limited to the respiratory tract.

Bibliography

National Asthma Education and Prevention Program. Expert Panel Report 3. Guidelines for the Diagnosis and Management of Asthma. Available at: www.nhlbi.nih.gov/guidelines/asthma/asthsumm.pdf. Accessed July 27, 2012.

Item 34   Answer: B
Educational Objective: Evaluate the radiation risk of CT scanning.

A high-resolution CT scan is the best test to evaluate the interstitial infiltrates identified on chest radiograph. The pattern of infiltrates with restrictive pulmonary function indicates a differential that includes idiopathic pulmonary fibrosis, nonspecific interstitial pneumonia, cryptogenic organizing pneumonia, and hypersensitivity pneumonia among others, and CT would help narrow the differential. Although unnecessary and repetitive CT scans are a concern, a CT scan of the chest confers an effective dose of radiation in the range of 5 to 7 millisieverts (mSv) and is comparable to the amount of radiation a person receives from ambient solar radiation over 1 year. A CT study confers about 40 times the radiation of a single posteroanterior chest radiograph (0.1-0.2 mSv). Although the risk is small, evidence from epidemiologic studies supports that the dose of radiation associated with two or three CT scans results in increased risk of cancer. The use of CT has risen dramatically in the past couple of decades, and prudent use of repetitive CT is advised.

Although MRI scanning is not associated with radiation exposure, it has a limited role in lung imaging. Chest MRI requires longer imaging times and is more susceptible to artifact, and the resolution is not ideal for assessing parenchymal disorders. It is therefore not a preferred imaging method for most lung diseases.

PET is based on the uptake of radiolabeled 18-fluorodeoxyglucose in metabolically active areas of the lung associated with inflammation or malignancy. It is frequently coupled with CT scanning (PET-CT) to provide further anatomic localization. Although PET scanning without CT is associated with minimal radiation exposure, it would not lead to clinically meaningful information in this patient.

Ventilation/perfusion scanning is a nuclear medicine study involving the concurrent injection and inhalation of a radiotracer. It has been used primarily in the diagnosis of pulmonary embolism by indicating areas of ventilation and perfusion mismatch. However, this study would not be indicated or helpful in this patient.

KEY POINT

- The risk associated with radiation from a CT of the chest is small, and the risk is usually acceptable when a CT study is the most appropriate test.

Bibliography

Smith-Bindman R, Lipson J, Marcus R, et al. Radiation dose associated with common computed tomography examinations and the associated lifetime attributable risk of cancer. Arch Intern Med. 2009;169(22):2078-2086. [PMID: 20008690]

Item 35   Answer: C
Educational Objective: Diagnose vocal cord dysfunction.

The most appropriate next step in management is laryngoscopy. Patients with vocal cord dysfunction (VCD) have inspiratory and expiratory wheezing, respiratory distress, and anxiety. During attacks, VCD can be difficult to distinguish from asthma. Potential clues include sudden onset and abrupt termination of the attacks, lack of response to asthma therapy, prominent neck discomfort, lack of hypoxemia, and lack of hyperinflation on chest radiography. The distinction between the two conditions can be more difficult when patients have asthma as well as VCD. Laryngoscopy in symptomatic patients can reveal characteristic adduction of the vocal cords during inspiration. Alternatively, a flow-volume loop (in which the patient is asked to take a deep breath and then exhale while the inspiratory and expiratory flows are recorded) may be useful. In patients with VCD, the inspiratory limb of the flow-volume loop is "cut off" owing to narrowing of the extrathoracic airway (at the level of the vocal cords) during inspiration. The expiratory flows are preserved. Recognizing VCD is essential to avoid treating patients with repeat courses of systemic corticosteroids and other therapies for severe asthma while delaying the start of therapies targeted at VCD. These include speech therapy, relaxation techniques, and treatment of underlying causes such as anxiety, postnasal drip, and gastroesophageal reflux.

Chest radiograph in patients with acute asthma is not indicated unless the patient does not respond to initial therapy, has severe exacerbations, has clinical evidence of a concurrent illness (such as fever to suggest pneumonia, or crackles and leg edema to suggest heart failure), has evidence of a complication (subcutaneous air, asymmetric breath sounds that may suggest pneumothorax), or requires hospitalization.

Intravenous magnesium sulfate can be considered in acute asthma exacerbations, but it has no role in treating VCD.

There is no indication for antibiotics in this patient even if an acute asthma exacerbation were suspected.

KEY POINT

- Potential clues for vocal cord dysfunction include sudden onset and abrupt termination of attacks, lack of response to asthma therapy, prominent neck discomfort, and lack of hypoxemia.

Bibliography

Benninger C, Parsons JP, Mastronarde JG. Vocal cord dysfunction and asthma. Curr Opin Pulm Med. 2011;17(1):45-49. [PMID: 21330824]

Item 36   Answer: A
Educational Objective: Treat ventilatory failure caused by opioids.

The most appropriate next step in managing this patient's encephalopathy is to administer a higher dose of naloxone. This patient's nonfocal neurologic examination, pinpoint pupils, shallow respirations, respiration rate less than 12/min, and hypothermia are all highly suggestive of opioid intoxication. Given the high suspicion for opioid intoxication, this patient should be treated with additional naloxone. Escalating doses, typically 0.4 mg to 1 mg, are used every few minutes until the patient has adequate spontaneous ventilation and airway protection. Once this is achieved, the patient should be closely monitored for recurrent excess somnolence, in which case repeat dosing or naloxone infusion is indicated. Patients who do not respond to a total dose of 5 to 10 mg should undergo evaluation for alternative causes of encephalopathy.

Immediate endotracheal intubation and initiation of invasive mechanical ventilation are not necessary at this time. There is no evidence of aspiration or severe hypoxemia, and it is likely that this patient's ventilatory failure can be rapidly reversed with naloxone.

Hypoglycemia is unusual in patients not taking insulin or other hypoglycemic agents. Most patients do not experience symptoms of hypoglycemia until the blood glucose level is less than 60 mg/dL (3.3 mmol/L), more often less than 40 to 55 mg/dL (2.2 to 3.1 mmol/L). This patient's blood glucose is at an acceptable level, and the administration of intravenous glucose is not necessary.

A noncontrast CT of the head is used to evaluate for intracranial hemorrhage in patients with possible stroke. This patient has encephalopathy without focal neurologic deficits, which makes stroke much less likely than opioid intoxication.

KEY POINT

- Patients with suspected opioid intoxication should receive the opioid antagonist naloxone to rapidly reverse excess sedation.

Bibliography

Dahan A, Aarts L, Smith TW. Incidence, Reversal, and Prevention of Opioid-induced Respiratory Depression. Anesthesiology. 2010;112(1):226-238. [PMID: 20010421]

Item 37   Answer: D
Educational Objective: Assess risk for recurrent pulmonary embolism.

The most appropriate next step in management is to restart anticoagulation. Patients with a first unprovoked episode of deep venous thrombosis (DVT) or pulmonary embolism (PE) should receive anticoagulation for a period of 3 months and then be evaluated for the risks/benefits of anticoagulation cessation. This patient is relatively young and otherwise healthy, and he has done well during a 3-month course of anticoagulation for a recent episode of idiopathic PE (that is, unprovoked PE). However, he is now back to work at his sedentary occupation. Results of a D-dimer assay performed after a period of anticoagulation therapy have been shown to be predictive of thrombotic recurrence. The assay must be done 3 to 4 weeks after warfarin therapy is stopped. An elevated high-sensitivity D-dimer assay result predicts an increased risk for recurrence by at least fourfold compared with a normal result. Thus, a positive assay provides further impetus to continue long-term anticoagulation, whereas a normal assay might lead to cessation of therapy because of an altered risk/benefit ratio for continued anticoagulation. Because this patient has no history or findings that raise the risk of anticoagulation, it would be appropriate to restart anticoagulation for an indefinite period.

Measuring the B-type natriuretic peptide level might be helpful if there were concern for pulmonary hypertension due to an acute PE or to chronic thromboembolic disease; however, neither seems likely in this patient. Moreover, a normal result would not eliminate the indication for restarting anticoagulation.

Venous Doppler ultrasonography of the legs may be useful if there is concern for DVT. However, even if the study is negative, restarting anticoagulation is still appropriate for the reasons noted above.

Although a normalized D-dimer on a repeat test in 1 month would be reassuring, deferring anticoagulation may place the patient at ongoing risk for PE and DVT.

- Results of a D-dimer assay performed after a period of anticoagulation therapy have been shown to be predictive of thrombotic recurrence.

Bibliography

Guyatt GH, Akl EA, Crowther M, Gutterman DD, Schünemann HJ; American College of Chest Physicians Antithrombotic Therapy and Prevention of Thrombosis Panel. Executive summary: Antithrombotic Therapy and Prevention of Thrombosis, 9th ed: American College of Chest Physicians Evidence-Based Clinical Practice Guidelines. Chest. 2012;141(2 suppl):7S-47S. [PMID: 22315257]

Item 38   Answer: A

Educational Objective: Treat inadequately controlled asthma.

The most appropriate treatment is to add a long-acting β_2-agonist inhaler. This patient has been doing well until her recent exacerbation. Her asthma is now moderate persistent based on the Expert Panel Report (EPR) guidelines (daily symptoms of asthma and nocturnal awakenings more than once per week), and the symptoms are not well controlled on a moderate dose of inhaled corticosteroids. The EPR guidelines recommend the addition of a long-acting β_2-agonist in such a patient because this has been proved to lead to greater improvement in asthma control compared with doubling the dose of inhaled corticosteroids. The systemic side effects of inhaled corticosteroids are relatively uncommon but do occur in patients on high-dose therapy (particularly long-term, high-dose therapy). These effects include adrenal suppression, glaucoma, cataracts, osteopenia, and skin thinning. Therefore, the lowest dose consistent with disease control should always be used. Finally, therapy by metered-dose inhaler with various agents is essential in asthma. Patients should be shown the proper technique for using inhalers, and any patients with poorly controlled disease should be evaluated for the proper inhaler technique.

Ipratropium enhances the bronchodilator effect of β_2-agonists when given for acute asthma exacerbations; however, its use for long-term control of asthma is not generally recommended. Recent studies by the Asthma Clinical Research Network demonstrated that the addition of a long-acting anticholinergic drug (tiotropium) was equivalent to the addition of a long-acting β_2-agonist in patients with asthma whose symptoms are inadequately controlled with inhaled corticosteroids alone.

Although macrolide antibiotics are beneficial in treating atypical respiratory tract infections (which can be associated with asthma exacerbations and asthma-like symptoms), their routine use in treatment of asthma is not recommended and has not been shown to improve asthma control.

- Guidelines recommend the addition of a long-acting β_2-agonist to medium-dose corticosteroids in patients with moderate persistent asthma because this has been proved to lead to greater improvement in asthma control compared with doubling the dose of inhaled corticosteroids.

Bibliography

National Asthma Education and Prevention Program. Expert Panel Report 3. Guidelines for the Diagnosis and Management of Asthma. Available at: www.nhlbi.nih.gov/guidelines/asthma/asthsumm.pdf. Accessed July 27, 2012.

Item 39   Answer: D

Educational Objective: Treat an acute exacerbation of idiopathic pulmonary fibrosis.

The most appropriate treatment is to initiate narcotics to palliate shortness of breath without pursuit of mechanical ventilation. Multiple retrospective series of patients with idiopathic pulmonary fibrosis (IPF) who have been intubated and mechanically ventilated for acute respiratory failure have demonstrated extremely poor outcomes. Two recent studies demonstrated in-hospital mortality rates of 86% and 97% in this patient population. This patient has evidence of an acute exacerbation of IPF without a known cause. He has been treated for several days with further evidence of clinical worsening. The likelihood of recovery is remote and, as a result, the most recent evidence-based guidelines recommend reducing unnecessary suffering and not pursuing mechanical ventilation in this patient population.

Initiating antifungal treatment in addition to this patient's broad-spectrum antibiotics is not appropriate because he has no clear evidence of bacterial or fungal infection, given the lack of consistent findings on his imaging studies and negative sputum culture. Acute exacerbations of IPF are typically treated with antibiotics empirically without obvious evidence of infection; this patient has already been treated with broad coverage for several days without evidence of improvement.

Evidence is limited for the efficacy of high-dose corticosteroids in patients with an acute exacerbation of IPF. Pathology specimens from patients with an acute exacerbation most often demonstrate a background of usual interstitial pneumonia with scattered areas of hyaline membranes. There have been occasional reports of organizing pneumonia as the predominant pathologic feature; corticosteroids may be of benefit when organizing pneumonia is present. However, this patient has already been treated with corticosteroids for 7 days, and the likelihood of clinical response to additional corticosteroids is low.

Nebulized albuterol is not appropriate in this patient because the physiologic abnormality in IPF is restrictive lung disease. The use of bronchodilators would be of little clinical benefit in this situation.

> **KEY POINT**
>
> - Patients with acute exacerbations of idiopathic pulmonary fibrosis have a remote likelihood of recovery; therefore, the most recent evidence-based guidelines recommend reducing unnecessary suffering and not pursuing mechanical ventilation in this patient population.

Bibliography

Raghu G, Collard HR, Egan JJ, et al; ATS/ERS/JRS/ALAT Committee on Idiopathic Pulmonary Fibrosis. An official ATS/ERS/JRS/ALAT statement: idiopathic pulmonary fibrosis: evidence-based guidelines for diagnosis and management. Am J Respir Crit Care Med. 2011;183(6):788-824. [PMID: 21471066]

Item 40   Answer: C

Educational Objective: Treat hypoxemic respiratory failure with continuous positive airway pressure.

The most appropriate next step in management is continuous positive airway pressure (CPAP). This patient's presentation is most consistent with hypoxemia due to postoperative atelectasis. Obesity, which reduces end-expiratory lung volumes, coupled with curtailed diaphragmatic excursion from upper abdominal surgery, places patients undergoing bariatric surgery at increased risk of postoperative atelectasis. The diminished basilar breath sounds on examination correlate with the low lung volumes noted on chest radiograph, which also revealed linear opacities consistent with platelike atelectasis. Previous trials found that CPAP reduces the need for intubation and risk of pneumonia in patients with hypoxemia complicating abdominal surgery and lung resection.

Bronchoscopy can be useful in the evaluation and management of postoperative lobar or complete-lung atelectasis, which is typically caused by mucus plugging. Generally, chest physiotherapy is considered first-line treatment with bronchoscopy reserved for refractory cases. However, this patient's basilar, platelike atelectasis is due to shallow inspiration with collapse of distal airways rather than mucus plugging and would not be amenable to bronchoscopic intervention.

Administering continuous albuterol by nebulizer would be appropriate if this patient were having an asthma exacerbation; however, the absence of wheezes and accessory muscle use on examination and the presence of atelectasis rather than hyperinflation on chest radiograph make it much less likely that asthma is the cause of this patient's hypoxemia.

Naloxone might be appropriate if this patient's hypoxemia were due to hypoventilation from the residual sedating effects of operative sedation and analgesia. However, this patient is alert, and his arterial blood gas studies indicate acute hypoxemic rather than hypercapnic failure.

> **KEY POINT**
>
> - Continuous positive airway pressure reduces the need for intubation and risk of pneumonia in patients with hypoxemia complicating abdominal surgery and lung resection.

Bibliography

Squadrone V, Coha M, Cerutti E, et al; Piedmont Intensive Care Units Network (PICUN). Continuous positive airway pressure for treatment of postoperative hypoxemia: a randomized controlled trial. JAMA. 2005;293(5):589-595. [PMID: 15687314]

Item 41   Answer: B

Educational Objective: Manage immunizations in a patient with COPD.

The most appropriate immunization regimen for this patient is influenza and pneumococcal vaccines now. Pneumococcal vaccine may be administered concurrently with other vaccines, such as the influenza vaccine, but at a separate site. Waiting for the next scheduled routine visit to administer the pneumococcal vaccine carries a risk of not administering the vaccine in a timely fashion and the possibility of failing to administer the vaccine at all. Influenza and pneumococcal vaccines are recommended for patients with COPD. Influenza vaccine is recommended annually for all adults. High-dose influenza vaccine is an option for patients 65 years and older. Pneumococcal vaccine is recommended for adults 65 years and older. Pneumococcal vaccine is recommended for all adults regardless of age if they have the following chronic conditions: chronic lung disease (including asthma), chronic liver disease, diabetes mellitus, cirrhosis, chronic alcoholism, functional or anatomic asplenia, immunocompromising conditions (including chronic kidney failure or the nephritic syndrome), cochlear implants, or cerebrospinal fluid leaks. Other indications are smokers and residents of nursing homes or long-term care facilities. One-time revaccination is indicated after 5 years for persons aged 19 to 64 years with the nephritic syndrome or chronic kidney failure, functional or anatomic asplenia, and immunocompromising conditions. One-time revaccination is recommended for patients who were vaccinated 5 or more years ago and were less than 65 years of age at the time of primary vaccination. The 7-valent pneumococcal polysaccharide vaccine seems to induce a superior immune response than the 23-valent-pneumococcal polysaccharide vaccine. Data suggest that influenza vaccination, but not pneumococcal vaccination, is associated with reduced all-cause mortality.

KEY POINT

- Influenza and pneumococcal vaccines are recommended for patients with COPD and can be administered at the same time but at different sites.

Bibliography

Centers for Disease Control and Prevention (CDC). Recommended adult immunization schedule—United States, 2011. MMWR Morb Mortal Wkly Rep. 2011;60(4):1-4. [PMID: 21381442]

Item 42   Answer: B

Educational Objective: Diagnose pulmonary embolism as the cause of respiratory failure in a patient with COPD.

The most appropriate next step in management is to obtain a CT angiogram of the chest. Physicians caring for patients with apparent COPD exacerbations should also consider other common causes of acute dyspnea, including heart failure, pulmonary embolism (PE), and pneumonia. Hypoxemia is generally mild in patients with COPD exacerbation and readily improves with supplemental oxygen. This patient, however, continues to have marginal oxygenation despite a significant amount of supplemental oxygen, which should prompt consideration of other causes of respiratory distress. PE is relatively common in patients with COPD who are hospitalized for increased dyspnea; some (but not all) published studies found more severe hypoxemia among patients with COPD and PE compared with those with an exacerbation alone. This patient has no findings that support the diagnosis of heart failure, pneumonia, or other apparent cause of her clinical findings. Therefore, CT angiography should be performed to evaluate for PE prior to attributing her symptoms to an exacerbation of her COPD.

Aminophylline is a theophylline derivative that causes bronchodilation. It was previously used extensively in the treatment of acute bronchospasm, but it is currently a second-line agent that is infrequently used for the treatment of COPD exacerbations. Addition of this medication to the combination of inhaled bronchodilators and systemic corticosteroids carries a significant risk of gastrointestinal and cardiovascular side effects.

An echocardiogram might be appropriate in a patient with a history of heart failure, but the absence of pleural effusions, pulmonary infiltrates, inspiratory crackles, or suggestive electrocardiographic findings in this patient makes it unlikely that a cardiac cause is responsible for her severe hypoxemia.

Antibiotics are indicated in the treatment of COPD exacerbations for critically ill patients and patients with a combination of increased dyspnea, increased sputum production, and increased sputum purulence. However, this patient is experiencing increased dyspnea alone and does not have an infiltrate on her chest radiograph to suggest pneumonia; further evaluation for the cause of her severe hypoxemia should take precedence.

KEY POINT

- Physicians caring for patients with an apparent COPD exacerbation should also consider other common causes of acute dyspnea, including heart failure, pulmonary embolism, and pneumonia.

Bibliography

Rizkallah J, Man SF, Sin DD. Prevalence of pulmonary embolism in acute exacerbations of COPD: a systematic review and metaanalysis. Chest. 2009;135(3):786-793. [PMID: 18812453]

Item 43   Answer: C

Educational Objective: Manage hypertensive emergency.

The initial target blood pressure for this patient should be approximately 185/110 mm Hg. He has evidence of hypertensive encephalopathy characterized by changes in the level of consciousness. Other findings may include focal neurologic deficits and visual field defects. Retinal hemorrhages, exudates, or papilledema may also be present on examination. Too rapid and aggressive lowering of the blood pressure can result in additional end-organ hypoperfusion, compounding the damage to key organs. Patients who present in hypertensive crisis usually have chronic hypertension, and the blood pressure should be treated adequately but should never be decreased to a normal level. In general, the mean arterial pressure should be lowered by no more than 25% in the first hour of treatment and subsequently decreased to systolic levels of 160 mm Hg and diastolic levels between 100 and 110 mm Hg in the next 2 to 6 hours. More rapid blood pressure lowering may be attempted if there is evidence of myocardial ischemia, left ventricular failure with pulmonary edema, acute aortic dissection, intracranial and subarachnoid hemorrhages, pheochromocytoma, and preeclampsia/eclampsia.

KEY POINT

- In patients with hypertensive emergency, the mean arterial pressure should generally be lowered by no more than 25% in the first hour of treatment.

Bibliography

Marik PE, Rivera R. Hypertensive emergencies: an update. Curr Opin Crit Care. 2011;17(6):569-580. [PMID: 21986463]

Item 44   Answer: B

Educational Objective: Treat exercise-induced bronchospasm.

The most appropriate treatment is an inhaled short-acting β_2-agonist 15 minutes before exercise. This patient has mild intermittent asthma with daytime symptoms occurring mainly with exercise. He has no nighttime symptoms. He has no significant limitation other than exercise-induced symptoms, which are typical for mild intermittent asthma. He has a normal physical examination and normal baseline spirometry with a significant drop in FEV_1 following intense exercise. Recommended therapy for this patient is a short-acting β_2-agonist (step 1 of the Expert Panel Report) as needed. Use of a β_2-agonist 10 to 15 minutes before exercise prevents exercise-induced bronchospasm in most patients.

Exercise-induced asthma can be controlled in the majority of patients; therefore, avoidance of physical activity is neither recommended nor necessary.

Inhaled corticosteroids are recommended for patients with more frequent symptoms (more than twice daily, often with weekly nighttime symptoms) and are not necessary for this patient.

A physical conditioning program may help reduce the minute ventilation requirement during exercise and could help patients such as this one; however, the use of an inhaled β_2-agonist will result in more predictable and faster results.

KEY POINT

- Use of a short-acting β_2-agonist 10 to 15 minutes before exercise prevents exercise-induced bronchospasm in most patients.

Bibliography

Parsons JP, Mastronarde JG. Exercise-induced asthma. Curr Opin Pulm Med. 2009;15(1):25-28. [PMID: 19077702]

Item 45   Answer: A

Educational Objective: Diagnose lymphangioleiomyomatosis.

The most likely diagnosis is lymphangioleiomyomatosis (LAM). LAM is a rare cystic lung disease that occurs sporadically in women of childbearing age or in association with tuberous sclerosis. Although the disease is rare and often initially diagnosed as emphysema, spontaneous pneumothorax and/or chylothorax in a young woman with dyspnea and chest radiography demonstrating hyperinflation should prompt consideration of LAM. Suspicion of LAM should lead to high-resolution CT, which can be diagnostic in conjunction with additional clinical criteria, with findings of diffuse, thin-walled, small cysts as seen in this patient's imaging study. LAM occurs secondary to smooth muscle cells that infiltrate the lung with inactivating tuberous sclerosis complex gene mutations. These mutations result in constitutive activation of the mammalian target of rapamycin (mTOR) signaling pathway. Sirolimus is an immunosuppressant medication that blocks mTOR activation of downstream kinases. A recent preliminary investigation evaluating the use of sirolimus in the treatment of pulmonary disease secondary to LAM demonstrated a

significant decrease in the decline in the FEV_1 of patients who were taking the drug. This suggests that there is now a potential therapy for lung disease secondary to LAM. As a result, referral to a center with expertise is appropriate for this rare disease.

Organizing pneumonia typically presents with symptoms over 4 to 6 weeks and not more than 6 months in duration. In addition, the radiographic findings in organizing pneumonia show patchy airspace disease with consolidation and ground-glass opacities but no cystic changes.

Respiratory bronchiolitis–associated interstitial lung disease (RB-ILD) is a form of bronchiolitis that occurs in most smokers and is occasionally severe enough to cause clinical symptoms and characteristic radiographic abnormalities. High-resolution CT shows a pattern of centrilobular nodules with air-trapping and scattered ground-glass attenuation. This patient's history and CT findings are not consistent with this disorder.

Characteristic CT findings in sarcoidosis are a pattern of reticulonodular abnormalities in a central distribution along the bronchovascular lymphatic vessels associated with bilateral hilar and mediastinal lymphadenopathy. These findings are not present in this patient.

KEY POINT

- Lymphangioleiomyomatosis is a rare cystic lung disease that occurs sporadically in women of childbearing age or in association with tuberous sclerosis; characteristic findings include diffuse, thin-walled, small cysts on CT.

Bibliography

McCormack FX, Inoue Y, Moss J, et al; National Institutes of Health Rare Lung Diseases Consortium; MILES Trial Group. Efficacy and safety of sirolimus in lymphangioleiomyomatosis. N Engl J Med. 2011;364(17):1595-1606. [PMID: 21410393]

Item 46   Answer: D

Educational Objective: Manage acute pulmonary embolism with unfractionated heparin.

The most appropriate next step in management is unfractionated heparin. This patient has documented acute pulmonary emboli. Although she had a period of hypotension on presentation, she is now normotensive but tachycardic following fluid administration. There is right ventricular dilatation, borderline pulmonary hypertension, and an elevated B-type natriuretic peptide level, suggesting she is at risk for hemodynamic complications. Thus, anticoagulation with unfractionated heparin is indicated at this time. Unfractionated heparin is typically administered in a fixed-dose, weight-adjusted manner via continuous intravenous infusion. Activated partial thromboplastin time (aPTT) should be monitored and the dose should be adjusted appropriately.

The primary indication for thrombolysis with agents such as alteplase in pulmonary embolism is persistent

Answers and Critiques

CONT.

hypotension and hemodynamic instability. Because this patient stabilized with fluid resuscitation, there is no current indication for thrombolysis. Thrombolytic agents could, however, be used if the patient's status deteriorates. Available data suggest that this strategy (anticoagulation with escalation to thrombolytic therapy if further deterioration occurs) can be used with very acceptable outcomes.

Although low-molecular-weight heparin (LMWH) would provide therapeutic anticoagulation and is convenient, particularly for treatment of thrombotic disease in ambulatory patients, dosing is more difficult in patients with significant kidney impairment, and the anticoagulant effect of LMWH is more difficult to assess than unfractionated heparin. Additionally, because these agents are long acting and not readily reversible, their use would be problematic if the patient became hypotensive and a decision was made to treat with thrombolytic agents or clot extraction.

Thrombus extraction, either surgically or by catheter, is not appropriate in this patient. Like thrombolytic therapy, extraction is best reserved for emboli causing hemodynamic instability. Extraction should be used in situations where thrombolytic agents would be used but are contraindicated. Moreover, the segmental and multifocal distribution of this patient's clots is not ideal for such an approach.

KEY POINT

- **When treating acute pulmonary embolism, unfractionated heparin may be preferred in situations where rapid reversal of anticoagulation may be required.**

Bibliography

Todd JL, Tapson VF. Thrombolytic therapy for acute pulmonary embolism: a critical appraisal. Chest. 2009;135(5):1321-1329. [PMID: 19420199]

Item 47   Answer: B

Educational Objective: Recognize appropriate treatment to reduce the duration of invasive mechanical ventilation in a patient with acute respiratory distress syndrome.

The intervention most likely to reduce the duration of this patient's mechanical ventilation is scheduled doses of furosemide. Although this patient's hypoxemia is due to acute respiratory distress syndrome (ARDS) rather than cardiogenic edema, diuresis can shorten the duration of mechanical ventilation. A large study of patients with ARDS and normal blood pressure and kidney function found that patients treated with aggressive diuresis spent less time on a ventilator without increased risk of nonpulmonary organ failure compared with patients who were given usual care. This patient's weight gain, peripheral edema, pleural effusions, and relatively elevated central venous pressure suggest she will respond well to furosemide.

The early use of paralytic agents such as cisatracurium in patients with severe lung injury (arterial PO_2/FIO_2 <120 mm Hg [16.0 kPa]) has been shown to improve mortality and shorten the duration of mechanical ventilation, but this strategy has not yet been widely adopted. This patient is already 6 days into her illness and does not have severe hypoxemia.

Prone positioning improves oxygenation in most patients with ARDS, primarily by facilitating the recruitment of flooded and collapsed alveoli in posterior, dependent regions of the lung. Although previous trials did not demonstrate improved mortality, a recent meta-analysis suggests prone positioning may improve survival in the most severely affected patients. Prone positioning is not indicated in the current scenario given this patient's relatively mild hypoxemia and readiness for ventilator weaning.

Previous trials of inhaled nitric oxide in ARDS demonstrated improved oxygenation but no mortality benefit.

KEY POINT

- **Aggressive diuresis may decrease the length of required mechanical ventilation in patients with acute respiratory distress syndrome who have normal blood pressure and kidney function.**

Bibliography

Wiedemann HP, Wheeler AP, Bernard GR, et al; National Heart, Lung, and Blood Institute Acute Respiratory Distress Syndrome (ARDS) Clinical Trials Network. Comparison of two fluid-management strategies in acute lung injury. N Engl J Med. 2006;354(24):2564-2575. [PMID: 16714767]

Item 48   Answer: A

Educational Objective: Manage nutrition in a patient with extensive burns.

The most desired approach to nutritional support in this patient is to place a nasogastric feeding tube and initiate enteral nutrition. Patients with burns require many special nutritional considerations that are intended to supply the needs of their hypermetabolic state, prevent mucosal breakdown and infection in the gut, prevent the loss of lean body mass, and assist in wound healing. Enteral feeding through the stomach is preferred if it can be tolerated, as it maintains the integrity of the entire gastrointestinal tract by avoiding disuse atrophy. It is typically amenable to long-term use, which may be required during recovery from a severe burn injury. Most patients with burns, and even those with airway injury, can tolerate placement of an enteral feeding tube.

Although this patient's nutritional needs could likely be met with the use of a jejunal feeding tube, there is no clear indication for this intervention because the upper gastrointestinal system is not impaired, and this patient would benefit from continuing its use. Jejunal feeding systems are sometimes used in patients in whom there is concern about possible reflux and aspiration of gastric contents.

However, no clear benefit of postpyloric tube placement has been shown in terms of either nutritional or reflux and aspiration outcomes. A percutaneous feeding tube carries a high risk of infection in a patient whose abdominal skin is not intact.

Total parenteral nutrition through central venous access is associated with high risk for infection, particularly in patients with extensive burn injuries. Other potential issues associated with central parenteral nutrition include maintenance of access, atrophy of the gastrointestinal tract, trace element deficiency, and high costs and maintenance requirements, particularly for long-term treatment. Thus, parenteral nutrition should only be given if enteral options have been tried and failed or were not tolerated.

Parenteral nutrition through peripheral access is limited in its nutritional value because of the difficulty in providing an adequate volume of high-concentration fluids through a noncentral catheter. In addition to access issues, infection risk, and costs, peripheral parenteral nutrition would likely not be adequate to meet this patient's increased nutritional needs associated with her burn injury.

KEY POINT

- Enteral feeding is the desired means of nutritional support if it can be tolerated in most patients with critical illness; most patients with burns, and even those with airway injury, can tolerate placement of an enteral feeding tube.

Bibliography

Martindale RG, McClave SA, Vanek VW, et al; American College of Critical Care Medicine; A.S.P.E.N. Board of Directors. Guidelines for the provision and assessment of nutrition support therapy in the adult critically ill patient: Society of Critical Care Medicine and American Society for Parenteral and Enteral Nutrition: Executive Summary. Crit Care Med. 2009;37(5):1757-1761. [PMID: 19373044]

Item 49   Answer: D

Educational Objective: Diagnose idiopathic pulmonary fibrosis.

The most likely diagnosis is idiopathic pulmonary fibrosis (IPF). Patients typically present with progressive dyspnea of greater than 6 months' duration and a dry, hacking cough. Digital clubbing is present in 30% of patients. In addition, this patient has several risk factors for the development of IPF, including his smoking history, previous work as a carpenter (extensive organic dust exposure), and his age (increased prevalence of IPF with increasing age). His CT scan discloses the classic findings of definitive IPF, with basal and peripheral disease with septal thickening, evidence of honeycomb changes, traction bronchiectasis, and no evidence of ground-glass opacities or nodules.

This patient does not have COPD because spirometry demonstrates a normal FEV_1/FVC ratio. Although this can be seen in patients with significant air-trapping, the physical examination also reveals inspiratory crackles, which are not characteristic of COPD. This in conjunction with the CT findings rules out COPD.

This patient does not have heart failure because there are no symptoms of orthopnea, paroxysmal nocturnal dyspnea, or lower extremity edema. In addition, there is no S_3 or jugular venous distention on examination. Although septal lines can be seen in patients with heart failure on CT scan, honeycomb changes are not a finding of pulmonary edema.

Hypersensitivity pneumonitis is an allergic, inflammatory lung disease that is also called extrinsic allergic alveolitis. It results from exposure to airborne allergens that cause a cell-mediated immunologic sensitization. Most patients exposed to an inhalational antigen develop symptoms within 4 to 12 hours. This patient's 12-month history of progressive dyspnea and cough and lack of exposure history are not compatible with this diagnosis.

KEY POINT

- Idiopathic pulmonary fibrosis is characterized by progressive dyspnea and cough for more than 6 months and dry inspiratory crackles; classic CT findings include basal and peripheral disease with evidence of honeycomb changes without evidence of ground-glass opacities or nodules.

Bibliography

Raghu G, Collard HR, Egan JJ, et al. An official ATS/ERS/JRS/ALAT statement: Idiopathic pulmonary fibrosis: Evidence-based guidelines for diagnosis and management. Am J Respir Crit Care Med. 2011;183(6):788-824. [PMID: 21471066]

Item 50   Answer: D

Educational Objective: Diagnose obstructive lung disease in a patient who works as a coal miner.

The most appropriate diagnostic test to perform next is pulmonary function testing, specifically with measurement of spirometry, lung volumes, and DLCO. Exposure to coal dust in occupational settings may lead to a spectrum of clinical conditions ranging from asymptomatic deposition of coal particles without an inflammatory response (anthracosis) to complicated pulmonary disease with massive pulmonary fibrosis caused by the activation of inflammatory mediators in response to inhaled coal dust. Impairment of lung function in individuals exposed to coal dust is also significantly accelerated in smokers. Autopsy studies have shown that the extent of emphysema was significantly greater in ever-smokers who were miners in comparison with the never-smoker, non-miner population. In addition, the extent of emphysema was sixfold greater in those who were never-smoker miners compared with never-smoker non-miners. Documentation of declines in FEV_1 in coal miners provides strong evidence for the development of obstructive lung disease in workers exposed to significant coal dust. As a result, symptomatic patients should undergo pulmonary function testing to identify obstructive physiology, whether or not they have a smoking history. This allows for earlier interventions such as bronchodilator therapy, avoidance of further exposure, and the opportunity for continued monitoring.

In asymptomatic patients with a history of coal exposure in whom baseline radiographs have been obtained, radiographic studies should be repeated every 5 years to monitor for progressive lung disease. These studies should be performed more frequently in patients who develop symptoms. However, initiating routine surveillance alone in this symptomatic patient without further evaluation would not be appropriate.

Although coal miners are at increased risk for interstitial lung diseases, this patient presents with bronchitic symptoms and a normal chest radiograph. Before pursuing CT imaging, pulmonary function testing should be performed to differentiate between obstructive and restrictive physiology.

The role of PET scanning for the diagnosis and surveillance of lung disease associated with coal exposure has not been established. Because of its high sensitivity for detection of inflammation, its use in assessing malignancy in coal-exposed patients is limited owing to high false-positive rates.

KEY POINT

- Studies have shown that workers exposed to significant coal dust have a high risk for the development of obstructive lung disease.

Bibliography

Kuempel ED, Wheeler MW, Smith RJ, Vallyathan V, Green FH. Contributions of dust exposure and cigarette smoking to emphysema severity in coal miners in the United States. Am J Respir Crit Care Med. 2009;180(3):257-264. [PMID: 19423717]

Item 51   Answer: B

Educational Objective: Manage impending respiratory failure with endotracheal intubation in a patient with asthma.

The most appropriate next step in management is endotracheal intubation. This patient has a life-threatening asthma exacerbation despite aggressive treatment with a short-acting β_2-agonist and should be intubated and placed on invasive mechanical ventilation. Most patients with asthma present with acute respiratory alkalosis. This patient's combination of mild respiratory acidosis and severe respiratory distress indicate impending respiratory arrest.

Continuous nebulized bronchodilator therapy may be appropriate for patients with moderate levels of bronchospasm in an acute care setting. However, it is not an appropriate intervention in a patient with evidence of severe respiratory compromise.

This patient's severe exacerbation can be attributable at least in part to the recent absence of inhaled corticosteroids in her baseline asthma regimen, and her severe exacerbation should be treated with systemic corticosteroids. Because corticosteroids require 4 to 6 hours to have a clinical effect, they should be administered as soon as possible, but they are not the primary intervention in this patient who requires more immediate stabilization.

This patient is likely anxious, but her distress is appropriate for the severity of her illness; providing sedation with lorazepam poses substantial risk of exacerbating her acute respiratory acidosis without benefit to her bronchospasm.

KEY POINT

- Patients with life-threatening asthma exacerbation despite aggressive treatment with short-acting β_2-agonists should be intubated and placed on invasive mechanical ventilation.

Bibliography

National Heart, Lung, and Blood Institute, National Asthma Education and Prevention Program. Expert Panel Report 3: guidelines for the diagnosis and management of asthma: full report 2007. Available at: www.nhlbi.nih.gov/guidelines/asthma/asthgdln.pdf. Accessed July 27, 2012.

Item 52   Answer: A

Educational Objective: Prevent high-altitude illness.

The most appropriate management is acetazolamide. This patient had a clinical picture consistent with acute mountain sickness (AMS), a form of high-altitude illness, during her last trip to a significant elevation. The key feature of AMS is headache, along with fatigue, nausea, and sleep disturbance (usually due to high-altitude periodic breathing [HAPB], an altitude-associated respiratory change). The most effective method of prevention is to gradually ascend to the target elevation. When that is not possible, acetazolamide, starting 24 to 48 hours before ascent, is the most effective therapy to prevent AMS and HAPB. Acetazolamide works via several different mechanisms to stabilize ventilation, improve oxygenation, counteract fluid retention, and induce a mild metabolic acidosis, all of which accelerate acclimatization and improve acute symptoms associated with the transition to high altitudes. Prophylaxis should be reserved for patients who are at risk for altitude-related illness (particularly those with a history of altitude-related illness) or patients with cardiopulmonary disease.

Dexamethasone is the drug treatment of choice for established mountain sickness or cerebral edema. Because of its side-effect profile, it is a second choice for prophylaxis after acetazolamide.

The effect of acetazolamide on preventing HAPB is independent of its diuretic action. Therefore, other

Answers and Critiques

diuretics like furosemide would not be expected to alleviate HAPB.

Zolpidem may be effective for insomnia related to travel but will not prevent HAPB.

> **KEY POINT**
> - When gradual ascent to the target elevation is not feasible, acetazolamide is the most effective therapy to prevent acute mountain sickness and high-altitude periodic breathing.

Bibliography
Teppema LJ, Balanos GM, Steinback CD, et al. Effects of acetazolamide on ventilatory, cerebrovascular, and pulmonary vascular responses to hypoxia. Am J Respir Crit Care Med. 2007;175(3):277-281. [PMID: 17095745]

Item 53   Answer: C
Educational Objective: Diagnose delirium in the intensive care unit.

The most likely diagnosis is delirium. Delirium is an acute state of confusion that may manifest as a reduced level of consciousness, cognitive abnormalities, perceptual disturbances, or emotional disturbances. It is common in the intensive care unit and should be controlled to ensure patients' safety and to allow appropriate evaluation. Delirium is classified according to psychomotor behavior as hyperactive, hypoactive, and mixed. Pure hyperactive delirium, which accounts for less than 5% of cases of intensive care unit delirium, is characterized by increased psychomotor activity with agitated behavior. Hypoactive or quiet delirium, which accounts for approximately 45% of cases, is characterized by reduced psychomotor behavior and lethargy. Mixed delirium, which accounts for approximately 50% of cases, alternates unpredictably between a hyperactive and a hypoactive manifestation.

An acute stroke is unlikely to cause fluctuating neurologic or cognitive deficits. A hemorrhagic stroke may certainly evolve, producing progressively worsening deficits, but alternating agitation and somnolence would not be typical.

There is no evidence for respiratory failure in this patient. Her arterial blood gas studies and vital signs are normal.

This patient has not been receiving opioids long enough to develop physical dependence and thus be at risk for withdrawal.

Fluctuating mental status would be an unlikely result of a recurrent pulmonary embolism. The interruption of this patient's anticoagulation for a period of a few hours for her hip reduction increases the risk of a recurrent embolism; however, this patient does not have hypoxemia or respiratory distress, which would most likely be evident if she had a recurrent embolism.

> **KEY POINT**
> - Delirium, defined by fluctuating mental status, is common in the intensive care unit and should be controlled to ensure patients' safety and to allow appropriate evaluation.

Bibliography
Schiemann A, Hadzidiakos D, Spies C. Managing ICU delirium [erratum in Curr Opin Crit Care. 2011;17(3):315]. Curr Opin Crit Care. 2011;17(2):131-140. [PMID: 21301333]

Item 54   Answer: C
Educational Objective: Treat mild persistent asthma.

The most appropriate treatment is to add a low-dose inhaled corticosteroid (ICS). This patient has mild persistent asthma; she has symptoms more than 2 days per week but not daily and she wakes up once a week but not nightly. The preferred therapy for this patient is a low-dose ICS added to an as-needed short-acting β₂-agonist. Alternatives to ICS include a leukotriene receptor antagonist or theophylline.

Adding a long-acting β_2-agonist is not recommended for patients with asthma who are not already receiving ICS therapy.

Providing combination long-acting β_2-agonist and ICS therapy is not indicated at this point. Based on the Expert Panel Report 3 guidelines and an FDA black box warning, patients should be started on ICS first. Long-acting β_2-agonists should be added only if medium-dose ICS therapy fails to control symptoms.

Scheduled use of albuterol is not recommended, because it might mask ongoing airway inflammation and the need to provide anti-inflammatory therapy with ICS.

Allergen immunotherapy is an option for some patients, but its benefits are mostly for those with allergic rhinitis and would not be recommended for patients with mild persistent asthma.

> **KEY POINT**
> - The preferred therapy for mild persistent asthma is a low-dose inhaled corticosteroid added to an as-needed short-acting β_2-agonist.

Bibliography
National Asthma Education and Prevention Program. Expert Panel Report 3. Guidelines for the Diagnosis and Management of Asthma. Available at: www.nhlbi.nih.gov/guidelines/asthma/asthsumm.pdf. Accessed July 27, 2012.

Item 55   Answer: C
Educational Objective: Diagnose pulmonary arterial hypertension.

The most appropriate diagnostic test is right heart catheterization. A substantial proportion of patients with pulmonary arterial hypertension have delays in diagnosis of their condition. Younger patients are particularly vulnerable to such delays. This patient's pulmonary hypertension and clinical presentation are highly suggestive of pulmonary arterial hypertension, likely of the idiopathic variety given the negative evaluation and a history that is inconsistent with obstructive sleep apnea. This diagnosis can only be confirmed by right heart catheterization. Moreover, assessment of responsiveness to vasodilator agents can be tested during the procedure, providing information that may be essential to management.

This patient's clear lung fields and her symptoms out of proportion to her stable pulmonary function tests are evidence against an interstitial lung process as the cause of her symptoms. Little is likely to be gained from a high-resolution CT scan.

Although chronic thromboembolic pulmonary hypertension is consistent with this patient's history and examination, ventilation/perfusion lung scans are typically quite abnormal with major lobar and segmental mismatched perfusion defects. A pulmonary angiogram as an isolated study is therefore not indicated.

This patient is unlikely to have obstructive sleep apnea as a cause for her underlying pulmonary hypertension given her negative history of snoring or daytime somnolence and her normal BMI. Because of the low pretest probability for obstructive sleep apnea, a sleep study will be a low-yield test.

Transesophageal echocardiography is not indicated because it is unlikely to add appreciable new information to the recent transthoracic study.

KEY POINT

- **Right heart catheterization is essential to confirm the diagnosis of pulmonary hypertension by direct measurement of mean pulmonary artery pressure.**

Bibliography

Brown LM, Chen H, Halpern S, et al. Delay in recognition of pulmonary arterial hypertension: factors identified from the REVEAL Registry. Chest. 2011;140(1):19-26. [PMID: 21393391]

Item 56   Answer: B

Educational Objective: Diagnose a posterior mediastinal mass.

The patient most likely has a neurilemmoma (or schwannoma), a benign neoplasm arising from neural tissue and characteristically located in the posterior mediastinum. The mediastinum lies between the two pleural surfaces in the center of the chest and is divided into anterior, middle, and posterior compartments. These categories are helpful clinically in determining a differential diagnosis for masses arising in this area. Lesions located in the anterior mediastinum include thyroid tumors, thymic tumors, and lymphomas. Middle mediastinal tumors include bronchogenic cysts,

pericardial cysts, and lymphadenopathy. Posterior mediastinal masses are generally limited to growths of neural tissue (as in this patient) or esophageal tumors or cysts. Neurilemmomas are encapsulated tumors made entirely of benign neoplastic Schwann cells. They are the most common tumor of peripheral nerves and may occur in the chest. Patients with mediastinal tumors may present with cough, venous distention, hoarseness, back pain, or chest pain; they may also be asymptomatic. Imaging with CT, MRI, and sometimes additional studies such as a thyroid scan or endoscopic ultrasound are used for further characterization. Removal is usually done if symptoms occur or the diagnosis is in question.

KEY POINT

- **The anatomic location within the mediastinum is helpful in focusing the differential diagnosis of lesions arising in this area.**

Bibliography

Ponce FA, Killory BD, Wait SD, Theodore N, Dickman CA. Endoscopic resection of intrathoracic tumors: experience with and long-term results for 26 patients. J Neurosurg Spine. 2011;14(3):377-381. [PMID: 21250809]

Item 57   Answer: A

Educational Objective: Diagnose hypoxemia in a patient with a falsely elevated oxygen saturation reading on pulse oximetry.

The most appropriate diagnostic test is to obtain arterial blood gas studies. This patient presents with a COPD exacerbation. With her history of smoking and the presence of somnolence, there is a high chance that she has arterial hypoxemia and probably alveolar hypoventilation with carbon dioxide retention. Both are best evaluated by obtaining arterial blood gas studies. The presence of a normal oxygen saturation by pulse oximetry does not exclude arterial hypoxemia in this patient, particularly given her ongoing smoking; the presence of carboxyhemoglobin would result in a falsely elevated reading by pulse oximetry. Her low-normal pulse oximetry value also does not exclude significant carbon dioxide retention due to alveolar hypoventilation, and an assessment of her arterial blood gases would be necessary to evaluate this possibility.

A chest CT scan is unnecessary in this patient and is not likely to add important information.

A complete blood count might be helpful in this patient because it could show increased hemoglobin (due to long-standing hypoxemia), but it is not likely to be useful acutely.

An echocardiogram is not necessary in this patient; however, it would likely show elevated pressures on the right side given the patient's severe COPD and likely cor pulmonale.

- Carboxyhemoglobinemia can cause a falsely elevated oxygen saturation reading via pulse oximetry; if there is uncertainty about adequacy of the patient's oxygenation, arterial blood gas studies should be obtained.

Bibliography

Global Strategy for Diagnosis, Management, and Prevention of COPD. December 2011. Available at: www.goldcopd.org. Accessed July 27, 2012.

Item 58   Answer: C
Educational Objective: Manage dyspnea in a patient with end-stage COPD.

The most appropriate management is to administer morphine sulfate. Dyspnea is one of the most common symptoms encountered in palliative care. It is most often the result of direct cardiothoracic pathology, such as pleural effusions, heart failure, COPD, pulmonary embolism, pneumonia, or lung metastases. Patients with underlying lung disease on bronchodilator therapy should have this therapy continued to maintain comfort. Opioids are effective in reducing dyspnea in patients with underlying cardiopulmonary disease and malignancy. In patients already receiving opioids, using the breakthrough pain dose for dyspnea and increasing this dose by 25% if not fully effective may be helpful. A 5-mg dose of oral morphine given four times daily has been shown to help relieve dyspnea in patients with end-stage heart failure. Low-dose (20-mg) extended-release morphine given daily has been used to relieve dyspnea in patients with advanced COPD.

If severe anemia is uncovered as a cause of dyspnea, a blood transfusion may help relieve symptoms. However, this patient has adequate oxygen carrying capacity, so a blood transfusion is not indicated.

In contrast to opioids, benzodiazepines have not demonstrated consistent benefit in treating dyspnea; however, they may have a special use in patients with dyspnea caused by anxiety.

Oxygen may be useful in relieving dyspnea in terminally ill patients with hypoxemia, but a meta-analysis suggests that it has limited use in symptom relief in patients without hypoxemia. Increasing the flow of oxygen provides no added value in patients already receiving oxygen with adequate oxygenation.

- Opioids are effective in reducing dyspnea in patients with end-stage COPD.

Bibliography

Mahler DA, Selecky PA, Harrod CG, et al. American College of Chest Physicians consensus statement on the management of dyspnea in patients with advanced lung or heart disease. Chest. 2010;137(3):674-691. [PMID: 20202949]

Item 59   Answer: B
Educational Objective: Diagnose neuromuscular respiratory failure.

The bedside vital capacity is the most appropriate test to assess impending respiratory failure in a patient with neuromuscular weakness. In the intensive care unit, serial bedside measurements of vital capacity and maximum negative inspiratory force are used to assess the need for mechanical ventilation in patients with neuromuscular disease. Patients with vital capacity less than 20 mL/kg, patients who cannot generate more than 30 cm H_2O of negative inspiratory force, or patients with declining values are at high risk for ventilatory failure.

Serial measurement of arterial blood gas levels may not be a sufficiently sensitive predictor of ventilatory failure in patients with neuromuscular weakness.

A chest radiograph would likely reveal low lung volumes and basilar atelectasis. However, these findings are much less indicative of the risk for developing respiratory failure than measurement of respiratory muscle function.

The rapid shallow breathing index is used to predict whether patients can be successfully weaned from invasive mechanical ventilation and does not have a role in assessing the need for intubation in patients presenting with acute respiratory failure.

- **The bedside vital capacity and maximal inspiratory pressure are the most appropriate tests to assess impending respiratory failure in patients with neuromuscular weakness.**

Bibliography

Mehta S. Neuromuscular disease causing acute respiratory failure. Respir Care. 2006;51(9):1016-1021; discussion 1021-1023. [PMID: 16934165]

Item 60   Answer: A
Educational Objective: Diagnose asbestosis.

The most likely diagnosis is asbestosis. Asbestosis refers to bilateral interstitial fibrosis of the lung parenchyma caused by inhalation of asbestos fibers. Asbestosis is diagnosed in a patient with findings of pulmonary fibrosis and an exposure history to asbestos with an appropriate latency period (at least 10-15 years). This patient worked in a shipyard at a time when personal protections were not used. CT imaging in asbestosis characteristically reveals bilateral peripheral- and basal-predominant septal line thickening with evidence of diffuse pleural thickening and calcified pleural plaques, as shown (see next page). Ninety percent of asbestos-induced pleural abnormalities are due to pleural plaques (well-circumscribed lesions) and diffuse pleural thickening. Pleural plaques alone are rarely associated with symptomatic disease and are most often seen as an incidental finding on chest radiograph. Diffuse pleural thickening, on the other hand, is much more likely to be associated with symptoms and other clinical findings, including breathlessness

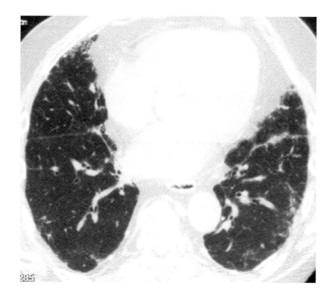

and restrictive pulmonary physiology. Patients with diffuse pleural thickening may develop hypercapnic respiratory failure as their lungs become encased by a thick pleural rind that prevents the lungs from expanding. An association between occupational exposure to asbestos and lung cancer is also well established; cigarette smoke and asbestos have a synergistic (multiplicative) effect on the risk for lung cancer.

This patient has a normal cardiac examination and a chronically progressive history over the last 14 months. This in conjunction with the CT findings makes heart failure a less likely diagnosis for the patient's symptoms. Although crackles are heard on pulmonary examination, this is a common finding in patients with pulmonary fibrosis and should not be interpreted as evidence of pulmonary edema.

Hypersensitivity pneumonitis occurs more acutely after exposure to an antigen and often results in fever, flulike symptoms, and cough that will wax and wane with the exposure. Radiographic findings are typically mid- and upper-lung predominant, rather than basal predominant, with evidence of centrilobular micronodules and without pleural plaques.

Although idiopathic pulmonary fibrosis (IPF) can cause parenchymal findings as described in this patient, it is typically diagnosed in patients with interstitial lung disease in whom no other cause may be found. In this patient, the exposure history identifies a plausible cause for the development of fibrosis, and his radiographic findings are consistent with the likely diagnosis. Therefore, it is highly unlikely that this patient has IPF.

KEY POINT

- Asbestosis is diagnosed in a patient with findings of pulmonary fibrosis and an extensive exposure history to asbestos with a latency period of at least 10 to 15 years.

Bibliography

Paris C, Thierry S, Brochard P, et al; National APEXS Members. Pleural plaques and asbestosis: dose- and time-response relationships based on HRCT data. Eur Respir J. 2009;34(1):72-79. [PMID: 19129281]

Item 61   Answer: D

Educational Objective: Manage an exacerbation of COPD with noninvasive positive pressure ventilation.

The most appropriate additional management is noninvasive positive pressure ventilation (NPPV). This patient's acute COPD exacerbation warrants a trial of NPPV. NPPV reduces mortality, the need for intubation, and the length of hospital stay in selected patients. It also improves respiratory acidosis and decreases respiration rate and severity of breathlessness. Patients with moderate to severe dyspnea, moderate to severe acidosis (pH <7.35) and/or hypercapnia, and respiration rate greater than 25/min benefit from NPPV. Exclusion criteria for NPPV are respiratory arrest, cardiovascular instability (hypotension, arrhythmias, and myocardial infarction), change in mental status, uncooperativeness, high aspiration risk, viscous or copious secretions, recent facial or gastroesophageal surgery, craniofacial trauma, fixed nasopharyngeal abnormalities, burns, and extreme obesity. Severe acidosis (pH <7.25) and respiration rate greater than 35/min are indications for intubation rather than NPPV. Failure of an initial trial of NPPV is also an indication for intubation.

Positive airway pressure is the treatment of choice for most patients with obstructive sleep apnea. Continuous positive airway pressure (CPAP), which provides a constant fixed-level pressure throughout the respiratory cycle, is used for most patients. CPAP does not provide ventilatory support and would not be helpful in treating hypoxic ventilatory failure, as in this patient.

Increasing oxygen alone is not an appropriate treatment option because the patient's oxygen saturation is adequate. Oxygen therapy is indicated for patients who have hypoxemia, arterial P_{O_2} less than 55 mm Hg (7.3 kPa), or oxygen saturation of 88% or lower.

KEY POINT

- In patients with COPD exacerbations characterized by acute hypercapnic respiratory failure, noninvasive positive pressure ventilation reduces mortality, the need for intubation, and the length of hospital stay.

Bibliography

Khilnani GC, Banga A. Noninvasive ventilation in patients with chronic obstructive airway disease. Int J Chron Obstruct Pulmon Dis. 2008;3(3):351-357. [PMID: 18990962]

Item 62   Answer: C

Educational Objective: Evaluate lung cancer in a patient with an abnormal PET scan.

The most appropriate next step in management is mediastinal lymph node sampling. This patient has a mediastinal mass and sputum cytology that is positive for squamous cell carcinoma. The next step is to determine the stage of the cancer. Unlike conventional CT scanning, PET-CT scanning provides metabolic rather than anatomic data and is able to detect likely tumor activity in lymph nodes of normal size. The areas of increased activity on this patient's PET-CT scan likely represent tumor involvement of these lymph nodes. However, because false-positive results do occur with PET-CT, the next step in management is to establish a pathologic stage with mediastinal node sampling. Endobronchial ultrasound–guided node sampling, if available, is a less invasive method than mediastinoscopy; it also has a lower cost, does not require general anesthesia or a skin incision, and has a comparably high yield. Endobronchial ultrasonography provides real-time imaging of the mediastinal nodes as directed by the PET-CT and enables the operator to see the needle in the node at the time of sampling. Yields of over 90% for the paratracheal and subcarinal nodes and negative predictive values of over 90% have been reported.

CT-guided needle aspiration would likely establish the diagnosis but not the stage; this modality would yield information about the primary tumor but not the mediastinal lymph nodes. Therefore, a second procedure would be needed to determine the stage.

The purpose of staging is to determine the prognosis and guide therapy. Understanding the extent of disease allows determination of appropriate surgical or medical interventions. Surgical resection of the primary tumor with curative intent without knowledge of the extent of local or regional involvement or metastatic disease would not be appropriate. Surgical intervention for the purpose of diagnosis and staging was common before development of less invasive approaches; it may still be useful for this purpose if other modalities are not successful. Similarly, without staging it is not possible to determine whether a medical approach to treatment would be the most appropriate.

KEY POINT

- **Endobronchial ultrasound–guided lymph node sampling has a high yield and is less invasive than surgery for staging of lung cancer.**

Bibliography

Silvestri GA, Gould MK, Margolis ML, et al; American College of Chest Physicians. Noninvasive staging of non-small cell lung cancer: ACCP evidenced-based clinical practice guidelines (2nd edition). Chest. 2007;132(3 suppl):178S-201S. [PMID: 17873168]

Item 63   Answer: C

Educational Objective: Manage lack of response to appropriate COPD therapy by checking inhaler technique.

The most appropriate management is to check the patient's inhaler technique. This patient has moderate (stage 2) COPD and is on an appropriate medication regimen that includes a long-acting anticholinergic agent and a long-acting β_2-agonist. The patient is adherent to this regimen. The most appropriate next step is to check the inhaler technique. Inhaler therapy is very important in the treatment of COPD. Several drug- and patient-dependent factors, including age, eyesight, finger dexterity, degree of lung function, cognitive function, breathing pattern, inhaler technique, drug formulation, and device-related variables, affect the drug's distribution and clinical outcomes. Patient-dependent factors also change over time. It is very important to ensure that the inhaler technique is correct (see www.acpfoundation.org/materials-and-guides/video/short-video-health-tips-for-patients/how-to-use-an-inhaler.html).

Adding an inhaled corticosteroid is not an appropriate option for this patient before checking his inhaler technique.

Oxygen therapy is a major component of treatment for patients with very severe COPD. It is usually prescribed for patients who have an arterial P_{O_2} less than or equal to 55 mm Hg (7.3 kPa) or oxygen saturation less than or equal to 88% with or without hypercapnia or who exhibit an arterial P_{O_2} of 56 to 59 mm Hg (7.4 to 7.8 kPa) or oxygen saturation less than 89% with one or more of the following: pulmonary hypertension, evidence of cor pulmonale or edema as a result of right-sided heart failure, or hematocrit greater than 56%. This patient has none of these indications for oxygen therapy.

Restarting prednisone is not appropriate at this time because this patient was adequately treated with a short course of a systemic corticosteroid. Long-term corticosteroids are not recommended because of lack of evidence of benefit and many side effects.

KEY POINT

- **If a patient is not responding to appropriate therapy for COPD, inhaler technique should be assessed before therapy is adjusted.**

Bibliography

Fromer L, Goodwin E, Walsh J. Customizing inhaled therapy to meet the needs of COPD patients. Postgrad Med. 2010;122(2):83-93. [PMID: 20203459]

Item 64   Answer: A

Educational Objective: Diagnose an acute exacerbation of idiopathic pulmonary fibrosis.

This patient has an acute exacerbation of idiopathic pulmonary fibrosis (IPF). IPF was previously believed to be marked by a progressive, steady decline in pulmonary function. However, it is now clear that there are some patients who develop an acute exacerbation of IPF. Diagnostic criteria include unexplained worsening or development of dyspnea in less than 30 days, high-resolution CT showing new bilateral ground-glass opacity and/or consolidation superimposed on a background of findings consistent with usual interstitial pneumonia, and no evidence of alternative causes. The only intervention shown to improve survival in selected patients with IPF is lung transplantation. Surgical lung biopsy specimens from these patients have consistently shown superimposed diffuse alveolar damage on a background of usual interstitial pneumonia. Short-term prognosis is poor, and medical therapy is not effective. This patient's age of 62 years and absence of comorbid illness make him an excellent candidate for transplantation.

Although diffuse alveolar hemorrhage (DAH) can result in a CT scan with diffuse ground-glass opacities, this diagnosis is confirmed based on the findings of the bronchoalveolar lavage fluid, which will be progressively bloody in a patient with DAH. This patient's bronchoalveolar lavage fluid was clear, and this rules out DAH.

Pneumocystis jirovecii pneumonia (PJP) is unlikely because this patient is not on immunosuppressant medications that would put him at risk for this complication. In addition, the cytopathology examination of the bronchoalveolar lavage fluid was negative. Diagnosis of PJP is based on documentation of the presence of the organism in respiratory secretions.

Pulmonary edema due to tachycardia is not a likely cause of this patient's clinical presentation. His elevated heart rate and findings of crackles on examination are likely due to his underlying pulmonary disease. Additionally, there is no evidence of left ventricular dysfunction, including an S_3, jugular venous distention on examination, or elevation of the B-type natriuretic peptide level.

KEY POINT

- Diagnostic criteria for an acute exacerbation of idiopathic pulmonary fibrosis include unexplained worsening or development of dyspnea in less than 30 days, high-resolution CT showing new bilateral ground-glass opacity and/or consolidation superimposed on a background of findings consistent with usual interstitial pneumonia, and no evidence of alternative causes.

Bibliography

Collard HR, Moore BB, Flaherty KR, et al; Idiopathic Pulmonary Fibrosis Clinical Research Network Investigators. Acute exacerbations of idiopathic pulmonary fibrosis. Am J Respir Crit Care Med. 2007;176(7):636-643. [PMID: 17585107]

Item 65   Answer: C

Educational Objective: Treat a patient with stage IIB lung cancer who is a surgical candidate.

The most appropriate next step in management is surgical resection. This patient has a presumed diagnosis of lung cancer on the basis of a growing nodule that is now a large mass. The mass has uptake on PET and there is no associated lymphadenopathy identified on CT or PET. Owing to the size of the mass, the clinical stage is T3N0M0 or IIB.

Surgery, if feasible, is the treatment with the best long-term survival. Although this patient has mild COPD, her pulmonary function appears optimal on her current therapy, and there are no significant comorbidities that would prohibit surgery. For patients with an FEV_1 of less than 80% of predicted, calculating the predicted postoperative pulmonary function helps identify which patients are otherwise acceptable surgical candidates. The postoperative predicted pulmonary function is calculated by subtracting the approximate percentage of lung function to be lost with surgical removal (segment, lobe, or pneumonectomy) from the preoperative function. If the postoperative predicted FEV_1 and D_{LCO} are greater than 40% of the predicted normal, surgery is generally well tolerated.

Chemotherapy has shown improved survival for patients with resected IIB disease as adjuvant therapy, but it should not be used before surgery as a neoadjuvant therapy.

Radiation therapy is an option for localized disease, but it would not be preferred over surgery for a lesion of this size.

Although obtaining tissue for diagnosis, prognosis, and staging is pursued in a majority of patients with possible lung cancer, a primary surgical approach with avoidance of the added risks associated with transthoracic needle biopsy is preferable for this patient, given the high probability that a lesion of this size in this clinical setting is a malignancy and that surgical resection with curative intent is considered possible.

KEY POINT

- Surgery is the treatment with the best long-term survival for patients with lung cancer who have favorable tumor characteristics and no medical contraindications to the procedure.

Bibliography

Scott WJ, Howington J, Feigenberg S, Movsas B, Pisters K; American College of Chest Physicians. Treatment of non-small cell lung cancer stage I and stage II: ACCP evidence-based clinical practice guidelines (2nd edition). Chest. 2007;132(3 suppl):234S-242S. [PMID: 17873171]

Item 66   Answer: C

Educational Objective: Manage early septic shock.

Empiric antibiotic therapy should be initiated within 1 hour of recognition of sepsis after cultures have been taken from the blood and other suspected sites of infection. This patient has septic shock, most likely from a urinary source. The goals of sepsis management are to treat infection and optimize tissue perfusion. This is accomplished by controlling sources of infection, instituting early and appropriate antibiotic therapy, optimizing oxygen delivery by correcting hypoxia, using crystalloids to maintain adequate preload, starting vasoactive agents to maintain perfusion pressure for persistent hypotension despite administration of fluids, and transfusion of erythrocytes if oxygen delivery is inadequate despite the previous measures. Initial resuscitation should begin early and be aggressive. Inadequate initial antibiotic therapy is independently associated with poor outcomes, and initial empiric therapy should include agents with activity against all probable pathogens.

Transfusion is recommended if the central venous oxygen saturation is less than 70% after adequate fluid challenge or if the hematocrit is below 30%, but it would not be appropriate at this time. This patient has not yet received an adequate fluid challenge, and his hematocrit is 33%.

Vasopressor therapy should be considered only when aggressive volume resuscitation fails to bring mean arterial pressure to greater than 65 mm Hg. This patient has not yet received an adequate volume challenge. If the patient remains hypotensive after a fluid challenge, norepinephrine would be a better choice than dopamine because dopamine has been associated with a higher rate of cardiac arrhythmias.

Traditionally, a pulmonary artery catheter has been used to guide hemodynamic resuscitation; however, at least four international landmark studies have shown that neither pulmonary artery catheters nor specific protocols that incorporate data from such catheters yield superior outcomes in most patients. In addition, these catheters have more risk associated with their use compared with central venous pressure transduction from a simple central line.

KEY POINT

- Empiric antibiotic therapy should be initiated within 1 hour of recognition of sepsis after cultures have been taken from the blood and other suspected sites of infection.

Bibliography

Rivers E, Nguyen B, Havstad S, et al; Early Goal-Directed Therapy Collaborative Group. Early goal-directed therapy in the treatment of severe sepsis and septic shock. N Engl J Med. 2001;345(19):1368-1377. [PMID: 11794169]

Item 67   Answer: D

Educational Objective: Treat neuroleptic malignant syndrome.

The most appropriate treatment is intravenous fluids and benzodiazepines such as lorazepam. This patient has neuroleptic malignant syndrome (NMS), an idiosyncratic reaction to neuroleptic antipsychotic agents. It is characterized by muscle rigidity, hyperthermia, and autonomic dysregulation. Potent "typical" neuroleptics such as haloperidol are most commonly implicated, but all neuroleptic agents have been associated with the syndrome. Treatment efforts are supportive and are aimed at controlling hyperthermia, rigidity, and dehydration. Benzodiazepines should be administered for agitation, and the neuroleptic agent should be stopped. The syndrome is commonly associated

with dehydration, but the association is not fully understood. In addition to intravenous fluids and benzodiazepines, recommended therapies, if indicated, include cooling techniques such as cooling blankets, ice packs, or lavages; blood pressure control with nitroprusside or other intravenous vasodilators; antiarrhythmic agents; and heparin to prevent deep venous thrombosis. Lithium should be discontinued along with the other neuroleptic medications. Concomitant use of lithium is a risk factor for NMS, as is dehydration. In patients who require ongoing neuroleptic therapy, neuroleptic agents should be restarted after a waiting period of at least 2 weeks. A low-potency agent should be used at a low dose and should be titrated upward slowly. Concomitant lithium therapy and dehydration should be avoided. These patients should be monitored closely for recurrent NMS.

There is insufficient evidence to support the use of either acetaminophen or aspirin for treatment of hyperthermia due to NMS.

There is no evidence to support the use of neuromuscular blocking agents such as atracurium in NMS. In some severe cases, electroconvulsive therapy has been used, along with associated anesthesia and paralysis. Succinylcholine is usually avoided owing to the risk of malignant hyperthermia, but there has not been an observed excess of this rare complication in patients with NMS.

Mechanical ventilation is not appropriate because respiratory failure is not an imminent threat. Some patients with NMS may have respiratory failure owing to rigidity, seizures, or fatigue, and ventilatory support and/or airway control would be appropriate for those patients.

Although this patient has significantly elevated blood pressure, he has not yet been treated for NMS. If his blood pressure remains in this range or increases following initiation of hydration and benzodiazepine treatment, more aggressive antihypertensive therapy, possibly with nitroprusside or other intravenous agents, would be appropriate.

KEY POINT

- Treatment of neuroleptic malignant syndrome consists of stopping the neuroleptic agent, maintaining blood pressure stability, replacing fluid volume, lowering the elevated temperature as in malignant hyperthermia, and administering benzodiazepines for agitation.

Bibliography

Strawn JR, Keck PE, Caroff SN. Neuroleptic malignant syndrome. Am J Psychiatry. 2007;164(6):870-876. [PMID: 17541044]

Item 68   Answer: B

Educational Objective: Manage very severe COPD with long-term oxygen therapy.

The most appropriate next step in management is long-term oxygen therapy (LTOT). This patient's oxygen saturation is

86% breathing ambient air. Indications for LTOT are an arterial P_{O_2} of less than or equal to 55 mm Hg (7.3 kPa) or an oxygen saturation of less than or equal to 88% when breathing ambient air. In patients who qualify for continuous therapy because of resting hypoxemia, duration of oxygen treatment should be greater than 15 hours per day and preferably longer. The use of long-term oxygen therapy in patients with chronic respiratory failure improves survival and has a beneficial effect on hemodynamics, hematologic characteristics, exercise capacity, mental status, general alertness, motor speed, and hand grip. Studies have shown that delivering oxygen during exercise can increase the duration of endurance and/or reduce the intensity of breathlessness at the end of exercise. The Nocturnal Oxygen Therapy Trial (NOTT) showed that continuous supplemental oxygen therapy is better than nocturnal oxygen therapy alone in enhancing survival. The role and effectiveness of supplemental oxygen are less clear in patients with pulmonary disease who have normal oxygenation at rest and desaturation with exertion or nocturnally.

There is no indication for antibiotics or prednisone because this patient has no evidence of an acute exacerbation or bronchospasm.

This patient may benefit from undergoing pulmonary rehabilitation again, because data show that repeating pulmonary rehabilitation has benefits. However, given her resting hypoxemia, the most appropriate next step in management is LTOT.

KEY POINT

- **In patients with COPD, indications for long-term oxygen therapy are an arterial P_{O_2} of less than or equal to 55 mm Hg (7.3 kPa) or an oxygen saturation of less than or equal to 88%.**

Bibliography

Stoller JK, Panos RJ, Krachman S, Doherty DE, Make B; Long-term Oxygen Treatment Trial Research Group. Oxygen therapy for patients with COPD: current evidence and the long-term oxygen treatment trial. Chest. 2010;138(1):179-187. [PMID: 20605816]

Item 69   Answer: D

Educational Objective: Diagnose obesity hypoventilation syndrome.

The most likely diagnosis is obesity hypoventilation syndrome (OHS). OHS is characterized by daytime hypercapnia (arterial P_{CO_2} >45 mm Hg [6.0 kPa]) that is thought to be a consequence of diminished ventilatory drive and capacity related to extreme obesity. It is estimated that nearly one third of persons with a BMI of 35 or higher and one half with a BMI of 50 or higher exhibit sleep-related hypoventilation. Pulmonary hypertension and polycythemia are commonly associated with OHS. Obstructive sleep apnea (OSA) often coexists with OHS, and polysomnography is usually required to (1) determine the extent of OSA and (2) to titrate positive airway pressure

therapy. Continuous positive airway pressure (CPAP) is often effective first-line therapy; however, resistant hypoventilation and hypoxemia may necessitate the addition of supplemental oxygen or bilevel positive airway pressure. Clinical trials comparing different treatment options are currently lacking, but weight loss (possibly including surgical intervention) should be universally recommended.

Cheyne-Stokes breathing is a form of central sleep apnea characterized by a crescendo-decrescendo ventilatory pattern. It is most commonly seen in men with advanced left ventricular dysfunction who are typically older and thinner than this patient.

Long-standing, severe COPD may lead to carbon dioxide retention and hypercapnia. However, despite this patient's modest smoking history, he does not have a history or clinical picture consistent with a diagnosis of COPD to account for his symptoms and findings.

Pulmonary function testing can demonstrate restrictive physiology in parenchymal disorders such as interstitial lung disease (ILD) as well as in obesity, where there are limitations in chest wall movement. However, although hypercapnia defines OHS, such a finding is unusual in ILD until the disease reaches a very advanced stage.

KEY POINT

- **Obesity hypoventilation syndrome is characterized by daytime hypercapnia (arterial P_{CO_2} >45 mm Hg [6.0 kPa]) that is thought to be a consequence of diminished ventilation related to extreme obesity.**

Bibliography

Mokhlesi B, Kryger MH, Grunstein RR. Assessment and management of patients with obesity hypoventilation syndrome. Proc Am Thorac Soc. 2008;5(2):218-225. [PMID: 18250215]

Item 70   Answer: A

Educational Objective: Diagnose acute respiratory distress syndrome.

The most likely cause of this patient's hypoxemia is acute respiratory distress syndrome (ARDS). This patient has septic shock owing to a bladder infection that has triggered ARDS. Sepsis is one of the most common causes of ARDS, and onset within 48 to 72 hours after risk factor exposure is typical. The diagnosis of ARDS is most often made from clinical criteria that have recently changed. The 2012 Berlin consensus definition for ARDS updated the diagnostic criteria, classified the severity, and eliminated the term acute lung injury (ALI). The need for objective assessment (echocardiogram or pulmonary arterial wedge pressure) to exclude cardiogenic edema as a cause for ARDS is no longer required in patients with a known ARDS risk factor. Acuity of onset is now defined as 1 week, and chest CT is an accepted imaging modality to recognize bilateral alveolar opacities. ARDS is now classified into mild, moderate, and severe based on the severity of hypoxemia, and the term ALI is no longer used.

Escherichia coli pneumonia is unlikely because hematogenous spread of infection to the lungs is unusual even in bacteremic patients. Sepsis-induced ARDS is much more likely.

Heart failure should be clinically excluded as the cause of acute bilateral alveolar infiltrates in patients being evaluated for ARDS. This patient's young age, normal central venous pressure, and absence of cardiomegaly on chest radiograph all make heart failure unlikely.

Idiopathic acute eosinophilic pneumonia is characterized by infiltration of the lung parenchyma by eosinophils. Patients present with fever, nonproductive cough, dyspnea, and bilateral infiltrates. Peripheral eosinophilia may not be present early in the course of illness, but prominent eosinophilia is present in bronchoalveolar lavage fluid. Idiopathic acute eosinophilic pneumonia, however, is rare and would be unlikely in a patient presenting with gram-negative infection and sepsis.

KEY POINT

- Acute respiratory distress syndrome is usually diagnosed on clinical criteria, which include acute development of hypoxemic respiratory failure with radiographic evidence of bilateral alveolar opacities that are not caused by heart failure.

Bibliography

ARDS Definition Task Force, Ranieri VM, Rubenfeld GD, Thompson BT, et al. Acute respiratory distress syndrome: the Berlin Definition. JAMA. 2012;307(23):2526-33. [PMID: 22797452]

Item 71   Answer: D

Educational Objective: Diagnose a malignant pleural effusion.

The most appropriate next step in the evaluation of this patient's pleural effusion is to repeat thoracentesis and repeat pleural fluid cytology. This patient is a former smoker and presents with concerning symptoms of cough, hoarseness, and unexplained weight loss, as well as imaging studies that demonstrate a unilateral pleural effusion with an ipsilateral lung mass suspicious for bronchogenic carcinoma with pleural metastasis. Initial evaluation is with thoracentesis, because positive cytology for non–small cell carcinoma will effectively establish a diagnosis and simultaneously establish the malignancy as stage IV. This patient's pleural fluid analysis shows a lymphocyte-predominant exudate, which could be consistent with a malignant pleural effusion; however, pleural fluid cytology is negative. The overall sensitivity of pleural fluid cytology averages 60%, with 65% of positive results obtained on the initial sampling. An additional 27% are identified on the second sampling, and 5% on the third. Diagnostic yield does not increase appreciably after the

third sampling. Repeat thoracentesis is the appropriate evaluation owing to the sequential increase in diagnostic yield up until the third sampling.

Although a diagnosis may be established by bronchoscopic sampling, staging will be incomplete and additional procedures will be required.

Closed pleural biopsy, although effective diagnostically in diffuse pleural diseases such as tuberculosis, has lower sensitivity than cytology in the diagnosis of malignant pleural disease owing to the typically sporadic distribution of pleural metastatic lesions. If a diagnosis is not established with serial thoracentesis, it would be reasonable to consider thoracoscopic pleural biopsy.

There is little suspicion for lymphoma in this patient, so pleural fluid flow-cytometry is not indicated.

KEY POINT

- In patients with pleural effusions that are suspicious for non–small cell lung cancer, diagnostic yield increases with repeat thoracentesis and cytology (65% of positive results obtained on the initial sampling, 27% on the second, and 5% on the third).

Bibliography

Garcia LW, Ducatman BS, Wang HH. The value of multiple fluid specimens in the cytological diagnosis of malignancy. Mod Pathol. 1994;7(6):665-668. [PMID: 7991525]

Item 72   Answer: B

Educational Objective: Evaluate for autoimmune disease in a patient with nonspecific interstitial pneumonia.

The most appropriate next step in management is to repeat studies to evaluate for possible connective tissue disease. The pulmonary histopathologic finding of nonspecific interstitial pneumonia (NSIP) has been associated with undifferentiated connective tissue disease. In one study, greater than 80% of patients met diagnostic criteria for undifferentiated connective tissue disease at the time of their presentation with NSIP. However, patients without evidence of autoimmune disease at presentation may subsequently develop symptoms and signs of systemic disease. A more recent study showed that over 50% of patients with a diagnosis of idiopathic NSIP developed evidence of an underlying autoimmune disease over an average of 22 months. This patient presents with new evidence of arthritis. Given her pulmonary history and increasing joint pain symptoms, there should be high suspicion for an underlying connective tissue disease. The association of NSIP with autoimmune disease may reflect a common pathophysiology, and establishing the diagnosis of associated connective tissue disease informs the follow-up and treatment of both disorders.

Bronchoalveolar lavage is frequently abnormal in patients with NSIP and may be helpful in excluding other diseases such as infection or malignancy. However, with biopsy-proven disease, this procedure would not be expected to contribute additional information.

A repeat lung biopsy would not be indicated with a prior adequate study and stable clinical picture.

Although continued observation of this patient's lung disease may be appropriate, further evaluation of her joint symptoms in the context of her known pulmonary diagnosis is indicated.

KEY POINT

- **For patients with idiopathic nonspecific interstitial pneumonia, follow-up should include screening for the development of systemic symptoms because systemic connective tissue disease can present after the development of lung involvement.**

Bibliography

Romagnoli M, Nannini C, Piciucchi S, et al. Idiopathic nonspecific interstitial pneumonia: an interstitial lung disease associated with autoimmune disorders? Eur Respir J. 2011;38(2):384-391. [PMID: 21273390]

Item 73   Answer: C
Educational Objective: Treat severe asthma.

The most appropriate treatment is to initiate omalizumab. This patient has severe asthma that appears to be refractory to high-dose inhaled corticosteroid and long-acting β_2-agonist therapy. Treatment with omalizumab has been shown to reduce the frequency of exacerbations, improve quality of life, and decrease the need for inhaled and systemic corticosteroid therapy. Omalizumab is recommended for patients with severe asthma who have evidence of allergies, have an elevated IgE level, and remain symptomatic despite optimizing therapy with combination therapy of high-dose inhaled corticosteroids and a long-acting β_2-agonist. Because this therapy can be associated with serious anaphylactoid reactions, it should be started only by providers who are skilled at monitoring and treating these complications. The cost of omalizumab can exceed several thousand dollars per month; therefore, the decision to initiate therapy should be made after consideration of the potential benefits (mainly reduction in exacerbations) and drawbacks (need for scheduled injections, cost, and anaphylaxis). Because response to this treatment is highly variable, continued treatment may not be justified if there is no clear improvement after 6 months of initiating omalizumab.

Treatment of patients with severe asthma using methotrexate and azathioprine is associated with modest benefit and significant side effects; therefore, these agents are not recommended.

Tumor necrosis factor α inhibitors have been evaluated for the treatment of asthma because of their ability to suppress inflammation. However, they have not been shown to decrease the frequency of exacerbations or improve pulmonary function. Therefore, they are not recommended for asthma therapy.

KEY POINT

- **Omalizumab is recommended for patients with severe asthma who have evidence of allergies, have an elevated IgE level, and remain symptomatic despite optimizing therapy with combination therapy of high-dose inhaled corticosteroids and a long-acting β_2-agonist.**

Bibliography

Hanania NA, Alpan O, Hamilos DL, et al. Omalizumab in severe allergic asthma inadequately controlled with standard therapy: a randomized trial. Ann Intern Med. 2011;154(9):573-582. [PMID: 21536936]

Item 74   Answer: A
Educational Objective: Diagnose a pleural effusion due to heart failure.

The most likely cause of this patient's pleural effusion is heart failure. This patient presents with classic findings of decompensated heart failure. In this patient, pleural fluid analysis is consistent with an exudate by total protein criteria only (pleural fluid to serum total protein ratio of 0.51), with a transudative lactate dehydrogenase ratio. Pleural fluid differentiation into transudative or exudative categories by modified Light criteria is almost 100% sensitive but only 83% specific for an exudative process, and specificity further declines in the setting of a transudative process with concurrent diuretic therapy, such as in this patient. In this setting, determining the albumin or total protein gradient is useful in confirming the clinical suspicion that the effusions are in fact due to heart failure alone. A serum to pleural fluid albumin gradient greater than 1.2 g/dL (12 g/L) or a serum to pleural fluid total protein gradient greater than 3.1 g/dL (31 g/L) are equally consistent with a transudative process under these circumstances.

Pleural effusions due to malignancy tend to be unilateral with exudative chemical characteristics, and up to two thirds are lymphocyte predominant. The effusion in this patient is most consistent with a transudate, in which case the lymphocyte predominance is of no clinical significance.

Pneumonia is associated with an exudative pleural effusion, which is not present in this patient. In addition, the absence of fever reduces the probability of a parapneumonic effusion. Although the results of the pleural fluid analysis may increase or decrease the posttest probability that the effusion is exudative, a low clinical suspicion of an exudate should not be affected by borderline test results.

Pleural effusions due to pulmonary embolus are small and unilateral, with 86% resulting in only blunting of the costophrenic angle. Pleural fluid analysis is not helpful in establishing the diagnosis; however, it is almost always consistent with an exudative process.

Bibliography

Romero-Candeira S, Fernández C, Martín C, Sánchez-Paya J, Hernández L. Influence of diuretics on the concentration of proteins and other components of pleural transudates in patients with heart failure. Am J Med. 2001;110(9):681-686. [PMID: 11403751]

Item 75   Answer: E

Educational Objective: Manage severe COPD with smoking cessation in a patient who is otherwise a candidate for lung transplantation.

The most appropriate next step in management is to advise this patient to quit smoking. He meets criteria for possible lung transplantation based on the severity of his COPD. However, substance addiction (alcohol, tobacco, or narcotics) that is current or active within the last 6 months is an absolute contraindication to lung transplantation. This patient is still smoking and therefore should be advised to quit. Transplantation in patients with COPD should be considered if deterioration continues despite appropriate, maximal medical therapy in patients without clear contraindications to the procedure. The BODE (BMI, Obstruction, Dyspnea, Exercise) index is a method for assessing severity of COPD and is based on health care quality-of-life measures and independent predictors of disease-related mortality. A BODE score of greater than 5 is an indication for referral for evaluation for lung transplantation. Transplantation is indicated in patients with a BODE index of 7 to 10 and at least one of the following: history of hospitalization for exacerbation associated with hypercapnia; pulmonary hypertension, cor pulmonale, or both despite oxygen therapy; FEV_1 of less than 20% of predicted and either D_{LCO} of less than 20% of predicted or homogeneous distribution of emphysema. Referral for lung transplantation would be appropriate for this patient only if he stops smoking.

This patient's oxygenation is adequate; therefore, increasing the oxygen is not appropriate, especially in a patient with a history of acute hypercapnia. Oxygen therapy is indicated for patients who have hypoxemia, arterial

PO_2 less than 55 mm Hg (7.3 kPa), or arterial oxygen saturation of 88% or lower.

Patients with an FEV_1 of less than 20% of predicted and either a D_{LCO} of less than 20% of predicted or homogeneously distributed emphysema are considered high risk for lung volume reduction surgery (LVRS). Because this patient's FEV_1 and D_{LCO} are less than 20% of predicted, this patient is not an ideal candidate for LVRS.

Pulmonary rehabilitation is very effective in patients with advanced COPD, and repeated courses or continuous pulmonary rehabilitation has value. However, it is not a definitive treatment for patients with severe disease who would otherwise be eligible for lung transplantation.

Bibliography

Kreider M, Kotloff RM. Selection of candidates for lung transplantation. Proc Am Thorac Soc. 2009;6(1):20-27. [PMID: 19131527]

Item 76   Answer: A

Educational Objective: Treat a patient with acute respiratory distress syndrome by optimizing positive end-expiratory pressure.

The most appropriate treatment is to increase positive end-expiratory pressure (PEEP) to 10 cm H_2O. This patient has acute respiratory distress syndrome (ARDS) with persistent hypoxemia. Increasing PEEP, FIO_2, and inspiratory to expiratory ratio will all improve oxygenation. PEEP improves oxygenation by recruiting atelectatic alveoli, increasing static compliance, and decreasing shunt. However, at high levels PEEP can lead to barotrauma, low cardiac output, and hypotension. Multiple clinical trials comparing differing levels of PEEP have found no significant differences in survival between higher and lower levels of PEEP; however, there were improvements in some secondary clinical endpoints, especially in the sickest patients with ARDS. Current recommendations are to use an amount of PEEP that achieves an FIO_2 of less than 0.6 and does not cause hypotension.

Increasing the respiration rate will increase the minute ventilation and elimination of carbon dioxide, but it will have no effect on oxygenation.

Increasing tidal volume may transiently improve oxygenation but will result in a tidal volume higher than 6 mL/kg of ideal body weight (IBW). Survival is improved when patients with ARDS are ventilated with a tidal volume of 6 mL/kg of IBW.

Nitric oxide is a pulmonary vasodilator that, when aerosolized, will improve ventilation/perfusion matching and modestly (and transiently) improve oxygenation;

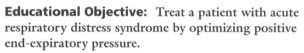

CONT.

however, it has no demonstrated impact on important patient outcomes such as survival.

KEY POINT

- For patients with acute respiratory distress syndrome, current recommendations for mechanical ventilation are to choose a level of positive end-expiratory pressure (PEEP) that achieves an FIO$_2$ of less than 0.6 and does not cause hypotension.

Bibliography

Putensen C, Theuerkauf N, Zinserling J, Wrigge H, Pelosi P. Meta-analysis: ventilation strategies and outcomes of the acute respiratory distress syndrome and acute lung injury [erratum in Ann Intern Med. 2009;151(12):897]. Ann Intern Med. 2009;151(8):566-576. [PMID: 19841457]

Item 77   Answer: D

Educational Objective: Manage Löfgren syndrome.

The most appropriate management is observation. This patient presents with classic Löfgren syndrome. Sarcoidosis is a multiorgan inflammatory disease characterized by tissue infiltration by mononuclear phagocytes, lymphocytes, and noncaseating granulomas. An estimated 90% of patients have pulmonary involvement at the time of presentation. Sarcoidosis commonly involves the eyes and skin; the central nervous system, heart, and gastrointestinal tract are less commonly involved. Most patients require a tissue diagnosis, but there are some exceptions that do not warrant histologic confirmation such as Löfgren syndrome (fever, erythema nodosum, polyarthralgia, and hilar lymphadenopathy) and Heerfordt syndrome (uveitis, parotid gland enlargement, and fever). More than 80% of patients with sarcoidosis who present with Löfgren syndrome have spontaneous resolution.

Bronchoscopy with transbronchial biopsy, video-assisted thoracoscopic biopsy, and high-resolution CT scan of the chest are not warranted at this time because the cost/benefit analysis of further evaluation does not favor this approach. As mentioned above, more than 80% of patients will have spontaneous resolution.

KEY POINT

- Most patients with suspected sarcoidosis require a tissue diagnosis, but there are some classic clinical presentations of known sarcoid syndromes (such as Löfgren syndrome) that do not warrant histologic confirmation.

Bibliography

Hamzeh N. Sarcoidosis. Med Clin North Am. 2011;95(6):1223-1234. [PMID: 22032436]

Item 78   Answer: A

Educational Objective: Manage upper airway obstruction due to angioedema associated with ACE inhibitor use.

The most appropriate next step in management is endotracheal intubation. This patient is experiencing angioedema, likely triggered by use of an ACE inhibitor, and should be intubated immediately because he is at high risk of asphyxiation due to upper airway edema. The absence of signs and symptoms of an allergic reaction, such as urticaria, pruritus, bronchospasm, and hypotension, is typical of ACE inhibitor–associated angioedema. Although angioedema is most often reported within 1 week of starting or increasing the dose of the medication, it can occur after years of use. The risk of recurrence with continued exposure to ACE inhibitors is substantial, and patients should be switched to an alternative medication.

Methylprednisolone and epinephrine are useful in the treatment of upper airway obstruction triggered by croup and anaphylactic reactions, but they do not have a clear role in the treatment of angioedema associated with ACE inhibitors. This patient's airway is severely compromised, and there is insufficient time to delay intubation in order to allow a trial of therapy.

Noninvasive positive pressure ventilation may decrease the patient's work of breathing and help splint the upper airway open, but it does not adequately secure the airway and should not be used to manage upper airway obstruction regardless of the cause.

KEY POINT

- ACE inhibitor–associated angioedema is characterized by the absence of signs and symptoms of an allergic reaction (such as urticaria, pruritus, bronchospasm, and hypotension); endotracheal intubation should be considered if severe upper airway edema is present.

Bibliography

Malde B, Regalado J, Greenberger PA. Investigation of angioedema associated with the use of angiotensin-converting enzyme inhibitors and angiotensin receptor blockers. Ann Allergy Asthma Immunol. 2007;98(1):57-63. [PMID: 17225721]

Item 79   Answer: D

Educational Objective: Exclude pulmonary embolism with a D-dimer test in a low-risk patient.

The most appropriate next step in management is measurement of peak flow. This patient has a strong family history of asthma and a remote personal history of asthma. She has wheezing and pharyngeal injection on examination, which could reflect a viral respiratory infection or reflux triggering bronchospasm as the cause of her dyspnea. Thus, assessment for airflow obstruction is appropriate. Despite a history of recent surgery and symptoms of acute onset of dyspnea, this patient's pulmonary embolism (PE) risk score determined by either the Wells or Revised Geneva scoring systems suggests a low probability of PE. Immunologic D-dimer assays are particularly sensitive for detecting the presence of intravascular thrombosis. In this patient with a low PE risk score, the normal D-dimer level effectively excludes PE; therefore, further testing for PE, either by CT angiography or by duplex ultrasound of the legs (to identify deep venous thrombosis as a source for PE), is not indicated.

Although abdominal surgery (particularly an open procedure) is associated with an increased risk for perioperative pulmonary complications, there is no suggestion by history or physical examination of an ongoing abdominal process as a cause of this patient's respiratory symptoms that would indicate the need for abdominal imaging.

KEY POINT

- **In clinically stable patients with a low pretest probability of pulmonary embolism using the Wells or Revised Geneva scores, a normal D-dimer assay effectively excludes an acute thrombotic process and eliminates the need for further testing.**

Bibliography

Moores LK, King CS, Holley AB. Current approach to the diagnosis of acute nonmassive pulmonary embolism. Chest. 2011;140(2):509-518. [PMID: 21813530]

Item 80   Answer: B
Educational Objective: Manage septic shock.

The most appropriate next step in management is diagnostic paracentesis to identify a potential source of infection. This patient's physical examination findings are characteristic of distributive shock. Both liver failure and sepsis can present with this form of shock; however, septic shock should be assumed first and excluded as a cause. The patient's distributive shock with a profound alteration of mental status meets criteria for the systemic inflammatory response syndrome (SIRS) (altered temperature, tachycardia, hyperventilation, and abnormal leukocyte count). The combination of organ dysfunction and SIRS is diagnostic of severe sepsis. In addition to aggressive intravenous fluid therapy and empiric broad-spectrum antibiotic therapy, identifying the source of potential infection is the next step in management. The ascites associated with this patient's chronic liver disease represents a potential source that should be evaluated for evidence of infection. Identification of a source is important in guiding the choice of appropriate empiric antibiotic coverage and focusing longer-term antibiotic therapy once an organism has been identified. This patient's worsening liver failure and new-onset encephalopathy can be precipitated by infection.

An abdominal CT scan is not helpful in the diagnosis of bacterial peritonitis, and direct examination of the ascitic

fluid is necessary to assess this as a potential source of infection. Imaging for other potential abdominal sources of infection may be indicated if no other cause is found once peritonitis is excluded.

Vasopressors such as dopamine are recommended for patients with septic shock and a mean arterial blood pressure (MAP) of less than 65 mm Hg following an adequate trial of intravenous fluids. This patient's current blood pressure is adequate, and vasopressor medications are currently not indicated.

Corticosteroid therapy is not recommended in the setting of septic shock unless the patient's endocrine or corticosteroid history warrants treatment or there is suspicion of undetected adrenal insufficiency. This patient has no clear history of chronic or intermittent corticosteroid use and has not had an adequate trial of volume expansion.

KEY POINT

- **The primary goals of sepsis management are infection source control and early antibiotics.**

Bibliography

Dellinger RP, Levy MM, Carlet JM, et al; International Surviving Sepsis Campaign Guidelines Committee; American Association of Critical-Care Nurses; American College of Chest Physicians; American College of Emergency Physicians; Canadian Critical Care Society; European Society of Clinical Microbiology and Infectious Diseases; European Society of Intensive Care Medicine; European Respiratory Society; International Sepsis Forum; Japanese Association for Acute Medicine; Japanese Society of Intensive Care Medicine; Society of Critical Care Medicine; Society of Hospital Medicine; Surgical Infection Society; World Federation of Societies of Intensive and Critical Care Medicine. Surviving Sepsis Campaign: international guidelines for management of severe sepsis and septic shock: 2008 [erratum in Crit Care Med. 2008;36(4):1394-1396]. Crit Care Med. 2008;36(1):296-327. [PMID: 18158437]

Item 81   Answer: D
Educational Objective: Diagnose COPD with spirometry.

The most appropriate management is to perform spirometry. A clinical diagnosis of COPD should be considered in any patient who has dyspnea, chronic cough or sputum production, and/or a history of risk factors for the disease. In symptomatic patients, spirometry is helpful for determining whether the symptoms are due to respiratory disease or other conditions. COPD is diagnosed when spirometry demonstrates airflow obstruction characterized by a reduction of the FEV_1/FVC and the FEV_1.

In patients who have symptoms suggestive of asthma but normal spirometry, bronchial challenge testing can help establish the presence of airway hyperresponsiveness. Spirometry is obtained after inhalation of increasing concentrations of an inhaled medication that promotes bronchoconstriction to determine the effect on FEV_1. A bronchial challenge is not appropriate in this patient because his symptoms do not suggest asthma and he has not yet had spirometry.

CT of the chest without contrast is not a good initial choice because it is expensive, carries radiation risk, and does not address the diagnosis of COPD. CT scan could be useful if there was concern for lung cancer or if the patient was being evaluated for lung volume reduction surgery. However, the most important first step is to make a diagnosis of COPD with spirometry.

DLCO is a measurement of the rate of diffusion of carbon monoxide across the alveolar-capillary membrane. A DLCO value greater than or equal to 80% of predicted is considered normal. DLCO is used to determine the possible presence of parenchymal lung disease and pulmonary vascular disease. DLCO is normal in conditions associated with abnormal spirometry measurements and lung volumes but normal lung parenchyma (such as asthma or neuromuscular disease). It may be abnormal in patients with COPD but does not add additional diagnostic value in patients with symptoms compatible with COPD and abnormal spirometry.

KEY POINT

- COPD is diagnosed in patients with compatible symptoms and when spirometry demonstrates airflow obstruction characterized by a reduction of the FEV_1/FVC and the FEV_1.

Bibliography

Qaseem A, Wilt TJ, Weinberger SE, et al; American College of Physicians; American College of Chest Physicians; American Thoracic Society; European Respiratory Society. Diagnosis and management of stable chronic obstructive pulmonary disease: a clinical practice guideline update from the American College of Physicians, American College of Chest Physicians, American Thoracic Society, and European Respiratory Society. Ann Intern Med. 2011;155(3):179-191. [PMID: 21810710]

Item 82   Answer: B

Educational Objective: Manage acute respiratory distress syndrome with the appropriate plateau pressure.

The most appropriate next step in management is to decrease the tidal volume. The plateau pressure must be decreased to prevent overstretching the lung. The use of low (6 mL/kg predicted weight) rather than standard (12 mL/kg predicted weight) tidal volumes reduces the mortality rate from acute respiratory distress syndrome (ARDS) from 40% to 30%. Elevated plateau pressures were associated with increased mortality in the ARDS Clinical Network trial. In the study, the tidal volume was initially set at 6 mL/kg of ideal body weight (IBW) and was subsequently reduced stepwise by 1 mL/kg IBW if necessary to maintain a plateau pressure less than 30 cm H_2O. The application of this lung-protective ventilator strategy often requires permissive hypercapnia as well as

the use of a high FIO_2 to maintain adequate oxygenation in patients with severe ARDS. Permissive hypercapnia is not harmful to the patient; some evidence suggests that mild hypercapnia may decrease the degree of ventilator-induced lung injury.

Decreasing the respiration rate or increasing the FIO_2 would not affect the elevated plateau pressure, and increasing positive end-expiratory pressure would increase the plateau pressures further. All of these measures would negate the improved mortality rate associated with the lung-protective ventilatory strategy.

KEY POINT

- In patients with acute respiratory distress syndrome, a lung-protective strategy of low tidal volume (6 mL/kg predicted weight) and plateau pressure less than 30 cm H_2O is associated with reduced mortality.

Bibliography

Petrucci N, Iacovelli W. Lung protective ventilation strategy for the acute respiratory distress syndrome. Cochrane Database Syst Rev. 2007;18;(3):CD003844. [PMID: 17636739]

Item 83   Answer: B

Educational Objective: Diagnose cough-variant asthma.

The most appropriate diagnostic test is a bronchial challenge test. This patient has chronic cough. Asthma, postnasal drip, and gastroesophageal reflux are the most common diagnoses for patients with chronic cough and a normal chest radiograph. This patient has episodic cough triggered by cold air and hyperventilation. The symptoms are suggestive of cough-variant asthma. Bronchial challenge testing in such a patient can exclude asthma if negative and suggest cough-variant asthma if positive. Such testing is indicated when asthma is suspected despite routine spirometry failing to show evidence of bronchospasm. Patients with underlying asthma typically have bronchial hyperresponsiveness and will have an exaggerated response to agents that promote bronchoconstriction. Diagnostic criteria are based on the degree of airway obstruction triggered by inhalation of these medications relative to baseline. The diagnosis of cough-variant asthma should be confirmed with clinical response to usual asthma therapy.

Although it is important to consider pertussis in patients with acute or subacute cough, this patient has had cough for nearly 1 year and has no recent symptoms to suggest acute infection. Furthermore, he has already received two courses of antibiotics, including drugs from two classes that should have been effective against *Bordetella pertussis*.

Bronchoscopy should be reserved for patients with an abnormal chest radiograph or who are at higher risk of lung cancer (long-standing history of smoking, older age).

A chest CT scan in a young nonsmoker with a clear chest radiograph would be unlikely to reveal any useful information; it is therefore not indicated.

KEY POINT

- Bronchial challenge testing in patients with suspected cough-variant asthma can exclude asthma if negative and suggest cough-variant asthma if positive.

Bibliography

Dicpinigaitis PV. Chronic cough due to asthma: ACCP evidence-based clinical practice guidelines. Chest. 2006;129(1 suppl):75S-79S. [PMID: 16428696]

Item 84   Answer: D
Educational Objective: Treat pulmonary metastases from colorectal carcinoma.

The most appropriate treatment is surgical resection. The lung is a common site for metastatic disease from a treated colorectal carcinoma. Following treatment for stage II disease, posttreatment surveillance usually consists of periodic history and physical examination with serial assay of the serum concentrations of the tumor marker carcinoembryonic antigen, annual surveillance CT scans, and colonoscopy to detect metachronous primaries. The majority of recurrent disease appears within 5 years of treatment. Metastases to the lung from colorectal carcinoma may be multiple and tend to be smoothly bordered and without evidence of calcification. Resection is the primary treatment for metastatic colorectal carcinoma limited to the lung; many patients experience long-term survival with this intervention alone, including those with multiple pulmonary sites of metastasis. The efficacy of additional chemotherapy and/or radiation therapy directed toward the area of metastasis following surgical resection is not clear, but these interventions are frequently considered factoring in the age and general health of the patient and the potential long-term effects of these treatments.

With the exception of nonresectable disease, chemotherapy and radiation therapy are not considered primary treatment for colorectal pulmonary metastatic disease.

Hospice care is not appropriate for this patient before viable therapeutic options are pursued.

KEY POINT

- In patients with colorectal carcinoma with metastatic disease to the lung, surgical resection is the primary treatment and is associated with good long-term survival.

Bibliography

Hornbech K, Ravn J, Steinbrüchel DA. Outcome after pulmonary metastasectomy: analysis of 5 years consecutive surgical resections 2002-2006. J Thorac Oncol. 2011;6(10):1733-1740. [PMID: 21869715]

Item 85   Answer: D
Educational Objective: Treat severe COPD.

The most appropriate next step in treatment is to add roflumilast. This patient, who has severe COPD and a history of multiple exacerbations, is on all appropriate medication regimens for severe COPD, so roflumilast is an appropriate addition to the treatment regimen. Roflumilast is an oral phosphodiesterase-4 inhibitor recently approved for use in patients with severe and very severe COPD associated with chronic bronchitis and a history of frequent exacerbations. It is an anti-inflammatory agent and not a strong bronchodilator and therefore is not indicated for treatment of acute COPD exacerbations; however, it provides a measurable but modest improvement in FEV_1 independent of the patient's smoking status or use of concomitant medications. It is not intended for the treatment of primary emphysema. Common side effects of roflumilast include diarrhea, weight loss, nausea, headache, backache, decreased appetite, dizziness, and occasionally neuropsychiatric symptoms such as depression and suicidality. Roflumilast is expensive and should be considered as add-on therapy in highly selected patients. There are no data comparing theophylline and roflumilast, but theophylline does not have the same indications as roflumilast and has a worse side-effect profile.

Long-term use of oral corticosteroids is not recommended owing to their limited, if any, benefit and serious side effects such as osteoporosis, glaucoma, and adrenal suppression.

This patient's oxygenation is adequate, so there is no indication for long-term oxygen therapy at this time. Oxygen therapy is indicated for patients who have hypoxemia, arterial PO_2 less than 55 mm Hg (7.3 kPa), or arterial oxygen saturation of 88% or lower.

Mucolytics such as *N*-acetylcysteine have been used for many years in oral and inhaled forms to thin mucus and assist in expectoration of secretions associated with chronic bronchitis. However, there is little evidence documenting effectiveness in improving lung function or clinical outcomes in patients with stable COPD or in acute exacerbations.

KEY POINT

- Roflumilast is an oral phosphodiesterase-4 inhibitor recently approved for use in patients with severe and very severe COPD associated with chronic bronchitis and a history of frequent exacerbations.

Bibliography

Calverley PM, Rabe KF, Goehring UM, Kristiansen S, Fabbri LM, Martinez FJ; M2-124 and M2-125 study groups. Roflumilast in symptomatic chronic obstructive pulmonary disease: two randomised clinical trials [erratum in Lancet. 2010;376(9747):1146]. Lancet. 2009;374(9691):685-694. [PMID: 19716960]

Item 86   Answer: B

Educational Objective: Manage carbon monoxide toxicity.

The most appropriate management is hyperbaric oxygen therapy, if available. This patient has carbon monoxide (CO) toxicity. The serial blood gas analyses show that she is recovering; with time and adequate oxygen, her carboxyhemoglobin levels will continue to decrease. However, the high levels measured on her arrival in the emergency department put her at risk for developing delayed neurocognitive impairment often associated with carbon monoxide poisoning. Hyperbaric oxygen therapy will greatly speed the clearance of carboxyhemoglobin and has been shown to reduce the incidence of delayed neurocognitive impairment. Whether hyperbaric oxygen therapy is available or not, administration of 100% high-flow oxygen through a nonrebreather mask will also help clear the carboxyhemoglobin more quickly.

In victims of smoke inhalation, a blood lactic acid level of 90 mg/dL (10.0 mmol/L) or greater is sensitive and specific for cyanide poisoning. Because this patient had a lactic acid level of 41 mg/dL (4.6 mmol/L), cyanide poisoning is unlikely. If inhaled cyanide toxicity is suspected, the correct antidote is sodium thiosulfate.

Mechanical ventilation is not appropriate because there is no indication that respiratory failure is imminent. Evidence of airway thermal injury or suspicion of low-solubility toxin inhalation could require intubation for airway protection and/or therapeutic intervention, but this patient has no sign of airway compromise.

Pulse oximetry is unreliable in the presence of carboxyhemoglobin and will indicate a falsely reassuring oxygen saturation. Even if more accurate co-oximetry is used to monitor oxyhemoglobin levels as this patient improves, allowing the patient to clear the carboxyhemoglobin slowly in the absence of oxygen therapy will put her at increased risk for neurocognitive impairment.

KEY POINT

- In patients with carbon monoxide toxicity and high levels of carboxyhemoglobin, hyperbaric oxygen therapy greatly speeds the clearance of carboxyhemoglobin and has been shown to reduce the incidence of delayed neurocognitive impairment.

Bibliography
Garrabou G, Inoriza JM, Morén C, et al. Hyperbaric oxygen therapy for carbon monoxide poisoning. Intensive Care Med. 2011;37(10):1711-1712. [PMID: 21667143]

Item 87   Answer: D

Educational Objective: Reduce lung cancer risk with smoking cessation.

Smoking cessation is the most important and effective intervention to reduce the risk of lung cancer and dying of lung cancer. Lung cancer risk for a current smoker with a 40-pack-year history is approximately 20 times that of someone who has never smoked. This patient's risk by age 70 years would be approximately halved if he quit now compared with if he continues smoking. Although there is some evidence that decreasing the amount of tobacco use in heavy smokers may decrease overall risk slightly, this reduction is not as great as is seen with complete abstention. Therefore, this patient should be encouraged to continue efforts to quit smoking.

Randomized trials have not shown mortality benefit of screening for lung cancer with chest radiography.

Randomized trials in the United States of β-carotene supplementation in both men and women smokers failed to show a decreased mortality rate due to lung cancer. In one Finnish study, β-carotene supplementation in smokers resulted in an 18% increase in the incidence of lung cancer and an 8% increase in overall mortality.

Because of their ability to reverse squamous metaplasia, retinoids have been evaluated for possible chemoprevention in smokers, particularly those with cellular abnormalities on sputum sampling. However, multiple clinical trials have failed to demonstrate a significant benefit from their use as an agent for chemoprevention.

KEY POINT

- Primary prevention for lung cancer consists of smoking cessation, never starting smoking, and avoidance of second-hand smoke.

Bibliography
Chandler MA, Rennard SI. Smoking cessation. Chest. 2010;137(2):428-35. [PMID: 2013328]

Item 88   Answer: B

Educational Objective: Treat cocaine-induced chest pain.

The most appropriate treatment is intravenous diltiazem and lorazepam. This patient is having acute chest pain associated with cocaine use. Cocaine raises blood pressure, heart rate, and myocardial oxygen requirements. It can also induce spasm of the coronary circulation even if there is no preexisting coronary artery stenosis. Patients with chest pain in the setting of cocaine use should be evaluated and managed as any other patient with chest pain (except for the use of β-blockers; see discussion in the following paragraphs). Calcium channel blockers and benzodiazepines are safe in this setting and are effective in lowering the heart rate, blood pressure, and myocardial oxygen demand.

Alteplase infusion is not appropriate because the patient does not meet criteria for thrombolytic therapy, which is usually used only in cases of ST-elevation myocardial infarction. Because there is no ST-segment elevation on this patient's electrocardiogram, alteplase would not be appropriate.

The use of β-blockers in patients with cocaine-induced chest pain is controversial because of the pharmacologic concern that they may leave the patient with unopposed α-mediated vasoconstriction, leading to increased blood pressure and myocardial ischemia. Although β-blockade is considered beneficial in most patients with possible ischemic cardiac disease, in this scenario a calcium channel blocker should be used to decrease the blood pressure and heart rate and lower myocardial oxygen demand.

Intravenous nitroprusside is not appropriate because this patient's presentation is not consistent with a hypertensive urgency, aortic dissection, or other acute need to lower the blood pressure primarily. The blood pressure is elevated, but it is in a range consistent with the patient's cocaine ingestion and agitation.

KEY POINT

- Calcium channel blockers and benzodiazepines are safe in patients with cocaine-associated chest pain and are effective in lowering the heart rate, blood pressure, and myocardial oxygen demand.

Bibliography

McCord J, Jneid H, Hollander JE, et al; American Heart Association Acute Cardiac Care Committee of the Council on Clinical Cardiology. Management of cocaine-associated chest pain and myocardial infarction: a scientific statement from the American Heart Association Acute Cardiac Care Committee of the Council on Clinical Cardiology. Circulation. 2008;117(14):1897-1907. [PMID: 18347214]

Item 89   Answer: A

Educational Objective: Diagnose pulmonary embolism using CT angiography.

The most appropriate next step in management is CT angiography (CTA). This patient has an intermediate to high probability of having a pulmonary embolism (PE) as assessed by one of the validated risk stratification systems (Wells or Revised Geneva scores). Therefore, the diagnosis of PE should be pursued by further testing. In this patient, CTA is the preferred method of diagnosis given his structurally abnormal lungs and lack of contraindications to this study. CTA findings of filling defects within the segmental or larger pulmonary arteries are specific for PE.

D-dimer testing is very sensitive for the detection of thromboembolic disease; in patients with a low probability for deep venous thrombosis or PE, a negative study is helpful in excluding the need for further testing. However, D-dimer testing is less helpful in patients with an intermediate to high probability of disease, which is an indication for definitive testing; D-dimer testing should not be obtained in these situations.

Lower-extremity compression ultrasonography is sometimes used to assess for evidence of thrombotic disease in patients with suspected PE when chest imaging is unavailable or if there are contraindications to chest imaging. If thrombotic disease is detected, treatment is similar to that of PE. However, in this patient with intermediate to high probability of PE and no contraindication to chest imaging, CTA is the most appropriate study.

Ventilation/perfusion scanning is typically more difficult to interpret than CTA in patients with an intermediate risk of PE and in those with structurally abnormal lungs. However, it remains a diagnostic option for PE in patients with contraindications to CTA (such as kidney failure and pregnancy).

KEY POINT

- Pulmonary CT angiography is the preferred method of diagnosis in patients with intermediate to high probability of pulmonary embolism when the test is available and there are no contraindications to radiocontrast dye administration; D-dimer testing in these patients is not appropriate.

Bibliography

Agnelli G, Becattini C. Acute pulmonary embolism. N Engl J Med. 2010;363(3):266-274. [PMID: 20592294]

Item 90   Answer: C

Educational Objective: Manage nutrition in critical illness.

The most appropriate next step in management is to increase the rate of the current nutritional preparation. The enteral route is generally well tolerated with a low complication rate. Because this patient has not demonstrated intolerance of enteral nutrition, the best management is to advance his enteral nutrition to goal. Enteral feeding should be initiated at an infusion rate of 15 to 30 mL/h and incrementally increased. Reasonable goals are 25 kcal/kg/d for calories and 2 g/kg/d for protein. The enteral feeding rate should be titrated to meet these needs given his increased metabolic requirements. There is consensus that nutritional support improves nutritional outcomes, such as body weight and mid-arm muscle mass. However, there is disagreement regarding whether nutrition improves important clinical outcomes, such as duration of mechanical ventilation, length of stay, and mortality rates. The goals of nutritional support include combating the adverse effects of malnutrition and modulating the underlying disease.

Parenteral nutrition is associated with more complications, particularly infectious complications, and has not been proved superior to enteral nutrition. Parenteral nutrition is indicated for patients in whom an enteral feeding trial fails or who have contraindications to enteral feeding.

Several nutrients, including glutamine, arginine, and omega-3 fatty acids (known as immunonutrition), influence immunologic responses. Use of immunonutrition is

CONT.

controversial, has not shown clear benefit, and is generally not recommended.

Use of a lipid suspension would increase calories delivered but would not be favorable to the nitrogen balance.

KEY POINT

- When possible, enteral feeding is preferred over parenteral routes in critically ill patients.

Bibliography

Martindale RG, McClave SA, Vanek VW, et al; American College of Critical Care Medicine; A.S.P.E.N. Board of Directors. Guidelines for the provision and assessment of nutrition support therapy in the adult critically ill patient: Society of Critical Care Medicine and American Society for Parenteral and Enteral Nutrition: Executive Summary. Crit Care Med. 2009;37(5):1757-1761. [PMID: 19373044]

Item 91   Answer: B

Educational Objective: Manage a severe asthma exacerbation.

The most appropriate next step in management is to admit to the intensive care unit (ICU). This patient is experiencing a severe asthma exacerbation, as evidenced by her severely decreased FEV_1, tachypnea, and accessory muscle use. In addition, her low peak expiratory flow indicates that she is not responding rapidly to aggressive treatment with short-acting β_2-agonists. The initial response to bronchodilators appears to be a better predictor of overall clinical course than a patient's pretreatment presentation. The newest National Asthma Education and Prevention Program guidelines recommend ICU admission for symptomatic patients with even mild carbon dioxide retention (arterial PCO_2 ≥42 mm Hg [5.6 kPa]) or severely decreased pulmonary function tests despite aggressive bronchodilator treatment (persistent FEV_1 or peak expiratory flow <40% of predicted).

The patient has no historical or physical examination findings to support an infectious cause of her respiratory symptoms. Antibiotics are not routinely indicated in the management of asthma exacerbations.

Although this patient remains at risk of deterioration, she is not confused, retaining carbon dioxide, or showing signs of severe respiratory muscle fatigue; therefore, she does not need intubation at this time. However, she may be a suitable candidate for administration of adjunctive therapies such as magnesium sulfate, helium-oxygen mixtures, and/or noninvasive positive pressure ventilation.

Laryngoscopy is useful in the diagnosis of paradoxical vocal cord motion, which, like asthma, presents with dyspnea and wheezing. However, patients with vocal cord dysfunction typically present with preserved expiratory flows and inspiratory stridor. Performing direct laryngoscopy could also precipitate respiratory arrest in this patient given her tenuous respiratory status.

KEY POINT

- The National Asthma Education and Prevention Program guidelines recommend intensive care unit admission for symptomatic patients with an arterial PCO_2 of greater than or equal to 42 mm Hg (5.6 kPa) or persistent FEV_1 or peak expiratory flow less than 40% of predicted despite aggressive bronchodilator treatment.

Bibliography

Lazarus SC. Clinical practice. Emergency treatment of asthma. N Engl J Med. 2010;363(8):755-764. [PMID: 20818877]

Item 92   Answer: C

Educational Objective: Diagnose Lambert-Eaton paraneoplastic syndrome.

A diagnosis of small cell lung cancer is the best explanation for this mediastinal mass in a former smoker with probable myasthenic syndrome (Lambert-Eaton syndrome). Approximately 50% of patients with Lambert-Eaton syndrome will have small cell lung cancer, and about 3% of those with small cell lung cancer will develop Lambert-Eaton syndrome. Lambert-Eaton myasthenic syndrome is a rare neuromuscular junction transmission disorder caused by antibodies directed against presynaptic voltage-gated P/Q-type calcium channels. Patients typically report progressive proximal limb weakness, and most have symptoms of dysautonomia, such as dry eyes, dry mouth, constipation, and erectile dysfunction. Lambert-Eaton myasthenic syndrome should be considered in any patient with findings of proximal limb weakness and absent deep tendon reflexes on neurologic examination. Facilitation (improvement of deep tendon reflexes and muscle strength after brief isometric exercise) may also be noted on neurologic examination. Electromyography testing and positive assays for P/Q-type calcium channel antibodies establish the diagnosis.

Myasthenic syndrome is not associated with carcinoid tumor, fibrosing mediastinitis, or thymoma. Pulmonary carcinoid tumors most typically present as centrally located endobronchial lesions or as well-circumscribed solitary pulmonary nodules, not mediastinal masses. The CT appearance of fibrosing mediastinitis is an infiltrative mediastinal process obliterating fat planes; a focal mass may or may not be present. Thymoma is associated with myasthenia gravis and presents as an anterior mediastinal mass, which is inconsistent with the clinical and radiographic findings of this patient.

KEY POINT

- Lambert-Eaton myasthenic syndrome is strongly associated with small cell lung cancer.

Bibliography

Payne M, Bradbury P, Lang B, et al. Prospective study into the incidence of Lambert Eaton myasthenic syndrome in small cell lung cancer. J Thorac Oncol. 2010;5(1):34-38. [PMID: 19934775]

Item 93   Answer: A

Educational Objective: Diagnose α_1-antitrypsin deficiency.

The most appropriate next step in management is measurement of the α_1-antitrypsin (AAT) level. This patient's symptoms and spirometry findings are consistent with COPD. In this young patient with COPD, AAT deficiency is a likely cause. AAT is an antiproteolytic enzyme that neutralizes neutrophil elastase. AAT deficiency results in excessive amounts of neutrophil elastase in the lung, which destroys elastin and causes early-onset obstructive pulmonary disease, typically panacinar emphysema with basilar predominance. Some patients with AAT deficiency may develop liver and skin disorders. AAT deficiency should be evaluated in selected patients with COPD because of the availability of specific therapy. AAT deficiency should be considered in patients with persistent airflow obstruction (particularly those diagnosed with COPD at age 45 years or younger), nonsmokers with emphysema, patients with predominantly basilar lung disease, and patients with chronic liver disease.

Inhaled corticosteroids may be indicated in patients with severe COPD in addition to a long-acting bronchodilator, but they should not be used as monotherapy in any stage of COPD.

Sweat chloride testing is the diagnostic test for cystic fibrosis. Bronchiectasis and purulent sputum are hallmarks of this disease. However, this patient has no evidence of bronchiectasis on CT scan. Patients with this degree of airflow obstruction and no purulent sputum would not have cystic fibrosis.

Genotyping for the most common AAT alleles is usually performed in patients who have documented deficiency of AAT, but it is premature to perform genotyping before documenting AAT deficiency.

KEY POINT

- α_1-Antitrypsin deficiency should be evaluated in selected patients with COPD because of the availability of specific therapy.

Bibliography

Silverman EK, Sandhaus RA. Clinical practice. Alpha1-antitrypsin deficiency. N Engl J Med. 2009;360(26):2749-2757. [PMID: 19553648]

Item 94   Answer: B

Educational Objective: Diagnose deep venous thrombosis using Duplex venous ultrasonography of the legs.

The most appropriate and cost-effective evaluation is duplex ultrasonography of the legs. This patient has acute-onset dyspnea with no objective evidence of a cause. His examination findings (except for tachycardia), electrocardiogram, and troponin levels are normal. His history and examination findings do not suggest a pneumonic process, and the chest radiograph is normal. His age and the presence of tachycardia yield a modified Geneva score of 6, indicating a moderately high probability of pulmonary embolism (PE) as the cause of his dyspnea. The Wells scoring system would also yield a moderately high (>4) probability if the clinician believed that PE was at least as likely as any other diagnosis. This patient's leg fracture was more than 1 month ago and contributes no points to the Wells or Geneva scores; however, the history of fracture should raise the clinician's suspicion for deep venous thrombosis (DVT) or PE. Because DVT is an important consideration given the history of recent leg fracture, the most appropriate approach is duplex ultrasonography of the legs.

CT angiography is not appropriate at this time because it may unnecessarily expose the patient to radiographic contrast dye and radiation if a venous study of the legs identifies DVT. Such a result would also save the cost of the more expensive CT angiography, because treatment for DVT/PE would be the same in this clinical setting and CT angiography would be unnecessary. If the venous study is negative, then CT angiography would be an appropriate next step.

An echocardiogram is not indicated at this time, because the clinical scenario does not suggest an acute cardiac event. Any assessment of pulmonary vascular hypertension related to PE should be deferred at least until that diagnosis is more firmly established.

In the setting of a moderate or high probability of DVT/PE using the Wells or Revised Geneva scores, such as in this patient, there is no role for D-dimer testing. A normal D-dimer level does not substantially lower the likelihood of the diagnosis, and more definitive testing would still be needed.

KEY POINT

- Because of the close relationship between lower-extremity deep venous thrombosis and pulmonary embolism, compression ultrasonography of the legs to detect evidence of clots has an important role in evaluating patients with a high pretest probability of acute pulmonary embolism.

Bibliography

Douma RA, Mos IC, Erkens PM, et al; Prometheus Study Group. Performance of 4 clinical decision rules in the diagnostic management of acute pulmonary embolism: a prospective cohort study. Ann Intern Med. 2011;154(11):709-718. [PMID: 21646554]

Item 95   Answer: C

Educational Objective: Manage very severe COPD with lung volume reduction surgery.

The most appropriate next step in management is evaluation for lung volume reduction surgery (LVRS), an extensive surgical procedure in which parts of the lung are resected, leading to reduction of hyperinflation, improvement of mechanical efficiency of respiratory muscles, and improvement of expiratory flow rate. LVRS should be considered in patients with severe COPD on maximal medical therapy who have completed pulmonary rehabilitation and meet the following criteria: (1) presence of bilateral emphysema on CT scan; (2) postbronchodilator total lung capacity greater than 150% and residual volume greater than 100% of predicted; (3) maximum FEV_1 no greater than 45% of predicted; and (4) arterial PCO_2 no more than 60 mm Hg (8.0 kPa) and arterial PO_2 of at least 45 mm Hg (6.0 kPa) breathing ambient air. This patient is a good candidate for LVRS because he has predominant upper lobe emphysema and meets criteria without having significant hypercapnia or hypoxia. LVRS is highly invasive, expensive, and associated with substantial morbidity and mortality; therefore, it is indicated only in highly selected patients.

This patient's oxygenation is adequate on his current regimen, and his clinical symptoms are likely not due to hypoxia; therefore, increasing his oxygen is not necessary at this time.

Long-term oral corticosteroid therapy has been shown to have limited, if any, benefits in chronic, stable COPD and would not be indicated as a next step in treatment of this patient.

This patient recently completed pulmonary rehabilitation for the second time. Although maintenance pulmonary rehabilitation may be helpful and should be recommended, it is not a definitive therapy for his severe, symptomatic lung disease.

KEY POINT

- **Lung volume reduction surgery is an extensive surgical procedure in which parts of the lung are resected, leading to reduction of hyperinflation, improvement of mechanical efficiency of respiratory muscles, and improvement of expiratory flow rate; it is recommended only in highly selected patients with COPD.**

Bibliography

Berger RL, Decamp MM, Criner GJ, Celli BR. Lung volume reduction therapies for advanced emphysema: an update. Chest. 2010;138(2):407-417. [PMID: 20682529]

Item 96   Answer: C

Educational Objective: Diagnose cryptogenic organizing pneumonia.

The most likely diagnosis is cryptogenic organizing pneumonia (COP). The radiographic description of bilateral, diffuse, alveolar opacities in the presence of normal lung volume is most consistent with that of bronchiolitis obliterans organizing pneumonia (BOOP). COP is the idiopathic form of BOOP. Patients with COP often present with signs and symptoms consistent with community-acquired pneumonia and may be treated at least once with antibiotics for this presumed diagnosis. However, the failure to respond to treatment and the development of a subacute process suggest a noninfectious diffuse parenchymal lung disease. Many underlying conditions, including certain infectious diseases, collagen vascular diseases, and drug-induced reactions, are associated with BOOP histopathology and best respond to specific treatment of the primary disease process. The vast majority of patients have symptoms for less than 3 months, and very few have symptoms for more than 6 months. Prognosis is typically favorable with a good response to systemic corticosteroids. Recurrences are fairly common with a tapering of corticosteroids, but they typically respond to an increase in therapy and slow subsequent taper.

Subacute or chronic pulmonary emboli may present with progressive dyspnea and hypoxia over weeks to months without systemic symptoms such as fever or chills. However, this patient has no clear risk factors for hypercoagulability (except tobacco use), and chest imaging in patients with chronic pulmonary emboli is often normal or shows minimal parenchymal findings, unlike in this patient.

COPD rarely develops in a 32-year-old patient, and it presents with a more insidious onset of shortness of breath. Chest examination will reveal severely decreased breath sounds with or without wheezing and a prolonged inspiratory to expiratory ratio. In addition, COPD primarily affects the airways, resulting in a chest radiograph that demonstrates a lack of parenchymal opacities and hyperinflation.

Lymphangioleiomyomatosis is a rare cystic lung disease that is associated with pneumothoraces and is almost exclusively diagnosed in women.

KEY POINT

- **Cryptogenic organizing pneumonia presents with cough and other symptoms suggestive of community-acquired pneumonia, but the diagnosis should be considered when symptoms and clinical findings persist despite one or more courses of antibiotics.**

Bibliography

Drakopanagiotakis F, Paschalaki K, Abu-Hijleh M, et al. Cryptogenic and secondary organizing pneumonia: clinical presentation, radiographic findings, treatment response, and prognosis. Chest. 2011;139(4):893-900. [PMID: 20724743]

Item 97   Answer: E

Educational Objective: Treat pulmonary embolism with anticoagulation in a patient with kidney disease.

The most appropriate treatment is unfractionated heparin plus warfarin. This patient has documented acute pulmonary embolism but also has kidney disease. She is hemodynamically stable and is oxygenating well. It is appropriate to begin anticoagulation, and unfractionated heparin would be the anticoagulant of choice owing to her chronic kidney disease. Warfarin should be started simultaneously in preparation for her ongoing management.

Thrombolytic therapy such as alteplase should be reserved for patients with persistent hypotension (defined as a systolic blood pressure <90 mm Hg or a drop in systolic pressure of >40 mm Hg) owing to the high risk of bleeding complications and lack of efficacy in clinical trials of hemodynamically stable patients. This patient is hemodynamically stable and thus the risks of thrombolysis outweigh the benefits.

Argatroban, a direct thrombin inhibitor that is particularly useful for heparin-induced thrombocytopenia, might be considered because it is cleared by the liver and is not affected by kidney disease. However, it predictably raises the INR and may create some difficulty in managing warfarin when the two drugs are administered simultaneously.

Low-molecular-weight heparin and synthetic Xa inhibitors such as fondaparinux are contraindicated in the setting of advanced kidney disease (creatinine clearance below 30 mL/min/1.73 m^2) because of unreliable pharmacokinetics in the setting of impaired kidney function.

KEY POINT

• Low-molecular-weight heparin and fondaparinux are contraindicated in the setting of advanced kidney disease.

Bibliography
Guyatt GH, Akl EA, Crowther M, Gutterman DD, Schuünemann HJ; American College of Chest Physicians Antithrombotic Therapy and Prevention of Thrombosis Panel. Executive summary: Antithrombotic Therapy and Prevention of Thrombosis, 9th ed: American College of Chest Physicians Evidence-Based Clinical Practice Guidelines. Chest. 2012;141(2 suppl):7S-47S. [PMID: 22315257]

Item 98   Answer: B

Educational Objective: Manage air travel in a patient with COPD.

The most appropriate management is a hypoxia altitude simulation test (HAST), which can be used to predict in-flight hypoxemia in patients with COPD. Patients with cardiopulmonary disease are at risk for complications from air travel owing to their limited ability to compensate for the effects of decreased cabin pressure. Air travel can cause significant oxygen desaturation in patients with COPD that is worsened by in-flight physical activity. During HAST, the patient breathes a hypoxic gas mix for 20 minutes. The aim is to predict hypoxemia at the lowest allowable cabin pressure, equivalent to an altitude of 2500 meters (8000 feet). The American Thoracic Society and European Respiratory Society guidelines recommend a HAST for patients with COPD who have comorbidities, previous in-flight symptoms, recent exacerbation(s), or hypoventilation on oxygen administration. The Aerospace Medical Association and Canadian Thoracic Society consider an arterial Po$_2$ of less than 70 mm Hg (9.3 kPa) at sea level an indication for HAST. In-flight oxygen therapy is recommended if arterial Po$_2$ during HAST decreases to less than 50 mm Hg (6.7 kPa). If arterial Po$_2$ is greater than 55 mm Hg (7.3 kPa), the patient does not require in-flight supplemental oxygen. If HAST arterial Po$_2$ is 50 to 55 mm Hg (6.7 to 7.3 kPa), the test is considered borderline, and measurement of HAST arterial Po$_2$ during activity may be performed.

Exercise stress test, 6-minute walk test, and pulmonary function tests are part of a pulmonary rehabilitation program or are used to evaluate dyspnea or changes in symptoms. These tests do not play a role in predicting in-flight hypoxia.

KEY POINT

• A hypoxia altitude simulation test can be used to predict in-flight hypoxia in patients with COPD.

Bibliography
Dine CJ, Kreider ME. Hypoxia altitude simulation test. Chest. 2008;133(4):1002-1005. [PMID: 18398121]

Item 99   Answer: A

Educational Objective: Evaluate a ground-glass pulmonary nodule.

The most appropriate management is follow-up CT scan in 1 year. Ground-glass opacity (GGO) refers to a radiographic finding that is characterized by focal (including nodular) or diffuse partial (not solid) opacification of the lung parenchyma; the underlying vasculature is visible and is not associated with an air-bronchogram pattern. Additional follow-up is recommended for this patient because GGOs may represent slow-growing invasive adenocarcinomas or adenocarcinoma in situ (formerly known as bronchioloalveolar cell carcinomas). Other entities in the differential diagnosis of GGOs include focal atelectasis, fibrosis, inflammation, and atypical alveolar hyperplasia. Although most lung cancers that present as nodules are solid and have doubling times of 50 to 150 days, GGO may represent a slow-growing adenocarcinoma with a doubling time of over 400 days. The possibility that the GGO is a slow-growing adenocarcinoma requires that follow-up be extended beyond the typical 2 years recommended for a solid nodule. The optimal duration of follow-up remains unclear, but some practitioners recommend extending follow-up to at least 5 years. Identification of slow-growing adenocarcinomas or adenocarcinoma in situ may not be evident by a change in size but rather by a change in their radiographic appearance (becoming part solid); such a change is a strong indicator that the nodule is malignant.

The low density of GGOs causes low 18-fluorodeoxyglucose uptake on PET-CT scan, which results in a high number of false negatives unless the lesion has become solid. Therefore, PET-CT scan would not be appropriate in this patient.

Resection is not indicated at this time because the nodule may be benign or may be an indolent adenocarcinoma in situ and may not be clinically significant. Continuing observation rather than performing an invasive procedure is the best course of action.

A needle biopsy is generally not indicated for a stable nodule and is not recommended for a GGO owing to the difficulty in pathologic interpretation (difficulty in determining invasion in a small sample of a lesion of this character).

KEY POINT

- Ground-glass–appearing pulmonary nodules require more than 2 years of follow-up with CT because they may represent slow-growing adenocarcinoma in situ (formerly known as bronchioloalveolar cell carcinomas).

Bibliography

Godoy MC, Naidich DP. Subsolid pulmonary nodules and the spectrum of peripheral adenocarcinomas of the lung: recommended interim guidelines for assessment and management. Radiology. 2009;253(3):606-622. [PMID: 19952025]

Item 100   Answer: D
Educational Objective: Manage a complicated parapneumonic effusion with thoracostomy tube placement.

The most appropriate next step in management of this patient's pleural effusion is to initiate antibiotics for community-acquired pathogens and anaerobes and place a thoracostomy tube. This patient presents with community-acquired pneumonia and a complicated parapneumonic effusion. Her pleural fluid analysis is consistent with an exudate, which is clinically most consistent with a complicated parapneumonic effusion. Factors shown to correlate with a more complicated course include large effusions (greater than one half of a hemithorax), especially those with areas of loculation; positive pleural fluid Gram stain or culture; pleural fluid glucose less than 60 mg/dL (3.3 mmol/L); or pleural fluid pH less than 7.2. If any of these criteria are met, thoracostomy tube placement should be pursued.

Although this patient may require surgical intervention to control her pleural-space infection, the majority of patients improve without the need for surgery; therefore, evaluation for surgical decortication is not indicated at this time.

Although most uncomplicated parapneumonic effusions resolve with treatment of the underlying pneumonia, this patient has evidence of a complicated effusion, which is best treated with more aggressive therapy. Thoracostomy tube placement should be pursued rather than observation with repeat chest radiography in 1 week.

Similarly, this patient's complicated parapneumonic effusion is unlikely to be adequately addressed by serial therapeutic thoracentesis alone, and a thoracostomy tube should be placed.

KEY POINT

- Parapneumonic effusions with complicating factors (greater than one half of a hemithorax, septations and areas of loculation, pleural fluid pH less than 7.2, glucose level less than 60 mg/dL [3.3 mmol/L], or positive pleural fluid Gram stain or culture) should be treated with antibiotics and pleural drainage.

Bibliography

Davies HE, Davies RJ, Davies CW; BTS Pleural Disease Guideline Group. Management of pleural infection in adults: British Thoracic Society Pleural Disease Guideline 2010. Thorax. 2010;65(suppl 2):ii41-53. [PMID: 20696693]

Item 101   Answer: E
Educational Objective: Diagnose sarcoidosis.

The most likely diagnosis is sarcoidosis. Sarcoidosis is an idiopathic disorder that most often involves the lungs and is characterized by non-necrotizing granulomatous inflammation that may involve lymph nodes and the lung parenchyma. Upper-lobe predominance is the characteristic distribution of the infiltrates in the lungs on chest imaging; this is often most apparent on the lateral view. Despite rather extensive radiographic abnormalities, patients with sarcoidosis may have normal or minimally abnormal pulmonary function testing as another clue to the diagnosis. The diagnosis of sarcoidosis requires histopathologic demonstration of organ involvement with noncaseating granulomatous inflammation in conjunction with the appropriate clinical and radiographic findings and the exclusion of other diseases.

Asbestosis, cryptogenic organizing pneumonia, heart failure, and idiopathic pulmonary fibrosis are unlikely in this patient because these diseases typically have lower lung zone predominance. In addition, this patient provides no occupational history that is consistent with asbestos exposure. The patient does not have physical examination findings consistent with heart failure (S_3, jugular venous distention, crackles) or idiopathic pulmonary fibrosis (bibasilar "Velcro" inspiratory crackles). Patients with cryptogenic organizing pneumonia most typically present subacutely with cough, fatigue, and low-grade fever often mistaken for pneumonia.

KEY POINT

- Sarcoidosis is characterized by upper-lobe predominance of infiltrates in the lungs on chest imaging; this is often most apparent on the lateral view.

Bibliography

Iannuzzi MC, Rybicki BA, Teirstein AS. Sarcoidosis. N Engl J Med. 2007;357(21):2153-2165. [PMID: 18032765]

Item 102   Answer: A

Educational Objective: Treat hypoventilation related to neuromuscular weakness.

The most appropriate treatment is noninvasive positive pressure ventilation (NPPV) in the form of bilevel positive airway pressure (BPAP). BPAP employs independently set inspiratory positive airway pressure and expiratory positive airway pressure that directly augment ventilation. Nocturnal BPAP therapy decreases nocturnal P_{CO_2}, daytime P_{CO_2}, and daytime sleepiness. This patient has hypercapnic respiratory failure related to amyotrophic lateral sclerosis (ALS), which is an indication for nocturnal ventilatory support. Ventilatory respiratory failure refers to inadequate alveolar ventilation, and the primary manifestation of ventilatory failure is hypercapnia. NPPV in the form of BPAP has been shown to improve quality of life and may prolong survival in patients with ALS who use it regularly. Although polysomnography is not mandatory to initiate NPPV, it is often helpful to precisely titrate pressures.

Obstructive sleep apnea (OSA) is common in patients with ALS, but this patient's documented awake hypercapnia suggests chronic hypercapnic respiratory failure. Nocturnal continuous positive airway pressure (CPAP) maintains upper airway patency but does not augment ventilation. Isolated OSA without hypercapnia can be managed with CPAP, but BPAP is needed because of this patient's hypoventilation.

In patients with hypercapnic respiratory failure, particularly in the setting of neuromuscular weakness, supplemental oxygen can further depress ventilation and acutely increase blood carbon dioxide tensions. If supplemental oxygen is used in this setting, it should be used in conjunction with positive pressure ventilation such as BPAP.

Tracheostomy is occasionally performed in patients with advanced disease who cannot tolerate noninvasive ventilation or who have problems managing oral secretions. Because of the invasiveness of the intervention, complexity of home management, and progressive nature of ALS, such surgery should be preceded by a thorough discussion of the goals of care.

KEY POINT

- Bilevel positive airway pressure is effective for treating hypercapnic respiratory failure related to neuromuscular weakness.

Bibliography

Hardiman O. Management of respiratory symptoms in ALS. J Neurol. 2011;258(3):359-365. [PMID: 21082322]

Item 103   Answer: A

Educational Objective: Manage acute respiratory distress syndrome with the appropriate tidal volume.

The most appropriate tidal volume is 300 mL. The physiologic hallmark of acute respiratory distress syndrome (ARDS) is hypoxemia, which is typically corrected with mechanical ventilation combined with supplemental oxygen and positive end-expiratory pressure (PEEP). Limiting atelectrauma (lung injury that is presumed to arise from repetitive opening and closing of alveoli) and barotrauma may limit the potential for disruption of the alveolar capillary membrane by the ventilator, often referred to as ventilator-associated lung injury. This can be achieved by delivering tidal volumes of limited size, minimizing plateau pressure, optimizing PEEP, and reducing F_{IO_2} to less than 0.6. Survival is improved when patients with ARDS are ventilated with a tidal volume of 6 mL/kg of ideal body weight (IBW). IBW rather than actual body weight should be used to calculate tidal volume. In patients who are overweight or edematous, using actual body weight will typically result in inappropriately large tidal volumes. A low tidal volume mechanical ventilation strategy is now the standard of care for ARDS. The ARDS Clinical Network trial found a significant reduction in mortality (from 40% to 30%) in the group treated with lower tidal volumes. The tidal volume was set at 6 mL/kg IBW and was subsequently decreased stepwise by 1 mL/kg IBW as necessary to maintain a plateau pressure of no more than 30 cm H_2O. The minimal tidal volume was 4 mL/kg IBW. Ideal body weight is calculated as 50.0 kg (110.2 lb) + 2.3 kg (5.1 lb) for each inch over 60 inches (152.4 cm) in men and 45.5 kg (100.3 lb) + 2.3 kg (5.1 lb) for each inch over 60 inches (152.4 cm) in women.

Higher tidal volumes would result in more ventilator-induced lung injury and worse patient outcomes and are therefore not appropriate.

KEY POINT

- Survival is improved when patients with acute respiratory distress syndrome are ventilated with a tidal volume of 6 mL/kg of ideal body weight.

Bibliography

Patroniti N, Isgrò S, Zanella A. Clinical management of severely hypoxemic patients. Curr Opin Crit Care. 2011;17(1):50-56. [PMID: 21157316]

Item 104   Answer: C

Educational Objective: Diagnose high-altitude periodic breathing.

The most likely diagnosis is high-altitude periodic breathing (HAPB), which is characterized by cyclic central apneas and hyperpneas during sleep that are associated with ascension to high altitude. HAPB is a form of high-altitude illness; it involves changes in respiratory neural signaling in response to hypobaric conditions that result in hypoxemia, thereby stimulating ventilation, which is further destabilized with the response to the respiratory alkalosis that occurs during sleep. These changes lead to a form of periodic breathing that occurs with acute altitude changes but resolves with eventual acclimatization. Its prevalence increases with the degree of elevation and typically does not occur at altitudes less than 2500 meters (approximately 8200 feet). Symptoms include repeated awakenings from sleep, sometimes with a sense of dyspnea, and fatigue related to poor sleep quality.

Although nocturnal symptoms are common in asthma, this patient has no cough or wheeze and does not have a history of asthma.

An extreme and serious manifestation of acute mountain sickness is high-altitude cerebral edema, where encephalopathy (characterized by altered mental status) and ataxia occur in response to vasogenic brain swelling. These findings are not present in this patient.

High-altitude pulmonary edema results from lung capillary leak thought to occur in response to hypoxia. This patient has dyspnea that is characteristic of exercise at altitude, but she does not have cough, sputum, or any examination findings to suggest pulmonary edema.

KEY POINT

- High-altitude periodic breathing is characterized by cyclic central apneas and hyperpneas during sleep that are associated with ascension to altitude; symptoms include repeated awakenings from sleep, sometimes with a sense of dyspnea, and fatigue related to poor sleep quality.

Bibliography

Schoene RB. Illnesses at high altitude. Chest. 2008;134(2):402-416. [PMID: 18682459]

Item 105   Answer: D

Educational Objective: Diagnose chronic thromboembolic pulmonary hypertension.

The most appropriate next step in diagnosis is a ventilation/perfusion scan. This patient has a clinical picture consistent with chronic thromboembolic pulmonary hypertension (CTEPH), characterized by recurrent, small pulmonary emboli occurring over an extended period of time leading to increased pulmonary artery pressure and a gas transfer defect. Onset of this process may date back to this patient's surgery and postoperative pulmonary symptoms, which may have represented a pulmonary embolism but were diagnosed as pneumonia. As many as 50% of patients with CTEPH may not report a previously known episode of diagnosed acute deep venous thrombosis or pulmonary embolism. A ventilation/perfusion scan is the preferred method of diagnosis for CTEPH because it detects the characteristic matching defects more reliably than other imaging options. Pulmonary angiography permits direct observation of the pulmonary vasculature and assessment of pulmonary hemodynamics if other studies are inconclusive. Treatment is with long-term anticoagulation and possibly pulmonary endarterectomy in patients with severe functional impairment.

Although CT angiography is generally the preferred diagnostic method for suspected acute pulmonary embolus, it is more sensitive for larger, more proximal thrombi than are seen in most patients with CTEPH. It may have a role in localizing a thrombus and assessing accessibility if surgical endarterectomy is being considered.

A D-dimer study would likely be positive, but this test would not be adequate to establish the diagnosis of CTEPH.

Lower-extremity duplex ultrasonography might detect a source of chronic venous thromboembolic disease, but additional testing would be needed to definitively diagnose CTEPH even if the test was positive. A negative study would not exclude the diagnosis.

KEY POINT

- Ventilation/perfusion scanning is the preferred initial diagnostic study in patients suspected of having chronic thromboembolic pulmonary hypertension.

Bibliography

Fedullo P, Kerr KM, Kim NH, Auger WR. Chronic thromboembolic pulmonary hypertension. Am J Respir Crit Care Med. 2011;183(12):1605-1613. [PMID: 21330453]

Item 106   Answer: C

Educational Objective: Manage septic shock.

The most appropriate next step in management is to start vasopressor therapy with norepinephrine. This patient presents with a clinical picture consistent with sepsis, likely due to a urinary tract infection. The goals of sepsis management are to treat infection and optimize tissue perfusion. This is accomplished by starting early and appropriate antibiotic therapy and using crystalloids to maintain an adequate preload. If an initial fluid challenge of 1000 mL of crystalloid fails to achieve an adequate blood pressure, defined as a mean arterial pressure of greater than or equal to 65 mm Hg or central venous pressure of 8 to 12 mm Hg, initiation of a vasoactive agent is indicated to ensure that tissue perfusion is maintained. The mean arterial pressure is calculated with the following equation:

$$([2 \times \text{diastolic blood pressure}] + \text{systolic blood pressure}) \div 3$$

Despite an initial 1000-mL normal saline bolus, this patient's mean arterial pressure remains below 65 mm Hg. The recommended vasopressors for initial treatment are dopamine or norepinephrine, administered centrally.

Although erythrocyte transfusions act as colloidal substances and may be useful in resuscitation when oxygen-carrying capacity is impaired (such as with acute blood loss), this patient's measured hemoglobin level appears adequate to maintain tissue oxygenation without the need for erythrocyte transfusion. Transfusion for volume expansion in the absence of another clear indication is not appropriate.

Intravenous hydrocortisone in stress doses is indicated only in situations when hypotension remains unresponsive to adequate fluid resuscitation and vasopressor therapy, or if there is concern for possible underlying adrenal insufficiency.

Although patients with sepsis frequently have significant fluid requirements owing to hemodynamic instability, increasing the infusion rate is not an effective means to acutely restore intravascular volume and by itself would not be adequate to optimize tissue perfusion.

KEY POINT

- Vasopressor therapy is indicated to maintain a mean arterial pressure of greater than or equal to 65 mm Hg or central venous pressure measurement of 8 of 12 mm Hg in patients with sepsis who have failed to respond to an initial crystalloid fluid challenge.

Bibliography

Dellinger RP, Levy MM, Carlet JM, et al; International Surviving Sepsis Campaign Guidelines Committee; American Association of Critical-Care Nurses; American College of Chest Physicians; American College of Emergency Physicians; Canadian Critical Care Society; European Society of Clinical Microbiology and Infectious Diseases; European Society of Intensive Care Medicine; European Respiratory Society; International Sepsis Forum; Japanese Association for Acute Medicine; Japanese Society of Intensive Care Medicine; Society of Critical Care Medicine; Society of Hospital Medicine; Surgical Infection Society; World Federation of Societies of Intensive and Critical Care Medicine. Surviving Sepsis Campaign: international guidelines for management of severe sepsis and septic shock: 2008 [erratum in Crit Care Med. 2008;36(4):1394-1396]. Crit Care Med. 2008;36(1):296-327. [PMID: 18158437]

Item 107   Answer: A

Educational Objective: Manage a patient with a preoperative COPD exacerbation.

The most appropriate management is to delay surgery. This patient's acute COPD exacerbation should be treated before his elective surgical procedure. Bronchodilator therapy is a cornerstone of management of COPD exacerbations, and he should be treated more aggressively than his current as-needed regimen, with continuation of his current anticholinergic medication. Corticosteroids and antibiotics may also be indicated depending on the severity of his exacerbation. Postoperative pulmonary complications may be prevented by treating patients with COPD who are clinically symptomatic before the anticipated procedure, with postponement of the surgery until the patient returns to baseline if necessary. Lung infections, atelectasis, and/or increased airflow obstruction are among the major postoperative pulmonary complications that can result in acute respiratory failure; therefore, pulmonary function should be optimized before surgical intervention in those with known lung disease. Upper abdominal and thoracic surgery in particular is associated with increased risk of postoperative pulmonary complications. Smoking, age, poor general health status, and COPD severity are important risk factors. Early mobilization, deep breathing, and incentive spirometry in the perioperative period may decrease the risk of pulmonary complications.

This patient has stable COPD and had pulmonary function testing done 4 months ago. Because his diagnosis has been established, repeating pulmonary function tests will not help with perioperative management of this patient.

Roflumilast is a phosphodiesterase-4 inhibitor that is indicated for possible chronic treatment of patients with severe and very severe COPD with a history of recurrent exacerbations. It is not used for treatment of acute exacerbations.

This patient has an increased risk of perioperative complications, so nonintervention is not appropriate in this patient with a COPD exacerbation before anticipated surgery.

KEY POINT

- Elective surgery should be postponed if a patient with stable COPD has an exacerbation.

Bibliography

Global Strategy for Diagnosis, Management, and Prevention of COPD. December 2011. Available at: www.goldcopd.org. Accessed July 27, 2012.

Item 108   Answer: B

Educational Objective: Diagnose carcinoid tumor.

The most likely diagnosis is a carcinoid tumor. Carcinoid tumor in the lung is a low-grade malignancy consisting of cells of neuroendocrine origin. They account for only about 2% of all tumors in the lung and have no association with smoking. Owing to the tendency for carcinoid tumors to have an endobronchial location, patients frequently present with hemoptysis or evidence of bronchial obstruction resulting in atelectasis or focal bronchiectasis, consistent with the clinical presentation in this patient. The CT shown (see below) reveals a smoothly bordered tumor at the level

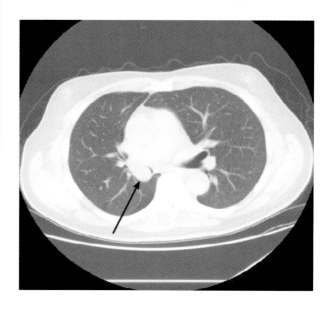

of the bronchus intermedius (*arrow*). There is complete obstruction distally and collapse of the lung distally. A carcinoid tumor is the most likely tumor to present in a young never-smoker with evidence of a smoothly bordered endobronchial obstruction and a history of recurrent pneumonia. Treatment for carcinoid tumor is surgical resection when possible. For typical carcinoid, 5-year survival is about 90%.

Carcinomas tend to grow too quickly to cause endobronchial obstruction resulting in recurrent pneumonia and focal bronchiectasis, with recurrent episodes of pneumonia over the course of years. Small cell and squamous cell cancers frequently cause bronchial obstruction but would be exceedingly rare in a young never-smoker. Adenocarcinoma is the most common cell type in a never-smoker but is an infrequent cause of endobronchial obstruction.

KEY POINT

- Although uncommon, a carcinoid tumor is the most likely neoplasm to present in a young never-smoker with evidence of endobronchial obstruction and a history of recurrent pneumonia.

Bibliography

Cao C, Yan TD, Kennedy C, Hendel N, Bannon PG, McCaughan BC. Bronchopulmonary carcinoid tumors: long-term outcomes after resection. Ann Thorac Surg. 2011;91(2):339-343. [PMID: 21256263]

Index

Note: Page numbers followed by f and t denote figures and tables, respectively. Test questions are indicated by Q.

A — NAME AND ADDRESS (Please complete.)

Last Name _____ First Name _____ Middle Initial _____

Address _____

Address cont. _____

City _____ State _____ ZIP Code _____

Country _____

Email address _____

ACP
AMERICAN COLLEGE OF PHYSICIANS
INTERNAL MEDICINE | Doctors for Adults

Medical Knowledge Self-Assessment Program® 16

TO EARN *AMA PRA CATEGORY 1 CREDITS*™ YOU MUST:

1. Answer all questions.
2. Score a minimum of 50% correct.

==

TO EARN *FREE* SAME-DAY *AMA PRA CATEGORY 1 CREDITS*™ ONLINE:

1. Answer all of your questions.
2. Go to **mksap.acponline.org** and access the appropriate answer sheet.
3. Transcribe your answers and submit for CME credits.
4. You can also enter your answers directly at **mksap.acponline.org** without first using this answer sheet.

To Submit Your Answer Sheet by Mail or FAX for a $10 Administrative Fee per Answer Sheet:

1. Answer all of your questions and calculate your score.
2. Complete boxes A–F.
3. Complete payment information.
4. Send the answer sheet and payment information to ACP, using the FAX number/address listed below.

B — Order Number
(Use the Order Number on your MKSAP materials packing slip.)

C — ACP ID Number
(Refer to packing slip in your MKSAP materials for your ACP ID Number.)

COMPLETE FORM BELOW ONLY IF YOU SUBMIT BY MAIL OR FAX

Last Name _____ First Name _____ MI ____

Payment Information. Must remit in US funds, drawn on a US bank.

The processing fee for each paper answer sheet is $10.

☐ Check, made payable to ACP, enclosed

Charge to ☐ **VISA** ☐ MasterCard ☐ AMERICAN EXPRESS ☐ DISCOVER

Card Number _____

Expiration Date _____ / _____ Security code (3 or 4 digit #s) _____
            MM   YY

Signature _____

Fax to: 215-351-2799

Mail to:
Member and Customer Service
American College of Physicians
190 N. Independence Mall West
Philadelphia, PA 19106-1572

Questions?
Go to **mskap.acponline.org** or email **custserv@acponline.org**

1 Ⓐ Ⓑ Ⓒ Ⓓ Ⓔ   46 Ⓐ Ⓑ Ⓒ Ⓓ Ⓔ   91 Ⓐ Ⓑ Ⓒ Ⓓ Ⓔ   136 Ⓐ Ⓑ Ⓒ Ⓓ Ⓔ
2 Ⓐ Ⓑ Ⓒ Ⓓ Ⓔ   47 Ⓐ Ⓑ Ⓒ Ⓓ Ⓔ   92 Ⓐ Ⓑ Ⓒ Ⓓ Ⓔ   137 Ⓐ Ⓑ Ⓒ Ⓓ Ⓔ
3 Ⓐ Ⓑ Ⓒ Ⓓ Ⓔ   48 Ⓐ Ⓑ Ⓒ Ⓓ Ⓔ   93 Ⓐ Ⓑ Ⓒ Ⓓ Ⓔ   138 Ⓐ Ⓑ Ⓒ Ⓓ Ⓔ
4 Ⓐ Ⓑ Ⓒ Ⓓ Ⓔ   49 Ⓐ Ⓑ Ⓒ Ⓓ Ⓔ   94 Ⓐ Ⓑ Ⓒ Ⓓ Ⓔ   139 Ⓐ Ⓑ Ⓒ Ⓓ Ⓔ
5 Ⓐ Ⓑ Ⓒ Ⓓ Ⓔ   50 Ⓐ Ⓑ Ⓒ Ⓓ Ⓔ   95 Ⓐ Ⓑ Ⓒ Ⓓ Ⓔ   140 Ⓐ Ⓑ Ⓒ Ⓓ Ⓔ

6 Ⓐ Ⓑ Ⓒ Ⓓ Ⓔ   51 Ⓐ Ⓑ Ⓒ Ⓓ Ⓔ   96 Ⓐ Ⓑ Ⓒ Ⓓ Ⓔ   141 Ⓐ Ⓑ Ⓒ Ⓓ Ⓔ
7 Ⓐ Ⓑ Ⓒ Ⓓ Ⓔ   52 Ⓐ Ⓑ Ⓒ Ⓓ Ⓔ   97 Ⓐ Ⓑ Ⓒ Ⓓ Ⓔ   142 Ⓐ Ⓑ Ⓒ Ⓓ Ⓔ
8 Ⓐ Ⓑ Ⓒ Ⓓ Ⓔ   53 Ⓐ Ⓑ Ⓒ Ⓓ Ⓔ   98 Ⓐ Ⓑ Ⓒ Ⓓ Ⓔ   143 Ⓐ Ⓑ Ⓒ Ⓓ Ⓔ
9 Ⓐ Ⓑ Ⓒ Ⓓ Ⓔ   54 Ⓐ Ⓑ Ⓒ Ⓓ Ⓔ   99 Ⓐ Ⓑ Ⓒ Ⓓ Ⓔ   144 Ⓐ Ⓑ Ⓒ Ⓓ Ⓔ
10 Ⓐ Ⓑ Ⓒ Ⓓ Ⓔ   55 Ⓐ Ⓑ Ⓒ Ⓓ Ⓔ   100 Ⓐ Ⓑ Ⓒ Ⓓ Ⓔ   145 Ⓐ Ⓑ Ⓒ Ⓓ Ⓔ

11 Ⓐ Ⓑ Ⓒ Ⓓ Ⓔ   56 Ⓐ Ⓑ Ⓒ Ⓓ Ⓔ   101 Ⓐ Ⓑ Ⓒ Ⓓ Ⓔ   146 Ⓐ Ⓑ Ⓒ Ⓓ Ⓔ
12 Ⓐ Ⓑ Ⓒ Ⓓ Ⓔ   57 Ⓐ Ⓑ Ⓒ Ⓓ Ⓔ   102 Ⓐ Ⓑ Ⓒ Ⓓ Ⓔ   147 Ⓐ Ⓑ Ⓒ Ⓓ Ⓔ
13 Ⓐ Ⓑ Ⓒ Ⓓ Ⓔ   58 Ⓐ Ⓑ Ⓒ Ⓓ Ⓔ   103 Ⓐ Ⓑ Ⓒ Ⓓ Ⓔ   148 Ⓐ Ⓑ Ⓒ Ⓓ Ⓔ
14 Ⓐ Ⓑ Ⓒ Ⓓ Ⓔ   59 Ⓐ Ⓑ Ⓒ Ⓓ Ⓔ   104 Ⓐ Ⓑ Ⓒ Ⓓ Ⓔ   149 Ⓐ Ⓑ Ⓒ Ⓓ Ⓔ
15 Ⓐ Ⓑ Ⓒ Ⓓ Ⓔ   60 Ⓐ Ⓑ Ⓒ Ⓓ Ⓔ   105 Ⓐ Ⓑ Ⓒ Ⓓ Ⓔ   150 Ⓐ Ⓑ Ⓒ Ⓓ Ⓔ

16 Ⓐ Ⓑ Ⓒ Ⓓ Ⓔ   61 Ⓐ Ⓑ Ⓒ Ⓓ Ⓔ   106 Ⓐ Ⓑ Ⓒ Ⓓ Ⓔ   151 Ⓐ Ⓑ Ⓒ Ⓓ Ⓔ
17 Ⓐ Ⓑ Ⓒ Ⓓ Ⓔ   62 Ⓐ Ⓑ Ⓒ Ⓓ Ⓔ   107 Ⓐ Ⓑ Ⓒ Ⓓ Ⓔ   152 Ⓐ Ⓑ Ⓒ Ⓓ Ⓔ
18 Ⓐ Ⓑ Ⓒ Ⓓ Ⓔ   63 Ⓐ Ⓑ Ⓒ Ⓓ Ⓔ   108 Ⓐ Ⓑ Ⓒ Ⓓ Ⓔ   153 Ⓐ Ⓑ Ⓒ Ⓓ Ⓔ
19 Ⓐ Ⓑ Ⓒ Ⓓ Ⓔ   64 Ⓐ Ⓑ Ⓒ Ⓓ Ⓔ   109 Ⓐ Ⓑ Ⓒ Ⓓ Ⓔ   154 Ⓐ Ⓑ Ⓒ Ⓓ Ⓔ
20 Ⓐ Ⓑ Ⓒ Ⓓ Ⓔ   65 Ⓐ Ⓑ Ⓒ Ⓓ Ⓔ   110 Ⓐ Ⓑ Ⓒ Ⓓ Ⓔ   155 Ⓐ Ⓑ Ⓒ Ⓓ Ⓔ

21 Ⓐ Ⓑ Ⓒ Ⓓ Ⓔ   66 Ⓐ Ⓑ Ⓒ Ⓓ Ⓔ   111 Ⓐ Ⓑ Ⓒ Ⓓ Ⓔ   156 Ⓐ Ⓑ Ⓒ Ⓓ Ⓔ
22 Ⓐ Ⓑ Ⓒ Ⓓ Ⓔ   67 Ⓐ Ⓑ Ⓒ Ⓓ Ⓔ   112 Ⓐ Ⓑ Ⓒ Ⓓ Ⓔ   157 Ⓐ Ⓑ Ⓒ Ⓓ Ⓔ
23 Ⓐ Ⓑ Ⓒ Ⓓ Ⓔ   68 Ⓐ Ⓑ Ⓒ Ⓓ Ⓔ   113 Ⓐ Ⓑ Ⓒ Ⓓ Ⓔ   158 Ⓐ Ⓑ Ⓒ Ⓓ Ⓔ
24 Ⓐ Ⓑ Ⓒ Ⓓ Ⓔ   69 Ⓐ Ⓑ Ⓒ Ⓓ Ⓔ   114 Ⓐ Ⓑ Ⓒ Ⓓ Ⓔ   159 Ⓐ Ⓑ Ⓒ Ⓓ Ⓔ
25 Ⓐ Ⓑ Ⓒ Ⓓ Ⓔ   70 Ⓐ Ⓑ Ⓒ Ⓓ Ⓔ   115 Ⓐ Ⓑ Ⓒ Ⓓ Ⓔ   160 Ⓐ Ⓑ Ⓒ Ⓓ Ⓔ

26 Ⓐ Ⓑ Ⓒ Ⓓ Ⓔ   71 Ⓐ Ⓑ Ⓒ Ⓓ Ⓔ   116 Ⓐ Ⓑ Ⓒ Ⓓ Ⓔ   161 Ⓐ Ⓑ Ⓒ Ⓓ Ⓔ
27 Ⓐ Ⓑ Ⓒ Ⓓ Ⓔ   72 Ⓐ Ⓑ Ⓒ Ⓓ Ⓔ   117 Ⓐ Ⓑ Ⓒ Ⓓ Ⓔ   162 Ⓐ Ⓑ Ⓒ Ⓓ Ⓔ
28 Ⓐ Ⓑ Ⓒ Ⓓ Ⓔ   73 Ⓐ Ⓑ Ⓒ Ⓓ Ⓔ   118 Ⓐ Ⓑ Ⓒ Ⓓ Ⓔ   163 Ⓐ Ⓑ Ⓒ Ⓓ Ⓔ
29 Ⓐ Ⓑ Ⓒ Ⓓ Ⓔ   74 Ⓐ Ⓑ Ⓒ Ⓓ Ⓔ   119 Ⓐ Ⓑ Ⓒ Ⓓ Ⓔ   164 Ⓐ Ⓑ Ⓒ Ⓓ Ⓔ
30 Ⓐ Ⓑ Ⓒ Ⓓ Ⓔ   75 Ⓐ Ⓑ Ⓒ Ⓓ Ⓔ   120 Ⓐ Ⓑ Ⓒ Ⓓ Ⓔ   165 Ⓐ Ⓑ Ⓒ Ⓓ Ⓔ

31 Ⓐ Ⓑ Ⓒ Ⓓ Ⓔ   76 Ⓐ Ⓑ Ⓒ Ⓓ Ⓔ   121 Ⓐ Ⓑ Ⓒ Ⓓ Ⓔ   166 Ⓐ Ⓑ Ⓒ Ⓓ Ⓔ
32 Ⓐ Ⓑ Ⓒ Ⓓ Ⓔ   77 Ⓐ Ⓑ Ⓒ Ⓓ Ⓔ   122 Ⓐ Ⓑ Ⓒ Ⓓ Ⓔ   167 Ⓐ Ⓑ Ⓒ Ⓓ Ⓔ
33 Ⓐ Ⓑ Ⓒ Ⓓ Ⓔ   78 Ⓐ Ⓑ Ⓒ Ⓓ Ⓔ   123 Ⓐ Ⓑ Ⓒ Ⓓ Ⓔ   168 Ⓐ Ⓑ Ⓒ Ⓓ Ⓔ
34 Ⓐ Ⓑ Ⓒ Ⓓ Ⓔ   79 Ⓐ Ⓑ Ⓒ Ⓓ Ⓔ   124 Ⓐ Ⓑ Ⓒ Ⓓ Ⓔ   169 Ⓐ Ⓑ Ⓒ Ⓓ Ⓔ
35 Ⓐ Ⓑ Ⓒ Ⓓ Ⓔ   80 Ⓐ Ⓑ Ⓒ Ⓓ Ⓔ   125 Ⓐ Ⓑ Ⓒ Ⓓ Ⓔ   170 Ⓐ Ⓑ Ⓒ Ⓓ Ⓔ

36 Ⓐ Ⓑ Ⓒ Ⓓ Ⓔ   81 Ⓐ Ⓑ Ⓒ Ⓓ Ⓔ   126 Ⓐ Ⓑ Ⓒ Ⓓ Ⓔ   171 Ⓐ Ⓑ Ⓒ Ⓓ Ⓔ
37 Ⓐ Ⓑ Ⓒ Ⓓ Ⓔ   82 Ⓐ Ⓑ Ⓒ Ⓓ Ⓔ   127 Ⓐ Ⓑ Ⓒ Ⓓ Ⓔ   172 Ⓐ Ⓑ Ⓒ Ⓓ Ⓔ
38 Ⓐ Ⓑ Ⓒ Ⓓ Ⓔ   83 Ⓐ Ⓑ Ⓒ Ⓓ Ⓔ   128 Ⓐ Ⓑ Ⓒ Ⓓ Ⓔ   173 Ⓐ Ⓑ Ⓒ Ⓓ Ⓔ
39 Ⓐ Ⓑ Ⓒ Ⓓ Ⓔ   84 Ⓐ Ⓑ Ⓒ Ⓓ Ⓔ   129 Ⓐ Ⓑ Ⓒ Ⓓ Ⓔ   174 Ⓐ Ⓑ Ⓒ Ⓓ Ⓔ
40 Ⓐ Ⓑ Ⓒ Ⓓ Ⓔ   85 Ⓐ Ⓑ Ⓒ Ⓓ Ⓔ   130 Ⓐ Ⓑ Ⓒ Ⓓ Ⓔ   175 Ⓐ Ⓑ Ⓒ Ⓓ Ⓔ

41 Ⓐ Ⓑ Ⓒ Ⓓ Ⓔ   86 Ⓐ Ⓑ Ⓒ Ⓓ Ⓔ   131 Ⓐ Ⓑ Ⓒ Ⓓ Ⓔ   176 Ⓐ Ⓑ Ⓒ Ⓓ Ⓔ
42 Ⓐ Ⓑ Ⓒ Ⓓ Ⓔ   87 Ⓐ Ⓑ Ⓒ Ⓓ Ⓔ   132 Ⓐ Ⓑ Ⓒ Ⓓ Ⓔ   177 Ⓐ Ⓑ Ⓒ Ⓓ Ⓔ
43 Ⓐ Ⓑ Ⓒ Ⓓ Ⓔ   88 Ⓐ Ⓑ Ⓒ Ⓓ Ⓔ   133 Ⓐ Ⓑ Ⓒ Ⓓ Ⓔ   178 Ⓐ Ⓑ Ⓒ Ⓓ Ⓔ
44 Ⓐ Ⓑ Ⓒ Ⓓ Ⓔ   89 Ⓐ Ⓑ Ⓒ Ⓓ Ⓔ   134 Ⓐ Ⓑ Ⓒ Ⓓ Ⓔ   179 Ⓐ Ⓑ Ⓒ Ⓓ Ⓔ
45 Ⓐ Ⓑ Ⓒ Ⓓ Ⓔ   90 Ⓐ Ⓑ Ⓒ Ⓓ Ⓔ   135 Ⓐ Ⓑ Ⓒ Ⓓ Ⓔ   180 Ⓐ Ⓑ Ⓒ Ⓓ Ⓔ

MKSAP®16

Medical Knowledge Self-Assessment Program®

Nephrology

Welcome to the Nephrology section of MKSAP 16!

Here, you will find updated information on the clinical evaluation of kidney function, fluids and electrolytes, acid-base disorders, hypertension, chronic tubulointerstitial disorders, glomerular diseases, genetic disorders and kidney disease, acute kidney injury, kidney stones, the kidney in pregnancy, and chronic kidney disease. All of these topics are uniquely focused on the needs of generalists and subspecialists *outside* of nephrology.

The publication of the 16th edition of Medical Knowledge Self-Assessment Program heralds a significant event, culminating 2 years of effort by dozens of leading subspecialists across the United States. Our authoring committees have strived to help internists succeed in Maintenance of Certification, right up to preparing for the MOC examination, and to get residents ready for the certifying examination. MKSAP 16 also helps you update your medical knowledge and elevates standards of self-learning by allowing you to assess your knowledge with 1,200 all-new multiple-choice questions, including 108 in Nephrology.

MKSAP began more than 40 years ago. The American Board of Internal Medicine's examination blueprint and gaps between actual and preferred practices inform creation of the content. The questions, refined through rigorous face-to-face meetings, are among the best in medicine. A psychometric analysis of the items sharpens our educational focus on weaknesses in practice. To meet diverse learning styles, we offer MKSAP 16 online and in downloadable apps for PCs, tablets, laptops, and smartphones. We are also introducing the following:

High-Value Care Recommendations: The Nephrology section starts with several recommendations based on the important concept of health care value (balancing clinical benefit with costs and harms) to address the needs of trainees, practicing physicians, and patients. These recommendations are part of a major initiative that has been undertaken by the American College of Physicians, in collaboration with other organizations.

Content for Hospitalists: This material, highlighted in blue and labeled with the familiar hospital icon (🏥), directly addresses the learning needs of the increasing number of physicians who work in the hospital setting. MKSAP 16 Digital will allow you to customize quizzes based on hospitalist-only questions to help you prepare for the Hospital Medicine Maintenance of Certification Examination.

We hope you enjoy and benefit from MKSAP 16. Please feel free to send us any comments to mksap_editors@acponline.org or visit us at the MKSAP Resource Site (mksap.acponline.org) to find out how we can help you study, earn CME, accumulate MOC points, and stay up to date. I know I speak on behalf of ACP staff members and our authoring committees when I say we are honored to have attracted your interest and participation.

Sincerely,

Patrick Alguire, MD, FACP
Editor-in-Chief
Senior Vice President
Medical Education Division
American College of Physicians

Nephrology

Committee

Gerald A. Hladik, MD, Editor[1]
Doc J. Thurston Distinguished Professor of Medicine
University of North Carolina Kidney Center
Training Program Director, Division of Nephrology
The University of North Carolina at Chapel Hill
Chapel Hill, North Carolina

Virginia U. Collier, MD, MACP, Associate Editor[2]
Hugh R. Sharp, Jr. Chair of Medicine
Christiana Care Health System
Newark, Delaware
Professor of Medicine
Jefferson Medical College of Thomas Jefferson University
Philadelphia, Pennsylvania

Gabriel Contreras, MD, MPH[2]
Professor of Clinical Medicine
University of Miami
Miller School of Medicine
Division of Nephrology and Hypertension
Miami, Florida

Melanie Hoenig, MD[1]
Assistant Professor
Harvard Medical School
Renal Division
Beth Israel Deaconess Hospital
Joslin Clinic
Boston, Massachusetts

James Paparello, MD[2]
Associate Professor
Department of Medicine, Nephrology
Northwestern University
Chicago, Illinois

Raymond R. Townsend, MD[2]
Professor of Medicine
Department of Medicine, Renal Division
Perelman School of Medicine
University of Pennsylvania
Philadelphia, Pennsylvania

Suzanne Watnick, MD[1]
Associate Professor of Medicine
Training Program Director, Nephrology
Division of Nephrology and Hypertension
Portland VA Medical Center and

Oregon Health and Science University
Portland, Oregon

Editor-in-Chief

Patrick C. Alguire, MD, FACP[1]
Senior Vice President, Medical Education
American College of Physicians
Philadelphia, Pennsylvania

Deputy Editor-in-Chief

Philip A. Masters, MD, FACP[1]
Senior Medical Associate for Content Development
American College of Physicians
Philadelphia, Pennsylvania

Senior Medical Associate for Content Development

Cynthia D. Smith, MD, FACP[2]
American College of Physicians
Philadelphia, Pennsylvania

Nephrology Clinical Editor

Virginia U. Collier, MD, MACP[2]

Nephrology Reviewers

Robert J. Anderson, MD, MACP[1]
Pieter Cohen, MD, FACP[1]
Frantz Duffoo, MD, FACP[1]
Robert T. Means, Jr., MD, FACP[2]
Ileana L. Piña, MD, MPH[2]
Steven Ricanati, MD, FACP[1]
Mark D. Siegel, MD, FACP[2]

Nephrology Reviewer Representing the American Society for Clinical Pharmacology & Therapeutics

Carol Collins, MD[1]

Nephrology ACP Editorial Staff

Megan Zborowski[1], Staff Editor
Sean McKinney[1], Director, Self-Assessment Programs
Margaret Wells[1], Managing Editor
Linnea Donnarumma[1], Assistant Editor

ACP Principal Staff

Patrick C. Alguire, MD, FACP[1]
Senior Vice President, Medical Education

D. Theresa Kanya, MBA[1]
Vice President, Medical Education

Sean McKinney[1]
Director, Self-Assessment Programs

Margaret Wells[1]
Managing Editor

Valerie Dangovetsky[1]
Program Administrator

Becky Krumm[1]
Senior Staff Editor

Ellen McDonald, PhD[1]
Senior Staff Editor

Katie Idell[1]
Senior Staff Editor

Randy Hendrickson[1]
Production Administrator/Editor

Megan Zborowski[1]
Staff Editor

Linnea Donnarumma[1]
Assistant Editor

John Haefele[1]
Assistant Editor

Developed by the American College of Physicians

---

1. Has no relationships with any entity producing, marketing, re-selling, or distributing health care goods or services consumed by, or used on, patients.

2. Has disclosed relationships with entities producing, marketing, re-selling, or distributing health care goods or services consumed by, or used on, patients. See below.

Conflicts of Interest

The following committee members, reviewers, and ACP staff members have disclosed relationships with commercial companies:

Virginia U. Collier, MD, MACP
Stock Options/Holdings
Celgene, Pfizer, Merck, Schering-Plough, Abbott, Johnson and Johnson, Medtronic, McKesson, Amgen

Gabriel Contreras, MD, MPH
Speakers Bureau
Roche

Robert T. Means, Jr., MD
Consultantship
Beckman Coulter

James Paparello, MD
Other
Medtronic

Ileana L. Piña, MD
Employment
Case Western Reserve University
Research Grants/Contracts
NIH
Consultantship
FDA, GE HealthCare, Solvay
Speakers Bureau
AstraZeneca, Novartis, Otuska

Mark D. Siegel, MD, FACP
Research Grants/Contracts
Altor Bioscience, Bristol-Myers Squibb, Pfizer
Consultantship
Siemens

Cynthia D. Smith, MD, FACP
Stock Options/Holdings
Merck and Company

Raymond R. Townsend, MD
Consultantship
Pfizer, Novartis, Nicox, Medtronic
Speakers Bureau
ASN, ASH
Research Grants/Contracts
NIH

Acknowledgments

The American College of Physicians (ACP) gratefully acknowledges the special contributions to the development and production of the 16th edition of the Medical Knowledge Self-Assessment Program® (MKSAP® 16) made by the following people:

Graphic Services: Michael Ripca (Technical Administrator/Graphic Designer) and Willie-Fetchko Graphic Design (Graphic Designer).

Production/Systems: Dan Hoffmann (Director, Web Services & Systems Development), Neil Kohl (Senior Architect), and Scott Hurd (Senior Systems Analyst/Developer).

MKSAP 16 Digital: Under the direction of Steven Spadt, Vice President, ACP Digital Products & Services, the digital version of MKSAP 16 was developed within the ACP's Digital Product Development Department, led by Brian Sweigard (Director). Other members of the team included Sean O'Donnell (Senior Architect), Dan Barron (Senior Systems Analyst/Developer), Chris Forrest (Senior Software Developer/Design Lead), Jon Laing (Senior Web Application Developer), Brad Lord (Senior Web Developer), John McKnight (Senior Web Developer), and Nate Pershall (Senior Web Developer).

The College also wishes to acknowledge that many other persons, too numerous to mention, have contributed to the production of this program. Without their dedicated efforts, this program would not have been possible.

Introducing the MKSAP Resource Site (mksap.acponline.org)

The MKSAP Resource Site (mksap.acponline.org) is a continually updated site that provides links to MKSAP 16 online answer sheets for print subscribers; access to MKSAP 16 Digital, Board Basics® 3, and MKSAP 16 Updates; the latest details on Continuing Medical Education (CME) and Maintenance of Certification (MOC) in the United States, Canada, and Australia; errata; and other new information.

ABIM Maintenance of Certification

Check the MKSAP Resource Site (mksap.acponline.org) for the latest information on how MKSAP tests can be used to apply to the American Board of Internal Medicine for Maintenance of Certification (MOC) points.

RCPSC Maintenance of Certification

In Canada, MKSAP 16 is an Accredited Self-Assessment Program (Section 3) as defined by the Maintenance of Certification Program of The Royal College of Physicians and Surgeons of Canada (RCPSC) and approved by the Canadian Society of Internal Medicine on December 9, 2011. Approval of Part A sections of MKSAP 16 extends from July 31, 2012, until July 31, 2015. Approval of Part B sections of MKSAP 16 extends from December 31, 2012, to December 31, 2015. Fellows of the Royal College may earn three credits per hour for participating in MKSAP 16 under Section 3. MKSAP 16 will enable Fellows to earn up to 75% of their required 400 credits during the 5-year MOC cycle. A Fellow can achieve this 75% level by earning 100 of the maximum of 174 *AMA PRA Category 1 Credits*™ available in MKSAP 16. MKSAP 16 also meets multiple CanMEDS Roles for RCPSC MOC, including that of Medical Expert, Communicator, Collaborator, Manager, Health Advocate, Scholar, and Professional. For information on how to apply MKSAP 16 CME credits to RCPSC MOC, visit the MKSAP Resource Site at mksap.acponline.org.

The Royal Australasian College of Physicians CPD Program

In Australia, MKSAP 16 is a Category 3 program that may be used by Fellows of The Royal Australasian College of Physicians (RACP) to meet mandatory CPD points. Two CPD credits are awarded for each of the 174 *AMA PRA Category 1 Credits*™ available in MKSAP 16. More information about using MKSAP 16 for this purpose is available at the MKSAP Resource Site at mksap.acponline.org and at www.racp.edu.au. CPD credits earned through MKSAP 16 should be reported at the MyCPD site at www.racp.edu.au/mycpd.

Continuing Medical Education

The American College of Physicians is accredited by the Accreditation Council for Continuing Medical Education (ACCME) to provide continuing medical education for physicians.

The American College of Physicians designates this enduring material, MKSAP 16, for a maximum of 174 *AMA PRA Category 1 Credits*™. Physicians should claim only the credit commensurate with the extent of their participation in the activity.

Up to 16 *AMA PRA Category 1 Credits*™ are available from December 31, 2012, to December 31, 2015, for the MKSAP 16 Nephrology section.

Learning Objectives

The learning objectives of MKSAP 16 are to:
- Close gaps between actual care in your practice and preferred standards of care, based on best evidence
- Diagnose disease states that are less common and sometimes overlooked and confusing
- Improve management of comorbid conditions that can complicate patient care
- Determine when to refer patients for surgery or care by subspecialists
- Pass the ABIM Certification Examination
- Pass the ABIM Maintenance of Certification Examination

Target Audience

- General internists and primary care physicians
- Subspecialists who need to remain up-to-date in internal medicine
- Residents preparing for the certifying examination in internal medicine
- Physicians preparing for maintenance of certification in internal medicine (recertification)

Earn "Same-Day" CME Credits Online

For the first time, print subscribers can enter their answers online to earn CME credits in 24 hours or less. You can submit your answers using online answer sheets that are provided at mksap.acponline.org, where a record of your MKSAP 16 credits will be available. To earn CME credits, you need to answer all of the questions in a test and earn a score of at least 50% correct (number of correct answers divided by the total number of questions). Take any of the following approaches:

1. Use the printed answer sheet at the back of this book to record your answers. Go to mksap.acponline.org, access the appropriate online answer sheet, transcribe your answers, and submit your test for same-day CME credits. There is no additional fee for this service.

2. Go to mksap.acponline.org, access the appropriate online answer sheet, directly enter your answers, and submit your test for same-day CME credits. There is no additional fee for this service.

3. Pay a $10 processing fee per answer sheet and submit the printed answer sheet at the back of this book by mail or fax, as instructed on the answer sheet. Make sure you calculate your score and fax the answer sheet to 215-351-2799 or mail the answer sheet to Member and Customer Service, American College of Physicians, 190 N. Independence Mall West, Philadelphia, PA 19106-1572, using the courtesy envelope provided in your MKSAP 16 slipcase. You will need your 10-digit order number and 8-digit ACP ID number, which are printed on your packing slip. Please allow 4 to 6 weeks for your score report to be emailed back to you. Be sure to include your email address for a response.

If you do not have a 10-digit order number and 8-digit ACP ID number or if you need help creating a username and password to access the MKSAP 16 online answer sheets, go to mksap.acponline.org or email custserv@acponline.org.

Disclosure Policy

It is the policy of the American College of Physicians (ACP) to ensure balance, independence, objectivity, and scientific rigor in all of its educational activities. To this end, and consistent with the policies of the ACP and the Accreditation Council for Continuing Medical Education (ACCME), contributors to all ACP continuing medical education activities are required to disclose all relevant financial relationships with any entity producing, marketing, re-selling, or distributing health care goods or services consumed by, or used on, patients. Contributors are required to use generic names in the discussion of therapeutic options and are required to identify any unapproved, off-label, or investigative use of commercial products or devices. Where a trade name is used, all available trade names for the same product type are also included. If trade-name products manufactured by companies with whom contributors have relationships are discussed, contributors are asked to provide evidence-based citations in support of the discussion. The information is reviewed by the committee responsible for producing this text. If necessary, adjustments to topics or contributors' roles in content development are made to balance the discussion. Further, all readers of this text are asked to evaluate the content for evidence of commercial bias and send any relevant comments to mksap_editors@acponline.org so that future decisions about content and contributors can be made in light of this information.

Resolution of Conflicts

To resolve all conflicts of interest and influences of vested interests, the ACP precluded members of the content-creation committee from deciding on any content issues that involved generic or trade-name products associated with proprietary entities with which these committee members had relationships. In addition, content was based on best evidence and updated clinical care guidelines, when such evidence and guidelines were available. Contributors' disclosure information can be found with the list of contributors' names and those of ACP principal staff listed in the beginning of this book.

Hospital-Based Medicine

For the convenience of subscribers who provide care in hospital settings, content that is specific to the hospital setting has been highlighted in blue. Hospital icons (🏥) highlight where the hospital-only content begins, continues over more than one page, and ends.

Educational Disclaimer

The editors and publisher of MKSAP 16 recognize that the development of new material offers many opportunities for error. Despite our best efforts, some errors may persist in print. Drug dosage schedules are, we believe, accurate and in accordance with current standards. Readers are advised, however, to ensure that the recommended dosages in MKSAP 16 concur with the information provided in the product information material. This is especially important in cases of new, infrequently used, or highly toxic drugs. Application of the information in MKSAP 16 remains the professional responsibility of the practitioner.

The primary purpose of MKSAP 16 is educational. Information presented, as well as publications, technologies, products, and/or services discussed, is intended to inform subscribers about the knowledge, techniques, and experiences of the contributors. A diversity of professional opinion exists, and the views of the contributors are their own and not those of the ACP. Inclusion of any material in the program does not constitute endorsement or recommendation by the ACP. The ACP does not warrant the safety, reliability, accuracy, completeness, or usefulness of and disclaims any and all liability for damages and claims that may result from the use of information, publications, technologies, products, and/or services discussed in this program.

Publisher's Information

Unauthorized Use of This Book Is Against the Law

MKSAP 16 ISBN: 978-1-938245-00-8
(Nephrology) ISBN: 978-1-938245-10-7

Printed in the United States of America.

For order information in the U.S. or Canada call 800-523-1546, extension 2600. All other countries call 215-351-2600. Fax inquiries to 215-351-2799 or email to custserv@acponline.org.

Errata and Norm Tables

Errata for MKSAP 16 will be available through the MKSAP Resource Site at mksap.acponline.org as new information becomes known to the editors.

MKSAP 16 Performance Interpretation Guidelines with Norm Tables, available July 31, 2013, will reflect the knowledge of physicians who have completed the self-assessment tests before the program was published. These physicians took the tests without being able to refer to the syllabus, answers, and critiques. For your convenience, the tables are available in a printable PDF file through the MKSAP Resource Site at mksap.acponline.org.

Table of Contents

Nephrology High-Value Care Recommendations

The American College of Physicians, in collaboration with multiple other organizations, is embarking on a national initiative to promote awareness about the importance of stewardship of health care resources. The goals are to improve health care outcomes by providing care of proven benefit and reducing costs by avoiding unnecessary and even harmful interventions. The initiative comprises several programs that integrate the important concept of health care value (balancing clinical benefit with costs and harms) for a given intervention into various educational materials to address the needs of trainees, practicing physicians, and patients.

To integrate discussion of high-value, cost-conscious care into MKSAP 16, we have created recommendations based on the medical knowledge content that we feel meet the below definition of high-value care and bring us closer to our goal of improving patient outcomes while conserving finite resources.

High-Value Care Recommendation: A recommendation to choose diagnostic and management strategies for patients in specific clinical situations that balances clinical benefit with cost and harms with the goal of improving patient outcomes.

Below are the High-Value Care Recommendations for the Nephrology section of MKSAP 16.

- Kidney ultrasonography is safe, not dependent upon kidney function, noninvasive, and relatively inexpensive and may be used to diagnose urinary tract obstruction, cysts, and mass lesions as well as to assess kidney size and cortical thickness (see Item 90).
- Although home blood pressure monitors are usually not reimbursed by insurers, their relatively low cost (usually less than $100) and reasonable accuracy have made them attractive components to the management of hypertension.
- There is wide variability in the cost of antihypertensive medications; newer and more expensive agents have not been shown to be significantly safer or more effective than many older, well-established medications that are available in generic form.
- Fixed combinations of antihypertensive medications offer less dosing flexibility and are often substantially more expensive than prescribing the component medications independently.
- Lifestyle modifications, including weight loss, reduction of dietary sodium intake, aerobic physical activity of at least 30 minutes a day at least three times a week, and a reduction in alcohol consumption, are a relatively cost-effective way to reduce high blood pressure (see Item 6 and Item 102).
- Only consider evaluating for secondary causes of hypertension when there is onset at a young age, no family history, no risk factors, rapid onset of significant hypertension, abrupt change in blood pressure in a patient with previously good control, or a concomitant endocrine abnormality (see Item 43, Item 58, Item 62, Item 91, and Item 107).
- The benefit of ultrafiltration for fluid removal over adequately dosed diuretics is unproved, especially when the risk of the procedure (central line placement) and increased hypotension are considered.
- Rasburicase is considerably more expensive than allopurinol and is therefore used primarily in patients with high risk for tumor lysis syndrome or if excessively high uric acid levels occur in the context of chemotherapy (see Item 3).
- Plain abdominal radiography has no role in the acute diagnosis of kidney stones (see Item 21 and Item 75).
- Cinacalcet is currently the only calcimimetic agent available; this agent is very expensive, and its role in patients with chronic kidney disease has not yet been defined (see Item 42).
- There is no role for the routine measurement of erythropoietin levels in patients with chronic kidney disease (see Item 105).
- Hospice services are infrequently utilized for patients with end-stage kidney disease who choose to avoid or withdraw from dialysis but would be a potential benefit.

Clinical Evaluation of Kidney Function

Glomerular Filtration Rate

Glomerular filtration rate (GFR) is the parameter most frequently used to assess kidney function and monitor disease progression. GFR can be estimated by mathematical equations based on the serum creatinine level or, in special circumstances, by methods such as creatinine clearance measurement or radionuclide kidney clearance scanning.

Estimation of Glomerular Filtration Rate

Serum Indicators of Kidney Function

Measurement of the serum creatinine level has historically been used to evaluate kidney function. The relationship between GFR and serum creatinine is not linear, but inversely proportional (**Figure 1**). A 50% reduction in GFR results in a doubling of the serum creatinine level once steady state conditions are attained. At high levels of GFR, small changes in the serum creatinine level may reflect large changes in GFR. At low levels of GFR, large changes in the serum creatinine level reflect relatively smaller changes in GFR. In patients who become functionally anephric (for

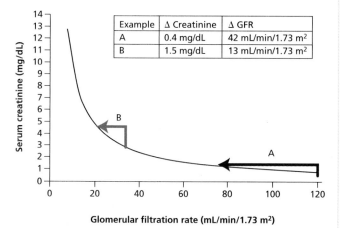

Example	Δ Creatinine	Δ GFR
A	0.4 mg/dL	42 mL/min/1.73 m²
B	1.5 mg/dL	13 mL/min/1.73 m²

FIGURE 1. The relationship between serum creatinine and glomerular filtration rate. Example A illustrates that a small increase in the serum creatinine level in the reference range (in this case, 0.8 to 1.2 mg/dL [70.7-106 micromoles/L]) reflects a relatively large change in GFR (120 to 78 mL/min/1.73 m²). Example B illustrates that a relatively greater increase in the serum creatinine level (in the high range of 3.0 to 4.5 mg/dL [265-398 micromoles/L]) reflects a proportionately smaller change in GFR (35 to 22 mL/min/1.73 m²). GFR = glomerular filtration rate.

example, from profound acute kidney injury), the serum creatinine level typically increases 1.0 to 1.5 mg/dL (88.4-133 micromoles/L) per day.

Although serum creatinine is one of the most commonly used markers of GFR, it is an imperfect measure of kidney function. Reduction of muscle mass, as seen in amputees and patients with malnutrition or muscle wasting, can result in a lower serum creatinine level without a corresponding change in GFR. Younger persons, men, and black persons often have higher muscle mass and higher serum creatinine levels at a given level of GFR compared with older persons with decreased muscle mass. Patients with advanced liver disease produce lower levels of precursors of serum creatinine and often have muscle wasting, with a correspondingly lower serum creatinine level at a particular level of GFR. Finally, serum creatinine overestimates kidney function in elderly persons, especially women.

Certain medications, including cimetidine and trimethoprim, block tubular secretion of creatinine and result in a higher serum creatinine level without a change in GFR. The nephrotic syndrome is associated with increased tubular secretion of creatinine, leading to overestimation of GFR. The colorimetric assay for serum creatinine cross-reacts with cefoxitin, flucytosine, and acetoacetate, leading to falsely high values. Elevated bilirubin levels interfere with the colorimetric assay, resulting in falsely low values of serum creatinine.

Serum cystatin C is an alternative marker of GFR that is less influenced by age, gender, muscle mass, and body weight compared with serum creatinine. Serum cystatin C is more sensitive in identifying milder decrements in kidney function than serum creatinine. Serum levels, however, are affected by thyroid status, inflammation, diabetic status, and corticosteroid use. The clinical utility of serum cystatin C remains to be established, and it is not clear whether serum cystatin C will replace the serum creatinine level as a marker of GFR.

Blood urea nitrogen (BUN) is derived from the metabolism of proteins. Although widely used, BUN concentration is a poor marker of kidney function for several reasons: it is not produced at a constant rate; it is reabsorbed along the tubules; and alterations in kidney blood flow markedly influence tubular reabsorption and excretion. BUN should not be used in isolation to predict kidney function. Urea clearances significantly underestimate GFR but may be useful in estimating GFR when it is less than 15 mL/min/1.73 m². **Table 1** outlines several factors unrelated to the kidney that can affect BUN and serum creatinine levels.

TABLE 1. Factors Altering Blood Urea Nitrogen and Serum Creatinine Levels Independent of Kidney Function

	Decreased	Increased
Blood urea nitrogen	Muscle wasting; protein malnutrition; cirrhosis	Poor kidney perfusion (volume depletion, chronic heart failure, cirrhosis); gastrointestinal bleeding; hyperalimentation; hypercatabolic states
Serum creatinine	Decreased muscle mass; cirrhosis	Tubular secretion blocked (trimethoprim, cimetidine); interference of assay (ketones, bilirubin, flucytosine, cephalosporins); overproduction (creatine ingestion, rhabdomyolysis, sustained exercise)

Methods for Estimating Glomerular Filtration Rate

The National Kidney Foundation Kidney Disease Outcomes Quality Initiative (NKF KDOQI) recommends the use of mathematical equations to estimate GFR (**Table 2**). These equations should only be used when the serum creatinine level has been stable for at least 24 to 48 hours.

The Modification of Diet in Renal Disease (MDRD) study equation has been validated in multiple populations with chronic kidney disease (CKD); however, this equation frequently underestimates GFR when it is greater than 60 mL/min/1.73 m^2. The Chronic Kidney Disease Epidemiology (CKD-EPI) Collaboration equation performs better at higher (normal) values of GFR.

Accurate estimation of GFR is important for appropriate adjustment of drug dosing, particularly in the elderly population and in patients with kidney disease. Historically, drug dosing guidelines were developed based on the estimated creatinine clearance derived from the Cockcroft-Gault equation. This equation takes into account lean body weight, age, and gender. Simulation studies show a high concordance rate between the estimates via the Cockcroft-Gault and MDRD study equations for drug dosing.

Most clinical laboratories employ the MDRD study equation to estimate GFR, and higher levels of GFR are reported as ">60 mL/min/1.73 m^2." This practice raises concern because physicians may ignore other signs or symptoms of CKD, such as proteinuria, after erroneously assuming that the GFR is normal. Conversely, the benefits of labeling a patient with a stable GFR around 55 mL/min/1.73 m^2 (apart from guiding appropriate drug dosing) as having stage 3 CKD when there are no other signs of kidney disease remain unclear.

Estimation equations are less accurate when there are extremes in age and weight, in the setting of pregnancy, and in patients who have undergone amputation or have underlying cirrhosis. In these circumstances, a 24-hour urine collection for creatinine clearance should be used to estimate GFR. Because creatinine is secreted by renal tubules, creatinine clearance overestimates GFR. Inaccuracies arise with over- or undercollection of urine. Observed creatinine excretion can be compared with expected excretion to assess the accuracy of the sample. The expected excretion of creatinine is 20 to 25 mg/kg/24 h (177-221 mmol/kg/24 h) for men and 15 to 20 mg/kg/24 h (133-177 mmol/kg/24 h) for women.

GFR can be measured very precisely using radionuclide kidney clearance scanning, which measures clearance of radiolabeled iothalamate or diethylenetriamine pentaacetic acid (DTPA). The complexity and cost of these methods limit use in clinical practice, but they may be of value when there is a need to precisely measure GFR.

KEY POINTS

- Most clinical laboratories employ the Modification of Diet in Renal Disease study equation to estimate the glomerular filtration rate (GFR), and higher levels of GFR are often reported as ">60 mL/min/1.73 m^2."

- Observed creatinine excretion can be compared with expected excretion to assess the accuracy of a 24-hour urine collection.

- Glomerular filtration rate can be measured very precisely using radionuclide kidney clearance scanning.

Interpretation of the Urinalysis

Dipstick analysis and microscopic examination of the urine are indicated in the clinical evaluation of kidney function for both acute and chronic kidney disease (**Table 3, on page 4**). The sample is best collected without contamination, which requires a "clean catch" midstream collection or a bladder catheterization. The specimen should ideally be examined within 1 hour of being produced to minimize the breakdown of formed elements.

Urine Dipstick

Specific Gravity

Specific gravity is the ratio of the weight of urine to an equal quantity of the weight of water. The typical range is 1.005 to 1.030 but can vary depending on hydration status and the capacity of an individual's kidneys to maximally dilute and concentrate the urine. **Table 4 (on page 4)** illustrates the approximate urine osmolality that corresponds to a given value of urine specific gravity.

pH

Ingestion of a typical high-protein American diet results in consumption of a high "acid-ash" content and the need to

TABLE 2.	Methods for Estimating Kidney Function		
Method		**Considerations**	**Application**
Modification of Diet in Renal Disease (MDRD) Study Equation[a]			
GFR = 175 × (Scr)$^{-1.154}$ × (age)$^{-0.203}$ × 0.742 (if female) or × 1.212 (if black)		Most accurate when eGFR is 15-60 mL/min/1.73 m^2	Chronic kidney disease when GFR is 15-60 mL/min/1.73 m^2
		Underestimates GFR when GFR >60 mL/min/1.73 m^2	
		Less accurate in populations with normal or near normal GFR, extremes of age and weight, amputees, in pregnancy, and cirrhosis	
Chronic Kidney Disease Epidemiology (CKD-EPI) Collaboration Study Equation[a]			
GFR = 141 × min(Scr/K,1)$^\alpha$ × max(Scr/K,1)$^{-1.209}$ × 0.993^{age} × 1.018 (if female) × 1.159 (if black)[b]		Superior to CGE and MDRD equations in patients with eGFR <60 mL/min/1.73 m^2	More accurate than MDRD equation in elderly population
Cockcroft-Gault Equation (CGE)			
CrCl = $\dfrac{(140 - age) \times (weight\ in\ kg) \times (0.85\ if\ female)}{(72 \times Scr)}$		Most accurate when eGFR is 15-60 mL/min/1.73 m^2	Improved accuracy when age is <65 years
		Underestimates GFR in obesity	
		Overestimates GFR when BMI <25	
Creatinine Clearance			
$\dfrac{Ucr\ (mg/dL) \times 24\text{-hour urine volume (mL/24 h)}}{Scr\ (mg/dL) \times 1440\ (min/24\ h)}$		Overestimates GFR 10%-20%	Use in pregnancy, extremes of age and weight, amputees, and cirrhosis
		Incomplete or excessive 24-hour urine collections limit accuracy	
Serum Cystatin C			
		Levels are affected by thyroid status, inflammation, and corticosteroids	More accurate in elderly population and patients with cirrhosis
Radionuclide Kidney Clearance Scanning			
Iothalamate GFR scan

Diethylenetriamine pentaacetic acid (DTPA) GFR scan | | Most precise method and expensive | Kidney donor evaluation if GFR is borderline for donation; research; prediction of GFR following nephrectomy |

CrCl = creatinine clearance; eGFR = estimated glomerular filtration rate; GFR = glomerular filtration rate; Scr = serum creatinine (mg/dL); Ucr = urine creatinine (mg/dL).

[a]Mathematical equations recommended by the National Kidney Foundation Kidney Disease Outcomes Quality Initiative for estimation of GFR.

[b]K is 0.7 for women and 0.9 for men; α is -0.329 for women and -0.411 for men; min = the minimum of Scr/K or 1; max = the maximum of Scr/K or 1.

excrete the acid load, primarily via the kidneys. The urine in this case is relatively more acidic, ranging from 5.0 to 6.0. An alkaline pH of 7.0 or greater can occur in strict vegetarians, patients with distal renal tubular acidosis, or those with infections caused by urease-splitting organisms, including *Proteus* and *Pseudomonas* species.

Albumin

Albumin is the predominant protein detected on urine dipstick. The urine dipstick detects albumin excretion graded as trace (5-30 mg/dL), 1+ (30 mg/dL), 2+ (100 mg/dL), 3+ (300 mg/dL), and 4+ (>1000 mg/dL). Highly alkaline urine specimens can produce false-positive results.

The sulfosalicylic acid (SSA) test is a simple bedside test that can be used to detect the presence of albumin and other proteins such as urine light chains. Recent exposure to radiocontrast can result in false-positive results. The diagnosis of myeloma cast nephropathy should be raised in patients with acute kidney injury when the urine dipstick reads negative or trace for protein but shows increased positivity for protein by the SSA test, reflecting the presence of urine light chains or immunoglobulins not detected by the urine dipstick.

TABLE 3. Findings on Urinalysis

	Reference Range	Comments
Dipstick		
Specific gravity	1.005-1.030	Low with dilute urine; high with concentrated urine or hypertonic product excretion such as contrast dye
pH	5.0-6.5	Elevated with low acid ingestion, inability to excrete acid load (renal tubular acidosis), urease-splitting organisms
Blood	None	False positives with myoglobin or intravascular hemolysis
Albumin	None to trace	Most dipsticks detect primarily albumin but not other proteins; trace positive can be normal in a concentrated specimen
Glucose	None	Positive when plasma glucose level exceeds 180 mg/dL (10.0 mmol/L)
Ketones	None	Positive for acetoacetic acid, not acetone or β-hydroxybutyrate
Nitrites	None	Detects nitrite converted from dietary nitrate by bacteria; normally, no nitrites are present in urine
Leukocyte esterase	None	Detects the presence of leukocytes in the urine; positive test requires at least 3 leukocytes/hpf
Microscopy		
Erythrocytes	0-3/hpf	Urine microscopy should be performed to evaluate erythrocyte morphology
Leukocytes	0-3/hpf	Lower levels can be abnormal
Casts	None or hyaline	Hyaline casts are indicative of poor kidney perfusion but can be benign or reversible; other casts are indicative of intrinsic injury
Crystals	None	Most common include calcium oxalate, calcium phosphate, uric acid, and struvite; occur when urine is supersaturated with a specific substance

TABLE 4. Relationship Between Urine Specific Gravity and Urine Osmolality[a]

	Maximally Dilute		Isosmotic	Concentrated	Maximally Concentrated
Urine osmolality (mosm/kg H_2O)	50-100	200	300	600-900	1200
Urine specific gravity	1.002	1.005	1.010	1.020	1.030

[a]These correlations are not valid when solutes such as glucose or radiocontrast, which disproportionately increase the specific gravity relative to osmolality, are present in the urine.

Glucose

Glycosuria typically occurs when the plasma glucose concentration is greater than 180 to 200 mg/dL (10.0-11.1 mmol/L). Proximal tubular dysfunction, such as that observed in proximal renal tubular acidosis, may result in glycosuria in the absence of hyperglycemia.

Ketones

Ketones are associated with diabetic ketoacidosis, salicylate toxicity, isopropyl alcohol poisoning, and states of starvation such as alcoholic ketoacidosis. Because the urine dipstick detects acetoacetate but not β-hydroxybutyrate, ketotic patients with β-hydroxybutyrate as the only ketone body do not display a positive urine dipstick for ketones; this scenario may occur in patients with alcoholic ketoacidosis. Drugs such as captopril or levodopa have sulfhydryl groups that can result in a false-positive urine dipstick for ketones.

Blood

The urine dipstick detects both free hemoglobin and intact erythrocytes via peroxidase activity. One to three erythrocytes/hpf are usually required for positive results.

Other substances with peroxidase activity can cause false-positive reactions, including myoglobin, bacteria expressing peroxidase activity, hypochlorite, rifampin, chloroquine, and certain forms of iodine. Ascorbic acid can cause a false-negative result. Urine myoglobin levels can be measured to confirm myoglobinuria in patients with rhabdomyolysis.

Leukocyte Esterase and Nitrites

Leukocyte esterase is an enzyme present in leukocytes. When approximately 3 leukocytes/hpf are present in the urine, the urine dipstick is usually positive for leukocyte esterase. Nitrites result from the conversion of nitrates to nitrites, which occur in urinary tract infections (UTIs) caused by gram-negative organisms, including *Escherichia coli*, *Klebsiella pneumoniae*, and *Proteus* and *Pseudomonas* species. False-negative results for nitrites can occur in the setting of a UTI when the infecting organism is gram-positive, such as *Enterococcus* species. The presence of both leukocyte esterase and nitrites on urine dipstick is highly suggestive of a UTI; the absence of both has a high negative predictive value for a UTI.

Bilirubin
Conjugated bilirubin is not usually present in the urine of patients with normal serum bilirubin levels. The presence of conjugated bilirubin is suggestive of severe liver disease or obstructive jaundice. False-positive results occur with chlorpromazine, and false-negative results occur with ascorbic acid.

Urobilinogen
Urobilinogen is produced in the gut from the metabolism of bilirubin and is then reabsorbed and excreted in the urine. A positive urine dipstick for urobilinogen usually results from hemolytic anemia or hepatic necrosis but not from obstructive causes.

KEY POINTS

- Albumin is the predominant protein that is detected on urine dipstick.
- The presence of both leukocyte esterase and nitrites on urine dipstick is highly suggestive of a urinary tract infection (UTI); the absence of both has a high negative predictive value for a UTI.

Urine Microscopy
Microscopic assessment of the urine sediment is indicated for patients with abnormalities on urine dipstick, acute kidney injury, suspicion for glomerulonephritis, or newly diagnosed CKD. Cells, casts, and crystals are possible findings in a patient with kidney disease.

Leukocytes
Pyuria refers to excess leukocytes in the urine and is defined as 4 or more leukocytes/hpf. The most common cause of pyuria is a UTI. Sterile pyuria refers to the presence of leukocytes in the urine in the setting of a negative urine culture. *Mycobacterium tuberculosis* infection is an important infectious cause of sterile pyuria. Acute interstitial nephritis is often caused by antibiotics, NSAIDs, or proton pump inhibitors and is associated with sterile pyuria and low-grade proteinuria. Kidney stones and kidney transplant rejection can also cause sterile pyuria.

Eosinophils
Urine eosinophils are visualized via Wright or Hansel stains. The presence of eosinophils in the urine can be indicative of an allergic reaction, atheroembolic disease, rapidly progressive glomerulonephritis, small-vessel vasculitis, UTI, prostatic disease, or parasitic infections. Poor sensitivity and specificity limit the utility of assays for urine eosinophils in the diagnosis of interstitial nephritis.

Erythrocytes
Erythrocytes in the urine can originate at any location along the genitourinary tract, from the glomerulus to the urethra. Assessment of erythrocyte morphology is a key component in the evaluation of hematuria (see Clinical Evaluation of Hematuria). Isomorphic erythrocytes are of the same size and shape and usually arise from a urologic process such as a tumor, stone, or infection. Conversely, dysmorphic erythrocytes demonstrate varying sizes and shapes. Acanthocytes, one form of dysmorphic erythrocytes, are characterized by vesicle-shaped protrusions (**Figure 2**). Although some types of dysmorphic erythrocytes can be caused by pH or osmolality shifts, this is not true of acanthocytes. Acanthocytes and erythrocyte casts are most commonly present in glomerulonephritis but occasionally can be seen in severe interstitial nephritis and acute tubular necrosis. Such findings on microscopy should prompt an assessment for proteinuria and impaired kidney function.

Microscopic hematuria can be variously defined as the presence of 2 to 4 erythrocytes/hpf in a spun urine sediment, with lower cut-off values corresponding to increased sensitivity but decreased specificity. There is no lower limit that can exclude significant pathology, and the reference range needs to be interpreted within the clinical context. For example, 3 erythrocytes/hpf has greater significance in a patient with a long history of smoking at increased risk for urothelial malignancy.

Casts
Urine casts consist of a matrix comprised of Tamm-Horsfall mucoprotein, which may contain cells, cellular debris, or

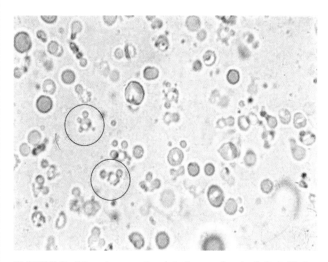

FIGURE 2. Urine microscopy demonstrating acanthocytes, indicated in the red circles. Acanthocytes, one form of dysmorphic erythrocytes, are characterized by vesicle-shaped protrusions.

Courtesy of J. Charles Jennette, MD.

lipoprotein droplets. Casts are formed within the tubular lumen and are therefore cylindrical, conforming to the shape of the tubule. Documentation of particular types of casts is instrumental in the diagnostic evaluation of acute and chronic kidney disease. Hypovolemia may lead to low urine flow rates and the presence of hyaline casts composed of Tamm-Horsfall mucoprotein alone. Tubular injury may lead to deposition of pigmented epithelial tubular debris in the proteinaceous matrix of the cast, with the formation of pigmented granular (muddy brown) casts. Erythrocyte casts are found primarily in patients with glomerulonephritis. Tubulointerstitial inflammation of the kidney, including pyelonephritis, can lead to the formation of leukocyte casts.

Crystals

Table 5 highlights the crystals commonly observed in the urine, along with morphology and associated conditions.

Certain medications, including sulfa drugs, calcium carbonate, intravenous acyclovir, and indinavir, can also result in crystals in the urine.

Measurement of Albumin and Protein Excretion

Protein detected by urine dipstick or by the SSA test should always be quantified, and the NKF KDOQI recommends measurement of the urine protein–creatinine ratio on randomly obtained samples to quantify proteinuria (**Table 6**). This ratio correlates with daily protein excretion. A ratio of 2 mg/mg, for example, indicates a daily protein excretion of approximately 2 grams per 1.73 m² per day. A ratio of less than 0.2 mg/mg is considered normal. Nephrotic-range proteinuria is defined as a urine protein–creatinine ratio greater than 3.5 mg/mg, and, when comprised of albumin, is indicative of underlying glomerular disease. A urine

TABLE 5. Urine Crystals		
Type	**Morphology/Shape**	**Associated Conditions**
Calcium oxalate	Envelope Dumbbell Needle	Hypercalciuria Hyperoxaluria Calcium oxalate stones Ethylene glycol poisoning
Calcium phosphate	Prism Needle Star-like clumps	Distal renal tubular acidosis Urine pH above 6.5 Tumor lysis syndrome Acute phosphate nephropathy
Uric acid	Rhomboid Needle Rosette	Diabetes mellitus Obesity Gout Hyperuricemia Tumor lysis syndrome Urine pH below 6.0
Magnesium ammonium phosphate (struvite)	Coffin-lid	Chronic urinary tract infection with urease-producing organisms
Cystine	Hexagonal	Cystinuria

TABLE 6. National Kidney Foundation Kidney Disease Outcomes Quality Initiative Definitions of Proteinuria and Albuminuria				
	Urine Collection Method	**Normal**	**Microalbuminuria**	**Albuminuria or Clinical Proteinuria**
Total Protein	24-Hour excretion (varies with method)	<300 mg/24 h	–	>300 mg/24 h
	Spot urine dipstick	<30 mg/dL	–	>30 mg/dL
	Spot urine protein–creatinine ratio (varies with method)	<0.2 mg/mg	–	>0.2 mg/mg
Albumin	24-Hour excretion	<30 mg/24 h	30-300 mg/24 h	>300 mg/24 h
	Spot urine albumin-specific dipstick	<3 mg/dL	>3 mg/dL	–
	Spot urine albumin–creatinine ratio	<30 mg/g	30-300 mg/g	>300 mg/g

Modified from American Journal of Kidney Diseases. 39(2 Suppl 1). K/DOQI clinical practice guidelines for chronic kidney disease: evaluation, classification, and stratification. Part 4: Definition and classification of stages of chronic kidney disease. S46-S75. [PMID: 11904577] Copyright 2002, with permission from Elsevier.

protein–creatinine ratio less than 2 mg/mg may indicate either tubulointerstitial disease or glomerular disease. At least two samples on different days should be collected to confirm the diagnosis of proteinuria.

Proteinuria is most commonly comprised of albumin, but other proteins, including kidney-derived low-molecular-weight proteins, monoclonal immunoglobulins and light chains, myoglobin, and hemoglobin, may be present. If monoclonal immunoglobulins are found, it is important to further characterize the proteinuria using urine immunofixation. Low-molecular-weight proteinuria is more common in tubulointerstitial disease, whereas a predominance of albuminuria favors a glomerular process.

The American Diabetes Association (ADA) recommends annual testing to assess urine albumin excretion by measuring the urine albumin–creatinine ratio in patients with type 1 diabetes mellitus of 5 years' duration and in all patients with type 2 diabetes starting at the time of diagnosis. Microalbuminuria is defined by the ADA as a urine albumin–creatinine ratio of 30 to 300 mg/g; diagnosis requires an elevated urine albumin–creatinine ratio on two of three random samples obtained over 6 months.

Patients at increased risk for kidney disease, particularly those with diabetes or hypertension, should be screened for proteinuria. Quantitation of urine protein excretion is important to assess prognosis and cardiovascular risk and to follow response to therapy. Patients with diabetes and microalbuminuria, for example, are at increased risk for progression and cardiovascular disease. Use of ACE inhibitors or angiotensin receptor blockers in patients with proteinuric kidney disease or in diabetic patients with microalbuminuria delays progression of kidney disease, underscoring the importance of early detection.

Transient proteinuria is common and is associated with febrile illnesses or rigorous exercise and requires no further evaluation. Orthostatic proteinuria occurs when proteinuria increases during the day and decreases at night when the patient is recumbent; this benign condition, more common in adolescents, can be assessed via a split urine collection. This test should be obtained in patients younger than 30 years of age who have persistent proteinuria.

Clinical Evaluation of Hematuria

Hematuria may be a sign of a life-threatening process and thus merits careful clinical evaluation (**Figure 3**). More than 3 erythrocytes/hpf constitutes hematuria and is a common finding on urinalysis. The most common causes are kidney stones and UTIs. A single episode in older patients or those at risk should prompt a full evaluation of the upper and lower urinary tract. In low-risk patients who are younger than 40 years old, a repeat urinalysis should be performed to establish hematuria.

Gross hematuria is more commonly associated with malignancy than microscopic hematuria. Red-colored urine is more common with urinary tract bleeding, whereas brown- or tea-colored urine is more common in glomerulonephritis.

Careful examination of the urine sediment is indicated to document erythrocyte morphology and whether there are concurrent erythrocyte casts. Erythrocytes with normal morphometry on urine microscopy are associated with urologic causes of hematuria, whereas dysmorphic erythrocytes or acanthocytes are associated with nephrologic causes of hematuria, usually of glomerular origin (see Erythrocytes).

The presence of hematuria should raise suspicion for genitourinary tract malignancies in patients with risk factors. The U.S. Preventive Services Task Force currently does not recommend screening urinalysis for asymptomatic adults for purposes of bladder cancer screening. Recent evidence, however, demonstrated an adjusted hazard ratio of 18.5 for the development of end-stage kidney disease in patients found to have microscopic hematuria in a large unselected cohort of adolescents and young adults followed for 21 years, raising the question whether routine screening with urine dipstick should be recommended in adolescents and adults.

Risk factors for urologic malignancy or features of systemic vasculitis should be sought in the medical history. Risk factors for bladder cancer include smoking, male gender, and age over 40 years. The presence of isomorphic hematuria in this setting warrants cystoscopy and upper urinary tract imaging. Conversely, the presence of acanthocytes, erythrocyte casts, and proteinuria warrants prompt nephrologic consultation for possible kidney biopsy.

Urinary tract imaging is important in the evaluation of hematuria to identify or exclude specific causes. The choice of imaging modality for evaluating the upper urinary tract depends on the risk factor profile of a given patient and the estimated GFR (**Table 7, on page 9**). CT urography is the test of choice for high-risk patients with well-preserved GFR. MR urography may be helpful when the estimated GFR is in the range of 30 to 60 mL/min/1.73 m^2. Ultrasonography is warranted in patients less than 40 years old with no risk factors for urologic malignancy. Noncontrast abdominal helical CT is indicated when there is suspicion for nephrolithiasis. Intravenous pyelography has low sensitivity for urologic tumors or stones and is no longer recommended. In patients who have hematuria with a negative upper urinary tract evaluation, visualization of the lower urinary tract is typically accomplished by cystoscopy to assess for lower ureteral, bladder, or urethral causes. Cytologic studies may also be indicated for detecting possible malignancies not identified on imaging or direct visualization.

Urologic follow-up for patients with an initial negative evaluation for isomorphic hematuria is guided by risk factors, with more aggressive surveillance for those with increased risk for urologic malignancy. The choice of studies and optimal timing have yet to be determined. The American Urological Association opinion-based protocol is outlined in Figure 3.

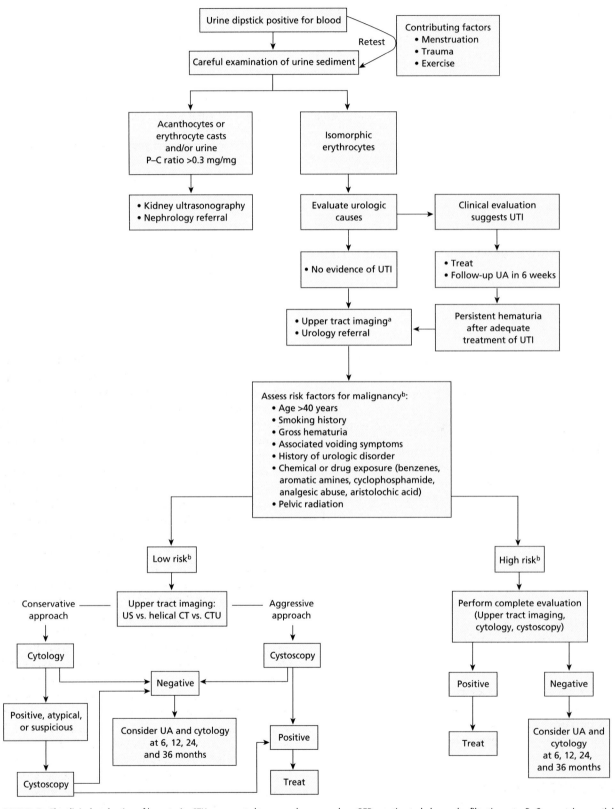

FIGURE 3. The clinical evaluation of hematuria. CTU = computed tomography urography; eGFR = estimated glomerular filtration rate; P–C = protein–creatinine; UA = urinalysis; US = ultrasonography; UTI = urinary tract infection.

[a]See Table 7 for imaging studies used in the evaluation of hematuria.

[b]Modified with permission from Urology. 57(4). Grossfeld GD, Litwin MS, Wolf JS, et al. Evaluation of asymptomatic microscopic hematuria in adults: the American Urological Association best practice policy–part II: patient evaluation, cytology, voided markers, imaging, cystoscopy, nephrology evaluation, and follow-up. 604-610. 2001, [PMID: 11306357] with permission from Elsevier.

TABLE 7. Imaging Used in the Evaluation of Hematuria

Study	Advantages	Disadvantages
CT urography (CTU)	High sensitivity (100%) and specificity (97%)	High radiation dose (2 × IVP)
		Risk of CIN
		Contraindicated in pregnancy
MR urography	Useful in eGFR range of 30-60 mL/min/1.73 m^2	Contraindicated when eGFR <30 mL/min/1.73 m^2 (gadolinium)
		Less sensitive than CTU for smaller cancers and stones
Ultrasonography	No contrast	Limited sensitivity, especially for lesions <2 cm
	No radiation exposure	
	Useful in setting of pregnancy	
	Lower cost	
Intravenous pyelography (IVP)	Less radiation than CTU	Risk of CIN
		Low sensitivity (40%-65%)

CIN = contrast-induced nephropathy; eGFR = estimated glomerular filtration rate.

Hematuria in patients with an underlying bleeding diathesis or on anticoagulation requires evaluation and should not be attributed to the coagulopathy until other causes are excluded.

KEY POINTS

- Microscopic assessment of the urine sediment is indicated for patients with abnormalities on urine dipstick, acute kidney injury, suspicion for glomerulonephritis, or newly diagnosed chronic kidney disease.

- The most common cause of pyuria is a urinary tract infection.

- Isomorphic erythrocytes are of the same size and shape and usually arise from a urologic process such as a tumor, stone, or infection.

- Acanthocytes and erythrocyte casts are most commonly present in glomerulonephritis but occasionally can be seen in severe interstitial nephritis and acute tubular necrosis.

- The most common causes of hematuria are kidney stones and urinary tract infections, but the presence of hematuria should raise suspicion for genitourinary tract malignancies in patients with risk factors.

Imaging Studies

Assessment of kidney disease often includes imaging of the kidneys and urinary tract. Kidney ultrasonography is safe, not dependent upon kidney function, noninvasive, and relatively inexpensive. Because it does not require contrast, ultrasonography does not place patients at risk for contrast-induced nephropathy. This is often the first imaging study used to evaluate the structure of the upper genitourinary tract. Ultrasonography can be used to diagnose urinary tract obstruction, cysts, and mass lesions as well as to assess kidney size and cortical thickness. Doppler ultrasonography can detect renal artery stenosis when performed by experienced technicians.

Abdominal CT with contrast offers better resolution and characterization of kidney mass lesions or cysts than ultrasonography; however, contrast can be harmful to patients with an estimated GFR of less than 60 mL/min/1.73 m^2. CT urography is the test of choice for the evaluation of urologic bleeding in patients at high risk for bladder cancer with an estimated GFR above 60 mL/min/1.73 m^2.

Noncontrast abdominal helical CT is more accurate than ultrasonography in identifying nephrolithiasis and may be more useful in obese patients in whom technical problems may arise during general ultrasonography. Plain abdominal radiography of the kidneys, ureters, and bladder (KUB) can identify non-uric acid–containing kidney stones, although CT offers greater contrast resolution to detect nephrolithiasis.

MRI of the kidneys can accurately identify mass lesions and cysts. Gadolinium enhancement can be useful to determine whether a mass lesion has malignant features. MR angiography, which usually employs gadolinium, is useful in the diagnosis of renal artery stenosis. Gadolinium, however, has been associated with nephrogenic systemic fibrosis in patients with stage 4 and stage 5 CKD, acute kidney injury, and in patients following kidney and liver transplantation and should be avoided in these populations.

Radionuclide kidney clearance scanning is the gold standard for quantifying GFR and renal plasma flow. These studies are very accurate and are useful in the evaluation of renal plasma flow and function of transplanted kidneys, the assessment of the functional significance of renovascular disease, the presurgical assessment of kidney function before nephrectomy, and the functional significance of hydronephrosis in patients with possible urinary tract obstruction.

KEY POINTS

- Because it does not require contrast, ultrasonography does not place patients at risk for contrast-induced nephropathy and is often the first imaging study used to evaluate the structure of the upper genitourinary tract.
- MRI of the kidneys can accurately identify mass lesions and cysts.
- Radionuclide kidney clearance scanning is the gold standard for quantifying the glomerular filtration rate and renal plasma flow.

Kidney Biopsy

In patients with kidney disease, a kidney biopsy provides tissue that can be used for diagnosis, prognosis, treatment, and surveillance. Indications include suspected glomerular pathology such as glomerulonephritis and the nephrotic syndrome, acute kidney injury of unclear cause, and kidney transplant dysfunction. Biopsies are usually performed under direct visualization with ultrasonographic or CT guidance.

Contraindications include bleeding diatheses, active infection of the genitourinary system, hydronephrosis, atrophic kidneys, and uncontrolled hypertension. Relative contraindications include a solitary kidney, severe anemia, and chronic anticoagulation. Risks include pain within the first few days after biopsy; gross hematuria that can result in urinary obstruction; bleeding with the need for transfusion in approximately 5% of patients; potential nephrectomy in less than 0.3% of patients; and death in less than 0.1%.

KEY POINTS

- Indications for kidney biopsy include suspected glomerular pathology such as glomerulonephritis and the nephrotic syndrome, acute kidney injury of unclear cause, and kidney transplant dysfunction.
- Contraindications to kidney biopsy include bleeding diatheses, active infection of the genitourinary system, hydronephrosis, atrophic kidneys, and uncontrolled hypertension.

Fluids and Electrolytes

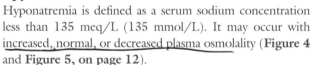

Osmolality and Tonicity

Under normal physiologic conditions, plasma osmolality is determined by the concentration of sodium and its accompanying anions; plasma glucose; and blood urea nitrogen (BUN).

Osmolality can be directly measured with an osmometer or calculated using the following equation:

$$\text{Plasma Osmolality (mosm/kg } H_2O) = 2 \times \text{Serum Sodium (meq/L)} + \text{Plasma Glucose (mg/dL)}/18 + \text{BUN (mg/dL)}/2.8$$

The serum osmolal gap is the difference between the measured and calculated plasma osmolality; a value greater than 10 mosm/kg H_2O is considered elevated and reflects the presence of unmeasured solutes.

Under conditions of normal health, the effective osmolality is maintained in the range of 275 to 295 mosm/kg H_2O. Effective osmolality is tightly regulated, thereby maintaining constant intracellular volume. Changes in effective osmolality are sensed by osmoreceptors near the hypothalamus. A 1% to 2% increase in effective osmolality causes release of antidiuretic hormone ([ADH]; also known as arginine vasopressin), which results in increased reabsorption of water in the collecting ducts. Physiologic, nonosmotic release of ADH also occurs in response to true hypovolemia. Nonphysiologic ADH secretion causes the syndrome of inappropriate antidiuretic hormone secretion (SIADH). **H**

KEY POINT

- A serum osmolal gap greater than 10 mosm/kg H_2O is considered elevated and reflects the presence of unmeasured solutes.

Disorders of Serum Sodium

Hyponatremia

Hyponatremia is defined as a serum sodium concentration less than 135 meq/L (135 mmol/L). It may occur with increased, normal, or decreased plasma osmolality (**Figure 4** and **Figure 5, on page 12**).

Causes

Pseudohyponatremia

Pseudohyponatremia is a laboratory artifact that may be observed in patients with hyperglobulinemia or severe hyperlipidemia. Although this artifact is now less common with the use of ion-specific electrodes, it remains a problem in laboratories using indirect potentiometry to assess the amount of sodium in a specific sample volume; an increase in the solid phase of a specimen displaces and decreases the effective volume analyzed for sodium content, leading to reporting of an artificially low serum sodium level. Visible lipemia is usually present with hyperlipidemia-associated pseudohyponatremia but may be absent in patients with high levels of cholestasis-associated lipoprotein-X. Measured osmolality is normal in pseudohyponatremia; the increased osmolal gap cannot be accounted for by an increase in glucose, BUN, or other solutes such as mannitol, sorbitol, or glycine.

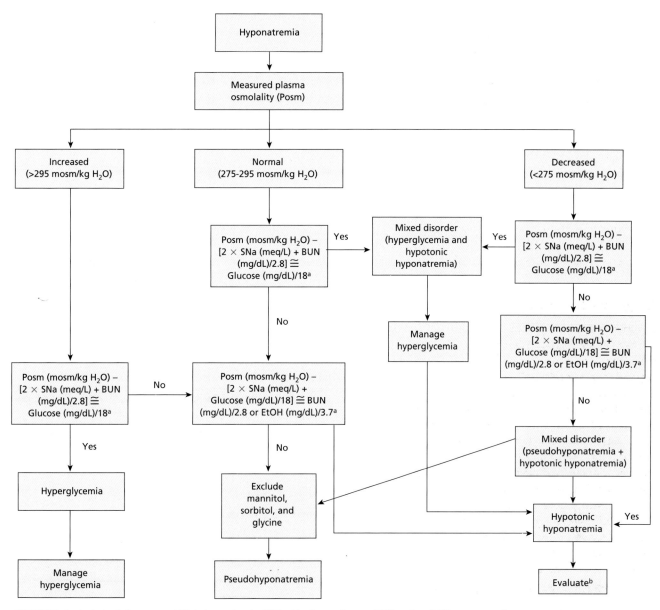

FIGURE 4. Analysis of plasma osmolality in hyponatremia. BUN = blood urea nitrogen; EtOH = ethanol; SNa = serum sodium.

[a]Difference may vary by approximately 5 mosm/kg H_2O due to unmeasured osmoles that are normally present in the serum.

[b]See Figure 5 for the evaluation of hypotonic hyponatremia.

Hypotonic Hyponatremia

Hypotonic hyponatremia is the most common form of hyponatremia. It may occur in patients with normal, increased, or decreased extracellular fluid (ECF) volumes. Measured plasma osmolality is usually low but may be normal or increased in the presence of elevated BUN, glucose, or an exogenous solute such as alcohol.

Hypertonic Hyponatremia

Hypertonic hyponatremia is caused by marked hyperglycemia or exogenously administered solutes such as mannitol or sucrose. Hyperglycemia causes the translocation of water from

the intracellular to the ECF compartment, which results in a decrease in the serum sodium level by approximately 1.6 meq/L (1.6 mmol/L) for every 100 mg/dL (5.6 mmol/L) increase in the plasma glucose above 100 mg/dL (5.6 mmol/L).

Isosmotic Hyponatremia

Isosmotic hyponatremia may occur as a result of pseudohyponatremia or when two or more disorders are present simultaneously. For example, a patient with hyponatremia due to SIADH who subsequently develops hyperglycemia will have a normal measured plasma osmolality when the increase in osmolality resulting from increased glucose counterbalances the initial

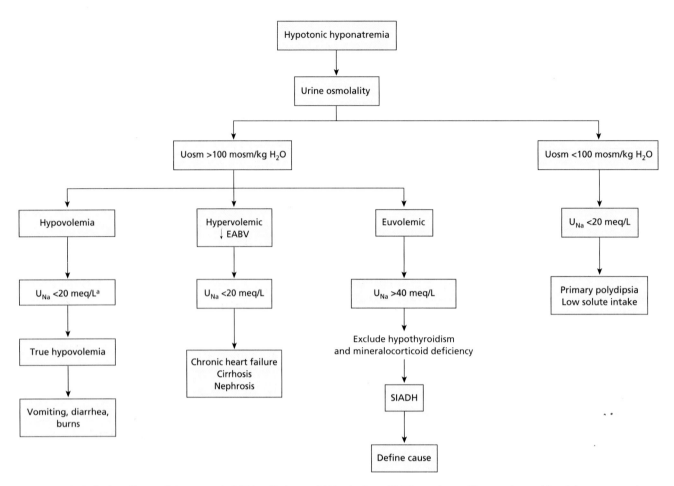

☞ **FIGURE 5.** Evaluation of hypotonic hyponatremia. EABV = effective arterial blood volume; SIADH = syndrome of inappropriate antidiuretic hormone secretion; U_{Na} = urine sodium concentration; Uosm = urine osmolality.

[a]Exceptions include diuretic therapy, mineralocorticoid deficiency, cerebral salt wasting, osmotic diuresis, and salt wasting nephropathy.

decrement in osmolality that resulted from SIADH-associated water retention. Absorption of isosmotic irrigating solutions such as glycine or sorbitol also can cause isosmotic hyponatremia.

Evaluation

The first step in the evaluation of hyponatremia is to check plasma osmolality (see Figure 4). If pseudohyponatremia is suspected, plasma osmolality will be normal, and documentation of elevated levels of cholesterol, triglycerides, or serum total protein will lend support to the diagnosis. The plasma sodium concentration is normal in pseudohyponatremia when measured with blood gas analyzers equipped with direct potentiometry.

The cause of hypotonic hyponatremia can be established by patient history, volume status, urine osmolality, and urine sodium level (see Figure 5).

Hypotonic Hyponatremia with an Appropriately Low Urine Osmolality

Patients with primary polydipsia and hyponatremia typically present with urine osmolality less than 100 mosm/kg H_2O in the presence of hypotonicity. Because water excretion is in part solute dependent, severe limitations in solute intake decrease free water excretion, and hyponatremia may develop in this setting with only modest increases in fluid intake. This syndrome is termed *beer potomania* when observed in patients with chronic alcohol abuse and low solute intake.

Hypotonic Hyponatremia with an Inappropriately High Urine Osmolality

Urine osmolality greater than 100 mosm/kg H_2O in the setting of hypotonic hyponatremia reflects non-osmotic ADH secretion due to true hypovolemia, decreased effective arterial blood volume (EABV), or nonphysiologic ADH release. Total body water and ECF volume are increased in SIADH; however, this increase cannot be detected clinically by physical examination, principally because two thirds of the excess water is retained in the intracellular fluid compartment. Increased ECF volume leads to increased sodium excretion resulting from increased kidney perfusion and decreased sodium uptake in the proximal nephron.

CONT.

Consequently, the urine sodium concentration is greater than 40 meq/L (40 mmol/L) when dietary sodium intake is adequate (>80 meq/d).

Reset osmostat is a syndrome that may occur in patients with quadriplegia, tuberculosis, advanced age, pregnancy, and psychiatric disorders. These patients can be distinguished from those with SIADH by documenting excretion of dilute urine following a water load. Stability of the serum sodium under conditions of variable fluid intake is a clue to the diagnosis.

It is often difficult to differentiate between mild hypovolemia with appropriate osmotically stimulated ADH release and SIADH by physical examination and urinary indices, particularly when solute intake is decreased and urine sodium values are equivocal. Clinical history and interpretation of serum and urine levels of urea and uric acid may help in the diagnostic evaluation (**Table 8**). An increase in the serum sodium concentration after infusion of 1 liter of normal saline favors a diagnosis of hypovolemia but should only be attempted in asymptomatic patients when the diagnosis remains uncertain. Hypothyroidism and adrenal insufficiency should be excluded in patients with euvolemic hyponatremia. **Table 9** summarizes the causes of SIADH.

Patients with hyponatremia secondary to non-osmotic ADH secretion include those with true hypovolemia as well as patients with decreased EABV who have heart failure, the nephrotic syndrome, or cirrhosis. The urine sodium concentration is usually less than 20 meq/L (20 mmol/L) in this setting. Exceptions include patients on active diuretic therapy or those with kidney sodium wasting as may occur

TABLE 8. Serum and Urinary Indices in the Syndrome of Inappropriate Antidiuretic Hormone Secretion and Hypovolemia

Favors SIADH

Urine sodium >40 meq/L (40 mmol/L)

FE_{Na} >1%

Serum uric acid <4 mg/dL (0.24 mmol/L)

FE_{UA} >10%

BUN <10 mg/dL (3.6 mmol/L)

FE_{UN} >50%

Favors Hypovolemia

Urine sodium <20 meq/L (20 mmol/L)

FE_{Na} <1%

Serum uric acid >6 mg/dL (0.35 mmol/L)

FE_{UA} <10%

BUN >15 mg/dL (5.4 mmol/L)

FE_{UN} <35%

BUN = blood urea nitrogen; FE_{Na} = fractional excretion of sodium; FE_{UA} = fractional excretion of uric acid; FE_{UN} = fractional excretion of urea; SIADH = syndrome of inappropriate antidiuretic hormone secretion.

TABLE 9. Causes of the Syndrome of Inappropriate Antidiuretic Hormone Secretion

Central nervous system disorders
  Hemorrhage[a]
  Infections
  Inflammatory disorders
  Guillain-Barré syndrome
  Multiple sclerosis
  Mass lesions[a]
Drugs
  3,4-Methylenedioxymethamphetamine (also known as ecstasy)[a]
  Antipsychotic medications
  Carbamazepine
  Chlorpropamide
  Clofibrate
  Cyclooxygenase-2 inhibitors[a]
  Cyclophosphamide
  Desmopressin[a]
  Ifosfamide
  Nicotine
  NSAIDs[a]
  Opiates[a]
  Phenothiazines
  Selective serotonin reuptake inhibitors[a]
  Serotonin norepinephrine reuptake inhibitors[a]
  Tricyclic antidepressants
  Vasopressin[a]
  Vincristine
Endurance exercise
Familial disorders
Infections
  HIV infection
  Rocky Mountain spotted fever
Postoperative setting
  Anesthesia[a]
  Nausea[a]
  Pain[a]
Pulmonary disorders
  Infections[a]
  Inflammatory disorders
  Positive pressure mechanical ventilation[a]
  Respiratory failure
Tumors
  Gastrointestinal tract tumors
  Genitourinary tract tumors
  Lymphomas
  Respiratory tract tumors[a]
  Sarcomas
  Small cell carcinoma[a]
  Thymomas

[a]Most common causes.

CONT.

in mineralocorticoid deficiency, cerebral salt wasting, chronic kidney disease (CKD), or following cisplatin chemotherapy. Cerebral salt wasting is a syndrome of hypotonic hyponatremia that may complicate subarachnoid hemorrhage or neurosurgery. Increased levels of B-type natriuretic peptide result in kidney sodium wasting and hypovolemic hyponatremia.

Clinical Presentation

Acute hyponatremia is defined as the onset of hypotonicity in less than 24 hours. Risk factors include postoperative administration of hypotonic fluids, the use of thiazide diuretics, the use of the illicit drug 3,4-methylenedioxymethamphetamine (also known as ecstasy), overhydration associated with extreme exercise, and primary polydipsia. Increased neuronal cell volume may result in neurologic symptoms and the high mortality seen in patients with severe hypotonic hyponatremia.

Patients with symptomatic hyponatremia may initially have nonspecific symptoms such as nausea, fatigue, and headache. Cerebral edema most commonly occurs in patients in whom the serum sodium level decreases by more than 10 meq/L (10 mmol/L) over 1 to 3 days. As cerebral edema worsens, symptoms may progress to obtundation, seizures, coma, hypoxia, and respiratory arrest.

Chronic hyponatremia develops over 72 hours or more, and patients are less likely to have symptomatic cerebral edema. Chronic hypotonicity stimulates extrusion of intracellular solutes and leads to a reduction in cell volume toward normal. Overly rapid correction of hyponatremia in these patients is more likely to induce osmotic demyelination syndrome (see Treatment, Osmotic Demyelination Syndrome). Many patients with chronic hyponatremia develop superimposed acute symptomatic hyponatremia in the setting of acute illness such as concomitant hypovolemia.

Recent evidence suggests that patients with mild degrees of chronic hyponatremia (serum sodium level of 125-135 meq/L [125-135 mmol/L]) without overt symptoms of cerebral edema may have subtle neurocognitive deficits that can only be detected with careful neurocognitive and functional testing. These patients have an increased risk of falls, hip fracture, and osteoporosis. The benefits of implementing measures to correct the serum sodium level to greater than 135 meq/L (135 mmol/L) in these patients remain an area of investigation.

KEY POINTS

- Patients with symptomatic hyponatremia may initially have nonspecific symptoms such as nausea, fatigue, and headache.
- As cerebral edema worsens in patients with symptomatic hyponatremia, symptoms may progress to obtundation, seizures, coma, hypoxia, and respiratory arrest.

Treatment

Treatment of patients with hyponatremia depends on the cause as well as the presence and severity of symptoms.

Symptomatic Hyponatremia

Patients with symptoms of cerebral edema merit more rapid correction. Symptomatic patients with SIADH warrant treatment with hypertonic saline, whereas patients with hyponatremia secondary to true hypovolemia can be treated with normal saline. The safety of vasopressin receptor antagonists (vaptans) in symptomatic patients has yet to be validated. These agents are contraindicated in patients with hypovolemic hyponatremia. Treatment should continue until symptoms resolve, and serum sodium correction should not exceed 10 meq/L (10 mmol/L) within the first 24 hours or 18 meq/L (18 mmol/L) within the first 48 hours. Recent evidence suggests that acutely increasing the serum sodium concentration by 4 to 6 meq/L (4-6 mmol/L) within the first 24 hours is sufficient for most patients with symptomatic hyponatremia. Patients with acute hypotonic hyponatremia complicated by seizures or coma should be treated with 100 mL or 2 mL/kg bolus infusions of 3% saline, which can be repeated up to two times if needed.

Close monitoring of the serum sodium level at least every 2 to 4 hours is indicated during the initial phase of therapy. Patients with SIADH and highly concentrated urine may develop worsening hyponatremia with infusion of normal saline due to excretion of urine with increased tonicity relative to serum ("desalination") and retention of infused water; therefore, 3% saline is preferred for treatment of symptomatic patients with SIADH. Patients with hyponatremia due to volume depletion or SIADH often exhibit water diuresis during therapy, which can result in overly rapid correction. Correction of concurrent hypokalemia may also induce overly rapid correction. When this occurs, the serum sodium concentration can be corrected back to the target level with use of 5% dextrose in water and/or desmopressin.

Osmotic Demyelination Syndrome

Correction of acute hyponatremia that exceeds 10 meq/L (10 mmol/L) within the first 24 hours and 18 meq/L (18 mmol/L) within the first 48 hours of therapy has been associated with onset of the osmotic demyelination syndrome (ODS). These values should be considered upper limits of correction rather than goals of therapy. Clinical features of ODS include progressive quadriparesis, speech and swallowing disorders, coma, and "locked-in" syndrome. Neurologic deficits are often irreversible; therefore, preventive measures are essential.

Asymptomatic Hyponatremia

Treatment of patients with asymptomatic hyponatremia depends on the underlying cause (**Table 10**). Fluid restriction is essential in patients with SIADH or hypervolemic

TABLE 10. Management of Asymptomatic Hypotonic Hyponatremia

Etiology	Management
True hypovolemia	Correct etiology of hypovolemia
	Isotonic saline
Syndrome of inappropriate antidiuretic hormone secretion (SIADH)	Treat underlying cause
	Discontinue offending drugs
	Fluid restriction
	Furosemide
	Demeclocycline
	Vasopressin receptor antagonists (vaptans)
	Ensure adequate solute and protein intake
Hypervolemic hyponatremia (chronic heart failure, cirrhosis, nephrosis)	Treat underlying cause
	Fluid and sodium restriction
	Furosemide
	Vasopressin receptor antagonists (vaptans)

(handwritten annotation near Demeclocycline: "decrease collecting tubule response to ADH")

CONT.

hyponatremia. Total intake, including both oral and intravenous, must be less than total output (including insensible losses) in order to cause a rise in the serum sodium level.

Hypertonic hyponatremia due to hyperglycemia will correct as plasma glucose levels fall with insulin therapy, leading to movement of water back into the intracellular compartment. No further intervention for hyponatremia per se is warranted for pseudohyponatremia, and hyperlipidemia and hyperproteinemia should be evaluated and treated as indicated.

KEY POINTS

- Hypertonic saline is indicated for symptomatic patients who have the syndrome of inappropriate antidiuretic hormone secretion.
- Patients with hyponatremia secondary to true hypovolemia can be treated with normal saline.
- Recent evidence suggests that acutely increasing the serum sodium concentration by 4 to 6 meq/L (4-6 mmol/L) over the first 24 hours is sufficient for most patients with symptomatic hyponatremia.
- Fluid restriction is essential in patients with asymptomatic hyponatremia who have the syndrome of inappropriate antidiuretic hormone secretion or hypervolemic hyponatremia.

Hypernatremia

Hypernatremia is defined as a serum sodium concentration greater than 145 meq/L (145 mmol/L). Hypernatremia is a common disorder in critically ill patients and is associated with high morbidity and mortality. The cause can usually be ascertained from evaluating the history and volume status, in conjunction with determination of the urine volume and urine osmolality (**Table 11**).

Causes
Inadequate Water Intake
Thirst and water intake protect against the development of hypernatremia. Failure to adequately replace water loss is the most common cause of hypernatremia. Hypernatremia is often observed in elderly patients or infants with impaired mentation or functional impairment that precludes access to water. Hypothalamic lesions may interfere with the thirst response, resulting in marked hypernatremia.

Hypotonic Fluid and Pure Water Loss
Urinary and gastrointestinal fluid losses are usually hypotonic, causing a rise in the serum sodium concentration in the absence of compensatory fluid intake. Gastrointestinal losses, diuretic therapy, and osmotic diuresis cause hypernatremia in association with hypovolemia.

Patients with diabetes insipidus are typically able to replace urinary water losses by drinking, and the serum sodium level is usually only slightly increased unless water intake is impaired. Causes of diabetes insipidus include decreased release of ADH (central diabetes insipidus); ADH resistance (nephrogenic diabetes insipidus); and metabolism of ADH by circulating vasopressinase (gestational diabetes insipidus) (**Table 12**). Adipsic diabetes insipidus results in severe hypernatremia in patients with central nervous system lesions involving both the posterior pituitary gland and hypothalamic thirst center.

Assessment of Polyuria
Polyuria in adults is defined by an increase in urine volume above 3 L/24 h and is often accompanied by hypernatremia. The differential diagnosis of polyuria includes diabetes insipidus, primary polydipsia (which, unlike other causes of polyuria, results in hyponatremia), and osmotic diuresis.

TABLE 11. Causes and Clinical Findings in Hypernatremia

Cause	Volume Status	Urine Volume	Urine Osmolality (mosm/kg H_2O)
Hypotonic Fluid Loss			
Gastrointestinal losses (vomiting, nasogastric suction, diarrhea)	Hypovolemic	Decreased	>600
Diuretics (except osmotic diuretics)	Hypovolemic	Variable	~150
Osmotic diuresis (hyperglycemia; urea [high protein diet or enteral feeding, relief of urinary tract obstruction, recovery phase of acute tubular necrosis])	Hypovolemic	Increased	>300
Pure Water Loss			
Insensible water losses (skin, respiratory tract) that are not replaced (impaired mentation, stroke, hypothalamic lesion, functional impairment limiting access to fluids)	Normal	Decreased	>600
Diabetes insipidus	Normal	Increased	<200
Hypertonic Fluid Gain			
Administration or ingestion of sodium chloride, hypertonic saline, or sodium bicarbonate	Hypervolemic	Increased	>300

TABLE 12. Causes of Diabetes Insipidus

Central diabetes insipidus
  Autoimmune hypophysitis (idiopathic)[a]
  Malignancy (metastatic or primary)[a]
  Neurosurgery[a]
  Trauma
  Infiltration (sarcoidosis, histiocytosis X, lymphocytic hypophysitis, granulomatosis with polyangiitis [also known as Wegener granulomatosis], IgG4 disease)[a]
  Following correction of supraventricular tachycardia
  Hypoxic encephalopathy
  Anorexia nervosa
  Sheehan syndrome
  Familial
Nephrogenic diabetes insipidus
  Lithium[a]
  Other medications (demeclocycline, cidofovir, foscarnet, didanosine, amphotericin B, ifosfamide, ofloxacin)[a]
  Electrolyte disorders (hypercalcemia, hypokalemia)[a]
  Sickle cell nephropathy
  Urinary tract infection
  Amyloidosis
  Sjögren syndrome
  Nephronophthisis
  Cystinosis
Gestational diabetes insipidus (placental vasopressinase)

[a]Most common causes.

Patients with central diabetes insipidus are more likely to present with abrupt onset of polyuria.

Urine osmolality during osmotic diuresis is usually greater than 300 mosm/kg H_2O, whereas it usually is less than 200 mosm/kg H_2O in diabetes insipidus and primary polydipsia. Urine osmolality occasionally rises above 200 mosm/kg H_2O in hypovolemic patients with partial central diabetes insipidus. The serum sodium concentration is typically less than 138 meq/L (138 mmol/L) in primary polydipsia and greater than 142 meq/L (142 mmol/L) in diabetes insipidus. Water deprivation testing demonstrates an increase in urine osmolality to approximately 600 mosm/kg H_2O in primary polydipsia. Urine osmolality remains less than 200 mosm/kg H_2O in patients with diabetes insipidus with water deprivation. Administration of desmopressin results in a rise in urine osmolality to approximately 600 mosm/kg H_2O in central diabetes insipidus and in gestational diabetes insipidus but not in nephrogenic diabetes insipidus. Unlike ADH, desmopressin is not metabolized by pregnancy-related vasopressinase.

Treatment
Patients with circulatory collapse should initially be treated with sufficient isotonic saline to correct organ hypoperfusion. Isotonic saline boluses should be avoided in the absence of shock given the risk of associated cerebral edema, and hypotonic solutions such as 5% Dextrose in water are preferred. Hypernatremia should be corrected at a rate no more than 10 meq/L (10 mmol/L) per day to avoid cerebral edema. The water deficit can be estimated by the following equation:

$$\text{Total Body Water } [0.6 \text{ in Men and } 0.5 \text{ in Women} \times \text{Body Weight (kg)}] \times [(\text{Serum Sodium}/140 \ [\text{or target serum sodium}]) - 1]$$

This equation does not account for urinary, gastrointestinal, and insensible losses; it is also inaccurate because of the error inherent in estimating total body water. Furthermore, this calculation estimates the water deficit relative to total body

CONT. sodium and only represents the amount of free water needed to correct the hypernatremia and not the total body volume deficit. The serum sodium concentration should therefore be monitored carefully during correction.

A patient with a serum sodium level of 160 meq/L (160 mmol/L) weighing approximately 70 kg (154 lb) presenting with hypotension and circulatory shock, for example, should receive bolus therapy with isotonic saline until shock is resolved. Therapy is then directed toward correcting the hyponatremia based on estimating the water deficit (Total Body Water = 0.5 × 70 kg = 35 L; water deficit necessary to correct serum sodium to 150 meq/L = 35 L × [160/150 – 1] = 2.33 L). 5% Dextrose in water could then be infused at a rate of approximately 100 mL/h over the first 24 hours, measuring the serum sodium every 3 to 4 hours to permit appropriate adjustment of the infusion rate.

Polyuria caused by central or gestational diabetes insipidus is treated with intranasal desmopressin. Thiazide diuretics increase proximal sodium and water reabsorption and can be employed to decrease urine volume in nephrogenic diabetes insipidus.

If possible, lithium should be discontinued in patients with severe nephrogenic diabetes insipidus, particularly when associated with progressive lithium-related interstitial kidney disease. If lithium must be continued, amiloride (which blocks uptake into apical sodium channels in the collecting duct epithelium) can be used to limit tubular uptake and toxicity. Careful monitoring of lithium levels is warranted when diuretics are used, because hypovolemia increases proximal lithium reabsorption, thereby increasing serum lithium levels. [H]

KEY POINTS

- Causes of hypernatremia include hypotonic fluid loss, pure water loss, diabetes insipidus, and hypertonic fluid gain.
- Gastrointestinal losses, diuretic therapy, and osmotic diuresis cause hypernatremia in association with hypovolemia.
- Hypernatremia should be corrected at a rate no more than 10 meq/L (10 mmol/L) per day to avoid cerebral edema.

[H] Disorders of Serum Potassium
Hypokalemia

Hypokalemia is defined as a serum potassium concentration less than 3.5 meq/L (3.5 mmol/L). The differential diagnosis includes cellular redistribution, kidney or gastrointestinal tract losses, and decreased intake. Hypokalemia manifests with abnormal skeletal and cardiac muscle cell function related to alterations in action potential generation or changes in renal tubular cell function (**Table 13**). Symptoms generally do not occur until the serum potassium concentration decreases to less than 3 meq/L (3 mmol/L).

TABLE 13. Clinical Manifestations of Hypokalemia
Cardiac
Arrhythmias
Premature atrial beats
Atrial tachycardia
Sinus bradycardia
Atrioventricular block
Junctional tachycardia
Premature ventricular beats
Ventricular tachycardia
Ventricular fibrillation
Electrocardiographic changes
Depressed ST segment
Decreased T wave amplitude
Increased U wave amplitude
Skeletal muscle
Muscle cramps
Ascending muscle weakness
Respiratory muscle weakness
Paralysis
Rhabdomyolysis
Smooth muscle dysfunction and ileus
Glucose intolerance
Kidney
Increased ammoniagenesis and alkalosis
Impaired urinary concentration
Hypokalemic nephropathy

Evaluation

The evaluation of hypokalemia begins with a thorough history. Diuretics are the most common cause of hypokalemia. Assessment of factors that alter the cellular distribution of serum potassium should then be considered (**Figure 6**).

Pseudohypokalemia, a laboratory artifact caused by intracellular uptake of serum potassium in patients with marked leukocytosis, is a diagnostic consideration in patients with myeloproliferative disorders. β_2-Agonists, epinephrine, insulin, vitamin B_{12} repletion, and systemic alkalosis also can result in increased intracellular uptake of serum potassium, as can toxicity due to barium, chloroquine, quetiapine, and risperidone. Hypokalemic periodic paralysis is a rare syndrome that presents with acute episodic muscle weakness, often following a high carbohydrate meal or strenuous exercise. Hypokalemic periodic paralysis presents as either a familial syndrome or as an acquired form due to interferon therapy or thyrotoxicosis. Persons of Asian or Mexican descent are at increased risk for this syndrome.

After excluding conditions that cause cellular redistribution, the diagnosis of hypokalemia is established by history

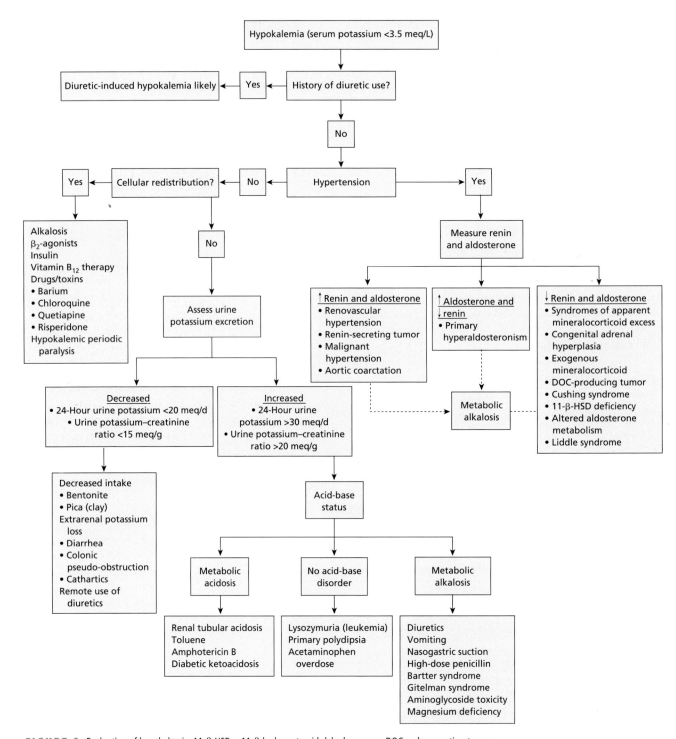

FIGURE 6. Evaluation of hypokalemia. 11-β-HSD = 11-β-hydroxysteroid-dehydrogenase; DOC = deoxycorticosterone.

and assessment of urine potassium excretion, blood pressure, and acid-base status. Urine potassium excretion is determined by the amount of potassium secreted in the cortical collecting duct (CCD). Aldosterone, enhanced lumen-negative voltage, and increased tubular flow and sodium delivery to the CCD increase urine potassium excretion.

Potassium depletion due to gastrointestinal losses decreases kidney potassium excretion to levels less than 20 meq/L (20 mmol/L) per day. In hypokalemic patients, a 24-hour urine potassium excretion above 30 meq/L (30 mmol/L) per day suggests ongoing urine potassium losses. Random values of urine potassium can be used to assess the kidney response to hypokalemia but must be corrected for the degree of urinary concentration. This can be achieved by calculating the urine potassium–creatinine ratio, which when expressed in meq/g creatinine, is derived from the following equation:

$$\text{Urine Potassium–Creatinine Ratio (meq/g)} =$$
$$\text{Urine Potassium (meq/L)} \times 100 \, [(\text{mg} \times \text{L})/(\text{dL} \times \text{g})] \div$$
$$\text{Urine Creatinine (mg/dL)}$$

A urine potassium–creatinine ratio above 20 meq/g is characteristic of kidney potassium wasting, whereas a value below 15 meq/g reflects cellular redistribution, decreased intake, or extrarenal potassium loss. Patients with kidney potassium wasting can be divided into those with or without hypertension. Plasma renin activity and aldosterone levels are then used to differentiate causes of hypokalemia associated with hypertension. The cause of hypokalemia in patients with normal or low blood pressure is diagnosed based on acid-base status and urine sodium and chloride levels (see Figure 6).

Hypokalemia commonly occurs with concomitant metabolic alkalosis. Diuretics, vomiting, and nasogastric suction are frequent causes that are also associated with urine potassium loss. Bartter and Gitelman syndromes are congenital disorders presenting with hypokalemic metabolic alkalosis resulting from abnormalities in the loop diuretic–sensitive sodium-potassium-chloride cotransporter in the thick ascending limb and the thiazide diuretic–sensitive sodium-chloride cotransporter in the distal tubule. Aminoglycosides such as gentamicin, when given for prolonged courses, can induce a Bartter-like syndrome resulting from activation of the calcium-sensing receptor in the thick ascending limb, thereby inhibiting the sodium-potassium-chloride cotransporter in the thick ascending limb.

Treatment

A decrease in the serum potassium concentration from 4 to 3 meq/L (4 to 3 mmol/L) is associated with a potassium deficit of approximately 100 meq when there is no change in cellular distribution. However, a linear relationship between the serum potassium concentration and the total body potassium deficit is not observed below serum levels of 3 meq/L (3 mmol/L), and careful monitoring of the serum potassium concentration during repletion is therefore indicated to avoid iatrogenic hyperkalemia.

Patients with large potassium deficits, particularly when associated with cardiac or skeletal muscle dysfunction, should be treated with intravenous potassium chloride at a maximum rate of 20 meq/h infused at a concentration no greater than 40 meq/L (40 mmol/L). Addition of sodium bicarbonate and/or glucose to intravenous solutions, which cause increased intracellular uptake of potassium, should be avoided during initial therapy of symptomatic hypokalemia.

Oral supplementation is appropriate for asymptomatic patients or for those with mild symptoms. Potassium citrate can be used for patients with concomitant metabolic acidosis due to renal tubular acidosis. Potassium-sparing diuretics are helpful for patients with conditions associated with chronic kidney potassium wasting but should be avoided when there is concomitant metabolic acidosis. Magnesium depletion frequently accompanies hypokalemia, and correction of magnesium deficits may limit urine potassium loss. 🄷

KEY POINTS

- Hypokalemia manifests with abnormal skeletal and cardiac muscle cell function related to alterations in action potential generation or changes in renal tubular cell function.

- Diuretics are the most common cause of hypokalemia.

- In patients with hypokalemia, a urine potassium–creatinine ratio above 20 meq/g is characteristic of kidney potassium wasting, whereas a value below 15 meq/g reflects cellular redistribution, decreased intake, or extrarenal potassium loss.

- Patients with large potassium deficits, particularly when associated with cardiac or skeletal muscle dysfunction, should be treated with intravenous potassium chloride at a maximum rate of 20 meq/h infused at a concentration no greater than 40 meq/L (40 mmol/L).

Hyperkalemia

Hyperkalemia is defined as a serum potassium concentration greater than 5 meq/L (5 mmol/L). Risk factors include underlying acute or chronic kidney disease and decreased renin-angiotensin-aldosterone activity. Clinical manifestations include ascending muscle weakness, electrocardiogram (ECG) changes, and life-threatening cardiac arrhythmias and paralysis when the hyperkalemia is severe.

Evaluation

The initial goal is to establish whether hyperkalemia is life-threatening through the history and physical examination and analysis of the ECG. As the serum potassium level rises, the ECG most commonly reveals peaked T waves with a shortened QT interval initially, followed by an increased PR interval and QRS duration, decreased P wave amplitude, and eventually a sinoventricular pattern heralding ventricular standstill. The presence of ECG changes warrants emergency therapy (see Treatment).

The initial evaluation of hyperkalemia also includes assessment for cellular redistribution (**Figure 7**). In the absence of symptoms or ECG changes, pseudohyperkalemia should be considered. Severe leukocytosis (leukocyte count >120,000/microliters [120×10^9/L]) and thrombocytosis

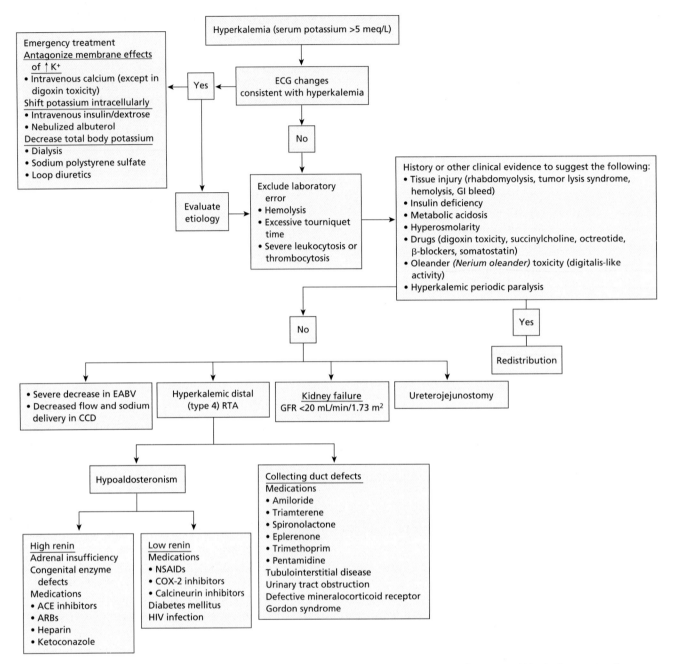

FIGURE 7. Evaluation of hyperkalemia. ARB = angiotensin receptor blocker; COX = cyclooxygenase; EABV = effective arterial blood volume; ECG = electrocardiography; GFR = glomerular filtration rate; GI = gastrointestinal; K = potassium; RTA = renal tubular acidosis.

(platelet count >600,000/microliters [600 × 10^9/L]) can result in the release of intracellular potassium in serum specimens. The diagnosis of pseudohyperkalemia due to thrombocytosis is established by documenting a simultaneous normal plasma (heparinized sample) potassium level. Pseudohyperkalemia related to leukocytosis is diagnosed by repeating a serum potassium measurement in a sample carefully transported to the laboratory without agitation immediately following phlebotomy. Measurement of whole blood

potassium in uncentrifuged specimens using ion-specific electrodes also confirms the diagnosis.

Hyperkalemia may also occur as a result of mechanical trauma or a prolonged tourniquet time during venipuncture, and a serum potassium measurement should be repeated in asymptomatic patients with no apparent risk factors for hyperkalemia or ECG changes.

Due to increased release of aldosterone and resultant enhanced kidney potassium excretion, the serum potassium

CONT.

concentration remains in the normal range in healthy adults with potassium intake as high as 280 meq/d (280 mmol/d), well above the average daily intake of 70 meq (70 mmol) in a typical Western diet. Dietary intake of potassium contributes to the pathogenesis of hyperkalemia only in patients with a kidney defect in potassium secretion, usually resulting from a defect in the renin-angiotensin-aldosterone system or a glomerular filtration rate (GFR) less than 20 mL/min/1.73 m². Hyperkalemia that occurs above this level of GFR indicates that there is a defect in potassium secretion in the CCD (see Figure 7).

The capacity of the kidney to excrete potassium in the setting of hyperkalemia can be evaluated by calculating the transtubular potassium gradient (TTKG), which estimates the ratio of the potassium level in the CCD to that in the peritubular capillary. The TTKG is calculated by the following equation:

$$TTKG = [Urine\ Potassium \div (Urine\ Osmolality / Plasma\ Osmolality)] \div Serum\ Potassium$$

The TTKG should be greater than 10 in hyperkalemia under normal physiologic conditions. A TTKG less than 10 in a hyperkalemic patient indicates a kidney defect in potassium excretion.

Various drugs interfere directly or indirectly with CCD potassium secretion. Blockade of the renin-angiotensin-aldosterone system with drugs, particularly use of combination therapy such as an ACE inhibitor and spironolactone in CKD, frequently induces hyperkalemia. Hyporeninemic hypoaldosteronism most commonly occurs in patients with long-standing diabetes mellitus or HIV infection. Injury to the CCD epithelium because of chronic tubulointerstitial disease, sickle cell nephropathy, or urinary tract obstruction impairs potassium secretion and leads to hyperkalemia. Factors resulting in decreased mineralocorticoid activity, including congenital or acquired adrenal insufficiency as well as inherited mineralocorticoid receptor defects, may be associated with hyperkalemia. Hyperkalemia may also develop as a complication of ureterojejunostomy because of increased absorption of urine potassium in the jejunal bypass limb.

Treatment

Patients with symptomatic hyperkalemia or those with a rapidly rising serum potassium level and/or ECG manifestations should receive prompt treatment under continuous cardiac monitoring. Intravenous calcium chloride or calcium gluconate antagonizes the depolarization effects of hyperkalemia and should be administered every 5 minutes until ECG changes resolve. Intravenous calcium is contraindicated in patients with digoxin toxicity, because it potentiates adverse electrophysiologic effects. Treatment directed toward increasing intracellular uptake of potassium should then be initiated. Intravenous insulin (with intravenous glucose when the plasma glucose level is <250 mg/dL [13.9 mmol/L]) is the most efficient intervention that enhances intracellular potassium uptake. This effect begins within 10 minutes and is sustained

for 4 to 6 hours. High-dose nebulized albuterol (10-20 mg) is additive to the action of insulin, with a peak effect at 90 minutes. Sodium bicarbonate may be used to treat hyperkalemia when complicated by metabolic acidosis but has minimal efficacy in patients with end-stage kidney disease.

The use of intravenous calcium, insulin, sodium bicarbonate, and nebulized albuterol is only a temporizing measure. Definitive therapy must include measures that decrease total body potassium. Sodium polystyrene sulfate in sorbitol has historically been used to decrease total body potassium in patients with hyperkalemia. However, preparations containing sorbitol have been implicated in gastrointestinal necrosis and bleeding; therefore, use of the sorbitol-free preparation is preferred. Hemodialysis is indicated when hyperkalemia is severe, particularly in patients with severe kidney failure.

Mild to moderate hyperkalemia can often be controlled through dietary potassium restriction to less than 2500 mg/d. Hypovolemia and urinary tract obstruction, when present, should be corrected. Contributing medications such as NSAIDs and cyclooxygenase-2 inhibitors should be strictly avoided. Medications that inhibit the activity of the renin-angiotensin-aldosterone system such as ACE inhibitors or spironolactone may require dose reduction or discontinuation when the serum potassium level remains above 5.5 meq/L (5.5 mmol/L). Patients with a GFR less than 30 mL/min/1.73 m² require closer monitoring of the serum potassium level (every 7 to 10 days after initiating or increasing the dose of renin-angiotensin-aldosterone system inhibitors such as ACE inhibitors). Loop diuretics can be used to promote decreased total body potassium in patients with CKD or chronic heart failure. **H**

KEY POINTS

- Clinical manifestations of hyperkalemia include ascending muscle weakness, electrocardiogram changes, and life-threatening cardiac arrhythmias and paralysis when the hyperkalemia is severe.
- Dietary intake of potassium contributes to the pathogenesis of hyperkalemia only in patients with a kidney defect in potassium secretion, usually resulting from a defect in the renin-angiotensin-aldosterone system or a glomerular filtration rate less than 20 mL/min/1.73 m².
- Intravenous insulin (with intravenous glucose when the plasma glucose level is <250 mg/dL [13.9 mmol/L]) is the most efficient intervention that enhances intracellular potassium uptake.
- Mild to moderate hyperkalemia can often be controlled through dietary potassium restriction to less than 2500 mg/d.
- Medications that inhibit the activity of the renin-angiotensin-aldosterone system may require dose reduction or discontinuation when the serum potassium level remains above 5.5 meq/L (5.5 mmol/L).

Disorders of Serum Phosphate

Hypophosphatemia

Hypophosphatemia is defined as a serum phosphate concentration less than 2.5 mg/dL (0.81 mmol/L) and is most common in patients with a history of chronic alcohol use, critical illness, and malnutrition. Most patients with hypophosphatemia are asymptomatic, but symptoms of weakness may manifest at levels less than 2 mg/dL (0.65 mmol/L). Serum phosphate levels less than 1 mg/dL (0.32 mmol/L) may result in respiratory muscle weakness, hemolysis, and rhabdomyolysis.

Evaluation

The causes of hypophosphatemia are summarized in **Table 14**. In most cases, the cause is evident from the history. If the diagnosis remains unclear, urine phosphate excretion can be assessed by obtaining a 24-hour urine phosphate excretion or by calculating the fractional excretion of phosphate from a random urine specimen.

When hypophosphatemia is due to increased cellular uptake or extrarenal phosphate loss, the 24-hour urine phosphate excretion is less than 100 mg/dL (32.3 mmol/L) and the fractional excretion of phosphate is less than 5%.

Treatment

Hypophosphatemia usually resolves with treatment of the underlying cause. Phosphate supplementation is indicated for symptomatic patients and for those with chronic phosphate

TABLE 14. Causes of Hypophosphatemia
Kidney phosphate wasting
Acetaminophen poisoning
Vitamin D deficiency or resistance
Hyperparathyroidism
Osmotic diuresis
Oncogenic osteomalacia
Kidney transplantation
Proximal (type 2) renal tubular acidosis (Fanconi syndrome)
Tenofovir
Ifosfamide
Hypophosphatemic rickets
Chronic diarrhea
Decreased absorption
Vitamin D deficiency or resistance
Phosphate binders and antacids
Decreased intake
Intracellular uptake
Refeeding syndrome
Treatment of diabetic ketoacidosis with insulin
Parathyroidectomy (hungry bone syndrome)
Respiratory alkalosis

wasting. Oral phosphate supplementation is preferred because of the risk of hypocalcemia and acute kidney injury associated with intravenous phosphate infusions. Intravenous phosphate supplementation is indicated for symptomatic patients with serum phosphate levels less than 1 mg/dL (0.32 mmol/L). Serum phosphate and calcium levels should be monitored every 6 hours during intravenous therapy, and doses of phosphate should be restricted to 80 mmol over 12 hours.

Hyperphosphatemia

Hyperphosphatemia is defined as a serum phosphate concentration greater than 4.5 mg/dL (1.45 mmol/L). Hyperphosphatemia most commonly occurs in patients with advanced CKD but may also occur when there is increased cell turnover, cell injury, or exogenous phosphate administration. The cause is usually apparent from the clinical history. Patients with CKD are treated with phosphate binders taken with meals to limit intestinal absorption of phosphate. Patients with acute phosphate nephropathy or tumor lysis syndrome with severe hyperphosphatemia (serum phosphate >10 mg/dL [3.23 mmol/L]) and concomitant oliguria may warrant initiation of hemodialysis.

KEY POINTS

- Hypophosphatemia is most common in patients with a history of chronic alcohol use, critical illness, and malnutrition.
- Serum phosphate levels less than 2 mg/dL (0.65 mmol/L) may cause symptomatic weakness, and levels less than 1 mg/dL (0.32 mmol/L) may result in respiratory muscle weakness, hemolysis, and rhabdomyolysis.
- Intravenous phosphate supplementation is indicated for symptomatic patients with serum phosphate levels less than 1 mg/dL (0.32 mmol/L).

Acid-Base Disorders

General Approach

Because of the importance of maintaining a stable metabolic milieu, the systemic pH is carefully controlled through both renal and respiratory mechanisms. Disturbances in acid-base balance lead to predictable responses that serve to limit the magnitude of change of blood pH. The cause of acid-base disturbances is often apparent by examining data from an arterial blood gas study (pH and PCO_2) and venous electrolyte measurement (primarily serum bicarbonate) in the context of a given clinical situation.

Primary acid-base disorders are classified as respiratory or metabolic. Respiratory acidosis is defined as an arterial PCO_2 above the normal range, with a value below normal representing respiratory alkalosis. Metabolic acidosis is defined as

CONT.

a serum bicarbonate level below the normal range, with a value above normal representing metabolic alkalosis.

Analysis involves identification of the likely dominant acid-base disorder, followed by an assessment of the secondary, compensatory response. The expected compensatory responses to primary acid-base disturbances are listed in **Table 15**. When measured values fall outside the range of the predicted secondary response, a mixed acid-base disorder is present; multiple acid-base disturbances may coexist in a single patient. The correct diagnosis of respiratory acid-base disorders, particularly when associated with a second disorder, often requires correlation with the clinical history.

Metabolic Acidosis

Metabolic acidosis occurs when there is loss of serum bicarbonate, decreased excretion of acid, imbalance between production and consumption of endogenous acids, or ingestion or intravenous administration of exogenous acids.

Evaluation

When metabolic acidosis is present, it should be further characterized by analysis of the anion gap. The anion gap is useful in assessing whether the decreased serum bicarbonate is due to the presence of an additional unmeasured acid (such as lactate or an ingested acid) that will raise the anion gap, or a loss or lack of production of serum bicarbonate in which the serum chloride increases to maintain electroneutrality, in which case the anion gap is normal. Based on this analysis, a metabolic acidosis is classified as being either an *increased anion gap* or a *normal anion gap* metabolic acidosis. The anion gap is calculated from the following equation:

Anion Gap = Serum Sodium (meq/L) − [Serum Chloride (meq/L) + Serum Bicarbonate (meq/L)]

The normal reference range for the anion gap is approximately 8 to 10 meq/L ± 2 meq/L (8-10 mmol/L ± 2 mmol/L), which may vary among laboratories and individuals. Because albumin is an unmeasured anion, changes in the serum albumin level can affect the magnitude of the expected anion gap. For every 1 g/dL (10 g/L) decrease in serum albumin, for example, the expected or "normal" anion gap falls by approximately 2.3 meq/L (2.3 mmol/L). The presence of unmeasured cations such as cationic light chains also decreases the anion gap. H

KEY POINTS

- Metabolic acidosis occurs when there is loss of serum bicarbonate, decreased excretion of acid, imbalance between production and consumption of endogenous acids, or ingestion or intravenous administration of exogenous acids.
- The anion gap is used to characterize the nature of a metabolic acidosis.
- The presence of a low serum albumin level or unmeasured cations such as cationic light chains results in a decreased anion gap.

Classification

Mixed Metabolic Disorders

Additional analysis is required when an increased anion gap metabolic acidosis is present to determine whether the serum bicarbonate level was normal before the development of the acidosis or if there was a preexisting metabolic abnormality before the acidosis creating the anion gap occurred. This is done by calculating the corrected bicarbonate based on the change in the anion gap (termed the *delta anion gap* or *delta gap*), which estimates the serum bicarbonate level

TABLE 15.	Compensation in Acid-Base Disorders
Condition	**Expected Compensation**
Metabolic acidosis	Acute: $P_{CO_2} = (1.5)[H_{CO_3}] + 8$
	Chronic: $P_{CO_2} = [H_{CO_3}] + 15$
	Failure of the P_{CO_2} to decrease to expected value = complicating respiratory acidosis; excessive decrease of the P_{CO_2} = complicating respiratory alkalosis
	Quick check: P_{CO_2} = value should approximate last two digits of pH
Metabolic alkalosis	For each ↑ 1 meq/L in [H_{CO_3}], P_{CO_2} ↑ 0.7 mm Hg
Respiratory acidosis	Acute: 1 meq/L ↑ [H_{CO_3}] for each 10 mm Hg ↑ in P_{CO_2}
	Chronic: 3.5 meq/L ↑ [H_{CO_3}] for each 10 mm Hg ↑ in P_{CO_2}
	Failure of the [H_{CO_3}] to increase to the expected value = complicating metabolic acidosis; excessive increase in [H_{CO_3}] = complicating metabolic alkalosis
Respiratory alkalosis	Acute: ↓ 2 meq/L [H_{CO_3}] for each 10 mm Hg ↓ in P_{CO_2}
	Chronic: 4-5 meq/L ↓ [H_{CO_3}] for each 10 mm Hg ↓ in P_{CO_2}
	Failure of the [H_{CO_3}] to decrease to the expected value = complicating metabolic alkalosis; excessive decrease in [H_{CO_3}] = complicating metabolic acidosis

that existed in the absence of the increased anion gap acidosis. The corrected bicarbonate is calculated from the following equation:

$$\text{Corrected Bicarbonate} = 24 \text{ meq}/\text{L} - \Delta \text{ Anion Gap (meq/L)}$$

(in which Δ anion gap is the increase in the anion gap above normal)

If the measured bicarbonate is greater than the corrected bicarbonate, it suggests that a concomitant metabolic alkalosis may be present in addition to the increased anion gap metabolic acidosis. If the measured serum bicarbonate is less than the corrected bicarbonate, a concomitant normal anion gap metabolic acidosis is likely present in addition to the increased anion gap metabolic acidosis.

This approach is limited by the assumption that organic acids are buffered 1:1 by bicarbonate. Because buffering also occurs through intracellular uptake of protons, an increase in the measured bicarbonate to a level greater than the corrected bicarbonate may reflect intracellular buffering rather than metabolic alkalosis. The ratio of the change in anion gap to the change in bicarbonate can be used to account for the effect of intracellular buffering. A ratio of less than 1 may reflect the presence of concurrent normal anion gap metabolic acidosis, whereas a ratio of greater than 2 may indicate the presence of metabolic alkalosis.

Anion Gap Metabolic Acidosis

The differential diagnosis of increased anion gap metabolic acidosis is shown in **Table 16**.

Lactic Acidosis

Lactic acidosis, the most common form of increased anion gap metabolic acidosis, is defined as a serum lactate level greater than 4 mg/dL (0.44 mmol/L). Type A lactic acidosis occurs when tissue hypoperfusion is apparent, whereas type B lactic acidosis occurs in the absence of hypoperfusion. Lactic acidosis associated with acetaminophen toxicity is caused by direct hepatic injury as well as by a metabolite that uncouples oxidative phosphorylation. Lactic acidosis frequently accompanies severe asthma in which high doses of β_2-agonists and corticosteroids as well as respiratory alkalosis all contribute to increased lactic acid production.

Treatment of lactic acidosis is directed toward reversing or removing the underlying cause as well as supportive measures such as fluid resuscitation in patients with hypovolemic shock. Sodium bicarbonate therapy, targeting an arterial pH of approximately 7.2, should be considered when the arterial pH is less than 7.1, particularly in patients with cardiovascular compromise.

Propofol-Related Infusion Syndrome

Administration of intravenous propofol in doses exceeding 4 mg/kg/h for more than 48 hours can induce type B lactic

TABLE 16. Causes of Increased Anion Gap Metabolic Acidosis
Advanced acute and chronic kidney disease
Alcoholic ketoacidosis
Diabetic ketoacidosis
D-Lactic acidosis
Diethylene glycol poisoning
Ethylene glycol poisoning
Type A lactic acidosis (hypoperfusion or hypoxia)
Anemia (severe)
Carbon monoxide poisoning
Cardiogenic shock
Septic shock
Hemorrhagic shock
Hypoxia
Type B lactic acidosis (no hypoperfusion or hypoxia)
Medications or toxins
Acetaminophen poisoning
Cyanide
Ethylene glycol
Linezolid
Mangosteen juice
Metformin
Methanol
Nucleoside reverse transcriptase inhibitors (stavudine, didanosine)
Propylene glycol
Propofol
Salicylates
Thiamine deficiency
Systemic disease
Liver failure
Malignancy
Glucose 6-phosphatase dehydrogenase deficiency
Pyroglutamic acidosis
Salicylate toxicity

acidosis and a syndrome characterized by rhabdomyolysis, hyperlipidemia, and J-point elevation on electrocardiogram. Once recognized, propofol should be discontinued. Treatment is supportive, and hemodialysis may be required for severe acidosis and kidney failure.

D-Lactic Acidosis

Accumulation of the D-isomer of lactic acid can occur in patients with short-bowel syndrome following jejunoileal bypass or small-bowel resection. In these patients, excess carbohydrates that reach the colon are metabolized to D-lactate. Symptoms include intermittent confusion, slurred speech, and ataxia. This condition may be mistaken for a neurologic syndrome. Neurologic symptoms may be mediated by as yet unidentified toxins produced by bacteria in the colon rather than D-lactate. Laboratory studies show increased anion gap metabolic acidosis with normal serum lactate levels, because the D-isomer is not measured by conventional laboratory assays for lactate. Diagnosis should be considered in patients with an unexplained increased anion gap metabolic acidosis in the appropriate clinical context and is confirmed by specifically measuring D-lactate. Therapy consists of antibiotics directed toward bowel flora such as metronidazole or neomycin as well as restriction of dietary carbohydrates.

Diabetic Ketoacidosis

Diabetic ketoacidosis usually presents with an increased anion gap metabolic acidosis, but it may also present with normal anion gap metabolic acidosis in the absence of hypovolemia due to excretion of ketoacids in the urine. Insulin deficiency, increased catecholamines, and glucagon result in incomplete oxidation of fatty acids, which leads to the production of acetoacetate and β-hydroxybutyrate. The presence of ketoacids can be measured using the nitroprusside assay or by directly measuring serum assays for specific ketoacids. Because the nitroprusside assay detects only acetone and acetoacetate (and not the predominant ketoacid β-hydroxybutyrate), the results can be falsely negative in the presence of severe ketoacidosis.

Administration of insulin is critical in reversing the underlying cause, and intravenous fluids are indicated to correct volume deficits. Serum potassium levels need to be followed closely with careful repletion because patients are typically potassium depleted, and serum levels will fluctuate with correction of the serum pH. Sodium bicarbonate therapy to correct the metabolic acidosis is controversial because ketoacidosis will reverse with insulin administration, and sodium bicarbonate therapy may slow recovery or lead to a rebound metabolic alkalosis following recovery. Therefore, sodium bicarbonate therapy is generally reserved for patients with a pH less than 7.0, metabolic instability due to acidosis, or life-threatening hyperkalemia potentially corrected by sodium bicarbonate administration. Although phosphate depletion is common, there is no evidence that intravenous repletion is beneficial in the absence of severe symptoms, and resumption of oral intake is usually sufficient to correct the deficit.

Alcoholic Ketoacidosis

Alcoholic ketoacidosis presents with an increased anion gap metabolic acidosis and ketosis in patients with chronic ethanol abuse. It often follows a period of poor caloric intake. Nausea, vomiting, and hypovolemia are common. Increased levels of circulating catecholamines result in mobilization of fatty acids and ketoacidosis. The predominant ketoacid is β-hydroxybutyrate, thereby limiting the sensitivity of the nitroprusside assay.

Intravenous glucose administration or resumption of caloric intake reverses the ketoacidosis by stimulating insulin release, resulting in decreased fatty acid mobilization and decreased hepatic release of ketoacids. Hypovolemia, when present, should be corrected with intravenous normal saline.

Ethylene Glycol and Methanol Toxicity

Ethylene glycol and methanol poisoning are highly lethal intoxications that present with severe increased anion gap metabolic acidosis usually associated with an osmolal gap greater than 10 mosm/kg H_2O (see Fluids and Electrolytes, Osmolality and Tonicity). The acidosis is due to acid metabolites of the parent compound as well as lactic acidosis. The increase in the osmolal gap results from elevated levels of the parent alcohol; patients presenting after complete metabolism of the parent alcohol may have a normal osmolal gap. Simultaneous ingestion of ethylene glycol or methanol with ethanol may delay the onset of acidosis and symptoms because ethanol inhibits alcohol dehydrogenase, thereby limiting the breakdown of the parent alcohol to toxic metabolites. Clinical manifestations of ethylene glycol and methanol poisoning include inebriation early in the course to obtundation, seizures, coma, and cardiovascular collapse.

Patients with ethylene glycol toxicity may have flank pain or oliguria resulting from calcium oxalate precipitation in the renal tubules. Clinically, the calcium oxalate precipitation manifests as acute kidney injury often accompanied by hypocalcemia, nephrocalcinosis on abdominal radiograph, and calcium oxalate crystals in the urine sediment. Cardiovascular collapse and pulmonary edema may ensue.

Methanol toxicity may result in impaired vision that can progress to blindness, abdominal pain, and pancreatitis. Retinal toxicity is mediated by formic acid. Physical examination may demonstrate mydriasis or an afferent pupillary defect. Approximately 10% to 20% of patients who survive methanol poisoning have permanent visual impairment. Methanol can induce putaminal injury, and survivors may develop secondary parkinsonism.

Diagnosis of ethylene glycol and methanol toxicity is usually established on clinical grounds in patients with severe anion gap metabolic acidosis and increased osmolal gap. Serum levels are not rapidly available in most hospital laboratories, and treatment must be instituted before confirmatory levels are available. Increased anion gap acidosis associated with a serum bicarbonate level less than 10 meq/L (10 mmol/L) and an osmolal gap greater than 25 mosm/kg H_2O should raise suspicion for ethylene glycol or methanol poisoning. A normal osmolal gap, however, does not exclude the diagnosis.

Treatment includes supportive measures to optimize ventilation and organ perfusion. Fomepizole, a competitive inhibitor of alcohol dehydrogenase that prevents the formation of toxic acid metabolites, is indicated once the diagnosis is suspected. Hemodialysis should be initiated

CONT.

when there is significant high anion gap metabolic acidosis or evidence of end-organ injury such as kidney failure or neurologic symptoms. Acidemia is known to facilitate the cellular uptake of toxic metabolites, and sodium bicarbonate therapy should be administered to maintain the pH above 7.3 until hemodialysis can be initiated. Intravenous folic acid should be administered in suspected methanol poisoning, and pyridoxine and thiamine should be given in ethylene glycol poisoning to facilitate metabolism of the parent alcohol to nontoxic compounds.

Propylene Glycol Toxicity

Propylene glycol is a solvent used as a vehicle for numerous intravenously administered medications. Toxicity has been reported in association with the use of high-dose lorazepam. It is more likely to occur when propylene glycol levels exceed 25 mg/dL or when the osmolal gap is greater than 12 mosm/kg H_2O. Laboratory findings include increased anion gap metabolic acidosis and concomitant increased osmolal gap. The metabolic acidosis is principally due to L-lactic and D-lactic acidosis, the acid metabolites of propylene glycol. Acid-base status and plasma osmolality should be carefully monitored in patients receiving lorazepam at doses greater than 1 mg/kg/d. The syndrome is unlikely to develop if the 24-hour lorazepam dose is limited to less than 166 mg/d in adults.

Most patients improve with discontinuation of the intravenous infusion. Early initiation of hemodialysis is indicated for patients with kidney failure or severe metabolic acidosis. The use of fomepizole in propylene glycol toxicity is unproved, although theoretically it would inhibit generation of toxic metabolites.

Salicylate Toxicity

Ingestion of as little as 10 to 30 grams of aspirin in an adult can result in lethal salicylate toxicity. Toxicity can also develop from ingestion or mucocutaneous exposure to salicylate-containing preparations such as methyl salicylate (oil of wintergreen). Salicylate toxicity commonly presents with abnormalities in acid-base balance, the most common in adults being respiratory alkalosis, which occurs in response to stimulation of the medullary respiratory center. With more severe intoxication, increased anion gap metabolic acidosis develops both as a result of the salicylate anion and concomitant lactic and ketoacidosis.

Clinical manifestations are primarily due to intracellular toxicity of salicylic acid rather than acid-base abnormalities. Early manifestations include tinnitus, confusion, tachypnea, and, occasionally, low-grade fever. Nausea, vomiting, and resultant metabolic alkalosis may develop as a result of direct gastric mucosal toxicity as well as stimulation of medullary chemoreceptors. Neurologic dysfunction is mediated by salicylate-induced cellular toxicity and neuroglycopenia and manifests as mental status changes that can progress to cerebral edema and fatal brainstem herniation. Acute lung injury and noncardiogenic pulmonary edema have been reported in older adults, particularly in the setting of chronic salicylate exposure. Large ingestions may cause hepatic injury and impaired vitamin K metabolism, resulting in increases in the prothrombin time and INR.

Treatment of salicylate poisoning includes judicious volume expansion and sodium bicarbonate therapy to maintain the arterial pH between 7.45 and 7.6. Urine alkalinization also promotes urine excretion of salicylic acid, and sodium bicarbonate infusions should be adjusted to maintain urine pH above 7.5. Supplemental intravenous glucose, 100 mL of 50% dextrose in adults, should be provided when mental status changes are present to treat neuroglycopenia irrespective of the plasma glucose level. The serum salicylate level, arterial blood gases, and venous electrolytes should be monitored at least every 2 hours until clinical and laboratory manifestations and toxic drug levels resolve.

Intubation should be avoided whenever possible because of the risk of inducing a decrease in arterial pH, thereby enhancing intracellular salicylic acid uptake. Hypokalemia should be corrected, because it interferes with urine alkalinization. Indications for hemodialysis include impaired mental status, cerebral edema, serum salicylate levels above 80 mg/dL (5.8 mmol/L), severe metabolic acidosis, pulmonary edema, and kidney failure.

Pyroglutamic Acidosis

Pyroglutamic acidosis is a cause of increased anion gap acidosis in patients receiving therapeutic doses of acetaminophen on a chronic basis. Clinical manifestations are limited to mental status changes and increased anion gap acidosis. The syndrome most commonly occurs in patients with critical illness, poor nutrition, liver disease, or chronic kidney disease as well as in persons on a vegetarian diet. Chronic treatment with acetaminophen in these conditions can cause disruption of the γ-glutamyl cycle and accumulation of pyroglutamic acid (also called 5-oxoproline). Diagnosis can be confirmed by measuring urine levels of pyroglutamic acid. Treatment includes discontinuation of acetaminophen, volume expansion with isotonic saline and glucose, and possibly N-acetylcysteine to replace depleted glutathione stores.

Acidosis in Acute and Chronic Kidney Disease

Metabolic acidosis in patients with acute and chronic kidney disease is mediated by two mechanisms: decreased ammonia buffer synthesis when the glomerular filtration rate (GFR) decreases to less than 45 mL/min/1.73 m^2, causing normal anion gap metabolic acidosis; and retention of sulfates, phosphates, and organic acids when the GFR decreases below 15 mL/min/1.73 m^2, resulting in an increased anion gap metabolic acidosis. H

- Lactic acidosis, the most common form of increased anion gap metabolic acidosis, is defined as a serum lactate level greater than 4 mg/dL (0.44 mmol/L).

- Ethylene glycol and methanol poisoning are characterized by a severe increased anion gap metabolic acidosis associated with an osmolal gap greater than 10 mosm/kg H_2O.

- Fomepizole, an inhibitor of alcohol dehydrogenase that prevents the formation of toxic acid metabolites, is indicated for patients with ethylene glycol and methanol toxicity.

Normal Anion Gap Metabolic Acidosis

Normal anion gap metabolic acidosis may be due to failure of the kidney to excrete the daily fixed acid load, gastrointestinal loss of bicarbonate, diversion of urine through a gastrointestinal conduit, or retention of hydrogen ions derived from organic anions that are excreted in the urine as sodium salts. The cause is often apparent from the history. When the cause remains unclear, analysis of urine acid excretion may be helpful in making a specific diagnosis.

The normal kidney response to acidemia is characterized by an increase in urine ammonium excretion from a baseline of approximately 0.5 meq/kg/d to approximately 3 meq/kg/d. This response occurs in patients with a normal GFR in the absence of concomitant hyperkalemia over the course of 3 to 5 days. Thus, if urine ammonium excretion is elevated, the kidney response is appropriate and the cause of the acidosis is likely due to a non-kidney cause, whereas low urine excretion suggests a primary kidney defect. Because urine ammonium is not easily measured, two methods are used to estimate urine acid secretion: the urine anion gap and the urine osmolal gap.

The urine anion gap uses the urine sodium (Na^+), potassium (K^+), and chloride (Cl^-) concentration values and is defined as:

$$\text{Urine Anion Gap} = [Na^+] + [K^+] - [Cl^-]$$

If significant urine NH_4^+ is present, the urine anion gap will be negative because urine NH_4^+ is a positive ion and is not directly measured. If present, increased negatively charged ions (primarily Cl^-) will also be present in the urine in order to maintain electrical neutrality. As the negative ions are directly measured, and the known positive ions in the urine are subtracted from this measurement, the presence of more negative than positive ions in the urine (a negative anion gap) infers that another positively charged ion must be present, specifically NH_4^+. Therefore, a negative urine anion gap indicates appropriate tubular ammonium excretion and acidification of the urine in the presence of a metabolic acidosis. Conversely, if the urine anion gap is 0 or positive, it is unlikely

that significant urine NH_4^+ is present, indicating that there has been an inadequate renal response to the acidosis.

If the urine osmolal gap is used, the urine ammonium may be estimated by dividing the urine osmolal gap by two:

$$\text{Urine Ammonium (meq/L)} \cong \text{Urine Osmolal Gap (mosm/kg } H_2O)/2$$

$$\text{Urine Osmolal Gap} = \text{Measured Urine Osmolality} - \text{Calculated Urine Osmolality}$$

$$\text{Calculated Urine Osmolality (mosm/kg } H_2O) = 2 \\ (\text{Urine Sodium [meq/L]} + \text{Urine Potassium [meq/L]}) + \\ \text{Urine Urea (mg/dL)}/2.8 + \text{Urine Glucose (mg/dL)}/18$$

The urine osmolal gap is not an accurate marker of urine ammonium excretion when there is a urinary tract infection due to a urea-splitting organism or when a solute such as an alcohol or mannitol is present in the urine.

Patients with predominantly extrarenal loss of bicarbonate exhibit urine ammonium levels above 80 meq/L, whereas ammonium levels in individuals with a primary kidney defect remain less than 30 meq/L (**Figure 8**). In patients with metabolic acidosis due to renal tubular dysfunction, the various causes of renal tubular acidosis (RTA) may be defined and evaluated based on the serum potassium level and urine pH (**Figure 9, on page 29**).

Proximal (Type 2) Renal Tubular Acidosis

Metabolic acidosis in proximal (type 2) RTA is caused by a reduction of bicarbonate reabsorption in the proximal tubule, which initially leads to bicarbonaturia. Once a new steady state is established at a lower serum bicarbonate level, the urine is then devoid of bicarbonate and the urine pH is less than 5.5. Proximal RTA is rarely an isolated finding and is usually associated with Fanconi syndrome, which is characterized by other signs of proximal tubular dysfunction such as low-molecular-weight proteinuria, phosphaturia, or glycosuria (**Table 17**). Mild hypokalemia is usually present as a consequence of secondary hyperaldosteronism. 1α-Hydroxylase activity is often decreased, leading to 1,25-dihydroxy vitamin D deficiency, hypocalcemia, and osteomalacia. Distal urine acidification is preserved; therefore, urine pH is less than 5.5 in the presence of systemic acidemia.

In patients with proximal RTA, correction of the metabolic acidosis is usually difficult because of urine bicarbonate wasting that occurs with alkali therapy. The efficacy of alkali therapy may be enhanced through the addition of a thiazide diuretic, which enhances proximal bicarbonate absorption. When induced by a medication, discontinuation of the offending agent is indicated when possible.

Hypokalemic Distal (Type 1) Renal Tubular Acidosis

Hypokalemic distal (type 1) RTA is a defect in distal urine acidification related to a primary tubular disorder or to injury

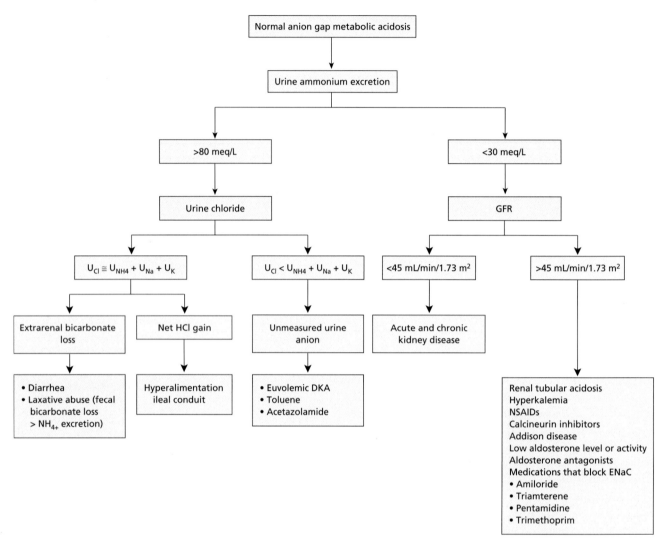

FIGURE 8. Evaluation of normal anion gap metabolic acidosis. DKA = diabetic ketoacidosis; ENaC = epithelial sodium channel on apical surface of principal cells in collecting duct; GFR = glomerular filtration rate; HCl = hydrochloric acid; NH_{4+} = ammonium; U_{Cl} = urine chloride concentration (meq/L); U_K = urine potassium concentration (meq/L); U_{Na} = urine sodium concentration (meq/L); U_{NH4} = ammonium concentration (meq/L).

TABLE 17. Causes of Proximal (Type 2) Renal Tubular Acidosis
Medications
Tenofovir
Ifosfamide
Amyloidosis
Multiple myeloma
Kidney transplantation
Heavy metal toxicity
Cadmium
Copper
Lead
Mercury
Cystinosis
Wilson disease

of the tubular epithelium, resulting in impaired excretion of hydrogen ions (**Table 18**). Decreased secretion of hydrogen ions leads to lumen-negative voltage, urine pH greater than 6.0, kidney potassium wasting, and hypokalemia. Calcium-phosphate kidney stones and nephrocalcinosis develop because of increased urine pH and decreased levels of urine citrate. Correction of the potassium deficit should precede correction of acidosis to avoid exacerbating hypokalemia. Acidosis should be corrected by the use of supplemental alkali in the form of potassium citrate at a dose of 1 meq/kg/d. Potassium-sparing diuretics are relatively contraindicated because of associated metabolic acidosis.

Hyperkalemic Distal (Type 4) Renal Tubular Acidosis
Hyperkalemic distal (type 4) RTA occurs in two distinct forms (see Figure 9). The first type, often associated with hypoaldosteronism, is characterized by urine pH less than 5.5.

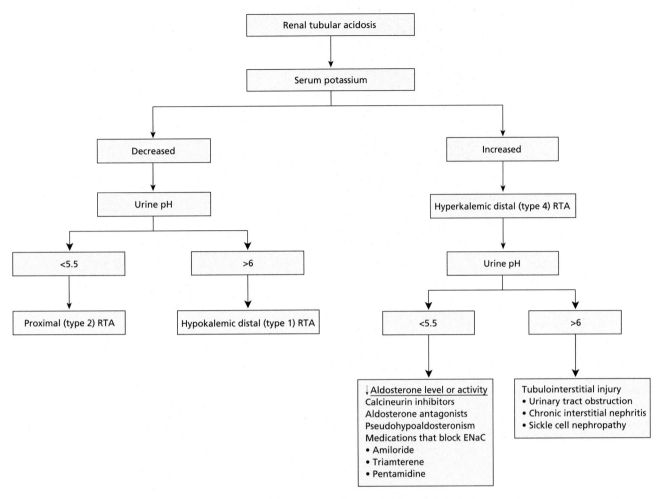

FIGURE 9. Evaluation of renal tubular acidosis. ENaC = epithelial sodium channel on apical surface of principal cells in collecting duct; RTA = renal tubular acidosis.

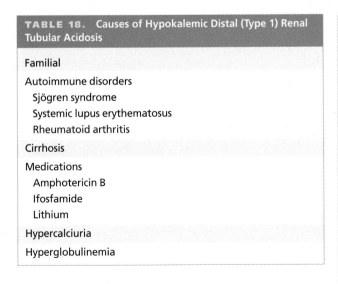

TABLE 18. Causes of Hypokalemic Distal (Type 1) Renal Tubular Acidosis
Familial
Autoimmune disorders
Sjögren syndrome
Systemic lupus erythematosus
Rheumatoid arthritis
Cirrhosis
Medications
Amphotericin B
Ifosfamide
Lithium
Hypercalciuria
Hyperglobulinemia

CONT.

Hyperkalemia results in impaired generation of ammonia and metabolic acidosis. Treatment of hyperkalemia in these patients corrects the acidosis. Management includes correcting the hyperkalemia, treating the underlying cause, and either reducing the dose or discontinuing contributing medications. Replacement of mineralocorticoids with fludrocortisone is indicated for patients with Addison disease. Dietary potassium restriction to approximately 2500 mg/d is a useful adjunct, and patients should be referred for dietary counseling.

The second type is associated with tubulointerstitial injury involving the collecting duct, as may occur in sickle cell nephropathy or urinary obstruction, which impairs urine acidification to a greater degree, resulting in urine pH levels above 6.0. Treatment of hyperkalemia in patients with these disorders does not correct the acidosis. Treatment includes relief of urinary obstruction when present, dietary potassium restriction, and sodium bicarbonate therapy to correct the serum potassium to approximately 23 meq/L (23 mmol/L).

Mixed Forms of Renal Tubular Acidosis
Defects in carbonic anhydrase result in combined proximal and distal RTA. An acquired form can develop in patients treated with topiramate, which inhibits carbonic anhydrase in the proximal and distal tubule. Topiramate is associated with an increased

risk of calcium phosphate stones because of the high urine pH (greater than 6.0 despite acidemia) and hypocitraturia. **H**

KEY POINTS

- In patients with proximal (type 2) renal tubular acidosis, correction of the metabolic acidosis is usually difficult because of urine bicarbonate wasting that occurs with alkali therapy.

- Treatment of hypokalemic distal (type 1) renal tubular acidosis involves correction of the potassium deficit followed by alkali therapy.

- Management of hyperkalemic distal (type 4) renal tubular acidosis includes correcting the hyperkalemia, treating the underlying cause, and either reducing the dose or discontinuing contributing medications.

Metabolic Alkalosis

Metabolic alkalosis is caused by net loss of acid or retention of serum bicarbonate. Metabolic alkalosis can be classified as either occurring with normal extracellular fluid volume, hypovolemia, or decreased effective arterial blood volume (EABV) and increased extracellular fluid volume (heart failure, cirrhosis, nephrosis) or occurring with increased extracellular fluid volume and hypertension (**Figure 10**). Metabolic alkalosis, when associated with increased extracellular fluid volume and hypertension, is saline-resistant. Metabolic alkalosis associated with true hypovolemia responds to correction of the volume deficit with isotonic saline and is categorized as saline-responsive.

Urine sodium and chloride levels can help distinguish the various causes of metabolic alkalosis (see Figure 10). Metabolic alkalosis is commonly associated with increased

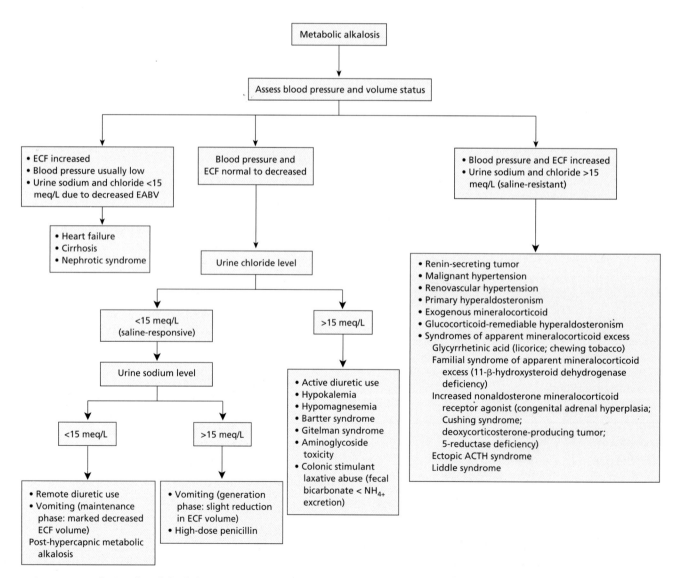

FIGURE 10. Evaluation of metabolic alkalosis. ACTH = adrenocorticotropic hormone; EABV = effective arterial blood volume; ECF = extracellular fluid; NH$_{4+}$ = ammonium.

CONT.

aldosterone or aldosterone-like activity and is usually accompanied by concomitant hypokalemia. The differential diagnosis of saline-responsive metabolic alkalosis includes vomiting, loss of gastric secretions through nasogastric suction, diuretic use, and post-hypercapnic alkalosis.

Treatment of saline-responsive metabolic alkalosis is directed toward correcting volume, sodium, chloride, and potassium deficits as well as reversing the underlying cause. Hypokalemia and symptomatic hypovolemia associated with diuretic-induced metabolic alkalosis are treated with potassium chloride supplementation and intravenous isotonic saline. Patients with severe metabolic alkalosis and symptomatic edema and decreased EABV as a consequence of severe chronic heart failure or cirrhosis can be treated with acetazolamide.

Bartter and Gitelman syndromes are rare inherited defects in kidney sodium and chloride handling that mimic the effects of loop and thiazide diuretics, respectively. Bartter syndrome typically presents in childhood, whereas Gitelman syndrome usually presents in late childhood or adulthood. Hypomagnesemia is frequently present. Symptoms include muscle cramps, postural hypotension, and weakness. Infusion of saline does not correct the alkalosis because of continued urine sodium and chloride losses. Laboratory abnormalities generally persist even with aggressive replacement of electrolytes; therefore, treatment should be directed toward ameliorating symptoms. Patients should be instructed to maintain a diet high in sodium and potassium. Amiloride is a useful adjunct for persistent symptomatic hypokalemia.

Metabolic alkalosis associated with hypertension results in increased urine sodium and chloride levels consequent to volume expansion and resultant decreased kidney sodium and chloride reabsorption. Diagnosis is established through measuring plasma renin and aldosterone levels. The most common form of saline-resistant metabolic alkalosis is primary hyperaldosteronism, which is characterized by increased aldosterone production, suppressed renin, and hypertension. Primary hyperaldosteronism may be due to either unilateral or bilateral adrenal gland hypersecretion of aldosterone (see MKSAP 16 Endocrinology and Metabolism). Therapy with aldosterone antagonists such as spironolactone can be used to control blood pressure and correct increased aldosterone production and hypokalemia. Patients with unilateral hypersecretion are candidates for unilateral adrenalectomy, especially when hypertension and metabolic abnormalities are resistant to medical therapy.

Syndromes of apparent mineralocorticoid excess present with hypertension and hypokalemic metabolic alkalosis and low plasma renin and aldosterone levels (**Figure 11**).

KEY POINTS

- Saline-responsive metabolic alkalosis is characterized by true hypovolemia and responds to correction of the volume deficit with isotonic saline.

- Treatment of saline-responsive metabolic alkalosis is directed toward correcting volume, sodium, chloride, and potassium deficits as well as reversing the underlying cause.

Respiratory Acidosis

Respiratory acidosis usually results from decreased effective ventilation, leading to hypercapnia and retention of hydrogen ions. Respiratory acidosis can also result from intrinsic lung pathology or from processes that impede ventilation (**Table 19**).

Clinical Manifestations and Diagnosis

When severe, respiratory acidosis can impair mentation, increase cerebral blood flow, and result in cerebral edema, asterixis, decreased cardiac contractility, or cardiac arrhythmias. Neurologic effects of hypercapnia may decrease respiratory drive, further exacerbating the acidosis.

An elevation in the measured or expected arterial P_{CO_2} is the hallmark of respiratory acidosis and results in secondary hyperbicarbonatemia due to increased proximal bicarbonate reabsorption. In the first several hours, the serum bicarbonate level increases by 1 meq/L (1 mmol/L) for every 10 mm Hg (1.3 kPa) increase in P_{CO_2}. After 3 to 5 days, the serum bicarbonate level increases by 3.5 meq/L (3.5 mmol/L) for every 10 mm Hg (1.3 kPa) increase in P_{CO_2}.

TABLE 19. Causes of Respiratory Acidosis
Upper airway obstruction
Impaired pulmonary capillary CO_2 exchange
Pulmonary parenchymal disease
Obstructive lung disease
Pulmonary edema
Thromboembolic disease
Respiratory muscle weakness
Muscle fatigue due to increased work of breathing
Hypokalemia
Hypophosphatemia
Neuromuscular disease
Inadequate response of the medullary respiratory center
Asthma
Central hypoventilation syndrome
Chronic obstructive lung disease
Suppression of the medullary respiratory center
Hypercapnia
Myxedema coma
Central nervous system depressants
Increased tissue CO_2 production
Extreme exercise
Seizures
Severe heart failure
Hyperalimentation in mechanically ventilated patients

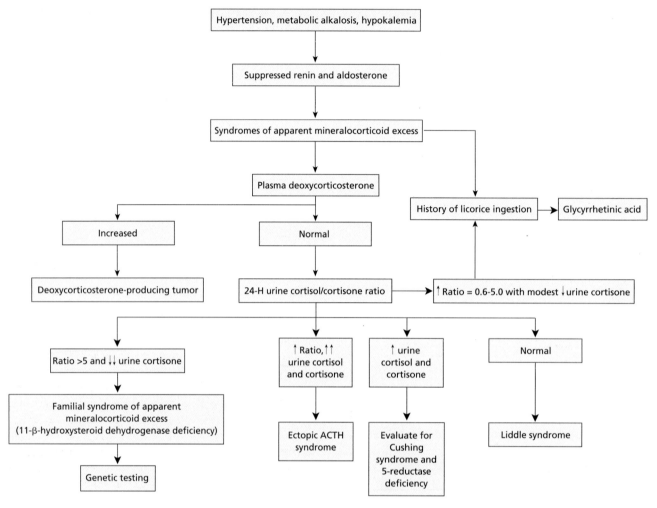

FIGURE 11. Evaluation of syndromes of apparent mineralocorticoid excess. ACTH = adrenocorticotropic hormone.

Treatment

Treatment of respiratory acidosis should initially focus on correcting hypoxia. Supplemental oxygen may decrease ventilatory drive in some patients with chronic respiratory acidosis, but this should not deter correction of hypoxia. Mechanical ventilation should be considered in patients in whom correction of hypoxia decreases the arterial pH to less than 7.2. When mechanical ventilation is required, the Pco_2 should be slowly decreased to minimize the magnitude of post-hypercapnic metabolic alkalosis, which will persist in the setting of hypovolemia. Infusion of isotonic saline and discontinuation of diuretics when possible may be necessary to correct the alkalosis. Patients with significant edema and persistent post-hypercapnic alkalosis can be treated with acetazolamide.

Respiratory Alkalosis

Respiratory alkalosis is a common acid-base disorder associated with a high mortality. Salicylate poisoning is the most important cause of respiratory alkalosis. Salicylate poisoning should be suspected in patients with mental status changes, tachypnea, and respiratory alkalosis often with concomitant increased anion gap metabolic acidosis (see Metabolic Acidosis, Anion Gap Metabolic Acidosis, Salicylate Toxicity). The causes of respiratory alkalosis are listed in **Table 20**.

Mixed respiratory alkalosis and lactic acidosis should raise suspicion for sepsis or severe liver disease. Respiratory alkalosis results in secondary hypobicarbonatemia due to decreased proximal tubular reabsorption of bicarbonate. The serum bicarbonate level decreases by 2 meq/L (2 mmol/L) in the first few hours and by 4 to 5 meq/L (4-5 mmol/L) after 3 to 5 days for every 10 mm Hg decrease in Pco_2. The anion gap is frequently increased as a result of increased albumin anionic charge and increased lactate production. Ionized calcium levels may fall due to increased binding of calcium to albumin.

Respiratory alkalosis is known to decrease cerebral blood flow, and hyperventilation can be employed in the treatment of cerebral edema. Symptoms of respiratory alkalosis include circumoral and extremity paresthesias and dizziness, which can progress to carpopedal spasm and tetany with more severe levels of alkalosis.

TABLE 20.	Causes of Respiratory Alkalosis

Anxiety

Medications
  Salicylates
  Medroxyprogesterone
  Theophylline

Advanced liver disease

Sepsis

Hypoxia
  Cyanotic heart disease
  Chronic heart failure
  Pulmonary parenchymal disease
  High altitude exposure

Pregnancy

Subarachnoid hemorrhage

Thoracic stretch receptor stimulation
  Asthma
  Pulmonary fibrosis
  Pneumonia
  Pulmonary edema
  Pulmonary embolism

CONT.

Management is directed toward identifying and treating the underlying cause. Anxiety-related respiratory alkalosis can be treated with a closed bag rebreathing system, which results in a rise in the P_{CO_2}. 🄷

KEY POINTS

- An elevation in the measured or expected arterial P_{CO_2} is the hallmark of respiratory acidosis and results in secondary hyperbicarbonatemia due to increased proximal bicarbonate reabsorption.

- Treatment of respiratory acidosis should initially focus on correcting hypoxia; although supplemental oxygen may decrease ventilatory drive in some patients with chronic respiratory acidosis, this should not deter correction of hypoxia.

- The most important cause of respiratory alkalosis is salicylate poisoning, which should be suspected in patients with mental status changes, tachypnea, and respiratory alkalosis often with concomitant increased anion gap metabolic acidosis.

- Management of respiratory alkalosis is directed toward identifying and treating the underlying cause.

Hypertension

Epidemiology

Hypertension is a common finding among adults and is the greatest contributor to cardiovascular disease, premature death, and disability from cardiovascular diseases worldwide. Hypertension, along with coronary artery disease, accounts for most incident heart failure outcomes. Hypertension also is the leading cardiovascular risk factor for stroke as well as stroke recurrence.

Prevalence increases with age and is associated with numerous comorbidities, including diabetes mellitus and chronic kidney disease. Hypertension is controlled in approximately 50% of U.S. adults diagnosed with the condition, with control rates lower in younger (18-39 years of age) and Hispanic patients.

Associated Complications

End-Organ Damage

The principal target organs affected by hypertension are the brain, the heart wall and coronary circulation, and the kidneys. The mechanisms by which hypertension mediates damage to these organs involve changes in vessel walls and linings.

Brain

In the upright position, blood pressure is lower in the brain than in the heart or kidneys. The brain has an obligate blood flow requirement at all times. Consequently, the brain has a remarkable ability to regulate blood flow across a wide range of arterial pressures. Damage to the brain as a result of elevated blood pressure may lead to hemorrhage into brain tissue from rupture of tiny Charcot-Bouchard aneurysms, progressive narrowing and occlusion of small vessels resulting in lacunar infarction, promotion of major vessel (carotid, middle cerebral arteries) atherosclerosis with brain infarction, and dementia.

Heart

Because the heart generates the blood pressure through muscular contraction, elevated blood pressure levels function as a pathophysiologic stimulus to thickening of the heart muscle itself (left ventricular hypertrophy). To a certain degree, such adaptation is well tolerated, but as the heart wall thickens progressively, the subendocardial layers experience relative ischemia, potentially generating an arrhythmogenic focus or the development of pump failure. Hypertension also promotes atherosclerosis in the coronary artery circulation.

Kidney

The kidney, like the brain, is an extensive vascular bed. Although the kidneys represent less than 1% of body weight, they receive approximately 20% of the cardiac output. Dealing with this high level of blood flow requires an exquisite adaptation in the vascular resistance of the kidneys. This organ, like the brain, adapts well across a large range of blood pressure levels. Unlike the brain, the circulation to the kidney allows the mean arterial pressure to penetrate very deeply into the microcirculation of the kidney. As a result, the delicate capillary structure in the glomerulus is at risk when there is a failure in the upstream autoregulation of vascular resistance.

Hypertension tends to accelerate the course of primary kidney disorders, including glomerulonephritis and diabetic nephropathy. Hypertension is the second most common cause of end-stage kidney disease in the United States.

Cardiovascular Risk

In isolation, elevated blood pressure is a modest but important component of overall cardiovascular risk. Numerous studies indicate that this risk from elevated blood pressure has no specific pressure-defined cut-off point. Additionally, elevated blood pressure levels enhance the cardiovascular risk of other factors, including diabetes, dyslipidemia, obesity, and cigarette smoking.

There are two basic ways in which elevated blood pressure contributes to cardiovascular risk. First, elevated blood pressure can result in heart wall thickening as an adaptation to the increased afterload as well as remodeling of the blood vessel wall in response to the elevated pressure, leading to vascular hypertrophy. The second way is through enhancement of proatherosclerotic influences. Elevated blood pressure levels interact specifically with increased cholesterol, diabetes, and a host of proinflammatory cytokines, contributing to the loss of vascular lumen patency. The unique susceptibility of the heart wall and the heart circulation to elevated blood pressure levels contributes to its prominence as the most commonly affected target organ of the hypertensive process.

KEY POINT

- Hypertension is the greatest contributor to cardiovascular disease, premature death, and disability from cardiovascular diseases worldwide.

Evaluation

The evaluation of a patient with high blood pressure is directed toward determining if the blood pressure is elevated as a secondary phenomenon, if there are other cardiovascular risk factors present, and if there is evidence of target organ damage.

History

Patient history can help determine the duration of blood pressure elevation and evaluate for symptoms that may indicate the presence of a provoking cause or clues to the presence of target organ damage. Several common over-the-counter and prescription drugs can influence blood pressure (**Table 21**). It is useful to ask about alternative or herbal medications, because patients may not consider them to have significant pharmacologic actions.

Physical Examination

Physical examination should focus on the target organs: the brain, heart, kidney, retina, and peripheral pulses. Neurologic damage from hypertension is evidenced by focal neurologic findings, such as gait or motor function impairment. Some

Type	Agent	Mechanism(s)
OTC	Black licorice (European)	Mineralocorticoid activity enhancement; sodium retention
OTC	Ethanol	Adrenergic stimulation
OTC	NSAIDs	Sodium retention
Rx	Calcineurin inhibitors (e.g., cyclosporine)	Vasoconstriction; sodium retention
Rx	Selective serotonin or norepinephrine reuptake inhibitors	Adrenergic stimulation
Rx	Erythrocyte simulation agents (e.g., erythropoietins)	Vasoconstriction
Rx	Highly active antiretroviral therapies	Not clear
Rx	Sympathomimetics; appetite suppressants; decongestants; vigilance enhancers (e.g., amphetamines)	Vasoconstriction; sodium retention
Rx	Vascular endothelial growth factor antagonists (e.g., bevacizumab)	Vasoconstriction (endothelial dysfunction)
Rx	Corticosteroids (e.g., prednisone)	Sodium retention; weight gain
Rx	Oral contraceptives	Increased renin-angiotensin system activity; sodium retention
–	Caffeine	Adrenergic stimulation
–	Cocaine; 3,4-methylenedioxymethamphetamine (ecstasy); recreational drugs	Adrenergic stimulation

TABLE 21. Over-The-Counter and Prescription Agents that Increase Blood Pressure

OTC = over the counter; Rx = prescription.

patients will have changes on central nervous system imaging, such as lacunar infarction or white matter disease, which are usually attributed to hypertension.

Changes in retinal arteriolar appearance can be used to classify blood pressure and to gauge the degree of target organ impairment. Hemorrhage, exudate, and cotton wool spots suggest advanced degrees of retinopathy secondary to hypertension.

On cardiac and pulmonary examinations, the presence of an S_4 heart sound, detection of left ventricular enlargement, and evidence of possible left ventricular failure may indicate cardiac end-organ damage from hypertension.

In patients with autosomal dominant polycystic kidney disease, enlarged kidneys may be palpable on physical examination; high blood pressure is a frequent component of this disorder. Auscultation of the renal circulation may reveal systolic or diastolic bruits, which may suggest potentially restricted renal arterial flow, a possible secondary cause of hypertension.

Adequacy of the large-vessel circulation to the lower extremities may be assessed by calculating the ratio of ankle and brachial systolic blood pressures (the ankle-brachial index); a ratio of less than 0.9 suggests circulatory disease.

Laboratory Studies

The initial laboratory evaluation of a patient with high blood pressure includes a complete blood count, electrolyte panel, fasting lipid profile, fasting glucose, an estimate of glomerular filtration rate, and a urinalysis. Elevated levels of hemoglobin or hematocrit reflect increased blood viscosity, which can contribute to elevated blood pressure. Reduced kidney function, manifested by a decrease in estimated glomerular filtration rate, is an indicator of target organ damage and may also implicate the kidney as a factor causing high blood pressure. Reductions in serum potassium concentration may be evidence of aldosterone excess. Elevated plasma glucose levels signal the presence, or a tendency toward, diabetes, which has substantial cardiovascular risk implications. The fasting lipid profile may show an atherogenic dyslipidemia. A urinalysis showing blood or protein can reflect target organ damage to the kidney or point to a kidney-related process contributing to blood pressure increase.

12-Lead electrocardiography (ECG) is needed to evaluate for cardiac changes associated with hypertension and to provide a baseline for comparison in the future to determine adequacy of blood pressure therapy. On ECG, cardiac damage from hypertension is manifested by left ventricular hypertrophy and possibly the presence of Q waves.

KEY POINT

- The evaluation of a patient with elevated blood pressure should address the presence of secondary factors that increase blood pressure, other cardiovascular risk factors, and target organ damage.

Blood Pressure Measurement

Despite its critical importance as a vital sign, surprisingly few health care workers receive formal training in proper blood pressure measurement. Errors in positioning the patient, incorrect cuff size relative to arm circumference, and interferences such as recent caffeine intake or cigarette smoking contribute to variability in blood pressure measurement.

Office Measurement

Accuracy and reliability in measuring blood pressure in the clinic setting are of great importance (**Table 22**). Following a standard approach reduces the variability in blood pressure measurement. There is evidence that blood pressure measurements by physicians tend to be higher than by other health care personnel in the same patient in the same setting. Repeated measurements, possibly by different physicians, may be helpful in obtaining accurate data when making treatment decisions. The increasing use of devices that allow patients to have repeated blood pressure measurements without a health care worker present may obviate some of this variability. Additionally, obtaining clinical information from different sources, such as home blood pressure measurements, may be useful in better informing physicians about the true level of blood pressure or adequacy of treatment.

Ambulatory Blood Pressure Monitoring

Ambulatory blood pressure monitoring (ABPM) is an effective means of assessing blood pressure over 24 hours and away from a health care setting. ABPM typically takes blood pressure measurements every 15 to 20 minutes during daytime hours and every 30 to 60 minutes during the night. It is important to emphasize to the patient the need to complete

TABLE 22. Accurate Office Blood Pressure Measurement

Caffeine, exercise, and smoking should be avoided by the patient ≥30 minutes before measurement

The patient should be seated quietly for 5 minutes (in a chair, not the examination table) with feet on the floor

The patient's arm should be supported at heart level

The auscultatory method is preferred

Use the correct cuff size for accuracy (cuff bladder encircles at least 80% of the patient's arm)

Cuff should be inflated to an adequate pressure (approximately 20-30 mm Hg above the systolic pressure) to avoid measurement error from an auscultatory gap and then deflated at a rate of 2 mm Hg per second

Record systolic (onset of first sound) and diastolic (disappearance of sound) pressures

Average two or more measurements

Data from the U.S. Department of Health and Human Services. Seventh Report of the Joint National Committee on Prevention, Detection, Evaluation, and Treatment of High Blood Pressure. www.nhlbi.nih.gov/guidelines/hypertension/jnc7full.htm. Accessed June 8, 2012.

the diary correctly so that the hours of sleep can be incorporated into the ABPM report.

Research using ABPM increasingly shows that nighttime blood pressure measurements appear to provide the greatest information regarding cardiovascular risk. Cardiovascular risk is more closely associated with nighttime blood pressure levels than office-based measurement or those of the cumulative daytime hours (**Figure 12**). In addition, patients with the greatest variability in blood pressure during the 24 hours of monitoring are at greater risk of cardiovascular target organ damage.

Although ABPM is approved only for the indication of white coat hypertension, it is specifically used to diagnose both white coat hypertension and masked hypertension. **Figure 13** shows the permutations of clinic and ambulatory blood pressure monitoring (see Classification).

Electronic Blood Pressure Measurement

With the nearly complete disappearance of mercury-based blood pressure measurements, electronic devices are increasingly used to measure blood pressure. Most of these devices work on oscillometric principles. The cuff is inflated while electronically monitoring the brachial pulse and its disappearance. On deflation, sensors detect increasing amplitude in the brachial pulsation and measure the mean arterial pressure. From this value, the systolic and diastolic values are usually inferred. Typically, the systolic blood pressure reported by these devices is slightly lower than the real value as measured intra-arterially, and the diastolic blood pressure reads slightly higher than the intra-arterial pressure. Although the solid-state

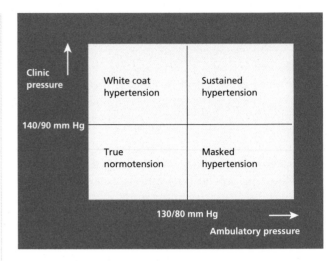

FIGURE 13. Classification of blood pressure when there may be discordance between clinic/office values and ABPM values. Blood pressures are dichotomized (either above or below 140/90 mm Hg clinic/office or above or below 130/80 mm Hg by ABPM). For example, if a patient has an office blood pressure of 150/94 mm Hg and an ABPM value of 142/88 mm Hg, the patient is in the category labeled "sustained hypertension." ABPM = ambulatory blood pressure monitoring.

technology in these devices maintains a reasonable degree of calibration over time, it is good clinical practice to periodically compare the results from these instruments with a device of known accuracy to ensure their precision and reliability. The accuracy of wrist and finger blood pressure monitors has not been well established. These devices in particular should be compared with a known, reliable instrument if they are to be

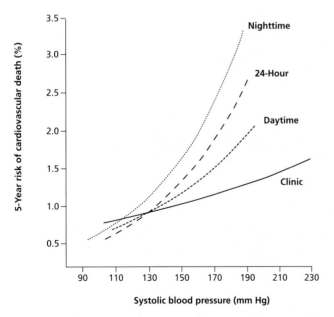

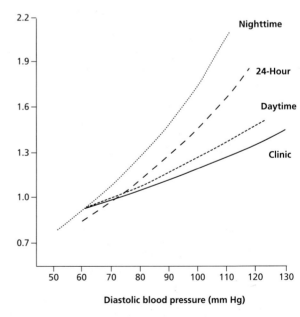

FIGURE 12. The relationships between office systolic and diastolic blood pressures and 5-year cardiovascular risk, alongside ambulatory blood pressure measurements shown as 24-hour averaged, daytime averaged, and nighttime averaged systolic and diastolic levels in 5292 subjects.

used in making treatment decisions. There is a substantial range in cost depending on the presence of memory, the ability to program for multiple blood pressure measurements, the ability to connect to the Internet for downloading data, and the presence of printing capabilities.

Home Blood Pressure Monitoring

Approximately 50% of patients with hypertension measure their blood pressure at home. Although blood pressure monitors are usually not reimbursed by insurers, their relatively low cost (usually less than $100) and reasonable accuracy have made them attractive components to the management of hypertension. Specific recommendations have been published detailing how to incorporate home pressure measurements into overall blood pressure care. For example, two measurements in the morning between 7 AM and 10 AM and two measurements in the evening between 7 PM and 10 PM for 7 consecutive days are recommended. Values from the first day are discarded, and the readings from the subsequent 6 days are averaged. If the average is less than 125/76 mm Hg, the patient is said to be not hypertensive, and drug treatment can be deferred. If the value exceeds 135/85 mm Hg, hypertension is likely present. For values falling between these two ranges (125-135/76-85 mm Hg), ABPM is recommended. If the 24-hour value is greater than 130/80 mm Hg, antihypertensive treatment is reasonable.

Other Settings for Electronic Blood Pressure Management

Internet-based blood pressure management protocols have been developed, sometimes termed "eBP." Patients with access to a computer with Internet connectivity are able to upload home blood pressure readings to a designated health care provider who reviews the data and coordinates communication between the patient and physician. This strategy is particularly useful in patients whose blood pressures are not at target when measured in the office setting; it also allows

patients to more actively participate in their own care. Existing data suggest that achieving a target blood pressure level in patients with uncontrolled hypertension taking multiple medications is nearly twice as likely when enrolled in this type of program.

KEY POINTS

- Errors in positioning the patient, incorrect cuff size relative to arm circumference, and interferences such as recent caffeine intake or cigarette smoking contribute to variability in blood pressure measurement.

- Ambulatory blood pressure monitoring provides the best estimate of cardiovascular risk from hypertension, particularly when nighttime blood pressure measurements are considered.

- Electronic devices that measure blood pressure may report the systolic blood pressure as slightly lower than the real value as measured intra-arterially and the diastolic blood pressure as slightly higher than the intra-arterial pressure.

Classification

The Seventh Report of the Joint National Committee on Prevention, Detection, Evaluation, and Treatment of High Blood Pressure (JNC 7) guidelines remain the current U.S. standard for the evaluation, classification, and management of hypertension (**Table 23**). As of publication, the Eighth Report reflecting current research data is in progress. Blood pressure is classified utilizing both the systolic and diastolic components, and the categories are determined by the higher value of either the systolic or the diastolic blood pressure.

Classification of hypertension is based on an average of two or more seated blood pressure readings obtained more than 1 minute apart at two or more visits. It is important to check the blood pressure more than once during the same visit and to recheck this within several weeks to a month

TABLE 23. Classification of Hypertension		
Classification[a]	Office Blood Pressure (mm Hg)	24-Hour ABPM (mm Hg)[b]
Normal	<120/80	<125/75
Prehypertension	120-139/80-89	(125-130/75-80)
Stage 1 hypertension	140-159/90-99	>130/80
Stage 2 hypertension	≥160/100	–

ABPM = ambulatory blood pressure monitoring.

[a]When discordant values are found in the blood pressure values (for example, office blood pressure measurement of 136/94 mm Hg), the higher classification category of the two values (in this case, the diastolic value of 94 mm Hg) is used to classify the blood pressure (stage 1 hypertension in this example). Classification should use blood pressure data obtained in at least duplicate readings on at least two occasions.

[b]These are values averaged over the full 24 hours. The values inside the parentheses are inferred because ABPM is not used for the diagnosis of prehypertension. Once ABPM values exceed 130/80 mm Hg, they are not further parsed into stage 1 and 2.

Data from Chobanian AV, Bakris GL, Black HR, et al. Seventh Report of the Joint National Committee on Prevention, Detection, Evaluation, and Treatment of High Blood Pressure. Hypertension. 2003;42(6):1206-1252. [PMID: 14656957] and Kikuya M, Hansen TW, Thijs L, et al. Diagnostic thresholds for ambulatory blood pressure monitoring based on 10-year cardio-vascular risk. Circulation. 2007;115(16):2145-2152. [PMID: 17420350] (depending on the clinical severity) before acting on the information.

In a large meta-analysis encompassing more than 1 million patient years, it was found that the level of blood pressure below which no risk from blood pressure could be inferred was 115/75 mm Hg. This meta-analysis also established the current clinical dictum that for every increase in systolic pressure of 20 mm Hg or diastolic pressure of 10 mm Hg, cardiovascular risk doubles.

KEY POINTS

- The Seventh Report of the Joint National Committee on Prevention, Detection, Evaluation, and Treatment of High Blood Pressure guidelines define normal blood pressure as less than 120/80 mm Hg and hypertension as 140/90 mm Hg or higher.
- Classification of hypertension is based on an average of two or more seated blood pressure readings obtained more than 1 minute apart at two or more visits.

Prehypertension

The prehypertension category established by the JNC 7 designates a group at high risk for progression to hypertension, in whom lifestyle modifications may be preemptive (see Table 23). Studies such as the Trial of Preventing Hypertension (TROPHY) have shown that about two thirds of patients diagnosed as prehypertensive will develop stage 1 hypertension during 4 years of follow-up. This finding argues strongly for implementation of lifestyle modifications in this population. At present, there is no evidence that drug therapy, more extensive blood pressure

monitoring, or further work are needed when managing prehypertension.

Essential Hypertension

Pathogenesis

The pathogenesis of essential hypertension remains poorly elucidated and likely results from the complex interaction of multiple factors. **Figure 14** illustrates a useful concept of how different physiologic processes work together to regulate the blood pressure. Given the crucial need to preserve organ blood flow, these processes are redundant and designed to overlap if failure of one occurs.

The pathogenic processes of essential hypertension can be divided into those based on genetic mechanisms and those in which environmental influences play a role. Isolated genetic mutations inherited in mendelian fashion probably account for less than 1% of hypertension. To date, single gene mutations found to influence blood pressure meaningfully are relatively few in number and almost all relate to mechanisms that govern sodium excretion by the kidney. Genetic studies underscore the primary importance of sodium handling in blood pressure control, as most single gene mutations that have a significant impact on blood pressure levels are in sodium-handling pathways. Recently, genetic influences are thought to be many in number (polygenic), with each accounting for only a fraction of increased blood pressure. Attempts to integrate these genetic polymorphisms into the different physiologic pathways known to influence blood pressure may help in the understanding of the roles that genes play in blood pressure control.

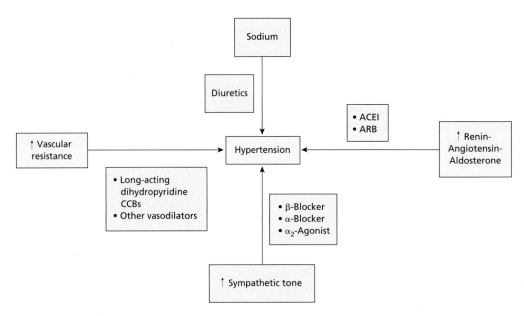

FIGURE 14. Schema for understanding major physiologic processes influencing blood pressure levels and main mechanistic pathways by which antihypertensive drugs work. ACEI = angiotensin-converting enzyme inhibitor; ARB = angiotensin receptor blocker; CCB = calcium channel blocker.

Complex environmental exposures also influence blood pressure levels. These include sodium intake, socioeconomic stress, cigarette smoking, various drug exposures, obesity, and the occurrence of comorbidities such as diabetes and chronic kidney disease (CKD), all of which alter the processes of normal blood pressure regulation.

Secondary forms of hypertension have been helpful in understanding the pathogenesis of elevated blood pressure (see Secondary Hypertension).

A substantial area of interest in the pathogenesis of hypertension relates to the relationship of the endothelium to the underlying vascular smooth muscle, which is represented as the "vascular resistance" component of Figure 14. The production and release of the vasodilator nitric oxide at the endothelial level plays a clear regulatory role on the underlying vascular smooth muscle tone. Abnormalities in nitric oxide generation or its inactivation by oxidative stresses underlie the findings of endothelial dysfunction, which is often found before the onset of hypertension.

Management

Blood Pressure Goals

According to the JNC 7, in the absence of comorbidities or compelling indications, the blood pressure goal in patients younger than 80 years is 140/90 mm Hg. For patients aged ≥80 years, the recommendation is a systolic blood pressure goal of less than 150 mm Hg based on the Hypertension in the Very Elderly Trial (HYVET) (see Special Populations, Older Patients). In patients with diabetes and most patients with CKD, the blood pressure goal set by the American Diabetes Association and the National Kidney Foundation remains at less than 130/80 mm Hg.

Strong evidence exists that treating systolic pressures ≥160 mm Hg in patients aged 60 years or older or diastolic values ≥90 mm Hg in those aged 30 years or older reduces cardiovascular outcomes (cardiovascular death, myocardial infarction, heart failure, fatal and nonfatal stroke). In those with isolated systolic blood pressure elevations between 140 and 159 mm Hg (inclusive) or in those younger than 30 years of age, there is scant evidence of benefit, although most guidelines support lifestyle modifications and initiation of drug therapy if systolic blood pressures greater than 140 mm Hg persist.

Lifestyle Modifications

Several nondrug approaches are useful in lowering blood pressure. The most effective measure to reduce blood pressure is weight loss if the patient is overweight. The second most effective measure is a reduction in salt (sodium chloride) intake, followed by an increase in aerobic physical activity of at least 30 minutes a day at least 3 days per week. Lastly, a reduction in alcohol consumption helps reduce blood pressure.

Other approaches, including potassium, magnesium, and calcium supplementation, fish oil, garlic usage, and green tea consumption, have had variable success in managing hypertension. Although they do not appear harmful, these approaches typically do not have robust data to recommend their widespread use in the management of prehypertension and hypertension.

Choosing an Antihypertensive Agent

Many patients with hypertension find it difficult to lose weight or to adjust their dietary intake and physical activity status to effectively control their blood pressure. Drug treatment is recommended when blood pressure remains above 140/90 mm Hg in patients younger than 80 years of age. In patients aged 80 years or older, a systolic blood pressure of 150 mm Hg is recommended as the threshold for treatment initiation. See **Table 24** for indications, contraindications, and side effects for antihypertensive agents. There is wide variability in the cost of antihypertensive medications; newer and more expensive agents have not been shown to be significantly safer or more effective than many older, well-established medications that are available in generic form.

A large, recent meta-analysis suggests that the five main classes of antihypertensive agents (ACE inhibitors, angiotensin receptor blockers [ARBs], β-blockers, calcium channel blockers, and diuretics), when used effectively to treat elevated blood pressure, can be relied upon to reduce target organ damage. Choosing an agent involves a decision-making process that takes into account the patient's demographics such as age and ethnicity, the cost of the drug, and the anticipated side-effect profile.

The chief mechanism of action of medications in each class of antihypertensive agents is interference at the point of at least one defined process in the control of blood pressure (see Figure 14). The usual response to monotherapy is a reduction in systolic pressure ranging from 12 to 15 mm Hg and diastolic pressure ranging from 8 to 10 mm Hg.

A few caveats about antihypertensive treatment have arisen in recent years. α-Blockers such as prazosin are not recommended as first-line therapy because they have not been shown to produce the cardiovascular benefit noted, for example, with diuretics. Secondly, β-blockers (particularly atenolol) given to older patients with hypertension do not produce as much reduction in stroke as other classes. It is not known if this concern also applies to newer β-blockers such as nebivolol or α-β blockers such as carvedilol. Finally, heart failure and stroke are the target organ damages most benefited by long-term antihypertensive therapy.

When single-agent treatment is initiated, most agents exert their effect at a given dose by 2 to 4 weeks. Consequently, follow-up visits for blood pressure assessment and possible drug titration are usually scheduled at 2- to 4-week intervals to assess adequacy of treatment.

Combination Therapy

In patients whose goal blood pressure requires reductions of systolic pressure more than 20 mm Hg and diastolic pressure

TABLE 24. Compelling Indications, Contraindications, and Side Effects for Antihypertensive Medications

Class of Medication	Compelling Indications	Contraindications	Side Effects
Thiazide diuretics	Heart failure; advanced age; volume-dependent hypertension; low-renin hypertension; systolic hypertension	Gout	Hypokalemia; hyperuricemia; glucose intolerance; hypercalcemia; impotence
Aldosterone antagonists	Primary hyperaldosteronism; resistant hypertension; sleep apnea	Reduced GFR; hyperkalemia	Hyperkalemia; increased creatinine level; painful gynecomastia; menstrual irregularities; gastrointestinal distress
ACE inhibitors	Heart failure; left ventricular dysfunction; proteinuria; diabetic nephropathy; chronic kidney disease; post–myocardial infarction	Pregnancy; hyperkalemia	Cough; angioedema; hyperkalemia; potential increased creatinine level in patients with bilateral renal artery stenosis; rash; loss of taste; leukopenia (captopril)
Angiotensin receptor blockers	Same as ACE inhibitors; useful when ACE inhibitors are not tolerated	Pregnancy; hyperkalemia	Angioedema (rare); hyperkalemia; potential increased creatinine level in patients with bilateral renal artery stenosis
Calcium channel blockers	Systolic hypertension; cyclosporine-induced hypertension; angina; coronary heart disease	Heart block (for nondihydropyridine calcium channel blockers verapamil and diltiazem)	Headache; flushing; gingival hyperplasia; edema; constipation
β-Blockers	Angina; heart failure; post–myocardial infarction; migraine; tachyarrhythmias	Asthma and COPD; heart block	Bronchospasm; bradycardia; heart failure; impaired peripheral circulation; insomnia; fatigue; decreased exercise tolerance; hypertriglyceridemia
α-Blockers	Prostatic hyperplasia	Orthostatic hypotension	Headache; drowsiness; fatigue; weakness; postural hypotension

GFR = glomerular filtration rate.

more than 10 mm Hg, current JNC 7 recommendations indicate that combination therapy can be used, which can shorten the time to achieve the blood pressure goal, increase the likelihood of achieving the goal, and reduce the number of visits needed for drug titrations.

Combination drug therapy is often more desirable than giving agents at maximum dose in stepwise fashion, because, in most cases, the majority of the antihypertensive effect is manifest at approximately half the manufacturer's maximum recommended dose, and increasing the dose to the maximum usually only produces a few millimeters of Hg more blood pressure reduction but risks greater side-effect occurrence.

Combination drug treatment approaches can be used to intervene in different blood pressure control processes (see Figure 14). Added benefit occurs when a known side effect of one class (for example, edema associated with calcium channel blockers) can be offset by the use of a class such as ACE inhibitors, which provide additional antihypertensive benefit (and offset the edema due to calcium channel blockers). Both the JNC 7 and the International Society for Hypertension in Blacks espouse the use of combination drug therapy approaches, which reduce the time needed to achieve control and improve the overall likelihood of achieving target blood pressure levels.

Until recently, no data supported superiority of one combination drug approach. However, the Avoiding Cardiovascular Events through Combination Therapy in Patients Living With Systolic Hypertension (ACCOMPLISH) trial demonstrated that despite identical blood pressure control, a regimen combining an ACE inhibitor with a calcium channel blocker was superior to a regimen of an ACE inhibitor with a diuretic in hypertensive patients at high cardiovascular risk.

Many fixed combinations of antihypertensive medications are available. Although these may be more convenient for patients who have achieved a stable, effective dose, they tend to offer less dosing flexibility and are often substantially more expensive than prescribing the component medications independently.

KEY POINTS

- Lifestyle modifications, including weight loss, reduction of dietary sodium intake, aerobic physical activity of at least 30 minutes a day at least three times a week, and a reduction in alcohol consumption, can help reduce high blood pressure.

- Drug treatment is recommended when blood pressure remains above 140/90 mm Hg in patients younger than 80 years of age; in those aged 80 years and older, a systolic blood pressure of 150 mm Hg is recommended as the threshold for treatment initiation.

- In patients whose goal blood pressure requires reductions of systolic pressure more than 20 mm Hg and diastolic pressure more than 10 mm Hg, combination therapy can be used, which can shorten the time to achieve the blood pressure goal, increase the likelihood of achieving the goal, and reduce the number of visits needed for drug titrations.

Secondary Hypertension

Secondary hypertension accounts for less than 10% of all forms of high blood pressure and typically emanate from the kidney (vascular and parenchymal origins) or the adrenal gland (cortex or medulla). Secondary hypertension is important to recognize, because it often points to specific mechanisms elevating blood pressure, which guide therapy.

Because most cases of elevated blood pressure are essential, most patients with hypertension do not require evaluation for an underlying cause. However, clinical factors that raise the possibility of secondary hypertension include onset at a young age in patients with no family history of hypertension or other risk factors, or a rapid onset of significant hypertension or an abrupt change in blood pressure in patients with previously well-controlled hypertension. Most commonly, resistant hypertension suggests a possible underlying contributing factor to the blood pressure elevation (see Resistant Hypertension). Additionally, any patient with other symptoms or findings associated with a possible secondary cause (such as an endocrine abnormality) may warrant further investigation.

Kidney Disease
Epidemiology
Kidney disease is the most common cause of secondary hypertension. Depending on the degree of functional kidney impairment, up to 90% of patients with advanced kidney failure or patients on dialysis have hypertension.

Pathophysiology
The processes by which impaired kidney function raises blood pressure are complex. Because the kidney is the primary regulator of sodium balance, disorders of sodium metabolism rank high among the pathogenic processes. The kidney also is a target organ of the hypertensive process, which makes adequate control of blood pressure in patients with hypertension associated with kidney failure essential.

Management
The first step in the management of hypertension in patients with CKD is to determine the presence or absence of proteinuria. When proteinuria is present, most guidelines recommend the use of either an ACE inhibitor or ARB, because these agents seem to have particular benefit for both proteinuria reduction and blood pressure control. The current target blood pressure level in patients with CKD is less than 130/80 mm Hg. When significant proteinuria is present (>500 mg/24 h), the target level is less than 125/75 mm Hg. In the absence of proteinuria, no specific antihypertensive agent class has proved to be superior in lowering blood pressure or reducing target organ damage.

When treating patients with CKD, it is common to see an increase in the serum creatinine level as blood pressure falls. In most cases, an increase of up to 25% is an acceptable trade-off for blood pressure control. When the serum creatinine level increases beyond this, for example, to levels two or three times baseline value, it is reasonable to reassess the aggressiveness of the diuretic regimen (if one is used) or to consider the possibility of bilateral renal arterial disease, particularly when patients are treated with an ACE inhibitor or ARB (see Renovascular Hypertension).

KEY POINTS

- Secondary hypertension accounts for less than 10% of all forms of high blood pressure and typically emanates from the kidney or the adrenal gland.

- Kidney disease is the most common cause of secondary hypertension; depending on the degree of functional kidney impairment, up to 90% of patients with advanced kidney failure or patients on dialysis have hypertension.

Renovascular Hypertension
Epidemiology

Renovascular hypertension is an increase in blood pressure due to significant narrowing of one or both of the renal arteries resulting in abnormal vasoregulatory responses by the kidney because of a perceived decrease in the adequacy of renal blood flow. True renovascular hypertension is found in only 1% to 2% of all patients with hypertension but may have a higher prevalence in those with known atherosclerotic vascular occlusive disease.

Pathophysiology
The renin-angiotensin system is activated when blood flow to the kidney is significantly reduced, with pathologic consequences such as renovascular hypertension occurring only when there is substantial luminal obstruction (>75%).

Narrowing of the renal arteries occurs either as part of generalized atherosclerosis or in the form of fibromuscular dysplasia. In the former, atherosclerotic risk factors are typically present, foremost among them being cigarette smoking, often with a modest impairment in kidney function. Fibromuscular dysplasia is more often found in younger patients, particularly women. Whereas atherosclerosis tends to affect the proximal portion of the renal artery, fibromuscular dysplasia is usually found more distally. Both forms of renovascular disease may be associated with midepigastric bruits. Unilateral renal lesions are thought to elevate blood pressure through renin-mediated mechanisms, whereas bilateral (or unilateral with a single functioning kidney) forms of vascular disease have a strong component of sodium excess in causing blood pressure elevation.

Renal artery stenosis is best demonstrated by angiography (conventional kidney angiography or CT of the renal arteries); however, these studies involve contrast, which may precipitate acute kidney injury in susceptible persons. Alternatives include MR angiography, often using gadolinium, or renal Doppler studies. In patients with reduced kidney function (<30 mL/min/1.73 m^2) in whom neither iodinated nor gadolinium contrast is desirable, a renal Doppler study is a reasonable screening consideration.

Management

Considerable debate exists on how to manage renovascular disease in patients with hypertension. In young patients with fibromuscular dysplasia, percutaneous transluminal kidney angioplasty is considered low risk and deemed the treatment of choice given the high likelihood of both technical success and meaningful blood pressure improvement.

The management of atherosclerotic renovascular disease is much more controversial. Several recent trials, including Angioplasty and Stenting for Renal Artery Lesions (ASTRAL) and Stent Placement in Patients with Atherosclerotic Renal Artery Stenosis and Impaired Renal Function (STAR), do not support an angioplasty intervention, although ongoing trials may provide further guidance regarding appropriate therapy. Current recommendations for the treatment of atherosclerotic renovascular disease support aggressive risk factor management (blood pressure control, antihyperlipidemic therapy, smoking cessation techniques), with angioplasty or surgical intervention reserved for those with refractory hypertension despite extensive treatment or progressive diminution in kidney function.

Patients with bilateral renal artery disease (or unilateral disease in a single functioning kidney) are at risk of a worsening of kidney function when treated with drugs that interfere with the renin-angiotensin system such as ACE inhibitors or ARBs. This is particularly true in the presence of aggressive diuretic use and should be suspected in those with known atherosclerotic vascular occlusive disease, especially when serum creatinine values rise much more than 25% from baseline.

Aldosterone Excess

Aldosterone excess may be present in up to 10% of patients with new-onset hypertension. Many patients found to have elevated serum aldosterone levels display normal serum potassium and bicarbonate levels. Diagnosis can be aided by a 24-hour urine collection for aldosterone, plasma renin activity measurement, and an imaging study. See MKSAP 16 Endocrinology and Metabolism for a detailed discussion of primary hyperaldosteronism.

Pheochromocytoma

Pheochromocytomas and paragangliomas increase blood pressure through secretion of norepinephrine and epinephrine. Diagnosis requires a high degree of suspicion, with confirmation of excess catecholamine production either by 24-hour urine collection for catecholamine and metanephrine excretion or by plasma metanephrine measurement. Definitive therapy for these tumors is surgical removal. See MKSAP 16 Endocrinology and Metabolism for a detailed discussion of pheochromocytoma. **H**

KEY POINTS

- Percutaneous transluminal kidney angioplasty is considered the treatment of choice for young patients with fibromuscular dysplasia.
- Current recommendations for the treatment of atherosclerotic renovascular disease support aggressive risk factor management (blood pressure control, antihyperlipidemia therapy, smoking cessation techniques), with angioplasty or surgical intervention reserved for those with refractory hypertension despite extensive treatment or progressive diminution in kidney function.

White Coat Hypertension

Patients with white coat hypertension have elevated blood pressure measurements in the office setting but normal measurements (for example, daytime blood pressure $<130/80$ mm Hg) outside the office, accompanied by the absence of target organ damage. ABPM is considered the gold standard for diagnosing white coat hypertension. Pharmacologic management of white coat hypertension has not been shown to reduce morbid events or produce cardiovascular benefit.

Masked Hypertension

Masked hypertension is characterized by blood pressure that is higher at home than in the office setting, which is confirmed by ambulatory blood pressures that are greater than 130/80 mm Hg despite office blood pressures of less than 140/90 mm Hg. There are no clear guidelines to pursue the diagnosis of masked hypertension; ABPM does not carry a formal indication for this diagnosis but may be useful in establishing this blood pressure pattern. An increasing number of studies suggest that the cardiovascular risk of masked hypertension approaches that of sustained hypertension.

Resistant Hypertension

Resistant hypertension occurs when blood pressure measurements consistently exceed the blood pressure goal despite taking three antihypertensive drugs (one of which is a diuretic). This occurs in approximately 10% to 15% of patients with hypertension. Evaluation includes confirmation that the blood pressure is truly high outside of the office, with verification that good technique, including correct cuff size, was used in blood pressure measurement. There should also be a search for factors that might potentially lead to suboptimal control, such as high salt intake or use of drugs such as NSAIDs, and consideration of potentially modifiable pathogenic factors, such as aldosterone excess and obstructive sleep apnea. Resistant hypertension is one of the most common reasons for referral to a hypertension specialist.

KEY POINTS

- Patients with white coat hypertension have elevated blood pressure measurements in the office setting but normal measurements outside the office.
- Ambulatory blood pressure monitoring is considered the gold standard for diagnosing white coat hypertension.
- Resistant hypertension is defined as blood pressure above goal despite the administration of three antihypertensive drugs, one of which is a diuretic.

Special Populations

Women

To date, women show similar blood pressure responses to men in randomized clinical trials. Before menopause, women have lower blood pressures than similarly aged men. This tends to reverse after menopause, and black women tend to have the highest blood pressures. In women of childbearing potential who have hypertension, ACE inhibitors and ARBs should be avoided because of the risk of fetal malformations. Women tend to develop hypokalemia more often when treated with diuretics and have a greater risk of hyponatremia when treated with thiazide diuretics.

Patients with Diabetes Mellitus

Patients with diabetes mellitus and hypertension are at substantial cardiovascular risk. Managing high blood pressure is an effective way to reduce this risk, but debate exists regarding goal blood pressure levels. The American Diabetes Association and the National Kidney Foundation currently recommend target blood pressure levels of less than 130/80 mm Hg, regardless of age. In the recently completed Action to Control Cardiovascular Risk in Diabetes (ACCORD) trial,

the intensive therapy group randomly assigned to the lower blood pressure goal (<120 mm Hg systolic) did not experience an improvement in the primary outcome despite systolic blood pressures that were 14 mm Hg lower than the values achieved in the standard therapy group. Stroke, however, was significantly reduced in the lower blood pressure goal group. On the other hand, the increased medication requirement to achieve the intensive therapy goal blood pressures resulted in more side effects, including worse kidney function.

Black Patients

Black patients tend to experience enhanced target organ damage at any level of blood pressure compared with most other groups, particularly white patients. The reasons for this are not clear, but the intense search for genetic predisposition continues to attract much attention. Cardiovascular complications are more frequent in black patients, and black patients are approximately fourfold more likely to experience end-stage kidney disease compared with white patients.

The African American Study of Kidney Disease and Hypertension (AASK), performed in black patients with long-standing hypertension and mild proteinuria, demonstrated that the ACE inhibitor ramipril was superior to the β-blocker metoprolol and the calcium channel blocker amlodipine in slowing kidney disease progression in black patients with impaired kidney function caused by hypertension.

Other recommendations for the management of high blood pressure in black patients were released in the International Society on Hypertension in Blacks (ISHIB) consensus statement. ISHIB defines treatment goals in black patients based upon either the *absence* of target organ damage (primary prevention), in which the blood pressure goal is less than 135/85 mm Hg, or the *presence* of target organ damage (secondary prevention), in which the blood pressure goal is less than 130/80 mm Hg.

Older Patients

The pattern of blood pressure elevation in older patients is typically characterized by a prominent systolic blood pressure. This relates in large part to the significant role of vascular stiffness in the blood pressure increases of older patients, which in addition to raising systolic pressure, also leads to a decline in the diastolic pressure. Clinical trials have documented the value of reducing elevated systolic pressures when they exceed 160 mm Hg. Although a target blood pressure of 140/90 mm Hg is generally accepted for most patients, there are less data on patients over the age of 80 years to guide therapy. The Hypertension in the Very Elderly Trial (HYVET) enrolled patients at least 80 years of age and used a target systolic blood pressure of 150 mm Hg. The trial demonstrated decreased mortality and heart failure with active drug therapy; therefore, treatment to this blood pressure goal appears reasonable for persons over age 80 years.

patients who are aged 60 to 79 years, the 140/90 blood pressure goal (in the absence of comorbidities such as diabetes, coronary artery disease, or CKD) remains reasonable if it can be achieved without significant side effects, particularly orthostatic hypotension, of which elderly patients are more prone to than other populations. Reducing a systolic blood pressure that is above 160 mm Hg systolic results in less stroke and less cardiovascular disease. There is concern regarding lowering an already low diastolic blood pressure in patients with existing coronary artery disease. In this regard, a "J-curve" is thought to exist, in which an *increase* in cardiovascular events occurs below a certain threshold of blood pressure. Current recommendations are to avoid lowering the diastolic blood pressure below 70 mm Hg in those with active coronary disease at any age.

KEY POINTS

- In women of childbearing potential who have hypertension, ACE inhibitors and angiotensin receptor blockers should be avoided because of the risk of fetal malformations.

- For patients with diabetes mellitus, current recommendations indicate a target blood pressure goal of less than 130/80 mm Hg.

- A target systolic blood pressure goal of 150 mm Hg or less appears reasonable for patients aged 80 years or older.

- Current recommendations are to avoid lowering the diastolic blood pressure below 70 mm Hg in those with active coronary disease at any age.

Chronic Tubulointerstitial Disorders

Pathophysiology and Epidemiology

Pathologic processes that affect the tubules and/or the interstitium of the kidney are termed *tubulointerstitial disorders*.

In their chronic form, these disorders develop over months to years from long-term exposures or systemic processes and are associated with a slow decline in kidney function. Glomerular and vascular renal lesions can be accompanied by secondary chronic tubulointerstitial nephritis. In contrast, acute interstitial nephritis develops over days to weeks and is associated with acute kidney injury.

Acute interstitial nephritis may evolve into chronic tubulointerstitial nephritis. Glomerular and vascular structures are subsequently involved, with fibrosis and scarring throughout the kidney. The degree of fibrosis is predictive of progression to end-stage kidney disease (ESKD), and 10% to 20% of incident ESKD is attributed to tubulointerstitial disease.

For further discussion of acute interstitial nephritis, see Acute Kidney Injury.

KEY POINT

- Chronic tubulointerstitial disorders develop over months to years from long-term exposures or systemic processes and are associated with a slow decline in kidney function.

Clinical Manifestations

The pathophysiology of chronic tubulointerstitial disorders gives insight to the clinical manifestations of these diseases. Ongoing tubulointerstitial damage leads to the defects listed in **Table 25**.

Diagnosis and Evaluation

The clinical diagnosis of chronic tubulointerstitial disease is often one of exclusion. History and physical examination should address conditions that may be associated with this disorder. A careful review of medications is essential (**Table 26**).

Laboratory values can show anemia as a result of damage to the erythropoietin-producing cells in the kidney. Urinalysis can be bland or reveal sterile pyuria, with minimal hematuria. Urine protein excretion (usually low-molecular-weight protein rather than albumin) is typically less than 2 g/24 h. Kidney ultrasound can show small, atrophic kidneys consistent with

TABLE 25. Clinical Manifestations of Chronic Tubulointerstitial Disorders	
Abnormality[a]	**Cause**
Decline in glomerular filtration rate	Obstruction of tubules; damage to microvasculature; fibrosis and sclerosis of glomeruli
Proximal tubular damage (Fanconi syndrome)	Incomplete absorption and renal wasting of glucose, phosphates, bicarbonate, and amino acids
Non–anion gap metabolic acidosis	Proximal and distal renal tubular acidosis; decreased ammonia production
Isosthenuria and polyuria	Decreased concentrating and diluting ability
Proteinuria	Decreased tubular protein reabsorption (usually <2 g/24 h)
Hyperkalemia	Defect in potassium secretion (hyperkalemic distal renal tubular acidosis)

[a]The degree of these abnormalities depends on the extent and location of injury.

TABLE 26. Causes of Chronic Tubulointerstitial Disorders

Autoimmune disorders
  Anti–tubular basement membrane antibody-mediated tubulointerstitial nephritis
  Sarcoidosis
  Sjögren syndrome
  Systemic lupus erythematosus
  Tubulointerstitial nephritis with uveitis

Balkan endemic nephropathy

Heavy metal nephropathy
  Lead
  Cadmium
  Mercury

Hereditary tubulointerstitial nephritis
  Medullary cystic disease (type II is associated with hyperuricemia and gout)
  Mitochondrial disorders

Infection-related
  Polyoma BK virus (posttransplantation; most common following kidney transplantation)
  Brucellosis
  Cytomegalovirus
  Epstein-Barr virus
  Fungal infections
  Legionella species
  Mycobacterium tuberculosis
  Toxoplasmosis

Malignancy-related
  Leukemia
  Lymphoma
  Myeloma cast nephropathy
  Plasmacytomas

Medication-induced
  Analgesic nephropathy (highest toxicity with combination therapy)
  Calcineurin inhibitors (secondary tubulointerstitial injury consequent to arteriolopathy)
  Chinese herb nephropathy (aristolochic acid)
  Cyclooxygenase-2 inhibitors
  Lithium
  NSAIDs
  Prolonged exposure to any medication that can cause acute interstitial nephritis
    5-Aminosalicylates (e.g., mesalamine)
    Allopurinol
    Cephalosporins
    Fluoroquinolones
    H_2 blockers
    Indinavir
    Penicillins
    Proton pump inhibitors
    Rifampin
    Sulfonamides

Secondary tubulointerstitial injury due to glomerular and vascular disorders

Urinary tract obstruction

chronic kidney disease (CKD). Indications for biopsy include unclear etiology of disease, with potential for a change in therapy based on biopsy results.

Causes

The causes of primary chronic tubulointerstitial disorders often lead to progressive CKD (see Table 26).

Immunologic Diseases

Sjögren Syndrome

Chronic tubulointerstitial disease occurs in 25% to 50% of patients with Sjögren syndrome and is typically seen within the first several years of the disease. Interstitial nephritis may precede the onset of extrarenal manifestations. A decreased glomerular filtration rate (GFR), urinary concentrating defects, and renal tubular acidosis are also common. Glomerular disease, such as membranous or membranoproliferative nephropathies, is less common and occurs later in the disease course. Corticosteroid therapy may improve the course of disease.

Sarcoidosis

Noncaseating granulomatous interstitial nephritis is the classic renal lesion of sarcoidosis, although tubulointerstitial nephritis without granulomas is also common. Other associated disorders can lead secondarily to chronic tubulointerstitial nephritis, including hypercalcemia, nephrocalcinosis, and nephrolithiasis from increased 1,25-dihydroxy vitamin D levels. Polyuria is common in these patients. Corticosteroid therapy can lead to renal recovery if viable tissue remains.

Systemic Lupus Erythematosus

Tubulointerstitial nephritis in patients with systemic lupus erythematosus most commonly occurs in conjunction with glomerular disease. In more than 50% of patients, biopsy specimens reveal immune complex deposits in tubular basement membranes. Tubulointerstitial disease without glomerular involvement is rare but displays clinical manifestations similar to those listed in Table 25. More extensive tubulointerstitial involvement is a poor prognostic marker. Therapy is aimed at treating the underlying glomerular lesions and other systemic manifestations of the disease.

Infectious Diseases

Infectious organisms are associated with tubulointerstitial nephritis via direct infiltration or a reactive systemic inflammatory response. Patients predisposed to infection-related tubulointerstitial damage include those with preexisting kidney disease (such as kidney transplant recipients) or those with impaired immune system function (such as patients on chemotherapy or chronic immunosuppressant medications or those with advanced HIV infection). Organisms include *Mycobacterium tuberculosis*, Epstein-Barr virus, cytomegalovirus, and polyoma BK virus (in kidney transplant recipients).

Malignancy

Malignancies associated with chronic tubulointerstitial nephritis include multiple myeloma and lymphoproliferative disorders. In multiple myeloma, kidney dysfunction is present in more than 50% of patients at the time of initial presentation. Myeloma cast nephropathy is common and is caused by precipitation of Bence-Jones protein with Tamm-Horsfall mucoprotein in the renal tubule acutely, which causes direct tubular toxicity, with multinucleated giant cells present in the tubular walls and interstitium. This leads to tubular obstruction and injury and acute kidney injury. Predisposing factors for kidney involvement in multiple myeloma include volume depletion and hypercalcemia. A more chronic process with tubular dysfunction associated with myeloma light chain deposition may occur over months to years and lead to proximal renal tubular acidosis and electrolyte and concentration abnormalities resembling the Fanconi syndrome. Therapy includes treatment of hypercalcemia, correction of volume depletion, and treatment of the underlying plasma cell dyscrasia (see Glomerular Diseases and Acute Kidney Injury).

Lymphomatous or leukemic infiltration is present in up to 50% of patients with lymphoproliferative disorders on postmortem examination. Patients present with non–nephrotic-range proteinuria, sterile pyuria, and kidneys that appear large on imaging studies. Therapy directed at the malignancy can lead to a decrease in kidney size and improvement in function.

Medications

Analgesics

A strong association exists between chronic tubulointerstitial nephritis and long-term use of combination analgesics such as aspirin, phenacetin, and caffeine. The incidence and prevalence of analgesic nephropathy have diminished over the past two decades, coinciding with the removal of phenacetin and other analgesic mixtures as over-the-counter pain relievers. Data suggest that there is an association between chronic daily acetaminophen use and CKD, although a causal relationship has not been established. The epidemiologic data supporting the association between analgesic nephropathy and NSAIDs are not as robust; however, exposure to large quantities may result in CKD.

Studies suggest that nephrotoxicity is dose-dependent, with clinically evident disease appearing after chronic, high-dose use of NSAIDs for 5 or more years. There is a female predominance, and the kidney manifestations are nonspecific, including sterile pyuria, mild proteinuria, reduced GFR, and urinary concentrating defects. Hypertension and anemia are characteristic of patients with more advanced disease. Early diagnosis is important, because kidney function can stabilize or moderately improve if analgesics are discontinued before advanced disease occurs.

Analgesic nephropathy is associated with genitourinary tract malignancies, which develop in up to 10% of patients. In patients with analgesic nephropathy and hematuria, upper urinary tract imaging, urine cytology, and cystoscopy are recommended.

Calcineurin Inhibitors

Chronic use of calcineurin inhibitors such as cyclosporine or tacrolimus is associated with kidney disease, especially in transplant recipients and in those with autoimmune disorders. Chronic vasoconstriction causes kidney fibrosis and scarring as well as direct tubular and vascular toxicity. Toxicity is dose-dependent. Hyperkalemic distal renal tubular acidosis is common.

Lithium

Long-term lithium exposure can result in chronic tubulointerstitial nephritis. Repeated toxicity and high chronic lithium levels can result in worsening dysfunction. Other kidney manifestations include decreased GFR, partial nephrogenic diabetes insipidus, and incomplete distal renal tubular acidosis. Lithium is reabsorbed along the nephron at sites where sodium is reabsorbed, resulting in ubiquitous uptake along the renal tubules. Amiloride blocks lithium uptake at the epithelial sodium channel and attenuates nephrogenic diabetes insipidus. Discontinuation of lithium may reverse some of the underlying kidney damage and should be considered if a patient's underlying disorder is controlled with other medications.

Lead

Lead nephropathy is an underrecognized cause of chronic tubulointerstitial disorders. Lead is taken up by the proximal tubule, leading to direct toxic tubulointerstitial effects, including Fanconi syndrome, decreased urine uric acid excretion, and interstitial fibrosis. Patients who are hypertensive, are prone to (saturnine) gout, and have a decreased GFR should be asked about past lead exposure.

Serum lead levels are a poor marker for lead nephropathy, because more than 90% of body lead resides in the bone. Calcium disodium ethylenediaminetetraacetic acid (EDTA) mobilization testing with 24-hour urine lead excretion should be performed if lead toxicity is suspected. Levels of more than 600 micrograms (2.9 micromoles) in 24 hours are diagnostic.

Hyperuricemia

The association of hyperuricemia and CKD has been demonstrated; however, causality has neither been proved nor refuted. In one study of more than 21,000 persons, those with a serum uric acid level of 7.0 to 8.9 mg/dL (0.413-0.525 mmol/L) had double the risk of incident kidney disease, and those with levels of more than 9.0 mg/dL (0.531 mmol/L) had triple the risk. Some epidemiologic studies also have demonstrated hyperuricemia to be a marker of worse cardiovascular outcomes.

The kidney is the primary organ for uric acid excretion. With a pKa of 5.4, uric acid exists in its non-ionized form in acidic urine and exists as urate salts in the more alkaline environments of the interstitium and blood. Chronic urate nephropathy may result in tubulointerstitial nephritis from deposition of sodium urate crystals in the medullary interstitium. The chronic inflammatory response leads to interstitial fibrosis and CKD. Many patients believed to have urate nephropathy may have a form of hereditary interstitial kidney disease (type II medullary cystic disease).

Although allopurinol can be used to lower serum uric acid levels, it is unclear if treatment of asymptomatic hyperuricemia results in improved outcomes. If a patient has clinical gout and hyperuricemia, uric acid–lowering therapy should be more strongly considered.

Obstruction

Obstructive uropathy results from functional or structural obstruction to urinary flow anywhere along the urinary tract. Obstruction and reflux of urinary flow can result in an inflammatory response in the interstitium and eventual ischemic atrophy. The most common obstructive causes are benign prostatic hyperplasia in men and disorders of the reproductive system (including malignancy) in women. Prompt diagnosis via radiographic imaging studies is indicated to prevent the long-term sequelae of CKD. Obstruction that is present for more than 6 to 12 weeks typically results in irreversible damage.

KEY POINTS

- Patients predisposed to infection-related tubulointerstitial damage include those with preexisting kidney disease or those with impaired immune system function.

- Kidney manifestations of analgesic nephropathy include sterile pyuria, mild proteinuria, reduced glomerular filtration rate, and urinary concentrating defects.

- The most common obstructive causes of chronic tubulointerstitial diseases are benign prostatic hyperplasia in men and disorders of the reproductive system (including malignancy) in women.

͏ement

Rapid assessment and treatment of underlying causes of chronic tubulointerstitial disorders may slow down progression to ESKD or may result in some degree of reversibility. However, once chronic damage has occurred, significant reversibility is unlikely. Steps for practitioners to take include discontinuation of drugs and removal of exogenous toxins; diagnosing immunologic, infectious, or malignant disease; ensuring obstruction is not present; treating the underlying cause; and consideration for immunosuppressive therapy in consultation with a nephrologist.

KEY POINT

- Rapid assessment and treatment of underlying causes of chronic tubulointerstitial disorders may slow down progression to end-stage kidney disease or may result in some degree of reversibility.

Glomerular Diseases

Pathophysiology

The kidneys contain approximately two million ultrafiltration units known as nephrons, each comprised of two components: the glomerulus and the renal tubule. The glomerulus is the primary filtration unit of the kidney and is composed of a tuft of capillaries between the afferent and efferent arterioles of the renal circulation. The glomerular capillaries are supported by the mesangium, which is made of specialized mesangial cells and a surrounding structural matrix. The glomerular capillary has three distinct components: an inner layer of endothelial cells, the capillary basement membrane, and an outer layer of visceral epithelial cells known as podocytes, which wrap around the capillaries, leaving small slits (slit diaphragm) between these projections (foot processes). Together these components form a selective filtration barrier (**Figure 15**).

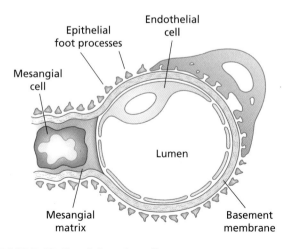

FIGURE 15. Normal glomerular capillary.

The glomerular capillary tufts are almost completely surrounded by a cup-like sac composed of a single layer of parietal epithelial cells called the Bowman's capsule that is continuous with the renal tubule. Filtrate from the glomerular capillaries is collected in this space and then passes to the renal tubule, which is the primary location for the processing of the glomerular filtrate.

Damage to the glomerulus may alter glomerular capillary permselectivity and result in proteinuria, the clinical hallmark of glomerular diseases. It also may alter the continuity of the filtration barrier, manifesting as glomerular hematuria. Extensive damage to glomeruli is associated with a progressive decline in the glomerular filtration rate (GFR), leading to advanced chronic kidney disease (CKD) and possibly end-stage kidney disease (ESKD).

Clinical Manifestations

Glomerular diseases are frequently characterized by different patterns of clinical presentation, including the nephrotic syndromes, in which significant leakage of plasma proteins is predominant, and the nephritic syndromes (also called glomerulonephritis), in which there is passage of both plasma proteins and cells (erythrocytes and leukocytes) from the glomerulus into the renal tubule. Because certain diseases tend to follow specific patterns, these characterizations may be useful in understanding the potential causes of a clinical kidney disorder. However, these classifications are not exclusive because some conditions may present with either pattern, others may have features of both, and some disorders may progress from one pattern to the other. Kidney biopsy is usually essential in making a correct diagnosis and guiding therapy.

Glomerular diseases may also be designated by their clinical time course. Rapidly progressive glomerulonephritis (RPGN) is a form of the nephritic syndrome characterized by the rapid loss of kidney function over weeks to months compared with other forms of glomerular disease, which may be more chronic or slowly progressive.

The Nephrotic Syndrome

The nephrotic syndrome is characterized by heavy proteinuria, defined as a urine protein–creatinine ratio of greater than 3.5 mg/mg or a timed urine protein collection of greater than 3.5 g/24 h. Hypoalbuminemia and edema are hallmark findings of the nephrotic syndrome. Other clinical manifestations, such as hyperlipidemia or coagulation abnormalities, are related to losses of proteins other than albumin or caused by increased protein synthesis (**Table 27**).

The Nephritic Syndrome

Compared with the nephrotic syndrome in which there is primarily protein leakage across the glomeruli, the nephritic syndrome involves injury to or inflammation within the glomerulus that allows the passage of protein, erythrocytes, and leukocytes into the renal tubule. The resulting damage may be associated

TABLE 27. Clinical Manifestations of Urine Protein Losses and Associated Altered Protein Synthesis in the Nephrotic Syndrome

Urine Protein Losses

Proteins	Clinical Manifestations
Albumin	Edema
High-density lipoprotein	Atherosclerosis
Heparan sulfate	Atherosclerosis
α1-Acid glycoprotein	Atherosclerosis
Complement component factor B	Infections
Immunoglobulin (IgG)	Infections
Antithrombin III; proteins S and C	Thrombosis
Coagulation factors IX, XI, and XII	Bleeding
Iron-binding protein	Anemia
Erythropoietin	Anemia
Vitamin D–binding proteins	Osteomalacia
Thyroid-binding protein and thyroxine	Hypothyroidism

Altered Protein Synthesis

Proteins	Clinical Manifestations
Insufficient synthesis of albumin	Hypoalbuminemia
Increased synthesis of apolipoprotein B; LDL cholesterol	Atherosclerosis
Increased synthesis of fibrinogen	Thrombosis
Increased synthesis of coagulation factors V, VII, VIII, and X	Thrombosis
Increased synthesis of α_2-globulins and β-globulins	Unknown
Increased synthesis of immunoglobulin IgM	Unknown

with decreased glomerular filtration, decreased kidney function, and abnormal blood pressure regulation. Thus, the nephritic syndrome is characterized by proteinuria, hematuria, pyuria, and, frequently, decreased kidney function and hypertension.

RPGN, a severe form of acute nephritis, is a nephrologic emergency characterized by a rapid decline in kidney function that can lead to advanced CKD and ESKD in weeks to months if untreated. The histologic correlate of RPGN is the crescent. Crescents develop in Bowman's space following glomerular capillary rupture with extravasation of inflammatory cells, macrophages, and fibrin resulting in parietal cell proliferation that takes on a characteristic crescent shape on microscopy. Prompt diagnosis and initiation of therapy in RPGN are essential to optimize clinical outcomes and decrease the risk of progression to ESKD. **H**

KEY POINTS

- The nephrotic syndrome is characterized by heavy proteinuria (a urine protein–creatinine ratio >3.5 mg/mg); hypoalbuminemia, edema, and hyperlipidemia are common clinical findings.

- The nephritic syndrome is characterized by proteinuria, hematuria, pyuria, and, frequently, decreased kidney function and hypertension.

- Rapidly progressive glomerulonephritis is a nephrologic emergency characterized by a rapid decline in kidney function that can lead to advanced chronic kidney disease and end-stage kidney disease in weeks to months if untreated.

Conditions that Cause the Nephrotic Syndrome

Disorders presenting with the nephrotic syndrome may occur as a primary condition or may be a secondary manifestation of another disease process. Table 28 lists the causes of the nephrotic syndrome.

Major Causes of the Nephrotic Syndrome with Kidney-Limited Disease

Focal Segmental Glomerulosclerosis

Epidemiology and Pathophysiology

Focal segmental glomerulosclerosis (FSGS) is the leading cause of primary nephrotic syndrome and is the most common primary glomerular disease leading to ESKD in the United States. FSGS may be primary, familial, or secondary to HIV infection (see HIV-Associated Nephropathy),

TABLE 28. Nondiabetic Causes of the Nephrotic Syndrome in Adults[a]

Condition	Frequency as a Cause of Primary Nephrotic Syndrome	Comments
Focal segmental glomerulosclerosis	36%-80%	Most common cause of primary nephrotic syndrome in the United States
		Predilection for black persons
		Five subtypes: not otherwise specified; perihilar variant; tip variant; cellular variant; collapsing variant (may be associated with HIV infection, heroin use, parvovirus infection, or pamidronate exposure)
		Familial forms
		Morbid obesity
		Decreased kidney mass (congenital kidney dysplasia, reflux nephropathy)
Membranous glomerulopathy	18%-41%	Primary form (most common worldwide): antiphospholipase A_2 receptor autoantibodies can be found in 75% of cases
		May be associated with or secondary to:
		Systemic lupus erythematosus
		Infections: hepatitis B and C virus infections; syphilis; malaria
		Medication exposure: penicillamine; NSAIDs; anti-TNF therapy; tiopronin
		Mercury or gold exposure
		Malignancies: bladder, breast, colon, lung, pancreas, prostate, stomach carcinoma; carcinoid; sarcomas; lymphomas; leukemias
		Thyroid disease
		Highest predilection for renal vein thrombosis among all causes of the nephrotic syndrome
Minimal change glomerulopathy	9%-16%	Most common cause of primary nephrotic syndrome in children
		May be associated with or secondary to:
		Atopic diseases
		Mononucleosis
		Malignancies: Hodgkin lymphoma and carcinomas
		Medication exposure: NSAIDs; interferon; pamidronate; lithium; rifampin
Fibrillary glomerulopathy	<1%	May be associated with malignancy
Immunotactoid glomerulopathy	<1%	May be associated with chronic lymphocytic leukemia or B-cell lymphomas
Amyloidosis	2%	AL (light chains) or AH (heavy chains) amyloidosis may be primary or associated with myeloma
		AA amyloidosis is usually associated with inflammatory conditions such as rheumatoid arthritis, familial Mediterranean fever, chronic infections, or malignancies
		Familial forms
Monoclonal immunoglobulin deposition disease	<1%	Frequently associated with multiple myeloma
Membranoproliferative glomerulonephritis[b]	25%-30%	May present with features of the nephrotic syndrome, the nephritic syndrome, or both

TNF = tumor necrosis factor.

[a]See Table 29 for the clinical stages of diabetic nephropathy.

[b]See Table 30 for causes of the nephritic syndrome.

morbid obesity, reflux nephropathy, and heroin use. Primary FSGS is postulated to be in part mediated by lymphocytes that release cytokines, leading to increased permeability and injury to the glomerular capillary bundle and podocytes.

Risk factors associated with progression of FSGS to ESKD include black race, proteinuria greater than 2 g/24 h, elevated serum creatinine levels, low GFR, BMI greater than 27, hypertension at onset, lack of remission, and relapse during follow-up.

Clinical Manifestations
Primary FSGS frequently presents as the nephrotic syndrome and is commonly accompanied by kidney failure, hematuria, and hypertension. FSGS may also present as asymptomatic subnephrotic proteinuria. Progressive CKD is common.

Diagnosis
Diagnosis of primary FSGS is confirmed by kidney biopsy, with light microscopy showing scarring or sclerosis involving some (focal) glomeruli, which are affected only in a portion of the glomerular capillary bundle (segmental).

Management
Management of FSGS using ACE inhibitors or angiotensin receptor blockers (ARBs) to a target blood pressure of less than 130/80 mm Hg is indicated to forestall progression and reduce proteinuria. At disease onset, patients with nephrotic-range proteinuria should be considered for treatment with immunosuppressive regimens such as corticosteroids or calcineurin inhibitors. Of patients with primary FSGS, 39% to 45% become frequently relapsing corticosteroid-dependent or corticosteroid-resistant, and a calcineurin inhibitor can achieve remission in up to 70% of these patients; however, 60% of patients can relapse after reducing or stopping these agents. Many of these patients require chronic immunosuppressive therapy, which may also include cyclophosphamide, mycophenolate mofetil, and rituximab.

Response to treatment is the most important factor that influences prognosis. Up to 90% of patients with complete remission, 78% with partial remission, and 40% with persistent nephrotic-range proteinuria remain free of ESKD within 10 years of disease onset.

Membranous Glomerulopathy
Epidemiology and Pathophysiology
Membranous glomerulopathy is the second leading cause of primary nephrotic syndrome. Primary membranous glomerulopathy has a predilection to develop more frequently in adults older than 50 years. Untreated, approximately two thirds of patients with membranous glomerulopathy undergo spontaneous complete or partial remission, and one third of

patients have a persistent or progressive disease that may result in ESKD within 10 years of onset.

Primary membranous glomerulopathy is an in situ immune complex disease in which immunoglobulins of the IgG class react with constitutive or planted antigens in the outer aspect of the glomerular basement membrane.

Membranous glomerulopathy can also be secondary to other conditions such as systemic lupus erythematosus, hepatitis B and C virus infections, malaria, malignancies, and medications such as NSAIDs.

Risk factors associated with progressive CKD in patients with membranous glomerulopathy include male gender, age greater than 50 years, elevated serum creatinine levels, low GFR, hypertension, and findings of secondary glomerulosclerosis and chronic tubulointerstitial changes on kidney biopsy. Because of the high rate of spontaneous remission of membranous glomerulopathy, persistent proteinuria of ≥4 g/24 h for more than 6 months and a decline in the slope of GFR over time are the most important risk factors associated with progression of membranous glomerulopathy to advanced CKD.

Clinical Manifestations
Membranous glomerulopathy usually presents as the nephrotic syndrome, although some patients may have asymptomatic subnephrotic proteinuria. Many patients have normal kidney function at the time of presentation. Membranous glomerulopathy has the highest prevalence of renal vein thrombosis compared with other causes of the nephrotic syndrome.

Diagnosis
Diagnosis of membranous glomerulopathy requires kidney biopsy, which shows diffuse thickening of the glomerular capillary wall on light microscopy and intramembranous electron-dense deposits initially located in the subepithelial aspect of the glomerular basement membrane on electron microscopy.

Management
Because of the potential toxicity of immunosuppressive therapies and the high rate of spontaneous remission, the clinical features and risk for disease progression should determine the most appropriate treatment in patients with primary membranous glomerulopathy (**Figure 16**). Treatment of hyperlipidemia also is recommended, with frequent (every 1-3 months) monitoring of proteinuria and GFR.

Remission is the most important factor that predicts the renal survival in patients with primary membranous glomerulopathy. Most patients with complete remission and 90% with partial remission remain free of advanced CKD or ESKD compared with 45% with persistent nephrotic syndrome within 10 years of disease onset.

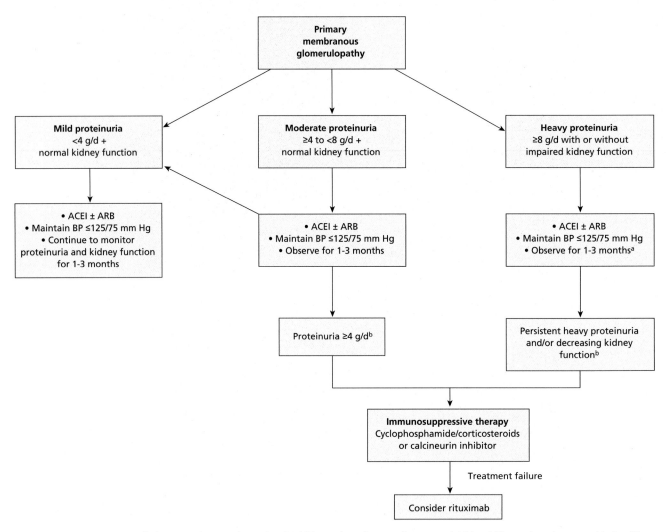

FIGURE 16. Management of primary membranous glomerulopathy. ACEI = angiotensin-converting enzyme inhibitor; ARB = angiotensin receptor blocker; BP = blood pressure.

[a]Decreasing kidney function or complication: start treatment early.

[b]Introduction of risk reduction strategies, including treatment of hyperlipidemia and consideration for prophylactic anticoagulation if patient is at low risk for bleeding and has a serum albumin level of less than 2.8 g/dL (28 g/L).

Modified with permission of the American Society of Nephrology, from J Am Soc Nephrol. Management of membranous nephropathy: when and what for treatment. Cattran D. 2005;16:1188-1194. [PMID: 15800117]; permission conveyed through Copyright Clearance Center, Inc.

Minimal Change Glomerulopathy
Epidemiology and Pathophysiology
Minimal change glomerulopathy ([MCG]; also known as minimal change disease) is associated with atopic diseases and lymphomas. It is believed to be a disorder of lymphocytes, which release immunoglobulins and cytokines that alter glomerular capillary permselectivity.

Clinical Manifestations
MCG usually presents with significant proteinuria and its consequences as the major clinical finding. Progressive CKD due to MCG is rare.

Diagnosis
Diagnosis of MCG is confirmed with kidney biopsy. Light and immunofluorescence microscopy are normal (minimal change), with electron microscopy demonstrating characteristic fusion and effacement of podocyte (visceral epithelial cell) foot processes.

Management
Most patients with MCG are responsive to daily or alternate-day prednisone, 1 mg/kg/d or 2 mg/kg every other day for 8 to 16 weeks, with complete remission achieved in approximately 70% of cases. Of those who respond to corticosteroids,

73% relapse at least one time, with most responding again to corticosteroids.

Approximately 28% of patients with MCG develop a frequently relapsing corticosteroid-dependent disease, and 25% can develop a corticosteroid-resistant disease. Immunosuppressive agents may be required in these patients.

Fibrillary and Immunotactoid Glomerulopathies
Epidemiology and Pathophysiology
Fibrillary and immunotactoid glomerulopathies are rare glomerular diseases that cause less than 1% of cases of the nephrotic syndrome in adults. Fibrillary glomerulopathy is characterized by the finding of randomly arranged fibrils with a diameter between 18 and 22 nm on electron microscopy that stain for complement and immunoglobulin, suggesting that it is an immune complex–mediated disease.

Immunotactoid glomerulopathy is characterized by the presence of organized microtubular structures with a diameter between 30 and 80 nm in the mesangium and along the subendothelial and/or subepithelial aspects of the glomerular basement membrane. In more than 60% of cases, it is associated with lymphoproliferative disorders.

Clinical Manifestations
Both fibrillary and immunotactoid glomerulopathy present in middle aged to older persons with the nephrotic syndrome, accompanied by hematuria and hypertension. Progression of kidney failure is common, with more than 50% of patients having ESKD within 10 years despite treatment.

Diagnosis
Diagnosis of both fibrillary and immunotactoid glomerulopathy is made on electron microscopy of kidney biopsy specimens showing the characteristic findings of each disorder. Assessment for the potential presence of diseases associated with these kidney findings is appropriate.

Management
No controlled trials on treatment for either disorder have been performed. Corticosteroids, cytotoxic agents, and plasmapheresis have been used, although kidney failure may progress despite therapy. Response to the treatment of an underlying lymphoproliferative disorder in immunotactoid glomerulopathy is associated with overall patient survival. ∎

KEY POINTS

- Of patients with primary focal segmental glomerulosclerosis, 39% to 45% become frequently relapsing corticosteroid-dependent or corticosteroid-resistant; many of these patients require chronic immunosuppressive therapy.

- Because of the potential toxicity of immunosuppressive therapies and the high rate of spontaneous remission, the clinical features and risk for disease progression should determine the most appropriate treatment in patients with primary membranous glomerulopathy

- Treatment with daily or alternate-day prednisone is indicated for patients with minimal change glomerulopathy.

Systemic Diseases that Cause the Nephrotic Syndrome
Diabetic Nephropathy
Epidemiology and Pathophysiology
Diabetic nephropathy is the most common glomerulopathy, developing in approximately 35% of patients with type 1 or type 2 diabetes mellitus. American Indian, Mexican-American, and black patients have a higher risk for developing diabetic nephropathy compared with white patients. Other risk factors include poor glycemic control, hypertension and/or family history of hypertension, cigarette smoking, family history of kidney involvement, and older age of onset of diabetes.

In the United States, diabetic nephropathy constitutes approximately 44% of new cases of ESKD: 6% due to type 1 diabetes and 38% due to type 2 diabetes. Hyperglycemia, hypertension, and albuminuria and/or proteinuria are modifiable risk factors associated with progressive CKD.

Hyperglycemia promotes the formation of advanced glycosylation end products in the kidney tissue and other target organs, which stimulate oxidative stress pathways conducive to damage. Glomerular hyperfiltration mediated by nitric oxide, the renin-angiotensin-aldosterone system, natriuretic peptides, and other vasoactive pathways also are important in the pathogenesis and progression of diabetic nephropathy.

Clinical Manifestations
Diabetic nephropathy results in characteristic structural changes to the kidney, including expansion of the mesangium, thickening of the basement membrane, and sclerosis of the glomeruli. Clinical manifestations typically include progressive proteinuria, a decline in kidney function, and hypertension, although the findings at presentation depend on the clinical stage at the time of diagnosis, which may be delayed, particularly in type 2 diabetes. Acute nephritic syndrome is an uncommon manifestation and should raise suspicion of concurrent glomerulonephritis.

Diagnosis
Detection of early-stage diabetic nephropathy and microalbuminuria requires annual measurement of the urine albumin–creatinine ratio for patients who have had type 1 diabetes

CONT.

for 5 years or more and for all patients with type 2 diabetes beginning at the time of diagnosis.

Longitudinal studies of high-risk patients with type 1 diabetes have delineated five clinical stages based on changes in GFR, degree of albuminuria, and development of hypertension (**Table 29**). These stages also appear to apply to type 2 diabetes except that nephropathy may occur earlier and progress more quickly, and hypertension may develop before nephropathy. However, not all patients may progress in a step-wise progression; microalbuminuria has been noted to regress in younger patients with aggressive glycemic and blood pressure control, and some patients may develop CKD without significant albuminuria. The mechanisms underlying kidney disease in these patients are not well defined.

Management

Treatment of patients with microalbuminuria or overt proteinuria in diabetic nephropathy includes tight glycemic control and careful management of hypertension with preferential use of ACE inhibitors or ARBs. In type 1 and 2 diabetic patients with microalbuminuria, randomized controlled trials indicate that achieving a hemoglobin A_{1c} of approximately 7% significantly decreased the risk of developing overt proteinuria. In type 1 or type 2 diabetic patients with nephropathy and hypertension, treatment with ACE inhibitors or ARBs significantly reduces the risk of progression compared with other antihypertensive agents. The optimal blood pressure target in type 1 and 2 diabetic patients with established nephropathy is less than 130/80 mm Hg.

Lower blood pressures may further decrease the risk of developing overt proteinuria, although more aggressive treatment is associated with potential adverse effects, including the sudden elevation of serum creatinine or reduction in the GFR, hypotension, and syncope.

Amyloidosis

Epidemiology and Pathophysiology

Amyloidosis is caused by the pathologic deposition of a protein with an altered structure that polymerizes into an insoluble form (amyloid) that is deposited into the tissues. More than 20 types of amyloidosis are classified according to the precursor protein that aggregates to form amyloid deposits. In AL amyloidosis, the most common form, the precursor protein is a monoclonal light chain, usually of the lambda isotype. AH amyloidosis results from increased production and tissue deposition of truncated monoclonal heavy chains. In AA amyloidosis, the precursor protein is amyloid AA protein, an acute phase reactant released in chronic inflammatory states such as rheumatoid arthritis, tuberculosis, and osteomyelitis. Up to 20% of patients with AL amyloidosis have a coexisting multiple myeloma or other lymphoproliferative disease.

Clinical Manifestations

AL amyloidosis is a systemic disease, and the kidney is one of the most prominently affected organs, in addition to the heart, lungs, and gastrointestinal tract. Virtually every kidney compartment can be affected by amyloidosis, but glomerular lesions predominate, resulting in the nephrotic syndrome. AL

TABLE 29. Clinical Stages of Diabetic Nephropathy in Patients with Type 1 Diabetes Mellitus		
Clinical Stage	**Manifestations**	**Occurrence**
Stage 1: Hyperfiltration	Supernormal GFR Albuminuria <30 mg/d Normal blood pressure Large kidneys on ultrasound	Within the first 5 years after onset of diabetes
Stage 2: Microalbuminuric	Normal or high GFR Albuminuria from 30-300 mg/d Prehypertension or hypertension	5-15 years after onset of diabetes
Stage 3: Overt Proteinuric	Normal or decreasing GFR Albuminuria >300 mg/d (overt proteinuria) Hypertension	10-20 years after onset of diabetes
Stage 4: Progressive	Decreasing GFR Nephrotic syndrome Hypertension	15-25 years after onset of diabetes
Stage 5: End-Stage Kidney Disease	GFR <15 mL/min/1.73 m^2 Difficult to control hypertension	20-30 years after onset of diabetes

GFR = glomerular filtration rate.

CONT.

amyloidosis has a poor prognosis with a short median survival ranging between 5 and 34 months after onset of the disease. AL amyloidosis survivors with kidney involvement generally have progressive CKD leading to ESKD within 5 years of onset. The prognosis in patients with AA amyloidosis is determined by its cause and in general is more favorable than AL amyloidosis.

Diagnosis
Definitive diagnosis of amyloidosis requires histologic confirmation. A fat pad aspirate is a minimally invasive and high-value diagnostic method for suspected amyloidosis; kidney biopsy should be considered when either fat pad aspirate or a rectal biopsy is nondiagnostic. On kidney biopsy, light microscopy reveals amorphous material effacing varying proportions of glomeruli, vessels, or interstitium that demonstrate green birefringence with the Congo red stain on polarized microscopy. Immunofluorescence microscopy demonstrates specific staining for monoclonal light or heavy chains or amyloid AA protein. The diagnosis of AL or AH amyloidosis warrants further evaluation for possible underlying multiple myeloma, including serum and urine protein electrophoresis and immunoelectrophoresis.

Management
For appropriate patients (younger patients with relatively well-preserved organ function), autologous hematopoietic stem cell transplantation may be considered. A regimen of low-dose melphalan and corticosteroids is often employed for patients who are not deemed candidates for autologous hematopoietic stem cell transplantation. The newer agents bortezomib and lenalidomide show promise and are being evaluated in ongoing clinical trials.

Multiple Myeloma
Epidemiology and Pathophysiology
Multiple myeloma is a plasma cell dyscrasia that results in neoplastic proliferation and production of a monoclonal immunoglobulin. Although multiple myeloma may cause kidney injury through different mechanisms (see Chronic Tubulointerstitial Disorders and Acute Kidney Injury), the glomerular manifestations of myeloma include amyloidosis, membranoproliferative glomerulonephritis, and deposition of light and heavy chains resulting in monoclonal immunoglobulin deposition disease.

Clinical Manifestations
The degree of kidney failure at presentation may range from mild to severe. Proteinuria is variable but generally mild, with less than 25% of patients presenting with nephrotic-range proteinuria.

Diagnosis
Kidney biopsy is recommended to confirm suspected myeloma-related kidney disease and to exclude other kidney disorders.

Management
Carefully administered intravenous fluids to establish euvolemia and maintain high urine output are used to treat dehydration, hypercalcemia, and hyperuricemia, if present. Use of plasmapheresis to remove the monoclonal immunoglobulin remains an area of controversy. Systemic chemotherapy to treat the underlying myeloma is indicated.

HIV-Associated Nephropathy
Epidemiology and Pathophysiology
HIV-associated nephropathy (HIVAN), a form of collapsing focal segmental glomerulosclerosis, occurs in approximately 3.5% to 12% of patients with HIV infection. HIVAN has a predilection to develop in black persons who are HIV positive and is currently the third leading cause of ESKD in black persons between the ages of 20 and 64 years. Other glomerular lesions seen less commonly in patients with HIV infection include IgA nephropathy, immune complex–mediated glomerulonephritis, membranoproliferative glomerulonephritis, lupus-like glomerulonephritis, membranous glomerulopathy, thrombotic microangiopathy, minimal change glomerulopathy, and amyloidosis.

Clinical Manifestations
HIVAN classically presents as the nephrotic syndrome accompanied by progressive kidney failure and large kidneys on ultrasound. HIVAN more commonly occurs in patients with advanced HIV infection but can also be seen early in infection. Hypertension and edema are uncommon.

Diagnosis
Diagnosis of HIVAN is often made on clinical grounds in patients with advanced HIV infection and typical clinical features. Patients with a rapid decline in kidney function, hypocomplementemia, dysmorphic hematuria or erythrocyte casts, or abnormal serologic studies such as cryoglobulins merit further evaluation with kidney biopsy. Because HIVAN is rare in white persons and those of Northwest European descent, biopsy should be more strongly considered in these persons if HIVAN is suspected. Light microscopic features on HIVAN include collapsing focal segmental glomerulosclerosis.

Management
Combination antiretroviral therapy is indicated and has reduced the incidence of progression to ESKD. ACE inhibitors and ARBs should be used to treat hypertension and proteinuria.

Hepatitis B Virus–Associated Kidney Disease

Epidemiology and Pathophysiology

Hepatitis B virus (HBV)–associated kidney disease is most prevalent in endemic areas, such as Asia, sub-Saharan Africa, the South Pacific, and the Middle East, and is less common in North America and Western Europe. HBV-associated kidney disease affects approximately 16% to 56% of patients with HBV infection.

The most common form of kidney disease associated with HBV infection is membranous glomerulopathy, although it may also be associated with membranoproliferative glomerulonephritis and polyarteritis nodosa (see Conditions that Cause the Nephritic Syndrome, Hepatitis B Virus–Associated Kidney Disease). Membranous glomerulopathy is particularly common in children infected with hepatitis B. It is believed that deposition of hepatitis B antigen-antibody immune complexes in the subepithelial membrane is responsible for the increased glomerular permeability and membranous glomerulopathy.

Clinical Manifestations

HBV glomerulopathy may occur in patients with serologically proven active hepatitis B, although clinically significant hepatitis may not be present. Patients with membranous glomerulopathy usually present with typical findings of the nephrotic syndrome.

Diagnosis

Diagnosis of HBV-associated kidney disease includes serologic studies for the presence of active HBV infection and kidney biopsy results consistent with membranous glomerulopathy. Complement levels may be low in HBV-associated kidney disease.

Management

Spontaneous resolution may occur, particularly in children. Remission is less common in adults, with some patients developing progressive kidney disease.

The use of an ACE inhibitor or ARB for proteinuria and/or blood pressure control is appropriate. Treatment of the underlying hepatitis infection with antiviral agents appears to be of benefit in treating the associated kidney disease. However, the use of immunosuppressive agents for treatment of severe membranous glomerulonephritis is less clear in the presence of active HBV infection.

KEY POINTS

- Detection of early-stage diabetic nephropathy and microalbuminuria requires annual measurement of the urine albumin–creatinine ratio for patients who have had type 1 diabetes for 5 years or more and for all patients with type 2 diabetes beginning at the time of diagnosis.
- Treatment of patients with microalbuminuria or overt proteinuria in diabetic nephropathy includes tight glycemic control and careful management of hypertension with preferential use of ACE inhibitors or angiotensin receptor blockers.
- Up to 20% of patients with AL amyloidosis have a coexisting multiple myeloma or other lymphoproliferative disease.

Conditions that Cause the Nephritic Syndrome

Table 30 lists the causes of the nephritic syndrome.

IgA Nephropathy

Epidemiology and Pathophysiology

IgA nephropathy, the most common primary glomerulonephritis, is an immune complex disease in which IgA antigen-antibody complexes are deposited primarily in the mesangium. IgA nephropathy may primarily involve only the kidney or may be secondarily associated with other conditions such as HIV infection, chronic liver disease, inflammatory bowel disease, or celiac disease. IgA nephropathy is the renal

Disorder	Frequency as a Cause of Primary Nephritic Syndrome[a]	Serum Complement Pattern
IgA nephropathy	25%-30%	Normal
Lupus nephritis	20%	Low C3 and C4
Pauci-immune crescentic glomerulonephritis	15%-25%	Normal
Membranoproliferative glomerulonephritis	6%-10%	Low C3 and/or low C4
Thrombotic microangiopathy	5%-8%	Low C3 in some persons
Postinfectious glomerulonephritis	4%-8%	Low C3
Anti–glomerular basement membrane antibody disease	3%	Normal
C3 glomerulopathy	<1%	Low C3

TABLE 30. Causes of the Nephritic Syndrome

[a]Based on biopsy series and therefore may not reflect true prevalence.

CONT.

lesion of Henoch-Schönlein purpura, a systemic vasculitis most commonly seen during childhood.

Primary IgA nephropathy occurs at any age and has a predilection to develop in men who are white or Asian. Approximately 20% to 30% of patients have progressive disease that can lead to ESKD within 10 to 20 years of onset. Risk factors associated with progressive CKD include younger age at onset; hypertension; proteinuria ≥1 g/24 h; elevated serum creatinine levels; low GFR; and secondary glomerulosclerosis, chronic tubulointerstitial changes, and crescents on biopsy. Persistent proteinuria (≥1 g/24 h) and hypertension are two modifiable risk factors that increase the risk of progression to advanced CKD.

Clinical Manifestations

Most patients with IgA nephropathy are asymptomatic at presentation, with only microscopic hematuria and proteinuria discovered on evaluation of the urine. A common presentation of primary IgA nephropathy is recurrent gross hematuria occurring synchronously with an episode of respiratory ("synpharyngitic hematuria") or gastrointestinal infection. This may be associated with acute kidney injury precipitated by occlusion of tubular lumina by erythrocytes and erythrocyte casts. Less frequently, patients may present with the nephrotic syndrome or RPGN.

Diagnosis

Diagnosis is confirmed by kidney biopsy, which demonstrates mesangioproliferative glomerulonephritis with IgA-dominant mesangial immune deposits on immunofluorescence microscopy.

Management

Patients who have IgA nephropathy and a low risk for progressive disease should be treated with ACE inhibitors or ARBs, with the goal to maintain urine protein excretion to less than 1 g/24 h. Hypertension is common in patients with IgA nephropathy, and optimal treatment to a blood pressure goal of less than 130/80 mm Hg is recommended. Immunosuppressive therapy should be considered for patients with persistent proteinuria (usually >1 g/24 h), progressive kidney dysfunction, or histologic findings (such as crescents) indicative of more aggressive disease.

For patients at highest risk for progressive disease, pulse and oral corticosteroids as well as alkylating regimens such as cyclophosphamide followed by azathioprine with ACE inhibitors and/or ARBs have shown a significant reduction in the risk for ESKD. Patients with milder disease are often treated with omega-3 fatty acids.

Membranoproliferative Glomerulonephritis
Epidemiology and Pathophysiology

Membranoproliferative glomerulonephritis (MPGN) most often is secondary to immune complex formation in response to chronic antigen stimulation. Traditionally, when the source of the antigen has been identified, the glomerulonephritis has been categorized as secondary MPGN I. Causes include hepatitis C virus infection (see Hepatitis C Virus–Associated Glomerulonephritis); other chronic indolent infections such as hepatitis B, syphilis, subacute bacterial endocarditis, osteomyelitis, and mastoiditis; autoimmune diseases (lupus and Sjögren); essential cryoglobulinemia (types I and II); and malignancies (carcinomas, sarcomas, lymphomas, and leukemias).

When the source of the chronic antigen cannot be identified, the process has been historically termed *primary MPGN*, with one of three histopathologic phenotypes: MPGN I, MPGN II (dense deposit disease), and MPGN III. Some cases of primary MPGN with immune complex deposition are also likely related to chronic antigen stimulation from an as yet undefined autoimmune, infectious, or neoplastic process. However, other cases are immune complex negative, develop as a consequence of abnormalities in complement regulation, and are more properly classified as C3 glomerulopathy.

Clinical Manifestations

MPGN most commonly manifests as the nephritic syndrome but may also present with heavy proteinuria, referred to as a mixed nephritic-nephrotic picture. MPGN may follow a more indolent course but may also present as an RPGN. The most important factors associated with progression of primary MPGN to advanced CKD include decreased GFR, heavy proteinuria, hypertension, and crescents and chronic tubulointerstitial disease on biopsy.

Diagnosis

Diagnosis of MPGN requires a kidney biopsy demonstrating the characteristic pathologic findings. Immunofluorescence microscopy in addition to electron microscopy may be helpful in appropriately classifying and determining the cause of the disease.

Management

Corticosteroids with immunosuppressive agents and antiplatelet agents may be beneficial in the management of primary MPGN, but more than 50% of patients progress to advanced CKD. Treatment of secondary MPGN I is directed toward the underlying cause. **H**

KEY POINTS

- IgA nephropathy may primarily involve only the kidney or may be secondarily associated with other conditions such as HIV infection, chronic liver disease, inflammatory bowel disease, or celiac disease.

- Causes of membranoproliferative glomerulonephritis include hepatitis C virus infection, other chronic indolent infections, autoimmune diseases, essential cryoglobulinemia, and malignancies.

Hepatitis C Virus–Associated Glomerulonephritis

Epidemiology and Pathophysiology

Hepatitis C virus–associated glomerulonephritis (HCV-GN) is an immune complex disease that occurs in as many as 21% of patients who have HCV infection. It most commonly presents as MPGN and mixed cryoglobulinemia and is characterized by an indolent course in one third of patients, remission in another third, and a relapsing course in the remaining patients, with potential progression to advanced CKD.

The pathogenesis of HCV-GN involves viral infection of B lymphocytes that synthesize polyclonal or monoclonal antibodies with or without a cryoprecipitating property. Circulating immune complexes are usually IgG-IgM complexes, which are often cryoglobulins, with or without HCV viral proteins that are deposited in the glomeruli. The virus also directly infects the kidney tissue.

Clinical Manifestations

HCV-GN usually manifests as the nephritic syndrome. Other manifestations include combined nephrotic-nephritic syndrome, isolated proteinuria with hematuria, RPGN, and acute and chronic kidney failure. In patients with HCV infection, HCV-GN can also be a component of a systemic cryoglobulinemic vasculitis with involvement of the skin, peripheral nerves, and musculoskeletal system.

Diagnosis

Most patients with HCV-GN have low complement levels, particularly C4, and a positive rheumatoid factor. Diagnosis is confirmed by kidney biopsy, which demonstrates the pattern of membranoproliferative glomerulonephritis with or without capillary cryoglobulin deposition on light microscopy.

Management

Combination therapy with peginterferon and ribavirin (when GFR is >50 mL/min/1.73 m^2) is indicated for patients with HCV-GN who have relatively well-preserved kidney function. Triple therapy using the protease inhibitors telaprevir or boceprevir in combination with peginterferon and ribavirin (when GFR is >50 mL/min/1.73 m^2) is indicated for patients with hepatitis C genotype I. Rituximab may benefit patients with associated hepatitis C–related cryoglobulinemia.

Hepatitis B Virus–Associated Kidney Disease

Epidemiology and Pathophysiology

HBV infection may be associated with MPGN and polyarteritis nodosa. MPGN is believed to result from deposition of virally associated antigen-antibody complexes in the subendothelial space and mesangium. Polyarteritis nodosa (PAN), a systemic medium- to large-vessel necrotizing vasculitis that occurs in up to 5% of patients with HBV infection, may also be induced by deposition of antigen-antibody immune complexes in blood vessel walls. PAN may specifically affect the medium-sized renal arteries (lobar, lobular, arcuate, and interlobular), while sparing capillaries and venules. The acute arterial injury is characterized by fibrinoid necrosis and infiltration of inflammatory cells with thrombosis, infarction, and inflammatory aneurysms.

Clinical Manifestations

HBV-associated nephritis typically presents with subnephrotic-range proteinuria and hematuria, usually without erythrocyte casts; hypertension and decreased kidney function are common. Complement levels may be low. The clinical course may be variable, with some patients having a rapidly progressive course and others developing a more chronic glomerulonephritis with a remitting-relapsing pattern. Patients with PAN typically present with fever, abdominal pain, arthralgia, and weight loss that develop over days to months. PAN also usually involves other organ systems, including the skin, muscles, nerves, gastrointestinal tract, and arterial ischemia.

Diagnosis

Diagnosis is based on demonstration of active HBV infection and compatible kidney biopsy results, although demonstration of specific antigen deposition in the kidney is not readily available. PAN is diagnosed by biopsy of affected organs or radiographically with conventional angiography, CT angiography, or MR angiography.

Management

Treatment of patients with HBV-associated kidney disease involves antiviral therapy for HBV infection. In patients with RPGN, brief courses of corticosteroids are sometimes used. In PAN, glucocorticoids with or without plasma exchange are often used in addition to treatment of the HBV infection. The optimal duration of antiviral therapy for HBV-associated kidney disease has not been established. ◪

KEY POINTS

- Hepatitis C virus–associated glomerulonephritis is an immune complex disease that most commonly presents as membranoproliferative glomerulonephritis and mixed cryoglobulinemia.
- Hepatitis B virus infection may be associated with membranoproliferative glomerulonephritis and polyarteritis nodosa.

Postinfectious Glomerulonephritis

Epidemiology and Pathophysiology

Acute postinfectious glomerulonephritis (PIGN) is an immunologic disease triggered by acute, usually self-limited, infections. Many bacteria, viruses, and parasites can cause PIGN; the most common microbes are nephritogenic strains of streptococci and staphylococci. PIGN has traditionally

CONT.

been associated with streptococcal infections of the throat and/or skin, particularly in children; however, this etiology has been declining in developed countries with more aggressive treatment of these infections. PIGN secondary to staphylococcal infections has increased, particularly in adults with diabetes, chronic liver disease, and other immunocompromised conditions.

Clinical Manifestations
PIGN presents with acute nephritis with rapid onset of edema, hypertension, oliguria, and erythrocyte casts in the urine sediment. Less commonly, PIGN manifests as RPGN or as persistent mixed nephritic-nephrotic syndrome that may progress to advanced CKD. Symptoms typically begin to remit after several weeks, with hematuria usually resolving over the course of 3 to 6 months. Proteinuria may persist 6 months or longer.

Diagnosis
Diagnosis of PIGN is usually made clinically in patients with acute onset of nephritis ≥1 week following an acute pyogenic infection. Confirmation of recent streptococcal infection by culture or an increase in anti-streptococcal antibodies such as anti-streptolysin O or anti-DNAse B lends further support to the diagnosis. C3 levels are decreased, and C4 levels are usually normal. Kidney biopsy is reserved for patients with atypical features such as progressive kidney dysfunction or when the clinical findings fail to remit at the expected rate.

Management
Early treatment of bacterial infections with appropriate antibiotics can prevent or lessen the severity of PIGN.

Management of established PIGN is supportive, aiming to control the manifestations of the disease, particularly volume overload with diuretics, antihypertensives, and, if necessary, dialysis. Corticosteroids with or without immunosuppressive agents are occasionally used but without evidence of proven benefit.

Lupus Nephritis
Epidemiology and Pathophysiology
Kidney involvement is common in patients with systemic lupus erythematosus (SLE). The cumulative incidence of lupus nephritis is higher in Asian, black, and Hispanic patients compared with white patients.

Lupus nephritis is an immune complex–mediated disease typically occurring in patients with readily identifiable extrarenal manifestations of SLE. Involvement of the renal vasculature is also common, ranging from indolent vascular immune deposits to fibrinoid necrosis and thrombotic microangiopathy. Nephritogenic anti–double-stranded DNA antibodies play a critical role in the pathogenesis of lupus nephritis.

Lupus nephritis can be divided into six distinct histologic categories (**Table 31**). Classes I and II have a similar indolent course and are common in white patients. Classes III and IV, and class V when combined with class III or IV, are severe, leading to permanent, chronic damage; these classes are more frequent in black, Hispanic, and Asian patients. Class V, alone without class III or IV, may have an indolent prolonged course but also can have a severe course, particularly when occurring with resistant nephrotic syndrome. Class VI is the result of permanent damage secondary to severe lupus nephritis. The categorization of lupus nephritis is not a continuum of the same disease, and most patients remain with

TABLE 31. International Society of Nephrology/Renal Pathology Society 2003 Classification of Glomerulonephritis in Systemic Lupus Erythematosus

Class	Histopathology	Comments
I	Minimal mesangial glomerulonephritis	Normal in light microscopy, but immune-complex deposits with immunofluorescence microscopy and/or electro-dense deposits by electron microscopy; good prognosis
II	Mesangial proliferative glomerulonephritis	Mesangial hypercellularity on light microscopy; mesangial immune-complex deposits; good prognosis
III	Focal proliferative glomerulonephritis	Involves <50% of all glomeruli with intracapillary proliferation, segmental or global active lesions; subendothelial immune-complex deposits; bad prognosis without adequate management
IV	Diffuse proliferative glomerulonephritis	Involves ≥50% of all glomeruli with intracapillary proliferation, segmental or global active lesions; subendothelial immune-complex deposits; bad prognosis without adequate management
V	Membranous glomerulonephritis	Characterized by thickening of the basement membrane, subepithelial immune-complex deposits. It can occur in combination with class III or IV; bad prognosis without adequate management
VI	Advanced sclerosing glomerulonephritis	≥90% of glomeruli globally sclerosed without residual activity; the results of progressive unresponsive severe glomerulonephritis

Modified with permission of the American Society of Nephrology, from The classification of glomerulonephritis in systemic lupus erythematosus revisited. Weening JJ, D'Agati VD, Schwartz MM, et al. J Am Soc Nephrol. 2004;15(2):241-250. [PMID: 14747370], Copyright 2004.

CONT.

the same class; however, transformation may be observed from one class to another.

Clinical Manifestations

Kidney manifestations often develop concurrently or shortly following the onset of SLE. Risk factors for progressive kidney disease are male gender; black and Hispanic ethnicity; young age; crescents in more than 50% of the glomeruli and high chronicity index on biopsy; initial high serum creatinine levels that do not normalize with treatment; the nephrotic syndrome that does not undergo remission with treatment; relapse; hypertension; noncompliance; anemia; and the presence of antiphospholipid antibodies.

Diagnosis

Diagnosis of lupus nephritis is suggested by proteinuria (>500 mg/24 h) or cellular casts (erythrocytes or leukocytes) in the urine sediment of patients fulfilling the formal criteria for the diagnosis of SLE (see MKSAP 16 Rheumatology). Most patients with active lupus nephritis have low complement levels. Kidney biopsy is indicated to define both the histologic subtype and the degree of disease activity and chronicity essential for planning appropriate therapy.

Management

Treatment with ACE inhibitors or ARBs is indicated for proteinuria in patients with class I or II lupus nephritis. Extrarenal manifestations may require treatment with corticosteroids or quinine derivatives. Patients with the proliferative classes III, IV, and V in combination with III or IV require immunosuppressive agents to induce remission, prevent relapse, and reduce the risk of progressive CKD without substantial adverse events. Several treatment regimens for induction and maintenance have been shown to be effective.

Without adequate management, classes III, IV, or class V combined with class III or IV generally are progressive, with a probability of ESKD as high as 50% to 70% after 5 to 10 years of diagnosis. However, overall survival in SLE patients with severe lupus nephritis has improved to more than 80% over the past two decades, which is likely attributable to the rational use of effective immunosuppressive therapy as well as the availability of dialysis and kidney transplantation. **H**

KEY POINTS

- Postinfectious glomerulonephritis presents with acute nephritis with rapid onset of edema, hypertension, oliguria, and erythrocyte casts in the urine sediment.
- In patients with lupus nephritis, kidney biopsy is indicated to define both the histologic subtype and the degree of disease activity and chronicity essential for planning appropriate therapy.

Anti–Glomerular Basement Membrane Antibody Disease

H

Epidemiology and Pathophysiology

Anti–glomerular basement membrane (GBM) antibody disease is mediated by an autoantibody to the GBM. Antigen-antibody complexes develop along the extent of the GBM, leading to an influx of inflammatory cells and mediators and resulting in necrotizing crescentic glomerulonephritis. The disease may be renal-limited, in which case it is called anti–GBM nephritis. When both the lung and the kidney are involved, it is referred to as Goodpasture syndrome.

Anti-GBM antibody disease is found in approximately 15% of patients who manifest RPGN. Younger patients are more likely to present with Goodpasture syndrome with both diffuse pulmonary hemorrhage and glomerulonephritis, whereas older patients may have only glomerulonephritis. Anti-GBM antibody disease is generally severe, with approximately 60% to 70% of patients rapidly progressing to ESKD within a few months after onset. At presentation, serum creatinine levels of more than 5.0 mg/dL (442 micromoles/L), oliguria, crescents in more than 80% of glomeruli (particularly of the circumferential and fibrous types), and a high degree of tubular atrophy and interstitial fibrosis observed on biopsy are risk factors associated with poor kidney survival. Patient survival is approximately 75% to 90% after 1 year of presentation. Risk factors associated with high mortality include sepsis as well as severe kidney and pulmonary manifestations.

Clinical Manifestations

Anti-GBM antibody disease usually manifests as RPGN. Nephrotic-range proteinuria is rare. Pulmonary manifestations often develop concurrently or shortly before and/or after onset of the glomerulonephritis. Hemoptysis is a common pulmonary manifestation usually seen in the context of moderate to severe respiratory failure, with patchy or diffuse alveolar infiltrates.

Diagnosis

Anti-GBM antibody disease can be rapidly confirmed by kidney biopsy, which shows diffuse necrotizing crescentic glomerulonephritis with linear staining of the GBM with fluorescein-tagged anti-IgG antibodies on immunofluorescence microscopy. The presence of circulating antibodies of the IgG type specific for the GBM may be useful in the diagnosis of this disease.

Management

The combined use of plasmapheresis using albumin replacement for 1 to 2 weeks with cyclophosphamide and corticosteroids for 3 to 6 months is more effective at inducing remission when instituted early during the disease for both kidney and lung manifestations. Although relapse is rare, azathioprine maintenance for 1 to 2 years is recommended.

Small- and Medium-Vessel Vasculitis
Epidemiology and Pathophysiology
A group of vasculitis-related conditions that may affect the kidney is termed *pauci-immune crescentic glomerulonephritis* (PICG). The three major disease entities associated with PICG are granulomatosis with polyangiitis (also known as Wegener granulomatosis), microscopic polyangiitis, and Churg-Strauss syndrome. These diseases are the most common form of crescentic glomerulonephritis and are defined pathologically by the absence of glomerular immune complexes or anti–GBM antibodies on immunofluorescence microscopy. ANCA detected in most patients is pathogenic. PICG may occur as a renal-limited process or as an element of systemic small-vessel vasculitis. Patients with granulomatous inflammation (often involving the respiratory tract) and PICG are categorized as having granulomatosis with polyangiitis; those without granulomatous inflammation and systemic vasculitis are classified as having microscopic polyangiitis; and those with concurrent asthma and eosinophilia have Churg-Strauss syndrome.

PICG associated with granulomatosis with polyangiitis or microscopic polyangiitis is an aggressive disorder, with approximately 43% of patients progressing to ESKD within 12 months after onset. Risk factors associated with poor renal survival include oliguria, crescents in more than 80% of glomeruli (particularly of the circumferential and fibrous types), and a high degree of tubular atrophy and interstitial fibrosis. Patient survival is more than 75% 2 years after presentation. Risk factors associated with high mortality include older age, severe kidney and pulmonary involvement, and the development of sepsis.

Clinical Manifestations
PICG usually presents as RPGN (glomerular hematuria, proteinuria, pyuria, hypertension, signs of hypervolemia, and a rapid decline of GFR).

Diagnosis
Kidney biopsy shows necrotizing crescentic glomerulonephritis or necrotizing vasculitis of microscopic vessels such as the small arteries, arterioles, capillaries, or venules. Proteinase 3- or myeloperoxidase-ANCA, as determined by enzyme-linked immunoassay, is positive in approximately 90% of patients with granulomatosis with polyangiitis, 70% of patients with microscopic polyangiitis, and 50% of patients with Churg-Strauss syndrome, lending further support for the diagnosis.

Management
Treatment with immunosuppressive agents is indicated to induce remission, prevent relapse, and reduce the risk of ESKD and mortality. Induction with cyclophosphamide and corticosteroids followed by long-term maintenance therapy with azathioprine and corticosteroids is highly effective in inducing remission and preventing relapse in patients with moderate disease. Patients with severe kidney injury may also benefit from plasmapheresis using albumin replacement. The use of rituximab for patients with PICG and moderate small-vessel vasculitis has shown an equivalent efficacy and safety compared with regimens of immunosuppressive agents with corticosteroids in patients with relatively well-preserved kidney function. Rituximab is generally reserved for patients who cannot tolerate or refuse therapy with cyclophosphamide.

Cryoglobulinemic Vasculitis
Epidemiology and Pathophysiology
Cryoglobulinemia is characterized by the presence of temperature-sensitive monoclonal immunoglobulins, which may precipitate and deposit in vessel walls most prominently in the skin and glomerular capillaries, eliciting an inflammatory response, systemic vasculitis, and glomerulonephritis. Cryoglobulinemic vasculitis is most often associated with hepatitis C virus infection but has also been reported in patients with HIV infection, lymphoproliferative disorders, and plasma cell dyscrasias.

Clinical Manifestations
Extrarenal manifestations of cryoglobulinemia may include cutaneous vasculitis and Raynaud phenomenon. Cryoglobulinemia-associated kidney disease findings may vary based on the degree of immune complex and thrombotic disease, but most patients have progressive disease within 3 to 5 years of diagnosis.

Diagnosis
In cryoglobulinemia, kidney biopsy demonstrates a membranoproliferative pattern on light microscopy, with curved microtubular aggregates of cryoglobulins in the subendothelial zone on electron microscopy.

Management
Cryoglobulinemia is treated by addressing the underlying cause, and plasmapheresis and immunosuppressive agents may be indicated to remove and decrease the production of cryoglobulins.

Thrombotic Microangiopathy
Epidemiology and Pathophysiology
Thrombotic microangiopathy is a systemic disease that is usually characterized by thrombocytopenia and microangiopathic hemolytic anemia, which commonly involves the kidney. The causes of thrombotic microangiopathy are listed in **Table 32**.

Thrombotic thrombocytopenic purpura (TTP) is associated with decreased activity of the von Willebrand factor–cleaving protease (now termed a disintegrin and metalloprotease with a thrombospondin type 1 motif, member 13 [*ADAMTS13*]). In addition, inhibitory antibodies can be

TABLE 32. Causes of Thrombotic Microangiopathy
Infectious agents
Enteric pathogens
Escherichia coli O157:H7
Escherichia coli O104:H4
Campylobacter jejuni
Yersinia, Shigella, and *Salmonella* species
HIV infection
Mycoplasma pneumoniae
Legionella species
Coxsackie A and B viruses
Systemic disorders
Systemic lupus erythematosus
Thrombotic thrombocytopenic purpura
Hemolytic uremic syndrome
The antiphospholipid syndrome
Systemic sclerosis
Malignant hypertension
Neoplasms
Medications
Clopidogrel
Ticlopidine
Calcineurin inhibitors
Mitomycin C
Vinblastine
Cisplatin
Bleomycin
Cytosine arabinoside
Gemcitabine
Daunorubicin
Quinine
Vaccinations
Yellow fever
Influenza
Measles-mumps-rubella
Organ transplantation

CONT.

produced, resulting in ultra-large von Willebrand factor multimers that promote thrombosis.

Hemolytic uremic syndrome (HUS) is typically caused by enteric pathogens such as the *Escherichia coli* O157:H7 strain and is characterized by the binding of Shiga-like toxin to the endothelium, causing activation of inflammatory pathways and platelets and resulting in thrombosis. Atypical HUS is defined by the absence of diarrhea or Shiga toxin–producing infection and is associated with HIV infection, streptococcal pneumonia, and a number of genetic disorders resulting from abnormalities in complement regulation.

Clinical Manifestations

TTP and HUS are forms of thrombotic microangiopathy that share a similar clinical presentation of fever, hemolytic anemia, consumptive thrombocytopenia, neurologic findings, and kidney failure.

In other forms of thrombotic microangiopathy, clinical manifestations may occur that are related to the underlying disorder. Scleroderma renal crisis, for example, presents in patients with signs of systemic sclerosis often accompanied by severe hypertension and progressive kidney disease.

Diagnosis

Diagnosis is often made based on clinical findings of microangiopathic hemolytic anemia and acute kidney injury. Kidney biopsy is often not possible due to severe thrombocytopenia. If the diagnosis remains uncertain, patients with acceptable coagulation parameters may be candidates for kidney biopsy.

Management

Treatment of thrombotic microangiopathy varies according to its cause. Plasma exchange therapy with immunosuppressive agents is indicated for most adults with TTP, HUS, and SLE. Plasma exchange, however, is generally not indicated for patients with thrombotic microangiopathy that develops following transplantation or cancer chemotherapy. Aggressive control of blood pressure with antihypertensive agents such as ACE inhibitors or ARBs is indicated in patients with systemic sclerosis and malignant hypertension. Treatment with anticoagulation, glucocorticoids, and plasma exchange with or without intravenous immune globulin is recommended for patients with catastrophic antiphospholipid syndrome and associated thrombotic microangiopathy. Eculizumab, a monoclonal antibody directed toward complement component C5, has been approved for treatment of atypical HUS in adults. However, it is very expensive, and its role in treatment of HUS has not yet been established. **H**

KEY POINTS

- When both the lung and the kidney are involved, anti–glomerular basement membrane antibody disease is referred to as Goodpasture syndrome.

- Pauci-immune crescentic glomerulonephritis associated with granulomatosis with polyangiitis (also known as Wegener granulomatosis) or microscopic polyangiitis is treated with immunosuppressive agents to induce remission, prevent relapse, and reduce the risk of end-stage kidney disease and mortality.

- Cryoglobulinemic vasculitis is most often associated with hepatitis C virus infection but has also been reported in patients with HIV infection, lymphoproliferative disorders, and plasma cell dyscrasias.

- Thrombotic thrombocytopenic purpura and hemolytic uremic syndrome are forms of thrombotic microangiopathy that share a similar clinical presentation of fever, hemolytic anemia, consumptive thrombocytopenia, neurologic findings, and kidney failure.

Genetic [ ]
Kidney [ ]

Kidney C[ ]

End-stage kid[ ]
disorders in a[ ]
the genetic a[ ]
cystic disord[ ]

Autoso[ ]
Disease[ ]

Autosom[ ] D) is
the mos[ ] nited
States, A[ ] o 10%
of pati[ ] mes 16
(PKD[ ] 5% and
15% [ ]

Scr[ ]

Scr[ ] formed by
ki[ ] ngs include
la[ ] oth kidneys.
[ ] r all types of
[ ] omatic adults
[ ] efits of screen-
[ ] erienced coun-

[ ] absence of cysts
[ ] egative rate of 2%.
[ ] is not conclusive.
[ ] e 30 is specific for

[ ]nent

[ ]lude kidney enlarge-
[ ]. Urinary concentrat-
[ ] production are com-
[ ] is common and usually
[ ]ade. ESKD occurs, on

average, at age 54 in patients with *PKD1* and age 74 in those with *PKD2*.

In more than 50% of patients with ADPKD, recurrent pain localized to the flank or back occurs, which can result from kidney enlargement, bleeding, infection, and stones. Hematuria usually indicates cyst rupture and is commonly self-limited, resolving within a week. If it persists, radiographic imaging is indicated. The incidence of renal cancers is the same as in the general population.

Infections are most commonly due to infected cysts and acute pyelonephritis caused by gram-negative organisms that ascend from the urinary tract. Treatment of cyst infection requires antibiotics that are capable of penetrating the cyst such as a fluoroquinolone or trimethoprim-sulfamethoxazole.

In patients with ADPKD, kidney stones are predominantly composed of uric acid, with most others comprised of calcium oxalate. Short-term therapy includes analgesics and hydration. Hypertension is common in patients with ADPKD, and treatment with an ACE inhibitor or an angiotensin receptor blocker to a blood pressure target of less than 130/80 mm Hg is indicated. Low-grade proteinuria is typically present and is tubular in origin. Nephrotic-range proteinuria should raise suspicion for an additional glomerular process.

Cardiovascular disease is the most common cause of death in patients with ADPKD; therefore, modifiable cardiovascular risk factors should be treated aggressively. Extrarenal manifestations include diverticulosis; hernias; cysts in the pancreas, spleen, thyroid, and seminal vesicles; and cysts in the liver in approximately 40% of patients. Intracranial cerebral aneurysms (ICAs) occur in approximately 8% of patients with ADPKD; experts recommend screening for ICAs using MR angiography of the cerebral arteries in patients with a positive family history of ICAs.

Therapies under investigation include rapamycin and vasopressin receptor antagonists to slow the progression of ADPKD. Increased fluid intake should be encouraged to suppress excess plasma vasopressin secretion to possibly inhibit cyst growth.

Kidney Cystic Disorders			
Di[ ]		Gene Mutation	Clinical Features
ADPKD	AD	*PKD1*; *PKD2*	Cerebral aneurysm; mitral valve prolapse; extrarenal (hepatic) cysts; kidney stones; diverticulitis
ARPKD	AR	*PKHD1*	Presents in infancy; hypertension; hepatic fibrosis
Tuberous Sclerosis	AD	*TSC1*; *TSC2*	Angiofibromas; angiolipomas; hamartomas
MCKD I; MCKD II	AD	Unknown; uromodulin abnormalities	Hyperuricemia and gout in MCKD II; progress variably to ESKD between ages 20 and 70 years

AD = autosomal dominant; ADPKD = autosomal dominant polycystic kidney disease; AR = autosomal recessive; ARPKD = autosomal recessive polycystic kidney disease; ESKD = end-stage kidney disease; MCKD = medullary cystic kidney disease.

- Kidney manifestations of autosomal dominant polycystic kidney disease include kidney enlargement, back or flank pain, hematuria, infections, kidney stones, hypertension, and low-grade proteinuria.

- Treatment of hypertension with an ACE inhibitor or angiotensin receptor blocker to a blood pressure target of less than 130/80 mm Hg is indicated for patients with autosomal dominant polycystic kidney disease.

- Extrarenal manifestations of autosomal dominant polycystic kidney disease include diverticulosis; hernias; cysts in the liver, pancreas, spleen, thyroid, and seminal vesicles; and intracranial cerebral aneurysms.

Autosomal Recessive Polycystic Kidney Disease

Autosomal recessive polycystic kidney disease (ARPKD) is a rare inherited disorder caused by mutations in the *PKHD1* gene, which encodes for fibrocystin on chromosome 6. More severe disease presents earlier in life; massive kidney enlargement due to cystic dilation of the renal tubules may be seen at birth. Progressive kidney failure is common, with hepatic fibrosis and portal hypertension being more pronounced in patients presenting after infancy. Most patients present with hypertension and growth retardation.

There are no specific treatments to delay the progression of ARPKD. Dialysis and kidney or kidney-liver transplantation are appropriate therapies. Parents of children with ARPKD should be counseled about the 1 in 4 chance of disease in future children.

Tuberous Sclerosis Complex

Clinical Manifestations

Tuberous sclerosis complex (TSC) is an autosomal dominant disorder resulting from mutations in the *TSC1* or *TSC2* gene. This neurocutaneous disorder involves many organ systems and is characterized by benign hamartomas of the kidney, brain, skin, or other organs.

The most common kidney manifestations are kidney cysts and angiomyolipomas. Angiomyolipomas occur in 75% of patients and are detected by CT or MRI. Complications include pain and hemorrhage, which can be benign or, rarely, can result in kidney failure or death. Renal cell carcinoma is much less common, occurring in 1% to 2% of adults with the disorder. Ultrasonographic surveillance is recommended to monitor lesion growth and malignant transformation.

Diagnosis

Diagnostic criteria require either the presence of at least two major features or one major feature and two minor features. Major criteria include facial angiofibromas, three or more hypomelanotic macules, kidney angiomyolipomas, and retinal hamartomas. Minor criteria include nonrenal hamartomas, multiple kidney cysts, and various dental abnormalities such as pits on dental enamel and gingival fibromas.

Management

Everolimus has shown promise in reducing kidney angiomyolipomas but is not yet an established therapy. Other interventions include arterial embolization of angiomyolipomas, which can decrease the risk of bleeding, pain, and concern for malignancy.

Medullary Cystic Kidney Disease

The medullary cystic kidney diseases (MCKD I and MCKD II) are rare autosomal dominant disorders that often appear during the teenage years. The causative mutation is unknown, but most cases result from mutations in the gene for uromodulin, also called Tamm-Horsfall mucoprotein.

Types I and II have similar clinical manifestations, including impaired kidney function, mild urinary concentrating defects, minimal proteinuria, and a benign urine sediment. On ultrasonographic imaging, medullary cysts can be seen but are not present in most cases. Diagnosis is often suspected based on clinical findings and family history and can be confirmed by genetic testing.

Optimal treatment strategies are not clear, aside from the general management of CKD. Allopurinol should be considered for patients with hyperuricemia and gout.

- Hepatic fibrosis and portal hypertension are more pronounced in patients who present with autosomal recessive polycystic kidney disease after infancy.

- The most common kidney manifestations of tuberous sclerosis complex are angiomyolipomas and kidney cysts.

Noncystic Disorders

Alport Syndrome

Alport syndrome, also termed hereditary nephritis, is an inherited glomerular disease arising from mutations in genes that code for $\alpha 3$, $\alpha 4$, or $\alpha 5$ chain of type IV collagen. This disease is X-linked in 80% of patients, autosomal recessive in 15%, and autosomal dominant in 5%. Alport syndrome most commonly occurs in men, and women usually have a milder form of disease.

Alport syndrome is characterized by sensorineural hearing loss, ocular abnormalities, microscopic hematuria, and a family history of kidney disease and deafness. These signs and symptoms are due to disruption of the basement membrane in the affected organ. Proteinuria, hypertension, and CKD usually develop over time. ESKD commonly occurs between the late teenage years and the fourth decade of life. The autosomal dominant form may manifest somewhat later.

Diagnosis is confirmed by either skin or kidney biopsy, which reveals the absence of type IV collagen. Expression of type IV collagen can be variable in women owing to lyonization of the X chromosome.

There are no specific therapies for Alport syndrome. Kidney transplantation is the optimal treatment for ESKD, and patients have no risk for disease recurrence. However, approximately 5% of patients develop anti–glomerular basement membrane antibody disease after transplantation.

Thin Glomerular Basement Membrane Disease

Thin glomerular basement membrane disease, also known as benign familial hematuria, is a set of heterogeneous conditions that result in hematuria. Some are heterozygous mutations that encode for α3 and α4 chains of type IV collagen. Up to 5% of the population may be affected. This disease is characterized by microscopic or macroscopic hematuria, which often initially occurs in childhood, as well as a family history suggestive of the condition. Long-term prognosis is excellent, with rare progression to CKD. Blood pressure control and drugs to decrease proteinuria are reasonable goals in this population.

Fabry Disease

Fabry disease is a rare X-linked disorder of α-galactosidase A deficiency, an error of the glycosphingolipid pathway. Clinical manifestations arise from the progressive deposit of globotriaosylceramide (Gb3) in lysosomes.

This disease should be considered in young men with urinary concentrating defects, proteinuria, or CKD. Other manifestations include premature coronary artery disease, severe neuropathic pain, telangiectasias, and angiokeratomas.

Screening for Fabry disease is recommended for family members of affected patients. Enzyme replacement therapy with recombinant human α-galactosidase A is effective.

KEY POINTS

- Alport syndrome is characterized by sensorineural hearing loss, ocular abnormalities, microscopic hematuria, and a family history of kidney disease and deafness.

- Thin glomerular basement membrane disease is characterized by microscopic or macroscopic hematuria, which often initially occurs in childhood, as well as a family history suggestive of the condition.

- Clinical manifestations of Fabry disease include urinary concentrating defects, proteinuria, chronic kidney disease, premature coronary artery disease, severe neuropathic pain, telangiectasias, and angiokeratomas.

Acute Kidney Injury

Pathophysiology and Epidemiology

Acute kidney injury (AKI) indicates recent-onset damage to the kidneys. As opposed to chronic kidney disease (CKD), which by definition is present for 3 months, AKI occurs within hours to weeks. Kidney injury refers to the impaired ability of the kidneys to perform their normal physiologic functions: maintaining electrolyte and volume balance and homeostasis. Patients with AKI may recover some or all of the lost kidney function.

Multiple pathophysiologic mechanisms can lead to AKI, which can be grouped into three categories: prerenal, intrinsic, or postrenal. The likelihood of the cause of injury depends on the clinical setting. Prerenal causes occur more commonly in outpatient settings, and intrinsic causes are more common in the hospital. Prerenal kidney injury and intrinsic kidney injury due to ischemia are part of a spectrum, with ischemic intrinsic kidney injury a possible outcome in severe prerenal kidney injury. The incidence of AKI is estimated at 1% of patients who present to the hospital. Among hospitalized patients, the incidence can range from 7% to up to 50% of patients in the intensive care unit.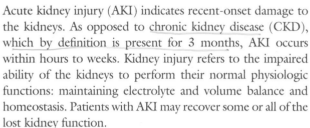

KEY POINTS

- Acute kidney injury indicates recent-onset damage to the kidneys and occurs within hours to weeks.

- The three categories of acute kidney injury are prerenal, intrinsic, and postrenal; the likelihood of the cause of injury depends on the clinical setting.

Definition and Classification

The Acute Dialysis Quality Initiative initially developed the RIFLE criteria to help clarify the definition of AKI. Subsequently, the Acute Kidney Injury Network (AKIN) modified and simplified these criteria (**Table 34**). AKI can be defined by either an increase in serum creatinine or a decline in urine output, with different stages defined by the amount of elevation in serum creatinine or decrease in urine output.

Clinical Manifestations and Diagnosis

The underlying cause of AKI (such as hypovolemia or vasculitis) often determines the symptoms. Excluding the symptoms attributable to the underlying diagnosis, the symptoms from AKI are variable and dependent on the severity of the kidney insult. Many patients have AKI without any symptoms; in these cases, the episode of AKI is recognized only by laboratory test results. If the AKI is severe, symptoms of uremia (malaise, anorexia, nausea, vomiting) can occur. There may be decreased urine output, which may go unnoticed by

TABLE 34. Acute Kidney Injury Network Criteria for the Classification of Acute Kidney Injury

Stage	Serum Creatinine Criteria	Urine Output Criteria
1	Cr ↑ by 1.5-2× or Cr ↑ by 0.3 mg/dL (26.5 μmol/L) or more	<0.5 mL/kg/h for 6 h
2	Cr ↑ by 2-3×	<0.5 mL/kg/h for 12 h
3	Cr ↑ by more than 3× or Cr increase of 0.5 mg/dL, with baseline Cr ≥4 mg/dL (354 μmol/L)	<0.3 mL/kg/h for 24 h (or anuria for 12 h)

Cr = serum creatinine.

Data from Bellomo R, Ronco C, Kellum JA, Mehta RL, Palevsky P; Acute Dialysis Quality Initiative Workgroup: Acute renal failure-definition, outcome measures, animal models, fluid therapy and information technology needs: the Second International Consensus Conference of the Acute Dialysis Quality Initiative (ADQI) Group. Crit Care. 2004;8(4):R204-R212. [PMID:15312219]

the patient. Symptoms from volume overload (edema, dyspnea) and electrolyte abnormalities (muscle weakness, palpitations/arrhythmias) may also occur.

Diagnosis of AKI relies on an accurate history and physical examination as well as laboratory tests, including urine studies and imaging. A complete history includes both a full review of systems to evaluate for systemic diseases that can cause AKI and a detailed review of recent historical events that could cause kidney damage or compromise blood flow to the kidneys. The presence of diseases that damage the kidneys over time (diabetes mellitus, hypertension, vascular disease) helps identify patients at higher risk for kidney damage. A history of AKI is associated with future development of CKD as well as a predisposition to future AKI.

The diagnostic evaluation for AKI includes a review of recent serum creatinine levels, repeat kidney function studies, urine electrolytes and osmolality, and a urinalysis. **Figure 17** shows the typical urine microscopy and urine chemistry findings for the classes of AKI.

When testing for measures of kidney function, special mention should be made concerning certain medications. Trimethoprim-sulfamethoxazole or histamine H_2 receptor blockers can cause a rise in serum creatinine that may be interpreted as AKI. This rise is due to decreased tubular secretion of creatinine and is reversible when the medications are discontinued.

The urine sodium, fractional excretion of sodium (FE_{Na}), and urine osmolality help differentiate between prerenal and intrinsic causes of AKI (see Figure 17), particularly oliguric AKI, with oliguria defined as urine output less than 500 mL/d. Prerenal causes of AKI are associated with kidney retention of sodium, a low FE_{Na}, and elevated urine osmolality. Recent diuretic use can alter the urine sodium, making urine sodium and FE_{Na} less reliable in assessing for a prerenal cause; the fractional excretion of other substances (urea, uric acid) may be more accurate in this setting. **Table 35** shows how to calculate a fractional excretion and lists which tests are useful in the presence of diuretics. Multiple calculators for fractional excretion are available online.

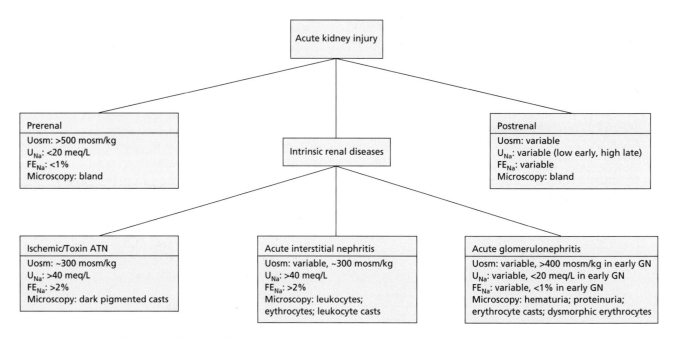

FIGURE 17. Urine findings associated with acute kidney injury. ATN = acute tubular necrosis; FE_{Na} = fractional excretion of sodium; GN = glomerulonephritis; U_{Na} = urine sodium; Uosm = urine osmolality.

TABLE 35. Fractional Excretion of Various Solutes in Oliguric Acute Kidney Injury[a]

Fractional Excretion of	Level Suggesting Prerenal Acute Kidney Injury	Altered by Diuretics
Sodium	<1%	Yes
Urea	<35%	No
Uric acid	<10%	No

[a]Calculation of fractional excretion of substance X:

(Urine Concentration of X/Plasma Concentration of X) ÷ (Urine Concentration of Creatinine/Plasma Concentration of Creatinine)

Preexisting kidney disease may also alter urine sodium handling and decrease the effectiveness of fractional excretion calculations at differentiating prerenal azotemia from other intrinsic AKI causes.

Although glomerulonephritis can cause a low urine sodium and a low FE_{Na}, glomerulonephritis is better differentiated from prerenal causes of kidney injury by blood, protein, and/or casts found in the urine. Urinalysis findings of blood, protein, dysmorphic erythrocytes, or erythrocyte casts suggest a glomerular insult. The urine sediment in prerenal kidney injury and obstructive kidney injury is often bland. Pigmented granular casts suggest acute tubular necrosis or rhabdomyolysis.

In patients with AKI, it is important to use imaging to look for obstructive causes. Ultrasonography is the preferred test because it does not involve radiation or contrast. A noncontrast CT can also evaluate for obstruction but exposes the patient to radiation. The use of contrast agents in patients with AKI is discussed in the Contrast-Induced Nephropathy section.

KEY POINTS

- Patients with suspected acute kidney injury (AKI) should undergo a complete history to evaluate for systemic diseases as well as a detailed review of recent historical events that could cause AKI.
- Urine studies and urinalysis findings can help differentiate between prerenal and intrinsic causes of acute kidney injury.
- In patients with acute kidney injury, ultrasonography is the preferred test to look for obstructive causes because it does not involve radiation or contrast.

Causes
Prerenal Azotemia
Prerenal azotemia results from hypovolemia and low blood flow to the kidney. In the classic setting of hypovolemia, the kidneys sense both the lower blood pressure in the afferent arteriole and the lower solute and urine flow rate through the juxtaglomerular apparatus; as a result, activation of the renin-angiotensin-aldosterone system leads to increased tubular

reabsorption of sodium. In prerenal azotemia, the tubules are still functional; therefore, the urine sodium is low, which reflects the reabsorption of sodium from the tubular urine. Increased water reabsorption under the influence of increased antidiuretic hormone results in concentrated urine and decreased urine output. The typical urine studies for prerenal azotemia are listed in Figure 17.

Prerenal azotemia is often associated with a high blood urea nitrogen (BUN)–creatinine ratio. In the tubules, urea is reabsorbed via urea transporters, whereas creatinine is secreted. In patients with prerenal azotemia, both BUN and creatinine can increase, but BUN often increases disproportionately more than creatinine, as the slow flow through the tubules allows more time for BUN to be reabsorbed (decreasing BUN clearance and increasing the BUN) and creatinine to be secreted (increasing creatinine clearance, particularly when compared with BUN clearance). Antidiuretic hormone also increases the expression of urea transporters, thereby further enhancing urea reabsorption in states of hypovolemia.

Prerenal azotemia is the most common cause of AKI in the outpatient setting. The kidney functions properly in patients with prerenal azotemia, and appropriate treatment with hydration should result in a quick recovery. The cause is usually evident from the history, which may reveal poor oral intake, increased volume losses (such as from diarrhea, vomiting, or diuretics), or both poor intake and increased losses. Symptoms such as dizziness and lightheadedness may accompany the hypovolemia. The physical examination may be notable for signs of volume depletion with decreased skin turgor, a low blood pressure, tachycardia, and orthostasis; however, these findings are not sensitive, and laboratory tests are indicated to confirm the diagnosis.

Treatment with 0.9% saline should reverse the prerenal state in patients with true volume depletion. Patients can also have prerenal physiology (a sodium avid kidney) in the setting of a decreased effective arterial blood volume from decompensated heart failure, cirrhosis, or the nephrotic syndrome. In these conditions, the kidney retains salt and water even though the patient has an increased total body volume and edema. For this type of prerenal azotemia, correction of the underlying disease is indicated (see Hepatorenal Syndrome and Cardiorenal Syndrome).

KEY POINTS

- Prerenal azotemia is the most common cause of acute kidney injury in the outpatient setting.
- The kidney functions properly in patients with prerenal azotemia, and appropriate treatment with hydration should result in a quick recovery.

Intrinsic Kidney Diseases

Acute Tubular Necrosis
Acute tubular necrosis (ATN) is the most common cause of intrinsic kidney disease causing AKI. ATN usually occurs after

CONT.

an ischemic event or exposure to nephrotoxic agents. Prerenal azotemia, if severe and prolonged, can cause ischemic ATN. Urine studies typically reveal high urine sodium, high FE_{Na}, and isosthenuria (defined as a urine osmolality near 300 mosm/kg H_2O, which is similar to the plasma osmolality) (see Figure 17). Urinalysis classically shows dark, pigmented, granular (muddy brown) casts (**Figure 18**), renal tubular epithelial cells, or epithelial cell casts that result from tubular damage. Otherwise, the urine is often bland, with minimal or no blood or protein.

The diagnostic approach to ATN begins with identifying when the serum creatinine level began to increase or when the urine output began to decrease. Then, the clinical course during the days preceding the kidney injury is evaluated for kidney insults. Events that might compromise kidney perfusion, such as a decrease in blood pressure, an arrhythmia, or hypoxia, should be sought. If the patient underwent surgery or a procedure, the operative note and anesthesia record may reveal a hemodynamic kidney insult not evident in other parts of the chart. A history or chart review for administration of nephrotoxic agents is also necessary (**Table 36**). Even if an ischemic or toxic insult is not found, some kidney insults may be multifactorial in nature and the cause not readily apparent.

Certain patients are at risk for ATN due to impaired autoregulation of kidney blood flow that makes the kidney more susceptible to injury. **Table 37** lists clinical features associated with impaired autoregulation. In these patients, even modest decrements in blood pressure may result in ischemic kidney injury because of impaired autoregulation. A patient accustomed to higher blood pressures may have an autoregulatory range higher than normal. Such a patient may develop ischemic ATN with a drop in blood pressure even though the blood pressure is considered to be within a normal range. Low kidney blood flow may also increase susceptibility to nephrotoxic agents.

Standard treatment of ATN involves maintaining an adequate perfusion pressure, discontinuing potential nephrotoxic agents, and adjusting the dose of renally excreted medications

TABLE 36. Common Agents that Cause Direct Tubular Toxicity
Antibiotics
Aminoglycosides
Amikacin
Gentamicin
Kanamycin
Streptomycin
Tobramycin
Amphotericin B
Pentamidine
Foscarnet
Tenofovir
Intravenous dye
NSAIDs
Chemotherapy
Cisplatin
Carboplatin
Ifosfamide
Herbal medications/exposures (toxicity may be tubular damage from chronic interstitial disease)
Aristolochia/aristolochic acid
Germanium
Heavy metals/lead

for the current level of kidney function. Data on the use of ACE inhibitors (and angiotensin receptor blockers) in patients with ATN are limited; these agents generally are discontinued because they may compromise perfusion through their effects on renal blood flow.

Recovery from ATN is variable and depends on the severity of the initial insult. Mild ATN usually resolves quickly if the inciting insult is corrected. Severe ATN can lead to dialysis-dependent kidney failure; patients with this condition may regain kidney function after weeks to months, although the longer the time on dialysis the less likely recovery becomes. If a patient is oliguric, one of the first signs of kidney recovery is a spontaneous increase in urine output. In general, nonoliguric kidney injury has a better prognosis than oliguric kidney injury. Although diuretics may be useful to manage volume status in patients with oliguric kidney failure, a response to diuretics does not mean patients have a greater likelihood of kidney recovery than oliguric patients who do not respond to diuresis; thus, diuretics should not be used in AKI except to treat volume overload. Low-dose dopamine has not been shown to be beneficial in expediting renal recovery from ATN.

Contrast-Induced Nephropathy

Iodinated contrast can induce vasospasm and cause ischemic injury or direct damage to the kidneys. Contrast-induced nephropathy (CIN) is defined as either an increase in serum

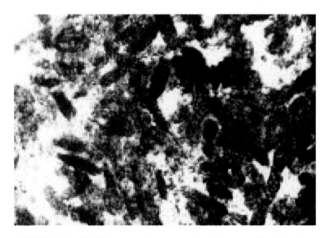

FIGURE 18. Muddy brown casts seen on urine microscopy in a patient with acute tubular necrosis.

TABLE 37. Clinical Features Associated with Impaired Renal Autoregulation and Increasing Susceptibility to Ischemic Acute Tubular Necrosis

Clinical History
Older age (>70 years old)
History of vascular disease/atherosclerosis/renal artery stenosis
Long-standing hypertension
Chronic kidney disease/nephrosis
Diabetes mellitus
Liver disease/hepatorenal syndrome
Heart failure

Medications
Agents that affect the renin-angiotensin system
ACE inhibitors
Angiotensin receptor blockers
Renin inhibitors
Agents that affect prostaglandin synthesis
NSAIDs
Cyclooxygenase-2 inhibitors

Data from Abuelo JG. Normotensive ischemic acute renal failure. N Engl J Med. 2007;357(8):797-805. [PMID: 17715412]

CONT.

creatinine of 0.5 mg/dL (44.2 micromoles/L) or an increase in serum creatinine of 25% from baseline at 48 hours after contrast administration.

Risk factors for severe kidney damage from contrast are summarized in **Table 38**. Physicians should assess the need for the contrast study in terms of the patient's risk. Although CIN may occur in persons with normal baseline kidney function, the risk of contrast-associated injury is substantially higher in patients with preexisting acute or chronic kidney disease, and contrast studies in these patients should be approached with caution. A calculator that estimates a patient's risk for developing CIN is available at www.zunis.org/Contrast-Induced %20Nephropathy%20Calculator2.htm. This calculator was validated in patients undergoing cardiac catheterization and may overestimate risk in other circumstances. Although it provides a limited range of risk categories, it can provide a starting point to discuss risk of CIN with patients. If the contrast study is not necessary or if useful information can be obtained without contrast exposure (for example, with non-contrast studies or ultrasonography), avoiding contrast is the safest option in all patients.

If contrast administration is unavoidable, minimizing the risk of contrast is the priority. Several guidelines have been published, and the main points are listed in **Table 39**. Optimizing hemodynamics is recommended, and the intravenous fluids of choice are normal saline or isotonic sodium bicarbonate. There is no clear evidence supporting one of these fluid choices over the other. Finally, the use of a low or iso-osmolar iodinated contrast is recommended. High osmolar contrast has an osmolality of 2000 mosm/kg H_2O, and there is evidence that it is the most nephrotoxic. Low osmolar (osmolality of 600-800 mosm/kg H_2O) and iso-osmolar (osmolality of approximately 300 mosm/kg H_2O) contrast are thought to be safer than high osmolar contrast. There is no clear difference in CIN risk between low and iso-osmolar agents, and a lack of consensus suggests a small real difference between the two options. N-acetylcysteine has been shown in some studies to prevent a rise in serum creatinine after contrast administration. Because it has minimal toxicity, N-acetylcysteine is used as prophylaxis to prevent CIN, although efficacy of N-acetylcysteine for CIN prevention is not proved.

TABLE 38. Predictors of Severe Contrast-Induced Nephropathy[a]

Initial serum creatinine
Chronic heart failure
Diabetes mellitus
Urgent/emergent procedure
Intra-aortic balloon pump (preprocedure)
Age ≥80 years

[a]The predictors are in order of relative weight. Severe contrast nephropathy in this study was defined as ≥50% increase in serum creatinine, ≥2 mg/dL (177 µmol/L) rise in serum creatinine, or the requirement of dialysis postprocedure.

Reprinted from American Heart Journal. 155(2). Brown JR, DeVries JT, Piper WD, et al; Northern New England Cardiovascular Disease Study Group. Serious renal dysfunction after percutaneous coronary interventions can be predicted. 260-266. 2008, [PMID: 18215595] with permission from Elsevier.

TABLE 39. Approach to the Prevention of Contrast-Induced Nephropathy

Use a noncontrast study if possible:
  Noncontrast CT or MRI
  Ultrasonography

If contrast needed, minimize the dye volume:
  Biplanar imaging if angiography
  Avoid left ventriculography with cardiac catheterization
  Use a low or iso-osmolar iodinated contrast agent

Hydration with normal saline or isotonic fluid with sodium bicarbonate in patients without volume overload (particularly if GFR <60 mL/min/1.73 m²):
  Hold NSAIDs and metformin
  Hold diuretics in patients without volume overload

Oral *N*-acetylcysteine may be beneficial and is not harmful

GFR = glomerular filtration rate.

Forty-eight hours after contrast administration, the serum creatinine level should be measured to determine if any kidney damage has occurred. An increase in serum creatinine should be followed with repeat measurements to determine the severity of the damage. Fortunately, the increase in serum creatinine may only be a transient phenomenon. A persistently increasing creatinine should prompt evaluation for other possible contributors to the kidney damage as well as close follow-up for any complications of impaired kidney function or the possible need for kidney replacement therapy.

In patients with preexisting kidney failure, MRI is frequently used instead of contrast imaging. However, the MRI contrast agent gadolinium has been associated with nephrogenic systemic fibrosis, an irreversible condition seen primarily in patients with an estimated glomerular filtration rate (GFR) of less than 30 mL/min/1.73 m². Therefore, except under very specific clinical situations, MRI with gadolinium contrast should be avoided in patients with abnormal kidney function (see Chronic Kidney Disease, Management, Special Considerations, Imaging).

Pigment Nephropathy

Pigment nephropathy refers to kidney damage from either hemoglobin or myoglobin present in excessive concentrations in the renal tubules. Both are thought to damage the kidney through multiple mechanisms: they may induce ischemia, block tubules, and cause direct toxic damage to the tubules. The patient history is usually remarkable for a precipitating cause for the hemolysis in hemoglobin-induced pigment nephropathy or muscle damage in rhabdomyolysis.

Hemolysis, the destruction of erythrocytes, causes release of excessive amounts of hemoglobin along with other erythrocyte contents into the circulation. When the level of erythrocyte destruction overwhelms normal clearance mechanisms, adequate hemoglobin may be delivered to the renal tubule to cause damage. Rhabdomyolysis is muscle damage leading to release of intracellular muscle contents into the circulation, including the heme pigment myoglobin, which when present in adequate amounts can cause kidney damage.

Laboratory values in hemolysis-induced kidney disease are consistent with massive hemolysis (anemia, increased lactate dehydrogenase, decreased haptoglobin) and kidney failure (increased creatinine). In rhabdomyolysis, laboratory test results are notable for an increased creatine kinase and serum and/or urine markers of increased myoglobin consistent with muscle damage, as well as increased creatinine due to kidney damage. Because of increased release of creatine kinase from damaged muscle, the creatine kinase increase can be dramatic in rhabdomyolysis.

Evaluation of the urine can be particularly helpful in identifying pigment nephropathy. The urine dipstick tests positive for blood in the urine in the presence of either hemoglobin or myoglobin but does not differentiate between hemoglobin and myoglobin. The urine sediment, however, may not reveal blood cells. The discrepancy between the urine dipstick identifying blood and the urine microscopy showing no erythrocytes suggests hemoglobin- or myoglobin-induced kidney injury. The classic urine sediment in pigment nephropathy shows dark (pigmented) granular casts (see Figure 18). Complications of rhabdomyolysis include hypocalcemia, hyperphosphatemia, hyperuricemia, metabolic acidosis, acute muscle compartment syndrome, and limb ischemia.

Treatment of pigment nephropathy consists of reversing the underlying cause (hemolysis or rhabdomyolysis) and intravenous fluids to dilute and possibly promote excretion of the pigment through the kidneys. The goal urine output is 200 to 300 mL/h. Whether bicarbonate-containing fluid is better than other fluid options (normal saline) is not established. Administration of intravenous fluid as soon after the injury as possible is important. Electrolytes must be monitored because alkalosis and hypocalcemia or acidosis can develop, depending on the type of fluid given and the degree of tubular injury. Treatment is then supportive, monitoring for compartment syndrome, further kidney damage, and hyperkalemia while avoiding nephrotoxins and assessing for complications of kidney failure and potential dialysis needs. Patients with suspected compartment syndrome require urgent surgical consultation to evaluate for possible fasciotomy. There is no evidence to support using dialysis to help remove hemoglobin or myoglobin; the decision to initiate dialysis is based on clinical and metabolic needs only.

Acute Interstitial Nephritis

Although some systemic diseases such as multiple myeloma or autoimmune diseases may cause acute interstitial nephritis (AIN), AIN typically is caused by a hypersensitivity reaction to a medication (**Table 40**). The clinical presentation of AIN is variable and in part dependent on the underlying medication. The classic presentation of AIN is fever, rash, and

TABLE 40.	Causes of Acute Interstitial Nephritis
Medications	
Antibiotics	
β-Lactams	
Fluoroquinolones	
Sulfonamides	
Antivirals	
Indinavir	
Abacavir	
Analgesics	
NSAIDs	
Cyclooxygenase-2 inhibitors	
Gastrointestinal	
Proton pump inhibitors	
5-Aminosalicylates	
Herbal medications	
Chinese herb nephropathy	
Heavy metals (germanium; lead)	
Miscellaneous	
Allopurinol	
Phenytoin	
Autoimmune Disorders	
Systemic lupus erythematosus	
Sarcoidosis	
Tubulointerstitial nephritis and uveitis (TINU syndrome)	
Systemic Diseases	
Sarcoidosis	
HIV infection	
Multiple myeloma	
Leukemia	
Lymphoma	

Thrombotic Microangiopathy

Thrombotic thrombocytopenic purpura (TTP) and hemolytic uremic syndrome (HUS) are two forms of thrombotic microangiopathy that can cause AKI. In TTP and HUS, obstruction of small blood vessels due to endothelial activation, intimal expansion, and thrombi causes kidney injury, which can range from chronic and smoldering to acute and oliguric. The urine sediment may be bland or show blood and protein and therefore mimic glomerulonephritis. Treatment is dictated by the underlying etiology and may range from supportive care for most cases of Shiga-like toxin–associated (typical) HUS to plasma exchange for idiopathic TTP. For further discussion of thrombotic microangiopathy, see the Glomerular Diseases chapter.

Other Syndromes of Acute Kidney Injury

Vancomycin may be associated with nephrotoxicity, possibly mediated through extra osmoles introduced during the manufacturing process, causing osmotic nephropathy. A similar mechanism of kidney injury has been reported with certain IgG preparations. The evidence for vancomycin-induced AKI is limited, but care should be taken to dose this medication appropriately for a patient's body weight and GFR.

Phosphate nephropathy has been described in patients using oral phosphorus bowel preparations. Phosphate deposition in the renal tubules can occur, particularly in patients with CKD or who are dehydrated, resulting in kidney injury that can be permanent and lead to a need for dialysis. Oral phosphorus bowel preparations should not be given to patients with CKD and probably are best avoided. High-dose vitamin C, orlistat, carambola juice (star fruit), and gastric bypass surgery can cause acute oxalate nephropathy. ■

KEY POINTS

- Acute tubular necrosis usually occurs after an ischemic event or exposure to nephrotoxic agents and is commonly associated with muddy brown casts on urinalysis and a fractional excretion of sodium greater than 2%.

- Contrast-induced nephropathy is defined as either an increase in serum creatinine of 0.5 mg/dL (44.2 micromoles/L) or an increase in serum creatinine of 25% from baseline at 48 hours after contrast administration.

- Interventions to decrease the incidence and severity of contrast-induced nephropathy include minimizing the amount of iodinated contrast used, optimizing hemodynamics, and using a low or iso-osmolar iodinated contrast.

- Acute interstitial nephritis typically is caused by a hypersensitivity reaction to a medication; the clinical presentation is variable and in part dependent on the underlying medication.

eosinophilia in a patient with an elevated serum creatinine level, but this presentation is found in only 10% of patients.

Diagnosis is most often made by a history of exposure to a drug with a high likelihood of causing AIN. AIN usually occurs after 7 to 10 days of drug exposure; however, prior exposure to a drug may result in a more sudden onset. The urine may show leukocytes and leukocyte casts with negative urine cultures (sterile pyuria) and erythrocytes.

The mainstay of AIN treatment is discontinuation of the offending agent. The symptoms usually resolve, and the serum creatinine level decreases soon after stopping the medication. Recovery may sometimes be prolonged. Evidence for using corticosteroids in patients with AIN is limited. Corticosteroids are often considered in patients with severe or prolonged AIN, particularly when kidney biopsy results confirm a significant component of acute inflammation. If used, corticosteroids seem to be more effective the earlier they are initiated.

Postrenal Disease

Urinary obstruction is an important reversible cause of AKI. AKI results from obstruction that affects both kidneys (or obstruction of a single kidney or a unilaterally functioning kidney). Because relief of obstruction can reverse kidney injury and prevent chronic damage, timely diagnosis of urinary obstruction is essential. Urinary obstruction can be asymptomatic and can be associated with no noted change in urine output. Bladder outlet obstruction should be excluded by bladder ultrasonography or catheterization. Without evidence of outlet obstruction, kidney imaging, typically ultrasonography, should be performed in all patients with AKI. Findings in the medical history, such as pelvic tumors or irradiation, congenital urinary abnormalities, kidney stones, genitourinary infections, procedures or surgeries, or prostatic enlargement, should increase suspicion for obstruction. In obstruction, the urinalysis is bland. Urine electrolytes are variable; in early obstruction, the urine sodium and FE_{Na} may be low, but in late obstruction, the urine sodium and FE_{Na} may be high, indicative of tubular damage. Because of impaired kidney potassium, acid, and water excretion, hyperkalemic metabolic acidosis and hyponatremia can be present. Kidney ultrasonography or noncontrast CT can be used to identify obstruction, although early obstruction and obstruction with concomitant dehydration or retroperitoneal fibrosis may be missed. Diuretic radionuclide kidney clearance scanning is often used to more definitively evaluate for obstruction if other imaging is equivocal. Treatment by removing or bypassing the obstruction is most effective if implemented early.

KEY POINT

- Without evidence of outlet obstruction, kidney imaging, typically ultrasonography, should be performed in all patients with acute kidney injury.

Acute Kidney Injury in Specific Clinical Settings

Critical Care

Increased intra-abdominal pressure (IAP) may cause AKI. Although the pathophysiology is not completely elucidated, contributing deleterious processes likely include a depressed cardiac output, decreased renal blood flow (both arterial and venous), and increased pressure on the ureter.

Intra-abdominal hypertension is defined as an IAP ≥12 mm Hg. IAP can be estimated by measuring the bladder pressure through a bladder catheter. Abdominal compartment syndrome (ACS) is new organ dysfunction with an IAP greater than 20 mm Hg. ACS should be suspected in patients with oliguria or increasing serum creatinine level who have had abdominal surgery, who have received massive fluid resuscitation, who have a tense abdomen, or who have liver disease with ascites. Diagnosis of ACS is made by measuring bladder pressures to confirm the high IAP in the setting of organ dysfunction. Although medical treatment (diuresis, dialysis, management of ascites) can be tried, surgical decompression of the abdomen is often necessary to definitively treat ACS.

KEY POINTS

- Abdominal compartment syndrome is defined by new organ dysfunction in the setting of an intra-abdominal pressure greater than 20 mm Hg.
- Surgical decompression of the abdomen is often necessary to definitively treat abdominal compartment syndrome.

Cardiovascular Disease

Cardiorenal Syndrome

There is an intricate physiologic interaction between the heart and the kidneys. Cardiorenal syndrome occurs when one organ system dysfunction affects another. Cardiorenal syndrome is divided into five types: acute heart failure compromising kidney function (AKI), chronic heart failure causing CKD, AKI compromising heart function acutely, CKD contributing to chronic heart disease, and concomitant cardiac and kidney dysfunction caused by another process (such as sepsis).

Treatment of any type of cardiorenal syndrome focuses on reversing (if possible) any specific underlying cause or improving the compromised organ function, usually through improving hemodynamic parameters. The difficulty in treating cardiorenal syndrome is the delicate balance between fluid removal and hemodynamics, specifically kidney perfusion. Diuretics may be used, and if not successful, ultrafiltration or dialysis may be indicated. Diuretic boluses seem to be as effective as diuretic drips for diuresis as long as adequate doses are used. Isolated ultrafiltration has shown greater fluid removal compared with diuretics in some studies. However, the benefit of this therapy over adequately dosed diuretics is unproved, especially when the risk of the procedure (central line placement) and increased hypotension are considered.

Atheroembolic Disease

Atherosclerotic plaque dislodgement from arterial walls during invasive procedures or spontaneously can cause cholesterol embolization and result in systemic findings, including kidney injury. Atheroembolic disease usually occurs in patients with vascular disease risk factors (hypertension, hyperlipidemia, smoking, older age, diabetes) or known atherosclerotic disease (bruits on examination, history of coronary artery disease, arterial stents, or bypass procedures) who undergo intra-arterial intervention. Soon after the procedure, a livedo reticularis rash may appear. Evidence of emboli (blue digits or ischemic tips of digits) may be noted, particularly downstream from the instrumented vessels. A Hollenhorst plaque (a cholesterol plaque in the retinal artery or its branches) may be noted on funduscopic examination. An

CONT.

increase in the serum creatinine level indicates AKI, and eosinophilia is found in two thirds of patients. Hypocomplementemia may also be seen. Although intravenous contrast can also cause an increase in serum creatinine, contrast should not cause the other clinical findings associated with atheroembolic disease.

In high-risk patients, avoiding invasive vascular procedures is the best prevention. Devices that are deployed downstream to catch plaque are sometimes used but are not always effective. There is no proven treatment once the disease has occurred; however, therapy, including statins, treatment of hypertension, and aspirin, should be initiated for secondary prevention of cardiovascular disease.

KEY POINTS

- Cardiorenal syndrome is divided into five categories based on the interactions of abnormal renal and cardiac physiology.

- Treatment of cardiorenal syndrome focuses on reversing any specific underlying cause or improving the compromised organ function.

- Atheroembolic disease usually occurs in patients with vascular disease risk factors or known atherosclerotic disease who undergo intra-arterial intervention.

- There is no proven treatment for atheroembolic disease; however, therapy should be initiated for secondary prevention of cardiovascular disease.

Liver Disease

Hepatorenal syndrome (HRS), kidney dysfunction occurring in the setting of liver disease without another identifiable etiology, is believed to be due to altered vasoregulation arising from changes in the splanchnic circulation. HRS is essentially a diagnosis of exclusion; hypotension/shock, hypovolemia, and renal parenchymal damage should be ruled out before making the diagnosis. The urine sodium is often low in HRS because the kidney senses decreased blood volume and avidly retains sodium and water. Diagnostic criteria are listed in **Table 41**.

TABLE 41. Diagnostic Criteria for Hepatorenal Syndrome in Cirrhosis

Liver disease: cirrhosis with ascites

Kidney disease: serum creatinine level >1.5 mg/dL (133 μmol/L)

Kidney function not improved by fluid challenge: diuretics held and albumin 1 g/kg given for 2 days (maximum 100 g/d)

No other etiology for kidney dysfunction: shock not present; no precipitating/current nephrotoxins

No evidence of parenchymal kidney disease (proteinuria, hematuria, or abnormal kidney ultrasound)

Modified from Gut. Diagnosis, prevention and treatment of hepatorenal syndrome in cirrhosis. Salerno F, Gerbes A, Ginès P, Wong F, Arroyo V. 56(9):1310-1318, [PMID: 17389705] Copyright 2008 with permission from BMJ Publishing Group.

There are two types of HRS. Type I HRS, in which acute liver failure leads to AKI, is severe, progresses rapidly, and requires intensive care monitoring. Type II HRS is found in chronic liver disease, usually with refractory ascites. The hemodynamic derangements from the liver disease result in splanchnic vasodilation and reduced renal blood flow, causing a slow progressive decline in kidney function.

Management of both types of HRS consists of reversing any precipitating causes (gastrointestinal bleeding, peritonitis, other infections) and optimizing hemodynamics. The use of albumin in patients with cirrhosis and spontaneous bacterial peritonitis has been shown to reduce mortality and the incidence of HRS. A liver transplant is definitive therapy and can be curative for both types. Midodrine and octreotide have shown some promise in treating type II HRS, although evidence is limited. Vasopressin analogs, such as terlipressin, are being investigated as potential therapies for HRS.

KEY POINTS

- Hepatorenal syndrome is kidney dysfunction occurring in the setting of liver disease without another identifiable etiology.

- The use of albumin in patients with cirrhosis and spontaneous bacterial peritonitis has been shown to reduce mortality and the incidence of hepatorenal syndrome.

Malignancy

Tumor Lysis Syndrome

Tumor lysis syndrome refers to the release of intracellular contents from breakdown of tumor cells and release of their contents into the circulation. Manifestations include AKI and arrhythmias resulting from the release of potassium, phosphorus, and uric acid. The cell death can be spontaneous with highly proliferative malignancies but more commonly is induced by chemotherapy. Patients with tumor lysis syndrome present with hyperkalemia, hyperuricemia, and hyperphosphatemia and may require urgent medical intervention. Precipitation of uric acid and calcium phosphate crystals in the renal tubules may result in AKI, often with oliguria.

Treatment of tumor lysis syndrome begins with recognizing the at-risk patient. Those with fast-growing tumors, a high tumor burden, or a tumor highly responsive to treatment are at increased risk. Once the patient with increased risk is identified, treatment with intravenous fluid is recommended. Intravenous hydration with saline is preferred given the risk of metabolic alkalosis and possible precipitation of phosphorus at higher urine pH associated with sodium bicarbonate therapy. Allopurinol, a xanthine oxidase inhibitor, can be given prophylactically to reduce uric acid formation, and rasburicase, a urate oxidase that catalyzes the degradation of uric acid, can be used to actively lower uric acid levels. Rasburicase is considerably more expensive than allopurinol and is therefore used primarily in patients with high risk for

CONT.

tumor lysis syndrome or if excessively high uric acid levels occur in the context of chemotherapy. If kidney function is compromised, the patient must be assessed closely for the need for dialysis. Early initiation of continuous dialysis may be beneficial in tumor lysis syndrome with decreased kidney function and oliguria to prevent accumulation of potassium, phosphorus, uric acid, and the extra volume given to prevent and treat tumor lysis syndrome.

Chemotherapy-Induced Disease

Chemotherapy, besides precipitating tumor lysis syndrome, can also cause direct kidney injury. Platinum-based therapies can cause nonoliguric AKI with magnesium and potassium wasting, similar to aminoglycosides. Ifosfamide can also cause acute tubular injury. Prolonged use of nitrosoureas can cause chronic interstitial disease. Vascular endothelial growth factor inhibitors are known to induce proteinuria usually secondary to thrombotic microangiopathy. To minimize toxicity, the doses of renally excreted agents should be adjusted for GFR.

Myeloma Cast Nephropathy

Kidney involvement is common in multiple myeloma, with up to 25% of patients having kidney insufficiency at the time of diagnosis. Kidney failure may be the presenting finding. There is a correlation of the presence of kidney disease, its severity, and its response to therapy with overall survival in multiple myeloma.

Myeloma-related kidney disease occurs through several mechanisms. Myeloma-related hypercalcemia may cause a decreased GFR and an increased serum creatinine level. Certain glomerular diseases (membranoproliferative glomerulonephritis, cryoglobulinemia, and amyloidosis) may also result from monoclonal light chain deposition in the glomeruli (see Glomerular Diseases). Light chains may also accumulate in the tubules and form complexes with Tamm-Horsfall mucoprotein, leading to development of tubular casts (myeloma cast nephropathy) with obstruction, direct tubular injury, and AKI (see Chronic Tubulointerstitial Disorders).

In patients with myeloma cast nephropathy, urine examination is generally bland, and the urine dipstick typically does not reveal albuminuria. However, the addition of sulfosalicylic acid to the urine will precipitate all nonalbumin proteins, including light chains. Serum and urine protein electrophoresis with immunofixation can identify and quantify the monoclonal immunoglobulin.

Treatment of myeloma cast nephropathy requires reducing the burden of the paraproteins. Chemotherapy for multiple myeloma reduces paraprotein production; plasmapheresis to remove excess paraproteins is controversial. Autologous stem cell transplantation may be a treatment option for appropriate patients. Kidney transplantation has been successful in patients with multiple myeloma who have achieved full remission, but recurrence of light chain nephropathy and kidney failure has been reported.

HIV Infection

Patients with HIV infection have a high incidence of prerenal AKI thought to be due to volume depletion, concomitant liver disease, and hypoperfusion with infections. HIV infection is associated with some parenchymal diseases (HIV nephropathy, interstitial/infiltrative diseases, immune complex–mediated nephritis), which can present as AKI (see Glomerular Diseases). Medications used to treat HIV infection can cause AKI. Indinavir and atazanavir can cause AKI from obstruction, although using lower doses should cause less crystalluria. Tenofovir is absorbed by the proximal tubule and can also cause AKI and proximal renal tubular acidosis. Kidney biopsy should be considered in patients with HIV infection who have unexplained AKI. H

KEY POINTS

- Tumor lysis syndrome refers to the release of intracellular contents from breakdown of tumor cells and release of their contents into the circulation.

- Management of tumor lysis syndrome consists of early recognition, intravenous hydration with saline, medication to lower uric acid levels, and dialysis if needed to control the metabolic abnormalities.

- Myeloma cast nephropathy is associated with tubular obstruction, tubular injury, and acute kidney injury.

- Kidney biopsy should be considered in patients with HIV infection who have unexplained acute kidney injury.

Kidney Stones

Kidney stones are common, and the lifetime incidence has increased to nearly 10% in the United States. An initial kidney stone was most commonly seen in patients in their 30s and 40s; however, epidemiologic data now suggest that there has been an increase in nephrolithiasis in younger patients, which may coincide with the increase in metabolic syndrome and obesity in younger Americans.

The constituents of urine are typically insoluble at concentrations excreted each day, but several urine proteins and inhibitors limit stone formation. However, this balance is easily disrupted by low urine volume, anatomic abnormalities that cause urine stasis, medications, supplements, and dietary and metabolic factors.

Types of Kidney Stones

Calcium Stones

Calcium-containing stones account for nearly 80% of all kidney stones. Most calcium-containing stones are composed of calcium oxalate, which is relatively insoluble in acid urine; 10% are composed of calcium phosphate, which is insoluble in alkaline urine.

Risk Factors

Hypercalciuria

Hypercalciuria is the most common metabolic factor associated with calcium oxalate kidney stones. Hypercalciuria may occur in the setting of hypercalcemia, in which the filtered load of calcium is increased, as seen in primary hyperparathyroidism, sarcoidosis, and vitamin D excess. More frequently, the cause of hypercalciuria is not identified and is called idiopathic hypercalciuria, a disorder that is commonly familial.

Management of idiopathic hypercalciuria includes thiazide diuretics, which promote reabsorption of calcium by inducing mild hypovolemia and increased proximal tubular calcium reabsorption. A diet low in sodium increases the effectiveness of thiazide diuretics. Patients should not limit calcium intake, which paradoxically appears to increase urine calcium. Instead, patients should aim for age-appropriate calcium intake.

Hyperoxaluria

Excess oxalate excretion can also contribute to calcium oxalate stones. Excessive intake of dietary oxalate (chocolate, spinach, green and black tea) can lead to hyperoxaluria.

Enteric hyperoxaluria occurs in the setting of gastrointestinal malabsorption when free fatty acids bind to calcium, allowing free oxalate to be absorbed in the colon. This is particularly common in patients who undergo Roux-en-Y gastric bypass procedures for obesity; these patients have an increased risk of nephrolithiasis. Oral calcium carbonate in doses up to 4 g/d is used for patients with enteric hyperoxaluria to bind oxalate within the gastrointestinal tract.

Primary hyperoxaluria is an autosomal recessive disorder in which excess oxalate is produced, leading to deposition of calcium oxalate in the kidneys and other organs. The increased urine excretion of oxalate can lead to calcium oxalate kidney stones. Calcium oxalate can also deposit in the kidney parenchyma, blood vessels, and other major organs. Treatment includes increased fluid intake, avoidance of food with high oxalate content, and the use of pyridoxine (vitamin B_6) to limit the formation of oxalate.

Hypocitraturia

Reduced urine citrate can occur in settings of metabolic acidosis (such as distal renal tubular acidosis) when there is increased proximal absorption of urine citrate. A high protein diet also promotes proximal reabsorption of citrate. Citrate normally chelates calcium and limits the formation of calcium oxalate in the urine. If urine citrate is reduced, patients may take potassium citrate supplements.

Struvite Stones

Less than 10% of patients with kidney stones have struvite stones, which are composed of magnesium ammonium phosphate (struvite) and calcium carbonate apatite. Infections caused by urease-splitting organisms such as *Proteus* and *Klebsiella* species hydrolyze urea to ammonium, which alkalinizes the urine and leads to precipitation of phosphate ion complexes.

Without adequate treatment, the process tends to promulgate, and the stones may form "staghorn" shapes that fill the kidney pelvis. Antibiotic therapy and stone removal are the mainstays of therapy for struvite stones.

Uric Acid Stones

Uric acid stones cause approximately 10% of kidney stones. Uric acid is insoluble in an acid pH, but remarkably few patients develop uric acid stones. Patients who develop uric acid stones typically have low urine volume or hyperuricosuria. The latter may result from a high protein diet or rapid purine metabolism as in tumor lysis syndrome. Other risk factors include gout, conditions associated with uric acid overproduction, diabetes mellitus, the metabolic syndrome, and chronic diarrhea. Alkalinization of the urine and increased fluid intake are essential for management of uric acid stones. In addition, allopurinol can be used if the patient has gout or when urine uric acid excretion exceeds 1 g/24 h (5.9 mmol/d).

Cystine Stones

Cystine stones are an exceedingly rare cause of nephrolithiasis seen in patients with cystinuria. In this autosomal recessive disorder, patients lack the proximal tubular transporter for dibasic amino acids, including cystine. Cystine stones occur because cystine is insoluble in an acid pH. Crystals have a telltale hexagon shape. Without treatment, stones can be large.

Treatment is directed at alkalinization of the urine and use of agents that can chelate cystine with a sulfhydryl group such as penicillamine or the better-tolerated tiopronin.

KEY POINTS

- Hypercalciuria is the most common metabolic factor associated with calcium oxalate kidney stones.
- Management of idiopathic hypercalciuria includes thiazide diuretics, and calcium intake should not be limited, which paradoxically appears to increase urine calcium.
- Struvite stones may develop in patients with infections caused by urease-splitting organisms such as *Proteus* and *Klebsiella* species.
- Patients who develop uric acid stones typically have low urine volume or hyperuricosuria.

Clinical Manifestations

Patients with kidney stones usually present with colicky flank pain; however, pain may be localized along the path of the urinary tract to the groin, penis, or testicle, or it may be abdominal. On occasion, it may mimic an acute abdomen. When stones reach the bladder, irritative symptoms such as urinary urgency and frequency may occur. Patients may experience severe paroxysmal pain, nausea, and vomiting.

Diagnosis

Physical examination is important to identify other conditions. Urinalysis usually demonstrates hematuria. If crystals are present in the urine, this may be helpful in determining the composition of the kidney stones but is not diagnostic. Laboratory studies are indicated to evaluate kidney function, electrolyte levels, and the possible presence of coincident infection.

Imaging studies aid in the diagnosis of nephrolithiasis and help guide management based on the size and location of the stone. Noncontrast abdominal helical CT is the gold standard for diagnosing nephrolithiasis. This study can identify every type of kidney stone throughout its path in the urinary tract and may be able to suggest the type of stone present. Plain abdominal radiography has no role in acute diagnosis but may be used to assess the stone burden in patients with known radiopaque stones. Ultrasonography may identify stones in the kidneys but does not detect ureteral stones and may not detect early hydronephrosis. **H**

KEY POINTS

- Patients with kidney stones usually present with colicky flank pain; however, pain may be localized along the path of the urinary tract to the groin, penis, or testicle, or it may be abdominal.

- Noncontrast helical CT is the gold standard for diagnosing nephrolithiasis and can identify every type of kidney stone throughout its path in the urinary tract and may be able to suggest the type of stone present.

Acute Management

Patients with kidney stones whose pain can be controlled with oral analgesia and who can achieve oral hydration with a goal of at least 2 L of urine output daily can be managed conservatively with close follow-up. Because knowledge of stone type is helpful in management, patients should be instructed to strain their urine, and recovered stones should be sent for chemical analysis if the stone type and risk factors have not yet been established. Medical expulsive therapy with the α-blocker tamsulosin or a calcium channel blocker such as nifedipine has been shown to accelerate the passage of small stones. Utilization of these agents to facilitate stone passage is off label but common practice. Head-to-head comparisons show similar efficacy, but most clinicians prefer to use tamsulosin to avoid hypotension. With these strategies, more than 90% of small stones (<5 mm) pass spontaneously. In contrast, stones that are more than 7 mm are unlikely to pass without intervention (**Figure 19**). If urgent decompression of the collecting system is needed because of concerns of infection, bilateral obstruction, or obstruction of a solitary kidney, then percutaneous nephrostomy or ureteral stenting should be performed; the appropriate procedure is determined by the location of the stone and the clinical condition of the patient.

Patients who do not have an urgent indication for urologic intervention may still require intervention if the stone does not pass after a period of observation. The American Urological Association recommends careful counseling regarding all technical options. Extracorporeal shock wave lithotripsy is a widely used, noninvasive strategy used to treat symptomatic calculi located in the proximal ureter or within the kidney. Although generally well tolerated, tissue injury

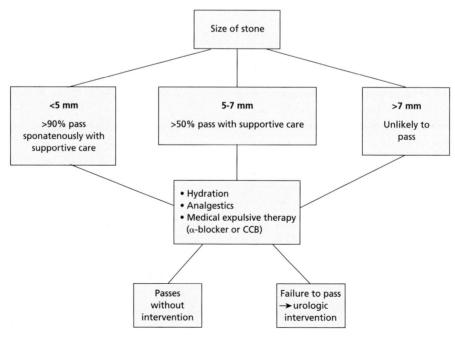

FIGURE 19. Acute management of symptomatic kidney stones.

CONT.

can occur, and several studies have found new-onset hypertension following treatment. This association, however, is controversial. On occasion, very large complex stones require intervention with percutaneous nephrolithotomy.

In contrast, stones located in the distal ureter are usually accessible by directed therapy guided by ureteroscopy. During ureteroscopy, "intracorporeal" lithotripsy can be performed using lasers, ultrasonography, or other techniques. Stone fragments can be snared in baskets, or ureteral stents may be placed to facilitate stone fragment passage.

Risk Factor Evaluation and Subsequent Treatment

Historically, clinicians have been taught to look for the cause after the second kidney stone; however, in 1988, the NIH consensus conference on this topic suggested that an evaluation be pursued after the first stone. This assessment includes urinalysis and measurement of serum electrolytes, blood urea nitrogen, creatinine, calcium, phosphorus, and uric acid.

Analysis of passed stones and evaluation of the cause of kidney stones using a 24-hour urine collection are also recommended to guide management of kidney stones. Because the evaluation of the constituents of urine requires different preservatives, more than one collection may be required unless a special collection kit is utilized. Each 24-hour urine collection must include urine creatinine to assure a complete collection and facilitate comparison of future collections. Collections should also measure urea (to assess dietary protein intake), calcium, phosphate, citrate, oxalate, uric acid, and sodium. A radiologic assessment of "stone burden" should be performed at the onset of treatment, at 1 year, and, if negative, every 2 to 4 years thereafter. This can be done with kidney ultrasonography or plain radiography of the abdomen if stones are radiopaque.

After evaluation, patients should be counseled with general advice on how to prevent new stone formation as well as specific measures directed at identified metabolic abnormalities (**Table 42**). Without intervention, recurrence is common. Approximately 40% of patients have another stone within 5 years and nearly double that at 20 years.

KEY POINTS

- Medical expulsive therapy with the α-blocker tamsulosin or a calcium channel blocker such as nifedipine has been shown to accelerate the passage of small kidney stones.

- Extracorporeal shock wave lithotripsy is a widely used, noninvasive strategy used to treat symptomatic calculi located in the proximal ureter or within the kidney.

- Stones located in the distal ureter are usually accessible by directed therapy guided by ureteroscopy.

- Analysis of passed stones and evaluation of the cause of kidney stones using a 24-hour urine collection are recommended to guide management of kidney stones.

The Kidney in Pregnancy

Normal Physiologic Changes in Pregnancy

Hemodynamic Changes

During normal pregnancy, blood pressure lowers as a result of peripheral vasodilation and relative loss in response to vasoconstrictive hormones such as angiotensin II and vasopressin. These changes begin shortly after the first missed menstrual period and plateau in the middle of the second trimester. Concurrently, the plasma volume increases steadily because of increasing renal sodium and water retention. The increase in plasma volume leads to an increase in renal plasma flow and glomerular filtration rate (GFR). The increase in GFR results in a decrease in the serum creatinine level from the normal prepregnancy value of 0.8 mg/dL (70.7 micromoles/L) to 0.5 mg/dL (44.2 micromoles/L). The increased GFR may result in a small increase in proteinuria in healthy women and more substantial increases in women with preexisting proteinuria.

Changes in the Urinary Tract

Coincident with the increase in plasma volume, maternal hormones cause dilatation of the renal pelvis, calices, and ureters that may be mistaken for kidney obstruction. The dilated urinary system may be more prone to ascending pyelonephritis; therefore, standard practice includes a urine culture on the first prenatal visit and treatment of asymptomatic bacteriuria (>100,000 colony-forming units/mL). Finally, the incidence of kidney stones is slightly greater during the third trimester.

Changes in Acid-Base Regulation

Maternal hormones affect the configuration of the thoracic cage and stimulate ventilation, causing an increase in tidal volume and relative hyperventilation. The resulting hypocapnia, with an average arterial Pco_2 of 30 mm Hg (4.0 kPa), favors carbon dioxide transfer from the fetus to the maternal circulation. The kidney responds secondarily with increased bicarbonate excretion, resulting in a serum bicarbonate level of 18 to 20 meq/L (18-20 mmol/L) and a serum pH of 7.4 to 7.45 throughout pregnancy.

Changes in Water Homeostasis

Although both sodium and water retention occur, which increase plasma volume during pregnancy, water retention exceeds sodium retention. The decrease in the osmotic threshold for suppression of arginine vasopressin and thirst leads to a decline in the serum sodium level of approximately 4 meq/L (4 mmol/L), matched by a decrease in the plasma osmolality of 8 to 10 mosm/kg H_2O.

TABLE 42. Prevention of New Kidney Stone Formation

Stone Type	Risk Factor	Treatment	Therapeutic Targets/Comments
General stone advice		Increase fluid intake	>2 L/d
		Low sodium diet	<100 meq/d (100 mmol/d)
		Low protein diet	0.8-1 g/kg/d
		Dietary calcium intake	Age-appropriate calcium intake
Calcium (primarily calcium oxalate except with high urine pH, which predisposes to calcium phosphate)	Idiopathic hypercalciuria	Thiazide diuretics	Chlorthalidone, 12.5-25 mg daily or hydrochlorothiazide, 25 mg twice daily
	Hypocitraturia	Potassium citrate	20-30 meq twice daily
	Enteric hyperoxaluria	Calcium carbonate or citrate	1-2 g with meals
		Avoid high oxalate foods	e.g., chocolate, spinach
		Cholestyramine	4 g with meals
	Primary hyperoxaluria (urine oxalate >80 g/d)	Increase fluid intake	>3 L/d
		Avoid high oxalate foods	e.g., chocolate, spinach
		High-dose pyridoxine	5-20 mg/kg/d
	High urine pH	Correct metabolic acidosis	Serum bicarbonate 22-24 meq/L (22-24 mmol/L); keep urine pH <6.6
Uric acid	Urine pH <6.0	Potassium citrate or bicarbonate	40-80 meq/d (40-80 mmol/d): titrate to urine pH of 6.1-7.0
	Hyperuricosuria (>1000 mg/d [59 mmol/d])	Allopurinol	100-300 mg/d
Struvite	Urinary tract infection	Urologic interventions: percutaneous nephrolithotomy; surgery	Complete removal of all stone material
		Aggressive treatment of infection when present	Antibiotics as indicated
		Urease inhibitor (acetohydroxamic acid)	Rarely used due to toxicity
Cystine	Cystinuria	Potassium citrate or bicarbonate	Urine pH >7.0; 3-4 meq/kg/d (3-4 mmol/kg/d)
		Chelating agents	Tiopronin; penicillamine (captopril if hypertension)

KEY POINTS

- Pregnancy is normally associated with a lowering in blood pressure, a small increase in proteinuria, and a decrease in the serum creatinine level.
- Maternal hormones cause dilatation of the renal pelvis, calices, and ureters that may be mistaken for kidney obstruction.

Hypertensive Disorders Associated with Pregnancy

Chronic Hypertension

The normal systemic vasodilation seen early in pregnancy typically results in blood pressure values that are lower than those of nongravid women; therefore, women with chronic hypertension may have normal or low blood pressure during pregnancy.

When hypertension is noted before the 20th week of gestation, it is most consistent with a new diagnosis of chronic hypertension. There is no evidence that tight control of hypertension during pregnancy will prevent preeclampsia; instead, antihypertensive therapy is warranted only to limit maternal end-organ damage in those with severe hypertension. Therefore, most experts recommend that blood pressure should be maintained below 150/100 mm Hg and possibly lower in the setting of chronic kidney disease (CKD). If treatment is necessary, it is important to note that all antihypertensive agents cross the placenta. Methyldopa and labetalol appear to be the safest choices, whereas ACE inhibitors, angiotensin receptor blockers (ARBs), and likely renin inhibitors are not safe (**Table 43**). Women of child-bearing age who require blockade of the renin-angiotensin system for control of blood pressure and proteinuria should be counseled regarding the risk of birth defects should they become pregnant; these agents should be discontinued if conception is possible or anticipated.

Because many healthy women receive regular medical care for the first time during pregnancy, this may also be the first time that chronic hypertension is diagnosed. Such hypertension may be essential or secondary. CKD is the most common cause of secondary hypertension. Renovascular hypertension is another important cause of hypertension in young women, but diagnosis is particularly difficult during pregnancy when renin, angiotensin, and aldosterone are all normally elevated to achieve the sodium retention required to increase the plasma volume. Similarly, the diagnosis of primary hyperaldosteronism is challenging.

KEY POINTS

- Antihypertensive therapy is warranted only to limit maternal end-organ damage in pregnant patients with severe hypertension.
- In pregnant patients, blood pressure should be maintained below 150/100 mm Hg and possibly lower in the setting of chronic kidney disease.
- Blockade of the renin-angiotensin system should be discontinued before conception because of the risk of birth defects.

Gestational Hypertension

Gestational hypertension refers to hypertension that develops after 20 weeks of pregnancy in the absence of proteinuria or other maternal end-organ damage. Blood pressure should return to normal within 6 weeks of delivery; if the blood pressure remains high, it is more consistent with chronic hypertension. Some women with gestational hypertension may have undiagnosed chronic hypertension masked by the early decline in blood pressure seen in the first trimester that returned to prepregnancy values after 20 weeks. Up to 45% of women initially diagnosed with gestational hypertension develop preeclampsia, and the risk is greatest if the hypertension develops remote from term.

Preeclampsia

Preeclampsia is characterized by new-onset hypertension accompanied by the development of proteinuria. This condition can develop any time after 20 weeks of pregnancy. New generalized edema also may occur but is not part of the diagnostic criteria, because edema is common during uncomplicated pregnancy. Severe disease is characterized by thrombocytopenia, heavy proteinuria, rising serum creatinine levels, and elevated liver chemistry test results. Risk factors for preeclampsia include a family history of preeclampsia, nulliparity, multiple gestations, obesity, CKD, chronic hypertension, diabetes mellitus, and thrombophilia (such as antiphospholipid antibodies).

Pathophysiology

The broad spectrum of clinical manifestations and predisposing factors associated with preeclampsia suggest that it is a heterogeneous disorder. Nevertheless, increasing evidence suggests a cascade of events following insufficient maternal uterine vascular response to the placenta and placental ischemia. In addition, anti-angiogenic factors made by the placenta circulate in high levels shortly before the development of preeclampsia. Measurement of these factors may soon aid in the early diagnosis of preeclampsia.

TABLE 43. Management of Hypertension During Pregnancy

Medication	Role in Management	Comments
Methyldopa	First line for gestational/chronic hypertension	May cause thirst, nausea, drowsiness
Labetalol	First line for acute/severe hypertension; first line for gestational/chronic hypertension	Increasingly preferred over methyldopa because of side-effect profile; may cause headache
Sustained-release nifedipine	Second line for chronic hypertension (less long-term experience than labetalol)	Avoid short-acting agents; avoid with magnesium
Hydralazine	Second line for acute/severe hypertension; third line for chronic management	Frequent dosing impractical for chronic treatment; lupus-like syndrome may occur in chronic setting
β-Blockers	Third line for chronic management	Conflicting data on atenolol safety; metoprolol appears to be safe
Thiazide diuretics	Third line for chronic management; may continue if patient taking prior to pregnancy	Theoretical concern for decrease in maternal plasma volume but no deleterious effects reported; hypokalemia may occur
ACE inhibitors; angiotensin receptor blockers; renin inhibitors	Contraindicated in pregnancy	Early exposure associated with cardiac anomalies; late exposure associated with kidney agenesis

Clinical Manifestations

Preeclampsia may be complicated by fetal injury (including fetal growth restriction) and maternal end-organ damage. Patients with preeclampsia may develop headache, visual disturbances, nausea, and vomiting. Variants include HELLP (hemolysis, elevated liver enzymes, low platelet count) and eclampsia (the development of seizures).

Prevention and Treatment

Many agents have been advocated to decrease the risk of preeclampsia; however, at present, only low-dose aspirin appears to modestly reduce risk. The definitive treatment of preeclampsia is delivery; in women at or near term, induction of labor is appropriate. Women who have mild disease and are remote from term can be managed with close monitoring of the mother and fetus, bed rest, and antihypertensive therapy for systolic blood pressures greater than 150 to 160 mm Hg. Antenatal corticosteroids can be given to promote fetal lung maturity if delivery is anticipated before the 34th week of gestation. Magnesium sulfate is the antiepileptic drug of choice and can be administered intrapartum or immediately postpartum in severe preeclampsia to prevent seizures. The clinical manifestations of preeclampsia typically resolve in the postpartum period, although resolution of hypertension may take longer with higher blood pressures. Similarly, higher proteinuria levels take longer to resolve.

KEY POINTS

- Gestational hypertension refers to hypertension that develops after 20 weeks of pregnancy in the absence of proteinuria or other maternal end-organ damage.
- Preeclampsia is characterized by new-onset hypertension accompanied by proteinuria and can develop any time after 20 weeks of pregnancy.
- Low-dose aspirin appears to modestly reduce the risk of preeclampsia.
- The definitive treatment of preeclampsia is delivery; in women at or near term, induction of labor is appropriate.
- Women with mild preeclampsia who are remote from term can be managed with close monitoring of the mother and fetus, bed rest, and antihypertensive therapy.
- In patients with severe preeclampsia, magnesium sulfate can be administered intrapartum or immediately postpartum to prevent seizures.

Kidney Disease in the Pregnant Patient

Women with CKD need significant counseling before considering pregnancy. Data suggest that women whose serum creatinine level is greater than 1.4 mg/dL (124 micromoles/L, stage 3 CKD or higher) have a significantly greater risk of complications from pregnancy, including preeclampsia and a significant decline in kidney function. In addition, there is a far greater risk of preterm delivery and intrauterine growth restriction.

Diabetes Mellitus

Patients with diabetes mellitus or gestational diabetes typically have excellent outcomes if they are able to maintain tight glycemic control. Women with diabetes and albuminuria who are treated with ACE inhibitors or ARBs must discontinue these agents before conception because of their teratogenic effects. In pregnant patients with albuminuria and hypertension who require treatment, specific calcium channel blockers have been shown to have a renoprotective effect and are considered safe for use in pregnancy (see MKSAP 16 Endocrinology and Metabolism).

Systemic Lupus Erythematosus

Patients with active systemic lupus erythematosus (SLE) have a high risk of maternal and fetal complications. Some of these complications relate to the autoimmune profile of the mother. In the setting of antiphospholipid antibodies, miscarriages and hypertensive disorders are common. In contrast, other autoantibodies increase the risk of neonatal lupus erythematosus. In addition, pregnancy may result in an exacerbation of SLE. Patients who receive cyclophosphamide or mycophenolate mofetil for nephritis should be counseled to avoid pregnancy. Therapy during pregnancy is ideally limited to corticosteroids and azathioprine.

Management of End-Stage Kidney Disease During Pregnancy

Pregnancy is very uncommon in women who are undergoing dialysis. Most of these patients have anovulatory cycles and decreased libido related to kidney failure and comorbid conditions. When pregnancy does occur, care should focus on adequacy of dialysis with goals greater than those for nonpregnant persons. Goals include maintaining normal electrolytes, lowering blood urea nitrogen levels (<40-45 mg/dL [14.3-16.1 mmol/L]), and maintaining adequate nutrition, with little fluctuation in weight or blood pressure. To achieve this end, hemodialysis is increased from an average of 12 hours per week to more than 20 hours per week. Peritoneal dialysis confers additional challenges, as the uterus grows and assumes an increasing amount of space in the abdomen; near term, it is difficult to achieve sufficient clearance without nearly continuous exchanges.

In contrast, successful pregnancy is increasingly common after kidney transplantation. Women should be counseled to wait 1 to 2 years after transplantation when they are on a stable medication regimen. In addition, women who take mycophenolate mofetil must shift to alternative agents, because this medication is not safe in pregnancy. There is experience with calcineurin inhibitors, azathioprine, and corticosteroids, but there are limited data for sirolimus. During pregnancy, transplant recipients may be more prone to anemia, glucose intolerance, hypertension, infection, and preeclampsia. There also is an increased risk of fetal complications, including intrauterine growth restriction, congenital anomalies, hypoadrenalism (if the mother is taking corticosteroids), and infections.

KEY POINTS

- Women with diabetes mellitus and albuminuria who are treated with ACE inhibitors or angiotensin receptor blockers must discontinue these agents before conception because of their teratogenic effects.

- Hemodialysis is increased from an average of 12 hours per week to more than 20 hours per week in pregnant patients with end-stage kidney disease.

- Kidney transplant recipients should wait 1 to 2 years after transplantation before conceiving.

Chronic Kidney Disease

Pathophysiology and Epidemiology

Chronic kidney disease (CKD) is abnormal kidney function persisting for more than 3 months. Abnormal kidney function can be defined by either a decreased glomerular filtration rate (GFR) or by anatomic or structural abnormalities. CKD is functionally classified according to the degree of impairment in the GFR (**Table 44**). This classification system may overestimate the prevalence of CKD (particularly stages 1 and 2) but allows patients with CKD to be appropriately identified and evaluated.

Approximately 13% of the U.S. population has CKD. It generally has been thought that once the kidney is damaged, kidney disease will progress over time and require dialysis because of the increased work of the remaining nephron mass; however, patients with stages 1 through 4 CKD are more likely to die than to progress to kidney replacement therapy.

Screening

Recognizing patients at risk for CKD is imperative in a disease that can be asymptomatic. **Table 45** lists relevant medical history and predisposing risk factors that should prompt screening for CKD. In particular, evaluation for diseases that can damage the kidneys directly or can cause damage through their treatment is indicated. A family history of CKD is a risk factor, as more evidence points to an inherited predisposition to CKD. A history of acute kidney injury (AKI) is recognized as a risk for future AKI and CKD. Various genitourinary abnormalities also can cause CKD.

Screening for CKD includes measurement of the serum creatinine level, estimation of GFR, and urinalysis to evaluate for blood, protein, and casts. Kidney imaging (usually ultrasonography) should be considered, particularly if the serum

Stage[a]	GFR, mL/min/1.73 m²	Description	U.S. Population, %
1	≥90	Normal or increased GFR with other evidence of kidney damage	2
2	60-89	Slight decrease in GFR, with other evidence of kidney damage	3
3[b]	30-59	Moderate decrease in GFR, with or without other evidence of kidney damage	8
3A	45-59		
3B	30-44		
4	15-29	Severe decrease in GFR, with or without other evidence of kidney damage	0.4
5	<15	Established end-stage kidney disease	0.2

TABLE 44. Expanded Classification System for Chronic Kidney Disease

GFR = glomerular filtration rate.

[a]Suffixes are used to further describe the stages (for example, stage 2P, stage 3T):

"P" denotes the presence of proteinuria defined as a urine albumin–creatinine ratio greater than 30 mg/g or a urine protein–creatinine ratio greater than 0.5 mg/mg.

"T" denotes a patient with a functioning transplant.

"D" denotes a patient on dialysis (usually stage 5D).

[b]Stage 3 is sometimes divided in stages 3A and 3B to recognize the increased rate of cardiovascular complications in stage 3B compared with stage 3A. In persons older than 70 years of age, an estimated GFR between 45 to 59 mL/min/1.73 m², if stable over time and without any other evidence of kidney damage, is unlikely to be associated with complications related to chronic kidney disease.

National Institute for Health and Clinical Excellence (2008). Adapted from CG 73 Chronic kidney disease: early identification and management of chronic kidney disease in adults in primary and secondary care. London: NICE. Available from: www.nice.org.uk/cg73. Reproduced with permission.

TABLE 45. Medical History and Historical Features Associated with Chronic Kidney Disease

Medical History/Possible Causes of CKD

Causing Direct Kidney Damage	Important Historical Features
Diabetes mellitus	Duration
Hypertension	Duration
Glomerulonephritis	Autoimmune disease history
Multiple myeloma	History of treatment
AKI episodes	Episodes of kidney failure; dialysis
Chronic viral infections	History of hepatitis B, hepatitis C, or HIV

Kidney Damage from Treatment	Important Historical Features
Cancer	History of chemotherapy use
Chronic pain	Pain medications and duration used
Infections	Antibiotics used

Genitourinary Abnormalities	Important Historical Features
Kidney stones	Flank pain; hematuria
Kidney cancer	Kidney surgery/resection
Obstruction	Voiding issues; prostate issues; endometrial/pelvic cancers
Ureteral reflux	Urine infections; kidney infections

Exposures	Important Historical Features
Contrast	Repeat imaging studies/angiography
Heavy metals	Exposure history
Herbal supplements	Nonprescription/OTC use

Increased Risk

Increased Predisposition	Important Historical Features
Patient demographics	Older age (>70 years); obesity (BMI >30)
Family history	Family history of dialysis, proteinuria, kidney failure, or genetic kidney diseases (such as polycystic kidney disease)
Prior AKI even if baseline serum creatinine level is normal	Episodes of kidney failure; dialysis; prolonged hospitalizations; sepsis
Kidney transplant	Immunosuppressive drug use; episodes of rejection
Liver disease	Hepatitis; alcohol use

AKI = acute kidney injury; CKD = chronic kidney disease; OTC = over the counter.

creatinine level or urinalysis is abnormal or if there is suspicion of a structural abnormality.

Clinical Manifestations

The ability of the kidney to compensate for lost function can result in delayed presentation of clinical kidney disease; minimal or no symptoms may be present. The symptoms of CKD can be vague and include dysgeusia, pruritus, anorexia, fluid retention, fatigue, and impaired cognitive function. Pericarditis, serositis, gastrointestinal bleeding, encephalopathy, and uremic neuropathy typically do not develop until the GFR falls below 10 to 15 mL/min/1.73 m².

KEY POINTS

- Chronic kidney disease is characterized by a decreased glomerular filtration rate or by anatomic or structural abnormalities that have persisted for more than 3 months.

- Many conditions, including diabetes mellitus, hypertension, cancer, genitourinary abnormalities, and autoimmune diseases, are associated with chronic kidney disease.

- In patients with risk factors for chronic kidney disease, screening includes measurement of the serum creatinine level, estimation of glomerular filtration rate, and urinalysis to evaluate for the presence of blood, protein, and casts.

- The symptoms of chronic kidney disease include dysgeusia, pruritus, anorexia, fluid retention, fatigue, and impaired cognitive function.
- Pericarditis, serositis, gastrointestinal bleeding, encephalopathy, and uremic neuropathy typically do not develop until the glomerular filtration rate falls below 10 to 15 mL/min/1.73 m².

Management

Prevention of Progression

The approach to delaying or halting kidney disease progression involves an accurate diagnosis of the cause of CKD. If the diagnosis is not evident from the history, physical examination, laboratory studies, and imaging, a kidney biopsy may be appropriate.

Specific therapy to treat the underlying cause should then be instituted, such as treatment of an autoimmune disease, glomerulonephropathy, or interstitial nephritis. If treatment specific to the underlying cause of CKD is not indicated, management to delay kidney disease progression focuses on blood pressure control, cardiovascular risk reduction, use of sodium bicarbonate therapy, avoidance of further insults to the kidney, and proteinuria reduction.

Hypertension

Blood pressure control has been shown to delay CKD progression. The Seventh Report of the Joint National Committee on Prevention, Detection, Evaluation, and Treatment of High Blood Pressure (JNC 7) recommends a target blood pressure of less than 130/80 mm Hg for patients with kidney disease (as of publication, the eighth report reflecting current research data is in progress). **Figure 20** gives an algorithmic approach to the management of hypertension in patients with CKD.

Certain agents may help preserve kidney function beyond their blood pressure–lowering effect. ACE inhibitors have been shown to delay progression in patients with moderate to severe kidney disease and are particularly beneficial in patients with proteinuric (>1000 mg/24 h) CKD. Angiotensin receptor blockers (ARBs) may have effects on CKD progression similar to ACE inhibitors; the evidence is more limited, but growing.

Serum potassium levels should be monitored in patients taking ACE inhibitors or ARBs. If hyperkalemia develops, dietary potassium restriction, discontinuation of NSAIDs or other contributing medications, and the addition of loop or thiazide diuretics can be implemented to facilitate continuation of angiotensin blockade whenever possible.

The serum creatinine level should also be followed for progressive increases. A small increase in the serum creatinine level (<30% increase from baseline) can occur and may be a marker of effective renoprotection: decreased glomerular pressure causes an increase in the serum creatinine level, but the lower glomerular pressure results in less kidney damage over time. If the serum creatinine level increases by more than 30% after initiating an ACE inhibitor or ARB, evaluation for other sources of the decline in kidney function, such as bilateral renal artery stenosis, may be appropriate. If no other cause of AKI is apparent, the ACE inhibitor or ARB should be discontinued. If the serum creatinine level has increased to less than 30% from baseline but stabilizes, the benefits of renoprotection from the ACE inhibitor or ARB generally favor continuation of angiotensin blockade for most patients.

In patients in whom the GFR is marginal (such as <20 mL/min/1.73 m²), discontinuation of the ACE inhibitor or ARB has been shown in one observational study to delay progression to end-stage kidney disease (ESKD) in patients with advanced diabetic nephropathy on average by 1 year. ACE inhibitors or ARBs can be resumed in patients who do not show improvement in kidney function after discontinuation in the absence of other contraindications such as hyperkalemia. After initiating ACE inhibitor or ARB therapy, the GFR should be monitored closely in the following months. If a patient has a progressive decline in GFR in the months after starting ACE inhibitor or ARB therapy, and this rate of decline is faster than prior to initiation of the medication, the patient may have underlying vascular disease. The risk of accelerated CKD progression on angiotensin blockade in such patients likely outweighs the potential benefits.

Diuretics are effective agents for blood pressure control in patients with CKD and should be used in patients with edema. These agents generally require higher doses in patients with CKD to be effective. If a patient has CKD and uncontrolled blood pressure on hydrochlorothiazide, switching to a loop diuretic should be a first consideration. The addition of a thiazide to a loop diuretic such as furosemide can result in enhanced diuresis. Adequate dosing of loop and thiazide diuretics should increase potassium excretion, which lowers serum potassium levels and allows for more liberal use of other agents that block the renin-angiotensin-aldosterone system (such as ACE inhibitors, ARBs, or spironolactone).

The ACCOMPLISH trial demonstrated that combination therapy with a dihydropyridine calcium channel blocker and an ACE inhibitor was superior in preserving kidney function in patients with CKD compared to an ACE inhibitor with a thiazide diuretic. In the absence of edema, this combination is appropriate for patients requiring two agents to achieve target blood pressures. Spironolactone can also be a particularly effective antihypertensive agent in patients with resistant hypertension, but the serum potassium level must be monitored closely, particularly in patients with CKD who take ACE inhibitors or ARBs. Spironolactone is generally well tolerated in patients with an estimated GFR greater than 45 mL/min/17.3 m² and a baseline serum potassium level less than 4.5 meq/L (4.5 mmol/L).

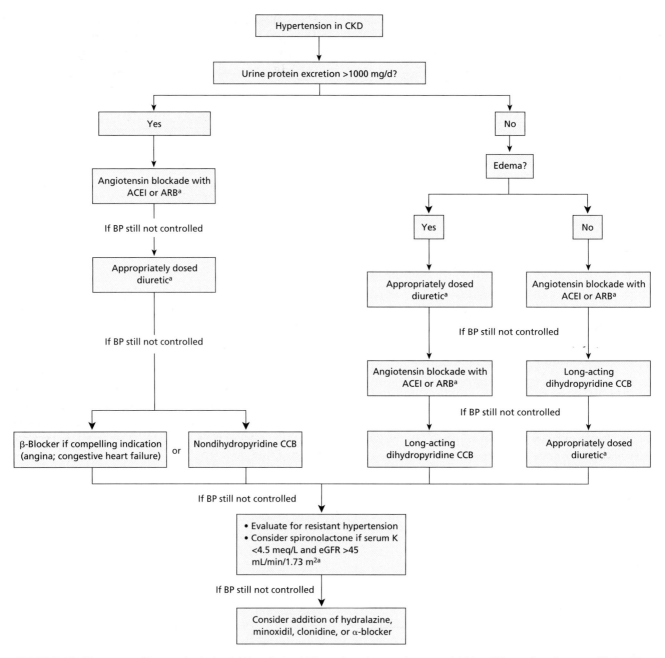

FIGURE 20. Management of hypertension in chronic kidney disease. ACEI = angiotensin-converting enzyme inhibitor; ARB = angiotensin receptor blocker; BP = blood pressure; CCB = calcium channel blocker; CKD = chronic kidney disease; eGFR = estimated glomerular filtration rate; K = potassium.

aMonitor serum potassium and creatinine levels. If serum potassium is greater than 5 meq/L (5 mmol/L), implement dietary potassium restriction, discontinue contributing agents such as NSAIDs, and consider increasing diuretic dose.

The peripheral vasodilators hydralazine and minoxidil are usually reserved for more refractory hypertension, which is more likely to occur in patients with CKD. Hydralazine or minoxidil should only be used as part of a multidrug regimen. Before initiating a peripheral vasodilator, the antihypertensive regimen should consist of an appropriate diuretic regimen and β-blockade to prevent edema and reflex tachycardia.

Metabolic Acidosis

Metabolic acidosis commonly develops in patients with CKD due to the loss of the ability of the kidney to regenerate bicarbonate. A delay in CKD progression with alkali therapy has been shown in several studies. The largest study involved more than 100 patients with stage 4 CKD who had baseline serum bicarbonate levels of 16 to 20 meq/L (16-20 mmol/L); those who received oral sodium bicarbonate

(600 mg, three times a day, with dose adjusted to achieve a serum bicarbonate level of at least 23 meq/L [23 mmol/L]) had a slower decline in GFR. Despite increased sodium intake, there was no difference in blood pressure or evidence of volume overload. Alkali treatment was given in addition to standard care, which included blood pressure control and ACE inhibitors. Alkali-treated patients also have been shown to have improved nutritional parameters. The low cost and low side-effect profile of this therapy make it an attractive treatment.

Nephrotoxins

An important part of preserving kidney function is avoiding the potentially harmful administration of medications that can damage kidney function. In patients with kidney disease, avoidance of certain over-the-counter medications, herbal supplements, nephrotoxic medications, or medications that can raise blood pressure is indicated (**Table 46**). Prescribed medications need to be dosed appropriately for the patient's GFR.

Iodinated contrast should be avoided if possible in patients with kidney disease, especially when the estimated GFR is less than 60 mL/min/1.73 m^2 (see Special Considerations, Imaging).

Proteinuria

Greater degrees of proteinuria have been associated with a more rapid decline of kidney function in diabetic and nondiabetic kidney disease. Proteinuria reduction is generally thought to be beneficial for the preservation of GFR in kidney disease. Blood pressure should first be lowered to a target of 130/80 mm Hg, preferentially using agents that block angiotensin (ACE inhibitors or ARBs). Spironolactone also has been shown to reduce proteinuria in patients with diabetes. The ONTARGET study showed that adding an ARB (telmisartan) to an ACE inhibitor (ramipril) reduced proteinuria but actually worsened renal outcomes in patients over the age of 55 years who have diabetes and end-organ damage or atherosclerotic vascular disease. This study, however, did not include many patients with high degrees of proteinuria. In general, using an ACE inhibitor and ARB in combination is not recommended, but in high-risk (heavy proteinuria) patients, this combination is under investigation.

Protein Restriction

Protein restriction has been shown to delay kidney disease progression in animals. Evidence in humans remains unclear; studies indicate a small but insignificant improvement in the rate of decrease of GFR in protein-restricted patients who have CKD. A protein restriction of 0.6 to 0.8 g/kg/d to delay CKD progression can be instituted in very adherent patients. Body weight and serum albumin levels should be followed to ensure adequate nutrition. When used, protein restriction should be used in combination with measures proved to forestall progression, such as hypertension control or angiotensin blockade.

TABLE 46.	Over-the-Counter Medications to Avoid in Patients with Chronic Kidney Disease
Agent	**Potential Adverse Effects**
NSAIDs	Hemodynamic changes due to prostaglandin inhibition; interstitial nephritis
Decongestants	Increased blood pressure
Herbal supplements	
Aristolochia/aristolochic acid	Tubular atrophy and interstitial fibrosis
Chromium	Chronic interstitial nephritis
Creatine	Chronic interstitial nephritis; rhabdomyolysis; AKI
Germanium	Tubular injury and degeneration
Ma Huang/Ephedra	Increased blood pressure; rhabdomyolysis; AKI
Salt substitutes	High in potassium
Gastrointestinal medications	
Laxatives/enemas	
Sodium phosphate	Elevated serum phosphate levels
Magnesium hydroxide	Elevated serum magnesium levels
Magnesium citrate	Elevated serum magnesium levels
Antacids/antidyspepsia agents	
Aluminum and magnesium hydroxide	Elevated serum magnesium and aluminum levels
Sodium bicarbonate, potassium bicarbonate, and citric acid	Elevated serum sodium and potassium levels

AKI = acute kidney injury.

Complications

In addition to measures to prevent kidney disease progression, efforts should be undertaken to recognize and manage complications specific to CKD.

Cardiovascular Disease

CKD is associated with an increased risk of cardiovascular disease, specifically, myocardial infarction, stroke, peripheral vascular disease, and cardiovascular death. This risk is greater in patients with CKD than in the general population, even after adjusting for traditional risk factors such as hypertension and diabetes. The risk of cardiovascular events (and death and hospitalizations) has been shown to increase steadily with increased CKD stage (or decreased GFR) when GFR was stratified into stages 3A, 3B, 4, and 5 (see Table 44). Addressing cardiovascular risk is a management priority in patients with CKD. Patients with CKD are more likely to experience cardiovascular complications and death than to progress to ESKD and the need for kidney replacement therapy.

Lifestyle modification, including smoking cessation, exercise, and weight loss in overweight patients, may have benefit in delaying kidney disease progression and should be implemented to help reduce cardiovascular risk. Other treatment targets (hypertension, dyslipidemia, and coronary artery disease) are discussed in the next sections.

Hypertension

The prevalence of hypertension is higher in patients with CKD than in the general population. The prevalence of hypertension in the general adult population is almost 25%. The prevalence increases with increasing stage of kidney disease—from approximately 35% in stage 1 to more than 80% in stages 4 and 5. Although patients with CKD often have been excluded from hypertension trials, the cardiovascular benefit of lowering blood pressure found in the general population is also likely true for patients with CKD.

The treatment of hypertension in patients with CKD is discussed in the Prevention of Progression section. A preference for agents that inhibit angiotensin (ACE inhibitors and ARBs) is reasonable, as these agents can also delay CKD progression (particularly when proteinuria is present) and have been shown in some studies to reduce cardiovascular mortality.

Dyslipidemia

No consistent pattern of lipid abnormalities has been identified in patients with CKD. Alterations in apolipoproteins have been noted before the serum cholesterol levels change, and a decrease in HDL cholesterol and increase in triglycerides has been reported as CKD progresses. The variability of lipid levels in CKD may reflect the underlying cause of the CKD. Although treatment of dyslipidemia with statins has not been shown to delay CKD progression, lowering cholesterol levels with statins reduces cardiovascular risk. Statins may also reduce proteinuria and have beneficial anti-inflammatory and vascular effects.

A 2009 Cochrane review of statins in patients with CKD showed reduced cardiovascular mortality in those with stages 3 and 4 CKD, and the incidence of side effects was similar in the CKD population to the general population. Although effective in patients with stages 1 through 4 CKD, large studies have not shown a mortality benefit to statin use in the dialysis CKD population.

Coronary Artery Disease

The prevalence of coronary artery disease in patients with CKD is estimated at 40% to 65%. The event rate for myocardial infarction is higher in CKD patients without diabetes than in non-CKD patients with diabetes. A portion of the increased cardiovascular risk in patients with CKD may be attributable to decreased use of appropriate medications, perhaps because of concern about a higher rate of side effects. ACE inhibitors, aspirin, and statins are less likely to be used in patients with CKD. These agents should not be withheld on the basis of a diagnosis of CKD; in fact, treatment with these medications may benefit the CKD population more than the general population. CKD may also cause some confusion with diagnostic blood tests. The levels of cardiac enzymes in the blood, specifically creatine kinase, B-type natriuretic peptide, and troponin, may be elevated in those with CKD relative to patients with normal kidney function, particularly in patients on dialysis. These elevated levels should not be attributed to CKD alone without an appropriate evaluation.

Coronary artery bypass grafting can be beneficial in selected patients with CKD and should be considered for appropriate patients, although these patients have a higher risk of postoperative AKI. The risk of kidney disease requiring dialysis in a patient with CKD undergoing heart surgery can be estimated by a calculator available online at www.zunis.org/Need%20For%20Dialysis%20After%20Heart%20Surgery%20Calculator.htm.

Chronic Kidney Disease-Mineral Bone Disorder

The kidney plays a critical role in calcium and phosphorus homeostasis; as kidney function deteriorates, adaptations occur that maintain normal serum calcium levels. Yet these accommodations may lead to a spectrum of adverse consequences, including serious bone disease and extraskeletal vascular calcification. The term *chronic kidney disease-mineral bone disorder* (CKD-MBD) has been adopted to reflect these abnormalities. The 2009 Kidney Disease Improving Global Outcomes (KDIGO) guidelines on the evaluation and treatment of CKD-MBD are available at www.kdigo.org/guidelines/mbd/index.html.

Calcium and Phosphorus Homeostasis

Cholecalciferol (vitamin D_3) is synthesized in the skin with exposure to ultraviolet light and can also be obtained from fortified dietary sources. Vitamin D deficiency is common, particularly in the setting of CKD. Vitamin D is hydroxylated in the liver and then in the kidney into calcitriol (1,25-dihydroxy vitamin D). Calcitriol promotes absorption of dietary calcium and phosphorus in the gastrointestinal tract. As the kidney loses the ability to hydroxylate vitamin D, the plasma level of calcitriol often decreases as the GFR declines, which prompts an increase in the parathyroid hormone (PTH) level via both direct and indirect mechanisms, termed *secondary hyperparathyroidism*. Low calcitriol levels can result in hypocalcemia, leading to a compensatory increase in serum PTH levels.

Vitamin D deficiency removes the inhibitory effect of calcitriol on the vitamin D receptor of parathyroid cells.

PTH liberates calcium and phosphorus from bone and limits urine calcium excretion; routine serum calcium levels may be normal as the PTH levels increase due to increased mobilization of calcium from bone (**Figure 21**).

Reduced kidney function leads to a decrease in phosphate filtration and increases in serum phosphorus levels. This also results in an increased release of PTH, which inhibits proximal tubular reabsorption of phosphorus and results in increased phosphorus excretion. Yet when the GFR is reduced, this effect is limited; the concurrent PTH-driven liberation of phosphorus from bone increases the filtered load of phosphate and exacerbates the hyperphosphatemia. A vicious cycle may ensue in which hyperparathyroidism worsens steadily in response to hypocalcemia and hyperphosphatemia.

Laboratory Abnormalities

A large multicenter observational study noted that an elevation in PTH level is often the first detectable change associated with CKD-MBD, which may occur very early in the course of CKD; therefore, KDIGO guidelines recommend testing for MBD beginning with stage 3 CKD.

Assessment includes measurement of serum calcium and phosphorus levels and measurement of PTH levels using the "intact" assay that measures active PTH hormone in two sites (fragments of the PTH molecule are cleared by the kidney

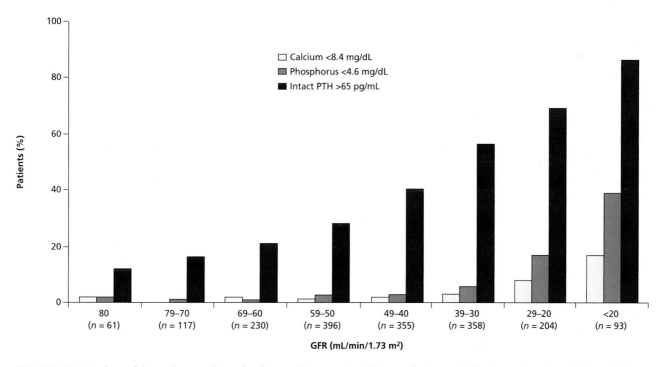

FIGURE 21. Prevalence of abnormal serum calcium, phosphorus, and intact parathyroid hormone by glomerular filtration rate in patients with chronic kidney disease. GFR = glomerular filtration rate; PTH = parathyroid hormone.

and may be elevated in CKD). Calcidiol (25-hydroxy vitamin D) should be measured because it has a long half-life and reflects both nutritional intake and skin synthesis. Alkaline phosphatase also may be used as an adjunct to interpret testing; however, if levels are elevated, a liver source should be excluded. If the PTH is in normal range and kidney function is stable, annual measurements of calcium, phosphorus, and PTH should suffice; however, if the patient's kidney function declines or if the patient requires treatment, then calcium, phosphate, and PTH should be monitored every 3 months.

Vascular Calcification

Severe vascular calcification appears to play a significant role in the risk of cardiovascular disease in patients with CKD. Whereas patients with atherosclerosis develop calcification in the intima of arteries, even young patients with CKD can develop medial vascular calcifications. This pathology leads to a decrease in vascular compliance, which is associated with hypertension, left ventricular hypertrophy, and reduced end-organ perfusion. Although calcification was thought to be the result of a simple physicochemical relationship of the high calcium and phosphorus product, it now appears that the mineral imbalance initiates a complex response with damage to the vascular smooth muscle cells and perhaps phenotypic transformation of these cells into osteoblast-like cells. As the bone is demineralized, the vasculature becomes more calcified. Calcific uremic arteriolopathy (calciphylaxis) is the most severe form of this process and involves the small cutaneous arteries. This disorder is characterized by ischemic and painful skin ulceration and is associated with a high mortality rate. It is not yet clear whether improved calcium and phosphorus control will translate to a reduction in vascular calcification and an improvement in clinical outcomes in patients with CKD.

Renal Osteodystrophy

Renal osteodystrophy refers to the skeletal complications associated with CKD. Bone disease may result in bone pain or fractures. Although there are several patterns of pathology, all patterns confer a markedly increased risk of fracture. The most common forms of renal osteodystrophy are osteitis fibrosa cystica, osteomalacia, and adynamic bone disease; patients may also have a mixed disorder or additional conditions such as osteoporosis or amyloidosis. Distinction between these types of bone disease can only be made by bone biopsy, which is generally reserved for patients with unexplained findings when pathology may help guide therapy. Instead, treatment decisions are generally based on biochemical profiles.

Osteitis fibrosis cystica describes the high-turnover bone disease associated with chronic secondary hyperparathyroidism. Patients typically are asymptomatic but may develop bone pain and have an increased risk of fractures. Classic radiograph findings include subperiosteal bone reabsorption, especially in the distal clavicles and the phalanges. Treatment includes maintaining serum calcium and phosphorus levels in the normal range through use of phosphate binders as well as use of calcitriol or other 1,25-dihydroxy vitamin D analogs or cinacalcet to maintain serum PTH levels at target levels.

Osteomalacia is characterized by decreased bone mineralization at the newly formed osteoid in sites of bone turnover. This disorder can occur in children with vitamin D deficiency and is called rickets when the unfused growth plates are also involved. Although vitamin D deficiency is common in CKD, this form of bone pathology is unusual and is typically associated with an additional abnormality. In the past, the most common etiology was aluminum toxicity, which is taken up by bone and leads to abnormal bone mineralization. Avoidance of aluminum in over-the-counter and prescribed medications as well as limitation of aluminum in water supplies and in phosphate-binding agents has greatly decreased the incidence of this disorder. Treatment of aluminum toxicity requires prolonged chelation therapy.

Adynamic bone disease is characterized by low turnover of bone with both reduced bone formation and resorption. Although the pathophysiology is poorly understood, it appears to be associated with oversuppression of PTH. This may be seen in the setting of excessive treatment with vitamin D and calcium or following parathyroidectomy. Patients typically have PTH levels below 100 pg/mL (100 ng/L), bone pain, and fractures. Alkaline phosphatase levels are usually not elevated. A decrease or discontinuation of vitamin D analogs and calcium-based binders is indicated.

Patients with CKD can also develop osteoporosis; however, the diagnosis may be more difficult in the setting of CKD because bone mineral density studies in patients with either osteoporosis or CKD-MBD may demonstrate reduction in bone density and cannot reliably determine risk for fracture nor differentiate osteoporosis from other pathology. For this reason, it is currently recommended that patients with mild kidney impairment (stages 1 or 2 CKD) be treated for suspected osteoporosis like the general population. Patients with stage 3 CKD should be evaluated for evidence of secondary hyperparathyroidism. If these biochemical markers are normal, they can also be treated like the general population for osteoporosis.

In contrast, when the estimated GFR is less than 30 mL/min/1.73 m^2, the focus of therapy should be on correcting secondary hyperparathyroidism. Bisphosphonates are cleared by the kidney and have not been adequately tested in patients with reduced kidney function. In this setting, the dose must be reduced or stopped altogether. Furthermore, because the mechanism of action is to inhibit osteoclast reabsorption, bisphosphonates may subsequently limit new bone formation and result in adynamic bone disease. Other antiresorptive agents used in the treatment of osteoporosis such as raloxifene have not been extensively studied in patients with reduced kidney function.

Treatment

The initial goal in the treatment of CKD-MBD is correction of hyperphosphatemia and hypocalcemia. Hyperphosphatemia can be treated by dietary phosphate restriction and oral medications that bind dietary phosphate in the gastrointestinal tract. The goal of therapy is to maintain the serum phosphorus level in the normal range. Aluminum salts work well to bind phosphate, but long-term use results in neurologic, skeletal, and hematologic toxicity. Calcium salts (carbonate and acetate) also can serve to bind phosphate; however, large doses are needed, and recent concerns regarding their role in vascular calcification have prompted clinicians to select newer and more costly noncalcium-, nonaluminum-based agents such as sevelamer and lanthanum. However, this shift has not yet produced any clear clinical improvements.

Patients with vitamin D deficiency should receive supplemental vitamin D. If vitamin D levels are robust and the phosphate level is normal, but the PTH level is elevated above target levels, active vitamin D analogs should be initiated. The National Kidney Foundation guidelines suggest graded PTH goals based on the level of kidney function; in stage 3 CKD, the goal should be at the upper limit of normal, whereas in stage 5 CKD, the goal could be much higher. In contrast, the KDIGO guidelines suggest aiming for normal values at all stages of CKD with more permissive rises once a patient begins dialysis. Both sets of guidelines are opinion-based, and both agree that vitamin D analogs should be discontinued in the setting of hypercalcemia or hyperphosphatemia.

In contrast to vitamin D analogs, calcimimetic agents modulate the calcium-sensing receptor on the parathyroid cells and increase the signal of extracellular ionized calcium. As a result, these agents "mimic" calcium at the receptor and decrease PTH release. There is currently one calcimimetic available, cinacalcet, which is FDA approved only for use in patients who are on dialysis. This agent is very expensive, and its role in patients with CKD has not yet been defined.

Anemia

Anemia is common in patients with CKD and usually occurs when the estimated GFR falls below 30 mL/min/1.73 m². Erythropoietin is made by interstitial peritubular fibroblasts of the kidney. Patients with reduced kidney function may have low erythropoietin levels, but erythropoietin resistance also occurs. When patients with reduced kidney function develop anemia, evaluation for other causes is appropriate; in particular, relative iron deficiency is common. If iron stores are adequate and other causes have also been eliminated, the anemia can be attributed to CKD. There is no role for the routine measurement of erythropoietin levels in this setting because this expensive test does not aid in the diagnosis or guide treatment decisions.

The erythropoiesis-stimulating agents (ESAs) epoetin and darbepoetin have been found to limit the development of left ventricular hypertrophy and the need for blood transfusions as well as to improve quality-of-life markers in patients on dialysis. Although target hemoglobin levels were never established, standard practice was to treat patients to a target hemoglobin level of 11 to 12 g/dL (110-120 g/L). In recent years, a number of trials have investigated outcomes when

ESAs have been dosed to achieve normal hemoglobin levels. A large randomized trial of men with cardiovascular disease on hemodialysis was terminated early due to a trend toward increased mortality in the normal hemoglobin group. Investigators suspected that this was related to hemoconcentration and hyperviscosity in patients undergoing hemodialysis. Targeting a normal hematocrit was also studied in patients with CKD in three large randomized trials. These trials did not demonstrate benefit in cardiovascular morbidity or mortality from the higher target hemoglobin level. In addition, one study suggested that patients with higher hemoglobin targets were more likely to have adverse outcomes, and another found nearly a doubling in the risk of strokes. Subsequent analyses have shown that decreased responsiveness to ESAs, and therefore, higher pharmacologic doses, also conferred a worse prognosis.

Multiple recent trials on the use of ESAs in the treatment of anemia associated with cancer suggest that ESAs may increase the risk of tumor growth and shorten survival in patients with cancer. For this reason, the FDA has issued a warning, and patients with cancer can only use ESAs with appropriate counseling and enrollment in a monitoring program.

ESAs should be considered for patients with symptomatic anemia attributable to erythropoietin deficiency when the hemoglobin level is less than 10 g/dL (100 g/L). Patients with CKD must be carefully counseled about the risks of ESAs, which include increased risk of thrombotic and cardiovascular events as well as increased blood pressure. In addition, clinicians should explain that the targets for hemoglobin are lower than those used in the past, and that patients must be monitored regularly to titrate the dose to a target hemoglobin level of 10 to 11 g/dL (100-110 g/L).

KEY POINTS

- Complications associated with chronic kidney disease include cardiovascular disease, chronic kidney disease-mineral bone disorder, and anemia.

- Patients with chronic kidney disease may develop renal osteodystrophy that manifests as osteitis fibrosa cystica, osteomalacia, and adynamic bone disease.

- The initial goal in the treatment of chronic kidney disease-mineral bone disorder is correction of hyperphosphatemia and hypocalcemia.

- Anemia of chronic kidney disease is a diagnosis of exclusion; erythropoietin levels are not diagnostic and should not be pursued.

- Erythropoiesis-stimulating agents should be considered for patients with symptomatic anemia attributable to erythropoietin deficiency when the hemoglobin level is less than 10 g/dL (100 g/L).

- Erythropoiesis-stimulating agent therapy requires careful monitoring to titrate the dose to target hemoglobin levels of 10 to 11 g/dL (100-110 g/L).

Special Considerations

Special considerations for patients with CKD include medication dosing, medication selection, imaging, and vascular access. Medications that are renally excreted should be dosed based on the GFR of the patient. When intravenous or new medications are started, levels should be monitored if possible to avoid toxic levels and to ensure appropriate therapeutic levels. Non-nephrotoxic medications should be used when possible, and intravenous contrast should be avoided unless necessary. Fluid and electrolyte replacement should be administered carefully because patients with CKD can have impaired renal excretion of sodium, potassium, phosphorus, and magnesium.

Imaging

Iodinated contrast used in imaging studies can cause AKI in patients who have CKD and should be avoided. Alternatives include ultrasonography, noncontrast studies, plain radiography, and MRI (see Clinical Evaluation of Kidney Function, Imaging Studies). If a radiocontrast study is necessary, minimizing the amount of contrast and optimizing patient hemodynamics are cornerstones of treatment. Optimizing kidney perfusion entails avoiding hypovolemia, optimizing cardiac function (particularly in patients with heart failure), and discontinuing agents that can compromise kidney perfusion such as ACE inhibitors, ARBs, renin inhibitors, or NSAIDs. *N*-acetylcysteine is frequently given to prevent contrast-induced nephropathy; although the benefit may not be robust, *N*-acetylcysteine is associated with minimal risk. Once a patient with minimal urine output is on dialysis, iodinated contrast administration is thought to be safe.

The MRI contrast agent gadolinium is associated with nephrogenic systemic fibrosis (NSF) and should be avoided in patients with CKD, particularly those with a GFR less than 30 mL/min/1.73 m^2. NSF manifests as cutaneous plaques, papules, and nodules with a brawny wooden texture that start symmetrically in legs and may then involve the arms and trunk with sparing of the face. NSF usually occurs within a few months of gadolinium exposure but may take years to appear (or be recognized). In addition to skin and periarticular fibrosis, the heart, lungs, skeletal muscle, and diaphragm can also be affected. Patients with NSF often have a progressive course, resulting in worsening morbidity (from limited mobility and pain) and ultimately death. Although reversal with kidney transplantation has been reported, the best treatment is prevention. H

Vaccination

Patients with CKD are considered to have impaired immune systems. Vaccination should be addressed aggressively in patients with CKD because potential outcomes include dialysis and kidney transplantation. Providing vaccination before transplantation or dialysis may result in a superior immune response.

Annual influenza vaccination, as well as vaccination against *Streptococcus pneumoniae* at the time of CKD diagnosis and at 5-year intervals, is indicated. Hepatitis B vaccine series is recommended for patients with progressive CKD. Live virus vaccines are contraindicated in transplant recipients and should be avoided 3 months before planned transplantation. The role of the live varicella zoster vaccine in progressive CKD is not yet clear.

Hospitalization

Patients with CKD may ultimately need dialysis, and maintaining vein patency will make future arteriovenous hemodialysis access creation (fistula or graft) possible. Veins can be protected by avoiding intravenous lines and blood draws as much as possible. Use of the hands for veins for blood draws and peripheral intravenous lines is preferred. Peripherally inserted central catheter lines and subclavian central access should be avoided, and internal jugular central venous access is preferred if central access is needed to limit the risk of subsequent subclavian vein stenosis. Avoiding central veins, if possible, is preferred. Minimizing phlebotomy protects veins and reduces the potential for anemia. For patients on hemodialysis, phlebotomy can be done with their dialysis, which can spare these patients unnecessary venipuncture. H

KEY POINTS

- The MRI contrast agent gadolinium is associated with nephrogenic systemic fibrosis and should be avoided in patients with chronic kidney disease, particularly those with a glomerular filtration rate less than 30 mL/min/1.73 m^2.

- Vaccination should be addressed aggressively in patients with chronic kidney disease because the response to vaccination is superior before dialysis or transplantation.

- In patients with chronic kidney disease, avoiding intravenous lines and venipuncture in the arms is helpful to preserve veins for future dialysis access; use of the hands for venipuncture and peripheral intravenous lines is preferred.

Treatment of End-Stage Kidney Disease

Despite efforts to slow CKD progression, sometimes the residual renal mass is insufficient, and kidney function continues to decline. Discussions regarding the decline in kidney function and modalities of kidney replacement therapy should begin at least 1 year before the patient is likely to need kidney replacement therapy. When the estimated GFR approaches 20 mL/min/1.73 m^2, referral to a transplant center is appropriate, and more comprehensive "options teaching" should occur.

Transplantation is the treatment of choice for ESKD because the mortality and morbidity are far lower than with other modalities of kidney replacement therapy. Patients can undergo preemptive transplantation before initiating dialysis, which has a better prognosis than transplantation after dialysis. Preemptive transplantation is usually performed using a living donor but sometimes a patient may receive a kidney from a deceased donor. Nevertheless, many patients may not be appropriate candidates for transplantation or may not have an appropriate donor. Instead, they will need to pursue dialysis and, if appropriate, wait for a kidney while undergoing dialysis (**Table 47**).

Recent studies have shown that there is no benefit from early initiation of dialysis when kidney function is above an estimated GFR ≥12 mL/min/1.73 m². Patients should wait until they have uremic symptoms, electrolyte abnormalities that cannot be managed easily with medications, or evidence of malnutrition. Dialysis is typically initiated when the estimated GFR is between 8 and 11 mL/min/1.73 m²; most patients will be symptomatic at this level. Management of volume overload often necessitates earlier initiation compared with patients who can tolerate extra volume.

KEY POINTS

- Discussions regarding the decline in kidney function and modalities of kidney replacement therapy should begin at least 1 year before the patient is likely to need kidney replacement therapy.

- Kidney transplantation is the treatment of choice for patients with end-stage kidney disease.

- Patients can undergo preemptive kidney transplantation before initiating dialysis, which has a better prognosis than transplantation after dialysis.

- Dialysis should be initiated in patients with uremic symptoms, electrolyte abnormalities that cannot be easily managed with medications, uncontrollable volume overload, or evidence of malnutrition.

Dialysis

Hemodialysis

The most common modality for dialysis in the United States is hemodialysis. Hemodialysis is typically done three times a week for 4 hours. Longer nocturnal strategies, which are employed six times a week, are gaining popularity. In anticipation of hemodialysis, patients should be referred for vascular access. Ideally, an autologous arteriovenous fistula is created by anastomosing a vein to an artery. The vein becomes thickened or "arterialized" and is then able to sustain repeated cannulation when dialysis is needed. If there are no appropriate veins, a synthetic conduit can be used, but these are more likely to develop thrombosis or infection. Finally, if initiation of dialysis is more urgent and the patient does not have access, a catheter can be placed. Large-gauge tunneled catheters are typically placed in the internal jugular vein rather than the subclavian vein because the latter may lead to subclavian venous stenosis and limit venous return of future arteriovenous access on the ipsilateral side. Catheters are easy to use but have a high rate of infection.

Because treatments are usually only three times a week, patients must adhere to a strict diet and limit sodium, potassium, and fluids between treatments. During dialysis, volume, electrolytes, anemia, and bone disease are carefully managed.

Peritoneal Dialysis

Peritoneal dialysis, in which the peritoneum is used as a dialysis membrane, is an alternative to hemodialysis for most patients with ESKD. Patients with heart failure tolerate peritoneal dialysis well because there are smaller fluid shifts than during hemodialysis, but patients who have had prior extensive abdominal surgeries may have too much scarring to utilize this modality. A catheter is placed in the peritoneum and tunneled through the abdominal wall. The incision requires 1 month to heal, and the patient receives training to perform exchanges. Peritoneal dialysis can be done by manually instilling and removing the dialysis fluid (an exchange), or a cycling

TABLE 47.	Kidney Transplantation and Graft Survival[a]					
Transplantation	**Comment**	**1-Year Graft Survival**	**1-Year Patient Survival**	**5-Year Graft Survival**	**5-Year Patient Survival**
Living donor (related or unrelated)	Elective surgery may allow avoidance of dialysis	97%	99%	81%	91%
Deceased donor	Waiting time varies by blood type but typically >4 years for type O	93%	96%	72%	84%
Extended criteria Deceased donor	Shorter wait time; may include donors >60 years or those with hypertension; history of cerebrovascular accident or serum creatinine level >1.5 mg/dL (133 µmol/L)	86%	92%	57%	72%

[a]1-year data is from 2007 and 5-year data is from 2002 to 2007.

Data from Axelrod DA, McCullough KP, Brewer ED, Becker BN, Segev DL, Rao PS. Kidney and pancreas transplantation in the United States, 1999-2008: the changing face of living donation. Am J Transplant. 2010;10(4 Pt 2):987-1002. [PMID: 20420648]

CONT.

machine can be utilized during the night that is programmed to perform exchanges automatically. In both techniques, fluid with a high concentration of dextrose is instilled into the peritoneum. Diffusion and convection aid in the movement of water, urea, and electrolytes into the dialysate, which is then drained and discarded. This modality offers independence for patients able to participate in their own care and more gradual shifts in electrolytes and fluid, but it may worsen control of diabetes from absorption of the dextrose in the peritoneal fluid. **H**

Management without Dialysis

Patients may decide not to participate in dialysis or may decide to stop dialysis after initiation ("withdrawal"). In these cases, the decision should be explored with the assistance of the patient's nephrologist. Patients who have been established on dialysis and then choose to stop typically survive less than 2 weeks; the progression to death is painless, and patients typically drift into a coma before death. If patients with a very low estimated GFR decide to continue on a protein-restricted diet without dialysis, the course can be much slower but similarly painless. Hospice services are infrequently utilized for patients with ESKD who choose to avoid or withdraw from dialysis but would be a potential benefit.

Complications of Dialysis

Cardiovascular Disease

Cardiovascular disease is the leading cause of death in patients on dialysis. The increased risk is multifactorial, but conventional cardiovascular risk factors do not fully explain the excess risk. Additional factors may be present in the uremic milieu, including mediators of inflammation, sympathetic nerve activity, disturbed mineral balance, and endothelial dysfunction. In addition, electrolyte abnormalities associated with intermittent hemodialysis make patients more susceptible to arrhythmias and sudden death. **H**

Acquired Renal Cystic Disease

Patients with CKD commonly develop multiple small bilateral cysts in the kidneys that may be noted incidentally on imaging. Although cysts may be seen before dialysis, the incidence increases as the number of months or years on dialysis increases. Most cysts are asymptomatic, but on occasion, patients may develop hematuria or flank pain. The most serious complication of acquired renal cystic disease is the development of renal cell carcinoma. The incidence of renal cell carcinoma is not clear, but some experts recommend screening after 3 to 5 years of dialysis.

KEY POINT

- Patients on dialysis have an increased risk for cardiovascular disease and acquired renal cystic disease.

Kidney Transplantation

Kidney transplants can be from living or deceased donors. A living donor may be a relative, unrelated but emotionally related, or altruistic. Donor evaluation includes age-appropriate screening tests, kidney imaging, and assessment of kidney function and proteinuria. Donors are typically excluded if they have diabetes or hypertension. Recent studies show that carefully screened donors have no greater risk of ESKD than the general population.

Careful screening of the potential recipient is also essential. There are multiple potential barriers to transplantation, including ischemic heart disease, substance abuse, malignancy, and infection. In addition, cognitive, behavioral, and financial issues must be addressed.

Immunosuppressive Therapy
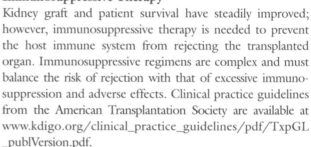
Kidney graft and patient survival have steadily improved; however, immunosuppressive therapy is needed to prevent the host immune system from rejecting the transplanted organ. Immunosuppressive regimens are complex and must balance the risk of rejection with that of excessive immunosuppression and adverse effects. Clinical practice guidelines from the American Transplantation Society are available at www.kdigo.org/clinical_practice_guidelines/pdf/TxpGL _publVersion.pdf.

Initial treatment includes induction immunosuppressive therapy because this is the period when the risk of acute rejection is greatest. Induction therapy may include T-cell–depleting antibodies or antibodies that block the IL-2 receptor. Maintenance therapy typically includes a calcineurin inhibitor and an antiproliferative agent with or without corticosteroids. Combination therapy with low doses of several agents that have different mechanisms of action may allow improved efficacy with less toxicity (**Table 48**).

Risks of Transplantation
Infection

Polyoma BK virus is an increasingly recognized cause of graft nephropathy. Screening with polymerase chain reaction testing and urine cytology is recommended in the first year and when there is a decline in kidney function. Definitive diagnosis requires kidney biopsy. When BK nephropathy occurs, reduction of immunosuppression to the minimum level possible to avoid rejection is required.

Cytomegalovirus (CMV) remains an important pathogen in the posttransplant period. Risk of infection depends on the serology of the donor and the recipient and is greatest when the donor is positive for CMV but the recipient is negative. Chemoprophylaxis with valganciclovir decreases the risk of infection. Patients with acute CMV infection may have a nonspecific febrile syndrome or more serious illness with enteritis, pneumonitis, or hepatitis. CMV infection is also associated with both acute and chronic rejection.

TABLE 48. Maintenance Immunosuppressive Therapy for Kidney Transplantation			
Class	**Medication**	**Mechanism**	**Adverse Effects**
Anti-inflammatory	Prednisone	Inhibits T-cell activation by blocking IL-1, IL-6, IL-2, and IFN synthesis	Glucose intolerance; avascular necrosis; cataracts; hypertension; central obesity; bone loss
Calcineurin inhibitor	Tacrolimus and cyclosporine	Inhibits calcineurin activity necessary for transcription of genes that activate T cells	Both agents are nephrotoxic; tacrolimus: causes more glucose intolerance and neurologic toxicity (tremors, headaches); cyclosporine: causes more hypertension, hirsutism, and gingival hyperplasia
Antimetabolite	Mycophenolate mofetil and azathioprine	Blocks T- and B-cell proliferation by interrupting purine synthesis	Mycophenolate mofetil: nausea, diarrhea, leucopenia, anemia, viral infections; azathioprine: leukopenia, thrombocytopenia, hepatitis, susceptibility to infection and cancer (particularly squamous cell)
Inhibits rapamycin	Sirolimus	Blocks IL-2 dependent T-cell proliferation	Leukopenia; hyperlipidemia; proteinuria; glucose intolerance; decreased wound healing; pneumonitis; infertility

IFN = interferon; IL = interleukin.

CONT.

Transplant recipients also are at increased risk of urinary tract infection in the first 6 months following transplantation. Prophylaxis with trimethoprim-sulfamethoxazole is usually recommended. This strategy also provides prophylaxis for *Pneumocystis jirovecii* pneumonia, and many centers will continue prophylaxis for the latter indefinitely. In addition, prophylaxis to prevent oral and esophageal candidiasis is recommended in the immediate posttransplant period.

Cancer
Kidney transplant recipients are at an increased risk for post-transplant lymphoproliferative disease (PTLD), which is often related to the Epstein-Barr virus. Reduction or withdrawal of immunosuppressive therapy may be sufficient to address PTLD, but some patients may require additional strategies to control the disease.

The incidence of squamous cell carcinoma of the skin is increased, particularly in those with long exposure to azathioprine, and all patients with CKD should be counseled to limit exposure to ultraviolet light.

Special Considerations in Transplant Recipients
Disease Recurrence
Several primary kidney diseases may recur in the transplanted kidney; the most concerning is primary focal segmental glomerulosclerosis. In this situation, the nephrotic syndrome may recur early in the posttransplant period but may respond to plasmapheresis. Thrombotic microangiopathy may also recur, particularly in the setting of calcineurin inhibitors, and may respond to withdrawal of these agents and use of plasma exchange. Diabetic nephropathy and IgA nephropathy may also recur as a late complication.

Cardiovascular Disease
The predilection for cardiovascular disease in patients with CKD continues after transplantation. Lipid abnormalities are common; however, they can be difficult to manage because use of calcineurin inhibitors together with statins increases the risk for rhabdomyolysis. Pravastatin and fluvastatin appear to have the lowest risk of myopathy and are not metabolized by CYP3A4; however, many transplant teams still prefer atorvastatin because it is the only statin that also lowers triglycerides and in low doses still has a low risk of myopathy.

Bone Disease
Although kidney transplantation may improve CKD-MBD, it may not completely resolve. Persistent posttransplant hyperparathyroidism is common and can manifest with hypophosphatemia and progressive decline in bone density. In addition, exposure to corticosteroids may lead to rapid bone loss or avascular necrosis.

Vaccinations
Ideally, patients should receive appropriate vaccinations before transplantation. At 6 months posttransplantation, a routine vaccination schedule can be resumed with the annual influenza vaccine, pneumococcal pneumonia vaccine every 5 years, and the tetanus vaccine every 10 years. Live vaccines such as varicella zoster, bacillus Calmette-Guérin, and oral polio are contraindicated after transplantation.

Nonadherence
Nonadherence is common and is associated with a high risk of rejection and graft loss. The most common reasons for nonadherence include side effects and costs of medications. Inadequate social support, substance use, and poor follow-up with transplant specialists are also important risk factors. This is best addressed by a team approach, which includes education, monitoring, detection, and intervention.

- Immunosuppression with both induction and maintenance therapy is needed in kidney transplant recipients to prevent the host immune system from rejecting the transplanted organ.

- Kidney transplant recipients have an increased risk for infection, cardiovascular disease, and malignancy as well as recurrence of their original kidney disease.

- Nonadherence by kidney transplant recipients is associated with a high risk of rejection and graft loss; the most common reasons include side effects and costs of medications.

Bibliography

Clinical Evaluation of Kidney Function

Brown RS. Has the time come to include urine dipstick testing in screening asymptomatic young adults? JAMA. 2011;306(7):764-765. [PMID: 21846861]

Chou R, Dana T. Screening adults for bladder cancer: a review of the evidence for the U.S. preventive services task force. Ann Intern Med. 2010;153(7):461-468. [PMID: 20921545]

Glassock RJ, Winearls C. Screening for CKD with eGFR: doubts and dangers. Clin J Am Soc Nephrol. 2008;3(5):1563-1568. [PMID: 18667744]

Guy M, Newall R, Borzomato J, Kalra PA, Price C. Use of a first-line urine protein-to-creatinine ratio strip test on random urines to rule out proteinuria in patients with chronic kidney disease. Nephrol Dial Transplant. 2009;24(4):1189-1193. [PMID: 18987264]

Levey AS, Stevens LA, Schmid CH, et al; CKD-EPI (Chronic Kidney Disease Epidemiology Collaboration). A new equation to estimate glomerular filtration rate. Ann Intern Med. 2009;150(9): 604-612. [PMID: 19414839]

Melamed ML, Bauer C, Hostetter TH. eGFR: is it ready for early identification of CKD? Clin J Am Soc Nephrol. 2008;3(5):1569-1572. [PMID: 18667739]

National Kidney Foundation. K/DOQI clinical practice guidelines for chronic kidney disease: evaluation, classification, and stratification. Am J Kidney Dis. 2002;39(2 Suppl 1):S1-S266. [PMID: 11904577]

Stevens LA, Schmid CH, Greene T, et al. Comparative performance of the CKD Epidemiology Collaboration (CKD-EPI) and the Modification of Diet in Renal Disease (MDRD) Study equations for estimating GFR levels above 60 mL/min/1.73 m2. Am J Kidney Dis. 2010;56(3):486-495. [PMID: 20557989]

Vivante A, Afek A, Frenkel-Nir Y, et al. Persistent asymptomatic isolated microscopic hematuria in Israeli adolescents and young adults and risk for end-stage renal disease. JAMA. 2011;306(7):729-736. [PMID: 21846854]

Fluids and Electrolytes

Alshayeb HM, Showkat A, Babar F, Mangold, Wall BM. Severe hypernatremia correction rate and mortality in hospitalized patients. Am J Med Sci. 2011;341(5):356-360. [PMID: 21358313]

Fenske W, Maier SKG, Blechschmidt A, Allolio B, Störk S. Utility and limitations of the traditional diagnostic approach to hyponatremia: a diagnostic study. Am J Med. 2010;123(7):652-657. [PMID: 20609688]

Liamis G, Milionis HJ, Elisaf M. Medication-induced hypophosphatemia: a review. QJM. 2010;103(7):449-459. [PMID: 20356849]

Sterns RH, Hix JK, Silver S. Treatment of hyponatremia. Curr Opin Nephrol Hypertens. 2010;19(5): 493-498. [PMID: 20539224]

Unwin RJ, Luft FC, Shirley DG. Pathophysiology and management of hypokalemia: a clinical perspective. Nat Rev Nephrol. 2011;7(2):75-84. [PMID: 21278718]

Weir MR, Rolfe M. Potassium homeostasis and renin-angiotensin-aldosterone system inhibitors. Clin J Am Soc Nephrol. 2010;5(3):531-548. [PMID: 20150448]

Acid-Base Disorders

Adrogué HJ, Madias NE. Secondary responses to altered acid-base status: the rules of engagement. J Am Soc Nephrol. 2010;21(6):920-923. [PMID: 20431042]

Gennari FJ, Weise WJ. Acid-base disturbances in gastrointestinal disease. Clin J Am Soc Nephrol. 2008;3(6):1861-1868. [PMID: 18922984]

Kraut JA, Kurtz I. Toxic alcohol ingestions: clinical features, diagnosis, and management. Clin J Am Soc Nephrol. 2008;3(1):208-225. [PMID: 18045860]

Kraut JA, Madias NE. Metabolic acidosis: pathophysiology, diagnosis and management. Nat Rev Nephrol. 2010;6(5):274-285. [PMID: 20308999]

Hypertension

American Diabetes Association. Standards of medical care in diabetes—2011. Diabetes Care. 2011;34(Suppl 1):S11-S61. [PMID: 21193625]

Bangalore S, Messerli FH, Wun CC, et al; Treating to New Targets Steering Committee and Investigators. J-curve revisited: an analysis of blood pressure and cardiovascular events in the Treating to New Targets (TNT) Trial. Eur Heart J. 2010;31(23):2897-2908. [PMID: 20846991]

Beckett NS, Peters R, Fletcher AE, et al; HYVET Study Group. Treatment of hypertension in patients 80 years of age or older. N Engl J Med. 2008;358(18):1887-1898. [PMID: 18378519]

Calhoun DA, Jones D, Textor S, et al; American Heart Association Professional Education Committee. Resistant hypertension: diagnosis, evaluation, and treatment: a scientific statement from the American Heart Association Professional Education Committee of the Council for High Blood Pressure Research. Circulation. 2008;117(25):e510-e526. [PMID: 18574054]

Chobanian AV, Bakris GL, Black HR, et al; Joint National Committee on Prevention, Detection, Evaluation, and Treatment of High Blood Pressure. National Heart, Lung, and Blood Institute; National High Blood Pressure Education Program Coordinating Committee. Seventh report of the Joint National Committee on Prevention, Detection, Evaluation, and Treatment of High Blood Pressure. Hypertension. 2003;42(6):1206-1252. [PMID: 14656957]

ACCORD Study Group, Cushman WC, Evans GW, Byington RP, et al. Effects of intensive blood-pressure control in type 2 diabetes mellitus. N Engl J Med. 2010;362(17):1575-1585. [PMID: 20228401]

Egan BM, Zhao Y, Axon RN. US trends in prevalence, awareness, treatment, and control of hypertension, 1988-2008. JAMA. 2010;303(20):2043-2050. [PMID: 20501926]

Flack JM, Sica DA, Bakris G, et al; International Society on Hypertension in Blacks. Management of high blood pressure in blacks: an update of the International Society on Hypertension in Blacks consensus statement. Hypertension. 2010;56(5):780-800. [PMID: 20921433]

Green BB, Cook AJ, Ralston JD, et al. Effectiveness of home blood pressure monitoring, Web communication, and pharmacist care on hypertension control: a randomized controlled trial. JAMA. 2008;299(24):2857-2867. [PMID: 18577730]

Jamerson K, Weber MA, Bakris GL, et al; ACCOMPLISH Trial Investigators. Benazepril plus amlodipine or hydrochlorothiazide for hypertension in high-risk patients. N Engl J Med. 2008;359(23):2417-2428. [PMID: 19052124]

Law MR, Morris JK, Wald NJ. Use of blood pressure lowering drugs in the prevention of cardiovascular disease: meta-analysis of 147 randomised trials in the context of expectations from prospective epidemiological studies. BMJ. 2009;338:b1665. [PMID: 19454737]

Pickering TG, Miller NH, Ogedegbe G, Krakoff LR, Artinian NT, Goff D; American Heart Association; American Society of Hypertension; Preventive Cardiovascular Nurses Association. Call to action on use and reimbursement for home blood pressure monitoring: executive summary: a joint scientific statement from the American Heart Association, American Society of Hypertension, and Preventive Cardiovascular Nurses Association. Hypertension. 2008;52(1):1-9. [PMID: 18497371]

Rossi GP, Bernini G, Caliumi C, et al; PAPY Study Investigators. A prospective study of the prevalence of primary aldosteronism in 1,125 hypertensive patients. J Am Coll Cardiol. 2006;48(11):2293-2300. [PMID: 17161262]

Chronic Tubulointerstitial Disorders

Appel GB. The treatment of acute interstitial nephritis: more data at last. Kidney Int. 2008;73(8):905-907. [PMID: 18379525]

Bendz H, Schön S, Attman PO, Aurell M. Renal failure occurs in chronic lithium treatment but is uncommon. Kidney Int. 2010;77(3):219-224. [PMID: 19940841]

Menè P, Punzo G. Uric acid: bystander or culprit in hypertension and progressive renal disease? J Hypertens. 2008;26(11):2085-2092. [PMID: 18854744]

Glomerular Diseases

ACCORD Study Group, Cushman WC, Evans GW, Byington RP, et al. Effects of intensive blood-pressure control in type 2 diabetes mellitus. N Engl J Med. 2010;362(17):1575-1585. [PMID: 20228401]

de Boer IH, Rue TC, Hall YN, Heagerty PJ, Weiss NS, Himmelfarb J. Temporal trends in the prevalence of diabetic kidney disease in the United States. JAMA. 2011;305(24):2532-2539. [PMID: 21693741]

Dooley MA, Jayne D, Ginzler EM, et al; ALMS Group. Mycophenolate versus azathioprine as maintenance therapy for lupus nephritis. N Engl J Med. 2011;365(20):1886-1895. [PMID: 22087680]

Duckworth W, Abraira C, Moritz T, et al; VADT Investigators. Glucose control and vascular complications in veterans with type 2 diabetes [errata in N Engl J Med. 2009;361(10):1024-1025 and N Engl J Med. 2009;361(10):1028]. N Engl J Med. 2009;360(2):129-139. [PMID: 19092145]

Jayne DR, Gaskin G, Rasmussen N, et al; European Vasculitis Study Group. Randomized trial of plasma exchange or high-dosage methylprednisolone as adjunctive therapy for severe renal vasculitis. J Am Soc Nephrol. 2007;18(7):2180-2188. [PMID: 17582159]

Sethi S, Nester CM, Smith RJ. Membranoproliferative glomerulonephritis and C3 glomerulopathy: resolving the confusion. Kidney Int. 2012;81(5):434-441. [PMID: 22157657]

Waldman M, Crew RJ, Valeri A, et al. Adult minimal-change disease: clinical characteristics, treatment, and outcomes. Clin J Am Soc Nephrol. 2007;2(3):445-453. [PMID: 17699450]

Working Group of the International IgA Nephropathy Network and the Renal Pathology Society, Cattran DC, Coppo R, Cook HT, et al. The Oxford classification of IgA nephropathy: rationale, clinicopathological correlations, and classification. Kidney Int. 2009;76(5):534-545. [PMID: 19571791]

Genetic Disorders and Kidney Disease

Curatolo P, Bombardieri R, Jozwiak S. Tuberous sclerosis. Lancet. 2008;372(9639):657-668. [PMID: 18722871]

Gubler MC. Inherited diseases of the glomerular basement membrane. Nat Clin Pract Nephrol. 2008;4(1):24-37. [PMID: 18094725]

Haas M. Alport syndrome and thin glomerular basement membrane nephropathy: a practical approach to diagnosis. Arch Pathol Lab Med. 2009;133(2):224-232. [PMID: 19195966]

Kashtan CE, Segal Y. Genetic disorders of glomerular basement membranes. Nephron Clin Pract. 2011;118(1):c9-c18. [PMID: 21071975]

Pei Y, Obaji J, Dupuis A, et al. Unified criteria for ultrasonographic diagnosis of ADPKD. J Am Soc Nephrol. 2009;20(1):205-212. [PMID: 18945943]

Torres VE, Harris PC. Autosomal dominant polycystic kidney disease: the last 3 years. Kidney Int. 2009;76(2):149-168. [PMID: 19455193]

Walz G, Budde K, Mannaa M, et al. Everolimus in patients with autosomal dominant polycystic kidney disease. N Engl J Med. 2010;363(9):830-840. [PMID: 20581392]

Acute Kidney Injury

Abu-Alfa AK, Younes A. Tumor lysis syndrome and acute kidney injury: evaluation, prevention, and management. Am J Kidney Dis. 2010;55(5 Suppl 3):S1-S13. [PMID: 20420966]

Bosch X, Poch E, Grau JM. Rhabdomyolysis and acute kidney injury. N Engl J Med. 2009;361(1):62-72. [PMID: 19571284]

Coiffier B, Altman A, Pui CH, Younes A, Cairo MS. Guidelines for the management of pediatric and adult tumor lysis syndrome: an evidence-based review [erratum in J Clin Oncol. 2010;28(4):708]. J Clin Oncol. 2008;26(16):2767-2778. [PMID: 18509186]

European Association for the Study of the Liver. EASL clinical practice guidelines on the management of ascites, spontaneous bacterial peritonitis, and hepatorenal syndrome in cirrhosis. J Hepatol. 2010;53(3):397-417. [PMID: 20633946]

Felker GM, Lee KL, Bull DA, et al; NHLBI Heart Failure Clinical Research Network. Diuretic strategies in patients with acute decompensated heart failure. N Engl J Med. 2011;364(9):797-805. [PMID: 21366472]

Hutchison CA, Bradwell AR, Cook M, et al. Treatment of acute renal failure secondary to multiple myeloma with chemotherapy and extended high cut-off hemodialysis. Clin J Am Soc Nephrol. 2009;4(4):745-754. [PMID: 19339414]

Perazella MA, Markowitz GS. Drug-induced acute interstitial nephritis. Nat Rev Nephrol. 2010;6(8):461-470. [PMID: 20517290]

Ronco C, Haapio M, House AA, Anavekar N, Bellomo R. Cardiorenal syndrome. J Am Coll Cardiol. 2008;52(19):1527-1539. [PMID: 19007588]

Scolari F, Ravani P. Atheroembolic renal disease. Lancet. 2010;375(9726):1650-1660. [PMID: 20381857]

Shah-Khan F, Scheetz MH, Ghossein C. Biopsy-proven acute tubular necrosis due to vancomycin toxicity. Int J Nephrol. 2011;2011:436856. [PMID: 21716699]

Kidney Stones

American Urological Association. Management of ureteral calculi: EAU/AUA nephrolithiasis panel (2007). Available at www.auanet.org/content/guidelines-and-quality-care/clinical-guidelines.cfm. Accessed July 3, 2012.

Eisner BH, Eisenberg ML, Stoller ML. Relationship between body mass index and quantitative 24-hour urine chemistries in patients with nephrolithiasis. Urology. 2010;75(6):1289-1293. [PMID: 20018350]

Goldfarb DS. In the clinic. Nephrolithiasis. Ann Intern Med. 2009;151(3):ITC2. [PMID: 19652185]

Krambeck AE, Rule AD, Li X, Bergstralh EJ, Gettman MT, Lieske JC. Shock wave lithotripsy is not predictive of hypertension among community stone formers at long-term followup [erratum in J Urol. 2011;185(3):1161]. J Urol. 2011;185(1):164-169. [PMID: 21074794]

Maalouf NM, Tondapu P, Guth ES, Livingston EH, Sakhaee K. Hypocitraturia and hyperoxaluria after Roux-en-Y gastric bypass surgery. J Urol. 2010;183(3):1026-1030. [PMID: 20096421]

Taylor EN, Fung TT, Curhan GC. DASH-style diet associates with reduced risk for kidney stones. J Am Soc Nephrol. 2009;20(10):2253-2259. [PMID: 19679672]

Worcester EM, Coe FL. Clinical practice. Calcium kidney stones. N Engl J Med. 2010;363(10):954-963. [PMID: 20818905]

The Kidney in Pregnancy

Berks D, Steegers EA, Molas M, Visser W. Resolution of hypertension and proteinuria after preeclampsia. Obstet Gynecol. 2009;114(6):1307-1314. [PMID: 19935034]

Lykke JA, Langhoff-Roos J, Sibai BM, Funai EF, Triche EW, Paidas MJ. Hypertensive pregnancy disorders and subsequent cardiovascular morbidity and type 2 diabetes mellitus in the mother. Hypertension. 2009;53(6):944-951. [PMID: 19433776]

Noori M, Donald AE, Angelakopoulou A, Hingorani AD, Williams DJ. Prospective study of placental angiogenic factors and maternal vascular function before and after preeclampsia and gestational hypertension. Circulation. 2010;122(5):478-487. [PMID: 20644016]

Podymow T, August P. Update on the use of antihypertensive drugs in pregnancy. Hypertension. 2008;51(4):960-969. [PMID: 18259046]

Seely EW, Ecker J. Clinical practice. Chronic hypertension in pregnancy. N Engl J Med. 2011;365(5):439-446. [PMID: 21812673]

Steegers EA, von Dadelszen P, Duvekot JJ, Pijnenborg R. Pre-eclampsia. Lancet. 2010;376(9741):631-644. [PMID: 20598363]

Chronic Kidney Disease

Axelrod DA, McCullough KP, Brewer ED, Becker BN, Segev DL, Rao PS. Kidney and pancreas transplantation in the United States, 1999-2008: the changing face of living donation. Am J Transplant. 2010;10(4 Pt 2):987-1002. [PMID: 20420648]

Bakris GL, Sarafidis PA, Weir MR, et al; ACCOMPLISH Trial investigators. Renal outcomes with different fixed-dose combination therapies in patients with hypertension at high risk for cardiovascular events (ACCOMPLISH): a prespecified secondary analysis of a randomised controlled trial. Lancet. 2010;3;375(9721):1173-1181. [PMID: 20170948]

Bomback AS, Kshirsagar AV, Amamoo MA, Klemmer PJ. Change in proteinuria after adding aldosterone blockers to ACE inhibitors or angiotensin receptor blockers in CKD: a systematic review. Am J Kidney Dis. 2008;51(2):199-211. [PMID: 18215698]

Cooper BA, Branley P, Bulfone L, et al; IDEAL Study. A randomized controlled trial of early versus late initiation of dialysis. N Engl J Med. 2010;363(7):609-619. [PMID: 20581422]

de Brito-Ashurst I, Varagunam M, Raftery MJ, Yaqoob MM. Bicarbonate supplementation slows progression of CKD and improves nutritional status. J Am Soc Nephrol. 2009;20(9):2075-2084. [PMID: 19608703]

Drawz P, Rahman M. In the clinic. Chronic kidney disease. Ann Intern Med. 2009;150(3):ITC2-1-ITC2-15. [PMID: 19189903]

Fellström BC, Jardine AG, Schmieder RE, et al; AURORA Study Group. Rosuvastatin and cardiovascular events in patients undergoing hemodialysis [erratum in N Engl J Med. 2010;362(15):1450]. N Engl J Med. 2009;360(14):1395-1407. [PMID: 19332456]

Go AS, Chertow GM, Fan D, McCulloch CE, Hsu CY. Chronic kidney disease and the risks of death, cardiovascular events, and hospitalization. N Engl J Med. 2004;351(13):1296-1305. [PMID: 15385656]

Gordon PL, Frassetto LA. Management of osteoporosis in CKD Stages 3 to 5. Am J Kidney Dis. 2010;55(5):941-956. [PMID: 20438987]

Ibrahim HN, Foley R, Tan L, et al. Long-term consequences of kidney donation. N Engl J Med. 2009;360:459-469 [PMID: 19179315]

Kidney Disease: Improving Global Outcomes (KDIGO) CKD-MBD Work Group. KDIGO clinical practice guideline for the diagnosis, evaluation, prevention, and treatment of chronic kidney disease-mineral and bone disorder (CKD-MBD). Kidney Int Suppl. 2009;(113):S1-S130. [PMID: 19644521]

Kidney Disease: Improving Global Outcomes (KDIGO) Transplant Work Group. KDIGO clinical practice guideline for the care of kidney transplant recipients. Am J Transplant. 2009;9(Suppl 3):S1-S155. [PMID: 19845597]

Mann JF, Schmieder RE, McQueen M, et al; ONTARGET Investigators. Renal outcomes with telmisartan, ramipril, or both, in people at high vascular risk (the ONTARGET study): a multicentre, randomised, double-blind, controlled trial. Lancet. 2008;372(9638):547-553. [PMID: 18707986]

Navaneethan SD, Nigwekar SU, Perkovic V, Johnson DW, Craig JC, Strippoli GF. HMG CoA reductase inhibitors (statins) for dialysis patients. Cochrane Database Syst Rev. 2009;(3):CD004289. [PMID: 19588351]

Navaneethan SD, Pansini F, Perkovic V, et al. HMG CoA reductase inhibitors (statins) for people with chronic kidney disease not requiring dialysis. Cochrane Database Syst Rev. 2009;(2):CD007784. [PMID: 19370693]

Palmer SC, Hayen A, Macaskill P, et al. Serum levels of phosphorus, parathyroid hormone, and calcium and risks of death and cardiovascular disease in individuals with chronic kidney disease: a systematic review and meta-analysis. JAMA. 2011;305(11):1119-1127. [PMID: 21406649]

Pfeffer MA, Burdmann EA, Chen CY, et al; TREAT Investigators. A trial of darbepoetin alfa in type 2 diabetes and chronic kidney disease. N Engl J Med. 2009;361(21):2019-2032. [PMID: 19880844]

Solomon SD, Uno H, Lewis EF, et al; Trial to Reduce Cardiovascular Events with Aranesp Therapy (TREAT) Investigators. Erythropoietic response and outcomes in kidney disease and type 2 diabetes. N Engl J Med. 2010;363(12):1146-1155. [PMID: 20843249]

U.S. Food and Drug Administration. FDA Drug Safety Communication: erythropoiesis-stimulating agents (ESAs): procrit, epogen and aranesp. www.fda.gov/Drugs/DrugSafety/PostmarketDrugSafetyInformationforPatientsandProviders/ucm200297.htm. Accessed July 3, 2012.

Wright JT Jr, Bakris G, Greene T, et al; African American Study of Kidney Disease and Hypertension Study Group. Effect of blood pressure lowering and antihypertensive drug class on progression of hypertensive kidney disease: results from the AASK trial. JAMA. 2002;288(19):2421-2431. [PMID: 12435255]

Nephrology Self-Assessment Test

This self-assessment test contains one-best-answer multiple-choice questions. Please read these directions carefully before answering the questions. Answers, critiques, and bibliographies immediately follow these multiple-choice questions. The American College of Physicians is accredited by the Accreditation Council for Continuing Medical Education (ACCME) to provide continuing medical education for physicians.

The American College of Physicians designates MKSAP 16 Nephrology for a maximum of 16 *AMA PRA Category 1 Credits*™. Physicians should claim only the credit commensurate with the extent of their participation in the activity.

Earn "Same-Day" CME Credits Online

For the first time, print subscribers can enter their answers online to earn CME credits in 24 hours or less. You can submit your answers using online answer sheets that are provided at mksap.acponline.org, where a record of your MKSAP 16 credits will be available. To earn CME credits, you need to answer all of the questions in a test and earn a score of at least 50% correct (number of correct answers divided by the total number of questions). Take any of the following approaches:

> ➢ Use the printed answer sheet at the back of this book to record your answers. Go to mksap.acponline.org, access the appropriate online answer sheet, transcribe your answers, and submit your test for same-day CME credits. There is no additional fee for this service.

> ➢ Go to mksap.acponline.org, access the appropriate online answer sheet, directly enter your answers, and submit your test for same-day CME credits. There is no additional fee for this service.

> ➢ Pay a $10 processing fee per answer sheet and submit the printed answer sheet at the back of this book by mail or fax, as instructed on the answer sheet. Make sure you calculate your score and fax the answer sheet to 215-351-2799 or mail the answer sheet to Member and Customer Service, American College of Physicians, 190 N. Independence Mall West, Philadelphia, PA 19106-1572, using the courtesy envelope provided in your MKSAP 16 slipcase. You will need your 10-digit order number and 8-digit ACP ID number, which are printed on your packing slip. Please allow 4 to 6 weeks for your score report to be emailed back to you. Be sure to include your email address for a response.

If you do not have a 10-digit order number and 8-digit ACP ID number or if you need help creating a username and password to access the MKSAP 16 online answer sheets, go to mksap.acponline.org or email custserv@acponline.org.

CME credit is available from the publication date of December 31, 2012, until December 31, 2015. You may submit your answer sheets at any time during this period.

Directions

*Each of the numbered items is followed by lettered answers. Select the **ONE** lettered answer that is **BEST** in each case.*

Item 1

A 41-year-old woman is evaluated during a follow-up visit for high blood pressure. She is a vegetarian and does not smoke cigarettes. She feels well except for an occasional tension headache. She takes no medications.

On physical examination, blood pressure is 162/100 mm Hg, which is similar to the values measured at her initial visit. Other vital signs are normal. BMI is 21. The remainder of the examination is unremarkable.

Laboratory studies reveal normal electrolytes, complete blood count, fasting glucose, and fasting lipid profile as well as normal kidney function.

Electrocardiogram is unremarkable.

Which of the following is the most appropriate next step in the management of this patient's hypertension?

(A) Combination drug therapy
(B) Lifestyle modifications
(C) Single-drug therapy
(D) Reevaluate patient in 2 weeks

Item 2

A 52-year-old woman is evaluated for a 2-day history of right flank pain, mild nausea, and fever. She has autosomal dominant polycystic kidney disease.

On physical examination, the patient appears ill. Temperature is 38.6 °C (101.4 °F), blood pressure is 149/94 mm Hg, pulse rate is 92/min, and respiration rate is 20/min. BMI is 26. Abdominal examination reveals right costovertebral angle tenderness on palpation; the abdomen is nondistended, and bowel sounds are normal.

Laboratory studies reveal a leukocyte count of 13,000/µL (13×10^9/L), a serum creatinine level of 1.9 mg/dL (168 µmol/L), and negative urine culture results.

On kidney ultrasound, the left kidney is 16.2 cm, and the right kidney is 16.9 cm; multiple bilateral intraparenchymal cysts are noted.

Which of the following is the most appropriate treatment for this patient?

(A) Amoxicillin
(B) Cephalexin
(C) Ciprofloxacin
(D) Nitrofurantoin

Item 3

A 51-year-old man is being followed in the hospital after receiving chemotherapy for acute myeloid leukemia 1 day ago. Kidney function was normal at the start of his treatment, which consisted of normal saline at a rate of 200 mL/h and rasburicase on the day of chemotherapy. He reports no symptoms except for some fatigue and nausea. He has no shortness of breath or fever.

On physical examination, the patient is afebrile. Blood pressure is 122/70 mm Hg, pulse rate is 72/min, and respiration rate is 12/min. BMI is 25. Some bruising is noted on the skin. There is no jugular venous distention. Heart rate is regular. Lungs are clear to auscultation. There is no edema.

Urine output has been around 50 mL/h.

Laboratory studies:

Albumin	3.2 g/dL (32 g/L)
Blood urea nitrogen	14 mg/dL (5.0 mmol/L)
Calcium	9 mg/dL (2.3 mmol/L)
Serum creatinine	1.0 mg/dL (88.4 µmol/L) (baseline: 0.9 mg/dL [79.6 µmol/L])
Electrolytes	
Sodium	139 meq/L (139 mmol/L)
Potassium	5.2 meq/L (5.2 mmol/L)
Chloride	100 meq/L (100 mmol/L)
Bicarbonate	25 meq/L (25 mmol/L)
Phosphorus	5.7 mg/dL (1.84 mmol/L)
Uric acid	7.1 mg/dL (0.42 mmol/L)

Which of the following is the most appropriate next step in management?

(A) Add sodium bicarbonate to intravenous fluid at current rate
(B) Add sodium polystyrene sulfonate
(C) Increase intravenous saline rate
(D) Substitute allopurinol for rasburicase

Item 4

A 31-year-old woman is seen to discuss treatment of her progressive chronic kidney disease resulting from membranoproliferative glomerulonephritis. She has had a steady decline in kidney function and is approaching the need for kidney replacement therapy. Her identical twin sister has agreed to donate a kidney but is currently pregnant, and donation will likely not be possible for at least a year. She is otherwise doing well and is actively involved in her medical care. In discussing future treatment options, she has expressed a desire to pursue peritoneal dialysis should kidney replacement therapy be needed before the availability of the transplant from her sister. Medications are epoetin alfa, sevelamer, amlodipine, and sodium bicarbonate.

On physical examination, blood pressure is 126/78 mm Hg. BMI is 24. Cardiac examination is normal without a rub. Lungs are clear. Abdominal examination is normal, with no evidence of prior surgery. There is no asterixis. Trace edema is present.

Laboratory studies reveal a blood urea nitrogen level of 88 mg/dL (31.4 mmol/L), a serum creatinine level of 4.7 mg/dL (415 µmol/L), and a urine protein–creatinine ratio of 3.3 mg/mg.

In counseling this patient, which of the following is the most appropriate recommendation for management?

(A) Plan for hemodialysis when needed
(B) Plan for peritoneal dialysis when needed

(C) Pursue a deceased donor kidney transplant

(D) Start either form of dialysis now

Item 5

A 20-year-old woman is evaluated for a 4-week history of fatigue, polyarthritis, oral ulcers, and edema. Her medical history is unremarkable, and she takes no medications.

On physical examination, blood pressure is 165/100 mm Hg; other vital signs are normal. There are ulcers on the hard palate and buccal mucosa. Symmetric swelling, erythema, and tenderness of the metacarpophalangeal and proximal interphalangeal joints are noted. There is 2+ pitting edema of the lower extremities.

Laboratory studies:

Hemoglobin	10.8 g/dL (108 g/L)
Leukocyte count	2000/μL (2.0 × 10⁹/L)
Platelet count	110,000/μL (110 × 10⁹/L)
Albumin	3.4 g/dL (34 g/L)
Serum creatinine	1.4 mg/dL (124 μmol/L)
Urinalysis	15-20 erythrocytes/hpf; 10-15 leukocytes/hpf; erythrocyte casts
Urine protein–creatinine ratio	2.8 mg/mg

Which of the following is the most likely diagnosis?

(A) Focal segmental glomerulosclerosis

(B) IgA nephropathy

(C) Postinfectious glomerulonephritis

(D) Proliferative lupus nephritis

Item 6

A 50-year-old man returns for a follow-up visit to discuss his blood pressure results. At his new patient office visit 6 weeks ago, his blood pressure was 138/82 mm Hg, and the evaluation was otherwise unremarkable. At his follow-up visit 2 weeks later, his blood pressure was 136/85 mm Hg. He does not smoke cigarettes or use alcohol or drugs. Family history is significant for his mother who has hypertension. He takes no medications.

On physical examination today, blood pressure is 135/84 mm Hg; other vital signs are normal. BMI is 26. The remainder of the examination, including cardiac and pulmonary examinations, is normal.

Laboratory studies:

Complete blood count	Normal
Serum creatinine	Normal
Electrolytes	Normal
Glucose	Normal
Total cholesterol	192 mg/dL (4.97 mmol/L)
LDL cholesterol	145 mg/dL (3.76 mmol/L)
HDL cholesterol	38 mg/dL (0.98 mmol/L)
Triglycerides	Normal

Electrocardiogram is normal.

In addition to lifestyle modifications, which of the following is the most appropriate next step in the management of this patient's blood pressure?

(A) Ambulatory blood pressure monitoring

(B) High-sensitivity C-reactive protein measurement

(C) Hydrochlorothiazide

(D) Recheck blood pressure in 1 year

Item 7

A 56-year-old man is evaluated in the emergency department after his wife found him unconscious. She reports that he has a history of alcohol abuse. Upon arrival, he has a generalized seizure that resolves spontaneously. He is treated with lorazepam, thiamine, and a 1-L bolus of 5% dextrose-0.9% saline.

On physical examination, the patient is thin, disheveled, and somnolent. Temperature is 35.8 °C (96.4 °F), blood pressure is 100/50 mm Hg, pulse rate is 110/min, and respiration rate is 18/min. Repeat examination 30 minutes later reveals an increased level of consciousness and normal strength. The remainder of the examination is normal.

Laboratory studies:

	Initial	30 Minutes Later
Blood urea nitrogen	56 mg/dL (20 mmol/L)	42 mg/dL (15 mmol/L)
Serum creatinine	1.6 mg/dL (141 μmol/L)	1.5 mg/dL (133 μmol/L)
Electrolytes		
Sodium	133 meq/L (133 mmol/L)	135 meq/L (135 mmol/L)
Potassium	3.5 meq/L (3.5 mmol/L)	3.4 meq/L (3.4 mmol/L)
Chloride	92 meq/L (92 mmol/L)	97 meq/L (97 mmol/L)
Bicarbonate	16 meq/L (16 mmol/L)	20 meq/L (20 mmol/L)
Ethanol	88 mg/dL (19 mmol/L)	–
Glucose	90 mg/dL (5.0 mmol/L)	102 mg/dL (5.7 mmol/L)
Osmolality	320 mosm/kg H₂O	–
Arterial blood gas studies (ambient air):		
pH	7.15	7.30
Pco₂	40 mm Hg (5.3 kPa)	37 mm Hg (4.9 kPa)
Po₂	86 mm Hg (11.4 kPa)	92 mm Hg (12.2 kPa)
Urinalysis	pH 5.4; trace protein; 1+ ketones; few hyaline casts	–

Which of the following is the most appropriate next step in management?

(A) Fomepizole
(B) Hemodialysis
(C) Sodium bicarbonate
(D) Supportive care

Item 8

A 55-year-old woman is evaluated during a routine visit. She was diagnosed with chronic kidney disease 3 years ago. For the past year, she has had increasing fatigue. She reports no shortness of breath or chest pain. Medications are lisinopril, furosemide, calcium acetate, ferrous sulfate, and a multivitamin.

On physical examination, temperature is normal, blood pressure is 100/70 mm Hg, pulse rate is 76/min, and respiration rate is 14/min. BMI is 30. Abdominal examination is normal. A stool specimen is negative for occult blood.

Laboratory studies:

Hemoglobin	8.9 g/dL (89 g/L) (1 year ago: 11 g/dL [110 g/L])
Mean corpuscular hemoglobin	30 pg
Mean corpuscular hemoglobin concentration	33 g/dL (330 g/L)
Mean corpuscular volume	91 fL
Reticulocyte count	1% of erythrocytes
Serum creatinine	2 mg/dL (177 µmol/L)
Ferritin	250 ng/mL (250 µg/L)
Transferrin saturation	33%
Folate	Normal
Vitamin B_{12}	Normal

Which of the following is the most appropriate intervention for this patient's management?

(A) Add ascorbic acid
(B) Add an erythropoiesis-stimulating agent
(C) Perform a blood transfusion
(D) Switch from oral to intravenous iron therapy

Item 9

A 42-year-old man hospitalized for recurrent variceal bleeding is evaluated 48 hours after admission for severe metabolic alkalosis. He has a 4-year history of alcoholic cirrhosis. He received endoscopic therapy for the varices. In the first 24 hours following admission, he required six units of packed red blood cells and four units of fresh frozen platelets to maintain hemodynamic stability. Today he feels confused but otherwise reports no symptoms. Medications are nadolol, octreotide, and intravenous ciprofloxacin.

On physical examination, temperature is normal, blood pressure is 100/70 mm Hg, and pulse rate is 96/min. BMI is 20. Cardiopulmonary examination is normal. Ascites is noted. There is 2+ presacral edema and 2+ leg edema.

Laboratory studies:

	On Admission	Hospital Day 2
Serum creatinine	1.2 mg/dL (106 µmol/L)	–
Electrolytes		
Sodium	138 meq/L (138 mmol/L)	136 meq/L (136 mmol/L)
Potassium	3.8 meq/L (3.8 mmol/L)	5.0 meq/L (5.0 mmol/L)
Chloride	105 meq/L (105 mmol/L)	85 meq/L (85 mmol/L)
Bicarbonate	21 meq/L (21 mmol/L)	38 meq/L (38 mmol/L)
Urine chloride	–	<5 meq/L (5 mmol/L) (normal range for men, 25-371 meq/L [25-371 mmol/L])
Arterial blood gas studies (ambient air):		
pH	–	7.52
P_{CO_2}	–	48 mm Hg (6.4 kPa)

Which of the following is the most appropriate management?

(A) Add acetazolamide
(B) Add furosemide
(C) Add isotonic saline
(D) Discontinue octreotide

Item 10

A 26-year-old man is evaluated for a 3-day history of fever, lower abdominal pain, tenesmus, hematochezia, and watery diarrhea. Seven months ago, he underwent a cadaveric kidney transplantation. At the time of transplantation, the transplant donor was seropositive for cytomegalovirus, and the patient was seronegative for this virus. Current medications are tacrolimus, mycophenolate mofetil, prednisone, and trimethoprim-sulfamethoxazole. Valganciclovir was discontinued 1 month ago after 6 months of prophylaxis as per standard protocol.

On physical examination, temperature is 38.8 °C (101.8 °F), blood pressure is 100/70 mm Hg, pulse rate is 104/min, and respiration rate is 18/min. BMI is 24. Cardiopulmonary examination is normal. Abdominal examination reveals increased bowel sounds but no tenderness to palpation. There is no organomegaly.

Laboratory studies:

Leukocyte count	2100/µL (2.1×10^9/L)
Alanine aminotransferase	72 units/L
Aspartate aminotransferase	60 units/L
Serum creatinine	1.4 mg/dL (124 µmol/L)

Chest radiograph is normal.

Which of the following is the most likely diagnosis?

(A) *Clostridium difficile* infection
(B) Cytomegalovirus infection

(C) Mycophenolate mofetil toxicity

(D) Tacrolimus toxicity

Item 11

A 62-year-old man is evaluated for a 1-month history of low-grade back pain, generalized weakness, and progressive fatigue. He also notes dyspnea with exertion. He has had no joint aches, fevers, or cough.

On physical examination, temperature is 36.9 °C (98.5 °F), blood pressure is 124/70 mm Hg, pulse rate is 69/min, and respiration rate is 14/min. There are no rashes or bruises on the skin. There are no enlarged lymph nodes. Cardiac examination is unremarkable. Lungs are clear. Abdominal examination is benign with no masses. Some tenderness is noted on the back along the spine. There is no edema. Neurologic examination is intact.

Laboratory studies:

Hemoglobin	8.1 g/dL (81 g/L)
Leukocyte count	6800/µL (6.8 × 10⁹/L) with normal differential
Platelet count	124,000/µL (124 × 10⁹/L)
Albumin	3.5 g/dL (35 g/L)
Blood urea nitrogen	59 mg/dL (21.1 mmol/L)
Calcium	11.1 mg/dL (2.8 mmol/L)
Serum creatinine	7.5 mg/dL (663 µmol/L) (5 years ago: 1.0 mg/dL [88.4 µmol/L])
Electrolytes	
Sodium	138 meq/L (138 mmol/L)
Potassium	4.5 meq/L (4.5 mmol/L)
Chloride	110 meq/L (110 mmol/L)
Bicarbonate	23 meq/L (23 mmol/L)
Glucose	102 mg/dL (5.7 mmol/L)
Phosphorus	6.4 mg/dL (2.07 mmol/L)
Total protein	8.1 g/dL (81 g/L)
Urinalysis	Specific gravity 1.018; pH 6.5; trace protein; 0-3 erythrocytes/hpf; 6-10 leukocytes/hpf; no casts
Urine protein–creatinine ratio	3.3 mg/mg

Chest radiograph is unremarkable. Kidney ultrasound shows no evidence of urinary obstruction.

Which of the following is the most appropriate diagnostic study to evaluate this patient's kidney injury?

(A) ANCA testing

(B) Kidney biopsy

(C) Parathyroid hormone measurement

(D) Serum and urine electrophoresis

Item 12

An 81-year-old woman is evaluated during a follow-up visit for a 3-year history of hypertension. She feels relatively well. She does not smoke cigarettes. She appears to be adherent to her medication regimen, which consists of maximum doses of chlorthalidone, enalapril, amlodipine, and carvedilol.

On physical examination, seated blood pressure is 158/68 mm Hg, and pulse rate is 68/min; other vital signs are normal. BMI is 26. A systolic crescendo-decrescendo murmur is noted at the right upper sternal border. The carotid upstrokes are normal, and no bruits are heard. Trace pedal edema is noted.

Laboratory studies reveal normal electrolytes, complete blood count, fasting glucose, and fasting lipid profile as well as normal kidney function.

Which of the following is the most appropriate next step in management?

(A) Ambulatory blood pressure monitoring

(B) Echocardiography

(C) Hydralazine

(D) Urine metanephrine measurement

Item 13

A 75-year-old man is evaluated for a 3-week history of increasing abdominal girth. He has alcoholic liver disease with cirrhosis. He is not a candidate for liver transplantation at this time because of recent alcohol use and medical non-adherence. His only medication is propranolol.

On physical examination, the patient is alert and oriented. Temperature is 36.2 °C (97.2 °F), blood pressure is 106/58 mm Hg, pulse rate is 58/min, and respiration rate is 16/min. BMI is 20. There are no focal neurologic deficits. There is no asterixis. Abdominal examination reveals shifting abdominal dullness. There is 1+ lower extremity edema.

Laboratory studies:

Albumin	2.0 g/dL (20 g/L)
Blood urea nitrogen	8 mg/dL (2.9 mmol/L)
Serum creatinine	1.6 mg/dL (141 µmol/L)
Electrolytes	
Sodium	119 meq/L (119 mmol/L)
Potassium	3.6 meq/L (3.6 mmol/L)
Chloride	87 meq/L (87 mmol/L)
Bicarbonate	21 meq/L (21 mmol/L)
Glucose	95 mg/dL (5.3 mmol/L)
Osmolality	250 mosm/kg H₂O
Urine studies:	
Osmolality	156 mosm/kg H₂O (normal range, 300-900 mosm/kg H₂O)
Potassium	5 meq/L (5 mmol/L) (normal range for men, 11-99 meq/L [11-99 mmol/L])
Sodium	<5 meq/L (5 mmol/L) (normal range for men, 18-301 meq/L [18-301 mmol/L])

A diagnostic paracentesis reveals findings consistent with transudative ascites; the ascitic fluid absolute neutrophil count is 50/µL.

Which of the following is the most appropriate management for this patient's hyponatremia?

(A) 3% Saline

(B) Conivaptan

(C) Demeclocycline
(D) Fluid restriction

Item 14

A 27-year-old woman seeks preconception counseling. She has IgA nephropathy established by kidney biopsy. She feels well, has no other medical problems, and takes no medications.

On physical examination, temperature is normal, blood pressure is 138/88 mm Hg, pulse rate is 68/min, and respiration rate is 16/min. Cardiovascular and pulmonary examinations are normal.

Serum creatinine level 1 year ago was 1.2 mg/dL (106 µmol/L). Urinalysis today shows 10-20 erythrocytes/hpf and 1+ protein.

Which of the following should be done next to further assess the maternal and fetal risk of pregnancy outcome?

(A) Measure IgA levels
(B) Measure serum creatinine level
(C) Obtain 24-hour ambulatory blood pressure measurement
(D) Repeat kidney biopsy

Item 15

An 81-year-old man is evaluated for progressive fatigue. Nine months ago, he was diagnosed with giant cell arteritis; at that time, prednisone, omeprazole, risedronate, and vitamin D were initiated. His symptoms improved, and the prednisone was tapered. Five months ago he began to feel more fatigued. Evaluation was unremarkable other than the urinalysis, which was positive for leukocytes and leukocyte esterase. He was treated with ciprofloxacin without improvement of his symptoms. A subsequent urine culture was negative.

On physical examination, temperature is 37.3 °C (99.1 °F), blood pressure is 151/65 mm Hg, pulse rate 98/min, and respiration rate is 14/min. The remainder of the examination is unremarkable.

Laboratory studies:
Hemoglobin	10.7 g/dL (107 g/L)
Leukocyte count	8700/µL (8.7 × 10⁹/L) (65% neutrophils, 23% lymphocytes, 11% monocytes, and 1% eosinophils)
Platelet count	198,000/µL (198 × 10⁹/L)
Blood urea nitrogen	51 mg/dL (18.2 mmol/L)
Serum creatinine	3.1 mg/dL (274 µmol/L) (baseline: 1.1 mg/dL [97.2 µmol/L])
Lactate dehydrogenase	80 units/L
Urinalysis	Specific gravity 1.014; pH 6.0; trace protein; + leukocyte esterase; occasional leukocytes; rare erythrocytes; occasional hyaline casts

Which of the following is the most likely diagnosis?

(A) Acute interstitial nephritis
(B) Acute tubular necrosis
(C) Glomerulonephritis
(D) Thrombotic thrombocytopenic purpura

Item 16

A 58-year-old man is evaluated for a 6-month history of lower extremity edema and a weight gain of 12 kg (26 lb). He has frothy urine but reports no burning while urinating or blood in the urine. The patient is black. Medical history is otherwise unremarkable, and he takes no medications.

On physical examination, blood pressure is 155/105 mm Hg; other vital signs are normal. BMI is 30. There is 3+ pitting edema of the lower extremities. The remainder of the examination is unremarkable.

Laboratory studies:
Albumin	2.4 g/dL (24 g/L)
Complement (C3 and C4)	Normal
Serum creatinine	1.6 mg/dL (141 µmol/L)
Total cholesterol	280 mg/dL (7.25 mmol/L)
LDL cholesterol	170 mg/dL (4.40 mmol/L)
HDL cholesterol	35 mg/dL (0.91 mmol/L)
Triglycerides	250 mg/dL (2.83 mmol/L)
Serum protein electrophoresis	Normal
Rheumatoid factor	Negative
Antinuclear antibodies	Negative
Hepatitis B surface antigen	Negative
Hepatitis C virus antibodies	Negative
HIV antibodies	Negative
Rapid plasma reagin	Negative
Urinalysis	1-3 erythrocytes/hpf; 1-3 leukocytes/hpf
Urine protein–creatinine ratio	7.4 mg/mg

A kidney biopsy is performed.

Which of the following is the most likely diagnosis?

(A) Focal segmental glomerulosclerosis
(B) IgA nephropathy
(C) Lupus nephritis
(D) Postinfectious glomerulonephritis

Item 17

A 23-year-old woman is evaluated in the emergency department for a 2-month history of progressive leg weakness. She has been unable to ambulate for 1 day. She reports no diarrhea or weight loss. Medical history is remarkable for Sjögren syndrome. She takes no medications.

On physical examination, vital signs are normal. BMI is 22. Diffuse weakness is noted most prominently in the legs, graded at 3/5. There is no muscle atrophy or tenderness.

Laboratory studies:

Albumin	4.5 g/dL (45 g/L)
Blood urea nitrogen	13 mg/dL (4.6 mmol/L)
Calcium	9.1 mg/dL (2.3 mmol/L)
Serum creatinine	1.1 mg/dL (97.2 µmol/L)
Electrolytes	
Sodium	141 meq/L (141 mmol/L)
Potassium	1.9 meq/L (1.9 mmol/L)
Chloride	117 meq/L (117 mmol/L)
Bicarbonate	14 meq/L (14 mmol/L)
Magnesium	2.2 mg/dL (0.91 mmol/L)
Phosphorus	3.5 mg/dL (1.13 mmol/L)
Total protein	8.9 g/dL (89 g/L)
Urine anion gap	Positive
Urinalysis	Specific gravity 1.014; pH 7.0; no blood; trace protein; no glucose; no leukocyte esterase; no nitrites

Kidney ultrasound shows nephrocalcinosis bilaterally.

Which of the following is the most likely diagnosis?

(A) Gitelman syndrome
(B) Hypokalemic distal (type 1) renal tubular acidosis
(C) Laxative abuse
(D) Proximal (type 2) renal tubular acidosis

Item 18

A 28-year-old man is found to have blood in the urine on testing related to an insurance physical examination. Family history is significant for his father who died of metastatic bladder cancer at the age of 55 years. The patient takes no medications.

On physical examination, temperature is 36.9 °C (98.4 °F), blood pressure is 138/85 mm Hg, pulse rate is 72/min, and respiration rate is 12/min. BMI is 28. The remainder of the examination is normal.

Urinalysis reveals no protein, 5-10 erythrocytes/hpf (all of which are isomorphic), and 0-2 leukocytes/hpf.

Which of the following is the most appropriate diagnostic test to perform next?

(A) CT urography
(B) Cystoscopy
(C) Repeat urinalysis
(D) Urine culture
(E) Urine cytology

Item 19

A 55-year-old woman is evaluated for a possible kidney transplant. She has end-stage kidney disease secondary to systemic lupus erythematosus (SLE). Her SLE has been quiescent since initiating hemodialysis 11 months ago. She feels well and has a stable weight and appetite. She has no arthritis, rashes, or other symptoms attributable to SLE. She reports voiding a minimal amount of urine once or twice a day.

On physical examination, vital signs are normal. Cardiopulmonary examination is normal. Abdominal examination is unremarkable.

Laboratory studies reveal a hemoglobin level of 10.8 g/dL (108 g/L), a leukocyte count of 8700/µL (8.7 × 10^9/L) with a normal differential, and a normal platelet count.

Kidney ultrasound reveals a complex-appearing mass suspicious for a renal neoplasm in the right kidney.

Which of the following is the most appropriate imaging study to perform next?

(A) CT with contrast
(B) Intravenous pyelography
(C) MRI with gadolinium
(D) Positron emission tomography

Item 20

A 59-year-old man is evaluated in the emergency department for a 3-month history of arthralgia, edema of the lower extremities, rash, and weakness. Medical history is remarkable for injection drug use.

On physical examination, blood pressure is 148/100 mm Hg. There is a diffuse, palpable erythematous rash. The lower extremities are notable for numbness, weakness, and 2+ pitting edema.

Laboratory studies on admission:

Hemoglobin	9.3 g/dL (93 g/L)
Leukocyte count	10,500/µL (10.5 × 10^9/L)
Platelet count	230,000/µL (230 × 10^9/L)
C3	Normal
C4	Decreased
Serum creatinine	1.8 mg/dL (159 µmol/L)
Lactate dehydrogenase	250 units/L
Cryoglobulin	Positive
Rheumatoid factor	Positive
Antinuclear antibodies	1:80
ANCA	Negative
Anti–glomerular basement membrane antibodies	Negative
Hepatitis B surface antibodies	Positive
Hepatitis B surface antigen	Negative
Hepatitis C virus antibodies	Positive
HIV antibodies	Negative
Peripheral blood smear	Erythrocytes of normal size and shape without schistocytosis
Urinalysis	Erythrocyte casts; leukocyte casts

Kidney biopsy results show a membranoproliferative glomerulonephritis with capillary microthrombi and diffuse IgM immune deposition in the capillary loops.

Which of the following is the most likely cause of this patient's kidney findings?

(A) Hepatitis B virus infection
(B) Hepatitis C virus infection

(C) Polyarteritis nodosa

(D) Thrombotic microangiopathy

Item 21

A 51-year-old man is evaluated for unilateral flank pain and a low-grade fever of several days' duration. He reports no nausea or vomiting. He has not experienced urinary changes such as hesitancy or frequency. He has a 10-year history of hyperlipidemia managed with simvastatin.

On physical examination, temperature is 37.8 °C (100.0 °F), blood pressure is 159/93 mm Hg, pulse rate is 92/min, and respiration rate is 12/min. BMI is 26. Abdominal examination reveals a soft and nondistended abdomen, normal bowel sounds, no masses, and mild diffuse tenderness, which is slightly worse in the right flank and right upper quadrant.

Laboratory studies:

Hemoglobin	14.1 g/dL (141 g/L)
Leukocyte count	11,500/µL (11.5 × 10⁹/L)
Urinalysis	pH 5.5; 2+ blood; trace protein; 1+ leukocyte esterase; 5-10 erythrocytes/hpf; 2-5 leukocytes/hpf; no nitrites

Hemoglobin 14.1 g/dL (141 g/L)

Leukocyte count 11,500/µL (11.5×10^9/L)

Urinalysis pH 5.5; 2+ blood; trace protein; 1+ leukocyte esterase; 5-10 erythrocytes/hpf; 2-5 leukocytes/hpf; no nitrites

Which of the following is the most appropriate test to perform next?

(A) Abdominal MRI

(B) Abdominal radiography of the kidneys, ureters, and bladder

(C) Intravenous pyelography

(D) Kidney ultrasonography

(E) Noncontrast abdominal helical CT

Item 22

A 47-year-old woman is evaluated during a follow-up visit for diabetic nephropathy. She also has chronic kidney disease, hypertension, retinopathy, and mild neuropathy. She has been well and is maintaining a healthy lifestyle. Medications are glyburide, amlodipine, and gabapentin.

On physical examination, blood pressure is 124/80 mm Hg. Cardiac examination is normal without a rub. Lungs are clear. Abdominal examination is unremarkable. Trace edema is present.

Laboratory studies:

Bicarbonate	17 meq/L (17 mmol/L)
Blood urea nitrogen	88 mg/dL (31.4 mmol/L)
Calcium	8.4 mg/dL (2.1 mmol/L)
Serum creatinine	3.1 mg/dL (274 µmol/L)
Phosphorus	4.5 mg/dL (1.45 mmol/L)
Potassium	4.8 meq/L (4.8 mmol/L)
Sodium	134 meq/L (134 mmol/L)
Uric acid	8 mg/dL (0.47 mmol/L)
Estimated glomerular filtration rate	16 mL/min/1.73 m²

Based on the laboratory studies, which of the following is the most appropriate addition to this patient's chronic kidney disease therapeutic regimen?

(A) Allopurinol

(B) Noncalcium-containing phosphate binder

(C) Sodium bicarbonate therapy

(D) Sodium polystyrene

Item 23

A 51-year-old woman is evaluated during a follow-up visit for hypertension. Her office blood pressure measurements are high; however, her home readings range from 118 to 140 mm Hg systolic and 82 to 88 mm Hg diastolic, averaging 126/84 mm Hg. She has no known cardiovascular disease. She consumes a heart-healthy diet, exercises regularly, and does not smoke cigarettes.

Using the patient's home device, blood pressure measurements are 150/86 mm Hg and 147/83 mm Hg. BMI is 25. Other vital signs are normal. The remainder of the examination is unremarkable.

Within the past 10 months, she has had normal chemistry laboratory test results and a normal electrocardiogram.

Ambulatory blood pressure monitoring is ordered, and results show an average 24-hour systolic blood pressure of 127 mm Hg and an average 24-hour diastolic blood pressure of 82 mm Hg; the average daytime pressure is less than 130/80 mm Hg, and the average nighttime pressure is less than 120/70 mm Hg (all values normal).

Which of the following is the most appropriate next step in management?

(A) Continue home blood pressure measurements

(B) Initiate chlorthalidone

(C) Order echocardiography

(D) Order a plasma aldosterone-plasma renin activity ratio

(E) Order a spot urine albumin–creatinine ratio

Item 24

A 41-year-old woman is evaluated for urinary frequency and some urgency. She reports no dysuria. Medical history is notable for chronic hepatitis C virus infection unresponsive to treatment and nephrolithiasis. She also has HIV infection that is well controlled with atazanavir, tenofovir, emtricitabine, and ritonavir.

On physical examination, the patient is comfortable and in no distress. Temperature is normal, blood pressure is 132/78 mm Hg, and pulse rate is 80/min. There are no rashes. Cardiac and pulmonary examinations are normal. Abdominal examination reveals no tenderness or flank pain.

Laboratory studies:

Blood urea nitrogen	27 mg/dL (9.6 mmol/L)
Calcium	9.2 mg/dL (2.3 mmol/L)
Serum creatinine	1.6 mg/dL (141 µmol/L) (6 months ago: 0.9 mg/dL [79.6 µmol/L])

Electrolytes
Sodium	138 meq/L (138 mmol/L)
Potassium	3.4 meq/L (3.4 mmol/L)
Chloride	108 meq/L (108 mmol/L)
Bicarbonate	18 meq/L (18 mmol/L)
Glucose	104 mg/dL (5.8 mmol/L)
Phosphorus	2.3 mg/dL (0.74 mmol/L)
CD4	625/µL
HIV RNA viral load	Undetectable
Hepatitis C viral load	250,000 units/L

Urine studies:
Creatinine	85 mg/dL (normal range for women, 15-327 mg/dL)
Sodium	70 meq/L (70 mmol/L) (normal range for women, 15-267 meq/L [15-267 mmol/L])
Fractional excretion of sodium	1%
Urinalysis	Specific gravity 1.008; pH 6.5; 1+ blood; 1+ protein; 1+ glucose; 1-3 erythrocytes/hpf; 1-2 leukocytes/hpf; no casts

Kidney ultrasound shows no hydronephrosis.

Which of the following is the most likely cause of this patient's acute kidney injury?

(A) Hepatitis C virus–associated glomerulonephritis
(B) HIV-associated focal segmental glomerulosclerosis
(C) Nephrolithiasis
(D) Tenofovir-induced toxicity

Item 25

A 26-year-old man is evaluated in the emergency department after being found on the floor in his apartment by friends who had not seen him in several days.

On physical examination, the patient is somnolent and minimally responsive. Temperature is 37.2 °C (98.9 °F), blood pressure is 92/54 mm Hg, pulse rate is 118/min, and respiration rate is 14/min with 97% oxygen saturation on ambient air. BMI is 25. Skin is mottled and edematous on the posterior surface of the legs, buttocks, and back. He withdraws from painful stimuli. Pupils are reactive. Neurologic examination reveals no focal or lateralizing findings. The remainder of the examination is normal.

Laboratory studies:
Blood urea nitrogen	174 mg/dL (62.1 mmol/L)
Calcium	7.8 mg/dL (2.0 mmol/L)
Creatine kinase	125,000 units/L
Serum creatinine	8.3 mg/dL (734 µmol/L)

Electrolytes
Sodium	151 meq/L (151 mmol/L)
Potassium	5.8 meq/L (5.8 mmol/L)
Chloride	121 meq/L (121 mmol/L)
Bicarbonate	19 meq/L (19 mmol/L)
Glucose	94 mg/dL (5.2 mmol/L)
Phosphorus	8.5 mg/dL (2.75 mmol/L)

Urinalysis	Specific gravity 1.012; pH 6.5; 3+ blood; 1+ protein; 0-5 erythrocytes/hpf; 1-3 leukocytes/hpf; dark granular casts
Toxicology screening	Pending

During the 3 hours he has been in the hospital, total urine output has been 60 mL.

Electrocardiogram reveals sinus tachycardia with normal intervals and no ST- or T-wave changes.

Which of the following is the most appropriate treatment for this patient?

(A) Hemodialysis
(B) Intravenous mannitol
(C) Rapid infusion of intravenous 0.9% saline
(D) Rapid infusion of intravenous 5% glucose

Item 26

A 52-year-old man is hospitalized for ganciclovir-resistant cytomegalovirus encephalitis. Therapy with foscarnet is initiated. He has advanced AIDS and does not currently take antiretroviral medications.

On physical examination, the patient is lethargic and oriented only to person. Temperature is 37.8 °C (100.0 °F), blood pressure is 136/56 mm Hg, pulse rate is 102/min, and respiration rate is 14/min. BMI is 17. During the first week of hospitalization, the serum sodium level increases from 143 meq/L (143 mmol/L) on admission to 156 meq/L (156 mmol/L); during this time, he has been receiving intravenous hydration with 0.9% saline.

Laboratory studies:

	On Admission	Day 7
Blood urea nitrogen	10 mg/dL (3.6 mmol/L)	15 mg/dL (5.4 mmol/L)
Serum creatinine	0.6 mg/dL (53 µmol/L)	1.2 mg/dL (106 µmol/L)
Glucose	88 mg/dL (4.9 mmol/L)	75 mg/dL (4.2 mmol/L)
Sodium	143 meq/L (143 mmol/L)	156 meq/L (156 mmol/L)
Plasma osmolality	300 mosm/kg H_2O	326 mosm/kg H_2O
Urine osmolality	186 mosm/kg H_2O (normal, 300-900 mosm/kg H_2O)	190 mosm/kg H_2O (normal, 300-900 mosm/kg H_2O)
Urine output	–	3020 mL/d

Following administration of desmopressin, the urine osmolality increases to 614 mosm/kg H_2O.

Which of the following is the most likely diagnosis?

(A) Central diabetes insipidus
(B) Cerebral salt wasting
(C) Nephrogenic diabetes insipidus
(D) Osmotic diuresis

Item 27

A 74-year-old woman is evaluated for a 2-month history of fatigue, anorexia, and a 6-kg (13.2-lb) weight loss. She was treated with chemotherapy for ovarian cancer 6 months ago. She also has hypertension managed with hydrochlorothiazide.

On physical examination, temperature is 36.2 °C (97.2 °F), blood pressure is 132/75 mm Hg without postural changes, pulse rate is 86/min without postural changes, and respiration rate is 14/min. BMI is 23. There are no neurologic findings. Estimated central venous pressure is less than 5 cm H_2O. Cardiac and pulmonary examinations are normal. There is no peripheral edema.

Laboratory studies:

Blood urea nitrogen	5 mg/dL (1.8 mmol/L)
Serum creatinine	0.4 mg/dL (35.4 µmol/L)
Electrolytes	
Sodium	128 meq/L (128 mmol/L)
Potassium	3.8 meq/L (3.8 mmol/L)
Chloride	90 meq/L (90 mmol/L)
Bicarbonate	25 meq/L (25 mmol/L)
Glucose	60 mg/dL (3.3 mmol/L)
Osmolality	266 mosm/kg H_2O
Cortisol (8 AM)	20 µg/dL (552 nmol/L) (normal range, 5-25 µg/dL [138-690 nmol/L])
Thyroid-stimulating hormone	1.3 µU/mL (1.3 mU/L)
Urine studies:	
Osmolality	50 mosm/kg H_2O (normal range, 300-900 mosm/kg H_2O)
Potassium	15 meq/L (15 mmol/L) (normal range for women, 17-164 meq/L [17-164 mmol/L])
Sodium	12 meq/L (12 mmol/L) (normal range for women, 15-267 meq/L [15-267 mmol/L])

Which of the following is the most likely cause of this patient's hyponatremia?

(A) Hypovolemia
(B) Low solute intake
(C) Measurement error (pseudohyponatremia)
(D) Primary adrenal insufficiency

Item 28

A 61-year-old woman is evaluated for the recent finding of a low estimated glomerular filtration rate (GFR). Laboratory studies performed by her previous physician revealed a serum creatinine level of 1.0 mg/dL (88.4 µmol/L), and the estimated GFR using the Modification of Diet in Renal Disease study equation was 56 mL/min/1.73 m².

She feels well and is active, exercising 5 days a week. She has no pertinent personal or family history. Medications are calcium carbonate and a daily multivitamin.

On physical examination, the patient appears younger than her age and is muscular. Vital signs and the remainder of the examination are normal.

Dipstick urinalysis results show no significant findings.

Which of the following is the most appropriate diagnostic test to perform next?

(A) 24-Hour urine collection for creatinine clearance
(B) Estimate GFR using the Chronic Kidney Disease Epidemiology Collaboration equation
(C) Estimate GFR using the Cockcroft-Gault equation
(D) Radionuclide kidney clearance scanning

Item 29

A 54-year-old woman is evaluated during a follow-up visit for a 15-year history of type 2 diabetes mellitus and a 10-year history of hypertension and hyperlipidemia. She is overweight and has been unsuccessful with weight loss. Medications are metformin, glipizide, irbesartan, hydrochlorothiazide, and simvastatin.

On physical examination, blood pressure is 154/82 mm Hg, and pulse rate is 88/min. BMI is 28. Cardiovascular examination is normal. The remainder of the examination is noncontributory.

Laboratory studies reveal a serum potassium level of 4.9 meq/L (4.9 mmol/L) and an estimated glomerular filtration rate of >60 mL/min/1.73 m². A urine albumin–creatinine ratio performed 3 months ago was 15 mg/g.

In addition to reinforcing lifestyle modifications, which of the following is the most appropriate next step in management?

(A) Add diltiazem
(B) Add furosemide
(C) Add lisinopril
(D) Add spironolactone

Item 30

A 36-year-old woman is evaluated during a follow-up visit for three episodes of nephrolithiasis that occurred during the past year. Each episode was treated with analgesics in an acute care setting. She had uncomplicated passage of the stones, although none was recovered for analysis. Her father and brother have a history of kidney stones. Her only medication is a multivitamin.

On physical examination, blood pressure is 126/78 mm Hg, and pulse rate is 96/min. BMI is 27. There is no costovertebral angle tenderness. The remainder of the examination is unremarkable.

Laboratory studies:

Blood urea nitrogen	15 mg/dL (5.4 mmol/L)
Calcium	8.9 mg/dL (2.2 mmol/L)
Serum creatinine	0.8 mg/dL (70.7 µmol/L)
Parathyroid hormone	Normal
Urine studies:	
Calcium excretion	379 mg/24 h (9.5 mmol/24 h)
Citrate excretion	521 mg/24 h (normal range, 320-1240 mg/24 h)
Oxalate excretion	26 mg/24 h (296 µmol/24 h) (normal range, 9.7-40.5 mg/24 h [111-462 µmol/24 h])
Uric acid excretion	359 mg/24 h (2.12 mmol/24 h)
Urine volume	1500 mL/24 h

Radiographs of the kidneys, ureters, and bladder show a 6-mm calcification in the lower pole of the right kidney.

In addition to recommending adequate fluid intake, which of the following is the most appropriate next step in management?

(A) Calcium-restricted diet
(B) Chlorthalidone
(C) Potassium chloride supplements
(D) Sodium citrate

Item 31

A 66-year-old man is evaluated for a 3-year history of chronic kidney disease (CKD). Medical history is significant for gout and hypertension, both of which were diagnosed at the same time as his CKD. He is retired as an industrial worker in a battery factory. His weight is stable, and his appetite is good. He has no history of drug abuse and does not smoke cigarettes. Medications are hydrochlorothiazide, amlodipine, and allopurinol. He does not take over-the-counter medications or remedies.

On physical examination, temperature is 36.9 °C (98.4 °F), blood pressure is 128/72 mm Hg, pulse rate is 82/min, and respiration rate is 13/min. BMI is 30. There are no rashes. There is no joint swelling or pitting edema of the extremities.

Laboratory studies:

Bicarbonate	21 meq/L (21 mmol/L)
Blood urea nitrogen	18 mg/dL (6.4 mmol/L)
Calcium	8.9 mg/dL (2.2 mmol/L)
Serum creatinine	1.9 mg/dL (168 µmol/L)
Glucose	95 mg/dL (5.3 mmol/L)
Lead	16 µg/dL (0.77 µmol/L) (normal range, <25 µg/dL [1.2 µmol/L])
Phosphorus	3.4 mg/dL (1.10 mmol/L)
Uric acid	5.8 mg/dL (0.34 mmol/L)
Urinalysis	pH 5.5; trace protein; + glucose; 0 erythrocytes/hpf; 1-3 leukocytes/hpf; no ketones
Urine protein–creatinine ratio	0.4 mg/mg

Which of the following is the most appropriate diagnostic study to perform next?

(A) Chelation mobilization testing
(B) Erythrocyte protoporphyrin measurement
(C) Long bone radiography
(D) Peripheral blood smear

Item 32

A 53-year-old man is hospitalized for treatment of osteomyelitis of the foot resulting from a chronic diabetic ulcer. Medical history is significant for type 1 diabetes mellitus, hypertension, and chronic kidney disease with a baseline serum creatinine level of 3.2 mg/dL (283 µmol/L) and an estimated glomerular filtration rate of 19 mL/min/1.73 m². The ulcer was surgically debrided, and

a deep culture of the bone grew an *Escherichia coli* species sensitive only to piperacillin-tazobactam.

Although maintaining peripheral intravenous access was difficult, he responded well to antibiotic therapy, and his current examination shows a clean and dry healing surgical site. The remainder of the physical examination is unremarkable except for a baseline dense lower extremity sensory neuropathy. Kidney function is unchanged from admission. Continued intravenous antibiotics to complete a 4-week course are planned following discharge.

Which of the following is the most appropriate route of access for ongoing antibiotic administration for this patient?

(A) Left internal jugular temporary dialysis catheter
(B) Left subclavian catheter
(C) Peripheral intravenous access
(D) Right peripherally inserted central catheter

Item 33

A 40-year-old man is evaluated during a follow-up visit for high blood pressure. Three weeks ago, his blood pressure was 150/94 mm Hg. He has no knowledge of prior blood pressure measurements. He has no history of cardiovascular disease. He takes no medications.

On physical examination, temperature is 37.1 °C (98.8 °F), blood pressure is 148/96 mm Hg seated and 156/100 mm Hg standing, pulse rate is 82/min, and respiration rate is 18/min. BMI is 27. Funduscopic examination shows arteriolar narrowing with two arteriovenous crossing defects ("nicking"). The remainder of the examination is unremarkable.

Initial laboratory studies, including serum electrolyte levels, complete blood count, lipid profile, and urinalysis, are normal. Normal kidney function is noted.

Which of the following is the most appropriate next step in management?

(A) Atenolol
(B) Electrocardiography
(C) Home blood pressure monitoring
(D) Plasma aldosterone-plasma renin activity ratio

Item 34

A 54-year-old man is evaluated during a follow-up visit for five previous episodes of nephrolithiasis. Two of these stones were composed primarily of uric acid. After his third episode, potassium citrate was initiated. Medical history is notable for type 2 diabetes mellitus, hypertension, and hyperlipidemia. He does not have a known history of gout. He eats a fairly high protein diet, and his fluid intake is inconsistent. Other medications are metformin, metoprolol, amlodipine, atorvastatin, and aspirin.

On physical examination, blood pressure is 136/82 mm Hg, and pulse rate is 68/min. BMI is 32. There is no costovertebral angle tenderness. The remainder of the examination is unremarkable.

Laboratory studies:

Blood urea nitrogen	15 mg/dL (5.4 mmol/L)
Calcium	8.5 mg/dL (2.1 mmol/L)
Serum creatinine	1.1 mg/dL (97.2 µmol/L)
Uric acid	7.8 mg/dL (0.46 mmol/L)
Urine studies:	
Calcium excretion	220 mg/24 h (5.5 mmol/24 h)
Citrate excretion	400 mg/24 h (normal range, 320-1240 mg/24 h)
Oxalate excretion	26 mg/24 h (296 µmol/24 h) (normal range, 9.7-40.5 mg/24 h [111-462 µmol/24 h])
Uric acid excretion	710 mg/24 h (4.19 mmol/24 h)
Urinalysis	Specific gravity 1.025; pH 6.2; no blood, protein, or leukocyte esterase
Urine volume	1600 mL/24 h

In addition to increased fluid intake and dietary changes, which of the following is the most appropriate treatment for this patient?

(A) Acetazolamide
(B) Allopurinol
(C) Calcium carbonate
(D) Chlorthalidone

Item 35

A 64-year-old man is evaluated for an 8-week history of fatigue, dyspnea, a sore tongue, leg edema, and painful burning feet. He has never smoked cigarettes and does not drink alcohol or use illicit drugs. He takes no medications.

On physical examination, the patient is afebrile; blood pressure is 156/84 mm Hg, pulse rate is 100/min, and respiration rate is 20/min. BMI is 22. Macroglossia and multiple ecchymoses are present. Jugular venous distention is noted. There is an S_3 at the cardiac apex. Crackles are heard at the posterior lung bases. Hepatomegaly is noted. There is 3+ pitting edema of the lower extremities. There is diminished sensation in the feet bilaterally.

Laboratory studies:

Hemoglobin	11.2 g/dL (112 g/L)
Hemoglobin A_{1c}	5.8%
Albumin	2.0 g/dL (20 g/L)
Calcium	9.2 mg/dL (2.3 mmol/L)
Serum creatinine	1.5 mg/dL (133 µmol/L)
Total protein	8.0 g/dL (80 g/L)
Urinalysis	0-3 erythrocytes/hpf; 3-5 leukocytes/hpf
Urine protein–creatinine ratio	8.9 mg/mg

Electrocardiogram reveals sinus tachycardia and low voltage. Chest radiograph reveals cardiomegaly and vascular congestion.

Which of the following is the most likely diagnosis?

(A) AL amyloidosis
(B) Diabetic nephropathy

(C) Polyarteritis nodosa
(D) Primary membranous glomerulopathy

Item 36

A 22-year-old man is evaluated for hypertension and hypokalemic metabolic alkalosis. He is asymptomatic. He does not have a history of licorice ingestion. He does not use NSAIDs, illicit drugs, alcohol, or tobacco products. Medications are amlodipine and benazepril.

On physical examination, temperature is 37.1 °C (98.8 °F), blood pressure is 164/98 mm Hg, pulse rate is 70/min, and respiration rate is 14/min. BMI is 29. The remainder of the examination is normal.

Laboratory studies:

Blood urea nitrogen	10 mg/dL (3.6 mmol/L)
Serum creatinine	0.7 mg/dL (61.9 µmol/L)
Electrolytes	
Sodium	142 meq/L (142 mmol/L)
Potassium	3.0 meq/L (3.0 mmol/L)
Chloride	102 meq/L (102 mmol/L)
Bicarbonate	34 meq/L (34 mmol/L)
Aldosterone	<4 ng/dL (110 pmol/L)
Plasma renin activity	<0.6 ng/mL/h (0.6 µg/L/h) (normal range, 0.6-4.3 ng/mL/h [0.6-4.3 µg/L/h])
24-Hour urine free cortisol	Normal
Urinalysis	Specific gravity 1.012; pH 6.0; no blood, protein, casts, or cells

Kidney ultrasound reveals normal-sized kidneys without hydronephrosis.

Which of the following is the most likely diagnosis?

(A) Liddle syndrome
(B) Pheochromocytoma
(C) Primary hyperaldosteronism
(D) Renovascular hypertension

Item 37

An 80-year-old woman is hospitalized for a 1-week history of progressive weakness, nausea, and anorexia. She lives independently but has become bedridden and confused during the past 3 days. She has hypertension managed with enalapril as well as chlorthalidone, which was initiated 2 weeks ago.

On physical examination, the patient is lethargic and unable to recognize family members. Temperature is 37.3 °C (99.2 °F), blood pressure is 160/86 mm Hg, pulse rate is 68/min, and respiration rate is 14/min. BMI is 20. Cardiac and pulmonary examinations are normal. Neurologic examination shows no focal deficits. There is no edema, ascites, or evidence of hypovolemia.

Laboratory studies are consistent with hypotonic hyponatremia; her serum sodium level is 110 meq/L (110 mmol/L). Therapy with 3% saline is initiated, and her mentation rapidly improves to baseline.

H **CONT.** Laboratory studies 10 hours after admission:

Serum sodium	121 meq/L (121 mmol/L)
Urine sodium	48 meq/L (48 mmol/L); 82 meq/L (82 mmol/L) on admission (normal range for women, 15-267 meq/L [15-267 mmol/L])
Urine osmolality	206 mosm/kg H_2O; 486 mosm/kg H_2O on admission (normal range, 300-900 mosm/kg H_2O)
Urine output	Approximately 400 mL/h since admission

Which of the following is the most appropriate treatment for this patient?

(A) 0.9% Saline
(B) 5% Dextrose in water
(C) Fluid restriction
(D) Tolvaptan

H **Item 38**

A 75-year-old man is hospitalized for community-acquired pneumonia and is treated with antibiotics and intravenous normal saline. His fever resolves and his breathing improves after 2 days. On day 3, he is preparing for discharge but reports his breathing has not returned to baseline. His dyspnea, although improved since admission, is particularly noticeable on exertion. Medical history is remarkable for hypertension, hyperlipidemia, and ischemic cardiomyopathy with an ejection fraction of 25%. Current medications are moxifloxacin, hydrochlorothiazide, metoprolol, lisinopril, simvastatin, and aspirin.

On physical examination, temperature is 36.4 °C (97.5 °F), blood pressure is 115/64 mm Hg, pulse rate is 102/min, and respiration rate is 18/min. Jugular venous pulsation is elevated. Cardiac examination reveals an S_3; there are no murmurs. Pulmonary examination reveals mild basilar crackles. There is trace lower extremity edema.

Laboratory studies:

Blood urea nitrogen	45 mg/dL (16.1 mmol/L)
Serum creatinine	1.9 mg/dL (168 µmol/L) (2 days ago: 1.3 mg/dL [115 µmol/L])
Electrolytes	
Sodium	133 meq/L (133 mmol/L)
Potassium	3.6 meq/L (3.6 mmol/L)
Chloride	102 meq/L (102 mmol/L)
Bicarbonate	23 meq/L (23 mmol/L)
Urinalysis	Specific gravity 1.019; pH 6.0; 0-1 erythrocytes/hpf; 0-1 leukocytes/hpf; occasional hyaline casts; no other casts

Which of the following is the most appropriate treatment?

(A) Administer a 500-mL bolus of normal saline
(B) Begin intravenous furosemide
(C) Increase lisinopril
(D) Increase metoprolol

Item 39

A 72-year-old man is evaluated during a follow-up visit for difficult-to-control hypertension. He has diabetes mellitus and stage 4 chronic kidney disease (CKD). A review of his laboratory studies shows his serum creatinine level has gradually increased over the past 3 years, consistent with progression of his CKD. He has been on the same antihypertensive regimen for years and takes hydrochlorothiazide, 25 mg/d; lisinopril, 40 mg/d; amlodipine, 10 mg/d; and metoprolol, 100 mg/d (long acting). He adheres to his medication regimen and reports no side effects. He is not taking any over-the-counter medications. He eats a low salt diet and exercises 20 to 30 minutes daily.

On physical examination, the patient is afebrile. Blood pressure is 162/74 mm Hg, and pulse rate is 62/min, without orthostatic changes. There is no elevation in jugular venous pressure. Cardiac examination is normal with no murmurs. Lungs are clear. There is trace edema of the lower extremities.

Laboratory studies:

Serum creatinine	3.2 mg/dL (283 µmol/L)
Potassium	4.7 meq/L (4.7 mmol/L)
Estimated glomerular filtration rate	24 mL/min/1.73 m²
Urine albumin–creatinine ratio	650 mg/g

Which of the following is the most appropriate adjustment to this patient's hypertensive medication regimen?

(A) Add clonidine
(B) Add hydralazine
(C) Add valsartan
(D) Change hydrochlorothiazide to furosemide

Item 40

A 34-year-old woman is evaluated for urinary frequency. She has no dysuria, fever, chills, or sweats. She is otherwise healthy, and her only medication is a daily multivitamin.

On physical examination, temperature is 37.1 °C (98.7 °F), blood pressure is 149/95 mm Hg, pulse rate is 72/min, and respiration rate is 18/min. BMI is 23. The remainder of the examination is normal.

Dipstick urinalysis shows a pH of 5.5, 1+ blood, 1+ protein, and negative leukocyte esterase. The urine microscopy is shown (see next page).

Which of the following diagnostic tests is most appropriate to perform next?

(A) Kidney biopsy
(B) Kidney ultrasonography and cystoscopy
(C) Urine culture
(D) Urine protein–creatinine ratio and serum creatinine measurement

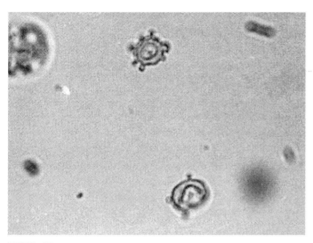

ITEM 40

Item 41

A 32-year-old woman is evaluated during a new patient visit. She is healthy, exercises regularly without symptoms, and takes no medications. Medical history is unremarkable. Family history is notable for her father and paternal aunt who both have hypertension and chronic kidney disease. There is no family history of polycystic kidney disease. Her father began dialysis when he was 50 years old and now has a kidney transplant.

Physical examination and vital signs are normal.

Which of the following should be done to screen for chronic kidney disease?

(A) 24-Hour urine collection for creatinine clearance
(B) Kidney ultrasonography
(C) Radionuclide kidney clearance scanning
(D) Serum creatinine, estimated glomerular filtration rate, and urinalysis

Item 42

A 68-year-old woman is evaluated following the results of a dual-energy x-ray absorptiometry measurement obtained at a hospital system–sponsored health fair, which revealed a T score of –3.0 in the lumbosacral spine and –3.2 in the left hip. She has chronic kidney disease. Her only medication is a calcium supplement, 1000 mg/d.

On physical examination, blood pressure is 124/80 mm Hg. BMI is 24. The remainder of the examination is unremarkable.

Laboratory studies:

Calcium	9.1 mg/dL (2.3 mmol/L)
Serum creatinine	2.4 mg/dL (212 µmol/L)
Phosphorus	4.5 mg/dL (1.45 mmol/L)
Intact parathyroid hormone	65 pg/mL (65 ng/L)
25-hydroxyvitamin D	38 ng/mL (95 nmol/L)
Estimated glomerular filtration rate	26 mL/min/1.73 m^2

In addition to recommending physical activity, which of the following is the most appropriate next step in management?

(A) Add cinacalcet
(B) Add risedronate
(C) Add sevelamer
(D) Discontinue the calcium supplement
(E) Maintain current therapeutic regimen

Item 43

A 75-year-old woman is evaluated during a follow-up visit for escalating hypertension. She has a 54-pack-year history of smoking; she quit 5 years ago after she had a transient ischemic attack. She is adherent to her medication regimen, which consists of a β-blocker, a calcium channel blocker, and a diuretic. Six months ago her blood pressure was 148/82 mm Hg, and three months ago it was 158/90 mm Hg.

On physical examination, temperature is normal, blood pressure is 174/96 mm Hg, and pulse rate is 60/min. BMI is 20. Cardiopulmonary examination reveals bilateral carotid bruits as well as midline and bilateral epigastric bruits. An S$_4$ gallop is noted. There is trace pedal edema.

Laboratory studies reveal a serum creatinine level of 1.7 mg/dL (150 µmol/L), an estimated glomerular filtration rate of 29 mL/min/1.73 m^2, and a negative urine dipstick.

Which of the following is the most appropriate next step in management?

(A) Add an ACE inhibitor
(B) Increase the β-blocker dose
(C) Obtain Doppler ultrasonography of the renal arteries
(D) Obtain kidney angiography

Item 44

An 83-year-old woman is hospitalized for a total knee replacement to manage her osteoarthritis. She also has hypertension and stage 3 chronic kidney disease. Current medications are amlodipine, fondaparinux, and celecoxib for postoperative pain. She is allergic to opioids, which cause delirium.

On physical examination, temperature is 36.0 °C (96.8 °F), blood pressure is 142/65 mm Hg, pulse rate is 80/min, and respiration rate is 15/min. BMI is 28. On postoperative day 3, her serum potassium level has increased from 4.2 meq/L (4.2 mmol/L) to 6.2 meq/L (6.2 mmol/L). A stool specimen is negative for occult blood.

Laboratory studies (postoperative day 3):

Hemoglobin	12.2 g/dL (122 g/L)
Leukocyte count	6700/µL (6.7 × 10^9/L)
Platelet count	396,000/µL (396 × 10^9/L)
Blood urea nitrogen	22 mg/dL (7.9 mmol/L)
Serum creatinine	1.2 mg/dL (106 µmol/L)
Electrolytes	
Sodium	136 meq/L (136 mmol/L)
Potassium	6.2 meq/L (6.2 mmol/L)
Chloride	106 meq/L (106 mmol/L)
Bicarbonate	20 meq/L (20 mmol/L)

Glucose	90 mg/dL (5 mmol/L)
Osmolality	288 mosm/kg H_2O
Estimated glomerular filtration rate	52 mL/min/1.73 m^2
Urine studies:	
Creatinine	100 mg/dL (normal range for women, 15-327 mg/dL)
Osmolality	576 mosm/kg H_2O (normal range, 300-900 mosm/kg H_2O)
Potassium	30 meq/L (30 mmol/L) (normal range for women, 17-164 meq/L [17-164 mmol/L])

Electrocardiogram reveals tall, symmetric, peaked T waves.

Which of the following is the most likely cause of this patient's hyperkalemia?

(A) Adrenal hemorrhage
(B) Celecoxib toxicity
(C) High potassium diet
(D) Pseudohyperkalemia

Item 45

An 18-year-old woman is evaluated for a 6-month history of progressive weakness and a 5-kg (11-lb) weight loss. She reports increased fatigue and myalgia following exercise during the past 2 months.

On physical examination, the patient is thin. Temperature is 36.4 °C (97.6 °F), blood pressure is 110/60 mm Hg, pulse rate is 96/min, and respiration rate is 18/min. BMI is 18. The remainder of the examination is unremarkable.

Laboratory studies:

Blood urea nitrogen	4 mg/dL (1.4 mmol/L)
Serum creatinine	0.5 mg/dL (44.2 µmol/L)
Electrolytes	
Sodium	135 meq/L (135 mmol/L)
Potassium	3.1 meq/L (3.1 mmol/L)
Chloride	108 meq/L (108 mmol/L)
Bicarbonate	18 meq/L (18 mmol/L)
Urine studies:	
Creatinine	120 mg/dL (normal range for women, 15-327 mg/dL)
Sodium	22 meq/L (22 mmol/L) (normal range for women, 15-267 meq/L [15-267 mmol/L])
Potassium	15 meq/L (15 mmol/L) (normal range for women, 17-164 meq/L [17-164 mmol/L])
Chloride	45 meq/L (45 mmol/L) (normal range for women, 20-295 meq/L [20-295 mmol/L])
Urea	112 mg/dL (normal range for women, 132-1629 mg/dL)
Osmolality	290 mosm/kg H_2O (normal range, 300-900 mosm/kg H_2O)
Urinalysis	Specific gravity 1.012; pH 5.8; no blood, protein, glucose, leukocyte esterase, ketones, or nitrites

Which of the following is the most likely cause of this patient's acid-base disorder?

(A) Diuretic abuse
(B) Hypokalemic distal (type 1) renal tubular acidosis
(C) Laxative abuse
(D) Surreptitious vomiting

Item 46

A 54-year-old woman is evaluated for an abnormal electrocardiogram obtained at a local health screening fair. She has no cardiovascular symptoms or risk factors and takes no medications.

On physical examination, blood pressure is 136/80 mm Hg; other vital signs are normal. The remainder of the examination is unremarkable.

Laboratory studies, including complete blood count, serum creatinine, electrolytes, and lipids, are normal.

The electrocardiogram demonstrates voltage criteria for left ventricular hypertrophy. A follow-up echocardiogram confirms the presence of symmetric left ventricular hypertrophy without evidence of aortic valve disease or resting outflow gradient.

Which of the following is the most appropriate next step in management?

(A) 24-Hour ambulatory blood pressure monitoring
(B) Cardiac MRI
(C) Chlorthalidone
(D) Coronary artery calcium score

Item 47

A 19-year-old woman is hospitalized for acute kidney injury (AKI) associated with bloody diarrhea that developed after she returned from a trip to South America. She also has nausea, vomiting, abdominal pain, fever, chills, and decreased urine output. Medical history is otherwise unremarkable, and she takes no medications.

On physical examination, temperature is 37.8 °C (100.0 °F), blood pressure is 135/90 mm Hg, and pulse rate is 110/min. The oral mucosa is dry. There is diffuse abdominal pain with guarding. The remainder of the physical examination is normal.

Laboratory studies:

Haptoglobin	8 mg/dL (80 mg/L)
Hemoglobin	5.2 g/dL (52 g/L)
Leukocyte count	20,000/µL (20 × 10^9/L)
Platelet count	36,000/µL (36 × 10^9/L)
Reticulocyte count	7.8%
Serum creatinine	5.7 mg/dL (504 µmol/L)
Lactate dehydrogenase	2396 units/L
Peripheral blood smear	Many schistocytes
Urinalysis	Many erythrocytes and erythrocyte casts
Urine protein–creatinine ratio	0.5 mg/mg

Which of the following is the most likely cause of this patient's acute kidney injury?

(A) Acute tubular necrosis
(B) Hemolytic uremic syndrome
(C) Postinfectious glomerulonephritis
(D) Scleroderma renal crisis

Item 48

A 28-year-old woman is evaluated during a follow-up visit. A life insurance examination revealed proteinuria. She is otherwise healthy and has no pertinent personal or family history.

On physical examination, temperature is 36.1 °C (97.0 °F), blood pressure is 110/64 mm Hg, pulse rate is 72/min, and respiration rate is 12/min. BMI is 23. The remainder of the examination is normal.

Laboratory studies today:

Serum creatinine	0.8 mg/dL (70.7 µmol/L)
Estimated glomerular filtration rate	>60 mL/min/1.73 m²
24-Hour urine collection for protein	200 mg/24 h
Urinalysis	1+ protein; 0-2 erythrocytes/hpf; 0 leukocytes/hpf

Which of the following is the most appropriate next step in management?

(A) Kidney biopsy
(B) Repeat 24-hour urine collection for protein
(C) Split urine collection
(D) Spot urine protein–creatinine ratio
(E) Reassurance

Item 49

A 47-year-old man is evaluated during a follow-up visit for stage 3 chronic kidney disease attributed to type 2 diabetes mellitus and hypertension. He feels well and has no complaints. Medications are fosinopril, amlodipine, and glipizide.

On physical examination, blood pressure is 148/82 mm Hg, and pulse rate is 80/min. BMI is 25. There is no jugular venous distention. Cardiac and pulmonary examinations are unremarkable. There is no edema.

Laboratory studies:

Blood urea nitrogen	45 mg/dL (16.1 mmol/L)
Calcium	9.0 mg/dL (2.3 mmol/L)
Serum creatinine	1.7 mg/dL (150 µmol/L)
Electrolytes	
Sodium	139 meq/L (139 mmol/L)
Potassium	4.3 meq/L (4.3 mmol/L)
Chloride	101 meq/L (101 mmol/L)
Bicarbonate	22 meq/L (22 mmol/L)
Phosphorus	4.3 mg/dL (1.39 mmol/L)
Parathyroid hormone	69 pg/mL (69 ng/L)
Estimated glomerular filtration rate	41 mL/min/1.73 m²
Urine protein–creatinine ratio	0.17 mg/mg

Which of the following changes to this patient's therapeutic regimen should be made next?

(A) Add sodium bicarbonate
(B) Begin activated vitamin D therapy
(C) Increase antihypertensive therapy
(D) No change

Item 50

A 33-year-old man is evaluated for nausea, anorexia, diarrhea, and weight loss. He has recurrent testicular germ cell cancer and is undergoing chemotherapy with vinblastine, ifosfamide, and cisplatin. He reports no tinnitus, dyspnea, or confusion. Other medications are ondansetron and aspirin as needed.

On physical examination, the patient appears thin, with bitemporal wasting. Temperature is 36.4 °C (97.6 °F), blood pressure is 128/84 mm Hg, pulse rate is 82/min, and respiration rate is 16/min. BMI is 22. There is no edema. The remainder of the examination is unremarkable.

Laboratory studies:

Albumin	3.9 g/dL (39 g/L)
Alkaline phosphatase	126 units/L
Blood urea nitrogen	22 mg/dL (7.9 mmol/L)
Calcium	8.5 mg/dL (2.1 mmol/L)
Serum creatinine	1.3 mg/dL (115 µmol/L)
Electrolytes	
Sodium	141 meq/L (141 mmol/L)
Potassium	3.4 meq/L (3.4 mmol/L)
Chloride	112 meq/L (112 mmol/L)
Bicarbonate	19 meq/L (19 mmol/L)
Glucose	82 mg/dL (4.6 mmol/L)
Magnesium	2.1 mg/dL (0.87 mmol/L)
Phosphorus	2 mg/dL (0.65 mmol/L)
Urinalysis	Specific gravity 1.012; pH 5.0; no blood; trace protein; 1+ glucose
Fractional excretion of phosphate	20% (Normal, <5%)

Which of the following is the most likely cause of this patient's hypophosphatemia?

(A) Malnutrition
(B) Oncogenic osteomalacia
(C) Primary hyperparathyroidism
(D) Proximal (type 2) renal tubular acidosis

Item 51

A 25-year-old man is evaluated for dark urine and decreased urine output. He reports a 5-day history of an upper respiratory infection with a dry cough, runny nose, sore throat, and low-grade fever that he has treated with over-the-counter NSAIDs. He also notes mild diffuse myalgia and bilateral flank pain but reports no vomiting, diarrhea, or burning while urinating.

On physical examination, blood pressure is 135/88 mm Hg. The pharynx is erythematous but without exudate. Shotty neck lymphadenopathy is noted. There is 1+ pitting edema.

Laboratory studies:

Hemoglobin	9.8 g/dL (98 g/L)
Leukocyte count	9800/µL (9.8 × 10⁹/L) with normal differential
Platelet count	258,000/µL (258 × 10⁹/L)
C3	100 mg/dL (1000 mg/L)
C4	Normal
Creatine kinase	95 units/L
Serum creatinine	2.3 mg/dL (203 µmol/L)
Antistreptolysin O antibodies	Negative
Urine myoglobin	Negative
Urinalysis	Dark red–appearing urine with >100 erythrocytes/hpf; 2-3 leukocytes/hpf; no bacteria

Kidney ultrasound shows normal-sized kidneys and no evidence of obstruction.

Which of the following is the most likely cause of this patient's acute kidney injury?

(A) Analgesic toxicity
(B) IgA nephropathy
(C) Postinfectious glomerulonephritis
(D) Rhabdomyolysis

Item 52

An 86-year-old man is hospitalized for heart failure. He has coronary artery disease that is managed with pravastatin, metoprolol, nitroglycerin, and aspirin.

On physical examination, temperature is 37.1 °C (98.8 °F), blood pressure is 105/60 mm Hg, pulse rate is 98/min, and respiration rate is 18/min. BMI is 31. Jugular venous distention, an S₃, pulmonary crackles, and pedal edema are noted.

After initial clinical improvement following the first day of treatment with furosemide and enalapril, he develops increased abdominal distention, vomiting, and watery diarrhea.

Laboratory studies:

	On Admission	Hospital Day 3
Blood urea nitrogen	26 mg/dL (9.3 mmol/L)	12 mg/dL (4.3 mmol/L)
Serum creatinine	1.3 mg/dL (115 µmol/L)	1.2 mg/dL (106 µmol/L)
Electrolytes		
Sodium	136 meq/L (136 mmol/L)	134 meq/L (134 mmol/L)
Potassium	3.8 meq/L (3.8 mmol/L)	2.8 meq/L (2.8 mmol/L)
Chloride	98 meq/L (98 mmol/L)	94 meq/L (94 mmol/L)
Bicarbonate	30 meq/L (30 mmol/L)	28 meq/L (28 mmol/L)
Urine studies:		
Creatinine	–	120 mg/dL (normal range for men, 22-392 mg/dL)
Potassium	–	16 meq/L (16 mmol/L) (normal range for men, 11-99 meq/L [11-99 mmol/L])

Abdominal radiographs reveal colonic dilatation from the cecum to the splenic flexure with preservation of haustral markings. CT scan of the abdomen shows no evidence of mechanical obstruction.

A nasogastric tube is placed to gravity drain, with drainage of 300 mL.

Which of the following is the most likely cause of this patient's hypokalemia?

(A) Colonic pseudo-obstruction
(B) Furosemide
(C) Nasogastric fluid loss
(D) Redistribution

Item 53

A 19-year-old man is evaluated for a 3-day history of lower extremity and periorbital edema that developed 3 weeks after an upper respiratory tract infection. He is otherwise in good health and takes no medications.

On physical examination, blood pressure is 150/94 mm Hg; other vital signs are normal. There is 2+ pitting leg edema.

Laboratory studies:

Blood urea nitrogen	35 mg/dL (12.5 mmol/L)
C3	Decreased
Serum creatinine	2 mg/dL (177 µmol/L)
Antistreptolysin O antibodies	Elevated
Anti-DNase B antibodies	Elevated
Throat culture	Negative for group A β-hemolytic streptococcus
Urinalysis	30-35 erythrocytes/hpf; 1-2 erythrocyte casts/hpf
Urine protein–creatinine ratio	2.2 mg/mg

Which of the following is the most appropriate treatment for this patient?

(A) Cyclosporine
(B) Intravenous pulse methylprednisolone followed by prednisone
(C) Plasmapheresis followed by cyclophosphamide with prednisone
(D) Prednisone and cyclophosphamide for 6 months
(E) Supportive care

Item 54

A 63-year-old woman is evaluated for a 4-week history of lower extremity edema and a weight gain of 3 kg (6.6 lb). She reports no burning while urinating or blood in the urine but has noticed frothy urine. She also has a 20-year history of hypertension and a 14-year history of type 2 diabetes mellitus and hyperlipidemia, all of which have been well controlled. Medications are lisinopril, metformin, and simvastatin.

On physical examination, blood pressure is 135/85 mm Hg. Retinal examination is normal. Bilateral edema of the legs is noted. Six months ago, blood pressure was 125/70 mm Hg, hemoglobin A_{1c} level was 6.2%, total cholesterol level was 155 mg/dL (4.01 mmol/L), and urine albumin–creatinine ratio was less than 30 mg/g.

Laboratory studies today:

Albumin	3.3 g/dL (33 g/L)
Blood urea nitrogen	21 mg/dL (7.5 mmol/L)
Complement (C3 and C4)	Normal
Total cholesterol	282 mg/dL (7.30 mmol/L)
Serum creatinine	0.7 mg/dL (61.9 µmol/L)
Glucose	96 mg/dL (5.3 mmol/L)
Cryoglobulin	Negative
Serum protein electrophoresis	Normal
Rheumatoid factor	Negative
Antinuclear antibodies	Negative
Hepatitis B surface antigen	Negative
Hepatitis C virus antibodies	Negative
HIV antibodies	Negative
Urinalysis	4+ protein; 0-5 leukocytes/hpf
Urine protein–creatinine ratio	7 mg/mg

Percutaneous kidney biopsy results show diffuse thickening of the glomerular basement membrane. There is no increase in cellularity or evidence of active inflammation. Immune staining reveals diffuse granular deposits of IgG and C3 along the basement membrane, and electron microscopy confirms numerous subepithelial electron-dense deposits with moderate podocyte foot process effacement.

Which of the following is the most likely diagnosis?

(A) Diabetic nephropathy
(B) Membranous lupus nephritis
(C) Minimal change glomerulopathy
(D) Primary membranous glomerulopathy

Item 55

A 48-year-old man is evaluated during a follow-up visit for urinary frequency. He reports no hesitancy, urgency, dysuria, or change in urine color. He has not experienced fevers, chills, sweats, nausea, vomiting, diarrhea, or other gastrointestinal symptoms. He feels thirsty very often; drinking water and using lemon drops seem to help. He has a 33-pack-year history of smoking. He has hypertension, chronic kidney disease, and bipolar disorder. Medications are amlodipine, lisinopril, and lithium. He has tried other agents in place of lithium for his bipolar disorder, but none has controlled his symptoms as well as lithium.

On physical examination, temperature is 37.3 °C (99.2 °F), blood pressure is 142/75 mm Hg, pulse rate is 82/min, and respiration rate is 14/min. BMI is 29. There are no rashes. There is no pitting edema of the extremities.

Laboratory studies:

Serum creatinine	1.9 mg/dL (168 µmol/L)
Serum sodium	143 meq/L (143 mmol/L)

Urine osmolality	206 mosm/kg H_2O (normal range, 300-900 mosm/kg H_2O)
Urinalysis	Specific gravity 1.009; pH 5.5; trace protein; 0 erythrocytes/hpf; 0-2 leukocytes/hpf
Urine cultures	Negative

Which of the following is the most appropriate treatment intervention for this patient?

(A) Amiloride
(B) Fluid restriction
(C) Prednisone
(D) Tolvaptan

Item 56

A 65-year-old man is hospitalized following emergent surgery for peritonitis consequent to a perforated diverticulum. A sigmoid colectomy and diverting colostomy are performed. He has stage 4 chronic kidney disease due to autosomal dominant polycystic kidney disease. He also has hypertension treated with amlodipine.

On physical examination, temperature is 38.1 °C (100.5 °F), blood pressure is 150/95 mm Hg, pulse rate is 102/min, and respiration rate is 18/min. BMI is 31. On abdominal examination, the colostomy site is well perfused; bowel sounds are present.

Postoperatively, the serum potassium level increases from 4.8 meq/L (4.8 mmol/L) on admission to 6.9 meq/L (6.9 mmol/L); the serum creatinine level increases from 5.4 mg/dL (477 µmol/L) on admission to 6.4 mg/dL (566 µmol/L); and the urine output decreases to 50 mL over the initial 8 hours postoperatively and does not improve following a fluid challenge.

Laboratory studies:

Hemoglobin	8.6 g/dL (86 g/L)
Leukocyte count	15,900/µL (15.9×10^9/L)
Platelet count	206,000/µL (206×10^9/L)
Blood urea nitrogen	86 mg/dL (30.7 mmol/L)
Serum creatinine	6.4 mg/dL (566 µmol/L)
Electrolytes	
Sodium	135 meq/L (135 mmol/L)
Potassium	6.9 meq/L (6.9 mmol/L)
Chloride	101 meq/L (101 mmol/L)
Bicarbonate	17 meq/L (17 mmol/L)

Electrocardiogram reveals tall, symmetric, peaked T waves and a shortened QT interval.

In addition to intravenous calcium and insulin-dextrose, which of the following is the most appropriate treatment?

(A) Furosemide
(B) Hemodialysis
(C) Sodium bicarbonate
(D) Sodium polystyrene sulfonate

Item 57

A 42-year-old man is evaluated in the emergency department for increased confusion. Earlier in the day, he visited a homeopathic practitioner for his psoriasis; he was treated with cream and a body wrap for 1 hour. He subsequently developed nausea and vomiting. He reports feeling "out of his body" and hearing water in his ears. He also has hypertension and type 2 diabetes mellitus complicated by proteinuria. Medications are enalapril and metformin.

On physical examination, the patient is irritable, anxious, and intermittently somnolent but easily aroused. Temperature is 37.6 °C (99.7 °F), blood pressure is 160/100 mm Hg, pulse rate is 106/min standing, and respiration rate is 20/min. BMI is 40. Erythematous plaques are noted on the scalp, back, and extensor surfaces of the elbows and knees. There are no focal neurologic findings.

Laboratory studies:

Hemoglobin	14.4 g/dL (144 g/L)
Leukocyte count	6300/µL (6.3×10^9/L)
Blood urea nitrogen	15 mg/dL (5.4 mmol/L)
Serum creatinine	1.3 mg/dL (115 µmol/L)
Electrolytes	
Sodium	145 meq/L (145 mmol/L)
Potassium	3.6 meq/L (3.6 mmol/L)
Chloride	109 meq/L (109 mmol/L)
Bicarbonate	22 meq/L (22 mmol/L)
Glucose	158 mg/dL (8.8 mmol/L)
Lactic acid	7.2 mg/dL (0.8 mmol/L)
Osmolality	308 mosm/kg H_2O
Arterial blood gas studies (ambient air):	
pH	7.51
PCO_2	35 mm Hg (4.7 kPa)
PO_2	96 mm Hg (12.8 kPa)
Urinalysis	Specific gravity 1.024; pH 6.0; trace blood; 2+ protein; 1+ glucose; trace leukocyte esterase; no ketones, nitrites, cells, or formed elements

Which of the following is the most likely cause of this patient's clinical presentation?

(A) Metformin toxicity
(B) Methanol toxicity
(C) Salicylate toxicity
(D) Sepsis

Item 58

A 27-year-old woman is evaluated during a follow-up visit for high blood pressure that manifested 4 months after she began taking an oral contraceptive pill. Despite stopping the oral contraceptive pill, her blood pressure has remained high. She states that she feels well. Medical history is otherwise unremarkable, and she takes no medications.

On physical examination, blood pressure measurements are 150 to 166 mm Hg systolic and 100 to 108 mm Hg diastolic without orthostasis; other vital signs are normal. There is a bruit in the right epigastric region. The remainder of the examination is unremarkable.

Kidney function is normal, and urinalysis is unremarkable.

A kidney angiogram is shown.

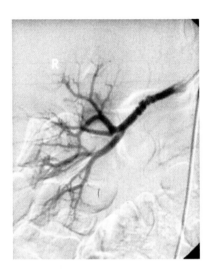

Which of the following is the most appropriate next step in management?

(A) ACE inhibitor
(B) Calcium channel blocker/ACE inhibitor combination
(C) Percutaneous transluminal kidney angioplasty
(D) Surgical revascularization

Item 59

A 28-year-old man is evaluated during a follow-up visit for Alport syndrome. He feels well and reports no fever, chills, or gastrointestinal symptoms. He has good exercise tolerance with normal fatigue levels with usual activity. He also has hypertension, and his kidney function has been declining steadily. Family history is notable for a brother who has chronic kidney disease and an uncle who has undergone kidney transplantation; his sister is healthy. Medications are furosemide, amlodipine, erythropoietin, and losartan.

On physical examination, the patient appears mildly fatigued. He wears hearing aids and eyeglasses. Temperature is 36.8 °C (98.1 °F), blood pressure is 138/88 mm Hg, pulse rate is 72/min, and respiration rate is 14/min. BMI is 23. His lungs are clear to auscultation. There is no edema. The remainder of the examination is unremarkable.

Laboratory studies:

Hemoglobin	10.1 g/dL (101 g/L)
Serum creatinine	5.4 mg/dL (477 µmol/L)
Estimated glomerular filtration rate	13 mL/min/1.73 m²
Spot urine protein–creatinine ratio	1.7 mg/mg

Kidney ultrasound performed last year revealed hyperechoic kidneys; the right kidney is 8.9 cm, and the left kidney is 9.1 cm.

Which of the following is the best management option?

(A) Add everolimus
(B) Begin hemodialysis
(C) Evaluate for kidney transplantation
(D) Switch losartan to lisinopril

Item 60

A 59-year-old man is evaluated for worsening kidney function. He was hospitalized 24 hours ago with a diabetic foot ulcer and associated cellulitis of 4 weeks' duration. He also has chronic diabetic kidney disease, hypertension, and type 2 diabetes mellitus. Medications are metformin, insulin glargine, lisinopril, and piperacillin-tazobactam.

On physical examination, blood pressure is 160/100 mm Hg (3 months ago: 130/78 mm Hg); other vital signs are normal. BMI is 30. An area of erythema extends about 3 cm around a 3- × 3-mm ulcer on the right heel. The involved area is tender and warm. There is 2+ pedal edema.

Laboratory studies:

Albumin	2.4 g/dL (24 g/L)
Complement (C3 and C4)	Decreased
Serum creatinine	4.1 mg/dL (362 μmol/L) (2 weeks ago: 1.4 mg/dL [124 μmol/L])
Urine studies:	
Urine sodium	15 meq/L (15 mmol/L) (normal range for men, 18-301 meq/L [18-301 mmol/L])
Urinalysis	25 erythrocytes/hpf; 1-2 erythrocyte casts/hpf
Urine albumin–creatinine ratio	1500 mg/g

Which of the following is the most likely cause of this patient's acute kidney injury?

(A) Diabetic nephropathy
(B) IgA nephropathy
(C) Postinfectious glomerulonephritis
(D) Primary membranous glomerulopathy

Item 61

A 34-year-old woman is scheduled to have a kidney biopsy. She has a 5-year history of systemic lupus erythematosus and a 3-year history of hypertension. Medications are prednisone, hydrochlorothiazide, atenolol, lisinopril, calcium carbonate, and a daily multivitamin.

On physical examination, blood pressure is 172/96 mm Hg, and pulse rate is 92/min. BMI is 26. A malar rash is present. There is no jugular venous distention. Cardiac examination reveals no murmurs, rubs, or gallops. Lungs are clear to auscultation. There is trace lower extremity edema.

Laboratory studies:

Hemoglobin	10.4 g/dL (104 g/L)
Platelet count	110,000/μL (110 × 10⁹/L)
Serum creatinine	1.1 mg/dL (97.2 μmol/L) (1 year ago: 0.9 mg/dL [79.6 μmol/L])

Urinalysis	1+ blood; 2+ protein; 2-5 erythro-cytes/hpf; 0-2 leukocytes/hpf

Kidney ultrasound from 1 week ago reveals normal-sized kidneys without hydronephrosis or other anatomic abnormalities.

Which of the following is a contraindication to kidney biopsy in this patient?

(A) BMI greater than 25
(B) Daily prednisone treatment
(C) Hemoglobin level less than 11 g/dL (110 g/L)
(D) Uncontrolled hypertension

Item 62

A 51-year-old man is evaluated for a 1-year history of uncontrolled hypertension. He has not responded to treatment with metoprolol and clonidine. He has no family history of hypertension. He has never smoked cigarettes and has no other medical problems. Current medications are maximum doses of chlorthalidone, lisinopril, and amlodipine.

On physical examination, seated blood pressure is 160/94 mm Hg, and pulse rate is 76/min. The remainder of the examination is unremarkable.

Laboratory studies reveal a serum creatinine level of 1.1 mg/dL (97.2 μmol/L), a potassium level of 4.1 meq/L (4.1 mmol/L), and an estimated glomerular filtration rate of >60 mL/min/1.73 m².

Which of the following is the most appropriate next step in management?

(A) Discontinue chlorthalidone; begin furosemide
(B) Discontinue lisinopril; begin aliskiren
(C) Obtain kidney Doppler ultrasonography
(D) Obtain a plasma aldosterone-plasma renin activity ratio

Item 63

A 62-year-old man is hospitalized after being found on the floor of his apartment by a neighbor. The patient is confused and can provide only minimal history and says that he was involved in a fight several days ago. He states that he has high blood pressure and high cholesterol but does not know the names of his medications. The neighbor notes that the patient has a history of alcohol abuse.

On physical examination, the patient is thin, disheveled, and malodorous. He is sleepy but arousable, and he is able to move all extremities but has pain when doing so. Numerous bruises and mild lacerations are seen on his body. He is oriented only to his name. Temperature is 37.3 °C (99.2 °F), blood pressure is 165/85 mm Hg, pulse rate is 102/min, and respiration rate is 18/min. There is no icterus; mucous membranes are dry. Cardiac examination is normal. Lungs are clear to auscultation. The abdomen is soft with diffuse, mild tenderness and no distention. There is no peripheral edema. The cranial nerves appear intact.

Laboratory studies:

Hemoglobin	9.3 g/dL (93 g/L)
Leukocyte count	6500/µL (6.5×10^9/L)
Platelet count	113,000/µL (113×10^9/L)
Blood urea nitrogen	85 mg/dL (30.3 mmol/L)
Calcium	8.3 mg/dL (2.1 mmol/L)
Creatine kinase	15,832 units/L
Serum creatinine	4.5 mg/dL (398 µmol/L)
Electrolytes	
Sodium	145 meq/L (145 mmol/L)
Potassium	5.1 meq/L (5.1 mmol/L)
Chloride	103 meq/L (103 mmol/L)
Bicarbonate	21 meq/L (21 mmol/L)
Phosphorous	5.8 mg/dL (1.87 mmol/L)
Liver chemistry tests	Normal
Serum ethanol	0 mg/dL
Urine studies:	
Creatinine	115 mg/dL (normal range for men, 22-392 mg/dL)
Sodium	85 meq/L (85 mmol/L) (normal range for men, 18-301 meq/L [18-301 mmol/L])
Fractional excretion of sodium	5.7%
Urinalysis	Specific gravity 1.015; pH 6.5; 3+ blood; no ketones; trace leukocyte esterase; 5-10 erythrocytes/hpf; 0-3 leukocytes/hpf; rare hyaline casts; several granular casts

Which of the following is the most likely diagnosis?

(A) Acute interstitial nephritis
(B) Hepatorenal syndrome
(C) Intra-abdominal compartment syndrome
(D) Pigment nephropathy

Item 64

A 30-year-old woman is evaluated for a 2-month history of lower extremity edema and a weight gain of 3 kg (7 lb). Medical history is unremarkable, and she takes no medications.

On physical examination, blood pressure is 132/82 mm Hg; other vital signs are normal. There is 3+ pitting leg edema. The remainder of the examination is unremarkable.

Laboratory studies:

Albumin	3.1 g/dL (31 g/L)
Blood urea nitrogen	19 mg/dL (6.8 mmol/L)
Serum creatinine	0.7 mg/dL (61.9 µmol/L)
Total cholesterol	237 mg/dL (6.14 mmol/L)
LDL cholesterol	147 mg/dL (3.81 mmol/L)
Hepatitis B surface antigen	Negative
Hepatitis C virus antibodies	Negative
HIV antibodies	Negative
Rheumatoid factor	Negative
Antinuclear antibodies	Negative
Antistreptolysin O antibodies	Negative
Urinalysis	3+ protein; 0-3 erythrocytes/hpf; 0-5 leukocytes/hpf
Urine protein–creatinine ratio	3.7 mg/mg

Kidney biopsy results reveal changes consistent with membranous glomerulopathy and no evidence of mesangium involvement, secondary glomerulosclerosis, or chronic tubulointerstitial changes.

Which of the following is the most appropriate treatment for this patient?

(A) ACE inhibitor and statin
(B) Calcineurin inhibitor
(C) Corticosteroids
(D) Cyclophosphamide
(E) Mycophenolate mofetil

Item 65

A 46-year-old man is hospitalized for a subarachnoid hemorrhage after collapsing shortly after developing a severe headache. He has stage 2 chronic kidney disease due to autosomal dominant polycystic kidney disease. He also has hypertension managed with enalapril.

Mechanical ventilation is initiated, and a ventriculostomy drain is placed. Sedation is maintained with propofol and morphine, and he is treated with fosphenytoin for seizure prophylaxis.

On physical examination, temperature is 35.8 °C (96.4 °F), blood pressure is 126/70 mm Hg, and pulse rate is 96/min. Cardiac and pulmonary examinations are normal.

Laboratory studies:

	Initial	Day 3
Blood urea nitrogen	42 mg/dL (15.0 mmol/L)	52 mg/dL (18.6 mmol/L)
Creatine kinase	45 units/L	1885 units/L
Serum creatinine	1.4 mg/dL (124 µmol/L)	2.3 mg/dL (203 µmol/L)
Electrolytes		
Sodium	140 meq/L (140 mmol/L)	135 meq/L (135 mmol/L)
Potassium	4.8 meq/L (4.8 mmol/L)	6.2 meq/L (6.2 mmol/L)
Chloride	104 meq/L (104 mmol/L)	99 meq/L (99 mmol/L)
Bicarbonate	25 meq/L (25 mmol/L)	14 meq/L (14 mmol/L)
Glucose	125 mg/dL (6.9 mmol/L)	146 mg/dL (8.1 mmol/L)
Lactic acid	14 mg/dL (1.5 mmol/L)	50 mg/dL (5.5 mmol/L)
Urinalysis	–	pH 5.4; 1+ blood; 1+ protein; no ketones; few granular casts; no cells

The patient's serum is noted to be lipemic in appearance.

Which of the following is the most likely cause of this patient's laboratory findings?

(A) Fosphenytoin
(B) Propofol
(C) Propylene glycol
(D) Pyroglutamate

Item 66

An 82-year-old woman is evaluated in the emergency department for a 1-week history of progressive fatigue and shortness of breath. She lives independently, but her family reports that during the past month she has had increased difficulty walking because of low back pain, for which she self-medicates with aspirin. She also has COPD managed with ipratropium.

On physical examination, temperature is 37.6 °C (99.7 °F), blood pressure is 146/82 mm Hg, pulse rate is 86/min, and respiration rate is 24/min. BMI is 23. Tachypnea and increased respiratory effort are noted. Gag reflex is intact. The remainder of the examination is unremarkable.

Laboratory studies:

Blood urea nitrogen	42 mg/dL (15.0 mmol/L)
Serum creatinine	1.3 mg/dL (115 µmol/L)
Electrolytes	
Sodium	138 meq/L (138 mmol/L)
Potassium	3.4 meq/L (3.4 mmol/L)
Chloride	106 meq/L (106 mmol/L)
Bicarbonate	~18 meq/L (18 mmol/L)
Glucose	86 mg/dL (4.8 mmol/L)
Salicylate	62 mg/dL (4.5 mmol/L) (therapeutic range, 10-25 mg/dL [0.72-1.8 mmol/L])
Arterial blood gas studies (ambient air):	
pH	7.42
P_{CO_2}	29 mm Hg (3.9 kPa)
P_{O_2}	68 mm Hg (9.0 kPa)
Urinalysis	Specific gravity 1.024; pH 5.2; no blood, protein, leukocyte esterase, ketones, or nitrites

Chest radiograph shows no infiltrates or edema.

Which of the following is the most appropriate treatment?

(A) Acetazolamide
(B) Hemodialysis
(C) Mechanical ventilation
(D) Sodium bicarbonate infusion

Item 67

A 48-year-old woman is evaluated in the emergency department for fatigue, diffuse weakness, and lightheadedness. Her symptoms developed after attending an outdoor music festival, where she was exposed to the sun most of the day.

She has a 2-year history of systemic lupus erythematosus; her last flare occurred 6 months ago. She also has hypertension, which is well controlled with hydrochlorothiazide. Other medications are hydroxychloroquine and as-needed ibuprofen. She took ibuprofen before arriving at the emergency department.

On physical examination, temperature is 37.1 °C (98.7 °F), blood pressure is 97/52 mm Hg, pulse rate is 98/min, and respiration rate is 12/min. When standing, blood pressure is 90/45 mm Hg, and pulse rate is 108/min. No rashes or edema are present. Cardiac and pulmonary examinations are normal.

Laboratory studies:

Blood urea nitrogen	21 mg/dL (7.5 mmol/L)
Serum creatinine	1.1 mg/dL (97.2 µmol/L) (baseline: 0.7 mg/dL [61.9 µmol/L])
Electrolytes	
Sodium	143 meq/L (143 mmol/L)
Potassium	4 meq/L (4 mmol/L)
Chloride	108 meq/L (108 mmol/L)
Bicarbonate	26 meq/L (26 mmol/L)
Urine studies:	
Sodium	34 meq/L (34 mmol/L) (normal range for women, 15-267 meq/L [15-267 mmol/L])
Creatinine	23 mg/dL (normal range for women, 15-327 mg/dL)
Urea	118 mg/dL (normal range for women, 132-1629 mg/dL)
Fractional excretion of sodium	1.2%
Fractional excretion of urea	27.4%
Urinalysis	Specific gravity 1.025; pH 6.5; trace blood; trace protein; occasional nondysmorphic erythrocytes; 3-5 hyaline casts; no renal tubular epithelial cells

Which of the following is the most likely diagnosis?

(A) Acute interstitial nephritis
(B) Acute tubular necrosis
(C) Lupus nephritis
(D) Prerenal azotemia

Item 68

A 45-year-old woman is evaluated as a new patient. She recently emigrated from Romania. She has chronic kidney disease (CKD). She also has hypertension, which was diagnosed at the same time as her CKD. Family history includes a cousin with CKD. She reports no urinary symptoms. Her only medication is captopril.

On physical examination, temperature is 37.7 °C (99.8 °F), blood pressure is 138/67 mm Hg, pulse rate is 72/min, and respiration rate is 12/min. BMI is 22. There are no rashes. Cardiac examination reveals normal heart sounds and no murmurs. The abdomen is nontender and without masses. There is trace pitting edema to the ankles.

Laboratory studies:

Serum creatinine	2.8 mg/dL (248 µmol/L)
Electrolytes	
Sodium	138 meq/L (138 mmol/L)
Potassium	4.9 meq/L (4.9 mmol/L)
Chloride	109 meq/L (109 mmol/L)
Bicarbonate	21 meq/L (21 mmol/L)
Urinalysis	pH 5.5; no blood; trace protein; no glucose; + leukocyte esterase; no nitrites; 0-1 erythrocytes/hpf; 2-5 leukocytes/hpf; rare granular and waxy casts
Urine cultures	Negative

Kidney ultrasound reveals small kidneys bilaterally without hydronephrosis or hydroureter.

Which of the following is the most likely diagnosis?

(A) Analgesic nephropathy
(B) Balkan nephropathy
(C) Hypertensive nephropathy
(D) IgA nephropathy

Item 69

A 76-year-old woman is evaluated in the emergency department for a 1-day history of nausea, vomiting, weakness, and confusion. Today, she has difficulty walking and has fallen several times.

On physical examination, the patient appears chronically ill; she is unable to stand without assistance because of generalized weakness. Temperature is 36.2 °C (97.2 °F), blood pressure is 130/78 mm Hg, pulse rate is 68/min without postural changes, and respiration rate is 18/min. BMI is 19. Neurologic, cardiac, and pulmonary examinations are normal. There is no peripheral edema.

Laboratory studies:

Albumin	3.6 g/dL (36 g/L)
Blood urea nitrogen	10 mg/dL (3.6 mmol/L)
Serum creatinine	0.9 mg/dL (79.6 µmol/L)
Electrolytes	
Sodium	120 meq/L (120 mmol/L)
Potassium	3.6 meq/L (3.6 mmol/L)
Chloride	83 meq/L (83 mmol/L)
Bicarbonate	27 meq/L (27 mmol/L)
Glucose	105 mg/dL (5.8 mmol/L)
Osmolality	255 mosm/kg H_2O
Total protein	9.1 g/dL (91 g/L)
Urine studies:	
Osmolality	408 mosm/kg H_2O (normal, 300-900 mosm/kg H_2O)
Potassium	32 meq/L (32 mmol/L) (normal range for women, 17-164 meq/L [17-164 mmol/L])
Sodium	90 meq/L (90 mmol/L) (normal range for women, 15-267 meq/L [15-267 mmol/L])

Which of the following is the most appropriate treatment?

(A) 0.9% Saline infusion
(B) 3% Saline infusion
(C) Furosemide
(D) Tolvaptan

Item 70

A 25-year-old woman comes for a preconception evaluation. She has a history of hypertension that is well controlled with lisinopril. Medical history is otherwise unremarkable.

On physical examination, blood pressure is 134/86 mm Hg in both upper extremities; other vital signs are normal. Results of the cardiovascular examination are unremarkable. There is no edema, cyanosis, digital clubbing, or radial artery–femoral artery pulse delay.

Laboratory studies reveal normal electrolytes, complete blood count, thyroid-stimulating hormone level, kidney function, and urinalysis.

An electrocardiogram is normal.

In addition to starting a prenatal vitamin, which of the following medication adjustments should be made before this patient proceeds with pregnancy?

(A) Discontinue lisinopril
(B) Substitute labetalol for lisinopril
(C) Substitute losartan for lisinopril
(D) Substitute spironolactone for lisinopril

Item 71

A 60-year-old man is evaluated as a new patient. He was diagnosed with type 2 diabetes mellitus during a health insurance evaluation 6 months ago. At that time, metformin was initiated. Medical history is otherwise unremarkable.

On physical examination, blood pressure is 145/94 mm Hg; other vital signs are normal. BMI is 29. The remainder of the examination is unremarkable.

Laboratory studies:

Hemoglobin A_{1c}	6.8%
Blood urea nitrogen	10 mg/dL (3.6 mmol/L)
Serum creatinine	0.9 mg/dL (79.6 µmol/L)
Glucose	126 mg/dL (7 mmol/L)
Urinalysis	Normal
Urine albumin–creatinine ratio	20 mg/g

Electrocardiogram reveals left ventricular hypertrophy.

Which of the following is the most appropriate next step in management?

(A) Add an ACE inhibitor
(B) Add a β-blocker
(C) Add a calcium channel blocker
(D) Add a diuretic
(E) Continue current regimen

Item 72

A 71-year-old man is evaluated during a follow-up visit 6 months after undergoing a kidney transplant because of ANCA-associated vasculitis. His postoperative course was uncomplicated, and his serum creatinine level was 1.3 mg/dL (115 µmol/L) at discharge. Over the past 3 months, his serum creatinine level has steadily increased. Current medications are tacrolimus, mycophenolate mofetil, metoprolol, and trimethoprim-sulfamethoxazole.

On physical examination, blood pressure is 110/64 mm Hg. BMI is 19. Cardiac examination is normal without rubs. Lungs are clear. There is a left brachiocephalic arteriovenous fistula with a palpable thrill and audible bruit. Abdominal examination is notable for a well-healed incision at the right lower quadrant; the kidney graft is nontender, and there is no bruit. There is no lower extremity edema.

Laboratory studies:

Blood urea nitrogen	42 mg/dL (15 mmol/L)
Serum creatinine	1.9 mg/dL (168 µmol/L)
Tacrolimus level (trough)	9 ng/mL (9 µg/L) (target, 8-10 ng/mL [8-10 µg/L])
Polymerase chain reaction	Positive for polyoma BK virus in the blood and urine
Urinalysis	1+ blood; 1+ protein; 1+ leukocyte esterase; 8-10 nondysmorphic erythrocytes/hpf; 4-8 leukocytes/hpf; rare leukocyte casts; no bacteria

Kidney biopsy results demonstrate an inflammatory interstitial infiltrate with evidence of tubulitis and scattered intranuclear viral inclusions in the tubular epithelial cells.

Which of the following is the most appropriate next step in management?

(A) Add acyclovir
(B) Add ganciclovir
(C) Add muromonab-CD3
(D) Decrease immunosuppression

Item 73

A 59-year-old woman is evaluated during a routine follow-up visit. She was recently diagnosed with type 2 diabetes mellitus and hyperlipidemia. She feels well. Medications are metformin, atorvastatin, and aspirin.

Physical examination findings and vital signs are normal. BMI is 27.

Laboratory studies reveal a serum creatinine level of 0.9 mg/dL (79.6 µmol/L), an estimated glomerular filtration rate of >60 mL/min/1.73 m^2, and normal urinalysis results.

Which of the following is the most appropriate diagnostic test to perform next?

(A) 24-Hour urine collection for protein
(B) Kidney ultrasonography
(C) Spot urine albumin–creatinine ratio
(D) No additional testing

Item 74

A 59-year-old man is evaluated during a follow-up visit for hypertension. He also has diabetes mellitus and stage 3 chronic kidney disease. One month ago, his dose of lisinopril was increased. Other medications are metoprolol, felodipine, and furosemide.

On physical examination, blood pressure is 158/75 mm Hg, and pulse rate is 70/min. There is dependent edema. The remainder of the examination is unremarkable.

Laboratory studies:

Serum creatinine	2.2 mg/dL (194 µmol/L)
Electrolytes	
Sodium	139 meq/L (139 mmol/L)
Potassium	5.3 meq/L (5.3 mmol/L)
Chloride	103 meq/L (103 mmol/L)
Bicarbonate	24 meq/L (24 mmol/L)

In addition to a low potassium diet, which of the following is the most appropriate treatment for this patient?

(A) Add sodium polystyrene sulfonate
(B) Add spironolactone
(C) Discontinue lisinopril
(D) Increase furosemide

Item 75

A 45-year-old man is evaluated for abdominal pain that began the previous night. The pain was intermittent and crampy. Over the course of the day, the pain has worsened and now radiates to the scrotum on the right side. He vomited once and reports anorexia. Medical history is notable for prostatitis 2 years ago and an appendectomy. He takes no medications.

On physical examination, the patient appears ill and is curled up on the examination table. Temperature is 37.9 °C (100.3 °F), blood pressure is 140/92 mm Hg, and pulse rate is 98/min. Cardiac and pulmonary examinations are normal. There is abdominal guarding. Genital examination is notable for the absence of penile discharge; there are normal-sized testes without tenderness. Rectal examination reveals normal tone and a smooth, nontender prostate. There is no edema.

Laboratory studies:

Leukocyte count	11,500/µL (11.5 × 10^9/L)
Blood urea nitrogen	15 mg/dL (5.4 mmol/L)
Serum creatinine	1.2 mg/dL (106 µmol/L)
Urinalysis	pH 5.0; + blood; no protein, glucose, bilirubin, or leukocyte esterase; 10-15 erythrocytes/hpf; 1-3 leukocytes/hpf

Which of the following is the most appropriate imaging study to determine the cause of this patient's pain?

(A) Abdominal radiography of the kidneys, ureters, and bladder
(B) Intravenous pyelography
(C) Noncontrast abdominal helical CT
(D) Testicular ultrasonography

Item 76

A 55-year-old woman is evaluated for a 6-month history of increased fatigue and decreased exercise tolerance. History is notable for HIV infection. Medications are trimethoprim-sulfamethoxazole, atazanavir, emtricitabine, and tenofovir.

On physical examination, temperature is 36.0 °C (96.8 °F), blood pressure is 146/80 mm Hg, pulse rate is 86/min, and respiration rate is 18/min. BMI is 28. Mild diffuse weakness is noted.

Laboratory studies:

Albumin	3.8 g/dL (38 g/L)
Blood urea nitrogen	12 mg/dL (4.3 mmol/L)
Calcium	8.1 mg/dL (2.0 mmol/L)
Serum creatinine	1.3 mg/dL (115 µmol/L)
Electrolytes	
Sodium	140 meq/L (140 mmol/L)
Potassium	2.9 meq/L (2.9 mmol/L)
Chloride	114 meq/L (114 mmol/L)
Bicarbonate	16 meq/L (16 mmol/L)
Glucose	105 mg/dL (5.8 mmol/L)
Phosphorus	1.8 mg/dL (0.58 mmol/L)
Venous blood gas studies:	
pH	7.32
P_{CO_2}	36 mm Hg (4.8 kPa)
Urine studies:	
Urinalysis	Specific gravity 1.012; pH 5.1; no blood; trace protein; 1+ glucose; no ketones, nitrites, or leukocyte esterase
Urine protein–creatinine ratio	0.525 mg/mg

Kidney ultrasound shows no nephrocalcinosis.

Which of the following is the most appropriate management?

(A) Discontinue tenofovir
(B) Discontinue trimethoprim-sulfamethoxazole
(C) Measure serum lactate level
(D) Order a stool laxative screen

Item 77

A 66-year-old woman is evaluated in the hospital for acute kidney injury 4 days following a partial colectomy for perforated diverticulitis. She had no intraoperative hypotension but has required a total of 15 L of intravenous fluids to maintain her blood pressure. Urine output has gradually diminished, and she is now oliguric with an indwelling bladder catheter in place. She received one dose of tobramycin postoperatively; additional medications are vancomycin and imipenem.

On physical examination, the patient is intubated and sedated. Temperature is 37.2 °C (98.9 °F), blood pressure is 91/52 mm Hg, pulse rate is 108/min, and respiration rate on ventilation is 14/min. BMI is 35. Cardiac examination is notable for tachycardia, with a regular rate and no murmur. Pulmonary examination is normal. Abdominal examination reveals a tense and distended abdomen, with hypoactive bowel sounds. The abdominal wall is edematous. There is pitting edema of the legs.

Laboratory studies:

Blood urea nitrogen	45 mg/dL (16.1 mmol/L)
Serum creatinine	Preoperative: 0.9 mg/dL (79.6 µmol/L); postoperative day 4: 2.9 mg/dL (256 µmol/L)
Fractional excretion of sodium	1.5%
Urinalysis	Specific gravity 1.011; pH 6.0; trace erythrocytes/hpf; 1-2 leukocytes/hpf; occasional granular casts

Kidney ultrasound reveals normal-sized kidneys and no hydronephrosis.

Which of the following is the most likely cause of this patient's kidney failure?

(A) Abdominal compartment syndrome
(B) Aminoglycoside nephrotoxicity
(C) Prerenal acute kidney injury
(D) Urinary obstruction

Item 78

A 53-year-old woman is evaluated for a 3-month history of swelling of the face, hands, and feet. She has untreated hepatitis C virus infection. She takes lithium for bipolar disorder. She has no additional symptoms.

On physical examination, temperature is normal, blood pressure is 134/93 mm Hg, pulse rate is 71/min, and respiration rate is 18/min. Bilateral periorbital edema and swelling of the hands and legs are noted. The remainder of the examination is unremarkable.

Laboratory studies:

Complete blood count	Normal
Albumin	1.6 g/dL (16 g/L)
Blood urea nitrogen	28 mg/dL (10 mmol/L)
Complement (C3 and C4)	Normal
Serum creatinine	1.5 mg/dL (133 µmol/L)
Cryoglobulin	Negative
Serum protein electrophoresis	Normal
Rheumatoid factor	Negative
Hepatitis B surface antigen	Negative
Hepatitis C virus antibodies	Positive with low RNA titer
HIV antibodies	Negative
Antinuclear antibodies	Negative
Urinalysis	4+ protein; 4-7 erythrocytes/hpf; 4-7 leukocytes/hpf
24-Hour urine collection of protein	14 g/24 h

Ultrasound shows normal-sized kidneys.

Percutaneous kidney biopsy results show glomeruli of normal size and cellularity, with patent capillary lumina. Diffuse fusion of podocyte foot processes is noted on electron microscopy. Immunofluorescence studies show no immune deposits.

Which of the following is the most likely cause of this patient's nephrotic syndrome?

(A) Hepatitis C virus–associated glomerulonephritis
(B) Lupus nephritis

(C) Membranous glomerulopathy

(D) Minimal change glomerulopathy

Item 79

A 50-year-old man is seen during a follow-up visit 2 days after he was evaluated in the emergency department for renal colic. Records from the emergency department show a normal metabolic profile, and a noncontrast CT scan revealed a 4-mm stone in the distal left ureter. He continues to have pain controlled with oxycodone.

On physical examination, vital signs are normal. Mild left costovertebral angle tenderness is noted. The remainder of the examination is unremarkable.

Which of the following is the most appropriate next step in management?

(A) 24-Hour urine collection for calcium, oxalate, and uric acid

(B) Extracorporeal shock wave lithotripsy

(C) Repeat noncontrast CT

(D) Tamsulosin

(E) Ureteroscopy and intracorporeal lithotripsy

Item 80

A 74-year-old man was hospitalized 3 days ago for extensive, nonpurulent cellulitis of the right lower extremity and is now being evaluated for acute kidney injury. He has hypertension, hyperlipidemia, and peripheral vascular disease. His hypertension has been poorly controlled; his last office blood pressure measurement was 165/92 mm Hg. Medications are lisinopril, metoprolol, hydrochlorothiazide, amlodipine, pravastatin, and aspirin. On admission, cefazolin was initiated.

The patient is now afebrile, and his blood pressure has not exceeded 118/60 mm Hg since admission. There is no evidence of orthostasis. The cellulitis has improved since admission.

Since admission, his serum creatinine level has progressively increased from 1.5 mg/dL (133 µmol/L) to 2.7 mg/dL (239 µmol/L).

Other laboratory studies are as follows:

Urine sodium	45 meq/L (45 mmol/L) (normal range for men, 18-301 meq/L [18-301 mmol/L])
Fractional excretion of sodium	2.3%
Fractional excretion of urea	51%
Urinalysis	Specific gravity 1.015; trace protein; no erythrocytes or leukocytes; occasional granular casts

Kidney ultrasound is normal.

Which of the following is the most likely cause of this patient's acute kidney injury?

(A) Acute interstitial nephritis

(B) Cholesterol emboli

(C) Normotensive ischemic acute kidney injury

(D) Prerenal azotemia

Item 81

A 54-year-old woman is evaluated during a follow-up visit for recurrent kidney stones. She underwent successful gastric bypass surgery for obesity approximately 1 year ago. Steady weight loss has occurred, and her BMI has decreased from 38 to 33. However, she has had two episodes of nephrolithiasis since the time of her surgery and most recently passed another kidney stone. None of the stones has been available for analysis. Medical history is notable for type 2 diabetes mellitus and hypertension. Medications are metoprolol and glyburide.

On physical examination, blood pressure is 125/78 mm Hg. The remainder of the examination is unremarkable.

Urine studies:

Calcium excretion	Normal
Citrate excretion	Normal
Oxalate excretion	High
Uric acid excretion	Normal
Urinalysis	Specific gravity 1.025; pH 5.0; no blood; 2-4 erythrocytes/hpf; many envelope-shaped crystals
Urine volume	1300 mL/24 h

In addition to increased fluid intake, which of the following is the most appropriate next step in management?

(A) Calcium carbonate supplements

(B) Chlorthalidone

(C) Potassium citrate

(D) Tamsulosin

Item 82

A 47-year-old man is evaluated during a routine follow-up visit. He has chronic kidney disease from IgA nephropathy and hypertension and has been treated with lisinopril, resulting in stable proteinuria and blood pressures in the 125/75 mm Hg range. He reports doing well except for a 1-week flu-like syndrome for which he has treated himself with an over-the-counter cold preparation and analgesic medication. His symptoms have improved, and he reports no apparent blood in his urine, arthritis, or fever.

On physical examination, blood pressure is 152/85 mm Hg, and pulse rate is 82/min. BMI is 25. There are no rashes. The ears are clear, and the nasal and oropharyngeal mucosa are slightly edematous and erythematous with a minimal amount of discharge. Cardiac and pulmonary examinations are normal. There is no arthritis or edema.

Urine protein is less than 1 g/24 h and unchanged from baseline.

Laboratory studies:

Electrolytes	Normal
Serum creatinine	1.7 mg/dL (150 µmol/L) (unchanged from baseline)
Urinalysis	pH 5.5; no leukocytes; 5-10 erythrocytes/hpf; no casts or epithelial tubular cells

Which of the following is the most appropriate next step in managing this patient's blood pressure?

(A) Add losartan
(B) Begin prednisone
(C) Discontinue over-the-counter medications
(D) Increase lisinopril

Item 83

A 68-year-old man is hospitalized for a 3-month history of dark brown–colored urine, malaise, and an unintentional 6.8-kg (15-lb) weight loss. He has felt febrile during this time period. He reports no urinary hesitancy, frequency, dysuria, nausea, vomiting, or diarrhea. He has not had any abdominal pain, fullness, or gastrointestinal symptoms. He has type 2 diabetes mellitus and hypertension. Medications are glipizide and lisinopril. He has a 40-pack-year history of smoking.

On physical examination, the patient appears fatigued and has periorbital edema. Temperature is 37.6 °C (99.6 °F), blood pressure is 162/93 mm Hg, pulse rate is 88/min, and respiration rate is 16/min. BMI is 29. Cardiac examination reveals no murmurs, rubs, or gallops. Lungs are clear to auscultation. The abdomen is nontender and nondistended, and bowel sounds are normal. There is 1+ pitting edema of the extremities.

Laboratory studies:

Hemoglobin	11.8 g/dL (118 g/L)
Albumin	3.4 g/dL (34 g/L)
Serum creatinine	3.2 mg/dL (283 µmol/L) (6 months ago: 1.6 mg/dL [141 µmol/L])
Urinalysis	1+ blood; 1+ protein; 5-10 erythrocytes/hpf; 50% acanthocytes; erythrocyte casts

Which of the following is the most likely diagnosis?

(A) Acute interstitial nephritis
(B) Acute tubular necrosis
(C) Polyarteritis nodosa
(D) Rapidly progressive glomerulonephritis

Item 84

A 63-year-old woman is evaluated during a follow-up visit for a 3-year history of type 2 diabetes mellitus and hypertension. Her diabetes has been well controlled on a twice daily dose of metformin. She takes lisinopril, 20 mg/d, for her hypertension; her blood pressure measurements are typically around 125/75 mm Hg.

On physical examination, vital signs recorded by a medical assistant show a temperature of 37.3° C (99.2 °F), blood pressure of 154/78 mm Hg, and pulse rate of 82/min. BMI is 32. The remainder of the examination is normal.

Laboratory studies reveal normal electrolytes, complete blood count, fasting lipid profile, and urine albumin–creatinine ratio as well as normal kidney function; hemoglobin A_{1c} level is 7.1%.

Which of the following is the most appropriate next step in management?

(A) Add hydrochlorothiazide
(B) Ambulatory blood pressure monitoring
(C) Increase lisinopril
(D) Repeat blood pressure measurement

Item 85

A 30-year-old woman is evaluated during a prenatal visit. She is 18 weeks pregnant, and this is her first pregnancy. She has a history of borderline hypertension, and her blood pressure measurements since conception have been in the range of 120 to 130/80 to 90 mm Hg without antihypertensive therapy. She adheres to a low sodium diet; a dietary assessment shows adequate amounts of dietary calcium. Family history is notable for her mother who had preeclampsia at 37 weeks' gestation. She takes prenatal vitamins.

Urinalysis is negative for protein.

Which of the following interventions may reduce this patient's risk of preeclampsia?

(A) Low-dose aspirin
(B) Methyldopa
(C) Oral calcium supplement
(D) Oral magnesium supplement
(E) Reduce blood pressure to less than 120/80 mm Hg

Item 86

A 57-year-old man is evaluated for a 20-year history of hypertension. He reports a 4.5-kg (10-lb) weight gain during the past 6 months. The patient is black. He does not smoke cigarettes. His only medication is low-dose chlorthalidone.

On physical examination, seated blood pressure is 146 to 150/88 mm Hg, and pulse rate is 78/min. BMI is 29. The remainder of the examination is unremarkable.

Laboratory studies reveal a serum creatinine level of 1.7 mg/dL (150 µmol/L), an estimated glomerular filtration rate of 51 mL/min/1.73 m², and a urine protein–creatinine ratio of 0.45 mg/mg.

Which of the following is the most appropriate next step in managing this patient's hypertension?

(A) Add amlodipine
(B) Add metoprolol
(C) Add ramipril
(D) Increase the chlorthalidone dose

Item 87

A 65-year-old man is evaluated in the emergency department for a 4-month history of fatigue and sinus symptoms and a 1-week history of low-grade fever, worsening fatigue, and hemoptysis. His medical history is otherwise unremarkable.

On physical examination, temperature is 37.9 °C (100.3 °F), blood pressure is 153/89 mm Hg, pulse rate is 95/min, and respiration rate is 22/min. Periorbital edema is noted. There is dried blood in the nares. Pulmonary examination reveals crackles and moderate respiratory distress. There is 1+ pitting edema of the lower extremities.

Laboratory studies on admission:

Hemoglobin	9.8 g/dL (98 g/L)
Leukocyte count	12,000/µL (12×10^9/L)
Bicarbonate	14 meq/L (14 mmol/L)
Blood urea nitrogen	70 mg/dL (25 mmol/L)
Serum creatinine	6.7 mg/dL (592 µmol/L) (3 months ago: 1.3 mg/dL [115 µmol/L]; 1 year ago: 0.7 mg/dL [61.9 µmol/L])
Potassium	6.1 meq/L (6.1 mmol/L)
p-ANCA	1:1240
Anti–glomerular basement membrane antibodies	Negative
Blood cultures	Negative
Sputum cultures	Negative
Arterial blood gas studies (ambient air):	
pH	7.32
P_{CO_2}	30 mm Hg (4.0 kPa)
P_{O_2}	75 mm Hg (10.0 kPa)
Urinalysis	2 erythrocytes/hpf; many erythrocyte casts

Chest radiograph reveals infiltrates in the lung fields.

Kidney biopsy results reveal diffuse necrotizing crescentic glomerulonephritis with a pauci-immune pattern.

Broad-spectrum antibiotics and intermittent hemodialysis support are initiated. He is transferred to the intensive care unit and placed on noninvasive positive-pressure ventilation for worsened respiratory failure.

Which of the following is the most appropriate induction therapy?

(A) Cyclophosphamide and corticosteroids
(B) Mycophenolate mofetil and corticosteroids
(C) Plasmapheresis
(D) Plasmapheresis, cyclophosphamide, and corticosteroids

Item 88

A 17-year-old teenager is evaluated during a follow-up visit. His mother states that he struggles in school and was held back a grade. Family history includes a first-degree cousin with cognitive impairment and a grandmother who died of "kidney failure." He takes no medications.

On physical examination, the patient appears generally well. Temperature is 37.1 °C (98.7 °F), blood pressure is 149/94 mm Hg, pulse rate is 72/min, and respiration rate is 16/min. BMI is 23. The patient wears eyeglasses but has no obvious ophthalmic lesions. There is poor dentition, including pitted tooth enamel and gum lesions. Several hypomelanotic lesions are present on the back and shoulders.

Laboratory studies reveal a serum creatinine level of 1.9 mg/dL (168 µmol/L), and urinalysis results are normal.

On kidney ultrasound, the left kidney is 9.8 cm, and the right kidney is 10.2 cm; there are two cystic lesions in each kidney.

Which of the following is the most likely diagnosis?

(A) Autosomal dominant polycystic kidney disease
(B) Autosomal recessive polycystic kidney disease
(C) Fabry disease
(D) Tuberous sclerosis complex

Item 89

A 67-year-old man is evaluated following a recent diagnosis of type 2 diabetes mellitus.

On physical examination, blood pressure is 134/84 mm Hg; other vital signs are normal. BMI is 30. The remainder of the examination is unremarkable.

Laboratory studies:

Hemoglobin A_{1c}	7.8%
Blood urea nitrogen	15 mg/dL (5.4 mmol/L)
Serum creatinine	1.0 mg/dL (88.4 µmol/L)
Urinalysis	No protein; 3+ glucose; 0-2 erythrocytes/hpf; 0-3 leukocytes/hpf

In addition to therapeutic lifestyle changes, which of the following is the most appropriate next step in management?

(A) Estimated glomerular filtration rate using the Modification of Diet in Renal Disease study equation
(B) Urine albumin–creatinine ratio in 5 years
(C) Urine albumin–creatinine ratio now
(D) Urine protein–creatinine ratio in 5 years
(E) Urine protein–creatinine ratio now

Item 90

A 69-year-old man is evaluated during a new patient visit. Medical history includes a 23-year history of hypertension as well as several kidney stones 15 years ago. Family history includes his mother who began dialysis at age 72 years for unknown reasons and died of "kidney disease" 5 years later. Medications are lisinopril, furosemide, and aspirin.

On physical examination, temperature is 36.9 °C (98.4 °F), blood pressure is 134/72 mm Hg, pulse rate is 72/min, and respiration rate is 14/min. BMI is 29. The remainder of the physical examination is normal.

Laboratory studies:

Hemoglobin	12 g/dL (120 g/L)
Serum creatinine	1.9 mg/dL (168 µmol/L) (1 year ago: 1.8 mg/dL [159 µmol/L]; 6 years ago: 1.4 mg/dL [124 µmol/L])
Estimated glomerular filtration rate	37 mL/min/1.73 m²
Urinalysis	2+ protein; 0-2 erythrocytes/hpf; 2-4 leukocytes/hpf
Urine cultures	No growth

Which of the following is the most appropriate diagnostic test to perform next?

(A) Abdominal CT with contrast
(B) Kidney biopsy
(C) Kidney ultrasonography
(D) Radionuclide kidney clearance scanning

Item 91

A 61-year-old man is evaluated for a 3-year history of hypertension. He also has pedal edema that is undetectable when he wakes up in the morning and worsens throughout the day. He feels tired and has slowly gained approximately 4.5 kg (10 lb) during the past 3 years. He does not smoke cigarettes. Medications are hydrochlorothiazide, losartan, and amlodipine.

On physical examination, the average blood pressure is between 128 and 134/70 mm Hg, which is similar to readings obtained during the past 3 years. Other vital signs are normal. BMI is 28. There are no abdominal bruits, and the distal pulses are normal. There is trace pedal edema bilaterally.

Laboratory studies:

Serum creatinine	1.6 mg/dL (141 μmol/L) (1 year ago: 1.5 mg/dL [133 μmol/L]; 3 years ago, before treatment: 1.2 mg/dL [106 μmol/L])
Estimated glomerular filtration rate	53 mL/min/1.73 m²
Urinalysis	1+ protein; no blood; no cells; otherwise unremarkable

Which of the following is the most likely cause of this patient's elevation in serum creatinine level?

(A) Angiotensin receptor blocker therapy
(B) Glomerulonephritis
(C) Inadequate blood pressure control
(D) Renovascular disease

Item 92

A 50-year-old man is hospitalized for progressively worsening right and left flank pain of 3 weeks' duration. Associated symptoms include anorexia, malaise, fever, and joint pain. He has no other medical problems and takes no medications.

On physical examination, the patient appears chronically ill. Temperature is 38.6 °C (101.5 °F), blood pressure is 168/94 mm Hg, and pulse rate is 66/min. There are no abnormal skin findings. Cardiopulmonary examination is normal. There is tenderness to deep abdominal palpation and percussion of the flanks, which is not concordant with the perceived abdominal pain level of 10 of 10.

Laboratory studies:

Erythrocyte sedimentation rate	101 mm/h
Serum creatinine	1.8 mg/dL (159 μmol/L) (1 year ago: 0.9 mg/dL [79.6 μmol/L])

ANCA	Negative
Hepatitis A total antibodies	Negative
Hepatitis B surface antigen	Positive
Hepatitis B surface antigen IgM antibody	Positive
Hepatitis B surface antigen IgG antibody	Negative
Hepatitis C virus antibodies	Negative
Urinalysis	3+ blood; 1+ protein; many erythrocytes; no dysmorphic erythrocytes; no casts

Kidney angiogram reveals multiple aneurysms and stenotic lesions of renal artery branches bilaterally.

Which of the following is the most likely diagnosis?

(A) Giant cell arteritis
(B) Granulomatosis with polyangiitis
(C) Polyarteritis nodosa
(D) Takayasu arteritis

Item 93

A 78-year-old woman is evaluated for increased fatigue. Two weeks ago, she was hospitalized for fever, chills, and weakness occurring 10 days following aortic valve replacement. At that time, blood cultures grew vancomycin-resistant *Enterococcus faecalis*, and intravenous linezolid was initiated. She has type 2 diabetes mellitus and hypertension. Medications are linezolid, amlodipine, enalapril, warfarin, and acetaminophen.

On physical examination, temperature is 37.3 °C (99.2 °F), blood pressure is 146/50 mm Hg, pulse rate is 96/min, and respiration rate is 24/min. BMI is 38. Cardiac examination is consistent with findings associated with a normal functioning prosthetic aortic valve. The lung fields are clear. The remainder of the examination is normal.

Laboratory studies:

Hemoglobin	10.4 g/dL (104 g/L)
Leukocyte count	7000/μL (7.0 × 10⁹/L)
Blood urea nitrogen	10 mg/dL (3.6 mmol/L)
Serum creatinine	0.7 mg/dL (61.9 μmol/L)
Electrolytes	
Sodium	143 meq/L (143 mmol/L)
Potassium	4.8 meq/L (4.8 mmol/L)
Chloride	106 meq/L (106 mmol/L)
Bicarbonate	9 meq/L (9 mmol/L)
Glucose	196 mg/dL (14.2 mmol/L)
Lactic acid	126 mg/dL (14 mmol/L)
Ketones	Negative
Arterial blood gas studies (ambient air):	
pH	7.23
P_{CO_2}	22 mm Hg (2.9 kPa)
P_{O_2}	98 mm Hg (13.0 kPa)

Which of the following is the most likely diagnosis?

(A) Diabetic ketoacidosis
(B) Pyroglutamic acidosis

(C) Sepsis

(D) Type B lactic acidosis

Item 94

A 26-year-old man is evaluated for a 6-month history of fatigue. He is subsequently diagnosed with hypokalemic metabolic alkalosis. He takes no medications.

On physical examination, temperature is 36.6 °C (97.9 °F), blood pressure is 110/64 mm Hg, pulse rate is 78/min, and respiration rate is 14/min. BMI is 20. Cardiac and pulmonary examinations are normal. There is no edema. The remainder of the examination is unremarkable.

Laboratory studies:

Blood urea nitrogen	12 mg/dL (4.3 mmol/L)
Serum creatinine	0.8 mg/dL (70.7 µmol/L)
Electrolytes	
Sodium	142 meq/L (142 mmol/L)
Potassium	2.9 meq/L (2.9 mmol/L)
Chloride	100 meq/L (100 mmol/L)
Bicarbonate	32 meq/L (32 mmol/L)

Which of the following is the most appropriate diagnostic test to perform next?

(A) Plasma aldosterone and renin levels

(B) Serum magnesium level

(C) Urine chloride level

(D) Urine osmolal gap

Item 95

A 71-year-old woman is hospitalized for chest pain. She has diabetes mellitus, hypertension, hyperlipidemia, and chronic kidney disease. Medications are lisinopril, rosuvastatin, as-needed furosemide, carvedilol, insulin, and aspirin.

On physical examination, the patient is afebrile; blood pressure is 118/50 mm Hg, and pulse rate is 70/min. There is no jugular venous distention. Cardiac examination is normal, with no murmurs or S_3. The lungs are clear. Abdominal examination is unremarkable. There is trace edema of the lower extremities, which is her baseline.

Laboratory studies:

Hematocrit	33%
Serum creatinine	3.1 mg/dL (274 µmol/L)
Electrolytes	Normal
Estimated glomerular filtration rate	19 mL/min/1.73 m²

Adenosine thallium scan reveals an area of reversible ischemia in the left anterior descending artery distribution. Cardiac catheterization is scheduled. Her lisinopril is held prior to the procedure.

Which of the following interventions will decrease this patient's risk for contrast-induced nephropathy?

(A) Hydration with isotonic saline

(B) Hydration with isotonic saline with mannitol diuresis

(C) Oral hydration

(D) Prophylactic hemodialysis

Item 96

A 68-year-old man is evaluated during a follow-up visit for chronic kidney disease. He also has hypertension, dyslipidemia, and COPD. His kidney function has remained stable, with an estimated glomerular filtration rate ranging from 30 to 40 mL/min/1.73 m². Medications are metoprolol, lisinopril, aspirin, atorvastatin, and albuterol and ipratropium inhalers.

On physical examination, blood pressure is 120/75 mm Hg, pulse rate is 80/min, and respiration rate is 14/min. There is no jugular venous distention. Cardiac examination reveals regular heart sounds and no murmur. The lungs are tympanitic with good air movement but mild diffuse expiratory wheezes. There is no lower extremity edema.

Laboratory studies:

Hemoglobin	10.5 g/dL (105 g/L)
Blood urea nitrogen	52 mg/dL (18.6 mmol/L)
Calcium	8.2 mg/dL (2.1 mmol/L)
Total cholesterol	179 mg/dL (4.64 mmol/L)
LDL cholesterol	115 mg/dL (2.98 mmol/L)
HDL cholesterol	42 mg/dL (1.09 mmol/L)
Triglycerides	110 mg/dL (1.24 mmol/L)
Serum creatinine	2.2 mg/dL (194 µmol/L)
Electrolytes	
Sodium	141 meq/L (141 mmol/L)
Potassium	4.9 meq/L (4.9 mmol/L)
Chloride	105 meq/L (105 mmol/L)
Bicarbonate	23 meq/L (23 mmol/L)
Phosphorus	4.5 mg/dL (1.45 mmol/L)
Parathyroid hormone	135 pg/mL (135 ng/L)
Estimated glomerular filtration rate	31 mL/min/1.73 m²
Urine albumin–creatinine ratio	235 mg/g

Which of the following interventions is most likely to prevent premature mortality?

(A) Begin 1,25-dihydroxy vitamin D

(B) Begin sodium bicarbonate replacement therapy

(C) Increase atorvastatin

(D) Increase lisinopril

Item 97

A 38-year-old woman is evaluated during a follow-up visit. She has a history of well-controlled hypertension and type 1 diabetes mellitus. She is at 16 weeks' gestation with her first pregnancy. Prior to conception she was taking lisinopril, which was discontinued in anticipation of the pregnancy, and labetalol was initiated. Other medications are insulin glargine, insulin lispro, and a prenatal vitamin.

On physical examination, she appears in good health. Blood pressure is 135/80 mm Hg. There is no edema. The remainder of the physical examination is normal.

Laboratory studies reveal a serum creatinine level of 0.7 mg/dL (61.9 µmol/L) and a urine protein–creatinine ratio of 0.8 mg/mg.

Which of the following is the most appropriate step in the management of this patient's hypertension?

(A) Add methyldopa
(B) Change labetalol to losartan
(C) Increase labetalol dose
(D) Continue current medication regimen

Item 98

An 82-year-old woman is evaluated during a follow-up visit for a 25-year history of hypertension. She feels well and has had no end-organ damage due to her blood pressure. Medications are maximal therapeutic daily doses of indapamide and lisinopril, which she tolerates well.

On physical examination, seated blood pressure is 146/68 mm Hg with a regular pulse rate of 72/min; after standing for 1 minute, blood pressure is 140/72 mm Hg with no change in pulse rate. The remainder of the examination is unremarkable.

Laboratory studies reveal normal electrolytes and kidney function.

Which of the following is the most appropriate next step in managing this patient's blood pressure?

(A) Add amlodipine
(B) Add metoprolol
(C) Discontinue indapamide; begin hydrochlorothiazide
(D) No change in management

Item 99

A 48-year-old man is evaluated during a follow-up visit for chronic kidney disease attributed to hypertensive nephrosclerosis. One week ago, he began to have dyspnea with exertion with increasing frequency. Episodes typically begin when he is walking, and he needs to sit for the symptoms to resolve. Occasionally the dyspnea is accompanied by nausea. He has no chest pain. He has never smoked and does not drink alcoholic beverages. Medications are lisinopril and lovastatin.

On physical examination, blood pressure is 142/86 mm Hg. BMI is 29. There is no jugular venous distention. Cardiac examination is normal. Lungs are clear. There is 1+ edema.

Laboratory studies (obtained 1 week ago):

Blood urea nitrogen	36 mg/dL (12.9 mmol/L)
Serum creatinine	2.1 mg/dL (186 µmol/L)
Total cholesterol	168 mg/dL (4.35 mmol/L)
LDL cholesterol	100 mg/dL (2.59 mmol/L)
HDL cholesterol	38 mg/dL (0.98 mmol/L)
Estimated glomerular filtration rate	41 mL/min/1.73 m^2
Urine protein–creatinine ratio	0.9 mg/mg

Electrocardiogram shows changes compatible with left ventricular hypertrophy.

Which of the following is the most appropriate next step in management?

(A) Begin an albuterol inhaler
(B) Begin furosemide
(C) Obtain spirometry
(D) Refer to the emergency department

Item 100

A 32-year-old man is evaluated for a recent diagnosis of autosomal dominant polycystic kidney disease (ADPKD) by kidney ultrasound. His mother had polycystic kidney disease, hypertension, and kidney failure requiring hemodialysis, and she died of a stroke. The patient also has hypertension that is managed with metoprolol and losartan.

On physical examination, blood pressure is 132/82 mm Hg, and pulse rate is 64/min. There is no flank pain or lower extremity edema. The remainder of the examination is unremarkable.

Laboratory studies reveal a serum creatinine level of 1.2 mg/dL (106 µmol/L) and a urine protein–creatinine ratio of 0.15 mg/mg; microscopic urinalysis reveals 5-10 erythrocytes/hpf.

Which of the following is the most appropriate next step in management?

(A) 24-Hour urine collection for protein
(B) Cerebral artery MR angiography
(C) Genotype testing for ADPKD subtype
(D) Noncontrast abdominal CT

Item 101

A 38-year-old woman is evaluated during a follow-up visit for stage 3 chronic kidney disease and hypertension secondary to polycystic kidney disease. Her only medication is lisinopril. Her daily dietary calcium intake is restricted to 1000 mg.

On physical examination, blood pressure is 124/80 mm Hg. Cardiopulmonary examination is normal. Abdominal examination is notable for bilateral palpable kidneys. The remainder of the examination is normal.

Laboratory studies:

Calcium	8.2 mg/dL (2.1 mmol/L)
Serum creatinine	1.7 mg/dL (150 µmol/L)
Phosphorus	4.3 mg/dL (1.39 mmol/L)
Intact parathyroid hormone	163 pg/mL (163 ng/L)
25-hydroxyvitamin D	12 ng/mL (30 nmol/L)
Estimated glomerular filtration rate	34 mL/min/1.73 m^2

Which of the following is the most appropriate next step in management?

(A) Begin calcitriol (1,25-dihydroxy vitamin D)
(B) Begin calcium carbonate
(C) Begin cholecalciferol (vitamin D$_3$)
(D) Begin sevelamer
(E) Continue current regimen

Item 102

A 21-year-old man is evaluated during a follow-up visit. He was initially evaluated at a student health center for flu-like symptoms and was found to have a blood pressure of 144/90 mm Hg. At his first office visit 3 weeks ago, his blood pressure was 136/83 mm Hg seated (average of three readings). Medical history is unremarkable. He takes no medications.

On physical examination today, blood pressure is 133/79 mm Hg seated (average of three readings); other vital signs are normal. The remainder of the examination is normal.

Which of the following is the most likely diagnosis?

(A) Masked hypertension
(B) Normotension
(C) Prehypertension
(D) White coat hypertension

Item 103

A 33-year-old woman is evaluated for hypertension. She is at 17 weeks' gestation with her second pregnancy. Her first pregnancy was complicated by hypertension at term. She has not followed up in the 4 years since the delivery of her first child. She has no allergies. Family history is notable for her father who has diabetes mellitus and hypertension. Her only medication is prenatal vitamins.

On physical examination, she appears well. Blood pressure is 140/90 mm Hg, and pulse rate is 90/min. Lungs are clear. The abdomen has a gravid uterus. Reflexes are normal. There is trace edema. The remainder of the examination is unremarkable.

Laboratory studies reveal a serum creatinine level of 1.7 mg/dL (150 μmol/L), 1+ protein on urinalysis, and a urine protein–creatinine ratio of 0.5 mg/mg.

Which of the following is the most likely diagnosis?

(A) Chronic kidney disease and hypertension
(B) Gestational hypertension
(C) The nephrotic syndrome
(D) Preeclampsia

Item 104

A 72-year-old woman is hospitalized for a 3-day history of fever, chills, and malaise. Three months ago, she had a complete heart block necessitating placement of a dual-chamber pacemaker.

On physical examination, temperature is 37.4 °C (99.3 °F), blood pressure is 128/56 mm Hg, pulse rate is 96/min, and respiration rate is 16/min. BMI is 26. A grade 3/6 holosystolic murmur is heard best along the left sternal border and is louder during inspiration.

Echocardiogram reveals a 1-cm vegetation on the tricuspid valve.

Blood cultures grow vancomycin-resistant *Enterococcus*. Intravenous vancomycin and gentamicin are initiated. On day 3, the patient develops increased agitation and paranoid delusions; quetiapine is initiated.

Laboratory studies:

	On Admission	10 Days Later
Blood urea nitrogen	26 mg/dL (9.3 mmol/L)	24 mg/dL (8.6 mmol/L)
Serum creatinine	0.8 mg/dL (70.7 μmol/L)	1.3 mg/dL (115 μmol/L)
Electrolytes		
Sodium	142 meq/L (142 mmol/L)	138 meq/L (138 mmol/L)
Potassium	5 meq/L (5 mmol/L)	2.9 meq/L (2.9 mmol/L)
Chloride	105 meq/L (105 mmol/L)	93 meq/L (93 mmol/L)
Bicarbonate	25 meq/L (25 mmol/L)	32 meq/L (32 mmol/L)
Urine studies:		
Chloride	–	96 meq/L (96 mmol/L) (normal range for women, 20-295 meq/L [20-295 mmol/L])
Creatinine	–	80 mg/dL (normal range for women, 15-327 mg/dL)
Potassium	–	40 meq/L (40 mmol/L) (normal range for women, 17-164 meq/L [17-164 mmol/L])
Sodium	–	103 meq/L (103 mmol/L) (normal range for women, 15-267 meq/L [15-267 mmol/L])
Urine potassium–creatinine ratio	–	50 meq/g

Which of the following is the most likely cause of this patient's electrolyte disorder?

(A) Gentamicin toxicity
(B) Primary hyperaldosteronism
(C) Quetiapine toxicity
(D) Vancomycin toxicity

Item 105

A 65-year-old woman is evaluated during a follow-up visit for long-standing diabetic nephropathy and hypertension. She feels well but reports mild dyspnea with exertion. Medications are lisinopril, metoprolol, hydrochlorothiazide, neutral protamine Hagedorn (NPH) insulin, and regular insulin.

On physical examination, blood pressure is 138/78 mm Hg, and pulse rate is 65/min. Cardiac examination is normal. Lungs are clear. The remainder of the examination is unremarkable.

Laboratory studies:

Hematocrit	29%
Leukocyte count and differential	Normal

Mean corpuscular volume	88 fL
Platelet count	Normal
Reticulocyte count	0.5% of erythrocytes
Serum creatinine	2.3 mg/dL (203 µmol/L)
Estimated glomerular filtration rate	21 mL/min/1.73 m²
Peripheral blood smear	Consistent with normocytic anemia

Which of the following is the most appropriate next step in the management of this patient's anemia?

(A) Discontinue lisinopril
(B) Initiate erythropoiesis-stimulating agents
(C) Measure serum erythropoietin level
(D) Measure serum iron stores

Item 106

A 67-year-old man is evaluated in the hospital for an increasing serum creatinine level. He was hospitalized for pneumonia 2 days ago and is improving on levofloxacin therapy. He has experienced no episodes of hypotension during the hospitalization. His only other medication is prazosin for benign prostatic hyperplasia.

On physical examination, blood pressure is 144/75 mm Hg, and pulse rate is 64/min. BMI is 34. Cardiac and pulmonary examinations are normal. The abdomen is non-tender, with normal bowel sounds and some suprapubic fullness. Urine output was 1200 mL in the past 24 hours.

Laboratory studies:

Serum creatinine	1.9 mg/dL (168 µmol/L) (1.2 mg/dL [106 µmol/L] on admission)
Potassium	5.7 meq/L (5.7 mmol/L) (4.5 meq/L [4.5 mmol/L] on admission)
Urinalysis	Specific gravity 1.011; pH 6.0; trace leukocyte esterase; 0-3 erythrocytes/hpf; 0-5 leukocytes/hpf

Which of the following is the most appropriate diagnostic test to perform next?

(A) Fractional excretion of sodium
(B) Kidney biopsy
(C) Kidney ultrasonography
(D) Serum creatine kinase level measurement

Item 107

A 20-year-old woman is evaluated in the hospital after a tonsillectomy because her blood pressure increased from 122/72 mm Hg before anesthesia induction to 210/126 mm Hg during induction. Her heart rate increased from 70/min to 106/min when her blood pressure increased. Intravenous nitroglycerin was initiated to lower her blood pressure. Other than occasional palpitations, her medical history, family history, and review of systems were unremarkable.

On physical examination 2 hours later, the patient is awake and alert. The nitroglycerin was discontinued 30 minutes ago. Current blood pressure is 118/76 mm Hg, and heart rate is 80/min. Other than a fresh tonsillectomy scar, the remainder of the examination is normal.

Which of the following is the most appropriate next step in management?

(A) CT of the adrenal glands
(B) Catheter-based kidney angiography
(C) Plasma metanephrine measurement
(D) Transthoracic echocardiography

Item 108

A 68-year-old man is hospitalized for acute kidney injury secondary to a bladder outlet obstruction. He also has benign prostatic hyperplasia, hypertension, chronic kidney disease, and bipolar disorder previously treated with lithium. Medications are doxazosin, valproate, and enalapril (held on admission).

On admission, serum creatinine level is 6.2 mg/dL (548 µmol/L); 6 months ago, it was 1.5 mg/dL (133 µmol/L). After placement of a bladder (Foley) catheter, 800 mL of urine drained immediately. Urine volume increased to 130 mL/h over the initial 48 hours of hospitalization.

On physical examination, temperature is 37.3 °C (99.2 °F), blood pressure is 160/60 mm Hg, pulse rate is 68/min, and respiration rate is 14/min. BMI is 30. Cardiopulmonary examination is normal. There is 1+ lower extremity edema.

Laboratory studies on day 3 of admission:

Blood urea nitrogen	86 mg/dL (30.7 mmol/L)
Serum creatinine	3.4 mg/dL (301 µmol/L)
Electrolytes	
Sodium	148 meq/L (148 mmol/L)
Potassium	5.2 meq/L (5.2 mmol/L)
Chloride	117 meq/L (117 mmol/L)
Bicarbonate	18 meq/L (18 mmol/L)
Glucose	106 mg/dL (5.9 mmol/L)
Urine studies:	
Osmolality	326 mosm/kg H₂O (normal, 300-900 mosm/kg H₂O)
Potassium	35 meq/L (35 mmol/L) (normal range for men, 11-99 meq/L [11-99 mmol/L])
Sodium	40 meq/L (40 mmol/L) (normal range for men, 18-301 meq/L [18-301 mmol/L])
Urinalysis	Specific gravity 1.012; pH 5.0; no blood; trace protein; no glucose

Kidney ultrasound reveals hydronephrosis bilaterally and cortical thinning bilaterally.

Which of the following is the most appropriate management?

(A) 0.45% Sodium chloride
(B) 5% Dextrose in water
(C) Desmopressin
(D) Water deprivation test

Answers and Critiques

Item 1   Answer: A

Educational Objective: Manage newly diagnosed stage 2 hypertension.

Combination drug therapy is indicated for this patient with newly diagnosed stage 2 hypertension. The Seventh Report of the Joint National Committee on Prevention, Detection, Evaluation, and Treatment of High Blood Pressure (JNC 7) guidelines classify stage 2 hypertension as a systolic blood pressure of ≥160 mm Hg or a diastolic blood pressure of ≥100 mm Hg. According to the JNC 7, in the absence of comorbidities or compelling indications, the blood pressure goal in patients younger than 80 years is 140/90 mm Hg. In patients whose blood pressure goal requires reductions of systolic pressure more than 20 mm Hg and of diastolic pressure more than 10 mm Hg, the JNC 7 indicates that combination therapy can shorten the time needed for medication adjustment and increase the likelihood of achieving the blood pressure goal, while reducing the number of visits needed for drug titrations. Initial treatment with two antihypertensive agents is therefore warranted in this patient who has blood pressure measurements at least 22/10 mm Hg above goal.

Several nondrug approaches are useful in lowering blood pressure, including weight loss if the patient is overweight, salt reduction, physical activity of at least 30 minutes per day at least 3 days per week, and a reduction in alcohol consumption. However, lifestyle modifications alone in this patient with a normal BMI who has good health habits will likely not adequately lower her blood pressure to the targeted goal.

Monotherapy is unlikely to be effective in patients whose blood pressure is more than 20 mm Hg above the blood pressure goal. This patient has newly diagnosed stage 2 hypertension, with blood pressure measurements that are unlikely to be controlled with a single agent.

A follow-up visit in 2 to 4 weeks to reevaluate this patient is also indicated; however, this is in addition to initiating treatment for her stage 2 hypertension.

KEY POINT

- **Initial treatment with two antihypertensive agents may be warranted in patients whose blood pressure is more than 20 mm Hg above the blood pressure goal.**

Bibliography

Rosendorff C, Black HR, Cannon CP, et al; American Heart Association Council for High Blood Pressure Research; American Heart Association Council on Clinical Cardiology; American Heart Association Council on Epidemiology and Prevention. Treatment of hypertension in the prevention and management of ischemic heart disease: a scientific statement from the American Heart Association Council for High Blood Pressure Research and the Councils on Clinical Cardiology and Epidemiology and Prevention [erratum in Circulation. 2007;116(5):e121]. Circulation. 2007;115(21):2761-2788. [PMID: 17502569]

Item 2   Answer: C

Educational Objective: Treat infected cysts in a patient with autosomal dominant polycystic kidney disease.

Ciprofloxacin is appropriate treatment for this patient with probable infected kidney cysts. She has autosomal dominant polycystic kidney disease (ADPKD) and now has flank pain and fever. Patients with ADPKD can have infected cysts without any abnormal findings on urinalysis or culture because the infected cyst(s) may not communicate with the rest of the urinary tract. With high suspicion of an infected cyst (flank pain and fever), treatment should consist of an antibiotic with an appropriate antimicrobial coverage spectrum for urinary tract pathogens and with good cystic penetration, such as ciprofloxacin. In this case, treatment should be continued for 2 to 4 weeks.

In patients with ADPKD, nitrofurantoin, cephalosporins, or penicillins are not considered appropriate antibiotic choices given their poor cystic penetration. Patients with ADPKD who have cystic hemorrhage can have flank pain and low-grade fever that may mimic infection; however, this patient's degree of fever with an elevated leukocyte count is out of proportion for what would be expected for a ruptured hemorrhagic cyst, suggesting infection.

KEY POINT

- **Patients with autosomal dominant polycystic kidney disease can have infected kidney cysts without abnormal findings on urinalysis or culture.**

Bibliography

Sallée M, Rafat C, Zahar JR, et al. Cyst infections in patients with autosomal dominant polycystic kidney disease. Clin J Am Soc Nephrol. 2009;4(7):1183-1189. [PMID: 19470662]

Item 3   Answer: C

Educational Objective: Prevent tumor lysis syndrome.

An increase in the intravenous saline rate is appropriate. This patient with acute myeloid leukemia received chemotherapy 1 day ago and is at risk for tumor lysis syndrome. Manifestations include acute kidney injury and arrhythmias resulting from the release of potassium, phosphorus, and uric acid from cells. The cell death can be spontaneous with highly proliferative malignancies but more commonly is induced by chemotherapy. Patients with untreated tumor lysis syndrome present with hyperkalemia, hyperuricemia, and hyperphosphatemia. Optimal treatment to prevent tumor lysis syndrome is intravenous fluids to promote a faster urine flow rate. The goal intravenous fluid rate is up to 3000 mL/m²/d, around 6 L/d in this patient. Although his initial intravenous fluid rate was reasonable, his high phosphorus and potassium levels suggest that cell breakdown is occurring, and an increased rate of saline infusion will help promote potassium excretion and decrease the solubility of phosphorus and uric acid by increasing urine volume. In this patient, an increased intravenous fluid with normal saline at a rate of 250 mL/h would be appropriate. The use of a loop diuretic to maintain urine flow is also reasonable in selected patients.

Although intravenous fluid with sodium bicarbonate has the benefit of alkalinizing the urine and therefore increasing uric acid clearance, it also increases the risk of calcium phosphorus precipitation, which can increase damage to the kidneys, and is not appropriate for this patient with a high serum phosphorus level.

Sodium polystyrene sulfonate can be used to treat this patient's hyperkalemia but will not improve his urine flow.

Rasburicase is generally preferred to allopurinol for prophylaxis of tumor lysis syndrome because of differences in mechanism. Rasburicase directly breaks down uric acid and minimizes xanthine accumulation, whereas allopurinol does not. Because this patient's serum uric acid levels appear to be adequately controlled with rasburicase, there would be no benefit of treatment with allopurinol.

KEY POINT

- Optimal treatment to prevent tumor lysis syndrome is intravenous fluids to promote a faster urine flow rate.

Bibliography
Howard SC, Jones DP, Pui CH. The tumor lysis syndrome. N Engl J Med. 2011;364(19):1844-1854. [PMID: 21561350]

Item 4   Answer: B

Educational Objective: Evaluate options for kidney replacement therapy in a patient with chronic kidney disease.

Planning for pretransplant peritoneal dialysis is indicated. This patient has advanced chronic kidney disease, with an estimated glomerular filtration rate of 11 mL/min/1.73 m². She has a genetically identical kidney donor in the future, but it is unlikely that she will be able to wait a year without kidney replacement therapy. Thus, an interim plan is needed. She is otherwise healthy, independent, and appears able to participate in peritoneal dialysis. She has never had abdominal surgery, and her BMI is normal. She

is an ideal candidate for peritoneal dialysis, and this modality will also allow her to preserve her independence and more easily transition to a life with end-stage kidney disease. Recent studies have shown that peritoneal dialysis offers similar outcomes to hemodialysis, and that there is no particular advantage to utilizing hemodialysis versus peritoneal dialysis in eligible patients who require pretransplant dialysis.

Compared with live donors, organs from deceased donors from the extended donor criteria pool have a far inferior renal allograft survival rate. These donors are of older age or have died of stroke or had a history of hypertension or reduced kidney function at the time of death. Utilization of an extended donor criteria kidney would be ill-advised for a young healthy recipient and a poor utilization of organs from the extended donor pool.

Preemptive dialysis has not been shown to be beneficial, and posttransplant outcomes appear to be worse with a longer duration of dialysis before transplant occurs. Therefore, the preferred method of kidney replacement therapy should be started when indicated by clinical circumstances, if needed, before transplant.

KEY POINT

- Peritoneal dialysis can preserve independence and allow a better transition to life with end-stage kidney disease.

Bibliography
Mehrotra R, Chiu YW, Kalantar-Zadeh K, Bargman J, Vonesh E. Similar outcomes with hemodialysis and peritoneal dialysis in patients with end-stage renal disease. Arch Intern Med. 2011;171(2):110-118. [PMID: 20876398]

Item 5   Answer: D

Educational Objective: Diagnose proliferative lupus nephritis.

The most likely diagnosis is proliferative lupus nephritis. This patient likely has systemic lupus erythematosus (SLE) based on her small-joint symmetric polyarthritis, oral ulcers, cytopenias, and kidney disease. Kidney disease is very common in patients with SLE. Patients satisfy this SLE criterion by having a 24-hour urine protein excretion greater than 500 mg/24 h, urinalysis showing more than 10 erythrocytes/hpf, erythrocyte or leukocyte casts in a sterile urine sample (proven by culture), or by kidney biopsy. Findings of proliferative lupus nephritis may include new-onset hypertension or edema typically associated with high titers of anti–double-stranded DNA antibodies and hypocomplementemia, proteinuria, hematuria, and erythrocyte and granular casts in the urine. Kidney biopsy is usually needed to make the diagnosis of lupus nephritis and to classify the pattern of glomerular disease. Kidney manifestations of lupus nephritis often develop concurrently or shortly following the onset of SLE in black, Hispanic, and Asian persons. Black patients who have SLE are commonly affected with severe lupus nephritis.

Focal segmental glomerulosclerosis (FSGS) is the leading cause of primary nephrotic syndrome, with a predilection for black patients. Patients with primary FSGS usually present with microscopic hematuria, hypertension, and kidney insufficiency. This patient has the nephritic syndrome, with erythrocyte casts in the urine sediment, which is very uncommon in patients with FSGS.

IgA nephropathy may only involve the kidney or can be secondarily associated with conditions such as HIV infection, chronic liver disease, inflammatory bowel disease, or celiac disease. It is not associated with SLE. IgA nephropathy has a predilection to develop in white or Asian men.

Postinfectious glomerulonephritis (PIGN) is an immunologic disease triggered by an infection, which is followed by the release of immunoglobulins and activation of complement proteins that are deposited in the glomeruli, activating cytokine inflammatory pathways. PIGN accounts for approximately 6% of the nephritic syndrome cases. PIGN cannot explain this patient's polyarthritis, oral ulcers, or cytopenias.

KEY POINT

- Findings of proliferative lupus nephritis may include new-onset hypertension or edema typically associated with high titers of anti–double-stranded DNA antibodies and hypocomplementemia, proteinuria, hematuria, and erythrocyte and granular casts in the urine.

Bibliography

Contreras G, Lenz O, Pardo V, et al. Outcomes in African Americans and Hispanics with lupus nephritis. Kidney Int. 2006;69(10):1846-1851. [PMID: 16598205]

Item 6   Answer: D
Educational Objective: Manage prehypertension.

This patient has prehypertension, and rechecking his blood pressure in 1 year is indicated. The prehypertension category established by the Seventh Report of the Joint National Committee on Prevention, Detection, Evaluation, and Treatment of High Blood Pressure (JNC 7) designates a group at high risk for progression to hypertension, in whom lifestyle modifications may be preemptive. Although this is not considered a mild form of hypertension, it is a category used to define persons considered at increased risk for the development of true hypertension. Increasing age and family history are also associated with an increased risk of eventually developing hypertension requiring treatment. Given his mild overweight and borderline lipid profile, this patient should be aggressively counseled on lifestyle intervention to improve his diet, increase his aerobic exercise capacity, and lose weight. His blood pressure should then be rechecked in 1 year.

Ambulatory blood pressure monitoring is indicated for patients with suspected white coat hypertension, to monitor patients with difficult-to-control blood pressure or those with significant symptoms such as hypotension on therapy, or if autonomic dysfunction is suspected. None of these situations is present in this patient.

C-reactive protein is a marker of inflammation that is increasingly associated with cardiovascular events and may eventually be useful in stratifying persons with cardiovascular risk. However, its use in prehypertension risk assessment has not been established.

This patient has not met the diagnostic criteria for sustained hypertension; therefore, initiation of long-term medical treatment is not appropriate.

KEY POINT

- Lifestyle modifications and a repeat blood pressure measurement in 1 year are indicated for patients with prehypertension.

Bibliography

Chobanian AV, Bakris GL, Black HR, et al; National Heart, Lung, and Blood Institute; Joint National Committee on Prevention, Detection, Evaluation, and Treatment of High Blood Pressure; National High Blood Pressure Education Program Coordinating Committee. The Seventh Report of the Joint National Committee on Prevention, Detection, Evaluation, and Treatment of High Blood Pressure: the JNC 7 report [erratum in JAMA. 2003;290(2):197]. JAMA. 2003;289(19):2560-2572. [PMID: 12748199]

Item 7   Answer: D

Educational Objective: Treat a patient who has lactic acidosis.

Supportive care is appropriate for this patient who presents with a mixed acid-base disorder after having a probable alcohol withdrawal seizure. He has an anion gap metabolic acidosis and his arterial P_{CO_2} is greater than the level expected, which is consistent with a concurrent respiratory acidosis. The increased anion gap acidosis is most likely due to a seizure-related lactic acidosis with concurrent alcoholic ketoacidosis; the improvement in acid-base status with volume repletion and supplemental glucose supports this diagnosis. His respiratory acidosis is consistent with a postictal state and alcohol use. Treatment of seizure-related lactic acidosis is directed toward controlling and preventing further seizures along with supportive measures such as adequate volume repletion.

Fomepizole, a competitive inhibitor of alcohol dehydrogenase, is indicated for patients with methanol or ethylene glycol ingestion to minimize their conversion to toxic metabolites. Both ingestions are associated with an elevated osmolal gap, calculated by the following equation:

$$\text{Osmolal Gap} = \text{Measured Plasma Osmolality} - \text{Calculated Plasma Osmolality, where,}$$

$$\text{Plasma Osmolality (mosm/kg H}_2\text{O)} = 2 \times \text{Serum Sodium (meq/L)} + \text{Plasma Glucose (mg/dL)}/18 + \text{Blood Urea Nitrogen (mg/dL)}/2.8\ (+ \text{Ethanol [mg/dL]}/3.7,\ \text{if present})$$

CONT.

The osmolal gap in this patient, when accounting for the contribution of ethanol, is less than 10; therefore, the use of fomepizole is not indicated.

Hemodialysis should be considered in patients with suspected ethylene glycol or methanol poisoning, severe propylene glycol toxicity, or severe isopropyl alcohol poisoning. This patient's improvement with supportive measures alone argues against toxic alcohol ingestion. The absence of calcium oxalate crystals also decreases the likelihood of ethylene glycol toxicity.

Supplemental sodium bicarbonate can be administered in persistent severe acidemia (pH <7.15), with the goal of maintaining the pH above 7.15, but is not indicated in this patient with evidence of improving acidosis.

KEY POINT

- Management of lactic acidosis is directed toward controlling the underlying cause along with supportive measures.

Bibliography

Rachoin JS, Weisberg LS, McFadden CB. Treatment of lactic acidosis: appropriate confusion. J Hosp Med. 2010;5(4):E1-E7. [PMID: 20394011]

Item 8 Answer: B

Educational Objective: Manage anemia associated with chronic kidney disease.

This patient has anemia associated with chronic kidney disease (CKD), and the most appropriate intervention is initiation of an erythropoiesis-stimulating agent (ESA). Anemia may develop in patients with stages 3 and 4 CKD and is primarily caused by reduced production of erythropoietin. Anemia is associated with decreased quality of life, left ventricular hypertrophy, and cardiovascular complications in patients with CKD. ESAs are indicated for patients with CKD who have hemoglobin levels less than 10 g/dL (100 g/L), but other causes of anemia, including iron deficiency, hemoglobinopathies, vitamin B_{12} deficiency, and gastrointestinal blood loss, should be considered before beginning this therapy. Because use of ESAs to correct hemoglobin levels to the normal range may be associated with an increased risk for cardiovascular events, ESAs should not be initiated in patients with hemoglobin levels greater than 12 g/dL (120 g/L). The FDA therefore recommends that patients with CKD who have not yet started dialysis have a hemoglobin level less than 10 g/dL (100 g/L) before initiating an ESA and supports a target hemoglobin level of 10 to 11 g/dL (100-110 g/L) during maintenance therapy.

Although ascorbic acid has been shown to augment oral iron absorption, there are no convincing data suggesting that the addition of this agent is worth the cost or increase in gastrointestinal side effects.

Blood transfusion is generally avoided in patients with chronic anemia in the absence of critical tissue ischemia, for example, chest pain and neurologic symptoms. This intervention can sensitize persons to HLA antigens, which may complicate the potential for kidney transplantation.

Because this patient's iron levels are adequate, switching from oral to intravenous iron therapy would not help to improve her anemia and is associated with an increased risk of anaphylaxis.

KEY POINT

- Initiation of an erythropoiesis-stimulating agent is indicated for patients with anemia associated with chronic kidney disease who have hemoglobin levels less than 10 g/dL (100 g/L); however, other causes of anemia, including iron deficiency, hemoglobinopathies, vitamin B_{12} deficiency, and gastrointestinal blood loss, should be considered before beginning this therapy.

Bibliography

U.S. Food and Drug Administration. FDA modifies dosing recommendations for erythropoiesis-stimulating agents. FDA News & Events Web site. Available at www.fda.gov/NewsEvents/Newsroom/ PressAnnouncements/ucm260670.htm. Updated June 24, 2011. Accessed July 23, 2012.

Item 9 Answer: A

Educational Objective: Manage metabolic alkalosis.

The addition of acetazolamide is indicated for this patient with significant metabolic alkalosis and hypervolemia. Metabolism of citrate contained in the blood products administered to this patient resulted in production of excess bicarbonate and metabolic alkalosis. Patients with normal kidney function and renal perfusion ordinarily can excrete excess bicarbonate, and the serum bicarbonate typically only increases by 1 to 2 meq/L (1-2 mmol/L), even with a very high filtered load of bicarbonate. Decreased renal blood flow in patients with cirrhosis, conversely, impairs kidney bicarbonate excretion because of increased proximal tubular reabsorption of filtered bicarbonate, leading to retention of the increased bicarbonate load and metabolic alkalosis. Acetazolamide promotes bicarbonate excretion and is the best therapeutic option for this patient with hypervolemia because it ameliorates both the metabolic alkalosis and sodium overload.

Furosemide facilitates sodium chloride but not bicarbonate excretion. Although this would result in increased sodium excretion, it might exacerbate the metabolic alkalosis if the patient becomes hypovolemic and develops further compromise of renal perfusion. This would lead to increased tubular bicarbonate reabsorption as well as enhanced bicarbonate generation in the cortical collecting duct.

Isotonic saline is unlikely to correct renal hypoperfusion in patients with cirrhosis and ascites who have underlying renal vasoconstriction and renal sodium avidity and therefore would not promote excretion of the increased bicarbonate load. Most of the infused sodium chloride would be retained because of increased tubular sodium chloride reabsorption, thereby aggravating the ascites and fluid overload.

In patients with active variceal bleeding, splanchnic vasoconstrictors such as octreotide are commonly used as an adjunctive treatment to endoscopic therapy. Infusions are typically continued for 3 to 5 days. Despite widespread use, octreotide is not associated with decreased mortality. This agent is not associated with metabolic alkalosis, and discontinuation of octreotide will not correct this patient's metabolic alkalosis.

KEY POINT

• Acetazolamide promotes bicarbonate excretion and can be used to ameliorate metabolic alkalosis in patients with hypervolemia and sodium overload.

Bibliography
Galla JH. Metabolic alkalosis. J Am Soc Nephrol. 2000;11(2):369-375. [PMID: 10665945]

Item 10   Answer: B
Educational Objective: Diagnose cytomegalovirus infection in a kidney transplant recipient.

The most likely diagnosis is cytomegalovirus (CMV) infection. Despite advances in immunosuppressive therapy and infection prophylaxis, more than 50% of kidney transplant recipients develop at least one infection during the first year after transplantation. CMV infection is particularly common in these patients. CMV infection is often suspected when patients have leukopenia and fevers during the posttransplant period. Viremia is best detected by polymerase chain reaction (PCR), a fast, sensitive, and reliable technique compared with serology, culture, or early antigen or CMV antigenemia detection. CMV infection can result in CMV disease, with organ involvement manifesting as retinitis, pneumonia, encephalitis, hepatitis, and gastrointestinal tract ulceration.

This patient underwent kidney transplantation 7 months ago and discontinued his CMV prophylaxis therapy 1 month ago as per standard protocol. Kidney transplantation from a donor who is seropositive for CMV to a recipient who is seronegative for this virus places the recipient at high risk for developing this condition. Furthermore, this patient's fever, leukopenia, and diarrhea are consistent with CMV infection, and his elevated liver chemistry studies raise suspicion for CMV-related hepatitis. Diagnosis of CMV infection is confirmed with a positive serum PCR test for viremia, and disease is confirmed by the presence of mucosal ulcers or erosion and CMV inclusion bodies seen on a biopsy specimen from the wall of the bowel obtained during colonoscopy.

Clostridium difficile infection may cause diarrhea and fever but does not explain this patient's leukopenia or elevated aminotransferase levels.

Mycophenolate mofetil can cause diarrhea and leukopenia but is rarely associated with elevated liver chemistry studies and does not explain this patient's fever. In addition, toxicity associated with mycophenolate mofetil usually occurs after a recent dosage change.

Tacrolimus toxicity can cause diarrhea but does not manifest as fever, leukopenia, or abnormal findings on liver chemistry studies.

KEY POINT

• Cytomegalovirus infection is particularly common in kidney transplant recipients and may manifest as fever, leukopenia, and diarrhea.

Bibliography
Helanterä I, Lautenschlager I, Koskinen P. The risk of cytomegalovirus recurrence after kidney transplantation. Transpl Int. 2011;24(12):1170-1178. [PMID: 21902725]

Item 11   Answer: D
Educational Objective: Diagnose multiple myeloma as a cause of acute kidney injury.

Serum and urine electrophoresis are indicated for this patient with probable multiple myeloma. Multiple myeloma, a plasma cell neoplasm resulting in the production of abnormal immunoglobulin (paraprotein), can present with bone pain, anemia, hypercalcemia, and kidney injury. Multiple mechanisms of kidney injury are involved in multiple myeloma, with kidney injury usually resulting from precipitation of paraproteins in the kidney. A clinical clue to the diagnosis is the presence of an elevated total urine protein, which quantifies both the albumin and non-albumin protein (paraprotein) present, when a urine dipstick (which measures only albumin) indicates only small amounts or no protein present. Similarly, the addition of sulfosalicylic acid to the urine in a patient with a urinary paraprotein will precipitate the proteins present with an increase in turbidity, while the urine dipstick shows minimal or no proteinuria. Serum and urine electrophoresis can identify the presence of the paraprotein in the blood and urine and can indicate the need for a bone marrow biopsy to confirm the hematologic diagnosis.

ANCA vasculitis can cause an elevated serum creatinine level, anemia, and fatigue, and it often occurs in patients over 60 years old. Anemia with vasculitis can be severe, particularly with lung hemorrhage. However, the urine sediment associated with vasculitis is active, with significant hematuria and dipstick-positive proteinuria, which is not present in this patient.

Kidney biopsy is indicated when there is kidney injury of unclear etiology. Kidney biopsy is not required for a diagnosis of multiple myeloma and is not indicated initially in the evaluation of this patient's acute kidney injury.

Although this patient has hypercalcemia, hyperparathyroidism does not adequately explain his degree of kidney injury; therefore, measurement of the parathyroid hormone level is not a useful diagnostic study in the context of myeloma-related hypercalcemia.

KEY POINT

- Kidney injury commonly accompanies multiple myeloma and may be associated with a discrepancy between the measured and urine dipstick protein quantifications.

Bibliography

Palumbo A, Anderson K. Multiple myeloma. N Engl J Med. 2011;364(11):1046-1060. [PMID: 21410373]

Item 12   Answer: A

Educational Objective: Diagnose resistant hypertension.

Ambulatory blood pressure monitoring is the most appropriate next step in management. This patient meets the diagnostic criteria for resistant hypertension, which is defined as blood pressure that remains above goal despite treatment with the optimal dosages of three antihypertensive agents of different classes, including a diuretic. Patient characteristics more likely to be associated with resistant hypertension include older age, BMI greater than 30, higher baseline blood pressure, diabetes mellitus, and black race. However, before this diagnosis is made, it is necessary to establish that this patient's blood pressure is truly high outside of the office. Ambulatory blood pressure monitoring can differentiate true resistant hypertension from a white coat effect that misleadingly suggests resistance to therapy. Once resistant hypertension is verified, a search for identifiable factors that may be modified is appropriate, including high salt intake, concurrent use of drugs such as NSAIDs, and the presence of other potentially exacerbating medical conditions such as obstructive sleep apnea.

Although potentially useful in assessing this patient's murmur or other suspected structural heart disease, echocardiography is not specifically indicated for evaluation of her hypertension.

The addition of another antihypertensive agent may be required for adequate blood pressure control but should be initiated only after resistant hypertension is diagnosed and other complicating factors are excluded.

In patients with resistant hypertension, consideration of possible secondary causes, such as assessment for catecholamine excess, may be indicated, but only after documentation that the diagnosis of resistant hypertension has been confirmed.

KEY POINT

- Resistant hypertension is defined as blood pressure that remains above goal despite treatment with the optimal dosages of three antihypertensive agents of different classes, including a diuretic.

Bibliography

Calhoun DA, Jones D, Textor S, et al. Resistant hypertension: diagnosis, evaluation, and treatment. A scientific statement from the American Heart Association Professional Education Committee of

the Council for High Blood Pressure Research. Hypertension. 2008;51(6):1403-1419. [PMID: 18391085]

Item 13   Answer: D

Educational Objective: Manage asymptomatic hyponatremia.

At this time, the most appropriate management for this patient's hyponatremia is fluid restriction. The absence of neurologic findings suggests that this patient's hyponatremia is chronic, and rapid correction is therefore not indicated. Asymptomatic hyponatremia in patients with cirrhosis is a poor prognostic marker, and the benefits of correcting hyponatremia in asymptomatic patients who are not candidates for imminent liver transplantation are not clear. Thus, ongoing observation of the serum sodium concentration and mental status while implementing fluid restriction is indicated. Some experts recommend implementing fluid restriction only when the serum sodium level is less than 120 meq/L (120 mmol/L) or as a component of therapy in patients with neurologic symptoms attributed to hyponatremia.

Hypertonic (3%) saline is only indicated in the presence of neurologic symptoms or for correction of hyponatremia when the serum sodium level is less than 130 meq/L (130 mmol/L) immediately preceding liver transplantation; however, care should be taken to avoid increasing the serum sodium level above 8 to 10 meq/L (8-10 mmol/L) per day given the increased risk for osmotic demyelination syndrome.

Conivaptan blocks both the V_2 and V_{1a} receptors, the latter of which can decrease blood pressure and increase the risk of variceal bleeding in patients with cirrhosis and is therefore relatively contraindicated in this group.

Demeclocycline can be used to manage asymptomatic hyponatremia due to the syndrome of inappropriate antidiuretic hormone secretion (SIADH). This patient does not have SIADH, as indicated by the presence of edema, ascites, and low urine sodium concentration. Furthermore, demeclocycline exhibits increased nephrotoxicity in those with underlying liver disease and is contraindicated in these patients.

KEY POINT

- Fluid restriction is indicated for the management of asymptomatic hyponatremia in patients with cirrhosis when the serum sodium level is less than 120 meq/L (120 mmol/L) or as a component of therapy in patients with neurologic symptoms attributed to hyponatremia.

Bibliography

Ginès P, Guevara M. Hyponatremia in cirrhosis: pathogenesis, clinical significance, and management. Hepatology. 2008;48(3):1002-1010. [PMID: 18671303]

Item 14   Answer: B

Educational Objective: Assess the risk of pregnancy outcome in a patient with reduced kidney function.

Serum creatinine level measurement is indicated for this patient with IgA nephropathy who is considering pregnancy. The degree of baseline kidney injury, as estimated by the glomerular filtration rate (GFR) or serum creatinine level, is most useful in assessing risk for subsequent pregnancy outcome. Women with chronic kidney disease (CKD) have a greater risk of complications of the pregnancy and adverse outcomes for the fetus. Reduced kidney function imparts a greater risk for eclampsia and preeclampsia and also a possible irreversible decline in kidney function during pregnancy, intrapartum, or after delivery. When serum creatinine is used to estimate kidney function in women, a normal value is nearly always less than 1.0 mg/dL (88.4 micromoles/L) (although many laboratories may report a higher normal range) because women have less muscle mass than men, and serum creatinine is a breakdown product of muscle. When the serum creatinine value for a woman is more than 1.4 mg/dL (124 micromoles/L), this correlates with an estimated GFR of less than 60 mL/min/1.73 m^2, and the patient has CKD stage 3 or higher. In women with kidney dysfunction at this stage or higher, there is an increased risk for fetal growth restriction, preeclampsia, preterm delivery, and perinatal death, as well as for loss of more than 25% of existing kidney function in the mother. Women who have milder impairments in kidney function or proteinuria may be at greater risk for complications from pregnancy than healthy women but are less likely to have significant kidney impairment as a consequence of pregnancy. Proteinuria associated with CKD may worsen with pregnancy, but the degree of proteinuria present at the time of pregnancy does not predict the risk for pregnancy-associated complications.

Although abnormal glycosylations of IgA may play an important role in the pathogenesis of IgA nephropathy, measurement of IgA levels plays no role in the management of IgA nephropathy nor does it have any implications for pregnancy.

Hypertension associated with CKD is an important factor in pregnancy in women with CKD and needs to be carefully controlled during pregnancy, although the presence of hypertension alone is not predictive of pregnancy outcome. This patient has prehypertension but does not need a 24-hour ambulatory blood pressure determination to further assess the risk of pregnancy.

Pregnancy complications and outcome appear similar with kidney disease of different causes, although the need to actively treat an underlying medical illness associated with the kidney disease may be a contributing factor in pregnancy outcome. Nevertheless, the patient's diagnosis is known, and a repeat kidney biopsy to assess for histologic progression is unnecessary and potentially dangerous.

Bibliography

Williams D, Davison J. Chronic kidney disease in pregnancy. BMJ. 2008;336(7637):211-215. [PMID: 18219043]

Item 15   Answer: A

Educational Objective: Diagnose acute interstitial nephritis.

This patient most likely has acute interstitial nephritis (AIN), which is typically caused by a hypersensitivity reaction to a medication. The clinical presentation of AIN is variable and in part dependent on the precipitating medication. The classic presentation of AIN is fever, rash, and eosinophilia in a patient with an elevated serum creatinine level, but this presentation is found in only 10% of cases. Diagnosis is most often made by a history of exposure to a drug that has a high likelihood of causing AIN. AIN usually occurs after 7 to 10 days of drug exposure; however, prior exposure to a drug may result in a more sudden onset. Urinalysis may show leukocytes and leukocyte casts with negative urine cultures (sterile pyuria) and/or erythrocytes. The mainstay of AIN treatment is discontinuation of the offending agent. This patient has leukocytes in the urine and takes the proton pump inhibitor (PPI) omeprazole, which most likely induced the AIN because PPI-induced AIN often has a subacute presentation.

This patient is taking a bisphosphonate, which can cause acute tubular necrosis (ATN). Bisphosphonate-induced ATN occurs mainly with intravenous administration. The urine sediment in this case is also more consistent with AIN than ATN, which is associated with muddy brown casts but not leukocytes.

Giant cell arteritis typically affects large blood vessels, not the small blood vessels in the kidney. Although small-vessel vasculitis can affect the kidneys and large vessels, this patient's urine sediment is not consistent with a glomerulonephritis (dysmorphic erythrocytes, erythrocyte casts, and proteinuria).

Numerous medications can cause thrombotic thrombocytopenic purpura (TTP), including cancer chemotherapeutic agents, cyclosporine, tacrolimus, quinine, and ticlopidine but not prednisone, omeprazole, or risedronate. Manifestations of the thrombotic microangiopathies include acute kidney injury that is usually accompanied by microangiopathic hemolytic anemia and thrombocytopenia. This patient's normal lactate dehydrogenase level and urine sediment with leukocytes are not consistent with TTP.

KEY POINT

- Diagnosis of acute interstitial nephritis (AIN) is most often made by a history of exposure to a drug that has a high likelihood of causing AIN and a urinalysis that typically shows leukocytes, leukocyte casts, and erythrocytes.

Bibliography

Praga M, González E. Acute interstitial nephritis. Kidney Int. 2010;77(11):956-961. [PMID: 20336051]

Item 16   Answer: A

Educational Objective: Diagnose focal segmental glomerulosclerosis.

The most likely diagnosis is focal segmental glomerulosclerosis (FSGS). This condition is the most common cause of idiopathic nephrotic syndrome in adults and the most common cause of the nephrotic syndrome in black adults. FSGS also is the most common primary glomerular disease that causes end-stage kidney disease in the United States. Patients with primary (idiopathic) FSGS usually present with microscopic hematuria, hypertension, and kidney disease. Secondary FSGS results from other disease processes that cause glomerular hypertrophy and hyperfiltration and is also associated with some infections, toxin exposures, or atheroembolic disease. These patients have minimal edema and rarely have the full spectrum of the nephrotic syndrome. This patient's presentation of the full spectrum of the nephrotic syndrome (nephrotic-range proteinuria, hypoalbuminemia, severe edema, and hyperlipidemia) is most consistent with primary FSGS. Diagnosis of primary FSGS is confirmed by kidney biopsy, with light microscopy showing scarring or sclerosis involving some (focal) glomeruli, which are affected only in a portion of the glomerular capillary bundle (segmental).

IgA nephropathy has a predilection to develop in men who are white or Asian and is very uncommon in black persons. Patients with IgA nephropathy may present after an upper respiratory tract infection and may have microscopic or frequently gross hematuria. Proteinuria is typically mild, and rapid progression to kidney failure is uncommon. IgA nephropathy is characterized by deposits of IgA primarily in the mesangium on immunofluorescence on kidney biopsy.

Systemic lupus erythematosus (SLE) may cause various kidney disorders, primarily due to immune complex deposition. Lupus nephritis has a predilection for young women, and this patient has no clinical or serologic evidence of SLE.

Postinfectious glomerulonephritis usually presents as the nephritic syndrome and results from immune complex deposition in the kidney after streptococcal or staphylococcal infections. This patient has no history of a preceding infection.

KEY POINT

- Patients with primary focal segmental glomerulosclerosis typically present with the nephrotic syndrome, microscopic hematuria, hypertension, and kidney disease.

Bibliography

Swaminathan S, Leung N, Lager DJ, et al. Changing incidence of glomerular disease in Olmsted County, Minnesota: a 30-year renal biopsy study. Clin J Am Soc Nephrol. 2006;1(3):483-487. [PMID: 17699249]

Item 17   Answer: B

Educational Objective: Diagnose hypokalemic distal (type 1) renal tubular acidosis.

This patient most likely has hypokalemic distal (type 1) renal tubular acidosis (RTA), a disorder characterized by normal anion gap metabolic acidosis and hypokalemia. Causes of hypokalemic distal RTA include autoimmune disorders such as Sjögren syndrome, systemic lupus erythematosus, or rheumatoid arthritis; drugs such as lithium or amphotericin B; hypercalciuria; and hyperglobulinemia. The kidney's ability to excrete hydrogen ions in response to acidemia in hypokalemic distal RTA is impaired, resulting in an inappropriately alkali pH of the urine in the presence of a systemic acidosis. The persistently increased pH encourages the development of kidney stones. Therefore, the pH above 6.0 in the setting of acidemia and the presence of nephrocalcinosis in this patient support the diagnosis of hypokalemic distal RTA.

Gitelman syndrome is an autosomal recessive syndrome characterized by hypokalemic metabolic alkalosis, not acidosis as noted in this patient. Blood pressure is normal to low, and hypomagnesemia is common. The defect is due to inactivating mutations in the gene for the thiazide-sensitive sodium chloride cotransporter in the distal convoluted tubule, and the electrolyte profile is analogous to that induced by thiazide diuretics.

Laxative abuse may also present with a hypokalemic normal anion gap metabolic acidosis. Patients with increased gastrointestinal losses of bicarbonate and potassium have intact kidney tubular function resulting in a compensatory increase in urine ammonium production, indicating increased acid secretion by the kidney. Urine ammonium may be estimated by calculating the urine anion gap, with a negative urine anion gap suggesting increased acid secretion and a positive urine anion gap indicating decreased acid secretion. This patient's urine anion gap is positive and is therefore not consistent with laxative abuse.

Proximal (type 2) RTA, a defect in regenerating bicarbonate in the proximal tubule, is characterized by a normal anion gap metabolic acidosis, hypokalemia, glycosuria (in the setting of normal plasma glucose), low-molecular-weight proteinuria, and renal phosphate wasting.

ONT.

However, distal urinary acidification mechanisms are intact, and the urine pH is less than 5.5 in the absence of alkali therapy. Proximal RTA is not associated with nephrocalcinosis or nephrolithiasis. This patient's normal urinalysis, high urine pH, and nephrocalcinosis are inconsistent with proximal RTA.

> **KEY POINT**
>
> - Hypokalemic distal (type 1) renal tubular acidosis is characterized by normal anion gap metabolic acidosis, hypokalemia, a urine pH greater than 6.0, and nephrocalcinosis.

Bibliography

Comer DM, Droogan AG, Young IS, Maxwell AP. Hypokalaemic paralysis precipitated by distal renal tubular acidosis secondary to Sjögren's syndrome. Ann Clin Biochem. 2008;45(Pt 2):221-225. [PMID: 18325192]

Item 18   Answer: C
Educational Objective: Diagnose hematuria.

A repeat urinalysis is appropriate for this low-risk patient with possible hematuria. Evaluation should ensure that a patient does not have any of the known risk factors, including a smoking history, occupational exposure to chemicals or dyes, history of gross hematuria, age older than 40 years, history of a urologic disorder, history of irritative voiding symptoms, history of urinary tract infection, analgesic abuse, or pelvic irradiation. In a patient under 40 years old, more than 3 erythrocytes/hpf on two or more occasions constitutes hematuria and is a common finding on urinalysis. A single episode in older patients or those at risk should initiate a full evaluation of the upper and lower urinary tract. This patient has had hematuria documented on one occasion; thus, urinalysis should be repeated before further evaluation, despite his family history. A family history of bladder cancer does not increase the patient's risk of developing a malignancy unless both family members have been exposed to similar toxins.

If hematuria is established after the repeat urinalysis, this patient should then be evaluated for its cause. Bleeding in patients with persistent hematuria may originate anywhere along the genitourinary tract, and the location of the bleeding must be identified in order to determine the next steps in evaluation. Therefore, differentiating between glomerular and nonglomerular hematuria by urine microscopy is important. Glomerular hematuria is characterized by the presence of dysmorphic erythrocytes or acanthocytes on urine microscopy, and hematuria associated with the presence of erythrocyte casts is specifically indicative of glomerulonephritis. Nonglomerular hematuria refers to blood in the urine that originates outside of the glomerulus. This condition is associated with isomorphic erythrocytes that usually appear normal on urine microscopy. The most common causes of asymptomatic nonglomerular hematuria are urinary tract infections and kidney stones. Renal or bladder cancer may also cause non-glomerular hematuria. An appropriate evaluation for persistent nonglomerular hematuria in this patient may begin with upper urinary tract imaging. The American Urological Association recommends CT, ultrasonography, or intravenous urography and notes that CT urography is the best choice if available. This should be followed by cystoscopy and possibly urine cytology.

Urine culture is unlikely to be helpful in this patient in the absence of dysuria or voiding symptoms and no leukocytes on urinalysis.

> **KEY POINT**
>
> - In patients younger than 40 years, the finding of more than 3 erythrocytes/hpf on urinalysis should be confirmed on two or more occasions to establish the diagnosis of hematuria.

Bibliography

Margulis V, Sagalowsky AI. Assessment of hematuria. Med Clin North Am. 2011;95(1):153-159. [PMID: 21095418]

Item 19   Answer: A
Educational Objective: Evaluate a patient for malignancy before kidney transplantation.

CT with contrast is indicated to exclude malignancy in this patient before kidney transplantation. Imaging with contrast is often needed to definitively characterize a renal lesion. In this patient with minimal residual kidney function who is on hemodialysis, CT with contrast will provide the most conclusive imaging with the least risk to the patient. Although she still produces urine, it is a minimal amount and is not likely contributing significantly to the clearance she is obtaining with hemodialysis. Avoidance of nephrotoxins is preferred in patients with chronic kidney disease who are not on dialysis and in dialysis patients with significant kidney function. However, in this patient with minimal residual kidney function who is on dialysis, the benefits of using contrast outweigh the risk of additional nephrotoxicity.

Intravenous pyelography outlines the anatomy of the urinary collecting system. Although it may demonstrate a filling defect indicative of a mass, intravenous pyelography does not help differentiate malignant from nonmalignant lesions and is also associated with a significant dose of contrast.

The use of gadolinium in MRI should be avoided in patients with a glomerular filtration rate of less than 30 mL/min/1.73 m^2. Nephrogenic systemic fibrosis (NSF) is a fibrosing skin disease caused by an inflammatory reaction to gadolinium that accumulates in the body due to kidney failure. NSF usually occurs within a few months of gadolinium exposure and typically presents with edema and thickened skin in the extremities that ultimately limits mobility and can be associated with pruritus and pain. NSF is progressive and can affect visceral organs and lead to death.

There are no effective treatments for NSF; prevention is the best course of action.

Positron emission tomography (PET) shows metabolic activity of tissue. Because of the high level of baseline metabolic activity in the kidney, PET cannot definitively exclude malignancy.

KEY POINT

- Contrast imaging should be avoided in patients with chronic kidney disease when possible; however, iodinated contrast can be given with less risk from nephrotoxicity in patients with minimal residual kidney function who are on dialysis.

Bibliography

Krajewski KM, Giardino AA, Zukotynski K, Van den Abbeele AD, Pedrosa I. Imaging in renal cell carcinoma. Hematol Oncol Clin North Am. 2011;25(4):687-715. [PMID: 21763963]

Item 20   Answer: B

Educational Objective: Diagnose hepatitis C virus–associated glomerulonephritis.

The most likely cause of this patient's kidney findings is hepatitis C virus–associated glomerulonephritis (HCV-GN). This immune complex disease can occur in as many as 21% of patients with HCV infection. HCV-GN usually manifests as the nephritic syndrome. Other manifestations may include combined nephrotic-nephritic syndrome, isolated proteinuria with hematuria, rapidly progressive glomerulonephritis, and acute and chronic kidney failure. HCV-GN can also be a component of a systemic cryoglobulinemic vasculitis with involvement of the skin, peripheral nerves, and musculoskeletal system. Most patients with HCV-GN have low complement levels, particularly C4, and a positive rheumatoid factor. Mildly positive antinuclear antibodies can also be seen. Diagnosis is confirmed by kidney biopsy, which demonstrates the pattern of membranoproliferative glomerulonephritis with or without capillary cryoglobulin deposition on light microscopy. This patient has mixed cryoglobulinemia associated with HCV infection: palpable purpura, arthralgia, peripheral neuropathy, hypocomplementemia, a positive rheumatoid factor, and the typical biopsy pattern of membranoproliferative glomerulonephritis with cryoglobulin deposition associated with HCV-GN.

Immune complex glomerulonephritis can be associated with hepatitis B virus infection. This patient shows evidence of previous hepatitis B virus exposure but not active infection, making this an unlikely cause of his kidney disease.

Polyarteritis nodosa is a systemic necrotizing vasculitis that primarily affects medium-sized arteries and is commonly associated with hepatitis B virus infection. It may be associated with HCV infection, affect the kidneys, and involve other organ systems. However, kidney biopsy results typically show evidence of vasculitis without immune complex deposition in the glomeruli.

Thrombotic microangiopathy is characterized by microangiopathic anemia and thrombocytopenia. Additionally, the deposition of immunoglobulins and/or complement components associated with HCV-GN on biopsy is not seen in thrombotic microangiopathy.

KEY POINT

- Diagnosis of hepatitis C virus–associated glomerulonephritis is confirmed by kidney biopsy, which demonstrates the pattern of membranoproliferative glomerulonephritis with or without capillary cryoglobulin deposition on light microscopy.

Bibliography

Roccatello D, Fornasieri A, Giachino O, et al. Multicenter study on hepatitis C virus-related cryoglobulinemic glomerulonephritis. Am J Kidney Dis. 2007;49(1):69-82. [PMID: 17185147]

Item 21   Answer: E

Educational Objective: Evaluate a patient with probable kidney stones using noncontrast abdominal helical CT.

The most appropriate test to perform next in this patient is a noncontrast abdominal helical CT. This patient has new-onset gradual abdominal and flank pain and a urinalysis revealing hematuria with low-grade pyuria, all of which are associated with kidney stones. Most kidney stones are radiopaque and are easily visualized on abdominal radiography of the kidneys, ureters, and bladder (KUB), which is inexpensive, noninvasive, and widely available. However, false-negative results may occur in patients with small stones, radiolucent stones that are composed of uric acid or related to use of indinavir, and interference of the overlying bowel. Noncontrast abdominal helical CT is the gold standard for diagnosing kidney stones. This study reveals urinary tract obstruction with hydronephrosis, detects stones as small as 1 mm in diameter, and helps evaluate other potential causes of abdominal pain and hematuria. However, noncontrast abdominal helical CT is expensive and has a higher radiation exposure than other imaging studies.

MRI does not visualize stones; therefore, a negative study cannot exclude the diagnosis of nephrolithiasis.

KUB can be used to follow stone burden but should not be used diagnostically because of possible false-negative results.

Intravenous pyelography has a high sensitivity and specificity in the diagnosis of kidney stones. However, this study requires bowel preparation and the use of intravenous iodinated contrast agents, which are contraindicated in patients with acute kidney injury and chronic kidney disease.

Kidney ultrasonography is often available when other modalities are not and is less expensive than CT; it can show both radiolucent and radiopaque stones but is best for visualizing the kidney and renal pelvis. However, its lower sensitivity and specificity are often associated with the need for additional confirmatory imaging studies that may negate any cost savings.

Bibliography

Goldfarb DS. In the clinic. Nephrolithiasis. Ann Intern Med. 2009;151(3):ITC2. [PMID: 19652185]

Item 22   Answer: C

Educational Objective: Manage metabolic acidosis in a patient with chronic kidney disease.

The addition of sodium bicarbonate therapy is indicated to treat metabolic acidosis in this patient with chronic kidney disease (CKD). Derangements in laboratory study results are common in patients with progressive CKD. As the estimated glomerular filtration rate (GFR) declines, more frequent assessment is needed to adjust medications and limit consequences of CKD. The metabolic acidosis that results from CKD is a common complication and typically develops when the GFR is less than 25 mL/min/1.73 m². Chronic metabolic acidosis has several adverse consequences, including exacerbation of bone disease as bone serves to buffer the pH. Chronic metabolic acidosis may also have adverse effects that impact thyroid hormone, growth hormone, muscle strength, and cardiovascular disease. Management of metabolic acidosis with oral sodium bicarbonate has been found to slow progression of CKD.

High uric acid levels have been associated with CKD progression, and there is increasing interest in the use of allopurinol to slow CKD progression; however, to date, there has not been conclusive evidence to support widespread use of allopurinol in patients without other indications for its use.

Noncalcium-containing phosphate binders such as sevelamer or lanthanum carbonate have been promoted to treat hyperphosphatemia without increasing the calcium phosphate product. The treatment of hyperphosphatemia is recommended in the management of secondary hyperparathyroidism. This strategy helps limit renal osteodystrophy, but it has not been proved to slow progression of CKD and is not indicated in this patient with a phosphorus level within the normal range.

Sodium polystyrene can be used to treat significant hyperkalemia in patients with CKD when other strategies such as dietary restriction, cessation of agents that block the renin-angiotensin system, or diuretics have failed. Sodium polystyrene, however, plays no role in halting progression of CKD and is otherwise not indicated in this patient with a potassium level of 4.8 meq/L (4.8 mmol/L).

Bibliography

De Brito-Ahurst I, Varagunam M, Raftery MJ, Yaqoob MM. Bicarbonate supplementation slows progression of CKD and improves nutritional status. J Am Soc Neph. 2009;20(9):2075-2084. [PMID: 1960873]

Item 23   Answer: A

Educational Objective: Manage white coat hypertension.

This patient has white coat hypertension with no evidence of target organ damage and should therefore continue home blood pressure measurements and return for a follow-up visit in 6 months. White coat hypertension is characterized by at least three separate office blood pressure measurements above 140/90 mm Hg and at least two sets of measurements below 140/90 mm Hg obtained outside the office, accompanied by the absence of target organ damage. Ambulatory blood pressure monitoring is considered the gold standard for diagnosing this condition. Patients with white coat hypertension have a lower risk for cardiovascular events compared with those with sustained hypertension but also have a greater risk for developing sustained hypertension than those without this condition and should be carefully monitored, including with home blood pressure measurements.

Pharmacologic treatment of white coat hypertension has not been shown to reduce morbid events or produce cardiovascular benefit and is therefore inappropriate for this patient.

This patient has normal laboratory test results and a normal electrocardiogram and therefore is at low cardiovascular risk; ordering further tests such as echocardiography or a spot urine albumin–creatinine ratio to screen for microalbuminuria is not necessary at this time.

A plasma aldosterone-plasma renin activity ratio would be appropriate if primary hyperaldosteronism were a consideration. This patient is not hypertensive, and this test is not indicated at this time.

Bibliography

Verdecchia P, Angeli F. The natural history of white-coat hypertension in the long term. Blood Press Monit. 2005;10(2):65-66. [PMID: 15812252]

Item 24   Answer: D

Educational Objective: Diagnose acute kidney injury in a patient with HIV infection.

The most likely cause of acute kidney injury (AKI) in this patient with HIV infection is tenofovir-induced toxicity. Patients with HIV infection have an increased risk of AKI, and medications used to treat HIV infection can cause AKI. In this patient, medication toxicity from the antiretroviral agent tenofovir is the most likely cause of her elevated serum creatinine level. Tenofovir is associated with nephrotoxicity thought to be due to mitochondrial damage to renal tubular cells. It may cause changes similar to those seen in the Fanconi syndrome: glycosuria despite a normal plasma glucose level, mild proteinuria consistent with proximal tubular damage, and a low serum bicarbonate level without an elevated anion gap. Phosphaturia can also cause a low serum phosphorus level. When identified, tenofovir kidney injury is treated by discontinuing the drug. Most patients show recovery in kidney function over weeks to months, although permanent injury is possible.

Hepatitis C virus–associated kidney disease is an immune complex disorder that occurs in association with active hepatitis C virus infection and leads to the development of glomerulonephritis. This disorder typically manifests as the nephritic syndrome and is associated with significant hematuria and proteinuria, neither of which is found in this patient.

HIV infection is associated with some parenchymal diseases (HIV-associated nephropathy, interstitial/infiltrative diseases, immune complex–mediated nephritis), with a collapsing form of focal segmental glomerulosclerosis (FSGS) being the most common. This form of kidney disease typically presents in patients with a high HIV viral load and is characterized by the nephrotic syndrome with high levels of urine protein, which is not present in this patient.

Although the antiretroviral agent atazanavir is associated with kidney stones, this patient has no symptoms of urinary obstruction, and the urinalysis is more consistent with proximal tubular damage.

KEY POINT

- Although patients with HIV infection are at increased risk for acute kidney injury (AKI) from a number of causes, medications are a leading etiology of AKI in this patient population.

Bibliography

Izzedine H, Harris M, Perazella MA. The nephrotoxic effects of HAART. Nat Rev Nephrol. 2009;5(10):563-573. [PMID: 19776778]

Item 25   Answer: C

Educational Objective: Manage rhabdomyolysis.

Treatment using rapid infusion of intravenous 0.9% saline is indicated for this patient with rhabdomyolysis. Rhabdomyolysis develops when muscle injury leads to the release of myoglobin and other intracellular muscle contents into the circulation. Rhabdomyolysis most commonly develops after exposure to myotoxic drugs, infection, excessive exertion, or prolonged immobilization. Diagnosis should be considered in patients with a serum creatine kinase level above 5000 units/L who demonstrate blood on urine dipstick testing in the absence of significant hematuria. Complications of rhabdomyolysis include hypocalcemia, hyperphosphatemia, hyperuricemia, metabolic acidosis, acute muscle compartment syndrome, and limb ischemia.

Although dialysis may ultimately be necessary if this patient does not respond to intravenous saline, there are no acute hemodialysis needs at this time. Although he is hyperkalemic, he has no electrocardiogram changes, and increasing sodium delivery with intravenous fluids through the renal tubules should help renal potassium excretion. If the potassium does not improve after a trial of intravenous fluids or the patient develops volume overload, dialysis may need to be initiated.

Although mannitol may promote renal tubular flow, it might also lead to further hypovolemia and has not been shown superior to hydration in the treatment of rhabdomyolysis.

This patient's hypernatremia indicates a free water deficit, and his history and examination suggest a hypovolemic hypernatremia. Rapid infusion of 5% glucose in water will help correct this patient's water deficit but will not expand the patient's volume and promote urine flow as effectively as sodium-containing intravenous fluid.

KEY POINT

- Intravenous fluid with saline is the treatment of choice for rhabdomyolysis.

Bibliography

Better OS, Abassi ZA. Early fluid resuscitation in patients with rhabdomyolysis. Nat Rev Nephrol. 2011;7(7):416-422. [PMID: 21587227]

Item 26   Answer: A

Educational Objective: Diagnose central diabetes insipidus.

The most likely diagnosis is central diabetes insipidus. A urine osmolality of less than 200 mosm/kg H_2O in the setting of increased effective plasma osmolality and polyuria is compatible with a diagnosis of diabetes insipidus. This patient has risk factors for both central (cytomegalovirus encephalitis) and nephrogenic (foscarnet therapy) diabetes insipidus. The only way to distinguish these disorders is through observation of the response to desmopressin. Urine osmolality will increase above 600 mosm/kg H_2O after administration of desmopressin in patients with central diabetes insipidus, indicative of the normal tubular response to the antidiuretic hormone (ADH) analog. Conversely, the urine osmolality will remain below 300 mosm/kg H_2O in patients with nephrogenic diabetes insipidus. The observed increase in urine osmolality to 614 mosm/kg H_2O in this patient establishes the diagnosis of central diabetes insipidus.

Cerebral salt wasting may give rise to sodium depletion, hyponatremia, and hypovolemia but usually does not cause hypernatremia or polyuria. Hypovolemia causes non-osmotic release of ADH, leading to a concentrated urine, retention of ingested or intravenously administered water, and hyponatremia. The initial urine osmolality below 200 mosm/kg H_2O, absence of hypovolemia on physical examination, and high serum sodium level in this patient are not consistent with cerebral salt wasting.

The urine osmolality should be greater than 300 mosm/kg H_2O in patients undergoing an osmotic diuresis. The urine osmolality in this patient was consistently less than 200 mosm/kg H_2O, thus excluding this diagnosis.

KEY POINT

- **Distinguishing between central diabetes insipidus and nephrogenic diabetes insipidus involves observation of the patient's response to desmopressin.**

Bibliography

Loh JA, Verbalis JG. Disorders of water and salt metabolism associated with pituitary disease. Endocrinol Metab Clin North Am. 2008;37(1):213-234. [PMID: 18226738]

Item 27   Answer: B

Educational Objective: Identify the cause of hypotonic hyponatremia.

This patient has hypotonic hyponatremia due to low solute intake. Her history of anorexia and weight loss, in conjunction with clinical euvolemia and both low plasma and low urine osmolality and sodium, supports this diagnosis. Because some solute excretion by the kidney is required for urinary water excretion, this patient's low solute intake is limiting her ability to excrete free water, leading to hypotonic hyponatremia as her water intake exceeds her ability to excrete urinary water.

The absence of physical examination findings suggesting hypovolemia, including postural changes in blood pressure and pulse, decreases the likelihood of hypovolemic hyponatremia in this patient. In patients with hypovolemia, urine osmolality typically exceeds 400 mosm/kg H_2O, which reflects increased tubular water resorption under the influence of antidiuretic hormone.

Pseudohyponatremia is characterized by a low serum sodium concentration due to measurement in a falsely large volume; an interfering substance displaces the liquid component of the sample, similar to ice cubes in a pitcher. The most common space-occupying substances are lipids and paraproteins. Measured plasma osmolality is normal in pseudohyponatremia and cannot be accounted for by increases in other solutes such as glucose, urea, or alcohols. The low measured plasma osmolality and the absence of an osmolal gap are consistent with hypotonic hyponatremia and exclude the diagnosis of pseudohyponatremia.

Hyponatremia is found in most patients with primary adrenal insufficiency, reflecting both mineralocorticoid deficiency and increased vasopressin secretion caused by cortisol deficiency. The absence of hypotension, hypovolemia, hyperkalemia, and a relatively high morning serum cortisol level does not support a diagnosis of primary adrenal insufficiency.

KEY POINT

- **Low solute intake can cause hypotonic hyponatremia.**

Bibliography

Berl T. Impact of solute intake on urine flow and water excretion. J Am Soc Nephrol. 2008;19(6):1076-1078. [PMID: 18337482]

Item 28   Answer: B

Educational Objective: Estimate the glomerular filtration rate in a low-risk, healthy person.

Estimation of the glomerular filtration rate (GFR) using the Chronic Kidney Disease Epidemiology Collaboration (CKD-EPI) equation is indicated. The Modification of Diet in Renal Disease (MDRD) study equation underestimates GFR at higher (normal) values. Thus, when the value of this equation is >60 mL/min/1.73 m², the recommendation is to report it as such, rather than the exact value. The MDRD study included patients with CKD who had lower muscle mass than the general population; therefore, this equation may underestimate GFR in healthy, low-risk persons who have a normal or increased muscle mass. The CKD-EPI equation has reduced this bias, which was shown in the NHANES study, in which median estimated GFR was 94.5 mL/min/1.73 m² using the CKD-EPI equation versus 85 mL/min/1.73 m² using the MDRD study equation. Additionally, in large cohort studies, patients reclassified from stage 3 CKD via the MDRD study equation to no CKD via the CKD-EPI equation were at similar risk for cardiovascular events as those not classified as having CKD. This patient has stage 3 CKD according to the MDRD study equation but does not have CKD when using the CKD-EPI equation (estimated GFR of 61 mL/min/1.73 m²). Although this value is still low, it is likely more accurate. The patient should be counseled to continue maintaining a healthy lifestyle, minimizing cardiovascular risk factors. Many Web sites (such as www.nephron.com) are available that allow physicians to easily calculate these values.

The Cockcroft-Gault method of assessing kidney function also tends to underestimate GFR at higher values and would not be expected to yield more accurate information than the MDRD study equation compared with the CKD-EPI equation.

Experts now recommend use of either a 24-hour urine collection for creatinine clearance or radionuclide kidney

Answers and Critiques

clearance scanning to obtain a precise estimation of kidney function, which is needed in circumstances such as the evaluation of living donor kidney transplant candidates. Properly collecting a 24-hour urine specimen is difficult, and over- or undercollection of a sample provides an inaccurate estimation of the GFR. Radionuclide kidney clearance scanning is more invasive and more expensive than an estimated GFR. This patient does not require a precise measurement of her kidney function because such a measurement is unlikely to change prognosis or treatment.

KEY POINT

- The Chronic Kidney Disease Epidemiology Collaboration equation performs better at higher (normal) values of glomerular filtration rate.

Bibliography

Levey AS, Stevens LA. Estimating GFR using the CKD Epidemiology Collaboration (CKD-EPI) creatinine equation: more accurate GFR estimates, lower CKD prevalence estimates, and better risk predictions. Am J Kidney Dis. 2010;55(4):622-627. [PMID: 20338463]

Item 29   Answer: A

Educational Objective: Manage hypertension in a patient with type 2 diabetes mellitus.

The addition of the calcium channel blocker diltiazem is indicated to manage hypertension in this patient who also has type 2 diabetes mellitus. Patients with diabetes and hypertension are at substantial cardiovascular risk. Managing high blood pressure is an effective way to reduce this risk, but debate exists regarding goal blood pressure levels. The American Diabetes Association and the National Kidney Foundation currently consider a target blood pressure goal of less than 130/80 mm Hg to be appropriate for most patients with diabetes, regardless of age, although modifications to this goal are reasonable based on individual patient characteristics and tolerance and side effects of antihypertensive treatment. This patient's blood pressure is substantially above this target; therefore, the use of diltiazem or a β-blocker is reasonable.

Thiazide diuretics are not effective in patients with an estimated glomerular filtration rate of less than 30 mL/min/1.73 m²; these patients require a loop diuretic such as furosemide for effective volume control. This patient has no indication for a loop diuretic either on the basis of kidney function or signs of volume overload.

In most patients with hypertension in the absence of microalbuminuria, combined therapy with an ACE inhibitor and an angiotensin receptor blocker is not indicated because the risk of hyperkalemia and decreased kidney function outweighs the benefit. A calcium channel blocker such as diltiazem will be equally effective in controlling the blood pressure without the added risk.

Spironolactone is useful in patients who remain hypertensive despite three-drug therapy at optimal dosages. This patient does not meet this criterion. Furthermore, spironolactone can cause an increase in the serum potassium level, which is undesirable in this patient whose potassium level is near the upper limit of the normal range.

KEY POINT

- The target blood pressure goal for most patients with hypertension and diabetes mellitus is less than 130/80 mm Hg; this goal may need to be appropriately modified based on patient characteristics and response to therapy.

Bibliography

The American Diabetes Association. Standards of Medical Care–2012. Diabetes Care. 2012;35(suppl 1):S11-S63. [PMID: 22187469]

Item 30   Answer: B

Educational Objective: Manage hypercalciuria in a patient with nephrolithiasis.

In addition to recommending adequate fluid intake, treatment with a thiazide diuretic such as chlorthalidone is indicated for this patient with hypercalciuria and probable calcium oxalate nephrolithiasis. Hypercalciuria, defined as a urine calcium level greater than 300 mg/24 h (7.5 mmol/24 h), is the most common metabolic factor associated with calcium oxalate kidney stones. This patient has low urine volume and idiopathic hypercalciuria, which occurs in the setting of a normal serum calcium level and no other clear cause. Idiopathic hypercalciuria is associated with a family history of nephrolithiasis, as noted by this patient who also recently passed kidney stones. Imaging was performed in this patient to assess the stone burden or stones that have already formed within the kidney before the onset of treatment. This imaging strategy, appropriately done with plain radiography for radiopaque calcium oxalate stones, is important because if symptoms of nephrolithiasis develop during treatment, physicians can then determine whether these are related to stones that were present before therapy or new stones that developed despite treatment. The mainstay of therapy is a thiazide diuretic such as chlorthalidone, which can promote distal reabsorption of calcium.

A calcium-restricted diet is not advised for this patient; paradoxically, a low calcium diet is associated with an increase in nephrolithiasis. In addition, chronically limiting calcium intake may have long-term implications on bone mineral density and eventual fracture risk.

Potassium supplements may be needed to offset potassium loss caused by thiazide diuretics, although this is not a primary treatment for calcium oxalate nephrolithiasis. If potassium supplementation is needed, potassium citrate, rather than potassium chloride, would be preferable because the citrate also serves to chelate calcium and limit crystallization.

Alkalinization of the urine may help increase the solubility of calcium oxalate; however, potassium citrate is usually prescribed rather than sodium citrate. Sodium increases urine calcium and may exacerbate this patient's tendency to hypercalciuria. Also, significant alkalinization may lead to calcium phosphate stones because these are less soluble in an alkaline pH.

KEY POINT

- **The mainstay of therapy for idiopathic hyper-calciuria is a thiazide diuretic.**

Bibliography

Worcester EM, Coe FL. Clinical practice. Calcium kidney stones. N Engl J Med. 2010;363(10):954-963. [PMID: 20818905]

Item 31   Answer: A

Educational Objective: Diagnose lead nephrotoxicity.

Chelation mobilization testing is the most appropriate next diagnostic study for this patient. Lead may be the cause of this patient's kidney injury based on his exposure history and other clinical and laboratory findings consistent with lead toxicity (hypertension and gout). Chronic kidney disease (CKD) resulting from lead typically occurs from chronic lead exposure, often in industrial settings, resulting in high blood levels. However, because more than 90% of the total body lead burden resides in the bones, blood levels may not be an adequate indicator of lead exposure over time, particularly if the acute exposure has been discontinued, as in this patient. Therefore, his normal blood lead level does not exclude lead as a potential cause of his CKD. Administration of the chelating agent calcium disodium ethylenediaminetetraacetic acid (EDTA), which mobilizes lead deposited in the tissues, is measured in the urine and can be used to assess for previous lead exposure. If this study reveals a high degree of lead excretion, chelation can then be used as therapy. Lead nephrotoxicity causes a chronic tubulointerstitial nephritis resulting in low-grade proteinuria, with rare leukocytes and erythrocytes in the urine sediment. Other kidney findings result in a Fanconi-like syndrome, with glycosuria in the setting of normoglycemia, hyperuricemia, hypophosphatemia, and aminoaciduria.

Erythrocyte protoporphyrin levels increase with active lead exposure but do not reflect the total body lead burden and are not helpful in detecting significant past lead exposure.

Lead lines seen on long bone radiographs are caused by increased density of the metaphysis of growing bones because of lead exposure and are therefore seen primarily in growing children exposed to high levels of lead; this testing is not effective in diagnosing lead exposure in adults.

The finding of basophilic stippling of erythrocytes on a peripheral blood smear is seen in lead toxicity. However, this finding is also seen in other conditions, such as megaloblastic anemia, and is not adequately specific for use in diagnosing lead toxicity.

KEY POINT

- **In patients with suspected lead nephrotoxicity, chelation mobilization testing may be required in those with normal blood lead levels.**

Bibliography

Ekong EB, Jaar BG, Weaver VM. Lead-related nephrotoxicity: a review of the epidemiologic evidence. Kidney Int. 2006;70(12):2074. [PMID: 17063179]

Item 32   Answer: C

Educational Objective: Recognize risk factors for damaging veins in patients with chronic kidney disease.

An attempt should be made to continue the use of peripheral intravenous access for antibiotic administration in this patient. In patients with chronic kidney disease who may eventually require hemodialysis, preservation of the patency of the central venous system is an important consideration in medical management. Stenosis of the central veins may render a patient's arm unsuitable for placement of a temporary dialysis catheter or an arteriovenous fistula or graft, which is the preferred access for long-term hemodialysis. Central vein stenosis most commonly results from endothelial damage due to mechanical trauma associated with centrally placed venous catheters.

There is currently no indication for placement of a temporary dialysis catheter in this patient given his stable kidney function; they also impart a significantly increased risk of central vein injury. Additionally, it is preferable to use a dedicated hemodialysis catheter for kidney replacement therapy and not for other interventions such as infusion of intravenous fluids or antibiotics.

Rates of stenosis depend on the type and location of the central catheter being used and the duration it is in place. Catheters in the subclavian position may have stenosis rates as high as 50%, whereas those in the right internal jugular position tend to have the lowest rate of stenosis (10%) because their anatomic location leads to less mechanical trauma. If central access is necessary in a high-risk patient, use of the right internal jugular vein is preferred.

Although they are inserted peripherally, peripherally inserted central catheter (PICC) lines may also cause central vein stenosis as well as thrombosis and occlusion of the peripheral veins, which may complicate the placement of long-term hemodialysis access. If a PICC line is used, it should only be placed after a multidisciplinary discussion between the nephrologist and access team in order to choose a site that will best preserve future dialysis access sites.

- Patients with chronic kidney disease may ultimately need dialysis, and maintaining vein patency will make future arteriovenous hemodialysis access creation (fistula or graft) possible.

Bibliography

Hoggard J, Saad T, Schon D, Vesely TM, Royer T; American Society of Diagnostic and Interventional Nephrology, Clinical Practice Committee; Association for Vascular Access. Guidelines for venous access in patients with chronic kidney disease. A Position Statement from the American Society of Diagnostic and Interventional Nephrology, Clinical Practice Committee and the Association for Vascular Access [erratum in Semin Dial. 2009;22(2):221-222]. Semin Dial. 2008;21(2):186-191. [PMID: 18364015]

Item 33   Answer: B

Educational Objective: Evaluate a patient with high blood pressure.

Electrocardiography is the most appropriate next step for this patient with high blood pressure. The evaluation of a patient with high blood pressure is directed toward determining if the blood pressure is elevated as a primary phenomenon or is secondary to another cause, if there are other cardiovascular risk factors present, and if there is evidence of target organ damage. Electrocardiography is a means of assessing for the presence of cardiac effects of sustained blood pressure elevation. On electrocardiogram, cardiac damage from hypertension is manifested by the presence of left ventricular hypertrophy and possibly Q waves. These findings also indicate high risk for cardiovascular events. Measures of kidney function are also used to evaluate for possible end-organ damage due to sustained hypertension. The European Society of Hypertension guidelines also recommend evaluation for microalbuminuria, but guidelines from the Seventh Report of the Joint National Committee on Prevention, Detection, Evaluation, and Treatment of High Blood Pressure (JNC 7) advocate that this testing remain optional. Measurement of lipids is useful in assessing for other cardiovascular risks.

Drug treatment is recommended when blood pressure remains above 140/90 mm Hg in patients younger than 80 years of age. However, β-blockers such as atenolol are no longer universally recommended as first-line agents in the absence of a compelling indication. JNC 7, the European Society of Hypertension, and the World Health Organization/International Society of Hypertension guidelines continue to recommend these agents for patients with a history of myocardial infarction and heart failure.

Home blood pressure monitoring is reasonable if white coat hypertension is suspected; however, it is more important to finish the initial evaluation of this patient, which lacks an electrocardiography. This patient's retinal arteriolar changes support target organ effect of blood pressure, particularly in this patient who is young, making white coat hypertension less likely.

Secondary hypertension should be considered in patients with hypertension who have atypical clinical features (onset at a young age, absent family history, severe hypertension) and are resistant to antihypertensive therapy. Spontaneous hypokalemia is strongly suggestive of primary hyperaldosteronism, and the plasma aldosterone-plasma renin activity ratio (ARR) is a screening test for primary hyperaldosteronism. This patient has no features suggestive of a secondary cause of hypertension, including hypokalemia, and screening with an ARR is not needed.

- Evaluation of a patient with high blood pressure includes determining if the blood pressure is elevated as a secondary phenomenon, if there are other cardiovascular risk factors present, and if there is evidence of target organ damage.

Bibliography

American College of Physicians. In the clinic. Hypertension. Ann Intern Med. 2008;149(11):ITC6(1-15). [PMID: 19047024]

Item 34   Answer: B

Educational Objective: Treat a patient who has uric acid stones.

Allopurinol is indicated for this patient who has recurrent uric acid stones despite alkalinization of the urine. Patients who develop uric acid stones typically have low urine volume or hyperuricosuria. The latter may result from a high protein diet (as in this patient) or rapid purine metabolism as in tumor lysis syndrome. Other risk factors include gout, conditions associated with uric acid overproduction, diabetes mellitus, the metabolic syndrome, and chronic diarrhea. This patient also has inconsistent fluid intake, a relatively high urine uric acid level, and low urine volume, all of which are significant risk factors for development of uric acid nephrolithiasis. Treatment with potassium citrate to alkalinize the urine is often sufficient to decrease the risk for recurrent stones, with the goal of increasing the urine pH to greater than 6.0. This patient continues to have recurrent uric acid nephrolithiasis despite his urine pH being appropriately alkaline. In addition to encouraging more aggressive daily oral hydration and a diet with limited animal protein, seafood, and yeast, the next appropriate step in management is to begin a xanthine oxidase inhibitor to lower uric acid production and urine excretion.

Acetazolamide can alkalinize the urine, but chronic use may lead to a metabolic acidosis and is therefore not typically used for this purpose. Instead, efforts at increasing the urine alkalinization, if necessary, would focus on the dose and frequency of potassium citrate.

Calcium carbonate is often utilized for high urine oxalate excretion from enteric hyperoxaluria, which is not seen in this patient.

A thiazide diuretic such as chlorthalidone is not appropriate for this patient, because thiazide diuretics tend to increase the serum uric acid level and could increase his propensity to develop gout.

KEY POINT

- In addition to urine alkalinization, treatment with allopurinol is indicated for patients who have recurrent uric acid stones.

Bibliography

Goldfarb DS. In the clinic. Nephrolithiasis. Ann Intern Med. 2009;151(3):ITC2. [PMID: 19652185]

Item 35   Answer: A

Educational Objective: Diagnose AL amyloidosis.

The most likely diagnosis is AL amyloidosis, which most frequently affects the kidneys and the heart. Kidney involvement usually is manifested by the nephrotic syndrome with progressive worsening of kidney function. Amyloid deposition in the heart results in rapidly progressive heart failure caused by restrictive cardiomyopathy. Hepatomegaly commonly occurs and is caused by congestion from right-sided heart failure or by amyloid infiltration. A painful, bilateral, symmetric, distal, sensory neuropathy that progresses to motor neuropathy is the usual neurologic manifestation in AL amyloidosis. Amyloidosis is classified according to the type of protein deposited. AL amyloidosis is the most common type of systemic amyloidosis in the United States. The precursor protein is a monoclonal light chain, usually of the lambda isotype. In patients with suspected amyloidosis, a fat pad aspirate with Congo red staining is a minimally invasive and high-value diagnostic test. A rectal biopsy is another diagnostic option, and kidney biopsy should be considered if these studies are nondiagnostic. Serum and urine protein electrophoresis with immunoelectrophoresis is used to detect the monoclonal light chain in this disease. Up to 20% of patients with AL amyloidosis also have a coexisting multiple myeloma or other lymphoproliferative disease.

Although diabetes mellitus may lead to proteinuria and decreased kidney function, this patient does not have evidence of underlying diabetes, and this diagnosis would not explain his other clinical findings.

Patients with polyarteritis nodosa typically present with fever, abdominal pain, arthralgia, and weight loss that develop over days to months. Two thirds of these patients have mononeuritis multiplex, and one third have hypertension, testicular pain, and cutaneous involvement, including nodules, ulcers, purpura, and livedo reticularis. Polyarteritis nodosa is not associated with heart failure, hepatomegaly, macroglossia, or the nephrotic syndrome.

Although primary membranous glomerulopathy is more common than AL amyloidosis, only the latter manifests as a systemic disease. Macroglossia, systolic heart failure, peripheral neuropathy, and elevated serum total protein levels are not seen in primary membranous glomerulopathy.

KEY POINT

- AL amyloidosis most frequently affects the kidneys and the heart; kidney involvement usually is manifested by the nephrotic syndrome with progressive worsening of kidney function.

Bibliography

Zhu X, Liu F, Liu Y, et al. Analysis of clinical and pathological characteristics of 28 cases with renal amyloidosis. Clin Lab. 2011;57(11-12):947-952. [PMID: 22239026]

Item 36   Answer: A

Educational Objective: Diagnose Liddle syndrome.

The most likely diagnosis is Liddle syndrome, a rare autosomal dominant disorder that presents with early-onset hypertension often accompanied by metabolic alkalosis and hypokalemia. The syndrome results from an activating mutation of the epithelial sodium channel in the cortical collecting duct. The findings of hypertension, hypokalemia, metabolic alkalosis, and suppressed renin and aldosterone levels are consistent with a syndrome of apparent mineralocorticoid excess. 24-Hour urine free cortisol is normal in this patient, which excludes familial syndrome of apparent mineralocorticoid excess, congenital adrenal hyperplasia, Cushing syndrome, and 5-reductase deficiency. Patients with Liddle syndrome are treated with amiloride or triamterene, which directly inhibits sodium uptake through the epithelial sodium channel.

The absence of headaches, sweating, and palpitations in this patient with findings consistent with a syndrome of apparent mineralocorticoid excess argues against the diagnosis of pheochromocytoma.

Primary hyperaldosteronism is unlikely because the serum aldosterone level is suppressed as a result of the primary kidney sodium retention and expansion of the extracellular fluid volume.

Renin and aldosterone levels are elevated in patients with renovascular hypertension, which is defined as hypertension caused by narrowing of one or more of the renal arteries. Underperfusion and ischemia of the kidneys lead to stimulation of the renin-angiotensin system. This patient does not have the findings associated with renovascular hypertension.

KEY POINT

- Liddle syndrome is a rare autosomal dominant disorder that presents with early-onset hypertension and is often accompanied by metabolic alkalosis, hypokalemia, and suppressed renin and aldosterone levels.

Bibliography

Lin SH, Yang SS, Chau T. A practical approach to genetic hypokalemia. Electrolyte Blood Press. 2010;8(1):38-50. [PMID: 21468196]

Item 37   Answer: B

Educational Objective: Manage overcorrection of hypotonic hyponatremia.

The most appropriate treatment for this patient is 5% dextrose in water. This patient has hypotonic hyponatremia associated with altered mentation, which typically warrants prompt correction with 3% saline. However, the increase in her serum sodium level following treatment exceeds the recommended initial target of 4 to 6 meq/L (4-6 mmol/L) over the first 24 hours. The high urine volume and decreasing urine osmolality following hypertonic saline administration reflect a rapid water diuresis and suggest that the serum sodium level will likely continue to increase, placing the patient at increased risk for osmotic demyelination syndrome (ODS). Therefore, hypotonic solutions such as 5% dextrose in water should be administered with close follow-up of the serum sodium level, with the goal of maintaining the serum sodium level in the range of 114 to 116 meq/L (114-116 mmol/L) in the first 24 hours.

Administration of 0.9% saline would result in continued increases in the serum sodium level in this patient undergoing a water diuresis, thereby placing her at risk for ODS.

Fluid restriction is indicated to manage hyponatremia due to the syndrome of inappropriate antidiuretic hormone secretion but would exacerbate overly rapid correction of the serum sodium level in this patient who is undergoing a water diuresis and has a rapidly rising serum sodium level.

Tolvaptan, a V_2 receptor antagonist, inhibits the activity of the antidiuretic hormone, thereby decreasing water uptake in the collecting ducts and promoting a water diuresis. This agent would augment the increase in the serum sodium level, exacerbating overcorrection of hyponatremia in this patient.

KEY POINT

- When overcorrection of the sodium concentration has occurred in the management of euvolemic hypotonic hyponatremia, administration of 5% dextrose in water is appropriate to lower the serum sodium level.

Bibliography

Sterns RH, Hix JK. Overcorrection of hyponatremia is a medical emergency. Kidney Int. 2009;76(6):587-589. [PMID: 19721422]

Item 38   Answer: B

Educational Objective: Manage cardiorenal syndrome.

Initiation of intravenous furosemide is appropriate for this patient with cardiorenal syndrome. There is intricate physiologic interaction that occurs between the heart and the kidneys, and the term cardiorenal syndrome is used when one organ system dysfunction affects another. This patient's cardiorenal syndrome was likely precipitated by the intravenous fluid therapy given during his 3-day hospitalization. In the setting of baseline chronic kidney disease and heart failure, sodium excretion is impaired, and patients have difficulty managing the increased sodium load effectively, even if only maintenance rates of normal saline are administered. Impaired sodium excretion can lead to volume overload that, in turn, leads to decreased cardiac output based on the limited ability of the heart to compensate for an increase in preload. Treatment to enhance sodium excretion by the kidneys should be initiated, and an intravenous loop diuretic is appropriate for this patient. Although there is often some hesitancy to give diuretics to patients with a rising serum creatinine level, intravenous furosemide is appropriate in this setting of volume overload.

Administering more intravenous fluid is often a reflexive response to a rising serum creatinine level. However, in the setting of volume overload, this treatment may worsen this patient's medical condition.

Although ACE inhibitors are useful in managing chronic heart failure, increasing the lisinopril dose at this time will not immediately address the volume overload, which is precipitating this patient's symptoms.

Increasing the metoprolol dose would address a heart rate that is high for chronic heart failure; however, a β-blocker should not be increased in acute decompensated heart failure. It also would not address the underlying issue of volume overload, which is driving this patient's pathophysiology and increased pulse rate.

KEY POINT

- Diuretics may be indicated in the setting of a rising serum creatinine level for patients with cardiorenal syndrome.

Bibliography

Ronco C, Haapio M, House AA, Anavekar N, Bellomo R. Cardiorenal syndrome. J Am Coll Cardiol. 2008;52(19):1527-1539. [PMID: 19007588]

Item 39   Answer: D

Educational Objective: Manage hypertension in a patient with chronic kidney disease.

Switching from hydrochlorothiazide to furosemide is indicated to manage resistant hypertension in this patient with chronic kidney disease (CKD). Resistant hypertension is defined as blood pressure that remains above goal despite treatment with the optimal dosages of three antihypertensive agents of different classes, including a diuretic. If a patient has CKD and uncontrolled blood pressure on hydrochlorothiazide, switching to a loop diuretic should be a first consideration. Although this patient takes antihypertensive medications from four different classes, his blood pressure measurements remain high. Hydrochlorothiazide is likely ineffective in this patient with an estimated glomerular filtration rate (GFR) of less than 30 mL/min/1.73 m². Therefore, changing hydrochlorothiazide to the loop diuretic furosemide dosed twice daily is appropriate. His edema on examination as well as his high blood pressure and lack of orthostasis indicate he is not hypovolemic and may be hypervolemic. Adding a loop diuretic has the added benefit of keeping the serum potassium level low because hyperkalemia is often a complication in patients with CKD.

Most patients with CKD and hypertension are hypervolemic, and a diuretic should be added to multidrug regimens in order to control hypertension. Adding a diuretic is preferred to adding drugs from other classes because the addition of an effective diuretic is likely to be more efficacious, associated with fewer side effects, and offers the convenience of single or twice daily dosing compared with other options, including hydralazine and clonidine.

Adding the angiotensin receptor blocker valsartan to an ACE inhibitor such as lisinopril may increase the chance of hyperkalemia and has not been shown to improve outcomes. In fact, the incidence of hyperkalemia and need for dialysis due to hyperkalemia may be higher in patients on both ACE inhibitors and angiotensin receptor blockers.

KEY POINT

- **Thiazide diuretics are less effective antihypertensive agents than loop diuretics in patients with an estimated glomerular filtration rate of less than 30 mL/min/1.73 m².**

Bibliography

Sarafidis PA, Bakris GL. Resistant hypertension: an overview of evaluation and treatment. J Am Coll Cardiol. 2008;52(22):1749-1757. [PMID: 19022154]

Item 40   Answer: D
Educational Objective: Diagnose glomerular hematuria.

The most appropriate diagnostic tests to perform next are a urine protein–creatinine ratio and a serum creatinine measurement to determine the degree of proteinuria and level of kidney function. This patient has microscopic hematuria that appears glomerular in origin. Glomerular hematuria on urine microscopy is characterized by the presence of dysmorphic erythrocytes or acanthocytes, which are erythrocytes that retain a ring shape but have "blebs" protruding from their membrane, giving them a characteristic shape (compared with acanthocytes in the blood, in which the membrane protrusions appear to have a "spiked" shape). Significant hematuria may also be associated with the presence of erythrocyte casts. These findings are highly associated with a glomerular etiology of bleeding and are specifically suggestive of glomerulonephritis. Urine microscopy in patients with glomerular disease also may detect intact erythrocytes; however, these are less specific for glomerular disease.

After determining this patient's degree of proteinuria and level of kidney function, a further evaluation for glomerular disease may include complement levels, a hepatitis panel, and blood cultures as well as testing for antinuclear antibodies, ANCA, anti–glomerular basement membrane antibodies, and antistreptolysin O antibodies. Depending on the serologic test results, this patient may undergo a kidney biopsy to determine the cause of the glomerulonephritis.

If this patient's asymptomatic microscopic hematuria were nonglomerular in origin, ultrasonography would be appropriate; she will likely not require a cystoscopy.

There is no indication that this patient has a urinary tract infection (negative leukocyte esterase and absent leukocytes on microscopic urinalysis); therefore, a urine culture is not indicated.

KEY POINT

- **Glomerular hematuria on urine microscopy is characterized by the presence of dysmorphic erythrocytes or acanthocytes, and significant hematuria may also be associated with the presence of erythrocyte casts; these findings are specifically suggestive of glomerulonephritis.**

Bibliography

Cohen RA, Brown RS. Microscopic hematuria. N Engl J Med. 2003;348(23):2330-2338. [PMID: 12788998]

Item 41   Answer: D
Educational Objective: Screen for chronic kidney disease.

This patient should be screened for chronic kidney disease (CKD) with a serum creatinine measurement, estimated glomerular filtration rate (GFR), and urinalysis. Recognizing patients at risk for CKD is imperative in a disease that can be asymptomatic. Certain medical history, including diabetes mellitus and hypertension, and predisposing risk factors should prompt screening for CKD. In particular, evaluation for diseases that can damage the kidneys directly (such as scleroderma) or can cause damage through their treatment (such as cisplatin) is indicated. A family history of CKD is a risk factor, as more evidence points to an inherited predisposition to CKD. A history of acute kidney injury (AKI) is recognized as a risk for future AKI and CKD. Various genitourinary abnormalities also can cause CKD. Screening for CKD includes measurement of the

Answers and Critiques

serum creatinine level and estimation of GFR as well as urinalysis to evaluate for blood, protein, and casts. Although evidence is lacking that targeted screening improves clinical outcomes, the National Kidney Foundation guidelines recommend targeted screening for CKD. Guidelines, however, do not support screening of the general population for kidney disease.

A 24-hour urine collection for creatinine clearance is generally used to obtain a precise estimation of kidney function, which is needed in circumstances such as the evaluation of living donor kidney transplant candidates. It is not a screening test for CKD because of the difficulty in obtaining the specimen correctly and its inconvenience.

Kidney imaging (usually ultrasonography) should be considered if the serum creatinine level or urinalysis is abnormal. Except for patients with a family history of polycystic kidney disease, it is not an initial screening study for CKD.

Radionuclide kidney clearance scanning is considered the gold standard for estimating GFR in healthy persons and in those with AKI. However, use of these studies is limited because of cost, lack of widespread availability, and operator technical difficulties.

KEY POINT

- **Patients with a family history of chronic kidney disease should be screened for the disease.**

Bibliography

Drawz P, Rahman M. In the clinic. Chronic kidney disease. Ann Intern Med. 2009;150(3):ITC2-1-ITC2-15. [PMID: 19189903]

Item 42   Answer: E

Educational Objective: Manage chronic kidney disease–mineral bone disorder.

This patient should maintain her current therapeutic regimen without changes. Use of bisphosphonates such as risedronate in patients with chronic kidney disease (CKD) is controversial for several reasons. Firstly, patients with reduced glomerular filtration rate (GFR) were excluded from most studies on the safety and efficacy of these agents. Also, because bisphosphonates adhere to bone mineral, they may lead to adynamic bone disease. Finally, bone disease is common in patients with CKD, but bone mineral density studies are not able to differentiate osteoporosis from other bone disorders that do not respond to treatment with a bisphosphonate. When administered, a significant percentage of bisphosphonates is taken up by bone and blocks osteoclast activity. The remainder is excreted unchanged by the kidney by both glomerular filtration and active secretion in the proximal tubule. For this reason, the dose must be reduced in patients with stage 3 CKD. When the GFR is less than 30 mL/min/1.73 m^2, most experts agree that these agents should be discontinued altogether unless there is a compelling indication or a bone biopsy is performed that confirms the presence of osteoporosis and there are indications to treat with a bisphosphonate, such as a fracture.

Cinacalcet is a calcimimetic used to manage secondary hyperparathyroidism in patients who cannot tolerate vitamin D analogs because of a tendency to develop hypercalcemia. Currently, it is only FDA approved for patients who have end-stage kidney disease. This patient does not have significant secondary hyperparathyroidism. For patients with stage 4 CKD, the target for intact parathyroid hormone is to maintain the parathyroid hormone at the normal range; this patient's level is at the upper limit of normal at 65 pg/mL (65 ng/L).

Sevelamer is used to treat patients with kidney disease who have high serum phosphorus levels. This agent is not indicated at this point because the patient's serum phosphorus level is normal.

Data are lacking on the most appropriate dose of calcium supplementation. High doses should be avoided; however, this patient takes 1000 mg/d, which is within the recommendations to keep total dietary calcium, calcium supplements, or calcium-containing phosphate binders below 2 grams daily.

KEY POINT

- **Bisphosphonates generally should not be used in patients with an estimated glomerular filtration rate of less than 30 mL/min/1.73 m^2.**

Bibliography

Gordon PL, Frassetto LA. Management of osteoporosis in CKD stages 3 to 5. Am J Kidney Dis. 2010;55(5):941-956. [PMID: 20438987]

Item 43   Answer: C

Educational Objective: Manage renovascular hypertension.

Doppler ultrasonography of the renal arteries is indicated for this patient with probable renovascular hypertension. Underperfusion and ischemia of the kidneys lead to stimulation of the renin-angiotensin system, with sodium retention and increased volume contributing to hypertension. Identification of renal artery stenosis and subsequent renal revascularization only improves hypertension in patients with an anatomic lesion that is hemodynamically significant and sufficiently severe to activate the renin-angiotensin system. Therefore, evaluation of renal artery stenosis in patients with suspected atherosclerotic renovascular hypertension should only be considered in patients with accelerated, resistant hypertension and possibly in those with evidence of atherosclerosis whose serum creatinine levels acutely increase after treatment with renin-angiotensin system blockers. This patient has accelerated, drug-resistant hypertension (blood pressure that exceeds the target goal despite taking three antihypertensive drugs, one of which is a diuretic). Doppler ultrasonography of the renal arteries offers a noninvasive estimate of renal artery patency and kidney size.

The addition of an ACE inhibitor to this patient's medication regimen could increase her serum creatinine level if she has significant bilateral renovascular disease and is therefore not indicated.

Increasing the β-blocker dose is not warranted because this patient's pulse rate is 60/min, and such an increase may result in symptomatic bradycardia.

Kidney angiography is the gold standard for the diagnosis of renal artery stenosis but is invasive and associated with several risks, including a large load of contrast dye that may precipitate acute kidney injury in susceptible persons. In addition, in an atherosclerotic aorta, the angiography catheter may disrupt a plaque with subsequent release of cholesterol emboli.

KEY POINT

- Evaluation of renal artery stenosis in patients with suspected atherosclerotic renovascular hypertension should only be considered in patients with accelerated, resistant hypertension and possibly in those with evidence of atherosclerosis whose serum creatinine levels acutely increase after treatment with renin-angiotensin system blockers.

Bibliography

Dworkin LD, Cooper CJ. Clinical practice. Renal-artery stenosis. N Engl J Med. 2009;361(20):1972-1978. [PMID: 19907044]

Item 44   Answer: B

Educational Objective: Identify the cause of hyperkalemia.

Celecoxib toxicity is the most likely cause of this patient's hyperkalemia. Regulation of kidney potassium excretion is dependent upon the renin-angiotensin-aldosterone system. NSAIDs such as celecoxib are known to inhibit renin synthesis, resulting in hyporeninemic hypoaldosteronism, decreased potassium excretion, and hyperkalemia. The ability of the kidney to excrete potassium in hyperkalemic patients can be assessed by calculating the transtubular potassium gradient (TTKG), an index that estimates the ratio of potassium in the cortical collecting duct to that in the peritubular capillaries. The TTKG is calculated by the following equation:

TTKG = [Urine Potassium ÷ (Urine Osmolality/Plasma Osmolality)] ÷ Serum Potassium

In general, the TTKG in a patient on a normal diet is 8 to 9 and should be greater than 10 in hyperkalemic states, reflecting excretion of excess potassium. This patient's TTKG of 2.5 is consistent with a defect in kidney potassium excretion in the presence of a high serum potassium level. The temporal relationship of starting celecoxib

in the postoperative period and documentation of impaired potassium excretion strongly supports celecoxib toxicity as the cause for this patient's impaired potassium excretion and hyperkalemia.

Patients with bilateral adrenal hemorrhage, which leads to adrenal insufficiency and loss of glucocorticoid and mineralocorticoid activity, typically present with other clinical features such as hypotension, flank pain, fever, or nausea, which are not present in this patient.

High potassium intake is a rare cause of hyperkalemia in patients with normal kidney function and an intact renin-angiotensin-aldosterone system. The TTKG would be expected to be above 10 when dietary intake is the only factor contributing to the hyperkalemia.

Thrombocytosis can induce pseudohyperkalemia, typically when the platelet count exceeds 400,000/microliters (400×10^9/L), but the electrocardiogram changes of hyperkalemia as noted in this patient exclude this diagnosis.

KEY POINT

- NSAIDs such as celecoxib are known to inhibit renin synthesis, resulting in hyporeninemic hypoaldosteronism, decreased potassium excretion, and hyperkalemia.

Bibliography

Nyirenda MJ, Tang JI, Padfield PL, Seckl JR. Hyperkalaemia. BMJ. 2009;339:b4114. [PMID: 19854840]

Item 45   Answer: C

Educational Objective: Identify laxative abuse as the cause of a normal anion gap metabolic acidosis.

This patient with normal kidney function has a normal anion gap metabolic acidosis most likely caused by laxative abuse. The cause of a normal anion gap metabolic acidosis may be characterized by assessing the kidney's ability to excrete an acid load. Excreted acid results in urine ammonium, although these levels are difficult to measure directly. However, urine ammonium excretion may be estimated through assessment of the urine osmolal gap, which is calculated using the following equation:

Urine Ammonium Level (meq/L) $\cong$ Urine Osmolal Gap (mosm/kg H$_2$O)/2

Urine Osmolal Gap = Measured Urine Osmolality − Calculated Urine Osmolality

Calculated Urine Osmolality (mosm/kg H$_2$O) =
2 (Urine Sodium [meq/L] + Urine Potassium [meq/L]) + Urine Urea (mg/dL)/2.8 + Urine Glucose (mg/dL)/18

Because urine ammonium is not directly measured, its presence in the urine represents excreted acid and will increase the measured urine osmolality, whereas the estimated urine osmolality will not reflect the presence of this cation. Patients with predominantly extrarenal losses of bicarbonate have urine ammonium levels above 80 meq/L, whereas those with a primary kidney defect have urine ammonium levels of less than 30 meq/L. This patient's urine osmolal gap is as follows: $290 - (2 \times (22 + 15) + 112/2.8 + 0/18) = 176$. Because the urine ammonium level is approximately one half the urine osmolal gap, or 88 meq/L, this value reflects an appropriate kidney response to the acidemia.

Laxative abuse can lead to chronic diarrhea, resulting in a normal anion gap metabolic acidosis. This occurs when colonic bicarbonate loss exceeds increased ammonium excretion stimulated by acidemia and potassium depletion. The increased urine ammonium excretion observed in this patient with hypokalemia is most consistent with laxative abuse. The urine ammonium level is usually greater than 80 meq/L in diarrheal acidosis unless there is concomitant hypovolemia.

Diuretic abuse and surreptitious vomiting can cause hypokalemic metabolic alkalosis, which is inconsistent with the hypokalemic metabolic acidosis observed in this patient.

Hypokalemic distal (type 1) renal tubular acidosis is associated with marked impairment of urine ammonium excretion due to tubular acidification defects. Unlike this patient, urine ammonium levels would be expected to be less than 30 meq/L despite systemic acidosis.

KEY POINT

- Laxative abuse can lead to chronic diarrhea, resulting in a normal anion gap metabolic acidosis.

Bibliography

Gennari FJ, Weise WJ. Acid-base disturbances in gastrointestinal disease. Clin J Am Soc Nephrol. 2008;3(6):1861-1868. [PMID: 18922984]

Item 46   Answer: A
Educational Objective: Diagnose masked hypertension.

The most appropriate next step in management is to obtain 24-hour ambulatory blood pressure monitoring. Masked hypertension is the most likely cause of this patient's unexplained left ventricular hypertrophy. Masked hypertension is characterized by a normal office blood pressure measurement and high ambulatory blood pressure measurement. This condition may affect up to 10 million persons in the United States. Patients with masked hypertension have a definite increased risk for cardiovascular events compared with patients with normal office and ambulatory blood pressure measurements. Suspicion for masked hypertension is usually raised when the physician is informed of discrepancies between office and home blood pressure readings or the discovery of unexplained findings such as left ventricular hypertrophy. Ambulatory blood pressure monitoring can be used to confirm this diagnosis.

If a diagnosis of hypertrophic cardiomyopathy is suspected despite nondiagnostic echocardiography, cardiac MRI can detect focal areas of ventricular hypertrophy and small areas of scarring, which would support the diagnosis. Echocardiographic findings of hypertrophic cardiomyopathy include asymmetric hypertrophy of the ventricle with preserved systolic function but abnormal diastolic function. This patient's echocardiographic findings are not compatible with hypertrophic cardiomyopathy, and cardiac MRI is not indicated.

There are no clinical trials addressing treatment of masked hypertension. However, treatment is indicated for patients with an elevated average 24-hour ambulatory blood pressure measurement. Initiation of chlorthalidone may be appropriate if masked hypertension is diagnosed with 24-hour ambulatory blood pressure measurement.

The coronary artery calcium (CAC) score correlates with cardiovascular risk but is not a direct measure of the severity of luminal coronary disease, and CAC scores are not indicated for routine screening. CAC measurement may be considered in asymptomatic patients with an intermediate risk of coronary artery disease (10%-20% 10-year risk) because a high CAC score (>400) is an indication for more intensive preventive medical treatment. This patient has no indication for CAC scoring, and it cannot explain the patient's left ventricular hypertrophy.

KEY POINT

- Masked hypertension is characterized by a normal office blood pressure measurement and high ambulatory blood pressure measurement.

Bibliography

Cuspidi C, Negri F, Sala C, Mancia G. Masked hypertension and echocardiographic left ventricular hypertrophy: an updated overview. Blood Press Monit. 2012;17(1):8-13. [PMID: 22183044]

Item 47   Answer: B
Educational Objective: Diagnose hemolytic uremic syndrome.

The most likely cause of this patient's acute kidney injury (AKI) is hemolytic uremic syndrome (HUS), which is caused by some strains of *Escherichia coli*, including the O157:H7 strain that produces Shiga-like toxin (also known as verotoxin). Shiga-like toxin is effective against small blood vessels such as those found in the digestive tract and the kidneys; one specific target for the toxin is the vascular endothelium of the glomerulus, causing cell death, breakdown of the endothelium, hemorrhage, and activation of platelets and inflammatory pathways resulting in intravascular thrombosis and hemolysis. In developing countries, enteric pathogen infections usually develop after ingesting contaminated food or water. This patient manifests the classic triad of microangiopathic hemolytic anemia (anemia, elevated reticulocyte count and lactate dehydrogenase level, low haptoglobin level, and schistocytes on the peripheral blood smear), thrombocytopenia, and AKI in the setting of dysentery caused by an enteric pathogen.

Acute tubular necrosis is an unlikely diagnosis in a patient with microangiopathic hemolytic anemia, thrombocytopenia, and evidence of glomerular damage (erythrocyte casts in the urine). Patients with acute tubular necrosis are more likely to present with muddy brown casts.

Postinfectious glomerulonephritis more commonly occurs after streptococcal and staphylococcal infections and characteristically has a latency period of 7 to 120 days before the onset of AKI. Postinfectious glomerulonephritis is not associated with microangiopathic hemolytic anemia.

Scleroderma renal crisis (SRC) occurs almost exclusively in patients with early diffuse cutaneous systemic sclerosis. This condition is characterized by the acute onset of severe hypertension, kidney failure, and microangiopathic hemolytic anemia. SRC is not associated with bloody diarrhea, and the absence of skin findings makes this diagnosis unlikely.

KEY POINT

- Patients with hemolytic uremic syndrome typically present with the classic triad of microangiopathic hemolytic anemia, thrombocytopenia, and acute kidney injury.

Bibliography

Zipfel PF, Heinen S, Skerka C. Thrombotic microangiopathies: new insights and new challenges. Curr Opin Nephrol Hypertens. 2010;19(4):372-378. [PMID: 20539230]

Item 48   Answer: C
Educational Objective: Diagnose orthostatic proteinuria.

A split urine collection is an appropriate initial evaluation for sustained, isolated proteinuria. Protein excretion may vary based on time of collection and, in a small percentage of children and young adults, with posture. Orthostatic (postural) proteinuria refers to protein excretion that increases during the day but decreases at night during recumbency. Diagnosis of orthostatic proteinuria is established by comparing the urine protein excretion during the day with findings from a separate urine collection obtained during the night. An 8-hour nighttime urine collection containing ≤50 mg of protein is required for diagnosis. Typically, urine protein excretion is less than 1 g/24 h but can rarely be greater than 3 g/24 h. Orthostatic proteinuria is benign and has not been associated with long-term kidney disease. Other benign causes of transient or isolated proteinuria include febrile illnesses and rigorous exercise. Transient or isolated proteinuria is typically benign and does not warrant further evaluation.

Kidney biopsy is recommended when histologic confirmation is needed to help diagnose kidney disease, implement medical therapy, or change medical treatment. Kidney biopsy is used predominantly in patients with glomerular disease, and the most common indications for kidney biopsy include the nephrotic syndrome, acute glomerulonephritis, or kidney transplant dysfunction. It is inappropriate to consider a kidney biopsy before excluding benign causes of proteinuria such as orthostatic proteinuria.

A repeat 24-hour urine collection for protein is unnecessary for this patient who already has a urine dipstick that is positive for albuminuria and a previous 24-hour urine collection (gold standard test) positive for proteinuria.

A spot urine protein–creatinine ratio does not necessarily add more information to an accurately collected 24-hour urine collection.

More than 95% of adults will excrete less than 130 mg/24 h of protein in the urine, and the normal value is defined as less than 150 mg/24 h. Reassurance in this case is incorrect because if orthostatic proteinuria is not established as the cause of the patient's proteinuria, this may be an indication of early kidney dysfunction.

KEY POINT

- A split urine collection is an appropriate initial evaluation for sustained, isolated proteinuria.

Bibliography

Naderi AS, Reilly RF. Primary care approach to proteinuria. J Am Board Fam Med. 2008;21(6):569-574. [PMID: 18988725]

Item 49   Answer: C
Educational Objective: Manage chronic kidney disease.

This patient's antihypertensive therapy should be increased to decrease his average blood pressure readings. Blood pressure control has been shown to delay chronic kidney disease (CKD) progression and reduces cardiovascular risk. Current recommended levels of blood pressure control in patients with CKD are less than 130/80 mm Hg. Sodium restriction is an effective means of controlling blood pressure in all patients with CKD and hypertension. Diuretics are reasonable initial therapy for hypertension in patients with nonproteinuric CKD, particularly if they have edema. Angiotensin blockade (ACE inhibitors or angiotensin receptor blockers) is particularly beneficial in patients with proteinuric CKD. Nondihydropyridine calcium channel blockers also have an antiproteinuric effect, although dihydropyridine calcium channel blockers may be more potent antihypertensives. Delaying CKD progression in patients without proteinuria should focus more on blood pressure control than on the specific agent. In this patient with nonproteinuric CKD, hypertension, and no edema, increasing either of his current antihypertensive agents is reasonable to achieve a desired blood pressure goal.

Administration of sodium bicarbonate has recently been shown to delay CKD progression in patients with stage 4 and 5 disease and initial serum bicarbonate levels of 15 to 20 meq/L (15-20 mmol/L). This patient has stage 3 CKD and a serum bicarbonate level of 22 meq/L (22 mmol/L).

Although this patient has evidence of secondary hyperparathyroidism with a slightly elevated parathyroid hormone (PTH) level, his calcium and phosphorus levels are within normal limits. It would be reasonable to start a 2- to 4-month trial of a low phosphate diet and repeat his laboratory studies. A phosphate binder can be considered if dietary modification does not help or if his phosphorus level increases. Initiating activated vitamin D therapy at this level of PTH is not indicated.

KEY POINT

- **Blood pressure control to a goal of less than 130/80 mm Hg is a key intervention for delaying progression of chronic kidney disease.**

Bibliography

de Galan BE, Perkovic V, Ninomiya T, et al; ADVANCE Collaborative Group. Lowering blood pressure reduces renal events in type 2 diabetes. J Am Soc Nephrol. 2009;20(4):883-892. [PMID: 19225038]

Item 50   Answer: D

Educational Objective: Identify the cause of hypophosphatemia.

This patient's hypophosphatemia is likely due to kidney phosphate wasting caused by proximal (type 2) renal tubular acidosis (RTA) due to ifosfamide nephrotoxicity. Ifosfamide, a synthetic analog of cyclophosphamide, is associated with considerable nephrotoxicity because of direct tubular injury. It commonly induces proximal RTA and other findings that resemble those seen in the Fanconi syndrome (glucosuria and renal phosphate, uric acid, and amino acid wasting) due to tubular dysfunction. Ifosfamide renal toxicity may be minimized primarily by limiting the cumulative dose, if possible. In most patients, tubular function returns to near normal with time after discontinuation of the drug, although in some patients there may be persistent tubular function defects requiring ongoing treatment.

Hypophosphatemia is defined as a serum phosphate concentration less than 2.5 mg/dL (0.81 mmol/L) and is most common in patients with a history of chronic alcohol use, critical illness, and malnutrition. When the cause of hypophosphatemia is uncertain, urine phosphate excretion can be assessed by calculating the fractional excretion of phosphate (FE_{PO4}) from a random urine specimen by the following formula:

$$FE_{PO4} = (\text{Urine Phosphate} \times \text{Serum Creatinine} \times 100) \div$$
$$(\text{Serum Phosphate} \times \text{Urine Creatinine})$$

An FE_{PO4} of less than 5% suggests increased cellular uptake or extrarenal phosphate loss as the cause of the low serum phosphate, whereas a value greater than 5% is consistent with renal phosphate wasting, as seen in this patient, which is consistent with ifosfamide-induced nephrotoxicity.

This patient's history of nausea and anorexia raises the possibility of malnutrition as the cause of the hypophosphatemia; however, the FE_{PO4} should be less than 5% when there is inadequate intake.

Oncogenic osteomalacia is a form of acquired hypophosphatemia associated with kidney phosphate wasting usually seen in patients with small, slow-growing mesenchymal tumors usually located in the craniofacial extremities. Other manifestations of proximal tubular dysfunction, such as glycosuria as noted in this patient, are not characteristic of oncogenic osteomalacia, arguing against this diagnosis. Recent evidence has implicated the phosphaturic hormone fibroblast growth factor-23 (FGF-23) in the pathogenesis of this disorder.

Primary hyperparathyroidism, when severe, can induce hypophosphatemia by inhibiting proximal reabsorption of phosphate. Hypercalcemia generally precedes onset of hypophosphatemia in primary hyperparathyroidism, and glycosuria with normoglycemia as noted in this patient would not be present.

KEY POINT

- **A fractional excretion of phosphate greater than 5% in patients with hypophosphatemia is consistent with renal phosphate wasting.**

Bibliography

Liamis G, Milionis HJ, Elisaf M. Medication-induced hypophosphatemia: a review. QJM. 2010;103(7):449-459. [PMID: 20356849]

Item 51   Answer: B

Educational Objective: Diagnose IgA nephropathy.

The most likely cause of this patient's gross hematuria complicated with acute kidney injury (AKI) is IgA nephropathy. Gross hematuria associated with an episode of respiratory or gastrointestinal infection can be the first clinical presentation of primary IgA nephropathy, which can precipitate AKI. Infections activate mucosal defenses and the production of IgA antibodies, which are deposited in the glomeruli, causing injury and bleeding. The mechanism of AKI is thought to be the combination of several factors: acute tubular necrosis due to tubular obstruction by erythrocyte casts, free hemoglobin and/or iron direct toxicity to tubular epithelium mediated by lipid peroxidation and free radical formation, and hemoglobin being a scavenger of nitric oxide whose reduction results in vasoconstriction and decreased oxygen supply. Patients who have IgA nephropathy presenting with AKI associated with macroscopic hematuria commonly have a good prognosis, with spontaneous recovery after cessation of the hematuria; however, factors such as macroscopic hematuria for more than 10 days, age greater than 50 years, severely decreased glomerular filtration rate (GFR), and severity of tubular damage on kidney biopsy increase the risk of chronic kidney disease. The presence of glomerular crescents on kidney biopsy has also been linked to an unfavorable prognosis and requires the use of immunosuppressive agents in addition to supportive therapy.

NSAIDs, particularly when taken in high doses, may be associated with decreased kidney function and AKI. However, injury is typically not due to glomerular damage, and gross hematuria is an uncommon manifestation of analgesic kidney injury.

Patients with postinfectious glomerulonephritis (PIGN) secondary to streptococcal or staphylococcal infections can present with dark urine and AKI. In this case, this diagnosis is unlikely in the absence of a latency period between the infection and the onset of the kidney disease. Additionally, PIGN usually is accompanied by low complement levels and elevated antistreptolysin O antibodies when associated with streptococcal infections.

Rhabdomyolysis develops when muscle injury leads to the release of myoglobin and other intracellular muscle contents into the circulation, which may lead to AKI. Although this patient may have had muscle pain associated with his respiratory infection, his normal creatine kinase level and negative urine myoglobin exclude this diagnosis.

KEY POINT

- **Gross hematuria associated with an episode of respiratory or gastrointestinal infection can be the first clinical presentation of primary IgA nephropathy.**

Bibliography

Gutiérrez E, González E, Hernández E, et al. Factors that determine an incomplete recovery of renal function in macrohematuria-induced acute renal failure of IgA nephropathy. Clin J Am Soc Nephrol. 2007;2(1):51-57. [PMID: 17699387]

Item 52   Answer: A

Educational Objective: Identify colonic pseudo-obstruction as the cause of hypokalemia.

This patient's hypokalemia is most likely caused by colonic pseudo-obstruction. He has hypokalemia without an obvious concurrent acid-base disorder. Random values of urine potassium can be used to assess the kidney response to hypokalemia but must be corrected for the degree of urinary concentration. This can be achieved by calculating the urine potassium–creatinine ratio (meq/g), which is calculated as follows:

$$\text{Urine Potassium (meq/L)} \times 100\,[(mg \times L)/(dL \times g)] \div \text{Urine Creatinine (mg/dL)}$$

A urine potassium–creatinine ratio above 20 meq/g is consistent with kidney potassium wasting, whereas a value below 15 meq/g suggests extrarenal potassium loss, cellular

redistribution, or decreased intake. This patient's urine potassium–creatinine ratio is 13 meq/g, thus indicating either extrarenal losses of potassium or redistribution. Colonic pseudo-obstruction is associated with up-regulation of potassium channels in the colon, resulting in secretory diarrhea, intestinal potassium loss, and hypokalemia.

Furosemide can cause hypokalemia through direct blockade of potassium uptake in the thick ascending loop of Henle as well as through induction of hypovolemia and secondary hyperaldosteronism. The urine potassium–creatinine ratio, however, should be greater than 20 meq/g, reflecting ongoing urine potassium loss, and not less than 15 meq/g as noted in this patient.

Vomiting and nasogastric suction can induce urine potassium losses by increasing delivery of sodium bicarbonate to the cortical collecting duct, as well as through secondary hyperaldosteronism when there is concurrent hypovolemia. Potassium levels are relatively low in gastric fluid (5-10 meq/L [5-10 mmol/L]), and potassium depletion in patients undergoing nasogastric suction is primarily due to urine potassium losses.

This patient's history does not suggest potassium redistribution (shift of potassium from the extracellular to the intracellular space), and the serum bicarbonate level of 28 meq/L (28 mmol/L) would not be predicted to cause alkalemia to a degree sufficient to shift potassium into cells and cause severe hypokalemia.

KEY POINT

- **Colonic pseudo-obstruction is associated with up-regulation of potassium channels in the colon, resulting in secretory diarrhea, intestinal potassium loss, and hypokalemia.**

Bibliography

Sandle GI, Hunter M. Apical potassium (BK) channels and enhanced potassium secretion in human colon. QJM. 2010;103(2):85-89. [PMID: 19892809]

Item 53   Answer: E

Educational Objective: Manage poststreptococcal glomerulonephritis.

The most appropriate treatment for this patient with poststreptococcal glomerulonephritis is supportive care with antihypertensive agents and diuretics for his hypertension and fluid retention. Poststreptococcal glomerulonephritis, a form of postinfectious glomerulonephritis, is an immunologic disease triggered by an infection, which is followed by the release of immunoglobulins and activation of complement proteins that are deposited in the glomeruli, activating cytokine inflammatory pathways. Acute nephritic syndrome is the typical manifestation of postinfectious glomerulonephritis, regardless of the offending organism, and is characterized by rapid onset of edema, hypertension, oliguria with low urine sodium, and erythrocyte casts in the urine sediment. Most patients with a typical presentation for poststreptococcal glomerulonephritis do not require a kidney biopsy to establish the diagnosis. A biopsy should be considered if the course or findings are atypical for poststreptococcal glomerulonephritis or if there is no clear history or documentation of a prior streptococcal infection. Early treatment of bacterial infections with appropriate antibiotics can prevent or lessen the severity of postinfectious glomerulonephritis. Management of established postinfectious glomerulonephritis is supportive, aiming to control the manifestations of the disease, particularly volume overload with diuretics, antihypertensives, and, if necessary, dialysis.

Less commonly, postinfectious glomerulonephritis can manifest as rapidly progressive glomerulonephritis (RPGN) or as persistent nephritic-nephrotic syndrome that may progress to advanced chronic kidney disease. The management of postinfectious glomerulonephritis presenting as RPGN or persistent nephritic-nephrotic syndrome can require intravenous pulse methylprednisolone, prednisone, cyclophosphamide, cyclosporine, and/or plasmapheresis. However, this patient is in the early course of the disease, and it is premature to consider these aggressive measures for a condition that will most likely resolve spontaneously.

KEY POINT

- **Management of poststreptococcal glomerulonephritis is primarily supportive, with attention to blood pressure and volume control.**

Bibliography

Nadasdy T, Hebert LA. Infection-related glomerulonephritis: understanding mechanisms. Semin Nephrol. 2011;31(4):369-375. [PMID: 21839370]

Item 54   Answer: D

Educational Objective: Diagnose primary membranous glomerulopathy in a patient with long-standing diabetes mellitus.

This patient most likely has primary membranous glomerulopathy, which usually manifests as the nephrotic syndrome, although some patients may have asymptomatic proteinuria. Microscopic hematuria and an absence of erythrocyte casts are common. Factors such as the baseline serum creatinine level and degree of proteinuria determine the rate of disease progression. Membranous glomerulopathy is usually primary but may occur secondary to conditions such as hepatitis B or C virus infection, malaria, syphilis, systemic lupus erythematosus, diabetes mellitus, or rheumatoid arthritis; use of drugs such as NSAIDs, captopril, or penicillamine; and malignancies of the breast, colon, stomach, kidney, or lung. Membranous glomerulopathy is confirmed by kidney biopsy showing characteristic diffuse glomerular membrane thickening without cellular infiltration, and coarsely granular deposits of IgG and C3 along the capillary loops by immunofluorescence microscopy. Electron microscopy shows moderate podocyte foot

process effacement consistent with changes leading to protein leakage from the glomerulus.

It is unlikely to see sudden onset of the nephrotic syndrome as the first manifestation of diabetic nephropathy, and this patient has well-controlled diabetes and no prior evidence of microalbuminuria or microvascular complications such as retinopathy or neuropathy.

Membranous lupus nephritis is unlikely without the diagnosis of lupus, a disease that is more commonly seen in younger women and shows a different pattern of immune complex deposition than in membranous glomerulopathy.

Minimal change glomerulopathy is more common in children and is not an immune complex glomerulonephritis. Minimal change glomerulopathy is characterized by normal light and immunofluorescence microscopies but with effacement of podocyte foot processes on electron microscopy.

KEY POINT

- **Primary membranous glomerulopathy typically manifests as the nephrotic syndrome, and diagnosis is confirmed by kidney biopsy.**

Bibliography

Tarrass F, Anabi A, Zamd M, et al. Idiopathic membranous glomerulonephritis in patients with type 2 diabetes mellitus. Hong Kong J Nephrol. 2005;7(1):34-37.

Item 55   Answer: A

Educational Objective: Manage chronic tubulointerstitial nephritis associated with lithium use.

Amiloride is appropriate for this patient. Long-term lithium exposure can result in chronic tubulointerstitial nephritis. High chronic lithium levels and repeated episodes of lithium toxicity can result in worsening dysfunction. Specific kidney manifestations include a decreased glomerular filtration rate and incomplete distal renal tubular acidosis. Lithium often causes a partial nephrogenic diabetes insipidus, resulting in high urine output and an inability to concentrate the urine. Lithium is reabsorbed along the nephron at sites where sodium is reabsorbed, accumulating in renal tubular cells. In patients with lithium-associated nephrotoxicity, this agent should be discontinued and another appropriate medication used in its place. However, this patient has been unable to do so. In such patients, medication levels should be followed closely so that they are maintained in the therapeutic range. If the agent must be continued, other steps should be considered to mitigate the ongoing damage by the medication. Amiloride directly blocks the epithelial sodium channel and decreases lithium uptake, resulting in less long-term damage.

Restricting water intake will only result in a free water deficit and possible hypernatremia, rather than a decrease in urine output or improvement in kidney function and is therefore not indicated for this patient.

The chronic damage that occurs with lithium is not improved with prednisone, which may be used for patients with acute tubulointerstitial nephritis if there is no improvement after discontinuation of the offending/inciting agent.

Indications for tolvaptan include hypervolemic or euvolemic hyponatremia, chronic heart failure, cirrhosis, and the syndrome of inappropriate antidiuretic hormone secretion. This medication is not used to treat partial nephrogenic diabetes insipidus.

> **KEY POINT**
> - Long-term lithium exposure can result in chronic tubulointerstitial nephritis; if lithium cannot be discontinued, amiloride is indicated to decrease lithium uptake, resulting in less long-term damage.

Bibliography

Grünfeld JP, Rossier BC. Lithium nephrotoxicity revisited. Nat Rev Nephrol. 2009;5(5):270-276. [PMID: 19384328]

Item 56   Answer: B

Educational Objective: Treat a patient who has hyperkalemia.

In addition to intravenous calcium and insulin-dextrose, hemodialysis is appropriate for this patient who has significant hyperkalemia with evidence of cardiac conduction abnormalities, which warrants emergency treatment. Hyperkalemia is defined as a serum potassium concentration greater than 5 meq/L (5 mmol/L). Risk factors include underlying acute or chronic kidney disease and decreased renin-angiotensin-aldosterone activity. Clinical manifestations include ascending muscle weakness, electrocardiographic changes, and life-threatening cardiac arrhythmias and paralysis when the hyperkalemia is severe. Intravenous calcium and insulin-dextrose are temporizing measures to decrease the arrhythmogenic effect of excessive potassium on the myocardium, and definitive therapy ultimately requires potassium removal. The presence of concurrent acute kidney injury (AKI) and recent gastrointestinal surgery in this patient favors use of hemodialysis.

The efficacy of furosemide in promoting a kaliuresis would likely be impaired in this patient with AKI and low urine output and is not considered a reliable method to address this degree of life-threatening hyperkalemia.

Sodium bicarbonate has limited efficacy in the management of hyperkalemia in the setting of end-stage kidney disease or severe AKI. In these populations, the hypokalemic response is often minimal and delayed by several hours, insufficient to bring about a clinically meaningful decrease in the serum potassium level. Conversely, patients with hyperkalemia, hypovolemia, and metabolic acidosis usually respond well to hydration with sodium bicarbonate.

Use of the cation exchange resin sodium polystyrene sulfonate is contraindicated in those who have had recent bowel surgery because these patients are at risk for intestinal necrosis. The risk of this complication appears to be increased in preparations formulated with sorbitol.

> **KEY POINT**
> - Sodium polystyrene sulfonate is contraindicated in the treatment of hyperkalemia in patients with recent bowel surgery.

Bibliography

Elliott MJ, Ronksley PE, Clase CM, Ahmed SB, Hemmelgarn BR. Management of patients with acute hyperkalemia. CMAJ. 2010;182(15):1631-1635. [PMID: 20855477]

Item 57   Answer: C

Educational Objective: Diagnose salicylate toxicity.

This patient most likely has salicylate toxicity. The differential diagnosis of combined increased anion gap metabolic acidosis and respiratory alkalosis includes salicylate toxicity, liver disease, and sepsis. Although intentional or accidental ingestion of aspirin is the most common route of salicylate exposure, toxicity may also occur with cutaneous exposure to salicylate-containing compounds such as oil of wintergreen, which is the most likely source of exposure in this case. Symptoms may include mental status changes, nausea, fever, vomiting, and tinnitus. Pulmonary edema is more common in chronic intoxication, particularly in the elderly population. The anion gap is slightly increased at 14 in this patient, likely reflecting increased serum levels of salicylate. The diagnosis is confirmed by measuring the serum salicylate level.

Metformin toxicity can cause severe lactic acidosis in patients with acute kidney injury on chronic therapy who have an estimated glomerular filtration rate less than 30 mL/min/1.73 m^2, particularly in the setting of critical illness or following acute overdose. This patient's normal serum lactate level excludes this diagnosis.

Methanol poisoning typically presents with an increased anion gap metabolic acidosis and concomitantly increased osmolal gap but does not cause a primary respiratory alkalosis. The osmolal gap, normally less than 10 mosm/kg H$_2$O, is calculated using the following equation:

$$\text{Osmolal Gap} = \text{Measured Plasma Osmolality} - \text{Calculated Plasma Osmolality, where}$$

$$\text{Plasma Osmolality (mosm/kg H}_2\text{O)} = 2 \times \text{Serum Sodium (meq/L)} + \text{Plasma Glucose (mg/dL)}/18 + \text{Blood Urea Nitrogen (mg/dL)}/2.8$$

The osmolal gap in this patient is less than 10 (308 – [(145 × 2) + 158/18 + 15/2.8] = 4), making this diagnosis much less likely.

Sepsis is less likely in this patient given the absence of other features of sepsis such as leukocytosis, lactic acidosis, or hypotension.

- Although ingestion of aspirin is the most common route of salicylate exposure, toxicity may also occur with cutaneous exposure to salicylate-containing compounds such as oil of wintergreen.

Bibliography

Pearlman BL, Gambhir R. Salicylate intoxication: a clinical review. Postgrad Med. 2009;121(4):162-168. [PMID: 19641282]

Item 58   Answer: C

Educational Objective: Manage renovascular hypertension secondary to fibromuscular dysplasia.

Percutaneous transluminal kidney angioplasty is indicated for this patient with renovascular hypertension secondary to fibromuscular dysplasia, a nonatherosclerotic, noninflammatory renovascular disease. Renovascular hypertension due to fibromuscular dysplasia is most commonly caused by medial fibroplasia of the renal artery. On angiogram, the characteristic finding of fibromuscular dysplasia is the "string of beads" appearance of the involved artery, which is apparent in this patient's angiogram. Fibromuscular dysplasia is a disease of unknown cause and most commonly involves the renal and carotid arteries. Hypertension caused by fibromuscular dysplasia is more common in women and usually affects patients between 15 and 30 years of age. Catheter-based kidney angiography is the most accurate method to diagnose this condition. This study is indicated for patients whose clinical presentation raises strong suspicion for fibromuscular disease–related hypertension, such as those with severe resistant hypertension and high plasma renin activity. Revascularization with kidney angioplasty may be performed at the same time as diagnostic angiography. The young age of many patients with fibromuscular dysplasia, such as this 27-year-old woman, reduces the risk of complications from this procedure.

The high likelihood of both technical success and meaningful blood pressure improvement from kidney angioplasty makes drug therapy in this young patient unnecessary at this time.

Surgical revascularization is not first-line treatment for this patient given the higher morbidity. Surgery should be reserved for patients who do not respond to kidney angioplasty or who have arterial anatomy too complex for kidney angioplasty.

- Management of renovascular hypertension secondary to fibromuscular dysplasia may involve revascularization with kidney angioplasty.

Bibliography

Olin JW, Sealove BA. Diagnosis, management, and future developments of fibromuscular dysplasia. J Vasc Surg. 2011;53(3):826-836.e1. [PMID: 21236620]

Item 59   Answer: C

Educational Objective: Manage end-stage kidney disease and Alport syndrome.

Evaluation for kidney transplantation is appropriate for this patient. He has end-stage kidney disease (ESKD) based on his estimated glomerular filtration rate (GFR) of 13 mL/min/1.73 m^2. He also has Alport syndrome, an X-linked disease affecting basement membranes due to a collagen protein synthesis defect. Clinical disease is characterized by sensorineural hearing loss, ocular abnormalities, and a family history of kidney disease and deafness. Patients with this disease can have proteinuria and hematuria, leading to ESKD in the second or third decade. There are no specific therapies for Alport syndrome. Kidney transplantation is the treatment of choice for patients with Alport syndrome and ESKD because the underlying disease does not recur in the transplanted kidney, and patients are relatively young at the time when kidney replacement therapy is indicated.

Everolimus is a derivative of sirolimus that is used as an immunosuppressant and also has a role in the treatment of several types of malignancies. It also has been shown to slow cyst progression in patients with autosomal dominant polycystic kidney disease and possibly slow tumor growth in patients with tuberous sclerosis complex. However, it has no known benefit in Alport syndrome.

Although this patient has ESKD with a very low GFR, he has no clear uremic signs or symptoms; therefore, hemodialysis should not be initiated at this time.

There is some evidence suggesting that angiotensin blockade with either an angiotensin receptor blocker (ARB) or ACE inhibitor may decrease protein excretion and slow the progression of kidney disease in Alport syndrome. This patient is already being treated with an ARB, and there would be no benefit of changing this to an ACE inhibitor such as lisinopril.

- Kidney transplantation is the treatment of choice for patients with Alport syndrome and end-stage kidney disease because the underlying disease does not recur in the transplanted kidney.

Bibliography

Gubler MC. Inherited diseases of the glomerular basement membrane. Nat Clin Pract Nephrol. 2008;4(1):24-37. [PMID: 18094725]

Item 60   Answer: C

Educational Objective: Diagnose postinfectious glomerulonephritis.

The most likely cause of this patient's acute kidney injury (AKI) is postinfectious glomerulonephritis (PIGN). PIGN presents with acute nephritic syndrome characterized by rapid onset of edema, hypertension, oliguria, and erythrocyte casts in the urine sediment. Less commonly, PIGN can manifest as rapidly progressive glomerulonephritis or as persistent nephritic-nephrotic syndrome that may progress to advanced chronic kidney disease (CKD). Diagnosis of PIGN is confirmed when at least three of the following criteria are fulfilled: clinical or laboratory evidence of infection preceding the onset of the disease; low serum complement levels; an exudative-proliferative glomerulonephritis pattern by light microscopy; C3-dominant or co-dominant glomerular staining by immunofluorescence microscopy; and subepithelial humps by electron microscopy. This patient had a documented stable baseline serum creatinine level of 1.4 mg/dL (123.8 micromoles/L) within the first 2 weeks of the infectious event onset before the onset of AKI 2 weeks later accompanied by hypocomplementemia due to activation of both the classic and alternative pathways. PIGN is confirmed by characteristic findings on kidney biopsy.

Diabetic nephropathy alone does not explain the onset of this patient's AKI. The natural history of progressive diabetic nephropathy in patients with type 2 diabetes mellitus is predictable, and decline of the glomerular filtration rate is no greater than 12 to 16 mL/min/1.73 m² per year.

Patients with IgA nephropathy may present with an episode of AKI and macroscopic or gross hematuria concomitantly with an infectious episode. However, there is no latency period between the infection and the AKI in IgA nephropathy. IgA deposition can be seen in PIGN associated with staphylococcal infections in which enterotoxins can act as superantigens, initiating an immunologic response.

Adult patients with primary membranous glomerulopathy frequently present with the nephrotic syndrome: timed urine protein collection of more than 3.5 g/24 h, edema, hypoalbuminemia, and hyperlipidemia. Another 30% to 40% of patients present with asymptomatic proteinuria, usually in the subnephrotic range. The urine sediment can reveal erythrocytes and granular casts, but erythrocyte casts are not a feature. Furthermore, complement levels are always normal.

KEY POINT

- The typical manifestation of postinfectious glomerulonephritis is a preceding infection associated with an acute nephritic syndrome, which is characterized by rapid onset of edema, hypertension, oliguria, and erythrocyte casts in the urine sediment.

Bibliography

Nasr SH, Share DS, Vargas MT, D'Agati VD, Markowitz GS. Acute poststaphylococcal glomerulonephritis superimposed on diabetic glomerulosclerosis. Kidney Int. 2007;71(12):1317-1321. [PMID: 17311069]

Item 61   Answer: D

Educational Objective: Identify hypertension as a contraindication to kidney biopsy.

Uncontrolled hypertension is a contraindication to kidney biopsy in this patient. She has systemic lupus erythematosus (SLE) and hypertension and is planning to undergo a kidney biopsy for suspected rapidly progressive glomerular disease. In patients with SLE, rapidly progressive glomerular disease left untreated can result in end-stage kidney disease. Thus, it is important to obtain an accurate tissue diagnosis as quickly as possible. However, severe hypertension can lead to increased rates of complications, such as post-biopsy hemorrhage. Although specific outcomes data establishing the optimal level of blood pressure control before kidney biopsy are not available, a measurement of less than 160/95 mm Hg is considered an appropriate level before proceeding to biopsy. Hypertension can be managed relatively quickly if present. Before the biopsy, the patient should be counseled to take all prescribed antihypertensive medications. All over-the-counter medications that may cause hypertension should be avoided, including certain cold remedies such as those containing phenylephrine. Patients can be prescribed a mild sedative (such as lorazepam) before the biopsy if they are anxious, which can also raise blood pressure. At the time of biopsy, if blood pressure is elevated, short-acting β-blockers (such as metoprolol) or centrally acting α-agonists (such as clonidine) can be prescribed. Blood pressure should be closely monitored before, during, and after the procedure.

Other contraindications to kidney biopsy include coagulopathy, thrombocytopenia, hydronephrosis, atrophic kidney, numerous kidney cysts, and acute pyelonephritis. The presence of a solitary kidney is a relative contraindication to percutaneous kidney biopsy because of the risk for nephrectomy due to uncontrolled bleeding. However, percutaneous kidney biopsy may be performed in this setting under direct visualization by laparoscopy. Kidney masses or renal cell carcinomas also are relative contraindications to kidney biopsy because they are associated with an increased risk of bleeding and spread of malignant cells through the biopsy tract.

A slightly increased BMI, chronic prednisone use, and mild anemia are not contraindications to kidney biopsy.

KEY POINT

- Uncontrolled hypertension is a contraindication for kidney biopsy.

Bibliography

Whittier WL, Korbet SM. Renal biopsy: update. Curr Opin Nephrol Hypertens. 2004;13(6):661-665. [PMID: 15483458]

Item 62   Answer: D

Educational Objective: Diagnose aldosterone excess in a patient with resistant hypertension.

Obtaining a plasma aldosterone-plasma renin activity ratio (ARR) is indicated for this patient. He has resistant hypertension, which is defined as blood pressure that remains above goal despite the administration of three antihypertensive drugs, one of which is a diuretic. A high proportion of patients with resistant hypertension have secondary hypertension due to primary hyperaldosteronism or renovascular hypertension; therefore, these conditions should be excluded in patients with resistant hypertension. Primary hyperaldosteronism is inconsistently associated with hypokalemia, and its absence in a patient with resistant hypertension should not influence the decision to screen for this condition. The ARR is a screening test for primary hyperaldosteronism. The normal range varies among institutions because renin and aldosterone assays may differ, but an ARR above 25 is generally considered abnormal. An elevated ARR alone is not diagnostic of primary hyperaldosteronism unless nonsuppressible or autonomous aldosterone excess is demonstrated by the presence of a urine aldosterone excretion of 12 micrograms/24 h (33.2 nmol/24 h) or higher obtained after correction of hypokalemia and adherence to a high-sodium diet for 3 days. In some patients, administering an intravenous saline infusion also may demonstrate nonsuppressible serum aldosterone levels. Both medical and surgical management have proved effective in the treatment of aldosterone excess.

The substitution of a loop diuretic such as furosemide for a thiazide diuretic is recommended in patients with difficult to control hypertension and chronic kidney disease or hypervolemic states. This patient has normal kidney function and no evidence of hypervolemia; therefore, the substitution is unlikely to affect his blood pressure.

Aliskiren is not a more effective antihypertensive agent than lisinopril. More importantly, evaluating for potential secondary causes of resistant hypertension is a more effective long-term strategy to control this patient's blood pressure than is switching to a new drug.

Atherosclerotic renovascular disease is usually associated with widespread atherosclerosis, peripheral vascular disease, cardiovascular disease, and ischemic target organ damage. This patient has no risk factors for renovascular hypertension; therefore, kidney Doppler ultrasonography is not warranted at this time.

KEY POINT

- **A high proportion of patients with resistant hypertension have secondary hypertension due to primary hyperaldosteronism or renovascular hypertension.**

Bibliography

Rossi GP. Diagnosis and treatment of primary aldosteronism. Rev Endocr Metab Disord. 2011;12(1):27-36. [PMID: 21369868]

Item 63   Answer: D

Educational Objective: Diagnose pigment nephropathy from rhabdomyolysis.

The most likely diagnosis is pigment nephropathy from rhabdomyolysis, which develops when muscle injury leads to the release of myoglobin and other intracellular muscle contents into the circulation. Nephrotoxicity results from kidney ischemia and tubular obstruction. Rhabdomyolysis most commonly develops after exposure to myotoxic drugs, infection, excessive exertion, or prolonged immobilization. Diagnosis should be considered in patients with a serum creatine kinase level above 5000 units/L. Another clue is heme positivity on urine dipstick testing in the absence of significant hematuria. The dipstick heme assay detects the presence of myoglobin. This patient presented with bruises and lacerations from a fight, and he was found immobile after consuming alcohol, all of which are risk factors for muscle damage and rhabdomyolysis. His high urine sodium and granular casts suggests intrinsic renal damage.

Patients with acute interstitial nephritis should have a suspicious medication exposure, which is not part of this patient's history.

Hepatorenal syndrome is associated with a significant history of liver disease and a low urine sodium, neither of which is seen in this patient.

Patients with intra-abdominal compartment syndrome usually have had surgery or massive volume resuscitation as well as a tense abdomen on physical examination, usually in a critical care setting.

KEY POINT

- **Rhabdomyolysis is a cause of intrinsic renal disease associated with high urine sodium, high fractional excretion of sodium, pigmented casts, and a history suggestive of muscle damage.**

Bibliography

Bosch X, Poch E, Grau JM. Rhabdomyolysis and acute kidney injury [erratum in N Engl J Med. 2011;364(20):1982]. N Engl J Med. 2009;361(1):62-72. [PMID: 19571284]

Item 64   Answer: A

Educational Objective: Manage primary membranous glomerulopathy.

The most appropriate treatment for this patient is an ACE inhibitor to control blood pressure and to reduce proteinuria as well as a statin to manage hyperlipidemia. This patient has primary membranous glomerulopathy, which frequently presents as the nephrotic syndrome and can be accompanied by hematuria, hypertension, kidney failure, and thromboembolic events. Observational studies have identified male gender, age older than 50 years, elevated serum creatinine level or low glomerular filtration rate (GFR), hypertension, secondary glomerulosclerosis, and chronic tubulointerstitial changes observed on biopsy at the time of diagnosis as risk factors associated with progressive chronic kidney disease (CKD). During follow-up or monitoring of kidney function, persistent proteinuria of ≥4 g/24 h for longer than 6 months and a decline in GFR over time are the most important risk factors associated with progression of primary membranous glomerulopathy to advanced CKD. In untreated primary membranous glomerulopathy, approximately two thirds of patients undergo spontaneous complete or partial remission, and only one third of patients have a persistent and/or progressive disease that may result in end-stage kidney disease within 10 years of onset. This patient has a low risk for disease progression, but she requires an ACE inhibitor to manage hypertension and proteinuria as well as a statin to manage hyperlipidemia. ACE inhibitors should be used cautiously in women of childbearing age, because these agents can be associated with severe congenital malformations.

Because of the potential toxicity of immunosuppressive therapies and the high rate of spontaneous remission of this disease, the clinical features and risk for disease progression should determine the most appropriate management in patients with primary membranous glomerulopathy. This patient has a low risk for CKD, and immunosuppressive agents should be initially avoided.

KEY POINT

- **Low-risk primary membranous glomerulopathy is managed with an ACE inhibitor and a statin.**

Bibliography

Cattran D. Management of membranous nephropathy: when and what for treatment. J Am Soc Nephrol. 2005;16(5):1188-1194. [PMID: 15800117]

Item 65   Answer: B

Educational Objective: Diagnose propofol-related infusion syndrome.

This patient most likely has propofol-related infusion syndrome, which is characterized by type B lactic acidosis, hypertriglyceridemia, rhabdomyolysis, and myocardial abnormalities seen as J-point elevation or a Brugada-like pattern on electrocardiogram. This rare syndrome occurs in approximately 1% of critically ill patients receiving propofol and most commonly occurs in those receiving doses above 4 mg/kg/h administered for more than 48 hours. The proposed mechanism involves the uncoupling of oxidative phosphorylation and energy production in mitochondria by propofol, coupled with the normal stress response to critical illness, to cause the characteristic findings of the syndrome. The findings of urine dipstick positivity for blood in the absence of hematuria consistent with rhabdomyolysis, lipemic serum, and unexplained anion gap acidosis in this critically ill patient receiving propofol support the diagnosis of propofol-related infusion syndrome. Treatment consists of discontinuing propofol and continued supportive care.

Fosphenytoin is not associated with significant metabolic abnormalities or an increased anion gap metabolic acidosis when appropriately dosed for kidney failure and potential drug interactions.

Propylene glycol is a solvent used in preparations of intravenous benzodiazepines (such as lorazepam and diazepam), and a lactic acidosis with an increased anion gap may occur in patients being treated with high doses of these medications, although the other findings in this patient are not associated with propylene glycol toxicity.

Pyroglutamic acidosis is usually observed in patients receiving therapeutic doses of acetaminophen in the setting of critical illness. Increased oxidative stress in patients receiving acetaminophen leads to depletion of glutathione stores, which disrupts the γ-glutamyl cycle and results in accumulation of pyroglutamic acid.

KEY POINT

- **Propofol-related infusion syndrome is characterized by lactic acidosis, rhabdomyolysis, hypertriglyceridemia, and myocardial abnormalities on electrocardiogram.**

Bibliography

Roberts RJ, Barletta JF, Fong JJ, et al. Incidence of propofol-related infusion syndrome in critically ill adults: a prospective, multicenter study. Crit Care. 2009;13(5):R169. [PMID: 19874582]

Item 66   Answer: D

Educational Objective: Treat a patient who has salicylate toxicity.

Sodium bicarbonate infusion is indicated for this patient with salicylate toxicity. Salicylate toxicity commonly presents with abnormalities in acid-base balance, the most common in adults being respiratory alkalosis, which occurs in response to stimulation of the medullary respiratory center. With more severe intoxication, increased anion gap metabolic acidosis develops both as a result of the salicylate anion and concomitant lactic and ketoacidosis. Early manifestations include tinnitus, confusion, tachypnea, and, occasionally, low-grade fever. Nausea and vomiting develop as a result of direct gastric mucosal toxicity. Management of salicylate poisoning depends on the magnitude of the serum salicylate level, the severity of clinical manifestations, and whether there is underlying kidney dysfunction. Alkalinization of the arterial pH to 7.5 to 7.6 is indicated to decrease intracellular uptake and toxicity of salicylic acid. Hydration and urine alkalinization to a pH of 7.5 to 8.0 will promote salicylate excretion. Follow-up serum salicylate levels, serum electrolyte levels, and acid-base parameters should be obtained at least every 2 hours to document improving clinical status. Hypokalemia, when present, should be corrected to prevent increased salicylate absorption in the distal tubule. Patients with impaired mentation warrant supplemental intravenous glucose to attenuate salicylate-induced neuroglycopenia.

CONT.

Although acetazolamide increases urine pH by decreasing proximal bicarbonate reabsorption, the use of this medication in salicylate toxicity is contraindicated because of the associated decrease in systemic pH, which promotes intracellular uptake of salicylic acid and toxicity.

Hemodialysis is indicated in patients with serum salicylate levels that exceed 80 mg/dL (5.8 mmol/L), altered mentation, pulmonary edema, advanced kidney disease, or when the clinical status worsens despite optimal medical therapy, none of which is present in this patient.

In the absence of absolute indications, mechanical ventilation should be avoided in patients with salicylate poisoning to avoid decreasing the systemic pH, thereby promoting intracellular uptake of salicylate and associated toxicity.

KEY POINT

- Management of salicylate toxicity depends on the magnitude of the serum salicylate level, the severity of clinical manifestations, and whether there is underlying kidney dysfunction.

Bibliography

Bora K, Aaron C. Pitfalls in salicylate toxicity. Am J Emerg Med. 2010;28(3):383-384. [PMID: 20223401]

Item 67   Answer: D

Educational Objective: Diagnose prerenal azotemia.

This patient most likely has prerenal azotemia. Prerenal azotemia generally occurs in patients with a mean arterial pressure below 60 mm Hg but may occur at higher pressures in patients with chronic kidney disease or in those who take medications, such as NSAIDs, that can alter glomerular hemodynamics. Patients with prerenal azotemia may have a history of decreased fluid intake accompanied by examination findings consistent with volume depletion. This patient was exposed to the sun for a prolonged period of time and took ibuprofen before going to the emergency department. She also takes hydrochlorothiazide daily for hypertension. Although her fractional excretion of sodium (FE_{Na}) is more than 1%, she is on a diuretic, which can increase the FE_{Na} even with prerenal azotemia. Because the fractional excretion of urea is less influenced by diuretics, it can be helpful in patients on diuretic therapy. It is calculated similarly to the FE_{Na} using the serum and urine urea levels. In prerenal azotemia, the fractional excretion of urea is below 35%, as in this patient. Finally, her urinalysis is concentrated, with hyaline casts and a high urine specific gravity.

Acute interstitial nephritis is most commonly caused by a hypersensitivity reaction to a medication. Urinalysis findings include leukocyte casts and eosinophils, neither of which is seen in this patient.

Acute tubular necrosis (ATN) is characterized by damage to the renal tubule due to a physiologic insult to the kidney such as hypoxia, toxins, or prolonged hypoperfusion. Kidney failure tends to be rapid, and the urine traditionally shows muddy brown casts. Although ATN may result from prolonged prerenal azotemia, this patient's clinical presentation and urinalysis are not consistent with this diagnosis.

This patient's lupus does not appear to be active, her urine is unremarkable for an active sediment (no dysmorphic erythrocytes or erythrocyte casts), and her urine protein is low in the setting of a concentrated urine, making lupus nephritis an unlikely diagnosis.

KEY POINT

- Patients with prerenal azotemia may have a history of decreased fluid intake accompanied by examination findings consistent with volume depletion.

Bibliography

Lameire N, Van Biesen W, Vanholder R. Acute renal failure. Lancet. 2005;365(9457):417-430. [PMID: 15680458]

Item 68   Answer: B

Educational Objective: Identify Balkan nephropathy as a cause of chronic tubulointerstitial nephritis.

The most likely diagnosis is Balkan nephropathy, a chronic tubulointerstitial condition of unclear cause found in patients from southeastern Europe (the Balkan region). It is thought to be caused by aristolochic acid, a plant alkaloid found in that region. Diagnostic criteria include epidemiologic criteria, decreased glomerular filtration rate, urine protein excretion of less than 1 g/24 h, and exclusion of other kidney diseases. There is an increased risk of urothelial cancers in these patients; therefore, physicians should have a high index of suspicion for these cancers. This patient has chronic kidney disease (CKD), minimal proteinuria, and a relatively benign urine sediment consistent with chronic tubulointerstitial disease. She is from Romania, which has areas with a very high incidence of Balkan nephropathy. She also has a cousin who has CKD and is possibly from the same area.

Analgesic nephropathy can result from exposure to large quantities of particular analgesics over years. This patient reports no history of high-dose exposure and is unlikely to have accumulated enough to result in analgesic nephropathy.

Hypertensive nephropathy can result after a long history of poorly controlled hypertension. Given her diagnosis of hypertension at the time of her CKD diagnosis, it is unlikely that her hypertension was poorly controlled for a prolonged period of time and is unlikely to be the cause of her CKD.

Patients with IgA nephropathy at this later stage of kidney disease are unlikely to exhibit no hematuria and only trace protein.

KEY POINT

- Balkan nephropathy is a chronic tubulointerstitial condition found in patients from southeastern Europe (the Balkan region) that is thought to be caused by aristolochic acid.

Bibliography

Stefanovic´ V, Polenakovic´ M. Fifty years of research in Balkan endemic nephropathy: where are we now? Nephron Clin Pract. 2009;112(2):c51-c56. [PMID: 19390202]

Item 69   Answer: B

Educational Objective: Treat a patient who has symptomatic hyponatremia.

This patient has symptomatic hypotonic hyponatremia, and a rapid increase in the serum sodium level using 3% saline infusion is indicated. The low plasma osmolality associated with a urine sodium level exceeding 40 meq/L (40 mmol/L) and urine osmolality greater than 200 mosm/kg H_2O in this patient without evidence of hypovolemia is most consistent with the syndrome of inappropriate antidiuretic hormone secretion (SIADH) as the cause of her hyponatremia. Infusion of 3% saline is used to treat patients who have SIADH with symptomatic hyponatremia because infusion of 0.9% (normal) saline can result in excretion of most of the infused sodium and retention of a significant portion of the infused water, leading to positive water balance and worsening hyponatremia. Because of its hypertonicity, 3% saline rapidly increases the serum sodium level but must be used with great caution to avoid overcorrection and the risk of central nervous system damage resulting from changes in plasma osmolality. Recent evidence suggests than an increase in the serum sodium level by approximately 4 to 6 meq/L (4-6 mmol/L) over the first 24 hours is sufficient in symptomatic patients. If the extracellular fluid osmolality rapidly normalizes in a patient with chronic hyponatremia, cell shrinkage may occur and can precipitate osmotic demyelination syndrome. Correction that exceeds the maximal limits of 10 meq/L (10 mmol/L) in the first 24 hours and/or 18 meq/L (18 mmol/L) in the first 48 hours should therefore be reversed with infusion of hypotonic intravenous solutions such as 5% dextrose in water and possibly concurrent administration of intravenous subcutaneous desmopressin.

Furosemide can be used as adjunctive management of hyponatremia caused by SIADH because this agent interferes with urinary concentration, thus increasing water excretion. However, the rapidity of correction expected with furosemide alone is insufficient to increase the serum sodium to an appropriate level in a symptomatic patient. Furosemide may be of benefit to patients with chronic asymptomatic hyponatremia due to SIADH, particularly

when the urine osmolality exceeds 400 mosm/kg H_2O, by causing excretion of a more dilute urine.

Tolvaptan, an oral V_2 receptor vasopressin antagonist, is approved to treat patients with asymptomatic euvolemic and hypervolemic hyponatremia. However, the safety of this agent in the management of symptomatic hyponatremia has yet to be established, and too rapid correction and overcorrection of the serum sodium level have been reported.

KEY POINT

- Patients with symptomatic hyponatremia due to the syndrome of inappropriate antidiuretic hormone secretion require a rapid increase in the serum sodium level using 3% saline infusion.

Bibliography

Sterns RH, Hix JK, Silver S. Treating profound hyponatremia: a strategy for controlled correction. Am J Kidney Dis. 2010;56(4):774-779. [PMID: 20709440]

Item 70   Answer: B

Educational Objective: Manage hypertension in a woman of childbearing age.

This patient has essential hypertension and should be switched from lisinopril to labetalol before pregnancy. Exposure to ACE inhibitors such as lisinopril during the first trimester has been associated with fetal cardiac abnormalities, and exposure during the second and third trimesters has been associated with neonatal kidney failure and death. Angiotensin receptor antagonists such as losartan have been associated with similar fetal toxicity as ACE inhibitors, most likely because of the dependence of the fetal kidney on the renin-angiotensin system. Therefore, both of these agents are pregnancy category X drugs and are contraindicated throughout pregnancy and in women planning to conceive.

Labetalol is a pregnancy risk category C drug and is commonly used during pregnancy owing to its combined α- and β-blocking properties and because it does not compromise uteroplacental blood flow. Methyldopa also is used extensively in pregnancy and is one of the only agents in which long-term follow-up of infants exposed in utero has proved to be safe. Furthermore, methyldopa is the only agent classified as a pregnancy category B drug. However, controlling blood pressure with single-agent methyldopa is often difficult, and many women are bothered by its sedating properties.

Cessation of antihypertensive therapy in a patient with hypertension is not recommended before pregnancy.

Aldosterone antagonists such as spironolactone have an antiandrogenic effect on the fetus when exposure occurs during the first trimester and should be avoided in women planning to conceive.

- ACE inhibitors, angiotensin receptor blockers, and aldosterone antagonists should be avoided during pregnancy and in women planning to conceive.

Bibliography

Cooper WO, Hernandez-Diaz S, Arbogast PG, et al. Major congenital malformations after first-trimester exposure to ACE inhibitors. N Engl J Med. 2006;354(23):2443-2451. [PMID: 16760444]

Item 71   Answer: A

Educational Objective: Prevent diabetic nephropathy in a patient with type 2 diabetes mellitus and hypertension.

An ACE inhibitor is indicated for this patient with type 2 diabetes mellitus who has hypertension and normal urine albumin excretion. Because of the increased risk of cardiovascular and kidney disease associated with diabetes, control of hypertension is essential in the management of patients with diabetes. Although the benefit of treatment of hypertension with ACE inhibitors has been well established in diabetic patients with albuminuria by preventing progression of proteinuria and subsequent decline in glomerular filtration rate, there is also evidence that interruption of the renin-angiotensin system may decrease the risk of developing microalbuminuria in hypertensive, type 2 diabetic patients. This effect of treating hypertension with an ACE inhibitor (or angiotensin receptor blocker [ARB]) in these patients with normal urine albumin excretion appears to be independent of the achieved blood pressure compared with similar hypertension control with other antihypertensive agents. In diabetes, glomerular hyperfiltration mediated by the renin-angiotensin-aldosterone system is very important in the pathogenesis and progression of diabetic nephropathy. The use of ACE inhibitors or ARBs reduces the glomerular hyperfiltration. This patient's blood pressure is greater than 140/90 mm Hg, and he is unlikely to reach his goal with lifestyle modifications alone. Therefore, he requires pharmacologic treatment, preferentially with an ACE inhibitor or ARB, for his hypertension until he reaches the American Diabetes Association recommended blood pressure goal of less than 130/80 mm Hg for patients with diabetes.

Other antihypertensives such as β-blockers, calcium channel blockers, and diuretics lower blood pressure but do not affect the glomerular hyperfiltration. Therefore, these antihypertensive classes are not first-line agents but may be considered for combination use if patients do not achieve their blood pressure goal with ACE inhibitor or ARB monotherapy or if they do not tolerate ACE inhibitors or ARBs.

- Prevention of diabetic nephropathy involves reducing the patient's risk of developing microalbuminuria, which is associated with progressive chronic kidney disease and cardiovascular events.

Bibliography

American Diabetes Association. Standards of medical care in diabetes–2012. Diabetes Care. 2012;35(suppl 1):S11-S63. [PMID: 22187469]

Item 72   Answer: D

Educational Objective: Manage polyoma BK virus–associated nephropathy in a kidney transplant recipient.

A decrease in immunosuppression is indicated for this patient with evidence of polyoma BK virus–associated nephropathy. This patient is a recent kidney transplant recipient and now has a decline in kidney function. Polyoma BK virus is an increasingly recognized cause of graft nephropathy. Although infection is asymptomatic in most persons, it often causes clinical disease in immunosuppressed patients. As the virus infects uroepithelial cells, viral activity in immunosuppressed kidney transplant patients is particularly problematic. Screening with polymerase chain reaction testing and urine cytology is recommended in the first year following transplantation and when there is a decline in kidney function. This patient is positive for polyoma BK virus, and his urinalysis is abnormal with erythrocytes, leukocytes, and some leukocyte casts, which is suggestive of interstitial nephritis. Kidney transplant biopsy provides the definitive diagnosis and shows evidence of polyoma BK virus–associated nephropathy with inflammation of the tubules and viral inclusions in the tubular epithelial cells. Initial treatment is directed at decreasing the immunosuppression. This patient's immunosuppression should be lowered by reducing the dose of either or both of his antirejection medications to as great a degree as possible without jeopardizing graft survival. This intervention may be adequate to control the activity of the infection.

If decreased immunosuppression is not effective, several agents show activity against polyoma BK virus, including fluoroquinolones, leflunomide, and cidofovir (off-label use). Most common antiviral agents, including ganciclovir and acyclovir, appear to have little activity against this virus.

Muromonab-CD3, a monoclonal antibody against the CD3 receptor on lymphocytes, acts to deplete lymphocytes and increase immunosuppression, which would likely exacerbate the infection rather than control it.

KEY POINT

- Screening for polyoma BK virus is recommended in kidney transplant recipients in the first year after transplantation and when there is a decline in kidney function.

Bibliography

Barraclough KA, Isbel NM, Staatz CE, Johnson DW. BK virus in kidney transplant recipients: the influence of immunosuppression. J Transplant. 2011;2011:750836. [PMID: 21766009]

Item 73   Answer: C

Educational Objective: Screen for chronic kidney disease in a patient with diabetes mellitus.

A spot urine albumin–creatinine ratio is indicated to evaluate this patient for chronic kidney disease (CKD). She has type 2 diabetes mellitus, a population that is at risk for CKD, and testing for microalbuminuria is appropriate. The National Kidney Foundation and the American Diabetes Association recommend annual testing to assess urine albumin excretion in patients with type 1 diabetes of 5 years' duration and in all patients with type 2 diabetes starting at the time of diagnosis by measuring the albumin–creatinine ratio. Microalbuminuria is defined as an albumin–creatinine ratio of 30 to 300 mg/g; diagnosis requires an elevated albumin–creatinine ratio on two of three random samples obtained over 6 months. Patients with diabetes and microalbuminuria are at increased risk for progression of CKD and cardiovascular disease. Use of ACE inhibitors or angiotensin receptor blockers delays progression in patients with proteinuric kidney disease or in patients with diabetes and microalbuminuria, underscoring the importance of early detection.

The gold standard for measuring urine protein excretion is a 24-hour urine collection. However, this test is cumbersome and unreliable if not collected correctly. Patients have a difficult time accurately collecting urine for 24 hours, in addition to keeping it on ice. Therefore, the National Kidney Foundation Kidney Disease Outcomes Quality Initiative (NKF KDOQI) recommends use of urinary ratios on random urine samples as an alternative method of estimating proteinuria in the clinical assessment of kidney disease. Furthermore, a 24-hour urine collection may not diagnose low-grade microalbuminuria.

Kidney ultrasonography can be performed once a diagnosis of CKD is made but should not be used to screen for CKD.

Although this patient has an estimated glomerular filtration rate of >60 mL/min/1.73 m^2 and normal urinalysis results, she has diabetes and should therefore be evaluated for CKD.

KEY POINT

- The National Kidney Foundation and the American Diabetes Association recommend annual testing to assess urine albumin excretion in patients with type 1 diabetes mellitus of 5 years' duration and in all patients with type 2 diabetes starting at the time of diagnosis by measuring the albumin–creatinine ratio.

Bibliography

KDOQI. KDOQI clinical practice guidelines and clinical practice recommendations for diabetes and chronic kidney disease. Am J Kidney Dis. 2007;49(2 suppl 2):S12-S154. [PMID: 17276798]

Item 74   Answer: D

Educational Objective: Manage hyperkalemia and hypertension in a patient with chronic kidney disease.

Increasing the furosemide dose is appropriate to manage hypertension and hyperkalemia in this patient with chronic kidney disease (CKD). Managing hypertension is indicated for all patients with kidney disease and is critical in the management of CKD regardless of the underlying etiology. Controlling blood pressure helps to decrease cardiovascular risk and may help to prevent progression to end-stage kidney disease. ACE inhibitors (such as lisinopril) or angiotensin receptor blockers (ARBs) are the preferred antihypertensive agents in patients with CKD, especially in those with proteinuria. ACE inhibitors and ARBs reduce efferent arteriolar resistance and lower intraglomerular pressure. The lower intraglomerular pressure is thought to be protective for the kidney but may be associated with a slight increase in the serum creatinine level. An increase in the serum creatinine of up to 30% after initiation of ACE inhibitors or ARBs is acceptable. Use of these agents also may cause hyperkalemia. Management of hyperkalemia using diuretics is preferred, especially in patients with hypertension. Diuretics are effective agents for blood pressure control in patients with CKD and are also useful in those with edema. Patients with CKD usually require higher diuretic doses to be effective. This patient remains hypertensive despite the increase in lisinopril dose. Increasing the furosemide dose should reduce intravascular volume, a common contributor to hypertension in patients with CKD and lower blood pressure.

Sodium polystyrene sulfonate can lower the serum potassium level but would have minimal effect on blood pressure and also causes gastrointestinal side effects.

Although spironolactone may help improve blood pressure control, its mechanism of aldosterone blockade will decrease urine potassium loss and may result in worsening hyperkalemia. Because of this, spironolactone should be used with caution in patients with CKD and in those on medications that may increase the serum potassium, and only with close monitoring of the serum potassium level.

Although discontinuing or lowering the ACE inhibitor (lisinopril) dose should help lower this patient's serum potassium level, these actions do not address the high blood pressure and likely would result in higher blood pressure.

KEY POINT

- In patients with chronic kidney disease, adding a diuretic, particularly a loop diuretic such as furosemide, can enhance the antihypertensive and antiproteinuric effects of antihypertensive agents and lower serum potassium concentration.

Bibliography

Ernst ME, Gordon JA. Diuretic therapy: key aspects in hypertension and renal disease. J Nephrol. 2010;23(5):487-493. [PMID: 20677164]

Item 75   Answer: C
Educational Objective: Diagnose nephrolithiasis using noncontrast abdominal helical CT.

Noncontrast abdominal helical CT is indicated for this patient with symptoms of renal colic. Distal ureteral stones may cause pain that radiates to the testicle in men or to the labia majora in women because the pain is referred from the ilioinguinal or genitofemoral nerves. A detailed physical examination, including that of the genitals, is appropriate. Noncontrast abdominal helical CT is the gold standard for diagnosing nephrolithiasis. This study can identify all types of kidney stones along the urinary tract with a sensitivity of more than 95% and is also able to detect associated urinary tract obstruction, if present.

Abdominal radiography of the kidneys, ureters, and bladder (KUB) is sometimes useful in the chronic management of patients with calcium-containing kidney stones. KUB can be used to follow the stone burden or to help with planning for surgical interventions. In the acute setting, KUB is not sufficiently sensitive or specific to guide management; patients may have bowel gas, extrarenal calcifications, or radiolucent stones that limit characterization.

Intravenous pyelography had previously been the standard imaging modality for nephrolithiasis, which utilizes intravenous contrast to characterize the anatomy, site, and size of stones, if present. However, this modality is rarely used currently because of the superiority of the images obtained by CT and the need for contrast exposure. It is also a more labor-intensive test that may require multiple delayed images.

Testicular ultrasonography is beneficial if testicular torsion is suspected and can identify other anatomic abnormalities of the testes, including tumors, hernia, abscess, or testicular rupture from trauma. However, the typical age range for testicular torsion is 12 to 18 years, and this patient's testicular examination is normal.

KEY POINT

- Noncontrast abdominal helical CT is the gold standard for diagnosing nephrolithiasis.

Bibliography

Coursey CA, Casalino DD, Remer EM, et al; Expert Panel on Urologic Imaging. ACR Appropriateness Criteria® acute onset flank pain–suspicion of stone disease. Guideline Summary. U.S. Department of Health and Human Services Web site. Available at www.guidelines.gov/content.aspx?id=32639&search=kidney+stone#Section420. Accessed July 24, 2012.

Item 76   Answer: A
Educational Objective: Manage proximal (type 2) renal tubular acidosis.

Discontinuation of tenofovir is appropriate. This patient has proximal (type 2) renal tubular acidosis (RTA) most likely related to tenofovir therapy for HIV infection. Her urine pH is less than 5.5, indicating preserved distal tubular function and urine acidification. Glycosuria in a patient with a normal glucose level, tubular-range proteinuria, and hypophosphatemia consequent to decreased proximal tubular reabsorption of phosphate, as observed in this patient, is most consistent with proximal RTA. The response to alkali therapy can serve as an important clue to the diagnosis. Patients with proximal RTA often require 10 to 15 meq/kg/d to correct the acidosis, whereas patients with distal RTA usually require only 1 to 2 meq/kg/d. The mechanism of kidney injury due to tenofovir is believed to be drug-related damage to mitochondrial DNA, noted most significantly in the renal tubules and causing tubular dysfunction. Patients taking tenofovir should therefore be monitored closely for evidence of kidney injury while on treatment. Drug withdrawal is indicated if nephrotoxicity is present; most patients show improvement in kidney function over weeks to months after stopping the medication, although permanent tubulointerstitial damage is possible.

The trimethoprim component of trimethoprim-sulfamethoxazole tends to cause hyperkalemia but not hypokalemia as noted in this patient. Trimethoprim, particularly in acid urine, blocks the epithelial sodium channel in the cortical collecting duct, leading to increased lumen positive potential, impaired potassium and proton secretion, hyperkalemia, and metabolic acidosis. This effect is more common with high doses of parenteral trimethoprim-sulfamethoxazole or when there is concomitant blockade of the renin-angiotensin-aldosterone system. Trimethoprim can also decrease the tubular secretion of creatinine, leading to a reversible increase in the serum creatinine level (usually up to approximately 0.5 mg/dL [44.2 micromoles/L]) that does not reflect a true decrease in glomerular filtration rate.

Lactic acid is a normal by-product of cellular metabolism, but when elevated due to overproduction or decreased metabolism, it causes an increased anion gap metabolic acidosis. Because the metabolic acidosis in this patient is associated with a normal anion gap, lactic acidosis as a cause of her acid-base disturbance is not likely.

Laxative abuse can cause normal anion gap metabolic acidosis when bicarbonate losses exceed hypokalemic-induced enhanced ammoniagenesis. This does not explain the glycosuria and hypophosphatemia consistent with proximal RTA seen in this patient.

KEY POINT

- Medications such as tenofovir can cause proximal (type 2) renal tubular acidosis, and discontinuation of the offending agent is indicated.

Bibliography

Unwin RJ, Luft FC, Shirley DG. Pathophysiology and management of hypokalemia: a clinical perspective. Nat Rev Nephrol. 2011;7(2):75-84. [PMID: 21278718]

Item 77   Answer: A

Educational Objective: Diagnose abdominal compartment syndrome.

This patient has abdominal compartment syndrome (ACS), which is defined by new organ dysfunction in the setting of a sustained, abnormal increase in the intra-abdominal pressure. Intra-abdominal pressure is normally between 0 and 5 mm Hg and is usually maintained in that range by the significant compliance of the abdominal wall. However, when a pathologic process (such as massive ascites, volume overload, or intra-abdominal or retroperitoneal hemorrhage) is present, the pressure may exceed the ability of the abdominal wall to compensate. Intra-abdominal hypertension is defined by sustained intra-abdominal pressures greater than 12 mm Hg; ACS occurs when the pressure exceeds 20 mm Hg and is accompanied by new organ dysfunction. The exact pathophysiology of ACS is uncertain, but high intra-abdominal pressure may adversely affect kidney function. Patients with a distended abdomen in the setting of aggressive fluid resuscitation and recent abdominal surgery should be evaluated for ACS. Measurement of the intravesicular pressure through a bladder catheter is the most common method for assessing the intra-abdominal pressure; although this value may not be identical to a directly measured intra-abdominal pressure, bladder pressure measurement appears to correlate adequately to be used in clinical decision making. Surgical decompression of the abdomen is often necessary to definitively treat ACS.

Aminoglycosides are well-known nephrotoxins. However, a single dose of tobramycin makes this a less likely cause of acute kidney injury (AKI), and aminoglycoside nephrotoxicity cannot account for this patient's increased intra-abdominal pressure.

Although kidney injury from ACS may appear prerenal because it is often associated with low blood pressures, the isosthenuric urine with a fractional excretion of sodium greater than 1% and the patient's unresponsiveness to fluids make this diagnosis less likely.

Although obstruction may have similar pathophysiology to ACS, the presence of an indwelling bladder catheter and lack of hydronephrosis on ultrasound suggest a different etiology of the AKI.

KEY POINT

- Abdominal compartment syndrome occurs when intra-abdominal pressure exceeds 20 mm Hg and is accompanied by new organ dysfunction.

Bibliography

De Waele JJ, De Laet I, Kirkpatrick AW, Hoste E. Intra-abdominal hypertension and abdominal compartment syndrome. Am J Kidney Dis. 2011;57(1):159-169. [PMID: 21184922]

Item 78   Answer: D

Educational Objective: Diagnose minimal change glomerulopathy.

Minimal change glomerulopathy (MCG) associated with lithium use is the cause of the nephrotic syndrome in this patient. MCG is usually idiopathic, but it also can be associated with atopic diseases; infections such as mononucleosis; malignancies such as Hodgkin lymphoma or carcinomas; and the use of NSAIDS, lithium, or rifampin. MCG usually presents as the nephrotic syndrome and may be accompanied by acute kidney injury, hematuria, and hypertension. Diagnosis is confirmed with kidney biopsy that reveals diffuse fusion and effacement of podocyte foot processes on electron microscopy with normal glomeruli by light and immunofluorescence microscopies. Lithium potentiates tumor necrosis factor– and interleukin-1–induced cytokines and cytokine receptor expression in T-cell hybridomas. It also accelerates interleukin-2 production in human T cells. These effects may have a role in podocyte toxicity and may explain why some patients develop massive proteinuria.

Lupus nephritis is unlikely in the absence of other findings associated with systemic lupus erythematosus and a negative antinuclear antibody titer.

Hepatitis C virus–associated glomerulonephritis, lupus nephritis, and membranous glomerulopathy always exhibit immune complex deposition on immunofluorescence microscopy.

KEY POINT

- Minimal change glomerulopathy is usually idiopathic, but it also can be associated with atopic diseases; infections such as mononucleosis; malignancies such as Hodgkin lymphoma or carcinomas; and the use of NSAIDS, lithium, or rifampin.

Bibliography

Jefferson JA, Nelson PJ, Najafian B, Shankland SJ. Podocyte disorders: Core Curriculum 2011. Am J Kidney Dis. 2011;58(4):666-677. [PMID: 21868143]

Item 79   Answer: D

Educational Objective: Treat a patient who has a kidney stone.

Treatment with tamsulosin is indicated for this patient who has a kidney stone that became symptomatic several days ago. The stone is of moderate size at 4 mm. Ninety percent of stones less than 5 mm pass spontaneously. In contrast, stones that are more than 10 mm are unlikely to pass without intervention. Although several days have passed, there is still a significant chance that he will pass the stone without surgical intervention. To increase the chance of stone passage, medical expulsive therapy using the α-blocker tamsulosin or a calcium channel blocker such as nifedipine should be employed. Tamsulosin is a very well-tolerated drug with mild side effects such as dizziness or rhinitis. This agent causes very little of the postural hypotension seen with other α_1-adrenergic antagonists and is generally better tolerated than a calcium channel blocker. Utilization of these agents for the facilitation of kidney stone passage is off label but common practice for stones less than 10 mm and well-controlled symptoms and is recommended by the American Urological Association and the European Association of Urology.

24-Hour urine collections are essential to identify specific abnormalities in urine composition and to tailor therapy for patients with a propensity to nephrolithiasis. Collections should be performed several weeks after stone passage when the patient is consuming his or her regular diet.

Patients who do not have an urgent indication for urologic intervention may still require intervention if the stone does not pass after a period of observation. The choice of intervention may depend on characteristics of the stone and practice of the particular center. Extracorporeal shock wave lithotripsy is a widely used, noninvasive strategy used to treat symptomatic calculi located in the proximal ureter or within the kidney.

Repeat imaging by noncontrast CT would expose the patient to more radiation without providing additional important diagnostic or prognostic information and is not indicated at this time.

Stones located in the distal ureter are usually accessible by directed therapy guided by ureteroscopy. During ureteroscopy, "intracorporeal" lithotripsy can be performed using lasers, ultrasonography, or other techniques. However, this intervention is premature at this time.

KEY POINT

- **Medical expulsive therapy using the α-blocker tamsulosin or a calcium channel blocker such as nifedipine is appropriate to increase the chance of passage of kidney stones less than 10 mm in patients with well-controlled symptoms.**

Bibliography

Parsons JK, Hergan LA, Sakamoto K, Lakin C. Efficacy of alpha-blockers for the treatment of ureteral stones. J Urol. 2007;177(3):983-987. [PMID: 17296392]

Item 80   Answer: C

Educational Objective: Diagnose normotensive ischemic acute kidney injury.

This patient most likely has normotensive ischemic acute kidney injury (AKI), which results when a patient with vascular risk factors and hypertension attains a blood pressure lower than usual measurements. If the new blood pressure is lower than the patient's range of renal autoregulation, an increased serum creatinine level due to renal hypoperfusion may result. This patient's medical history suggests underlying chronic kidney and vascular disease, which increase his risk for a normotensive ischemic insult. His lower blood pressure in the hospital may be the result of his infection, better adherence to medications, and/or diet. The findings of an elevated fractional excretion of sodium, fractional excretion of urea, granular casts on urinalysis, and normal kidney ultrasound are all consistent with this diagnosis.

Acute interstitial nephritis, which is most often caused by a hypersensitivity reaction to a medication, usually occurs after 1 week of exposure to the offending agent. This patient's lack of rash, fever, and leukocytes or erythrocytes on urinalysis also argues against this diagnosis.

Cholesterol crystal embolization may cause AKI in patients with aortic atherosclerotic plaques. This condition may occur spontaneously but most often develops after coronary or kidney angiography or aortic surgery. Anticoagulation with heparin, warfarin, or thrombolytic agents is believed to help incite this condition. It is associated with cutaneous and extrarenal manifestations and a bland urine sediment. Although this patient likely has underlying vascular disease, he has not had an invasive procedure or anticoagulation and lacks any of the associated skin or extrarenal manifestations of the syndrome, making this diagnosis less likely.

Patients with prerenal azotemia may have a history of fluid losses and decreased fluid intake accompanied by physical examination findings consistent with extracellular fluid volume depletion. Two findings make prerenal azotemia unlikely in this patient: fractional excretion of sodium above 2% and fractional excretion of urea above 50% (more reliable than fractional excretion of sodium for patients on diuretics). These findings are more consistent with acute tubular necrosis.

KEY POINT

- **Normotensive ischemic acute kidney injury can occur when patients with vascular risk factors and hypertension attain a blood pressure lower than their usual measurements.**

Bibliography

Abuelo JG. Normotensive ischemic acute renal failure. N Engl J Med. 2007;357(8):797-805. [PMID: 17715412]

Item 81   Answer: A

Educational Objective: Manage enteric hyperoxaluria in a patient who has a calcium oxalate stone.

Calcium carbonate supplements are indicated for this patient. Following gastric bypass surgery, she has developed kidney stones most likely caused by enteric hyperoxaluria. Her urinalysis shows the presence of characteristic calcium oxalate crystals in the urine sediment and a high specific gravity, which suggest that the urine is very concentrated. She also has a low urine volume of 1300 mL/24 h; patients with kidney stones should aim for at least 2000 mL of urine daily. Fatty acid malabsorption may occur following gastric bypass surgery and other causes of enteric hyperoxaluria. In this patient, oxalate absorption is increased because calcium, which normally binds to oxalate in the gut and limits oxalate absorption, binds to fatty acids. At the same time, the colon is exposed to insoluble bile salts and fatty acids, which increase the permeability to small molecules such as oxalate. Management of enteric hyperoxaluria includes a low fat diet and calcium carbonate supplementation to decrease oxalate absorption and excretion in the urine, coupled with aggressive oral hydration to decrease the concentration of the urine, both of which encourage stone formation.

Thiazide diuretics are useful to manage hypercalciuria because these agents promote reabsorption of urine calcium in the distal tubule. However, this patient's urine calcium level is normal.

Potassium citrate is useful in treating patients who have low urine citrate, which serves as an important inhibitor of crystallization by chelating urine calcium. Potassium citrate also is essential for treating patients with uric acid stones. This patient has both a normal urine citrate and uric acid excretion.

The α-blocker tamsulosin can be used to promote the movement of a stone along the ureter but will not affect the tendency to develop new stones.

KEY POINT

- **Management of enteric hyperoxaluria includes a low fat diet, calcium carbonate supplementation, and aggressive oral hydration.**

Bibliography
Kumar R, Lieske JC, Collazo-Clavell ML, et al. Fat malabsorption and increased intestinal oxalate absorption are common after Roux-en-Y gastric bypass surgery. Surgery. 2011;149(5):654-661. [PMID: 21295813]

Item 82   Answer: C

Educational Objective: Identify over-the-counter medication use as a cause of elevated blood pressure.

This patient should discontinue his over-the-counter medications and his blood pressure should be rechecked. He has chronic kidney disease (CKD) and may be taking an over-the-counter sinus decongestant, which often contains pseudoephedrine or phenylephrine, and/or an NSAID, medications that can elevate blood pressure. In the clinical setting of elevated blood pressure in a patient with previously well-controlled hypertension, exogenous factors such as new medications should be considered. Any suspicious medications should be stopped and the blood pressure followed for resolution.

The combination of an ACE inhibitor and an angiotensin receptor blocker (ARB) such as losartan to decrease the degree of proteinuria in patients with CKD is associated with significant adverse effects and unclear effects on kidney disease outcome. However, using combination therapy in patients with IgA nephropathy has not been studied extensively, and some clinicians use this intervention if the level of proteinuria and blood pressure are not adequately controlled with monotherapy. Dual treatment is not indicated in this patient, given his otherwise stable kidney function and lower level proteinuria.

Although an upper respiratory infection suggests a possible link to IgA nephropathy, the patient's urine studies do not support an exacerbation of IgA nephropathy. His serum creatinine level, microscopic hematuria, and proteinuria are at baseline; therefore, his increased blood pressure is not likely associated with worsening of his IgA nephropathy, and treatment with immunosuppression is not indicated.

ACE inhibitor or ARB therapy is a primary intervention to treat the proteinuria and hypertension frequently associated with IgA nephropathy. Increasing this patient's lisinopril dose may be appropriate if his blood pressure remains elevated, although exclusion of other causes of worsening blood pressure is important before making any dose adjustment, particularly given his previously effective blood pressure control and stable proteinuria.

KEY POINT

- **Over-the-counter medications can contribute to hypertension in patients with chronic kidney disease.**

Bibliography
Spence JD. Physiologic tailoring of treatment in resistant hypertension. Curr Cardiol Rev. 2010;6(2):119-123. [PMID: 21532778]

Item 83   Answer: D

Educational Objective: Diagnose rapidly progressive glomerulonephritis.

This patient most likely has rapidly progressive glomerulonephritis (RPGN), a clinical syndrome characterized by urine findings consistent with glomerular disease and rapid loss of kidney function over a period of days, weeks, or months. RPGN is most typically due to either anti–glomerular basement membrane antibody disease, immune complex deposition (for example, lupus nephritis),

CONT.

or an ANCA-positive vasculitis. Glomerulonephritis is characterized by hematuria, oliguria, hypertension, and kidney insufficiency caused by glomerular inflammation. Urinalysis usually reveals hematuria as well as cellular and granular casts, and proteinuria is typically present. This patient is subacutely ill with generalized symptoms of decline, poorly controlled hypertension, and periorbital and lower extremity edema. These findings, along with the presence of erythrocyte casts on urinalysis, make the diagnosis of RPGN most likely in this patient.

Acute interstitial nephritis may present with hematuria but more predominantly with pyuria and leukocyte casts. Furthermore, poorly controlled hypertension and periorbital edema are not in the typical constellation of symptoms associated with this disorder.

Acute tubular necrosis (ATN) is a common form of intrarenal disease that usually occurs after a sustained period of ischemia or exposure to nephrotoxic agents. More than 70% of patients with ATN have muddy brown casts in the urine. This patient's rapid clinical course, absence of risk factors for ATN, and presence of erythrocyte casts are inconsistent with ATN.

Polyarteritis nodosa is a vasculitis of medium-sized vessels. Clinical features include hypertension, variable kidney insufficiency, and, occasionally, kidney infarction bleeding caused by renal artery microaneurysm rupture. Urinalysis may show hematuria and subnephrotic proteinuria; however, because there is no inflammation or necrosis of glomeruli, erythrocyte casts are not seen.

KEY POINT

- Rapidly progressive glomerulonephritis is characterized by hematuria, oliguria, hypertension, and kidney injury caused by glomerular inflammation.

Bibliography
Mukhtyar C, Guillevin L, Cid MC, et al; European Vasculitis Study Group. EULAR recommendations for the management of primary small and medium vessel vasculitis. Ann Rheum Dis. 2009;68(3):310-317. [PMID: 18413444]

Item 84   Answer: D

Educational Objective: Identify the cause of a patient's change in blood pressure.

A repeat blood pressure measurement is indicated for this patient to ensure proper technique. Poor technique in measuring blood pressure is a common cause of apparent fluctuations in blood pressure, particularly in the ambulatory setting. The American Heart Association recommendations require 5 minutes of rest, bladder empty, back supported with feet on the floor (not in the supine position on an examination table), and proper cuff size, with the cuff bladder encircling at least 80% of the arm. In general, blood pressure also should not be measured through clothing and coats because this may lead to inaccuracies. In a hurried

situation, several of the requirements for blood pressure measurement can be violated, leading to errors in readings, as noted in this patient. Despite its critical importance as a vital sign, surprisingly few health care workers receive formal training in proper blood pressure measurement. Errors in positioning the patient, incorrect cuff size relative to arm circumference, intercurrent conversation, and interferences such as recent caffeine intake or cigarette smoking contribute to variability in blood pressure measurement. The increasing use of devices that allow patients to have repeated blood pressure measurements without a health care worker (physician or nurse) in the room may obviate some of this controversy, although these may also be associated with different forms of technical error.

It is important to make adjustments to a patient's antihypertensive regimen, regardless of setting, only if the blood pressure measurements on which those adjustments are being made are accurate and reflect evidence of sustained, inadequate control.

Ambulatory blood pressure monitoring is used to diagnose white coat hypertension and masked hypertension and to determine whether treatment of hypertension is adequate outside the office or hospital setting. However, it is not indicated in this patient with generally well-controlled blood pressure and a single abnormal determination.

KEY POINT

- Errors in positioning the patient, incorrect cuff size relative to arm circumference, intercurrent conversation, and interferences such as recent caffeine intake or cigarette smoking contribute to variability in blood pressure measurement.

Bibliography
Chobanian AV, Bakris GL, Black HR, et al; National Heart, Lung, and Blood Institute Joint National Committee on Prevention, Detection, Evaluation, and Treatment of High Blood Pressure; National High Blood Pressure Education Program Coordinating Committee. The Seventh Report of the Joint National Committee on Prevention, Detection, Evaluation, and Treatment of High Blood Pressure: the JNC 7 report. JAMA. 2003;289(19):2560-2572. [PMID: 12748199]

Item 85   Answer: A

Educational Objective: Prevent preeclampsia.

Low-dose aspirin (75 to 150 mg/d) is associated with a 10% to 15% relative risk reduction in preventing preeclampsia and reducing adverse maternal and fetal outcomes. Preeclampsia is defined as a systolic blood pressure ≥140 mm Hg or a diastolic blood pressure ≥90 mm Hg and a 24-hour urine protein excretion greater than 300 mg/24 h after the 20th week of gestation in a woman who did not have hypertension or proteinuria earlier in pregnancy. Clinical manifestations of preeclampsia may include headache, visual disturbances, liver dysfunction, and fetal growth restriction. The HELLP (hemolysis, elevated liver enzymes, low platelets) syndrome is a variant of preeclampsia. Several factors are associated with an increased risk of preeclampsia, including a personal history of preeclampsia, chronic hypertension, chronic kidney disease, and a family history of preeclampsia. This patient is at risk for preeclampsia because of her family history of preeclampsia, the fact that she is primiparous, and her personal history of borderline hypertension. Currently, only low-dose aspirin has been shown to modestly decrease the risk of preeclampsia, and most experts recommend this agent to women at risk.

Methyldopa is a first-line agent in the treatment of hypertension in the setting of pregnancy but has not been shown to decrease the risk of preeclampsia from chronic hypertension.

Calcium supplements reduce hypertension and preeclampsia modestly only in women consuming a baseline low-calcium diet.

Intravenous magnesium sulfate is used as an anticonvulsant to prevent eclampsia, but oral formulations of magnesium have not been shown to prevent either preeclampsia or eclampsia.

Reducing blood pressure to less than 120/80 mm Hg has not been shown to decrease the risk of preeclampsia. Instead, blood pressure goals are less stringent than those used for nonpregnant persons and are aimed primarily at limiting maternal end-organ damage during this finite period. Specific targets vary somewhat by professional society but generally aim for less than 150/100 mm Hg.

> **KEY POINT**
> - **Low-dose aspirin (75 to 150 mg/d) is associated with a 10% to 15% relative risk reduction in preventing preeclampsia and reducing adverse maternal and fetal outcomes.**

Bibliography
American College of Obstetricians and Gynecologists. ACOG Practice Bulletin No. 125: chronic hypertension in pregnancy. Obstet Gynecol. 2012;119(2 Pt 1):396-407. [PMID: 22270315]

Item 86   Answer: C

Educational Objective: Manage hypertension in a black patient with chronic kidney disease.

The addition of the ACE inhibitor ramipril is indicated for this black patient with hypertension, stage 3 chronic kidney disease (CKD), and proteinuria. Black patients tend to experience enhanced target organ damage at any level of blood pressure compared with most other groups, particularly white patients. Cardiovascular complications are also more frequent in black patients, and black patients are approximately fourfold more likely to experience end-stage kidney disease compared with white patients. These findings emphasize the need for aggressive blood pressure control in black patients, although the optimal level of control relative to other patient groups is unclear. Recommendations for high blood pressure management in black patients were released in the International Society on Hypertension

in Blacks (ISHIB) consensus statement. ISHIB defines treatment goals in black patients based on either the absence of target organ damage (primary prevention), in which the blood pressure goal is less than 135/85 mm Hg, or the presence of target organ damage (secondary prevention), in which the blood pressure goal is less than 130/80 mm Hg. In hypertensive patients with proteinuria, treatment with a renin-angiotensin system inhibitor (an ACE inhibitor or angiotensin receptor blocker) has been shown to decrease proteinuria and slow the progression of kidney disease. Despite the finding that black patients do not respond well to an ACE inhibitor as monotherapy for hypertension without proteinuria, the African American Study of Kidney Disease and Hypertension (AASK), performed in patients with long-standing hypertension and mild proteinuria, demonstrated that the ACE inhibitor ramipril slowed kidney disease progression in black patients with impaired kidney function caused by hypertension and is therefore an appropriate addition to this patient's treatment regimen.

In this same study, both metoprolol and amlodipine were inferior to ramipril for progression of kidney disease and are therefore not preferable agents to add to this patient's regimen.

The benefit of an ACE inhibitor in mitigating progression of kidney disease is due to hemodynamic changes within the glomerulus and other effects due to renin-angiotensin system blockade, in addition to treating systemic hypertension. While increasing this patient's dose of diuretic might successfully lower his blood pressure, he would not benefit from the treatment of his proteinuria associated with ramipril.

> **KEY POINT**
> - **In black patients with hypertensive kidney disease and proteinuria, treatment with the ACE inhibitor ramipril is appropriate for blood pressure control and to decrease kidney disease progression.**

Bibliography
Flack JM, Sica DA, Bakris G, et al; International Society on Hypertension in Blacks. Management of high blood pressure in blacks: an update of the International Society on Hypertension in Blacks consensus statement. Hypertension. 2010;56(5):780-800. [PMID: 20921433]

Item 87   Answer: D

Educational Objective: Manage severe ANCA vasculitis.

The most appropriate treatment for this patient with severe ANCA vasculitis is induction therapy with plasmapheresis, cyclophosphamide, and corticosteroids, followed by maintenance therapy with azathioprine and corticosteroids. Severe small-vessel vasculitis presenting as rapidly progressive glomerulonephritis (RPGN) is an emergency, and its early recognition is often missed. This patient had a progressive rise of the serum creatinine level to 6.7 mg/dL (592 micromoles/L), accompanied by respiratory manifestations for 4 months prior to hospitalization. Among the glomerular diseases that can manifest as RPGN, small-vessel vasculitis with ANCA positivity is the most frequent, occurring in 60% of patients with this disease. In patients with severe small-vessel vasculitis, induction therapy with plasmapheresis, cyclophosphamide, and corticosteroids, followed by maintenance therapy with azathioprine and corticosteroids, reduces the risk of end-stage kidney disease or mortality to 31% from the expected risk of 51%. Infection must be excluded before initiating the immunosuppressive therapy.

Induction therapy with cyclophosphamide and corticosteroids without plasmapheresis, followed by maintenance therapy with azathioprine and corticosteroids, is reserved for patients with moderately active vasculitis. Moderately active vasculitis usually manifests with a lesser degree of kidney disease (rise of serum creatinine to ≤5.8 mg/dL [513 micromoles/L] and/or no need for dialysis) without pulmonary hemorrhage.

Induction therapy with mycophenolate mofetil and corticosteroids, followed by maintenance therapy with mycophenolate mofetil and corticosteroids, has not been demonstrated to be effective in adequately designed trials.

The use of plasmapheresis alone to rapidly remove ANCAs can lead to a rebound production of these antibodies if cyclophosphamide with corticosteroids is not used.

KEY POINT

- **Induction therapy for severe ANCA vasculitis includes plasmapheresis, cyclophosphamide, and corticosteroids.**

Bibliography

Jayne DR, Gaskin G, Rasmussen N, et al; European Vasculitis Study Group. Randomized trial of plasma exchange or high-dosage methylprednisolone as adjunctive therapy for severe renal vasculitis. J Am Soc Nephrol. 2007;18(7):2180-2188. [PMID: 17582159]

Item 88   Answer: D

Educational Objective: Diagnose tuberous sclerosis complex.

This patient has a possible family history of kidney disease and a bilateral kidney cystic disorder, which most likely is tuberous sclerosis complex (TSC). TSC is most commonly manifested by angiomyolipomas or tubers of the skin, retina, kidneys, and other organs. Cognitive impairment, decreased visual acuity, and cystic lesions in the kidney can also be manifestations of the disease. Diagnostic criteria require either the presence of at least two major features or one major feature and two minor features. Major criteria include facial angiofibromas, three or more hypomelanotic macules (ash leaf spots), kidney angiomyolipomas, and

retinal hamartomas. Minor criteria include nonrenal hamartomas, multiple kidney cysts, and various dental abnormalities such as pits on dental enamel or gingival fibromas. This patient exhibits one major criterion (the presence of three or more hypomelanotic macules) and two minor criteria (dental enamel pits and possible gingival fibromas), making TSC a definitive diagnosis. Patients should have kidney ultrasonography at the time of diagnosis with repeat testing every 1 to 3 years if kidney lesions are found. In patients with TSC, 1% to 2% of adults can develop renal cell carcinoma and other concerning lesions that can result in hemorrhage. Some patients with TSC also have autosomal dominant polycystic kidney disease (ADPKD) because one of the TSC mutations is found on chromosome 16p (*TSC2*) that is immediately adjacent to the gene for ADPKD (*PKD1*).

The most common inherited cystic disease of the kidney is ADPKD; however, this patient's findings are most consistent with TSC. The number of kidney cysts seen on ultrasound that are required to establish a diagnosis of ADPKD varies based on the patient's age, PKD genotype, and whether a family history of ADPKD is present.

Tubular dilatation is the hallmark of autosomal recessive polycystic kidney disease and is associated with massive kidney enlargement at birth, abdominal masses, and respiratory distress. Difficult-to-control hypertension and growth retardation also are common.

Fabry disease is an X-linked disorder caused by deficiency of the α-galactosidase A enzyme and is not a cystic disease. Clinical manifestations include mild nephrotic-range proteinuria, slow deterioration in kidney function, cutaneous angiokeratomas, painful paresthesias of the hands, and premature coronary artery disease.

KEY POINT

- **Tuberous sclerosis complex is most commonly manifested by angiomyolipomas or tubers of the skin, retina, kidneys, and other organs.**

Bibliography

Curatolo P, Bombardieri R, Jozwiak S. Tuberous sclerosis. Lancet. 2008;372(9639):657-668. [PMID: 18722871]

Item 89   Answer: C

Educational Objective: Evaluate a patient for early diabetic nephropathy.

A urine albumin–creatinine ratio now is indicated to screen for diabetic nephropathy in this patient with newly diagnosed type 2 diabetes mellitus. Diabetic nephropathy is the most common glomerular disease and develops in approximately 35% of patients with type 1 and 2 diabetes. The American Diabetes Association guidelines specifically recommend annual measurement of the urine albumin excretion for patients who have had type 1 diabetes for 5 years or more and for all patients with type 2 diabetes beginning at the time of diagnosis. Screening for microalbuminuria usually involves obtaining a urine albumin–creatinine ratio on a first morning void urine sample, a random sample, or a timed urine collection. Microalbuminuria is confirmed when two of three samples obtained within a 6-month period reveal a urine albumin–creatinine ratio between 30 and 300 mg/g. Microalbuminuria is the first easily detectable sign of diabetic nephropathy and usually occurs 5 to 15 years after the diagnosis of diabetes. Approximately 10 to 15 years after the diagnosis of diabetes, macroalbuminuria (urine albumin–creatinine ratio above 300 mg/g) can be detected on urine dipstick and is accompanied by decreasing kidney function and increased blood pressure. Preventive measures in managing microalbuminuria include early initiation of an ACE inhibitor and/or angiotensin receptor blocker, adequate blood pressure control, blood glucose and lipid control, and smoking cessation, which reduce the risk of end-stage kidney disease and cardiovascular events.

The Modification of Diet in Renal Disease (MDRD) study equation was developed for patients with chronic kidney disease and has not been shown to accurately estimate kidney function in healthy persons or in diabetic patients with preserved glomerular filtration.

Waiting 5 years to screen for microalbuminuria is not appropriate in patients with type 2 diabetes because many patients may have diabetes for years before diagnosis, and earlier onset of diabetic nephropathy and faster progression of its clinical stages are common compared with type 1 diabetes.

The urine protein–creatinine ratio can be used in patients with overt proteinuria or later stages of diabetic nephropathy, neither of which is seen in this patient at this time.

KEY POINT

- A urine albumin–creatinine ratio is indicated to screen for diabetic nephropathy in patients with newly diagnosed type 2 diabetes mellitus.

Bibliography

Johnson SL, Tierney EF, Onyemere KU, et al. Who is tested for diabetic kidney disease and who initiates treatment? The Translating Research into Action for Diabetes (TRIAD) study. Diabetes Care. 2006;29(8):1733-1738. [PMID: 16873772]

Item 90   Answer: C

Educational Objective: Evaluate a patient with chronic kidney disease using ultrasonography.

Kidney ultrasonography is indicated for this patient with stage 3 chronic kidney disease (CKD), based on an estimated glomerular filtration rate (GFR) of 37 mL/min/1.73 m². He has not yet been evaluated for the cause of his CKD, which may have implications for therapy, including future transplantation. The patient's mother had known CKD, raising the possibility that there is a genetic

component to this patient's CKD. Kidney ultrasonography is often the first imaging choice to assess kidney disease because it is safe, not dependent upon kidney function, noninvasive, and relatively inexpensive. Because it does not require contrast dye, ultrasonography does not place patients at risk for contrast-induced nephropathy. Kidney ultrasonography can show small echogenic kidneys, elements of obstruction, or other chronic entities such as autosomal dominant polycystic kidney disease.

Abdominal CT can reveal information regarding causes of CKD and may be used for patients who are not suitable for ultrasonography (for example, unable to image because of obesity or large amounts of intestinal gas). However, CT is more costly than ultrasonography, exposes patients to additional radiation, and may involve use of intravenous iodinated contrast agents, which are associated with a risk for contrast-induced nephropathy in patients with an estimated GFR of less than 60 mL/min/1.73 m². Experts therefore recommend against the use of these agents in this population group.

Kidney biopsy is predominantly used in patients with glomerular disease. The most common indications for kidney biopsy include the nephrotic syndrome, acute glomerulonephritis, and kidney transplant dysfunction. None of these indications is present in this patient.

Radionuclide kidney clearance scanning can calculate GFR and renal plasma flow very accurately. However, its use is limited because of cost, lack of widespread availability, and operator technical difficulties. Estimating equations for GFR are reasonably accurate in patients with stage 3 CKD such as in this case; these equations can be calculated without the need for invasive studies and are generally preferred to radionuclide kidney clearance scanning.

KEY POINT

- Kidney ultrasonography is often the first imaging choice to assess kidney disease because it is safe, not dependent upon kidney function, noninvasive, and relatively inexpensive.

Bibliography

Drawz P, Rahman M. In the clinic. Chronic kidney disease. Ann Intern Med. 2009;150(3):ITC2-1-ITC2-15. [PMID: 19189903]

Item 91   Answer: A

Educational Objective: Identify the cause of kidney function decline in a patient with hypertension.

The increase in this patient's serum creatinine level is likely due to treatment with an angiotensin receptor blocker (ARB) for his essential hypertension. He has target organ damage to the kidneys that was present when treatment was initiated. A significant increase in serum creatinine occurs in some patients when an ARB is started, and similar changes are frequently noted with ACE inhibitors. Because of their mechanism of action, these medications tend to decrease the glomerular filtration rate and cause an increase in serum creatinine in patients with disorders in which intra-renal perfusion pressure is maintained by increased angiotensin, including hypertensive kidney disease, chronic kidney disease, heart failure, and renovascular disease. The rise in serum creatinine may be more pronounced in patients who have preexisting but unrecognized kidney injury before treatment is started, with the medication uncovering underlying kidney failure. However, these same effects may be protective against progression of kidney failure, and their use in these conditions may be beneficial if kidney function remains stable and there are no other complications of treatment, such as hyperkalemia.

The magnitude of proteinuria and otherwise unremarkable urine sediment on urinalysis do not suggest the presence of primary glomerular disease and are consistent with findings typically seen in patients with hypertensive kidney disease.

The patient's current level of blood pressure control appears adequate, and his increased serum creatinine level over the past 3 years likely does not reflect inadequate current blood pressure control.

Although this patient has several risk factors for vascular disease, he has no evidence of existing atherosclerotic disease by history or on examination, making renovascular causes of his kidney failure less likely.

KEY POINT

- Angiotensin receptor blockers and ACE inhibitors may lead to an increase in the serum creatinine level and may uncover previously undetected kidney dysfunction.

Bibliography

Taylor AA, Siragy H, Nesbitt S. Angiotensin receptor blockers: pharmacology, efficacy, and safety. J Clin Hypertens (Greenwich). 2011;13(9):677-686. [PMID: 21896150]

Item 92   Answer: C

Educational Objective: Diagnose polyarteritis nodosa.

This patient most likely has polyarteritis nodosa, a necrotizing vasculitis of the medium-sized arteries. The affected vessels are characterized by necrosis and inflammation in a patchy distribution. Approximately 50% of cases of polyarteritis nodosa are associated with hepatitis B virus infection, usually of recent acquisition; ANCA assays are almost always negative, particularly in patients with concomitant hepatitis B virus infection. Patients with polyarteritis nodosa typically present with fever, abdominal pain, arthralgia, and weight loss that develop over days to months. Two thirds of these patients have mononeuritis multiplex, and one third have hypertension, testicular pain, and cutaneous involvement, including nodules, ulcers, purpura, and livedo reticularis. In patients with a compatible clinical presentation, diagnosis is often confirmed by a biopsy from the skin

or a sural nerve. Radiographic imaging of the mesenteric or renal arteries can also be used to establish a definitive diagnosis of polyarteritis nodosa. Characteristic findings of this condition include aneurysms and stenoses of the medium-sized vessels.

Giant cell arteritis is a granulomatous vasculitis that most commonly affects the large and medium-sized arteries of the head and neck, including the temporal, ophthalmic, and posterior ciliary arteries. Subclinical involvement of the proximal and distal aorta also is common. Kidney involvement is not typical.

Granulomatosis with polyangiitis (also known as Wegener granulomatosis) is a necrotizing vasculitis that typically affects the respiratory tract and the kidneys. More than 70% of patients present with upper airway symptoms, particularly sinusitis. Kidney biopsy specimens reveal a pauci-immune crescentic glomerulonephritis; medium-sized artery aneurysms and stenosis are not found.

Takayasu arteritis is a large-vessel vasculitis associated with fever, arthralgia, myalgia, malaise, weight loss, and eventual vascular insufficiency. Diagnosis is made by demonstrating great-vessel narrowing visible on imaging studies, typically most marked at branch points in the aorta. This patient's short clinical course and involvement of medium-sized arteries is not compatible with Takayasu arteritis.

KEY POINT

- Characteristic angiographic findings of polyarteritis nodosa include aneurysms and stenoses of the medium-sized vessels.

Bibliography

Henegar C, Pagnoux C, Puéchal X, et al; French Vasculitis Study Group. A paradigm of diagnostic criteria for polyarteritis nodosa: analysis of a series of 949 patients with vasculitides. Arthritis Rheum. 2008;58(5):1528-1538. [PMID: 18438816]

Item 93   Answer: D

Educational Objective: Diagnose type B lactic acidosis.

The most likely diagnosis is type B lactic acidosis caused by linezolid toxicity. This patient has an anion gap metabolic acidosis associated with an increased serum lactate level. Type A lactic acidosis is associated with tissue hypoperfusion and hypoxia. The absence of shock or hypoxia in this patient is consistent with type B lactic acidosis. Type B lactic acidosis is often due to medication or toxin exposure and may also occur in patients with advanced malignancy, liver disease, or glucose-6-phosphate dehydrogenase deficiency. Linezolid is known to induce type B lactic acidosis by interfering with activity of the mitochondrial respiratory complex. Other medications known to induce type B lactic acidosis include acetaminophen overdose, metformin, the nucleoside reverse transcriptase inhibitors stavudine and didanosine, propofol, and salicylates. Lactic acidosis due to linezolid toxicity most commonly occurs after several weeks of therapy, although one third of reported cases occur within the first 2 weeks of therapy. Polymorphisms of mitochondrial DNA have been identified in affected persons. Onset of type B lactic acidosis warrants discontinuation of the offending agent (linezolid in this case), which leads to resolution of lactic acidosis in most patients. Those with end-stage kidney disease may benefit from intensification of dialysis to promote linezolid clearance.

Diabetic ketoacidosis presents with ketonemia, increased anion gap metabolic acidosis, and hyperglycemia with plasma glucose levels that usually exceed 300 mg/dL (16.7 mmol/L). This patient's modest degree of hyperglycemia and absence of detectable serum ketones argues against this diagnosis.

Pyroglutamic acidosis usually occurs in critically ill patients receiving therapeutic doses of acetaminophen. Patients present with unexplained increased anion gap metabolic acidosis due to the accumulation of pyroglutamic acid (also known as 5-oxoproline) as a consequence of impaired glutathione regeneration. Lactic acidosis is not a feature of pyroglutamic acidosis.

Although sepsis should always be considered in patients with lactic acidosis, the absence of leukocytosis, fever, tachycardia, and hypotension makes this diagnosis unlikely.

KEY POINT

- **Type B lactic acidosis is often due to medication or toxin exposure and may also occur in patients with advanced malignancy, liver disease, or glucose-6-phosphate dehydrogenase deficiency.**

Bibliography

Velez JC, Janech MG. A case of lactic acidosis induced by linezolid. Nat Rev Nephrol. 2010;6(4):236-242. [PMID: 20348931]

Item 94   Answer: C

Educational Objective: Evaluate a patient who has hypokalemic metabolic alkalosis.

Measurement of the urine chloride level is the most appropriate test to determine the cause of this patient's hypokalemic metabolic alkalosis. Metabolic alkalosis is caused by the net loss of acid or the retention of bicarbonate. The diagnostic evaluation of metabolic alkalosis begins with the clinical assessment of the volume status and blood pressure. Metabolic alkalosis that is associated with hypovolemia will correct with the administration of isotonic saline and volume expansion and is thus noted to be saline-responsive. When the metabolic alkalosis is associated with increased extracellular fluid volume and hypertension, it will not respond to isotonic saline and is termed saline-resistant. In this patient who does not have hypertension and has a normal or slightly decreased effective arterial blood

volume, the urine sodium and chloride levels can help distinguish the various causes of metabolic alkalosis. Patients with low urine chloride levels (<15 meq/L [15 mmol/L]; normal for men, 25-371 meq/L [25-371 mmol/L]) are usually either vomiting or have a decreased effective arterial blood volume from various causes, including prior use of diuretics or low cardiac output. Patients with high urine chloride levels (>15 meq/L [15 mmol/L]) most commonly are receiving active therapy with diuretics or, more rarely, may have a genetically based tubular disorder such as Bartter or Gitelman syndrome.

Plasma aldosterone and renin levels are most helpful in the diagnostic evaluation of metabolic alkalosis if there is associated hypertension. A plasma aldosterone-plasma renin activity ratio of 20 to 30 when the plasma aldosterone level is greater than 15 ng/dL (414 pmol/L) is highly suggestive of primary hyperaldosteronism, whereas suppression of both renin and aldosterone is consistent with syndromes of apparent mineralocorticoid excess. Plasma aldosterone and renin levels are elevated in patients with malignant hypertension, renin-secreting tumors, and renovascular hypertension.

Hypomagnesemia can lead to urine magnesium wasting and metabolic alkalosis and can be observed in patients with Bartter or Gitelman syndrome. However, serum magnesium measurement is not as helpful as the urine chloride value in distinguishing between the various causes of hypokalemic metabolic alkalosis.

The urine osmolal gap is a method of estimating urine ammonium excretion and is useful in the evaluation of normal anion gap metabolic acidosis. Ammonium excretion is variable in metabolic alkalosis and depends on numerous factors, including the magnitude of potassium depletion, protein intake, and volume status.

KEY POINT

- **The diagnostic evaluation of metabolic alkalosis begins with the clinical assessment of the volume status and blood pressure; urine sodium and chloride levels can help distinguish the various causes.**

Bibliography

Shin HS. Value of the measurement of urinary chloride in hypokalaemic metabolic alkalosis. Nephrology. 2010;15(1):133. [PMID: 20377781]

Item 95   Answer: A

Educational Objective: Assess the risk of contrast-induced nephropathy in a patient with chronic kidney disease.

Hydration with isotonic saline is indicated to decrease this patient's risk for contrast-induced nephropathy (CIN) associated with her cardiac catheterization. Patients with underlying kidney injury are particularly susceptible to additional kidney injury due to exposure of the renal tubule to nephrotoxic contrast media. Thus, avoidance of exposure to contrast in high-risk patients is preferable. However, in those who require contrast studies, use of low osmolar contrast agents and hydration to promote urine flow and avoid volume contraction has been shown to decrease the risk for CIN. There is some evidence that isotonic saline is preferable to hypotonic solutions for periprocedural hydration. Multiple studies have evaluated normal saline or intravenous fluids containing isotonic sodium bicarbonate as the prophylactic fluid. At this time, neither formulation appears significantly more effective than the other.

Although given to increase urine flow, diuresis with mannitol or a loop diuretic has not been shown to decrease the risk for CIN and may even increase the risk.

Oral hydration, with or without sodium loading, has not been shown to be more effective, and may be less effective, than intravenous hydration with isotonic saline.

Prophylactic hemodialysis has been evaluated as a method for removing nephrotoxic contrast agents in patients with existing kidney failure. No benefit has been shown, with possibly poorer outcomes, than with medical therapy.

KEY POINT

- Risk factors for contrast-induced nephropathy include poor baseline glomerular filtration rate and heart failure.

Bibliography
Solomon R, Dauerman HL. Contrast-induced acute kidney injury. Circulation. 2010;122(23):2451-2455. [PMID: 21135373]

Item 96   Answer: C

Educational Objective: Manage cardiovascular risk in a patient with chronic kidney disease.

An increase in the atorvastatin dose to lower the cholesterol level is indicated in this patient with chronic kidney disease (CKD). Besides therapies to delay CKD progression, treatment also includes managing the complications of CKD. Patients with CKD are at high risk for cardiovascular events, and the presence of CKD is considered a coronary heart disease equivalent in assessing risk and for guiding treatment. Although data about treatment of dyslipidemia with statins suggest no benefit in dialysis patients, statin therapy has been shown to reduce all-cause and cardiovascular deaths in patients with kidney disease not on dialysis. Statins may also reduce proteinuria and have beneficial anti-inflammatory and vascular effects. The goal for LDL cholesterol levels in patients with CKD is similar to those with significant coronary disease risk factors or known coronary artery disease, with a target of less than 100 mg/dL (2.59 mmol/L), and preferably less than 70 mg/dL (1.81 mmol/L).

Although treating secondary hyperparathyroidism is a management objective for patients with CKD, this patient's parathyroid hormone level is not far from a goal level for a patient with stage 3 CKD. Lowering parathyroid hormone levels has not been shown to improve mortality in patients with CKD.

The metabolic acidosis associated with CKD may have adverse effects, including worsening of bone disease. Sodium bicarbonate replacement therapy, typically to maintain a serum bicarbonate level ≥23 meq/L (23 mmol/L), is used in patients with CKD to treat kidney injury–associated metabolic acidosis and may delay kidney disease progression. It has not yet been shown to reduce mortality. Furthermore, this patient's serum bicarbonate level is adequate, and therapy is not indicated.

Increasing the ACE inhibitor dose in this patient with a blood pressure at target and a low level of proteinuria is unlikely to provide as much cardiovascular benefit as increasing the statin therapy.

KEY POINT

- Chronic kidney disease represents a cardiovascular risk factor, and management of dyslipidemia with statins can reduce cardiovascular risk in patients with chronic kidney disease.

Bibliography
Navaneethan SD, Pansini F, Perkovic V, et al. HMG CoA reductase inhibitors (statins) for people with chronic kidney disease not requiring dialysis. Cochrane Database Syst Rev. 2009;(2): CD007784. [PMID: 19370693]

Item 97   Answer: D

Educational Objective: Manage chronic hypertension in a pregnant patient.

For this pregnant patient with chronic hypertension, continuation of her current medication regimen is appropriate. Prior to conception, her medication was changed to labetalol, which is considered first-line therapy for the management of hypertension during pregnancy. This patient has a normal serum creatinine level but has proteinuria. She previously had been on an ACE inhibitor, which decreases proteinuria. Proteinuria is typically increased during pregnancy in patients with preexisting proteinuria. There is an increase in the glomerular filtration rate (GFR) related to the increase in plasma volume, yet this increase in GFR is not matched by an increase in tubular absorption of proteins; therefore, an increase in proteinuria follows. If this patient were not pregnant, strict blood pressure goals would be applied with blockade of the renin-angiotensin-aldosterone system. In contrast, blood pressure goals in pregnancy have not been rigorously tested; instead, management is focused on avoiding end-organ damage in the mother during this finite period. Although there are slight differences in the antihypertensive goals from various professional societies, most agree that the blood pressure should be less than 150/100 mm Hg. Currently, this patient's blood pressure is well within the target for management of chronic hypertension during pregnancy. Therefore, close monitoring and follow-up are indicated.

Although methyldopa is an acceptable medication with an established safety history for use in pregnancy, it frequently has a sedating effect and often needs to be given three times daily for an adequate antihypertensive effect. Furthermore, because this patient has achieved a reasonable blood pressure goal, there is no indication for add-on therapy at present.

Exposure to ACE inhibitors or angiotensin receptor blockers such as losartan during the first trimester has been associated with fetal cardiac abnormalities; exposure during the second and third trimesters has been associated with neonatal kidney failure and death. These agents are considered pregnancy category X drugs and should be held until after delivery.

There is no reason to increase the labetalol at this time because she is at a reasonable blood pressure goal and is tolerating the current dose well.

KEY POINT

- Close monitoring and follow-up are indicated for pregnant patients who have chronic hypertension with blood pressure measurements within target goals.

Bibliography

Seely EW, Ecker J. Clinical practice. Chronic hypertension in pregnancy. N Engl J Med. 2011;365(5):439-446. [PMID: 21812673]

Item 98   Answer: D

Educational Objective: Manage hypertension in a patient who is over the age of 80 years.

No change in management is required at this time. This 82-year-old woman has hypertension and currently takes indapamide and an ACE inhibitor; her blood pressure measurements have been less than 150 mm Hg systolic. The pattern of blood pressure elevation in older patients is typically characterized by a prominent systolic blood pressure. This relates in large part to the significant role of vascular stiffness in the blood pressure increases of older patients, which in addition to raising systolic pressure, also leads to a decline in the diastolic pressure. In the past, these physiologic changes were thought to be normal, and elevated blood pressures in older patients were not treated. However, it has been shown that treatment of blood pressure in aging patients does lead to improved cardiovascular outcomes. Although a target blood pressure of 140/90 mm Hg is generally accepted for most patients with hypertension, there are less data on patients over the age of 80 years to guide therapy. The Hypertension in the Very Elderly Trial (HYVET) enrolled patients at least 80 years of age and used a target systolic blood pressure of 150 mm Hg, which is assumed to be a reasonable goal for this population. HYVET also provided evidence affirming that treatment of

older patients with hypertension leads to fewer deaths and less heart failure with active drug therapy. This older patient with target blood pressure measurements does not require additional treatment, and a follow-up visit in 4 months is appropriate.

Adding an additional antihypertensive agent such as amlodipine or metoprolol to this patient's regimen is not appropriate because reducing the systolic value to less than 140 mm Hg in older patients has not been shown to be beneficial. Furthermore, an additional agent with a different mechanism of action may cause adverse effects in older patients who may not be able to compensate effectively for the physiologic changes induced by multiple medications.

This patient's current regimen of the diuretic indapamide and an ACE inhibitor appears to be reasonably effective; therefore, a diuretic substitution is unnecessary.

KEY POINT

- Treating hypertension in older patients has been shown to be effective in reducing death and adverse cardiovascular outcomes, although reducing the systolic blood pressure to less than 140 mm Hg has not been shown to be beneficial in this population.

Bibliography

Beckett NS, Peters R, Fletcher AE, et al; HYVET Study Group. Treatment of hypertension in patients 80 years of age or older. N Engl J Med. 2008;358(18):1887-1898. [PMID: 18378519]

Item 99   Answer: D

Educational Objective: Recognize the increased risk of cardiovascular disease in the setting of chronic kidney disease.

This patient should be sent promptly to the emergency department for evaluation and treatment of unstable angina. Patients with chronic kidney disease (CKD) who have acute coronary disease are less likely to have chest pain but are more likely to have atypical symptoms such as dyspnea or nausea. Recent evidence suggests that acute coronary disease is underrecognized and undertreated in patients with CKD. Although this patient is relatively young and has never smoked, the presence of both CKD and proteinuria are serious risk factors for cardiovascular disease. Even with well-controlled blood pressure and lipids, patients with CKD have a greater incidence of cardiovascular events and cardiovascular mortality compared with those with similar comorbid conditions. This finding has led many to consider nontraditional risk factors for cardiovascular disease that may play a role such as abnormal vascular calcification, inflammation, hyperhomocysteinemia, or neurohumoral activation. Because these nonconventional factors are poorly understood, efforts to manage traditional risk factors are of paramount importance.

Starting albuterol before establishing a cause of the patient's dyspnea is not appropriate.

Although patients with CKD may experience dyspnea due to volume overload, and a diuretic may be helpful in relieving symptoms, the patient's physical examination findings are not supportive of this diagnosis. More importantly, because exertional dyspnea can be an anginal equivalent in patients with CKD, this diagnosis should be evaluated before any other diagnosis is considered or treatment is undertaken.

If the patient's dyspnea is not due to coronary artery disease–related left ventricular dysfunction, a pulmonary evaluation that includes spirometry would be reasonable.

KEY POINT

- **Patients with chronic kidney disease have a greater incidence of cardiovascular events and cardiovascular mortality compared with those with similar comorbid conditions.**

Bibliography

Hage FG, Venkataraman R, Zoghbi GJ, Perry GJ, DeMattos AM, Iskandrian AE. The scope of coronary heart disease in patients with chronic kidney disease. J Am Coll Cardiol. 2009;53(23):2129-2140. [PMID: 19497438]

Item 100   Answer: B

Educational Objective: Screen for intracranial cerebral aneurysms in a patient with autosomal dominant polycystic kidney disease.

MR angiography of the cerebral arteries is appropriate for this patient with autosomal dominant polycystic kidney disease (ADPKD) and a family history of potential cerebral aneurysm rupture. Intracranial cerebral aneurysms occur in approximately 8% of patients with ADPKD. The most important risk factor for the development of an intracranial cerebral aneurysm is a family member with a known intracranial aneurysm, particularly in a first-degree relative with a previously ruptured aneurysm. Therefore, imaging to assess for the presence of an intracranial cerebral aneurysm is appropriate in this patient with ADPKD who has a family history of potential intracranial cerebral aneurysm rupture. MR angiography and high-resolution CT angiography are imaging options, having supplanted cerebral arteriography because of its invasiveness and risk of stroke associated with the procedure. MR angiography is adequately sensitive for detecting clinically significant aneurysms, although the use of gadolinium-based contrast agents in patients with moderate to severe kidney disease is contraindicated because of the risk of nephrogenic systemic fibrosis. The role of screening patients with ADPKD and no family history of cerebral aneurysm as well as the frequency of follow-up for high-risk screened patients without a cerebral aneurysm remain unclear.

This patient's laboratory studies already include a urine protein–creatinine ratio, which is a reasonable proxy for a 24-hour urine measurement of protein. Therefore, a 24-hour urine collection would not provide additional information relevant to long-term management.

Genotype testing is not routinely performed as part of the evaluation of ADPKD because it is expensive, difficult to obtain, and would not influence the initial management of this patient.

Abdominal CT is not necessary to confirm the diagnosis of ADPKD if the patient already has documentation of ADPKD by other imaging such as ultrasound.

KEY POINT

- **Screening for intracranial aneurysms is recommended for patients with autosomal dominant polycystic kidney disease who have a family history of potential intracranial cerebral aneurysm rupture.**

Bibliography

Pirson Y. Extrarenal manifestations of autosomal dominant polycystic kidney disease. Adv Chronic Kidney Dis. 2010;17(2):173-180. [PMID: 20219620]

Item 101   Answer: C

Educational Objective: Manage secondary hyperparathyroidism in a patient with chronic kidney disease.

The addition of cholecalciferol (vitamin D_3) is indicated for this patient with chronic kidney disease (CKD) who has vitamin D insufficiency. An elevation in the parathyroid hormone level is often the first detectable change associated with chronic kidney disease mineral bone disorder (CKD-MBD), which may occur very early in the course of CKD; therefore, the Kidney Disease Improving Global Outcomes (KDIGO) guidelines recommend testing for MBD beginning with stage 3 CKD. This evaluation typically begins with measurement of serum parathyroid hormone levels, vitamin D levels, and calcium and phosphorus concentrations. This patient's intact parathyroid hormone level is elevated, but there is evidence of vitamin D insufficiency. There is ongoing debate on the definition of vitamin D deficiency; nevertheless, suboptimal levels can contribute to secondary hyperparathyroidism. Before beginning a course of more expensive vitamin D analogs, it is appropriate to treat with the inactive forms of vitamin D, cholecalciferol or ergocalciferol, which may improve or correct the secondary hyperparathyroidism due to vitamin D insufficiency or deficiency.

If the intact parathyroid hormone level is elevated but the 25-hydroxy vitamin D level is more than 30 ng/mL (75 nmol/L), then an active oral vitamin D sterol such as calcitriol, alfacalcidol, or doxercalciferol should be utilized. Use of these agents requires careful monitoring to avoid hypercalcemia, vascular calcifications, or oversuppression of parathyroid hormone.

In the absence of vitamin D insufficiency or deficiency, calcium salts such as calcium carbonate can bind phosphorus in the gut and help control hyperphosphatemia of CKD.

Sevelamer is indicated to manage phosphate retention in patients with CKD who are unable to control hyperphosphatemia with oral calcium salts, cannot tolerate oral calcium, or develop hypercalcemia using calcium as a phosphate binder. However, this patient's serum phosphorus level is normal and does not require treatment with sevelamer.

KEY POINT

- **Underlying vitamin D insufficiency/deficiency can cause secondary hyperparathyroidism in patients with chronic kidney disease.**

Bibliography

Sprague SM, Coyne D. Control of secondary hyperparathyroidism by vitamin D receptor agonists in chronic kidney disease. Clin J Am Soc Nephrol. 2010;5(3):512-518. [PMID: 20133492]

Item 102   Answer: C
Educational Objective: Diagnose prehypertension.

This patient has prehypertension. Classification of hypertension is based on an average of two or more seated blood pressure readings obtained more than 1 minute apart at two or more visits. The prehypertension category established by the Seventh Report of the Joint National Committee on Prevention, Detection, Evaluation, and Treatment of High Blood Pressure (JNC 7) designates a group at high risk for progression to hypertension in whom lifestyle modifications may be preemptive. The JNC 7 definition of prehypertension is an average blood pressure reading of 120 to 139 mm Hg systolic or 80 to 89 mm Hg diastolic. Studies such as the Trial of Preventing Hypertension (TROPHY) have shown that about two thirds of patients diagnosed as prehypertensive will develop stage 1 hypertension during 4 years of follow-up.

Masked hypertension is characterized by blood pressure that is higher at home than in the office setting. Suspicion for masked hypertension is usually raised when the physician is informed of discrepancies between office and home blood pressure readings or findings that suggest the presence of undiagnosed hypertension such as left ventricular hypertrophy. Ambulatory blood pressure monitoring can be used to confirm this diagnosis.

Normotension is defined as a blood pressure measurement of less than 120/80 mm Hg.

White coat hypertension is characterized by at least three separate office blood pressure measurements above 140/90 mm Hg with at least two sets of measurements below 140/90 mm Hg obtained outside the office, accompanied by the absence of target organ damage. Ambulatory blood pressure monitoring is considered the gold standard for diagnosing this condition. This patient does not fit the criteria for the diagnosis of white coat hypertension.

KEY POINT

- **Patients with prehypertension (defined as an average blood pressure reading of 120 to 139 mm Hg systolic or 80 to 89 mm Hg diastolic) are at high risk for progression to hypertension, and lifestyle modifications in this patient population may be preemptive.**

Bibliography

Chobanian AV, Bakris GL, Black HR, et al; Joint National Committee on Prevention, Detection, Evaluation, and Treatment of High Blood Pressure; National Heart, Lung, and Blood Institute; National High Blood Pressure Education Program Coordinating Committee. Seventh report of the Joint National Committee on Prevention, Detection, Evaluation, and Treatment of High Blood Pressure. Hypertension. 2003;42(6):1206-1252. [PMID: 14656957]

Item 103   Answer: A
Educational Objective: Diagnose underlying chronic kidney disease and hypertension in a pregnant patient.

This patient is at 17 weeks' gestation and has underlying chronic kidney disease and hypertension. Because baseline proteinuria typically increases during pregnancy and edema is commonly seen during pregnancy, it is often difficult to determine whether a patient has an exacerbation of underlying kidney disease or a disorder associated with pregnancy. This patient describes hypertension complicating her first pregnancy. Currently, her blood pressure is elevated. During pregnancy, blood pressure levels typically decrease early in the first trimester and may remain lower than nonpregnant levels until term; therefore, when hypertension is present before 20 weeks' gestation, this represents chronic hypertension rather than a hypertensive disorder of pregnancy (gestational hypertension or preeclampsia). In addition, her serum creatinine level is elevated. The serum creatinine level typically falls during pregnancy because the increased plasma volume leads to an increase in glomerular filtration rate. She also has proteinuria noted on urine dipstick and confirmed by the urine protein–creatinine ratio. These findings suggest that the patient has chronic kidney disease and hypertension, which now complicate her second pregnancy.

Gestational hypertension refers to hypertension that develops after 20 weeks' gestation in the absence of proteinuria or other maternal end-organ damage. Up to 45% of women initially diagnosed with gestational hypertension develop preeclampsia, and the risk is greatest if the hypertension develops remote from term.

The nephrotic syndrome is characterized by a urine protein–creatinine ratio greater than 3.5 mg/mg, hypoalbuminemia, hyperlipidemia, lipiduria, edema, and hypercoagulability. This patient's urinalysis results show 1+ protein, which is likely to fall below the nephrotic range, and her urine protein–creatinine ratio suggests that the protein is less than 1 g/24 h.

Preeclampsia is characterized by new-onset hypertension accompanied by the development of proteinuria. This condition can develop any time after 20 weeks of pregnancy but usually occurs close to term.

KEY POINT

- Hypertension that occurs before 20 weeks' gestation suggests the presence of chronic hypertension and not a hypertensive disorder of pregnancy.

Bibliography

Yoder SR, Thornburg LL, Bisognano JD. Hypertension in pregnancy and women of childbearing age. Am J Medicine. 2009;122(10):890-895. [PMID: 19786154]

Item 104   Answer: A

Educational Objective: Identify gentamicin as the cause of hypokalemic metabolic alkalosis.

This patient's hypokalemic metabolic alkalosis is most likely caused by gentamicin toxicity. The differential diagnosis of hypokalemic metabolic alkalosis and normal to low extracellular fluid volume status includes diuretics, gastric fluid loss through vomiting or nasogastric suction, gentamicin toxicity, the inherited tubulopathies Gitelman and Bartter syndromes, and high-dose penicillin therapy. Exposure to greater than 1.2 grams of gentamicin is known to induce a Bartter-like syndrome. Aminoglycosides are divalent cations that can activate the calcium-sensing receptor in the thick ascending limb. Activation of the calcium-sensing receptor inhibits the sodium-potassium-chloride cotransporter in the thick ascending limb, mimicking the effect of loop diuretics and leading to hypokalemic metabolic alkalosis. The urine potassium–creatinine ratio of 50 meq/g is consistent with urine potassium losses due to tubular dysfunction caused by gentamicin toxicity.

This patient's elevated urine sodium, chloride, and potassium levels are consistent with primary hyperaldosteronism. However, the absence of hypertension as well as the acute onset of hypokalemic metabolic alkalosis temporally associated with gentamicin therapy makes this diagnosis unlikely.

Exposure to supratherapeutic doses of quetiapine has been reported to induce redistribution of potassium into the intracellular space and hypokalemia. The urine potassium–creatinine ratio should be less than 15 meq/g in this circumstance, and metabolic alkalosis is not an associated feature.

Vancomycin is associated with nephrotoxicity but is not known to induce hypokalemic metabolic alkalosis. Vancomycin-associated tubular injury most commonly results in hyperkalemia rather than hypokalemia.

KEY POINT

- Exposure to greater than 1.2 grams of gentamicin is known to induce a Bartter-like syndrome, which is associated with hypokalemic metabolic alkalosis.

Bibliography

Zietse R, Zoutendijk R, Hoorn EJ. Fluid, electrolyte and acid-base disorders associated with antibiotic therapy. Nat Rev Nephrol. 2009;5(4):193-202. [PMID: 19322184]

Item 105   Answer: D

Educational Objective: Diagnose anemia in chronic kidney disease.

Measurement of serum iron and ferritin concentrations and total iron-binding capacity (TIBC) to assess this patient's iron stores is indicated. She has normochromic normocytic anemia. Anemia is common in patients with chronic kidney disease (CKD) because of relative deficiency of erythropoietin, erythropoietin resistance, and shortened erythrocyte survival. The anemia of CKD is usually normochromic and normocytic with a low reticulocyte count. Anemia often occurs earlier in the course of kidney disease in patients with diabetic nephropathy compared with other kidney diseases. Before attributing anemia to CKD, it is important to exclude other etiologies. Iron deficiency is common in patients with CKD. Although most do not have an identifiable cause, patients with CKD are prone to ulcer disease and angiodysplasia-induced gastrointestinal blood loss, resulting in iron deficiency and eventually the development of microcytosis.

Patients with anemia should be evaluated for iron deficiency by serum iron and ferritin concentrations and TIBC. The serum iron concentration, a poor reflection of iron stores, is usually low in patients with iron deficiency; the TIBC is high; the percentage of transferrin saturation (iron/TIBC) is low; and the serum ferritin concentration is low. Because the serum ferritin concentration can increase in inflammatory states, ferritin may be normal or elevated in patients with iron deficiency, but a ferritin concentration of greater than 100 ng/mL (100 micrograms/L) excludes iron deficiency, and a ferritin level of less than 15 ng/mL (15 micrograms/L) confirms iron deficiency. If the results suggest iron deficiency, patients should be evaluated for blood loss, and iron should be prescribed.

ACE inhibitors can contribute to anemia in patients with marginal erythropoietin production; however, the benefit of ACE inhibitors in slowing progression of diabetic kidney disease outweighs this concern. Therefore, lisinopril should not be discontinued in this patient.

Initiation of erythropoiesis-stimulating agents should only be considered after patients have been evaluated for other causes of anemia and iron stores are adequate (ferritin >100 ng/mL [100 micrograms/L] and transferrin saturation >20%).

In patients with CKD, measurement of the serum erythropoietin level does not help to discriminate among other causes of anemia or to guide treatment decisions because CKD may be associated with reduced production of erythropoietin or erythropoietin resistance.

- The anemia of chronic kidney disease is a diagnosis of exclusion.

Bibliography

National Kidney Foundation. KDOQI clinical practice guidelines and clinical practice recommendations for anemia in chronic kidney disease (2006). Available at www.kidney.org/professionals/KDOQI/guidelines_anemia/index.htm. Accessed July 24, 2012.

Item 106   Answer: C
Educational Objective: Diagnose obstructive acute kidney injury.

Kidney ultrasonography is indicated for this patient with acute kidney injury (AKI) most likely caused by urinary obstruction. Because relief of obstruction can reverse kidney injury and prevent chronic damage, timely diagnosis is essential. Urinary obstruction can be asymptomatic and can be associated with no noted change in urine output. Because of the lack of definitive symptoms on presentation, kidney imaging, typically ultrasonography, should be considered in all patients with AKI, particularly when risk factors for obstruction are present. Medical history findings, including pelvic tumors or irradiation, congenital urinary abnormalities, kidney stones, genitourinary infections, procedures or surgeries, and prostatic enlargement, should increase suspicion for obstruction. Bladder ultrasonography can be done as a quick bedside procedure and may also diagnosis bladder obstruction; however, it will not reveal hydronephrosis or kidney anatomy.

In obstruction, the urinalysis is bland. Urine electrolytes are variable; in early obstruction, the urine sodium and fractional excretion of sodium (FE_{Na}) may be low, but in late obstruction, the urine sodium and FE_{Na} may be high, indicative of tubular damage. Because of impaired kidney excretion of potassium, acid, and water, hyperkalemic metabolic acidosis and hyponatremia can be present. The FE_{Na} is not helpful in obstruction, and the clinical information provided does not suggest a prerenal etiology of AKI should be entertained.

Kidney biopsy is performed to evaluate for kidney injury of unknown cause. In this patient with a history suggestive of obstruction, imaging to exclude obstruction should be done first.

Rhabdomyolysis is associated with an increased serum creatine kinase level and can cause elevated serum creatinine and potassium levels; however, the patient has no risk factors for rhabdomyolysis (crush injury, muscle pain, or medications known to cause rhabdomyolysis).

- Kidney imaging, typically ultrasonography, should be considered in all patients with acute kidney injury, particularly when risk factors for obstruction are present.

Bibliography

Licurse A, Kim MC, Dziura J, et al. Renal ultrasonography in the evaluation of acute kidney injury: developing a risk stratification framework. Arch Intern Med. 2010;170(21):1900-1907. [PMID: 21098348]

Item 107   Answer: C
Educational Objective: Diagnose pheochromocytoma.

Measurement of this patient's plasma metanephrine level is appropriate. The surge in this patient's blood pressure noted during anesthesia induction could reflect a stimulus to catecholamine release from a tumor such as a pheochromocytoma. Pheochromocytomas are relatively rare tumors composed of chromaffin cells derived from the neural crest that occur in 0.1% to 0.6% of persons with hypertension. Most pheochromocytomas predominantly secrete norepinephrine, which results in sustained or episodic hypertension. Major symptoms include diaphoresis, pallor, palpitations, and headaches; the classic triad of sudden severe headache, diaphoresis, and palpitations is highly suggestive of pheochromocytoma. Other symptoms may include weight loss and dyspnea. Clinical manifestations are variable, with hypertension (episodic or sustained) observed in more than 90% of patients. Other manifestations include arrhythmias (atrial and ventricular fibrillation) and catecholamine-induced cardiomyopathy. Diagnosis requires a high degree of suspicion, with confirmation of excess catecholamine production either by 24-hour urine collection for catecholamine and metanephrine excretion or by measurement of plasma metanephrine; the latter is easier to obtain and has good sensitivity and specificity. Definitive therapy for these tumors is surgical removal.

Elevated catecholamines typically prompt a tumor search by conventional imaging of the adrenal glands (such as CT or MRI) or the use of specialized nuclear scans such as iodine-131–metaiodobenzylguanidine (^{131}I-MIBG). CT or MRI should be obtained only after the diagnosis of pheochromocytoma is biochemically confirmed and is therefore not appropriate for this patient at this time.

Catheter-based kidney angiography can be harmful for this patient because pheochromocytomas occasionally secrete catecholamines in response to the iodinated contrast. Furthermore, severe hypertension associated with anesthesia induction is most compatible with pheochromocytoma, not renal artery stenosis.

Transthoracic echocardiography has many indications, most commonly for evaluating heart murmurs and left ventricular function. This patient has no obvious

CONT.

indication for transthoracic echocardiography, and this test will not be helpful in the evaluation of her recent episode of hypertension.

KEY POINT

- Pheochromocytoma can cause sustained or paroxysmal hypertension, diaphoresis, headache, and anxiety.

Bibliography

Prejbisz A, Lenders JW, Eisenhofer G, Januszewicz A. Cardiovascular manifestations of phaeochromocytoma. J Hypertens. 2011;29(11):2049-2060. [PMID: 21826022]

Item 108   Answer: B

Educational Objective: Manage hypernatremia.

The presence of significant hypernatremia indicates a relative deficit of water to sodium, and correction of the water deficit with 5% dextrose in water is indicated for this patient. The urine osmolality greater than 300 mosm/kg H_2O in this patient with polyuria is consistent with an osmotic diuresis. The diuresis that follows relief of urinary tract obstruction is predominantly due to excretion of retained solute. Urinary tract obstruction can lead to tubular injury and an associated concentrating defect. There is little evidence to guide the optimal rate of correction of hypernatremia, but a correction rate of 6 to 10 meq/L (6-10 mmol/L) per day is reasonable.

The presence of edema and hypernatremia in this patient is indicative of excess total body sodium; therefore, 0.45% sodium chloride is not indicated.

Desmopressin is indicated to treat patients with central diabetes insipidus and can also be employed as an adjunct in the management of nephrogenic diabetes insipidus, but the relatively high urine osmolality and high urine volume are most consistent with a solute diuresis.

Urine osmolality is generally less than 200 mosm/kg H_2O in patients with diabetes insipidus. A water deprivation test, which poses a risk of worsening hypernatremia, is therefore not indicated.

KEY POINT

- Correction of the water deficit using 5% dextrose in water is appropriate in patients with significant hypernatremia without evidence of hypovolemia or sodium depletion.

Bibliography

Pokaharel M, Block CA. Dysnatremia in the ICU. Curr Opin Crit Care. 2011;17(6):581-593. [PMID: 22027406]

Index

Note: Page numbers followed by f and t denote figures and tables, respectively. Test questions are indicated by Q.

Index

A | NAME AND ADDRESS (Please complete.)

Last Name   First Name   Middle Initial

Address

Address cont.

City   State   ZIP Code

Country

Email address

B | **Order Number**

(Use the Order Number on your MKSAP materials packing slip.)

C | **ACP ID Number**

(Refer to packing slip in your MKSAP materials for your ACP ID Number.)

ACP | AMERICAN COLLEGE OF PHYSICIANS
INTERNAL MEDICINE | Doctors for Adults

Medical Knowledge
Self-Assessment
Program® 16

TO EARN *AMA PRA CATEGORY 1 CREDITS*™ YOU MUST:

1. Answer all questions.
2. Score a minimum of 50% correct.

==

TO EARN *FREE* SAME-DAY *AMA PRA CATEGORY 1 CREDITS*™ ONLINE:

1. Answer all of your questions.
2. Go to **mksap.acponline.org** and access the appropriate answer sheet.
3. Transcribe your answers and submit for CME credits.
4. You can also enter your answers directly at **mksap.acponline.org** without first using this answer sheet.

To Submit Your Answer Sheet by Mail or FAX for a $10 Administrative Fee per Answer Sheet:

1. Answer all of your questions and calculate your score.
2. Complete boxes A–F.
3. Complete payment information.
4. Send the answer sheet and payment information to ACP, using the FAX number/address listed below.

COMPLETE FORM BELOW ONLY IF YOU SUBMIT BY MAIL OR FAX

Last Name   First Name   MI

Payment Information. Must remit in US funds, drawn on a US bank.

The processing fee for each paper answer sheet is $10.

☐ Check, made payable to ACP, enclosed

Charge to ☐ **VISA** ☐ *MasterCard* ☐ *AMERICAN EXPRESS* ☐ *DISCOVER*

Card Number _____

Expiration Date _____ / _____   Security code (3 or 4 digit #s) _____
         MM   YY

Signature _____

Fax to: 215-351-2799

Questions?
Go to **mskap.acponline.org** or email **custserv@acponline.org**

Mail to:
Member and Customer Service
American College of Physicians
190 N. Independence Mall West
Philadelphia, PA 19106-1572

1 Ⓐ Ⓑ Ⓒ Ⓓ Ⓔ
2 Ⓐ Ⓑ Ⓒ Ⓓ Ⓔ
3 Ⓐ Ⓑ Ⓒ Ⓓ Ⓔ
4 Ⓐ Ⓑ Ⓒ Ⓓ Ⓔ
5 Ⓐ Ⓑ Ⓒ Ⓓ Ⓔ

6 Ⓐ Ⓑ Ⓒ Ⓓ Ⓔ
7 Ⓐ Ⓑ Ⓒ Ⓓ Ⓔ
8 Ⓐ Ⓑ Ⓒ Ⓓ Ⓔ
9 Ⓐ Ⓑ Ⓒ Ⓓ Ⓔ
10 Ⓐ Ⓑ Ⓒ Ⓓ Ⓔ

11 Ⓐ Ⓑ Ⓒ Ⓓ Ⓔ
12 Ⓐ Ⓑ Ⓒ Ⓓ Ⓔ
13 Ⓐ Ⓑ Ⓒ Ⓓ Ⓔ
14 Ⓐ Ⓑ Ⓒ Ⓓ Ⓔ
15 Ⓐ Ⓑ Ⓒ Ⓓ Ⓔ

16 Ⓐ Ⓑ Ⓒ Ⓓ Ⓔ
17 Ⓐ Ⓑ Ⓒ Ⓓ Ⓔ
18 Ⓐ Ⓑ Ⓒ Ⓓ Ⓔ
19 Ⓐ Ⓑ Ⓒ Ⓓ Ⓔ
20 Ⓐ Ⓑ Ⓒ Ⓓ Ⓔ

21 Ⓐ Ⓑ Ⓒ Ⓓ Ⓔ
22 Ⓐ Ⓑ Ⓒ Ⓓ Ⓔ
23 Ⓐ Ⓑ Ⓒ Ⓓ Ⓔ
24 Ⓐ Ⓑ Ⓒ Ⓓ Ⓔ
25 Ⓐ Ⓑ Ⓒ Ⓓ Ⓔ

26 Ⓐ Ⓑ Ⓒ Ⓓ Ⓔ
27 Ⓐ Ⓑ Ⓒ Ⓓ Ⓔ
28 Ⓐ Ⓑ Ⓒ Ⓓ Ⓔ
29 Ⓐ Ⓑ Ⓒ Ⓓ Ⓔ
30 Ⓐ Ⓑ Ⓒ Ⓓ Ⓔ

31 Ⓐ Ⓑ Ⓒ Ⓓ Ⓔ
32 Ⓐ Ⓑ Ⓒ Ⓓ Ⓔ
33 Ⓐ Ⓑ Ⓒ Ⓓ Ⓔ
34 Ⓐ Ⓑ Ⓒ Ⓓ Ⓔ
35 Ⓐ Ⓑ Ⓒ Ⓓ Ⓔ

36 Ⓐ Ⓑ Ⓒ Ⓓ Ⓔ
37 Ⓐ Ⓑ Ⓒ Ⓓ Ⓔ
38 Ⓐ Ⓑ Ⓒ Ⓓ Ⓔ
39 Ⓐ Ⓑ Ⓒ Ⓓ Ⓔ
40 Ⓐ Ⓑ Ⓒ Ⓓ Ⓔ

41 Ⓐ Ⓑ Ⓒ Ⓓ Ⓔ
42 Ⓐ Ⓑ Ⓒ Ⓓ Ⓔ
43 Ⓐ Ⓑ Ⓒ Ⓓ Ⓔ
44 Ⓐ Ⓑ Ⓒ Ⓓ Ⓔ
45 Ⓐ Ⓑ Ⓒ Ⓓ Ⓔ

46 Ⓐ Ⓑ Ⓒ Ⓓ Ⓔ
47 Ⓐ Ⓑ Ⓒ Ⓓ Ⓔ
48 Ⓐ Ⓑ Ⓒ Ⓓ Ⓔ
49 Ⓐ Ⓑ Ⓒ Ⓓ Ⓔ
50 Ⓐ Ⓑ Ⓒ Ⓓ Ⓔ

51 Ⓐ Ⓑ Ⓒ Ⓓ Ⓔ
52 Ⓐ Ⓑ Ⓒ Ⓓ Ⓔ
53 Ⓐ Ⓑ Ⓒ Ⓓ Ⓔ
54 Ⓐ Ⓑ Ⓒ Ⓓ Ⓔ
55 Ⓐ Ⓑ Ⓒ Ⓓ Ⓔ

56 Ⓐ Ⓑ Ⓒ Ⓓ Ⓔ
57 Ⓐ Ⓑ Ⓒ Ⓓ Ⓔ
58 Ⓐ Ⓑ Ⓒ Ⓓ Ⓔ
59 Ⓐ Ⓑ Ⓒ Ⓓ Ⓔ
60 Ⓐ Ⓑ Ⓒ Ⓓ Ⓔ

61 Ⓐ Ⓑ Ⓒ Ⓓ Ⓔ
62 Ⓐ Ⓑ Ⓒ Ⓓ Ⓔ
63 Ⓐ Ⓑ Ⓒ Ⓓ Ⓔ
64 Ⓐ Ⓑ Ⓒ Ⓓ Ⓔ
65 Ⓐ Ⓑ Ⓒ Ⓓ Ⓔ

66 Ⓐ Ⓑ Ⓒ Ⓓ Ⓔ
67 Ⓐ Ⓑ Ⓒ Ⓓ Ⓔ
68 Ⓐ Ⓑ Ⓒ Ⓓ Ⓔ
69 Ⓐ Ⓑ Ⓒ Ⓓ Ⓔ
70 Ⓐ Ⓑ Ⓒ Ⓓ Ⓔ

71 Ⓐ Ⓑ Ⓒ Ⓓ Ⓔ
72 Ⓐ Ⓑ Ⓒ Ⓓ Ⓔ
73 Ⓐ Ⓑ Ⓒ Ⓓ Ⓔ
74 Ⓐ Ⓑ Ⓒ Ⓓ Ⓔ
75 Ⓐ Ⓑ Ⓒ Ⓓ Ⓔ

76 Ⓐ Ⓑ Ⓒ Ⓓ Ⓔ
77 Ⓐ Ⓑ Ⓒ Ⓓ Ⓔ
78 Ⓐ Ⓑ Ⓒ Ⓓ Ⓔ
79 Ⓐ Ⓑ Ⓒ Ⓓ Ⓔ
80 Ⓐ Ⓑ Ⓒ Ⓓ Ⓔ

81 Ⓐ Ⓑ Ⓒ Ⓓ Ⓔ
82 Ⓐ Ⓑ Ⓒ Ⓓ Ⓔ
83 Ⓐ Ⓑ Ⓒ Ⓓ Ⓔ
84 Ⓐ Ⓑ Ⓒ Ⓓ Ⓔ
85 Ⓐ Ⓑ Ⓒ Ⓓ Ⓔ

86 Ⓐ Ⓑ Ⓒ Ⓓ Ⓔ
87 Ⓐ Ⓑ Ⓒ Ⓓ Ⓔ
88 Ⓐ Ⓑ Ⓒ Ⓓ Ⓔ
89 Ⓐ Ⓑ Ⓒ Ⓓ Ⓔ
90 Ⓐ Ⓑ Ⓒ Ⓓ Ⓔ

91 Ⓐ Ⓑ Ⓒ Ⓓ Ⓔ
92 Ⓐ Ⓑ Ⓒ Ⓓ Ⓔ
93 Ⓐ Ⓑ Ⓒ Ⓓ Ⓔ
94 Ⓐ Ⓑ Ⓒ Ⓓ Ⓔ
95 Ⓐ Ⓑ Ⓒ Ⓓ Ⓔ

96 Ⓐ Ⓑ Ⓒ Ⓓ Ⓔ
97 Ⓐ Ⓑ Ⓒ Ⓓ Ⓔ
98 Ⓐ Ⓑ Ⓒ Ⓓ Ⓔ
99 Ⓐ Ⓑ Ⓒ Ⓓ Ⓔ
100 Ⓐ Ⓑ Ⓒ Ⓓ Ⓔ

101 Ⓐ Ⓑ Ⓒ Ⓓ Ⓔ
102 Ⓐ Ⓑ Ⓒ Ⓓ Ⓔ
103 Ⓐ Ⓑ Ⓒ Ⓓ Ⓔ
104 Ⓐ Ⓑ Ⓒ Ⓓ Ⓔ
105 Ⓐ Ⓑ Ⓒ Ⓓ Ⓔ

106 Ⓐ Ⓑ Ⓒ Ⓓ Ⓔ
107 Ⓐ Ⓑ Ⓒ Ⓓ Ⓔ
108 Ⓐ Ⓑ Ⓒ Ⓓ Ⓔ
109 Ⓐ Ⓑ Ⓒ Ⓓ Ⓔ
110 Ⓐ Ⓑ Ⓒ Ⓓ Ⓔ

111 Ⓐ Ⓑ Ⓒ Ⓓ Ⓔ
112 Ⓐ Ⓑ Ⓒ Ⓓ Ⓔ
113 Ⓐ Ⓑ Ⓒ Ⓓ Ⓔ
114 Ⓐ Ⓑ Ⓒ Ⓓ Ⓔ
115 Ⓐ Ⓑ Ⓒ Ⓓ Ⓔ

116 Ⓐ Ⓑ Ⓒ Ⓓ Ⓔ
117 Ⓐ Ⓑ Ⓒ Ⓓ Ⓔ
118 Ⓐ Ⓑ Ⓒ Ⓓ Ⓔ
119 Ⓐ Ⓑ Ⓒ Ⓓ Ⓔ
120 Ⓐ Ⓑ Ⓒ Ⓓ Ⓔ

121 Ⓐ Ⓑ Ⓒ Ⓓ Ⓔ
122 Ⓐ Ⓑ Ⓒ Ⓓ Ⓔ
123 Ⓐ Ⓑ Ⓒ Ⓓ Ⓔ
124 Ⓐ Ⓑ Ⓒ Ⓓ Ⓔ
125 Ⓐ Ⓑ Ⓒ Ⓓ Ⓔ

126 Ⓐ Ⓑ Ⓒ Ⓓ Ⓔ
127 Ⓐ Ⓑ Ⓒ Ⓓ Ⓔ
128 Ⓐ Ⓑ Ⓒ Ⓓ Ⓔ
129 Ⓐ Ⓑ Ⓒ Ⓓ Ⓔ
130 Ⓐ Ⓑ Ⓒ Ⓓ Ⓔ

131 Ⓐ Ⓑ Ⓒ Ⓓ Ⓔ
132 Ⓐ Ⓑ Ⓒ Ⓓ Ⓔ
133 Ⓐ Ⓑ Ⓒ Ⓓ Ⓔ
134 Ⓐ Ⓑ Ⓒ Ⓓ Ⓔ
135 Ⓐ Ⓑ Ⓒ Ⓓ Ⓔ

136 Ⓐ Ⓑ Ⓒ Ⓓ Ⓔ
137 Ⓐ Ⓑ Ⓒ Ⓓ Ⓔ
138 Ⓐ Ⓑ Ⓒ Ⓓ Ⓔ
139 Ⓐ Ⓑ Ⓒ Ⓓ Ⓔ
140 Ⓐ Ⓑ Ⓒ Ⓓ Ⓔ

141 Ⓐ Ⓑ Ⓒ Ⓓ Ⓔ
142 Ⓐ Ⓑ Ⓒ Ⓓ Ⓔ
143 Ⓐ Ⓑ Ⓒ Ⓓ Ⓔ
144 Ⓐ Ⓑ Ⓒ Ⓓ Ⓔ
145 Ⓐ Ⓑ Ⓒ Ⓓ Ⓔ

146 Ⓐ Ⓑ Ⓒ Ⓓ Ⓔ
147 Ⓐ Ⓑ Ⓒ Ⓓ Ⓔ
148 Ⓐ Ⓑ Ⓒ Ⓓ Ⓔ
149 Ⓐ Ⓑ Ⓒ Ⓓ Ⓔ
150 Ⓐ Ⓑ Ⓒ Ⓓ Ⓔ

151 Ⓐ Ⓑ Ⓒ Ⓓ Ⓔ
152 Ⓐ Ⓑ Ⓒ Ⓓ Ⓔ
153 Ⓐ Ⓑ Ⓒ Ⓓ Ⓔ
154 Ⓐ Ⓑ Ⓒ Ⓓ Ⓔ
155 Ⓐ Ⓑ Ⓒ Ⓓ Ⓔ

156 Ⓐ Ⓑ Ⓒ Ⓓ Ⓔ
157 Ⓐ Ⓑ Ⓒ Ⓓ Ⓔ
158 Ⓐ Ⓑ Ⓒ Ⓓ Ⓔ
159 Ⓐ Ⓑ Ⓒ Ⓓ Ⓔ
160 Ⓐ Ⓑ Ⓒ Ⓓ Ⓔ

161 Ⓐ Ⓑ Ⓒ Ⓓ Ⓔ
162 Ⓐ Ⓑ Ⓒ Ⓓ Ⓔ
163 Ⓐ Ⓑ Ⓒ Ⓓ Ⓔ
164 Ⓐ Ⓑ Ⓒ Ⓓ Ⓔ
165 Ⓐ Ⓑ Ⓒ Ⓓ Ⓔ

166 Ⓐ Ⓑ Ⓒ Ⓓ Ⓔ
167 Ⓐ Ⓑ Ⓒ Ⓓ Ⓔ
168 Ⓐ Ⓑ Ⓒ Ⓓ Ⓔ
169 Ⓐ Ⓑ Ⓒ Ⓓ Ⓔ
170 Ⓐ Ⓑ Ⓒ Ⓓ Ⓔ

171 Ⓐ Ⓑ Ⓒ Ⓓ Ⓔ
172 Ⓐ Ⓑ Ⓒ Ⓓ Ⓔ
173 Ⓐ Ⓑ Ⓒ Ⓓ Ⓔ
174 Ⓐ Ⓑ Ⓒ Ⓓ Ⓔ
175 Ⓐ Ⓑ Ⓒ Ⓓ Ⓔ

176 Ⓐ Ⓑ Ⓒ Ⓓ Ⓔ
177 Ⓐ Ⓑ Ⓒ Ⓓ Ⓔ
178 Ⓐ Ⓑ Ⓒ Ⓓ Ⓔ
179 Ⓐ Ⓑ Ⓒ Ⓓ Ⓔ
180 Ⓐ Ⓑ Ⓒ Ⓓ Ⓔ

MK